Encyclopedia of
Primary Prevention and Health Promotion

Encyclopedia of
Primary Prevention
and Health Promotion

Editors
Thomas P. Gullotta and Martin Bloom

Section Editors

Foundations
Thomas P. Gullotta and Martin Bloom

Early Childhood
Jonathan Kotch and Craig Blakely

Childhood
Lynne Bond

Adolescence
Gerald Adams and Thomas P. Gullotta

Adulthood
Martin Bloom

Older Adulthood
Colette Browne and Waldo Klein

Research Assistant
Jessica Ramos

A Sponsored Publication of the Child and Family Agency of Southeastern Connecticut

Kluwer Academic / Plenum Publishers
New York   Boston   Dordrecht   London   Moscow

Library of Congress Cataloging-in-Publication Data

The encyclopedia of primary prevention and health promotion/edited by Thomas P. Gullotta and Martin Bloom.
    p.   ; cm.
    Includes bibliographical references and index.
    ISBN 0-306-47296-1
        1. Health promotion—Encyclopedias.   2. Medicine, Preventive—Encyclopedias.   I. Gullotta, Thomas P., 1948–   II. Bloom, Martin, 1934–
    [DNLM: 1. Primary Prevention—Encyclopedias—English.   2. Health Promotion—Encyclopedias—English.   WA 13 E5655 2002]
    RA427.8 .E53 2002
    613′.03—dc21

                                                                                            2002030022

ISBN 0-306-47296-1

©2003 Kluwer Academic/Plenum Publishers, New York
233 Spring Street, New York, New York 10013

http://www.wkap.nl/

10   9   8   7   6   5   4   3   2   1

A C.I.P. record for this book is available from the Library of Congress.

Printed in the United States of America

Tom dedicates this effort to his muses, *pour la veiullieux femme et la jeune femme*, as inspiration and inspirational regarding all that is healthy and loving

Both editors offer this Encyclopedia
to the younger generations of
people beginning their work in primary prevention, and
in honor to the older generations who built this foundation

Contents

Introduction

Thomas P. Gullotta and Martin Bloom

Denis Diderot (1713–1784) directed the writing of the enormous *Encyclopedia, or Rational Dictionary of the Sciences, Arts, and Crafts* (in seventeen volumes published from 1751 to 1772, plus eleven volumes of plates). In his article on the *Encyclopedia*, Diderot states its general purpose for his 18th-century audience:

> To collect all the knowledge scattered over the face of the earth, to present its general outlines and structure to the men with whom we live, and to transmit this to those who will come after us, so that the work of the past centuries may be useful to the following centuries, that our children, by becoming more educated, may at the same time become more virtuous and happier, and that we may not die without having deserved well of the human race. (Reported in Gendzier, 1967, p. xv)

We have a more limited objective in presenting this *Encyclopedia of Primary Prevention and Health Promotion* to its 21st-century audience, even though it follows in the footsteps of many esteemed encyclopedias starting even before Diderot's. To our knowledge, no one has attempted what we present here, a full spectrum of the best available knowledge for action in primary prevention.

In the *Encyclopedia of Primary Prevention and Health Promotion*, we have attempted to collect the best available knowledge from many countries and to present its general content arranged in a standard format for ease of reading and cross-comparison. We did not collect the wisdom of the past centuries, because almost all empirically grounded and conceptually sophisticated theory and practice have been developed within the past few decades. This is not to deny our ancient heritage in preventive thinking and dreaming; rather, we now have enough solid research and sound theory to bring to contemporary programs what may be considered a fruitful direction for practice that was lacking only a short time ago.

Like Professor James A.H. Murray, the first general editor of the *Oxford English Dictionary* project that took from 1878 to 1928 to complete, we issued a general call for contributors, using list-servs, for the American Psychological Association, the American Public Health Association, the National Council on Family Relations, and other networks. We received a gratifying number of offers to help, from which we invited nearly 250 scholars, researchers, and practitioners from a dozen countries to provide these reviews of topics in primary prevention and health promotion. After several rounds of submission and revision—thanks again to the miracle of the Internet—we believe that the *Encyclopedia* represents a milestone in the history of primary prevention. This is the first time that this scale of information has been published in one easily accessible place.

In brief, the entries in the *Encyclopedia* represent the portals through which readers may enter an enormously and unexpectedly rich world of primary preventive thinking and action. From this wealth of knowledge, it becomes possible to locate the information needed to bring back to one's own situation the best available information to guide practice with hope of effective outcomes. With this best practice information available, readers can translate it into the strategies for addressing local concerns, with the confidence, as Mark Twain once said, of a Christian with four aces. That is, not only can we feel good about what we are about to do, but we can feel comfortable about doing it with the best information available. This does not guarantee success, but it increases our chances of being successful.

What we can do is to look at the world about us and make important decisions. It becomes possible, in some cases more than in others, to prevent predictable problems, to protect existing states of health and healthy functioning, and to promote desired goals and objectives for some population of people. This is the core meaning of primary prevention and health promotion.

There are two divisions within the *Encyclopedia*. Part I represents a set of basic entries that describe the foundations of contemporary preventive/protective/promotive theory, research, and practice. Study of these baker's dozen entries provides an overview of the structure of contemporary primary prevention and health promotion. These entries are:

- Definitions of Primary Prevention
- A Brief History of Primary Prevention
- Theories of Primary Prevention
- Evaluation of Primary Prevention Projects
- Principles of Effective Practice in Primary Prevention
- Ethics of Primary Prevention

followed by specific discussions on

- Consultation in Primary Prevention
- Achieving a Sustaining Ecological Future
- Primary Prevention with Minority Peoples
- Societal and Cultural Contributions in Primary Prevention
- Political Issues in Primary Prevention
- Financing Primary Prevention
- Primary Prevention at the Beginning of the 21st Century.

We believe that these foundation entries provide the grounding for the substantive entries that follow. One of the challenges of organizing this *Encyclopedia* was to design an arrangement of entries that is both self-standing and yet interrelated. We achieved this objective by the democracy of alphabetically ordered topics. Just remember that no one thinks less of Diderot's *Encyclopedia*, which has adjacent entries on Asparagus and Atheists; the reader simply has to come to such an encyclopedia knowing what he or she is looking for.

For many topics, we have a chronology of entries, those dealing with early childhood, childhood, adolescence, adulthood, and older adulthood—our five general developmental sections. For example, abuse is played out on different developmental stages with different actors and settings, but they are all still forms of abuse. Likewise, HIV/AIDS, antisocial behaviors, and nutritional issues continue to need addressing in developmentally differential ways. On the other hand, there are many positive aspects of life that are promoted across all age sections, such as creativity, self-esteem, and the various forms of competency and life skills. These too are addressed in developmentally differential ways. Some topics do not easily have chronological characteristics, and none are used.

Some topics contain overlapping subject matter, even when there is a clear topical focus under discussion.

The repetition usually offers different perspectives on related themes, often drawing on different literatures. The main point, however, is that if we could, we would have one 2000-page Grand Entry with its one hundred interrelated pieces each reflecting somewhat different ways of looking at the single entity, the whole of contemporary life. But such is not possible, and the best we can do is to make these interconnections ourselves as we read entries of personal interest. The Subject Index provides detailed suggested connections among entries.

Part II represents our best estimate of the 148 critical topics in primary prevention. Some are very familiar, such as the prevention of cancer, drug misuse, unwanted pregnancy, and violence. Others are less familiar because of how we construct our goals: We seek to promote positive goals based on the strengths that people possess, such as, marital satisfaction, positive peer relations, effective parenting, and resilience. Some readers may be disappointed in not finding certain topics in the *Encyclopedia*. We agree. Unfortunately, no one stepped forward to contribute these missing entries. We hope that in later editions, we will rectify these omissions.

Looking over the selections from Diderot's *Encyclopedia* (Gendzier, 1967), we observe only a few entries related to what we today would consider primary prevention. It may be worthwhile to reflect on one of them.

Inoculation, one entry reads, "is the prevailing term to designate the operation by which one artificially communicates smallpox for the purpose of preventing the danger and the ravages of that illness when contracted naturally" (Gendzier, 1967, p. 149). There is no discussion of the then-contemporary theory about inoculation because the facts were sufficiently well-known. However, what the author (Theodore Tronchin) proposes is an action plan to get this procedure instituted throughout the country. Then Trochin writes: "Inoculation, I repeat, will one day be prescribed in France, and the people will be astonished that it was not adopted sooner" (Gendzier, 1967, p. 150). However, history records that it was not easy to win the widespread approval of inoculation. And for primary prevention in our time, we may make the same prediction, that one day many of the strategies discussed in the *Encyclopedia* will be adopted on behalf of the betterment of people worldwide, and the people will be astonished that these measures were not adopted sooner.

STANDARD FORMAT USED IN SUBSTANTIVE ENTRIES

This *Encyclopedia* was constructed to facilitate its use by readers. This section explains the arrangement in the substantive entries (Part II) only, as the foundation entries (Part I) have their own unique format. We present here the outline authors were requested to follow as far as their content area permitted:

Introduction

This section presents in a few sentences what the topic in this entry is, and how it is handled, given the nature of the problem or potential being discussed.

Definitions

We asked authors to define unusual terms that were basic to the discussion of their topic. These terms are italicized for clarity.

Scope

Scope refers to three topics: the incidence of new cases, the prevalence of existing cases related to their topic, and relevant cost data. Cost data involve both human costs (to the people affected directly and indirectly) and economic costs (to society). Sometimes authors used rough indicators, as specific data were not available.

We encouraged international teams of authors for the substantive entries to achieve cross-cultural and cross-societal comparisons. While we were fortunate to enlist authors from a dozen countries, it was not always possible to present as much international information as is needed to see primary prevention in its global aspect.

Theories

We asked authors to describe the major theoretical guidelines regarding their own topic areas, on the widely held belief that theory-guided practice was more useful than practice without theory. Some authors described the theories they used with special reference to their own content areas, while others used general theories.

Research

We were concerned that information in the *Encyclopedia* be based on the best available empirical findings, and so asked authors to give a sense of the research base for their topic areas. Sometimes authors combined a discussion of theory-guided practice and empirically grounded practice; other times, these topics were kept separate.

Strategies

The most important part of these entries, and the part that was most difficult to construct, were the strategies guiding best practice. Sometimes research was lacking, so no information was available regarding how best to achieve a particular goal. However, knowing what we do not know provides the direction regarding what the next decade of research should address. At times, there was ample research and clear best practice models. Here the challenge was how to persuade users, such as school systems, governmental units, or parents in general, to make use of this "best available information." It is the sad case in many topic areas that some organizations go to the ineffective expedient (cheap, brief, attractively packaged programs) rather than to empirically documented strategies that work, which may require more expense, time, and energy, and yet provide a more likely successful outcome. The cost/benefit ratio favors these successful strategies.

We asked authors—we pleaded with them, as this request proved to be difficult for many—to provide information on three kinds of strategies: Strategies that Work, Strategies that Might Work, and Strategies that Do Not Work.

Strategies that Work

This category refers to those that have clear empirical support for their effectiveness. We asked authors to provide evidence that the strategies they recommended did in fact work. Some authors were able to use federal guidelines or professional society best practice models to identify exemplary programs. Other authors used a criterion of three or more well-designed and executed studies as their basis. Still other authors offered different criteria of effectiveness, which led to discussions with the editors regarding the soundness of these judgments, and often the placing of such programs in the promising category (Strategies that Might Work), rather than the strongly supported (Strategies that Work) category. When strategies that work were found, these became the best available information to guide practice in the field. These are precious pieces of information.

Strategies that Might Work

We recognize that in many areas of life, we simply do not yet have the solid kind of research that can be used to direct best practice. So we asked authors to look for promising programs, those that have not yet had the substantial research to document success, or which have partial success (and need further corrections to be more solidly supported). Sometimes, no direct research was available, and so authors borrowed evidence from related areas in which research was to be found and which might be adapted to a new population or circumstance. In principle, this evidence might be adapted to new preventive purposes. And lacking even indirect empirical evidence for successful strategies, authors were sometimes left to consider promising conceptual ideas that clearly need to be redesigned in tested practice situations.

Strategies that might work, or those that are promising, become the likely topics of the next generation of research in primary prevention, as we seek to expand our empirically grounded knowledge base and offer the public a variety of alternatives on how to achieve desired preventive, protective, or promotive goals.

Strategies that Do Not Work

We believe it is necessary to inform would-be users of prevention programs about strategies that have been used and found wanting, either because no evidence exists that they have been successful, or evidence exists that they have been not only unsuccessful but have been possibly harmful. No matter how good our intentions are in primary prevention, sometimes programs simply do not work, and the public deserves to know this. It was painful for authors to identify such strategies, but it will be a healthy exercise for the profession and society as a whole.

Synthesis

Finally, we asked authors to step back from their review of the literature of what theories and research are available as the bases of strategies that work, might work, and do not work, and to provide their expert judgment of what is likely to be the direction in a given area over the next decade. These are personal opinions. Some authors favored us with full-blown models of future strategies, or the principles by which such strategies could be known. Other times, authors could only wish for "more research" and "additional practice" to help move a topic area along. In this set of syntheses we can see the likely direction of primary prevention in the next decade, based on what works now, what looks promising, and in what we should stop investing limited funds.

References

We asked authors to keep references to a minimum of a page or two, as points of departure for additional study, but many authors found this request impossible to follow. So readers will find the number of references variable across entries. However, authors did comply with our request to make sure that references were recent, encompassing, or classic.

Overall—and we mean literally, overall of the 165 entries—we are optimistic for the future of primary prevention. There is an enormous amount of substantial research and a great deal of sophisticated theory available, and these have been put to work in many areas of primary prevention practice. We have entered the 21st century and it looks to be the century of primary prevention. This is not to say that progress has been, or will be, even; nor that there are not significant challenges to primary prevention in the future. But the growth of primary prevention knowledge, as reflected in the *Encyclopedia*, will convince open-minded people that, as Klein and Goldston (1977) phrased it a quarter-century ago, primary prevention is an idea whose time has come.

ACKNOWLEDGMENTS

A work of this magnitude owes acknowledgment to many people over long periods of time. We do not exaggerate when we begin with our great ancestors in primary prevention, such as Hippocrates for his pioneering work in public health and environmental issues, his inauguration of ethics in the helping professions, and his concern for observing closely the subject of his inquiry. However, were we to continue our acknowledgments this way, we would not be able to get to the content of the *Encyclopedia*. So we regretfully pass over the centuries of truly inspired work of which we all are the beneficiaries.

We acknowledge with grateful respect the labors our authors performed in these, first as the new manuscripts came in, and then as we requested modifications, a little more here, a little less there. Our authors showed grace under pressure, and we appreciate that. The *Encyclopedia* is truly a testament to their good work.

We report, with regret, that one contributor, Dr. Lori Irving, died unexpectedly, leaving a deeply saddened family and a wide network of friends of this productive young scholar.

We gladly acknowledge our section editors, Lynne Bond, Jonathan Kotch, Collette Browne, Waldo Klein, Craig Blakely, and Gerald Adams, who helped us to encourage, if not cajole our authors throughout this intensive process. Their long hours of work on early drafts and middle drafts and late drafts propelled this project into high gear, and we owe a great debt to them.

We acknowledge the ceaseless labors of Jessica Ramos, our Project Research Assistant, for her efforts in keeping in e-touch, time and again, with our hundreds of authors, section editors, and co-editors, during the various draft stages. We recognize the Board of Directors of Child and Family Agency who endorsed this project at its conception and whose leadership across the years has provided unwavering support for primary prevention and health promotion that made this monumental task possible.

We acknowledge the staff of Kluwer/Plenum, particularly, Mariclaire Cloutier, and the production staff, for their continuing support and enthusiasm for this project.

Finally, we offer some personal acknowledgments: Tom meditates about the influences that shaped his understanding of mental health—George Albee, Emory Cowen, Gerald Caplan, and many others, including one Wolf Welf Wulf von S___, a patient labeled as a schizophrenic, who long ago taught an undergraduate English major about dysfunctional *systems* when he was supposed to be learning about dysfunctional people. Martin wanders among the ancients, such as John Bellers, Robert Owen, and John Griscom, as well as in the 20th century for his inspiration for primary prevention. Most of all, Martin acknowledges with love Lynn, Bard, Vicki, Laird, Sara, Paul, and Beth—his inspirations.

References

Klein, D.C., & Goldston, S.E. (1977). Primary prevention: An idea whose time has come. *Proceedings of the Pilot Conference on Primary Prevention, April 24, 1976* (DHEW Publication No. ADM. 77-44). Washington, DC: GPO.

Gendzier, S.J. (Ed. and Trans.). (1967). *Denis Diderot's The Encyclopedia: Selections.* New York: J & J Harper Editions.

I. Foundation Topics in Primary Prevention and Health Promotion

Evolving Definitions of Primary Prevention

Martin Bloom and Thomas P. Gullotta

INTRODUCTION

Definitions matter! How we define a field of study strongly influences how we select research problems, choose variables to be studied, and interpret the data. Indirectly, these influence how users of our information construct their programs in the community. The definitions that have guided the field of primary prevention have been evolving. This does not necessarily mean changing for the better; they have simply changed to fit other systems of values. We will present the evolving definitions of primary prevention regarding the promotion of health and the prevention of illness and we will offer a working definition of the beginning of the 21st century. Briefly stated, primary prevention involves activities that (1) prevent predictable problems, (2) protect existing states of health or healthy functioning, and (3) promote desired goals for a population of people in three possible contexts: universally, as a basic utility for everyone's benefit; selectively, for groups at risk and with potential; and as indicated for groups at very high risk.

EARLY DEFINITIONS OF PRIMARY PREVENTION

The word *prevention* stems from Latin, meaning "to come before." It evolved from a core European definition by at least the 15th century (*Oxford English Dictionary*, 1971) with several meanings: "to anticipate," "to take precautions against [a danger or evil] and hence to evade that danger." "To avoid by timely action." Its Latin root is still central: "that which comes before or goes before something else," "antecedent," "anticipatory," "that which keeps from coming [about] or taking place." There is also a positive meaning to the word *prevent*: "to outdo, surpass, excel," "to hasten to bring about." The root word *prevent* was used in many domains, from the practical everyday usage (as in the folk aphorism, "an ounce of prevention ..." to legal, literary, theological, and political terms. There are some other historical usages that appear relevant to this discussion, such as *provent*, meaning "a coming forth," "[to] increase," which is something like the positive meaning of prevent. Likewise, in another positive variation, the word *promote* means "to move forward," "[to] advance."

The point in providing this linguistic excursion is to demonstrate that there are a number of valid and useful meanings of the core term. In a word, there is no single sovereign definition of "prevention" from its historical beginning, and there appears to be none today other than by asserting one's own definition. In spite of these misty beginnings, the term *primary prevention* has evolved among social scientists into five main patterns.

9

THE PUBLIC HEALTH/PREVENTIVE MEDICINE DEFINITION

Leavell and Clark (1953) provided a basic public health definition, within the classic terms of that field—host (population of potential victims), causal agents (and the vectors or carriers of these agents), and relevant environments. It would also be instructive to pair their definition with that of Mausner and Bahn (1974) who described the natural history of a disease from a medical perspective.

The first observation about Table 1 is that it is strongly dominated by a medical model with an emphasis on physical illness. Its terms provide little guidance for social or psychological problems, either in the sense of single underlying cause with clearly definable problems (symptoms), or with regard to standard and effective practices related to the problems. Moreover, this perspective stresses the pathological; there is no place in the definition for strengths or health, other than the lack of symptoms. Unlike the pure medical, the public health model focuses on populations at risk, rather than specific individuals having problems. It also means that other helping professions can be involved in prevention, and that preventive actions may be addressed to host, agent, and/or environment, thus multiplying the ways a preventable problem might be addressed.

A PREVENTIVE PSYCHIATRY DEFINITION

A second perspective was introduced by Caplan (1964) which combined concepts from the fields of epidemiology and psychiatry. This definition depends on the concepts of incidence (the rate of new cases in a population) and prevalence (the rate of cases with the existing problem in a population). Caplan distinguished three main terms: *Primary prevention* involved the lowering of the incidence for some specified mental disorder. *Secondary prevention* concerned reducing the disability rate due to a disorder by lowering the prevalence of the disorder in the community, that is, by lowering the number of new cases and shortening the duration of old cases. This connects primary prevention with the first, while secondary prevention focuses on the second. Logically, this means that secondary prevention includes primary prevention. *Tertiary prevention* involves reducing the rate of defective functioning in a community, or lowering the capacity remaining as a residue after the disorder has terminated. Tertiary prevention focuses on the latter, while primary and secondary prevention address the former. Again, logically, tertiary prevention thus includes the other two.

These terms—primary, secondary, and tertiary prevention—were widely used, and continue to be used. However, they are also commonly misused or confused, possibly because of the complex interrelationships among their meanings. Other critics point to the illogic of preventing something from occurring—that is, acting *before* a problem has occurred—when there is an already occurring (secondary prevention) or already occurred (tertiary prevention) condition.

A STRENGTHS-ORIENTED DEFINITION OF PRIMARY PREVENTION

The 1970s saw a reaction against the complex psychiatric definition and the medical/public health definitions, both of which were oriented toward pathology. The influential Vermont Conferences on the Primary Prevention of Psychopathology began in 1975 and produced important volumes on research and theory in primary prevention. President Jimmy Carter established the President's Commission on Mental Health (1978, p. 28), composed of a

Table 1. Public Health and Medical Perspectives

Stages of disease*	Preventive activities**
Stage of susceptibility The prerequisite conditions of the disease emerge, but are not yet operating as part of the disease entity.	*Health promotion* Furthering health and well-being through general measures (like education, nutrition, provision of social services), aimed at host populations in relevant environments. *Specific protections* Measures applicable to a particular disease in order to intercept the pathogenic agent.
Preclinical states No symptoms visible but analytic tools could reveal signs of pathogenic events. *Acute clinical stage* Manifest symptoms of which victim is aware.	*Early recognition and prompt treatment* • Screening and periodic exams of population at risk. • Disease control through standard medical practices. • Surveillance of pathogenic conditions in the environment.
Post-acute clinical stage [chronic] Residual effects of disease continue to be present and problematic, or remission of symptoms (but not of the disease).	*Disability limitations* Preventing or delaying the consequences of clinically advanced or noncurable disease in identified hosts.
Termination of clinical stage Patient rehabilitation to best level attainable.	*Rehabilitation* Affected persons brought back to useful place in society, so far as possible.

Notes:
 * Adapted from Mausner & Bahn (1974).
 ** Adapted from Leavell & Clark (1953).

group of leaders in the mental health field. The Task Force on Primary Prevention offered this description and definition of terms:

> Primary prevention in mental health is a network of strategies that differ qualitatively from the field's past dominant approaches. Those strategies are distinguished by several essential characteristics:
>
> 1. Most fundamentally, primary prevention is proactive in that it seeks to build adaptive strengths, coping resources, and health in people; not to reduce or contain already manifest deficit.
> 2. Primary prevention is concerned about total populations, and not about the provision of services on a case-by-case basis.
> 3. Primary prevention's main tools and models are those of education and social engineering, not therapy or rehabilitation, although some insights for its models and programs grow out of the wisdom derived from clinical experience.
> 4. Primary prevention assumes that equipping people with personal and environmental resources for coping is the best of all ways to ward off maladaptive problems, not trying to deal (however skillfully) with problems that have already germinated and flowered.

One outcome of this report was the establishment of a Center for Prevention in the National Institute of Mental Health (NIMH), and later at other governmental agencies. In turn, these developments led to the NIMH Centers for Prevention Research, established at universities across the United States.

Cowen (1973, 2000) introduced the concept of wellness enhancement and the basic philosophy that distinguished this approach from the "risk-driven, disease-prevention" notions of primary prevention. Effective enhancement of psychological wellness from the start is arguably just as effective as disease prevention (Durlak, 1997; Durlak & Wells, 1997), and both of these are more preferable than the costly, frustrating, and painful experience of treating victims one by one. The Diagnostic and Statistical Manuals (DSMs) over their several editions do not ever discuss health except as the absence of illness. Society and various vested interest groups are preoccupied with the individual and collective pathologies that are immediately and painfully present (juvenile delinquency, divorce, unemployment, etc.). Cowen (2000) points to recent research (Tolan & Guerra, 1994; Yoshikawa, 1994) suggesting that "effective early, comprehensive, family-oriented competence enhancement programs for preschoolers" were more effective in delinquency prevention than any specifically targeted adolescent program. In short, a promotive "jump-start" potentially has more protective value in forestalling diverse, maladaptive outcomes than later preventive interventions aimed at high risk groups, although Cowen and others argue for combining

both preventive and wellness-oriented approaches as best current wisdom.

Klein and Goldston (1977, p. 27) brought together another group of researchers in discussing "Primary prevention: An idea whose time has come." They offered this definition of terms, which also reflects a concern with both risk prevention and wellness enhancement:

> Primary prevention encompasses those activities directed to specifically identified vulnerable high-risk groups within the community who have not been labeled as psychiatrically ill and for whom measures can be undertaken to avoid the onset of emotional disturbance and/or enhance their level of positive mental health. Programs for the promotion of mental health are primarily educational rather than clinical in conception and operation with their ultimate goal being to increase people's capacities for dealing with crises and for taking steps to improve their own lives.

Bloom (1981) found a number of subtle variations in definitions of primary prevention. These included different models of causation (such as the underlying disease model or the environmental/learning model); different perspectives on timing of preventive efforts (from the long-before approach like wellness enhancement, to the just-before approaches, and even a shortly-after-a-problem-emerged approach); different preventive targets (from individuals per se, to specific at-risk groups, milestone occasions that everyone experiences, or whole populations in general); different modes of action (from preventing negative events or risks, to promoting positive events and strengths; from reactive prevention, to proactive prevention measures); different strategies of preventive efforts (from active strategies involving participant cooperation, to passive strategies where environmental changes were involved—think of the difference between buckling a seat belt or riding in a car with air cushions); and the awareness of the values involved or activated in conducting prevention programs (from a naive "all prevention is good" to a more critical "some prevention may be harmful to some people"). These subtle variations suggested little agreement in the core term, a state of affairs that many lamented (Mrazek & Haggerty, 1994, p. 19).

TYPES OF POPULATIONS AT RISK/MEDICAL DEFINITION

The United States Congress mandated the NIMH and other agencies within the Department of Health and Human Services, to provide a long-term agenda for prevention research. This task was given to the Institute of Medicine (IOM), and ultimately, a group of scholars (Mrazek & Haggerty, 1994) proposed a variation on the prior three models. *Prevention* was to be limited to those interventions designed to prevent the onset of disease. Following the writing of Gordon (1987) with regard to physical disease prevention, the term was further divided into three:

1. *Universal preventive interventions* are targeted to the general public or to a whole population group that has not been identified on the basis of individual risks (Mrazek & Haggerty, 1994, pp. 24–25). The intervention (like prenatal care or programs for the prevention of divorce) is defined as desirable for everyone in that group. While the individual costs and risks are low, and the intervention is effective and acceptable by the population, still the overall costs can be quite expensive (e.g., prenatal care for every child). This is something like Leavell and Clark's concept of health promotion, but the concept of promotion per se was intentionally removed because "…health promotion is not driven by an emphasis on illness, but rather by a focus on the enhancement of well-being" (Mrazek & Haggerty, 1994, p. 27). As such, promotion did not fit into this medical model.

2. *Selective preventive measures* for mental disorders are targeted to individuals or a subgroup of the population whose risks of developing mental disorders is higher than average (Mrazek & Haggerty, 1994, p. 25). Risk groups may be identified on the basis of biological, psychological, or social risk factors known to be associated with the onset of a mental disorder. Examples would be home visitation and infant child care for low birth-weight children of adolescent parents, preschool programs for children from an impoverished neighborhood with high unemployment rates, and support groups for elderly widows. This type of intervention is seen as most appropriate when costs are moderate and risks are minimal or nonexistent.

3. *Indicated preventive intervention* are used with high-risk people with minimal but detectable symptoms foreshadowing mental disorder, or biological makers indicating predisposition for mental disorder, but who do not meet DSM-III-R diagnostic levels at the current time (Mrazek & Haggerty, 1994, p. 25). An example would be a parent–child interaction training program for children identified by parents as having behavior problems. The kind of prevention program may be reasonable even if intervention costs are high and risks are involved. This is similar to Caplan's concept of secondary prevention, while Caplan's concept of tertiary prevention was discarded entirely.

Much has been written about this IOM definition (e.g., Cowen, 2000; Munoz, Mrazek, & Haggerty, 1996). The background of the origins of this definition involve a point of reference in the DSM-III-R, even with its limitations (Kirk & Kutchins, 1992; Kutchins & Kirk, 1997). It is, like the earlier medical definition, driven by considerations of illness. The business of mental health is mental illness, to borrow a phrase. As an illness-driven definition, the IOM definition is associated with genetic or biological causes for mental disorders that can potentially be treated with drugs under the directions of specialists. However, this potentiality is a double-edged sword from an ecological perspective in which many biopsychosocial factors contribute to any outcome. Over-emphasizing one solution (such as the use of medications) will lessen the attention given to other solutions involving psychological and social causes of the problem. If a set of genes is seen as the cause of a problem like depression or aggressiveness—and drugs are viewed as the solution—then parents, the schools, the community, the employment situation, cultural oppression, pollution, and other factors known to influence these social events, can be removed from public scrutiny. Another implication involves genetic engineering, even though the corpse of eugenics is hardly cold in the ground.

THE SOCIAL EXPERIENCE PERSPECTIVE

This perspective has many progenitors. Social learning theorists (Bandura, 1986) offered explanations on how people learned from their experiences and how they helped to construct those experiences. Social stress theorists (Bloom, 1985; Selye, 1976) linked various environmental pressures and stresses to resulting mental disorders. Holmes and Rahe (1967) introduced a stress scale that has been widely used and adapted. Albee (1983) has given this perspective its distinctive formulation in the form of an equation: The incidence of mental disorder is a function of organic factors plus social stresses plus social exploitation, reduced by the availability of personal competence, self-esteem, and social supports. Several others have suggested modifications in Albee's formulation, but the point is that these authors share a general biopsychosocial perspective. Every significant problem or potential is influenced by these factors. Ignore any one of them in the analysis of the problem or potential, and the overall formulation is weakened. Moreover, there is a clear acknowledgment of the strengths perspective (Saleebey, 1992) which means helping professionals can involve participants in their own health enhancement, building on their strengths and those of others in their environment.

What is missing from this formulation is the dark side of life, that people will die and thus need palliative care at some point; that people will get Alzheimer's disease and the prevention task involves helping the caretakers survive when there is no hope for the victims; and that people *en mass* may choose to do foolish things, like smoking or overeating, that endanger their lives in spite of knowledge to the contrary. It is very hard to be in primary prevention recognizing that nearly half of all current social health problems are preventable—and are not being prevented. The social experience perspective provides no sense of the proportion that each of the components contributes. This is not so much a failing, as it is the setting of the agenda for the future: to identify how and to what degree each factor is in fact active or activated in given situations, so as to know what preventive, protective, or promotive actions might be planned to help participants help themselves.

THE CONTINUING EVOLUTION IN THE DEFINITION OF PRIMARY PREVENTION

Nothing is certain except uncertainty. The process of defining primary prevention continues. We are in the awkward position of predicting what will be the next stage in the evolution of the term *primary prevention* for the coming decade in the 21st century. What we offer here is based on the principle that a definition of the core term of the *Encyclopedia of Primary Prevention* must serve many users and uses. Therefore, we offer the following discussion to be as inclusive as possible for the many points of view and the specialities involved in the day-to-day work of primary prevention as well as the foreseeable theorizing and research in this rapidly expanding field. We expect that the flow of federal grant dollars will largely continue to fund the genetic/biologically based medical model for the time being, while we hope for a counterbalancing trend that recognizes the social contributions to both health and illness, that is, to something like the social experience model.

What we propose is our current best guess of what practitioners in primary prevention need now and in the near future. In expanded form from our introductory statement, we offer the following:

> Primary prevention as the promotion of health and the prevention of illness involves actions that help participants (or to facilitate participants helping themselves, (1) to prevent predictable and interrelated problems, (2) to protect existing states of health and healthy functioning, and (3) to promote psychosocial wellness for identified populations of people. These consist of (a) whole populations in which everyone requires certain basic utilities of life; (b) selected groups of people at risk or with potential; and (c) indicated subgroups at very high risk. Primary prevention may be facilitated by increasing individual, group, organizational, societal, cultural, and physical environmental strengths and resources, while simultaneously reducing the limitations and pressures from these same factors.

Let us consider the major terms of this working definition:

"*Actions to help participants (or to facilitate participants helping themselves)*": This phrase suggests that participants may be helped by others (as educators supply students with information), but also that participants may be active in helping themselves (as in putting on a condom as a part of sexual activity), or both may be combined (as in sex education classes where people receive instruction and training in how to negotiate their mutual safety in the relationship).

"*Prevent predictable and interrelated problems*": This phrase requires knowledge about a future condition that will be problematic and that the individuals involved have characteristics known to be risk factors of that problem. Primary prevention is a knowledge-based applied science. Moreover, conditions that are problematic may run in clusters (such as early drinking and smoking may be related to problems in school). Primary prevention generally addresses the whole cluster of associated risks, as dealing only with one may not systematically affect the others. This is a systems perspective, and it also may involve multiple levels—persons, groups, communities.

"*Protecting existing states of health and healthy functioning*": This phrase recognizes that people have current strengths which become the bases of primary prevention efforts, that is, practitioners work with people's strengths and the constructive resources in the social and physical environment. Protection of healthy functioning requires knowledge of healthy states—physical, mental, and sociocultural (including spiritual) in a healthy environmental context—and what it requires to maintain them.

"*Promote psychosocial wellness*": This phrase assumes that an important part of primary prevention involves enhancing wellness in order that people may attain some desired state of well-being. Promotion is a positive activity in its own right, and is not simply a reduction of risk for illness. Well-being is a positive goal, and is not merely the absence of illness.

"*For identified populations of people*": This phrase implies a value statement that wellness must be relatively evenly enjoyed and that "wellness for some but not others" would be a contradiction of the democratic ideal (Rawls, 1971). We incorporate some of the IOM definition in distinguishing universal efforts (at whole populations needing basic utilities like clean water, decent education, and viable economic opportunities), selective efforts (at groups at risk for some specific predictable problem—but going beyond the IOM definition, at groups with specific potentials needing enhancement), and indicated groups at very high risk. This last-named group recognizes what we call a gray area between prevention and treatment; it is an area that we seek to minimize in the long run, by means of universal and selective efforts in primary prevention.

We also recognize the following assumptions in this working definition:

- Individual strengths and limitations may stem from biological, psychological (learned), and sociocultural influences in as yet unknown proportions. All of these individual-level factors can only take place in benign or supportive physical and social environments.

- Group strengths and limitations occur in families, support networks, and neighborhoods. All of these micro- or mezo-social factors imply that individual actors take action within social roles and contexts.
- Larger entities, like communities, states, nations, and cultures, are often involved in primary prevention because of the actions of various interest groups, planners, and policy makers. These macro-social entities take on a life of their own (traditions, norms, roles, etc.) that exist before and beyond the lives of the particular individuals who act as their agents.

The seemingly boundless physical environment is in fact being dangerously damaged and requires vision of peoples beyond national borders and short time periods in order to repair the damage and prevent future degradation. Included are both the microenvironments (such as children taking in secondhand smoke of parents), macroenvironments (such as parents working in polluted worksites), and universal environments (such as policies and actions directed toward global warming).

The word "simultaneously" implies that there may be situations in which it is insufficient merely to prevent some problem from occurring; one must simultaneously attempt to bring some desired state into existence in place of that predictable problem. This term also implies that all helping action is based on the existing strengths that people and environments have, so that where there are weaknesses in one, some other portion of the ecology can contribute its compensating service. This is a systems assumption that all aspects of a situation impinge on each other and that we have to attempt to view the whole system in order to grasp the workings of each element. Obviously, we have to compromise since we don't have omniscience; we must do the best we can with the tools at hand, while continuing the search for more knowledge.

We have tried to suggest a definition of primary prevention that will take us into the realities of the 21st century, which extend far beyond any one field of practice (like prevention of substance abuse or unwanted teen pregnancy), or in any one nation (as potentially preventable problems like HIV/AIDS, or global terrorism, know no borders). This is a definition for theorists, researchers, practitioners, and the public that is grounded in a humanistic ethical stance. It represents a goal to be attained, not a static reality. The working definition represents a functional approach, suggesting what has to be done to prevent, protect, and promote specific classes of events for individuals, groups, and environments.

Yet, the definitional problem is not solved. There are gray areas among prevention, treatment, and rehabilitation.

For example, a practitioner might treat an existing problem such as a traumatic date rape. At the same time, the same practitioner might provide education for the prevention of future rape situations. Likewise, this same practitioner might try to rehabilitate the victim to eventual healthy sexual relationships with a loved partner. What the practitioner does in action may rapidly move among prevention, treatment, and rehabilitation, regardless of the "separateness" of these three professional territories. In the future, this complex of primary prevention, treatment, and rehabilitation will likely require a coordinated team approach ultimately involving key players at all levels and across all nations. We have to recognize that what we do as individuals in one organization in one country has to be coordinated with the efforts of others people everywhere and for the indefinite future. Primary prevention must recognize the new global perspective. Multilevel and multisystem perspectives in primary prevention make conceptual sense and organizational chaos, unless we begin to train new generations of practitioners in almost every profession that their contributions count toward a universal objective of human well-being, not for the rich (nations) alone, not for the poor alone (to paraphrase Kahn & Kamerman, 1975), but for everyone.

Also see: History: Foundation; Theories: Foundation; Ethics: Foundation.

References

Albee, G.W. (1983). Psychopathology, prevention, and the just society. *Journal of Primary Prevention, 4*(1), 5–40.

Bandura, A. (1986). *Social foundations of thought and action: A social cognitive theory.* Englewood Cliffs, NJ: Prentice-Hall.

Bloom, B.L. (1985). *Stressful life events and research: Implications for primary prevention* (DHHS Publication No. ADM 85-1385). Washington, DC: GPO.

Bloom, M. (1981). *Primary prevention: The possible science.* Englewood Cliffs, NJ: Prentice-Hall.

Caplan, G. (1964). *Principles of preventive psychiatry.* New York: Basis Books.

Cowen, E.L. (1973). Social and community interventions. In P. Mussen & M. Rosenzweig (Eds.), *Annual Review of Psychology, 24,* 423–472.

Cowen, E.L. (2000). Psychological wellness: Some hopes for the future. In D. Cicchetti, J. Rappaport, I. Sandler, & R.P. Weissberg (Eds.), *The promotion of wellness in children and adolescents* (pp. 477–503). Washington, DC: CWLA Press.

Durlak, J.A. (1997). *Successful prevention programs for children and adolescents.* New York: Plenum.

Durlak, J.A., & Wells, A.M. (1997). Primary prevention programs for children and adolescents: A meta-analytic review. *American Journal of Community Psychology, 25,* 115–152.

Gordon, R. (1987). An operational classification of disease prevention. In J.A. Steinberg & M.M. Silverman (Eds.), *Preventing Mental Disorders* (pp. 20–26). Rockville, MD: Department of Health and Human Services.

Holmes, T.H., & Rahe, R.H. (1967). The social readjustment rating scale. *Journal of Psychosomatic Research, 11,* 213–218.

Kahn, A.J., & Kamerman, S.B. (1975). *Not for the poor alone: European social services*. Philadelphia: Temple University Press.

Kirk, S.A., & Kutchins, H. (1992). *The selling of DSM: The rhetoric of science in psychiatry*. New York: Aldine de Gruyer.

Klein, D., & Goldston, S. (1977). Primary prevention: An idea whose time has come. *Proceedings of the Pilot Conference on Primary Prevention*, April 24, 1976 (DHEW Publication No. ADM 77-447). Washington, DC: GPO.

Kutchins, H., & Kirk, S.A. (1997). *Making us crazy: DSM: The psychiatric bible and the creation of mental disorders*. New York: Free Press.

Leavell, H.R., & Clark, E.G. (Eds.). (1953). *Textbook of preventive medicine*. New York: McGraw-Hill.

Mausner, J.S., & Bahn, A.K. (1974). *Epidemiology: An introductory text*. Philadelphia: W.B. Saunders.

Mrazek, P.J., & Haggerty, R.J. (Eds.). (1994). *Reducing risks for mental disorders: Frontiers for preventive interventions*. Washington, DC: National Academy Press.

Munoz, R.F., Mrazek, P.J., & Haggerty, R.J. (1996). Institute of Medicine report on prevention of mental disorders: Summary and commentary. *American Psychologist, 51*, 1116–1122.

Oxford English Dictionary. (1971). New York: Oxford University Press.

President's Commission on Mental Health (1978). *Report to the President*. (Stock No. 040-000-00390-8). Washington, DC: GPO.

Rawls, J. (1971). *Theory of justice*. Cambridge, MA: Belknap Press of Harvard University Press.

Saleebey, D. (Ed.). (1992). *The strengths perspective in social work practice*. New York: Longman.

Selye, H. (1976). *Stress in health and disease*. Reading, MA: Butterworth.

Tolan, P.H., & Guerra, N.G. (1994). Prevention of delinquency: Current status and issues. *Applied and Preventive Psychology, 3*, 251–273.

Yoshikawa, H. (1994). Prevention as cumulative protection: Effects of early family support and education on chronic delinquency and its risks. *Psychological Bulletin, 115*, 28–54.

A Brief History and Analysis of Health Promotion

Jeffrey B. Bingenheimer, Paula B. Repetto, Marc A. Zimmerman, and James G. Kelly

INTRODUCTION

This entry provides a broad overview of the history of health promotion. The term *health promotion* has been defined in a variety of different ways (cf., Bloom, 1996; Kemm & Close, 1995; Nutbeam, 1998). We use the definition given by Green and Krueter (1999): "Any planned combination of educational, political, regulatory, community and organizational supports for actions and conditions of living that contribute to the health of individuals, groups, or communities" (p. 14). One appealing feature of this definition is its breadth. It encompasses health education and includes a wide range of human endeavors that are united by their common intention of improving health. Choosing such a broad definition of health promotion allows us to emphasize the diverse forms that efforts to promote health have taken through history, and to argue that health promotion, as it is currently practiced, is a product not only of scientific knowledge but also of contemporary social systems and institutions.

Rather than attempting a chronological presentation of all the important historical events in health promotion, this entry is organized around four themes. These themes are intended to provide a framework for understanding how and why health promotion has changed over time. The themes are: (1) the *prevalence and effects of diseases*; (2) *human theories of disease causation*; (3) the *technologies* available for preventing disease and promoting health; and (4) broader *social systems*. We discuss each of these factors in turn and, in the process, use for illustrative purposes many of the discrete historical events that one might expect to find in a more chronological presentation. Additionally, while much of the information we present is drawn from historical studies of health promotion in the United States and Western Europe, we also include information and examples pertaining to health promotion in other contexts as well.

HEALTH PROMOTION AND PATTERNS OF DISEASE

One of the most important factors shaping health promotion is the pattern of *disease prevalence*. Human societies differ markedly across time, place, and social category in the relative contribution that different diseases make to overall morbidity and mortality. Conditions that contribute the most to mortality of one social group at one place and time may be virtually non-existent in another. Smallpox, for example, was an important contributor to morbidity and mortality worldwide for centuries, but was eradicated by 1975 through a major vaccination campaign (Kemm & Close, 1995). These patterns of disease prevalence define in broad terms the situations to which health promotion efforts seek to respond.

Table 1 lists the top ten leading causes of death in the United States for the years 1900, 1950, and 1998. At the beginning of the 20th century, the three leading causes of death—pneumonia and influenza, tuberculosis, and diarrhea and enteritis—were caused by infectious agents, either viral or bacterial. Consequently, organized health promotion efforts in the early 20th century in the United States emphasized

Table 1. Ten Leading Causes of Death for the United States, 1900–1998

Rank	1900	1950	1998
1	Pneumonia and influenza	Diseases of the heart	Diseases of the heart
2	Tuberculosis	Cancer	Malignant neoplasms
3	Diarrhea and enteritis	Vascular lesions affecting the central nervous system	Cerebrovascular diseases
4	Heart diseases	Accidents	Chronic obstructive pulmonary disease
5	Intracranial lesions	Diseases of early infancy	Accidents and adverse effects
6	Nephritis	Pneumonia and influenza	Pneumonia and influenza
7	All accidents	Tuberculosis	Diabetes mellitus
8	Cancer	General arteriosclerosis	Suicide
9	Senility	Chronic and unspecified nephritis	Nephritis, nephrotic syndrome, and nephrosis
10	Diphtheria	Diabetes mellitus	Chronic liver disease and cirrhosis

Source: Murphy (2000).

the control of infectious diseases through strategies such as sanitary engineering and mass immunization campaigns. By the early 1950s, however, non-infectious, chronic diseases such as cardiovascular disease and cancer had replaced infectious diseases as the leading causes of mortality in the United States. As a result of these changes, health promotion at mid-century began to focus on factors thought to cause chronic diseases, especially individual behaviors such as diet, physical activity, tobacco smoking, and alcohol consumption. Some of these efforts may be beginning to pay off. Figure 1 reveals that the rate of mortality due to cardio-vascular disease has declined in the United States since the early 1970s. This decline may be attributable, in part, to health promotion efforts to persuade people to eat more fiber and less fat, to refrain from tobacco smoking, to engage in regular physical activity and to treat elevated blood pressure (Kemm & Close, 1995). As health promotion efforts successfully address a disease, the pattern of disease may shift. This interdependence of disease pattern and efforts to control and prevent them helps account for the dynamic nature of health promotion.

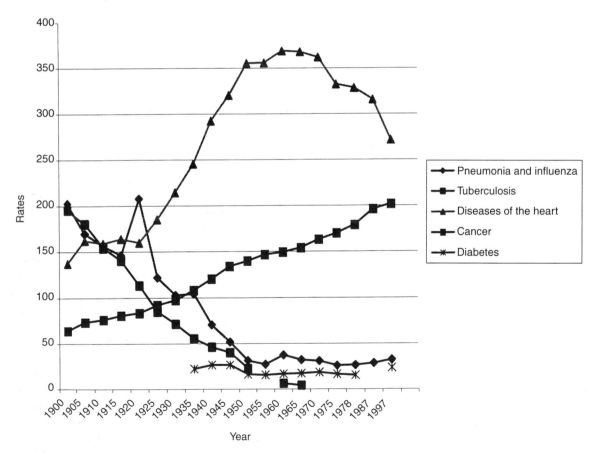

Figure 1. Mortality Rates per 100,000 for Some Specific Causes, United States, 1900–1997 (midyear estimates).
Source: CDC (2000); PAHO (1996); Murphy (2000).

Table 2. Leading Causes of Worldwide Mortality and Region-Specific Ranks, 1998

Cause of death	All countries	Africa	Americas	Eastern Mediterranean	Europe	Southeast Asia	Western Pacific
Ischemic heart disease	1	9	1	1	1	1	3
Cerebrovascular disease	2	7	2	5	2	4	1
Acute lower repiratory infections	3	3	3	2	4	2	4
HIV/AIDS	4	1	13	27	42	8	42
Chronic obstructive pulmonary disease	5	14	6	10	5	11	2
Diarrheal diseases	6	4	10	3	22	3	17
Perinatal conditions	7	5	7	4	13	5	10
Tuberculosis	8	11	19	7	23	6	9
Cancer of the trachia, bronchus, and lung	9	38	4	20	3	15	6
Road traffic accidents	10	12	5	9	8	7	12

Source: World Health Organization (1999).

Just as patterns of morbidity and mortality vary markedly over time, they also vary by place. Table 2 presents the leading causes of worldwide mortality in 1998, along with their region-specific ranks. These data reveal significant regional differences. Ischemic heart disease, for example, is the leading contributor to mortality worldwide and in several regions, but ranks third in the Western Pacific and ninth in Africa. HIV/AIDS, in contrast, ranks first in Africa, but fourth worldwide and forty-second in Europe and the Western Pacific. The infectious diseases that used to be the leading causes of death in the United States are still important contributors to mortality elsewhere. Diarrheal diseases rank as the third leading cause of death in Southeast Asia and the Eastern Mediterranean, and fourth in Africa. This geographic variation in the patterns of morbidity and mortality may be explained by a variety of factors, including climate, culture, and level of economic development. Geographic variation in health can also be found within countries. Within the United States, for instance, mortality rates are substantially elevated in impoverished inner city neighborhoods (Geronimus, Bound, & Waidmann, 1996; McCord & Freeman, 1990). The health promotion efforts found in different regions of the world and within a country, therefore, will reflect to some degree this geographic variation in the prevalence of diseases.

Patterns of disease burden also vary substantially across social categories, such as sex, socioeconomic position, and race/ethnicity. Table 3 presents the ten leading causes of death in the United States in 1998 for Whites, African Americans, and Latinos. This table reveals both similarities and differences. All three groups share the first two leading causes of death: diseases of the heart and malignant neoplasms. In contrast, HIV/AIDS ranks among the top ten only for African Americans, while suicide makes this list only for Whites. The accidents and adverse effects category ranks

Table 3. Ten Leading Causes of Death for Whites, African Americans, and Latinos in the United States, 1998

Rank	Whites	African Americans	Latinos
1	Diseases of the heart	Diseases of the heart	Diseases of the heart
2	Malignant neoplasms	Malignant neoplasms	Malignant neoplasms
3	Cerebrovascular diseases	Cerebrovascular diseases	Accidents and adverse effects
4	Chronic obstructive pulmonary disease	Accidents and adverse effects	Cerebrovascular diseases
5	Accidents and adverse effects	Diabetes mellitus	Diabetes mellitus
6	Pneumonia and influenza	Homicide and legal intervention	Pneumonia and influenza
7	Diabetes mellitus	HIV/AIDS	Homicide and legal intervention
8	Suicide	Pneumonia and influenza	Chronic liver disease and cirrhosis
9	Chronic liver disease and cirrhosis	Chronic obstructive pulmonary disease	Chronic obstructive pulmonary disease
10	Alzheimer's disease	Conditions originating in the perinatal period	Conditions originating in the perinatal period

Source: Murphy (2000).

highest for Latinos, partly because of the disproportionate involvement of members of this population in the agricultural labor force, where fatal accidents are relatively common (Mishra, Conner, & Magana, 1996). Similarly, Table 4 shows sex-specific mortality rates for several different cancer sites for males and females in the United States. Some of the differences that appear in this table have a clear genetic basis (e.g., uterine, cervical, and prostate cancer). Other differences, however, are based upon culturally defined expressions of gender. Lung and bronchus cancer death rates may be

Table 4. Death Rates by Sex for Selected Cancers in the United States, 1998 (per 100,000)

Cancer site	Female	Male
Oral	1.1	3.2
Colon and rectum	10.4	15.2
Breast	20.0	—
Prostate	—	15.9
Lung and bronchus	26.6	52.3
Uterus (cervix)	2.4	—
All sites	108.3	156.0

Source: Murphy (2000).

higher in males than in females because, until recently, tobacco smoking was more widespread among and more socially acceptable for men. Differences such as these in the distribution of diseases across social groups result in different health promotion priorities for different populations. This variability is also central for determining resource allocation and shaping health policy.

Yet, the ways in which patterns of disease prevalence shape health promotion are not always straightforward or completely rational. An example of this is how populations tend to respond to *epidemic* as opposed to *endemic* diseases. Several researchers (e.g., Duffy, 1990; Lupton, 1995) have noted that diseases characterized by sporadic outbreaks (e.g., bubonic plague, smallpox, yellow fever, and Asiatic cholera) provoked widespread panic and concerted public responses. In contrast, endemic diseases that contributed much more to morbidity and mortality (such as measles, scarlet fever, and enteric diseases) were taken for granted as a normal part of life. A major objective of the field of epidemiology, therefore, has been to describe more accurately the pattern of diseases so that treatment and prevention resources could be allocated most appropriately (Hennekens & Buring, 1987). A major step in this direction was the development in the early 20th century of reliable systems for the collection of vital records (Duffy, 1990).

More recently, epidemiologists have focused their attention not only on the distribution of health and disease, but also upon the determinants of ill health. Possible causes of disease may be called a correlate, fixed marker, risk factor, or causal risk factor depending upon the strength of the epidemiological evidence pointing to them as causes of disease (Kraemer, Kazdin, Offord, Kessler, Jensen, & Kupfer, 1997). More recent research has begun to focus on factors that decrease the likelihood of disease, identifying individual and community assets, and measuring social capital (Coleman, 1988; Kawachi, Kennedy, Lochner, & Prothrow-Stith, 1997; Zimmerman, 2000; Zimmerman & Arunkumar, 1994). Epidemiologists have attempted to quantify the cost of different diseases using increasingly sophisticated measures such as attributable risk, years of life lost, and quality adjusted life years (Hennekens & Buring, 1987; Lupton, 1995). Such efforts provide policy makers with information that will enable them to allocate treatment and prevention resources in ways that will be most beneficial.

This discussion of disease patterns shaping health promotion may appear to imply that all health promotion efforts are intended to reduce the prevalence or incidence of specific diseases. It should be noted, however, that health professionals (e.g., Green & Kreuter, 1999) often emphasize that the goals of health promotion include not only disease prevention, but also the promotion of positive physical, mental, and social well-being. Nevertheless, most contemporary health promotion work is oriented toward the prevention of specific diseases rather than the general promotion of well-being.

HEALTH PROMOTION AND THEORIES OF DISEASE

Just as health promotion has evolved in response to changes in the prevalence and incidence of different diseases, it has also been shaped by our changing theories of disease. Throughout history, societies have differed in the conditions they define as illnesses, in the names they give to these illnesses, and in their beliefs about the underlying causal processes that lead to the appearance of an illness in an individual or group. These ideas, which we refer to as *theories of disease*, have implications not only for how illnesses are treated and controlled once they appear, but also for how societies attempt to prevent them.

The oldest known theories of disease were *theurgical.* People ascribed illness and health to the actions of supernatural beings, including demons, spirits, and gods (Ellencweig & Yoshpe, 1984). Different societies had different theurgical theories of disease, each forming a part of an overall religious and cultural framework. In many cases, people interpreted epidemics as a form of divine retribution for sin. Theurgical theories of disease led to a variety of strategies for preventing illness, including prayer, the offering of sacrifices to placate wrathful spirits, and the encouragement of righteous living (Ellencweig & Yoshpe, 1984; Lupton, 1995). Although many alternatives to theurgical theories of disease now exist, many people still subscribe to these traditional views in some ways. Among people living in southern African countries, for instance, illnesses that take unusual forms or that are unresponsive to standard treatments are often attributed to witchcraft, sorcery, or evil spirits (Foser, 1981; Green, 1999). Similarly, in the United States, some people still view illness as the expression of God's judgment, as evidenced by the use of the phrase "Wrath of God

Syndrome" in the early 1980s to refer to what we now call HIV disease or AIDS (Treichler, 1988).

One of the earliest alternatives to theurgical theories of disease was the *humoral theory* (Ellencweig & Yoshpe, 1984). This theory was developed in ancient Greece during the Classical Era. It held that bodily health could be preserved by maintaining an appropriate balance among the four humors (blood, phlegm, black bile, and yellow bile), the four elements (earth, air, fire, and water), and four qualities (hot, cold, wet, and dry). A striking feature of the humoral theory is its emphasis on the interaction between individuals and their environments. Health promotion strategies based on the humoral theory, therefore, focused on monitoring the passage of exterior elements (e.g., food, water, air) into the body, and of interior elements (feces, blood, sweat, urine, semen) out of the body and into the environment (Lupton, 1995). In Europe, the fall of the Roman Empire brought about an abandonment of the humoral theory and a return to theurgical theories of disease. During this period, however, the humoral theory was disseminated throughout much of the Arab world where it was taught in medical schools and helped lead to the description of anthrax, leprosy, scabies, smallpox, measles, and bubonic plague as distinct conditions (Ellencweig & Yoshpe, 1984). Like theurgical theories of disease, the humoral theory is still influential today. Many people continue to believe that spending time in the cold (e.g., going outdoors without a jacket during the winter) is likely to cause someone to become ill, even though this belief conflicts with contemporary understandings of the transmission of viral and bacterial pathogens.

In medieval Europe, while theurgical theories of disease were predominant, various forms of *contagion theory* became influential. The basic proposition of contagion theory is that diseases are capable of being passed in some way from one person to another. Prior to the widespread acceptance of germ theory, theories of contagion were not specific about the underlying mechanisms of disease transmission. Nevertheless, people in medieval times understood that some diseases were contagious and developed disease prevention strategies based upon this understanding. Such strategies, including *quarantine* and *sequestration*, were intended to separate those who were sick from those who were not. During epidemics of bubonic plague, for instance, Italian cities regularly placed under quarantine merchant ships that came to port. In fact, the word quarantine is based upon the Italian for *forty days*, which is how long such ships were often made to wait before coming ashore (Musto, 1988). These practices were largely ineffective, however, because they did not deal with the main vector of plague transmission: rats and the lice that lived upon them.

Another theory of disease that arose in medieval Europe was the *miasma theory*. This theory held that disease was caused by the inhalation of or contact with damp, polluted, and malodorous air. It arose in part because of people's observation that plague and other epidemics tended to occur during the hot summer months when the air was humid and, especially in cities, filled with the odors of garbage, decomposing animals, and human waste (Cipolla, 1992; Duffy, 1990). People believed that miasmas emanating from diseased or decomposing bodies could lead to a variety of conditions, including syphilis, gangrene, scurvy, and fevers (Lupton, 1995). The *sanitary movement* of the 19th century, to which historians of health promotion generally point as the beginning of modern health promotion (e.g., Duffy, 1990; Rosen, 1993), was based largely upon the miasma theory of disease. This movement was led by upper-class, reform-minded men such as Chadwick in England, Villerme in France, and J.H. Griscom, Shattuck, and Banks in the United States (Aita & Crabtree, 2000; Duffy, 1990). These men believed that environmental conditions, particularly those that led to unpleasant odors, were responsible for the high mortality rates in the working class sections of emerging industrial cities. They therefore proposed not medical, but physical and social engineering solutions to deal with such problems as open sewers, poor drainage, and accumulated waste.

The next major development in theories of disease occurred in the late 19th century when the work of Pasteur and Koch led to the widespread acceptance of *germ theory* (Aita & Crabtree, 2000; Duffy, 1990). In fact, bacteria had been observed centuries earlier by the Dutch microscopist Leeuwenhoek. Pasteur's success in dealing with rabies and diseases affecting silkworms, however, gave great credence to the germ theory of disease, with profound implications for health promotion (Duffy, 1990). This theory provided a more detailed explanation of contagion. It also discredited the miasma theory while simultaneously providing support for many of the measures for which the sanitary reformers had argued, such as, the construction of modern sewers and the removal of waste from streets. Ironically, while the microbial revolution hastened the remediation of many of the environmental causes of infectious diseases, it also drew the attention of public health workers away from social issues such as poverty, inadequate housing, and the pollution of waterways, focusing it instead on the role of microorganisms in causing disease (Fee & Porter, 1992; Lupton, 1995). Consequently, health promotion turned its attention to the microscopic world, and for several decades in the late 19th and early 20th centuries, the chief health promotion strategies included vaccination and individual behavior change (e.g., promotion of personal cleanliness).

Not all health problems could be solved with vaccines or antibiotics. As many of the longstanding infectious diseases became less important in developed countries in the early 20th century, other conditions such as heart disease and cancer became more widespread. The causal mechanisms behind these diseases, however, could not be reduced to a single microbial agent. Moreover, interventions as simple as vaccination were not automatic, but required action on the part of individuals. For these reasons, by the middle of the 20th century the role of individual behaviors became a significant part of theories of disease, and changing behaviors became a priority for health promotion. At first, most health promotion efforts in this area were governed by a crude theory of behavior change: Provide knowledge, and people will change their behavior accordingly. In 1920, for instance, the motto of the Ontario Board of Health was "Let not the people perish for lack of knowledge" (Lupton, 1995, p. 40).

After World War II, however, social psychological theories of behavior became influential and led to the development of the Health Belief Model (Janz & Becker, 1984; Strecher & Rosenstock, 1997), the Theory of Planned Behavior (Ajzen & Fishbein, 1980; Montano, Kasprzyk, & Taplin, 1997), and other theories that emphasized the role of individual values, beliefs, and expectations in governing individual health-related behaviors. Subsequently, Social Cognitive Theory (Bandura, 1986, 1997; Baranowski, Perry, & Parcel, 1997) emphasized the idea that behaviors are often learned from others, and that changing behavior sometimes requires the acquisition of skills and the confidence that one can successfully carry out behaviors. While these models of human behavior differ in their specifics, they all share in common the theory that individual behavior is a critical determinant of health and therefore an appropriate focus for health promotion.

In recent decades, health promotion has begun to incorporate an *ecological theory* of disease, which views illness and health as the outcomes of processes operating at a variety of levels, ranging from genetic and pathogenic at the micro level to social structural at the macro level. One early expression of this ecological theory of disease was the report "A New Perspective on the Health of Canadians," published by Canadian Minister of National Health and Welfare, Marc Lalonde, in 1974. Lalonde argued in this report that four factors were largely responsible for health outcomes: individual biophysiological characteristics, environmental pollution, health care services, and individual lifestyle or behavior. Researchers have described different ecological models, but their common theme focuses on the interdependent connections across biological, individual, family/organizational, community, and policy levels that influence health and disease (e.g., Bloom, 1996; Kelly, Ryan, Altman, & Stelzner, 2000; McLeroy, Bibeau, Steckler, & Glanz, 1988; Stokols, 1992). Health promotion workers today focus their energies at a variety of levels. Some continue to emphasize the importance of individual behaviors, and seek to encourage

behavior change with strategies ranging from individual counseling to media advertising. Others point to larger social structural factors affecting health, such as, poverty and racism, and call for policy changes or work on grassroots organizing (Kaplan, Pamuk, Lynch, Cohen, & Balfour, 1996; Minkler, 1989; Williams, Yu, Jackson, & Anderson, 1997). While they emphasize different levels and work in different ways, most health promotion professionals today share an ecological theory of disease that emphasizes the complex interactions between individuals and their physical and social environments.

HEALTH PROMOTION AND CHANGE TECHNOLOGY

In addition to the prevalence of diseases and our theories about how and why they occur, a third factor shaping health promotion is the technology available for the prevention of disease. *Change technology* refers to the strategies and methods used in health promotion efforts. The development of change technologies is governed largely by our theories of disease. These theories provide direction to efforts to develop effective change technologies, suggesting points in the causal chain at which interventions could potentially prevent the disease from occurring. Effective health promotion technologies, however, do not follow automatically from theories of disease. In the case of HIV infection, for example, biomedical researchers have a very detailed understanding of the pathogenic interactions between the virus and human immune system, but have not yet been able to develop an effective vaccine. Change technologies take many forms, ranging from the microbiological to the macroeconomic. In this section, we highlight five broad strategies that have persisted over time. These five classes of change technology are: engineering the physical environment; biomedical interventions; mass communications; policy change and legislation; and social and behavioral interventions.

Perhaps the earliest type of health promotion interventions were those in which *engineering the physical environment* is used to provide people with healthy living conditions. The Romans selected building sites on the basis of Greek humoral theory, and built sophisticated water and sewer systems (Ellencweig & Yoshpe, 1984). Centuries later, sanitarians such as Chadwick pushed for improvements to the physical environment of the growing urban industrial areas of England, France, and the United States (Chave, 1984). Their efforts led to the construction of sewers, the creation of systems to supply people with clean water, waste removal systems, and codes governing the quality of housing (Duffy, 1990; Ellencweig & Yoshpe, 1984; Kemm & Close, 1995; Lupton, 1995). Such engineering efforts were not always simple. The technology for supplying clean water supplies, for example, developed quite slowly. While many large American cities had devised some water systems by the end of the 18th century, Philadelphia was the first to replace its wooden water mains with cast iron mains and lead service pipes in 1818. The development of effective filtration systems did not occur until the end of the 19th century (Duffy, 1990). More recent examples of engineering healthy physical environments include ventilation systems for modern buildings, the development of ergonomic work stations, the creation of sites for treating and storing hazardous waste, the use of fire-retardant materials in residential and commercial construction, and the fortification of the US grain supply with folic acid to prevent fetal neural tube defects (Hine, 1996).

Another important class of health promotion technologies includes *biomedical interventions.* Perhaps the most well-known such intervention is vaccination. Inoculation has existed for a surprisingly long time. A method of inoculating people against smallpox was developed in Greece and Turkey by the 17th century, and was discussed in British medical journals as early as 1714. This method involved taking pus from someone with active smallpox and inserting it in the arm of a healthy individual. It was used widely in colonial America; in fact, General Washington ordered that all troops in the Continental Army be inoculated against smallpox in 1776 (Duffy, 1990). In 1798, Jenner devised a method for vaccinating people against smallpox using the closely related cowpox virus. This method was much safer than inoculation, and soon became widespread in spite of strong opposition from some people (Duffy, 1990). Surprisingly, these technologies were developed prior to biomedical research into the functioning of the human immune system. Other immunizations were developed more recently: diphtheria in 1915, poliomyelitis in 1954, measles in 1963, hepatitis B in 1980, meningococcal in 1981, hepatitis A in 1994, and others (National Vaccine Advisory Committee, 1999). These vaccines have played a central role in the reduction in rates of many infectious diseases, including the eradication of smallpox worldwide. Other biomedical interventions include the prescription of drugs called beta blockers to prevent heart disease in people with high blood pressure and the nicotine patch to help people quit cigarette smoking (Hajek, West, Foulds, Nilsson, Burrows, & Meadow, 1999). The role of health promotion was not so much in the development of the vaccines or drugs themselves. Rather, it was in helping to develop strategies for getting people inoculated and educating patients about compliance to prescribed medication regimens.

A third class of health promotion technology is *mass communication.* In general, the purpose of health promotion efforts using mass communication techniques is to convey basic information or a persuasive message to a large number of people. The earliest forms of mass communication were print media, including newspapers and posters (Hovland, 1953). The development of the printing press and printing technology such as lithography made possible the widespread dissemination of health messages on paper. In the 1920s the French National Office of Social Hygiene developed a series of highly stylized color lithograph posters about syphilis. Each included some color illustration along with information or a persuasive message (Fox & Karp, 1988). With the introduction and dissemination of electronic media, such as radio, motion pictures, and television, new avenues of mass communication became available for health promotion. Beginning in the 1940s, electronic media were used by public health workers in efforts to change behaviors associated with cardiovascular disease (Finnegan & Viswanath, 1997; Maccoby & Farquhar, 1975; Solomon, 1982). The Minnesota Heart Health Program used media to communicate messages regarding cardiovascular disease risk factors to the public (Luepker, Murray, Jacobs, Mittelmark, Bracht, & Carlaw, 1994; Mittelmark, Luepker, Jacobs, Bracht, Carlaw, & Crow, 1986). While early attempts at using mass communications media to promote health may have been somewhat simplistic, recent decades have seen the emergence of sophisticated techniques for designing and implementing such campaigns. These techniques, sometimes referred to as *social marketing*, utilize a process model from commercial marketing to segment the target audience, select appropriate media channels, develop materials, and assess program effectiveness (Lefebvre & Rochlin, 1997). Additionally, some health promoters prefer to use mass communications techniques called *media advocacy* (Wallack, 1990). Whereas social marketing basically amounts to advertising health promotive behaviors, in media advocacy health promoters attempt to stimulate and influence the content of news media coverage of health-related policy issues. The goal, in most cases, is to frame the issues in ways that lead to the adoption or maintenance of public policies that are conducive to health.

Another change technology is *public policy and legislation.* Laws promoting health have a long history. An early example is the *quarantine.* During medieval times, it was the policy of Italian city governments to keep travelers from entering the cities during times when bubonic plague threatened (Cipolla, 1992; Lupton, 1995; Musto, 1988). This meant closing the city gates to foot traffic, suspending trade, and requiring ships to remain anchored in the harbor rather than landing ashore (Risse, 1988). A closely related policy is that of *sequestration*, or the isolation of infected individuals. Policies of isolating the sick have been used for plague, leprosy, yellow fever, cholera, tuberculosis, and other ailments (Musto, 1988). More recent examples of laws governing individual behavior in the interest of health include seat belt laws (Fields & Weinberg, 1994), speed limits and drunk driving laws (Farrell, 1989), and prohibitions against smoking in certain public places (Wakefield, Chaloupka, Kaufman, Orleans, Barker, & Ruel, 2000). Other laws target the behavior of corporations, municipalities, schools, and other groups. These include laws governing air quality and emissions (Browner, 1997), laws mandating the printing of the Surgeon General's warning on cigarette packages and advertisements (Davis & Kendrick, 1989), levying taxes on tobacco and alcohol purchases, and defining acceptable levels of toxins (e.g., arsenic) in drinking water.

Social and behavior interventions comprise a fifth type of health promotion technology. This class includes a wide range of efforts including individual level programs and community organizing strategies. An early example of behavioral interventions is health visiting. Health visiting has a long history, with examples dating back as far as the Roman Empire (Brainard, 1985). Beginning in the late 1800s, British health authorities employed women as health visitors. Their role was to visit the homes of poor people and provide them with instructions in child-rearing and household sanitation (Kemm & Close, 1995). Individual level behavioral interventions are extremely common today, focusing on a broad range of health behaviors and taking place in such diverse settings as homes, workplaces, schools, hospitals, churches, and elsewhere (Clark, Janz, Dodge, & Sharpe, 1992; Perry et al., 1996). Such programs are often guided by value-expectancy models and learning theories.

More recently, community-level and community-based social interventions to promote health have increased (Israel, Schultz, Parker, & Becker, 1998; Kelly et al., 2000). The broad goal of such interventions is to mobilize members of a community to bring about changes in some aspect of the physical or social environment that may be detrimental to health. Social interventions generally involve some type of community organizing (Rothman & Tropman, 1987). Specific applications use grassroots organizing, coalition building, lay health workers, consciousness raising, and culturally relevant practice (Caldwell, Zimmerman, Isichei, 2001; Israel et al., 1998; Minkler, 1997; Zimmerman, Ramirez-Valles, Suarez, de la Rosa, & Castro, 1997).

HEALTH PROMOTION AND SOCIAL INFLUENCES

The three factors discussed above—patterns of disease prevalence, theories of disease, and available technology of intervention—do not operate in isolation. Rather, it is through their dynamic interaction with one another that they take shape and exert their influence on health promotion. They also take place in a social context that influences health promotion on every level. *Social factors* refer to a wide range of phenomena including large-scale economic and political developments (e.g., the industrial revolution, the rise of modern nation-states); the features of specific social and historical contexts (e.g., social stratification, power relations); and the beliefs and values of individuals working to promote health (e.g., culture, social norms). These social factors shape health promotion indirectly by influencing patterns of disease prevalence, theories of disease, and available technologies of intervention. They also operate directly by helping to determine *who* develops and implements health promotion programs, *how* they do it, and *for whom.*

One of the ways in which social factors shape health promotion is by influencing the pattern of disease prevalence. A striking example of this is the effect of European exploration and colonization on the health of indigenous Americans in the decades following 1492. During these years, contact with Europeans led to outbreaks of infectious diseases, especially smallpox, among the native people. These epidemics wiped out as much as 30–50 percent of the indigenous population, causing major social upheavals and clearing the way for European conquest and colonization (Crosby, 1972). Similarly, European colonization in sub-Saharan Africa led to outbreaks of communicable disease among both the colonists and native populations (Hartwig & Patterson, 1978). Changes brought about by the colonial regimes, including labor migration, resettlement, forced labor camps, the development of towns, the construction of roads, and the introduction of bicycles, also contributed to the spread of infectious diseases like relapse fever (Azevodo, 1978; Good, 1978). More recently, the outbreak of major epidemics of HIV among urban gay men in the United States had its roots in social factors. These included the establishment of gay male communities in large American cities in the late 19th and early 20th centuries; the emergence in these communities of commercial sex establishments where men could easily find a large number of sex partners; and the sexual revolution of the 1960s and 1970s, which made casual sex with multiple partners more socially acceptable (D'Emilio, 1983). These social changes lay the groundwork for a variety of sexually transmitted disease epidemics, beginning with gonorrhea and syphilis in the 1960s and culminating in the first reported AIDS cases in 1981 (Rotello, 1997). In all of these cases, developments that were social, political, and economic in origin had profound effects on the distribution of disease.

Just as patterns of disease distribution are influenced by social forces, so too are the theories people use to understand these diseases. In the late 19th century, the two leading explanations of disease—contagion theory and miasma theory—were associated with different social, political, and economic interests. Contagion theory was generally favored by those who sought to preserve the traditional economic and social systems, while miasma theory was favored by those who advocated industrialization and commerce, and who saw the rise of capitalism as a sign of progress (Tesh, 1988).

Another interesting example of the effects of social factors on theories of disease is the rise during the last century of biomedicine as the ultimate arbiter of truth in matters of health and illness (Goldstein, 1992; Lupton, 1995). While biomedicine's success in treating a variety of illnesses provides a partial explanation for its current dominance, social factors played an equally important role. Three related developments were critical. The first was the formation by physicians and other health workers of professional organizations. The American Medical Association, for example, was founded in 1847 and by the early 1900s had become a powerful political force, influencing important policy decisions and commanding impressive resources (Duffy, 1990). At the same time, the early 20th century saw the emergence of modern welfare states, the power and legitimacy of which depended upon the perception of governments as acting to safeguard the health and well-being of their citizens (Ellencweig & Yoshpe, 1984). The third and perhaps most important development was the alliance that formed between the medical profession and welfare states in the middle of the 20th century (Duffy, 1990). This alliance provides legitimacy to welfare states, and benefits the medical profession in a variety of ways, not the least of which is by supporting medical research at a level that is unprecedented in human history. Thus, as much as biomedicine's technical success, its professional organization and alliance with modern welfare states helps to account for its current dominance in theories of disease causation.

Social factors also have direct effects on health promotion. They help determine (a) who develops and implements health promotion programs, (b) for whom such programs are developed, and (c) what form these interventions take. One example of the role of social factors in shaping who does health promotion can be found in the relationship between public health and medicine in Great Britain and the United States (Fee & Porter, 1991). In both countries, professional roles in health promotion were virtually non-existent at the beginning of the 19th century. In Great Britain, the public health movement began and gained momentum during the 1840s and 1850s—a time when there was an overabundance of physicians. In that context, many medical practitioners had a hard time earning a living providing fee-for-service care. They were therefore happy to enroll in coursework geared toward obtaining a Diploma in Public Health, which would virtually guarantee them full-time employment doing public health work for a local government. In contrast, in the United States the public health movement began 50 years later, when medical education had already been reorganized to restrict the number of physicians in training. Graduates

from medical school in the United States had little trouble earning impressive incomes through clinical practice. Public health training programs were therefore organized largely outside of medical schools, and attracted only a few physicians. Because of these differences, physicians in Great Britain continue to play a vital role in many aspects of health promotion, whereas in the United States health promotion is less closely connected to medicine. Health promotion in the United States has largely become the responsibility of professionals trained in fields such as public health, nursing, chemistry, engineering, and the social sciences (Fee & Porter, 1991).

Social factors also help determine for whom health promotion interventions are provided. A recent example of this is the failure of many public health institutions in the United States and elsewhere to take action during the early years of the HIV/AIDS epidemic. This failure has generally been attributed to the fact that those who first developed AIDS were mostly members of politically weak or socially stigmatized groups, including Haitians, injection drug users, and gay men (Perrow & Guillen, 1990; Shilts, 1987). Since the early years of the epidemic, much has changed. In particular, members of the hardest hit gay communities developed their own service organizations and became politically mobilized to advocate for more, and more effective, official responses to the epidemic (Crimp & Rolston, 1990; Kramer, 1989). Today, federal and state expenditures on HIV research, treatment, and prevention are so high that many people criticize them as being disproportionate to the effect of AIDS in the population, relative to other ailments such as cancer and cardiovascular disease. Nevertheless, in the mid-1990s the groups that accounted for some 83 percent of reported AIDS cases in the United States were gay men and injection drug users, but only a small proportion of federal HIV prevention dollars were targeted to these groups. Instead, much of the Centers for Disease Control's $584 million AIDS prevention budget in 1996 was earmarked for groups that face a relatively low risk of infection (Bennett & Sharpe, 1996). Thus, while epidemiological information about the relative burden of disease in different groups plays a role in determining who receives health promotion services, the allocation of such services continues to be shaped by political and social factors.

Social factors also help determine the content and procedures involved in health promotion efforts. The debate among health promotion experts in recent years between those who favor individual behavior change approaches versus those who advocate environmental and social change approaches serves to illustrate the political and social nature of health promotion interventions. Those who favor individual behavior change interventions argue that these approaches are most effective, and that individuals should be held responsible for their own health-related behaviors. A well-known statement of this position was provided by the president of the Rockefeller Foundation, who wrote, "The next major advances in the health of the American people will be determined by what the individual is willing to do for himself and for society at large" (Knowles, 1977, p. 1103). Similarly, a team of epidemiologists in the 1990s attempted to trace deaths in the United States to what they defined to be their actual causes. They concluded that individual behaviors such as tobacco use, diet, physical activity patterns, alcohol consumption, and sexual behaviors were among the most important factors needing to be addressed (McGinnis & Foege, 1993). Indeed, individual behavior change has been the focus of the federal health promotion strategy in countries ranging from the United States to Cuba for many years (Tesh, 1988).

Some critics, however, argue that individual behavior change strategies may not be the most effective approach (e.g., Labonte, 1986; Minkler, 1989). They trace the causes of disease to social conditions, and view individual behavior change efforts as socially unjust and victim blaming. Instead, they call for social change to reduce inequality, improve living conditions, and empower oppressed and marginalized groups, arguing that these approaches stand the best chance of bringing about improvements in health. Tesh (1988) has shown that both of these positions—those favoring individual behavior change approaches and those advocating social change—are integrally connected to more general ideological positions about social justice, the relationship of the individual to society, and the role of the state versus the market. In short, the broader social, economic, and political beliefs of those in health promotion lead to different prescriptions about how health promotion ought to be done.

The examples provided above only begin to reveal the pervasive role of political and social factors in shaping health promotion. Indeed, health promotion is an inherently social product, and thus can never be purely the product of objective science, if such a thing exists. Instead of wishing that health promotion were less subject to political and social influences, therefore, it may be useful to embrace the notion that health promotion is a social product, and then to consider the ways in which social factors may help shape health promotion for the common good.

One example of this is the role that local cultures—including the attitudes, beliefs, and practices of local people—can play in helping or hindering even the simplest health promotion efforts. Wellin (1955) investigated factors associated with Peruvian villagers' decision to boil their drinking water after being encouraged to do so by a health promotion worker. He discovered that there were indeed differences between those who boiled their water and those who did not, but these differences were not simple. Among water boilers as among non-boilers there were often different and even opposing motives for the same end-product behaviors. He discovered the subtle distinctions in ethnic identifications and socioeconomic standing that effected their decisions to boil water. The significance of Wellin's work is "that even the most taken-for granted items of action programs may be found, on scrutiny, to have linkages with unexpected parts of culture and to carry meanings that have consequences for a program's career" (Wellin, 1955, p. 100). This is the very kind of knowledge that is essential for the design and implementation of health promotion programs. Decades later a Catholic organization with a long history of implementing social programs in rural Honduras managed in a short period of time to get virtually all residents of several villages to begin boiling their drinking water. They did this by involving local housewives' organizations in the design of the program, and by connecting water boiling and other disease preventive actions to the larger social and economic concerns experienced by members of these communities (Minkler & Cox, 1980).

CONCLUSION

Health promotion is a centuries old tradition that has taken on different forms and focused on different issues over time. Patterns and theories of disease, change technologies, and social factors have all played a role in shaping the various health promotion efforts found throughout history. Health promotion efforts have consistently included a range of strategies from environmental to individual behavior change. Yet, the emphasis across time and from place to place has varied widely. As infectious diseases were controlled with environmental and medical interventions, the focus of health promotion shifted to health behavior change. The behavioral changes focused first on the rational mind approaches where knowledge was thought to be enough to motivate people to change risky behaviors, but we have learned that knowledge alone does not translate into behavior change. Thus, behavior change theories and their concomitant strategies blossomed, but disease prevalence and population health did not change much. More recently, health promotion has turned its attention to sociocultural context and community-level strategies of change. Today health promotion includes a range of activities that cut across the level of analysis with a theme of community involvement. As t he prevalence and theory of disease transforms, change technologies develop, and ever-changing social forces influence the context within which health promotion operates, so too will the focus and shape of health promotion develop. While lessons have been learned from the past, health promotion must help individuals, groups, and communities gain the skills and resources necessary so they can effectively prevent disease and enhance their own health. As health promotion develops in the years to come, a vital component of any effort will be to include communities and the individuals who live in them in the process of program development, implementation, and evaluation.

Also see: Financing: Foundation; Culture: Foundation; Society and Social Class: Foundation; Definition: Foundation.

References

Aita, V.A., & Crabtree, B. (2000). Historical reflections on current preventive practice. *Preventive Medicine, 30,* 5–16.

Ajzen, I., & Fishbein, M. (1980). *Understanding attitudes and predicting social behavior.* Englewood Cliffs, NJ: Prentice-Hall.

Azevodo, M.J. (1978). Epidemic disease among the Sara of Southern Chad. In G.W. Hartwig & K.D. Patterson (Eds.), *Disease in African history* (pp. 118–152). Durham: University Press.

Bandura, A. (1986). *Social foundations of thought and action: A Social Cognitive Theory.* Englewood Cliffs, NJ: Prentice-Hall.

Bandura, A. (1997). *Self-efficacy: The exercise of control.* New York: W.H. Freeman.

Baranowski, T., Perry, C.L., & Parcel, G.S. (1997). How individuals, environments, and health behavior interact: Social Cognitive Theory. In K. Glanz, F.M. Lewis, & B.K. Rimer (Eds.), Health behavior and health education: Theory, research, and practice (2nd ed., pp. 153–178). San Francisco: Jossey-Bass.

Bennett, A., & Sharpe, A. (1996). AIDS fight is skewed by federal campaign exaggerating risks: Most heterosexuals face scant peril but receive large proportion of funds; less goes to gays, addicts. *Wall Street Journal,* May 1, 1996.

Bloom, M. (1996). *Primary prevention practices.* Thousand Oaks, CA: Sage.

Brainard, A.M. (1985). *The evolution of public health nursing.* New York: Garland.

Browner, C.M. (1997). Smog and soot: updating air quality standards. *Public Health Reports, 112*(5), 366–367.

Caldwell, C.H., Zimmerman, M.A., & Isichei, P.A.C. (2001). Forging collaborative partnerships to enhance family health: An assessment of strengths and challenges in conducting community-based research. *Journal of Public Health Management and Practice, 7*(2), 1–9.

CDC. (2000). Ten Leading Causes of Death 1900–1978. In http://www.cdc.gov/nchs/data/lead0078.pdf

Chave, S.P. (1984). The Duncan memorial lecture. "Duncan of Liverpool—and some lessons for today." *Community Medicine, 6,* 61–71.

Cipolla, C.M. (1992). *Miasmas and disease; Public health and the environment in the pre-industrial age.* New Haven: Yale University Press.

Clark, N.M., Janz, N.K., Dodge, J.A., & Sharpe, P.A. (1992). Self-regulation of health behavior: The "Take PRIDE" program. *Health Education Quarterly, 19*(3), 341–354.

Coleman, J. (1988). Social capital and the creation of human capital. *American Journal of Sociology, 94,* S95–S120.

Crimp, D., & Rolston, A. (1990). *AIDS demographics.* Seattle: Bay Press.

Crosby, A.W. (1972). *The Columbian exchange: biological and cultural consequences of 1492.* Westport, CT: Greenwood Press.

Davis, R.M., & Kendrick, J.S. (1989). The Surgeon General's warnings in outdoor cigarette advertising: Are they readable? *Journal of the American Medical Association, 261*(1), 90–94.

D'Emilio, J. (1983). *Sexual politics, sexual communities: The making of a homosexual minority in the United States, 1940–1970.* Chicago: University of Chicago Press.

Duffy, J. (1990). *The sanitarians: A history of American public health.* Chicago: University of Illinois Press.

Ellencweig, A.Y., & Yoshpe, R.B. (1984). The definition of public health. *Public Health Reviews, 12,* 65–78.

Farrell, S. (1989). Policy alternatives for alcohol-impaired driving. *Health Education Quarterly, 16*(3), 413–427.

Fee, E., & Porter, D. (1991). Public health, preventive medicine, and professionalization: Britain and the United States in the nineteenth century. In E. Fee & R.M. Acheson (Eds.), *A history of education in public health: Health that mocks the doctors' rules* (pp. 15–43). New York: Oxford University Press.

Fee, E., & Porter, D. (1992). *Public health, preventive medicine and professionalization: England and America in the nineteenth century.* Cambridge: Cambridge University Press.

Fields, M., & Weinberg, K. (1994). Coverage gaps in child-restraint and seat-belt laws affecting children. *Accident Analysis & Prevention, 26*(3), 371–376.

Finnegan, J.R., & Viswanath, K. (1997). Communication theory and health behavior change. In K. Glanz, F.M. Lewis, & B.K. Rimer (Eds.), *Health behavior and health education: Theory, research, and practice* (2nd ed., pp. 313–341). San Francisco: Jossey-Bass.

Foser, G.B. (1981). Disease classification in rural Ghana: Framework and implications for health behaviour. *Social Science and Medicine, 15B*(4), 471–482.

Fox, D.M., & Karp, D.R. (1988). Images of plague: Infectious disease in the visual arts. In E. Fee & D.M. Fox (Eds.), *AIDS: The burdens of history* (pp. 172–189). Berkeley: University of California Press.

Geronimus, A.T., Bound, J., & Waidmann, T.A. (1996). Excess mortality among blacks and whites in the United States. *New England Journal of Medicine, 335,* 1552–1558.

Goldstein, M.S. (1992). *The health movement: Promoting fitness in America.* New York: Twayne.

Good, C.M. (1978). Man, milieu and the disease factor: Tick-borne relapsing fever in East Africa. In G.W. Hartwig & K.D. Patterson (Eds.), *Disease in African history.* Durham: Duke University Press, 46–87.

Green, E.C. (1999). *Indigenous theories of contagious disease.* Walnut Creek, CA: AltaMira Press.

Green, L.W., & Kreuter, M.W. (1999). *Health promotion planning: An educational and ecological approach.* Mountain View, CA: Mayfield.

Hajek, P., West, R., Foulds, J., Nilsson, F., Burrows, S., & Meadow, A. (1999). Randomized comparative trial of nicotine polacrilex, a transdermal patch, nasal spray, and an inhaler. *Archives of Internal Medicine, 159*(17), 2033–2038.

Hartwig, G.W., & Patterson, K.D. (1978). *Disease in African history: an introductory survey and case studies.* Durham, NC: Duke University Press.

Hennekens, C.H., & Buring, J.E. (1987). *Epidemiology in medicine.* Boston: Little, Brown.

Hine, R.J. (1996). What practitioners need to know about folic acid. *Journal of the American Dietetic Association, 96,* 451–452.

Hovland, C.I. (1953). *Communication and persuasion: Psychological studies of opinion change.* New Haven: Yale University Press.

Israel, B.A., Schultz, A.J., Parker, E.A., & Becker, A.B. (1998). Review of community-based research: Assessing partnership approaches to improve public health. *Annual Review of Public Health, 19,* 173–202.

Janz, N.K., & Becker, M.H. (1984). The Health Belief Model: A decade later. *Health Education Quarterly, 11*(1), 1–47.

Kaplan, G.A., Pamuk, E.R., Lynch, J.W., Cohen, R.D. & Balfour, J.L. (1996). Inequality in income and mortality in the United States: Analysis of mortality and potential pathways. *British Medical Journal, 312,* 999–1003.

Kawachi, I., Kennedy, B.P., Lochner, K., & Prothrow-Stith, D. (1997). Social capitol, income inequality, and mortality. *American Journal of Public Health, 87,* 1491–1498.

Kelly, J.G., Ryan, A.M., Altman, B.E., & Stelzner, S.P. (2000). Understanding and changing social systems: An ecological view. In J. Rappaport & E. Seidman (Eds.), *Handbook of community psychology* (pp. 133–159). New York: Kluwer Academic.

Kemm, J., & Close, A. (1995). *Health promotion: Theory and practice.* London: Macmillan.

Knowles, J.H. (1977). Responsibility for health. *Science, 198*(4322), 1103.

Kraemer, H.C., Kazdin, A.E., Offord, D.R., Kessler, R.C., Jensen, P.S., & Kupfer, D.J. (1997). Coming to terms with the terms of risk. *Archives of General Psychiatry, 54*(4), 337–343.

Kramer, L. (1989). *Reports from the holocaust: The making of an AIDS activist.* New York: St. Martin's Press.

Labonte, R. (1986). Social inequality and healthy public policy. *Health Promotion, 1,* 341–351.

Lalonde, M. (1974). A new perspective on the health of Canadians. Ottowa: Office of the Canadian Minister of National Health and Welfare.

Lefebvre, R.C., & Rochlin, L. (1997). Social marketing. In K. Glanz, F.M. Lewis, & B.K. Rimer (Eds.), *Health behavior and health education: Theory, research, and practice* (2nd ed., pp. 384–402). San Francisco: Jossey-Bass.

Luepker, R.V., Murray, D.M., Jacobs, D.R., Mittelmark, M.B., Bracht, N., & Carlaw, R. (1994). Community education for cardiovascular disease prevention: Risk factor changes in the Minnesota Heart Health Program. *American Journal of Public Health, 84*(9), 1383–1393.

Lupton, D. (1995). *The imperative of health: Public health and the regulated body.* Thousand Oaks: Sage.

Maccoby, N., & Farquhar, J.W. (1975). Communication for health: Unselling heart disease. *Journal of Communication, 25*(3), 114–126.

McCord, C., & Freeman, H.P. (1990). Excess mortality in Harlem. *New England Journal of Medicine, 322,* 173–177.

McGinnis, J.M., & Foege, W.H. (1993). Actual causes of death in the United States. *Journal of the American Medical Association, 270*(18), 2207–2212.

McLeroy, K.R., Bibeau, D., Steckler, A., & Glanz, K. (1988). An ecological perspective on health promotion programs. *Health Education Quarterly, 15*(4), 351–377.

Minkler, M. (1989). Health education, health promotion, and the open society: An historical perspective. *Health Education Quarterly, 16*(1), 17–30.

Minkler, M. (1997). *Community organizing and community building for health.* New Brunswick, NJ: Rutgers University Press.

Minkler, M., & Cox, K. (1980). Creating critical consciousness in health: Applications of Friere's philosophy and methods to the health care setting. *International Journal of Health Services, 10*(2), 311–322.

Mishra, S.I., Conner, R.F., & Magana, J.R. (1996). Migrant workers in the United States: A profile from the fields. In S.I. Mishra, R.F. Conner, & J.R. Magana (Eds.), *AIDS crossing borders: The spread of HIV among migrant Latinos* (pp. 1–24). Boulder, CO: Westview Press.

Mittelmark, M.B., Leupker, R.V., Jacobs, D.R., Bracht, N.F., Carlaw, R.W., & Crow, R.S. (1986). Community-wide prevention of cardiovascular disease: Education strategies of the Minnesota Heart Health Program. *Preventive Medicine, 15,* 1–17.

Montano, D.E., Kasprzyk, D., & Taplin, S.H. (1997). The Theory of Reasoned Action and the Theory of Planned Behavior. In K. Glanz, F. M. Lewis, & B.K. Rimer (Eds.), *Health behavior and health education: Theory, research, and practice* (2nd ed., pp. 85–112). San Francisco: Jossey-Bass.

Murphy, S. (2000). Deaths: Final data for 1998. *National Vital Statistics Report, 48*(11), 1–106.

Musto, D.F. (1988). Quarantine and the problem of AIDS. In E. Fee & D.M. Fox (Eds.), *AIDS: The burdens of history* (pp. 67–85). Berkeley: University of California Press.

National Vaccine Advisory Committee (1999). Lessons learned from a review of the development of selected vaccines. *Pediatrics, 104,* 942–950.

Nutbeam, D. (1998). Health promotion glossary. *Health Promotion International, 13,* 349–364.

PAHO. (1996). *Health conditions in the Americas.* Washington: WHO.

Perrow, C., & Guillen, M.F. (1990). *The AIDS disaster: The failure of organizations in New York and the nation.* New Haven: Yale University Press.

Perry, C.L., Williams, C.L., Veblen-Mortenson, S., Toomey, T., Komro, K.A., Anstine, P.S., et al. (1996). Project Northland: Outcomes of a community-wide alcohol use prevention program during early adolescence. *American Journal of Public Health, 86,* 956–965.

Risse, G.B. (1988). Epidemics and history: Ecological perspectives and social responses. In E. Fee & D.M. Fox (Eds.), *AIDS: The burdens of history* (pp. 33–66). Berkeley: University of California Press.

Rosen, G. (1993). *A history of public health.* Baltimore: Johns Hopkins University Press.

Rotello, G. (1997). *Sexual ecology: AIDS and the destiny of gay men.* New York: Dutton.

Rothman, J., & Tropman, J.E. (1987). Models of community organization and macro practice perspectives: Their mixing and phasing. In F.M. Cox, J.L. Erlich, J. Rothman, & J.E. Tropman (Eds.), *Strategies of community organization: Macro practice* (4th ed., pp. 3–26). Itasca, IL: F.E. Peacock.

Shilts, R. (1987). *And the band played on: Politics, people, and the AIDS epidemic.* New York: St. Martin's Press.

Solomon, D.S. (1982). Mass media campaigns for health promotion. *Prevention in Human Services, 2,* 115–128.

Stokols, D. (1992). Establishing and maintaining healthy environments: Toward a social ecology of health promotion. *American Psychologist, 47*(1), 6–22.

Strecher, V.J., & Rosenstock, I.M. (1997). The Health Belief Model. In K. Glanz, F.M. Lewis, & B.K. Rimer (Eds.), *Health behavior and health education: Theory, research, and practice* (2nd ed., pp. 41–59). San Francisco: Jossey-Bass.

Tesh, S.N. (1988). *Hidden arguments: Political ideology and disease prevention policy.* New Brunswick: Rutgers University Press.

Treichler, P.A. (1988). AIDS, gender, and biomedical discourse: Current contests for meaning. In E. Fee & D.M. Fox (Eds.), *AIDS: The burdens of history* (pp. 190–266). Berkeley: University of California Press.

Wakefield, M.A., Chaloupka, F.J., Kaufman, N.J., Orleans, C.T., Barker, D.C., & Ruel, E.E. (2000). Effect of restrictions on smoking at home, at school, and in public places on teenage smoking: Cross sectional study. *British Medical Journal, 321*(7257), 333–337.

Wallack, L. (1990). Improving health promotion: Media advocacy and social marketing approaches. In C. Atkin & L. Wallack (Eds.), *Mass communication and public health: Complexities and conflicts* (pp. 147–163). Newbury Park, CA: Sage.

Wellin, E. (1955). Water boiling in Peru. In B.J. Paul (Ed.), *Health, culture and community* (pp. 71–103). New York: Russell Sage Foundation.

Williams, D.R., Yu, Y., Jackson, J.S., & Anderson, N.B. (1997). Racial differences in physical and mental health: Socio-economic status, stress and discrimination. *Journal of Health Psychology, 2*(3), 335–351.

World Health Organization. (1999). *World health report.* Geneva, Switzerland: Author.

Zimmerman, M.A. (2000). Empowerment theory: Psychological, organizational and community levels of analysis. In J. Rappaport & E. Seidman (Eds.), *Handbook of Community Psychology* (Chap. 2, pp. 43–63). New York: Plenum Press.

Zimmerman, M.A., & Arunkumar, R. (1994). Resiliency research: Implications for schools and policy. *Social Policy Report, 8,* 1–18.

Zimmerman, M.A., Ramirez-Valles, J., Suarez, E., de la Rosa, G., & Castro, M.A. (1997). An HIV/AIDS prevention project for Mexican homosexual men: An empowerment approach. *Health Education & Behavior, 24,* 177–190.

Theories of Primary Prevention and Health Promotion

Morton M. Silverman

THE SPECTRUM OF INTERVENTION AND THE PLACE OF PREVENTION

Although there are a wide variety of interventions that may reduce the actual occurrence of a disease or disorder and thus in the most general sense are "preventive," not all of these efforts are appropriately labeled as prevention. Primary prevention should be accorded its own unique status, and secondary prevention given the more descriptive and appropriate label of early intervention. Similarly, treatment also should be accorded the separate and unique status it requires, rather than simply being lumped as merely another form of prevention.

The unique and defining features of prevention programs are (1) in their timing, (2) the levels of analysis that are targeted, and (3) the conditions that are the direct or indirect targets of change (Silverman & Felner, 1995). Given the "before-the-fact" nature of primary prevention, it could be argued that any intervention to reduce a specific behavior targeted at a group of individuals who have not yet demonstrated the behavior would qualify as prevention. Here the reasoning is that because they have not yet acted in a problematic way, they do not yet have the disorder. However, it is difficult to identify the specific point of "onset" for many socioemotional and health-related disorders.

A second critical feature of prevention programs relates to the level of analysis to which they are subjected. Prevention initiatives are targeted to populations or subpopulations, and the individuals who are the recipients of the intervention are selected based on their membership in the target group, rather than through a process of screening and selection based on individually specific characteristics (Cowen, 1983). Once interventions move to such screening and identification of conditions that are specific to discrete individuals, they have moved to early intervention and/or treatment. The targeting of populations is based on their exposure to conditions of risk (which are always population or subpopulation-level, never individual-level conditions) or the lack of exposure to important protective and developmentally enhancing conditions. In each local community, these conditions may be quite different, and careful analysis of the local community conditions is necessary for effective prevention program design. Although conditions that are stressful, that fail to promote the acquisition of important competencies, or that fail to provide necessary support are all ones that may predispose to or precipitate an adverse event, their specific manifestation in a local community requires attention and appropriate adaptation of "one-size-fits all programming."

The third defining feature for prevention efforts relates to what is targeted. In early intervention or treatment, there are clearly identifiable, highly individually specific conditions that need to be reversed or strengthened. These conditions are the direct targets of change and the evaluation of programming can follow from them, in that changes in these focal conditions will be apparent. In prevention, the first- and second-order targets of change are those conditions that lead to the focal conditions. *First-order targets of change*, or those conditions that are most directly targeted for change by the intervention, are the conditions of risk or protective factors to which all members of the population or subpopulation are exposed that have been identified as etiologically significant. *Second-order targets of change* are the levels of those vulnerabilities and competencies that result from exposure to the risk and protective factors of concern. Finally, through the modification of these critical elements of the etiological pathway, the incidence and prevalence of the targeted disorder or dysfunction will be affected (Felner & Lorion, 1985; Lorion, Price, & Eaton, 1989). Prevention applies to the systematic enhancement, disruption, alteration, or modification of the developmental processes (and conditions) that lead to well-being or to serious mental illness or social problems (Felner & Lorion, 1985).

Many of the advances in primary prevention have come as a result of advances in the related fields of public health and mental health (Albee, 1982; Cowen, 1983; Pardes, Silverman, & West, 1989). Our understanding of behavioral disorders has evolved alongside our understanding of disease entities and conditions as defined by public health and mental health researchers, theoreticians, clinicians, and epidemiologists. The major evolutions in related fields are:

1. *Epidemiology*—the definition and classification of disease processes; the identification and elaboration of risk factors; the modeling of causal relationships between and among risk and demographic variables; the accurate measurement and reporting of behavior in a defined population over time (surveillance)
2. *Treatment*—the evolution of techniques and technologies to effectively and efficiently treat individuals demonstrating early (and sometimes late) the signs and symptoms of distress and disorder
3. *Community mental health movement*—a recognition of the power and importance of the role of family,

community, schools, and workplace on the etiology, maintenance, and exacerbation of individual and group disturbance; the recognition of the powerful roles of ecology and environment in the development, expression, and maintenance of disordered social systems that express themselves as beliefs, attitudes, and behavior (Rappaport, 1987).

DEFINITIONS AND CONCEPTS OF PRIMARY PREVENTION

The concept of prevention has often been used broadly to refer to many different types of interventions and actions aimed at alleviating all manners of distress, illness, dysfunction, and disease in both individuals and larger populations, as well as promoting health and optimum social functioning. Unfortunately, few well-intentioned practitioners or investigators make the effort to define their terms precisely or link outcomes to specific interventions in advance of implementing programs. A brief review of definitions and concepts will set the stage for a fuller analysis of the strengths and limitations of existing models for the prevention of diseases and disorders in community settings. Different definitions and concepts will be presented to underscore their relevance to different targeted outcomes in different settings.

The field of public health has traditionally held twin goals: disease prevention and health promotion. Public health is grounded in the science of epidemiology. Hence, we will begin with the standard tripartite epidemiological definitions of prevention (Caplan, 1964) (Table 1). Primary prevention reduces the prevalence of a disorder or dysfunction by reducing the number of new cases (incidence) that appear in a defined population. Secondary prevention reduces the prevalence of a disorder by reducing the duration of a disorder or dysfunction in individuals who have expressed signs and symptoms of that disorder. One recent debate in the prevention research arena relates to the extent to which preventive interventions targeted at individuals identified as expressing early signs and symptoms of a significant disorder or dysfunction are classified as early secondary prevention or late primary prevention (Felner, Felner, & Silverman, 2000; Lorion et al., 1989). Tertiary prevention reduces recurring

Table 1. Epidemiological Definitions of Prevention

Prevalence = incidence × duration
Incidence = prevalence/duration
Primary prevention: reduce prevalence by reducing *incidence*
Secondary prevention: reduce prevalence by reducing *duration*
Tertiary prevention: reduce prevalence by reducing *reoccurrence*

episodes. Table 2 illustrates the various methods that are subsumed under the tripartite conceptualization of prevention.

The prevention spectrum can be understood in terms of a linear progression of activity from primary through tertiary interventions. Traditionally, primary prevention has predominantly focused on the modalities of education; motivational encouragement; social support; laws and policies; physical environmental changes; and the like. Early recognition, identification, and intervention has been seen to precede the secondary prevention efforts of assessment and referral for intervention. Concepts of tertiary prevention would be relevant to a discussion of suicidal behavior only to the extent to which individuals who have engaged in certain forms of

Table 2. Prevention Concepts Focus on Child and Adolescent Mental Health

Type	Goal	Methods	Examples
Primary	Reduce incidence	Disease/ disorder prevention	Prenatal and postnatal screening for genetic defects
			Counseling pregnant women on fetal alcohol syndrome
		Health promotion and enhancement	Alcohol and other drug use public education programs
			Parent education programs on child development and nutrition
		Health promotion (modifying agent/ environment)	Protection from hazardous environmental conditions (seat belts, lead, gun control)
			Labeling of alcoholic beverages
		Health maintenance	Educational programs on exercise, stress management, relaxation techniques
			Regular physical checkups, including mental status assessments
Secondary	Reduce prevalence	Early intervention and treatment	Early detection, referral, and treatment of adolescent drug abusers
			Screening and remediation for childhood emotional dysfunctions
Tertiary	Reduce disability/ dependence	Rehabilitation programs	Treatment services for youth in criminal detention facilities
		Community support programs	Shelter and programs for battered women and their children
		Treatment for the chronically ill	Integrating continuing care systems in the community

suicidal activity are amenable to receiving interventions that are designed to prevent recurrent episodes.

Albee (1979, 1980, 1982, 1983) introduced concepts of community-based prevention of psychological and emotional disorders by using concepts of social relations and psychological self-awareness. He redefined classical prevention terminology in terms of psychological variables (skills and self-definition) and social factors (social support and environmental stress).

Table 3 presents his concept of the incidence of mental disorder. One can reduce the incidence of a psychological disorder in the community, and thereby achieve the primary prevention of that disorder, by decreasing the destructive factors in the numerator, increasing the facilitative factors in the denominator, or doing both simultaneously.

Primary prevention efforts have some critical components, which include providing information, improving competencies, improving adjustment to stressors, and modifying environmental settings (ecology). The provision of information may be dynamic in nature or static over time. In short, strategies to disseminate information have many characteristics that involve issues of timing, intensity, frequency, duration, and targeting of specific messages to specific target groups. The improvement of personal competencies and social integration occurs at the individual, group, organizational, community, and societal levels. Improving the adjustment to stressors predominantly falls within the stress paradigms of stress management, stress reduction, and stress avoidance. Finally, issues of modifying one's environment include the full range of environmental factors such as noise, pollution, or lighting.

There exists a certain degree of tension between these different definitions, which is reflected in the types of preventive interventions recommended for the prevention of unwelcome behaviors. Epidemiological models emphasize measurable medical constructs, while others emphasize social, psychological, and economic factors.

The working definition of Primary Prevention and Health Promotion that has been adopted for the *Encyclopedia* is: "Primary prevention as the promotion of health and the prevention of illness involves actions that help participants (or to facilitate participants helping themselves, (1) to prevent predictable and interrelated problems, (2) to protect existing states of health and healthy functioning, and (3) to promote psychosocial wellness for identified populations of people. These consist of (a) whole populations in which

everyone requires certain basic utilities of life; (b) selected groups of people at risk or with potential; and (c) indicated subgroups at very high risk. Primary prevention may be facilitated by increasing individual, group, organizational, societal, cultural, and physical environmental strengths and resources, while simultaneously reducing the limitations and pressures from these same factors."

RISK AND PROTECTIVE FACTORS

Risk and protective factors and their interactions form an empirical base for prevention. Risk factors are associated with a greater potential for the development and expression of diseases and disorders, while protective factors are associated with reduced potential. Risk and protective factors encompass genetic, neurobiological, psychological, social, and cultural characteristics of individuals and groups and environmental factors. This expanding base of empirical evidence generates promising ideas about what can be changed or modified to prevent the appearance of a disease, disorder, or dysfunction.

Progress has been made toward the scientific understanding of mental and substance abuse disorders, and in developing interventions to treat these disorders. For example, increased understanding of brain systems regulated by neurotransmitters holds promise for understanding the biological underpinnings of depression, anxiety disorders, impulsiveness, aggression, and violent behaviors. Much remains to be learned, however, about the common social, economic, or cultural risk factors for mental disorders and substance abuse, suicide, and other forms of intentional violence including homicide, domestic violence, and child abuse, among other social problems (US Public Health Service, 1999).

Some of these contributory risk factors are modifiable and others are not. We lack the most efficient and effective interventions at this time to modify, alter or intervene with some of the modifiable risk factors. However, it remains a researchable question as to which risk factors are truly amenable to preventive interventions on a large-scale community or national basis.

THE GOALS OF PREVENTIVE INTERVENTIONS

Within the prevention field, as is typical of most other emerging and evolving fields of human study, there is a subtle language that is attempting to define the goals of prevention. The translation of primary and secondary prevention into operational terminology has resulted in a plethora of action verbs. Some of these operational terms to describe the

Table 3. George Albee's Definition of Incidence of Mental Disorders (1983)

$$\text{Incidence of mental disorders} = \frac{\text{organic factors} + \text{stress} + \text{exploitation}}{\text{coping skills} + \text{self-esteem} + \text{support groups}}$$

goals of prevention are: interfere, interrupt, delay, modulate, moderate, attenuate, eliminate, disrupt, divert, and reduce. Unfortunately, these terms are not synonymous and convey subtle differences in meaning as well as in outcome criteria, as measured by various evaluation standards. Thus, when evaluating the various prevention models, one must be clear about what *precisely* is being prevented, and what *precisely* is being measured, to determine to what extent the intervention has been successful at achieving that specific goal.

Another major consideration in the understanding of preventive intervention models is to decide what is encompassed under the term "primary prevention" as it relates to the mental health field. There are some who believe that primary prevention refers solely to the prevention of emotional disorders and dysfunctions as well as severe psychological and psychiatric illness. Others (Cowen, 1983) contend that primary prevention in mental health comprises both the prevention of psychological and emotional disorders and dysfunctions *as well as* the promotion of mental health and mental well-being. There are as many difficulties that arise in defining mental health and mental well-being—as anything other than the absence of disease and dysfunction—as there are in defining mental illness—as the absence of health. However, in the last decade, much has been published regarding the operational definitions of competence, optimum potential, stress immunity, coping, and other similar psychological constructs (including self-esteem and self-worth) that are determined to be essential ingredients of mental health and well-being (*American Psychologist*, 2000, *55*(1)).

What is the exact relationship between the prevention of mental disorder and the promotion of mental health? Some argue that it is not the *active* promotion of mental health, but the maintenance or protection of a safe and healthy familial, community and societal environment that is a guarantee against the expression of psychiatric illness. Although intellectually and philosophically intriguing, a full discussion of this conceptual debate is beyond the scope of this entry (Felner & Felner, 1989; Felner et al., 2000). Nevertheless, it is important to remember that when one evaluates models of prevention, one must look to see whether the models focus on disease prevention, health protection (maintenance), health promotion, or all three.

Another critical factor is to determine to what extent these models may be overlapping, mutually exclusive, enhancing, additive, or complementary. Again, we must return to our initial conceptual understanding of the etiology, pathophysiology, and expression of behaviors that we characterize as negative in nature, in order to evaluate the extent to which a model matches our view of reality.

Just as there is a subtle language for prevention, so there is for promotion. Such words as protecting, maintaining, enhancing, facilitating, encouraging, are terms that are used in the mental health promotion literature. As with its mirror image, the promotion field needs to specifically define its outcomes. Conceptually, the process of prevention entails breaking linkages along a pathological continuum from health to disease, while the process of promotion entails forging and strengthening linkages along a continuum of health maintenance to health promotion. These approaches remain conceptually different and practically important.

THE ANATOMY OF PREVENTION MODELS

When looking at a model for the primary prevention of a behavioral or emotional disorder, or a social problem, a model must account for the following variables: (1) it must be applicable to *specific settings* in which one would find groups of individuals at risk for the disorder; (2) it must be adaptable to various *developmental stages and phases* of groups of individuals, or be specifically focused on a target population known to be at high risk for the disorder; (3) it must be *adaptable to various settings* where groups of people congregate; (4) it must *specifically address the etiology, pathogenesis, or known risk factors* associated with the targeted disorder; (5) it must clearly *identify the goal of its activity*, that is, primary prevention, early intervention, secondary prevention, or pretreatment; (6) it must allow for the use of *multiple types of interventions* over time (Silverman & Koretz, 1989); (7) it must be *testable*, in that its components can be measured and easily defined.

The implication is that behavioral and psychological *processes* that are the prime targets of preventive efforts should be those deviations in normal developmental processes, experienced by the target population in a given social and physical context, that lead to the outcomes of concern. Felner et al. (2000) identified a critical set of tasks that must be addressed in the design of preventive efforts. These tasks are: (1) to assess the ways in which normal developmental processes have been disrupted in the target population; (2) to identify those socioeconomic or cultural conditions that lead to these disruptions and distortions; and (3) to create interventions whose goals are to modify or "correct" these distortions until they closely approximate those that lead to "healthy" development and healthy outcomes.

A viable model must address the who, what, when, and why of preventive interventions. An intervention must have significant components that address the fundamental properties of an intervention, such as frequency, duration, timing, intensity. For example, any model for the prevention of suicide must allow for many different types of interventions to coexist in a comprehensive, coordinated and collaborative program. The types of interventions that are currently being developed, implemented, and evaluated for the prevention of mental disorders and the promotion of mental health are quite broad (Table 4).

One must start by defining features of prevention that must be present in any model: (1) interventions are timed to be "before the fact," that is, before the expression of the targeted disorder or symptom, and hence directed at essentially "well" populations; (2) the level of analysis is at the population, group, or community level; (3) the focus of the change efforts are on preconditions, antecedent conditions, precipitating conditions, perpetuating conditions, etc. The first-order targets of change are the unfolding processes and conditions that lead to trajectories of well-being or disruption; (4) efforts are directed at promoting strengths, well-being, and positive developmental outcomes or reducing psychological maladjustment; and (5) a sensitivity to the physical, emotional, and psychological developmental stages of the targeted behavior must be present (Cowen, 1983; Felner et al., 2000). As Seidman (1987) states, "All loci of preventive interventions are before the fact, mass-oriented, and ultimately aimed at averting disorder and/or promoting wellness in individuals. Individuals are the immediate target of intervention only when they constitute a group or population of interest" (p. 9).

Primary prevention is not a prescribed program and it is not a manual. Prevention is interactive, and constantly evolving based on input from the many sectors it continuously monitors. Hence, it becomes very difficult to evaluate, and even to replicate, preventive interventions addressing behavioral dysfunctions, because they are in a constant state of evolution as they try to respond to changing transactional and ecological elements. Furthermore, many preventive interventions are not direct "assaults" on *sufficient conditions* that lead clearly to the expression of disorder, but more often are directed at *necessary conditions* that do not always develop into a clear expression of disease. In this way, preventive interventions may be more akin to immunization programs

Table 4. Examples of Preventive Interventions

1. Biological (drugs, nutrition, diet)
2. Physiological (relaxation therapy, exercise)
3. Cognitive/learning (problem-solving techniques)
4. Behavioral (stress reduction)
5. Social skills training and competency building (peer pressure resistance)
6. Ecological (family, workplace, church, community)
7. Psychoeducational (coping, adaptation, appraisal, and assessment)
8. Media (TV, radio, magazines, newspapers)
9. Social support/mutual help (sense of community)
10. Job training (maximizing employment skills)
11. Environmental (pollution control)
12. Political (prevent war/terrorism)
13. Legislative (mandatory seat belts)

that prepare an individual to withstand an assault by a sufficient condition that initiates disorder. Immunizations serve to protect and to enhance a population's ability to ward off the effects of environmental change, which may take the form of the introduction of a pathogen into the system.

A critical element for preventive interventions is that they must demonstrate comprehensiveness that may take the form of both horizontal elements and vertical elements. *Horizontal comprehensiveness* refers to interventions that occur at particular life stages and at critical risk periods (a linear, time-line perspective). *Vertical comprehensiveness* reflects a lifespan perspective that transcends any particular point in time. Programming must be comprehensive within life stages (horizontal), and programming must be complementary across life stages (vertical) (Felner et al., 2000).

MODELING THE PREVENTION OF BEHAVIOR DISORDERS AND THE PROMOTION OF HEALTHY OUTCOMES

The purpose of a model is to provide us with a theoretical construct upon which we can place our theories about the etiology, pathogenesis, salutogenesis, and expression of an illness or health. The purpose also provides us with a conceptualization of how, when, where, and why a particular preventive intervention might work to interrupt, disrupt, or prevent the presumed development and expression of an illness, or how a given promotive intervention will lead to a healthy outcome. Certain assumptions are automatically inherent in this statement. For instance, most existing medical models of illness suggest a linear progression for the development of the illness. Most existing theories suggest simple vectors or influence that heighten the "load" of an individual until they "break down" with the disorder (Silverman, 1996).

This conceptualization also assumes that these interventions, even if well-timed and of the appropriate duration, frequency, intensity, and so on, will have their permanent impact at the time of their initial introduction. However, we have learned many lessons from our infectious disease colleagues. Their techniques are clinical (antibiotics for the immediate attenuation or destruction of the offending agent), preventive (inoculations), and promotive (eradication of smallpox through infectious disease control measures).

One lesson relates to the concept of "booster shots" and "inoculations" that enhance or reestablish our immunity (already acquired through initial immunizations) to certain pathogens at times when we may be most likely to be exposed to them (by virtue of our choosing to be in environmental situations where the infectious disease is endemic). These booster shot "effects" are not necessarily felt or seen at the time of the inoculation. In fact, they may never be needed at all. If needed, time and place may separate the relationship between exposure to pathogen and prior preventive intervention. On the other hand, one must not assume that any preventive "inoculation," even if ideally delivered at an age-appropriate and an environmentally sensitive time, is sufficient for a lifetime of exposure to various risk factors that can promote, encourage, facilitate, or enhance the expression of behaviors or disorders (Silverman, 1996).

THE INTERFACE BETWEEN BEHAVIORAL ILLNESSES AND PREVENTION MODELS

One of the conceptual difficulties in developing preventive interventions based on sophisticated and intricate multicausal models of disease or disorder development (particularly transactional–ecological models), is that it becomes more difficult to analyze which factors are responsible for determining which interventions are most effective, at which time, and to what degree. It is the who, what, when, where, why, and how questions that constitute the level of analysis required to determine whether preventive interventions do, in fact, have an effect.

Inasmuch as most behavioral disorders are multicausal in etiology, so must preventive interventions be multifocal in terms of the behaviors and etiological agents they are designed to target. The more complex the model of disorder development, the more complex the nature of the preventive interventions to address the behaviors. The anatomy of the preventive intervention (structure, form) and its attendant characteristics (frequency, duration, timing, etc.) become essential components to the eventual success or failure of the effort.

Any serious discussion of preventive efforts directed at a particular disorder or dysfunction must first define those behaviors that: (1) define the targeted disorder to be prevented; (2) define the pathological continuum associated with the disorder; and (3) represent the frequently observed signs and symptoms found to be highly associated with the disorder under investigation. Effective prevention outcomes are predicated on intervening before the targeted disorder or illness becomes a reality. However, predicting future behavior, even in a psychiatrically ill population, is not easy to do, if not impossible. For example, a summary of the existing research literature suggests that approximately 10–15 percent of suicide attempters eventually die by suicide, while 30–40 percent of those who die by suicide have had a prior history of suicide attempts (Maris, 1992). Although these numbers suggest that there is a small, but significant, group of suicide attempters who warrant our attention and intervention, there is also a larger group of individuals for whom other markers are needed to identify their risk status for suicide.

There is a need for a comprehensive, multicausal, and nonspecific developmental pathways model (Felner & Felner, 1989). Such a model would account for the following: (1) most of the disorders we seek to prevent have a large number of common risk factors; (2) conditions that protect against one disorder generally also protect against many other disorders; (3) there are nonspecific personal vulnerabilities that increase a person's susceptibility to the onset of a wide array of dysfunctions. The pathways to most of the social, emotional, and adaptive difficulties with which we are concerned are generally complex and shared by more than one disorder (Coie et al., 1993; Felner et al., 2000).

Adequate preventive efforts at each developmental life stage are *necessary*, but not always *sufficient* conditions for obtaining both the short-term outcomes (keeping an individual on a developmentally sound trajectory of health) and long-term outcomes that we seek. It is the interplay between the necessary and sufficient conditions that have occupied the attention of behavioral scientists working in this field in the last decade.

CURRENT CONTROVERSIES IN THE PREVENTION OF MENTAL DISORDERS AND THE PROMOTION OF MENTAL HEALTH AND WELL-BEING

Before embarking on a review of prevention models, it is important to remember that there are current controversies in the preventive intervention field that limit the utility and applicability of these models to any particular target behavior.

Table 5 is a listing of basic assumptions in developing preventive interventions and developing prevention models. Any preventive endeavor assumes that there exists: (1) interrelationships among theories of disease expression; (2) epidemiologically established risk factors (both causative and correlational); (3) effective, efficacious, and efficient interventions specifically targeted at risk factors; (4) culturally sensitive and population-focused interventions that will be readily received and adopted; and (5) the existence of outcome measures that are sensitive and specific to measuring the outcomes that are linked to the specific interventions.

Table 5. Basic Assumptions about Prevention

We know:
1. How to define the risk condition/behavior
2. Who is at risk
3. How to identify who is at most risk
4. Why an individual is at risk
5. When an individual is at most risk
6. What situations/settings/behaviors place an individual at most risk
7. What interventions lower risk status
8. When interventions are to be applied to lower risk
9. What outcomes are to be measured

Table 6. Decision Points in Selecting Preventive Interventions

- Which points in the causal chain are particularly vulnerable to interruption?
- Which interventions are likely to contribute to the prevention of a large proportion of a disorder?
- Which interventions are likely to be effective across different (but related) types of disorders?
- What sorts of interventions will result in *immediate* reductions in such disorders?
- What sorts of interventions will result in *long-term* reductions in such disorders?
- Which of the potential interventions are *feasible* and most readily adopted?
- What are the costs of the various promising interventions, relative to their likely *effectiveness*?

Adapted from Third National Injury Control Conference (Department of Health and Human Services, 1992).

These conditions allow us to reach decision points about which preventive interventions to select (Table 6).

Conclusion

The lack of knowledge about the etiology, pathogenesis, and expression of a disorder or dysfunction limit the development and application of a preventive intervention. Controversy and confusion regarding the definition of the dysfunctional or disordered behavior also limit it. Prevention efforts are also hampered by poorly administered interventions. Prevention efforts are undermined when outcome measures, both formative and summative, are not clearly defined in advance of implementing the intervention. Prevention efforts are thwarted when there is imprecise language and unfocused thinking about targeting specific interventions at specific populations for specific purposes to prevent specific outcomes.

Prediction is based on statistical power and statistical methodologies. Good prediction assumes a high base rate of disorder in a particular population, such that the expression of the targeted behavior is not statistically random. When applying prevention concepts to psychiatric disorders, one must recognize the low base rate of certain psychiatric illnesses (Eisenberg, 1980). Hence a major strategic decision in developing preventive interventions for psychiatric disturbances is to target them at other related and more common risk factors that are highly correlated with the expression of the targeted behaviors.

For example, this argument has been used (Shaffer, 1989) to hypothesize that the highest likelihood of reducing the largest number of suicides in the community is to identify and appropriately treat all individuals with depressive illness. This argument is based on the high association between depressive illness and suicidal behavior. The problem with this otherwise logical and statistically sound approach is that if we adopt this perspective (1) prevention becomes individually focused, not group-focused; (2) prevention becomes synonymous with clinical treatment; (3) prevention becomes a very costly endeavor; and (4) although the socially beneficial effects are evident in treating all individuals in a community, the cost-effectiveness in terms of preventing suicide in this population is not high enough to warrant such an expensive effort solely for purposes of preventing suicidal behaviors.

PREVENTION MODELS

The development of efficacious preventive interventions is in its infancy. Those theoretical models that will be presented here are currently being researched and tested in community settings, and are constantly undergoing revisions and modifications as we gain feedback from evaluating their effectiveness.

Models have their limitations. Models only serve to suggest how, where, and when to intervene. Because they are an amalgam of theory, clinical data, hypothesis, and intuition, they are not perfect representations of the real world, that is, a real world populated by real people whose behaviors are multi-determined, multidirected, multi-intentioned, and multi-dependent on changing variables within a temporal context.

This section will focus on models of behavioral disorders, which are abstract constructs that aid us in visualizing theories of the etiology, pathogenesis, and expression of disorder as it applies to targeted populations. Ideally, they should account for all the known facts and all the critical elements. Once constructed, these models should suggest the type of preventive interventions that might be most effective, as well as efficient and efficacious, suggesting the appropriate timing, frequency, intensity, and duration of these interventions (the who, what, when, where, why, and how of interventions).

Public Health Models

Tripartite Causal Model

The traditional public health model of prevention evolved from the effective treatment of infectious diseases. Gruenberg, Lewis, and Goldston (1986) have stated that

> during the first half of the [20th] century, primary prevention was achieved with traditional public health approaches for at least two illnesses with psychiatric components: pellagra and general paresis. The discovery that infection with measles, during a woman's first trimester, puts the fetus at risk for brain dysfunction also resulted in the application of primary prevention techniques for women in their childbearing years. (Cited in Pardes et al., 1989, p. 405)

Pardes et al. (1989, p. 405) went on to say, that, "the application of public health methods to mental health problems has been a complex proposition. The classic public health model, conceptualizing illness in terms of host, agent, and environment, does not 'fit' most psychiatric disorders."

The classic tripartite model identifies three intersecting and overlapping circles of influence: host, agent, and environment. This model looks at disease development from a causal-etiological perspective in that assignment of contributing factors are in three spheres. This model does not readily allow for an understanding of the possible interactions that occur among these three sectors. It is when at least two (or three) of the spheres intersect that there is a high likelihood of the expression of an illness. A number of researchers have struggled with this model over the years in an attempt to apply it to the prevention of mental disorders and behavioral dysfunctions. Most have found this model to be lacking, in part because it reflects a linear view of the evolution of dysfunction and assumes that the timing of the onset of dysfunction is something that can be readily identified (Sameroff & Fiese, 1989).

Gordon's Operational Model

Robert Gordon (1983) has argued that the tripartite classification of prevention efforts (primary vs. secondary vs. tertiary) is an artifact of the mechanistic conceptions of health and disease that characterized early eras when biomedical research was almost exclusively a laboratory activity. The growth of epidemiological research has introduced more complex causal models that may restructure approaches to prevention.

Gordon maintained that the tripartite distinction does not separate preventive strategies that have different epidemiological justifications and that require different utilization strategies. A further problem is that, especially for the nonprofessional community, the terms imply a preferred priority when only a qualitative distinction is intended (Felner & Silverman, 1989).

The model offered by Gordon (1983) has an *intervention focus*, and is not based on causality or etiology. It defines preventive interventions as categories using an operational nomenclature, and thus serves as an alternative to the traditional triad of primary, secondary, and tertiary prevention. His three categories of interventions are universal procedures, selective procedures, and indicated procedures. This organization is based on how the target groups are identified. The Institute of Medicine (IOM) of the National Academy of Science commissioned a Committee on Prevention of Mental Disorders to prepare an integrated report of current research with policy-oriented and detailed long-term recommendations for a prevention research agenda for mental disorders

(Mrazek & Haggerty, 1994). They reviewed existing prevention models, definitions, and intervention approaches and concluded that Gordon's operational model held the most promise for reducing risks of mental disorders.

Universal preventive interventions are directed at an entire population and not specifically at subgroups presumed to be at greater risk. Health promotion and protection measures desirable for "essentially everybody" are classified here.

In this category fall all those measures that can be advocated confidently for the general public and that, in many cases, can be applied without professional advice or assistance. The benefits outweigh the costs and risks for everyone.

Selective interventions are directed at individuals who are at greater risk for diseases or disorders than the general population. These measures can be reasonably recommended, in terms of "the balance of benefits against risk and cost," for a relatively large subgroup "whose risk of becoming ill is above normal," because they have shared exposure to some epidemiologically established risk factors.

Indicated interventions are targeted at those relatively small groups who are found, by screening programs or other inquiries, to "manifest a risk factor, condition, or abnormality that identifies them, individually, as being at sufficiently high risk to require the preventive intervention" (Gordon, 1983, p. 28). As a society moves from universal procedures to indicated procedures, the cost of providing these procedures increases in terms of manpower, time, effort, and cost. In a reformulated model of prevention, both universal and selected interventions would continue to be included under the rubric of prevention.

Haddon's Injury Control Model

William Haddon, Jr. (1968, 1980) first expanded the public health model of pathogenesis to include an injury control approach. The Haddon Matrix provides an elegant framework that forces a consideration of structural interventions aimed at modifying the physical environment (e.g., the highway) and the vehicles of energy exchange (e.g., the automobile or firearm) as well as the human host or larger social environment (e.g., social norms about weapon ownership or family violence) (Runyan, 1993, p. 638). His model of pathogenesis includes 5 elements: host, environment, agent, vehicles, and vectors.

Haddon (1967, 1980) set forth ten unintentional injury control strategies to break the chain of injury causation. These strategies fall into the tripartite concept of primary, secondary, and tertiary prevention and deal respectively with the pre-injury, injury, and post-injury phases (Table 7) (Institute of Medicine, 1985; Department of Health and Human Services, 1992).

Table 7. Haddon's Ten Unintentional Injury Control Strategies: Breaking the Chain of Injury Causation

Primary prevention (*pre-injury phase*)
 1. Prevent the initial creation of the hazard
 2. Reduce the amount of hazard that is created
 3. Prevent release of a hazard that already exists

Secondary prevention (*injury phase*)
 4. Modify the rate of release or spatial distribution of the hazard from its source
 5. Separate, in time or space, the hazard from persons to be protected
 6. Interpose a barrier between the hazard and the person to be protected
 7. Modify contact surfaces and structures to reduce injury
 8. Strengthen the resistance of persons who might be injured by the hazard

Tertiary prevention (*post-injury phase*)
 9. Move rapidly to detect and limit damage that has occurred
10. Initiate immediate and long-term reparative actions

Source: W. Haddon, Jr. (1980).

The advantage of injury control modeling is that it allows for the identification of multiple causes that, in and of themselves, may be necessary, but not sufficient, to propel the individual to act in an unhealthy manner. Thus, one does not necessarily have to strongly believe or defend any one particular cause and limit one's interventions to only that cause. The modeling allows for the displaying of multiple causes and for an objective development and identification of the most cost-effective intervention. Furthermore, it allows for the identification of various methods to identify and break the chain of disease causation at its weakest link. The weakest link might be proximal or distal to the disorder and might involve passive or active countermeasures.

Haddon's approach places a primary emphasis on structural and environmental changes. Needless to say, this preventive intervention does not address motivation, psychological disorder, domestic disruption, socioeconomic disorder, or biological predilection.

Deficit Reduction Model

Another approach to understanding mental disorders and behavioral dysfunctions is to borrow from the clinical field and apply concepts of developmental psychopathology to the construction of models (Cicchetti, 1990). The *deficit reduction model* is a particularly popular conceptualization of disease. The focus is often on the problem residing within an individual and often residing as an internal construct with one's self-concept. This model places the locus of control within the individual. It suggests that there are psychological and psychiatric deficits that reside in an individual, and that prevention efforts need to be addressed at stemming the expression of these preexisting deficits.

Hence, the preventive intervention is to provide the individual with basic skills for survival. The skills have been variously categorized under numerous schema, but basically fall within the following broad categories: (1) cognitive skills/problem solving; (2) interpersonal and emotional coping skills; (3) behavioral skills; and (4) assertiveness training/peer-pressure resistance. Examples of *cognitive skills/problem-solving* include academic skills, information assessment and evaluation, and awareness of cognitive dissonance. Examples of *interpersonal and emotional coping skills* include self-regulation and monitoring, emotion and problem; focused coping styles, and acquired resiliencies and vulnerabilities (expectancies, self-esteem, self-concept, etc.). Examples of *behavioral skills* include refusal skills, peer interaction, and social skills. *Assertiveness training/peer-pressure resistance* are social skills which include values clarification and social support enhancement.

Competence-oriented models aim to increase specific social skills to produce "social inoculation" against life's problems. Social competence skills include communication skills and techniques of inoculation with prepared responses in advance of anticipated situations. Cognitive problem-solving skills also include decision-making skills. Cognitive skills also include critical thinking, good judgment, and common sense.

Interpersonal and emotional coping skills include management of "daily hassles" of living such as transient anxiety, loneliness, depression, disappointment, frustration, etc. Coping skills also include development of a repertoire of problem-solving tools and techniques, as well as psychological maneuvers to avoid situations that raise one's level of perturbation. Such coping skills might include stress management, stress reduction, and stress avoidance. Stress models recognize the importance of critical stressful life events as contributors to the etiology of mental disorders, and argue for the protective nature of social support to maintain individuals on trajectories of normal development.

Overall, this model assumes that there is a deficit that needs to be corrected in the individual, or in the group identified to be at high risk for the disorder. If one corrects the specific deficit, or set of deficits, then the disorder will not appear. The assumption is that there is a direct linkage between the identified deficit, which is being prevented, and the expression of the disorder. Such a model has its limitations if one assumes that behavior is multi-determined and is contingent on various factors and environments that are hard to predict in advance.

Enhancement/Wellness and Health Promotion Models

In the last decade, there has been a major refocusing of attention away from prevention of specific disorders and dysfunctions to the general enhancement of health and well-being. The argument is that a broader approach to the total being will result in the higher likelihood of an overall benefit. Again, however, the locus of control in this model is mainly within the individual. One can conceptualize a continuum of health behavior that includes health *destroying* behaviors (i.e., nicotine dependence; excessive alcohol intake) and health *defeating* behaviors (overworking, ignoring symptoms of stress and distress, poor attention to hygiene and sleep). The continuum then suggests that there are health behaviors that can *maintain* health (diet, exercise, nutrition, appropriate rest), *protect* health (immunization, use of seat belts), and *promote or enhance* health (avoidance of risk settings and situations, regular physical examinations).

A wellness model does lend itself to the identification of target groups for health enhancement, risk avoidance, and risk reduction. *Health enhancement* would be perceived as a primary prevention effort and would be directed at those who are free of any apparent risk factors (i.e., children, young adults, those individuals in transition). *Risk avoidance* would be targeted to those identified to be at risk for expression of the illness. Such groups might include individuals exposed to significant stressful life events. *Risk reduction* is reserved for those who have already expressed the signs and symptoms of the disorder and who are most at risk for continued difficulties.

Health promotion strategies rely on the belief that individuals clearly see the importance and relevance of changing or modifying their current behavior in order to "protect" themselves from some future unknown negative health outcome. Different health promotion strategies rely on different health behavior theories for their specific components.

One popular model is the social norms approach that posits that behavior is influenced by incorrect perceptions of how other members of our social group think and act. The theory predicts that overestimations of problem behavior will increase these problem behaviors while underestimations of healthy behaviors discourage individuals from engaging in them (Perkins & Berkowitz, 1986). Social norms interventions focus on peer influences that have been found to be more influential in shaping individual behavior than biological, personality, familial, religious, cultural or other influences (Berkowitz & Perkins, 1986). These peer influences are based more on what we think our peers believe or do ("the perceived norm") than on their real beliefs or actions ("the actual norm"). By presenting correct information about peer group norms, perceived peer pressure is reduced and individuals are more likely to express preexisting attitudes and beliefs that are health-promoting.

Most health behavior theories have at least six common elements which are essential for achieving behavioral change: (1) individuals must recognize a serious health problem and perceive that they are at risk for the development of this problem; (2) individuals must be motivated to act and have true intentions to change; (3) individuals must have knowledge and skills necessary to perform behavioral modifications; (4) individuals must believe that they can accomplish this change and perceive that they can take action in their own self-benefit (self-efficacy); (5) individuals must have access to models of behavior change and be able to select from among the models that best fit their view of themselves and the contingencies that must occur; and (6) there must be community and societal norms to support these behavioral changes.

The reality is that changing behavior is hard to do. Maintaining a new behavioral repertoire is also hard. Effecting change involves understanding the interplay among attitudes, beliefs, values, and knowledge in the target population. These multiple variables are complex and difficult to implement broadly.

Antecedent Conditions Model

A paradigmatic shift has occurred in our thinking about what should be the target of preventive interventions (Kuhn, 1970). This shift resulted in preventive intervention models that were based on modifying antecedent conditions that are related by correlation to an outcome rather than focusing exclusively on the outcome itself (Bloom, 1986). The assumption was that there is not a specific etiologic agent that is identifiable. This challenges the previously held concept of a universal, nonspecific vulnerability for illness. This model suggested that there are predisposing circumstances that are distal to the eventual outcome and that these *predisposing conditions* place an individual in a category of being generally vulnerable to a specific outcome. It is only when more proximal or *precipitating conditions* or circumstances "interact" with the general state of vulnerability that an individual expresses a negative outcome.

This model suggests that there are two distinct sets of conditions which are antecedent to the expression of negative behaviors—predisposing conditions and precipitating conditions (Felner & Silverman, 1989). These two conditions place individuals at increased risk and make them more vulnerable. Predisposing conditions are distal to the behavior itself, but are necessary to place an individual at risk. Predisposing conditions include poor cognitive skills, poor family functioning, and poor behavioral skills. Precipitating conditions are proximal conditions to the behavior and are often associated with the expression of the dysfunction in a temporal manner. Examples of precipitating conditions include poor affective skills, removal of social supports, hopelessness, and a sense of frustrated psychological needs. Precipitating conditions alone, without the presence of predisposing conditions, often will not lead to the expression of the dysfunction.

This model suggests that there are two loci for intervention. One is a more societal or community approach that eradicates or diminishes predisposing conditions for the entire population. The second level of intervention is for those who have already been identified as having experienced predisposing conditions. For this "at-risk" population, the approach is to eliminate or ameliorate those *precipitating* conditions that are proximally or temporally related to the expression of the disease.

This perspective finds that "an antecedent-condition model applies across a wide range of emotional and behavioral dysfunctions. These observers argue that nonspecific predisposing factors and precipitating conditions may be responsible for the expression of many disorders, moving away from the focus on specific risk factors to the possibility of a more universal potential for disturbance in various populations" (APA Task Force, 1990). Felner and Silverman (1989, p. 25) stated:

> At this point, a key debate in the prevention literature becomes salient if we are to decide how and who to move from "risk factors" to programs. We need to be clear on how we answer the questions (a) do we attempt to tailor primary prevention programs to the prevention of a specific disorder, or (b) do we develop programs which are effective in alleviating a number of conditions that are antecedent to a range of emotional and physical problems, including, but not limited to the target problem?
>
> The "specific disorder prevention" model rests heavily in a classic medical-public health paradigm which views diseases as caused by specific conditions that interact with individual vulnerabilities, again, specifiable. In contrast, the antecedent condition model argues that at least for a wide range of emotional and behavioral disorders, particularly those related to stress and other elements of the normal life-course, the specific etiology model is not appropriate.

This antecedent condition model is of interest because it can be combined with other models to strengthen its overall appeal as a comprehensive conceptualization for identifying and developing targeted areas for preventive interventions. The focus of preventive interventions is on the mechanism and processes from which disorder results, not on the disorder itself, and not on the individual who may not be ill or expressing the problem. The assumption is that negative outcomes may be healthy adaptations to disordered environments. Such a radical rethinking of causal and correlational factors in the evolution of disease and disorder has resulted in a shift in emphasis to ecological, transactional, and social/environmental domains (Felner & Felner, 1989).

Ecological Model

This model has evolved from the work of Barker (1968), Bronfonbrenner (1979), Kelly (1979), Rappaport (1987), and Vincent and Trickett (1983). The model suggests that individuals exist in a multilayered ecological system, and are constantly reacting to and responding to changes in the environment. They argue that the individual is in a dynamic interchange with both positive and negative factors that surround him/herself. It is this interaction that is at the heart of developing prevention programming. They argue that it is the individual's perception and degree of mastery with ecological factors that determines outcomes. Their model also argues that any targeted intervention at the individual, school, peer, family, community, or social/environmental level must transcend each setting to be effective. Hence, highly targeted interventions directed solely at a family unit will not be effective, because the individual does not solely exist within this framework. They believe that it is only through coordinated, comprehensive, and collaborative efforts that messages and interventions that sustain themselves over time can be delivered.

What is missing from these models is an accounting of the interactive nature of each component. The ecological model is basically a systems model that looks at interactions from a systems perspective. The model attempts to define and study the relation between the systems in the environment, such as society, and its impact on the individual. There are salient systems within the society which bear directly and indirectly on the individual. What is studied is how these systems and individual relate to each other, and the adaptive relevance of the individual's particular behavior.

Transactional Model

Sameroff and colleagues (Sameroff & Chandler, 1975; Sameroff, 1983; Sameroff & Fiese, 1989) and others (Lorion et al., 1989) have evolved the transactional model over time. They have proposed a transactional model that is developmental, dynamic, reciprocal, and interactional. Each interaction has feedback loops to other levels of the system. The contingencies and strengths of these vectors change over time and within time frames. This approach is developmentally focused and suggests that influences of an individual's greater environment (i.e., parents and society) shift with time, and with increasing degrees of maturity of the individual. The transactional model places the problem in the context of the dynamic transaction *between* the individual and the environment. The emphasis is on reciprocal effects and adaptive adequacies of individuals to their environments (dyadic and bidirectional).

Basically, this model outlines pathways to deviant behavior. It suggests that there is a transaction that occurs between the individual and a higher level, which changes over time. The model was initially developed to understand the transactional relationship between the child and his/her parent. The parent in this model is the mediator for all interactions between the child and other parts of his/her environment, such as the society at large. The analysis takes place at the transactional level, but provides no lens for understanding whether the subsequent behavior is deviant or not.

Transactional/Ecological Models

Felner and colleagues (Felner & Silverman, 1989; Felner & Felner, 1989; Felner, Adan, & Silverman, 1992; and Felner et al., 2000) and Seidman (1987, 1990) have attempted to integrate both the ecological models and the transactional models into a model which expands the level of analysis beyond microsystems, mesosystems, and macrosystems. The contribution of this model is to offer an alternative way of viewing the phenomena of the *interactions* between various parts of a total ecological and psychological system. Here, equal weight is placed not only on the transactions between child and parent, parent and society, and child and society, but also on an analysis of the interactions between various macrosystems.

A transactional/ecological model would lend credence to an analysis of the interaction between two society-level institutions in terms of how that interaction then subsequently may influence either the child or the parental system. Individuals may not always have a dyadic, bidirectional interaction with their environment. These relationships are not always reciprocal in nature. Furthermore, the model allows for analysis of interactions *between* persons in a population, and between many different settings. This model expands our focus to include the ways in which person–setting interactions are influenced by relationships between settings, as well as the broader, macrosystemic contexts in which they may be nested. Equal weight is given to understanding dyadic transactions and to the analysis of the impact of and interactions among various settings, mesosystems, and macrosystems that may significantly influence developmental pathways (Bronfonbrenner, 1979).

This model is based on the following assumptions: (1) disorders are secondary to deviations in normal developmental trajectories and processes; (2) some negative outcomes or behaviors may in fact be healthy adaptations to disordered conditions that precede the expression of the outcome; (3) the focus of preventive interventions is on the nature of the interactions (contexts) between the individual and their environment; (4) the locus of the disorder or the dysfunction is outside of the individual; and (5) a multicausal model of behavior and psychological development means an emphasis is placed on broad-based antecedent factors and processes. The focus of the model is on the contexts in which a behavior is adaptive or dysfunctional. Preventive interventions are directed at environments (ecologies), the interfaces between the individual and their environment (transactions), and the processes and contexts of the individual environment. The transactional–ecological model allows one to see that some apparently deviant behavior may in fact be adaptive within the context in which it occurs. Such a perspective might not always find negative behaviors to be maladaptive or "abnormal," given the particular setting in which they occur. The challenge would be to devise preventive interventions that change the settings if we are to influence the behaviors in that setting (context).

Felner and colleagues believe that this model also allows for mathematical modeling and assignment of weights to various interactions and transactions that occur in the natural environment. Along with the transactional model, this model shares the concept of a time frame and the fact that interactions and contexts change in time and over time. The model allows for some "future thinking" and allows for predicting the consequences of particular events, both in the past and the present, for subsequent behaviors. Such a model, then, meets one of the criteria for prevention, which is to be able to predict the occurrence of future events from existing data. Such a model also allows one to differentiate various components of the system and to potentially modify, alter, enhance, or decrease the potential effects of each component in the overall equation.

Conclusion

Prevention is predicated on prediction. None of us have proven to be good predictors of future human behavior. Our best predictions have been in the arena of violence prevention, that is, human aggression perpetrated on another (Flitcraft, 1992; Marzuk, Tardiff, & Hirsch, 1992). Even here the best predictive indicators are a history of past violent behavior and a family history of being a victim of violence.

Primary prevention has become a central goal among those concerned with a wide array of human conditions (Felner, Jason, Moritsugu, & Farber, 1983; Bloom, 1981). The Secretary of Health and Human Services labeled prevention as the nation's number one health priority for the 1990s (DHHS, 1990). The US Surgeon General has emphasized prevention activities in the mental health arena as we enter the 21st century. The reasons for prevention becoming a central priority on the national health agenda are quite clear. Simply put, after-the-fact treatment approaches have proven to be inadequate to the task of reducing the ever-rising levels of social and health problems confronting the nation.

Most of the interventions we have readily available (i.e., treatment) are expensive, time intensive, and not always effective. There will never be adequate levels of human or economic resources to address these dramatic levels of need if we rely on reconstructive and individually focused models of intervention (Albee, 1959; Sarason, 1981). As Albee (1982) reminds us, no epidemic was ever successfully brought under control or eliminated by treating those already affected.

A barrier to the successful mounting of prevention programs relates to arguments and misperceptions among professionals themselves (Broskowski & Baker, 1974). The scarce resource context of human services has led to issues of "turf." Treatment and prevention have often been set up, however inappropriately, as competitors. What is not understood is that if prevention efforts succeed there will be a decrease in demand for treatment such that extant levels of treatment resources may be more effective. Thus, prevention is not a competitor to treatment but an important ally. We are not arguing that prevention is somehow "better" than treatment when we argue for clarity and differentiation from treatment in the spectrum of intervention. Rather, we are simply arguing that such clarity will facilitate the creation of more systematic and useful knowledge bases and action strategies that will enhance both (Silverman & Felner, 1995). Prevention holds the promise of providing more good to more people, more effectively and more efficiently (Felner, Felner, & Silverman, 2000).

The field of prevention has evolved from a conceptual framework that included only three factors (host, environment, agent) and three levels of intervention (primary, secondary, tertiary) to one that allows for multifactorial considerations and multiple levels of intervention without assigning hierarchical value to them (Mrazek & Haggerty, 1994). Primary prevention has expanded to encompass disease prevention, health protection (or maintenance), and health promotion. It is in the arenas of health protection, health promotion, and health maintenance that human behavioral dynamics have become a focus of great interest and study.

In order to effectively mount a successful prevention program, it is incumbent to first measure the extent of the problem (epidemiology), identify who is at risk (risk assessment), decide how and where to target interventions (needs assessment), identify local resources and support networks (ecological assessment), and be prepared to provide immediate interventions for those identified at most risk (treatment) (Silverman & Koretz, 1989).

In the end, any one prevention model is not all-inclusive or definitive. No one model fits all contingencies, situations, or target outcomes. Most of the models suggest where to intervene, but do not ensure effectiveness, efficiency, or specificity. The models help direct one to points of entry, the identification of modifiable risk factors, and the most likely times to intervene. They do not tell us which interventions to use, in what dosages, at what intervals, at what intensities, or for what duration. The models provide testable hypotheses and alternative perspectives. Hence, they serve as catalysts which may transcend their current heuristic function.

A critical question is to what extent these prevention models may be overlapping, mutually exclusive, enhancing, additive, or complementary. Again, we must return to out initial conceptual understanding of the etiology, pathophysiology and expression of behaviors that we characterize as negative and maladaptive in nature, in order to evaluate the extent to which a model matches our view of reality. What is the context in which a behavior is expressed? What factors must be present, and in what degree, for a behavior to occur?

Another issue refers to the difference between elegant models and effective (and efficient) models. Given enough space to draw boxes, arrows, Venn diagrams, circles, and lines, most theoreticians can successfully produce a schematic representation of their perspectives. However, these overly complex and complicated representations are not necessarily translatable into effective programming. A usable or efficient model must be simple to understand, comprehend, and operationalize. Only then can it be effective.

The field of primary prevention must develop on two fronts simultaneously. First, it must create a series of reactive strategies focused on populations at risk for identifiable mental disorders and related negative behaviors. Determination of risk represents, in and of itself, a formidable challenge that will test both the predictive accuracy of state-of-the-art epidemiological strategies and the existing knowledge bases in the behavioral sciences. Risk determination is a statistical concept that is based on prediction and probability. In addition, risk determination must encompass an awareness and sensitivity to risk and protective factors in the development of psychopathology (Rutter, 1987; Rolf, Master, Cicchetti, Nuechterlein, & Weintraub, 1990; Kellam Brown, Rubin, & Ensminger, 1983) and social pathology and wellness.

Speculation about the etiology of dysfunction must be replaced by a rigorous understanding of its individual, familial, sociocultural, and environmental determinants. Simple-minded univariate conceptions of cause and effect must give way to complex transactional–ecological and diathesis–stress models of psychopathology, which will enable us to determine who is at risk for what dysfunction under what specific conditions (Felner & Silverman, 1989). Primary preventive efforts may then be designed either to modify the "whos," in order to fortify them against potential pathogens and pathological processes, or to modify the pathogenetic conditions, in order to remove them from the environment. We must accept the challenge of learning about the ecology of health and pathology, in order, ultimately, to engineer environments, social as well as physical, that minimize negative emotional states and promote positive adaptive coping styles.

The second front for primary prevention is toward promotive or proactive interventions, which focus, not on the alleviation of pathology per se, but on the development of positive, adaptive, adjustive capacities and skills as ends, in and of themselves. In essence, proactive efforts carry the promise of allowing the mental health professions to finally focus on that very outcome—mental health—and social well-being.

Regardless of whether the focus of the primary prevention activity is reactive or proactive, it is essential that it be characterized by specific actions directed at specific populations for specific purposes (Goldston, 1980). Each of these facets must be operationally defined so that the intervention process can be monitored and its impacts objectively assessed, be they reactive or proactive. It is equally important, given the population-focused nature of such efforts, that public health strategies of education, community organization, and coordination of the major social systems be integral components of the specific interventions affecting the target population (Silverman, 1985).

A FEW FINAL WORDS OF CAUTION

Critical to any effort to effect behavioral change over time is the accurate measurement of that change. The importance of incorporating formative and summative (process and outcome) evaluations into the total preventive intervention program cannot be sufficiently emphasized (Lorion, 1983). Before one embarks on a comprehensive, coordinated, collaborative, community-based suicide preventive intervention program, the policy planners and implementation teams must set reasonable and rational goals within reasonable and rational time frames, agree on reasonable formative and summative outcome measures, and promise to evaluate the intervention over time.

Also see: Primary Prevention, 21st Century: Foundation; Definition: Foundation; Effective Programming: Foundation.

References

Albee, G.W. (1959). *Mental health manpower trends*. NY: Basic Books.
Albee, G.W. (1979). Primary prevention. *Canada's Mental Health, 27*, 5–9.
Albee, G.W. (1980). A competency model must replace the defect model. In L.A. Bond & J.C. Rosen (Eds.), *Competence and coping during adulthood* (pp. 75–104). Hanover, NH: University Press of New England.
Albee, G.W. (1982). Preventing psychopathology and promoting human potential. *American Psychologist, 37*, 1043–1050.
Albee, G.W. (1983). The argument for primary prevention. In H.A. Marlowe, Jr. & R.B. Weinberg (Eds.), *Primary prevention: Fact or fallacy*. Tampa, FL: University of South Florida Press.
American Psychiatric Association (APA) Task Force on Prevention Research. (1990). Report of the APA Task Force on Prevention Research. *American Journal of Psychiatry, 147*, 1701–1704.
American Psychologist. (January, 2000). Happiness, excellence, and optimal human functioning [Special issue]. 55:1, pp. 5–183.
Barker, R.G. (1968). *Ecological psychology: Concepts and methods of studying the environment of human behavior*. Stanford, CA: Stanford University Press.
Berkowitz, A.D., & Perkins, H.W. (1986). Resident advisors as role models: A comparison of drinking patterns of resident advisers and their peers. *Journal of College Student Personnel, 27*, 146–153.
Bloom, M. (1981). *Primary prevention: The possible science*. NJ: Prentice-Hall.
Bloom, B.L. (1986). Primary prevention: An overview. In J.T. Barter & S.W. Talbott (Eds.), *Primary prevention in psychiatry: State of the art* (pp. 3–12). Washington, DC: American Psychiatric Press.
Bronfonbrenner, U. (1979). *The ecology of human development: Experiments by nature and design*. Cambridge: Harvard University Press.
Broskowski, A., & Baker, F. (1974). Professional, organizational, and social barriers to primary prevention. *American Journal of Orthopsychiatry, 44*(5), 707–719.
Caplan, G. (1964). *Principles of preventive psychiatry*. NY: Basic Books.
Cicchetti, D. (1990). Developmental psychopathology and prevention of serious mental disorders: Overdue detente and illustrations through the affective disorders. In P. Muehrer (Ed.), *Conceptual research models for preventing mental disorders* (pp. 215–254) (DHHS Publication No. ADM 90-1713). Rockville, MD: National Institute of Mental Health.
Coie, J.D., Watt, N.F., West, S.G., Hawkins, J.D., Asarnow, J.R., Markman, H.J., Ramey, S.L., Shure, M.B., & Long, B. (1993). The science of prevention: A conceptual framework and some directions for a national research program. *American Psychologist, 48*(10), 1013–1022.
Cowen, E.L. (1983). Primary prevention in mental health: Past, present and future. In R.D. Felner, L.A. Jason, J.N. Morisugu, & S.S. Farber (Eds.), *Preventive psychology: Theory, research and practice* (pp. 11–25). New York: Pergamon Press.
Department of Health and Human Services. (1990). *Healthy People 2000: National health promotion and disease prevention objectives* (DHHS Publication No. PHS 91-50212). Washington, DC: US Government Printing Office.
Department of Health and Human Services. (1992). *The Third National Injury Control Conference* (DHHS Publication No. 1992-634-666). Washington, DC: US Government Printing Office.
Eisenberg, L. (1980). Adolescent suicide: On taking arms against a sea of troubles. *Pediatrics, 66*, 315–319.
Felner, R.D., Adan, A.M., & Silverman, M.M. (1992). Risk assessment and prevention of youth suicide in school and educational contexts. In R.W. Maris, A.L. Berman, J.T. Maltsberger, & R.I. Yufit (Eds.), *Assessment and prediction of suicide* (pp. 420–447). New York: The Guilford Press.
Felner, R.D., & Felner, T.Y. (1989). Primary prevention programs in the educational context: A transactional–ecological framework and analysis. In L. Bond & B. Compas (Eds.), *Primary prevention and promotion in the schools* (pp. 13–49). Newbury Park, CA: Sage.
Felner, R.D., Jason, L.A., Moritsugu, J.N., & Farber, S.S. (1983). *Preventive psychology: Theory, research, and practice*. NY: Pergamon Press.

Felner, R.D., & Lorion, R.P. (1985). Clinical child psychology and prevention: Toward a workable and satisfying marriage. Proceedings: National Conference on Training Clinical Child Psychologists (pp. 41–95).

Felner, R.D., & Silverman, M.M. (1989). Primary prevention: A consideration of general principles and findings for the prevention of youth suicide. In Alcohol, drug abuse, and mental health administration. *Report of the secretary's task force on youth suicide, Vol. 3: Prevention and interventions in youth suicide* (pp. 23–30) (DHHS Publication No. ADM 89-1623). Washington, DC: US Government Printing Office.

Felner, R.D., Felner, T.Y., & Silverman, M.M. (2000). Prevention in mental health and social intervention: Conceptual and methodological issues in the evolution of the science and practice of prevention. In J. Rappaport & E. Seidman (Eds.), *Handbook of community psychology* (pp. 10–55). New York: Plenum Press.

Flitcraft, A.H. (1992). Violence, values, and gender. *Journal of American Medical Association, 267*(3), 3194–3195.

Goldston, S.E. (1980). An overview of primary prevention programming. In D.C. Klein & S.E. Goldston (Eds.), *Primary prevention: An idea whose time has come* (pp. 23–40) (DHHS Publication No. ADM 80-447). Washington, DC: US Government Printing Office.

Gordon, R.S. (1983). An operational classification of disease prevention. *Public Health Reports, 98*, 107–109.

Gruenberg, E.M., Lewis, C., & Goldston, S.E. (Eds.). (1986). *Vaccinating against brain syndromes: The campaign against measles and rubella.* New York: Oxford University Press.

Haddon, W., Jr. (1967). The prevention of accidents. In D.M. Clark & B. MacMahon (Eds.), *Preventive medicine.* Boston: Little, Brown.

Haddon, W., Jr. (1968). The changing approach to the epidemiology, prevention, and amelioration of trauma: The transition to approaches etiologically rather than descriptively based. *American Journal of Public Health, 58*, 1341–1348.

Haddon, W., Jr. (1980). Advances in the epidemiology of injuries as a basis for public policy. *Public Health Reports, 95*, 411–421.

Institute of Medicine. (1985). *Injury in America: A continuing public health problem.* Washington, DC: National Academy Press.

Kellam, S.G., Brown, C.H., Rubin, B.R., & Ensminger, M.E. (1983). Paths leading to teenage psychiatric symptoms and substance abuse: Developmental epidemiological studies in Woodlawn. In S.B. Guze, F.T. Earls, & J.E. Barrett (Eds.), *Childhood psychopathology and development* (pp. 17–51). New York: Raven Press.

Kelly, J.C. (Ed.). (1979). *Adolescent boys in high school: A psychological study of coping and adaptation.* Hillsdale, NJ: Eribaum.

Kuhn, T.S. (1970). *The structure of scientific revolutions* (2nd ed.). Chicago, IL: University of Chicago Press.

Lorion, R.P. (1983). Evaluating preventive interventions: Guidelines for the serious social change agent. In R.D. Felner, L.A. Jason, J.N. Moritsugu, & S.S. Farber (Eds.), *Preventive psychology: Theory, research, and practice* (pp. 251–268). New York: Pergamon Press.

Lorion, R.P., Price, R.H., & Eaton, W.W. (1989). The prevention of child and adolescent disorders: From theory to research. In D. Shaffer, I. Philips, N.B. Enzer, M.M. Silverman, V. Anthony (Eds.), *Prevention of mental disorders, alcohol and other drug use in children and adolescents* (pp. 55–96) (DHHS Publication No. ADM 89-1646). Washington, DC: US Government Printing Office.

Maris, R.W. (1992). The relationship of nonfatal suicide attempts to completed suicides. In R.W. Maris, A.L. Berman, J.T. Maltsberger, & R.I. Yufit (Eds.), *Assessment and prediction of suicide* (pp. 362–380). New York: Guilford Press.

Marzuk, P.M., Tardiff, K., & Hirsch, C.S. (1992). The epidemiology of murder–suicide. *Journal of American Medical Association, 267*(23), 3179–3183.

Mrazek, P.J., & Haggerty, R.J. (Eds.). (1994). *Reducing risks for mental disorders: Frontiers for preventive intervention research.* Washington, DC: National Academy Press.

Pardes, H., Silverman, M.M., & West, A. (1989). Prevention and the field of mental health: A psychiatric perspective. In L. Breslow, J.E. Fielding, & L.B. Lave (Eds.), *Annual Review of Public Health*, Vol. 10 (pp. 403–422). Palo Alto, CA: Annual Reviews.

Perkins, H.W., & Berkowitz, A.D. (1986). Perceiving the community norms of alcohol use among students: Some research implications for campus alcohol education programming. *International Journal of the Addictions, 21*(9/10), 961–976.

Rappaport, J. (1987). Terms of empowerment/exemplars of prevention: Toward a theory for community psychology. *American Journal of Community Psychology, 15*, 121–148.

Rolf, J., Masten, A.S., Cicchetti, D., Nuechterlein, K.H., & Weintraub, S. (Eds.). (1990). *Risk and protective factors in the development of psychopathology.* New York: Cambridge University Press.

Runyan, C.W. (1993). Progress and potential in injury control. *American Journal of Public Health, 83*, 637–639.

Rutter, M. (Ed.). (1987). *Developmental psychiatry.* Washington, DC: American Psychiatric Press.

Sameroff, A.J. (1983). Developmental systems: Contexts and evolution. *W. Keeson's History, Theory and Methods, vol. 1.* P.H. Mussen (Ed.), *Handbook of Child Psychology.* New York: Wiley.

Sameroff, A.J., & Chandler, A.J. (1975). Reproductive risk and the continuum of caretaking casualty. In F.D. Horowitz, E.M. Heatherington, S. Scarr-Salapatek, & G. Siegal (Eds.), *Review of child development research*, Vol. 4 (pp. 187–244). Chicago: University of Chicago Press.

Sameroff, A.J., & Fiese, B.H. (1989). Conceptual issues in prevention. In D. Shaffer, I. Philips, N.B. Enzer, M.M. Silverman, & V. Anthony (Eds.), *Prevention of mental disorders, alcohol, and other drug use in children and adolescents* (pp. 23–54) (DHHS Publication No. ADM 89-1646). Washington, DC: US Government Printing Office.

Sarason, S.B. (1981). *Psychology misdirected.* New York: Free Press.

Seidman, E. (1987). Toward a framework for primary prevention research. In J.A. Steinberg & M.M. Silverman (Eds.), *Preventing mental disorders: A research perspective* (pp. 2–19) (DHHS Publication No. ADM 87-1492). Washington, DC: US Government Printing Office.

Seidman, E. (1990). Pursuing the meaning and utility of social regularities for community psychology. In P. Tolan, C. Keys, F. Chertok, & L. Jason (Eds.), *Researching community psychology: Issues of theory and methods* (pp. 91–100). Washington, DC: American Psychological Association.

Shaffer, D. (1989). Prevention of psychiatric disorders in children and adolescents: A summary of findings and recommendations from project prevention. In D. Shaffer, I. Philips, N.B. Enzer, M.M. Silverman, & V. Anthony (Eds.), *Prevention of mental disorders, alcohol, and other drug use in children and adolescents* (pp. 443–456) (DHHS Publication No. ADM 89-1646). Washington, DC: US Government Printing Office.

Silverman, M.M. (1985). Preventive intervention research: A new beginning. In T.C. Owan (Ed.), *Southeast Asian mental health treatment, prevention, services, training, and research* (pp. 169–182) (DHHS Publication No. ADM 85-1399). Washington, DC: US Government Printing Office.

Silverman, M.M. (1996). Approaches to suicide prevention: A focus on models. In R.F. Ramsay & B.L. Tanney (Eds.), *Global trends in suicide prevention: Toward the development of national strategies for suicide prevention* (pp. 25–94). Mumbai, India: Tata Institute of Social Sciences.

Silverman, M.M., & Felner, R.D. (1995). Suicide prevention programs: Issues of design, implementation, feasibility, and developmental appropriateness. *Suicide and Life-Threatening Behavior, 25*(1), 92–104.

Silverman, M.M., & Koretz, D.S. (1989). Preventing mental health problems. In R.E. Stein (Ed.), *Caring for children with chronic illness: Issues and strategies* (pp. 213–229). New York: Springer Publishing Company.

Vincent, T.A., & Trickett, E.J. (1983). Preventive interventions and the human context: Ecological approaches to environmental assessment and change. In R. Felner, L. Jason, J. Moritsugu, & S. Farber (Eds.), *Preventive psychology: Theory, research, and practice* (pp. 67–86). New York: Pergamon Press.

US Public Health Service. (1999). *The Surgeon General's call to action to prevent suicide*. Washington, DC: Author.

The Evaluation of Prevention and Health Promotion Programs

Jacob Kraemer Tebes, Joy S. Kaufman, and Christian M. Connell

The evaluation of prevention and health promotion programs is one component of the broader field of evaluation research or social program evaluation. Evaluation research applies the practices and principles of social research to assess the conceptualization, design, implementation, effectiveness, and efficiency of social interventions (Rossi & Freeman, 1993). Prevention program evaluation is one component of evaluation research that draws on knowledge and traditions from several disciplines and fields of study, including public health, psychology, sociology, education, social work, social policy, and public administration.

Below we provide a summary of prevention program evaluation. We begin with a brief social and intellectual history of evaluation research and then summarize the prevention context for the field, including a brief history of prevention in America and a discussion of prevention science. Next, we summarize the phases of prevention program evaluation, and then discuss, in detail: pre-design considerations, data collection and analysis, and the use and dissemination of findings. We conclude by discussing current theories of knowledge which guide evaluation practice.

EVALUATION RESEARCH: A SUMMARY OF ITS SOCIAL AND INTELLECTUAL HISTORY

Although social program evaluation in America has its roots in applied social research dating back to the 1930s, the modern era of evaluation can be traced to the 1960s. This was the period of the Great Society in which federal social welfare programs were launched to reduce poverty and its consequences. Evaluation research emerged as a federally funded professional activity to monitor and assess the impact of anti-poverty programs in education, income maintenance, housing, health, and criminal justice (Shadish, Cook, & Leviton, 1991).

During this time, the field of evaluation research experienced considerable growth. A number of texts were developed for the evaluation of social programs (Campbell & Stanley, 1966; Reicken et al., 1974; Suchman, 1967; Weiss, 1972). In addition, evaluation journals such as *Evaluation Review* and *Evaluation and Program Planning*—begun in 1976 and 1978, respectively—were established to provide a scholarly forum for evaluation work, and the American Evaluation Association was formed to foster exchange among professionals.

Shadish et al. (1991) maintain that, since the field's emergence in the 1960s and 1970s and continuing through the present, evaluation practice has progressed through three stages. The first stage was characterized by application of scientific methods to the study of social interventions. The work of Donald C. Campbell and his colleagues exemplify this approach to evaluation (Campbell, 1969; Campbell & Stanley, 1966; Cook & Campbell, 1979). In this stage, scientist/quantitative methods derived from the laboratory were viewed as central to effective social program evaluation because they maximized one's opportunity for finding the "truth" about a given program (Shadish et al., 1991; Campbell, 1969). Experimental design was highly valued, with randomization of experimental conditions regarded as essential because it reduced threats to internal validity (i.e., the ability to make inferences about the causal relationship between two variables), thus enabling one to draw conclusions about a program's operation and its effects. In the absence of randomization, evaluators were encouraged to select quasi-experimental designs that minimized threats to validity, and in particular, internal validity.

The intellectual basis for this "experimenting society" (Campbell, 1969) stage of social program evaluation was logical empiricism (McGuire, 1986). Logical empiricism is the intellectual successor to 19th century logical positivism, in that it synthesized "... the rationalist deductive thesis and positivist inductive antithesis ... (so as to) maintain that knowledge representations should be, on the a priori side, validly deducible from a broader, empirically anchored theory, and on the a posteriori side, should have survived the jeopardy of disconfirmation by observations yielded by a new empirical test" (p. 279). This tradition has remained in the forefront of evaluation research, but is no longer the exclusive focus of practice and discourse among evaluators.

The second stage of evaluation research emerged in reaction to the perceived limitations and failures of its initial stage (Shadish et al., 1991). For some evaluators, it became apparent that managers, policy makers, and politicians often did not act on recommendations and results derived from carefully controlled, technically proficient, and scientifically rigorous studies. In part, this was because evaluations were not usually designed by keeping in mind how findings would be used; that is, how findings would change practice, inform policy, or address the needs of specific constituencies. Evaluations were also found lacking because they often did not incorporate the perspective of groups likely to be impacted by the findings, such as its stakeholders. Not only did this latter practice pose political problems for evaluators, but it made enlisting the support of stakeholders to implement solutions that were subsequently derived from the evaluation more difficult. In response, a number of alternative approaches to evaluation emerged (Shadish et al., 1991). Some evaluators focused on how evaluation results would be used by various stakeholders (Patton, 1978; Stake, 1975), others on how they would be incorporated into changing agency practices or services systems (Wholey, 1979), and still others on how they would inform thinking about programs and policies, including program theory (Weiss, 1972). There was also a general movement toward the use of qualitative approaches in evaluation. Such approaches were believed to help evaluators understand better the meanings, relationships, and processes embedded in the local context of a given program or service (Guba & Lincoln, 1981; Patton, 1980). This "second stage" intellectual tradition (Shadish et al., 1991) continues as a strong force in evaluation today (Patton, 1997; Stake, 1994; Weiss, 1997; Wholey, Hatry, & Newcomer, 1994).

Shadish et al.'s (1991) third stage of evaluation practice, which emerged in the 1980s and continues through the present, reflects the emergence of an integrative approach to social program evaluation. Cronbach (1982) was an early proponent of this view in his advocacy of "functional" evaluation, in which the evaluator selects an evaluation design and corresponding methods based on the purposes of the evaluation. In functional evaluation, evaluations can serve multiple purposes—the meanings a program has for various stakeholders; the assessment of cause and effect; or the generalization of inferences about the program across persons, settings, and times, to name just a few. In a critique of experimental approaches to program evaluation, Cronbach (1982, 1986) described internal as no longer the sine qua non (Campbell, 1969) of evaluation. In contrast, he argued that the role of the evaluator was to generalize to the domains of interest in any given evaluation. Cronbach (1982, 1986) maintained that if the primary purpose of an evaluation is to generalize one's findings to multiple contexts that have

relevance for policy, then external validity (i.e., generalizing to other persons, settings, or times) may take precedence over internal validity in a given design. Mark (1986) went further in recommending that evaluators should examine the different types of validity for their relevance to policy, and then prioritize among them on that basis, even if all threats to internal validity have not been ruled out. Tebes (2000) has argued that following such an approach is likely to increase scientific knowledge in prevention and advance public policy.

Peter Rossi and Howard Freeman are two other influential evaluators who have advocated a more integrative approach to evaluation research, as is evident in their textbook, *Evaluation: A Systematic Approach* (Rossi & Freeman, 1985, 1993; Rossi, Freeman, & Lipsey, 1999). Shadish et al. (1991) maintain that Rossi and Freeman's emphasis on comprehensive, tailored, and theory-driven evaluation provides an intellectual basis for integrating the previous two stages of the field. Comprehensive evaluations are those that assess the conceptualization, implementation, and impact of an intervention. Tailored evaluations emphasize conducting such assessments differentially based on whether a program is an innovation, a modification, or an ongoing program. And theory-driven evaluations involve developing and specifying a program model to guide the intervention and its evaluation. Not only do these varying objectives for evaluation encourage evaluators to use multiple methods in their designs—depending on the nature and purpose of the evaluation—they also advocate for the inclusion of stakeholders throughout the evaluation process. Furthermore, the use of multiple methods provides a rationale for integrating quantitative and qualitative methods into a single evaluation design, a practice that increasingly is viewed as essential to effective program evaluation (Sechrest & Sidani, 1995; Shadish, 1995).

EVALUATION RESEARCH AND PREVENTION

To provide a context for understanding the current status of evaluation research in prevention, we provide a brief history of prevention in America and discuss a recent trend in the field—the emergence of prevention science.

Prevention in Historic Perspective

The growth of prevention in America coincided with that of social program evaluation, beginning with its inclusion in the Report of President's Joint Commission on Mental Illness and Health in 1961. The 1961 Joint Commission Report advocated for the use of social and community-based interventions to prevent problems prior to the need for treatment (Levine & Perkins, 1987). This report was instrumental in the creation of the 1963 Community Mental Health Centers Act which represented a large-scale, federal initiative to translate recommendations from the report into action (Tebes, Kaufman, & Chinman, in press). The 1963 Act funded community mental health centers (CMHCs) not only to provide comprehensive clinical services, but also consultation and education services (i.e., prevention programming), within geographic "catchment areas" throughout the country. This usually required CMHCs to establish collaborative relationships with local communities to implement prevention programs and services, conduct needs assessments, and evaluate the effectiveness of innovative programs.

In the decades immediately following its passage, the Community Mental Health Centers Act of 1963 established an institutional basis for prevention and fostered the development and evaluation of preventive interventions. The growth in prevention was subsequently reflected in advocacy efforts by such groups as the National Mental Health Association (Long, 1989) and various professional associations. Prevention was also emphasized in the report of the President's Commission on Mental Health in 1978. The Commission recommended a larger federal role for prevention to train researchers and fund prevention research through establishment of an Office of Prevention Research at the National Institute of Mental Health (NIMH). The creation and continued funding of this office in 1982 led to a steady voice for prevention at the federal level (NIMH, 1998). During the intervening years, prevention and health promotion have also been advanced by other federal institutes or agencies, such as the National Institute on Drug Abuse, the National Institute on Alcohol Abuse and Alcoholism, the Department of Justice, the Department of Education, the Centers for Disease Control and Prevention, the National Cancer Institute, and the Center for Substance Abuse Prevention of the Substance Abuse and Mental Health Services Administration. Initiatives from these sources have stimulated state and private foundation efforts to advance prevention and health promotion services and related evaluation research.

The Emergence of Prevention Science

Over the past decade, a controversial development in prevention and health promotion activities has been the emergence of prevention science (Reiss & Price, 1996; Tebes et al., in press). Prevention science has reconceptualized research and practice from one which emphasizes social interventions that have a wide range of intended impacts on the individual or community to those that give priority to individual change in the prevention of psychiatric disorders (NIMH, 1996). Rather than classify preventive interventions as primary, secondary, or tertiary, prevention science identifies three types

of prevention activities: universal, selective, and indicated (Gordon, 1987; NIMH, 1996). Universal interventions target the general public or entire population groups regardless of risk status; selective interventions target individuals or population subgroups whose risk of developing the disorder may be higher than average; and, indicated interventions target high-risk individuals with detectable signs of the disorder—perhaps indicating a biological marker or a predisposition for the disorder—but who do not meet criteria for a psychiatric diagnosis (NIMH, 1996; Tebes et al., 2002). Thus, prevention is one end of a continuum of intervention that includes mental health treatment and extends through rehabilitation (Munoz, Mrazek, & Haggerty, 1996).

Risk reduction is the primary focus of intervention in prevention science, with risk defined as "those characteristics, variables, or hazards that, if present for a given individual, make it more likely that this individual, rather than someone selected from the general population, will develop a disorder" (NIMH, 1996, p. 6). Risk reduction is likely to be most effective when it is implemented in developmentally appropriate contexts which address the transactional nature of both risk and protection (Mrazek & Haggerty, 1994), and is informed by epidemiological data about the distribution of mental disorders and patterns of risk in a given population (Kellam, Koretz, & Moscicki, 1999; NIMH, 1996).

Another major emphasis of prevention science has been to conceptualize research and the evaluation of prevention programs and services as part of a broader "preventive intervention research cycle" (Mrazek & Haggerty, 1994; NIMH, 1996). This cycle consists of several phases beginning with the identification of a problem or disorder that is to be the target of intervention, followed by a review of risk and protective factors associated with the onset of that problem or disorder. Determining the efficacy of an intervention through pilot, confirmatory, and replication studies represents the next phase of the preventive intervention research cycle. Research on efficacy is guided by specification of a theoretical model, which is then tested through randomized controlled efficacy trials and replications. In the fourth phase, efficacious preventive interventions are implemented and evaluated for their effectiveness in real-world settings, if possible, under controlled conditions. In the cycle's final phase, effective preventive interventions are implemented and evaluated in the community. This phase often requires the establishment of partnerships between researchers and community members or among community stakeholders to ensure that such larger-scale interventions are implemented successfully. Researcher–stakeholder partnerships may also be essential to ensure that prevention program and service evaluations are attuned to local conditions, needs, and priorities (Tebes et al., 2002).

The growth of prevention science has also accelerated a movement, among state and federal funders, towards the implementation of science- or evidence-based approaches to intervention; that is, interventions that have been shown through systematic research to be effective (Morrisey, Wandersman, Seybolt, Nation, Crusto, & Davino, 1997). These approaches are aimed, in part, to reduce the gap between the positive impacts obtained in controlled prevention trials and the minimal observed effects found in much of prevention practice.

Criticisms of Prevention Science

The emergence of prevention science has not been without controversy. Critics have assailed its strong emphasis on the prevention of individual diagnosable mental disorders, its primary focus on risk reduction, and its prioritization of randomized trials as the sine qua non for prevention research (Tebes, 1997). Before prevention science came on the scene, prevention efforts were aimed at changing "problems-in-living" (Heller & Monahan, 1977) and related correlates that were associated with a variety of human problems—such as, poverty, unemployment, or social isolation—rather than on specific individual disorders. This broader focus for prevention was consistent with the prevailing *Zeitgeist* in which individual problems were viewed as being rooted in the social context. This original framework for prevention directed efforts beyond intra-individual and interpersonal processes to social processes and structures (Albee, 1996; Heller & Monahan, 1977). Within this latter perspective, mental disorders shared something in common with other problems-in-living; both were caused, exacerbated, or maintained by social factors, such as social institutions, community settings, the peer group, the school, and the family (Levine & Perkins, 1987; Price, 1974). This emphasis on the prevention of problems-in-living as rooted in individual responses to social structures and processes also made explicit the view that such problems were intrinsic to political systems and to the maldistribution of power within those systems (Rappaport, 1977). Some (Albee, 1996; Tebes, 1997; Tebes et al., in press) have argued that a prevention science that is focused on the prevention of individual mental disorders—defined within a classification system in which illnesses are diagnosed essentially in isolation from their sociopolitical context—is likely to devalue or dismiss claims about the social causes of problems-in-living and attempts to address them through social action.

Another criticism of prevention science is its primary focus on risk reduction. This is evident from recent reports from the Institute of Medicine (Mrazek & Haggerty, 1994) and the NIMH (1996, 1998). In both the reports, there is discussion of both risk and protective factor approaches to prevention. However, the emphasis is clearly on the prevention of risk as opposed to the promotion of protective processes let alone the enhancement of strengths. Such approaches, and the conceptual models that animate research and professional activity, are essential to addressing the complex ways in which both risks and protections interact to influence human behavior. Winett (1995, 1998) has articulated such a comprehensive framework in his description of the proactive-developmental-ecological perspective as the basis for health promotion. This perspective integrates prevention and health promotion practices in a manner that incorporates both individual and community-level variables of risk and protection.

A final criticism that has been made regarding prevention science is its emphasis on randomized experimental trials as the basis for generating knowledge. As is discussed in greater detail later, randomized trials are powerful designs for assessing the causal relationship among two or more variables. However, such designs also have significant limitations: (a) they place too high a priority on internal validity as opposed to external validity when evaluating an intervention (Cook & Shadish, 1994), and thus provide little guidance for translating findings into public policy (Cronbach, 1982); (b) they overemphasize outcomes as opposed to understanding processes among the variables of interest (Cook & Shadish, 1994); and (c) they fail to adequately take into account the local conditions of a given experiment (i.e., the characteristics of the experimental context) which influence the data obtained and the inferences drawn (Campbell, 1974; Tebes & Kraemer, 1991). This emphasis has discouraged investigators to use qualitative or other quantitative methods to study preventive interventions that may generate knowledge that complements that obtained in randomized trials. This issue is addressed further in a final section which discusses methodological pluralism in the evaluation of prevention programs.

PHASES IN THE EVALUATION OF PREVENTION PROGRAMS AND SERVICES

We consider evaluation to be a cluster of professional activities that can be understood in narrative terms as characterized by a beginning, a middle, and an end. The beginning phase of an evaluation includes activities that are completed prior to or in preparation for data collection and analyses. This may include the completion of a needs and resources assessment, a review of the scientific or professional literature, the involvement of key stakeholders in planning an evaluation, the completion of an evaluability assessment, the specification of a program theory and logic model, or the completion of a formative evaluation. Some of these activities may vary depending on whether the program is long-standing and well-established, is relatively new but has undergone some modification, or represents an innovation (Rossi & Freeman, 1993). It is also important to note that although this phase may include extensive data collection and analyses, the data gathered is usually collected to assist in the conceptualization, design, monitoring, or implementation of the program or its evaluation, rather than to describe, compare, or assess the impact of a specific program or service.

Every evaluation includes some systematic collection and analysis of data about a given intervention. This constitutes what might be viewed as the middle phase of an evaluation. Data may be gathered at one or several points in time, in one or more settings, and through the use of a variety of designs that may involve qualitative, quasi-experimental, or experimental methods. Data are analyzed based on the questions being addressed and the quality of the data available.

The final phase of an evaluation includes activities which focus on the use and dissemination of evaluation findings. Activities in this phase include: feedback and dissemination of evaluation findings to relevant stakeholders, completion of program materials for replication, and the use of evaluation findings to inform practice, program management, or policy development.

Although evaluation may be conceptualized within this narrative framework, in actual practice, it is more typical that activities carried out in a given phase often overlap with those planned or implemented in another phase. Below we describe evaluation activities by specific phases even though this distinction is admittedly arbitrary for purposes of explication.

BEGINNING AN EVALUATION: PRE-DESIGN CONSIDERATIONS

We discuss four types of evaluation activities in the early phase of an evaluation: needs and resources assessment, enhancing organizational and community capacity for evaluation, specifying the program theory and developing a logic model, and conducting a formative evaluation.

Needs and Resources Assessment

Program evaluators may be involved in the early stages of prevention program planning and development through implementation of a needs assessment. A needs assessment involves the systematic evaluation of the nature, depth, and scope of a social problem (Rossi & Freeman, 1993). Needs assessments are often used to develop programs to address social problems and needed resources (Murrell, 1977), and are most successful whey they include some understanding of the organizational context that influences how data is collected or interpreted (Price & Smith, 1985).

A wide range of methods may be used to conduct a needs assessment (Price & Smith, 1985; Rossi & Freeman, 1993). These include: (1) the analysis of archival data sources (e.g., publicly available sociodemographic and health statistics, continuously collected social indicators, indices of service use); (2) record reviews of client services intended to address a given problem; (3) quantitative or qualitative data collection methods (e.g., sample surveys, focus groups, community forums) of the general public, key informants (i.e., individuals who are knowledgeable about the problem), or community stakeholders (i.e., individuals who are affected by the problem in some important way or who may be invested in its solution, such as potential service recipients, their family members, service providers, funders, or community members); (4) the use of unobtrusive measures that pertain to the specified problem (Webb, Campbell, Schwartz, & Sechrest, 1966); and (5) conducting a large-scale needs assessment through the use of secondary data analysis—described by Gaber (2000) as a "meta-needs assessment." Each of these techniques has both advantages and disadvantages, and it is not uncommon to use a mix of approaches when conducting a thorough needs assessment.

In recent years, needs assessment data has also been supplemented by information about the nature and type of community resources or assets that may also be available to address a problem of concern. A systematic procedure has been developed to provide data about such resources that is known as community asset mapping (Allen, Cordes, & Hart, 1999). On one level, asset mapping represents the flip-side of needs assessment in identifying potential resources available in the community that may be underutilized or that could be mobilized to address a potential social problem. More importantly, however, asset mapping represents a philosophical departure from the usual practice of focusing mostly on a community's needs and problems to one which attempts to recognize, catalog, and capitalize on community strengths as resources toward problem resolution (Kretzmann & McKnight, 1996). Evaluators frequently combine these approaches to conduct a needs and resources assessment.

Following completion of a needs and resources assessment, evaluators often collaborate with stakeholders to define the scope of the social problem of interest and more clearly identify the particular targets of prevention programming. Targets may be defined as at-risk individuals or members of the general population, and may include specification of larger social units (e.g., groups, families) as well as geographical or politically related areas (e.g., neighborhoods, communities, regions) (Rossi & Freeman, 1993). Target definitions should incorporate an awareness of the incidence and prevalence of the social problem, and take into account issues of sensitivity (i.e., the likelihood of correctly identifying targets who should be included in a program) and specificity (i.e., the likelihood of correctly identifying those individuals who should be excluded from a program) when designing a program and its evaluation (Rossi & Freeman, 1993).

Enhancing Organizational and Community Capacity for Evaluation

A critical component in the success of any evaluation is the readiness of the program or service to be evaluated. One approach used to answer this question is to conduct an evaluability assessment (Horst, Nay, Scanlon, & Wholey, 1974; Wholey, 1983). Such an assessment is intended to enable the evaluator and relevant stakeholders to obtain a true picture of a program's operation that may be used to design and implement a subsequent evaluation. An evaluability assessment may be done with an existing program or service or with a coalition of several programs in a given community that target a specific problem (e.g., the prevention of adolescent substance abuse; teen pregnancy prevention).

Rossi and Freeman (1993) identify six iterative action steps for conducting evaluability assessments: (1) describe the program through the use of existing documents and materials; (2) interview key program leadership and staff to obtain details about program operations and activities; (3) observe (or "scout") the program in operation to obtain direct knowledge about it; (4) specify program elements and outcomes into a measurable program model; (5) identify the purpose of the evaluation and how it will be used by various stakeholders; and (6) obtain an organizational commitment, at multiple levels, to conduct the evaluation.

In recent years, several models have been proposed which extend the practice of evaluability assessment even further by identifying specific components for building organizational or community capacity to conduct evaluations (Linney & Wandersman, 1991; O'Sullivan & O'Sullivan, 1998; Wandersman, Imm, Chinman, & Kaftarian, 2000). Among the more ambitious of these approaches has been that proposed by Wandersman and his colleagues (Wandersman et al., 2000) in a manual entitled: *Getting to Outcomes: Methods and Tools for Planning, Evaluation and Accountability*. *Getting to Outcomes*, or GTO, provides methods and tools for program staff and management to design, plan, implement, and evaluate programs and policies. It addresses 10 accountability questions in planning and implementing a prevention program: needs and resources assessment; goal development; identification of best practices; assessment of program fit; assessment of organizational capacities; assessment of program plan; assessment of implementation; identification and collection of outcomes; development of a continuous quality improvement plan; and sustainability. The authors note that implementing GTO can be useful at any stage of prevention

programming at the agency or community coalition level for both preexisting programs and new programs, and may be particularly useful if reassessed over time.

An underlying principle in enhancing organizational or community capacity to conduct evaluations is a commitment to regarding service recipients and providers as well as other key stakeholders as partners in planning, implementing, and utilizing an evaluation. This is critical for at least two reasons. Involvement of stakeholders in an evaluation increases the likelihood of organizational buy-in for carrying it out and reduces organizational or community resistance to its implementation (O'Sullivan & O'Sullivan, 1998). More importantly, however, key stakeholders, such as front-line staff and consumers of services, are often the best informants for identifying outcomes and processes relevant to the assessment of program effectiveness and efficiency (Koch, Cairns, & Brunk, 2000; Patton, 1980; Tebes, Kaufman, Connell, & Ross, 2001).

Specifying the Program Theory and Developing a Logic Model

Although explicating the theory underlying a program may be part of an evaluability assessment, its utility in program evaluation is so essential that it deserves further consideration in its own right. Weiss (1997) defines a program theory as the set of assumptions and beliefs underlying a program that may be illustrated through a phased sequence of causes and effects. Evaluations based on a program theory are designed to illustrate not only whether and how much change has occurred, but also whether the sequence of steps leading to the observed changes are the expected mechanisms responsible for the change (Rossi and Freeman, 1985; Weiss, 1997). It is this information that is particularly useful to program planners and policy makers because it provides direction regarding program development and resource allocation.

The specification of the program theory into hypothesized causal links between program activities and outcomes is a logic model (Millar, Simeone, & Carnevale, 2001). Logic models link program inputs (resources) to specific planned program activities and expected proximal and distal outcomes (Hernandez, 2000; W.K. Kellogg Foundation, 2000). Logic models are often developed by program evaluators with input from staff who plan programs and from program leadership (Mohr, 1988). An evaluator who develops a logic model in collaboration with program leadership creates an opportunity not only for key personnel to understand the program's underlying theory more fully but also to develop an evaluation that is more likely to inform management decision making. This process of collaborative development of the logic model redefines the role of the evaluator to include that of facilitator and educator (Hernandez,

2000). The process of explicating a logic model also often helps staff view the evaluator as a partner who not only provides them with data about their program, but also challenges them in specifying what it is that they do, why they do it, and why they think it will make a difference.

Evaluations that are theory-driven often require more work prior to data collection on the part of evaluator because explicating the program theory and specifying the logic model can be tedious work. However, such work is essential in providing direction for subsequent data collection and analyses. Specification of a logic model focuses the evaluator's efforts more closely on the hypothesized mechanisms related to the intended outcomes and identifies potential measurement issues involving the links between theory, activities, and outcomes (Weiss, 1997). Theory-driven evaluations also provide additional challenges for the evaluator as feedback of data needs to occur frequently and in a timely manner for the results to have the intended impact on program development (Hernandez, 2000).

Conducting a Formative Evaluation

A formative evaluation is one type of process evaluation whose emphasis is on collecting data about various program components that may be useful in developing or modifying a program. Specifically, formative evaluations attempt to identify whether program activities are feasible given a particular target population and the settings in which activities take place, and how those activities are interpreted by program recipients and other stakeholders (Price & Smith, 1985; Scheirer, 1994). Formative evaluation is often considered as synonymous with process evaluation, even though the latter term describes a broader range of evaluation activities that include monitoring program implementation and assessing the relationship between intervention processes and outcomes (Scheirer, 1994).

Qualitative methods are the most common data collection procedures used in formative evaluations because these approaches allow greater flexibility for determining the meaning of various program components for individual stakeholders, and the fit between those components and stakeholders' "lived" experience. There are numerous examples of issues to be examined and approaches to be used in a formative evaluation. Service recipients may provide feedback in a focus group or community forum about the usefulness of a program activity or may state their preferences about different planned activities. A panel of experts may be asked to rate the value of program activities given their reading of the program's logic model. An ethnographer may observe the interactions of youth enrolled in a community prevention program to assess the developmental appropriateness of specific activities. And finally, evaluation staff

may conduct open-ended interviews with selected service providers to determine the difficulty of implementing various activities of the program. Such methods provide useful data about aspects of the program that may lead to its modification and subsequent evaluation (Scheirer, 1994).

THE MIDDLE OF AN EVALUATION: DATA COLLECTION AND ANALYSIS

Evaluation of prevention programs requires careful attention to design and methodology, which is one purpose of the evaluator's role. Prevention program evaluation differs from other scientific endeavors in that the fundamental goal is to provide reliable and credible information regarding: (a) the current status of a program; (b) its performance relative to a given standard; or (c) its effectiveness in ameliorating risk or promoting adaptation (Lipsey & Cordray, 2000; Sechrest & Figueredo, 1993; Snow & Tebes, 1991). Other important goals of an evaluation may also include obtaining a better understanding of the mechanisms underlying a program's success and the relative efficiency of that program in terms of costs and benefits.

Like other research endeavors, the conclusions drawn from a program evaluation may be either "weak" or "strong," and this determination is, in many ways, shaped by the degree to which the design and methodology were well-suited to address the questions of interest. Following Cronbach (1982), we believe that designs should be selected based on the purpose or function of the evaluation, and that the role of the evaluator is to weigh options and select the appropriate strategy given various resource constraints. Resource constraints include the economic costs and time commitment required of some experimental and quasi-experimental designs (Mowbray, Bybee, Collins, & Levine, 1998; US General Accounting Office, 1991), as well as factors that may impede data collection or limit the use of particular design approaches within a setting (Mowbray et al., 1998).

The Program Evaluation and Methodology Division of the US General Accounting Office (1991) recognizes three general categories of questions into which an evaluation may fall—descriptive, normative, or impact. A descriptive evaluation of a prevention program may be targeted at understanding participant characteristics or describing the current status of a particular program, while a normative evaluation may focus on the relationship between participant or program characteristics relative to existing benchmarks or stated objectives. Impact evaluations, on the other hand, address evaluation questions particular to program effects, trying to establish an understanding of cause-and-effect between the program of interest and participant outcomes. Descriptive and normative evaluations provide useful information about the current status of a program or its performance relative to accepted standards. Design approaches for such evaluations may include sample survey methods (e.g., cross-sectional, panel study, or criteria-referenced surveys), case study approaches, participant observation, participatory action research, or outcome monitoring. Impact assessments include a variety of quasi-experimental and true experimental designs that yield interpretable data about program effectiveness and efficiency. With the ever-increasing emphasis on identifying mechanisms that lead to specific program effects, many recent evaluators often integrate two or more of these types of designs—descriptive, normative, and impact—into a single evaluation.

Descriptive Designs and Approaches

Descriptive evaluation designs may include a variety of qualitative and quantitative methods that are used to assess the current status of a program. Such designs ordinarily do not focus on the program's performance relative to other programs or specific standards (as is the case for normative designs) nor do they emphasize program effectiveness (which is the focus of impact assessments). Below we describe some common descriptive designs.

Case Studies

Case studies represent a potentially useful evaluation approach for describing a particular intervention, for improving practice, and for revealing the perspective of stakeholders, including those whose voices are less likely to be heard (Stake, 1994). Stake (1978, 1994) pioneered the use of the case study approach to program evaluation, advocating the use of naturalistic observation, interviews with stakeholders, and reviews of program documents and records for use in evaluations. He believed that case studies of a given program should involve personalistic observation, an informal writing style, and descriptions that are holistic and contextual in nature.

Case studies can be conducted prospectively or retrospectively depending on the nature of the phenomena being studied. They require significant resources per case examined and can yield rich qualitative information, particularly in generating hypotheses about program implementation, processes, and impacts that can be examined more effectively using other methods (Shadish et al., 1991; Tebes & Kraemer, 1991). Merriam (1988) describes four essential features of case studies. They are: (1) particularistic—they focus on a particular situation, event, program, or phenomenon; (2) descriptive—the end product is a complete description of the phenomenon under study; (3) heuristic—they

illuminate the reader's understanding of the phenomenon under study; and (4) inductive—they rely on inductive reasoning, with hypotheses generated as data are collected. These features reflect the singular value of the case study approach—it provides a nuanced, contextualized understanding of human action as it unfolds at the level of the individual, the group, the organization, or the community—depending on one's focus. Fishman (1999) has argued that these advantages make the case study better-suited for advancing understanding about social problems and framing realistic solutions to those problems than the usual positivist approaches found in the social sciences.

Participant Observation

In participant observation the researcher interacts with informants in their natural setting and in the process works to collect systematic data in an unobtrusive manner (Taylor & Bogdan, 1998). Tebes and Kraemer (1991) summarize the main features of participant observation: (1) the observation is conducted in the natural setting; (2) the researcher can experience the phenomenon in its entirety; (3) hypotheses are generated as the data are collected; (4) the researcher maintains copious and detailed notes; and (5) participants are inform-ants and are seen as collaborators in the research process. Participant observation enables the researcher to observe phenomena as they occur within natural settings and to develop an experiential understanding of a particular setting. However, as a method it is time consuming and requires a high level of expertise on the part of the evaluator to limit informant reactivity and to minimize subjectivity in making causal inferences (Taylor & Bogdan, 1998; Tebes & Kraemer, 1991).

Participatory Action Research

Whyte (1989) describes participatory action research (PAR) as a powerful type of applied investigation that mutually benefits the researcher and those traditionally seen as "subjects" of a given study. In its purest form, participants (i.e., subjects) function as full partners who identify research questions and collaborate with the investigator in all phases of the evaluation process, including: design, data collection, analysis, dissemination, and utilization (Beamish & Bryer, 1999). Three characteristics distinguish PAR from other methodologies: (1) joint ownership of the research; (2) collaborative conduct of the research; and (3) immersion of the participants being studied in every stage of the research from design to outcome (Beamish & Bryer, 1999). PAR encourages participants and researchers to function as a team to develop mutual objectives and procedures for conducting the evaluation. PAR requires considerable time and effort

(Bruyere, 1993) to gain full participation and to develop consensus among diverse interests (Rogers & Palmer-Erbs, 1994).

Implementation Monitoring

Implementation monitoring is another form of process evaluation that refers to the collection of data on program activities as an intervention is carried out (Scheirer, 1994). Implementation monitoring may include measurement of activities, program quality, deviations from an intervention protocol, and the program's ability to reach its intended target group (Dignan & Carr, 1987; Hawe, Degeling, & Hall, 1990).

Implementation monitoring may also be useful as a component of a larger impact evaluation. In addition to tracking the nature, extent, and quality of a given intervention over time for individual participants, in such evaluations data is gathered on constructs hypothesized to be mechanisms of program impact (Price & Smith, 1985; Scheirer, 1994). This may create a link between program activities and intended program goals, thus providing a foundation for understanding outcome findings (Cunningham, Michielutte, Dignan, Sharp, & Boxley, 2000; Viadro, Earp, & Altpeter, 1997). In addition, when employed as part of an impact assessment, implementation monitoring provides a "manipulation check" for designs in which two or more groups may have differential exposure to a given intervention. This allows such findings about intervention processes to be used in subsequent analyses to help explain program outcomes, much as dosage or exposure to treatment indices are used in clinical or pharmaceutical trials. When the intervention processes assessed through program monitoring assessments are derived from specific theoretical assumptions, such evaluations may yield data about the mechanisms underlying the impact of the intervention (Scheirer, 1994). Thus, for example, a comprehensive, theory-driven process evaluation of a substance abuse prevention program for youth may monitor the nature and extent of curriculum exposure by individual participants, their level of involvement in various types of sessions, and the relationship between curriculum components received to hypothesized mediators (e.g., drug resistance strategies) of substance abuse prevention.

Normative Designs

Normative designs provide data about the performance of a program or service relative to a given standard or set of criteria (US General Accounting Office, 1991). Such "criterion-referenced" designs are very useful for determining whether the program's target population is being served as intended, whether services are being provided at the level of intensity or frequency planned, whether outcomes from service recipients meet a predetermined standard, and

whether program and managerial staff have the qualifications required. Normative designs are often used in organizations as one component of an agency quality assessment or quality assurance plan, or as part of agency performance improvement activities. Such criterion-referenced designs do not provide data that allows for inferences about program effectiveness or for determining whether program components were responsible for causing a particular outcome or effect; that is the focus of impact assessments using experimental or quasi-experimental designs. Below we describe the outcome monitoring design, an approach to data collection that has grown in popularity with the increasing emphasis on performance and accountability (Wandersman et al., 2000). To the extent that a program monitors the implementation of services relative to a given standard, implementation monitoring designs may also serve as a special type of normative design.

Outcome Monitoring

Also referred to as performance-based assessment, outcome monitoring involves the regular reporting of program outcomes that are tied to performance expectations for the program (Affholter, 1994). Outcome monitoring is an outgrowth of the trend toward results-based accountability that has gained favor among federal, state, and private funders of services (US General Accounting Office, 1991). Although one cannot make inferences about whether program activities were causally responsible for program outcomes independent of other factors experienced by service recipients, outcome monitoring provides a useful tool for program managers and policy makers to track program performance and to make more informed decisions about resource allocation (Affholter, 1994).

Typically, implementation of an outcome monitoring assessment involves having the evaluator collaborate with various stakeholders—funders, managers, providers, and service recipients—to identify key outcomes by service type. One or more outcome indicators which can be measured and tracked by program staff are then selected for the outcomes identified. This process usually also involves establishing performance standards for each outcome to indicate that a particular indicator has met criteria. Outcomes are then tracked at the individual client and/or program level, and then aggregated to provide some assessment of program performance.

Outcome monitoring is especially useful when incorporated as part of an agency's quality improvement or continuous performance improvement system because the infrastructure and commitment to collect outcome data on a periodic basis is already established through these agency operations. Issues to consider in designing an outcome monitoring plan include: (a) the extent to which different programs track the same types of outcomes (program managers and policy makers usually find it most useful to review data that tracks the same outcomes for programs with similar objectives and target populations served); (b) the number of outcomes to be monitored (in most instances, it is optimal to track only a few outcomes per program or service); and (c) the frequency with which outcomes are monitored (in most instances, programs track outcomes on a monthly, quarterly, or semi-annual basis depending on service objectives). Once data is collected on program outcomes, data should be shared not only with program leadership and policy makers, as appropriate, but also with line staff. This is important for two reasons. First, staff are more committed to assisting with the outcome monitoring process if they believe the results are being used to good purpose. And second, discussion of the results with staff may help explain why program performance did not meet expectations or may reveal ways in which the outcome monitoring approach did not capture what it was designed to do (Tebes et al., 2001).

Impact Assessments: Experimental and Quasi-Experimental Designs

Because impact evaluations involve the assessment of a cause-and-effect relationship between preventive or service programs and observed outcomes, the appropriate methodological choice is that of a field experiment, although data may be quantitative, qualitative, or a combination of the two (US General Accounting Office, 1991). Field experiments generally involve the use of an experimental or quasi-experimental design in which comparisons are made between participants exposed to a particular program of interest and an alternative group of participants that are not exposed to the prevention program.

Despite their limitations (Cook & Campbell, 1979; Murray, Moskowitz, & Dent, 1996), experimental designs still represent the gold-standard from which to draw valid and reliable causal statements about a given preventive intervention's effectiveness. The hallmarks of experimental design include random assignment to treatment and control conditions and rigorous control of conditions to minimize cross-group contamination effects. Random assignment to condition is recognized as the best means to address a number of common threats to internal validity including selection bias, sample maturation and history effects, instrumentation, and sampling effects associated with regression artifacts (Cook & Campbell, 1979; Keppel, 1991; Schalock & Thornton, 1988). Condition fidelity (i.e., maintaining distinction between a group exposed to a given prevention program and a comparison group not exposed) is also required for the evaluator to be able to make valid conclusions about

the effects of a particular program (Card, Greeno, & Peterson, 1992; US General Accounting Office, 1991). Below we describe several useful experimental and quasi-experimental designs to examine the impact of prevention programs.

The Repeated-Measures, Between-Groups Design

The basic experimental design employed by many program evaluations is the repeated-measures, between-groups design. Using this design, participants are randomly assigned to intervention and control groups; only the intervention group receives the programmatic independent variable, and both groups are pretested and posttested on the dependent variables of interest. This design allows the evaluator to examine variance on the dependent variables of interest between-groups (i.e., through the comparison of results for individuals exposed to the preventive intervention with those in the control group) as well as within-groups (i.e., over time). This is among the most common of *experimental* designs in program evaluation, although there are significant constraints on its use in many evaluation settings as will be discussed later. Snow and Tebes (1991) present a number of variations of this basic design relevant to the evaluation of prevention programs (in this case substance abuse prevention programs). The primary differences that exist among its variations involve the number and types of control groups, including the use of attention-placebo and graded intervention groups (i.e., with different or staggered intervention dosages), and the frequency and timing of measurement periods, from a simple pre–post design to multiple pre–post assessments on the dependent variables of interest (i.e., the repeated measures design with multiple pre- and posttest assessments). Although the variations may potentially increase the power and strength of conclusions drawn from prevention program evaluations, such enhanced designs may require significant resources in terms of time and money. In addition, designs with a large number of comparison groups or with multiple assessment periods may be subject to higher rates of differential attrition across groups, a factor that may have significant implications for the generalizability of findings (Snow & Tebes, 1991).

Program evaluation built around an experimental design allows the evaluator to be relatively confident in the validity of findings with respect to a program's effectiveness. As a result, a growing knowledge base has developed around the application of experimental methods, particularly randomization, to evaluation settings (see Boruch, 1997 for a detailed discussion of the issues related to its application in evaluation research). Research is also beginning to address the application of randomization procedures for evaluation of school- or community-wide initiatives through procedures like cluster random assignment (see Bloom, 1999 for an example of this discussion). There is, however, growing recognition of the limitations of the experimental method to prevention program evaluation in real-world contexts. Among the chief limitations is the requirement of randomized assignment, a requirement that may be difficult for either logistical or ethical reasons in a community setting or which may pose an extreme burden in cases where the community is the unit of analysis (Murray et al., 1996; Yin & Kaftarian, 1997). In some cases, despite efforts to follow an experimental design the evaluator may find that the design has been compromised either by cross-group contamination effects, differential attrition rates between condition, or by intentional sabotage of the experimental method (e.g., Devine, Brody, & Wright, 1997). In response to these challenges, many program evaluators choose, instead, to rely on quasi-experimental methods to draw conclusions on a prevention program's effectiveness.

The primary difference between quasi-experimental designs and experimental designs is in the level of control the evaluator can exercise over the independent variable under examination (i.e., assignment to treatment or control condition). Evaluations employing an experimental design are able to randomly assign participants (or larger social units like classrooms, schools, or communities) to receive either the preventive intervention or a suitable control or placebo condition, while evaluations employing a quasi-experimental design frequently rely on a nonequivalent (i.e., nonrandomly assigned) comparison group. A potential (though not exhaustive) list of quasi-experimental designs for evaluation of prevention programs includes: the non-equivalent comparison group design with repeated measures, simple and multiple time series designs, and the regression-discontinuity (RD) design.

The Nonequivalent Comparison Group Design, with Repeated Measures

The repeated measures design with a nonequivalent comparison group is among the most frequently employed quasi-experimental designs in the evaluation of prevention programs. This design resembles the repeated-measures between-group experimental design, except that assignment to condition is nonrandom. One reason for the popularity of this design in the evaluation literature is that it enables a program to be evaluated in a community setting in which random assignment might not be possible. The primary disadvantages of this design are that nonrandom assignment increases concerns about the internal validity of the evaluation and may lead to different conclusions than those drawn from comparable experimental designs. Lipsey and Wilson's

(1993) meta-analysis of over 300 educational and behavioral interventions suggests, for example, that even within a given intervention domain, results of randomized and nonrandomized control group designs can be quite divergent (although these differences may average out over a large number of studies). Shadish and colleagues (Heinsman & Shadish, 1996; Shadish & Ragsdale, 1996) report similar findings in a series of meta-analytic studies, although the authors suggest that nonrandomized designs can produce comparable results to that of randomized designs when appropriate statistical controls and attention to key methodological characteristics (e.g., use of internal versus external comparison groups, use of blocking in subject assignment, attention to activity level of the comparison group, etc.) are employed. Reynolds and Temple (1995) demonstrate a number of statistical approaches toward bias reduction using quasi-experimental estimates of compensatory preschool preventive interventions. The authors demonstrate that such techniques are very useful means of establishing program effectiveness when random assignment is not feasible.

The Simple and Multiple Time Series Design

The simple time series design involves multiple measures of a single group before and after the intervention being evaluated. The multiple time series design uses a similar measurement strategy, but combines the approach with the nonequivalent control group design. With either design, multiple measurements allow the evaluator to detect linear discontinuity following the intervention (either within or between groups for the multiple time series design). The latter design has been described as among the best options available for quasi-experimental designs (Campbell & Stanley, 1966), although threats to internal validity still remain and the requirement of multiple assessment periods poses a potential threat to external validity should differential attrition occur between groups or if intervention-testing and intervention-selection interactions are left uncontrolled. Forehand (1982) and McCleary and Hay (1980) address design and analysis issues related to time-series designs.

The Regression-Discontinuity Design

The RD design is a useful quasi-experimental design when random assignment to condition is not possible, and assignment to the program is based on a specified selection criteria related to the outcome of interest (e.g., low school performance is used to select into a program designed to boost school performance). The primary assumptions for use of the RD design include the following: (1) selection of individuals into a treatment condition is based on a cutoff score; (2) the relationship between outcome and selection criteria is known (e.g., linear, quadratic); and (3) changes in the relationship between the selection and outcome criteria across groups can be attributed to program assignment (Trochim, 1984). When these criteria are met, selection into a program that produces effects results in a discontinuity in the relationship between criterion and outcome that occurs between the two groups (Braden & Bryant, 1990; Marcantonio & Cook, 1994).

Analytic models for testing RD designs in evaluation are Analysis of Covariance (ANCOVA), in which the selection criteria scores are entered as a covariate, program placement as a main effect, and interactions are represented in the interaction between selection criteria and placement, although multiple regression may also be used to model the design. Although such designs are useful for conditions in which random assignment is not feasible and clear criteria for selection into a program exist, evaluators are cautioned against the use of RD designs when program assignment is not based on clear criteria, when the distribution of the dependent variable is highly skewed or abnormally distributed, when there is a small sample, or when the relationship between selection criteria and outcomes is weak or unclear (Braden & Bryant, 1990). Although this design has come under some criticism (e.g., Stanley, 1991), particularly when multiple regression models are used to evaluate outcomes, Reichardt and Trochim (1995) provide evidence of its applicability and conclude that the design is a strong one when circumstances limit the use of other experimental or quasi-experimental approaches to the evaluation of a program.

The above discussion of experimental and quasi-experimental evaluation designs presumes that interventions are conducted at the individual level, or that the potential for assignment to condition may be made at the person level. Increasingly, however, the community is the level at which prevention program evaluations are targeted, particularly in the substance abuse prevention and health promotion domains—although a similar challenge is present in school-level prevention programs within the educational domain. Community-based prevention programs pose a number of challenges for evaluators, in part because designs often employ a nested structure in which individuals are nested within social units (e.g., classrooms, schools) that may also be nested in broader groups (e.g., communities). From an analytic perspective, such designs require novel approaches to design or over-inflate Type I error and reduce the evaluation's power to detect meaningful differences (Murray & McKinlay, 1994). In the most extreme cases (i.e., when the community is the level of analysis) these problems are further compounded by the difficulty in recruiting enough communities to make assignment to condition possible. This may make it difficult to maintain fidelity to condition within an open community setting, and to determine the appropriate unit of measurement for the evaluation of a community

initiative (Yin & Kaftarian, 1997). A special section of the journal *Evaluation and Program Planning* addressed several strategies for evaluating such community-based programs, including: (1) comparison to statewide benchmark data (Furlong, Casas, Corral, & Gordon, 1997; Shaw, Rosati, Salzman, Coles, & McGeary, 1997); (2) use of a "non-equivalent, dependent variables design" (Cook & Campbell, 1979, p. 118) which a number of dependent variables were assessed at two time points (Rowe, 1997); (3) comparison of using multiple time series outcomes to statewide benchmark data (Gabriel, 1997); and (4) a cross-site evaluation design with multiple program and matched comparison communities (Saxe, Reber, Hallfors, Kadushin, Jones, Rindskopf, & Beveridge, 1997; Yin, Kaftarian, Ping, & Jansen, 1997).

Analysis of Experimental and Quasi-Experimental Data

Similar to evaluation design selection, the choice of statistical methodology should be shaped by the particular questions of interest within a particular evaluation, and should be a part of the evaluation planning process prior to its implementation. Particular evaluation designs are better suited to some types of analyses than others, and particular evaluation questions may be better suited to some analysis plans than others, so it is important to consider the questions of interest, the types of analyses that allow for an evaluation of these questions, and the designs that provide data for such analyses prior to implementation of the evaluation plan.

The range of analytic approaches available to evaluators of prevention programs, and the use of advanced or sophisticated statistical methods among evaluators, has grown tremendously in recent years. Lipsey and Cordray (2000) note that early evaluation analyses commonly employed an "intent-to-treat" model of analyses (Boruch, 1997) in which treatment effects, and the unit at which such groups were defined by randomization procedures, were the primary focus of analyses. Although this approach is still the primary focus of many outcome evaluations, Lipsey and Cordray note that more recently evaluators are utilizing sophisticated analysis strategies to incorporate elements of process evaluation data, program context, and program theory into the analysis of group differences. In addition, program evaluators are beginning to use growth modeling techniques to model those factors associated with individual and group change over time.

Analysis of Group Differences

Analysis of group differences is conducted to assess the degree to which two or more groups differ on dependent variables of interest, although they are also frequently used to assess the degree to which groups differ in terms of their response to the independent variable (i.e., the level of relative group change over time). Such analyses can be as simple or complex as warranted by the level of sophistication with which the evaluation questions were formed. At a basic level, the evaluator may examine data to look for between group differences on posttest data or for relative group differences on the level of change between pretest and posttest when groups are exposed to the prevention program between measurement periods. Girden (1992) provides a thorough discussion of analysis strategies related to Analysis of Variance (ANOVA) and ANCOVA procedures for detecting group differences on repeated measures designs such as pre–post and longitudinal time series designs. Although such approaches are common in the evaluation literature, critics have challenged the degree to which longitudinal service and prevention data conform to the assumptions necessary for such analyses (see Gibbons et al., 1993 for a thorough discussion of the limitations of such approaches). Multivariate ANOVA for repeated measures is one alternative strategy, while random effects regression models may overcome some problems with the analysis of multiple time series analyses including missing data problems inherent in such designs.

Lipsey and Cordray (2000) note that evaluation analyses are increasingly integrating process data with outcome data to treat dosage or exposure as a variable related to program outcomes. As an example of this approach, McGraw and Sellers (1996) examined teacher characteristics and curriculum implementation adherence as predictors of child outcomes in an evaluation of the Child and Adolescent Trial for Cardiovascular Health program, with evaluation results suggesting that teacher modifications appeared to strengthen some program outcomes above and beyond results attributed to the general curriculum effects. It is important for evaluators to be aware of the assumptions made by statistical tests, as well as the potential for regression artifacts to emerge when longitudinal or time-series data are analyzed with covariate or matched-group designs (see Campbell, 1996 for a thorough discussion of regression artifacts).

Although ANOVA and ANCOVA analyses are fairly common approaches toward assessing relative group change within the context of program evaluation, a growing number of evaluators are incorporating structural equation modeling (SEM) into program evaluation. SEM allows the evaluator to examine processes or mechanisms by which a program impacts outcomes of interest, and may be particularly useful within the context of theory-based program evaluation. The evaluator may specify critical mediating pathways between program participants and outcomes or test for moderating effects of subject characteristics on program outcomes. Hennessy and Greenberg (1999) used SEM to examine

causal mechanisms in a randomized experimental evaluation of a program to prevent or reduce risky sexual behavior in a female population. Petrosino (2000) discusses strategies for using SEM to examine mediators and moderators of program effects in the evaluation of children's programs.

Community- and school-based program evaluations also need to be aware of the effects of clustered or nested data on evaluation analyses. When the unit of randomization (or comparison) is different from the unit of interest—such as, when classrooms are assigned to prevention or control conditions but the evaluation is interested in assessing program effects at the individual level—analyses must incorporate the clustering effect of the randomization procedure on the data, particularly, if the number of subjects per cluster is unbalanced (Koepke & Flay, 1989). The problem occurs because standard analytic techniques assume that all observations are independent and fail to account for the variance in individual-level data due to higher intraclass correlations among participants within given subgroups (e.g., classrooms, schools, communities). Hedeker and colleagues have used random-effects regression modeling to assess effects of smoking cessation programs across samples clustered by classroom or school (Hedeker, Gibbons, & Flay, 1994) and worksite (Hedeker, McMahon, Jason, & Salina, 1994) and demonstrate the benefits of this approach over regression models that ignore clustering effects (e.g., individual-level analyses) or that aggregate individual data to examine cluster-level effects. Others have used this analytic model to analyze multisite evaluations of the D.A.R.E. program (Rosenbaum & Hanson, 1998), to evaluate educational programs (Bloom, Bos, & Lee, 1999), and to assess program impacts for health promotion programs (Woodruff, 1997).

Analysis of Growth Models

Growth modeling employs analytic techniques associated with the analysis of hierarchically structured data sets (i.e., hierarchical linear modeling or HLM) except that multiple time points of measurement are nested within individuals (rather than nesting individuals within sites as previously discussed with respect to nested data designs). As a result, this approach to evaluation analysis is particularly well-suited to Campbell and Stanley's (1966) replicated time series design in which multiple measures of the dependent variable are conducted over time with intervention-timing varying across cases to avoid confounding effects of maturation and history with program intervention exposure. Latent growth modeling (LGM) allow the evaluator to model the slope and intercept of the dependent variable of interest as latent constructs and then to look for individual and group characteristics that influence the slope or intercept. Hess (2000) provides a "primer" on the use of

LGM for program evaluation, identifying a number of recent applications of the method including growth models for drug and alcohol use (e.g., Andrew & Duncan, 1998; Curran, Stice, & Chassin, 1997; Duncan, Duncan, & Hops, 1998) and children's academic and social development (e.g., Schmitt, Sacco, Ramey, & Chan, 1999). Osgood and Smith (1995) employ HLM techniques to examine findings from the Boys Town Follow-up Study, controlling for the effects of history and maturation on findings, individual differences unrelated to program impact, and for interactions between individual differences and history effects. Lipsey and Cordray (2000) provide additional examples of this analytic approach to program evaluation.

Effect Size Estimates and Reporting Results

In addition to concern over appropriate analytic strategies, the field of prevention program evaluation has also begun to explore the limitations of statistical significance testing with regard to the detection and reporting of program effects. It is now largely understood by evaluators and social scientists that the detection of *statistically* significant findings does not necessarily equate with the detection of *clinically* significant findings (Thompson, 1993). Although statistical procedures may be used to evaluate the probability of an event, it is the work of the evaluator to make a judgment as to the value and importance of the finding with respect to the impact of a prevention program (Kellow, 1998). Toward that end, program evaluators are encouraged to make greater use of other indices to facilitate greater understanding of program effects and allow for cross-program comparisons of such effects. One strategy for allowing such comparisons is through the use of effect size estimates such as the standardized mean difference approach or proportion of variance explained (PVE) estimates (see Kellow, 1998 for a good introduction to these techniques). Such techniques provide additional information of the program's effects. The standardized mean difference approach, for example, converts group differences into percentage of improvement using the standard normal curve. The PVE approach, on the other hand, can be used to estimate the proportion of variance in the dependent variable that is explained by the independent variable. The R^2 one example of a PVE estimate that describes the impact of a program on changes in the outcomes of interest.

Cost–Outcome Analyses

One of the most important considerations in developing, maintaining, or terminating a prevention program is its cost. Cost–outcomes analyses refer to several different ways of assessing the costs of a program relative to its outcomes (Hargreaves, Shumway, Hu, & Cuffel, 1998). In most types of services research, one of three types of costing studies are conducted: cost-effectiveness analyses, cost–benefit analyses, and cost–utility analyses. Cost-effectiveness analyses are the most common type of cost–outcome study conducted in mental health or preventive services research. These involve studies in which outcomes are measured in units other than dollars, such as problem behaviors, achievement, or competencies, and then examined in relation to program costs. Cost–benefit analyses also assess program costs in relation to outcomes, but outcomes are expressed in monetary terms so that the comparison is made along a common metric. Finally, cost–utility analyses examine the value of outcomes whose costs are translated into "utilities" (e.g., units which correspond to a specified health state, ranging from death to optimal health) over a period of time, so as to allow comparison on a single, numerical outcome indicator (Hargreaves et al., 1998).

Cost–outcome evaluations face a number of complexities. One major issue confronting the evaluator is what perspective to use when estimating costs (Rossi & Freeman, 1993; Wolff, Helminiak, & Tebes, 1997). Cost estimation for a given program may assume any number of perspectives in accounting for costs, such as: a societal perspective (in which all costs attributable to a given program are estimated), a funder or governmental perspective (in which only those costs incurred by the program's funder, often the governmental agency, are estimated), or a target population perspective (in which only those costs incurred by program recipients are estimated). As is apparent, the complexity of estimating costs increases dramatically as one moves from the individual to the societal perspective (Sledge, Tebes, Wolff, & Helminiak, 1996).

Other challenges which face evaluators who conduct cost–outcome studies are difficulties encountered in estimating unit costs accurately (Wolff et al., 1997) and the inherent complexities in estimating costs prospectively (Hargreaves et al., 1998). Agency unit costing requires a number of complex operations, including: differentiating real and accounting costs, understanding and remediating the information systems for counting service units, and assuring that the resultant cost and unit measurement data are accurately matched (Tebes & Helminiak, 1999). Accurate mapping between costs and service units in a given program is often quite difficult because fiscal and agency MIS or service count data tend to be poorly integrated, if not totally, nonintegrated. Thus, cost estimation requires the careful alignment of relevant service and cost data, a task that, if done incorrectly, may result in estimations that are inaccurate by an order of magnitude (Wolff et al., 1997). As noted above, a related difficulty in cost estimation is conducting such studies prospectively. When estimating costs prospectively, not all costs are known, thus making it difficult to obtain data with which to even begin to estimate costs, particularly when one has adopted a societal costing perspective (Rossi & Freeman, 1993). For this reason, most cost–outcome evaluations are retrospective studies, although some researchers have described effective procedures for collecting cost data prospectively (Harrow & Lasater, 1996).

Two additional and related challenges for the cost–outcome evaluator are difficulties that involve: (a) translating social program benefits into monetary terms, as is found in cost–benefit analyses; and (b) translating costs into a common outcome metric, as is typical in cost–utility analyses (Hargreaves et al., 1998; Rossi & Freeman, 1993). In each type of analysis, there is often considerable disagreement among different stakeholders over how to value costs or benefits, respectively, in attempting to devise a common metric. As a result, it is often preferable for evaluators to conduct cost-effectiveness analyses and leave the assessment of the relative value of program outcomes in relation to costs to the individual judgments of stakeholders (Hurley, 1990).

ENDING AN EVALUATION: USE AND DISSEMINATION OF EVALUATION FINDINGS

A primary objective of evaluators is that the work they have completed will have some impact on practice, management, or policy. A critical consideration in an evaluation's impact is whether findings are actually used (Hendricks, 1994; Patton, 1980). Rossi and Freeman (1985) offer several ways for results to have an impact. The first involves the direct or instrumental use of evaluation results by stakeholders, and in particular, decision makers. When this occurs, programs or services are changed in accordance with the findings of an evaluation. A second use of evaluation findings is conceptual, in which findings influence how issues are considered, and thus, indirectly impact procedures, programming, or policy. Finally, Rossi and Freeman (1993) describe how evaluation findings may be used to persuade policy makers, such as politicians, to support or refute specific political positions, a form of use that also has an indirect impact on policy. For any of these uses, evaluation findings must be made accessible to an intended audience, rather than buried in long evaluation reports filled with jargon (Hendricks, 1994).

The involvement of key stakeholders in every step of the evaluation process is one way to increase the utilization of evaluation findings (Johnson, 1998; Patton, 1980). This involvement should be evident in: the design of the evaluation; the methodology employed to collect the data; the analyses completed; the dissemination of findings; and subsequent discussions of how the results may be used to improve programming or develop policy (Price & Smith, 1985). Continuous, multidirectional dissemination of information and results to program staff and service recipients—both during and after program delivery—has been found to increase use of evaluation findings by increasing evaluation relevance, attention to program modification, and stakeholder ownership of results (Johnson, 1998). Another related factor that may increase the use of evaluation findings is some personal contact between the evaluator and stakeholders that builds on opportunities for involvement (Price & Smith, 1985). Such contact strengthens the sense of collaboration between stakeholders and the evaluator, and also enables the evaluator to understand the cognitive styles of potential decision makers; thus, allowing feedback to be tailored to meet the needs of the intended audience (Rossi & Freeman, 1993).

The method by which evaluation findings are shared with key stakeholders is also critical to the utilization of findings (Hendricks, 1994; Price & Smith, 1985). The burden for communicating evaluation results effectively rests squarely on the evaluator, and a variety of approaches should be used to share findings. Evaluators should not save all of the information obtained for a final report, but rather should look for ways to share the evaluation findings throughout the process in both written form and in face to face meetings. Documents providing feedback should also be prepared for different target audiences, such as a report summarizing global findings to legislators, a report on specific process outcomes for a program director, and a report on program outcomes for consumers of services. Whenever possible, reports should pare findings down to key points, illustrate a particular feature of the evaluation, and be brief (Hendricks, 1994). If appropriate, they should also include recommendations to help facilitate discussion of program planning, management, or policy. Furthermore, when preparing a report, it is almost always useful to send a draft to stakeholders for a review before disseminating the findings publicly. This internal review enables stakeholders to add to the recommendations and place findings in context, and may prepare the evaluator for the subsequent public response. This practice also increases trust and may lead to discussions between evaluators and stakeholders of further evaluation activities to follow-up the report's findings. In our work, we have followed these procedures with success in numerous evaluations, often sharing results with stakeholders as we complete data analyses through an iterative process to help understand findings in context (Tebes & Kraemer, 1991; Tebes et al., 2001).

TOWARD A THEORY OF KNOWLEDGE FOR EVALUATION RESEARCH

All evaluation research ultimately rests on a theory of knowledge, one that Shadish et al. (1991) maintain addresses assumptions about the nature of reality (i.e., ontology), the justification of knowledge claims (i.e., epistemology), and the construction of knowledge (i.e., methodology). For most of its history, evaluation research has focused mostly on methodology, and specifically, on the application of various methods and analytical frameworks to the collection and interpretation of data. Other than the work of Scriven (1980) and Campbell and his colleagues (Campbell, 1969; Campbell, 1974; Campbell & Stanley, 1966; Cook & Campbell, 1979), who explicitly address this issue in much of their work, evaluation research has been guided by implicit theories of the nature of reality and the justification of knowledge claims.

In the earliest years of the field, the theory of knowledge that guided practice was logical empiricism (McGuire, 1983, 1986). The search for objective truth, the emphasis on internal validity and causal inference, and the use of experimental designs and quantitative methods are hallmarks of this initial era in evaluation research (Shadish et al., 1991). As noted earlier, this approach to evaluation remains a cornerstone of evaluation practice and is viewed by many evaluators as the most scientifically rigorous means for assessing a social intervention.

Approaches to evaluation practice that emerged in the decades immediately following this initial stage emphasized utilization of evaluation results, attention to local issues and concerns, stakeholder involvement, and the use of qualitative methods (Rossi & Freeman, 1993; Shadish et al., 1991). This approach also has flourished in the intervening years, and has been guided implicitly by a theory of knowledge based on contextualism.

Rosnow and Georgoudi (1986) define contextualism as "... the philosophical premise that all knowledge is perennially conceptual and conjectural and no method can conclusively demonstrate the truth. In short, the idea is that psychological knowledge is made concrete and is framed by relevant factors, relations, and conditions (the setting or context) within which, or among which, human acts and events unfold. Contextualism underscores the idea that human activity does not develop in a social vacuum, but rather it is rigorously situated within a sociohistorical and cultural context of meanings and relationship" (p. 4). Also known as transactionalism, constructivism, or perspectivism—depending upon which aspect of this philosophical position is emphasized—the primary objective of contextualism is to identify the various contexts in which a specific proposition is true or false (McGuire, 1986; Tebes, 1997). An underlying conjunctive premise of contextualism is that "all propositions are true" (in most contexts) just as "all propositions are false" (in most contexts). It is the work of science to determine which propositions are valid in which contexts (McGuire, 1983, 1986; Rosnow & Georgoudi, 1986).

Although contextualism has within it the potential to descend into extreme relativism and has proponents that eschew quantitative methods (Guba & Lincoln, 1981), such views are in the minority. Contextualism assumes that all knowledge claims are contextual, and that specification of local conditions and individual meanings is critical to understanding human events. The implications of contextualism for scientific inquiry and evaluation research is the validation of a pluralism of theories and methods, all of which have a legitimate basis for advancing knowledge (Jaeger & Rosnow, 1988). Contextualism acknowledges that "differing and complementary roles and functions of alternative theoretical and methodological perspectives should be recognized and utilized" (Jaeger & Rosnow, 1988, p. 69). These may include qualitative/humanistic approaches, such as ethnomethodology, narrative, and hermeneutics, as well as quantitative/scientistic approaches, such as behavior analysis, social experiments, and epidemiology (Tebes, 1997). Contextualist qua narrative approaches, for example, are likely to capture the intentional nature and developmental course of human events better than methods derived from logical empiricism. However, traditional scientific methods are likely to identify general conditions (e.g., risk or protective factors) which precede specific types of human action or causal relations under carefully specified local conditions. In combination, these methods are likely to yield more knowledge than either alone.

In the current era of evaluation research, in which aspects of both traditions are often integrated at a methodological level, both theories of knowledge are beginning to converge at the level of evaluation practice. In part, this is due to significant revisions to the logical empiricist position by some of its earlier advocates (Cook, 1985; Cook & Campbell, 1979). Cook (1985) has proposed a revision that he terms "postpositivist critical multiplism." Multiplism addresses some of the flaws of positivism as the basis for evaluation research. According to Cook (1985), multiplism accepts some of the earlier theory's assumptions: that social and psychological reality exist independent of the observer, and that they are knowable—albeit incompletely—through systematic observation using scientific methods. However, it also acknowledges the limitations of positivism: Social and psychological phenomena cannot be reduced to general laws through induction, and no one method is appropriate for the study of human phenomena. Multiplism advances the use of multiple methods—including qualitative approaches—and multiple theories about human phenomena because no one approach to knowledge construction can sufficiently capture reality. Multiplism also offers a conceptual framework for adopting evaluation practices that were eschewed in the field's initial stage, such as conducting research that incorporates the views of multiple stakeholders and designing evaluations that emphasize generalizability across multiple populations, settings, and times (Cook, 1985).

Both multiplism and contextualism are part of an emerging "pluralist revolution" (Humphreys, 1993) that emphasizes the benefits of theoretical and methodological pluralism in advancing knowledge about human behavior. As theories of knowledge, they provide useful conceptual frameworks for the major traditions within evaluation research—one emphasizing quantitative/scientistic methods, the other qualitative/humanistic methods—to guide evaluation practice.

Also see: Effective Programming: Foundation; Substances: Adolescence (Roona); Cost Benefit Analysis: Adulthood.

References

Affholter, D.P. (1994). Outcome monitoring. In J.S. Wholey, H.P. Hatry, & K.E. Newcomer (Eds.), *Handbook of practical program evaluation* (pp. 96–118). San Francisco: Jossey-Bass.

Albee, G.W. (1996). Revolutions and counterrevolutions in prevention. *American Psychologist, 51*, 1130–1133.

Allen, H., Cordes, H., & Hart, J. (1999). *Vitalizing communities: Building on assets and mobilizing for collective action.* Lincoln, NE: University of Nebraska-Lincoln.

Andrew, J.A., & Duncan, S.C. (1998). The effect of attitude on the development of adolescent cigarette use. *Journal of Substance Abuse, 10*, 1–7.

Beamish, W., & Bryer, F. (1999). Programme quality in Australian early special education: An example of participatory action research. *Child Care, Health and Development, 25*(6), 457–472.

Bloom, H.S. (1999). Using cluster random assignment to measure program impacts: Statistical implications for the evaluation of education programs. *Evaluation Review, 23*(4), 445–469.

Bloom, H.S., Bos, J.M., & Lee, S. (1999). Using cluster random assignment to measure program impacts: Statistical implications for the evaluation of education programs. *Evaluation Review, 23*(4), 445–469.

Boruch, R.F. (1997). *Randomized experiments for planning and evaluation: A practical guide.* Thousand Oaks, CA: Sage.

Braden, J.P., & Bryant, T.J. (1990). Regression discontinuity designs: Applications for school psychologists. *School Psychology Review, 19*(2), 232–240.

Bruyere, S. (1993). Participatory action research: An overview and implications for family members of individuals with disabilities. *Journal of Vocational Rehabilitation, 3*(2), 62–68.

Campbell, D.T. (1969). Reforms as experiments. *American Psychologist, 24*, 409–429.

Campbell, D.T. (1974). *Qualitative knowing in action research.* Kurt Lewin Award Address, Society for the Psychological Study of Social Issues, presented at the 82nd annual meeting of the American Psychological Association, New Orleans, LA.

Campbell, D.T. (1996). Regression artifacts in time-series and longitudinal data. *Evaluation and Program Planning, 19*(4), 377–389.

Campbell, D.T., & Stanley, J.C. (1966). *Experimental and quasi-experimental designs for research.* Skokie, IL: Rand McNally.

Card, J.J., Greeno, C., & Peterson, J.L. (1992). Planning an evaluation and estimating its cost. *Evaluation and Program Planning, 15*(4), 75–89.

Cook, T.D. (1985). Postpositivist critical multiplism. In L. Shotland & M.M. Mark (Eds.), *Social science and social policy* (pp. 21–62). Beverly Hills: Sage.

Cook, T.D., & Campbell, D.T. (1979). *Quasi-experimentation: Design and analysis issues for field settings.* Skokie, IL: Rand McNally.

Cook, T.D., & Shadish, W.R. (1994). Social experiments: Some developments over the past fifteen years. *Annual Review of Psychology, 45*, 545–580.

Cronbach, L.J. (1982). *Designing evaluations of educational and social programs.* San Francisco: Jossey-Bass.

Cronbach, L.J. (1986). Social inquiry by and for earthlings. In D.W. Fiske & R.A. Schweder (Eds.), *Meta theory in social science* (pp. 83–107). Chicago: University of Chicago Press.

Cunningham, L.E., Michielutte, R., Dignan, M., Sharp, P., & Boxley, J. (2000). The value of process evaluation in a community-based cancer control program. *Evaluation and Program Planning, 23*, 13–25.

Curran, P.J., Stice, E., & Chassin, L. (1997). The relation between adolescent alcohol use and peer alcohol use: A longitudinal random coefficients model. *Journal of Consulting and Clinical Psychology, 65*, 130–140.

Devine, J.A., Brody, C.J., & Wright, J.D. (1997). Evaluating an alcohol and drug treatment program for the homeless: An econometric approach. *Evaluation and Program Planning, 20*(2), 205–215.

Dignan, M.B., & Carr, P.A. (1987). *Program planning for health education and promotion.* Philadelphia: Lea & Febiger.

Duncan, T.E., Duncan, S.C., & Hops, H. (1998). Latent variable modeling of longitudinal and multilevel alcohol use data. *Journal of Studies on Alcohol, 59*, 399–408.

Fishman, D.B. (1999). *The case for pragmatic psychology.* New York: New York University Press.

Forehand, G.A. (Ed.). (1982). *Applications of time series analysis to evaluation.* San Francisco: Jossey-Bass.

Furlong, M.J., Casas, J.M., Corral, C., & Gordon, M. (1997). Changes in substance use patterns associated with the development of a community partnership project. *Evaluation and Program Planning, 20*(3), 299–305.

Gaber, J. (2000). Meta-needs assessment. *Evaluation and Program Planning, 23*(1), 139–147.

Gabriel, R.M. (1997). Community indicators of substance abuse: Empowering coalition planning and evaluation. *Evaluation and Program Planning, 20*(3), 335–343.

Gibbons, R.D., Hedeker, D., Elkin, I., Waternaux, C., Kraemer, H.C., Greenhouse, J.B., Shea, M.T., Imber, S.D., Sotsky, S.M., Watkins, J.T. (1993). Some conceptual and statistical issues in analysis of longitudinal psychiatric data. *Archives of General Psychiatry, 50*, 739–750.

Girden, E.R. (1992). *ANOVA repeated measures.* Thousand Oaks, CA: Sage.

Gordon, R. (1987). An operational classification of disease prevention. In J. Steinberg & M. Silverman (Eds.), *Preventing mental disorders: A research perspective* (pp. 20–26) (DHHS Publication No. ADM 87-1492). Rockville, MD: Alcohol, Drug Abuse, and Mental Health Administration.

Guba, E.G., & Lincoln, Y.S. (1981). *Effective evaluation: Improving the usefulness of evaluation results through responsive and naturalistic approaches.* San Francisco: Jossey-Bass.

Hargreaves, W.A., Shumway, M., Hu, T., & Cuffel, B. (1998). *Cost-outcome methods for mental health.* San Diego: Academic Press.

Harrow, B.S., & Lasater, T.M. (1996). A strategy for accurate collection of incremental cost data for cost-effectiveness analyses in field trials. *Evaluation Review, 20*(3), 275–290.

Hawe, P., Degeling, D., & Hall, J. (1990). *Evaluating health promotion: A health worker's guide.* Sydney: MacLennan & Petty.

Hedeker, D., Gibbons, R.D., & Flay, B.R. (1994). Random-effects regression models for clustered data with an example from smoking prevention research. *Journal of Consulting and Clinical Psychology, 62*(4), 757–765.

Hedeker, D., McMahon, S.D., Jason, L.A., & Salina, D. (1994). Analysis of clustered data in community psychology: With an example from a worksite smoking cessation project. *American Journal of Community Psychology, 22*(5), 595–615.

Heinsman, D.T., & Shadish, W.R. (1996). Assignment methods in experimentation: When do nonrandomized experiments approximate answers from randomized experiments? *Psychological Methods, 1,* 154–169.

Heller, K., & Monahan, J. (1977). *Psychology and community change.* Homewood, IL: Dorsey Press.

Hendricks, M. (1994). Making a splash: Reporting evaluation results effectively. In J.S. Wholey, H.P. Hatry, & K.E. Newcomer (Eds.), *Handbook of practical program evaluation* (pp. 549–575). San Francisco: Jossey-Bass.

Hennessy, M., & Greenberg, J. (1999). Bringing it all together: Modeling intervention processes using structural equation modeling. *American Journal of Evaluation, 20*(3), 471–480.

Hernandez, M. (2000). Using logic models and program theory to build outcome accountability. *Education and Treatment of Children, 23*(1), 24–40.

Hess, B. (2000). Assessing program impact using latent growth modeling: A primer for the evaluator. *Evaluation and Planning, 23*(4), 419–428.

Horst, P., Nay, J.N., Scanlon, J.W., & Wholey, J.S. (1974). Program management and the federal evaluator. *Public Administration Review, 34*(4), 300–308.

Humphreys, K. (1993). Expanding the pluralist revolution: A comment on Omer and Strenger (1992). *Psychotherapy, 30,* 176–177.

Hurley, S. (1990). A review of cost-effectiveness analyses. *Medical Journal of Australia, 153*(Suppl.), S20–3.

Jaeger, M.E., & Rosnow, R.L. (1988). Contextualism and its implications for psychological inquiry. *British Journal of Psychology, 79,* 63–75.

Johnson, R.B. (1998). Toward a theoretical model of evaluation utilization. *Evaluation and Program Planning, 21,* 93–110.

Kellam, S.G., Koretz, D., & Moscicki, E.K. (1999). Core elements of developmental epidemiologically-based prevention research. *American Journal of Community Psychology, 27,* 463–482.

Kellow, J.T. (1998). Beyond statistical significant tests: The importance of using other estimates of treatment effects to interpret evaluation results. *American Journal of Evaluation, 19*(1), 123–134.

Keppel, G. (1991). *Design and Analysis: A Researcher's Handbook* (3rd ed.). Englewood Cliffs, NJ: Prentice-Hall.

Koch, R., Cairns, J.M., & Brunk, M. (2000). How to involve staff in developing an outcomes-oriented organization. *Education and Treatment of Children, 23*(1), 41–47.

Koepke, D., & Flay, B.R. (1989). Levels of analysis. In M.T. Braverman (Ed.), *Evaluating health promotion programs: New directions for program evaluation* (pp. 75–87). San Francisco: Jossey-Bass.

Kretzmann, J., & McKnight, J. (1996). *Mobilizing community assets: Program for building communities from the inside out.* Chicago: ACTA Publications.

Levine, M., & Perkins, D.V. (1987). *Principles of community psychology.* New York: Oxford.

Linney, J.A., & Wandersman, A. (1991). *Prevention plus III: Assessing alcohol and other drug prevention programs at the school and community level.* Washington, DC: US Department of Health & Human Services.

Lipsey, M.W., & Wilson, D.B. (1993). The efficacy of psychological, educational, and behavioral treatment: Confirmation from meta-analysis. *American Psychologist, 48,* 1181–1209.

Lipsey, M., & Cordray, D.S. (2000). Evaluation methods for social intervention. *Annual Review of Psychology, 51,* 345–375.

Long, B.B. (1989). The Mental Health Association and prevention. *Prevention in Human Services, 6,* 5–44.

Marcantonio, R.J., & Cook, T.D. (1994). Convincing quasi-experiments: The interrupted time series and regression-discontinuity designs. In J.S. Wholey, H.P. Hatry, & K.E. Newcomer (Eds.), *Handbook of practical program evaluation* (pp. 133–154). San Francisco: Jossey-Bass.

Mark, M.M. (1986). Validity typologies and the logic and practice of quasi-experimentation. *New Directions for Program Evaluation, 31,* 47–66.

McCleary, R., & Hay, R.A. (1980). *Applied time series analysis for the social sciences.* Newbury Park, CA: Sage.

McGraw, S.A., & Sellers, D.E. (1996). Using process data to explain outcomes: An illustration from the Child and Adolescent Trial for Cardiovascular Health (CATCH). *Evaluation Review, 20*(20), 291–312.

McGuire, W.J. (1983). A contextualist theory of knowledge: Its implications for innovation and reform in psychological research. In L. Berkowitz (Ed.), *Advances in experimental social psychology* (pp. 1–47). New York: Academic Press.

McGuire, W.J. (1986). A perspectivist looks at contextualism and the future of behavioral science. In R.L. Rosnow & M. Georgundi (Eds.), *Contextualism and understanding in behavioral science* (pp. 271–303). New York: Pergamon.

Merriam, S. (1988). *Case study research in education.* San Francisco: Jossey-Bass.

Millar, A., Simeone, R.S., & Carnevale, J.T. (2001). Logic models: A systems tool for performance management. *Evaluation and Program Planning, 24,* 73–81.

Mohr, L.B. (1988). *Impact analysis for program evaluation.* Chicago: The Dorsey Press.

Morrisey, E., Wandersman, A., Seybolt, D., Nation, M., Crusto, C., & Davino, K. (1997). Toward a framework for bridging the gap between science and practice in prevention: A focus on evaluator and practitioner perspectives. *Evaluation and Program Planning, 20*(3), 367–377.

Mowbray, C., Bybee, D., Collins, M., & Levine, P. (1998). Optimizing evaluation quality and utility under resource constraints. *Evaluation and Program Planning, 21,* 59–71.

Mrazek, P.J., & Haggerty, R.J. (Eds.). (1994). *Reducing risks for mental disorder: Frontiers for preventive intervention research.* Washington, DC: Institute of Medicine, National Academy Press.

Muñoz, R.F., Mrazek, P.J., & Haggerty, R.J. (1996). Institute of Medicine report on prevention of mental disorders. *American Psychologist, 51,* 1116–1122.

Murray, D.M., & McKinlay, S.M. (1994). Design and analysis issues in community trials. *Evaluation Review, 18*(4), 493–514.

Murray, D.M., Moskowitz, J.M., & Dent, C.W. (1996). Design and analysis issues in community-based drug abuse prevention. *American Behavioral Sciences, 39,* 853–867.

Murrell, S.A. (1977). Utilization of needs assessment for community decision-making. *American Journal of Community Psychology, 5,* 461–468.

National Institute of Mental Health. (1996). *A plan for prevention research at the National Institute of Mental Health: A report by the National Advisory Mental Health Council* (NIH Publication No. 96-4093). Bethesda, MD: National Institutes of Health.

National Institute of Mental Health. (1998). *Priorities for prevention research at NIMH: A report by the National Advisory Mental Health Council* (NIH Publication No. 98-2079). Bethesda, MD: National Institutes of Health.

O'Sullivan, R.G., & O'Sullivan, J.M. (1998). Evaluation voices: Promoting evaluation from within programs through collaboration. *Evaluation and Program Planning, 21,* 21–29.

Osgood, D.W., & Smith, G.L. (1995). Applying hierarchical linear modeling to extended longitudinal evaluation: The Boys Town follow-up study. *Evaluation Review, 19*(1), 3–38.

Patton, M.Q. (1978). *Utilization-focused evaluation.* Beverly Hills: Sage.

Patton, M.Q. (1980). *Qualitative evaluation methods.* Beverly Hills, CA: Sage.

Patton, M.Q. (1997). *Utilization-focused evaluation* (3rd ed.). Beverly Hills: Sage.

Petrosino, A. (2000). Mediators and moderators in the evaluation of programs for children: Current practice and agenda for improvement. *Evaluation Review, 24*(1), 47–72.

Price, R.H. (1974). Etiology, the social environment, and the prevention of psychological dysfunction. In P. Insel & R. Moos (Eds.), *Health and the social environment* (pp. 74–89). Lexington, MA: Heath.

Price, R.H., & Smith, S.S. (1985). *A guide to evaluating prevention programs in mental health* (DHHS Publication No. ADM 85-1365). Washington, DC: US Government Printing Office.

Rappaport, J. (1977). *Community psychology.* New York: Holt, Rinehart & Winston.

Reichardt, C.S., & Trochim, W.M.K. (1995). Reports of the death of regression-discontinuity analysis are greatly exaggerated. *Evaluation Review, 19*(1), 39–64.

Reicken, H.W., Boruch, R.F., Campbell, D.T., Caplan, N., Glennan, T.K., Pratt, J.W., Rees, A., & Williams, W. (1974). *Social experimentation: A method for planning and evaluating social intervention.* New York: Academic Press.

Reiss, D., & Price, R.H. (1996). National research agenda for prevention research. The National Institute of Mental Health report. *American Psychologist, 51,* 1109–1115.

Reynolds, A.J., & Temple, J.A. (1995). Quasi-experimental estimates of the effects of a preschool intervention. *Evaluation Review, 19*(4), 347–373.

Rogers, E.S., & Palmer-Erbs, V. (1994). Participatory action research: Implications for research and evaluation in psychiatric rehabilitation. *Psychosocial Rehabilitation Journal, 18*(2), 3–12.

Rosenbaum, D.P., & Hanson, G.S. (1998). Assessing the effects of school-based drug education: A six-year multilevel analysis of Project D.A.R.E. *Journal of Research in Crime & Delinquency, 35*(4), 381–412.

Rosnow, R.L., & Georgoudi, M. (Eds.). (1986). *Contextualism and understanding in behavioral science. Implications for research and theory.* New York: Praeger.

Rossi, P.H., & Freeman, H.E. (1985). *Evaluation: A systematic approach* (3rd ed.). Newbury Park: Sage.

Rossi, P.H., & Freeman, H.E. (1993). *Evaluation: A systematic approach* (5th ed.). Newbury Park: Sage.

Rossi, P.H., & Freeman, H.E., & Lipsey, M. (1999). *Evaluation: A systematic approach* (6th ed.). Newbury Park: Sage.

Rowe, W.E. (1997). Changing ATOD norms and behaviors: A Native American community commitment to wellness. *Evaluation and Program Planning, 20*(3), 323–333.

Saxe, L., Reber, E., Hallfors, D., Kadushin, C., Jones, D., Rindskopf, D., & Beveridge, A. (1997). Think globally, act locally: Assessing the impact of community-based substance abuse prevention. *Evaluation and Program Planning, 20*(3), 357–366.

Schalock, R.L., & Thornton, C. (1988). *Program evaluation: A field guide for administrators.* New York: Plenum.

Scheirer, M.A. (1994). Designing and using process evaluation. In J.S. Wholey, H.P. Hatry, & K.E. Newcomer (Eds.), *Handbook of practical program evaluation* (pp. 40–68). San Francisco: Jossey-Bass.

Schmitt, N., Sacco, J.M., Ramey, S., & Chan, D. (1999). Parental employment, school climate, and children's academic and social development. *Journal of Applied Psychology, 84,* 737–753.

Scriven, M. (1980). *The logic of evaluation.* Inverness, CA: Edgepress.

Sechrest, L., & Figueredo, A.J. (1993). Program evaluation. *Annual Review of Psychology, 44,* 645–674.

Sechrest, L., & Sidani, S. (1995). Quantitative and qualitative methods: Is there an alternative? *Evaluation and Program Planning, 18*(1), 77–87.

Shadish, W.R. (1995). Philosophy of science and the quantitative–qualitative debates: Thirteen common errors. *Evaluation and Planning, 18*(1), 63–75.

Shadish, W.R., & Ragsdale, K. (1996). Random versus nonrandom assignment in controlled experiments: Do you get the same answer? *Journal of Consulting and Clinical Psychology, 64,* 1290–1305.

Shadish, W.R., Jr., Cook, T.D., & Leviton, L.C. (1991). *Foundations of program evaluation: Theories of practice.* Newbury Park, CA: Sage.

Shaw, R.A., Rosati, M.J., Salzman, P., Coles, C.R., & McGeary, C. (1997). Effects on adolescent ATOD behaviors and attitudes of a five-year community partnership. *Evaluation and Program Planning, 20*(3), 307–313.

Sledge, W.H., Tebes, J.K., Wolff, N., & Helminiak, T. (1996). Inpatient vs. crisis respite care: Part II—Service utilization and costs. *American Journal of Psychiatry, 153,* 1074–1083.

Snow, D.L., & Tebes, J.K. (1991). Experimental and quasi-experimental designs in prevention research. In C.G. Leukefeld & W. Bukoski (Eds.), *Drug abuse prevention intervention research: Methodological issues* (pp. 140–158) (NIDA Research Monograph 107). Washington, DC: US Government Printing Office.

Stake, R.E. (1975). An interview with Robert Stake on responsive evaluation. In R.E. Stake (Ed.), *Evaluating the arts in education: A responsive approach* (pp. 33–38). Columbus, OH: Merrill.

Stake, R.E. (1978). The case study method in social inquiry. *Educational Researcher, 7,* 5–8.

Stake, R.E. (1994). Case studies. In N.K. Denzin & Y.S. Lincoln (Eds.), *Handbook of qualitative research* (pp. 236–247). Thousand Oaks, CA: Sage.

Stanley, T.D. (1991). "Regression-disconuity design" by any other name might be less problematic. *Evaluation Review, 15*(5), 605–624.

Suchman, E. (1967). *Evaluative research.* New York: Russell Sage.

Taylor, S.J., & Bogdan, R. (1998). *Introduction to qualitative research methods* (3rd ed.). New York: John Wiley & Sons.

Tebes, J.K. (1997, May). *Self-help, prevention, and scientific knowledge.* Invited paper presented at the Self-Help Pre-Conference of the 5th Biennial Conference of the Society for Community Research and Action, Columbia, SC.

Tebes, J.K. (2000). External validity and scientific psychology. *American Psychologist, 55*(12), 1508–1509.

Tebes, J.K., & Kraemer, D.T. (1991). Quantitative and qualitative knowing in mutual support research: Some lessons from the recent history of scientific psychology. *American Journal of Community Psychology, 19,* 739–756.

Tebes, J.K., & Helminiak, T.H. (1999). Measuring costs and outcomes in mental health. *Mental Health Services Research, 1*(2), 119–121.

Tebes, J.K., Kaufman, J.S., Connell, C., & Ross, E. (2001, June). Designing an evaluation to inform public policy. In J.K. Tebes (Chair), *Real world contexts in program evaluation.* Symposium conducted at the Eighth Biennial Conference of the Society for Community Research and Action, Atlanta, GA.

Tebes, J.K., Kaufman, J.S., & Chinman, M.J. (2002). Teaching about prevention to mental health professionals. In D. Glenwick & L. Jason (Eds.), *Innovative approaches to the prevention of psychological problems.* New York: Springer.

Thompson, B. (1993). The use of statistical significance tests in research: Bootstrap and other alternatives. *Journal of Experimental Education, 61,* 361–377.

Trochim, W.M.K. (1984). *Research design for program evaluation: The regression discontinuity approach.* Beverly Hills, CA: Sage.

US General Accounting Office. (1991). *Program evaluation and methodology division: Designing evaluations.* Washington, DC: Author.

Viadro, C.I., Earp, A.L., & Altpeter, M. (1997). Designing a process evaluation for a comprehensive breast cancer screening intervention: Challenges and opportunities. *Evaluation and Program Planning, 20*(3), 237–249.

W.K. Kellogg Foundation. (2000). *Logic model development guide: Using logic models to bring together planning, evaluation and action.* Battle Creek, MI: Author.

Wandersman, A., Imm, P., Chinman, M., & Kaftarian, S. (2000). Getting to outcomes: A results-based approach to accountability. *Evaluation and Planning, 23*(3), 389–395.

Webb, E.J., Campbell, D.T., Schwartz, R.D., & Sechrest, L.B. (1966). *Unobtrusive measures: Nonreactive research in the social sciences.* Chicago: Rand McNally.

Weiss, C.H. (1972). *Evaluation research: Methods for assessing program effectiveness.* Englewood Cliffs, NJ: Prentice-Hall.

Weiss, C.H. (1997). How can theory-based evaluation make greater headway? *Evaluation Review, 21*(4), 501–524.

Wholey, J.S. (1979). *Evaluation: Promise and performance.* Washington, DC: Urban Institute.

Wholey, J.S. (1983). *Evaluation and effective public management.* Boston: Little, Brown.

Wholey, J.S., Hatry, H.P., & Newcomer, K.E. (Eds.). (1994). *Handbook of practical program evaluation.* San Francisco: Jossey-Bass.

Whyte, W.F. (1989). Advancing scientific knowledge through participatory action research. *Sociological Forum, 4*(3), 367–385.

Winett, R.A. (1995). A framework for health promotion and disease prevention programs. *American Psychologist, 50*(5), 341–350.

Winett, R.A. (1998). Prevention: A proactive-developmental-ecological perspective. In T.H. Ollendick & M. Hersen (Eds.), *Handbook of child psychopathology* (3rd ed., pp. 637–671). New York: Plenum Press.

Wolff, N., Helminiak, T.W., & Tebes, J.K. (1997). Getting the cost right in cost-effectiveness analyses. *American Journal of Psychiatry, 154*(6), 736–743.

Woodruff, S.I. (1997). Random-effects models for analyzing clustered data from a nutrition education intervention. *Evaluation Review, 21*(6), 688–697.

Yin, R.K., & Kaftarian, S.J. (1997). Introduction: Challenges of community-based program outcome evaluations. *Evaluation and Program Planning, 20*(3), 293–297.

Yin, R.K., Kaftarian, S.J., Ping, Y., & Jansen, M.A. (1997). Outcomes from CSAP's community partnership program: Findings from the national cross-site evaluation. *Evaluation and Program Planning, 20*(3), 345–355.

Effective Prevention and Health Promotion Programming

Joseph A. Durlak

Researchers and practitioners tend to specialize and the area of prevention is no different. Some strive to prevent drug use, mental health problems, learning difficulties, child maltreatment, and so on. Specialization encourages concentrated effort which is often needed to overcome obstacles impeding progress and to achieve scientific breakthroughs. However, if one steps back to observe efforts in several areas

Table 1. Generalizations about Effective Prevention and Health Promotion Interventions

Successful interventions
1. are research based and theory driven
2. recognize that multiple factors present at multiple levels influence adjustment
3. emphasize skill development and behavior change
4. are well-timed
5. use developmentally appropriate program materials and intervention techniques
6. take steps to insure good program implementation
7. are tailored and adapted for the target population and setting
8. are carefully evaluated.

simultaneously, it is possible to make several generalizations about the most successful interventions. These generalizations are important because they provide convergent validity to the primary prevention enterprise. If researchers and practitioners working independently are effective in achieving different preventive ends, but seem to share similar practices, then this commonality can be of great value in understanding successful interventions. This entry presents and explains eight generalizations that can be made about successful prevention programs based on an examination of the outcome research in several areas of prevention and health promotion: mental health, substance use, child maltreatment, learning difficulties, unintentional injuries, and the broad area of physical health which includes sexuality, pregnancy, AIDS, diet, nutrition, and exercise.

The eight generalizations are listed in Table 1. Each successful intervention does not necessarily reflect all eight features, each of which can be manifested somewhat differently depending on the specific target area and program goals. Although these generalizations are often related to each other during the conduct of the intervention, they are discussed separately to give each one its due. The generalizations presented here share several commonalities with schema presented by other authors (Dusenbury & Falco, 1995; Dusenbury, Falco, Lake, Brannigan, & Bosworth, 1997; Kirby et al., 1994; Payton, Wardlaw, Graczyk, Bloodworth, Tompsett, & Weissberg, 2000; Wandersman & Nation, in press).

GENERALIZATION ONE: EFFECTIVE INTERVENTIONS ARE THEORY DRIVEN AND RESEARCH BASED

Probably the most important over-arching ingredient of effective programs involves the extent to which the intervention is theory driven and research based. Good theory is fundamental to intervention because it offers guidance in answering the basic questions that any intervention should attempt to answer, namely, what, who, why, how, how long, which, and when (Gullotta, 1994). That is, theory offers a blueprint for determining what the program should contain (which components should it have and for how long should the program last), who should participate (as both recipients and providers of services), why the program might work (i.e., what processes should account for positive outcomes), and, finally, how to assess program impact (i.e., which types of outcomes are expected, and how and when should they be measured).

Theories advance scientific progress through their continual modification and evolution in the light of emerging data. That is why programs should be both theory driven and research based. Data from well-done research studies are essential for either confirming or disconfirming different facets of a theoretical framework and hence suggesting which theories need refinement, and which types of interventions should be supported and promoted. Empirical findings thus become extremely important in eventually developing cost-effective interventions, that is, those that yield good overall benefits relative to overall costs.

Prevention is a very young science compared to other established disciplines; over 95 percent of all controlled outcome studies have appeared since 1975. However, the relatively short history of prevention science has already witnessed substantial changes in prevention theories. Initially, many interventions attempting to prevent problems such as pregnancy, drug use, and risky sexual behavior and to enhance physical health were based on the theory that giving people accurate information would be the best way to change their behavior. Many of these early programs eventually came to be called information programs (or didactic programs). In other words, it was believed that if young people knew about the dangers of drug-taking, the serious implications of early pregnancies, or the importance of good diet and nutrition, they would change their behaviors accordingly. However, outcome studies from early information programs indicated that the theories guiding these interventions were incorrect (Durlak, 1997). Providing information did not prevent later negative outcomes. As a result, we now know that simply telling people what they should do is not an effective method of prevention. Some early programs also combined information with fear tactics, for example, by emphasizing to youth the negative consequences associated with sexual activity, drug use, and so on. These programs were also ineffective. Scaring young people is not a good preventive strategy either.

As it became clear that information programs were not effective, investigators turned to several other theories that were much more helpful in creating prevention programs that worked, which is how certain theories became prominent in prevention. No single theory is dominant in primary prevention. However, a few theories appear repeatedly in many successful programs. These theories sometimes take slightly different forms and receive different names and explanations, but, in general, the following are ascendant in prevention science: social cognitive theory, social learning theory, behavioral theory, the health belief model, and ecological theory. Sometimes successful programs use different parts of these theories in combination.

Social learning theory stresses the importance of modeling, behavioral practice, reinforcement, and environmental supports in developing and maintaining new habits and behaviors. *Social cognitive theory* emphasizes the importance of many of these same dimensions, but also focuses on the cognitive processes that promote change. For instance, social cognitive theories stress the importance of language in guiding behavior. These theories identify various cognitive strategies involving self-talk, self-reinforcement, and self-monitoring that can be used to help individuals internalize new skills and information, to solve interpersonal problems, to cope with stress or developmental challenges more effectively, and to use self-monitoring and self-reinforcement processes in making progress toward personal goals.

Behavioral theories stress the importance of environmental events and contingencies in shaping behavior. Antecedent conditions are important in prompting individuals to emit certain responses, and the consequences that follow responses exert a strong influence on whether that response will increase or decrease in frequency over time. Behavioral theory uses different combinations of prompting, shaping, and reinforcement schedules to increase desirable behaviors and/or decrease undesirable behaviors. The *health belief model* and its variants have been popular in the physical health area. The health belief model emphasizes that behavioral changes regarding health status result from an interplay between perceptions of the susceptibility and severity of different possible negative outcomes and beliefs that one can overcome potential obstacles and barriers and take the necessary action to prevent an undesirable outcome.

Finally, various *ecological theories* stress the fundamental importance of person–environment interactions and maintain that behavior cannot be separated from the context in which it occurs. Moreover, ecological theories assert that multiple environmental factors influence adjustment and these factors interact with each other to produce unique effects. As a result, preventive interventions for young people that are guided by ecological theories often attempt to involve parents and teachers as active participants because of the strong influence these significant others can have over youth. In other words, according to ecological theory, it is expected that if both parents and teachers become actively and positively involved in a prevention program, better results can be obtained then if none or only one of these groups participates. This is exactly what has been obtained in several prevention programs, most notably in programs to prevent academic, drug, and behavioral programs (Bloom, 1996; Durlak, 1995, 1997).

GENERALIZATION TWO: EFFECTIVE INTERVENTIONS RECOGNIZE THAT MULTIPLE FACTORS PRESENT AT MULTIPLE LEVELS INFLUENCE ADJUSTMENT

Although in medicine there is often a search for the pathogen or singular cause of a specific physical condition or problem, the situation is quite different in the behavioral and social sciences where the principle of multiple causality is widely accepted. The principle of multiple causality states that multiple factors contribute to the occurrence of any positive or negative outcome. The risk, protective, and positive factor paradigm offers a good way to understand the principle of multiple causality, and Table 2 lists several of the most prominent of these factors that have appeared in connection with successful interventions. The following discussion first focuses on risk and protective factors before introducing the notion of positive factors and their relationship to outcomes.

A *risk factor* is anything that is associated with an increased likelihood of a future negative outcome, while a *protective factor* is something associated with a decreased likelihood of a future negative outcome. Speaking first about risk factors, empirical evidence clearly indicates that multiple risk factors combine to produce negative outcomes. This is not to say that a single risk factor cannot be important, but by itself one factor does not completely account for later outcomes. Rather, it is the accumulation of risk factors that eventually leads to undesirable outcomes and the interaction and timing of these factors are also important. Furthermore, the influence of most risk factors is usually multiplicative, not additive, in nature. For instance, suppose you were comparing the functioning of several groups exposed to varying numbers of risk factors. Typically, there would not be much difference in adjustment between the groups exposed to one or two single risk factors versus the group exposed to none, but as the number of risk factors increases, there would be a substantial increase in the problems manifested by the affected group compared to the unexposed group. For example, three risk factors might increase the odds of poorer adjustment by five or sixfold in the exposed group (instead of only three times), and more than three factors might lead to ten times more problems in the affected group. Although we have less information on protective factors, the same principles hold: a single factor is insufficient to explain outcomes, the accumulation of protective factors produces the strongest effects, and so on. Moreover, the presence of protective factors reduces the effects of risk factors. The findings from several studies illustrate these

principles (Brown, Cohen, Johnson, & Salzinger, 1998; Fergusson & Lynsky, 1996).

There are several issues to keep in mind regarding risk and protective factors. First, most factors have nonspecific effects: two different factors can be associated with the same outcome while the same factor can lead to very different types of outcomes. In the latter case for instance, ineffective parenting has been associated with behavior and social problems, academic difficulties, or drug use in children and adolescents and, sometimes, with all three types of problems simultaneously. Second, the mechanism of action for different factors is unknown. We do not know exactly why or how different factors produce their effects. Third, all the relevant factors for different types of outcomes have not yet been identified. Fourth, the same factor can exert different factors depending on its timing, the circumstances in which it appears and the presence of other factors. Fifth, although in a few cases, risk and protection may exist along a single continuum (e.g., school quality as noted in Table 2), for the most part, risk and protective factors are not simply opposites of each other. For example, a decrease in harsh parenting (a family-level risk factor) does not necessarily mean an increase in parental warmth (a family-level protective factor).

Another critically important issue is that risk and protective factors exist at different levels of influence. Five different levels are commonly identified: the individual, family, peer group, social organization (e.g., school or work), and neighborhood or community. Several reviews describe factors present at multiple levels that combine to produce different outcomes (Bloom, 1996; Durlak, 1997; Hawkins et al., 1992).

There are many different types of risk and protective factors. Some are demographic characteristics (e.g., low-income levels, gender) which can help in identifying who might be at greater risk and thus merit intervention. Factors can also be repetitive behavior such as aggression, or a series of related behaviors emitted by one or more members of the social environment (e.g., harsh and punitive child-rearing practices). Some of these factors cannot be altered such as gender; others require sustained social and political effort to bring about change (e.g., income level), but many factors have been modified through intervention.

Most risk and protective factors are not all-or-none phenomena, but exist in degrees. For example, although these have yet to be determined precisely, there are believed to be threshold effects associated with different factors. For instance, extremely harsh parenting is a major risk factor for many negative outcomes, but mild punishment or punitiveness is not. A major focus in prevention research is devoted to identifying threshold effects and the relative influences of different risk and protective factors, how different factors

Table 2. Representative Risk, Protective, and Positive Factors at Different Levels of Influence

Level of influence	Type of factor		
	Risk	Protective	Positive
Individual	Difficult temperament Early adjustment problems	Easy temperament Personal/social skills (communication, coping, problem-solving)	Personal/social skills Self-efficacy
	Physical problems, disabilities		Sense of optimism Interpersonal bonds and attachments
Family life	Ineffective parenting (harsh, punitive, rejecting, hostile)	Effective parenting (warmth, clear communication, close monitoring)	Effective parenting
			High expectations and support Positive family environment (cohesive, organized, supportive)
	Marital discord Parental psychopathology	Marital satisfaction Parental well-being	Marital satisfaction Parental well-being
Peers	Peer bullying/victimization Peer rejection	Peer support Peer acceptance/inclusion	Peer support Positive and diverse role models
School life	Low quality schools (relating to instruction, organization, and teacher–student relations and expectations)	High quality schools	High quality schools
			Close family and community connections (parental involvement in school, good vocational opportunities in business sector, adequate school financing)
Community	High rates of crime, violence, unemployment	Effective social policies (relating to drugs, guns)	Respect for diversity
			Provision of social needs (health, child care, safety, housing)
	Accessibility of guns and drugs		
		Contact with mentors Supportive neighbors	Positive sense of community (e.g., belonging, influence, chance to participate)
	Mass media influences, promoting violence, drug use		
			Opportunities for growth: socially, spiritually, recreationally, vocationally, personally and in civic life Pro-family policies (e.g., family leave, flex time, child support)

Note: Stress can be present at any level of influence such that high stress levels, attempts to help individuals cope with stress, and efforts to create growth enhancing environments can exist as risk, protective, or positive factors, respectively, depending on the situation.
Source: Drawn from Bloom (1996), Durlak (1998a), Hawkins, Catalano & Miller (1992).

interact, and ascertaining when in the course of development their introduction is most critical.

Put another way, many successful programs focusing on risk and protective factors try to modify the components of the following equation:

$$A \quad X \quad B = \text{Problems},$$

where A represents the relevant multiple risk factors for a particular outcome that exist at different levels, B, the corresponding relevant multiple protective factors that exist at different levels, and X refers to how risk and protective factors interact to produce problems.

While risk and protection refer to the likelihood of negative outcomes, there is also the positive side of adjustment to consider. Much attention has been devoted to health promotion, a term which overlaps with several others such as positive psychology, empowerment, positive development, and wellness (Cicchetti, Rappaport, Sandler, & Weissberg, 2000; Cowen, 1994). The term, *positive factor*, has been used in this respect to refer to a factor that is associated with an increased likelihood of a future positive outcome such as enhanced well-being, better social skills, increased academic performance, and the like, as opposed to a protective factor which relates to a reduced chance of a future negative outcome (Durlak, 1997). Several positive factors that have been targeted in health promotion efforts are also listed in Table 2.

Health promotion is a broader area than prevention because it can involve any effort to enhance positive adjustment and functioning over the entire life span. The overlap between health promotion and traditional approaches to prevention becomes obvious when one sees in Table 2 that some protective and positive factors are identical. The general rationale for health promotion as a preventive strategy is that enhanced well-being will prevent later problems. In other words, whereas some preventionists see the personal and social competencies listed in Table 2 as important because they protect against later problems, health promotion advocates view some of these same competencies in a different light, as positive factors that lead to heightened overall health (e.g., higher self-esteem, greater life satisfaction, better school and work performance, and so on). Therefore, health promotion is not antithetical to a risk and protection paradigm because competencies are important in both approaches, but health promotion views competencies as the mediators of heightened well-being, and the reduction of any future problems as an important byproduct of this enhanced adjustment, as illustrated in Figure 1.

A health promotion approach is not limited to individual-level change, and recognizes the vital contribution of the social environment. That is, it is also important to modify schools, peer groups, and communities so that they are less stressful and more conducive to personal growth.

As the above discussion suggests, different preventive strategies can be pursued using the general risk, protective, and positive factor paradigm. For example, one can focus on eliminating risk factors, promoting protective factors, introducing positive factors, or try these strategies in some combination. Because risk, protective, and positive factors exist at multiple levels, the corresponding multilevel preventive interventions can be developed. One can try to influence individuals by working with them directly and also try to change their home, school, work, or community environment, thus targeting more of the relevant risk, protective, and positive factors that apply to the outcome in question. A few ambitious programs have successfully intervened at all five levels of influence (Bloom, 1996; Durlak, 1995, 1997; Institute of Medicine, 1994). Therefore, while successful programs may differ in specific procedure, scope, and purpose, they nevertheless share a common interest in changing multiple, multilevel influences on behavior.

GENERALIZATION THREE: EFFECTIVE PROGRAMS EMPHASIZE SKILL DEVELOPMENT AND BEHAVIOR CHANGE

The key to preventing negative outcomes is behavioral change, particularly in the learning of new skills and competencies. That is, prevention often works when people learn what to do, rather than what not to do. Often the new behaviors that develop in a person's repertoire become incompatible with negative or undesirable behaviors that could lead to poor outcomes. For instance, to prevent aggression, it is far better to teach children how to behave prosocially with others than to command them not to fight, or to punish them when they do.

In some areas such as drugs or sexuality, people do need accurate information to guide their behavior, yet knowledge by itself is insufficient. Simply changing attitudes or intentions is also insufficient; people need to develop new competencies and how to apply them. Furthermore, for new skills to develop, they must be systematically taught and one reason social learning and behavioral theories are frequently used in prevention programs is because they offer a proven and efficient way to develop new skills. For example, many programs have used the following sequence to develop new competencies in children. Target skills are broken down into their components. The skill is described and modeled either by the teacher or by a peer who is competent in that skill. The child is asked to perform the skill and receives immediate performance feedback. The cycle of modeling, practice, and feedback is continued until mastery is reached and training moves to the next skill in the sequence. Often this training occurs in small groups so the children can help each other improve and positive peer norms about the skill develop. Finally, new skills have to be continually practiced until they become habitual so it is important to develop supports and feedback in the social environment for newly learned skills. This is

Intervention → Increased personal & Heightened well-being → Fewer subsequent problems → Social competencies

Figure 1. Role of Personal and Social Competencies in Health Promotion Prevention Programs.

accomplished in multilevel interventions that involve classroom meetings, new school policies or events, and parent involvement. The following skills have been effectively developed in successful prevention programs: communication and assertiveness, friendship making, safe sexual practices, interpersonal problem solving and decision-making, goal setting, relaxation and other stress reduction techniques, different types of self-management practices related to self-instruction, self-monitoring, and self-reinforcement, and how to resist undue peer pressures (sometimes called refusal skills and often related to drug and sexuality issues). Social learning training techniques can produce initial mastery in 10–20 hr of training depending on the target skills and are applicable for all ages and groups (Cartledge & Milburn, 1980; Stephens, 1978).

GENERALIZATION FOUR: EFFECTIVE INTERVENTIONS ARE WELL-TIMED

Ideally, primary prevention should be delivered before most in the target population have any problems. It is unlikely that one can discover a population in which everyone is totally problem-free. For primary prevention, optimal timing depends on the usual emergence of different types of problems and research offers clues when to intervene. For instance, many youth begin experimenting with drugs or sexual behavior in the fifth or sixth grade; academic problems often need attention before children reach first grade; programs to prevent child maltreatment and unintentional injuries have found the most useful point to be at the time of the mother's pregnancy so that the physical health of the mother and child can be targeted and early child care and parenting practices can be modified (Olds & Kitzman, 1993). Peer bullying (i.e., physical threats or attacks) can begin as early as kindergarten (Olweus, 1994). As a result, successful prevention programs are delivered at a time when they can be effective and when most in the target population are problem-free.

Several key life transitions also present natural time points for intervention. Research has identified several potentially stressful and challenging transitions that can lead to later problems if the transition is not successfully negotiated. Major transitions include getting married or divorced, losing a job, changing schools, moving, a first pregnancy, and undergoing painful or anxiety-arousing medical and dental treatments. Preventive interventions have been successful in easing the passage of these transitions for affected individuals (Durlak & Wells, 1997; Jason et al., 1992; Olds & Kitzman, 1993; Pedro-Carroll & Cowen, 1985; Stanley, Markman, St. Peters, & Leber, 1995; van den Boom, 1995).

GENERALIZATION FIVE: EFFECTIVE INTERVENTIONS USE DEVELOPMENTALLY APPROPRIATE PROGRAM MATERIALS AND INTERVENTION TECHNIQUES

This principle is relevant for interventions targeting children and adolescents because there are some natural developmental limitations regarding what young people can understand and interpret, and what types of skills they can establish at different ages. For instance, complicated hypothetical, problem-solving strategies are unattainable for most young people until they reach the period of formal operational thought which does not develop until adolescence, and even during this developmental period, it takes time for such abilities to become established. A future time perspective is also a difficult concept for children (and some adolescents) to understand and to utilize, as youth are often affected by immediate, here-and-now issues and concerns.

Young children often learn best from concrete experiences so many programs de-emphasize lecture and verbal instruction and instead use an innovative blend of active learning strategies. These strategies typically involve a combination of games, exercises, small group discussions, coaching, and group projects designed to help youth personalize and internalize the basic program principles. Depending on the target population's age, puppets, movies, or videos are also used and the length of program sessions is adjusted in relation to the typical attention span of the audience. Small group discussions, exercises, and interactions help young people understand the impact of behavior on others and how others' needs, feelings, and rights should be recognized and respected; these are all developmental competencies that evolve over time.

Another way to make programs developmentally appropriate is to spread them out over successive years. Multiyear programs have the dual advantage of being able to reinforce previously established skills and to respond to young people's evolving needs. For instance, older youth need more help in responding to the many social pressures related to sexuality, particularly as their own sexual feelings are increasing and dating leads to greater interpersonal intimacy. Successful programs thus try to sequence their activities to target typical developmental issues and needs.

Understanding the target population's current life experiences and behaviors is another way to make programs developmentally appropriate and establish realistic program goals. A good example involves whether or not sexuality programs should stress sexual abstinence. The empirical evidence suggests that this issue is probably best decided based on the developmental status and activity of the target group. Sexual abstinence programs may have positive impact on youth who are not yet sexually active, but they have been largely ineffective in changing the behavior of sexually active youth (Christopher, 1995). In the latter case, findings indicate that sexually active youth need to learn safe sexual practices and can profit from access to effective contraceptive methods. Incidentally, effective sexuality programs that do provide access to contraception have not increased youths' levels of sexual activity, and have led to less risky sexual behavior related to possible pregnancy and sexually transmitted diseases (Christopher, 1995). This can be a reassuring finding for parents and others who may worry about possible unintended negative program effects.

Another example of developmental appropriateness has been the experience of successful child abuse programs. Many of these programs begin during pregnancy and conduct follow-up home visits after the child's birth. The initial focus is not on abusive practices but basic medical and child care activities because these are the types of services that new parents frequently need and are eager to receive. As the child develops, new parents are taught how to deal with common everyday problems relating to sleep, feeding, and infant stimulation. The home visiting feature of these programs also helps to individualize the intervention so parents learn what directly applies to their child and home situation (Olds & Kitzman, 1993).

GENERALIZATION SIX: EFFECTIVE INTERVENTIONS TAKE STEPS TO INSURE GOOD PROGRAM IMPLEMENTATION

Implementation refers to how well an intended program is actually put into practice (sometimes also called program adherence or program fidelity). Two important findings have emerged regarding the implementation of prevention programs (Durlak, 1998b). First, there are often large gaps between what programs look like on paper (i.e., what is intended) and what they look like in actual practice. Change agents may substantially modify certain program components, fail to complete certain parts of an intervention effectively, or omit some components entirely. In other words, the quantity or quality of program implementation is almost never 100 percent. Second, the level of program implementation does influence program outcomes. There have been several illustrations of programs that have failed to be effective because they were not well enough implemented in the first place, or that obtained better results when they were more effectively conducted (Durlak, 1998b).

The developers of prevention programs have used a combination of techniques to increase the level of program implementation. For example, they provide a clear rationale for the program, and specify the goals and procedures for different program components so that those adopting the program know what is expected. They produce user-friendly training materials to help others learn how to conduct the program and they monitor implementation once the program begins to deal with unanticipated problems.

GENERALIZATION SEVEN: EFFECTIVE INTERVENTIONS ARE TAILORED AND ADAPTED FOR THE TARGET POPULATION AND SETTING

At first glance, this generalization seems to contradict the previous one that interventions should be conducted with a high degree of fidelity to the original theory and plan. Many preventionists now recognize, however, that a natural balance exists between program implementation and program adaptation (Backer, 2000). There is almost always a need to modify a program in some way so that it fits well in a new setting. For instance, schools and communities are not the same in terms of their resources, needs, operating routines, and the populations they serve, so just because a particular program has worked in one setting does not mean the program could or should be conducted exactly in the same fashion in another locale. Of course, programs should not be changed so that their power to produce results is undermined. Therefore, it is important that program adaptation does not eliminate or undermine an intervention's essential components. Nevertheless, a good fit is important to increase the likelihood that a program will be maximally effective.

Although there is no natural recipe for blending program implementation and program adaptation to create the perfect balance, experience suggests several factors should be considered.

For example, suppose a program to prevent aggression in young children is proposed for a school system and it requires the active participation of teachers. That is, teachers will be expected to conduct most of the program in their regular classrooms. Although not comprehensive, the following issues are likely to be important not only in whether the school system will decide to try the program in the first place, but also how well the program will be implemented, and whether it will be maintained after a trial period. Some of the following points reproduce earlier comments about implementation to underscore the natural interplay between program implementation and adaptation.

1. Does the program address an important need in the eyes of the school community, particularly among teachers who will do the intervention and parents whose children will participate in the program?

2. What resources will be needed to conduct the program and how will these resources be provided or developed?
3. Are those proposing the program willing to provide the schools with meaningful input into how the program might have to be modified to fit the practical realities of the schools?
4. Will the teachers receive sufficient training in how to conduct the program?
5. Will consultants be available to provide personal and technical assistance to deal with any problems in program implementation that may arise once the program begins?
6. Is there agreement and acceptance about how the program will be evaluated and what will be done with the results of the evaluation?

Another aspect of program adaptation involves how to tailor interventions to insure their relevance for different cultural or ethnic groups. At this point, it does not appear that the most successful programs require substantial modification in terms of their core components. Rather, tailoring interventions effectively more typically involve changes in language, examples, and styles of presentation to suit the values and norms of the target audience. For instance, programs may use rap music and videos or stress specific cultural themes as a way to convey program principles and engage different target populations.

PRINCIPLE EIGHT: EFFECTIVE PROGRAMS ARE CAREFULLY EVALUATED

Both the science and practice of prevention are advanced when interventions are carefully evaluated because the results of such evaluations can weed out ineffective programs, eliminate unnecessary components of otherwise successful interventions and suggest ways to change programs to enhance their impact. In this way, each community can ultimately use its limited resources most efficiently to reach the most people. There is also an ethical obligation to evaluate programs because they involve people whose lives can be either positively or negatively affected. Fortunately, outcome research indicates that negative effects from prevention are rare (Durlak & Wells, 1997, 1998).

Programs can be evaluated in several ways depending on their scope and purpose, but good evaluations usually have several components. First, a design is chosen that is maximally sensitive to the program and its environmental context. Second, outcome measures are chosen that: (a) are clinically and socially meaningful (i.e., they assess important outcomes in people's lives such as school or job performance or level of clinical problems); (b) are psychometrically adequate, that is, that are reliable and valid for the task at hand; (c) address multiple aspects of functioning (usually functioning in several dimensions is evaluated such as at home, school, with peers, at work, and so on); and (d) assess both proximal (short-term) and distal (longer-term) effects of the intervention. Third, statistical analyses take into account such factors as the characteristics of the target population, attrition rates, and levels of program implementation. Fourth, it is important to obtain evidence for the theoretical basis of the intervention which can be done by assessing the processes that presumably lead to desired changes. For instance, if a theory says that drug use can be prevented by improving students' refusal skills (i.e., their ability to resist social pressures to take drugs), it is very important in a program evaluation to not only address drug use, but also to ascertain how students' refusal skills have been changed, and whether changes in refusal skills explain whatever changes have occurred in drug use. Often, it is the accumulation of data from numerous outcome studies that offers the most convincing evidence of intervention impact.

In sum, current research and practice make it possible to develop eight generalizations about successful preventive interventions. While this template might be modified as work on prevention continues, it has wide applicability in many areas of prevention, and can serve as a general schema for understanding the impact of effective programs.

Also see: Evaluation: Foundation; Cost Benefit Analysis: Adulthood; Primary Prevention 21st Century: Foundation.

References

Backer, T.E. (2000). The failure of success: Challenges of disseminating effective substance abuse prevention programs. *Journal of Community Psychology, 28,* 363–373.

Bloom, M. (1996). *Primary prevention practices.* Thousand Oaks, CA: Sage.

Brown, J., Cohen, P., Johnson, J.G., & Salzinger, S. (1998). A longitudinal analysis of risk factors for child maltreatment: Findings of a 17-year prospective study of officially recorded and self-reported child abuse and neglect. *Child Abuse and Neglect, 22,* 1065–1078.

Cartledge, G., & Milburn, J.F. (Eds.). (1980). *Teaching social skills to children: Innovative approaches.* NY: Pergamon.

Christopher, F.S. (1995). Adolescent pregnancy prevention. *Family Relations, 44,* 384–391.

Cicchetti, D., Rappaport, J., Sandler, I., & Weissberg, R.P. (2000). *The promotion of wellness in children and adolescents.* Washington, DC: Child Welfare League of America.

Cowen, E.L. (1994). The enhancement of psychological wellness: Challenges and opportunities. *American Journal of Community Psychology, 22,* 149–179.

Durlak, J.A. (1995). *School-based prevention programs for children and adolescents.* Thousand Oaks, CA: Sage.

Durlak, J.A. (1997). *Successful prevention programs for children and adolescents*. New York: Plenum.

Durlak, J.A. (1998a). Common risk and protective factors in successful prevention programs. *American Journal of Orthopsychiatry, 68,* 512–520.

Durlak, J.A. (1998b). Why program implementation is important. *Journal of Prevention and Intervention in the Community, 17,* 5–18.

Durlak, J.A., & Wells, A.M. (1997). Primary prevention mental health programs for children and adolescents: A meta-analytic review. *American Journal of Community Psychology, 25,* 115–152.

Durlak, J.A., & Wells, A.M. (1998). Evaluation of preventive intervention (secondary prevention) mental health programs for children and adolescents. *American Journal of Community Psychology, 26,* 775–802.

Dusenbury, L., & Falco, M. (1995). Eleven components of effective drug abuse prevention curricula. *Journal of School Health, 65,* 420–425.

Dusenbury, L., Falco, M., Lake, A., Brannigan, R., & Bosworth, K. (1997). Nine critical elements of promising violence prevention programs. *Journal of School Health, 67,* 409–414.

Fergusson, D.M., & Lynsky, M.T. (1996). Adolescent resiliency to family adversity. *Journal of Child Psychology and Psychiatry, 37,* 281–292.

Gullotta, T.P. (1994). The what, who, why, where, when, and how of primary prevention. *Journal of Primary Prevention, 15,* 5–14.

Hawkins, J.D., Catalano, R.F., & Miller, J.Y. (1992). Risk and protective factors for alcohol and other drug problems in adolescence and early adulthood: Implications for substance abuse prevention. *Psychological Bulletin, 112,* 64–105.

Institute of Medicine. (1994). *Reducing risks for mental disorders: Frontiers for preventive intervention research*. Washington, DC: National Academy Press.

Jason, L.A., Weine, A.M., Johnson, J.H., Warren-Sohlberg, L., Filippelli, L.A., Turner, E.Y., & Lardon, C. (1992). *Helping transfer students: Strategies for educational and social readjustment*. San Francisco: Jossey-Bass.

Kirby, D., Short, L., Collins, J., Rugg, D., Kolbe, L., Howard, L., Miller, B., Sonenstein, F., & Zabin, L.S. (1994). School-based programs to reduce sexual risk behaviors: A review of effectiveness. *Public Health Reports, 109,* 339–360.

Olds, D.L., & Kitzman, H. (1993). Review of research on home visiting for pregnant women and parents of young children. *The Future of Children, 3,* 53–92.

Olweus, D. (1994). Bullying at school: Basic facts and effects of a school-based intervention program. *Journal of Child Psychology and Psychiatry, 35,* 1171–1190.

Payton, J.W., Wardlaw, D.M., Graczyk, P.A., Bloodworm, M.R., Tompsett, C.J., & Weissberg, R.P. (2000). Social and emotional learning: A framework for promoting mental health and reducing risk behavior in children and youth. *Journal of School Health, 70,* 179–185.

Pedro-Carroll, J.L., & Cowen, E.L. (1985). The Children of Divorce Intervention Program: An investigation of the efficacy of a school-based prevention program. *Journal of Consulting and Clinical Psychology, 53,* 603–611.

Stanley, S.M., Markman, H.J., St. Peters, M., & Leber, B.B. (1995). Strengthening marriages and preventing divorce: New directions in prevention research. *Family Relations, 44,* 392–401.

Stephens, T.M. (1978). *Social skills in the classroom*. Columbus, OH: Cedars Press.

van den Boom, D.C. (1995). Do first-year intervention effects endure? Follow-up during toddlerhood of a sample of Dutch irritable infants. *Child Development, 66,* 1798–1816.

Wandersman, A., & Nation, M. (in press). What works in prevention: Principles of effective prevention programs. *American Psychologist*.

Ethical Considerations in Prevention

Michael B. Blank, Raymond P. Lorion, and Paul Root Wolpe

OVERVIEW

As David Stenmark prepared his Presidential address to what was then the Division of Community Psychology* of the American Psychological Association, he was approached by his daughter, Marci, and asked what he was writing and why. Carefully he explained his leadership role in the Division and that the talk provided an opportunity to review the discipline's commitment to identifying and responding to oppression; to avoiding disorder rather than waiting for its appearance; and to empower the disadvantaged rather than merely come to their assistance. After a few moments reflection, Marci looked at her father and asked: "Did those people ask you to do that for them?" The question is insightful and, in our view, as yet unanswered.

Our perspective originates within a public health framework. Public health scientists and service providers, genuinely concerned for the welfare of those who suffer from emotional and behavioral disorders, seek to prevent the onset of disorders, to mitigate the immediate and long-term consequences of illness, and promote optimal health for all. However noble that goal may be, Marci's question hovers overhead. For good or bad, public health interventions are designed and introduced intentionally to alter the lives of those whom they touch. By definition, the targets of preventive efforts do not present diagnosable disorders and most are unaware that they are at risk for such outcomes. Similarly, wellness and health promotion efforts, assuming that they operate as intended, alter the developmental experiences of those involved. Rarely, however, do the participants have any say in implementation of the intervention, or awareness of the intervention's intent, or perhaps even of its existence. Our purpose in this entry is to examine the legitimacy of that practice and to offer to the field suggestions for adding informed consent to recruitment and implementation procedures.

We raise these issues because we believe that heightened consideration must be paid to the ethics of implementing interventions to prevent disorder and promote health. Increased

* Subsequently renamed the Society for Community Research and Action. The story is based on the recollection of one of the authors (RPL).

health consumer sophistication, widespread publicity about claims of potential harms of public health interventions (such as vaccination), suspicion in certain subpopulations about the underlying motivations of public health activities, and other concerns demand a re-evaluation of the ethical underpinnings of our intervention efforts. Without more specific guidelines for the unique ethical challenges confronting us, we may find some of our efforts thwarted at the expense of the health and welfare of vulnerable members of society.

Similar views have been expressed by O'Neill (1989) and Davidson (1989), and by Lorion (1987) before them. Davidson (1989) related community psychology's risk for ethical lapses to four factors. First, our commitment to cultural relativism leaves us seemingly without absolute standards for determining right and wrong. In a sense, we assign to the setting in which we work the determination of what outcomes we should endorse and encourage and which we should seek to alter. Second, our work frequently mixes modes of intervention and conceptions of behavior. Thus, we seek to introduce changes at a systems level, yet continue to define problems at the individual level. Third, by remaining removed from directly intervening (e.g., consulting to a day-care center or to a center for victims of domestic violence), we are linked to the ethics of indirectly serving the public. Finally, most telling in the authors' view is the absence of a solid scientific basis for our interventions. Too often, we offer what we *believe* to be beneficial, or what we *succeed in negotiating* with relevant systems or settings, or what the recipients of our interventions are *willing to accept* rather than what solid science says is necessary. In effect, we allow others to determine how we will define, respond to, deliver and assess our interventions. Hardly a solid base from which to assure that an optimal intervention occurs!

INTRODUCTION

The need for new initiatives in public health ethics has been recognized. The Department of Health and Human Services, through the National Cancer Institute and its Cancer Prevention Fellowship Program offered its first fellowship in the Ethics of Public Health and Prevention in 2001. The new position offers ethicists, philosophers, physicians, and scientists an opportunity to study ethical issues in prevention research and their application in public health practice. Public health ethics, while closely linked to biomedical ethics, has unique concerns that require special emphasis and specialized research efforts. A prime example of this is the primary prevention of mental disorders and the promotion of mental health.

Consider, for example, the question of how one selects an outcome for a proposed intervention, that is, what specific condition(s) are to be prevented? Clearly, the seriousness of the disorder (in terms of distress, chronicity, secondary effects for the effected individual, family, friends, etc.) should be among the factors considered. For example, distinctions among chronic mental disorders such as autism or schizophrenia, transient affective disorders, emotional distress, and behavioral annoyances call for different ethical considerations in the design before interventions are implemented. Assuming that there is an adequate evidentiary basis for linking measurable risk factors with diagnosable disorders and that one can reasonably estimate the likelihood that the disorder would occur in the absence of the intervention, an intervention to avoid initial or recurring autism or schizophrenia seems justifiable. Of course, the stronger the evidence for effectiveness, the stronger the argument is for recruitment into the program. However, what if such evidence is weak? One must then examine in more detail the costs to the individual of participation (e.g., do known or foreseeable iatrogenic consequences exist?) or non-participation (e.g., what is the likelihood of an episode in the absence of intervention?).

Although complex, the above scenario is relatively straightforward. What if, however, the outcome to be avoided does not represent a recognized diagnosed disorder but rather represents an uncomfortable, unpleasant, or annoying temperament state? What if the rationale for preventing or reducing that state (e.g., alcohol consumption during adolescence; binge drinking) is that its presence over time has been identified as a risk factor for a subsequent diagnosable condition (e.g., alcoholism or substance abuse)? The ethical calculus becomes more complicated. First, one must consider how much weight to assign to distress experienced by the person with the problem, by members of that person's family, by teachers or other social agents, by peers, and so on. Does each have a say in whether the intervention is to be utilized? How solid a link must be established between the antecedent condition and the diagnosable problem? Since many end-state diagnosable conditions result from combinations of risks rather than from solitary risk factors, how substantial must the burden of risk be to justify program recruitment?

The latter question arises because a number of prevention programs are designed to reduce the occurrence of behaviors that may be illegal (e.g., adolescent drinking and drug use), immoral (e.g., bullying), or unhealthy (e.g., unprotected intercourse). If asked, most members of a community would prefer that the behaviors not occur, but in fact they are *not* mental disorders. Rather, they represent personal decisions which may offend, concern, annoy, or otherwise distress those around the individual and may even create legal, health, or emotional problems for the individual and others. They do not represent disorder defined either using diagnostic criteria or Wakefield's (1992, 1997) concept of "harmful dysfunction." So, by what ethical standards should we justify the introduction of such interventions in socially desirable ways? This raises the question of who ultimately decides which choices about attitudes or behaviors are allowed and which are not.

Antecedent to examining ethical guidelines for preventive interventions and wellness/health promotion activities, it is essential to develop a common understanding of these terms. In his classic work, *Principles of Community Psychiatry*, Caplan (1964) urged adoption by the mental health disciplines of existing public health distinctions among primary, secondary, and tertiary intervention strategies. Tertiary interventions, by definition, are targeted to individuals presenting evidence of a diagnosable disorder and have a measurable likelihood of experiencing specific sequelae. Secondary interventions are targeted to individuals displaying early signs of disorder or incipient indicants. Since the likelihood that the underlying pathogenic process will continue can be established epidemiologically, the risk of intervening and non-intervening can be specified. Primary prevention intends to act before even the earliest signs of disorder are present. Significant ethical issues arise for primary preventive interventions; many of these can be resolved only as the pathway from risk to disorder is elucidated and the relative costs of (non)intervention can be calculated.

The aforementioned three categories were established for viral and bacterial diseases. Gordon (1987) proposed an alternative set of categories that he believed more accurately reflected the characteristics of emotional and behavioral disorders. His rationale was simple. Many of those disorders had indistinguishable onsets and varying courses and preventive interventions differed more on targeting than etiological factors. Moreover, he recognized the need to consider costs, both financial and other indirect costs, in planning and implementing such interventions. Thus, he proposed that "universal" interventions (e.g., public service announcements against adolescent pregnancy or substance use) refer to those that are non-specifically targeted, very low in costs per individual reached, unlikely to be harmful and, by definition, extremely difficult to be assessed in terms of effectiveness. "Selective" interventions, by contrast, are targeted to segments of the population that are epidemiologically identified as having heightened risk for an outcome of concerns (e.g., children of alcoholic or drug-addicted parents; victims of domestic violence). These interventions tend to be more expensive, more intense, and thus, potentially more iatrogenic. They can, however, be assessed in terms of impact. Finally, "indicated" interventions are targeted to specific individuals whose risk is defined on the basis of signs of incipient or early-stage disorders. These interventions are the most expensive, intense, and potentially iatrogenic but more easily assessable. Gordon's categories were endorsed by the

Institute of Medicine's recent analysis of the state of prevention science and practice (Institute of Medicine, 1994).

Therefore, the definition of prevention that is accepted is important in determining the efficacy and effectiveness of prevention efforts. As Gordon notes, it is also relevant to understanding the risk associated with introducing such interventions. By definition, universal interventions do not allow opportunities for consent. Exposure to a billboard, a public service message on radio or television or an insert in a newspaper or magazine, arrives without warning. Their messages are generally assumed neutral at worst. Consider, however, the response of a ten-year-old girl confronting a poster that likens adolescent pregnancy to an "18 year prison sentence." She wonders whether her mother feels that way about her having been born when she was fourteen. Similarly, what thoughts might those posters engender in a sixteen-year-old who is eight months pregnant? The poster's intent is certainly noble. Are its designers and distributors responsible for anticipating all possible reactions and all possible responses to such reactions?

After reviewing the evolution of current thought regarding ethical challenges for prevention, we suggest that architects of preventive interventions are particularly vulnerable to violations of informed consent, beneficence, and non-maleficence. These result from ambiguity regarding the intended beneficiaries of intervention, the lack of a scientific base, and adherence to a system of values that reduces the likelihood of considering alternatives and worldviews that are inconsistent with our preconceptions. Consider the aforementioned poster example. To some the posters represent a step toward empowering otherwise vulnerable young girls. To others they represent an insult against what was considered a personal choice, or at the very least an unexpected blessing. Some will read into the poster a call to abstinence; to others a call for the termination of a pregnancy. Each of these seems a reasonable interpretation of a seemingly simple message delivered with the best of intention.

Consider also the increasing attention to the design and dissemination of interventions to promote health and wellness (e.g., Cicchetti, Rappaport, Sandler, & Weissberg, 2000). Health promotion has been contrasted with disease prevention and Rappaport (1981) has gone so far as to suggest that prevention of disease is paradoxical to promotion of wellness. This development resulted in the notion of psychological empowerment, a trend that has been juxtaposed with disease prevention, and, in our opinion, incorrectly distanced from methods of public health and epidemiology as methods of evaluating the impact of interventions. These interventions go beyond the commitment to protect against documented risks for disease and disorder and extend into a priori decisions about what is best for designated segments of the population and ways to alter their behaviors with or without their knowledge.

As a consequence of a felt need within the guild of community psychologists to distance themselves from community psychiatry, and later from clinical psychology and community mental health, there has been a denial of methods common in public health. This is often mistakenly described as a rejection of "the medical model" or embracing a strengths approach. However, it is our belief that the values of community psychology with regard to health promotion and wellness are not in conflict with the tenets of public health, and that the rejection of a public health approach puts the public at risk for interventions that fail to adhere to the foundational ethical principles of informed consent, beneficence, and non-maleficence.

The threat to foundational ethical principles is a result of ambiguity regarding the intended beneficiaries of intervention, the lack of an evidence base in our practice, and adherence to a system of values that reduces the likelihood of considering alternatives and worldviews that are inconsistent with our preconceptions. The latter bias is discussed in terms of Irving Janis' "groupthink" phenomenon, and a few antidotes are prescribed. We conclude that a clearer understanding of epidemiological trends in mental health and mental illness is essential to evaluate the impact of interventions and provide an evidentiary base for preventive practices. We also outline a few principles for the ethical practice of primary prevention.

PUBLIC HEALTH ETHICS

Much of the ideology surrounding primary prevention is based on the notion of prophylaxis rather than amelioration of illness. This has its roots in public health and was originally related to prevention of contagious diseases such as cholera. Since 1854, when Dr. John Snow removed the pump handle from a well on London's Broad Street, preventionists have argued that interventions can be successful in public health in the absence of a clear understanding of the underlying etiology of illness. After all, Snow did not know that cholera was caused by bacteria. At that time, several different companies were responsible for supplying water in different areas of the city. All he needed to recognize to prevent further outbreaks of illness was that people who drank the water supplied by the Southwark and Vauxall Company were eight to nine times more likely to become ill than were those living in other areas of London (Lillienfeld and Stolley, 1994). It should be appreciated, however, that Snow did precede his action with a careful analysis of how the disease was distributed among the population and what factors differentiated those who were or were not ill. His field work mirrored the procedures still relied on by epidemiologists throughout the world. The ethical question is how much must be known before action is taken and what factors determine how long one can wait to act before that information is gained. The most widely recognized application of these procedures relate to the occurrence of epidemic or endemic conditions. However, if Snow had maintained that it was unimportant to know how many cases of cholera there were in the community, who had it, and where they lived, he would have been hamstrung in his efforts to prevent it. Moreover, if Snow had simply counted the number of overall cases in London, he might very well have missed the link between contamination of a specific source and the occurrence of disease. He might even have mistakenly driven people who were not at risk because their water supply was safe, to seek water from a contaminated well or other source. The specificity of *where* he took action is as important as the specificity of the action he took. Broadly applied preventive interventions may exacerbate rather than reduce risks and may protect some (e.g., those served by Southwark and Vauxall) while placing others in peril. Clearly, the ethical practice of prevention requires an understanding of who is at risk, and who is not, and, in each case, why.

Epidemics are defined as outbreaks of illness that are in excess of what would normally be expected. While the underlying etiology of illness may or may not be understood, it is imperative that baseline rates of illness and their distribution be known in order to evaluate the outbreak of an epidemic. The importance of an understanding of case rates and distribution of illness also applies to mental health and mental illness. Proper consideration of the implications of epidemiological data can greatly enlarge our understanding and identifying loci for preventive efforts of many sorts.

Community psychology has its roots firmly planted in community psychiatry and public health. Impetus for the discipline's origin at the Swampscott Conference arose from concerns about how mental health practices and its service providers (primarily psychiatrists and psychologists) would need to change in response to passage of the Community Mental Health Centers Acts of 1963 and 1965 (Anderson, Bennet, Cooper, Hassol, Klein, & Rosenblum, 1966; Bloom, 1973). Since the Swampscott conference, there has been continuing debate regarding the relative importance of having a clear inductive understanding of the underlying causal chain for disease processes versus implementation of interventions that work, and deducing the mechanisms that account for effectiveness post hoc (Albee, 1986). This dynamic continues to play a central role in the planning, implementation, and evaluation of preventive interventions. We agree with Bloom (1973) that the separation from those roots has led to a denial by many of the disciplines' leaders over the past three decades of the importance of understanding the epidemiology of illness as a basis for evaluating the impact of preventive interventions.

That there were special ethical issues in community psychology, with its concomitant emphasis on interventions at the group and population levels, was recognized early on. In commenting on the new Ethical Principals for Psychologists of the American Psychological Association, Golann (1969) suggested that the principles were inadequate to the needs of community psychologists and their focus on prevention. Since that time, not much progress has been made in that regard. Pettifor (1986) analyzed the ethical principles for psychologists that were in place in both Canada and the United States almost two decades later and found that they continued to inadequately address issues surrounding informed consent and adverse events, among others.

O'Neill (1989) challenged the field by suggesting that much of the difficulty in developing adequate ethical standards for community psychologists was inherent in the ambiguity of the goals of primary prevention. Methods of measuring positive growth and development were and are poorly conceptualized and articulated. Circumstances often force psychologists to balance different values and beliefs among constituent groups, and to cope with unanticipated consequences. In order to deconstruct the competing features of an ethical problem and devise an appropriate course of action, psychologists must decide who are the targets of any intervention and what outcomes can be reasonably linked to the effort. Using vignettes of two interventions as illustration, O'Neill demonstrated how preventive efforts are often implemented in settings where the interests of constituent groups are ambiguous and inconsistent, and where radiating effects render the likelihood of iatrogenic effects more likely. Both examples involved community psychologists as advocates (in one instance for a shelter for battered women, and for a group seeking specialized day care in another). Both circumstances involved the psychologist getting caught between decision-makers and the groups for whom they were advocating, and both involved pressures to represent circumstances to decision-makers in a way that was favorable, although not necessarily accurate. These examples are illustrative of the special demands made of community psychologists, who frequently find themselves in situations where they are called upon to balance information both as scientist and advocate. By insisting that ethical decision-making be guided by an evidentiary base, O'Neill reflects earlier sentiment by Cowen (1973) and Lorion (1987). In contrast, other leaders in the field (e.g., Albee, 1986) expressed serious reservations about the limitations that would or could be placed on our interventions if we were required to justify them empirically.

There were a number of published comments to the charges inherent in O'Neill's vignettes. Heller (1989) followed up by describing a number of ethical dilemmas he encountered and emphasized that what we study and how we attempt to change communities reflect individual value systems as well as the collective values that we hold as community psychologists. These dilemmas are tricky. It is frequently the case that the interventionist is not clearly accountable to anyone. Further, due to limitations in our research methods, even programs with empirically demonstrable short-term impact have rarely been evaluated for longer term effects. Heller suggested that we should share our experiences with ethical dilemmas with each other in order to provide practitioners with input from their colleagues and to help others anticipate similar dilemmas in their own efforts. Alderfer's (1989) comments centered about promising more than we can deliver, that psychologists must be ever vigilant to pressure to provide unreasonably favorable expectations for effects or interpretations of outcomes. Bond (1989) suggested that an understanding of the social ecology of the setting and ways that scarce resources frame ethical dilemmas is necessary to avoid a situation where constituents end up "blaming" the interventionist. Davidson (1989) suggested that we often ignore ethical dilemmas. This is seen as a result of an over-reliance on a perception of cultural relativity, where conflicts are normalized. He also suggested that we frequently implement programs and then stand back, reflecting a confusion regarding a consultative role in intervention. He also reiterated the lack of sound scientific bases for many of our preventive efforts.

By contrast, Reinharz (1989) argued that the problems raised by O'Neill should have been anticipated and that what seem to be ethical dilemmas are rather the result of confusion about the proper role of the interventionist. He suggested that much of the pressure that generates role confusion is a result of communities failing to generate their own funding to support these prevention efforts. Since prevention practitioners are frequently providing funding through research or linking recipients with funding sources, they are often seen as the legitimate owners of the program when in fact they are not. Prevention practitioners may be faced with ethical conflicts surrounding the allocation of resources under these circumstances.

Pope (1989) suggested that ethical problems are inherent in preventive interventions because of difficulties in accommodating ethical principles to the values, concerns, and language of community psychology. He suggested that because of the continuous evolution of community psychology, clarification of assumptions and values is often elusive and precludes adopting any formal code of ethics. This frequently results in creative ethical decision-making, and increases the potential for unanticipated negative consequences of interventions. He emphasized the need to accept responsibility for unanticipated consequences of prevention efforts.

Riger (1989) attempted to reconceptualize these ethical dilemmas from a structural perspective. She viewed the problems discussed by O'Neill as lack of information that lead to unanticipated negative effects. She encouraged a perspective that frames dilemmas as struggles for increased political power. Community stakeholders often have conflicting needs and expectations. This results in interventions providing a focal point for previously existing conflict between stakeholders. Recognizing the role that interventions may play within existing power structures should allow prevention practitioners to improve the effectiveness of their efforts.

Another difficulty in ethical decision-making is that development of interventions frequently requires the psychologist to adopt a participant–observer or resident-researcher role. This is particularly true in rural areas where dual relationships are common. Wicker and Sommers (1993) consider the ethical issues in a resident-researcher model where community psychologists intervene in the very community where they live. They argue that due to specific local knowledge, resident-researchers can often make more informed decisions about research problems and methods. Because of community residence and longevity, more powerful longitudinal designs to assess change over time can be used. This should result in a better understanding of the impact of intervention and to assist in interpretation and further refinement implementation. However, some of the inherent difficulty in adopting the role of a participant–observer or resident-researcher includes the possibility of provincialism, avoiding perceptions of pursuing self-interest, unintended effects caused by the resident-researcher, and role conflicts. Watts (1993) outlined other ethical dilemmas inherent in the resident-researcher model. He suggests that the local knowledge and personal insight gained by the researcher is compatible with community psychology and action research, but that there would also be the temptation to use research data for personal gain. He reiterates the problems inherent in dual relationships—the difficulty in maintaining a balance between professional and personal life—and the problem of community factions. The resident-researcher must navigate between the Scylla of appeasing competing factions and the Charybdis of an artificial construction of consensus in the community. Throughout, the motivation for resident research must be carefully considered.

In her 1993 Presidential address to the Society for Community Research and Action, Irma Serrano-Garcia explored power and ethics (Serrano-Garcia, 1994). She reviewed ethical constructs including beneficence and non-maleficence in relationship to a model for community psychology based on power and influence, and explored the complex relationships between ethics and power. She argued that the APA ethical principles that guide psychology were incompatible with the goals of action research and social change and may actually serve to undermine the efforts of community psychologists, suggesting that in order to achieve those goals, the interaction between power and ethics would need to be reshaped.

Snow and his colleagues (Snow, Grady, & Goyette-Ewing, 2000) identified five critical ethical issues for community psychologists and preventive interventions. These included a need to be explicit regarding values and value conflicts, and clarity with regard to defining goals and processes. They discuss the diffuse nature of informed consent in prevention, especially regarding interventions with children. They also conclude that evidence regarding the ability of preventive intervention to prevent disease must be gathered objectively and used judiciously.

INFORMED CONSENT, BENEFICENCE, AND NON-MALEFICENCE

Informed consent flows directly from the ethical principle of individual autonomy and applies both to clinical practice and clinical research. The principle of autonomy recognizes the right of the recipient of any treatment to participate knowingly and voluntarily and to be the ultimate decision-maker regarding whether or not to participate (Appelbaum, Lidz, & Meisel, 1987). Typically, informed consent requires disclosure of the type of research or intervention to be provided, the known or anticipated risks and benefits of procedures, alternatives to participation, and in research, freedom to withdraw without adverse effects to any ongoing clinical care. The issue of participants' capacity for understanding is a separate but important issue from the provision of information, and is particularly germane to persons whose cognitive functioning is compromised due to mental illness or other factors.

While the actual term "informed consent" was first written into law in a 1957 California Supreme Court decision, *Salgo v. Leland Stanford Jr, the University Board of Trustees*, the concept is usually attributed to the Nuremberg Code as an outgrowth of the horrendous and inhumane experiments foisted upon unknowing individuals during the Nazi regime (Daugherty, 1999). Of particular relevance to the discussion of informed consent regarding preventive intervention are the concepts of *anticipated benefits* and *foreseeable risks* (Shore, 1996).

It is most frequently the case that preventive interventions are assumed to provide only positive benefits and at worst, to have no impact. However, determining the actual impact of preventive interventions on participants has proven most elusive. Purveyors of preventive interventions have been less than forthcoming about the potential negative consequences of participation, and have minimized the potential for harm inherent in such participation (Lorion, 1983). This is due to at least two complimentary forces. First, as proponents and advocates of preventive interventions, we have become accustomed to defending our methods and may fall into the trap of promising more than we can deliver. Second, we tend to underestimate the iatrogenic effects, such as labeling and other unintended negative consequences. In the next section, we use vaccination as an example of the promise and pitfall of preventive interventions.

There are special risks and burdens associated with implementing preventive interventions with children, who are legally unable to provide informed consent. In order to satisfy the principle of informed consent, agreement to participate must be voluntary, the person giving consent must be competent, and the consent must be given after a balanced disclosure of all relevant information (Mesiel, Roth, & Lidz, 1977). In most instances, parents or guardians serve as proxies for children, and while ideally their assent should be sought, children are assumed to lack the capacity to consent fully and are assumed to be more vulnerable than adults. Ethical practice requires that information regarding the nature of participation be provided to proxies, including expected benefits, known and expected risks, as well as a cost-benefit analysis. Competency requires that the person giving consent has a suitable appreciation of the information given, implying more than a simple factual or rote understanding. Further, the decision made must meet a standard of reasonableness.

Weithorn (1987) provided an excellent review of the legal and ethical issues involved with obtaining consent for prevention programming for children. She outlined many of the difficult issues involved with truly voluntary consent, and the difficulties inherent with having parents provide consent for their children. Since many preventive interventions for children are implemented in schools by teachers, distinctions between educational and mental health programming, between outcomes assessment that are part of an educational program or research, and between programs that have proven effectiveness or not, are frequently obscured. Weithorn emphasized how difficult it is to balance children's rights when conducting research into effectiveness for prevention programming. The principle of *autonomy*, or the ability for self-determination, is usually set aside for children as are privacy considerations.

Two other principles that are central to this discussion are beneficence and non-maleficence. *Beneficence* is simply the principle of biomedical ethics that states that we attempt to help people and leave them better off than when we found them. It is because of this principle that "no treatment" control groups are unethical where proven best practice standards exist, and it is incumbent upon the researcher to provide control that at least represents treatment-as-usual.

Non-maleficence means to do no harm, and it is this principle that frequently gets shortest shrift in prevention research. Oftentimes purveyors of prevention overestimate the anticipated benefits of their programs, but of even greater concern is the tendency to gloss over, minimize, or dismiss outright the potential negative effects of participation in prevention (Lorion, 1987). An example of the tendency to discount negative effects in prevention is given by the example of vaccination.

VACCINATION

There is little doubt that inoculation against infectious disease has proven to be one of the most effective measures in public health and preventive medicine (Schumacher, 1979). However, there are fundamental ethical questions related to this most effective preventive intervention. There are many parallels between vaccination programs and preventive interventions designed to prevent mental illness or promote mental health. First, inoculations are typically given to healthy children who are unable to give informed consent. Second, it is not immediately clear that the children themselves are the proximal beneficiaries of the vaccination program. Childhood diseases such as chicken pox, mumps, and measles actually are of relatively small risk to children. However, the inoculation of children against these diseases also serves to protect others, most notably frail adults, pregnant women and their fetuses, and the elderly. Another feature common to these preventive interventions is that vaccination programs are de facto compulsory, at least in the United States. Children cannot be enrolled in school in most states without providing evidence of up-to-date vaccinations.

There is widespread perception that vaccination programs are harmless, despite scientific evidence to the contrary, and public health officials are not forthcoming with information about the potential for such harm. An example of potential unintended negative consequences of inoculation programs is the recent findings about effects related to a preservative commonly found in vaccinations. Thimerosal (an antimicrobial containing 49.6 percent ethylmercury [etHg] by weight) is a very effective preservative that contains mercury and has been used in some vaccines and other products since the 1930s. Thimerosal is still the most widely used preservative in vaccines. The Food and Drug Administration (FDA) estimates that it is used in more than 30 licensed vaccines and biologics. The Food and Drug Administration (FDA) Modernization Act of 1997 called for a review of the use of mercury-containing biologics. Following shortly after the passage of this Act, in December 1998, the FDA requested manufacturers' data on vaccines that contain Thimerosal.

By 1999 there was widespread recognition that cumulative exposures to children vaccinated with these products typically exceeded the existing guidelines for intake of organic mercury. This prompted the US Public Health Service and the American Academy of Pediatrics to issue a joint statement urging that the administration of hepatitis B vaccine at birth be postponed until the second month of life. Subsequently, the National Vaccine Advisory Committee convened a public workshop at the National Institutes of Health (NIH) to examine the evidence for risks associated with these exposures. Although the data regarding the neurodevelopmental toxicity of mercury are extensive, the overall conclusion of the NIH meeting participants was that there was no extant evidence of a significant public health problem from Thimerosal-containing vaccines and therefore these exposures represented only a theoretical concern. Nonetheless, the participants urged that Thimerosal be removed from vaccines, and that screening analyses into the putative association of Thimerosal-containing vaccines be undertaken.

The preliminary findings of these screening analyses suggested a dose-response relationship between exposure to Thimerosal-containing vaccines and some neurologic developmental disorders (NDDs). Results from two HMOs using claims data found significant associations between exposure and several neurodevelopmental outcomes including ADHD, speech delay, language delay, stammering, tics, and other adverse developmental outcomes (Centers for Disease Control and Prevention, 1999). The data should be interpreted with caution since the study utilized claims data with nonspecific outcome measures. In addition, the use of claims data could reflect a health care-seeking bias. However, these findings represent a prime example of how seemingly innocuous preventive intervention can have widespread and potentially far-reaching negative effects.

There are several important points to be made of the Thimerosal example. First, it is important to note that the only reason that we are able to assess the potential negative effects of toxic agents is because there are known incidence and prevalence rates for neurodevelopmental diseases such as ADHD for the population. Second, even assuming that there was disclosure of the risks inherent in the vaccines themselves, it is unlikely that any disclosure of risks associated with the preservative contained in the vaccines were ever disclosed to parents prior to 1999, and probably not often thereafter. Third, expert panels do not agree and are not likely to agree in the future that there is any proven association between exposure to the prevention intervention and adverse developmental consequences. However, there is almost complete unanimity of opinion regarding the benefits of a public vaccination program. We certainly are not advocating for suspension of inoculation programs or even suggesting that the allegations of negative consequences are correct—only that they have some merit. What does concern us is the negative potential of the hegemony of a health policy that is seen as purely beneficial with no appreciable risk.

GROUP-THINK AND PREVENTION IN MENTAL HEALTH

The notion of "group-think" refers to a process of group dynamics. When we work together in groups we sometimes suffer illusions of righteousness and invincibility. Irving Janis (1972), in his book *Victims of Groupthink*, described his observations of phenomena of group leadership and member interaction that are characterized by inward-looking, self-regulating, and stereotypical behaviors that lead to distorted decision-making. Janis defines group-think as "a mode of thinking that people engage in when they are deeply involved in a cohesive group, when the members' strivings for unanimity override their motivation to realistically appraise alternative courses of action" (Janis, 1989, p. 117). He was dissecting the question of how a distinguished group of experts could collectively make decisions that in retrospect are clearly bad ones. He postulated that errors imbedded within group dynamics are not isolated, a notion that is quite consistent with that of social ecology. Janis used presidential decision-making for many examples to illustrate the myopic visions that emerged from group-think. He describes these as fiascoes or complete failures of reason in decision-making. These fiascoes included Franklin Roosevelt's failure to heed clear signals of impending attack before Pearl Harbor, Truman's ill-advised invasion of North Korea, Johnson's escalation of the Vietnam War, Nixon's Watergate break-in, and Reagan's Iran–Contra scandal cover-ups.

While decision-making regarding the planning and implementation of preventive interventions do not typically take place in the Oval Office, they are usually products of executive decision-making and, we maintain, also vulnerable to the excesses inherent in group-think dynamics. Symptoms of defective decision-making in executive groups associated with problems and mistakes in policy decisions stem from a variety of closely linked phenomena.

Frequently, decision-makers fail to adequately explore alternatives. Because an idea (e.g., prevention is better than treatment) has been focused on for so long, scant attention is given to other ideas. Rejected alternatives are seldom re-examined and go unheeded. That a "medical model" is antithetical to the "values" of community psychology is hardly ever challenged in our graduate programs. As a result, the group fails to consider all available objectives and the best course of action may not be chosen, indeed it may not even be considered.

Another outgrowth of group-think is that sufficient exploration of costs and risks of options may not be considered. For instance, an adolescent pregnancy prevention program is likely to include information about condom use and other methods of birth control. To focus on an abstinence-only approach would no doubt be seen as puritanical, wrong headed, and doomed to failure. However, the impact of implementation of interventions that may be in direct opposition to the values and teaching of parents who may adhere to a more traditional values system (those who frequently voice strong opposition to the intervention) is rarely considered. What is the impact on the parent–child dyad when one message is given at home and another by the preventionists? All too often this question is discounted or overlooked.

Another associated risk of group-think is that searches for new information can be superficial. As experts in our respective content areas, we may incorrectly assume that we are up-to-date on the current findings and literature, since it is our friends and colleagues who are publishing that literature. However, all possible data for the decision are rarely gathered and information that does not support the intended plan is given short shrift and dismissed, particularly if its source is not readily recognized as credible within a discipline. There is also selective and biased filtering of information as well as communicating that information to others. The group tends to exclude valuable items of information that are inconsistent with the prevailing zeitgeist or worldview.

A more contemporary example is given in Redding's (2001) call for sociopolitical diversity in psychology. He notes that while psychologists celebrate cultural diversity and castigate those who fail to embrace it, there is a notable lack of critical thought from a conservative political perspective within contemporary psychology. This liberal bias, as it is described, sometimes results in intellectually indefensible conclusions and recommendations for public policy that are heavy on advocacy sprinkled lightly with science. One poignant example that is given concerns adolescents and their legal competency, specifically in regard to making medical decisions like receiving an abortion on the one hand, and at what age they may be transferred to adult court and tried on the other. A review of the literature shows that psychological research on medical decision-making most often focuses on cognitive ability and concludes that adolescents have the capacity to make informed decisions early in their teen years. However, when we turn our lens toward the courts, most research concludes that because of a lack of social maturity, most teens up to age eighteen are not criminally culpable and should not be tried criminally as adults. Redding (2001) provides several other compelling examples for his liberal bias argument, however our intent here is not to attack liberalism or embrace conservatism. Our intention is to point out that within the universe of worldviews, liberal and conservative

differences in the United States are actually quite small, and academic psychology does not fairly represent even that attenuated range. Further, within academic psychology, it may be fair to opine that community psychology represents an even more restricted range in accepted values and ideology.

In sum, a uniformly like-minded group frequently fails to work out the details of implementation, monitoring, and contingency planning, and worst-case scenarios. They may also over-assume what is or is not possible. Consequences and risks are then more likely to be ignored or glossed over. Group-think can be avoided when precautions are taken. It is important to assign roles to individuals in the group so as to prevent confusion and arguments. Group leaders need to solicit and receive feedback and criticism from others regarding decisions. This feedback and examination process needs to be seen as a contributor to quality and not a gripe or complaint mechanism. The potential for holding grudges and punishment of critics must be avoided.

PREVENTIVE INTERVENTION ETHICAL GUIDELINES

This section presents an adaptation of the 1995 Code of Ethics from the National Association of Prevention Professionals and Advocates. We suggest that these principles provide a framework to continue the dialog surrounding ethical principals for prevention practitioners and provide some protections against the hegemony of prevailing beliefs at a given time and place.

Nondiscrimination

Prevention practitioners do not discriminate against service recipients or colleagues based on race, ethnicity, religion, national origin, sex, age, sexual orientation, economic condition, or physical, medical, or mental disability. Prevention practitioners should seek to broaden their understanding and acceptance of cultural and individual differences, and in so doing, render services and provide information that is culturally competent.

Competence

Prevention practitioners observe the Ethical Standards for Psychologists of the American Psychological Association and strive continually to improve personal competence and quality of service delivery, and discharge professional responsibility. Competence is derived from a synthesis of education and experience. It begins with the mastery of a body of knowledge and skill competencies. The maintenance of competence requires a commitment to learning and professional improvement that continues throughout one's professional life. Prevention practitioners should be diligent in discharging responsibilities. Diligence imposes the responsibility to render services carefully and promptly, to be thorough, and to observe applicable technical and ethical standards. Due care requires professionals to plan and supervise adequately and evaluate, to the extent possible, any professional activity for which they are responsible. Prevention practitioners should recognize the limitations and boundaries of competencies and not use techniques or offer services outside of those competencies. Prevention practitioners are responsible for assessing the adequacy of their own competence for the responsibility to be assumed and should seek outside assessments where possible.

When prevention practitioners have knowledge of unethical conduct or practice on the part of an agency or another professional, they have an ethical responsibility to report the conduct or practices to appropriate funding or regulatory bodies or to the public. Prevention practitioners should recognize the effect of impairment on professional performance and should be willing to seek appropriate treatment for themselves.

Integrity

In order to maintain and broaden public confidence, prevention practitioners perform all responsibilities with the highest sense of integrity. Personal gain and advantage should not subordinate service and public trust. Integrity can accommodate the inadvertent error and honest differences of opinion. It cannot accommodate deceit or subordination of principle. All evidence regarding known effects of proposed interventions should be presented fairly and accurately. This evidence should document and assign credit to all contributing sources used in published material or public statements. Prevention practitioners should not be associated directly or indirectly with any service, products, individuals, or organization in a way that is misleading.

Nature of Services

Services provided by prevention practitioners shall be respectful and non-exploitive. The potential for negative consequences that are known as well as the potential for those not yet known should be fully disclosed. Reasonable efforts to obtain informed consent from participants should always be made, and if the target is a minor child, guardian permission should be obtained. Interventions should use the media and other methods of informing the public to obtain "community consent." Forums that invite discussion and dissent should be available. Services should be provided in

a way that preserves the protective factors inherent in each culture and individual. Prevention practitioners should use formal and informal structures to receive and incorporate input from service recipients in the development, implementation, and evaluation of prevention services. Where there is suspicion of abuse of children or vulnerable adults, the prevention practitioner reports the evidence to the appropriate agency and follows up to ensure that appropriate action has been taken.

Confidentiality

Confidential information acquired during service delivery shall be safeguarded from disclosure, including—but not limited to—verbal disclosure, unsecured maintenance of records, or recording of an activity or presentation without appropriate releases. Prevention practitioners are responsible for knowing the confidentiality regulations relevant to their prevention specialty. Prevention practitioners should be proactive on public policy and legislative issues. The public welfare and the individual's right to services and personal wellness should guide the efforts of the general public and policy makers.

CONCLUSION

Ethical considerations in preventive interventions are complex. Efforts may have few or unproven benefits, or may even be harmful. Disclosure of these considerations should always be part of obtaining informed consent. However, there are many impediments to obtaining such consent. These include bias on the part of the prevention practitioner and capacity of the individual providing consent, as both parties need to be aware of any evidence-base for what are complex phenomena. It may be difficult for people to assimilate this information, particularly when children are the target population. We argue that evidence-based practice and a public health perspective can provide a guide through these competing interests for the prevention practitioner. Clinical practice guidelines may be helpful, but they frequently are related to providers' beliefs about practice and are not necessarily based on evidence. Adhering to public health principles and demanding epidemiological evidence can help solve these dilemmas. Research into the efficacy and effectiveness of prevention programs must commit to report and publish both positive and negative results in relation to known rates of disorders in the population. We should also make available balanced, evidence-based information that is comprehensible to the target population. We should increase our emphasis on the ethics of prevention. This can be accomplished in part by making decisions on the basis of relative reductions of morbidity or mortality and the use of evidence-based prevention practice guidelines rather than those based on authority or belief. Perhaps of greatest importance is the willingness to define outcomes in the measurable and countable terms of epidemiology and public health. This will allow us to finally develop an empirical base and standards against which to compare the effectiveness of preventive efforts.

Also see: Diversity: Foundation; Culture, Society, and Social Class: Foundation; Politics and Systems Change: Foundation.

References

Albee, G.W. (1986). Advocates and adversaries in prevention. In M. Kessler & S.E. Goldston (Eds.), *A decade of progress in primary prevention* (pp. 309–332). Hanover, NH: University Press of New England.

Alderfer, C.P. (1989). Commentary on "Responsible to whom? Responsible for what?" *American Journal of Community Psychology, 17*(3) June 1989, 347–354.

Applebaum, P.S., Lidz, C.N., & Meisel, A. (1987). *Informed consent: Legal theory and clinical practice*. New York: Oxford University Press.

Bennet, C.C., Anderson, L.S., Cooper, S., Hassol, L., Klein, D.C., & Rosenblum, G. (Eds.). (1966). *Community psychology: A report of the Boston conference on the education of psychologists for community mental health*. Boston: Boston University Press.

Bloom, B. (1973). *Community mental health: A historical and critical analysis*. Morristown, NJ: General Learning Press.

Bond, M.E. (1989). Ethical dilemmas in context: Some preliminary questions. *American Journal of Community Psychology, 17*(3) June 1989, 355–359.

Caplan, G. (1964). *Principles of community psychiatry*. New York: Basic Books.

Centers for Disease Control and Prevention. (1999). Thimerosal in vaccines: A joint statement of the American Academy of Pediatrics and the Public Health Service. *Morbidity and Mortality Weekly Review, 48,* 563–565.

Cicchetti, D., Rappaport, J., Sandler, I., & Weissberg, R. (Eds.). (2000). *The promotion of wellness in children and adolescence*. Thousand Oaks, CA: Sage.

Cowen, E.L. (1973). Social and community interventions. *Annual Review of Psychology, 24,* 423–472.

Daugherty, C. (1999). Impact of therapeutic research on informed consent and the ethics of clinical trials: A medical oncology perspective. *Journal of Clinical Oncology, 17*(5), 1601–1617.

Davidson, W.S. (1989). Ethical and moral dilemmas in community psychology: Tarnishing the angels' halo. *American Journal of Community Psychology, 17*(3), 385–389.

Golann, S.E. (1969). Emerging areas of ethical concern. *American Psychologist, 24*(4), 454–459.

Gordon, R. (1987). An operational classification of disease prevention. In J.A. Steinberg & M.M. Silverman (Eds.), *Preventing mental disorders: A research perspective* (pp. 20–26). Rockville, MD: DHHS.

Institute of Medicine. (1994). *Reducing risk for mental disorders: Frontiers for preventive intervention research*. Washington, DC: National Academy Press.

Heller, K. (1989). Ethical dilemmas in community intervention. *American Journal of Community Psychology, 17*(3), 367–378.

Janis, I. (1972). *Victims of Groupthink*, Boston: Houghton Mifflin.

Janis, I. (1989). *Crucial decisions: Leadership in policymaking and crisis management* (pp. 89–117). New York: Free Press.

Lillienfeld, D.E., & Stolley, P.D. (1994). *Foundations of epideliology* (3rd ed.). New York: Oxford University Press.

Lorion, R.P. (1983). Evaluating preventive interventions: Guidelines for the serious social change agent. In R.D. Felner, L.A. Jason, J.N. Moritsugu, & S.S. Farber (Eds.), *Preventive psychology: Theory and practice* (pp. 251–268). New York: Pergammon Press.

Lorion, R.P. (1987). The other side of the coin: The potential for negative consequences of prevention interventions: In J.A. Steinberg & M.M. Silverman (Eds.), *Preventing mental disorders: A research perspective*. DHHS Publication No. (ADM) 87-1492.

Meisel, A., Roth, L.H., & Lidz, C.W. (1977). Toward a model of the legal doctrine of informed consent. *American Journal of Psychiatry, 134,* 285–289.

O'Neill, P.T. (1989). Responsible to whom? Responsible to what? Some ethical issues in community intervention. *American Journal of Community Psychology, 17*(3), 323–341.

Pettifor, J.L. (1986). Ethical standards for community psychology. *Canadian Journal of Community Mental Health, 5*(1), 39–48.

Pope, K.S. (1989). A community psychology of ethics: Responding to "Responsible to whom? Responsible for what." *American Journal of Community Psychology, 17,* 343–346.

Rappaport, J. (1981). In praise of paradox: A social policy of empowerment over prevention. *American Journal of Community Psychology, 9,* 1–25.

Redding, R.E. (2001). Sociopolitical diversity in psychology: The case for pluralism. *American Psychologist, 56,* 205–215.

Riger, S. (1989). The politics of community intervention. *American Journal of Community Psychology, 17*(3), 379–383.

Reinharz, S. (1989). Taking on the roles of educator and mediator: Two means of preventing ethical conflicts for community psychologists when financial resources are scarce. *American Journal of Community Psychology, 17*(3), 391–396.

Schumacher, W. (1979). Legal/ethical aspects of vaccinations. International symposium on immunization: Benefit versus risk factors. *Developmental Biology Standards, 43,* 435–438.

Serrano-Garcia, I. (1994). The ethics of the powerful and the power of ethics. *American Journal of Community Psychology, 22*(1), 1–20.

Shore, D. (1996). Ethical principles and informed consent: An NIMH perspective. *Psychopharmacology Bulletin, 32*(1), 7–10.

Snow, D.L., Grady, K., & Goyette-Ewing, M. (2000). A perspective on ethical issues in community psychology. In J. Rappaport & E. Seidman (Eds.), *Handbook of community psychology* (pp. 897–917). New York, NY: Kluwer Academic/Plenum Publishers.

Wakefield, J.C. (1992). Disorder as harmful dysfunction: A conceptual critique of DSM-III—R's definition of mental disorder. *Psychological Review, 99*(2), 232–247.

Wakefield, J.C. (1997). Diagnosing DSM-IV—Part I: DSM-IV and the concept of disorder. *Behaviour Research and Therapy, 35*(7), 633–649.

Watts, R.J. (1993). "Resident research" and community psychology. *American Journal of Community Psychology, 21*(4), 483–486.

Wicker, A.W., & Sommers, R. (1993). The resident researcher: An alternative career model centered on community. *American Journal of Community Psychology, 21*(4), 469–482.

Weithorn, L.A. (1987). Informed consent for prevention research involving children: Legal and ethical issues. In J.A. Steinberg & M.M. Silverman (Eds.), *Preventing mental disorders: A research perspective*. DHHS Publication No. (ADM) 87-1492.

The Use of Consultation as a Foundation for Promoting Health and Preventing Problems

Joseph E. Zins and William P. Erchul

Consultation is a joint problem-solving process that can be applied to a variety of health-enhancing and problem prevention activities. It guides the identification, development, implementation, and evaluation of virtually all of the promotion and prevention strategies described in this volume. Through this collaborative process, participants share their expertise to benefit a third party (e.g., student, child, organization), with consultees (e.g., parent, teacher, agency director) usually being the primary agents who provide the intervention. The indirect manner in which primary prevention assistance is provided distinguishes consultation from other types of professional helping services.

Consultation has a long tradition and is widely practiced within most human service and health care fields (Gallessich, 1982). There generally is agreement on the major components of the process and on the procedures for delivering consultation services. As might be expected, however, there is variation regarding the specific definition of consultation within various disciplines and thus there are differences in some of the interpersonal and problem-solving aspects.

The focus of this entry is on human services consultation, although most concepts are applicable to consulting in other settings. It begins by defining consultation and then distinguishing it from other similar services. Next, three major approaches to consultation are described, along with the elements common to them. Following that section, the literature on the effectiveness of consultation as a means of promoting health and preventing problems is reviewed, and the entry concludes with suggestions for effective practice. Much of the discussion draws upon the work of Erchul and Martens (2002), Gutkin and Curtis (1999), and Zins and Erchul (2002).

DEFINITION

Over the years consultation has acquired many different meanings to professionals within various disciplines, and even those in the same discipline often define the term differently. Despite these variations, there is more agreement than disagreement about the essential ingredients.

Consultation is defined as a method of providing preventively oriented psychological and educational services in which consultants and consultees form cooperative partnerships and engage in a reciprocal, systematic, problem-solving process guided by ecobehavioral principles. The goal is to enhance and empower consultee systems, thereby promoting clients' well-being (Zins & Erchul, 2002). The core elements of consultation listed in the definition are common to most models as described below, although the discussion may be more closely assigned with the ecobehavioral model than any other.

MAJOR MODELS OF CONSULTATION

In this section three of the most commonly used models of consultation are described. There are a number of other models of consultation such as collaborative, conjoint, instructional, process, rational-emotive, and so forth, that have been put forth, but they share essentially the same characteristics and are far more similar than different (Erchul & Martens, 2002).

Behavioral Consultation

Behavioral consultation is based on contemporary theories of learning and behavioral psychology, although more recently ecological and social learning theories have been integrated into the model by many practitioners (thus, some use the term ecobehavioral). However, the major texts on the topic (e.g., Bergan & Kratochwill, 1990) continue to focus almost exclusively on proximal environmental variables, and give little consideration to more distal events (Gutkin & Curtis, 1999) and systems issues, thereby limiting its scope.

Behavioral consultation involves the following problem-solving steps that are conducted during structured interviews: problem identification, problem analysis, implementation, and evaluation. In an expansion of traditional behavioral consultation, Sheridan, Kratochwill, and Bergan (1996) developed an approach that follows the same steps, but the entire process is conducted with parents *and* teachers together. A primary contribution of the behavioral model is its adherence to methodological rigor and scientific precision. Indeed, for this reason, the majority of the research in consultation has focused on this model (Sheridan, Welch, & Orme, 1996).

Mental Health Consultation

Mental health consultation and its associated focus on prevention has its roots in the work of Caplan, as reflected in his 1970 seminal text and follow-up work (Caplan, 1970; Caplan & Caplan, 1993/1999). Although many aspects of ecobehavioral consultation are based on Caplan's pioneering work, there are differences in the two models.

Theoretically, mental health consultation is closely aligned with psychoanalytic theory, which accounts for its focus on more intrapersonal or person-centered issues. There are four overlapping types of mental health consultation: client-centered case consultation, consultee-centered case consultation, program-centered administrative consultation, and consultee-centered administrative consultation. As suggested by the terms, these approaches differ depending on whether the focus is on individual cases or programs. Likewise, they vary in terms of emphasizing prevention or remediation. Consultee-centered case consultation, for example, is directed toward "elucidating and remedying the shortcomings in the consultee's professional functioning ... [so as to] ... lead to an improvement in the consultee's professional planning and action, and hopefully to improvement in the client" (Caplan & Caplan, 1993/1999, p. 101). Even though mental health consultation has received much attention, little empirical support has been produced for it.

Organizational/Systems Consultation

There has been much less written about consultation designed to have an impact on large groups within an organization or on the entire organization, either of which could be the focus of organizational or systems consultation. Many preventionists, however, utilize this approach when implementing programs, and it has the advantage of allowing consultants to share their skills and knowledge with a larger number of individuals, thereby expanding their impact.

This model draws on a number of theoretical perspectives ranging from general systems theory (von Bertalanffy, 1968) to those specifically developed for use in human service organizations (e.g., French & Bell, 1980; Maher, Illback, & Zins, 1984). It involves a planned, systemic process of introducing new principles and practices into an organization, with the goal of effecting organizational improvement, effectiveness, and competence. Consultants can use diagnostic, process, individual, and/or technostructural interventions to assist the organization (Maher et al., 1984), or they can apply consultative principles to implement new programs. Targets might include a range of issues, such as designing an intervention in a youth organization to prevent bullying and harassment, or an organization development program in a public health agency to improve communication among staff.

ELEMENTS COMMON TO MOST MODELS

This section, based on the work of Zins and Erchul (2002), describes the major elements common to most

models of consultation, but it primarily reflects an ecobehavioral orientation (Gutkin, 1993). Some of the primary differences in models were identified in the preceding discussion.

Preventive-Orientation

Consultation has a dual focus. First, it provides a mechanism through which existing problems can be identified, addressed, and resolved. Second, rather than being simply reactive, it is intended to increase consultees' skills so that they can be proactive and more skillfully solve similar problems in the future or prevent their occurrence. Likewise, it may serve to alter environmental variables and setting events that elicit and maintain problematic behaviors or it can be focused on systems level concerns. Consequently, consultative procedures are intended to resolve current problems, while at the same time preventing them from becoming more severe or keeping additional ones from arising, and it may also address more large-scale issues. As discussed later, consultation's potential and promise as a prevention strategy in its own right has yet to be fully realized.

Cooperative Partnership

In contrast to the type of interactions that characterize many professional exchanges in which an expert primarily provides advice to another person or group without much involvement on their part, consultants and consultees work together as partners to solve problems. As a result, they are able to take advantage of the knowledge and expertise that each participant possesses, and thus develop more creative, thoughtful solutions to problems. It is highly desirable for them to establish a relationship characterized by trust, openness, genuine regard, and a sharing of responsibilities and expertise, as the success of the entire process depends on the ability of participants to interact and communicate effectively.

Reciprocal Interactions

The functioning of consultants, consultees, and clients results from the continuous and reciprocal interactions among behavioral, personal, and environmental factors. That is, they influence and are influenced by one another. During the interpersonal exchanges that constitute consultation, participants draw from available power bases (e.g., expert, referent, informational) and exert influence on one another. Their beliefs, attitudes, and behaviors can be altered as a result (Erchul & Raven, 1997), which in many cases helps to resolve the presenting problem or to prevent future ones from occurring.

Ecological/Systems Perspective

Training for many human service providers traditionally had a person-centered focus, and as a result, many practitioners give minimal consideration to addressing system level concerns that may influence the problem situation. However, as it has become clear that a broader range of factors may contribute to the development and maintenance of problems, ecological/systems theories are now used more often. For example, factors such as school climate, federal laws, community support, and teachers' instructional style, each may influence how a student performs in school. Likewise, the effective operation of a community mental health center depends not only on the skills of its managers and employees, but also on the level community involvement and financial support received. Ecological/systems perspectives particularly have been used to expand on traditional approaches in behavioral and organizational consultation.

Means of Empowerment

Consultants explicitly recognize that consultees and consultee systems already possess or readily can develop most competencies necessary to deal with child- and system-related problems when they are given the right opportunities and knowledge of available resources (Rappoport, 1981). As with the ecological/systems perspective, professionals who view their work as helping to empower others must change some of their long-standing beliefs about help giving.

Enhancement of Client Well-Being

Although consultation frequently focuses on improving consultees' skills and performance, changing their behavior, or modifying some aspect of the environment, the ultimate beneficiary of the efforts is always intended to be the client. The client could be an individual child, a family, a group within an organization, an entire organization, or even a community.

Systematic Problem-Solving Process

Consultation primarily involves having participants engage in joint problem solving. During the process, they proceed through an orderly, systematic sequence of steps, as shown in Table 1 and discussed below. Although the steps generally proceed sequentially, there is some flexibility in the order in which they occur. It is essential for consultants to be skilled in these techniques.

Establishing a cooperative partnership. Prerequisites to effective problem solving include adequate communication skills and development of a trusting partnership.

Table 1. Consultative Problem-Solving Process

Establishment of cooperative partnership
- Promote understanding of each other's roles and responsibilities
- Avoid the egalitarian virus.

Problem identification and analysis
- Define problem in behavioral terms and obtain agreement with consultee
- Collect baseline data regarding problem frequency, duration, and/or intensity and conduct task analysis as needed
- Identify antecedent determinants of the problem behavior
- Identify consequences that may maintain the behavior
- Assess other relevant environmental factors
- Identify all available resources.

Intervention development and selection
- Brainstorm range of possible interventions
- Evaluate the positive and negative aspects of the interventions
- Select intervention(s) from the alternatives generated.

Intervention implementation, evaluation, and follow-up
- Clarify implementation procedures and responsibilities
- Implement the chosen strategy
- Evaluate intended outcomes and any side effects
- Program generalization, plan maintenance, and develop appropriate fading procedures
- Recycle and follow-up as necessary.

Note: From Zins & Erchul (2002). Copyright 2002 by the National Association of School Psychologists. Reprinted by permission of the publisher.

Participants must be able to interact effectively and build trust in one another before they can solve problems.

Clarifying the problem. The first and most important step in actual problem solving is identification and clarification of the problem. Problems should be identified in objective, measurable terms to the extent possible so that progress in solving them can be assessed.

If the problem is not identified properly, efforts are likely to be directed toward solving the wrong problem. On the other hand, once it is correctly identified, there is a good chance that it will be resolved satisfactorily. It often takes a good amount of time to complete this process, particularly for external consultants, as a wide variety of contextual factors need to be understood.

Problem analysis. During this step participants try to understand the forces that are causing and maintaining the problem situation, as well as those that may be available to resolve it. Participants develop the best hypotheses about the problem possible. Taking a broad, ecological/systems perspective is important, as problems usually are the result of a complex interaction of multiple factors. Unless these various factors are considered, it is likely that a simplistic, ineffective problem solution will be developed.

Brainstorming and exploring intervention options. Once the problem has been defined and analyzed, the next step is to consider possible means of resolving it. At this stage using a very flexible, brainstorming approach is a helpful way to identify a vast array of potential solutions. Both consultants and consultees should contribute to the brainstorming process so that the most creative, thoughtful ideas can be generated.

Selecting an intervention. Once the list of potential solutions is developed, participants need to examine each for its feasibility, cost, likelihood of success, and consequences. Although there are always limited resources, it is common on the other hand to overlook potential resources that may be both effective and inexpensive (e.g., senior citizen volunteers, cooperative learning). Similarly, the issues of intervention acceptability needs to be considered, as consultees may be hesitant to implement a particular strategy because of its costs, perceived effectiveness, how much it disrupts routines, and so forth (Elliott, 1988). It is important to remember that even after an intervention has been selected, the list that was generated from the brainstorming should be maintained in the event the chosen intervention does not work.

Clarifying implementation procedures and responsibilities. A great deal of effort will have been put forth by this point in the consultative problem-solving process. For that reason, it is common to find that to save time or for other reasons, implementation procedures often are not specified in sufficient details. As a result, treatments that usually have been found to be effective may not work. The issue is not that the wrong treatment was implemented, but rather that it was not implemented correctly and/or that was provided for an insufficient amount of time. For these reasons it is advisable to develop a written plan of action and to explicitly make plans to follow-up once the intervention has been implemented as well as to establish a plan for monitoring the implementation process. Participants can then determine the extent to which the intervention is being implemented as planned, which has significant implications with respect to interpreting positive and negative outcomes. Even though monitoring the implementation process involves additional effort, there is danger that potentially useful interventions may be prematurely and inaccurately discontinued unless steps are taken in this regard (Durlak, 1998).

Implementing the strategy. The chosen strategy can now be put into action according to the plans and timelines developed. Consultants need to be available to consultees in the event that unforeseen problems arise or some changes in the environment occur. Also, consultants can provide support for consultees' efforts, as initially consultees may not receive much positive feedback in terms of seeing improvements in the problem situation.

Evaluating intervention effectiveness and follow-up. Consultants need to remain available as long as necessary. Eventually, however, their goal is to terminate their involvement in this particular problem situation.

During the first step it was emphasized that problems should be identified in objective, measurable terms. If that process occurred, then it should be possible at this point to evaluate progress toward resolving the problem, assuming that sufficient time has passed and improvements reasonably could be expected.

Other Issues

A few other aspects of the process need to be mentioned. First, the issues discussed during consultation must remain confidential (issues such as child abuse, drug use, etc., may be exceptions) if consultees are to develop a high level of trust in consultants. Second, consultants and consultees have "temporary" relationships, in that their work together ceases once the problem is resolved. Of course, they can resume their relationship if the problem emerges again or to address other concerns. In fact, it may be beneficial for consultants and consultees to have a series of consultative interactions, as the process often proceeds much more expeditiously when they become more proficient in working together.

Consultants can be internal or external to the system. Most schools, for example, employ counselors and special education teachers who may serve as consultants to the general education teachers, while a public advocacy agency may employ a consultant on a contractual basis to help it deal with the low morale of its employees or to evaluate a new program. Internal consultants tend to understand the workings of the organization and the people within it much better because of their more frequent interactions and continuous involvement. On the other hand, external consultants may have the advantage of being more objective in their perceptions of problems and may be less likely to feel pressured by organizational members to make certain decisions.

Finally, the term consultation often is used interchangeably with collaboration. Caplan and Caplan (1993/1999), however, describe collaboration as involving both direct (e.g., social skills training) and indirect (e.g., consultation) service. Similarly, consultation is distinguished from supervision in that it does not involve the evaluation of consultees' performance. It likewise differs from the expert advice giving commonly found in the medical fields, which involves a referral to an expert who examines the patient and then prescribes a recommendation for treatment. Thus, it is more of a direct service that usually involves little interaction between the professionals. In these fields consultation as used in this entry is most similar to consultation liaison. Finally, consultation employs many skills in interpersonal interactions similar to counseling. However, consultation focuses on work- or care-giving-related issues involving a third part, while counseling is directed toward solving personal or emotional problems.

REVIEW OF LITERATURE ON EFFECTIVENESS OF CONSULTATION AS A MEANS OF PROMOTING HEALTH AND PREVENTING PROBLEMS

The research base in consultation has continued to grow over the years despite the inherent difficulties in undertaking such investigations and the associated problems with the studies that have been conducted (Gresham & Noell, 1993). For example, when conducting research on the implementation and outcomes of a smoking prevention program, it is necessary to (a) examine the consultation process by which the program was developed and implemented, and (b) evaluate the outcomes of the prevention program with clients. Frequently, the consultative aspects are described only minimally, making it difficult to determine what was actually done. Further, consultees often carry out the actual preventive intervention, a process over which consultants have little control. Thus, this simple example makes it easy to recognize why there remains a need to improve the met' \odology, scope, quality, and quantity of consultation 1 search. Despite the shortcomings in the research, several meta-analyses and literature reviews that have examined consultation (e.g., Busse, Kratochwill, & Elliott, 1995; Medway & Updyke, 1985; Sheridan et al., 1996), provide a level of support for its effectiveness. Sheridan and her colleagues, for instance, conducted a comprehensive analysis of 46 school consultation outcome studies that were published between 1985 and 1995. They found that consultation produced at least some positive results in 67 percent of the studies reviewed, while 28 percent were neutral. The other 5 percent were negative. As noted earlier, behavioral consultation studies were most prevalent compared to mental health, organization, and various teaming strategies. They also noted that advances had been made in the use of experimental designs, multiple outcome measures, assessment of acceptability, and attention to social validity.

SYNTHESIS: SUGGESTIONS FOR EFFECTIVE PRACTICE

Consultation continues to be discussed frequently in the literature, yet it is common to find that what is actually meant by the term is not specified sufficiently. It is clear that there is a need for more precision when discussing the process, and this entry represents our efforts to define the term and to describe the elements of effective practice.

Philosophically, there continues to be a need to increase commitment to prevention and health promotion efforts, to adoption of ecological perspectives, and to development of true partnerships with consultees. These conceptualizations are consistent with the approach to consultation described, and they must take place if there is to be more support for prevention and promotion programs. Expanding practice to include more organizational consul-tation also would give human service providers additional opportunities to share their expertise and expand their influence.

Implementation is an area that has been given only minimal attention in the consultation, treatment, health promotion, and prevention literatures. More attention must be devoted to it because of its importance in determining the internal, external, construct, and statistical validity of the outcomes of these procedures (see Noell, Witt, Gilbertson, Ranier, & Freeland, 1997).

Finally, in recent years, use of the term evidence-based interventions has increased (e.g., Task Force on Promotion, 1995). Although there may be different points of view about what constitutes sufficient evidence to support a particular intervention, consultation clearly can be used to implement such procedures and programs.

Also see: Theories: Foundation; Politics and Systems Change: Foundation; Community Capacity.

References

Bergan, J.R., & Kratochwill, T.R. (1990). *Behavioral consultation in applied settings.* New York: Plenum.

Busse, R.T., Kratochwill, T.R., & Elliott, S.N. (1995). Meta-analysis for single-case outcomes: Applications to research and practice. *Journal of School Psychology, 33,* 269–285.

Caplan, G. (1970). *The theory and practice of mental health consultation.* New York: Basic Books.

Caplan, G., & Caplan, R.B. (1999). *Mental health consultation and collaboration.* Prospect Heights, IL: Waveland Press. (Original work published 1993.)

Durlak, J. (1998). Why program implementation is important. *Journal of Prevention and Intervention in the Community, 17,* 5–18.

Elliott, S.N. (1988). Acceptability of behavioral treatments: Review of variables that influence treatment selection. *Professional Psychology: Research and Practice, 19,* 68–80.

Erchul, W.P., & Martens, B.K. (2002). *School consultation: Conceptual and empirical bases of practice* (2nd ed.). New York: Kluwer Academic.

Erchul, W.P., & Raven, B.H. (1997). Social power in school consultation: A contemporary view of French and Raven's bases of power model. *Journal of School Psychology, 35,* 137–171.

French, W., & Bell, C.H. (1980). *Organization development* (2nd ed.). Englewood Cliffs, NJ: Prentice-Hall.

Gallessich, J. (1982). *The practice and profession of consultation.* San Francisco: Jossey-Bass.

Gresham, F.M., & Noell, G.H. (1993). Documenting the effectiveness of consultation outcomes. In J.E. Zins, T.R. Kratochwill, & S.N. Elliott (Eds.), *Handbook of consultation services for children* (pp. 249–273). San Francisco: Jossey-Bass.

Gutkin, T.B. (1993). Moving from behavioral to ecobehavioral consultation: What's in a name? *Journal of Educational and Psychological Consultation, 4,* 95–99.

Gutkin, T.B., & Curtis, M.J. (1999). School-based consultation theory and practice: The art and science of indirect service delivery. In C.R. Reynolds & T.B. Gutkin (Eds.), *The handbook of school psychology* (3rd ed., pp. 598–637). New York: John Wiley.

Maher, C.A., Illback, R.J., & Zins, J.E. (Eds.).(1984). *Organizational psychology in the schools.* Springfield, IL: Thomas.

Medway, F.J., & Updyke, J.F. (1985). Meta-analysis of consultation outcome studies. *American Journal of Community Psychology, 13,* 489–504.

Noell, G.H., Witt, J.C., Gilbertson, D.N., Ranier, D.D., & Freeland, J.T. (1997). Increasing teacher intervention implementation in general education settings through consultation and performance feedback. *School Psychology Quarterly, 12,* 77–88.

Rappoport, J. (1981). In praise of paradox: A social policy of empowerment over prevention. *American Journal of Community Psychology, 9,* 1–25.

Sheridan, S.M., Kratochwill, T.R., & Bergan, J.R. (1996). *Conjoint behavioral consultation: A procedural manual.* New York: Plenum.

Sheridan, S.M., Welch, M., & Orme, S.F. (1996). Is consultation effective? A review of outcome research. *Remedial and Special Education, 17,* 341–354.

Task Force on Promotion and Dissemination of Psychological Procedures. (1995). Training in and dissemination of empirically-validated psychological treatments. *The Clinical Psychologist, 48,* 3–23.

von Bertalanffy, L. (1968). *General systems theory.* New York: Braziller.

Zins, J.E., & Erchul, W.P. (2002). Best practices in school consultation. In A. Thomas & J. Grimes (Eds.), *Best practices in school psychology-IV* (pp. 625–644). Bethesda, MD: National Association of School Psychologists.

Achieving an Ecologically Sustainable Future

E. Scott Geller

The future of Earth is uncertain because of acid rain, global warming, damage to the protective ozone layer, worldwide misuse of land and water, and overpopulation. These problems can be alleviated through technological advances, but not solved. There is a crucial role for social and behavioral science in addressing our environmental crisis. In fact, the sustainability of Earth is inextricably dependent upon human behavior. Some of our behaviors degrade the environment, while other behaviors protect our environment. An ecologically sustainable future is contingent on the large-scale increase of environment-preserving behaviors and worldwide decrease of environment-destructive behaviors. This entry addresses the human element of environmental protection and sustainability by reviewing current theories and intervention approaches that need to be considered if the three main sources of the Earth's environmental problems are to be addressed—human overpopulation, overconsumption, and underconservation.

The following terms need to be defined.

Acid rain refers to invisible plumes of sulfur and nitrogen oxides in rain and clouds resulting from the burning of oil and coal.

Chlorofluorocarbons (*CFCs*) are ozone-destroying chemicals, such as Freon, which are used worldwide as solvents, as refrigerants in air-conditioning systems, and as foam-blowing agents for making insulation. They were once used as propellants in aerosol cans until that application was banned in the 1980s.

Dioxin is a carcinogenic chemical resulting from the burning of fossil fuels, the incineration of plastics and paper, the bleaching of paper with chlorine, and the manufacturing of various chlorine-containing chemicals such as pesticides.

Establishing condition refers to certain psychological state, expectancy, or mood caused by external operations, interpersonal relationships, or environmental conditions that influences behavior, analogous to food or social deprivation increasing a person's tendency to seek food or social attention.

Ecology is the science concerned with the relationship between organisms and their environment.

The greenhouse effect refers to the amount of Earth's heat radiated into space which is reduced by carbon dioxide (CO_2) produced when oil, gas, coal, or wood are burned, much as the glass roof in a greenhouse lets in warming sunlight but prevents warm air from escaping.

The ozone layer is a region of the upper atmosphere, between 10 and 20 miles in altitude, containing a high concentration of ozone that absorbs solar ultraviolet rays, thereby shielding Earth from radiation from the sun that could cause skin cancer in humans and similar damage to many crops and to the plankton that forms the base of the ocean food chain.

Some have claimed that our environmental crises have reached proportions of no repair (e.g., Ehrlich, Ehrlich, & Holdren, 1977), while others maintain a relentless optimism regarding planetary concerns. Some adopt a "business as usual" stance (as if environmental problems will correct themselves naturally); others assume high-technology engineering, physics, biology, and chemistry will find sufficient answers. Thus, we not only have a problem of environmental sustainability, but we also have a problem of human denial, helplessness, or apathy. Skinner (1987), defined this crisis elegantly and succinctly as follows:

> Most thoughtful people agree that the world is in serious trouble … fossil fuels will not last forever, and many other critical resources are nearing exhaustion; the earth grows steadily less habitable; and all this is exacerbated by a burgeoning population that resists control. The timetable may

not be clear, but the threat is real. That many people have begun to find a recital of these dangers tiresome is perhaps an even greater threat. (Skinner, 1987, p. 1)

According to Oskamp (2000) there are currently seven drastic dangers to the Earth's environment:

1. Global warming due to the greenhouse effect will result in an average warming of the Earth's surface air temperature by approximately 3.5 °F by the year 2100. Even an average increase of 1 or 2 °F can change regional climates, disrupt agriculture world-wide, and cause extensive melting of the polar ice-caps which in turn will raise ocean levels and cause flooding of vast areas of low-lying coastal communities worldwide.

2. Loss of the Earth's protective ozone layer as a result of the release of CFCs. This allows the penetration of excessive ultraviolet radiation that has damaging impact on human, animal, and plant health, as well as on world fisheries.

3. Destruction of tropical and temperate rain forests causing global climate change and the extinction of plant and animal species. This leads to flooding, land erosion, the clogging of streams and rivers, and rising temperatures. According to the eminent zoologist E.O. Wilson, continuing the current rate of deforestation could result in the extinction of more than 50 percent of the Earth's plant and animal species by the end of this century (cited in Oskamp, 2000).

4. Exhaustion of fisheries, agricultural land, and water supplies as a result of numerous unsustainable practices, including pollution from city sewers, factory toxic waste, and runoff of agricultural pesticides and fertilizers.

5. Acid rain which kills fish, plants, organisms in lakes and rivers, and destroys crops and forests.

6. Toxic pollution of air and water due to the burning of fossil fuels, mining with toxic chemicals, and farming with fertilizers and pesticides. In addition, contamination from manufacturing wastes and garbage landfills have made numerous water supplies unsafe to drink.

7. Exposure to toxic chemicals such as dioxin which are dangerous carcinogens cumulating to alarming levels in the body tissue of most Americans.

Psychological approaches to sustaining ecology are essentially founded in behaviorism and humanism. Behaviorists study overt behavior and its observable environmental, social, and physiological determinants. In contrast, humanists attempt to increase environmental preserving behavior by reasoning with people or appealing to guilt or "social conscience." In general, behaviorism offers the technology for changing behaviors and attitudes in pro-environment directions, whereas humanism offers the states or expectancies needed in people to increase their propensity to use behavioral technology for environmental protection.

THE ACTIVELY CARING MODEL

Geller (1995) integrated behavioral and humanistic perspectives by presenting basic behavior change techniques that have been shown to be effective in motivating environmentally responsible behavior (ERB) and proposing that certain psychological states or establishing conditions increase the probability that this technology will be applied to benefit the environment. In other words, the performance of ERB is dependent on people having certain person states. And, particular interpersonal and environmental factors (including education and training) can benefit these person states and thereby increase a person's propensity to actively care for ecology.

These person states are illustrated in Figure 1, and are variables discussed frequently by humanists but rarely by behaviorists. An integration of behaviorism and humanism is represented by the fact that operations and contingencies developed and evaluated by behaviorists can be used to influence these states defined and appreciated by humanists. It is proposed that these states (or establishing conditions) increase the occurrence of actively caring or altruistic behavior, which includes emitting ERBs and serving as

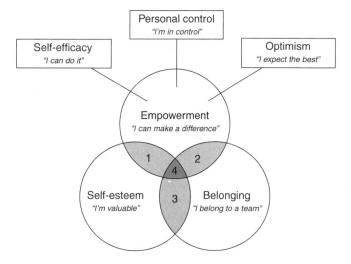

1. I can make valuable differences
2. We can make a difference
3. I'm a valuable team member
4. We can make valuable differences

Figure 1. The Actively Caring Model (adapted from Geller, 1995).

intervention agents to motivate others to also actively care for the environment.

COMPETENCE THEORY

Kaplan (2000) proposed that focusing on altruism as a key motive for ERB is problematic because it alludes to such behavior being sacrificial and beyond self-interest. Similarly, DeYoung (2000) theorized that presuming "humans are egocentric gain-maximizers" (p. 514) with no concern for ecological sustainability saps the potential internal motivation derived from ERB. Both these researchers and scholars offer a similar alternative perspective which relates to the theory that the human concern for competence is a primary source of motivation (White, 1959).

White argues that the desire for competence is self-initiating and self-rewarding, and the behaviors related to a sense of competence are highly focused activities that are inherently reinforcing. This notion is quite similar to self-efficacy theory (Bandura, 1997), and to the empowerment domain of the actively caring model described above, which in addition to self-efficacy, includes two other concepts directly linked to perceived competency—personal control (Rotter, 1966) and optimism (Seligman, 1991).

Kaplan (2000) refers to this alternative way of considering ERB as the Reasonable Person Model. He assumes people are motivated to know, to understand what is going on, to learn, to discover, and to participate. They work to avoid feeling incompetent or helpless. Given this, ERB should be discussed in the context of increasing competence, maintaining personal control, and avoiding helplessness. Since people are naturally motivated to make beneficial differences, it is not necessary to call on guilt or sacrifice to get people involved in procedures to preserve and protect our planet. Participating in efforts to sustain ecology provides opportunities to satisfy a basic human need—the need for competence.

COMMUNITY-BASED SOCIAL MARKETING

Recognizing the failure of information-intensive campaigns to foster ERB, McKenzie-Mohr (2000) proposed a community-based social marketing model for large-scale prevention of environmental problems. This approach merges principles from behavioral science and social marketing (see also Geller, 1989) to maximize the community-wide dissemination and impact of behavior-change techniques (as reviewed in the next section on evidence-based research).

The following procedural steps comprise the community-based social marketing approach: (1) select potential behaviors to target, which could be environment-destructive behaviors to decrease or ERBs to increase, (2) identify the various barriers associated with each of the potential actions, and decide whether resources and strategies are available to remove the barriers, (3) based on an analysis of barriers, decide which behavior(s) to target, (4) design an intervention process to overcome the barriers to the selected behavior(s), (5) pilot the behavior-change program on a small scale to identify the most cost-effective approach and refine specific strategies, (6) implement the refined intervention community-wide, and (7) evaluate changes in the target behavior, as well as actual environmental impact (e.g., decreases in electricity or water consumption) and participants' opinions of the program.

Following the first Earth Day in the Spring of 1970, behaviorists began applying behavior-change interventions to sustain ecology. They followed a simple Activator–Behavior–Consequence scheme, or ABC model, with the basic premise that activators direct behavior and consequences motivate behavior.

ACTIVATORS

Activators for environmental protection have taken the form of: (1) written or spoken messages (e.g., films, television commercials, promotional fliers, verbal reminders, and road signs); (2) awareness or education sessions; (3) modeling or demonstrations (e.g., on videotape or by live exemplars); (4) goal setting (to reach certain individual or group performance outcomes); (5) commitment techniques (by signing a promise card to emit certain behavior); and (6) engineering and design techniques that make the desired behavior more salient or convenient (e.g., adding decorated trash receptacles or recycling bins to the milieu).

The wealth of field research evaluating the impact of activator techniques on environment destructive and preserving behaviors is reviewed in several sources (e.g., Cone & Hayes, 1980; Dwyer, Leeming, Cobern, Porter, & Jackson, 1993; Geller, Winett, & Everett, 1982). Generally, activators alone (without consequences) have been effective at increasing environmental protective behaviors when the instructions have been behavior-specific and given in close physical and temporal proximity with opportunities to emit the target behavior, and when performing the behavior is relatively convenient (e.g., like turning off lights in unoccupied rooms, using a particular trash receptacle or recycling container, or purchasing drinks in returnable bottles).

When target behaviors are perceived as being relatively inconvenient to perform, behavior change interventions have usually required consequences to have substantial beneficial impact. A notable exception has been the application of "pledge card commitment" activators. Field researchers, for example, have markedly increased participation in community recycling programs by asking residents to sign cards promising their participation (e.g., Burn & Oskamp, 1986; Wang & Katzev, 1990).

CONSEQUENCES

Incentives and disincentives are activators that announce the availability of a rewarding or penalizing consequence, respectively, in order to motivate behavior change. Traditionally, local, state, and federal governments have used disincentives and penalties to motivate environment-preserving behaviors. These attempts to protect the environment usually take the form of ordinances or laws (e.g., fines for littering, illegal dumping, using excessive water, or for polluting land, water, or air); and to be effective, these disincentive/penalty interventions usually require extensive promotion (activators) and enforcement (consequences). Behaviorists have de-emphasized this approach, primarily because negative effect, feelings, or attitudes typically accompany attempts to mandate behavior change through disincentive/penalty tactics.

TYPES OF REWARD CONTINGENCIES

The reward contingencies implemented for environmental protection have been diverse. Some rewards have been given after the performance of a desired target behavior, whereas other rewards have been contingent upon a particular outcome (e.g., for reaching a designated level of environmental cleanliness, energy conservation, or water savings). The rewards themselves have varied widely, including such events as monetary rebates, verbal commendations, merchandise discount coupons, raffle tickets, self-photographs, soft drinks, and recognition on an "energy efficient" honor roll.

As reviewed in several documents (e.g., Cone & Hayes, 1980; Dwyer et al., 1993; Geller et al., 1982), most of the reward contingencies produced dramatic increases in the desired behaviors; but unfortunately the behaviors usually returned to pre-intervention baseline levels when the reward contingencies were withdrawn. However, most of the intervention phases in this research were relatively short term and likely did not allow sufficient time for natural consequences such as social approval, media recognition, or visible environmental improvement to gain control. Moreover, many of the rewarding consequences (e.g., raffle coupons for prizes donated by community merchants) were inexpensive enough to keep in place for long time periods. Indeed, in some cases it is cost effective to maintain a consequence strategy indefinitely. Many feedback strategies, for example, are cheap and effective, and do not have to be withdrawn.

FEEDBACK TECHNIQUES

Most of the feedback research for environmental protection addressed residential energy consumption, and the feedback was usually given to residents (e.g., see review by Winett, 1980). The more labor-intensive procedures included the delivery of feedback cards with amount of kilowatt hours or cubic feet of gas used (and the cost) for a particular time period. The technology is currently available to deliver this sort of feedback directly and automatically to homes equipped with appropriate displays. Analogous devices have been tested and have shown much promise for dramatic energy savings, including a hygrothermograph giving continuous readings of room temperatures and humidity, an electronic feedback meter with a digital display of electricity cost per hour, a special device with a light that illuminates whenever electricity use exceeds 90 percent of a household's peak level, and a fuel flow meter that displays continuous miles-per-gallon or gallons-per-hour consumption of gasoline during vehicle travel.

To achieve a sustainable ecology, large-scale changes in behavior are needed worldwide. As reviewed in the prior section, substantial research has demonstrated beneficial impact of applying the basic three-term contingency of applied behavior analysis (i.e., ABC). However, there have been few if any large-scale implementations of any of these behavior-change strategies for environmental protection. Thus, while the direct behavioral approach is clearly the most cost-effective strategy for increasing ERBs and decreasing environment-destructive behavior, it has not as yet produced large-scale environmental benefits. In this section, reasons for this lack of impact are considered, as well as ways to overcome these deficiencies.

WHO IS THE AUDIENCE?

There are a variety of possible reasons for the failure of the studies reviewed in the prior section to have any notable impact on environmental sustainability. Most obvious is the audience of these demonstration projects. The research is published in professional journals and books read almost exclusively by other psychologists. As such, the authors give convincing demonstrations of the efficacy of their behavior-change techniques to people who have little interest or influence in large-scale dissemination and application. In other words, the critical social marketing aspects of behavior-change technology have not been addressed (Geller, 1989).

Bailey (1991) commented on this dissemination problem as follows, "We have a great science (the experimental analysis of behavior) and a pretty good technology (applied behavior analysis) but no product development or marketing"

(p. 39). He explains further that "we do not value market-ing" and have "neglected to develop socially acceptable ter-minology for presenting our concepts to consumers... we have, in our zest for science and technology, taken the human concerns out of behavior analysis" (p. 39).

WHAT BEHAVIORS ARE TARGETED?

Another problem may be the selection of target behav-iors to change. Oskamp (2000), for example, identified over-population and overconsumption as the key threats to environmental sustainability, not litter control or recycling which have been prime targets for applied behavior analysts.

Stern and Gardner (1987) distinguish between curtail-ment behaviors (such as reducing consumption) and effi-ciency behaviors (which reduce the resource consumption of equipment and machinery). They emphasize that people can do more to save environmental resources by purchasing energy-efficient vehicles and water heaters than by carpool-ing or insulating their current water heater. Moreover, effi-ciency behaviors require a one-time purchase of an environmentally friendly product (from vehicles and major appliances to home heating and cooling systems), whereas curtailment behaviors typically involve repeating inconven-ient or sacrificial action (from carpooling and collecting recyclables to reducing water use and turning back thermo-stats). Behavior analysts have typically targeted curtailment behaviors rather than one-shot efficiency behaviors.

WHO SHOULD CHANGE?

Efficiency behavior requires efficiency options, and such avail-ability is greatly determined by organizations and government policy. Stern and Gardner (1987) emphasized "corporations make a greater direct contribution to environmental problems than individuals, and it is worth examining whether more can be done to alleviate these problems by modifying corporate rather than individual behavior" (p. 1050). Thirteen years later, Stern (2000) makes the same point, reminding us that "organ-izations usually do more to degrade the environment than indi-viduals and households" (p. 523), and "If manufacturers adopt 'greener' production technologies and product designs, this will further increase the potential to help solve environmental problems without sacrificing well-being" (p. 525).

CAN BEHAVIOR CHANGE BE MAINTAINED?

Another reason for the lack of environmental impact from behavioral technology is the fact that long-term maintenance and institutionalization of behavior-change strategies have rarely been studied. All of the applications of behavior analysis to change environment-related behavior have been short-term demonstration projects, conducted to show that a particular intervention procedure has a desired effect. Methods to sustain the environmental impact of a behavior-change technique have not been addressed. This is not critical for one-time efficiency behaviors, but is obvi-ously necessary for the regular repetition of curtailment behaviors.

Boyce and Geller (2001) addressed this challenge of response maintenance by reviewing the research literature related to applying behavior analysis techniques to improve occupational safety. They found no systematic study of fac-tors related to successful institutionalization of an effective behavior-change process. However, they did identify some variables conducive to sustaining a successful behavior-change process, and these have been verified by practitioners (McSween & Mathews, 2001). For example, the following factors contribute to the long-term impact of behavior-change interventions in industrial settings.

- Each level of an organization (from management to line workers) need education and training to under-stand the rationale behind an intervention, and to real-ize their specific roles in making the process work.
- Indigenous staff need to implement the intervention procedures and thus have substantial input into intervention design.
- A formal accountability system is required, which is best handled by an employee-manned steering com-mittee that monitors intervention results and devel-ops action plans for enhancing intervention impact.
- A formal procedure for collecting, reviewing, and using behavioral results is needed to support the accountability system and enable continuous improvement.
- Group and individual rewards are needed to support ongoing participation in the process, as well as to recognize exemplary achievements.

Although these conclusions were derived from large-scale applications of behavior analysis to improve safety performance in organizations, they are certainly relevant to sustaining environmental protection interventions, espe-cially in organizational settings which should be a prime tar-get (Stern, 2000; Stern & Gardner, 1987).

The direct behavior-change approach is most cost-effective over the short term, but may not be the best strategy for long-term environmental protection. The challenge of per-suading the right audience to adopt and maintain ERBs was addressed above. Now let us consider some inherent prob-lems with direct persuasion. Aronson (1999) suggests that indirect or self-persuasion is necessary for durable behavior change, and there is substantial empirical research to support this viewpoint.

DIRECT PERSUASION

Advertisers use direct persuasion. They show us people enjoying positive consequences or avoiding negative consequences by using their products. As such, they apply the ABC contingency discussed above to sell their wares or services. The activator (or "A" of the ABC contingency) announces the availability of a reinforcing consequence (the "C" of the ABC contingency) if the purchasing behavior is performed (the "B" of the ABC contingency). Advertisers are not requesting behavior that is inconvenient or difficult. Normally, the purpose of an advertisement is merely to persuade a consumer to select a certain brand of merchandise.

Environment-sustaining behavior is usually more inconvenient and requires more effort than switching brands at a supermarket. It often requires significant adjustment in a highly practiced and regular routine at work, at home, or on the road. Thus, adopting a pro-environment way of doing something might first require the elimination of an efficient and convenient habit that uses excessive environmental resources. Furthermore, participation in an environment-sustaining effort usually requires the regular performance of several inconvenient ERBs.

Consequently, direct persuasion might not be the most effective approach for increasing the frequency of ERBs. Since other people are not usually around to hold us accountable for selecting the most pro-environment behavior available, we need to hold ourselves accountable. We need to view ERB as consistent with our perception of ourselves. In other words, we need to perceive ourselves as ecology-sustaining people.

BEHAVIORAL SELF-PERCEPTION

Bem (1972) prefaces his behavioral presentation of self-perception theory with "... individuals come to 'know' their own attitudes, emotions, and other internal states by inferring them from observations of their own overt behavior and/or the circumstances in which this behavior occurs" (p. 2). In other words, we write mental scripts or make internal attributions about ourselves from our observations and interpretations of the various ABC contingencies that enter our life space. And, "... if external contingencies seem sufficient to account for the behavior, then the individual will not be led into using the behavior as a source of evidence for his self-attributions" (p. 19).

Thus, children who had the excuse of a severe threat for not playing with a "forbidden toy" did not internalize a rule, and therefore played with the forbidden toy when the threat contingency was removed (Lepper & Greene, 1978). Similarly, college students paid $20 for telling other students a boring task was fun did not develop a personal view that the task was enjoyable (Festinger & Carlsmith, 1959). The reinforcement contingency made their behavior incredible as a reflection of their belief or self-perception.

In contrast, participants who received a mild threat or low compensation (only $1) to motivate their behavior developed a self-perception consistent with their behavior. The children avoided playing with the forbidden toy in a subsequent situation with no threat, and the college students who lied for low compensation decided they must have liked the boring task. In theory, these participants viewed their behavior as a valid guide for inferring their private views, since their behavior was not under strong contingency control.

Much additional research supports the notion that self-persuasion is more likely when the extrinsic control of the ABC contingency is less obvious or perhaps indirect. In other words, when there are sufficient external consequences to justify the amount of effort required for an ERB, the performer does not develop an internal justification for the behavior. There is no self-persuasion (Aronson, 1999) and performing the behavior does not alter self-perception (Bem, 1972). Under these circumstances, the maintenance of ERB is unlikely, unless it is possible to keep a sufficient accountability system (e.g. incentives or disincentives) in place over the long term.

A substantial amount of environment-focused research has attempted to measure individual propensity to perform ERBs. The construct reflecting a person's natural internal motivation to protect the environment has been termed "environmental concern" (Weigel & Weigel, 1978), "ecological consciousness" (Ellis & Thompson, 1997), "proenvironmental orientation" (Dunlap & Van Liere, 1978), and "ecological worldview" (Dunlap, Van Liere, Mertig, & Jones, 2000). It might be theoretically useful to search for personality states and traits that relate to the performance of ERBs, but the practical utility of this approach for primary prevention is equivocal.

If a consistent pro-environment profile were identified (which has not happened yet), it might be possible to use this information to select behavior-change agents for community-wide promotion of ERBs. Or, if the individual difference variables were transient states (rather than permanent traits), it might be possible to move such states (or establishing conditions) in a pro-environment direction, as proposed by the actively caring model described earlier (see Figure 1). These possibilities are far removed from current reality, however, and given the need for immediate large-scale promotion of

ERBs, this approach should be abandoned for the systematic search of practical ways to directly and indirectly increase and institutionalize ERBs.

An integration or synthesis of the effective primary prevention strategies for ecological sustainability entails essentially a summary of the principal points in this entry relevant to intervention, from the significant theories and evidence-based research reviewed to the discussion of direct and indirect primary prevention strategies. Each of the theories is relevant for the development of large-scale and long-term community programs to increase ERBs and decrease environment-destructive behaviors. In addition, the various challenges discussed in disseminating and implementing a behavior-change process and maintaining its effects need to be considered when designing a far-reaching environmental protection program.

External contingencies are not usually available to motivate pro-environment behavior. Therefore, it is often necessary to implement an intervention process to motivate environment-protective behavior on a large scale. However, to promote self-persuasion and self-accountability, it is critical for the ABC contingency of applied behavior analysis to be strong enough to get the behavior started but not overly powerful to provide complete justification for the effort. But, of course, this is only relevant for curtailment behaviors, or pro-environment practices that need to be regularly repeated in order to have substantial beneficial impact on the environment. In the case of one-shot efficiency behaviors, a single application of the ABC contingency can motivate the purchase of certain equipment or machinery which saves environmental resources whenever it is used.

Thus, it seems achieving an ecologically sustainable future involves the following ten steps: (1) Define specific curtailment and efficiency ERBs; (2) Order this list from most to least critical with regard to environmental impact; (3) Identify barriers related to each ERB, and define ways to remove the barriers; (4) Decide on ERBs to target, considering resources available to remove barriers; (5) Develop and implement a process to instruct, support, and motivate the occurrence of the selected ERB(s); (6) If motivational contingencies must eventually be withdrawn, then make them only strong enough to get the behavior started but not powerful enough to provide complete justification for the effort and thereby hinder self-persuasion and feelings of personal responsibility for environmental protection; (7) Derive a marketing plan for large-scale dissemination and implementation of the behavior-change intervention; (8) Involve community leaders as much as possible in the various steps of the process, from selecting target ERBs and indentifying barriers to designing and evaluating the behavior-change process; (9) Use the competence motive to initiate and maintain participation by referring to the target ERB(s) as showing competence and personal control rather than self-sacrifice and altruism; and (10) Make allowances for potential impact of the actively caring person states in creating the kind of establishing conditions that can increase a person's propensity to perform an ERB.

Also see: Politics and Systems Change: Foundation; Theories: Foundation; History: Foundation.

References

Aronson, E. (1999). The power of self-persuasion. *American Psychologist, 54*, 875–884.

Bailey, J.S. (1991). Marketing behavior analysis requires different talk. In E.S. Geller (Ed.), *Science, theory, and technology: Varied perspectives* (pp. 37–40), *Monograph No. 6*, Lawrence, KS: Society for the Experimental Analysis of Behavior.

Bandura, A. (1997). *Self-efficacy: The exercise of control*. New York: W.H. Freeman.

Bem, D.J. (1972). Self-perception theory. In L. Berkowitz (Ed.), *Advances in experimental social psychology, Vol. 6* (pp. 1–60). New York: Academic Press.

Boyce, T.E., & Geller, E.S. (2001). Applied behavior analysis and occupational safety: The challenge of response maintenance. *Journal of Organizational Behavior Management, 21*(1), 31–60.

Burn, S.M., & Oskamp, S. (1986). Increasing community recycling with persuasive communication and public commitment. *Journal of Applied Social Psychology, 16*, 29–41.

Cone, J.D., & Hayes, S.C. (1980). *Environmental problem/behavioral solutions*. Monterey, CA: Brooks/Cole.

DeYoung, R. (2000). Expanding and evaluating motives for environmentally responsible behavior. *Journal of Social Issues, 56*, 509–526.

Dunlap, R.E., & Van Liere, K.D. (1978). The "new environmental paradigm": A proposed measuring instrument and preliminary results. *Journal of Environmental Education, 9*, 10–19.

Dunlap, R.E., Van Liere, K.D., Mertig, A.G., & Jones, R.E. (2000). Measuring endorsement of the new ecological paradigm: A revised NEP scale. *Journal of Social Issues, 56*, 425–442.

Dwyer, W.O., Leeming, F.C., Cobern, M.K., Porter, B.E., & Jackson, J.M. (1993). Critical review of behavioral interventions to preserve the environment: Research since 1980. *Environment and Behavior, 25*, 275–321.

Ehrlich, P.R., Ehrlich, A.H., & Holdren, J.P. (1977). *Ecoscience: Population, resources, environment*. San Francisco: Freeman.

Ellis, R.J., & Thompson, F. (1997). Culture and the environment in the Pacific Northwest. *American Political Science Review, 91*, 885–897.

Festinger, L., & Carlsmith, J.M. (1959). Cognitive consequences of forced compliance. *Journal of Abnormal and Social Psychology, 58*, 203–210.

Geller, E.S. (1989). Applied behavior analysis and social marketing: An integration for environmental preservation. *Journal of Social Issues, 45*, 17–36.

Geller, E.S. (1995). Integrating behaviorism and humanism for environmental protection. *Journal of Social Issues, 51*, 179–195.

Geller, E.S., Winett, R.A., & Everett, P.B. (1982). *Preserving the environment: New strategies for behavior change*. New York: Pergamon Press.

Kaplan, S. (2000). Human nature and environmentally responsible behavior. *Journal of Social Issues, 56*, 491–508.

Lepper, M.R., & Greene, D. (1978). *The hidden costs of reward: New perspectives on the psychology of human motivation*. Hillsdale, NJ: Erlbaum.

McKenzie-Mohr, D. (2000). Fostering sustainable behavior through community-based social marketing. *American Psychologist, 55*, 531–537.

McSween, T.E., & Mathews, G.A. (2001). Maintenance in organizational behavior management. *Journal of Organizational Behavior Management, 21*(1), 75–83.

Oskamp, S. (2000). A sustainable future for humanity? How can psychology help? *American Psychologist, 55*, 496–508.

Rotter, J.B. (1966). Generalized expectancies for internal versus external control of reinforcement. *Psychological Monographs, 80*(1).

Seligman, M.E. (1991). *Learned optimism.* New York: Alfred A. Knoff.

Skinner, B.F. (1987). *Upon further reflection.* Englewood Cliffs, NJ: Prentice-Hall.

Stern, P.C. (2000). Psychology and the science of human–environment interactions. *American Psychologist, 55*, 523–530.

Stern, P.C., & Gardner, G.T. (1987). Managing scarce environmental resources. In D. Stokols & I. Altman (Eds.), *Handbook of environmental psychology, Vol. 2* (pp. 1043–1088). New York: Wiley.

Wang, T.H., & Katzev, R. (1990). Group commitment and resource conservation: Two field experiments on promoting recycling. *Journal of Applied Social Psychology, 20*, 265–275.

Weigel, R.H., & Weigel, J. (1978). Environmental concern: The development of a measure. *Environment and Behavior, 10*, 3–15.

White, R.W. (1959). Motivation reconsidered: The concept of competence. *Psychological Review, 66*, 297–333.

Winett, R.A. (1980). An emerging approach to energy conservation. In D. Glenwick & L. Jason (Eds.), *Behavioral community psychology.* New York: Praeger.

Primary Prevention with Diverse Populations

Steven P. Schinke and Monica Matthieu

Diverse populations are demographically distinct groups of people who, by virtue of their ethnic–racial background, their lifestyle, or their particular physical, emotional, or social attributes, require and deserve specially designed *primary prevention programs*. Prevention programs for diverse populations may address any of the behaviors and states that typify primary prevention programs. These behaviors and states encompass such problems as substance abuse, physical and mental health, school performance, delinquency, pregnancy, sexually transmitted diseases, and the host of health, behavioral, and social problems that stimulate the development of primary prevention programs.

Moving beyond the reduction of problems, primary prevention for diverse populations also focuses on building new skill sets that are incompatible with problem behaviors. For example, good contemporary intervention programs exist through which prevention practitioners build on clients' racial pride, cultural symbols, traditions, and other attributes in the service of preventing such problems as violence and concurrently in promoting self-esteem and empowering clients in ways that would subsequently contribute to improved social performance, healthy development, and general well-being (cf. Okwumabua et al., 1999).

For members of diverse populations in particular, the promotion of strengths is as important or more important than problem behavior reduction in the design and implementation of primary prevention programs. Prevention programs, for example, can place emphasis on such targets as family life education—to help children live successfully in an oppressive or discriminatory culture, on physical health and exercise—for everyone, especially those who fall below the average on these health-promoting activities, and on creativity and intellectual talent—because poor schooling and supports for many mean that productivity from large numbers of talented and creative youth are being lost to society and themselves. In these and other ways, primary prevention programs for members of diverse populations can address a range of issues, not limited to the usual negative topics for prevention.

This entry offers a perspective on primary prevention with members of diverse populations. By defining three essential reasons for special programs aimed at members of diverse populations—*efficacy*, *efficiency*, and opportunities for drawing on *protective factors*—this entry makes an argument for giving careful attention to such programs. The authors illustrate programs that embody each of these three reasons. Finally, the entry provides conclusions and recommendations for prevention researchers, practitioners, and policy makers with an interest in the development and implementation of primary prevention programs for diverse populations.

Individuals who are members of diverse populations warrant expressly designed prevention programs for three reasons. Foremost is that prevention programs may be more *effective* when they are developed for a particular target group than when developed for a generic target group. This greater effectiveness may be due, in part, to the program's positive reception among members of the targeted diverse population, and due in part to the program's ability to aim at the particular risk and protective factors that characterize a diverse population.

The second reason to design primary prevention programs for diverse populations is that such programs are more *efficient* than generally aimed programs. Whereas the latter programs must necessarily consider all of the possible risks faced by all members of a heterogeneous population, the latter need only consider risks particular to the intended recipient population.

Finally, prevention programs for diverse populations can focus on common *protective factors* available to individual subpopulations. Quite simply, programs aimed at individual subgroups can draw and build upon a foundation of underlying strengths available to members of those subgroups. The considerable and myriad strengths of diverse populations allow prevention programs to enhance the accomplishment of positive goals and to help reduce the likelihood of predictable problems. The following sections discuss in detail each of these three reasons to justify the development of primary prevention programs for members of diverse populations.

EFFECTIVENESS

Results matter in prevention and must preoccupy program planners and policy makers when deciding how to approach a diverse population. Indeed, achieving better results is justification enough for designing prevention programs expressly for members of diverse populations. Data confirm the relative advantages of specially designed interventions relative to generic approaches to prevention with diverse populations.

Illustrative are findings from a New York City drug abuse prevention study that compared a culturally sensitive intervention, specifically developed for Black and Latino junior high students, with a conventional intervention program (Botvin, Schinke, Epstein, & Diaz, 1994). Whereas the latter program was already well researched and proven effective in a variety of settings with many types of youth populations, the former program was designed solely for purposes of the comparative study. From its origins, therefore, the culturally sensitive intervention drew upon cultural hallmarks of African American and Latino American experiences. The program incorporated stories and legends involving African and Spanish mythical characters into an intervention that taught youths problem-solving and decision-making relative to drug use opportunities, risks, and behaviors.

Youths were introduced to the culturally sensitive program in small group sessions and were engaged in the program via music, story telling, and role-play acting. Following this introductory material, youths took part in 15 small group exercises led by specially trained peer leaders about twice a week for 4 months. Group sessions allowed youths to further connect with the material through modeling, behavioral rehearsal, and practice sessions. Throughout the culturally sensitive intervention, youths were reminded of their African and Spanish heritage and its salience for contemporary drug use problems. For example, youths first observed, then practiced skills drawn from the lives of cultural figures who demonstrated appropriate responses to

various risky situations. These situations encompassed scenes from the lives of African and Spanish youths who overcame large obstacles in search of greater goals.

The conventional intervention program was a skills-based curriculum widely tested and shown effective with junior high students in school settings. Though not developed for minority populations, the conventional program nonetheless has been evaluated with diverse youth samples, including many members of Black, Latino, and other ethnic–racial minority groups. This curriculum also employed skills rehearsals and other cognitive–behavioral components parallel to the culturally sensitive intervention, and spanned approximately the same number of small group intervention sessions. Absent from the conventional intervention, however, were indicators of having African and Spanish origins, as was true for culturally sensitive intervention.

Outcome data comparing the two approaches accrued from a randomized clinical trial and longitudinal data collection. On outcome variables quantifying youths' behavioral intentions for alcohol and drug use, students in the culturally sensitive intervention and those in the conventional intervention reported lower future intentions to drink beer or wine after intervention delivery relative to their scores on the same measure prior to intervention. Whereas youths who received conventional intervention had lower intentions to drink hard liquor and use illicit drugs, youths who took part in the culturally sensitive program decreased their intentions to drink hard liquor. Both programs exerted a positive effect on the mediating variables of anti-alcohol and anti-illicit drug use attitudes and on general psychological tendencies of risk taking behaviors.

In a two-year follow-up study, both prevention programs showed overall positive results on alcohol and drug abuse variables relative to youths in a control group and to one another (Botvin, Schinke, Epstein, Diaz, Botvin, 1995). More than youths who received conventional intervention, however, youths in the culturally sensitive intervention group reported at two-year follow-up a reduction in future intentions to drink beer or wine. A significant decrease in the intentions to use liquor in the next year was also seen in both groups. Culturally sensitive intervention students also reported less frequency of drinking and drunkenness and lower amounts of alcohol consumed relative to convention intervention group youths. Finally, both interventions appeared to enhance the youths' antidrinking attitudes, their assertiveness regarding refusal of substance use, and their risk taking. Overall, the longitudinal data favored the culturally tailored approach on several key outcome variables.

Admittedly modest, findings from this comparative study support the added benefits of primary prevention programs designed for diverse populations. Particularly, in light of the two-year follow-up data, the study demonstrates that programs tailored for diverse populations may bring added value for members of those populations. Though the foregoing research stands alone as a comparative study of the added benefits of culturally sensitive interventions, as new empirical data accrue on other comparisons of prevention programs for diverse populations, the argument in favor of precisely designed programs may be strengthened on the basis of efficacy.

EFFICIENCY

Not unrelated to their ultimate effectiveness, prevention programs tailored for particular diverse populations are also efficient. Such efficiency results from program developers including in the intervention those risk factors and outcome problems most directly salient for diverse target populations. By investing a program with content that has special meaning for the specific target group and omitting content with less relevance, the program will respond more closely to the realities of the diverse population. What is more, such targeted programs can devote greater attention to the risks and outcomes that have particular meaning for the particular population. When programs focus on specific content for a specific group, they can concentrate their efforts and achieve potent results.

Illustrative of an efficient prevention program that also has achieved important outcome results is the Adolescent Training and Learning to Avoid Steroids (ATLAS) prevention program (Goldberg et al., 1996a,b). ATLAS is aimed at high school male athletes who are at risk for anabolic steroid use. Targeting one gender, a particular affiliated group, and a highly specific outcome behavior, ATLAS gives emphasis to variables that have meaning for its particular recipient population at a teachable moment in their lives. That teachable moment is the youths' desire to develop muscles for competing in sports. Rather than using steroids, the program advises young men to eat a diet balanced with proteins, fats, and carbohydrates. ATLAS warns youths about the dangers of anabolic steroid use, graphically demonstrating to them how steroids can, for example, reduce the size of their testicles. This population, gender, and lifestyle specific program illustrates how a precisely focused intervention can economically address a peculiar problem for members of a specific population.

The ATLAS prevention program tested for this study specifically targeted male varsity football players from two urban high schools that had similar total student enrollments, football win–loss records, family socioeconomic status, average parental education and student participation in school lunch program (Goldberg et al., 1996). One school received the 16-session ATLAS program while the other did not. The ATLAS program was completed in 1-hr sessions over 8 weeks—one session in the classroom with coaches and peer leaders and the other session in the school weight room by ATLAS weight lifting instruction staff. Additionally, the parents of ATLAS participants attended a single 1.5-hr meeting that provided programmatic information and nutrition material to assist the parents in helping the student athlete with their homework. To test program effects, a conditional regression model was utilized at post-intervention and long-term follow-up, with the posttest assessment adjusted for pretest levels for each participant.

Outcome results from implementation of the ATLAS program are impressive. After delivery of ATLAS, data on outcome variables covering knowledge, attitudes, intentions, body image, norms of steroid/drug use, skills, and beliefs of the adolescent student athletes revealed positive results in favor of the program relative to a control school football team. Athletes who received ATLAS had increased knowledge of steroid and drug effects, dietary supplements, and alternatives to steroid use. Additionally, the program changed students' attitudes about drugs in a positive direction, improved drug refusal skills, and lessened their intentions to use steroids. ATLAS program student athletes also reported improved body image, strength training self-efficacy, exercise and nutrition behaviors, and perception of athletic competence as a result of participation in the program. The study revealed positive program effects in the athletes' perception of other's use of steroids, and program recipients were less interested in trying steroids after the intervention.

Data on the ATLAS program demonstrate how a precisely focused program for members of a particular population can address those risk factors, problem behaviors, and strengths that directly touch the lives of the target population. By not needing to deal with issues extraneous to the target recipients, the prevention program achieved a level of parsimony that are not possible in programs aimed at a more general population or constellation of problem behaviors. Doubtless, the prevention literature will witness in the near future more examples of programs that limit their scope to only the salient factors for a specific minority population.

PROTECTIVE FACTORS

Protective factors are those theoretical and empirically supported variables that appear to help people avoid problems. Serving as innate and learned preventive features of our personalities, upbringing, and humanity, protective factors allow most children and youth to successfully bypass the myriad risks that get some into trouble. A homely example of a protective factor most of us possess is fear of heights. By respectfully avoiding high and dangerous places, we remove ourselves from the possibility of falling down. Illustrative of a learned protective factor is the ability to cross a busy street by waiting for the "Walk" light. Diverse populations also enjoy protective factors, often of a nature, magnitude, and scope that are disproportionate to the same protective factors in the larger population. Oftentimes, members of diverse populations are blessed with protective factors that are particular to their culture.

An example of such a culture in the context of prevention programming is that enjoyed by Native Americans. Native people in this country are uniquely situated to draw upon the culture they created prior to the Western immigration of Europeans .to America. Concurrently, Native Americans can draw upon the strengths afforded them by their pluralism—albeit largely involuntary—in surviving in the dominant European culture. Simultaneously exploiting the best of Native and European cultures, therefore, gives American Indians a set of competencies that are bicultural. Bicultural competence offers Native Americans protective factors that can be galvanized in the service of prevention.

A number of prevention programs have employed bicultural competence skills to develop effective interventions. One program, for example, taught Native youths to reach back to their traditional culture for such values as reverence of their bodies, worship of nature, and need for holistic balance as well as to take what is good about Western culture—appropriate assertiveness, educational advancement, and the harmonious diversity only possible in a heterogeneous society—for a combined set of cognitive and behavioral skills that can help them prevent their own and others' substance use (Schinke, Orlandi, Botvin, Gilchrist, Trimble, & Locklear, 1988).

Assertiveness provides an example of a skill set to help youths acquire cultural competencies. Albeit not generally positively regarded in Native American society, appropriate assertiveness can help youths refuse unreasonable requests from others to use tobacco, alcohol, and drugs. A bicultural approach to teaching Native youths skills for assertiveness therefore recognizes the American Indian value of non-confrontation while demonstrating the role of an assertive response to situations of peer and other pressure toward substance use. Through group exercises, youths can witness demonstrations of passive, aggressive, and assertive behavior, then can practice in role-plays how to present themselves in various pressure situations.

In a study by Schinke, Tepavac, and Cole (2000), Native American youths in the third through fifth grades in 27 tribal and public schools from 10 different reservations were divided into two intervention groups and one control group. One of the intervention groups received a weekly 50-minute instruction and cognitive and behavioral skills session totaling 15 sessions, and the other group received the same intervention as well as instruction that incorporated the youths' Native American heritage and values. The Native youths were taught problem-solving, personal coping and interpersonal communication skills within the context of contemporary Native American culture. This intervention also utilized role-playing to address modern day substance use risk situations, coaching from peer leaders on substance refusal skills, and community substance abuse prevention involvement to motivate students toward positive and healthy alternatives to substance use within their cultural traditions. The intervention programs were evaluated after 6 months, and every 12 months thereafter for 3 years with booster sessions semiannually to address increasing risks for youths with advancing age.

The results of the culturally competent intervention program shed light on the importance of protective factors in the usage of culturally specific prevention programs. The Native American youths were evaluated over the course of the 3.5-year study on reported use of smoked and smokeless tobacco, alcohol, and marijuana. With each substance, except cigarette smoking, all of the follow-up rates reveal significant decreases in current usage in both the skills training and culturally competent intervention group as compared to the control group. Specifically, both intervention groups show a decrease of 43 percent for smokeless tobacco, 24 percent for alcohol, and 53 percent for marijuana use over the rate of use for the control group in these Native American youth substance use prevention programs. Summative findings from process and outcome measures favor the culturally competent approach on several parameters with salience for youths and for risk factors under investigation in this research.

Logically, the ability to focus on protective factors and strengths relevant to the recipient group would be a valuable feature of prevention programs for diverse populations. Whether demarked by ethnic–racial background, sexual orientation, or other demographic background characteristic, members of diverse populations have great strengths that deserve inclusion in any primary prevention effort. Prevention program developers are wise to engage in the preliminary work that will discover those strengths for subsequent incorporation into the resulting program.

CONCLUSIONS AND RECOMMENDATIONS

Sadly, resource limitations and perhaps a lack of imagination have inhibited the development of an adequate number of prevention programs for diverse populations. The availability of prevention programs continues to be dominated by interventions developed for, tested with, and disseminated to majority culture and mixed populations. Snowden, Martinez, and Morris (2000) note that these diverse populations have different involvement and reactions to interventions that makes programming vital in targeting these groups. Accordingly, the dearth of programs for diverse populations becomes even more troubling when, as described and illustrated here, those programs are likely to be achieving high levels of effectiveness and efficiency. What is more, programs for diverse populations can address protective factors in a sensitive, parsimonious manner.

Programs aimed at members of diverse populations also stand a good chance of empowering the communities and institutions from which they arise. Prevention programs can achieve that end by creating an atmosphere of community and individual empowerment as members of those populations take an active role in addressing the problems they face. Engaging professionals, respected members of the community, and program recipients in the development of a program, allow preventionists to tap the vast potential of persons, institutions, and communities that otherwise are too often passive recipients (Snowden et al., 2000).

No matter how efficacious, prevention programs cannot be successful unless they are sustained. Programs that are not a part of the communities and organizations under whose auspices they are offered are unlikely to continue. Examples of such circumstances are programs implemented by outside developers, those are made possible by extraordinary, nonrecurring funds, and programs sponsored by a research or demonstration grant. Unlikely candidates for continued implementation are prevention programs and interventions not expressly designed for the target recipients. Accordingly, programs developed for diverse populations and by members of the host community, organization, or institution, have a strong probability of being embraced and used over time. Because programs for diverse populations are more likely than programs for general populations to originate from the places where members of those diverse populations live, work, and go to school, the former programs are also positioned better to be sustained over time.

Professionals involved in all dimensions of primary prevention programs—practitioners, theorists, and researchers—must become more sensitive to needs of diverse groups. In so doing, professionals can better embed science-based principles into primary prevention programs. Such sensitivity must begin with a thorough understanding of the research literature on the particular diverse population under consideration. Further, prevention professionals, if they are not already members of the target groups, should immerse themselves in the target culture, through exploratory work, focus groups, and ethnographic research, for example, to gain qualitative insights into the particular group.

Resources and strengths such as the family, religion/spirituality, and the use of indigenous healers are often overlooked as potential sources of cultural information on these diverse populations (Snowden et al., 2000). In addition, professionals can engage members of the target groups in designing, implementing, and evaluating primary prevention programs. In these ways, prevention professionals can better assure that programs intended for members of diverse populations truly serve the needs of those groups.

More research is needed to advance the science of prevention for diverse populations. Perhaps the advantages of expressly designed programs outlined in this paper—greater *efficacy*, *efficiency*, and focus on *protective factors*—will spur new work on responsive, culturally sound, and theory-based programs. Without question, innovative programs are solely needed for such populations as members of sexual orientation minority groups, women, and new immigrants to this country. Also woefully lacking are programs in languages other than English (cf. Muñoz, 2001; Muñoz, Marín, Posner, & Pérez-Stable, 1997). Additionally, research data on outcomes of those emerging grassroots programs must be available before the scientific community can embrace the programs and before the programs are ready for widespread dissemination. Together, researchers, practitioners, and members of specific target groups can carry out all ambitious agenda of new work to develop, test, and market primary prevention programs for all Americans, regardless of how they differ from the majority population.

Also see: Racial and Ethnic Disparities; Homophobia: All entries; Ethics: Foundations; Culture, Society, and Social Class: Foundation; Politics and Systems Change: Foundation.

References

Botvin, G.J., Schinke, S.P., Epstein, J.A., & Diaz, T. (1994). Effectiveness of culturally focused and generic skills training approaches to alcohol and drug abuse prevention among minority youths. *Psychology of Addictive Behaviors, 8*, 116–127.

Botvin, G.J., Schinke, S.P., Epstein, J.A., Diaz, T., & Botvin, E.M. (1995). Effectiveness of culturally focused and generic skills training approaches to alcohol and drug abuse prevention among minority adolescents: Two-year follow up results. *Psychology of Addictive Behaviors, 9*, 183–194.

Goldberg, L., Elliot, D.L., Clarke, G.N., MacKinnon, D.P., Zoref, L., Moe, E., Green, C., & Wolf, S.L. (1996a). The adolescent training and learning to avoid steroids (ATLAS) prevention program. *Archives of Pediatric and Adolescent Medicine, 150*, 713–721.

Goldberg, L., Elliot, D.L., Clarke, G.N., MacKinnon, D.P., Zoref, L., Moe, E., Green, C., Wolf, S.L., Greffrath, E., Miller, D.J., & Lapin, A. (1996b). Effects of a multidimensional anabolic steroid prevention intervention: The adolescent training and learning to avoid steroids (ATLAS) program. *Journal of the American Medical Association, 276*, 1555–1562.

Muñoz, R.F. (2001). On the road to a world without depression. *Journal of Primary Prevention, 21*, 325–338.

Muñoz, R.F., Marín, B.V.-O., Posner, S.F., & Pérez-Stable, E.J. (1997). Mood management mail intervention increases abstinence rates for Spanish-speaking Latino smokers. *American Journal of Community Psychology, 25*, 325–343.

Okwumabua, J.O. et al. (1999). Building self-esteem through social skills training and cultural awareness: A community-based approach for preventing violence among African American youth. *Journal of Primary Prevention, 20*(1), 61–74.

Schinke, S.P., Orlandi, M.A., Botvin, G.J., Gilchrist, L.D., Trimble, J.E., & Locklear, V.S. (1988). Preventing substance abuse among American Indian adolescents: A bicultural competence skills approach. *Journal of Counseling Psychology, 35,* 87–90.

Schinke, S.P., Tepavac, L., & Cole, K.C. (2000). Preventing substance use among Native American youth: Three-year results. *Addictive Behaviors, 25,* 387–397.

Snowden, L.R., Martinez, M., & Morris, A. (2000). Community psychology and ethnic populations. In J. Rappaport & E. Seidman (Eds.), *Handbook of Community Psychology* (pp. 833–855). New York: Kluwer Academic/Plenum.

The Contributions of Society, Culture, and Social Class to Emotional Disorder

George W. Albee

In this entry, I discuss the often negative contributions of society, culture, and social class to emotional disorders—in contrast to points of view that seek a brain defect for all mental illnesses.* Knowing the predominant environmental causes of emotional disorders can lead to effective programs of social change, rather than the brain defect point of view that essentially blames fate and exonerates society from making vital social changes.

Effective strategies for the primary prevention of mental/emotional disturbances depend to a significant degree on decisions on causation. There are currently two general positions: One is the social environmental approach, which will be presented in this entry. The other position emphasizes biological and physiological factors, as characterized by this statement: "All mental illness is caused by a brain defect" (Koplewicz, 1999). This biological point of view looks for genetic or physiologic risk factors for DSM-IV disorders (as listed in the Diagnostic and Statistical Manual of the

American Psychiatric Association, 2000). It also insists that only developmental studies with control groups aimed at reducing risk for DSM-IV disorders are scientific. Under criticism (see Albee, 1996c), this position by a group calling itself "prevention science" is changing somewhat.

An overriding problem is the lack of reliability for DSM-IV as Kutchins and Kirk (1997) have shown in delightful detail. Over the years, from the original DSM in 1955 to the present, specific mental illnesses have appeared, disappeared, have been added on request, deleted on demand, subjected to debate, and voted in or out. Meanwhile, an endless series of studies, preliminary reports, and authoritarian pronouncements about causation has appeared in the psychiatric journals and popular press, many of them fading without a trace.

But organic, brain-disease, defective-biology explanations persist because they support the ruling ideas of society. Closely linked historically to Calvinism (one is saved or damned from before birth) (see Rotenberg, 1975) and Social Darwinism (it is best for the human race if the strong survive and breed, and if the weak and defective do not), eugenics (Albee, 1996a) and biological arguments oppose "liberal" programs that support (with tax money) the poor, the exploited, the disadvantaged (see Albee, 1996a,b).

If, instead of brain disease, mental/emotional disorders result from the profound stresses in the social environment—child physical abuse, child sexual abuse, neglect, the miseries of poverty, bad housing, hunger and poor diet, from a society where women and poor minorities are exploited and victimized by more powerful (white) patriarchal forces controlling religion, jobs and wages, social roles, and mass media—then primary prevention would mean social change and a struggle for social justice (Albee, 1996c), ideas that a ruling elite finds threatening to their current status in society. This elite worries that such changes to increase social justice, such as child care, better schools, a higher minimum wage, would also increase taxes.

The latter half of the 19th century was a time of explosive successes in the search for the causes of diseases in humans. The invention of the microscope, perhaps more than any other development, led to the identification of the many specific microorganisms, each responsible for a separate disease. Other anatomical and physiological research identified defects in cellular and organic systems that resulted in identifiable diseases. Specific toxins in the environment, drinking water, air, were found to cause other specific diseases. As medical diagnoses became more reliable, treatment strategies could be developed and evaluated—the effectiveness of drugs to combat infections, the role of diet, especially of the newly discovered vitamins and minerals, the effectiveness of surgery and asepsis, all were evaluated against the criterion of their ability to reduce *prevalence*.

---

* In 1967 I was a participant in a symposium on "Industrialism, Behavioral Sciences, and Mental Health" at the InterAmerican Society of Psychology, in Mexico City. I prepared a long paper on "Social and cultural factors influencing disturbed behavior: The disappearance of sex in industrial society." Later I incorporated parts of that paper in a Distinguished Professional Contribution Award Invited address, "The Protestant Ethic, Sex, and Psychotherapy" which appeared in *The American Psychologist*, 1977, *32*(2), 150–161. In the current entry, I have used parts of both of these early papers, along with my later writings, especially Albee (1996a,b); all of these are used with permission of the American Psychological Association.

At the same time, the field of public health was making its own giant strides in efforts at reducing the *incidence* of specific diseases by changing the toxicity of the environment. Evidence that certain diseases were transmitted by drinking water contaminated with human and animal wastes led to major investments in sewage systems for sanitary disposal of waste. Water purification greatly reduced the incidence of diseases like cholera and typhoid. Pasteurization of milk, food sanitation, and refrigeration lowered the incidence of mortality, especially of children. Immunization techniques prevented millions of deaths by raising resistance. Enriched diets improved health and resistance.

However, research into the causes of mental disorders was far less successful. A few true diseases—like brain syphilis, hypothyroidism, and pellagra—were found. But most functional psychoses and neuroses defied the search for organic causes. Psychoanalysis and social epidemiology suggested that many emotional disorders were caused by disturbed early experience in interpersonal and social distress. But medicine has long insisted that eventually organic causes would be found.

The politically conservative medical position argued persistently against the emerging psychodynamic view of the origins of symptoms and denied the cultural origins of disturbance. Kraepelin (see Guse & Schmacke, 1980), the "great classifier" in psychiatry whose system provided the basis of the DSM system of American psychiatry, insisted on the *incomprehensibility* of symptoms and the pointlessness of socio-psychodynamics. German psychiatry added two more legs to the stool: the doctrine of *endogenous* origins, and *denial of society's responsibility* for causation. Eventually German psychiatrists with the Nazi's cooperated willingly in the murder of the nation's "defective" mental patients, seen as a hopeless drain (see Guse & Schmacke, 1980).

A great deal of research evidence (see Mirowsky & Ross, 1989) suggests that separate and discrete mental illnesses do not exist as objective entities with reliable separate markers as is the case for real diseases. And without reliable markers, the search for objective physical causes cannot be valid.

Considerable evidence suggests that complex patterns of behavior, whether bizarre, atypical, culturally approved, or culturally condemned, can be learned and sustained through patterns of social reinforcement. The laws of learning, of classical and instrumental conditioning, are well understood. From Watson to Skinner, it has been possible, particularly in the laboratory, to cause animals to learn complex patterns of both adaptive and maladaptive behavior simply by controlling reinforcement. Harlow's studies provide a model (Harlow, 1970).

The very strong possibility exists that many, if not most of the conditions that have been labeled "mental illnesses" are not caused by biological defects, microorganisms, or toxins, but rather are learned with a normal nervous system in a pathological social environment. Analogs of depression, social withdrawal, frenzied excitement, extreme suspiciousness, pathological aggression, bizarre sexuality, and self-preoccupation can all be learned.

Real physical illnesses are found to vary little from culture to culture, from one historical period to another, from one socioeconomic class to another, and even from male to female. (Obviously, there are diseases specific to males or to females—but most diseases are not sex-linked.) Whether the disease is strep throat, appendicitis, cancer, exothalmic goiter, malaria, or cataracts, it has identifiable symptoms and an objective marker—a blood test, x-ray, mass, discharge, etc.—that makes diagnosis objective and reliable. Severity of the disease may vary depending on factors like a long history leading to established widespread resistance. Syphilis was a mild disease among the Carib Indians, but when it was brought to Europe by Columbus' sailors, it became a raging epidemic among Europeans not previously exposed. Conversely, measles was deadly to Eskimos and Javanese when introduced by the resistant Europeans. Beri beri and kwashiorkor are more common among people with a poor diet. But despite differences in frequency and severity, these diseases are the same everywhere and can be reliably diagnosed. They have the same objective markers.

With mental/emotional disorders, the situation changes. Certain neuroses are present or absent if sexual stresses are high or low. The neuroses that are common in patriarchal societies that enforce strict sexual repression are often severe, and especially affect women. Depression is unknown in many tradition-directed societies where people do not have an internal conscience, and very common in puritanical conscience-laden cultures. Each successive immigrant group to America had high rates of "idiocy" and "lunacy" while they were poverty stricken, but the rate declined as succeeding generations achieved middle-class economic status (see Jarvis 1855 in Grob 1978; Albee, 1990a). Schizophrenia is much more common among the lowest social class, whichever ethnic group is at the bottom, and the rate declines as the class level of the group improves (Albee, 1996a; Hollingshead & Redlich, 1968).

The point is that the nature and content of most functional mental disorders varies with sociocultural conditions like sexual repression, the stresses of poverty, discrimination, sexism, religious orthodoxy, and patriarchy.

This is not a new observation. The "cultural relativity hypothesis" has been entertained for most of the past century. It was featured in the work of people like Ruth Benedict (1934), Franz Boas (1948) and Margaret Mead (1964) (see Albee, 1996b), all of whom tried to show that culture determined what behavior was considered normal or abnormal and that the same behavior was often judged normal in one culture and abnormal in another. Sexual behavior that was most commonly condemned by different cultures determined neurotic behavior. I will focus my attention on this area to illustrate the cultural relativity of mental diagnoses. The best source for my argument is the work of Riessman, Glazer, and Denny (1950).

Let me emphasize at the outset: if "mental disorders" have no marker, and if what is judged abnormal behavior in one society may be considered normal in another, then mental disorders differ in a profound way from real physical illnesses and it is *not* true that "mental illnesses are illnesses like any other." The implications for primary prevention are fundamental, nothing less than giving direction to our major efforts to prevent predictable problems, and to enhance the desired goals of people who are oppressed by their social environments.

Humans as we know them physically have inhabited the earth for something like the past million years. But civilization has existed for only the past six to eight thousand years, since the development of agriculture and the storage of surplus food freed us from the necessity of a nomadic food-gathering existence. If we liken the time that humans have been on earth to a 24-hr day, civilization has existed only for the past eight minutes. To understand the origins of human behavior, and especially disturbed behavior, we need to know what we were like during the 23 hr and 52 min we lived as nomadic wanderers, constantly struggling to survive in a hostile environment. We can be certain that a great deal of natural selection occurred. Those who were most intelligent and those with the most efficient orthosympathetic nervous system were best able to escape, or to overcome, the daily dangers of living. And those with the highest level sex drive produced more of the offspring who survived the high rate of infant mortality, and the endless daily threats to survival. If we scratch civilized people, we discover intelligent primordial people whose strong aggressive and sexual responses must be controlled enough to allow civilized communities to exist. And if we seek to explain disturbed behavior, we must examine the kinds of inner and outer controls erected to restrain aggression and sexuality. Freud's (1961) *Civilization and its discontents* is a good guide.

For most of the six to eight thousand years humans have lived in settled, civilized communities, they have had to control aggression, at least toward their in-group, but only relatively moderate restrictions have had to be placed on the sexual activity of young people. Most of these people lived in a tradition-directed agricultural society where children were an economic advantage, where the high death rate had to be balanced by a high birth rate, and where marriage, sex, and child-bearing ordinarily began shortly after puberty. Under these conditions, neurosis and sexual conflicts were (and *are* still, in many parts of the world) rare or unknown.

Psychological and social difficulties appear when individuals from a tradition-directed, controlling village society are forced, often because of population growth, to leave home, migrate to the city, and begin a new life working in the new urban-industrial factory as anonymous members of a society of strangers. In addition to the discovery that the traditional, ritualized patterns of behavior, from which one could not deviate back home, are now unenforced or inappropriate, often ridiculed, people also find themselves free of the danger of peer punishment, and so frequently exhibit relatively uncontrolled behavior that may take the form of crime, excessive use of alcohol, sexual abandon, personal irresponsibility, and neglect of family obligations. In the absence of external controls and without an internal conscience, there is little inhibition. Hogarth's sketches of London provide the illustration.

Industrializing nations must eventually move away from the values of tradition-directed society (that is composed primarily of a large number of rural agrarian people controlled by a small group of wealthy and powerful landowners) and toward an *inner-directed* society that gradually will be composed of a growing conscience-laden middle class whose task it is to further the essential goals of capital accumulation and the development of a productive and efficient industrial economy. Religions of restraint appear and dominate. In the process there occur certain dramatic changes in styles of living. These changes result in new personality structures and marked shifts in the patterns of emotional disturbances, with consequent changes in kinds of demand for intervention and care.

Epidemiological studies have found that the patterns of disturbed behavior we call *neuroses* are absent, or remarkably scarce, in agrarian peasant cultures (Albee, 1977; 1996b). In these societies, largely composed of people living on the land, sexual activity begins at an early age, marriage usually follows shortly after puberty, and there is little cultural demand for sexual repression. Sometimes a system of chaperonage protects young girls from the "uncontrollable lust" of the males of the society. But this is simply further evidence of the absence of inner control into the form of individual consciences. Thus, in Sicily, for example, males and females beyond the age of puberty are never left alone together under usual circumstances unless they are married, or unless they are siblings. Similar controls exist in most Islamic societies; girls and young women who defy convention may be subject to death from male relatives.

Such societies have been called "shame cultures" (Ausubel, 1958; Mead, 1964). Anthropologists suggest that forbidden or taboo behavior must be controlled externally in them. Individuals are born, live, and die within the same small social communities where they are known to everyone and where deviation from the proper role assigned by the culture is easily detected. Those few who deviate are subject to scorn, social censure, exclusion, and even banishment and death.

In the process of change from the agrarian tradition-directed shame culture, to an industrializing inner-directed guilt culture, a number of behavioral patterns and value systems must be revised, particularly by the developing middle class which is a new but essential part of the industrializing production-oriented society (Riessman et al., 1950). The most important requisite for this major societal change involves the repression of sexuality, postponement of marriage and child-bearing, and the replacement of early sexual activity with the accumulation of education, or capital, as the major activity of young upwardly mobile males. Women of the new middle class must be chaste and ignorant of sexuality.

To facilitate this process, it is necessary for the society to develop a *guilt* culture, where impulse control comes no longer externally, from the long-familiar members of the individual's own village society, but rather from a strict and tyrannical internalized conscience. In order to associate anxiety and guilt with sex, it becomes necessary that all sexual behavior, especially sexual interest and curiosity in children, be punished. Eventually, as generation succeeds generation, and religious beliefs are invented to rationalize social practices, sexual impulses acquire a load of anxiety. They are repressed, avoided, or otherwise twisted into unrecognizable forms. Sexual neuroses become common in the middle class. Freud's career and theories were based on the neuroses of repression.

Inevitably, the development of industrial capitalism (and probably industrial socialism as well) has resulted in severe strictures and repression of sexuality. Because of the urgency of the sex drive, as a consequence of a million years of evolution, which selected the most fecund for survival, repressions must go to great lengths and to surprising extremes.

It is improbable that an industrialized, production-oriented society can develop in the absence of a Victorian-like value system usually based on religion, which insists on purity, abstinence, and repression of sexual impulses by a strict internalized conscience. The burden of responsibility for control falls most often on (middle-class) women, but is passed on, eventually to children of both sexes.

It is instructive to study the attitudes of the middle class in Victorian England especially with regard to the sexual education of children and the proper sexual attitudes of middle-class English women. The topic has been discussed at length by Stephen Marcus (1984). He illustrates the new sexuality with extensive quotations from the leading sexual moralist of the 19th century, Dr. William Acton. This popular writer, a respected physician who specialized in diseases of the genito-urinary tract, wrote extensively about the proper control of sexuality. He stressed the importance of forbidding any kind of "sexual impression" from reaching the child who must be raised in total ignorance of anything sexual. He assured British parents that by shielding children from any exposure to sexual matters, they would grow up free of all sexual notions and feelings. He was speaking, of course, to the growing British middle class. He further assured his readers

that proper adult English women were not troubled with any sexual feelings; their only genuine passions involved responsibilities for family and children. Even sex in marriage was dangerous, and Dr. Acton warned about the effects of sexual excesses even within monogamous marriage. The only safe course, he advised, was continence brought about by the constant exercise of will power and control. Marcus points to a number of fascinating parallels between the social importance of thrift, of saving and accumulating capital, and parallel attitudes toward the saving of semen and the consequent importance of sexual thrift and the dangers of "spending." (Interestingly, the verb "spending" is the Victorian term for orgasm.) Success in an inner-directed industrializing society required saving not spending, work not play, and the earnest striving to attain long-term goals, rather than to succumb to the immediate temptations of the flesh.

Acton is not an exception in his views. Similar views are expressed in the 19th century essays of Thoreau and of Emerson, for example. Both of these New England essayists, widely respected for their wisdom and independent spirit, were full of sexual repressions and misconceptions. Thoreau expressed feelings of guilt over sexuality and was preoccupied with the struggle between virtue and vice. Sensuality, for him, was beastly. Delicately, Thoreau observed that degenerative energy, which, when we are loose, dissipates and makes us unclean; when we are continent, invigorates and inspires us. Chastity is the flowering of man; and what we call Genius, Heroism, Holiness, and the like, are but various fruits which succeed it. Man goes at once to God when the channel of purity is open (Thoreau, 1962). Emerson (1883) also argued that the sublime vision comes to the simple soul in a clean and chaste body.

In many tradition-directed shame cultures, there is often a surprisingly relaxed attitude toward (female) nudity. Women in Hawaii and the South Seas scandalized the missionaries. In the Victorian culture, on the other hand, middle-class women were instructed to do everything possible to make themselves sexless and unstimulating to men. The missionaries ordered the Hawaiian women (and those in Africa, India, Indonesia, ect.) to cover their sinful nudity. A consequence of this coincidence of industrialization and the strict over control of sexuality is the inevitable appearance of certain forms of psychopathology like hysteria, neurasthenia, and depression, more commonly in women, which were the result of guilt feelings gone out of control. The widespread prevalence of *hysteria* among middle-class women in Freud's Vienna, in Chariot's Paris, and throughout Western Europe during the latter part of the 19th century, was a clear-cut reflection of the repression and overcontrol of sexuality that was the cultural role for middle-class women. (Parenthetically, there was widespread male interest in pornography and prostitution satisfying unusual sexual desires—spanking in particular—reflecting a double standard of morality.) Many Victorian repressed middle-class men and women were unable to engage in healthy sexual relationships. Clearly, the sexual neurosis flourished in the middle class. Even today, London prostitutes advertise spanking, role-playing (nun or school girl), and S-M specialties.

The important point for our consideration is the interaction between the imposition of the cultural overcontrol of pleasure seeking that is essential for the hard work of industrialization, and the appearance of new and widespread forms of psychopathology. As behavioral scientists interested in prevention or alleviation of disturbed behavior, we must understand the relationship between social repression of strong human drives and resulting patterns of psychopathology. Explanations which attribute causation to brain disease and insist that "mental illness is an illness like any other" fail to account for the striking association between incidences of specific disorders and sociocultural conditions.

When there is little sexual repression, there is little neurosis. Leighton (1967) studying the Yoruba in Nigeria, found that it was extremely difficult to find a Yoruba word to describe the feelings meant by "depression." (Neither could they find a Yoruba term for senility.)

Victorian attitudes towards masturbation were extreme; their echoes linger on and have not disappeared in the United States. A survey was reported in the *Medical Tribune* (February 12, 1966) in which half of all students in five medical schools in the Philadelphia area, and 20 percent of the members of these medical school faculties, still expressed the belief that masturbation causes mental illness; many of these MDs are still in practice today.

An intriguing question is: Which comes first, the industrialization, or the changing set of guiding fictions about proper moral behavior? Or do these somehow interact and reinforce each other?

Perhaps a prerequisite to both industrialization and the development of the Protestant Ethic is a prior condition which questions established authority, and throws doubt on the concept of infallibility, whether it be sacred or secular. Once doubt has been created about the infallibility of established authority, then people will begin to search for new reasons to explain the mysteries of the world. This thesis would suggest that the development of industrialization can only follow the successful challenge of established authority, as occurred in the development of the Protestant Ethic. Certainly, the rise of skepticism of authority leads to the development of empirical scientific rationalism, which then leads to discovery and invention, which further accelerates the processes of production, and with a kind of interactive reinforcement that occurs in developing society.

According to economist Joseph Schumpeter (1942), rational thinking flowered for the first time in the West with the development of capitalism and industrialization. The complex process of converting natural resources into manufactured goods requires sustained attention, rational thinking, orderly planning, a system of record-keeping and accounting, and a sophisticated system of money, banking, and credit. All of these cognitive inventions are products of disciplined and independent human minds; and they lead to changed personality structures.

It has been suggested by the Freudians that these inventions and more obsessive personality traits, and the consequent preoccupation with production and trade of manufactured goods, results from the necessity for the stricter toilet training of children as people settled down to live closely together in fixed communities that grew larger. Many of the traits of orderliness, cleanliness, and obsessiveness have been referred to by Karl Abraham (1942) as "the Anal Character." While it may seem far-fetched to suggest that the need for increasingly strict toilet training in children resulted eventually in rebellion against authority, a compulsive interest in numbers and money, in thrift and trade, and that these traits led to the development of capitalism, there is certainly some historical and clinical evidence that this may be worth considering.

In order for capitalism to reach its full bloom, it was necessary that a whole new set of moral mystiques be developed—a new pattern of religious beliefs more consistent with the demands of rationalized production than was the earlier scholasticism. However, it is increasingly clear today that it is *not* capitalism which is responsible for these personality traits. We saw the same kinds of personality characteristics developing in socialist countries, even in countries where there is no Protestant religion, or in some cases, where there is no organized religion.

If it is the acceleration of industrial production that demands a Protestant-like (or Victorian) ethic, then we will find the development of a value system that stresses hard work and postponement of sexuality in any industrializing nation; conversely, we might predict the failure of industrialization in those nations where such changes in the guiding fictions do not occur.

To succeed in industrialization, the society must save, not spend; work, not play; strive earnestly for the attainment of long-term goals, not succumb to the temptations of the flesh. One example: The galloping industrialization that has occurred in northern Italy since World War II is not due to the discovery of new sources of power, or of raw materials, nor to new manufacturing processes, but to the change in the northern Italian personality. It is interesting to learn that the northern third of Italy now has the lowest birth rate of any comparable sized area in the world! Hard work, the accumulation of possessions, upward social mobility, thrift, and all of the other "virtues" of a Protestant morality have replaced "Amare, Cantare, Mangiare" as the order of the day! Lovemaking has been replaced with moneymaking. Singing has been replaced by counting and accounting; and even eating, as in most Protestant inner-directed countries, is no longer much fun. Fast food restaurants are a Protestant invention! An emphasis on industrial production is not compatible with a three-hour lunch-siesta routine, or with "girl watching," or with leisurely sociable eating. Machines are profitable only when they are in use. They demand constant planned and rationalized arrangements for the delivery of raw materials and for the accurate scheduling of work. Production schedules are not compatible with pleasure schedules. Guilt and duty replace fun and games before industrialization can proceed. Milano is about as exciting a city to visit as Pittsburgh or Detroit! On the other hand, Italy south of Rome (the Mezzogiorno) continues to be preoccupied with sex, siestas, and sin. The North actually wants to become separate from the South.

To choose another example closer to home: Modern Brazil has been trying to become an industrial country *before* developing a Protestant ethic. What more beautiful monument exists to Victorian aspirations than the capital city of Brasilia? Protestants *love* to sacrifice themselves for a hard life on the frontier. The exciting prospect of suffering, of starvation and danger (with the prospect of making one's fortune) draws the Protestant as a magnet. It is one of the substitutes for sex! But Brazil had found its beautiful capital, far off in the wilderness, cannot long hold legislators and civil servants. Instead, they rush back weekends to Rio for fun and games.

An interesting report from Chile bears on the thesis. Some years ago, the Santiago government tried to abolish the siesta in the middle of the day. It ordered government workers and factory workers to complete a straight shift, with just a brief pause for a sandwich at lunch. The widespread public resistance to the decree led to its being rescinded. But the fact that the government would make the attempt is clear testimony to the necessity for a shift from a pattern of living that fits the pleasures of people to a pattern of living that fits the need of the production machine. The midday siesta separates clearly the countries with a pleasure ethic from those with a work ethic (e.g., Hong Kong, Taiwan, Israel).

Both the kind, and the rate, of emotionally disturbed neurotic behavior are derived in significant measure from social and cultural conditions that are shaped and determined by the level of industrialization of a society. In the process of industrialization, the repressions of sexuality is necessary, so that time and energy may be devoted to serving the demands of an economy with a craving for manufactured goods. Eventually an interest in the production of these goods largely replaces an interest in sexuality by managers and the work-leaders in part because of the anxiety that has been conditioned to sexual impulses as a form of individual control. Anxiety avoidance is a major reinforcement.

The successes of capitalistic production are sowing the seeds of further major changes in modal, cultural personality. Production of manufactured goods rapidly outpaced consumption. The tight-lipped, saving-oriented, ascetic, sexually repressed American gothic couple portrayed by Grant Wood had to be replaced by impulse-yielding consumers who could be brain washed by skillful advertising to buy, buy, buy, charge, charge, charge. To be accepted by others was the new demand. Keeping up with the Jones required outspending them for unneeded consumer goods that are required for status.

As production expanded beyond all reasonable bounds, and as the middle class spread far down the social order to include the great mass of wage earners, a paradoxical situation developed—the ascetic Protestant ethic was incompatible with the high level of consumption required to use up the flood of goods produced.

The American character structure simply had to shift again. Now it was to be other people and their expectations and evaluations that determined behavior. The other-directed individual, uncertain of self and new identity, more eagerly seeks superficial friendship and approval or envy of peers. This person is likely to be a member of the new middle class of salaried government workers or salaried management. The social circle is wider than before and is more likely to include strangers. Control of behavior takes the form of neither shame nor guilt, but anxiety. The other-directed person is anxious to be accepted, to be liked, and to be seen as successful. As Riessman et al. (1950) put it, one's control is no longer a gyroscope but a radar device. Today, we might say it is the Internet. Another consequence of other-directedness is an increase in cosmopolitanism, which means that people are at home in a much wider range of situations while at the same time being at home nowhere. Travel must impress others, the more exotic, the better. One can be transferred from one upper-middle-class suburb to another without noticeable change. All live in houses of the same style, shop in the same suburban supermarkets, wear the same clothes, drive the same freeways, and shuffle the same papers, wherever the company sends them at home or abroad, in an increasingly global workplace.

Life for the other-directed woman becomes more difficult as her role becomes increasingly ambiguous as she achieves increasing equality with men. Riessman et al. (1950) point out that as the importance of occupational goals declines, the importance of sexuality increases, and sex must carry a much heavier load of meaning, to the point where it is often the significant area reassuring one of one's existence. As women become emancipated, they become more knowing consumers of sex, posing a greater challenge and also a greater threat to men. The Victorian husband could be smugly assured that his wife, raised in ignorance and totally inexperienced, could not evaluate his sexual performance. The current other-directed husband, on the other hand, is increasingly confronted with an experienced partner capable of reasonable evaluation. Guilt over sexuality is replaced by performance anxiety. The new modal neurosis is anxiety and depression. And Viagra helps the anxious male.

The winds of liberation were blowing for economic reasons. The reappearance of the pleasure principle as a way of life—the consumption ethic that had first been advocated by the freethinkers (Make Love, Not War)—was soon adopted by the capitalistic system itself as a way of disposing the surplus of manufactured goods. Small-town puritans and religious conservatives fought back for a time with the temperance movement and with the 18th Amendment. But the inexorable steamroller tactics of the manufacturing class and the values of the more cosmopolitan city dwellers triumphed. The repeal of the 18th Amendment signaled the end of the small-town, Protestant, ascetic domination of the American society. Daniel Bell (1976) describes the three social inventions that were primarily responsible for this revolution—mass production on an assembly line, the development of marketing techniques for creating strong artificial appetites, and the invention of installment credit. More recently, the credit card and Internet buying sealed the new model.

I find an ironic paradox. Capitalism, in order to sell its goods, has had to adopt a strategy that undermines its own ethic—yield to your impulses, buy labor-saving gadgets, indulge yourself, have fun, spend, don't save. Impulse buying, teenage charge accounts, installment credit—all of these are directly contrary to Franklin's advice and Calvin's ethic.

Advertising has become all pervasive. It is as destructive of the Protestant ethic as all else added together. By the time a child is six, she or he has watched as many hours of TV commercials probably having more psychological impact than a college education. Young people often have become immobilized couch potatoes, yielding to impulse buying of gadgets, disinterested in school or in learning, and often unhealthy and overweight.

With the loss of a functional conscience, the neuroses have declined. Self-centered pleasure seeking has caused an increased lack of concern for others' welfare. In many cases, this lack of empathy becomes psychopathic aggression as reflected in the rise in serious crime. The self-indulgence also takes the form of recreational drug use, teen alcohol consumption, and recreational sex without emotional commitment. Magazines for teenage young women regularly report on effortless ways to lose weight and techniques for attracting and pleasing young males. With easily available contraception, sex has become recreational, not procreational.

With a decrease in social cohesiveness, there is a growing and frantic contemporary search for identity. As the self-contained, inner-directed, career-oriented, middle-class individual is less frequent on the contemporary scene and is replaced with the status-seeking lotus eater, the only reality becomes the peer group. But the peer group is composed of the same self-indulgent individuals endlessly repeated like the television commercials. In fact, they are made of television commercials. We observe the death of the great Western religions, which as Daniel Bell points out, were all religions of restraint. As a result, we are informed that God is dead and new cults, creeds, and beliefs arise most of which glorify sensation and feeling, deny the importance of history and tradition, and reject the work of the intellect. The new gurus founding these cults attract people by emphasizing magic, ritual, and "now" sensory experiences.

The confusing, anchorless, goal-less young (and middle age) generations obtain relief from their anxiety and sense of meaningless through drugs and alcohol. Anxiety leads to psychosomatic disorders. From head to toe, people are urged to consume headache pills, acid reducers, digestion correctives, constipation/diarrhea tablets and remedies for hemorrhoids. New attractive abs and buns take only 8 minutes a day, and various dyes and unguents promise perpetual youth. Breasts can be re-contoured, fat sucked out, wrinkles smoothed, and wonder-of-wonders—erections manufactured on demand.

There is not yet an acceptable name for this new neurosis—the existential neurosis comes the closest, and anxiety neurosis, and depression. Others become sociopaths.

This entry has focused largely on the causative role of social forces like sexual repression in the development of industrial nations and, conversely, on the more recent encouragement of impulsive-yielding consumption of unneeded manufactured goods. The former produced the sexual neuroses of yesterday and the latter led to the self-centered pleasure seeking existential problems of today, resulting in anxiety, depression, and aggression.

In less detail, I suggest that the incidence of psychotic behavior has occurred in all societies, probably because these are patterns of uncontrolled behavior whose origins may be found very early in life in a failure to establish an objective hold on reality and a meaningful and unshakable relationship with others. Clearly, such problems are encountered more often among the very poor (in industrial societies). Whichever group has been poorest in America has reportedly had the highest rate of out-of-control behavior. But, and this is crucial, as each poverty group moved into the more economically secure middle class, its rate of "lunacy" declined and each new immigrant group moving in turn at the bottom now has the highest rate. This pattern has happened repeatedly (see Albee, 1977, 1996b; Marshall, 1996).

One additional social class related sociopolitical issue must be recognized. In the past quarter century, there has been a major change in the model explaining the origins of mental disorders. For many years, it was widely believed that child rearing and other social factors had a major influence on personality development and, especially, that early life trauma like child physical abuse, sexual abuse, neglect, early parental loss through death and divorce, and the stresses of poverty, sexism, racism, homophobia, exploitation, all increased the risk for later emotional disturbance (Albee, 1996a). This view has many of its origins in psychoanalysis and its psychodynamic variations. It has been the basis of much of social work, clinical psychology, and psychiatry.

This social view of causation has long been opposed by organic psychiatry and by political conservatives. With the swing of the US governmental administration toward a much more conservative position after 1980, and the appointment of organic psychiatrists to direct the national mental health effort, and with the rise of influential parent–citizen groups fiercely denying any role in causing distress in their children, and the increasing power of the pharmaceutical industry, the pendulum has swung to a major emphasis on biology, brain defect, and other endogenous factors as all-important causes. The current de-emphasis on psychotherapy and the renewed effort to force "out-patient commitment" and involuntary drug treatment reflects the power of the conservative position. And as many of the journals, the national and international mental health programs, and the psychiatric training programs all are powered by money from pharmaceutical firms, the organic view is heavily supported (Albee, 1996c; Marshall, 1996). In America, economic factors now dictate the thinking about causation and treatment.

If successful prevention of mental disorders requires the development of a rational, equalitarian, socially just society, we must be prepared for a bitter bloody battle with the ruling ideas promulgated by the ruling patriarchal exploiters.

Also see: Diversity: Foundation; Politics and Systems Change: Foundation; Sexual Harassment: Adulthood; Racial and Ethnic Disparities: Adulthood; Age Bias: Older Adulthood; History: Foundation.

References

Abraham, K. (1942). *Selected papers of Karl Abraham*. London: Hogarth Press.

Albee, G.W. (1977). The Protestant ethic, sex, and psychotherapy. *American Psychologist, 37*(2), 150–161.

Albee, G.W. (1990a). The answer is prevention. In P. Chance & T.G. Harris (Eds.), *The best of Psychology Today*. New York: McGraw-Hill.

Albee, G.W. (Ed.). (1996a). Social Darwinism and political models of mental/emotional problems. *Journal of Primary Prevention, 17*(1), 3–207.

Albee, G.W. (1996b). The psychological origins of the white male patriarchy. In G.W. Albee (Ed.), Social Darwinism and political models of mental/emotional problems. *Journal of Primary Prevention, 17*(1), 75–97.

Albee, G.W. (1996c). Revolutions and counterrevolutions in prevention. *American Psychologist, 51*, 1130–1133.

American Psychiatric Association. (2000). *Diagnostic and Statistical Manual of Mental Disorders* (4th ed.). Washington, DC.

Ausubel, D.P. (1958). Theory and problems of child development. NY: Grune & Straton.

Bell, D. (1976). *The cultural contradictions of capitalism*. New York: Basic Books.

Benedict, R. (1934). *Patterns of culture*. New York: Houghton Mifflin.

Boas, F. (1948). *Race, language, and culture*. New York: The Free Press.

Emerson, R.W. (1883). Education, and essay, and other selections. In *Ralph Waldo Emerson*. Boston: Houghton Mifflin.

Freud, S. (1961). *Civilization and its discontents*. New York: Norton.

Grob, G.N. (1978). *Edward Jarvis and the medical world of nineteenth century America*. Knoxville: University of Tennessee Press.

Guse, H.G., & Schmacke, N. (1980). Psychiatry and the origins of Nazism. *International Journal of Health Services, 10*(2), 177–196.

Harlow, H. (1970). The nature of love. *American Psychologist, 25*, 161–168.

Hollingshead, A.B., & Redlich, F.C. (1968). *Social class and mental illness*. New York: Wiley.

Koplewicz, H. (1999). *Statement by keynote speaker at the White House conference on mental health*.

Kutchins, H., & Kirk, S.A. (1997). *Making us crazy: The psychiatric bible and the creation of mental disorders*. New York: Free Press.

Leighton, A.H. (1967). Some notes on preventive psychiatry. *Canadian Psychiatric Association Journal, 12*, 43N–52.

Marcus, S. (1964). *The other Victorians*. New York: Basic Books.

Marshall, J.R. (1996). Science, "schizophrenia," and genetics: The creation of myths. In G.W. Albee (Ed.), Special issue on social Darwinism and political models of mental/emotional problems. *Journal of Primary Prevention, 17*(1), 99–115.

Mead, M. (1964). *Anthropology, a human science: Selected papers, 1939–1940*. Princeton, NJ: Van Nostrand.

Mirowsky, J., & Ross, C.E. (1989). *Social causes of psychological distress*. Hawthorne, NY: Aldine.

Riessman, D., Glazer, N., & Denny, R. (1950). *The lonely crowd*. New Haven, CT: Yale University Press.

Rotenberg, M. (1975). The Protestant ethic against the spirit of psychiatry: The other side of Weber's thesis. *British Journal of Sociology, 26*, 52–65.

Schumpeter, J. (1942). *Capitalism, socialism, and democracy*. New York: Harper.

Thoreau, H.D. (1962). *Walden and other writings* (p. 197). New York: Bantam Books.

The Political Context of Primary Prevention and Health Promotion

Milton F. Shore

Economic as well as humanitarian interests have moved the health and mental health fields away from a pathology/

treatment-based model focused on specialists curing illness to a model based on preventing disease and fostering directions for positive mental health, by emphasizing growth and development, mastery, and personal efficacy. However, as prevention and the promotion of mental health have become the direction for major interventions, they have come into conflict with deeply rooted and powerful vested interests. Most professionals in the field have been trained to treat client problems, and the established organizations tend to maintain the status quo. One need only mention the conflicts over the implementation of fluoridation in water to reduce tooth decay, the battle over installing seat belts in automobiles to reduce automobile injuries in crashes, and the fight over eliminating smoking to prevent many physical illnesses to illustrate the various political forces at work on any important issue. The theme of this entry is that the political context surrounds every substantive issue in primary prevention and health promotion, requiring that practitioners in these fields know both the specific content and the larger context in order to be effective.

Two major sets of events are in a collusion course. First, we are moving toward a greater understanding of primary prevention in mental health. We continue to expand our scope of activities—consider the range of topics in this *Encyclopedia*. Primary prevention is a strong presence in general health and mental health, social welfare, and education. It is becoming stronger in law, transportation, and urban planning.

However, with each advance in primary prevention, there are opposing economic and political forces whose self-interest would be harmed by the "ounce of prevention," rather than their "pound of cure." There are social and cultural forces that foster, stimulate, and exacerbate psychopathology. For example, there is considerable evidence that increases in stress produce a predictable rise in psychological problems. War, natural disasters, and terrorism are some visible sources of stress, but the more common garden variety of stresses such as divorce, death of a spouse, or job loss, have been recognized as increasing problems such as depression, drugs and alcohol addiction, and violence.

We know that poverty is related to psychological stress. For example, more than seventy years ago, we recognized that the elderly population in the United States was one of the poorest and sickest groups in the country. With extraordinary effort, there were major changes in American social policy, such as Social Security and Medicare, that have led to significant improvements in this segment of the population. A variety of political forces opposed these social policies as being harmful to the larger benefit of society. These same kinds of political forces oppose other social policies and programs that might offer improvements to other segments of society.

In the remainder of this entry, I would like to illustrate the political dimensions of primary prevention. These examples represent both the forces seeking to make the human condition more congenial and "user friendly," and the opposing forces seeking to maintain advantage for special groups within that family of man. Through these examples, I hope to illustrate both the large and small aspects of this political process, and ultimately, the place of prevention professionals in this political world.

The long-term effects of social policy on mental health: Born unwanted. As we know, decisions regarding abortion have in great part become political rather than health issues. In the middle of the last century, under Communist rule, Czechoslovakia had a policy that, since abortions were done legally under the national health service, a woman had to go before a committee to apply to have one. Most of the abortions were approved. For a number of reasons, however, the committee turned down some women who sought to abort. If the woman felt strongly about the decision of the committee she could appeal. If she lost the appeal, she would give birth to what has been called an "unwanted child." Since records were available, the psychological development of these "unwanted" children could be studied. They were followed and compared to a matched group of "wanted" children and to their siblings (to control for any large-scale environmental effects) (David, Dytrych, Matejcek, & Schuller, 1988). A 30-year follow-up study showed the effects of this social policy on the mental health of the children: the "unwanted" children grew up to have significantly more psychological problems (Kubicka, Matejcek, David, Dytrych, Miller, & Roth, 1995). The implications of the findings were so great that there was a change in social policy, with the availability of contraceptives increasing and education in family planning added to the school curriculum.

Empowering individuals to make institutional change: Pediatric hospitalization. Studies of attachment behavior in young children (ages 0–5) done over the last half century have consistently shown that young children who have been separated from their parents show severe psychological distress which can affect their development. A movie (Robertson, 1952) showed vividly how a normal two-year-old in the hospital for minor surgery developed iatrogenic emotional problems when separated from her parents. (A second movie of a child in a hospital with its mother showed no distress in the child.) To prevent such distress, major changes were needed not only in the physical structure of the pediatric hospital (a place for parents to remain with the child day and night) but also in the attitudes of the staff as well as in medical procedures. The resistance to change shown by the medical staff was great. Pediatricians and nurses feared that there would be an increase in infections and that parents would interfere with the children's medical care or bother staff. It was when mental health professionals teamed up with parents that the necessary changes took place. For example, parents (many of whom had witnessed their children's distress and regressed behavior when they came home after being alone in the hospital) listed hospitals that made it possible to stay with their child and suggested boycotting those that did not. Political pressure was put on hospitals to accommodate parents and a social movement for family-centered medical care was started. The National Institute of Mental Health (NIMH) gave legitimacy to this movement when it published a monograph, "Red is the Color of Hurting" (Shore, 1967) with contributions from a pediatrician, a nurse, a child psychiatrist, an anthropologist, and an architect. Over time the fears of the doctors and nurses have dissipated and today it is the rare hospital where parents cannot stay with their young child. In fact, family-centered medical care has become popular to the point where Congress passed the Family and Medical Leave Act which guarantees that a person will not lose their job if they take leave for family medical care (however, unlike in some other countries, the leave is unpaid).

Prevention and promotion in mental health: Social policy and the role of work. Despite Freud's belief that work was one of the major areas of human activity highly related to mental health, little attention has been paid to that area by mental health professionals. About forty years ago, the NIMH had a Center for the Study of Work and Mental Health whose aim was to study the meaning of work and the personal issues related to employment and work settings. At that time work was revived as a valuable intervention for those with severe and persistent mental illness. Concurrent with that revival was the use of work as a technique for successfully involving adolescent delinquent boys in psychotherapy (Shore and Massimo, 1991). More recently, however, work has been used as punishment for those on welfare who are required to participate in "workfare"—that is, usually low paying jobs without the provision of adequate child care, transportation, or benefits (in a manner reminiscent of indentured servitude).

The consequences of sudden job loss were first studied systematically by Jahoda (1982). A full issue of the *Journal of Social Issues* was devoted to the topic of the psychological impact of unemployment (Dooley and Catalano, 1988). Recognizing that individuals losing jobs are at high risk for poor physical health, depression, violence, alcoholism, drug addiction, and abusive behavior, Price and his colleagues (Price and Vinokur, 1995) developed a primary prevention program to assist those laid off through a variety of psychological interventions.

However, there is another area of work that has not been addressed—that of those about to enter the work force. Erik Erikson (1982) described how work is an important element in the formation of identity in late adolescence where stability and continuity become important issues. It has been found repeatedly that the 18–24-year-olds, the ages when young people enter the work force, have the highest rate of accidents, unwanted pregnancies, drug addiction, suicide, and crime and delinquency.

There is no doubt that the nature of work has changed over the years. These changes are not only in the huge rise in the number of service jobs, but also in the psychological aspects of the work world. No longer are we talking about a guaranteed job. The living wage movement, an effort to raise wages above the poverty level, is relatively small. The psychological changes are best illustrated in a cartoon from *The New Yorker* where a personnel officer says to a person applying for a job, "We expect little loyalty. In return, we offer little security." For those in the work force or entering the work force, temporary employment ("temping") has become a rite of passage with no benefits such as health care, retirement, or annual leave for vacation.

It has become clear that in order to promote mental health, a nation needs a national full-employment strategy. Such a strategy would cut across social and economic levels (many of those being laid off are middle-class employees in mid-career when they are planning families or making educational plans for their children). Such a program would have significant impact on the mental health of individuals and families. However, the systems of intersecting political entities that would be involved in this change make the hopes of attaining this goal daunting.

The political aspects of prevention: Declarations of Human Rights. Another perspective on the close tie between prevention and political forces is illustrated by the efforts of the United Nations to establish guarantees of universal rights. In 1959, the General Assembly of the United Nations passed the Declaration of the Rights of the Child (United Nations, 1959). The profound mental health implications of the document are obvious as the declaration states that the aim of such rights is "to the end that he (a child) may have a happy childhood." The rights include the banning of discrimination, special legal protections, increased opportunities for growth and development, guaranteed health care for mother and child, availability of special treatment if handicapped, and guaranteed education and play. Such rights, based on a scientific understanding of human growth and development, are separate from the treatment of mental illness, and form the foundation for universal prevention of much psychological dysfunction. The United States, recognizing the political implications of the document, is one of two nations in the world that is not a signatory to the document.

Affecting social change: The role of the mental health professional. Mental health professionals, aware that there is more to mental health than the treatment of mental disorders, recognize how social and political decisions affect mental health. There are two roles that mental health professionals can play in the political scene to bring about social change. One is that of *ombudsman* where the professional negotiates a way through the existing social system to make sure that the system responds appropriately to the needs of the individual. The other is change.

Conclusion. The field of primary prevention in mental health can challenge the basic structures of the social and political forces that shape a society. Those involved in prevention are particularly alert to the sources of stress in the society that can lead to psychological disorders. It is important that mental health professionals recognize that the mental health field is inherently political. Building on scientific knowledge, aware of the destructiveness of certain policies and institutions, and knowing the negative consequences of certain political decisions from a mental health perspective, the mental health professional is obligated to become vocal and visible in the political arena.

Also see: Culture, Society, and Social Class: Foundation; Racial and Ethnic Disparities: Adulthood; Ethics: Foundation; History: Foundation.

References

David, H.P., Dytrych, Z., Matejcek, Z., & Schuller, V. (1988). *Born unwanted: Developmental effects of denied abortion.* New York: Springer.

Dooley, D., & Catalano, R. (Eds.). (1988). Psychological effects of unemployment. *Journal of Social Issues, 44*(4).

Erikson, E. (1982). *The life cycle completed.* New York: Norton.

Jahoda, M. (1982). *Employment and unemployment: A social psychological analysis.* New York: Cambridge University Press.

Kubicka, L., Matejcek, Z., David, H.P., Dytrych, Z., Miller, W.B., & Roth, Z. (1995). Children from unwanted pregnancies in Prague, Czech Republic: Revisited at age 30. *Acta Psychiatrica Scandinavica, 91,* 361–369.

Price, R.H., & Vinokur, A.D. (1995). Supporting career transition in a time of organizational downsizing: The Michigan JOBS program. In M. London (Ed.), *Employees' careers and job creation: Developing growth-oriented human resource strategies and programs* (pp. 191–209). San Francisco: Jossey-Bass.

Robertson, J. (1952). *A two-year-old goes to the hospital* [film]. New York: New York University Film Library.

Shore, M.F. (Ed.). (1967). *Red is the color of hurting: Planning for children in the hospital* (DHEW Publication No. 1583). Washington, DC: US Government Printing Office.

Shore, M.F. (1998). Beyond self interest: Professional advocacy and the integration of theory, research, and practice. *American Psychologist, 53*(4), 474–479.

Shore, M.F., & Massimo, J.L. (1991). Contributions of an innovative psychoanalytic therapeutic program with adolescent delinquents to developmental psychology. In S.I. Greenspan & G.H. Pollack (Eds.), *The course of life: Vol. IV. Adolescence* (pp. 333–356). Madison, CT: International Universities Press.

United Nations. (1959). Declaration of the rights of the child. Proclaimed by General Assembly resolution 1386 (XIV), November 20.

Financing Primary Prevention and Health Promotion

Nancy Kennedy

INTRODUCTION

The technological advances in health care during the 20th and 21st centuries are so incredible that they seem to offer nirvana; nonetheless, this possibility remains illusory as no country is wealthy enough to support comprehensive, sophisticated health care for all of its population. Consequently, there are health care priorities in all countries and social, economic, cultural, and political forces determine the ranking of those priorities. Regardless of where health promotion and primary prevention are ranked, financing is critical. However, despite their importance for consumers, private and nonprofit health providers, public health organizations, and policy-makers, there is little discussion about the financing of health promotion and primary prevention.

The National Library of Medicine lists more than 21,000 published cost-effectiveness studies on health. Primary prevention is the subject of very few (Ramsey, 2000). This suggests that key stakeholders do not view health promotion and primary prevention as marketable products. It may also explain the fact that only one percent of the US total health expenditures goes for public health (Wall, 1998). In comparison to most other industrialized countries, the US government expends the least amount of public funds on health services (Anderson & Maxwell, 1994).

The umbrella for health promotion and primary prevention is public health. Thus, the topic of financing health promotion and primary prevention must be understood in the context of public health. A continued misunderstanding of public health contributes greatly to calculating the allocation of resources for health promotion and primary prevention. This historical discussion about public health in the United States is similar to that of other countries.

While public health and medicine have been inseparable throughout history, the two disciplines have different underpinnings and responsibilities. The inability to understand these differences has created misunderstandings, not the least of which is linguistic confusion.

Public health has had, and continues to have, an identity crisis. It has been almost fifty years since McGavran

(1953, p. 441) asked:

> What is public health? Is there a distinctive discipline of
> public health? These are simple questions, but the answers
> are not so simple. There are many leaders in public health
> who maintain that public health cannot be defined. If this be
> true, it is no wonder that with the changing times, there con-
> tinues to be increased misunderstanding of public health by
> the organized medical profession; and that there is apathy
> and indifference to public health on the part of the public
> and appropriating bodies of government.

PUBLIC HEALTH MODEL: PRIMARY PREVENTION

The public health model structures information within the framework of environmental, social, economic, and biological conditions affecting health or well-being. Like the medical model, one theoretical base is biological science. Other theoretical bases include the physical and social sciences, the humanities, and public health's two cornerstones—that is, epidemiology and biostatistics. Unlike the medical model, which is concerned with the individual, the public health model is focused on the health of the community. A major assumption of the public health model is that each person within the community has a right to an environment that promotes health and well-being. Public health seeks to promote health and minimize the causes of illnesses or disorders in populations by utilizing methods and activities that are designated as primary prevention, treatment, and rehabilitation (maintenance of restored health). In this entry, only primary prevention is described.

The dual goals of primary prevention are to promote health and well-being, and to prevent the occurrence of specific diseases, disorders, illnesses, or situations that may precipitate such. Examples of primary prevention activities that promote health and well-being include: pre-marital and preretirement advice (anticipatory guidance), seat belts and infant care seats (systems intervention), media campaigns, and antismoking classes (education). These activities are part of traditional school and community education agendas and are directed to problems of living—that is, those events, expected or unexpected, during life which in the absence of sufficient ability to cope, may lead to dysfunctional behavior, disease and/or disorder (Kennedy, 1999). Support for these efforts can be found at the individual, community, state, and federal level in programs to control access to tobacco, recreation programs, and disability payments.

The other major grouping of primary prevention activities involves specific protection. When a pathogen has been identified or a segment of population is acknowledged to have a higher statistical probability of developing an illness, disease, or disorder, prevention activities have been developed to

stop or delay the onset of the problem or lessen its impact. Examples include: immunization against diseases such as smallpox, rubella, or polio; industrial accident prevention including the wearing of hard hats or eye goggles; and highway safety prevention including the wearing of seat belts and use of car infant seats. Here, too, support for these efforts can be found at the individual, community, state, and federal level. Examples include pure food and drug laws, fluoridation, meat and restaurant inspection; surveillance system for identified infectious diseases and garbage collection.

Although primary prevention has a strong regulatory component in both health promotion and specific protection, the success of interventions is dependent upon resource allocation including financing. Holland and Stewart (1998, p. 278) have stressed the importance of public health practitioners influencing funding if public health is to be improved:

> They have to be able to influence the budget for public
> health activities order that the longer term issues are not
> omitted in favor of the clamant short-term demands. This is
> crucial to public health resource needs of clinical services.
> The latter nearly always takes precedence—treatment of
> individual patients seems far more immediate a priority than
> changes in health status for the future.

Influencing the budget cycle is critically important to ensure that public health funding is adequately supported. A decline in funding is associated with a decline in public health expertise and services, which becomes problematic when some public health crisis occurs in the absence of adequate response capability (Durham & Kill, 1999).

SOURCES OF FINANCING

The health system is shaped by the way the funds to maintain the system are collected, allocated, and distributed. Systems vary among countries, states, provinces within countries, and localities. There is no objective way to determine what the appropriate proportion of financing for health should be. The same applies to education, defense, and agriculture. The only common unit to measure returns from expenditure is social benefit calculated in financial terms. The main purpose of health promotion and specific protection is the production of the social benefit (i.e., health) (Cohen & Henderson, 1988). Even if the value of health can be determined, promotion of health and primary prevention is just one factor in determining health or wellness. Table 1 delineates sources of financing health services.

Tulchinsky and Varavikova (2000) describe three categories of funding sources, that is, public, private, and international cooperation. While this schema does not identify all possible funding sources, the variety of sources is illustrated. Most of the financial sources are indirect, for example,

Table 1. Sources of Financing Health Services

Public sources	Private sources	International cooperation
Federal state, and local Govt. general revenues, mainly from taxes; income, excise, resources, inheritance, value added, capital gains, property, special Social security tax Compulsory health insurance Lotteries Dedicated taxes Cigarettes, alcohol, gambling	Private health insurance Personal expenditures Private donations and wills Private foundations Voluntary community service User fees	United Nations affiliates Foundations Religious organizations Other nongovernmental organizations World Bank Government bilateral aid

Source: Tulchinsky & Varavikova (2000, p. 569).

general government funds including taxes, compulsory social insurance funds, voluntary insurance funds (both public and private), charitable funds, and grants from outside the country. The other category of financing is direct, that is, payments made by purchasers (i.e., consumers, employers, and/or government) in return for goods or services received. Included in Table 1 are the sources of financing health services, which includes medical care services, research, and public health. Thus, the terms "health care services" and "health expenditures" describe the sum of medical care and the subsection of public health services dedicated to individuals.

Concepts of cost and benefits are critical to understanding health financing. According to Cohen and Henderson (1988, p. 43):

> The key feature of both costs and benefits is value. In principle, a benefit is anything, which someone would be willing to pay something for, and a cost is anything, which someone would be willing to pay something to avoid. Whether or not payment is actually made is of no consequence to its value.

The main criterion for choice is maximizing benefits from available resources. Using resources one way means doing without the benefits that could have been obtained by using those same resources in another way. Thus, maximizing benefits means minimizing opportunity costs, which refers to the value of the sacrifice or of the benefit foregone (Cohen & Henderson, 1988). Costs and benefits are often classified as priced or unpriced. For example, volunteer labor and donated work space may be unpriced and considered "free" to a given program but are still the same "costs" from an economic and societal perspective (Ramsey, 2000).

The costs of providing these services require resources, for example, manpower and goods that could be used to meet other needs by individuals and communities.

Different measures are used in financing studies according to the type of research, for example, marginal analysis, elasticity. *Marginal analysis* is based on the principle that resources are scarce, and explicitly recognizes that all potentially preventable morbidity and mortality will never be achieved (Cohen & Henderson, 1988). *Elasticity* is measured as the proportionate change in aggregate demand resulting from a proportionate change in the variable of interest. To illustrate, when the price of cigarettes goes up, the demand (purchase) for cigarettes goes down among teenagers with limited incomes (Cohen & Henderson, 1988).

The key question for financing health promotion and specific protection is: Who pays for wellness or the pursuit of maximizing health? The improvement of health status is not possible without incurring cost (Schauffler, 2000). Throughout the years, the critical aspect in funding these programs is the ability to be creative and flexible in identifying and using different funding sources. With multiple financial sources, no single agency has responsibility for health promotion and primary prevention (Segal, 1998).

According to traditional economic theory, many primary prevention public health services, such as clean water, sanitation, food and restaurant inspection, are public goods. Obtaining these services individually would be impossible except for wealthiest as the costs are so exorbitant (Durham & Kill, 1999). Thus, it is socially desirable for the government to finance these services. Water fluoridation appears to be a profitable investment (Cohen & Henderson, 1988). The specific protection activities of primary prevention in the form of immunizations and well baby clinics are, in economic terms, merit goods as they produce externalities (Hsiao, 1995). *Externalities* are measured by recording items such as the dispensing of a vaccination or measuring the weights and heights of infants at designated times. In contrast, *internalities* such as improved mental health, increased resiliency, and enhanced self-concept are difficult to measure because of insufficient norms for different population segments. While the public benefits from government financing of such activities, the private sector also makes a substantial investment.

Any mechanism intended to provide economic support for health services aimed at *all* people seemingly must be organized through a national government. Governments can use the mechanisms of social or health insurance (depending upon the politics of the country) or general revenues to finance health care interventions (Roemer, 1977). However, some countries, notably the United States and Canada, have decentralized their public health programs and placed significant responsibility with more local levels of government usually on a cost-sharing basis (Gold, Ellwood, Davis, Liedschutz, Orland, & Cohen, 1995). The US experience with this approach is that dependency on local revenues results in a varying quality public health system because of changes in local funding priorities and shifting economic prosperity (Wall, 1998).

Government funding for health promotion and primary prevention in many countries, especially where health insurance predominates, is constrained by the demands of treatment and rehabilitative services as well as other sectors of the budget. The natural reaction to the need for additional governmental revenue is to raise tax rates, especially on products deemed harmful to health. Alcoholic beverages and tobacco products are frequently subject to a variety of federal, state, and local taxes while some local jurisdictions levy taxes on soft drinks, candy, chewing gum, or other high-sugar products (Cox, Williams, de Courten, Tuomilehto, & Zimmet, 2000; Ismail, Brodeur, Gagnon, Payette, Picard, & Hamalian, 1997; Jacobson & Brownell, 2000). Virtually every country has been taxing tobacco even before the health risks were well established, mainly because tobacco duty is an easy way to collect taxes and the demand for cigarettes does not seem to change dramatically for adults who smoke (Cohen & Henderson, 1988).

While policy-makers might assert that tobacco taxes are "costless" in comparison to programs that consume tangible resources, the smokers who pay these taxes know otherwise. In actuality, tax revenue is neither a cost nor a benefit, but a "transfer" (Cohen & Henderson, 1988). International and interstate comparisons reveal extraordinary variance in these excise taxes, reflecting contrasting values of health vis-à-vis producers of products (Center for Science in Public Interest [CSPI], 1991). Any increase in taxes reduces the amount of consumer surplus, and this is the cost of taxation, that is, the loss of personal revenue. Interestingly, one study from Switzerland suggests that non-smokers live longer but use medical services heavily during the last years of their life (Leu & Schaub, 1983). Elixhauser (1990) estimated that the price elasticity of the demand for cigarettes ranged from -1.4 for adolescents to $-.42$ for adults. In other words, every 10 percent increase in cigarette prices would result in a 4 percent decline in smoking initiation among adults and a 14 percent decline among adolescents. Thus, even with tobacco, an avowed worldwide public health problem, health economists have difficulty providing evidence to answer the age-old question: *Is an ounce of prevention worth a pound of cure?*

INTERNATIONAL PERSPECTIVE

International comparisons of financing health promotion and primary prevention are difficult because of varying definitions of public health and health expenditures, and because of the different values involved. A comparative international framework requires discussion of economic factors, sociopolitical factors, and historical/cultural influences (Roemer, 1977).

The most obvious example of economic factors is the wealth of the purchaser, whether that is a country or a consumer. This aside, there are other factors that impair the financing of health promotion and primary prevention such as outcomes tied to a narrow/short-term focus and reimbursement for medical necessity in preference to social necessity (Segal, 1998). In many countries, health promotion is a business supported not only by commercial vendors but also by health care facilities. The selling of health promotion can range from commercial strategies promoting the use of a particular product or program to the use of mass media by government and voluntary agencies for promoting health-related knowledge, attitude, and behavior change. Targeting health promotion at those who can afford to pay reinforces the belief that health is a commodity that can be bought and sold.

Interwoven with economic and historical/cultural factors are political and social forces that influence the financing of health promotion and primary prevention. For example, in controlled socialized countries such as China, public health has been considered the most important activity of the health sector (Pickett & Hanlon, 1990). In contrast over the past decade, New Zealand has experimented with several different public health configurations (Durham & Kill, 1999). As part of its reforms in 1991, the New Zealand government decided to separate the funding and management of population-based health strategies from personal health strategies, and to establish a Public Health Commission in 1993 which was terminated in 1995 (Durham & Kill, 1999). In addition to these political examples, there are social factors like religious organizations, schools, and workplaces that influence the design of the delivery system. Miller (1987, p. 2) described the church's role in health promotion:

> We cannot expect our current health care system to correct the ways we choose to exercise, eat, drink, or smoke. As a community of faith, we must move toward self-help, self-care, and prevention.

Of course, the specific health promotion activities of the church depend upon the religious affiliation. Despite Margaret Sanger's launching the "birth control" movement in 1914 in New York City, the World Health Organization did not consider a program in this field politically acceptable to launch until about 1965 and then only with the label of "human reproduction studies" (Roemer, 1977).

Historical/cultural factors are difficult to separate from economic and sociopolitical factors. Each source of financing in Table 1 has historical/cultural factors within a country and among countries. Culture is not restricted to racial, ethnic identification, or heritage; instead, culture is composed of the customs, beliefs, values, knowledge, and skills that guide people's behavior along shared paths (Kennedy, 1999). Indeed, cultures even define differently the concepts of health/wellness and disease/disorder.

When policy-makers undertake comparative studies on financing, expenditures are expressed relative to the gross national product (GNP), the gross domestic product (GDP), or the gross national expenditure (GNE). GNP and GDP are usually interchangeable and most frequently used for comparison. GNE is the value of all goods and services produced by a nation's economy, before the deduction of depreciation allowance for the consumption of durable capital goods, plus (earned) income and other funds (net transfers and borrowing) received from the rest of the world (Abel-Smith, 1963). Most studies examine health expenditures or health services (see Table 2) and not specifically health promotion and primary prevention.

Over a thirty-five-year period for the eight industrialized countries appearing in Table 2, the per capita health expenditures as a percentage GDP has increased more rapidly in the United States and Germany than in the other countries.

The 1961 World Health Organization (WHO) study of Ceylon, Chile, Czechoslovakia, Israel, Sweden, and the United States is essentially an economic study of health services with public health services differentiated from medical care services and research (Abel-Smith, 1963). I compared the health expenditures from this study with those reported in Table 2 and found that there was congruence with the two sets of figures for both Sweden and the United States (two countries that were included in both studies).

The public health services in the WHO study were further subdivided into services for populations, environmental regulatory services concerned with the elimination of

pathogens found in water, milk, sanitation, and so on, and other public health services including data on infrastructure and laboratory services. The GNE was selected as the most suitable measure of resources with which to compare total national expenditures on health. Not surprising, personal health care services represented at least 90 percent of current operating expenditures for the six countries (Abel-Smith, 1963). The role of environmental and other public health services was extremely small with Ceylon expending 4.1 percent of its health care budget on public health, Chile, 6.4 percent, Czechoslovakia, 3.4 percent, Israel, 1.9 percent, Sweden, 1.3 percent, and the United States, 0.8 percent.

The poorest country participating in the study, Ceylon, had the highest percentage of total current operating expenditures for environmental and other public health services (4.1 percent). In contrast, the richest country, the United States, had the lowest percentage for these services (0.8 percent) (Abel-Smith, 1963). One possible explanation for this discrepancy is that in 1963 the causes of morbidity and mortality in the United States were largely due to chronic diseases, while in Ceylon infectious diseases were more prevalent.

More recent approximate expenditures for public health relative to the total health budgets are available for three countries (Deeble, 1999; Lee & Paxman, 1997; New Zealand Ministry of Health, 1997; Wall, 1998)

- New Zealand 1.7%
- United States 1–3%
- Australia 2–3%

These expenditures consist of federal, state, and local revenues, as well as Medicaid payments, patient fees, and regulatory fees (Center for Studying Health Systems Change [CSHSC], 1996). These figures suggest that public health expenditures have more than doubled in the United States since the WHO study. Perhaps, these higher expenditures are the result of research demonstrating that 70 percent of today's illnesses or disorders in the United States and likely elsewhere are preventable (Kennedy, 1999).

Table 2. Per Capita Health Expenditures as Percentage of Gross Domestic Product for Selected Industrial Countries and Years

Country	1960	1970	1980	1990	1995
United States	5.1	7.1	8.9	12.2	13.6
Canada	5.5	7.1	7.3	9.2	9.7
France	4.2	5.8	7.6	8.9	9.9
Germany	4.3	5.7	8.1	8.2	10.4
Sweden	4.7	7.1	9.4	8.8	7.2
Japan	NA	4.4	6.4	6.0	7.2
Denmark	3.6	6.1	6.8	6.5	6.5
United Kingdom	3.9	4.5	5.6	6.0	6.9

Sources: Health United States: 1998, and Organization of Economic Cooperation and Economic Development (OECD) Health Data, 1998; Anderson, G.F. & Ponllier J.P., (1999) Health spending, access and outcomes: Trends in industrialized countries. *Health Affairs,* May/June, 178–192.

FEDERAL PERSPECTIVE IN THE UNITED STATES

Many public health professionals have observed that the United States does not have a health care system but rather a medical care system. The figures cited earlier would validate that observation. As the business of medicine flourished during most of the 20th century, public health was left out of the industry (Leviss, 2001). Medicine and medical care comprised the private sector and primary prevention and rehabilitation of the public health model became the responsibility of governmental entities.

At the federal level, public health programs in the United States were initiated by an act of Congress in 1798 "to provide for the relief of sick and disabled seamen" (Mullan, 1989). Less than a decade later, a National Health entity was established and shortly after that the federal government was given the authority to quarantine people to prevent epidemics.

The federal perspective in prevention is based on an assumption that most health problems are more effectively dealt with locally. As excerpted from the *Forward Plan for Health, FY 1977–1981* (1975), the Public Health Service's role in prevention is to:

- Identify and call public attention to the major causes of disease and death in the country and recommend alternative ways to prevent or control them.
- Assist states and localities and the private sector to improve their capacities to deal with these problems.
- Provide short-term technical and specialized assistance and training in prevention techniques and procedures.
- Promulgate uniform national prevention objectives, standards, and norms for planning programs and assessing progress.
- Provide funds to states and localities to carry out their prevention programs.
- Assure that all people have equal access to preventive programs and that the programs preserve each person's rights and freedom of choice.
- Compile and publish data on the nature, extent, and consequences of the principal causes of death and disease.
- Conduct and support research on the etiology of preventable diseases and on techniques for the prevention or control of the principal causes of such diseases.

The first federal "grant" program was created through the Public Health Service for venereal disease in 1918 although that program quickly ended with the close of World War I (Leviss, 2001). The 1935 passage of Title V and VI of the Social Security Act institutionalized federal funding for public health activities by creating "general health grants" to support state and local public health services (Mullan, 1989). In 1936, special grants were approved for maternal, child health, and disabled children. Federal grants totaling more than $63 million reached their zenith during the early 1950s (Leviss, 2001). A 1965 law established a Federal Water Pollution Control Administration that was moved from the Department of Health, Education and Welfare (HEW) to the Department of Interior. In 1970, this part of the Interior Department became the Environmental Protection Agency (EPA) (Mullan, 1989). Under President Reagan, many public health programs were reduced, eliminated, or combined in the form of block grants.

Two of the largest federal health programs, Medicaid and Medicare, have provided little support to state and local health departments (Leviss, 2001). Congress did, however, expand Medicaid coverage to pregnant women and children in the late 1980s, thereby providing some additional financing for traditional public health services (Joes, 1995). States continue to rely heavily on federal funding to support their public health departments and services. Due to their budgetary prominence, federal grants often drive programmatic policies and priorities at state and local levels (Leviss, 2001). In addition to federal grants, alcohol taxes generated $5.7 billion in federal receipts in FY 1990 (Cook & Moore, 1991).

STATE AND LOCAL PERSPECTIVE IN THE UNITED STATES

In the late 19th century, state boards of health developed across the United States (Mullan, 1989). Not surprisingly, because of communicable diseases, the growth of state and local health departments were inextricably linked with sanitary campaigns. As progress in this area was made, personal health services like maternal and child health emerged as important public health agendas (Kramer & Terris, 1949).

Recently, at a state level, the power of public health has been reduced as public health departments have merged with other departments like social services or been fractionalized (Leviss, 2001). What appears to be a deciding factor in this reorganization is the manner in which public health within a state is financed. Thus, organizational structure and programming follows funding rather than function. For example, the Women, Infants, and Children (WIC) nutrition program and other US Department of Agriculture nutrition funds account for the largest share of a state health departments' budgets with the Maternal and Child Health block grants (Title V) a distant second, followed by family planning (Title X) and other federal block grants and discretionary grants (Wall, 1998). Given this portfolio of funding, it is not surprising that two of every three dollars spent by a sample of states in a nationwide study went for personal health services or direct service provision (Public Health Foundation [PHF], 1996). Of the remaining funds for population-based health services, the largest amount (26 percent) was for enforcing laws and regulations to protect the health and safety of the public, while training (4 percent) and research (2 percent) received the smallest investments (PHF, 1996).

Over the past several years, most state public health departments have experienced annual increases in health financing in the range of 4–8 percent (Wall, 1998). These increases were the result of factors such as state tobacco taxes, enrolling Medicaid eligible individuals into managed care, widening the eligibility for participation in states' Children Health Insurance Programs (CHIP), reimbursing school-based health centers for services provided, better marketing of public health to state legislatures, and growth in federal funds reflecting the decentralization of many services, including public health (Santelli et al., 1998; Wall, 1998).

Many states organize public health systems around county health departments but there are exceptions. For example, large metropolitan areas like New York, Houston, and Los Angeles have city health departments and other variations exist (Wall, 1998). With the advent of managed care as the predominant health care organization and financing model within the United States, numerous changes in the health care system have resulted. For example, historically, Blue Cross and Blue Shield corporations have operated under state charters as tax-exempt status organizations in exchange for undertaking activities that benefit community health by expanding health insurance coverage and access to health care. However, during the 1990s, a significant number of BC/BS plans renegotiated their state characters and surrendered their tax-exempt status (Friedman, 1998).

While considerable negativity is associated with managed care, this way of managing insufficient financial resources has been critical for many states fiscally strained by having Medicaid account for approximately 27 percent of all state expenditures (National Governors' Association [NGA], 2001). While not often seen in practice, on paper the basic ideals and assumptions of managed care are health promotion, disease prevention, and successful self-management of chronic illness. These should result in cost-offsets, if not cost-effectiveness and cost-benefits (Kennedy, 1999).

The amount of funding provided by states to localities, the form it takes, and the requirements attached to it vary among states. State health departments provide both categorical grant funding and base funding for the provision of public health programs (Leviss, 2001). Some states dedicate part or all of their alcohol tax collections to financing the prevention and treatment of alcoholism. In addition, the last several years have yielded success after success for states seeking to recover funds spent on smokers through Medicaid plans, smokers with tobacco-related illnesses seeking damages, and nonsmokers pursuing their right to live and work in smoke-free environments (Cawood & Morrow, 2001).

Fiscal capacity measures the potential ability of state and local governments to finance public services (Gold et al., 1995). As contrasted with *fiscal effort*, or the amount of resources that are actually used, fiscal capacity determines the amount of resources that could be used to fund state and local services, including public health. While public health functions are carried out at all levels of government, the most visible activity occurs in more than 3000 county, city, and other municipal health departments throughout the states

(National Association of County and City Health Officials [NACCHO], 1998). Per capita personal income is the most widely used indicator of fiscal capacity as most taxes are paid from the income of states' residents (Gold et al., 1995). The property tax is the primary local source of revenue (PHF, 1996). Federal aid, including Medicaid, Medicare, block grants and discretionary funds, is another indicator of fiscal capacity (Gold et al., 1995). In addition, community hospitals contribute to local public health activities, especially by providing charitable services (Mays, 2001).

Table 3 delineates the sources of funds for local health departments in 12 states.

These particular states were selected by the Urban Institute's Health Policy Center in Washington, DC, because they illustrated diverse financing arrangements, varying degrees of privatization and different historical relationships between state and local entities (Wall, 1998). The largest share of funding, 40 percent on average, comes from the state, including federal pass-through funds. Typically, states allocate funds based on a formula although these vary considerably by state.

The second largest share of funding is local revenue. Looking at individual states reveals differences with regard to Medicaid. For example, local public health systems in the south have traditionally considered personal health services

Table 3. Sources of Funds for Local Health Departments, FY 1991, 1992, or 1993

State	Local[a] %	State[b] %	Federal[c] %	Medicaid[d] %	Medicare %	Other[e] %
MA	93	1	0	1	0	6
NJ	86	8	2	1	1	3
NY	27	26	3	18	14	12
MI	28	36	2	9	8	18
MN	26	27	4	11	6	25
WS	54	11	2	9	11	12
AL	9	19	5	25	32	10
FL	14	66	2	8	1	9
TX	51	38	3	2	0	6
CA	26	52	6	2	3	11
CO	50	27	2	5	5	11
WA	34	25	4	8	2	27
US	34	40	6	7	3	10

Source: National Association of County and City Health Officials (NACCHO), unpublished data.
Notes: The survey conducted by NACCHO asked local health departments to report revenues, for the most recent fiscal year for which data were available. Percentages are an average of those percentages reported by each health department (i.e., funding source proportions are not weighted by health department budget). Data for MS are not available.
[a] Includes city, township, town, and county sources.
[b] Includes pass-through funds from federal government and excludes Medicaid.
[c] Includes federal monies that are paid directly to the local health department, excluding Medicaid.
[d] Includes federal and state shares of Medicaid.
[e] Includes private foundations, health insurance, patient and regulatory fees, and other unspecified.

as their core mission because of the lack of access and short-age of private providers (Wall, 1998). This historical per-spective explains the high percentage of Medicaid and Medicare funding reflected in Table 3.

Nearly half of all local health departments maintain some type of alliance with managed care plans even though those plans may free-ride on public health services (NAACHO, 1998; Scutchfield, Harris, Koplan, Lawrence, Gordon, Violante, 1998). *Free-riding* occurs when health plan enrollees receive health care services from public health agen-cies that replace or reduce the need for such services from the plan (Mays, 2001). The likely services most apt to free-riding are primary prevention interventions such as immunizations, well-baby services, and health education services especially for Medicaid, Medicare and/or other patient populations who have established ties with public health clinics. Finally, the last source of public health income is derived from the fees and fines collected from their regulatory activities, such as licens-ing child care centers, inspecting eating establishments, and maintaining vital records like birth and death (Leviss, 2001).

After government, employers are the next most promi-nent health care payer in the United States (Levit et al., 1998). A recent survey found that 88 percent of major employers have introduced some form of disease prevention, health pro-motion, or early intervention to encourage healthy lifestyles among their salaried employees (Hewitt Associates, 1996). Today, most employers use a benefits or entitlement approach to health management and health care management (Moody & Turnock, 1998). To illustrate, benefit administrators might offer wellness programs to all employees and spend addi-tional resources on those employees who volunteer for such programs, such as purchasing memberships to fitness clubs. According to Chapman (1997), annual budgets for model worksite programs averaged $56.60 per employee for health promotion activities and $20.70 per employee for demand management activities. These figures might be underesti-mates because many companies do not include staff or facil-ity costs in their estimates. Nonetheless, these amounts pale in comparison to the approximate $4000 per year that employ-ers pay for each worker's health insurance (Lippman, 1997).

CONCLUSION

The measurement of the ultimate success in transforming the financing of health care systems in the United States and other countries is to focus on the continuum of care that begins with prevention, extends to treatment, and concludes with rehabilitation. The redesign and needed paradigm shift from a medical model to a population-based model is the major chal-lenge facing public health. Each element of the continuum is critical to avoid health system disintegration. Imagine for a moment the health consequences for a population without

safe drinking water or without access to a health care provider when ill, or services to restore functioning lost to a serious illness. Clearly, each element requires financing.

Financing for public health is difficult given the lack of understanding about what comprises public health. With cer-tain exceptions like HIV/AIDS or tuberculosis, and events like weather disasters or bioterrorism, public health is not in the spotlight. The sheer multitude and diversity of programs and services found under the auspices of public health are confusing to policy-makers and funders. Thus, fulfilling the full potential of public health suffers. As Leviss (2001) observed, "Federal and state funding has continued to follow specific programs and services of the day or of the year, and state and local public health agencies have continued to oper-ate in reactive as opposed to proactive modalities."

Managed care has dramatically changed the operation of medicine. Similarly, public health and its component parts, especially primary prevention, need to apply the principles of health care economics and marketing in order to survive as an important force in the continuum of care. Health promo-tion and primary prevention are not cost-free interventions. Financing is required and the amount of resources is a prime determinant of achievable outcomes. In spite of increasing costs for health insurance, Bodenhorn and Kemper (1997) report that most individuals who have insurance are willing to pay 5 percent more for coverage if their health plans pro-vided health promotion and disease management services. This desire might be realized as managed care companies provide evidence that health promotion and primary preven-tive interventions assist not only corporate image but also increase consumer satisfaction (Dwore, Murray, Parsons, & Gustafson, 2001).

The pay-offs from financing health promotion and pri-mary prevention are future-oriented and indistinct to many key stakeholders including policy-makers and consumers. Nevertheless, all of us are consumers as the resources for health promotion and primary prevention. When all of these resources have been tried without success to resolve "prob-lems of living," then the treatment and maintenance seg-ments need to be employed. Human resolve to seek healthy lifestyles is often forgotten when an extraordinary medical care exists. However, that system need not utilize resources for situations that require preventive interventions unless that is the appropriate venue of delivery. Other venues asso-ciated with resources for preventive intervention might be more appropriate, yielding not only lower fiscal costs but also better outcomes. Multiple examples exist of self-help and mutual support groups, peer networks, family strength-ening interventions, community-based programs and poli-cies and professional health promotion and primary prevention initiatives.

In conclusion, Lawrence (2001, p. 66) brings us full circle in this review of the financing of primary prevention:

> To compare alternative interventions for a population requires us to develop a language that reflects a communitarian or population-based ethic. Without the language—the framework embedded in our decisionmaking processes—we have nothing to guide us toward sound, ethical decisions that are in the best interests of the most people within a community or population. Even if we could operate with a population-based focus, we struggle with how to define the "greatest good." Is it reduction in mortality? Morbidity? Is it appropriateness of resource use to achieve the effect? Does it matter whether or not we are talking about people at the end of their productive lives or at the beginning? There is no agreement in our society, of course.

Public health, specifically health promotion and primary prevention, is an interdisciplinary field where health economists have often been on the periphery. In the past and currently, money has been the foremost concern of key stakeholders including consumers, providers, purchasers, and policymakers. Perhaps, the future cost-outcome analyses of health promotion and specific protection in public health needs to be "Willingness to Pay," that is, the amount society is willing to pay for a benefit that is priceless. This is the cost and benefit of producing health and well-being.

Also see: Cost Benefit Analysis: Adulthood; Evaluation: Foundation; Environment: Foundation; Political and Systems Change: Foundation.

References

Abel-Smith, B. (1963). *Paying for health services: A study of the costs and sources of finance in sex countries*, Geneva, Switzerland: World Health Organization.

Anderson, G.F., & Maxwell, S. (1994). The organization and financing of healthcare services. In R.J. Taylor & S. B. Taylor (Eds.), *The AUPHA manual of health services management (pp. 87–101)*. Gaithersburg, MD: Aspen Publishers, Inc.

Bodenhorn, K., & Kemper, L. (1997). *Spending for health*, Sacramento, CA: California Center for Health Insurance.

Cawood, J., & Morrow, T. (2001). Putting to use a clinical guideline for treating tobacco dependency. *Managed Care Interface*, 6, 79–83.

Center for Science in the Public Interest (CSPI). (1991). *State alcohol taxes: Case studies of the impact of higher excise taxes in 14 states and the district of Columbia. Raising revenues and reducing alcohol-related problems*. Washington, DC: The Center.

Center for Studying Health Systems Change (CSHSC). (1996). Tracking changes in the public health system, Washington, DC: CSHSC.

Chapman, L. (1997). Benchmarking best practices in workplace health promotion. *The Art of Health Promotion*, 11, 1–8.

Cohen, D.R., & Henderson, J.B. (1988). *Health, prevention, and economics*. Oxford, England: Oxford University.

Cook, P.J., & Moore, M.J. (1991). Taxation of alcoholic beverages. In M.E. Milton & G. Bloss (Eds.), *Economics and the prevention of alcohol-related problems (pp. 53–58)* (NIH Publication No. 93-3513). Rockville, MD: HHS.

Cox, H.S., Williams, J.W., de Courten, M.P., Tuomilehto, J., & Zimmet, P.Z. (2000). Decreasing prevalence of cigarette smoking in the middle income country of Mauritius: A questionnaire survey. *British Medical Journal*, 321(7257), 345–359.

Deeble, J. (1999). *Resource allocation in public health: an economic approach*. Melbourne, Australia: National Public Health Partnership-Secretariat.

Dwore, R.B., Murray, B.P., Parsons, R.P., & Gustafson, G. (2001). An opportunity for HMOs to use marketing to increase enrollee satisfaction. *Managed Care*, 1, 38–53.

Durham, G., & Kill, B. (1999). Public health funding mechanisms in New Zealand. *Australian Health Review*, 22(4), 100–117.

Elixhauser, A. (1990). The costs of smoking and the cost effectiveness of smoking cessation programs. *Journal of Public Health Policy*, Summer, 218–235.

Friedman, E. (1998). What price survival? The future of Blue Cross and Blue Shield. *Journal of the American Medical Association*, 279(23), 1863–1869.

Gold, S.T., Ellwood, D.A., Davis, E.I., Liedschutz, D.S., Orland, M.E., & Cohen, C. (1995). *State investments in education and other children's services: Fiscal profiles of the 50 states*. Prepared for the Finance Project, www.financeproject.com

Hewitt Associates. (1996). *Health promotion initiatives/managed health provided by major US employers in 1995: Based on practices of 1050 employers*. Lincolnshire, IL: Hewitt Associates.

Holland, W.W., & Stewart, S. (1998). Public health: Where should we be in ten years? *Journal of Epidemiology and Community Health*, 52, 278–279.

Hsiao, W.C. (1995). Abnormal economics in the health sector. *Health Policy*, 32, 125–139.

Ismail, A., Brodeur, J.M., Gagnon, P., Payette, M., Picard, D., & Hamalian, T. (1997). Restorative treatments received by children covered by a universal, publicly financed, dental insurance plan. *Journal of Public Health Dentistry*, 57(1), 11–18.

Jacobson, M., & Brownell, K. (2000). Small taxes on soft drinks and snack foods to promote health. *American Journal of Public Health*, 90(6), 854–857, 2000.

Joes, L. (1995). State by state approach to public health. *American Medical News*, 38(8), 1–2.

Kennedy, N.J. (1999). Behavioral medicine: Cost effectiveness of primary prevention. In T.P. Gullotta et al. (Eds.), *Children's health care: Issues for the year 2000 and beyond (pp. 229–282)*. Thousand Oaks, CA: Sage.

Lawrence, D.M. (2001). Priorities among recommended clinical preventive services. *American Journal of Preventive Medicine*, 21(1), 66–67.

Lee, P., & Paxman, D. (1997). Reinventing public health. *Annual Review of Public Health*, 18, 1–35.

Leu, R.E., & Schaub, T. (1983). Does smoking increase medical care expenditure? *Social Science and Medicine*, 17(23), 1907–1914, 1983.

Leviss, P.S. (2001). Financing the public's health. In L.F. Novick & G.P. Mays (Eds.), *Public health administration: Principles for population-based management (pp. 413–431)*. Gaithersburg, MD: Aspen.

Levit, D.R., Lazenby, H.C., Braden, B.R., et al. (1998). National health spending trends in 1996. *Health Affairs*, 17, 35–51.

Lippman, H. (1997). Another health cost explosion: It's not inevitable. *Business and Health*, 15, 27–32.

Mays, G.P. (2001). Organization of the public health delivery system. In L.F. Novick & G.P. Mays (Eds.), *Public health administration: Principles for population-based management (pp. 63–116)*. Gaithersburg, MD: Aspen.

McGavran, E.G. (December 1953). What is public health? *Canadian Journal of Public Health*, 44, 441–442.

Miller, J.T. (Sept/Oct 1987). Wellness programs through the church: Available alternative for health education. *Health Values*, 11(5).

Moody, C.M., & Turnock, B.J. (1998). Impact of Medicaid resources on core public health responsibilities of local health departments in Illinois. *Journal of Public Health Management and Practice*, 4(6), 69–78.

Mullan, F. (1989) *Plagues and Politics*. NY: Basic Books, Inc.

National Association of County and City Health Officials (NACCHO). (1998). National Profile of Local Health Departments, Washington, DC: NACCHO.

National Governors' Association (NGA) and National Association of State Budget Officers (NASBO). (2001). *The fiscal survey of states*, Washington, DC: NGA and NASBO.

New Zealand Ministry of Health. (1997). *Health expenditures trends in New Zealand, 1980–1998*, Wellington, New Zealand: Ministry of Health.

Pickett, G., & Hanlon, J.J. (1990). *Public health administration and practice*, Boston, MA: Times Mirror/Mosby College Publishing.

Public Health Foundation. (1996). *Measuring expenditures for essential public health services*. Report to the Office of Disease Protection and Health Promotion, DHHS.

Ramsey, S.D. (2000). Methods for reviewing economic evaluations of community preventive services: A cart without a horse? *American Journal of Preventive Medicine, 18*(1S), 15–17.

Roemer, M.I. (1977). *Systems of health care*, New York, NY: Springer.

Santelli, J., Vernon, M., Lowry, R., Osorio, J., DuShaw, M., Lancaster, M.S., Pham, N., Song, E., Ginn, E., & Kolbe, L.J. (1998). Managed care, school health programs, and adolescent services: Opportunities for health promotion. *Journal of School Health, 68*(10), 434–440.

Schauffler, H.H. (2000). The credibility of claims for the economic benefits of health promotion. In D. Caallahan (Ed.), *Promoting health behavior: How much freedom? Whose responsibility?* Washington, DC: Georgetown Press, 2000.

Scutchfield, F.D., Harris, J.R., Koplan, J.P., Lawrence, D.M., Gordon, R.L., & Violante, T. (1998). Managed care and public health. *Journal of Public Health Management and Practice, 4*(1), 1–11.

Segal, L. (1998). Health funding: The nature of distortions and implications for the health service mix. *Australian and New Zealand Journal of Public Health, 22*(2), 271–273.

Terris, M., & Kramer, N. (1949). Medical care activities of full-time health departments. *American Journal of Public Health, 39*(9), 1125–1129.

Tulchinsky, T.H., & Varavikova, E.A. (2000). *The new public health: An introduction for the 21st century*, San Diego, VA: Academic Press.

United States Department of Health, Education, and Welfare, Public Health Service. (June 1975). *Forward plan for health, FY 1977–1981*.

Wall, S. (1998). Transformations in public health systems. *Health Affairs, 17*(3), 64–80.

Primary Prevention at the Beginning of the 21st Century

Thomas P. Gullotta and Martin Bloom

As we complete this undertaking, two strong feelings emerge. First, of joy for bringing together this collection of entries on important topics and discovering how much the field has learned in just a few decades. Second, of humility in realizing how far we have yet to go, how restricted our theories, how limited our research base, how simplistic our practice. We celebrate the first feeling because this

Encyclopedia is an important accomplishment at this time for this young field of study and action. We can document that certain strategies are effective in preventing predictable problems, in protecting existing states of health, and in promoting desired goals. But we must never forget that we have a long way to travel to make the dream of primary prevention a reality for people everywhere.

By the end of the project, actually as we were re-reading all of the entries for the sixth time, we had an epiphany: Something was new, something enormously different. All of the separate pieces of theory, research, and practice were, of course, already present if one were persistent enough to scour a huge literature. However, the act of bringing them together in one place and reading them at one (well, several) sitting(s) gave rise to an emergent perception about the scope and potential of primary prevention at the beginning of the 21st century. We would like to summarize the nature of this insight along five dimensions:

THE COSTS OF PREVENTING PREDICTABLE PROBLEMS AND PROMOTING DESIRED GOALS

To begin, we understood from our front row seat what many contributors perceived from their individual research and practice efforts, that there are preventable problems and desired goals that should and can be attained. These problems and goals exist across the entire stage of human life. Everywhere we turned, we found important concerns that needed attention. One indicator of these is the monumental economic costs when unmet needs and unfulfilled objectives are ignored.

Consider this observation by the National Commission on Children (1991, pp. 126–127):

> Malnourishment, obesity, and the incidence of many illnesses are related to nutritional intake. Sexually transmitted diseases, accidents and injuries, and physical and mental impairments are directly attributable to early, unprotected sexual activity, drug and alcohol use, and delinquent behavior.... In fact, control of a limited number of risk factors...could prevent at least 40 percent of all premature deaths, one-third of all short-term disability cases, and two-thirds of all chronic disability cases. Changes in health behaviors can also reduce medical costs and limit losses in productivity. Illnesses attributable to smoking cost individuals and society more than $65 billion a year. The total cost of alcohol and drug abuse exceeds $110 billion each year.

This is a typical cost estimate for the several target areas identified in the quotation. Now, multiply these preventable costs by a conservative factor of 10 to account for the costs of the more than 100 other areas discussed in this

Encyclopedia and the potential preventable costs reach hundreds of billions of dollars a year—each year, every year. This imperfect estimate is difficult to grasp unless one has had the opportunity to look at cost estimates across the dozens of entries in the Encyclopedia.

THE SCOPE OF PRIMARY PREVENTION

Next, we began to appreciate in a new way the scope of preventable problems. To illustrate, investing in prevention will not mean the demise of either medical or mental health treatment services. Indeed, as Albee (Albee, 1983, 1985; Albee & Gullotta, 1986) and others (Surgeon General, 1999) have pointed out, epidemiological studies suggest that in any given year, 20 percent of the population of the United States are (to use the language of the health care industry) seriously emotionally ill. With an estimated US population of 288,000,000 individuals, this means that roughly 57,650,000 individuals are yearly in need of help. Yet, the treatment and rehabilitation capacity of the United States is but a tiny fraction of this number. If prevention was only to reduce this population of afflicted individuals by 20 percent or 11,530,000 cases a year, it would have exceeded the total treatment capacity for the United States for any given year. And this means that millions of children and adults would have avoided unnecessary pain and suffering (Yodanis & Godenzi, in this book). The implication of this example, multiplied by other entries in this encyclopedia, expands the scope of need and potential beyond what commonly has been recognized by policy planners and governments. We realized from this emerging understanding about the nature of preventable population problems and social goals that we need to consider *time* differently. Program planning and the evaluation of its success should not be measured in months or a year but in five, ten, or more years. The reason for this extended time perspective is not only about the life of a given project, but that one project will likely be integrated into a network of related preventive and promotive projects. This adds to the importance of portions of projects that generally get short shrift—the maintenance phase with booster sessions, the diffusion to a wide public, and the formation of connecting links·with other ongoing preventive projects. It is important not to close the door to health promotion, even after the primary prevention project is completed, because it is only then that the real work of health promotion and illness prevention really begins.

THEORIES IN PRIMARY PREVENTION

We always knew how important theories were to guide preventive and promotive thinking and action, but the insight we obtained from the wide-ranging discussions of working preventive theories illustrated throughout this *Encyclopedia* is how relatively few major theories have guided successful practice across a large public arena.

There are several obvious interpretations of this insight. One is that we need to generate more useful theories for primary prevention, and a second is that we already possess valuable understandings in our current theories.

A second theoretical insight involves the much larger number of micro theories or models that are brought to bear on particular preventive challenges. A new challenge for prevention writers and philosophers of science in the next decade will be to understand the use of large-scale theories versus special models, and is more useful in preventive practice.

A related insight is that however good some theories and practices may be, preventionists must be concerned with the political and socioeconomic climate within which a prevention program must fit.

RESEARCH IN PRIMARY PREVENTION

While research methodology and rigor varied considerably, we did find encouraging evidence that the field has and continues to make significant progress. Indeed, in areas like substance misuse and conduct disorder which have benefited from government and foundation funding over the past thirty years, the research base is comparable to the best available in any field.

However, this variability in the quality and quantity of primary prevention research is a concern for the field as a whole. The insight we obtained from viewing the enormous range of research presented on these pages is that we have reached a critical mass in methods and procedures, and that knowing about this body of rigorous research methods should stimulate new researchers to build on a solid foundation. Yet, knowing is not acting. The field of primary prevention needs the universities and relevant social, medical, and educational organizations to be receptive and inviting to keep forward momentum. This requires funding and other support from governments and foundations.

PRIMARY PREVENTION'S TECHNOLOGIES OR GENERAL STRATEGIES

To achieve illness prevention and health promotion, the field of primary prevention uses several general strategies or technologies (Gullotta, 1983, 1987, 1994). Time and again we discovered across topics that these general strategies are effective, but almost always in combinations, not singly. We present these five technologies and illustrate them by reference to entries in this *Encyclopedia*, but as we do so, notice how each strategy blends into the others, supporting and supported by them.

Education

The first general strategy is *education* in its various forms. The most often used of all prevention's technologies, alone it rarely, if ever, is effective. The reason for this is that while education increases knowledge only occasionally does it affect attitudes, and it almost never changes behavior which is influenced by a combination of thoughts, feelings, as well as perceptions of external influences. Thus, the tobacco user will acknowledge the hazards of tobacco use, might wish to give up the habit but rarely acts on that motivation. This said, education nevertheless plays an important role in health promotion and illness prevention in concert with other technologies. We might summarize this role as being necessary but not sufficient to achieve the full force of preventive/promotive services.

Education can take one of three forms. The first is *public information*. Examples can be found on the side of a cigarette package, an alcohol beverage bottle, or on the visor of an automobile. Information can be provided by means of print, radio, Internet, television, or film. It can be read, spoken, sung, or acted. In all instances the "teacher's" intention is to increase knowledge about a given subject and if possible, encourage feelings favorable to the teacher's point of view. Preventive educational messages may offer ways to achieve the goal which promotes health or prevents illness—often in the form of "Do as I say." But research is very clear that life is never that simple and the "student" often models the teacher in spite of the admonition not to "do as I do" (Evans & Getz, this volume).

A second and more specific form of education is *anticipatory guidance*. In this case, information is used to educate a group prior to some expected event (Wood, Macik, & Brown, this volume). Drawing on the folk wisdom that to be forewarned is to be forearmed, the group will be better prepared to cope with the circumstance and adapt to the demands the event may place on them. Common examples of anticipatory guidance are child birth preparation classes, children's visits to hospitals prior to elective surgery, and pre-retirement planning.

Education's third form is found in the personal self-management of behavior—or *self-instruction*. In this instance, the individual or group learns how to control emotional, neurological, and physical aspects of their behavior. The methods to achieve this outcome range from yoga, TM, biofeedback, to cognitive behavioral approaches.

Social Competency

Prevention's second tool is the promotion of *social competency*. To be socially competent requires that one belongs to a group, that the group values the membership of the individual, and that the individual makes a meaningful contribution to the group's existence. Socially competent people tend to possess the following individual characteristics: a positive sense of self-esteem, an internal locus of control, a sense of mastery or self-concept of ability, and an interest beyond themselves that extends to a larger group. Thus a feedback loop is established between belonging, valuing, and contributing and individual characteristics that is self-perpetuating.

Every effective prevention program contains exercises directed at nurturing these individual characteristics which are demonstrated in the ways in which groups embrace members, values its members, and affords its members opportunities to contribute to the welfare and well-being of the group (DuBois, in this volume; Rey, in this volume). This meaningful contribution can be as large as being president or as small as standing in a long line of many volunteering to donate blood on September 11, 2001. This value to the group can be that of the philanthropist or of the soup kitchen volunteer. This belonging is reflected in hundreds of ways, from displayed national flags, religious symbols, or emblems that represent school or club memberships, to songs and stories that celebrate the group's existence. To achieve the solidarity that is the essence of social competency requires not only education but prevention's next technology.

NATURAL CAREGIVING

Prevention's third technology is *natural caregiving*—a term Gullotta (1983) first used to draw a distinction between the services offered by mental health professionals and those afforded by others. Natural caregiving takes three different forms. The first is the *mutual self-help group* in which individuals are drawn together by some common experience. In the self-help group, members are both caregivers and care-receivers. Reliance is not on a professional, but on each other. Pathology is not the governing dynamic but rather muddling through life which can be best achieved by leaning on a companion who knows by experience only too well the stresses others are experiencing. Acknowledging the falls, celebrating the small successes and relying on each other for support and advice—good and bad, the mutual self-help group has no set office hours or answering service. Its members can as easily laugh as weep for themselves and each other. In the self-help group, members discover competency—the competency that goes with belonging, with being valued, and with being a contributing group member.

The phrase *indigenous trained caregiver* describes the second form of natural caregiving. These are people like ministers, teachers, and police officers that individuals turn to in time of need. While not trained as mental health professionals, their advice, comfort, and support enable many in society to lead healthy and productive lives.

In times of need, individuals turn first to friends and loved ones then to trained indigenous caregivers like the clergy, teachers, and the family doctor. Why—because the power of a single caring relationship over time is both nurturing and healing. As with other forms of caregiving, *indigenous caregiving* involves behaviors such as the sharing of knowledge, the sharing of experiences, compassionate understanding, companionship, and, when necessary, confrontation (Bloom, 1996; Cowen, 1982). The indigenous caregiver accepts responsibility for her or his life and ideally invests in the life (health) of at least one other individual.

Community Organization and Systems Intervention

Prevention's fourth general strategy is its most powerful. *Community organization and systems intervention* (COSI) are concerned with the promotion of a community's social capital. That is, how does a community interest its members to actively participate in the process of governance and how are inequities corrected. COSI addresses these issues in four ways. The first is *community development* and takes a variety of forms. The neighborhood civic association formed to be a local voice on zoning issues; the local recreation league created to afford after school opportunities; and the neighborhood watch started to deter crime are but three examples. In each example, a group of people with concerns about property, youth activities, or crime prevention draw together and act together to express their concerns and develop solutions in response to those concerns.

The second form COSI takes is *systems intervention*. The assumption is that every institution has dysfunctional elements within it that contribute to the needless suffering of individuals in society. Identifying those dysfunctional elements and correcting them is the purpose of this form of COSI. To illustrate, Tadmor (in this volume) describes her efforts to reform the medical practices used for children with cancer in one hospital. Policies and procedures that harmed children like restraining them to force compliance with the treatment regimen and separating them from parents during the treatment process were identified as dysfunctional and changed.

For the outsider, while the identification of these dysfunctional practices might appear obvious, they are not. Institutions whether schools, hospitals, social service agencies, child care centers, and larger entities like child protective services and other state departments develop unique internal cultures quite removed from the larger society. Staff within these institutional cultures often accept dysfunctional practices with a shrug of the shoulders and the aside that, "It's always been this way." These same staff will often resist change to the point of sabotage making this form of health promotion and illness prevention very difficult.

The final form COSI takes is *legislative changes and judicial action*. Drawing upon the earlier illustration of the difficulty that accompanies institutional change, it should be remembered that no legislative or judicial action benefits all. In these legislative and judicial contests, there are winners and losers. For example, while a universal family leave policy may be good for employees needing to care for loved ones, for the employer, preserving a job for someone who may not return to work is detrimental to their business. While restricting tobacco access can reduce billions of dollars in medical expenses a decade from now, it means a loss in income to tobacco growers and the tobacco industry today.

Legislative change and judicial action is a battleground where special interests strive to dominate the field. Rarely, does a matter near and dear to the heart of the preventionist succeed at first. But over time and with growing public impatience, seat belt laws do become enacted. Lead abatement standards are established. Tobacco laws restricting youth's access to cigarettes and other products are passed. Interestingly for us, it is often through the efforts of organizations like Mothers' Against Drunk Driving (MADD) and civil rights organizations whose origins reflect many of the characteristics of self-help groups that these laws capable of correcting injustice and improving public health are passed.

Redesign of the Physical Environment

The fifth general strategy focuses on the *redesign of our environment* to create a world in which equilibrium among species is achieved in harmony with the natural world. Consider Geller's (in this volume) provocative question on whether it is possible to achieve an ecologically sustainable future. Left untouched, life ending issues like global warming, the decline of the ozone layer, the destruction of life in the seas by overfishing, and toxic elements like PCBs threaten the existence of humankind and many other living species. Combining elements of prevention's other technologies like public awareness (education), government policy (legislative action), community development, and mutual self-help groups (like the Sierra Club, local historical and environmental societies and political action groups like Greenpeace), varying degrees of progress has been made in each of these areas. For example, efforts are being discussed to reduce fossil fuel consumption and steps taken to preserve forest land. International agreements have been reached on eliminating CFCs from aerosols and freon from cooling devices. International and local bodies have taken steps, albeit small and hesitant ones, to protect some water dwelling animals like the whale and in other instances to limit the catch of species like cod. In other instances, local bodies have insisted that fish ladders be built and even dams removed to enable fish to repopulate ancient fishing habitats. More interesting still is a recent decision that the Hudson River be dredged of cancer-causing PCBs that make current consumption of fish caught from that river ill-advised. From a global perspective to a local perspective of improving air quality by increasing mass transit and developing bikeways, this general strategy recognizes that earth should be an eden and not hell.

Thus, we come to see that when prevention's technology is fully utilized, a circle is completed. Education informs. Natural caregiving unites. Social competency enables, COSI is a means to achieving community change, and the physical environment can be made more benign, while at the same time maintaining its resources for future generations.

CLOSING THOUGHTS

Primary prevention and health promotion belong to the public. The heroes of health promotion and illness prevention are, first, the citizens who monitor their own health, encourage healthy behavior in others, and jealously protect the environment from assault. Second, there are institutional heroes in nonprofit organizations, government, and industry whose moral and humanistic efforts seek to prevent predictable problems, protect existing states of health and healthy functioning, and promote desired goals for populations of citizens.

However, there are institutions whose spokespersons do not hold the humanistic values that are part of primary prevention. Some of these engage in doublespeak that classifies the condiment, ketchup, as a vegetable, or practices circumlocution in which individuals with co-occurring emotional disorders are entitled to assistance for neither. The path to fulfillment of primary prevention's dreams, to prevent predictable problems, protect existing states of health, and promote desired goals, will be arduous and will need many friends and allies.

Preventionists, in their role as health care professionals, recognize that most often they cannot be the primary leaders in this alliance toward good health and effective social functioning. Rather, they contribute their skills as consultants and collaborators to improve a community's health and functioning. This said, as a member of a community in another role as taxpayer, mother, or father, they can and have on many occasions led efforts to improve a community's health.

Healthy communities are self-perpetuating entities that draw on internal group strengths and the collaboration with larger society to achieve local, national, and even international outcomes. These health outcomes are intrinsically interrelated, as ecological/systems theories suggest.

The epiphany as reflected in this encyclopedia tells us that we have vital information and skills to affect these desired changes. This may be the paradigm shift that brings to a new beginning point what Klein and Goldston (1976) stated a quarter of a century ago in their watershed monograph: *Primary Prevention: An Idea Whose Time Has Come.*

Also see: Effective Programming: Foundation; History: Foundation; Theories: Foundation; Evaluation: Foundation; Definition: Foundation.

References

Albee, G.W. (1983). Psychopathology, prevention, and the just society. *Journal of Primary Prevention, 4*(1), 5–40.

Albee, G.W. (1985). The argument for primary prevention. *Journal of Primary Prevention, 5*(4), 213–219.

Albee, G.W., & Gullotta, T.P. (1986). Facts and fallacies about primary prevention. *Journal of Primary Prevention, 6*(4) 207–218.

Bloom, M. (1996). *Primary prevention practices.* Thousand Oaks, CA: Sage.

Cowen, E.L. (1982). Help is where you find it: Four informal helping groups. *American Psychologist, 37,* 385–395.

DuBois, D.L. (2003). Promoting self-esteem in childhood. In T.P. Gullotta & M. Bloom (Eds.), *The encyclopedia of primary prevention and health promotion.* New York: Kluwer Academic/Plenum.

DuBois, D.L. (2003). Promoting self-esteem in adolescence. In T.P. Gullotta & M. Bloom (Eds.), *The encyclopedia of primary prevention and health promotion.* New York: Kluwer Academic/Plenum.

Evans, R.I., & Getz, J.G. (2003). Resisting health-risk behavior: The social inoculation approach and its extensions. In T.P. Gullotta & M. Bloom (Eds.), *The encyclopedia of primary prevention and health promotion.* New York: Kluwer Academic/Plenum.

Geller, E.S. (2003). Achieving an ecologically sustainable future. In T.P. Gullotta & M. Bloom (Eds.), *The encyclopedia of primary prevention and health promotion.* New York: Kluwer Academic/Plenum.

Gullotta, T.P. (1983, April). *Preventions developing technology.* Institute at the Annual American Orthopsychiatric Meeting, Boston, MA.

Gullotta, T.P. (1987). Preventions technology. *Journal of Primary Prevention, 7*(4), 176–196.

Gullotta, T.P. (1994). The what, who, why, where, when, and how of primary prevention. *Journal of Primary Prevention, 15*(1), 5–14.

National Commission on Children. (1991). *Beyond rhetoric: A new American agenda for children and families.* Washington, DC: US Government Printing Office.

Rey, J. (2003). The promotion of prosocial behavior in early childhood. In T.P. Gullotta & M. Bloom (Eds.), *The encyclopedia of primary prevention and health promotion.* New York: Kluwer Academic/Plenum.

Surgeon General (1999). *Mental health: A report of the surgeon general.* Washington, DC: US Government Printing Office.

Tadmor, C.S. (2003). The perceived personal control preventive intervention model: Reviewing past research—exploring future possibilities. In T.P. Gullotta & M. Bloom (Eds.), *The encyclopedia of primary prevention and health promotion.* New York: Kluwer Academic/Plenum.

Wood, D., Macik, F., & Brown, J. (2003). Physical health promotion in early childhood. In T.P. Gullotta & M. Bloom (Eds.), *The encyclopedia of primary prevention and health promotion.* New York: Kluwer Academic/Plenum.

II. Primary Prevention and Health Promotion Topics

A

Abuse, Early Childhood

Sharon G. Portwood and Julia J. Finkel

INTRODUCTION AND DEFINITION

Although awareness of child maltreatment as a serious social problem is becoming the norm in many countries, the field of child abuse prevention is young, and questions are more pervasive than answers. At the outset, prevention efforts have been complicated by the difficulty in reaching a consensual definition of key terms, including not only child maltreatment, but each of its four standard subcategories—physical abuse, psychological abuse, sexual abuse, and neglect (Miller-Perrin & Perrin, 1999). For example, researchers and practitioners have struggled to identify what caregiver behaviors should be prevented, as well as to develop useful and effective outcome measures to evaluate child abuse prevention programs.

SCOPE

In 1996, there were three million reports of child maltreatment in the United States; one million of these claims were substantiated (US Department of Health and Human Services, 1998). Over half of the cases substantiated by Child Protective Services were categorized as neglect, and fewer than 3 percent were sexual abuse cases (US Department of Health and Human Services, 1998). However, data from the Third National Incidence Study of Child Abuse and Neglect indicate that the incidence of child maltreatment may be higher than social service data suggest (Sedlak & Broadhurst, 1996). Self-report surveys also indicate that the rates of child maltreatment reported by social service agencies underestimate the extent of the problem (Miller-Perrin & Perrin, 1999).

Based on the available data, 31.2 percent of victims are children aged zero to four (US Department of Health and Human Services, 1998). The costs of physical abuse and neglect are particularly great for infants and young children, who are at greater risk of suffering brain dysfunction or death as a result of maltreatment.

It is difficult to compare rates of child maltreatment in the United States with rates in Canada since not only are data compiled and reported differently, but Canada does not have a single source for national data on child maltreatment (Locke, 2000). Nonetheless, according to a report from the Canadian Centre for Justice Statistics, in 1999, children under 18 were the victims of 24 percent of assaults as reported by a sample of police departments. Children were victimized by family members in 24 percent of these reports. On the other hand, two thirds of physical assaults of young children were committed by family members, as were 53 percent of sexual assaults (Locke, 2000).

THEORIES AND RESEARCH

Multiple theories exist to explain child maltreatment, many of which implicitly or explicitly underlie current prevention efforts. The broadest theories link child maltreatment to cultural and societal conditions (Miller-Perrin & Perrin,

1999). Some theorists propose that there is a spillover effect from acceptable forms of violence (e.g., violence on television) to unacceptable forms of violence (e.g., child maltreatment). Other researchers have proposed that the structure of the family creates a likely setting for violence. Family members spend a lot of time together, power differences exist, emotional interactions tend to be frequent, relationships between family members are difficult to break, and families are considered a private institution (Miller-Perrin & Perrin, 1999).

Theories involving social inequality and injustice are used to explain child maltreatment. These theories view child maltreatment within a social and ecological context, focusing on the resources and supports available to families (Garbarino & Crouter, 1978). According to strain theory, deviant behavior is more likely when people are denied access to resources (Miller-Perrin & Perrin, 1999).

Finally, child maltreatment theories link maltreatment to the implicit acceptance of violence against children in our society. Social bonding theorists and deterrence theorists believe the low social and legal costs of maltreatment support the message that child maltreatment is acceptable (Miller-Perrin & Perrin, 1999).

Environmental theories cite the relationship between child maltreatment and societal and cultural conditions, such as poverty, social isolation, racism, sexism, tolerance of violence (Daro, 1988). According to these theories, maltreatment would be decreased if resources (e.g., money, information) and supports (e.g., social support) for parents were increased, and systemic changes were made (Daro, 1988).

Theories of child maltreatment also focus on the family and the individual. Learning and behavioral theories link child maltreatment to a caregiver's lack of knowledge of child development or lack of child care skills (Daro, 1988). These theories suggest maltreatment could be prevented if caregivers had the knowledge and skills necessary to care for children appropriately (Daro, 1988).

The transactional model of child maltreatment views maltreatment as the result of interactions over time between the parent and the child within the family context (Wolfe, 1993). According to this theory, these interactions are the potential targets for prevention efforts (Wolfe, 1993). Research on attachment theory supports the assertion that interactions between caregivers and children that involve maltreatment lead to disorganized patterns of attachment (George, 1996).

Social learning theory is also used to understand child maltreatment (Miller-Perrin & Perrin, 1999). According to this theory, children who experience or witness violence are more likely to become violent themselves (Miller-Perrin & Perrin, 1999). Finally, theories involving caregiver psychopathology and behavioral characteristics of offenders have also been proposed (Daro, 1988). However, the specific relationships between particular psychological characteristics and child maltreatment are not clear (Miller-Perrin & Perrin, 1999).

Individual and family-oriented theories suggest prevention strategies such as parenting education classes, home visiting programs, and parent support groups (Daro, 1988). According to these theories, changes within particular families or individuals will prevent child maltreatment.

STRATEGIES THAT WORK

One of the most common approaches to child abuse prevention involves providing support and education to parents (Gomby, Culross, & Behrman, 1999). Ideally, interventions can be initiated early in the child's life, and even before the child's birth. Such parent education and support programs have many common components: (1) they seek to affect the parent–child relationship early in the child's life, before abuse can occur and before parents have established themselves in their parenting role and (2) they tend to be voluntary and to provide in-home services as well as case management support (Guterman, 1997). There are also a number of characteristics that differentiate programs. For example, programs vary in intensity and duration. Although most programs involve some form of home visiting, some programs also include group meetings or some other form of center-based support. The actual services provided also vary. Most programs provide parent education and guidance; however, they may contain a number of other components. For example, some programs provide assistance to families in meeting basic needs, cognitive/behavioral skills training, or training in infant cognitive stimulation. Finally, the training and education of service providers vary from program to program (Guterman, 1997).

Hundreds of parent education and support programs have been developed (Willis, Holden, & Rosenberg, 1992). One of the earliest, most comprehensive, best evaluated and most cited prevention programs of this type was the Prenatal/Early Infancy Project conducted by Olds and colleagues (Holden, Willis, & Corcoran, 1992). The program took place in rural Appalachia and included four treatment levels, to which participants were randomly assigned. The control group participated in pre-post data collection. A minimal intervention group received transportation assistance for attending doctor visits. A third group received prenatal nurse home visiting and transportation assistance. This program had positive effects on parenting attitudes and behavior, as well as on reports of child maltreatment (Holden et al., 1992).

Hawaii Healthy Start is a second example of a commonly cited parent education and support program (Duggan et al., 1999). Lay home visitors are the primary change agent. The role of the home visitor is to establish a trusting relationship with parents, to help parents address their needs and connect with resources, and to provide parenting education. The pilot evaluation of Hawaii Healthy Start indicated that few reports of child maltreatment were made on participating families during the first 3 years of the program. However, the evaluation did not include a control group, and the follow-up period was short. A well-designed and comprehensive evaluation of this program is currently underway. Initial results from the process evaluation indicate the program is rarely implemented as designed. For example, according to the design, home visitors are to visit parents weekly for most of the first year. However, the average number of contacts per year is 13. Nevertheless, initial results indicate improvements in maternal attitudes and self-reported use of harsh discipline (Duggan et al., 1999).

Parent education and support programs such as the Comprehensive Child Development Program and Parents and Teachers also provide good examples of this type of prevention program (Gomby et al., 1999). Unfortunately, carefully conceptualized and well-evaluated parent education and support programs are the exception rather than the rule.

STRATEGIES THAT MIGHT WORK

Reviews of evaluations of parent support programs indicate that, while some programs demonstrate success, many fail to provide evidence of the effectiveness of this technique (Gomby et al., 1999; Gough & Taylor, 1988). Inconsistent results may be due to a number of factors. First, evaluations may be poorly measuring outcomes (Gomby et al., 1999). Second, some programs are better than others. The factors that increase a program's likelihood of success need to be identified. Third, child abuse prevention may require change at levels beyond the individual. Even well-designed and well-implemented programs are unlikely to lead to substantial change if they are unsupported by their context.

Despite substantial evidence that community level factors affect child abuse and neglect, examples of community-based child abuse prevention programs are few and far between. One goal of many parent education and support programs is to enhance social support and to connect families to needed resources (Gomby et al., 1999). However, these aspects of parent-focused programs tend to be under-emphasized (Febbraro, 1994).

A few programs have been developed specifically to prevent child abuse at the community level. Dorchester CARES was a project designed to facilitate collaboration among existing service agencies, to maximize existing resources, to reduce service fragmentation, and to link families to preventive, neighborhood-centered services (Mulroy, 1997). It was expected that the project would reduce stress and social isolation by developing support networks. These changes were expected to strengthen parents and to reduce abuse. The program's conceptual framework was based on Bronfenbrenner's ecological paradigm. Project developers focused on the impact of societal, institutional, and other social-contextual factors on parenting. They also recognized the transactional nature of individual and environmental adaptation. The project was based on a vision of preventing child maltreatment through strengthening neighborhoods and families (Mulroy, 1997).

The program incorporated five areas of preventive services: (1) a family cooperative designed to provide basic necessities to community members; (2) a mentoring program; (3) a family nurturing program; (4) a home health visiting component for pregnant women; and (5) a home-based substance abuse program for parents (Mulroy, 1997). Process evaluation results stress the importance of working in cooperation with community members in order to ensure that the program meets the needs of the community (Mulroy, 1997).

A second example of a community-based effort to prevent child maltreatment is the North Lawndale Family Support Initiative (NLFSI) (Hay & Jones, 1994). The goals of the NLFSI are to increase community members' knowledge about child abuse and child abuse prevention, to provide life skills education in schools, provide parent education and support groups, and to increase the number of child abuse prevention services in the community. Although an outcome evaluation of this program is still underway, process evaluation data indicate that it is important to use positive language when describing child abuse prevention programs. Community members are much more supportive of a program focused on positive parenting than one focused on stamping out child abuse. Also, it is important to be very familiar with the community and to involve community members in the entire process of program development, implementation, and evaluation (Hay & Jones, 1994).

Although community level interventions to prevent child maltreatment are somewhat new phenomena, they provide an intuitively useful approach to the prevention of child maltreatment. Korbin and Coulton (1996) found that community members believe they can help prevent child maltreatment and are willing to do so when provided opportunities. Careful and detailed process and outcome evaluations of community-based programs will be extremely useful in establishing the efficacy and effectiveness of this approach.

Child maltreatment can also be prevented through system reform. Health care facilities have made institutional reforms directed toward the prevention of child maltreatment, and further health care reforms have been suggested. In response to research on attachment and early bonding, efforts were made to reform hospital childbirth practices (Garbarino, 1980). Although the period directly after birth may not be as crucial to the development of a bond between parent and child as was initially thought, reforming hospital practices to be more family centered is positive for other reasons. Family-centered childbirth includes preparing parents for childbirth, treating parents as active participants in the process, having the woman's partner present, using minimal medication, encouraging parent–child contact directly after delivery, having the baby stay in the mother's room, encouraging breast feeding, and encouraging visiting by family and friends. Such practices transform the birth of a child into a social event. It is thought that family-centered childbirth can help prevent maltreatment by providing new parents with an experience that results in feelings of social connectedness and social competence (Garbarino, 1980).

Other opportunities for reform in the health care system directed toward the prevention of child maltreatment focus on interactions between hospital staff and parents (Gough & Taylor, 1988; Wurtele, 1999). Prenatal services can be provided to pregnant women to help ensure adequate prenatal care, and to encourage healthy behavior. Perinatal prevention programs take advantage of the time new parents spend in the hospital after birth by providing education and referral services during this sensitive time period. Postpartum services that emphasize family planning can help families space their children appropriately and choose how many children to have. Well-child visits give health care professionals another opportunity to provide education, guidance, and referrals to parents. Health care providers can provide information on child development, handling common problems such as feeding difficulties, how to child proof, how to enhance children's development, how to choose child care, how to handle behavior problems, and how to discipline children without using violence. Health care staff can also help prevent neglect by helping families gain access to needed resources (Wurtele, 1999).

Health care workers are in a unique position in that they have access to almost all families at critical time periods. Reforms within the health care system could help prevent child maltreatment, but few of these reforms have been adopted or evaluated.

At the broadest level, child maltreatment takes place in the context of a violent, individualistic society that devalues children. Social problems such as poverty, oppression, and inequality cause a great deal of human suffering and are related to child maltreatment. Moreover, parenting is a role for which little preparation or support is provided (Febbraro, 1994). The role of caregiver is devalued, unsupported, and unrecognized (Febbraro, 1994).

The development of programs and policies that prevent maltreatment at the societal level has just begun (Hay & Jones, 1994). Public policy could be a powerful tool in the prevention of maltreatment. Health care reform focused on making health care affordable and accessible could help prevent infant mortality and medical neglect. The development of welfare policy that seeks to keep children out of poverty and insures the availability of affordable, quality child care would help to reduce the incidence of abuse and neglect (Hay & Jones, 1994).

There are not many programs that seek to prevent maltreatment by helping families escape poverty (Hay & Jones, 1994). Some programs encourage teen parents to return to school or obtain further training. This is a component absent from many programs working with older parents even though such parents often face more serious economic problems. Recently, programs have been developed to help parents obtain economic self-sufficiency. Initial evaluations of these programs suggest that they may be helpful in improving the economic situation of poor families. However, they require an intensive and long-term approach (Hay & Jones, 1994).

Child abuse prevention may be possible within the context of school reform (Hay & Jones, 1994). All schools could provide, and require students to take, classes in child development, family relations and/or parenting. Schools could also provide opportunities for students to interact with children (Hay & Jones, 1994). Ensuring all people grow up with some formal training in child development and parenting could be very helpful in preventing abuse.

Violence and the unrealistic portrayal of families in the media may contribute to child maltreatment (Hay & Jones, 1994). The media could be used to promote positive parenting and to discourage maltreatment. Public service announcements are one method currently used to help prevent maltreatment through the media, but their effectiveness has not been evaluated (Hay & Jones, 1994).

Although societal-level prevention efforts are currently limited, they provide direction for the future. Child maltreatment is a problem closely tied to our cultural context. By changing the social structure within which maltreatment is embedded, we can begin to lower the incidence of child maltreatment.

STRATEGIES THAT DO NOT WORK

There are approaches currently in use that do not seem to be effective. A prevention technique sometimes used with children as young as three or four involves teaching children to protect themselves from an abuser. There has been no evidence that these programs lead to a decline in victimization. Moreover, they promote the message that children are capable of protecting themselves from an abuser (Miller-Perrin & Perrin, 1999).

Even for programs that incorporate aspects of promising or model programs, evaluation results tend to be less positive when the program is implemented poorly (Guterman, 1997).

Unsuccessful programs also tend to be lacking in intensity, are short term, or are not comprehensive enough to achieve results (Guterman, 1997).

SYNTHESIS

Taken as a whole, data on current child abuse prevention programs indicate that future efforts must be based on a broader conceptualization of the problem of child maltreatment. The impact of the basic values and norms of our society on the treatment of children needs to be more carefully considered. Attitudes regarding violence, individualism, the importance and difficulty of parenting, and the value of the family need to be incorporated into theories and approaches to the prevention of child maltreatment.

References

Daro, D., & Gelles, R. (1992). Public attitudes and behaviors with respect to child abuse prevention. *Journal of Interpersonal Violence, 7*, 517–531.

Daro, D. (1988). *Confronting child abuse: Research for effective program design*. New York, NY: Free Press.

Duggan, A., McFarlane, E., Windham, A., Rohde, C., Salkever, D., Fuddy, L., Rosenberg, L., Buchbinder, S., & Sia, C. (1999). Evaluation of Hawaii's Healthy Start program. *The Future of Children, 9*, 66–90.

Febbraro, A. (1994). Single mothers "at-risk" for child maltreatment: An appraisal of person-centered interventions and a call for emancipatory action. *Canadian Journal of Community Mental Health, 13*, 47–60.

Garbarino, J. (1980). Changing hospital childbirth practices: A developmental perspective on prevention of child maltreatment. *American Journal of Orthopsychiatry, 50*, 588–597.

Garbarino, J., & Crouter, A. (1978). Defining the community context for parent–child relations: The correlates of child maltreatment. *Child Development, 49*, 604–616.

George, C. (1996). A representational perspective of child abuse and prevention. *Child Abuse and Neglect, 20*, 411–424.

Gomby, D.S., Culross, P.L., & Behrman, R.E. (1999). Home visiting: Recent program evaluations—Analysis and recommendations. *The Future of Children, 9*, 4–26.

Gough, D., & Taylor, J. (1988). Child abuse prevention: Studies of ante-natal and post-natal services. *Journal of Reproductive and Infant Psychology, 6*, 217–228.

Guterman, N. (1997). Early prevention of physical child abuse and neglect: Existing evidence and future directions. *Child Maltreatment, 2*, 12–34.

Hay, T., & Jones, L. (1994). Societal interventions to prevent child abuse and neglect. *Child Welfare, 73*, 379–403.

Holden, E., Willis, D., & Corcoran, M. (1992). Preventing child maltreatment during the prenatal/postnatal period. In D. Willis, E. Holden, & M. Rosenberg (Eds.), *Prevention of child maltreatment: Developmental and ecological perspectives* (pp. 193–224). New York, NY: John Wiley & Sons, Inc.

Korbin, J., & Coulton, C. (1996). The role of neighbors and the government in neighborhood-based child protection. *Journal of Social Issues, 52*, 163–176.

Locke, D. (2000). Violence against children and youth by family members. In V. Bunge & D. Locke (Eds.), *Family violence in Canada: A statistical profile*. Ottawa, Canada: Minister of Industry.

Miller-Perrin, C., & Perrin, R. (1999). *Child maltreatment: An introduction*. Thousand Oaks, CA: Sage.

Mulroy, E. (1997). Building a neighborhood network: Interorganizational collaboration to prevent child abuse and neglect. *Social Work, 42*, 255–264.

Sedlak, A., & Broadhurst, D. (1996). *Third National Incidence Study of Child Abuse and Neglect*. Washington, DC: US Government Printing Office.

US Department of Health and Human Services. (1998). *Child maltreatment 1996: Reports from the States to the National Child Abuse and Neglect Data System*. Washington, DC: US Government Printing Office.

Willis, D., Holden, E., & Rosenberg, M. (1992). Child maltreatment prevention: Introduction and historical overview. In D. Willis, E. Holden, & M. Rosenberg (Eds.), *Prevention of child maltreatment: Developmental and ecological perspectives* (pp. 1–14). New York, NY: John Wiley & Sons, Inc.

Wolfe, D. (1993). Prevention of child neglect: Emerging issues. *Criminal Justice and Behavior, 20*, 90–111.

Wurtele, S. (1999). Preventing child maltreatment: Multiple windows of opportunity in the health care system. *Children's Health Care, 28*, 151–165.

Abuse, Childhood

Sharon G. Portwood and Julia J. Finkel

INTRODUCTION

While there is widespread recognition of the problem of child maltreatment and the devastating consequences it can have for children, strategies for preventing the physical and sexual abuse and neglect of children between the ages of 5 and 12 are limited. Moreover, many current strategies have been criticized for placing the burden on children to prevent their own victimization and/or revictimization.

DEFINITIONS

Defining *child maltreatment* and each of its subcategories is a difficult task. While there is general agreement on what constitutes abuse or neglect in its extreme forms (e.g., intercourse with a child, punching a child in the face, or failure to feed a child for a week), the task of identifying maltreatment becomes more difficult when the act or omission is less extreme (e.g., parental nudity in front of a child, spanking, or failure to brush a child's hair for several days) (Portwood, 1999). Ambiguity in the definitions of types of child maltreatment causes a number of problems in research and practice; for example, it can be difficult to determine when maltreatment has occurred, and defining the effectiveness of a prevention strategy is complex.

Despite these definitional dilemmas, four categories of *child maltreatment* are generally recognized: physical abuse, psychological or emotional abuse, sexual abuse, and neglect (three of which are the subject of this entry). *Sexual abuse* consists of any sexual activity with a child where consent is not or cannot be given (Finkelhor, 1979). Whereas the critical factor in defining *abuse* tends to be a nonaccidental injury, *neglect* is characterized by negligent acts or omissions that harm or threaten harm to a child. Common subtypes of neglect include: *physical neglect*, which includes failure to provide for a child's basic physical needs, including food, shelter, or clothing; *emotional neglect*, which consists of inattention to a child's emotional needs; *medical neglect*, which refers to a caregiver's failure to provide prescribed medical treatment; and *educational neglect*, which can be defined as a caregivers' failure to comply with legal requirements for the education of children (Erickson & Egeland, 1996).

Broad definitions of child maltreatment also encompass exposure to domestic and/or community violence and sibling abuse, topics beyond the scope of this entry.

SCOPE

According to figures from the US Department of Health and Human Services (DHHS) (1998), three million reports of child maltreatment were made in 1996. One million of these claims were substantiated (i.e., deemed to be supported by credible evidence) by child protective service agencies. Of these victims, 4.6 percent were between the ages of 5 and 12; however, data from the Congressionally mandated Third National Incidence Study of Child Abuse and Neglect (Sedlak & Broadhurst, 1996), along with data from self-report surveys, indicate that the incidence of child maltreatment among this age group may be higher than social service data suggest (Miller-Perrin & Perrin, 1999).

Most data suggest that the risk of physical abuse and neglect decreases with age. For example, statistics consistently indicate that almost half of children victimized through physical abuse are age seven or younger (Miller-Perrin & Perrin, 1999). However, this decreased risk is not evidenced in self-report data, suggesting that it may not be the actual occurrence of abuse, but the risk of injury that dissipates as children age. The data further suggest that males are at slightly greater risk for physical abuse, particularly in regard to major acts of physical abuse (DHHS, 1998). In contrast, girls are at greater risk for sexual abuse (DHHS, 1998).

Contrary to other forms of maltreatment, the risk of sexual abuse appears to increase with age. Taken as a whole,

statistics indicate that the mean age of children reporting sexual abuse is between 9 and 11 years (Miller-Perrin et al., 1999). Although the majority of all sexual abuse cases, at least within the United States, occur within the 5- to 12-year age range, the majority of substantiated cases involving this group of children were neglect cases (DHHS, 1998). For all types of abuse and neglect, an adult known to the child is most likely to be the perpetrator (Miller-Perrin et al., 1999).

The costs of child maltreatment are substantial, including not only treatment for physical or emotional injuries sustained as an immediate result of the abuse, but also extending to chronic health and socioemotional difficulties. Research suggests that many problems emerge in childhood and continue well into adulthood, including drug or alcohol dependence and other deviant behaviors. Accordingly, the combined costs to public health, rehabilitation, criminal justice, and child welfare systems has been estimated to be in billions of dollars (Daro, 1988).

Although a direct cross-cultural comparison of the scope of the problem is not possible due to differences in compilation and reporting procedures, according to a report from the Canadian Centre for Justice Statistics, in 1999, Canadian children under 18 were the victims of 24 percent of assaults as reported by a sample of police departments. Overall, children were victimized by family members in 24 percent of reports; however, two thirds of physical assaults of young children were committed by family members, as were 53 percent of sexual assaults (Locke, 2000).

THEORIES

While child maltreatment can be viewed as an aggressive act and thus informed by traditional models of aggression, the special context in which most abuse occurs (i.e., the family) has focused most theories of child maltreatment on group and family processes. Overall, theories on the causes of child maltreatment have moved from a focus on the individual to an attempt to integrate multiple levels of analysis (Azar, Povilaitis, Lauretti, & Pouquette, 1998).

One popular group of theories views abuse as one end of a parenting continuum. These *developmentally based* models are essentially models of parenting adequacy, and thus have substantial import for the development of effective prevention strategies. *Perpetrator models* that, in the extreme, propose that offenders are psychotic or suffer from other psychological disorders were popular early explanations of child maltreatment (Azar et al., 1998). However, recently researchers have begun to explore perpetrator theories based on biological approaches. Some of the more promising perpetrator theories focus on parental social-cognitive disturbances, positing that such parental factors as a disturbed schema involving children, problem-solving deficits, and lack of perspective-taking ability may lead to maladaptive parenting. Other theories have focused on child victims, attempting to identify characteristics of abused children that may produce violent behavior in a vulnerable parent. However, cast as "victim blaming," such theories have not been widely accepted.

At the macrolevel, researchers have sought to identify a variety of social and cultural factors that contribute to child maltreatment. Foremost among these is a general tolerance for violent acts within the culture that may "spillover" into the home; for example, excessive exposure to violence through the media can contribute to a general acceptance of violence within the family environment. One marker of cultural standards in regard to physical violence against children is corporal punishment, leading some to suggest that a general acceptance of spanking as an appropriate form of discipline contributes, at least indirectly, to child maltreatment and to physical child abuse in particular (Miller-Perrin et al., 1999).

Strain theories have also developed around the notion that financial inequities within the societal structure place lower-income families, unemployed families, and families receiving governmental assistance, who experience high levels of stress and frustration, at higher risk of maltreatment.

More recent theories, rather than distinguishing among perpetrator, victim, and environmental factors, have proposed *multiple trajectories* to the development of abusive behavior that link these factors. One notable model is that of Belsky (1980), who suggests that the roots of maltreatment lie in multiple ecological systems, that is, what parents bring to parenthood, family factors, factors in the larger social setting, and cultural values and beliefs. A second model was outlined by Azar and Twentyman (1986), who identified five areas of parental skill deficit that contribute to an increased risk of abuse: "parenting skills (e.g., too narrow a repertoire), cognitive dysfunctions (e.g., unrealistic expectations regarding children), and impulse control, stress management, and social skills problems" (Azar et al., 1998, p. 9).

RESEARCH

Virtually all research on child maltreatment has been conducted since 1970. This research indicates that the origins and consequences of child maltreatment are complex. No single factor accounts for significant amounts of abuse. Research on the origins of maltreatment can be grouped into four categories: perpetrator characteristics, child characteristics, family characteristics, and the broader social context. In general, these factors vary by type of abuse, specifically physical abuse and neglect versus sexual abuse.

Physical Abuse and Neglect. Parental characteristics associated with physical abuse and neglect include substance abuse, and lack of involvement in community activities (Brown, Cohen, Johnson, & Salzinger, 1998). Abusive parents also tend to be single and young; they are less likely to be biological parents; they have lower self-esteem; their expectations of their children tend to be inappropriate; and they are less empathetic with their children (Milner, 1998). In general, five domains of parental disturbance can be considered: cognitive disturbances, deficits in parenting skill, problems with impulse control, difficulties with stress management, and social skill problems (Azar & Twentyman, 1986). Each of these deficits, alone or in combination, can play a role in more systemic difficulties that heighten the risk of abuse. For example, a parent's deficits in social skills may result in a smaller support network.

Child characteristics that have been associated with maltreatment include having a disability, a difficult temperament, psychiatric symptoms, or behavioral problems (Brown et al., 1998). However, when examining the behavior of both parents and children, the question of directionality arises, that is, to what degree and in what ways does negative parenting behavior contribute to negative behavior from the child or vice versa?

Family characteristics are also related to the rate of child maltreatment. Situations that contribute to the level of stress within a family, including illness, death of a family member, and larger than average family size have been established as risk factors for physical abuse (Miller-Perrin et al., 1999). Other family factors associated with child maltreatment include high levels of conflict, the occurrence of partner violence, social isolation, high levels of stress, and a lack of support (Milner, 1998). Parents who abuse their children tend to communicate less frequently with their children, and they demonstrate fewer positive parenting behaviors. Abusive parents also tend to report more violence in their family of origin (Milner, 1998). However, it is important to note that while "cycle of violence" theories have garnered a great deal of public attention, the majority of individuals abused as children (about 70 percent) do not grow up to be abusers (Miller-Perrin et al., 1999).

Child maltreatment rates are higher in communities with certain socioeconomic characteristics (Garbarino, Kostelny, & Grady, 1993). Communities where a larger proportion of residents live in poverty tend to have higher rates of maltreatment, as do communities with a larger proportion of African American or Latino residents. Communities with more female headed households, a higher unemployment rate, a lower percentage of wealthy residents, a lower median education level, more overcrowding, and a higher percentage of new residents tend to have higher rates of maltreatment as well (Garbarino et al., 1993). However, it is important to note that violence is by no means typical of all families that struggle financially, suggesting that other factors are at work.

Notable among these is social bonding/social isolation. Abusive parents have been found to have relatively fewer contacts with peer networks, immediate family, and other relatives (Miller-Perrin et al., 1999). Moreover, Emery and Laumann-Billings (1998) found that even in low-income neighborhoods, child maltreatment rates tend to be low when residents know one another, there is a sense of community pride, people are involved in community organizations, and residents feel that they can ask their neighbors for help.

Sexual Abuse. In regard to sexual abuse, the abuser tends to be male, to have interpersonal problems, and to be antisocial (Milner, 1998). Thus, it is perhaps not surprising that research on characteristics of sexual abusers has focused primarily on males and may not be generalizable to female perpetrators. The majority of this research has also been generated from a psychiatric model, assuming that the root cause of sexual abuse lies in the individual psychopathology of male abusers. As noted, there is some evidence to suggest that sexual abusers exhibit some antisocial tendencies, including a disregard for others and lack of impulse control, and/or deficits in heterosocial skills (Miller-Perrin et al., 1999). Other theories center on deviant sexual arousal, which prompts offenders to solicit sexual encounters with children. The as yet undetermined origins of this deviant sexual arousal are believed to be partially biological. However, this explanation does not appear adequate to explain incest. Instead, family dysfunction models posit that either the family or one of its adult members contributes to a context in which the sexual victimization of children is permitted or even encouraged.

Many early researchers focused on child characteristics in seeking explanations for sexual abuse, examining the victim's role in permitting or even encouraging the abuse. However, little evidence has been produced to support such a stance. While many victims of sexual abuse do exhibit sexualized behavior, most experts believe this to be a consequence rather than a cause of the abuse (Miller-Perrin et al., 1999).

In regard to family characteristics, poor parent–child relationships and marital conflict are associated with sexual abuse (Finkelhor, 1984). At the macrolevel, social and community factors, particularly social attitudes toward women and child pornography, appear to contribute to sexual abuse. Family environments in which incest occurs are particularly likely to be characterized by substantial power differentials between male and female members (Miller-Perrin et al., 1999). Unlike other forms of maltreatment, sexual abuse is not generally related to SES (Milner, 1998).

STRATEGIES THAT WORK

There is no evidence of specific prevention approaches that work in reducing maltreatment of children between the ages of 5 and 12. However, parent training and education models, which are more typically targeted at parents of younger children, may serve to benefit this population.

STRATEGIES THAT MIGHT WORK

Public awareness campaigns, media presentation, and speaker programs to voluntary organizations and civic groups may serve to increase public awareness of the problems associated with child maltreatment. Similarly, involvement of religious institutions may assist in preventing child maltreatment; however, efforts to assess such initiatives have been limited (National Research Council, 1993).

The most popular prevention approach related to this age group focuses on the children themselves. School-based programs aimed at teaching children to recognize, resist, and report abuse became popular in the United States during the 1980s. Despite the fact that children in this age group are at higher risk of neglect or physical abuse, the vast majority of these programs target the prevention of sexual abuse. Overall, they emphasize two goals: primary prevention (i.e., stopping abuse before it occurs) and detection (i.e., prompting children to disclose past and current abuse). Programs vary regarding the amount of time spent on lessons and on the details of the program content, utilizing films, skits, lectures, coloring books, songs, and/or puppet shows to convey lessons about sexual abuse, assertiveness, avoidance, and disclosure. However, these programs share the same core assumptions, specifically: (1) many children do not know what sexual abuse is; (2) children do not need to tolerate sexual touching; (3) adults want to know about children who experience sexual touching by adults; and (4) disclosure of sexual touching will help to stop it (National Research Council, 1993). Other key concepts typically incorporated into school-based sexual abuse prevention programs include: (1) children can control access to their own bodies; (2) there are different types of touches (e.g., good and bad); (3) children can and should tell others about touching (i.e., there should be no secrets about touching); and (4) supportive adults are available for children to tell about problems with touching (Conte, Rosen, & Saperstein, 1986).

Although school administrators, teachers, and parents have expressed enthusiasm for such programs, they have rarely been evaluated (Wurtele, 1998). Moreover, the limited evaluation data that are available suggest that while child participants in comprehensive school-based prevention programs demonstrate increased knowledge immediately following the program, these gains in knowledge tend to deteriorate over time (Finkelhor & Strapko, 1992). More importantly, there is no evidence of a reduction in the actual number of victimizations as a result of participation in these school-based programs.

While there is some evidence that these prevention programs may encourage disclosure, there is nothing to suggest that they help children resist abuse (Miller-Perrin et al., 1999).

Despite the popularity of child-focused sexual abuse prevention programs and some limited evidence of their success in achieving at least some of their goals, such programs have critics, and their inadequate evaluation has left unanswered questions. First, there is concern regarding the impact of these programs on children's developing sexuality. Parents and community members tend to oppose the use of correct names for body parts and open conversation using sexual terms (Melton, 1992). Moreover, programs focus on teaching children that sexual touch is bad. Both of these program characteristics could have an adverse impact on a child's ideas and attitudes regarding his or her body and sexuality (Melton, 1992).

A second problem with these programs is that the curricula are often confusing for children (Melton, 1992). Curriculum content must be developmentally appropriate to be understandable, but some concepts are difficult for all elementary-school-aged children to understand. For example distinguishing between "good touch" and "bad touch" can be confusing. This is not surprising considering the fact that many adults cannot decide exactly what constitutes "bad touch." Also, it is difficult for many children to understand that abusers can be familiar adults (Melton, 1992). Likewise, the self-defense and assertiveness training components of these programs are also difficult for children to understand and to use (Peled & Kurtz, 1994).

A third problem with child-focused prevention of sexual abuse is that such approaches may instill feelings of fear, vulnerability, and anxiety in children, while at the same time giving adults a false sense of security regarding children's safety (Adler & McCain, 1994). There have been few studies regarding the effect of these programs on children's sense of security, but results have been conflicting (Finkelhor & Strapko, 1992).

Finally, this type of prevention effort sends the message to children, teachers, parents, and society that children are responsible for preventing their own abuse (Melton, 1992). The idea that assertiveness training can prevent child sexual abuse may not only be inappropriate and potentially harmful to children, but also unrealistic; abusers are advantaged physically and cognitively, they tend to control access to resources, and they hold authority over children (Finkelhor & Strapko, 1992). Moreover, skills that arm children against attacks by a stranger may not transfer to assaults by a familiar and trusted adult. Although role playing and in vivo assessment situations may provide effective training for such situations, they raise important ethical issues that must be considered carefully before exposing children to these techniques (National Research Council, 1993).

While many child-focused programs have also tried to involve parents, the results have been disappointing; for example, in one study, only 39 of 116 parents attended parent education meetings (Berrick, 1988). Nonetheless, there are some studies to suggest that parents not only want to be involved, but are also effective in training their children about sexual abuse and successful protective skills (Miller-Perrin et al., 1999).

STRATEGIES THAT DO NOT WORK

It is popularly believed that strict criminal sanctions serve, in part, to reduce the occurrence of child maltreatment. However, there is no evidence that current laws have any deterrent effect. Moreover, there is some suggestion that legal procedures that lead to children's removal from their parents may be counterproductive, especially in cases involving parental offenders and mild to moderate forms of maltreatment. In regard to sexual abuse, Megan's Law (1996) has instituted requirements for sex-offender registration and community notification. This measure has remained controversial, due to the fact that most potentially dangerous individuals are not identified in the registry; as a result, parents may have a false sense of security not only that they are aware of the presence of any potential offenders in their community, but also that they can protect their children from these individuals.

SYNTHESIS

Recent reports indicate a decrease in the number of both reports and substantiated cases of child sexual abuse (down 26 and 31 percent, repectively, from 1992 to 1998) (Jones & Finkelhor, 2001). These data have prompted some to praise the success of current prevention efforts; however, as the study's authors note, given research suggesting that the results of these programs have not been as successful as had been hoped, this decline might instead reflect shifts in policy and attitudes making reporting not only less frequent, but also less likely to be taken seriously.

What seems clear is that the field of child abuse prevention is young, and current approaches are limited. Inadequate research and evaluation is a pervasive problem, and the failure to explore opportunities for prevention on multiple levels of analysis is a serious weakness. Although programs are usually based on general developmental or ecological theories, they are rarely grounded in a specific theory or set of theories of child abuse prevention. In addition, many studies fail to adhere to appropriate methodology; studies employing control groups, random assignment, adequate sample sizes, and a longitudinal design are needed. Appropriate proximal and distal outcome measures and process evaluation are also needed. At present, published evaluations of programs tend to provide little information about specific program content and even less information regarding the process by which the program achieved or failed to achieve desired effects.

Overall, there is concern that prevention efforts have had an insufficient focus on the specific type of maltreatment being addressed; current research suggests that different types of programs will be most effective for preventing particular types of maltreatment (Daro, 1988). Similarly, different approaches may be more effective with particular types of families. In addition, prevention programs must expand their focus beyond one particular system within the overall framework of systems that contribute to the occurrence of child maltreatment (e.g., individual, family, and macrosystem). Broader solutions to the problem need to be implemented and evaluated.

References

Adler, N., & McCain, J. (1994). Prevention of child abuse: Issues for the mental health practitioner. *Child and Adolescent Psychiatric Clinics of North America, 3,* 679–693.

Azar, S.T., & Twentyman, C.T. (1986). Cognitive behavioral perspectives on the assessment and treatment of child abuse. In P.C. Kendall (Ed.), *Advances in cognitive behavioral research and therapy* (Vol. 5, pp. 237–267). New York: Academic Press.

Azar, S.T., Povilaitis, T.Y., Lauretti, A.F., & Pouquette, C.L. (1998). The current status of etiological theories in intrafamilial child maltreatment. In J.L. Lutzker (Ed.), *Handbook of child abuse research and treatment* (pp. 3–30) New York: Plenum Press.

Belsky, J. (1980). Child maltreatment: An ecological integration. *American Psychologist, 35,* 320–335.

Berrick, J.D. (1988). Parental involvement in child abuse prevention training: What do they learn? *Child Abuse and Neglect, 12,* 543–553.

Brown, J., Cohen, P., Johnson, J., & Salzinger, S. (1998). A longitudinal analysis of risk factors for child maltreatment. *Child Abuse and Neglect, 22,* 1065–1078.

Conte, J.R., Rosen, C., & Saperstein, L. (1986). An analysis of programs to prevent the sexual victimization of children. *Journal of Primary Prevention, 6,* 141–155.

Daro, D. (1988). *Confronting child abuse: Research for effective program design.* New York: The Free Press.

Emery, R.E., & Laumann-Billings, L. (1998). An overview of the nature, causes, and consequences of abusive family relationships: Toward differentiating maltreatment and violence. *American Psychologist, 44,* 121–135.

Erickson, M.F., & Egeland, B. (1996). Child neglect. In J. Briere, L. Berliner, J.A. Bulkley, C. Jenny, & T. Reid (Eds.), *The APSAC handbook on child maltreatment* (pp. 4–20). Thousand Oaks, CA: Sage.

Finkelhor, D. (1979). *A sourcebook on child sexual abuse.* Newbury Park, CA: Sage.

Finkelhor, D. (1984). *Child sexual abuse: New theory and research.* New York: Free Press.

Finkelhor, D., & Strapko, N. (1992). Sexual abuse prevention education: A review of evaluation studies. In D. Willis, E. Holden, & M. Rosenberg (Eds.), *Prevention of child maltreatment: Developmental and ecological perspectives* (pp. 150–167). New York: John Wiley & Sons.

Garbarino, J., Kostelny, K., & Grady, J. (1993). Children in dangerous environments: Child maltreatment in the context of community violence. In D. Cicchetti & S. Toth (Eds.), *Child abuse, child development, and social policy* (pp. 167–189). Norwood, NJ: Ablex.

Jones, L., & Finkelhor, D. (January 2001). The decline in child sexual abuse cases. *OJJDP: Juvenile Justice Bulletin.* Washington, DC: US Department of Justice.

Locke, D. (2000). Violence against children and youth by family members. In V. Bunge & D. Locke (Eds.), *Family violence in Canada: A statistical profile.* Ottawa, Canada: Minister of Industry.

Megan's Law. (1996). Publication L. No. 104-145.

Melton, G. (1992). The improbability of prevention of sexual abuse. In D. Willis, E. Holden, & M. Rosenberg (Eds.), *Prevention of child maltreatment: Developmental and ecological perspectives* (pp. 168–189). New York: John Wiley & Sons.

Milner, J. (1998). Individual and family characteristics associated with intrafamilial child physical and sexual abuse. In P. Trickett & C. Schellenbach (Eds.), *Violence against children in the family and the community* (pp. 141–170). Washington, DC: American Psychological Association.

Miller-Perrin, C., & Perrin, R.D. (1999). *Child maltreatment: An introduction.* Thousand Oaks, CA: Sage.

National Research Council. (1993). *Understanding child abuse and neglect.* Washington, DC: National Academy Press.

Peled, T., & Kurtz, L. (1994). Child maltreatment: The relationship between developmental research and public policy. *The American Journal of Family Therapy, 22,* 247–262.

Portwood, S.G. (1999). Coming to terms with a consensual definition of child maltreatment. *Child Maltreatment, 4,* 56–68.

Sedlak, A., & Broadhurst, D. (1996). *Third National Incidence Study of Child Abuse and Neglect.* Washington, DC: US Government Printing Office.

US Department of Health and Human Services. (1998). *Child maltreatment 1996: Reports from the States to the National Child Abuse and Neglect Data System.* Washington, DC: US Government Printing Office.

Wurtele, S.K. (1998). School-based child sexual abuse prevention programs. In J.R. Lutzker (Ed.), *Handbook of child sexual abuse* (pp. 501–516). New York: Plenum.

Abuse and Neglect, Adolescence

Miriam Mulsow and Keri K. O'Neal

INTRODUCTION AND DEFINITIONS

Although the concepts of child abuse and maltreatment have been widely studied, problems with definitions still remain. Confusion over definitions may lead to individuals not recognizing their own behavior as abusive (Portwood, 1998), further complicated by differences in cultural norms. A widely accepted set of definitions of abuse comes from the National Incidence Study (NIS-3).

This study ...

> defines *physical abuse* as present when a child younger than age 18 years has experienced injury (harm standard) or risk of injury (endangerment standard) as a result of having been hit with a hand or other object or having been kicked, shaken, thrown, burned, stabbed, or choked by a parent or parent-substitute. *Physical neglect* refers to harm or endangerment as a result of inadequate nutrition, clothing, hygiene, and supervision. *Emotional abuse* includes verbal abuse, harsh non-physical punishments (e.g., being tied up), or threats of maltreatment, while *emotional neglect* covers failure to provide adequate affection and emotional support or permitting a child to be exposed to domestic violence. (Kaplan, Pelcovitz, & Labruna, 1999, p. 1214)

Sexual abuse is defined in the Child Abuse Prevention and Treatment Act (United States Congress, 1996) as the employment, use, persuasion, inducement, enticement, or coercion of any child to engage in, or assist any other person to engage in, any sexually explicit conduct or simulation of such conduct for the purpose of producing a visual depiction of such conduct, or as the rape, and in cases of caretaker or inter-familial relationships, statutory rape, molestation, prostitution, or other form of sexual exploitation of children, or incest with children.

SCOPE

Child Protective Services offices in 49 of 50 US states report that almost one million children were victims of substantiated abuse and neglect in 1997 (US Department of Health & Human Services, 1998). Other data suggest that the number may be even higher than that, with 2,815,600 children reportedly endangered and 1,553,800 of these reported harmed by abuse or neglect in 1993 (NIS-3, cited in Kaplan, Pelcovitz, & Labruna, 1999). Although male adolescents are more likely to be victims of homicides by their parents, female adolescents seem to experience more maltreatment, including physical abuse (Kaplan et al., 1999) and dating violence. The rate of severe violence among dating couples ranges from about 1 to 27 percent per year (Gelles, 2000). Emotional abuse and neglect are probably the most common forms of maltreatment in adolescence and occur at their highest frequency during this time (Kaplan et al., 1999). Further, the practice of selling adolescent girls into prostitution is perpetrated in many areas of the world (ECPAT International, 2001).

Worldwide statistics on child maltreatment are complicated by cultural variations in definitions of child maltreatment (Agathonos-Georgopoulou, 1992). Garbarino and Kostelny (1992) contend that maltreatment is a social judgment. An act is judged to be maltreatment "if it violates certain minimally recognized community standards" (Fortin & Chamberland, 1995, p. 277). For example,

adolescent initiation ceremonies occur in 55 percent of societies studied by Levinson (1989), with 47 percent of these using some form of painful initiation rites (e.g., female genital mutilation (FGM)). In all societies, however, there are behaviors considered inappropriate and abusive toward children (Levinson, 1989).

Cost of Maltreatment

Among the many consequences for adolescent victims of maltreatment are increased physical aggression, antisocial behavior, juvenile delinquency, inappropriate sexual behavior, substance abuse, poor school performance, weak social skills, and the intergenerational transmission of violence (Gelles, 2000). Further, adolescents who are sexually abused are at higher risk of being sexually abused as adults (Finkelhor and Yllo, 1985). In 1988, the total estimated cost to society for child maltreatment in the United States ranged from \$8.4–32.3 billion per year for hospitalization, rehabilitation, special education, foster care, social services, court expenses, and other expenses (Gelles, 2000).

THEORIES AND RESEARCH

Developmental-Ecological Model

Belsky's developmental-ecological model (1993) explains the etiology, or causes, of child maltreatment by discussing various "contexts of maltreatment" (p. 413), including the developmental context, the interactional context, and the broader community, cultural, and evolutionary context. Belsky explains that no single factor can account for the occurrence of child maltreatment but that it takes multiple factors interacting across these contexts to create a situation in which violence occurs. The developmental context includes factors within the parent such as childhood history of abuse, personality, and psychological resources, plus factors within the child such as age, physical health, and behavior. For example, abuse may occur when an impulsive, immature adolescent parent has an irritable, chronically ill infant. The interactional, or immediate context includes levels of parental responsiveness, negativity, affection, and hostility toward their children, punitive and power assertive disciplinary strategies, and parent–child reciprocity in aversive behaviors. The interaction between the adolescent parent in the previous example and the irritable infant may be exacerbated if there is a belief that the infant is intentionally defying the parent and if the infant responds to the parent's anger with increased irritability. The broader context includes factors within the community, such as availability of social support, the culture, and the historical, evolutionary context. For example, an adolescent mother who lives with her own mother may be less likely to abuse her child than an adolescent mother who is socially isolated and, therefore, has no one to help her with the responsibilities of parenting.

Social Learning Theory

Social learning theory proposes that child maltreatment results from parents using on their children the parenting methods they witnessed or experienced growing up. This learning may occur because of "modeling, direct reinforcement, coercion training (dependent on positive and negative reinforcement or negative reinforcement alone), and inconsistency training" (Belsky, 1993, p. 415). Inconsistency training occurs when the parenting style is so unpredictable that a child searches for any sort of consistency, even if that consistent behavior is negative. For example, an adolescent who is only able to gain attention from her father in the form of sexual abuse may crave even that attention and may learn to interpret sexual abuse as a sign of love.

Role Theory

The basic tenets of role theory posit that individual attitudes and perceptions are formed through cultural norms and expectations (Stryker & Statham, 1985). Moreover, societal attitudes act as guidelines for role enactment and subsequent behaviors. Taking a role theory perspective provides insight when considering the varying cultural definitions of what constitutes abuse. Societal norms determine roles and expectations that influence future behaviors. Further, role theory predicts that individuals are more likely to engage in behaviors that are positively sanctioned. Specifically, a positive sanction is established if few negative consequences result from the behavior. Therefore, the lack of negative consequences for acts of maltreatment and abuse will increase acceptance of such acts. One way in which adolescents learn about societal norms is through mass media. For example, typical music videos portray young women as objects to be used for males' sexual pleasure (Kalof, 1999). Is it surprising, then, that date rape among adolescents is widespread?

Conflict Theory/Feminist Theory

Conflict Theory and Feminist Theories share the idea that conflict is inevitable in any situation in which there is an imbalance of power such as a relationship in which one person is dominant while another is submissive (Steinmetz, 1988). In any family, there will be conflicting needs and interests. Violence may be used as a means of advancing one's interests when other methods fail. Families may be particularly vulnerable to violence when there is a perceived imbalance between the parents' authority and their power to bring about behaviors. Thus abuse may occur when parents of an adolescent perceive that they are losing their ability to control their child and are unwilling to relinquish that control.

Family Stress Theory

Family stress theory focuses on variations in families' reactions to and management of change (stressful life events), such as the transition from childhood to adolescence or the birth of a child, as well as little changes associated with the daily demands of life. Child maltreatment has long been linked to levels of family stress. Belsky (1993) proposes that "what determines whether child maltreatment takes place is the balance of stressors and supports ... when stressors ... outweigh supports, ... the probability of child maltreatment increases" (p. 413). Family stress theory includes the influence of resources on a family's ability to cope effectively with stressors. Parents with limited resources may resort to violence more readily. In addition, the peak in emotional abuse that occurs in adolescence has been attributed to the stressors involved in the transition from childhood to adolescence (Wurtele, 1999).

Abuse to Adolescents

Wurtele (1999) reports that physical abuse often, but not always, is a continuation of abuse begun in childhood. There are some categories of maltreatment, however, that are more commonly experienced by adolescents than by younger children. For example, adolescents are more vulnerable than younger children to homicides by fathers in addition to emotional abuse and sexual abuse (Barth, Derezotes, & Danforth, 1991; Kaplan et al., 1999; Wurtele, 1999). During adolescence, children are vulnerable to violent crime, abuse by peers, dating violence, genital mutilation, forced prostitution, and forced marriage.

Abuse by Adolescents

Mulsow and Murry (1996) discuss the risk of abuse by adolescent parents due to the overwhelming disadvantages with which they enter parenthood. For example, they experience increased stressors such as school dropout, low wages, unstable employment, poor childrearing skills, and single parenting. The resulting poverty and social isolation are associated with greater incidence of punitive parenting behavior (McLoyd, 1990). Approximately half of the adolescent mothers included in a study by Haskett, Johnson, and Miller (1994) were at risk of abusing their children. Those at greatest risk are young adolescents at the age of first birth with limited social support (Mulsow & Murry, 1996). Other abuse by adolescents includes dating violence, sexual abuse to children, and sibling violence (Barth et al., 1991).

Cultural Issues in Adolescent Abuse

Levinson (1989) argues that it is not practical to apply a distinct developmental stage of adolescence cross-culturally. For example, in the United States adolescence often stretches out through the college years and beyond. However, some cultures do not acknowledge a period known as adolescence and believe that an individual moves from childhood into adulthood.

A second issue involves whether a practice is abusive when it includes intentionally inflicted pain as part of an initiation ceremony (Levinson, 1989). The Role Theory perspective suggests that many involved would not label such acts as abuse, but as the only way to become an adult member of their society. FGM is such a practice. Some assert that FGM is an Islamic religious practice with which outsiders should not interfere. Barstow (1999), however, reports that this is not the case and in fact, religious leaders tend to view FGM as a custom rather than a theologically linked practice. In areas in which FGM is widespread, it is practiced not only by Muslims, but also by Christians, Jews, and others, and it is rare in many Islamic countries, including Iran, Iraq, Libya, and Saudi Arabia (Barstow, 1999). Further, Barstow (1999) asserts, slavery, the caste system in India, cannibalism, foot binding in China, and human sacrifice are all culturally linked practices that have been drastically reduced or eliminated due to "interference" that sought to improve the human condition.

In many cultures, the study of abuse and neglect has received little attention. Recently, however, scholars have begun to study rates of abuse and their impact on children. For example, a community survey in Hong Kong found that Chinese families showed slightly higher levels of severe violence when compared to US families (Tang, 1998). Subcultural influences also need to be considered in studying adolescent abuse. For example, a Latino adolescent in the United States who is sexually abused may be forced to marry the perpetrator, even if the sexual abuse involves severe coercion and violence (Romero, Wyatt, Loeb, Carmona, & Solis, 1999).

STRATEGIES: OVERVIEW

Prevention of abuse and neglect in adolescence involves both the prevention of abuse and neglect to adolescents and the prevention of child abuse or neglect that would have been perpetrated by adolescents. When discussing strategies that work well for preventing child abuse and

neglect, it must be understood that no strategy has been found to be highly successful in combating this problem (Gelles, 2000). There are strategies, however, that have produced some degree of improvement. Barth and associates (1991) indicate that a critical part of any preventive strategy is the opportunity for participants to practice new skills, for example, through role playing.

One problem faced by those conducting studies of child abuse prevention programs is how to measure outcomes. Among outcomes used are protective service reports, measures of aspects of parenting that have been linked to maltreatment, observing parent–child interactions, and medical reports such as emergency room visits (Guterman, 1997). There are problems with each of these. The most obvious choice, protective service reports, is problematic due to the fact that participants in a prevention program are commonly exposed to more mandated reporters for longer periods of time than are members of control groups. Therefore, participation in a prevention program, in some cases, increases the number of reports of suspected maltreatment (Guterman, 1997). Measuring parenting competency and observing parent–child interactions are both problematic because knowledge does not necessarily lead to action, and actions while being observed by researchers do not necessarily carry over into daily life. Medical reports are also problematic because there are conditions requiring medical intervention that do not involve maltreatment. For example, more emergency room visits for a child with asthma may be an indication of more competent parenting rather than of maltreatment (Mulsow & Murry, 1996). Prevention programs have shown widely varying levels of success based, in part, on what outcomes were chosen.

STRATEGIES THAT WORK

Home Visiting

Among the program types touted as most successful in combating abuse by adolescent parents are the various types of home visiting (Guterman, 1997). By definition, home visitation programs occur within the family's home, offering a variety of services that might not otherwise reach families in need. Home visitations provide parenting guidance, links to formal and/or informal supports in the community, and health education. Because programs are conducted in the home, visitors become aware of individuals' needs and may notice the early warning signs of stress and dysfunction (Wasik & Roberts, 1994). The most effective programs appear to start prenatally and continue through infancy, with frequent visits by trained paraprofessional staff, offered to low-income, single, adolescent mothers who are chosen demographically but not otherwise screened for high risk (Guterman, 1997; MacMillan, MacMillan, Offord, Griffith, & MacMillan, 1994). In addition, minority status may add to a parent's potential for success in a home visiting program (Guterman, 1997).

Reported success of home visiting programs depends on the outcomes used for evaluation. For example, Guterman (1997) reports that, among those he reviewed, only three out of ten home visiting programs using protective service reports as their outcome measure show positive intervention effects. However, when parent–child interactions or parenting attitudes are measured, half of the programs studied find positive intervention effects. When medical indicators are used as outcomes, four out of seven programs appear to be successful. Even using protective service reports, however, a fifteen year follow-up by Olds and associates (1997) shows that, among a group of high risk mothers who were adolescents at first birth, the control group has been almost twice as likely as the treatment group to be reported for child abuse or neglect.

Parenting Education

Some type of parenting education is included in most child abuse prevention programs (Guterman, 1997). In a meta-analytic review of parenting education programs O'Neal, West, Mulsow, and Willerton (2000) find conflicting results. Specifically, programs evaluated by using a number of child abuse cases among program participants appear to be less successful than those that examine parental competencies. In other words, while parents report more knowledge of appropriate techniques and may even be observed in the lab applying these techniques, an increase in parenting knowledge does not necessarily translate into a decrease in abuse or neglect (MacMillan et al., 1994). As with the home visiting interventions, however, some of this may be explained by a greater exposure to mandated reporters among families participating in parenting education programs.

School-Based Programs

According to Barth and colleagues, almost all school districts nationwide provide some education in the prevention of maltreatment to or by adolescents (Barth et al., 1991). School based programs, according to Johnson, "aim to convey knowledge and strategies that may help children protect themselves from abuse" (1994, p. 261). For example, adolescents may be taught to recognize and avoid or escape situations of potential violence. Violence prevention programs aimed at providing adolescents with nonviolent alternatives for conflict resolution have also shown moderate success (National Research Council, 1993). In addition, parenting programs offered through schools to provide adolescents with skills and knowledge to care for their own children have

resulted in improvements, especially when they are required for both boys and girls (Wurtele, 1999), are intensive, last at least one year (Barth et al., 1991), and include information on the health and behavioral consequences of abuse (Buzi, Smith, & Weinman, 1998).

Schools can provide a place where "parents and children can gather informally and enjoy each other" (Thompson & Wyatt, 1999, p. 191). Regardless of how impoverished a neighborhood may be, there will usually be a local school through which families can be offered services such as parent support groups, community referrals, after-school activities, and therapy (Thompson & Wyatt, 1999). After-school programs provide supervision and care for children who might otherwise be left alone or in unsafe situations. In addition, they remove the stressors on parents associated with providing care for their school-aged children. Further, school-based childcare programs both during and after school provide adolescent parents with the opportunity to complete their education, thus reducing stressors in these adolescents' families. Although most after-school programs target children ages 12 and younger, teen programs are provided in some, including the use of adolescents as tutors for younger children (Halpern, 1992). Outcome studies suggest that these programs work for the children who participate, but that by adolescence, many children are only occasional participants (Halpern, 1992).

Support Groups

Dunst and Trivette (1990) have defined social support as emotional, instrumental, material, or informational aid supplied by members of one's social networks. Today, the importance of a positive social support system to healthy child development is virtually uncontested in the social sciences (Belsky, 1993; Dunst and Trivette, 1990). Support groups are often incorporated into abuse prevention. A key component to many successful parenting programs is to provide families with both formal and informal support systems. In a community-based abuse prevention project, researchers find that participants appreciate the informal support provided by team members whose responses are accepting, nonthreatening and nonjudgmental (Onyskiw & Harrison, 1999).

STRATEGIES THAT MIGHT WORK

Screening and Treatment for Psychological Disorders in Parents

Belsky (1984) states that, among the determinants of parenting, the most important is parental psychological resources. Mulsow, O'Neal, and Murry (2001) indicate that those parents who suffer from moderate psychological disorders may lack the resources and coping skills to be able to apply preventive measures such as parenting training. Further, although parents with severe depression are more likely to be recognized and treated, moderate depression is more strongly associated with maltreatment (Christmas, Wodarski, & Smokowski, 1996; Zuravin, 1989). Kaplan and associates (1999) note that because high rates of depression, substance abuse, and antisocial behavior are found among abusive parents, diagnosis and treatment of these disorders in parents is needed. When these services are offered, emotional interactions between parents and children improve (Kaplan et al., 1999).

An area that has received much attention is the treatment of parental substance abuse as a means of prevention. Gelles (1997) reports that, although substance abuse is highly correlated with child maltreatment, it is unlikely that the substances cause the abuse. However, they may be used as a socially acceptable excuse for abusive behavior. With this in mind, there are strategies that target both the substance abuse and the improvement of parent–adolescent relationships. For example, Weinberg and associates report that structural-strategic family therapy involving all family members has been shown to be effective, as has multidimensional family therapy, and multisystemic family therapy (Weinberg, Rahdert, Colliver, & Glantz, 1998).

Policy Initiatives

As the awareness of abuse and neglect increases, so too does the call for policy initiatives. Unfortunately, these endeavors are often easier said than done. For example, in 1988, Article 9 of the Declaration of Korean Children's Rights was revised and declared that "Children should not be maltreated or abandoned and they should not be used for harmful or arduous labor" and Article 18, Section 9 of the Public Child Welfare Law made these abusive behaviors prohibited under penalty of fine or imprisonment (Doe, 2000). Although promising, the law has not been enforced.

There are similar initiatives underway to reduce the incidence of FGM and selling of adolescents into prostitution (Cohn, 1998). Barstow (1999) reports that "most of the countries in which [FGM] is practiced have passed legislation making the procedure a crime" (p. 509). Mackie (1996) suggests that FGM could be ended quickly through a combination of education about physiological consequences of FGM, information about international condemnation of the practice conveyed tactfully to practicing populations, and the creation of associations of parents who pledge not to perform FGM on their daughters or allow their sons to marry women to whom this has been done. Mackie states that footbinding in China was almost completely eliminated in one generation by use of these three steps.

The Stockholm Agenda for Action on child sexual abuse has been adopted by 122 governments worldwide. This agenda calls for governments to work together to end child prostitution, child pornography, and the trafficking of children for sexual purposes (ECPAT International, 2001). Whereas much work has been done in developing policy initiatives, it remains to be seen whether reductions in these practices have followed.

Teen Pregnancy Prevention Programs and Prenatal Care

Although not often thought of as a possible aide in reducing incidence of abuse and neglect, pregnancy prevention programs may be one of our best allies. An examination of the literature provides inconsistent findings related to consequences of early childbirth. Many of the short-term studies suggest that adolescent mothers have multiple hurdles not faced by those who delay birth. However, others argue that these differences are overstated (Brooks-Gunn & Furstenberg, 1989; Zabin & Hayward, 1993). Although these outcome variations exist, it is clear that some teen parents face risk factors that may lead to incidences of maltreatment. A primary concern is a lack of prenatal care. "Prematurity, congenital abnormalities, intrauterine growth retardation, and perinatal illness often impair parent–infant attachment, which can contribute to subsequent child abuse" (Darmstadt, 1990, p. 487). As Hamburg (1992) demonstrated, adolescent females have a greater chance than postadolescent females of giving birth to high-risk babies. Good prenatal care would alleviate many of the emotional, social, and physical problems associated with these high-risk births. Unfortunately, most pregnant adolescents—especially those 15 years and younger—receive inadequate or no care.

STRATEGIES THAT DO NOT WORK

Research has shown us that there are multiple, interacting causes of maltreatment (Belsky, 1993; National Research Council, 1993) and that targeting any one cause in isolation, while disregarding other problems, will not prevent maltreatment. Rather, targets for prevention need to be combined if strategies are to be effective. In addition, programs need to build on family strengths as well as correcting weaknesses in families (National Research Council, 1993). There are specific aspects of certain programs, however, that do not seem to work.

School-Based Programs That Are Left to Teacher Discretion or That Attempt to Involve Parents

Johnson (1994) reports that school-based primary prevention programs do not work when the implementation of these programs is left to teacher discretion and no support is provided for teachers in implementing these programs. Although many of these programs show disappointing results, Johnson states that most teachers do not implement the programs as they were intended but leave out essential sections on protective behaviors. Another form of school-based program that has not been successful is the sexual abuse prevention program that includes parents, because the few parents who do show up tend to be those who would have done a good job of preparing their children, anyway (National Research Council, 1993).

Culturally Insensitive Interventions

Programs that attempt to impose values, practices, or judgments of one group on another without considering the culture of and resources available to the recipient group are destined for failure, particularly when the targets of these programs are adolescents. "In no other age group is it so easy to alienate…" with programs that are not "developmentally and culturally synchronized with teenagers" (Barth et al., 1991, p. 203). For example, in some non-Western cultures, the free exchange of children across families is normal, as the entire community assumes responsibility for child rearing. The same sort of behavior in a Western culture might be seen as abandoning of one's children and thus, result in charges of child neglect (Agathonos-Georgopoulou, 1992). Imposing Western standards upon ethnic groups who share the standard of community child care may result in diminished rather than increased care. It is more socially acceptable, however, in Western cultures than in non-Western cultures for a parent of a disabled child to turn that child's lifelong care over to a large institution (Agathonos-Georgopoulou, 1992). Taking such children away from their families and communities to place them in institutions in non-Western cultures may, again, compromise the quality of care these children receive. Well-meaning people with unrecognized ethnocentric views may become involved in a wide range of programs, then not understand why they do not succeed. Cultural understanding, both within and across nations, is vital in order for any preventative strategy to be successful.

SYNTHESIS

The Coordination of Prevention Efforts

Most prevention programs target one problem at a time. For example, programs to prevent child maltreatment rarely include efforts to prevent substance abuse, despite the fact that substance abusers are more likely to abuse or neglect their children and maltreating parents are more likely than other parents to be substance abusers (Feig, 1998). If limited

resources available for prevention programs can be used in a more coordinated manner, multiple issues can be targeted simultaneously.

Home Visiting

Home visiting is an area that shows great promise for the prevention of abuse and neglect by adolescent parents. Traditionally, the primary targets for these programs have been adolescents judged to be high-risk who have just become mothers. Recently, more of these programs have begun to expand into offering prenatal services and to including fathers, grandparents, and others who provide support for new mothers. Findings from evaluations of home visiting programs support each of these changes. In addition, evaluations support the offering of services to those selected demographically rather than trying to identify individual high-risk mothers.

Prevention Funding

It is almost as popular among politicians and pundits to discuss the advantages of prevention over treatment as it is for these same people to recommend cuts in governmental funding for prevention programs. If we hope to be successful in preventing maltreatment, we will have to find ways to pay for prevention programs. In an environment of cutbacks in government spending, increased support from private sources such as foundations will be needed to fill some of the gap. In addition, researchers should continue efforts to educate politicians concerning the lower cost of prevention compared to later treatment and incarceration.

Measurement Issues

There is a need for more widely accepted methods of measuring abuse and neglect. First, definitions of the various types of abuse and neglect need to be clarified. Next, these definitions need to be widely disseminated and accepted. Even if ideal definitions are beyond our reach, agreement on working definitions for research purposes may be possible. Finally, measures that incorporate these definitions need to be developed or existing measures adapted. Consensus on ways to measure various types of maltreatment will make findings in this area more understandable and will make meta-analysis of studies more feasible.

Program Evaluation

Despite the widespread use of prevention programs worldwide, MacMillan and associates were only able to locate eleven standardized evaluations for their 1994 review. Even by 1999, Kaplan and colleagues mention the need for more well-designed studies. Evaluations of prevention programs should investigate not only whether improvements were seen, but also which aspects of the programs produced these improvements (MacMillan et al., 1994). For example, there are many governmental and non-governmental programs in place as of 2001 to prevent the use of FGM. Evaluations that tell us whether these programs are working and, if so, what parts of the programs are working will help us to direct limited resources into areas that are most likely to produce positive results.

Maltreatment is too complex of a problem to be solved by one program, regardless of its effectiveness. What are needed are systemic interventions, followed by thorough evaluations that include as many stakeholders as possible. These evaluations need to be published so that others can learn from the wisdom gained through both the successes and the failures of their predecessors.

Also see: Anger Regulation: Adolescence; Depression: Adolescence; Divorce: Adolescence; Family Strengthening: Adolescence.

References

Agathonos-Georgopoulou, H. (1992). Cross-cultural perspectives in child abuse and neglect. *Child Abuse Review, 1*, 80–88.

Barstow, D.G. (1999). Female genital mutilation: The penultimate gender abuse. *Child Abuse and Neglect, 23,* 501–510.

Barth, R.P., Derezotes, D.S., & Danforth, H.E. (1991). Preventing adolescent abuse. *Journal of Primary Prevention, 11*, 193–205.

Belsky, J. (1984). The determinants of parenting: A process model. *Child Development, 55*, 83–96.

Belsky, J. (1993). Etiology of child maltreatment: A developmental-ecological analysis. *Psychological Bulletin, 114*, 413–434.

Brooks-Gunn, J., & Furstenberg, F.F. (1989). Long-term implications of fertility-related behavior and family formation on adolescent mothers and their children. In K. Kreppner & R.M. Lerner (Eds.), *Family systems and life-span development* (pp. 319–339). Hillsdale, NJ: Erlbaum.

Buzi, R.S., Smith, P.B., & Weinman, M.L. (1998). Incorporating health and behavioral consequences of child abuse in prevention programs targeting female adolescents. *Patient Education and Counseling, 33*, 209–216.

Child Abuse Prevention and Treatment Act Amendments of 1996, Publication L. 104-235, Title I (section) 101, October 3, 1996, 110 Stat. 3063; codified at 42 USC.

Christmas, A.L., Wodarski, J.S., & Smokowski, P.R. (1996). Risk factors for physical child abuse: A practice theoretical paradigm. *Family Therapy, 23*, 233–248.

Cohn, J. (1998). Violations of human rights in children and adolescents: How can we safeguard rights for young human beings? *International Journal of Adolescent Medicine and Health, 10*, 185–192.

Darmstadt, G.L. (1990). Community-based child abuse prevention. *Social Work, 35*, 487–489.

Doe, S.S. (2000). Cultural factors in child maltreatment and domestic violence in Korea. *Children and Youth Services Review, 22*, 231–236.

Dunst, C.J., & Trivette, C.M. (1990). Assessment of social support in early intervention programs. In S.J. Meisels and J.P. Shonkoff (Eds.), *Handbook of early childhood intervention* (pp. 326–349). Cambridge, England: Cambridge University Press.

ECPAT International (2001). *1997–1998 Moving to Action. A second report on the implementation of the Agenda for Action adopted at the first World Congress against Commercial Sexual Exploitation of Children. Stockholm, Sweden, 28 August 1996.* Bangkok, Thailand: ECPAT International. Accessed at www.ecpat.net/projects/stockholm.htm

Feig, L. (1998). Understanding the problem: The gap between substance abuse programs and child welfare services. In R.L. Hampton, V. Senatore, & T.P. Gullotta (Eds.), *Substance abuse, family violence, and child welfare: Bridging perspectives* (pp. 62–95). Thousand Oaks, CA: Sage.

Finkelhor, D., & Yllo, K. (1985). *License to Rape.* New York: Simon and Schuster.

Fortin, A., & Chamberland, C. (1995). Preventing the psychological maltreatment of children. *Journal of Interpersonal Violence, 10*, 275–295.

Garbarino, J., & Kostelny, K. (1992). Child maltreatment as a community problem. *Child Abuse and Neglect, 16*, 455–464.

Gelles, R.J. (1997). *Intimate violence in families* (3rd ed.). Thousand Oaks, CA: Sage.

Gelles, R.J. (2000). Violence, abuse, and neglect in families. In P.C. McHenry & S.J. Price (Eds.), *Families and change: Coping with stressful events and transitions* (2nd ed., pp. 183–207). Thousand Oaks, CA: Sage.

Guterman, N.B. (1997). Early prevention of physican child abuse and neglect: Existing evidence and future directions. *Child Maltreatment, 2*, 12–34.

Halpern, R. (1992). The role of after-school programs in the lives of inner-city children: A study of the "Urban Youth Network." *Child Welfare*, pp. 215–230.

Hamburg, D.A. (1992). *Today's children: Creating a future for a generation in crisis.* New York: Time Books.

Haskett, M.E., Johnson, C.A., & Miller, J.W. (1994). Individual differences in risk of child abuse by adolescent mothers: Assessment in the perinatal period. *Journal of Child Psychology and Psychiatry and Allied Disciplines, 35*, 461–471.

Johnson, B. (1994). Teachers' role in the primary prevention of child abuse: Dilemmas and problems. *Child Abuse Review, 3*, 259–271.

Kalof, L. (1999). The effects of gender and music video imagery on sexual attitudes. *The Journal of Social Psychology, 139*, 22–45.

Kaplan, S.J., Pelcovitz, D., & Labruna, V. (1999). Child and adolescent abuse and neglect research: A review of the past 10 years. Part I: Physical and emotional abuse and neglect. *Journal of the American Academy of Child and Adolescent Psychiatry, 38*, 1214–1222.

Levinson, D. (1989). *Family violence in cross-cultural perspective.* Newbury Park, CA: Sage.

Mackie, G. (1996). Ending footbinding and infibulation: A convention account. *American Sociological Review, 61*, 999–1017.

MacMillan, H.L., MacMillan, J.H., Offord, D.R., Griffith, L., & MacMillan, A. (1994). Primary prevention of child physical abuse and neglect: A critical review. Part I. *Journal of Child Psychology and Psychiatry and Allied Disciplines, 35*, 835–856.

McLoyd, V.C. (1990). The impact of economic hardship on Black families and children: Psychological distress, parenting, and socioemotional development [Special issue: Minority children]. *Child Development, 61*, 311–346.

Mulsow, M., O'Neal, K., & Murry, V.M. (2001). Adult attention deficit hyperactivity disorder, the family, and child maltreatment. *Trauma, Violence, & Abuse: A Review Journal, 2*, 36–50.

Mulsow, M.H., & Murry, V.M. (1996). Parenting on edge: Economically stressed, single, African-American adolescent mothers. *Family Issues, 17*, 704–721.

National Research Council (1993). *Understanding child abuse and neglect: Panel on research on child abuse and neglect.* Washington, DC: National Academy Press.

Olds, D.L., Eckenrode, J., Henderson, C.R., Jr., Kitzman, H., Powers, J., Cole, R., Sidora, K., Morris, P., Pettitt, L.M., & Luckey, D. (1997).

Long-term effects of home visitation on maternal life course and child abuse and neglect. Fifteen-year follow-up of a randomized trial. *Journal of the American Medical Association, 278*, 637–43.

O'Neal, K., West, S., Mulsow, M., & Willerton, E. (2000, November). *A meta-analytic review of parenting programs designed to reduce the incidence of child maltreatment.* Paper presented at the annual meeting of the National Council on Family Relations, Minneapolis, MN.

Onyskiw, J.E., & Harrison, M.J. (1999). Formative evaluation of a collaborative community-based child abuse prevention project. *Child Abuse and Neglect, 23*, 1069–1081.

Portwood, S.G. (1998). The impact of individuals' characteristics and experiences on their definitions of child maltreatment. *Child Abuse and Neglect, 22*, 437–452.

Romero, G.J., Wyatt, G.E., Loeb, T.B., Carmona, J.V., & Solis, B.M. (1999). The prevalence and circumstances of child sexual abuse among Latina women. *Hispanic Journal of Behavioral Sciences, 21*, 351–365.

Steinmetz, S. (1988). Family violence: Past, present, and future. In M.B. Sussman & S.K. Steinmetz (Eds.), *Handbook of marriage and the family.* NY: Plenum Press

Stryker, S., & Statham, A. (1985). Symbolic interaction and role theory. In G. Lindzey & E. Aronson (Eds.), *Handbook of Social Psychology* (pp. 311–377). New York: Random House.

Tang, C.S. (1998). The rate of physical child abuse in Chinese families: A community survey in Hong Kong. *Child Abuse and Neglect, 22*, 381–391.

Thompson, R.A., & Wyatt, J.M. (1999). Current research on child maltreatment: Implications for educators. *Educational Psychology Review, 11*, 173–201.

US Department of Health and Human Services. (1998). *Child Maltreatment 1996: Reports from the States to the National Child Abuse and Neglect Data System.* Washington, DC: US Government Printing Office.

United States Congress. (1996). S. Res 919, 104th Congress (enacted).

Wasik, B.H., & Roberts, R.N. (1994). Survey of home visiting programs for abused and neglected children and their families. *Child Abuse and Neglect, 18*, 271–283.

Weinberg, N.Z., Rahdert, E., Colliver, J.D., & Glantz, M.D. (1998). Adolescent substance abuse: A review of the past 10 years. *Journal of the American Academy of Child and Adolescent Psychiatry, 37*, 252–261.

Wurtele, S.K. (1999). Preventing child maltreatment: Multiple windows of opportunity in the health care system. *Children's Health Care, 28*, 151–165.

Zabin, L.S., & Hayward, S.C. (1993). *Adolescent sexual behavior and childbearing.* Newbury Park, CA: Sage.

Zuravin, S.J. (1989). Severity of maternal depression and three types of mother-to-child aggression. *American Journal of Orthopsychiatry, 59*, 377–389.

Academic Success, Adolescence

Jodie L. Roth and Jeanne Brooks-Gunn

INTRODUCTION, DEFINITION, AND SCOPE

Adolescents' academic pursuits center on school. Their connections to school, motivation to achieve, course selection, and acquired knowledge and skills create a foundation for the future. Admission to higher education, and increasingly, jobs in the workplace, require a high school diploma. Graduation from high school, the most widely used measure of academic success during adolescence, signifies students' satisfactory completion of a set of required courses, and increasingly, passing scores on state proficiency tests. And with it, the assumption that students possess the reading, writing, and mathematical skills necessary for further schooling or entry-level jobs.

Academic Skills and High School Graduation

At the national level, standardized achievement test scores and high school graduation rates provide objective and comparable data on students who attain this level of academic success. The International Adult Literacy Survey measured basic literacy skills for young adults, ages 16–25, in 7 countries (Canadian Education Statistics Council, 2000). The tests measured three types of literacy: the knowledge and skills required to locate and use information contained in various formats, such as job applications or maps (document literacy); the skills and knowledge needed to understand and use information from texts (prose literacy); and the knowledge and skills necessary to apply arithmetic operations to numbers embedded in printed material, such as figuring a tip or balancing a checkbook (quantitative literacy).

Level 3 is considered the minimum level of skills for efficient day-to-day living in an advanced democratic country. In the United States, only 45 percent of the young adults scored at or above level 3 on the document scale, 46 percent on the prose scale, and 43 percent on the quantitative scale. Young adults in Canada performed substantially better. On the document scale, 67 percent scored at level 3 or above, 64 percent did so on the prose scale, and 61 percent on the quantitative scale. The only country other than the United States with a lower percentage of young adults reaching at least level 3 was Poland. Sweden showed the highest percentage, with 80 percent scoring at level 3 or above on the document and prose scales, and 77 percent on the quantitative scale (Canadian Education Statistics Council, 2000).

The Third International Mathematics and Science Study (TIMSS) provides international comparisons of students' mathematical and scientific skills for 4th, 8th, and 12th grade students. TIMSS scores represent the overall percent correct. American 12th graders scored below the average score for the 21 nations sampled in both mathematics and science in 1995. Eighth graders scored above the 41-nation average in science, but below the average in mathematics. Canadian adolescents in their final year of secondary school and in the 8th grade scored above the international mean in both subjects. Students in their final year of secondary school in the Netherlands scored the highest in mathematics and science. At the 8th grade level, students in Singapore earned the highest scores (National Center for Education Statistics, 1999).

Although some youth with limited skills do graduate from high school, poor achievement and school failure are common antecedents of dropping out of high school. Few adolescents drop out of school before the 10th grade, at least officially. The rates increase with age, and are highest for 18 and 19-year olds who are unable to graduate with their age-mates (Dryfoos, 1998). In 1996, 72 percent of American 18-year olds had graduated from high school, compared with 75 percent of Canadian 18-year olds. The percentage was higher in European countries. In Germany, for example, 86 percent of youth graduated from secondary school at the typical age for graduation (Canadian Education Statistics Council, 2000). The percentage of Americans with a high school diploma, however, increases with age; in 1998, 85 percent of young adults aged 18 to 24 received a high school diploma or its equivalent. The rates are similar for black young adults, but dramatically lower for Latino (63 percent; National Center for Education Statistics, 1999).

Consequences of Academic Failure

The consequences of not completing high school are well documented. The costs to individuals are typically calculated in economic terms. The lack of a high school diploma leads to fewer job prospects, lower salaries, and greater unemployment and welfare dependence (Baydar, Brooks-Gunn, & Furstenberg, 1993). And this trend can be expected to increase as the economy shifts to more high-tech jobs. Dropping out of high school is associated with other problem behaviors as well, including delinquency, substance abuse, and early child bearing. The economic costs to society for youth who do not graduate from high school include lost tax revenue as well as expenditures on welfare services. A large number of high school dropouts, alienated from school and undereducated, contribute to an unhealthy community environment (Benson, Leffert, Scales, & Blyth, 1998).

THEORIES AND RESEARCH

Adolescence, as a time of both risk and opportunity, poses a critical juncture for encouraging positive behaviors and developing competencies necessary for academic success. We draw on contextual developmental theory as well as the positive youth development framework to provide guidance for how to enhance adolescents' chances of academic success.

Adolescents live in various overlapping worlds, or contexts, including family, peers, school, workplace, neighborhood, community, region, and country. Models of development that stress both the multiple spheres of influence on human functioning as well as the connections among these spheres provide useful frameworks for understanding adolescents' behavior, including academic success. Such models—ecological systems theory (Bronfenbrenner & Morris, 1998) and developmental contextualism (Lerner, 1991)—offer a way of conceptualizing all the forces acting on an individual, as well as the relationships between and among individuals and contexts in their life. These contexts shape an adolescent through sustained, consistent, intersecting interactions (or lack of) with the adolescent (Bronfenbrenner & Morris, 1998).

This perspective highlights two beliefs about adolescent development. First, development is not unidirectional; development is truly dynamic—the individual and the environment, as well as their unique interactions, shape development. Second, this theoretical perspective emphasizes the plasticity of human development. The endpoint of development is not predetermined, either by genetic make-up or particular experiences. Individual's lives are best construed as probabilistic. The different contexts influencing adolescents' lives affect their academic success, including not only school and family (although these two have been the focus of most of the research), but peers and neighborhoods as well.

The largest body of research pertaining to academic success studies the pathways of school failure and dropping out of high school. Although school failure is best understood as a process rather than as a single event, the majority of this research looks for predictors of dropping out in the different contexts affecting adolescents. Youth who drop out of high school are disproportionally from lower socioeconomic strata, members of minority groups, and live in poorer communities (Rosenthal, 1998). Much of this research follows the developmental contextualist approach of seeking to identify the influences of different contexts in adolescent lives on their dropout behavior. Studies of the demographic, individual, familial, and school-level predictors of adolescents' high school dropout behavior consistently find academic achievement, typically assessed with standardized achievement tests or grade point average, to be one of the strongest predictors of dropping out of high school (Battin-Pearson, Newcomb, Abbott, Hill, Catalano, & Hawkins, 2000). Family characteristics found to play an important role in students' dropout behavior include financial (e.g., family income), social (e.g., family structure, family relationships), and human capital (e.g., parent education). How the family context interacts with the child's school context also plays a role in students academic success. Youth from families with poor relations with the school and a lack of parental involvement are more likely to drop out (Goldschmidt & Wang, 1999).

There are fewer studies focusing on school characteristics. A recent investigation of the influence of multiple contexts in adolescents' lives on dropping out early (by the 10th grade) or late (by the 12th grade) found that the percentage of students held back at least one grade and the percentage of misbehaving students in the class independently predicted both early and late dropout behavior

(Goldschmidt & Wang, 1999). A consistent finding in this literature is the effect of the perceived discipline climate at the school. Students are less likely to drop out from schools where the discipline is perceived to be fair (Rumberger, 1995). Research on academic achievement suggests that the school climate affects students interest in learning and achievement, particularly during middle school. For example, positive teacher regard and an emphasis on individual effort and improvement (intrinsic goals) were associated with an increase in academic achievement, as well as increases in academic values and feelings of academic competence in 8th grade (Roeser & Eccles, 1998). There is even less research on the role of peers on academic failure and dropping out of high school. Numerous researchers have shown that dropouts tend to have more deviant friends who also show potential for dropping out, but the mechanisms of this influence is largely unstudied (Battin-Pearson et al., 2000).

This line of research also finds that neighborhood poverty level affects student dropout behavior. Leventhal and Brooks-Gunn (2000) concluded in their review of the neighborhood literature that neighborhood socioeconomic status is positively associated with adolescents' achievement on basic skills tests, math performance, and grade point average, as well as on youths' chances of completing high school, attending college, and total years of schooling. However, the association between high neighborhood socioeconomic status and education attainment appears to be stronger for males than females and for European Americans than African Americans.

Supporting Academic Success

Research rooted in the contextual framework of adolescent development emphasizes the many influences on adolescents' lack of academic success. Research stemming from the positive development framework focuses on the factors that promote academic success. The positive youth development framework grew out of efforts in the prevention and intervention fields to improve youths' lives by shifting the focus from fixing problems to nurturing assets, or building competencies. Thus, navigating adolescence in healthy ways is best viewed as a continuous process, with earlier life experiences shaping later outcomes (Roth, Brooks-Gunn, Murray, & Foster, 1998).

Academic competence is considered part of the "five Cs" of healthy adolescent development: competence in academic, social, and vocational areas; confidence; connection to community, family, and peers; character; and caring and compassion (Lerner, Fisher, & Weinberg, 2000). This notion of academic success captures both the cognitive skills (such as literacy or mathematical abilities) as well as the noncognitive skills necessary for future adult success. For example, a substantial number of youth graduate from high school without adequate levels of literacy. However, graduation, in

and of itself, is important in terms of later life success. For these youth, other skills, such as the ability to persevere and work toward a goal, help them in later life (Baydar et al., 1993). Other noncognitive skills of import for academic success are orderliness, organization, conscientiousness, and motivation (Dunifon, Duncan, & Brooks-Gunn, 2001).

A commitment to learning also contributes to school success across all racial/ethnic groups (Scales, Benson, Leffert, & Blyth, 2000). Such a commitment can be fostered in the different contexts affecting adolescents' lives. For example, parents' involvement in their children's schooling, such as talking with their child about school, monitoring and helping with their homework, and providing support and high expectations contributes to school success (Roth & Brooks-Gunn, 2000).

STRATEGIES THAT WORK

Strategies to promote academic success among adolescents can be grouped into those that seek to improve the quality of education in the schools and those that attempt to augment schools' efforts in the home or community. The positive impact of effective schools for healthy development, including academic success, is a recurring finding from the resiliency research (Luthar, Cicchetti, & Becker, 2000). School reform takes many shapes—changes at the classroom level such as how teachers teach, what they teach, how learning is assessed, and how classrooms are organized, as well as changes in the larger school structure. They all aim to improve the quality of education, resulting in higher achievement for all students. Growing evidence supports the benefits of school-wide changes for improved educational outcomes for all students.

A decade ago, the Carnegie Corporation released the *Turning Points* report calling for changes in the structure and practice of middle school education based on the needs of young adolescents (Carnegie Council on Adolescent Development, 1989). Findings from over 420 schools participating in reform initiatives following the *Turning Points* recommendations show that fundamental changes in the structure and content of middle-grades education can produce substantial improvements in students' academic achievement and healthy development. Schools with the highest level of implementation of the recommendations showed the highest gains in students' mathematics, language, and reading achievement test scores, higher ratings of students' self-esteem (student-rated), and the lowest levels of student behavioral problems (teacher-rated) and students' self-reports of feelings of worry and fear (Felner, Jackson, Kasak, Mulhall, Brand, & Flowers, 1997).

Recently, the Carnegie Corporation released a follow-up, *Turning Points 2000*, with recommendations based on the experiences and research of the past 10 years on implementing their original reforms (Jackson & Davis, 2000). They call for a rigorous curriculum, grounded in public academic standards for what students should know and be able to do and how students learn best; instructional methods designed to prepare all students to achieve higher standards and become lifelong learners; teachers who are expert at teaching young adolescents and provided with targeted professional development opportunities; creating a climate of intellectual development and shared educational purpose; democratic school governance; safe and healthy school environments; and involving parents and communities.

Another approach of school reform focuses on specific programs for students most at risk of school failure, or dropout prevention programs. Programs that attempt to create a more supportive and personalized learning environment, often through a school-with-a-school approach, have met with success (Dynarski & Gleason, 1999). Career academies are one example of this approach. Career academies, an approach existing for more than 30 years, offer students an integrated academic and vocational curriculum, with occupational experiences through partnerships with employers and community organizations. Results from a longitudinal evaluation of nine sites, using random assignment, found that the Career Academies substantially improved high school outcomes—reduced dropout rates, improved attendance, increased academic course-taking, and increased likelihood of earning enough credits to graduate on time—for students at risk of dropping out. However, the Academies did not improve standardized math and reading achievement test scores. Participants received more interpersonal support, such as higher teacher expectations and more individualized attention, and had classmates who were more engaged in school (Kemple & Snipes, 2000).

Community-based youth development programs offer another approach for improving adolescents' academic success. Such efforts are varied in their approach, but typically encourage a strong commitment and connection to school. The encouragement can occur indirectly through program staffs' expectations for adolescents' achievement, as well as directly through homework assistance or staff contact with students' teachers and school personnel (Roth et al., 1998). Among the handful of well-evaluated youth development programs, all showed improvements in participants' school-related behaviors, such as grades, achievement test scores, and/or attitudes. For example, the Quantum Opportunities Program, a year-round, four-year, multiservice program for students from families receiving public assistance, provides students with educational support including tutoring, computer-assisted instruction, and homework help, as well as development and service activities. The explicit goals of the program are to foster academic and

social competencies. Results from the evaluation of the program, using random assignment, show that by the end of high school, participants displayed significant increases in academic skills and educational expectations. One year after the end of the program, program participants were significantly more likely to have earned their high school diploma (63 vs. 42 percent) and be in a postsecondary school (42 vs. 16 percent) (Hahn, Leavitt, & Aaron, 1994).

Recently, there has been an explosion in the number of mentoring programs aimed at improving students' school success and decreasing other problem behaviors. Few of these programs are rigorously evaluated; the Big Brothers/Big Sisters (BB/BS) program is a notable exception. The BB/BS program creates and supports one-to-one relationships between adult volunteers and youth living in single-parent households. The program does not specifically target problem behaviors. Instead, it offers a supportive environment and the caring of an adult friend intended to help youth develop positively. On an average, the youth and adult meet for three to four hours, three times per month for at least one year. The random assignment study of eight program sites found impressive results in participating youths' school-related behaviors, as well as their drug and alcohol use. After 18 months of participation, program youth earned higher grades, skipped half as many days of school, skipped fewer classes, and felt more competent about doing their schoolwork than did control youth (Tierney, Grossman, & Resch, 1995). The benefits of mentoring programs do not happen effortlessly. Effective mentoring relationships require an investment of time for a close, supportive relationship to develop, as well as adequate support, training, and guidance for the mentor from the program (Sipe, 1999).

These efforts share elements that contribute to their success in promoting academic achievement and high school graduation. A strong, positive relationship between teachers, or program staff, and adolescents is at the heart of their success. Adults who support adolescents' learning with high expectations, an understanding of the cognitive, social, and emotional changes that occur during adolescence, and a solid grasp of the subject matter, create a secure and positive learning environment that encourages and promotes adolescents' academic success (Dynarski & Gleason, 1999; Roth & Brooks-Gunn, 2000).

STRATEGIES THAT MIGHT WORK

Other types of after-school programs show promise for helping adolescents achieve academic success. Although the number and political support of after-school programs is burgeoning, few have documented results. Such programs are touted as an alternative to youth spending a large quantity of time alone or with peers in unsupervised, or inadequately supervised, activities during the after-school hours. Quality after-school programs can provide enriching age-appropriate activities that complement learning during the school day by combining academic, enrichment, cultural, and recreational activities. Evaluations of after-school programs show significant gains in participant's academic achievement, interest and ability in reading, improved attendance, increased engagement in school, and higher aspirations for the future (US Department of Education, 2000). However, many of the findings on the benefits of after-school programs are from studies with methodological flaws, such as the lack of a comparison or control group or the failure to collect preprogram measures. Furthermore, most examples of well-evaluated successful programs are for elementary school aged students; fewer academic enrichment after-school programs exist for adolescents.

Instead, adolescents' extracurricular activities tend to focus less on academic enrichment and more on sports or the arts. Still, adolescents' engagement in such activities is beneficial for their academic success. For example, after controlling for race and poverty status, 10th grade students who reported spending no time in school-sponsored activities were 57 percent more likely to drop out by their senior year compared to students spending 1–4 hours per week in extracurricular activities (Zill, Nord, & Loomis, 1995). Participation in extracurricular activities may provide an opportunity, outside of traditional classes, for students to develop a connection to school, or provide the motivation to maintain acceptable grades to participate.

Developing enjoyable, quality after-school activities for adolescents is a promising avenue for supporting their academic success. Successful programs share a focus on enriching learning opportunities by providing a challenging curriculum, coordinating learning with the regular school day, hiring enough qualified staff members, and coordinating and collaborating with the community. These elements are similar to those found in effective school reform efforts.

Community service requirements are gaining popularity in many middle and high schools as a way to increase youths' civic involvement, compassion, and personal growth, as well as contribute to the community. Despite its popularity and purported benefits, there are few longitudinal studies of the consequences of volunteering for adolescents. When studied longitudinally, many of the positive outcomes of volunteering, such as academic self-esteem, educational plans, and positive self-esteem, are no longer significant once selection into volunteering is controlled (Johnson, Beebe, Mortimer, & Snyder, 1998).

Service-learning programs, which combine community service requirements with classroom activities, receive widespread support for benefiting students, particularly those at risk of school failure and other risk behaviors. Again, there is scant quantitative research, but ample anecdotal or nonexperimental reports, supporting the benefits of these types of programs. There is some evidence, particularly for at-risk students, that service-learning opportunities improve academic performance and connectedness to school. Programs that include classroom activities that foster a connection between volunteer experiences and course content, and involve the opportunity for reflection, show the greatest benefits (Stukas, Clary, & Snyder, 1999).

The Teen Outreach Program is an exemplar of a (well-evaluated) service-learning program. Teen Outreach seeks to engage youth in a high level of structured, volunteer community service closely linked to classroom discussions of future life options with the goal of reducing rates of teenage pregnancy, school failure, and school suspension (Allen, Philliber, Herrling, & Kuperminc, 1997). Results from the experimental evaluation found substantially lower rates of pregnancy, school failure, and academic suspension for participants at the end of the nine-month program than compared with control students. More quality evaluation research might show that quality service-learning programs, either as part of the school day or an after-school program, promote students' academic success.

STRATEGIES THAT DO NOT WORK

The task of identifying strategies that fail to promote academic success for adolescents is hindered by the lack of published studies showing null results. Instead, we can draw on school practices that have been shown to lower students' academic achievement to highlight strategies that do not promote academic success. Tracking, or grouping students by ability, is one example of such a practice. Although most elementary schools use with-in class ability grouping, typically for reading and math lessons, middle and high school students are often tracked with students of similar ability throughout the day.

The practice of grouping students based on academic ability remains controversial. Parents of above-average students often believe that their child's learning is hindered by heterogeneous classes and many teachers find teaching classes with students of similar abilities easier to manage. However, there is a growing body of evidence that tracking leads to few achievement benefits and several negative effects. Tracking too often creates inequities in access to learning, particularly for low-income, African American and Latino students (Oakes, 1992). Lower-track students tend to receive inferior educational opportunities—less-experienced (and often less-capable) teachers, lower expectations, fewer resources, less demanding topics, and a greater focus on rote drill and basic skills—that hinder their motivation, learning, and life chances.

SYNTHESIS

School-wide reform efforts are difficult to implement. An evaluation of federal dropout prevention programs found that even with adequate funds, most recipients of school restructuring grants did little actual restructuring. Schools found it easier to add services than to change teaching and learning. In those that did, reforms were fragile, and easily undone with changes in the local political environment or leadership (Dynarski & Gleason, 1999). Still, promising approaches to creating middle and high schools that better promote academic success in all students, particularly those at greatest risk of school failure, exist, most notably community schools.

Community schools combine academics with full services for children and families in the community. Some community schools, such as the Beacon schools in New York City and San Francisco or the Lighted School Houses sponsored by the Mott Foundation, are community centers located in public school buildings, offering a range of activities and services to community residents of all ages during the nonschool hours. Others, such as the Children's Aid Society schools or COZI schools seek to provide activities and resources for the whole community while also improving the quality of education during the school day.

In New York City, the Children's Aid Society formed a partnership with the Board of Education to operate two middle and two elementary schools that were truly responsive to the needs of the impoverished community of Washington Heights. The Salome Urena Middle Academy (IS218) suggests what community schools can offer. Located in a new building designed to be a community school, with air conditioning and an attractive setting, IS218 is open up to 15 hours a day, 6 days a week, all year round. The school offers medical, dental, and mental health services; recreation; educational enrichment; teen programs; adult activities; a family resource center with social services; and parent education. With a restructured school day, built around four self-contained academies (schools-within-schools), the school offers more than just traditional education approaches with community services brought in. The goal is to have a seamless program without clear boundaries between what happens during the school day and what happens after school. Early results from the ongoing evaluation suggest a positive impact: improvements in attendance, substantial reductions in problem behaviors, and small increases in test scores (Dryfoos, 1998).

Community schools appear to draw on the best practices in educational reform and community-based service provision to create a new relationship between at-risk students and their families and the school. The promise lies in their efforts to affect change in the different spheres impacting adolescents' lives. Whether or not they live up to their promise in improving adolescents academic success remains to be seen.

Directions for the Future

Research on the pathways of academic failure shows the influences from the different spheres of adolescents' lives. Some of these spheres, such as school and family, are well understood. Others, such as the role of peers, neighborhoods, and societal factors (e.g., employment opportunities) are less well understood. Greater attention to the role of these spheres, both by themselves as well as their interaction with adolescents' schools and families would expand our comprehension of academic success and failure. In addition, little research has focused on pathways to success, rather than pathways to failure, when investigating academic outcomes. We know what contributes to failure, but we need to know more about what contributes to success for adolescents. Furthermore, current studies and evaluations of students "at-risk" for school failure are not consistent in their definition of "at-risk". Typically, "at-risk" status is assumed based on students' demographic backgrounds, not their competencies.

Our efforts to promote adolescents' academic success are further hindered by the lack of quality research on the effectiveness of interventions to promote academic success. This paucity pertains to both the types of interventions available and the quality of evaluation efforts. For example, we need to know more about how different bundles or package of components, as well as their intensity, influence adolescents' academic attitudes and behaviors. Evaluations of efforts with planned (systematic) variations of components would help move the field forward. Thus, future research on academic success during adolescence should focus on developing a broader picture of how academic success, and not only failure, develops for different groups of youth. On the applied side, better designed evaluations of a diverse set of intervention efforts are needed.

Also see: Creativity: Adolescence; Family Strengthening: Adolescence; Identity Promotion: Adolescence; Life Skills: Adolescence; Peer Relationships: Adolescence; Risk-Taking: Adolescence; School Dropouts: Adolescence; Self-Esteem: Adolescence; Social Competency: Adolescence; Social and Emotional Learning: Adolescence; Social Inoculation.

ACKNOWLEDGMENTS

We would like to thank the Canadian Institute for Advanced Research and the Robert Wood Johnson Foundation for their support in writing this paper.

References

Allen, J.P., Philliber, S., Herrling, S., & Kuperminc, G.P. (1997). Preventing teen pregnancy and academic failure: Experimental evaluation of a developmentally based approach. *Child Development, 64,* 729–742.

Battin-Pearson, S., Newcomb, M.D., Abbott, R.D., Hill, K.G., Catalano, R.F., & Hawkins, J.D. (2000). Predictors of early high school dropout: A test of five theories. *Journal of Educational Psychology, 92,* 568–582.

Baydar, N., Brooks-Gunn, J., & Furstenberg, F.F. (1993). Early warning signs of functional illiteracy: Predictors in childhood and adolescence. *Child Development, 64,* 815–829.

Benson, P.L., Leffert, N., Scales, P.C., & Blyth, D.A. (1998). Beyond the "village" rhetoric: Creating healthy communities for children and adolescents. *Applied Developmental Science, 2,* 138–159.

Bronfenbrenner, U., & Morris, P.A. (1998). The ecology of developmental process. In R.M. Lerner (Ed.), *Handbook of child psychology: Vol. 1. Theoretical models of human development* (5th ed., pp. 993–1028). New York: Wiley.

Canadian Education Statistics Council. (2000). *Education indicators in Canada: Report of the pan-Canadian education indicators program, 1999 [on-line].* Available: www.statcan.ca/english/freepub/81-582-XIE

Carnegie Council on Adolescent Development. (1989). *Turning points: Preparing American youth for the 21st century.* Washington, DC: Carnegie Council on Adolescent Development.

Dryfoos, J.G. (1998). *Safe passage: Making it through adolescence in a risky society.* New York: Oxford University Press.

Dunifon, R., Duncan, G.J., & Brooks-Gunn, J. (2001). As ye sweep, so shall ye reap. *American Economic Review, 91,* 150–154.

Dynarski, M., & Gleason, P. (1999). *How can we help? Lessons from federal drop-out prevention programs.* Princeton, NJ: Mathematica Policy Research. Available: www.mathematica-mpr.com

Felner, R.D., Jackson, A.W., Kasak, D., Mulhall, P., Brand, S., & Flowers, N. (1997). The impact of school reform for the middle years: Longitudinal study of a network engaged in Turning Points-based comprehensive school transformation. *Phi Delta Kappan, 78,* 528–532.

Goldschmidt, P., & Wang, J. (1999). When can schools affect dropout behavior? A longitudinal multilevel analysis. *American Educational Research Journal, 36,* 715–738.

Hahn, A., Leavitt, T., & Aaron, P. (1994). *Evaluation of the Quantum Opportunities Program (QOP): Did the program work?* Waltham, MA: Center for Human Resources, Brandeis University.

Jackson, A.W., & Davis, G.A. (2000). *Turning points 2000: Educating adolescents in the 21st century.* New York: Teachers College Press.

Johnson, M.K., Beebe, T., Mortimer, J.T., & Snyder, M. (1998). Volunteerism in adolescence: A process perspective. *Journal of Research on Adolescence, 8,* 309–332.

Kemple, J.J., & Snipes, J.C. (2000). *Career academies: Impacts on students' engagement and performance in high school.* New York: Manpower Demonstration Research Corporation.

Lerner, R.M. (1991). Changing organism–context relations as the basic process of development: A developmental–contextual perspective. *Developmental Psychology, 27,* 27–32.

Lerner, R.M., Fisher, C.B., & Weinberg, R.A. (2000). Toward a science for and of the people: Promoting the civil society through the application of developmental science. *Child Development, 71,* 11–20.

Leventhal, T., & Brooks-Gunn, J. (2000). The neighborhoods they live in: The effects of neighborhood residence on child and adolescent outcomes. *Psychological Bulletin, 126,* 309–337.

Luthar, S.S., Cicchetti, D., & Becker, B. (2000). The construct of resilience: A critical evaluation and guidelines for future work. *Child Development, 71,* 543–562.

National Center for Education Statistics. (1999). *The condition of education* [on-line]. Available: www/nces.ed.gov/pubs99/condition99

Oakes, J. (1992). Can tracking research inform practice? Technical, normative, and political considerations. *Educational Researcher, 21*(4), 12–21.

Roeser, R.W., & Eccles, J.S. (1998). Adolescents' perceptions of middle school: Relation to longitudinal changes in academic and psychological adjustment. *Journal of Research on Adolescence, 8,* 123–158.

Rosenthal, B.S. (1998). Non-school correlates of dropout: An integrative review of the literature. *Children and Youth Services Reviews, 20,* 413–433.

Roth, J.L., & Brooks-Gunn, J. (2000). What do youth need for healthy development?: Implications for youth policy. *Society for Research on Child Development Social Policy Report, 14*(1). Available: www.srcd.org/sprv14n1.pdf

Roth, J., Brooks-Gunn, J., Murray, L., & Foster, W. (1998). Promoting healthy adolescents: Synthesis of youth development program evaluations. *Journal of Research on Adolescence, 8*(4), 423–459.

Rumberger, R.W. (1995). Dropping out of middle school: A multilevel analysis of students and schools. *American Educational Research Journal, 32,* 101–121.

Scales, P.C., Benson, P.L., Leffert, N., & Blyth, D.A. (2000). Contribution of developmental assets to the prediction of thriving among adolescents. *Applied Developmental Science, 4,* 27–46.

Sipe, C.L. (1999). Mentoring adolescents: What have we learned? In J.B. Grossman (Ed.), *Contemporary Issues in Mentoring* (pp. 10–23). Philadelphia, PA: Public/Private Ventures.

Stukas, A.A., Clary, E.G., & Snyder, M. (1999). Service learning: who benefits and why. *Society for Research in Child Development Social Policy Report, 13*(4), 1–19.

Tierney, J.P., Grossman, J.B., & Resch, W.N.L. (1995). *Making a difference: An impact study of Big Brothers Big Sisters.* Philadelphia, PA: Public/Private Ventures.

US Department of Education. (2000). *Working for children and families: Safe and smart after-school programs.* Washington, DC: US Department of Education and US Department of Justice.

Zill, N., Nord, C.W., & Loomis, L.S. (1995). *Adolescent time use, risky behavior, and outcomes: An analysis of national data.* Rockville, MC: Westat.

Accident, Motor Vehicle, Adulthood

Thomas E. Boyce and E. Scott Geller

INTRODUCTION

This entry provides a current account of the status of driving safety, including a critical analysis of preventive strategies that have been attempted, as well as those that may be forthcoming to prevent injuries and deaths from motor vehicle crashes. Key terms are defined, the problem is identified, popular theories are discussed, and key research results reviewed. Preventive strategies are described and integrated into a comprehensive model for large-scale application.

DEFINITIONS

Baseline is a period of observation during which no attempt is made to change a target behavior. It serves as a control for comparison with the period during which a prevention strategy targets one or more behaviors.

Control group refers to participants who are not exposed to the experimental variable or prevention strategy; a group that remains in baseline.

Correlation is the relationship between two variables which has a particular strength and direction (direct and positive or inverse and negative).

Demographics are characteristics of human populations; vital statistics such as gender, ethnicity, and socioeconomic status.

Reliability is the consistency of a measure, determined by taking repeated measures of the same target or by having two independent observers record information from the same source.

Risk refers to the exposure to a situation or condition that increases the probability of injury or death to one or more persons.

Sensation-seeking is a desire for stimulation through physiological arousal, presumed to vary reliably among people as a personality characteristic predictive of risk-taking behavior.

SCOPE

On average 114 Americans die each day in motor vehicle crashes. This amounts to one death every 13 minutes (National Highway Traffic Safety Administration [NHTSA], 2001). In 1999, for example, 41,611 fatalities and 3.23 million serious injuries occurred in the United States as the result of vehicle collisions. In fact, motor vehicle crashes are the single leading cause of death and injury to Americans and are estimated to cost the nation an excess of $150.5 billion per year (NHTSA, 2001). The problem is less dramatic, but still severe in Canada. Specifically, nearly 3000 Canadians lost their lives and another 217,614 were injured in 1998 (Transport Canada, 2001). This amounts to 1.6 deaths and 121 injuries per 10,000 registered vehicles. In both the United States and Canada, the majority of vehicle crashes occur among drivers 25–34 years of age.

Despite injuries and fatalities occurring in epidemic proportions as a result of vehicle travel, large-scale changes in only a few driving behaviors can make a big difference. For example, substantial decreases in vehicle crashes in the United States occurred concomitant with reductions in the national speed limit (Evans, 1991). In addition, it is estimated that safety-belt use saved 10,414 lives in 1996 and 90,425 lives since 1975 (NHTSA, 2001). In fact, it has been predicted that a 1 percent increase in the use of safety belts in the United States can save 200 lives per year (Nichols, 1998). Given this, it is alarming that nationwide belt use in the United States is only 68 percent (Nichols, 1998), and many drivers choose to drive in ways that put themselves and others at risk for vehicle crashes and serious injury.

THEORIES

Personality-Based Theories

Most vehicle crashes can be attributed to driver behavior (Evans, 1991). More than a decade ago, an international symposium on "The Social Psychology of Risky Driving" offered innovative presentations of a person–situation–behavior approach to understanding at-risk driving and vehicle crashes. Theoretical formulations and research findings that risky driving (e.g., nonuse of safety belts, speeding, and alcohol-impaired driving) are components of a generic *risky driving syndrome* (Jessor, 1987) were supported by data presented at this symposium (Beirness & Simpson, 1988; Donovan, Umlauf, & Salzberg, 1988; Wilson & Jonah, 1988).

For example, Donovan et al. (1988) identified two clusters of risky drivers—those characterized by impulsivity, *sensation-seeking* (Zuckerman, 1994), and aggressive acting-out behavior versus those showing high levels of emotional distress, resentment, and an external perception of control. A third cluster of drivers exhibited the highest level of aggressiveness, competitive speeding, and driving for tension reduction. In addition, Wilson and Jonah (1988) found that traffic violations on people's driving records correlated directly with measures of the drivers' thrill-seeking and aggression, and an environmental variable—peer support. The researchers also showed substantial negative (or inverse) correlations between peer support and self-reports of other problem behaviors, including drug use, preferred vehicle speed, safety-belt nonuse, driving while intoxicated (DWI), and charges for nonvehicular offenses.

Personality and demographic differences between drivers have also predicted the occurrence of safe versus risky driving behaviors. For example, Wilson (1990) demonstrated that nonusers of safety belts were higher sensation seekers, more impulsive, and accumulated more traffic violations than moderate and consistent users of safety belts. Nonusers of safety belts were also more likely to be males, younger, and less educated than users of safety belts.

Sensation-seeking has also been shown to correlate positively with self-reports of (a) DWI, (b) driving faster than 20 mph above the speed limit, (c) racing with another vehicle, and (d) illegally passing another vehicle (Arnett, 1996). As with drivers not using vehicle safety belts, these behaviors were reported more prevalently by males than females and by those who scored higher on the *sensation-seeking* dimension.

Behavior-Focused Theory

Evans (1991) provides another perspective on risk taking and vehicle crashes. He distinguishes between driving ability (skill) and driving behavior (or what the driver does). He defines risky driving as any behavior that increases task difficulty, which in turn increases the probability of a vehicle conflict and therefore a collision.

According to Evans (1991), vehicle crashes occur when the driver is: (a) at fault, (b) not legally at fault, but could have avoided involvement, or (c) unavoidably involved, as in an "act of God." Accordingly, not using a safety belt is not considered a risky driving behavior, because although it increases the probability of death or serious injury in a crash, it does not increase the probability of a crash.* From Evans' perspective, collisions only occur as a result of two or more vehicles trying to occupy the same space (Evans, 1991). This is also the essence of the *traffic conflict technique* (TCT) for categorizing traffic crashes (Glauz & Miglets, 1980).

The *TCT* approach to transportation safety is based, in part, on the need for proactive rather than reactive strategies to reduce the probability of vehicle crashes.* It is believed that conflicts or near crashes severe enough to warrant driver avoidance reactions are powerful indicators of crash potential. Specifically, it is presumed that the greater number of near crashes that occur, the greater the probability a crash will eventually occur. However, it is also acknowledged that these events may not occur with enough frequency to allow for reliable assessment and prediction. This is a major problem with using archival crash data as a primary measure of driving safety. As a result, it is necessary to move further "upstream" and study driving behaviors leading to near crashes. Put simply, if safe driving behaviors can be increased, the vehicle conflicts, crashes, and resultant injuries and deaths will decrease.

In accordance with the principles of *applied behavior analysis* (Baer, Wolf, & Risley, 1968), behavior-focused theory presumes that risky driving is a function of its consequences. Therefore, to increase safe driving among those who know what to do but do not, a behavior-based prevention strategy needs to be motivational. Motivational contingencies need to be more powerful (soon, certain, and significant) than any other prevention strategy currently in place to increase the safe behavior. Thus, it can be argued that the most common and large-scale instructional strategies, often manifested as education/training programs or public service announcements, are irrelevant for many people whose behaviors are at risk.

For most risky drivers, the consequences of avoiding a crash or a moving violation are not soon, or certain enough to motivate behavior change. In contrast, the consequences of

risky driving (e.g., speeding) are soon, certain, and relatively significant (e.g., getting to one's destination faster). Therefore, to be effective, prevention efforts need to provide consequences that are more soon, probable, and significant than those already in place. In addition, these consequences need to be provided directly for specific safety-related driving behaviors. Rewarding safe behaviors directly is extremely difficult. Thus, the popular large-scale approach to reducing risky driving is the enforcement of safe-driving laws.

RESEARCH

The Relationship between Risky Driving and Vehicle Crashes

Research in the last decade has shown that risky driving is predictive of involvement in fatal vehicle crashes. For example, in the first of two studies, Rajalin (1994) reported that licensed drivers who had been involved in a fatal vehicle crash were more likely to have been convicted of a driving offense in the three-year period preceding the fatality than a control group of randomly selected licensed drivers who had not been involved in a fatal crash. These drivers were also more often responsible for the crash than were the control subjects. Furthermore, Rajalin demonstrated that excessive speed and loss of control (or driver error) typically caused running-off-the-road crashes, while inattention and judgment errors caused intersection crashes. Therefore, running-off-the-road crashes in particular involved risky driving behaviors. Finally, the drivers involved in fatal crashes were younger and more likely male than were the control drivers.

In a second study, high-risk drivers—those stopped by the police for a violation—were observed and interviewed to obtain behavioral measures of driving (Rajalin, 1994, Study 2). Police in unmarked cars observed speeding, close vehicle following, crossing of no-passing lines, and lane deviations (too close to the centerline). Subjects were 143 drivers stopped for traffic offenses and 138 control subjects selected from the same traffic flow. Drivers stopped by police were typically cited for speeding.

Results indicated that almost three times more control subjects had no prior traffic offenses in the past three years than did the risky drivers. Also, drivers stopped for a violation were younger, drove newer cars, more likely drove sports cars, and drove greater distances each year. In fact, the records of the risky drivers resembled those of the drivers in the first study who were involved in fatal crashes (Rajalin, 1994).

Similar findings were reported by Hunter, Stewart, Stutts, and Rodgman (1993) who showed that among North Carolina residents ($n=5,074$), drivers observed not using their safety belts experienced 35 percent more vehicle incidents and

---

* Some have argued, however, that using a safety belt increases the probability of someone sitting properly behind the wheel of a car, and in some situations, sitting behind the wheel can facilitate crash avoidance.

69 percent more driving convictions (as indicated by court records and actual accident reports) than those observed to use their safety belts. Collectively, this research suggests that identifying risky behaviors leading to critical incidents and then implementing strategies to reduce their occurrence could significantly decrease the number of traffic crashes and fatalities.

In-Vehicle Information Systems (IVIS)

To address the issue of predicting risk for a crash by observing driving behavior, recent research has investigated the viability of an *IVIS* to aid drivers in decision making during driving (Dingus et al., 1995; Janssen, 1994). The focus of this research has been to study the effects of collision avoidance warning, in-vehicle signing and warning displays, and routing and navigation systems on safe driving behaviors.

Boyce and Geller (2001a,b) studied how the *IVIS* technology could be used to unobtrusively assess on-going driver behavior at an individual level of analysis. An *IVIS* can record several driving behaviors at the same time, making it possible to study relationships among multiple driving behaviors. Some of these relationships could be informative with regard to understanding the *risky driving syndrome* and the development of more effective ways to improve driving safety.

The *IVIS* evaluated by Boyce and Geller (2001a) was termed a "Smart Car." The Smart Car is an instrumented vehicle capable of video recording and measuring on-going driving performance without a driver's knowledge. Computer-generated driving measures, in concert with real-time video recordings of the participants' driving, allow for unprecedented opportunities to perform a *behavior analysis* of driving performance in the context of normal traffic. Such methodology minimizes or avoids completely the problems related to the veracity of self-reports and driver reactivity to in-vehicle observers.

Boyce and Geller (2001a) developed and tested two approaches toward using the Smart Car to study on-going driving behaviors: (a) a time sampling or interval approach, and (b) a critical event approach. A primary purpose of that research was to define at-risk driving performance from electronic records of a Smart Car and to derive a methodology for reliable data coding from videotapes of multiple on-going driving behaviors. As expected, age was negatively related to risky driving. However, contrary to previous research, gender differences were not found. Interestingly, speeding, close vehicle following, and time spent performing behaviors unrelated to driving correlated significantly with one another. The failure to obtain gender differences may be an artifact of the reliance of previous research on self-reported measures of driving behavior (Boyce & Geller, 2001b).

The power of the technology described by Boyce and Geller (2001a) was demonstrated by its sensitivity to variability in driving safety. Specifically, behavioral variability decreased as participants got older. The authors argued that risky driving behaviors are "selected out" of a participant's repertoire over time, or that the participants themselves are "selected out" because of their risky driving. As such, the reduced variability among driving behaviors in older drivers may be a powerful real-world example of *selection by consequences* in a natural setting (Skinner, 1938). Knowledge that driving behavior may be a function of its consequences will aid in the development of effective strategies to improve driving and reduce the occurrence of vehicle crashes.

STRATEGIES THAT WORK

Community-Based Behavioral Science

Cost-effective injury prevention strategies are urgently needed in schools, industries, and throughout communities to reduce vehicle crashes and resultant injuries and fatalities. Over the past 30 years, applications of *behavior analysis* principles and procedures have been used often and successfully in community settings to develop primary prevention programs. An analysis of the environmental antecedents and consequences of behavior can enhance understanding of injury-causing behaviors and guide the development of an effective behavior-change process (Geller, 1998; Sleet, Hollenbach, & Hovell, 1986).

For example, behavior-based safety processes have successfully used: (a) participative education to increase the use of vehicle safety belts (Cope, Smith, & Grossnickle, 1986; Weinstein, Grubb, & Vautier, 1986), (b) behavioral feedback to decrease the frequency of traffic crashes (Evans, 1991), reduce driving speed (Van Houten & Nau, 1983) and increase safety-belt use (Grant, 1990), (c) pledge-card commitment to increase safety-belt use (Geller & Lehman, 1991), and (d) incentives/rewards to increase the use of safety belts (Campbell, Hunter, & Stutts, 1984; Roberts, Fanurik, & Wilson, 1988) and child safety seats (Roberts & Fanurik, 1986).

Ludwig & Geller (2000) observed certain safety-related behaviors of the delivery drivers for three pizza stores before, during, and after a goal-setting and feedback process was implemented at two stores. After baseline observations, employees at one store participated in an interactive discussion of driving safety and afterwards set a group goal for complete stops at intersections. One week later, the employees at a second store received a lecture on driving safety and were assigned a group goal for complete stops at intersections. The goal for participants at this site was the same as that set by the participants at the first site. A third site served as a no-treatment control. For four weeks following the participative goal setting at one site and assigned goals at the other, graphs were posted in the stores that tracked the daily percentages of employees making complete stops. This was considered group feedback.

At each of the stores receiving a prevention strategy, the percentage of complete stops at intersections increased significantly from baseline to intervention. Furthermore, turn-signal and safety-belt use (behaviors observed, but not targeted by the intervention) increased significantly at the store which received participative goal setting, but not at the store whose behavioral goal for complete stops had been assigned. None of the safety-related behaviors changed among the pizza deliverers at the control site.

This research demonstrated the relevance of transfer of training for transportation safety, suggesting that evaluation of behavior-based prevention strategies should measure changes in more than the target behaviors, and the type of prevention strategy can determine whether the beneficial effect of the strategy spreads to other behaviors. In the Ludwig and Geller evaluations, beneficial generalization of treatment was only found when the prevention program promoted interpersonal participation and employee empowerment, not when it was presented in a top-down format with minimal employee involvement.

STRATEGIES THAT MIGHT WORK

Behavior-Based Self-Management

Self-management (Watson & Tharp, 1997) is an improvement process whereby individuals use behavior-based prevention strategies to improve their own behavior. Specifically, individuals learn how to: (a) manipulate behavioral antecedents and consequences, (b) observe and record specific target behaviors, and (c) self-administer rewards for personal achievement. The practical benefits of self-management processes have been demonstrated in numerous clinical settings, including the reduction of alcohol consumption (Sobell & Sobell, 1995), weight control (Baker & Kirschenbaum, 1993), and smoking cessation (Curry, 1993; Shiffman, 1984).

Geller and Clarke (1999) investigated the viability of safety self-management as a strategy for increasing the safe-driving of short-haul truck drivers. Specifically, 12 male drivers from Site A (self-management) and 11 male drivers from Site B (control) were randomly selected to participate. During the week prior to implementing the self-management process, trained research assistants observed the driving behaviors of participants while riding in the passenger seat of the delivery truck. All employees at Site A ($n = 30$) were then asked to complete a self-observation checklist each day for a two-week period.

While on their sales routes, drivers recorded their specific driving behaviors. Self-observation forms were collected and graphed on a daily basis. A percent safe score was calculated for each participant's driving behaviors. These graphs were posted in a break room where employees gathered each day before and after their routes. Results indicated that overall safety did not improve in the control group (from 71.5 to 75.4 percent). In contrast, there was a significant increase in the overall safety among drivers in the self-management group (from 66.8 percent safe driving during baseline to 87.8 percent after self-management).

Overall, these results indicate that safety self-management can be an effective approach for increasing safe driving among professional drivers. While these findings are encouraging, further research is needed. It is noteworthy that the self-management process was effective despite some inaccuracy of self-observations recorded by the drivers. The inaccurate reporting of behavioral measures was presumed to result from participant reactivity to the prevention strategy. The technology developed by Boyce and Geller (2001a) could prevent measurement error due to participant reactivity.

STRATEGIES THAT DO NOT WORK

Drivers' Education

According to DePasquale and Geller (2001), it is assumed that students who participate in a drivers' education course will increase their safe driving behavior. However, data are not available to verify this assumption, partly because the primary dependent variables in such research are traffic violations and crash occurrences. As mentioned above, traffic crashes and violations are relatively rare events that do not lend themselves to a sensitive analysis.

Research does suggest that driver education programs may reduce violations of traffic laws, but there appears to be no significant relationship between driver education and subsequent crash records (Lund, Williams, & Zador, 1986). In fact, driver education programs may have the effect of licensing drivers at an earlier age. And, younger drivers are more at risk for experiencing vehicle crashes (Levy, 1990).

Without knowing whether students increase their performance of safe driving behaviors as a result of a driver education course, it is presumptuous to expect subsequent reductions in crash frequency (DePasquale & Geller, 2001). The likely effect of driver education courses is simply to increase a new driver's knowledge and confidence before they have sufficient physical maturity, skill, and judgment to drive defensively (Evans, 1991). Thus, it is likely that driver education fails to influence driving behavior in ways that increase skill and develop good judgment.

SYNTHESIS

Integrating Theory and Prevention Perspectives

Over two decades of behavior change research at corporate and community sites led to the development of the *multiple intervention level* (MIL) hierarchy depicted in Figure 1. This model is used to categorize behavior change approaches and evaluate the cost-effectiveness of successive prevention strategies to alter the behavioral patterns of large numbers of individuals (Geller, 1998).

An MIL approach to public health has critical implications for evaluating the cost-effectiveness of a behavior-based safety program to improve driving. Behavior-based safe driving programs generally involve the manipulation of behavioral antecedents and/or consequences. According to the MIL model, antecedent strategies such as education, training, policy, written prompts, and assigned goals are lower level prevention strategies reaching large numbers of people. Laws or disincentive/penalty programs, which threaten a negative consequence, are more intrusive when enforced and therefore are considered higher-level prevention strategies, reaching fewer people. More positive approaches such as individual feedback and incentive/reward programs are considered to be at the same level as disincentive/penalty programs.

More intrusive and individual-focused prevention strategies are needed for those not influenced by strategies designed to reach large numbers of people (e.g., fear appeals, policies, and public service announcements). More effective, higher-level prevention strategies are more labor intensive and therefore require people to become "change agents." That is, people already influenced by less-intrusive prevention strategies need to be trained and motivated to become change agents for the development and delivery of more intrusive strategies.

Boyce and Geller (1999) tested the utility of the MIL model as a heuristic to guide the design of large-scale

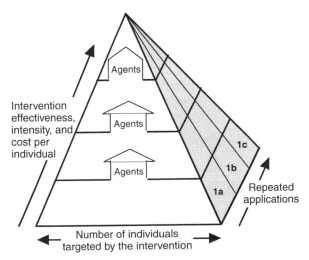

Figure 1. The Multiple Intervention Level Hierarchy.

behavior-change strategies by systematically implementing a series of prevention tactics over the course of two years in an attempt to increase safety-belt use among workers at a large industrial site. The strategies included: (a) written prompts, (b) a safety slogan contest and celebration, (c) assigned goals, (d) assigned goals plus feedback, (e) a voluntary promise card, and (f) a promise card plus rewards. Results indicated that safety-belt use remained relatively unchanged throughout the two-year study. Only a promise card plus reward process was successful at significantly increasing safety-belt use beyond the relatively high baseline (52 percent), presumably attained with the state belt-use law (BUL).

Overall, these data supported the MIL hierarchy (Geller, 1998). That is, one could argue that the antecedent strategies used to motivate safety-belt use were all first-level prevention strategies, no more powerful than the BUL in effect at the time of the study. The model predicts that the hard-core resisters, not influenced by the BUL, would not be influenced by repeated applications of lower-level strategies.

Fifteen years earlier, Geller, Davis, and Spicer (1983) implemented an incentive/reward process at the same industrial site, and increased safety-belt use from 17.4 to 50.6 percent among salary workers, and from 3.4 to 5.5 percent among hourly workers. As there was no BUL in 1982, the incentive/reward approach was enough to produce some desired behavior change. The baseline level of 52 percent belt use in Boyce and Geller (1999) was only slightly higher than the posttreatment levels obtained in 1982 among salary employees. This suggests that those workers not motivated to avoid the improbable fine of $25 were not likely to buckle up for the remote probability of winning a raffle drawing, the incentive/reward used by Boyce and Geller (1999). As predicted by the MIL hierarchy, these individuals apparently needed a more intrusive and intensive prevention strategy to motivate them to change.

The usefulness of the MIL model to predict behavior change can be interpreted in terms of potential for improvement (Gilbert, 1978). Specifically, it is presumed that behaviors occurring at lower rates have a greater potential for improvement and thus are more easily influenced. Therefore, low baseline rate behaviors may be influenced by lower level prevention efforts. That is, to get a 10 percentage point increase in the rate of a target behavior from 30 to 40 percent is easier than to get that same 10 percentage point increase from 70 to 80 percent. In other words, the 10 point change from 30 to 40 percent is a smaller proportion of the potential for improvement (14 percent of 70 available percentage points) than the same percentage point change from 70 to 80 percent (33 percent of a 30 percentage point potential for improvement). As a result, the former change should be easier to obtain than the latter.

It has been readily acknowledged in the behavioral science literature that the last few percentage points are the most difficult to reach. This is likely due to the failure of lower level prevention strategies to affect people who are still resisting behavior change at this point. Consistent with the MIL model, more intrusive prevention efforts are needed to affect these "hard-core resistors." Such a phenomenon may also help to explain the differential results obtained by Geller et al. (1983) versus Boyce and Geller (1999) in their efforts to increase safety-belt use at the same industrial site. In addition, it is becoming clear that the application of more intrusive prevention programs requires that change agents be trained and motivated to assist with the implementation of these behavior-change strategies. This defines a key challenge for subsequent psychological research and development in the critical domain of transportation safety.

Psychology has contributed significantly to identifying and improving the behavioral aspects of safe versus at-risk travel. But we've only cracked the tip of the "iceberg." Much more primary prevention research remains to be done in this domain. This entry summarized what we know at this point to develop large-scale prevention programs, and provided direction for critical follow-up research. But, there is substantial potential for improvement. It is hoped this realization will motivate more behavioral scientists to focus their research and prevention efforts on the serious public health problem of injury and death from vehicle crashes.

Also see: Injuries, Unintentional: Adolescence; Suicide: Adulthood.

References

Arnett, J.J. (1996). Sensation seeking, aggressiveness, and adolescent reckless behavior. *Personality and Individual Differences, 20,* 693–702.

Baker, R.C., & Kirschenbaum, D.S. (1993). Self-monitoring may be necessary for successful weight control. *Behavior Therapy, 24,* 377–394.

Beirness, D.J., & Simpson, H.M. (1988). Lifestyle correlates of risky driving and accident involvement among youth. *Alcohol Drugs, and Driving, 4*(3–4), 193–204.

Boyce, T.E., & Geller, E.S. (1999). Attempts to increase vehicle safety-belt use among industry workers: What can we learn from our failures? *Journal of Organizational Behavior Management, 19,* 27–44.

Boyce, T.E., & Geller, E.S. (2001). A behavior-based technology to measure driving safety with self-report or participant reactivity. *Journal of Applied Behavior Analysis, 34,* 39–53.

Boyce, T.E., & Geller, E.S. (2002). An instrumented vehicle assessment of problem behavior and driving style: Do young males take the most risks? *Accident Analysis and Prevention, 34,* 51–64

Campbell, R.J., Hunter, W.W., & Stutts, J.C. (1984). The use of economic incentives and education to modify safety-belt use behavior of high school students. *Health Education, 15,* 30–33.

Cope, J.G., Smith, G.A., & Grossnickle, W.F. (1986). The effect of variable-rate cash incentives on safety belt use. *Journal of Safety Research, 17,* 95–99.

Curry, S. (1993). Self-help interventions for smoking cessation. *Journal of Consulting and Clinical Psychology, 16,* 790–803.

DePasquale, J.P., & Geller, E.S. (2001). Intervening to improve driving instruction: Should behavioral feedback be delivered before or after a training session? *International Journal of Behavioural Safety, 1,* 1–14.

Dingus, T.A., McGhee, D.V., Hulse, M.C., Jahns, S., Manakkal, N., Mollenhauer, M.A., & Fleishman, R. (1995). *TravTek Evaluation Task C#—Camera Car Evaluation of the TravTek System.* Washington, DC: Federal Highway Administration, US Department of Transportation.

Donovan, D.M., Umlauf, R.L., & Salzberg, P.M. (1988). Derivation of personality subtypes among high-risk drivers. *Alcohol, Drugs, and Driving, 4*(3–4), 233–244.

Evans, L. (1991). *Traffic safety and the driver.* New York: Van Nostrand Reinhold.

Geller, E.S. (1998). *Applications of behavior analysis to prevent injuries from vehicle crashes* (2nd ed.). Cambridge, MA: Cambridge Center for Behavioral Studies.

Geller, E.S., & Clarke, S.W. (1999). Safety self-management: A key behavior-based process for injury prevention. *Professional Safety, 44*(7), 29–33.

Geller, E.S., Davis, L., & Spicer, K. (1983). Industry-based incentives for promoting seat-belt use: Differential impact on white-collar versus blue-collar employees. *Journal of Organizational Behavior Management, 5,* 17–29.

Geller, E.S., & Lehman, G.R. (1991). The buckle-up promise card: A versatile intervention for large-scale behavior change. *Journal of Applied Behavior Analysis, 24,* 91–94.

Gilbert, T.F. (1978). *Human competence: Engineering worthy performance.* New York: McGraw Hill.

Glauz, W.D., & Miglets, D.J. (1980). Application of traffic conflict analysis at intersections. *Transportation Research Board, 219,* 1–26.

Grant, B.A. (1990). Effectiveness of feedback and education in an employment-based seat belt program. *Health Education Research, 5*(2), 2–10.

Hunter, W.W., Stewart, J.R., Stutts, J.C., & Rodgman, E.A. (1993). Observed and self-reported seat belt wearing as related to prior traffic accidents and convictions. *Accident Analysis and Prevention, 25*(5), 545–554.

Janssen, W. (1994). Seat-belt wearing and driving behavior: An instrumented-vehicle study. *Accident Analysis and Prevention, 26,* 249–261.

Jessor, R. (1987). Risky driving and adolescent problem behavior: An extension of problem-behavior theory. *Alcohol, Drugs, and Driving, 3*(3–4), 1–11.

Levy, D.T. (1990). Youth and traffic safety: The effects of driving age, experience, and education. *Accident Analysis and Prevention, 22,* 327–334.

Ludwig, T.D., & Geller, E.S. (2000). Intervening to improve the safety of occupational driving: A behavior-change model and review of empirical evidence. *Journal of Organizational Behavior Management,* Special Issue, *19*(4), 1–124.

Lund, A.K., Williams, A.F., & Zador, P. (1986). High school driver education: Further evaluation of the DeKalb county study. *Accident Analysis and Prevention, 18,* 349–357.

National Highway Traffic Safety Administration (2001). *NHTSA Homepage* [On-line]. Available: www.nhtsa.gov

Nichols, J. (1998, May). *New opportunities: Can behavior analysis help with traffic safety?* Panel discussion at the 24th Annual Convention of the Association for Behavior Analysis, Orlando, FL.

Rajalin, S. (1994). The connection between risky driving and involvement in fatal accidents. *Accident Analysis and Prevention, 26*(5), 555–562.

Roberts, M.C., & Fanurik, D. (1986). Rewarding elementary school children for their use of safety-belts. *Health Psychology, 5,* 185–196.

Roberts, M.C., Fanurik, D., & Wilson, D. (1988). A community program to reward children's use of seat belts. *American Journal of Community Psychology, 16,* 395–407.

Shiffman, S. (1984). Coping with temptations to smoke. *Journal of Consulting and Clinical Psychology, 52,* 261–267.

Skinner, B.F. (1938). *The behavior of organisms*. Acton, MA: Copley.

Sleet, D.A., Hollenbach, K., & Hovell, M. (1986). Applying behavioral principles to motor vehicle occupant protection. *Education in Treating Children, 9*, 320–333.

Sobell, L.S., & Sobell, M.B. (1995). *Guided self-change case study: Lisa*. Toronto, Canada: Addiction Research Council.

Transport Canada (2001). Collision Statistics [On-line]. Available: www.tc.gc.ta/roadsafety/STATS

Van Houten, R., & Nau, P.A. (1983). Feedback interventions and driving speed: A parametric and comparative analysis. *Journal of Applied Behavior Analysis, 16*, 253–281.

Watson, D.L., & Tharp, R.G. (1997). *Self-directed behavior: Self-modification for personal adjustment* (7th ed.). Pacific Grove, CA: Brooks/Cole.

Weinstein, N.D., Grubb, P.D., & Vautier, J.S. (1986). Increasing seat belt use: An intervention emphasizing risk susceptibility. *Journal of Applied Psychology, 71*(2), 285–290.

Wilson, R.J. (1990). The relationship between seat belt non-use to personality, lifestyle and driving record. *Health Education Research: Theory and Practice, 5*(2), 175–185.

Wilson, R.J., & Jonah, B.A. (1988). The application of problem-behavior theory to the understanding of risky driving. *Alcohol, Drugs, and Driving, 4*(3–4), 181–192.

Zuckerman, M. (1994). *Behavioral expressions and biosocial bases of sensation seeking*. New York: Cambridge University Press.

Adoption, Childhood

Doreen Arcus and Theresa Milewski

INTRODUCTION

Children between the ages of 6 and 12 years living in adoptive families are a heterogeneous group. They include children adopted as infants in both open and closed arrangements as well as children adopted at later ages whose early years may have been marked by trauma or neglect and who may have had multiple placements along the way. Children may live in families with siblings who may or may not be related by biology. Race and ethnicity may vary across family members. Although adoption itself may be a protective factor for these children, considering the alternatives, it does carry challenges for children and families.

DEFINITIONS

Adoption means different things to different people. For some it is a legal transaction, the act of assuming legal responsibility for a minor child not born to them, and for others it is a lifelong process. Adoptions may be *public* through public or private child welfare agencies, *private* through businesses designed to arrange adoptions either domestically or internationally, or *independent* in which the birth parents typically are involved in selecting adoptive parents.

Adoptions vary in the degree to which they are *open* or *closed*. There may be minimal information about the birth parents (a relatively closed adoption), knowledge but not ongoing contact (semiopen, as in the older child, removed for protective reasons), or a full, ongoing relationship between all parties (open).

Adoptions of older children are often termed *special-needs adoptions*. This designation is used for cases that are, statistically speaking, more difficult to place due to older age, medical disabilities, minority group status, presence of a sibling group to be preserved, and certain physical, mental, or emotional needs. The use of the term *special-needs* to describe an adoption is sometimes confusing since the child need not have any special educational needs (e.g., learning or developmental disabilities) for the adoption to be so designated.

Not all adoptions last forever. *Disruption* is a failure of the relationship before it is legally finalized. *Dissolution* is a failure of the relationship after finalization. Disruption rates are estimated at 10–15 percent for children adopted at older ages, many of whom go on to subsequent successful placements (Rosenthal, 1993).

SCOPE

Complete data on the numbers of children living in adoptive families are not available; however, the numbers of children arriving for international adoptions and of children adopted through public agencies provide some indication of adoption prevalence.

Between 1990 and 1996, nearly 60,000 children from over 30 countries immigrated to the United States as orphans to be adopted, most of whom were adopted as infants or during early childhood. The largest number of children each year from 1950–1995 have come from Korea, except in 1991 when many western nations received an influx of children from Romanian orphanages, a cohort whose early institutional experiences were marked by extreme neglect. China and Russia have accounted for the greatest number of children since 1995 (US Department of State, 2000).

Adoptions through public agencies typically occur when biological parents are unable to care for their children and surrender their rights voluntarily, or when their parental rights are terminated by court action following histories of abuse and/or neglect. The median age of the 36,000 children adopted from the US public foster care system in 1998 was 6 years, 3 months. Nearly half (46 percent) of these children were Black, 38 percent White, and 13 percent Latino. They waited an average of 13 months for their adoptions following termination of parental rights, and 85 percent were adopted by nonrelatives, primarily married couples (66 percent) and single females (31 percent). Another 117,000 children with an average age of 8 years waited for adoption in 1998 and had been waiting an average of nearly 4 years in foster care (US Department of Health and Human Services, 2000).

Most families adopting children through public agencies receive ongoing subsidies for the care of those children, as did 86 percent of these families in 1998. The lifetime financial value of this societal investment to an 8-year-old who would otherwise remain in the public system has been estimated at more than six times the cost of long-term foster care (Rosenthal, 1993).

The contention that children who are adopted are at increased risk for adjustment or mental health problems is supported by the literature with important caveats. Brodzinsky and his colleagues were among the first to point out that, although school-aged children who had been adopted received higher ratings for psychological and school-related behavior problems and lower ratings for social competence and school achievement than a comparison group of nonadopted children, most of these children scored *in the normal range* on the rating instruments (Brodzinsky, Schecter, Braff, & Singer, 1984). More recently, Miller and colleagues analyzed a nationally representative school survey and found that 10–13-year-old adopted children showed moderately increased risk for substance use, skipping school, emotional distress, diminished hope for the future, health and physical problems, fighting, and lying to parents compared to nonadopted children, especially boys. Further analyses revealed that, although adopted children were more at risk they were markedly overrepresented in the extremes of the distributions; that is, among those children who did evidence problems in these areas, a much higher proportion of the adopted youth were among those with the most severe problems (Miller, Fan, Grotevant, Christensen, Coyl, & van Dulman, 2000).

Because of the multiplicity of paths by which school-aged children have come to adoption, the preplacement experiences of the child must be considered in examining the scope of the problems for which these children are at risk. Early risk factors, for example, have been found to be unrelated to children's socioemotional outcomes four to twelve years following the adoption among a low-risk—not transracial, international, or special needs—sample (Grotevant, Ross, Marchel, & McRoy, 1999). However, known or suspected histories of sexual abuse and physical abuse were present in 50 and 75 percent, respectively, of a sample of special-needs adoptees studied by Groze (1996). Even compared to other children whose adoptions were classified as special needs but who did not have a history of

abuse, higher proportions of abused children scored in the clinical range for internalizing and externalizing disorders, and engaged in less secure attachments to parents and family by parental report. These findings are supported by observations of children in foster care, among whom 60 percent of those who had been sexually abused displayed posttraumatic stress syndrome, with more severe cases among the 8–12-year-olds than among adolescents (Dubner & Motta, 1999). Unfortunately, although these data clearly demonstrate their importance, information about preplacement care and the experience of the child frequently is not available for, or included in, adoption studies.

THEORIES AND RESEARCH

Ecological Perspective

Strategies for promoting the healthy development of children in adoptive families during the school years (i.e., middle childhood) are informed by several theoretical perspectives. The broadest of these, an ecological view of human development, was developed by Bronfenbrenner (1979). This view places the developing child at the center of an active ecology comprised of nesting and interacting systems involving the child to more and less direct degrees. Influence is bidirectional—the child may influence the system as well as may be influenced by the system. Ecological transitions, that is, changes in any of the systems, are likely to be accompanied by changes in the child. As in the related family systems perspective, the focus is on interactive and interdependent contexts.

Arcus and McCartney (1989), for example, found more change in children's social behavior over a 14-month period among those whose family constellation changed with the addition of a younger sibling compared to those whose family structure had remained stable. Similar dynamics likely characterize families who adopt, although sibling adjustment has been understudied. When surveyed, foster parents indicated concern about the effects of foster placements on their biological children and the need for services to assist their children in coping (Poland & Groze, 1993), and it is likely that such concerns arise in adoptions of children from foster care as well.

Resources of the family and neighborhood may also be important considerations in adoption outcomes. Children with low IQ scores (one standard deviation or more below the mean) who were adopted between 4 and 6 years and who had histories of early abuse showed significantly elevated IQ scores (98 on average) when their adoptive families were in high socioeconomic strata (SES) compared to those living in lower SES (Duyme, Dumaret, & Tomkiewicz, 1999).

Finally, prevailing cultural views of adoption are relevant factors in the lives of children living in adoptive families, particularly as school-aged children grow in appreciation of their place in the larger social world. These views are reflected in surveys that find both support and skepticism about adoption across the general public, and newspaper articles, which cover negative over positive adoption outcomes by a 2 : 1 ratio (Freundlich, 1998; Waggenspack, 1998).

Attachment Perspective

A second important theoretical position relative to the development of children in adoptive families is attachment theory that holds that secure attachments between children and caregivers—especially in the early years—provide the basis for exploration of the world and healthy development (Bowlby, 1988). Clearly, attachments and losses are at the heart of the adopted child's experience, as well as the experience of other members of the adoptive family relative to the adoption and the circumstances that led to adopting in the first place (e.g., infertility). Adopted children are not likely to have had uninterrupted and positive relationships from the earliest days forward, and there is evidence that their subsequent social relationships are at risk. Attachment theory is a stage theory, that is, one that holds that successful development of later stages is dependent upon successful development in earlier ones. The invariant sequence of stages is key, rather than the absolute age at which they occur. Therefore, attachment theory, while it predicts difficulties for children who have not established secure and lasting attachments at an early age, does not predict doom. It is possible, although it may be more difficult, for primary attachments and subsequent positive relationships to develop at later ages or following traumatic loss.

Children adopted as infants have been found to be as likely to form secure attachments to their adoptive parents as biological children to their biological parents (Singer, Brodzinsky, Ramsay, Steir, & Waters, 1985). Even in a sample of children adopted in "special needs" circumstances, parents reported positive attachments to their children as evidenced in levels of trust, communication, respect, positive relations, and feelings of closeness. However, children adopted at later ages whose early years were marked by abuse, either physical or sexual, or both, evidenced substantial difficulties in attachment across all indices except for communication as indicated by their parents (Groze, 1996).

Clinical studies have characterized reactive attachment disorders of childhood as stemming from early negative reciprocal interactions (Levy & Orlans, 1998). When a child's needs are neglected or met harshly or abusively, the child learns to respond to a negative system and establishes angry, coercive patterns of interaction with others. Even

after the abusive relationship is terminated, and the child is moved to a nurturing, adoptive placement, behavior patterns that served important purposes during the child's early years may not disappear. New and complicated patterns can emerge from this insecure foundation. These patterns, while resistant to change, are not intractable and may respond to intervention designed to revisit the original trauma, revise the current patterns through establishing and modifying behaviors, and revitalize the child and family relationship to one of trust and respect (Bowlby, 1988; Terr, 1990).

Cognitive Perspective

Cognitive theories frame development in the middle childhood period by the child's cognitive competencies and information processing abilities. Memory storage and retrieval systems no longer depend on sensory experience but verbal mediation. Children from about 6 to 12 years are in Piaget's (1964) concrete operational stage of development. They can consider two aspects of a problem simultaneously, and are less egocentric and more logical, reflective, and analytic than in earlier stages. Thus, the adopted child begins to understand that being "chosen" by one set of parents means being "given up" by another and begins to conceive of the complexities of adoption and understand its inherent losses.

Research has shown that when adjustment problems are manifested by adoptees, they tend not to occur until around school age. Adopted infants and toddlers generally do not differ from nonadopted children but greater risks for problems such as aggression or depression emerge as the cognitive capacities of the 5–7-year-old child permit an understanding of the salience and implications of being adopted (Brodzinsky, 1993). In fact, by age 8 adopted children tend to develop considerable ambivalence about having been adopted (Singer, Brodzinsky, & Braff, 1982).

Biological Perspective

Biological contributions to the adopted child's development include genetic influences that reflect the family of origin. Genetically influenced traits, such as temperament or learning styles or disabilities may emerge during middle childhood with the social and academic demands of formal education. Attention deficit disorder, which is more prevalent among adopted than nonadopted children (Deutsch, Swanson, & Bruell, 1982), may complicate school performance, homework times, or participation in organized athletics.

Temperament research suggests that goodness of fit is an important concept in blending children and families, and it is likely that poor fit, rather than deficits in child or family per se, underlies many disrupted adoptions.

Children placed for adoption during middle childhood are more likely to have disrupted placements compared to children placed during the preschool years (Rosenthal, 1993). However, the presence of aggressive, hyperactive, or antisocial child behavior, a college-educated adoptive mother, and adoption by other than foster parents are risk factors as well (Barth & Berry, 1990). This combination of factors suggests that unrealistic expectations and the resultant poor fit may make a major contribution to the risk of disruption, and is consistent with the recent finding that people without personal knowledge of children in foster care may have "too high expectations" for them (Milewski, 2000).

Research has further shown that the link from genetic risk to observable behavior may be neither direct nor inevitable. Although numerous behavior genetic studies have suggested a substantial genetic effect on IQ and other indices of intelligence, adoption studies may overestimate that influence due to the restricted range in the profiles of adoptive parents compared to the general population (Stoolmiller, 1999).

Research examining genetic and environmental influences in social and emotional behavior indicates that genes and environments work together. O'Connor, Deater-Deckard, Fulker, Rutter, & Plomin (1998) observed two groups of adopted children from ages 7 to 12 years who varied in genetic risk for antisocial behavior based on their biological mother's history; their adoptive parents reported on the types of control and parenting they used to direct their children's behavior. The adoptive parents of children at genetic risk were more likely to use negative and coercive parenting practices than parents of low-risk children. In other words, the behavior of the child appeared to evoke responses from the parent that contributed to the child's externalizing behavior, although the evocative correlation did not explain all of the environmental effect. A review of 21 genetic studies further characterized the genes–behavior relation as mediated by environmental events, leading to the conclusion that a small number of adopted children appear to develop behavior problems when genetic predispositions are activated by environmental conditions (Peters, Atkins, & McKay, 1999).

STRATEGIES: OVERVIEW

Understanding what lies ahead for school-aged children is a key consideration in fostering their healthy development. Adequate preparation for the maturational changes of puberty and adolescence is particularly relevant for children in adoptive families. The emergence of sexual maturity brings up issues of reproduction and responsibility and provides the child a new perspective from which to consider his

or her birth parents and their inability to parent the child they produced. The development of formal operations and enhanced cognitive skills further permit the child to consider the entire logical system in which problems are embedded. Children who are adopted may begin to question the foundations of their life story as did this 13-year-old boy, "My life is very confusing to me. I have a lot of questions, like if they weren't ready to be parents, why did they decide to have kids in the first place?" Social development and the establishment of identity require that the adolescent integrate disparate sources of identity from his or her beginnings to the present. In anticipation of these developmental challenges, the middle childhood period can be used to gather information, normalize the process of adoption for creating families, and nurture the lines of communication.

STRATEGIES THAT WORK

Rosenthal (1993) suggests that strategies which *enhance flexibility* and *reduce rigidity* in adoptive families are likely to be associated with reduced risk for disruption, hence, more positive outcomes. Likewise, adequate *support* for adoptive families, particularly those adopting older children, has been associated with stability of the placement, and low levels of support with disruption (Rosenthal, 1993). In a cohort of special-needs adoptive families, Groze (1996) found significant relations between the degree of emotional support parents reported from their social networks and more positive outcomes, communication, and feelings of closeness to the child and each other.

Forty adoptive families were surveyed about the types of supports that were useful to them. They identified a variety of formal and informal sources, including access to family resource specialists and experienced adoptive parents, financial assistance, childcare, and respite care. Based on these parental suggestions, social and community service agencies should attempt to: (1) encourage potential adoptive parents to seek support and assistance from family members and other friends and associates, (2) encourage others to maintain support beyond the initial adoption period, (3) disseminate information about the availability of experienced adoptive parents and family resource specialists as well as increase the availability of such resources, (4) refer families to existing support groups, (5) facilitate the formation of new support groups for targeted needs, and (6) provide ongoing opportunities for families to learn about resources in the community (Kramer & Houston, 1998).

However, further research is needed to provide more information about the specific strategies that promote the healthy development of adopted children, with regard to both reducing rigidity and increasing support.

STRATEGIES THAT MIGHT WORK

Providing alternative family models, developmental information, careful preparation, and behavior management strategies will empower families to adapt and succeed (Berry & Barth, 1989; Kramer & Houston, 1998). The following discussion presents a number of promising approaches that need empirical testing.

Schools

The social relations of elementary school involve friends, classmates, teammates, and teachers. The same degree of intimacy should not characterize each relationship. Adopted children and their siblings should be prepared for questions about their family configuration that might be posed by any member of the school community. Developing a *"cover story"* is one way to have a response to inquiries that is honest without being invasive (Fahlberg, 1991). It is a brief, not particularly revealing, explanation of why a child is not living with his or her birth parents, for example, "My parents couldn't take care of me, so I needed a new family that could." A rehearsed cover story offers a script for children to use in situations that might be emotionally arousing and in which they might feel conflicted or confused. By providing a vehicle for negotiating such situations and the tools to protect his or her own privacy (e.g., "That's personal information and I'd rather not talk about it."), the cover story can contribute to a child's sense of agency and social competency.

Teachers should be *sensitive to classroom assignments* that might raise issues for adopted children. Consider the reaction of a youngster to a geography assignment he had been given. After telling his adoptive mother how many people lived in Seoul (the city in which he was born) as well as how many lived in all of Korea, he remarked, "I understand how you told me that my birth mother could not take care of me, but what was wrong with all those other billions of people?" (Pavao, 1998, p. 48). This example illustrates how easily an apparently innocuous assignment can carry emotional baggage for children in adoptive families, in this case prompting the child to contemplate not only the rejection of his birth mother but the rejection of an entire extended family and culture as well.

Teachers' sensitivity to such issues can also assist nonadopted children in other nontraditional families (e.g., stepfamilies or single parent families). The *"family orchard"* provides one approach to doing so as an alternative to the "family tree" assignment that typically appears in the genetics section of the elementary science curriculum. The family orchard "allows children to show the numerous trees that contributed to their being. It acknowledges the fact that

adoptive families are not totally unlike a stepfamily or a foster family in that they are complex; there is more than one set of mothers and fathers" (Pavao, 1998, p. 49). The orchard is an inclusive approach that alleviates the need to separate adopted children out for special assignments and illustrates the interaction of genes and environments that is supported by contemporary science.

Because there may be a higher incidence of Attention Deficit/Hyperactivity Disorder (ADHD) among children who are adopted, consideration should be given to the need for *special educational support services* to ensure that educational needs are met appropriately and minimize the risk of school failure and associated negative outcomes. For any child with a complicated history, it can be difficult to identify the extent to which behaviors are due to ADHD or to other issues. This is especially true for children who have been abused or neglected or who are transitioning to an adoptive placement from foster care. Nonetheless behaviors should be monitored carefully so that the appropriate forms of support can be put in place.

The effectiveness of attempts to *structure* the family for success by adhering to sibling issues in placement is difficult to document because placements are not random. Although Groze (1996) found that siblings in special-needs adoptions who were placed apart showed higher levels of anxiety and depression, which increased over time, and more reported social problems compared to those who had been placed together, he was unable to examine possible initial considerations that might explain these differences. Agencies may be more likely to separate those siblings whose histories were marked by the most abuse and whose own preplacement psychological and behavioral profiles were most disturbed so that each child could receive maximal individual attention in his or her adoptive family. Adoptive lore also suggests that displacing the ordinal position of children already placed in the family or "twinning" (bringing in a child who is the same age as a current member) is particularly disruptive to the family system; however, the literature does not directly address these issues.

How families construct their identity and the role that adoption plays in that construction is another area that might be useful in promoting healthy development. Kirk (1964) observed that adoptive families varied in the degree to which they distinguished between adoption and biology as ways to become a family on a continuum from *acknowledgement* to rejection of difference. Kirk argued that acknowledging differences was adaptive, allowing parents to cope with their adoptive parenthood and fostering better communication in the family. Rejection of differences was viewed as synonymous with repression and denial of the reality of adoptive parenting, inhibiting communication, and promoting poorer outcomes for the family and the child.

Brodzinsky (1987) offered an alternative nonlinear model. He suggested that acknowledgement was a healthy midpoint between rejection and insistence and that in this curvilinear model moderation was adaptive, and extreme views at either end (rejection or insistence of difference) were linked to poorer adjustment outcomes. The model, while intuitively appealing, remains untested perhaps, in part, because many commonly used statistical research tools rely on linear assumptions.

Further, acknowledgement may not be a unitary, cross-domain construct. Kaye (1990) observed families to vary in their distinctions about the adoptive experience depending on the area being considered. Those who did not distinguish in given areas (e.g., family roles) appeared not to be denying differences that in fact were there, but genuinely to feel few distinctions in these particular areas although there might be others (e.g., origins) in which they distinguished more strongly between adoptive and nonadoptive family experience. Hence, he concluded that failure to ascribe differences to the family because of adoption should not necessarily be interpreted as a lack of openness in discussing or dealing with adoption-related issues.

Grotevant, McRoy, Elde, and Fravel (1994) studied an aspect of acknowledgement, *openness* in adoption arrangement and the degree to which the parents showed interest in their adopted child's history or background. Between the ages of 4 and 12, children in this low-risk sample who had greater information about the adoption displayed higher cognitive levels of understanding adoption in general. There were, however, no relations between level of openness and the child's self-esteem, satisfaction with openness, or curiosity about the birth parents. The possibility that open lines of communication about the adoption will enhance the families' abilities to meet the challenges of adolescence will be explored in follow-up study. This possibility is suggested—assuming that children from less open families display more avoidant coping styles for adoption related stress—by earlier observations that avoidant coping was associated with negative and ambivalent feelings about being adopted among children aged 6–17 years (Smith & Brodzinsky, 1994).

The findings of Grotevant and colleagues may not generalize to special needs adoptions. Children adopted at later ages, for example, have knowledge about their preadoptive lives and family members that cannot be erased. In one study of 6–9-year-old children adopted from orphanages in the former Soviet Union, family communication and cohesion patterns were found to mediate the link between risk factors and child competence (McGuinness, 1999).

Specific strategies to encourage openness in communication about adoption include joint activities such as the creation and maintenance of a life book, life path, genogram, or ecomap (Fahlberg, 1991; Melina, 1998; Pavao, 1998). Each of these is a concrete representation of relationships and events that may include aspects of the child's life with both qualitative and quantitative information. Children's literature may also serve as a vehicle for reflection and discussion. Abandonment and the need for protection are prominent themes in children's fairy tales, and there are numerous children's books that address topics relevant to the experiences of adoptive families, some of which directly involve adoption (Banish, 1992; Krementz, 1988) and some of which do not (Blume, 1994).

STRATEGIES THAT DO NOT WORK

No rigorous research is available to indicate what strategies do not work in promoting the healthy development of children in adoptive families. However, experience over the years suggests that denial and secrecy about adoption is not a wise practice. Also, as Rosenthal (1993) suggests, families with rigidly defined roles and expectations may have more difficulty coping with the normal developmental changes in children's understanding of adoption over middle childhood. They will be challenged by children who have experienced trauma and begin to act out suppressed rage when, having spent enough time in a sufficiently safe environment, they are capable of doing so. These families will also find it more difficult to accommodate to the changes inherent in bringing an older child into the family unit.

SYNTHESIS

There are certain commonalities to the adoptive experiences of children—they all involve loss as well as the capacity to build new attachments and relationships. For children in the middle childhood period, the cognitive capacity to process and evaluate information as well as the social and academic demands of school also provide common stresses and potential sources of support. Beyond these shared attributes, adopted children and their parents and siblings bring tremendous individual differences to their experiences. What is particularly helpful for one child in a particular family may be much less helpful to another child with a different history and a different temperament in a different family with different values, challenges, and resources. What may also be helpful to one family at one time may be less helpful at another point in the child's development.

Based on our experience, we would add the following admonition to our review of the literature: Children speak with their behavior. This is especially important to remember for children with an early history of abuse or neglect who may have memories stored in ways that are not easily accessed at later ages given the cognitive changes of the 5–7-year period. Issues that are particularly confusing to the child or may be perceived as threatening to his or her current family and relationships may be too difficult or overwhelming to discuss. Changes in behavior may signal parents to attend to underlying issues. It is here that flexibility and the presence of a social and emotional support network can be particularly adaptive for parents and children alike.

No matter what changes and challenges adoptive families face during the middle childhood period, they are likely to pale in comparison to the challenges ahead in adolescence. Hence, families will do well not only to meet their children's presenting needs but to prepare for those to come as well. Even if families do not feel the need for support groups while their children are relatively young, for example, they may at a later time and will be better able to access such supports if they are aware of the appropriate resources in advance rather than needing to find them when life has become more difficult.

Early in the 20th century, the promotion of healthy development in children in adoptive families was believed to be fostered by secrecy and denial. At the beginning of the 21st century adoptions are considerably more open. Children and families bring complicated histories and relationships to their lives together, and the current state of the literature offers only limited guidance. Research that deals adequately with the complexity and diversity of circumstance in children living in adoptive families is, itself, in its youth. Like development, it will be a bidirectional process, informed as much by children and families as they are informed by it.

Also see: Anger Regulation: Childhood; Depression: Childhood; Family Strengthening: Childhood; Self-Esteem: Childhood; Social and Emotional Learning: Childhood; Peer Relationships: Childhood; Sport: Childhood.

References

Arcus, D., & McCartney, K. (1989). When baby makes four: Family influences on the stability of behavioral inhibition. In J.S. Reznick (Ed.), *Perspectives in behavioral inhibition* (pp. 197–218). Chicago: University of Chicago Press.

Banish, R. (1992). *A forever family.* New York: Harper.

Barth, R.P., & Berry, M. (1990). Preventing adoption disruption. *Prevention in Human Services, 9,* 205–222.

Berry, M., & Barth, R.P. (1989). Behavior problems of children adopted when older. *Children and Youth Services Review, 11,* 221–238.

Blume, J. (1994). *The pain and the great one.* New York: Bradbury Press.

Bowlby, J. (1988). *A secure base: Clinical applications of attachment theory.* London: Routledge.

Brodzinsky, D.M. (1987). Adjustment to adoption: A psychosocial perspective. *Clinical Psychology Review, 7,* 25–47.

Brodzinsky, D.M. (1993). Long term outcomes in adoption. *The Future of Children, 3,* 153–166.

Brodzinsky, D.M., Schecter, D.E. Braff, A.M., & Singer, L.M. (1984). Psychological and academic adjustment in adopted children. *Journal of Consulting and Clinical Psychology, 52,* 582–590.

Bronfenbrenner, U. (1979). *The ecology of human development.* Cambridge, MA: Harvard University Press.

Deutsch, C.K., Swanson, J.M., & Bruell, J.H. (1982). Overrepresentation of adoptees in children with attention deficit disorder. *Behavior Genetics, 12,* 231–237.

Dubner, A.E., & Motta, R.W. (1999). Sexually and physically abused foster care children and posttraumatic stress disorder. *Journal of Consulting and Clinical Psychology, 67,* 367–373.

Duyme, M., Dumaret, A.C., & Tomkiewicz, S. (1999). How can we boost IQ's of "dull children?": A late adoption study. *Proceedings of the National Academy of Sciences, 95,* 8790–8794.

Fahlberg, V.I. (1991). *A child's journey through placement.* Indianapolis, IN: Perspectives Press.

Freundlich, M. (1998). Adoption ambivalence: Americans support adoption—to a point. *Children's Voice, 4,* 5–8.

Grotevant, H.D., McRoy, R.G., Elde, C.L., & Fravel, D.L. (1994). Adoptive family dynamics: Variations by level of openness in the adoption. *Family Process, 33,* 125–146.

Grotevant, H.D., Ross, N.M., Marchel, M.A., & McRoy, R.G. (1999). Adaptive behavior in adopted children: Predictors form early risk, collaboration in relationships within the adoptive kinship network, and openness arrangements. *Journal of Adolescent Research, 14,* 231–247.

Groze, V. (1996). *Successful Adoptive Families.* Westport, CT: Praeger.

Kaye, K. (1990). Acknowledgement or rejection of differences. In D.M. Brodzinsky & M.D. Schechter (Eds.), *The psychology of adoption* (pp. 121–143). New York: Oxford University Press.

Kirk, H.D. (1964). *Shared fate.* NY: Free Press.

Kramer, L., & Huston, D. (1998). Supporting families as they adopt children with special needs. *Family Relations, 47,* 423–432.

Krementz, J. (1988). *How it feels to be adopted.* NY: Knopf.

Levy, T.M., & Orlans, M. (1998). *Attachment, trauma, and healing: Understanding and treating attachment disorder in children and families.* Washington, DC: Child Welfare League of America Press.

Melina, L.R. (1998). *Raising adopted children.* NY: HarperCollins.

McGuinness, T. (1999). Mitigating the effects of institutionalizations: Factors in adoptive families that make a difference. *Adoptive Families, 32,* 22–25.

Milewski, T.M.H. (2000). *Beliefs about children in foster care.* Unpublished Master's thesis, Department of Psychology, University of Massachusetts Lowell.

Miller, B.C., Fan, X., Grotevant, H.D. Christensen, M., Coyl, D., & van Dulman, M. (2000). Adopted adolescents' overrepresentation in mental health counseling: Adoptees' problems or parents' lower threshold for referral? *Journal of the American Academy of Child and Adolescent Psychiatry, 39,* 1504–1511.

O'Connor, T., Deater-Deckard, K., Fulker, D., Rutter, M., & Plomin, R. (1998). Genotype–environment correlations in late childhood and early adolescence: Antisocial behavioral problems and coercive parenting. *Developmental Psychology, 34,* 970–981.

Pavao, J.M. (1998). *The family of adoption.* Boston: Beacon Press.

Peters, B.R., Atkins, M.S., & McKay, M.M. (1999). Adopted children's behavior problems: A review of five explanatory models. *Clinical Psychology Review, 19,* 297–325.

Piaget, J. (1964). *Judgement and reasoning in the child.* Patterson, NJ: Littlefield, Adams.

Poland, D.C., & Groze, V. (1993). Effects of foster care placement on biological children in the home. *Child and Adolescent Social Work Journal, 10,* 153–164.

Rosenthal, J.A. (1993). Outcomes of adoptions of children with special needs. *The Future of Children, 3*, 77–88.

Singer, L.M., Brodzinsky, D.M., & Braff, A.M. (1982). Children's beliefs about adoption: A developmental study. *Journal of Applied Developmental Psychology, 3*, 285–294.

Singer, L.M., Brodzinsky, D.M., Ramsay, D., Steir, M., & Waters, E. (1985). Mother–infant attachment in adoptive families. *Child Development, 56*, 1543–1551.

Smith, D.W., & Brodzinsky, D.M. (1994). Stress and coping in adopted children: A developmental study. *Journal of Clinical Child Psychology, 23*, 91–99.

Stoolmiller, M. (1999). Implications of the restricted range of family environments for estimates of heritability and nonshared environment in behavior–genetic adoption studies. *Psychological Bulletin, 125*, 392–409.

Terr, L. (1990). *Too scared to cry*. New York: Basic.

US Department of Health and Human Services. (2000). Adoptions finalized in the federal fiscal year reported to AFCARS no later than May 16, 1999 (Retrieved from the World Wide Web 01/01 http://www.acf.dhhs.gov/programs/cb).

US Department of State. (2000). Orphans immigrating to the US: Countries of origin (Retrieved from the World Wide Web 01/01 http://travel.state.gov).

Waggenspack, B.M. (1998). The symbolic crises of adoption: Popular media's agenda setting. *Adoption Quarterly, 1*, 57–82.

Adoption, Adolescence

Kathleen Whitten

INTRODUCTION AND DEFINITIONS

About 1 million American children live with adoptive parents, and 2–4 percent of US families have an adopted child (Stolley, 1993). *Adoption*, in this entry, means the legal transfer of a child's parentage to an adult not biologically related to the child or to one of the child's biological parents. Stepparent adoption accounts for about half of US adoptions but it is a very different relationship (Kim, Hetherington, & Reiss, 1999). There is no national database on adoption and no central data collection on adopted children (Chandra, Abma, Maza, & Bachrach, 1999), so the numbers here likely do not represent all US adoptions. In spite of the number of adopted children in the United States, there is only a small body of scientific research on the effect of adoption on *adolescent adjustment*, meaning the ability to function well in most settings—home, school, and with peers. Further, there is no specific empirical evidence for the best ways to promote healthy growth of adopted children. Thus, this entry examines generic methods to promote healthy growth among adopted youth, based on two assumptions.

First, most adopted adolescents are not significantly different from nonadopted youth. Second, some adopted children are at higher risk for negative outcomes than nonadopted youth.

SCOPE

Adoption has changed considerably in the past 30 years. The percentage of infants born to unmarried women in the United States and placed for adoption dropped from 80 percent in 1970 to only 4 percent in 1983 (Cole & Donley, 1990) because unwed motherhood had become more socially acceptable. Effective contraception and legal abortion further reduced the number of North American and European infants placed for adoption. In 1992, the most recent year for which data are available, 15.5 percent of the children adopted in the United States were placed by public child welfare agencies with nonrelatives, while 37.5 percent were placed by private agencies or attorneys with nonrelatives. The remaining 42 percent were adopted by relatives (Flango & Flango, 1994).

Most domestic US adoptions since the mid-1980s have been "open," with various levels of contact between birth parents and adoptive parents, ranging from one exchange of photos and information about the baby to regular visits between families (Grotevant & McRoy, 1998). Adoptions from other countries by US, Canadian, and Western European couples have increased steadily. In the 1960s, US couples adopted about 1,500 children from other countries each year, but that number increased to 15,040 in 1999 (Joint Council on International Children's Services, 1999). Many international adoptions are considered *transracial*, although this term is difficult to define. It usually means families with members of different ethnic backgrounds, and recent trends include mixed-race children being adopted by mixed-race couples or mixed-race individuals (Whitten & Wilson, 1999).

THEORIES

The most commonly used theory on adoption and adjustment, the *stress and coping model* of adoption adjustment, assumes that "adopted children are at increased risk for various psychological and academic problems" (Brodzinsky, 1990, p. 3). According to this theory, a child's attitude toward adoption influences adjustment. Attitudes, in turn, come from the child's cognitive level, self-esteem, sense of mastery, sense of control, commitment, interpersonal trust, and values. These variables are indirectly influenced by genetics and prenatal experience, as well as environmental factors such as cultural and societal demands, social support, family demands, and placement history. The model assumes that a child's understanding of adoption changes over time. A transition phase might occur during the elementary school years when children realize that in order to be adopted, they had to be relinquished by their birth parents. Grief can accompany this realization. Children's coping with grief is supported or undermined by their relationship with their adoptive parents. Children whose parents acknowledge the differences between adoptive and biological families will have an easier adjustment, and children who successfully negotiate this phase of development between ages 6 and 11 should have better adjustment in adolescence.

A more inclusive *ecological model* of child development emphasizes interactions between the developing adolescent and various settings—the family, the family's environment, culture or society, and changes over time (Bronfenbrenner, 1979, 1986). The factor of time (chronosystem) (Bronfenbrenner, 1986) is important because the family is not an immutable object. It is a dynamic system that changes within itself and in response to outside influences (Bronfenbrenner, 1979). Adoption is defined by political and social processes and values, and is therefore shaped by cultural forces (Cole & Donley, 1990). Adoption is also a complex experience for children and their families, in which "the dynamic relationship between genes and experience is *played out in a cultural and interpretive context*" (Howe, 1997, p. 410, emphasis added).

Most research assumes that adoption is a "monolithic event that affects all major participants in the same, negative ways" (Demick & Wapner, 1988, p. 231). This assumption is flawed because the cultural context of adoption has changed radically since 1970. Responding to this misperception, the ecological perspective (Whitten, 2001) combines the individual emphasis of the stress and coping model of adoption adjustment with the ecological model's influences of the family and society. The culture surrounding adoption forms the macrosystem encompassing the family where the adolescent grows up (Bronfenbrenner, 1979). This system influences the institutions which create adoption policies, such as adoption agencies, state departments of social service, the US federal Immigration and Naturalization Service, and the Department of State. These institutions, the exosystem, determine many aspects of a child's adoption and subsequent life in an adoptive family, the microsystem (Bronfenbrenner, 1979). Other microsystems where the adolescent develops include neighborhood, school, and church. Research on family processes since the 1980s has shown the influence of these various systems on adolescent development, but they have not been considered in research on adoption and adjustment (Whitten, 2001).

RESEARCH

Studies of adoption's effect on adolescent adjustment often reach conflicting conclusions. In addition, different outcome measures make comparisons among studies difficult, and most research has important methodological weaknesses. Unfortunately, little scientific research has tried to differentiate the effects of selection into adoptive families from the consequences of being adopted (Rutter, 2000).

Some studies reported that adopted adolescents were "overrepresented" in groups of adolescents in mental health facilities compared to their proportion in the population (Brinich & Brinich, 1982; Jerome, 1986; Schechter, 1961; Simon & Senturia, 1966; Work & Anderson, 1971). Researchers interpreted these findings to mean that adoption constituted a risk for psychopathology. Adopted adolescents were more likely to be hospitalized for "adjustment disorder" than for serious mental illness (Weiss, 1985), or for generally less serious conditions than those of nonadopted children (Offord, Aponte, & Cross, 1969). However, in a recent study of children in mental health settings, adopted children were not overrepresented (Brand & Brinich, 1999).

Studies of children drawn from community samples also presented mixed results. While adopted children scored higher on average than nonadopted children on some measures of maladjustment (Brodzinsky, Radice, Huffman, & Merkler, 1987; Brodzinsky, Schechter, Braff, & Singer, 1984), most were within normal ranges. A recent study found that adopted adolescents were at higher risk than nonadopted youth, but effect sizes were small, especially for those living in two-parent families (Miller, Fan, Christensen, Grotevant, & Van Dulmen, 2000). In still another work, adopted adolescents were better adjusted than children born out-of-wedlock reared by their single mothers (Fergusson, Lynskey, & Horwood, 1995).

Prospective, longitudinal studies (Bohman, 1971; Bohman & Sigvardsson, 1980; DeFries, Plomin, & Fulker, 1994; Maughan & Pickles, 1990; Rhea & Corley, 1994; Wadsworth, DeFries, & Fulker, 1993) from Sweden, the United Kingdom, and the United States found no clear patterns in adopted children's adjustment. These studies were notable for their developmental perspective and for control of many adoption-related variables. European studies (Bohman, 1971; Bohman & Sigvardsson, 1980; Maughan & Pickles, 1990) found that maladjustment for adopted children peaked at age 11. However, differences between adopted and nonadopted adolescents disappeared with maturity—by age 23 (Bohman, 1971; Bohman & Sigvardsson, 1980; Maughan & Pickles, 1990).

On the other hand, the Texas Adoption Project reported that adopted children were better adjusted in some areas than biological children in the same families at the first interview but more poorly adjusted later (Loehlin, Willerman, & Horn, 1987). The Colorado Adoption Project studies of children at age 7 and 12 found differences between adopted and biological children, but they accounted for less than 5 percent of the variance on any given measure (DeFries, Plomin, & Fulker, 1994; Rhea & Corley, 1994; Wadsworth, DeFries, & Fulker, 1993).

Adjustment to adoption might vary with the child's age at placement (Rhea & Corley, 1994). Older age at placement could inhibit attachment to adoptive parents (Rila, 1997; Rutter, 2000). For internationally adopted children, the change in language could increase the risk of future problems for children adopted after they began to speak (Saetersdal & Dalen, 1991). However, other studies have found no risk for older age at placement (Brinich & Brinich, 1982). It has been speculated that negative reactions might come from preplacement care (Howe, 1997), with preplacement abuse or neglect a possibility (Logan, Morrall, & Chambers, 1998; O'Connor, Rutter, Beckett, Keaveney, Kreppner, and the ERA study team, 2000). In a study of Romanian orphans adopted in British Columbia, time in the orphanage was positively correlated with higher scores on the Child Behavior Checklist (CBCL) (Fisher, Ames, Chisholm, & Savoie, 1997). Another study of Romanian orphans found that children adopted after age 2 had lower IQ scores than those adopted before 6 months, but even within the most deprived group, the range of outcomes was wide (O'Connor et al., 2000).

Adopted adolescents' adjustment might be affected by three other factors. First, adopted siblings can provide a slight protective factor while biological children of the adoptive parents can double the risk of problem behaviors (Howe, 1997). However, Brodzinsky and Brodzinsky (1992) found no effect of siblings for adopted children. Second, open adoption has been proposed as an antidote to the closed adoptions common in the past because, "psychological problems are directly related to the secrecy or anonymity of the closed, traditional system of adoption" (Baran & Pannor, 1990, p. 318). The suspected connection between closed adoption and psychological problems has not been established (Grotevant & McRoy, 1998). Third, transracial adoption has been theorized to inhibit ethnic identity development and possibly cause behavior difficulties. However, research has found that transracially adopted children in Western Europe were not significantly different from controls in ethnically similar families on school achievement, behavior, and peer relationships (Cederblad, Hook, Irhammar, & Mercke, 1999).

STRATEGIES THAT WORK

Assuming adopted adolescents are like nonadopted youth, their healthy adjustment derives from the same influences. The healthiest adolescents have emotionally healthy parents with low-conflict marriages (Amato, 1993; Coyne, Kahn, & Gotlib, 1987). High-quality marriages are more likely to have shared parenting and similar parenting styles, so that parents have a good relationship with their children (Cummings & O'Reilly, 1997). Parenting styles and behavior management practices (Baumrind, 1993), the child's temperament (Rothbart & Ahadi, 1994) and its interaction with the parents' temperament (Rothbart & Ahadi, 1994) are all associated with positive adjustment. Authoritative parenting promotes healthy child development (Patterson & Bank, 1989; Maccoby, 1992), especially when it is combined with empathy and "emotion coaching" strategies (Gottman & DeClaire, 1997). In one of the few studies of the effect of religion on child outcomes, Brody, Stoneman, and Flor (1996) found that parental religiosity among rural African Americans was related to more cohesive family relationships, lower levels of interparental conflict and fewer externalizing and internalizing problems among adolescents. In a rare study of adoptive family processes, Rosnati and Marta (1997) found that a strong mother–child relationship was a protective factor for transracially adopted adolescents. Interventions that promote strong parent–child relationships strengthen the emotional health of youth. Developed in Australia, the Triple P—Positive Parenting Program is an example of such an effort. Several evaluations over 20 years have found it to be effective in helping parents promote children's positive behavior, and enhance parents' adjustment and functioning (Sanders, 1999). A second program worthy of consideration is Guerney's "Family Relationship Enhancement." Extensively studied in functional and dysfunctional families, it has been shown to increase empathic and expressive communications skills, general patterns of communication and relationship quality (Guerney, 1988).

STRATEGIES THAT MIGHT WORK

There is no empirical evidence for any of the following strategies. However, the strategies described here are supported by adoption theory and are in use in parts of the United States and Canada.

According to the stress and coping model of adoption adjustment, children adjust better to adoption if they develop a high degree of interpersonal trust (Brodzinsky, 1990). Adoptive parents can foster trust if they are open about their child's adoptive status, and provide details about the child's adoption when the child is mature enough for this information. The Stress and Coping Model also says that adolescents' sense of control and mastery promotes better adjustment. In an open adoption, the adolescent should have as much power and autonomy as legally possible in contacts with birth parents. If a search is possible, adoptive parents can support their adolescents in "searching" for birth parents or for information about them. Parents and professionals can help adopted adolescents feel empowered by working with other adults on adoption issues, particularly in ways that promote adoption as a desirable way to create a family. Older adolescents can be spokespeople for adoption. They can organize activities during National Adoption Month in November, make presentations to school groups, speak to adoptive parents' groups about their experience, and provide peer counseling for younger adopted children.

The ecological perspective on adoption and adjustment adds the influence of culture and forces outside the individual and family (Bronfenbrenner, 1979, 1987; Whitten, 2001). If adolescents feel isolated because of their adopted status, parents can help them connect with other adopted adolescents. Internationally adopted adolescents need help from adults to connect with others from the same country and, possibly, from the same orphanage. Some adolescents might want to meet adult adoptees from the same country. Adoption agencies can foster these connections through reunions and support groups for parents who have adopted children from the same country. Parents should also model this connection with other adoptive parents through local agencies, parents' groups, or even the Internet.* For adolescents who experience a loss of birth country, birth culture, and ethnic identity, parents can help them find "culture camps," connect with the culture of their birth country through local people, especially during major festivals (such as Tet Nguyen Dan or Chinese New Year), and attend language classes. Adolescents can also help plan trips back to their birth country and earn money to help pay for them.

The ecological perspective assumes that all institutions or settings where adolescents interact can have a positive influence. Parents can work with other adults on adoption issues, especially in school, church and adoptive families support groups. At school, parents might need to educate the adolescent's teachers on any issue the adolescent indicates is needed, such as "family tree" assignments or racial issues. The Center for Adoption Support and Education could be helpful in this regard. It provides a training program for teachers and parents, Support for Adoptive Families by Educators (S.A.F.E.), to promote an adoption-sensitive school (www.adoptionsupport. org). Parents can encourage the family's place of worship to recognize Adoption Month. They can participate in an

adoptive families group so their child has exposure to other similar families. Finally, parents can advocate for macrosystem-level adoption support, such as continuation of the federal adoption tax credit, approval of family leave for adoption, and federal funding for studies of adoption and adjustment.

STRATEGIES THAT DO NOT WORK

In the 1960s and 1970s, social work practice with adoptive families called for secrecy. Children were placed in ethnically matched homes, so families could pass as "normal." Case workers recommended that parents not tell children they were adopted until late adolescence, with the disastrous result that some adolescents discovered the secret by accident.

A current practice in the preplacement phase of adoption is education for parents about adoption risks. While some information about risks is useful, some practitioners overstate the probability of negative outcomes for adopted adolescents (Sharma, McGue, & Benson, 1998), which can prejudice parents and increase the probability of negative consequences for the child. The effect of case workers' communication with parents has not been empirically tested, but one study found a "genetic effect" for alcoholism and antisocial personality *only* when adoptive parents knew that their child's biological parent had the disorder (Riggins-Caspers, Cadoret, Panak, Lempers, Troughton, & Stewart, 1999).

SYNTHESIS

As there is no empirical evidence for the best interventions with adoptive families and their adolescents, there are many research opportunities in this area. First, basic research on adoption and adjustment is needed in order to develop empirically grounded interventions. Measuring the effect of changing time periods is a special challenge in a field where adolescent outcomes depend in part on changes in the social environment (Rushton & Minnis, 1997). The scientific method prescribes building on previous research, but culturally sensitive topics like adoption require caution in citing findings from the 1960s and 1970s.

Studies should examine continuous and time-limited maladjustment and healthy adjustment, with multiple occasions of measurement, to determine which aspects of a child's family and environment contribute to healthy development through adolescence and into adulthood. Potential strengths of adoptive families should be investigated for their effect on adolescent adjustment. Basic research is also needed into the effect of siblings, open adoption, and transracial placement. Research should continue to explore the effect of placement at different ages on attachment to adoptive parents, language

---

* For example, www.comeunity.com, www.fcvn.org, and www.adoptvietnam. org for Vietnamese adoption, for adopted children and birth parents (www.adoptioncrossroads.org), for general adoption information (www.calib.naic and www.adopting.com), and for research-based information (www.cyfc.umn.edu), be aware that sites might change or vanish during the life of the current edition of this Encyclopedia.

development, integration into adoptive culture, and retention of native culture and language.

Interventions to enhance general family functioning should be tested with adoptive families and their adolescents. Other interventions or programs specific to adoption should be tested, including the best ways to prepare prospective parents for adoptive parenthood, and the best ways to support them after their child arrives. The effect of parent–child communication about adoption should be investigated, particularly parent–child interaction about adoption at various ages, and parents' help with children's grief about adoption-related losses. Qualitative and quantitative assessments of parents' help for the child's search for birth parents (in "closed" adoptions) should be researched for their effect on adolescent outcomes. Parents' involvement with adoption-related issues should be assessed for its effect on the family and the adolescent. This could include work with schools, churches, or adoption support groups. Adolescents' involvement in adoption-related activities should be assessed for their effects on mental health outcomes. These can include acting as spokespersons for adoption, peer counseling, attending "culture camps," and participating in adoption-related support groups. Community-level and adoption agency-level programs should also be tested and evaluated.

If it takes a village to raise a child, it takes a world to promote the healthy development of adopted children. When all systems work together to promote their health, adopted children will have the best chance to develop into healthy adolescence and adulthood.

Also see: Anger Regulation: Adolescence; Depression: Adolescence; Family Strengthening: Adolescence; Self-Esteem: Adolescence; Peer Relationships: Adolescence; Risk-Taking: Adolescence.

References

Amato, P. (1993). Children's adjustment to divorce. *Journal of Marriage and the Family, 55*, 13–38.

Baran, A., & Pannor, R. (1990). Open adoption. In D.M. Brodzinsky & M.D. Schechter (Eds.), *The psychology of adoption* (pp. 316–331). New York: Oxford Press.

Baumrind, D. (1993). The average expectable environment is not good enough: A response to Scarr. *Child Development, 64*, 1299–1317.

Bohman, M. (1971). A comparative study of adopted children, foster children, and children in their biological environment born after undesired pregnancies. *Acta Paediatrica Scandinavia, 221*(Suppl.), 5–38.

Bohman, M., & Sigvardsson, S. (1980). A prospective, longitudinal study of children registered for adoption. *Acta Psychiatrica Scandinavia, 61*, 339–355.

Brand, A.E., & Brinich, P.M. (1999). Behavior problems and mental health contacts in adopted, foster, and nonadopted children. *Journal of Child Psychology and Psychiatry and Allied Disciplines, 40*, 1221–1229.

Brinich, P.M., & Brinich, E.B. (1982). Adoption and adaptation. *Journal of Nervous and Mental Disease, 160*, 489–494.

Brody, G.H., Stoneman, Z., & Flor, D. (1996). Parental religiosity, family process and youth competence in rural two-parent African-American families. *Developmental Psychology, 32*(4), 696–706.

Brodzinsky, D.M. (1990). A stress and coping model of adoption adjustment. In D.M. Brodzinsky & M.D. Schechter (Eds.), *The psychology of adoption* (pp. 3–24). New York: Oxford Press.

Brodzinsky, D.M., & Brodzinsky, A.B. (1992). The impact of family structure on the adjustment of adopted children. *Child Welfare, 71*(1), 69–76.

Brodzinsky, D.M., Radice, C., Huffman, L., & Merkler, K. (1987). Prevalence of clinically significant symptomatology in a nonclinical sample of adopted and nonadopted children. *Journal of Clinical Child Psychology, 16*, 350–356.

Brodzinsky, D.M., Schechter, M.D., Braff, A.M. & Singer, L.M. (1984). Psychological and academic adjustment in adopted children. *Journal of Consulting and Clinical Psychology, 52*, 582–590.

Bronfenbrenner, U. (1979). *The ecology of human development*. Cambridge: Harvard.

Bronfenbrenner, U. (1986). Ecology of the family as a context for human development: Research perspectives. *Developmental Psychology, 22*, 723–742.

Cederblad, M., Hook, B., Irhammar, M., & Mercke, A. (1999). Mental health in international adoptees as teenagers and young adults: An epidemiological study. *Journal of Child Psychology and Psychiatry, 40*(8), 1239–1248.

Chandra, A., Abma, J., Maza, P., & Bachrach, C. (1999, May 11). *Adoption, Adoption Seeking, and Relinquishment for Adoption in the United States*. National Center for Health Statistics, No. 306, Hyattsville, MD.

Cole, E.S., & Donley, K.S. (1990). History, values, and placement policy issues in adoption. In D.M. Brodzinsky & M.D. Schechter (Eds.), *The psychology of adoption* (pp. 42–61). New York: Oxford Press.

Coyne, J., Kahn, J., & Gotlib, I.H. (1987). Depression. In T. Jacob (Ed.), *Family Interaction and Pathology: Theories, Methods and Findings* (pp. 509–533). New York: Plenum Press.

Cummings, M.E., & O'Reilly, A.W. (1997). Fathers in family context: Effects of marital quality on child adjustment. In M. Lamb (Ed.), *The role of the father in child development* (3rd ed., pp. 49–65). New York: John Wiley.

DeFries, J.C., Plomin, R., & Fulker, D.W. (Eds.). (1994). *Nature and nurture during middle childhood*. Cambridge, MA: Blackwell.

Demick, J., & Wapner, S. (1988). Open and closed adoption: A developmental conceptualization. *Family Process, 27*, 229–249.

Fergusson, D.M., Lynskey, M., & Horwood, L.J. (1995). The adolescent outcomes of adoption: A 16-year longitudinal study. *Journal of Child Psychology and Psychiatry, 36*, 597–615.

Fisher, L., Ames, E.W., Chisholm, K., & Savoie, L. (1997). Problems reported by parents of Romanian orphans adopted to British Columbia. *International Journal of Behavioral Development, 20*(1), 67–82.

Flango, V., & Flango, C. (1994). *The flow of adoption information from states*. Williamsburg, VA: National Center for State Courts.

Gottman, J.M., & DeClaire, J. (1997). The heart of parenting: How to raise an emotionally intelligent child. New York: Simon & Schuster.

Grotevant, H.D., & McRoy, R.G. (1998). *Openness in adoption: Exploring family connections*. Thousand Oaks, CA: Sage.

Guerney, B.G. (1988). Family relationship enhancement: A skill training approach. In L.A. Bond & B.M. Wagner (Eds.), *Families in Transition: Primary Prevention Programs That Work. Primary Prevention of Psychopathology, 11*, pp. 99–134. Thousand Oaks, CA: Sage.

Howe, D. (1997). Parent-reported problems in 211 adopted children: Some risk and protective factors. *Journal of Child Psychology and Psychiatry, 38*(4), 401–411.

Jerome, L. (1986). Over representation of adopted children attending a children's mental health centre. *Canadian Journal of Psychiatry, 31*, 526–531.

Joint Council on International Children's Services. (1999). http://www.jcics.org.

Kim, J.E., Hetherington, E.M., & Reiss, D. (1999). Associations among family relationships, antisocial peers, and adolescents' externalizing behaviors: Gender and family type differences. *Child Development, 70*(5), 1209–1230.

Loehlin, J.C., Willerman, L., & Horn, J.M. (1987). Personality resemblance in adoptive families: A 10-year follow-up. *Journal of Personality and Social Psychology, 53*(5), 961–969.

Logan, F.A., Morrall, P.M.E., & Chambers, H. (1998). Identification of risk factors for psychological disturbance in adopted children. *Child Abuse Review, 7*(3), 154–164.

Maccoby, E. (1992). The role of parents in the socialization of children: A historical overview. *Developmental Psychology, 28*, 1006–1017.

Maughan, G., & Pickles, A. (1990). Adopted and illegitimate children growing up. In L. Robins & M. Rutter (Eds.), *Straight and devious pathways from childhood to adulthood* (pp. 36–61). Cambridge: Cambridge University Press.

Miller, B.C., Fan, X., Christensen, M., Grotevant, H.D., & Van Dulmen, M. (2000). Comparisons of adopted and nonadopted adolescents in a large, nationally representative sample. *Child Development, 71*(5), 1458–1473.

O'Connor, T., Rutter, M., Beckett, C., Keaveney, L., Kreppner, J., & the ERA study team. (2000). The effects of global severe deprivation on cognitive competence: Extension and longitudinal follow-up. *Child Development, 71*, 376–390.

Offord, D.R., Aponte, J.F., & Cross, L.A. (1969). Presenting symptomatology of adopted children. *Archives of General Psychiatry, 20*, 110–116.

Patterson, G.R., & Bank, L. (1989). Some amplifying mechanisms for pathologic processes in families. In M. Gunnar & E. Thelen (Eds.), *Minnesota symposium on child psychology: Vol. 22. Systems and development* (pp. 167–209). Mahwah, NJ: Erlbaum.

Rhea, S.A., & Corley, R.P. (1994). Applied issues. In J.C. DeFries, R. Plomin, & D.W. Fulker (Eds), *Nature and nurture during middle childhood* (pp. 295–309). Cambridge, MA: Blackwell.

Riggins-Caspers, K., Cadoret, R.J., Panak, W., Lempers, J.D., Troughton, E., & Stewart, M.A. (1999). Gene–environment interaction and the moderating effect of adoption agency disclosure on estimating genetic effects. *Personality and Individual Differences, 27*(2), 357–380.

Rila, B. (1997). The attachment disordered adoptee. In S.K. Rozia & A. Baran (Eds.), *Creating kinship*. Portland, ME: The Dougy Center.

Rosnati, R., & Marta, E. (1997). Parent–child relationships as a protective factor in preventing adolescents' psychosocial risk in inter-racial adoptive and nonadoptive families. *Journal of Adolescence, 20*, 617–631.

Rothbart, M.K., & Ahadi, S.A. (1994). Temperament and the development of personality. *Journal of Abnormal Psychology, 103*, 55–66.

Rushton, A., & Minnis, H. (1997). Annotation: Transracial family placements. *Journal of Child Psychology and Psychiatry, 38*(2), 147–159.

Rutter, M. (2000). Children in substitute care: Some conceptual considerations and research implications. *Children and Youth Services Review, 22*(9/10), 685–703.

Saetersdal, B., & Dalen, M. (1991). Intercountry adoptions in a homogeneous country. In H. Altstein & R.J. Simon (Eds.), *Intercountry adoption: A multinational perspective* (pp. 83–107). New York: Praeger.

Sanders, M.R. (1999). Triple P—Positive Parenting Program: Towards an empirically validated multilevel parenting and family support strategy for the prevention of behavior and emotional problems in children. *Clinical Child and Family Psychology Review, 2*(2), 71–90.

Schechter, M. (1961). Observations on adopted children. *Archives of General Psychiatry, 3*, 21–32.

Sharma, A.R., McGue, M.K., & Benson, P.L. (1998). The psychological adjustment of United States adopted adolescents and their nonadopted siblings. *Child Development, 69*(3), 791–802.

Simon, N.M., & Senturia, A.G. (1966). Adoption and psychiatric illness. *American Journal of Psychiatry, 122*, 858–868.

Stolley, K.S. (1993). Statistics on adoption in the United States. *The Future of Children: Adoption, 3*(1), 26–42.

Wadsworth, S.J., DeFries, J.C., & Fulker, D.W. (1993). Cognitive abilities of children at 7 and 12 years of age in the Colorado Adoption Project. *Journal of Learning Disabilities, 25*(9), 611–615.

Weiss, A. (1985). Symptomatology of adopted and nonadopted adolescents in a psychiatric hospital. *Adolescence, 20*, 763–774.

Whitten, K.L., & Wilson, M.W. (1999). Interracial families. In L. Balter (Ed.), *Parenthood in America: An encyclopedia*. Oxford: ABC-CLIO.

Whitten, K.L. (2001). *An ecological model of adoption and adjustment*. Presentation to the Biennial Meeting of the Society for Research in Child Development, Minneapolis, MN.

Work, H.H., & Anderson, H. (1971). Studies in adoption: Requests for psychiatric treatment. *American Journal of Psychiatry, 127*, 124–125.

African American Youth, Adolescence

Craig C. Brookins and Brigid Sackey

INTRODUCTION

The healthy development of African American youth may be influenced by a variety of social, psychological, political, and institutional forces. Among these are the stereotypical images and messages these youth received through mass media and educational systems, the denigration of African cultural values and practices on local and national levels, and the obstacles faced by families and communities in their efforts to counteract these oppressive forces. The promotion of health in the realms of physical, social, and psychological development for African American youth requires approaches that are historically and culturally grounded, explicitly focused on individual and community strengths, and necessarily address sociopolitical realities within the communities in which these groups reside (Brookins, 1996).

This approach is consistent with the *Youth Development and Empowerment* approach described by Kim, Crutchfield, Williams, and Hepler (1998) and designed to produce "fully prepared youth" capable of effectively coping with a diverse array of developmental challenges. Although it is recognized that the healthy development of youth is best accomplished when the antecedent child development period has been successful, this entry assumes that such development has taken place and focuses on youth that generally fall between the ages of 11 and 19 years. Achieving effective community structures that provide for the healthy development of youth will benefit all members of the community, promote community development, and ultimately result in a decrease in extant social problems.

DEFINITIONS

The sociopolitical context within which African American youth develop requires an understanding of key issues including optimal social and psychological development, oppression and sociopolitical development. *Optimal development* for African-descended youth, as is the case with youth of all ethnicities, requires environments where there is an alignment between familial and cultural values and the values of the societies in which they reside. These societal values are manifested in the familial, educational, religious, and political arenas of communities and affect youth in direct and indirect ways. In an optimal environment, the developmental needs for each member of the community, and at each stage of development (from infancy through old age), are met by appropriately designed community structures (Brookins, 1996; Myers et al., 1991). Optimal development therefore implies that given the proper ecological structure, the majority of individuals will develop in ways that will be healthy and successful.

African-descended youth often find themselves in oppressive environments that affect their optimal development. Oppression works on both sociopolitical and psychological levels. Sociopolitically, *oppression* is the "unjust exercise of power and the control of ideas and coveted resources in a way that produces and sustains social inequality" (Watts, Griffith, & Abdul-Adil, 1999). Psychologically, Bulhan (1985) uses a Fanonian theoretical framework to define oppression as essentially a form of violence to all aspects of the human psyche. An oppressive environment denies individuals and groups the ability to exert control over their space, time, energy, mobility, bonding, and identity. These six dimensions are what Bulhan (1985) suggests "define, determine, and substantiate the psyche" (p. 124). Over time, prolonged oppression may result in internalization of these external and suboptimal definitions of self that become manifested in a variety of dysfunctional behaviors. For youth, this often includes delinquent behavior, substance abuse, adolescent pregnancy, and violence (Geyen, 1993; Gibbs, 1989; Prothrow-Stith, 1990; Wilson, 1991).

SCOPE

A recent report by the Carnegie Corporation of New York (1995) documents the serious risks faced by adolescents in the United States. A variety of social indicators point to serious losses in the areas of education, and increases in unemployment, delinquency, substance abuse, adolescent pregnancy, and suicide rates (Gibbs, 1989). This higher prevalence for dysfunctional outcomes is particularly acute for African American youth in urban settings (Children's Defense Fund, 1991). Many of the problems these youth face have been partially attributed to the difficulties they encounter in making a successful transition from childhood, through adolescence, and into adulthood (Brookins, 1996). The ecological factors that place youth at risk for optimal development include inappropriate socialization practices (Hare & Hare, 1985; Spencer, 1990), an inability to participate in the economic structures of society (Muga, 1984; Ogbu, 1982; Oliver, 1989), and the peculiar effects of race, stereotyping, and prejudice (Spencer, 1987).

THEORIES

In order for youth to develop optimally within oppressive environments, community structures must exist that prevent this violence to the psyche, foster an optimal conceptual framework on which an individual's values and behavior can be based, and promote a culturally appropriate identity (Brookins & Robinson, 1995; Spencer, 1999). Three interrelated theoretical formulations are particularly useful as guiding strategies in these efforts: identity-focused cultural ecological orientations (Brookins, 1996; Spencer, 1999), sociopolitical development models (Watts et al., 1999), and youth empowerment models (Chinman & Linney, 1998; Kim et al., 1998).

Multiple theoretical orientations, by definition, are embedded within models that promote ecological approaches to promoting healthy development. Accordingly, Spencer (1999) presents the phenomenological variant of ecological systems theory (PVEST) that integrates culture, context, and normative developmental processes toward promoting healthy development broadly, and school adjustment more specifically. PVEST emphasizes the significance of identity processes to the development of youth who are psychologically healthy, contextually competent, have healthy relationships, and are academically successful. The *identity process* is defined as "... coming to understand oneself as a member of a society within a particular ethnic, cultural, religious, or political tradition" (Spencer, 1999, p. 48) and includes the development of interpersonal and intrapersonal competencies that effectively respond in a variety of contexts including those having oppressive elements to them as described earlier.

Brookins (1996) provides a similar identity-centered ecological model for promoting healthy development in African American youth. The adolescent developmental pathways paradigm (ADPP) arises out of theoretical formulations of identity that recognize the importance of cultural grounding and intellectual and social skill development. The ADPP is proposed as a model for community-based interventions designed to respond to the normal developmental needs of children and adolescents as they transition to adulthood. At its core, the ADPP assists the developing adolescent in attaching meaning to personal and group-based knowledge and experiences. Additionally, the ADPP recognizes the holistic nature of identity and self-concept and the need for youth to explore and develop commitments in a variety of identity domains (e.g., gender, occupation, social, spiritual).

According to Watts et al. (1999), sociopolitical development is the cognitive, cultural, and spiritual process that leads to and supports social and political action. It requires critical thinking and psychological empowerment skills that enables the individual to reduce internalized oppression and build a sense of self-efficacy. Watts and his colleagues propose a five dimensional profile of sociopolitical development in which the individual's awareness of oppression is limited or nonexistent (Acritical Stage) and, through proper intervention, can move to a point of awareness of the salience of oppression and the necessity of individual and collective action to combat it (Liberation Stage).

The sociopolitical development approach is consistent with the youth development and empowerment approach described by Kim et al. (1998) and designed to produce "fully prepared youth" capable of effectively coping with a diverse array of developmental challenges. Developed primarily for substance abuse prevention efforts the model integrates multiple social and psychological theoretical perspectives and promotes the development of youth as assets and resources to communities through the provision of meaningful social, economic, and public opportunity. These opportunities must be provided in an ecological context that includes adequate social support, high expectations, and consistent reinforcement from significant others, particularly caring adults in multiple settings such as the family, school, and other community institutions.

Similarly, Chinman and Linney (1998) propose a positive empowerment cycle model that emphasizes the need for opportunities within the adolescent's environment for engagement in positive and meaningful activities, learning useful and relevant skills, and receiving supportive feedback. These opportunities are believed to promote psychological empowerment by engaging adolescents in a process of normal and positive identity development.

RESEARCH

Although considerable empirical examination of these theoretical models remains to be conducted there have been some initial investigations. In a test of the PVEST, Spencer, Dupree, and Hartman (1997) have found empirical support for the relationship between adolescents' "intersubjective experiences" of their ecological context and some individual-level outcomes. Spencer and colleagues (1997) found that perceived stress (i.e., perceived unpopularity with peers, inferred negative teacher perceptions, parental monitoring) was predictive of negative learning attitude for African American adolescent males but not for females and perceived unpopularity with peers was a significant predictor of negative learning attitude for African American adolescent females. In a related study, Spencer (1999) reported these same stressor variables to be predictive of hypermasculinity in African American adolescent males. These findings acknowledge the role of the ecological context, at least as perceived by those embedded within it, on individual development and support intervention strategies that improve adolescents' experiences with and responses to their environment (i.e., mentoring, teacher training).

Although there is limited experimental data on the efficacy of identity-focused interventions, there is empirical support for the relationship of a healthy ethnic or racial identity to self-esteem (Phinney and Chavira, 1992; Smith, Walker, Fields, Brookins, & Seay, 1999), resistance to stress (Spencer, 1983), violence related behaviors (Ringwalt & Paschall, 1995), less risky sexual attitudes (Belgrave, Van Oss Marin, & Chambers, 2000), career aspirations and goal attainment (Smith et al., 1999), and academic achievement (Smith et al., 1999; Spencer, 1988).

Empirical data on the efficacy of identity-focused interventions is slowly beginning to emerge. Cherry, Belgrave, Jones, Kennon, Gray, and Phillips (1998) reported positive effects of an Africentric education and rites of passage program on the racial identity of African American fifth graders (Cherry et al., 1998). Two studies have also demonstrated a significant impact on the cultural and racial pride (a component of ethnic or racial identity) of African American adolescents as a result of their participation in culturally based rites-of-passage programs (Hargrove, 1997; Reddick-Gibson, 1999). It is clear, however, that additional experimental research is therefore warranted on interventions designed to effectively promote these variables.

Currently, only qualitative data exists that point to the potential efficacy of interventions promoting sociopolitical development on healthy outcomes for African American youth. Watts and Abdul-Adil (1997) demonstrated the potential of the effectiveness of an intervention developing critical consciousness (a component of sociopolitical development) in a sample of African American adolescent males. Systematic content analyses of an eight-session school-based intervention in which rap video, film, and other products of mass media were presented and discussed found critical consciousness of the sample youth to have been enhanced. Additional anecdotal data exists demonstrating the effectiveness of interventions promoting African American ethnic and cultural identity on frequency of after-school academic behavior and self-esteem (Ghee, Walker, & Younger, 1997), sexuality knowledge and attitudes, and achievement motivation (Brookins, 2001).

Chinman and Linney (1998) review a variety of empirical research studies that directly or indirectly support their positive empowerment cycle with regards to youths' participation in meaningful activities including employment, volunteer activities, educational interventions, community service, and mentoring.

STRATEGIES THAT WORK

Clear evidence is not yet available.

STRATEGIES THAT MIGHT WORK

As indicated earlier, although many culturally based programs that promote healthy development exist in African American communities (Ghee et al., 1997; Goddard, 1992; Shujaa, 1994; Warfield-Coppock, 1992), little empirical research exists that adequately document the effectiveness of the models identified or the correctness of the theories on which they are based. Each of the models identified above (ADPP, PVEST, sociopolitical development and youth empowerment), however, lend themselves to the operationalization of key constructs and empirical examination of the effectiveness of interventions on which they are based. Moreover, in addition to the reported efficacy of the identity-focused interventions identified above, there is empirical evidence on the positive impact of interventions that directly or indirectly utilize varying components of these ecologically oriented models. These interventions have been found to be effective in the areas of substance abuse prevention and juvenile delinquency (Blumenkrantz and Gavazzi, 1993) and achievement motivation and healthy sexual attitudes (Brookins, 2001).

There is fairly strong empirical support for programs that use adult or peer mentors to assist with the developmental processes of adolescence (Dennison, 2000; Thompson & Kelly-Vance, 2001; Tierney & Grossman, 2000). There is some evidence, however, that nonparental mentoring (a particularly popular strategy) most likely works indirectly through the enhancement of the parent–child relationship that it may promote (Rhodes, Grossman, & Resche, 2000).

STRATEGIES THAT DO NOT WORK

Given the relatively recent articulation of these models, little research exists as well to suggest areas that may not work. There does exist, however, cautionary evidence that must be taken into consideration when attempting to implement interventions based on these models. For instance, the data related to the PVEST model indicates gender differences in how adolescents perceive their environment that may lead to different outcomes (Spencer et al., 1997). Additionally, although employment may be a positively engaging activity for youth, such employment must be meaningful, promote requisite skills, and contribute to normative developmental needs (Greenberger & Steinberg, 1986).

SYNTHESIS

Promoting the healthy development of African American youth requires community structures that are driven by sound developmental and ecological theory. While developmental processes for African American youth have many commonalities with youth across the ethnic and racial spectrum, there are additional challenges these youth may face due to environments that are often developmentally antagonistic and oppressive. Consequently, community structures must be in place that allow youth to acquire the requisite skills and attitudinal dispositions (i.e., psychological empowerment, critical consciousness) to effectively counter these forces.

Each of the models recognizes the importance of the need for African American adolescents to develop a healthy ethnic (cultural) identity. Defined as a compendium of various characteristics such an identity includes attitudinal and behavioral strategies. Among these are context-specific self-esteem and self-efficacy, sociopolitical skills, and positive perceptions of the support offered by various components of their community (e.g., parents, peers, teachers).

Each of the models described in this entry have at their core an understanding of normative developmental processes that are consistently promoted by the community structures within which youth experiences are embedded (e.g., familial, educational, local community, religious). These models additionally recognize the need for efforts that move away from an individual deficit orientation to an individual and cultural strengths approach in which intervention is primarily aimed at community structure. While recognizing the diverse contexts (economic, geographic, historic) that are characteristic of African American communities, individually focused efforts within these models are designed to produce competencies in behavioral domains that will contribute to community change and development.

A key requirement for theory-driven intervention is that proposed models are based on implementable strategies. The literature is rich with descriptions of effective strategies in the area of violence prevention (Wilson-Brewer & Jacklin, 1990), the prevention of premature pregnancies in adolescents (Foster, Greene, & Smith, 1990; Franklin, Grant, Corcoran, Miller, & Bultman, 1997), mentoring (McPartland & Nettles, 1991), rites-of-passage (Brookins, 1996; Harvey & Coleman, 1997; Warfield-Coppock, 1992), and substance abuse prevention (Ringwalt & Paschall, 1995).

There remains a considerable need for empirical and experimental research on these proposed theoretical models and particularly on the further operationalization of ethnic identity constructs, the relationship between ethnic identity and positive developmental outcomes, the effectiveness of identity focused interventions on positive developmental outcomes, the role that youth perceptions play in determining developmental outcomes, and a further articulation of sociopolitical development as a relevant construct.

Also see: Family Strengthening: Adolescence; Peer Relationships: Adolescence; Racial and Ethnic Disparities: Adulthood; Risk-Taking: Adolescence; Social Competency: Adolescence; Social and Emotional Learning: Adolescence.

References

Belgrave, F.Z., Van Oss Marin, B., & Chambers, D.B. (2000). Cultural, contextual, and intrapersonal predictors of risky sexual attitudes among urban African-American girls in early adolescence. *Cultural Diversity and Ethnic Minority Psychology, 6*, 309–322.

Blumenkrantz, D.G., & Gavazzi, S.M. (1993). Guiding transitional events for children and adolescents through a modern day rite of passage. *Journal of Primary Prevention, 13*, 199–212.

Brookins, C.C. (1996). Promoting ethnic identity development in African-American youth: The role of rites of passage. *Journal of Black Psychology, 22*, 388–417.

Brookins, C.C. (2001). *A multiyear overview of youth development programs in Wake County, North Carolina.* Raleigh, NC: North Carolina State University.

Brookins, C.C., & Robinson, T.L. (1995). Rites-of-passage as resistance to oppression. *The Western Journal of Black Studies, 19*, 172–180.

Bulhan, H.A. (1985). *Frantz Fanon and the psychology of oppression.* New York: Plenum.

Carnegie Corporation of New York. (Ed.). (1995). *Great transitions: Preparing adolescents for a new century.* New York: Author.

Cherry, V.R., Belgrave, F.Z., Jones, W., Kennon, D.K., Gray, F.S., & Phillips, F. (1998). NTU: An Africentric approach to substance abuse prevention among African-American youth. *Journal of Primary Prevention, 18*, 319–339.

Children's Defense Fund. (1991). *The adolescent and young adult fact book.* Washington, DC: Author.

Chinman, M.J., & Linney, J.A. (1998). Toward a model of adolescent empowerment: Theoretical and empirical evidence. *Journal of Primary Prevention, 18*, 393–413.

Dennison, S. (2000). A win–win peer mentoring and tutoring program: A collaborative model. *Journal of Primary Prevention, 20*, 161–174.

Foster, H.W., Greene, L.W., & Smith, M.S. (1990). A model for increasing access: Teenage pregnancy prevention. *Journal of Health Care for the Poor and Underserved, 1*, 136–146.

Franklin, C., Grant, D., Corcoran, J., Miller, P.O.D., & Bultman, L. (1997). Effectiveness of prevention programs for adolescent pregnancy: A meta-analysis. *Journal of Marriage and the Family, 59*, 551–567.

Geyen, D.J. (1993). Understanding Black adolescent male violence. *Journal of Black Psychology, 19*, 493–496.

Ghee, K.L., Walker, J., & Younger, A.C. (1997). The RAAMUS academy: Evaluation of an edu-cultural intervention for young African-American males. *Journal of Prevention & Intervention in the Community, 16*, 87–102.

Gibbs, J.T. (1989). Black adolescents and youth: An update on an endangered species. In R.L. Jones (Ed.), *Black adolescents* (pp. 3–28). Berkeley, CA: Cobb & Henry.

Goddard, L.L. (1992). *An African centered model of prevention for African-American youth at high risk.* Rockville, MD: US Department of Health and Human Services.

Greenberger, E., & Steinberg, L.D. (1986). *When teenagers work: The psychological and social costs of adolescent employment.* New York: Basic Books.

Hare, N., & Hare, J. (1985). *Bringing the black boy to manhood: The passage.* San Francisco: Black Think Tank.

Hargrove, J.E., Jr. (1997). The significance of an Afrikan Rites of Passage on the development of an African-American male racial identity. *Dissertation Abstracts International: Section B: The Sciences and Engineering, 57*, 7249.

Harvey, A.R., & Coleman, A.A. (1997). An Afrocentric program for African-American males in the juvenile justice system. *Child Welfare, 76*, 197–211.

Kim, S., Crutchfield, C., Williams, C., & Hepler, N. (1998). Toward a new paradigm in substance abuse and other problem behavior prevention for youth: Youth development and empowerment approach. *Journal of Drug Education, 28*, 1–17.

McPartland, J.M., & Nettles, S.M. (1991). Using community adults as advocates or mentors for at-risk middle school students: A two-year evaluation of Project RAISE. *American Journal of Education, 99*(4), 568–586.

Muga, D. (1984). Academic sub-cultural theory and the problematic of ethnicity: A tentative critique. *The Journal of Ethnic Studies, 12*, 1–51.

Myers, L.J., Speight, S.L., Highlen, P.S., Cox, C.I. et al. (1991). Identity development and worldview: Toward an optimal conceptualization. *Journal of Counseling and Development, 70*, 54–63.

Ogbu, J.U. (1982). Cultural discontinuities and schooling. *Anthropology and Education Quarterly, 13*, 290–307.

Oliver, W. (1989). Black males and social problems: Prevention through Afrocentric socialization. *Journal of Black Studies, 20*, 15–39.

Phinney, J.S., & Chavira, V. (1992). Ethnic identity and self-esteem: An exploratory longitudinal study. *Journal of Adolescence, 15*, 271–281.

Prothrow-Stith, D. (1990). *Deadly consequences: How violence is destroying our teenage population and a plan to begin solving the problem.* New York: Harper-Collins.

Reddick-Gibson, F.L. (1999). *An evaluation of the B.U.I.L.D. rites of passage program on the attitudes and behaviors of adolescent African-American males.* Unpublished doctoral dissertation, University of Sarasota, Sarasota, FL.

Rhodes, J.E., Grossman, J.B., & Resche, N.L. (2000). Agents of change: Pathways through which mentoring relationships influence adolescents' academic adjustment. *Child Development, 71*, 1662–1671.

Ringwalt, C., & Paschall, M.J. (1995). Ethnic identity, drug use, and violence among African-American male adolescents. (N)

Shujaa, M.J. (Ed.). (1994). *Too much schooling, too little education: A paradox of Black life in White societies.* Trenton, NJ: Africa World Press.

Smith, E.P., Walker, K., Fields, L., Brookins, C.C., & Seay, R.C. (1999). Ethnic identity and its relationship to self-esteem, perceived efficacy and prosocial attitudes in early adolescence. *Journal of Adolescence, 22,* 867–880.

Spencer, M.B. (1983). Children's cultural values and parental child rearing strategies. *Developmental Review, 3,* 351–370.

Spencer, M.B. (1987). Black children's ethnic identity formation: Risk and resilience of castelike minorities. In J.S. Phinney & M.J. Rotheram (Eds.), *Children's ethnic socialization: Pluralism and development* (pp. 103–116). Newbury Park, CA: Sage.

Spencer, M.B. (1988). Self-concept development. *New Directions for Child Development, 42,* 59–72.

Spencer, M.B. (1990). Parental values transmission: Implications for the development of African-American children. In H.E. Cheatham & J.B. Stewart (Eds.), *Black families: Interdisciplinary perspectives* (pp. 111–130). New Brunswick, NJ: Transaction.

Spencer, M.B. (1999). Social and cultural influences on school adjustment: The application of an identity-focused cultural ecological perspective. *Educational Psychologist, 34,* 43–57.

Spencer, M.B., Dupree, D., & Hartmann, T. (1997). A phenomenological variant of ecological systems theory (PVEST): A self-organization perspective in context. *Development and Psychopathology, 9,* 817–833.

Thompson, L.A., & Kelly-Vance, L. (2001). The impact of mentoring on academic achievement of at-risk youth. *Children and Youth Services Review, 23,* 227–242.

Tierney, J., & Grossman, J.B. (2000). What works in promoting positive youth development: Mentoring. In M.P. Kluger & G. Alexander (Eds.), *What works in child welfare* (pp. 323–328). Washington, DC: Child Welfare League of America.

Warfield-Coppock, N. (1992). The rites of passage movement: A resurgence of African-centered practices for socializing African-American youth. *Journal of Negro Education, 61,* 471–482.

Watts, R.J., & Abdul-Adil, J. (1997). Promoting critical consciousness in young, African-American men. *Journal of Prevention & Intervention in the Community, 16,* 63–86.

Watts, R.J., Griffith, D.M., & Abdul-Adil, J. (1999). Sociopolitical development as an antidote for oppression—Theory and action. *American Journal of Community Psychology, 27,* 255–272.

Wilson, A.N. (1991). *Understanding black adolescent male violence.* Bronx, NY: Afrikan World Infosystems.

Wilson-Brewer, R., & Jacklin, B. (1990). Violence prevention strategies targeted at the general population of minority youth. *Public Health Reports, 106,* 270–271.

Age Bias, Older Adulthood

Bahira Sherif

INTRODUCTION

An increase in concern with *ageism*, which involves negative attitudes toward older adults, can be attributed to the aging of people in the United States, and the industrialized world in general. The number of older adults is increasing and will continue to increase more rapidly than the rest of the population for the foreseeable future. As the number of elderly increases exponentially, so does public concern with federal spending on retirement and medical care. This spending is, in the minds of many, further tied to the growing and "disproportionate" political power of the elderly. Ageism also has other ramifications, which makes it an important ethical and social issue. On an individual level, ageism can result in physical and mental decline as well as loss of self-esteem. On a societal level, ageism deprives society of a whole sector of productive creative older individuals who are pressured to retire. Ageism negates the value of knowledge and wisdom that is gained by individuals over the years.

DEFINITION

Ageism or *age bias* refers to the negative attitudes towards older adults. Ageism can be understood as "the process of systematically stereotyping and being prejudiced against all older individuals because they are old, just as racism and sexism accomplish this for skin color and gender" (Butler, 1995, p. 35). Ageism allows younger generations to see older people as different from themselves; thus they subtly cease to identify with their elders as human beings (Butler, 1995, p. 35). The concept of ageism, first coined by Butler in 1969, was subsequently popularized by Maggie Kuhn, a senior citizen who founded the Gray Panthers to fight against age discrimination after she was forced to retire from her job at the United Presbyterian Church (Ferraro, 1992).

Ageism encompasses two different concepts: *stereotypes* and *age discrimination*. *Stereotypes* are the compilation of ideas and beliefs attributed to people as a group or social category. They may incorporate some characteristics or attributes that accurately describe some people in the group but they always fail to capture the diverse qualities of the individuals in that group. *Age discrimination* refers to behaviors, not just beliefs, toward someone because of their age. Ageism is similar to sexism and racism in that it precludes looking at people as individuals and instead judges people by virtue of their membership in a social category. Currently, the most widely accepted definition of ageism is "prejudice and discrimination against older people based on the belief that aging makes people less attractive, intelligent and productive" (Ferraro, 1992, p. 296).

While all societies classify their members by age and sex and have different expectations for each category, it is argued that Americans have developed a set of prejudices and discriminations against elders that may be unequaled by any other society (Palmore, 1999). Prejudices range from the stereotype that most are senile or live in nursing homes to assumptions about their inability to work, their rigid morality, and supposedly nonexistent sexual lives. Ageism is evidenced in forms of discrimination that range from forced retirement, to the discounting of the opinions of older people by younger ones, to elder abuse.

The stereotyping and myths surrounding aging can, in part, be explained by a lack of knowledge and insufficient contact with a wide variety of older people. Ageism is, further, associated with a deep and profound dread of growing old in a society that values youth (Butler, 1995). Ageism is often perceived as an expedient method for society to relieve itself from the responsibility toward elderly individuals while protecting younger individuals from thinking about things they fear such as aging, illness, and death.

SCOPE

The last ten years have witnessed an increasing public and academic interest and concern with ageism in the United States. The most likely explanation for this recent concern revolves around the "aging of America." As the number of older individuals grows at a faster rate than the fertility rate, not just in the United States but in all industrialized nations including Japan, issues such as retirement, income security, and medical care have risen to the forefront. Further, as evidenced in the 2000 election, individuals over 65 are perceived as holding immense political power. While in 1900 just 4.1 percent of all Americans were 65 or older, by 2000 that figure had gone up to 12.8 percent and is expected to rise to 20 percent by 2030.

Two factors have contributed to this immense increase in the population of elderly: the aging of the cohort commonly referred to as the "baby boomers" as well as the growing longevity of the elderly. The end of World War II initiated a period of unprecedented economic prosperity which stimulated the greatest population spurt in the 20th century and led to the baby boom. Between 1946 and 1964, after which the birth rate began declining again, more than 75 million children were born—70 percent more than the number born in the preceding two decades (Siegel, 1993). At the peak of the baby boom in 1958, 4.2 million children were born in a single year compared to only 0.3 million in any year during the Great Depression (Congressional Budget Office, 1993). Today 4 out of every 10 Americans belong to the baby boom generation. The aging of the baby boomers is coinciding with another significant population trend: greater longevity among the very old. Between 1950 and 1994, the proportion of people aged 85 and over grew from 590,000 to 3.5 million, an increase of more than 600 percent. By 2040 the 85 and older population will

quadruple in size to nearly 14 million (Hobbs & Damon, 1996). Thus, the 21st century will be characterized by an unprecedented trend in history: older people will outnumber the number of births in all industrialized nations.

Costs

The costs of ageism are difficult to calculate, and the total is also related to individual values. The loss of productivity of retired workers who could and would contribute to the gross national product if there were no discrimination is difficult to quantify. However, approximately 5.4 million Americans 55 or older report that they are willing and able to work, but do not have jobs (Palmore, 1999). If 4 million of these individuals could contribute to the economy at about $15,000 per worker, this would amount to about $60 billion a year in gained productivity. One of the most significant consequences of ageism is the cost to the elderly populations themselves, brought on by residential segregation, disengagement of organizations, and unnecessary institutionalization. Further, it is impossible to estimate the loss of emotional involvement, knowledge, cultural traditions, expertise, and the actual experiences of aging that elderly individuals are unable, because of social and cultural constraints, to share with younger generations.

THEORIES AND RESEARCH

According to numerous authors, the elderly have been considered a social problem in the United States throughout the 20th century (Haber, 1994). From a historical perspective, ageism is explained by the intersection of economic changes with social institutions. Since the beginning of the century, the elderly have gone from being perceived as productive workers within society to a nonproductive status because of institutionalized retirement. Other developments include the move from an agricultural society where people were self-employed to an industrialized service oriented society where individuals were working for others, and the enormous growth in the number of older persons in more recent years. At times, societal changes have also profoundly affected elderly women and minorities to an even greater extent than older white men.

Issues of ageism can best be understood from a *social constructionist* perspective. Proponents of social constructionism do not perceive society as a set of structures distinct from people. Rather this view places humans as active agents who create the society in which they live. Individuals interpret their own experiences within this context. A social constructionist approach to ageism looks at the "situational, emergent and constitutive features of aging" and how social meanings of age arise change over time (Passuth & Bengtson,

1988, p. 3345; Lynott & Lynott, 1996). Seen through this perspective, ageism is a dynamic concept that changes over time and context.

Since the mid-1940s, researchers have concerned themselves with the issue of aging in the United States. Most early studies focused on the perceptions and stereotypes of the general public of older workers with the goal being to modify younger adults' perceptions of older individuals, as well as determining public support for older adults. More recently, ageism is being understood as undermining an older adult's sense of self-worth and that over time, the constant application of terms such as "senile" or "useless" or "disagreeable" to those over the age of 65 becomes a self-fulfilling prophecy (Palmore, 1999, p. 104). Many Americans, surrounded by an influx of these concepts, find the prospect of growing old, very unattractive. Retirement at 65 is for many the social boundary at which we regard individuals as having now begun the "formal" aging process. Thus, there is a certain dread that is associated with formal retirement when combined with the many negative images of aging in our society.

Issues of ageism can be related, in part to public policies with respect to the elderly (Binstock, 1996). For the most part, American public polices have been based on the concept of "compassionate ageism" (that the elderly are poor, frail, and deserving). Since 1978, this trend of compassion has been reversing itself. Now older individuals are often portrayed as being fairly well off, politically powerful, and selfish. Further, they are being scapegoated as draining the economy as younger generations try to solve societal problems, especially those related to health care costs. One repercussion was the creation of the 1985 Americans for Generational Equity Commission which sought to protect the country's economic resources for future generations by pointing out trends arising from the aging of the population. Concepts that are metaphors for this "equity" include justice between age groups, long-term care, increasing dependency ratios, and the political power of the aged (Binstock, 1992).

Ageism is related to a variety of demographic and economic factors in American society. However, research indicates that the most pervasive influence related to ageism is the mass media (Featherstone & Hepworth, 1990). Media documents the cultural resources our society draws upon to give meaning to old age and to shape societal customs. Negative stereotyping of the elderly exists in all forms of media including advertising, television, movies, children's books, magazines and even basic primary school readers (Vasil & Wass, 1993). Recent studies on the role of advertising illustrate that negative stereotypes were associated with increased age while positive stereotypes are more associated with younger adults (Hummert, 1994). Further, it was found that negative generalizations of older people used in

advertising actually harm the self-perception of older people, and distort the attitudes of the rest of society toward older adults. Supporters of this form of media argue that ageism is socially constructed and reflects society's perception of the elderly. When combined with a youth-oriented consumer culture, aging becomes necessarily unattractive, characterized by images that are weak, dependent, and nonsexual.

Similar issues arise in analysis of aging and the television industry. While television has become the most common source of entertainment and information in the world, depictions of the elderly have not changed. Already in the seventies, a variety of studies analyzed the relationship between depictions of aging and television (Vasil & Wass, 1993). They found that television perpetuated the myth of the "boring older adult whose inner life is unworthy of interest" and therefore not worth representing. More recent studies have found that the same perceptions as well as a lack of representation of older adults persisted in the nineties; less than 3 percent of all television characters depicted the elderly. Furthermore, men over 65 tended to be much more likely to be characterized as "middle aged" with jobs and an aura of respect. On the other hand, women over the age of 65 did not work outside the home and were usually depicted as "elderly" instead of middle aged as were the male characters. Elderly minorities were not at all depicted in the television industry, an extension of their lack of representation throughout the media. Ironically, all of these same studies reveal that the cohort with the highest television news usage was the "old old" who are often limited in their ability to be mobile and may use television as a means of keeping up with society. Thus, a negative television orientation toward the elderly potentially further influences the morale and increases both the health and security concerns of older adults.

Aspects of ageism also predominate in medical research, especially issues of health in older women. For example, although aging women predominate in terms of numbers, most medical research is based on male health problems and issues. Older women's health issues are further compounded by the tendency in a male-dominated society for women to be considered primarily as sexual objects which places them under constant pressure to appear young and attractive. This stress is thought to contribute to their health problems in later years. Additional physical and psychological stress comes from the societal expectation for women to be nurturers and caretakers for aging men (Culpepper, 1993).

STRATEGIES THAT WORK

Since the concept of ageism was introduced in the 1940s, there have been some gains on the part of the elderly. Perhaps most relevant in terms of public policy is the Age

Discrimination and Employment Act of 1967, amended in 1978, which ended mandatory retirement in the federal government and advanced it to age 70 in the private sector. In part, this policy has allowed for an increasing variability in the scheduling of work careers and work exits and in the pathways from work to retirement (O'Rand and Henretta, 1999). Further, there have been some societal advances in, and more attention to, the productive capabilities of older people as well as a stronger understanding that older individuals have satisfying personal and sex lives (Butler, 1995). The depiction of older people as "senile" because of problems of memory is being replaced by an understanding of the profound and most common form of what is popularly referred to as "senility," Alzheimer's disease. Senility is not seen any longer as an inevitable part of the aging experience, but instead as a disease or part of a group of diseases.

Until recently, knowledge about aging in the general public was limited to the role of older workers in the society. However, there is considerable evidence that interest in all aspects of aging among the general public, the mass media, the government, and academia is rapidly growing. Legislation and programs for the elderly have multiplied during the past 30 years. Further courses on aging in colleges and universities have quadrupled over the last 20 years. Studies of the effect of such courses have determined that the understanding of aging among young people before and after completing a course in gerontology, as well as projects that bring young people and the elderly together, changes age bias (Aday, 1996). These findings suggest that increased knowledge and exposure to elderly individuals work towards greatly reducing ageism. Further, there are dozens of contemporary books that address the subject of aging, many of them preoccupied with the concept of "positive aging" or, more recently, "successful aging." The proliferation of such books can be understood as attempts to counter the negativism of ageism to which the public is exposed on a day-to-day basis (Rowe and Kahn, 1998).

STRATEGIES THAT MIGHT WORK

There are several current trends that if continued will work to reduce ageism in our society: the increasing knowledge and research about aging; the increasing health and education of elders; the decreasing poverty of older adults; the growing federal austerity and the reductions of racism and sexism (Palmore, 1999).

Another significant trend to combat ageism has been the growing scientific research on aging. The Gerontological Society of America has grown from a few hundred members in the early 1960s to about 6,000 members currently. Also, there has been a proliferation of gerontological professional journals and books on the topic. This research has worked to combat ageism in two ways. First, it has served to dispel some of the myths that surround the biological aspects of aging by uncovering the scientific facts associated with the aging process. For example, a large body of research is dedicated to distinguishing between the normal aspects of aging in contrast with the consequences of disease and illness, as well as illustrating that aging is not as awful as is implied by negative stereotypes (Manton, Corder, & Stallard, 1993; Rowe and Kahn, 1998; Wetle, 1991). Second, the research has helped alert the general population how diseases of old age can be prevented or treated, how the aging process, itself can be slowed and longevity extended, and in a general way how to improve the quality of life for the elderly (Palmore, 1999). All of these factors increase general knowledge about aging and the elderly and work to reducing negative prejudice toward the aged.

Ageism is also being combated on a more macrolevel by actual biological changes in the elderly. As a large part of the scientific research on aging, through the extension of better medical care to all sectors of society through Medicare and Medicaid, and through an increasing emphasis in American society on preventive healthcare as well as healthier life styles, the elderly are becoming healthier. Further, in comparison to the existence of disabilities in the rest of the population, disabilities among those 65 and over have been steadily declining (Manton et al., 1993). This is serving to dispel the stereotype that aging causes disease, physical disabilities, and senility.

Not to be discounted are widespread societal changes that are affecting every sector of the population including the elderly. Increasingly, our society is becoming more literate. Literacy among elders has jumped from a minority in 1900 to more than 98 percent by 1989. This trend has reduced the generational education gap and challenges the stereotype of the illiterate or poorly educated older person. Also, it contributes to decreasing poverty, and aids in the acquisition of more wealth and high-level occupations among the elderly. While at the turn of the century the elderly represented the poorest group in our society, today there is less poverty among elders than among other groups in our society, and elders receive a disproportionately larger share of the national personal income (Palmore, 1999).

Another deterrent to ageism comes from declining racism and sexism in our society. Although, there have been many challenges to combating racism and sexism, there is general agreement that there has been much improvement over the last fifty years. These reductions contribute to combating ageism in significant ways. As a society we have become more aware of prejudice and discrimination in general and therefore are less likely to approve of it in other spheres. Further, legislation designed to stop racism and sexism may also have similar effects on ageism.

Despite all of these positive trends, there is little empirical evidence about actual reductions of ageism in our culture. Some studies claim that the last decade has witnessed a steady improvement in the attitudes toward the aged as a result of expanded education and increased media attention (Feathersone and Hepworth, 1990; Ferraro, 1992). Yet, this has been accompanied by a "new ageism" that envies the elderly for their economic progress and at the same time presents the poor elderly as being a tax burden and the non-poor elderly for draining Social Security. As images of the elderly as rich and powerful spread, it may be possible that this will result in a backlash where federal programs for the elderly are concerned. Nonetheless, given the growing size of the elderly population and their political power, this seems unlikely at the present time.

The greatest threat to ageism then remains in the potential of intergenerational conflict. As younger people may question some of the benefits that go to the elderly, elders may get defensive about their special privileges and attack anyone who may question them. Current special programs for elders will require a larger and larger portion of the government's budget, and younger people may rebel against this growing burden. Such a conflict would encourage a rapid growth in ageism, both among younger and older cohorts (Schlesinger & Kronebusch, 1994).

STRATEGIES THAT DO NOT WORK

Clear evidence is not yet available.

SYNTHESIS

Ageism is an increasingly significant issue because of the rapidly growing number of older people both in the United States and all other industrialized nations. Ageism costs us in terms of personal, economic, social, and cultural costs as well as violating basic democratic principles. The primary goal in describing aspects of ageism in American society is to reduce prejudice and discrimination toward the elderly. Ageism needs to be approached through developing both individual as well as societal strategies.

Age integration may be the single best strategy to bringing about a shift in attitudes and behaviors toward the elderly. Age integration would prevent one's age from determining entry, exit, and performance in education, work, and retirement. Age integration would reduce the structural lag that is created from the faster growth of the older population and would provide useful social roles for individuals of all ages. It would allow many individuals in their later years to be productive assets rather than burdens on the economy.

Furthermore, it would provide wider options for shaping the entire life course, reduce middle-aged burdens of work and family, protect against ageism, and enhance health and well-being that comes from all types of sustained active participation (Riley & Riley, 1994).

Many of the strategies that have been successful in reducing racism and sexism could also potentially be used to reduce ageism. Examples of individual actions include educating people about aging, avoiding ageist language or jokes, writing letters to editors and officials, boycotting, and voting for candidates opposed to ageism are potential means for eliminating ageism. In order to stimulate institutional changes, organized actions could include gathering and disseminating information about aging, lobbying for legislation opposed to ageism, legal actions, grievance procedures, boycotts, rent strikes, political campaigns, and passive resistance (Palmore, 1999). Further, organizations such as the American Association of Retired People (AARP) represent an important step in providing information about aging and aging-related services to the elderly themselves.

The uniqueness of old age as a stage in the life cycle of every human being must be recognized by all. The aged, in contrast to every other minority group, draw their entire population from the young who have been socialized as majority group members to accept negative stereotypes and feelings about old age. Yet, all individuals must be educated to recognize the inevitability of their own aging, and the recognition that they will ultimately benefit from whatever changes occur in the status of the elderly.

Also see: Crisis Intervention: Older Adulthood; Health Promotion: Older Adulthood; Life Challenges: Older Adulthood.

References

Aday, R. (1996). Changing children's perception of the elderly: The effects of intergenerational contact. *Gerontology and Geriatrics Education, 16*, 37–51.

Binstock, R. (1992). The oldest old and "intergenerational equity." In R. Suzman, D. Willis, & K. Manton (Eds.), *The oldest old*. New York: Oxford University Press.

Binstock, R. (1996). Continuities and discontinuities in public policy and aging. In V. Bengtson (Ed.), *Adulthood and aging* (pp. 308–324). New York: Springer.

Butler, R. (1995). Ageism. In G. Maddox (Ed.), *Encyclopedia of aging*. New York: Springer.

Congressional Budget Office. (1993). *Baby boomers in retirement: An early perspective*. Washington, DC: US Government Printing Office.

Culpepper, E. (1993). Ageism, sexism, and health care: Why we need old women in power. In G. Winslow & J. Walters (Eds.), *Facing limits: Ethics and health care for the elderly*. Boulder, CO: Westview Press.

Feathersone, M., & Hepworth, M. (1990). Images of ageing. In J. Bond & P. Coleman (Eds.), *Aging in society*. Newbury Park, CA: Sage.

Ferraro, K. (1992). Cohort changes in images of older adults. *The Gerontologist, 32*, 293–304.

Haber, C. (1994). And the fear of the poorhouse: Perceptions of old age impoverishment in Elderly Twentieth-century America. In D. Shenk & W. Achenbaum (Eds.), *Changing perceptions of aging and the aged* (pp. 75–84). New York: Springer.

Hobbs, F., & Damon, B. (1996). *65+ in the United States*. Washington, DC: US Bureau of the Census.

Hummert, M. (1994). Stereotypes of the elderly held by young, middle-aged and elderly adults. *Journal of Gerontology: Psychological Science, 49*, 249–250.

Lynott, R., & Lynott, P. (1996). Tracing the course of theoretical development in the sociology of aging. *The Gerontologist, 36*, 749–760.

Manton K., Corder, L., & Stallard, E. (1993). Estimates of change in chronic disability and institutional incidence and prevalence rates in the US elderly population from the 1982, 1984, and 1989 National Long Term Care Survey. *Journal of Gerontology, Social Sciences, 47* (Suppl.), S153–S166.

O'Rand, & Henretta, A.J. (1999). *Age and inequality. diverse pathways through later life*. Boulder, CO: Westview Press.

Palmore, E. (1999). *Ageism: negative and positive*. New York: Springer.

Passuth, P., & Bengtson, V. (1988). Sociological theories of aging: Current perspectives and future directions. In J. Birren & V. Bengtson (Eds.), *Emergent theories of aging* (pp. 333–355). New York: Springer.

Riley, M., & Riley, J. (1994). Age integration and the lives of older people. *The Gerontologist, 34*, 110–114.

Rowe, J., & Kahn, R. (1998). *Successful aging*. New York: Pantheon Books.

Schlesinger, M., & Kronebusch, K. (1994). Intergenerational tensions and conflict: Attitudes and perceptions about social justice and age-related need. In V. Bengtson & R. Harootyan (Eds.), *Intergenerational linkages: Hidden connections in American Society*. New York: Springer.

Siegel, J. (1993). *A generation of change: A profile of America's older population*. New York: Russel Sage Foundation.

Vasil, L., & Wass, H. (1993). Portrayal of the elderly in the media: A literature review and implications for educational gerontologists. *Educational Gerontology, 19*, 71–85.

Wetle, T. (1991). Successful aging: New hope for optimizing mental and physical well-being. *Journal of Geriatric Psychiatry, 24*, 3–21.

Aggressive Behavior, Childhood

Douglas C. Smith and Michael J. Furlong

INTRODUCTION

On a cold, windy morning in February in a suburb just outside Flint, Michigan, a six-year-old student at Buell Elementary School, armed with a .32-caliber handgun he had taken from his uncle's nightstand, shot and killed his first-grade classmate. According to some of his classmates and his teacher, the youngster had quarreled with the girl the previous day and was still angry on the day of the shooting. His motive was to exact revenge (APBnews.com, 2000).

Although serious acts of violence committed by children, such as the one described above, are exceedingly rare events, they represent a frightening awareness of the extent to which even very young children are capable of harmful and even lethal aggressive behavior when they have access to destructive weapons. Despite widely held perceptions of a rising tide of violence among children and youth, both in the United States and abroad, statistical data indicate a significant decline in serious acts of violence on school campuses and in surrounding communities (Dwyer, Osher, & Warger, 1998; US Departments of Education and Justice, 2000). Much more common, however, are less serious forms of aggression including teasing, bullying, fighting, and intimidation. This entry provides an overview of the development and manifestation of aggressive behavior in childhood with special emphasis on the prevention of such behaviors.

DEFINITIONS

Our focus is on common and relatively "normal" forms of aggressive behavior in childhood rather than on serious acts of violence. For purposes of this entry, *aggression* is defined as behavior that is intended to harm or injure another. The harm may be physical, social, emotional, or material. Some theorists (Dodge & Coie, 1987) have distinguished between *reactive* and *proactive* aggression or, in other words, aggression that occurs as an impulsive reaction to frustrating events versus aggression that is more carefully orchestrated to obtain a specific outcome. Other researchers (Crick & Grotpeter, 1995) have distinguished *physical* from *relational* aggression, the latter being designed to harm social relationships through exclusion, gossip, and spreading of negative "rumors." Such a distinction is thought to characterize one of the major differences between male and female forms of aggression in childhood and adolescence.

SCOPE

Data regarding the prevalence of so-called "low level" aggressive behavior among children are difficult to obtain, partially due to problems associated with accurate data collection, namely reliance upon children's self-reports. To overcome this, some researchers have relied upon reports from adults, particularly teachers, to understand the frequency, type, and intensity of aggressive behavior among young children.

Studies of the prevalence and incidence of aggressive behavior in childhood are further complicated by the different forms and functions of aggressive behavior during this age period (Coie & Dodge, 1998). Throwing tantrums, for example, is the most prevalent form of aggression during infancy and toddlerhood, occurring quite frequently in a sizeable proportion of children in response to discomfort or a need for attention. With the emergence of language, incidents of verbal aggression increase during the preschool years and then stabilize over time. As peer conflicts and conflicts over material possessions increase during early childhood, acts of physical aggression tend to increase, particularly among boys. During the elementary years, most children display fewer acts of aggression but a select few children become highly troublesome to both peers and adults. A form of childhood aggression experienced by elementary-age children is bullying that occurs in and out of school (Juvonen & Graham, 2001). As many as one in five children report being a chronic victim of a bully over time (Pellegrini, Bartini, & Brooks, 1999).

There is substantial evidence for the stability of different forms of aggressive behavior over time (Haapasalo & Tremblay, 1994; Olweus, 1979) and the fact that early patterns of aggressive behavior predict different manifestations of violence later in life including domestic violence, assault, and other criminal activities (Farrington, 1994). Loeber and Stouthamer-Loeber (1998) have pointed out, however, that a significant proportion of children decrease their overall prevalence of aggression from preschool to elementary school and from elementary school to middle school. Only those students manifesting more serious forms of aggressive behavior at an early age tend to continue to be aggressive in later years.

THEORIES AND RESEARCH

Contemporary models of aggressive behavior recognize that multiple factors operate in a cumulative and reciprocal fashion to promote aggression in children. Among these factors are the child's temperament, personal, and social skills, emotional intelligence, association with deviant peers, family functioning level, parents' child-rearing skills, school climate, and other community and ecological variables. Explanatory models of childhood aggression differ in the extent to which they ascribe primary influence to one or more of the above factors. In addition, these models seek to explain the stability of aggressive behavior over time and individual differences in aggression as a product of culture, gender, or ethnicity. Three major models of childhood aggression include the *social learning*, *information processing*, and *cognitive–neoassociationistic* models.

Social Learning

The social learning model, typified by the approach of Patterson and colleagues at the Oregon Social Learning Center (Patterson, Reid, & Dishion, 1992), places primary emphasis on the reciprocal nature of parent–child interactions in development of aggressive behavior. According to this view, it is within the context of everyday social exchanges between family members that verbal and physical patterns of aggression are learned. Such learning occurs through parental modeling of overly harsh, coercive, and inconsistent discipline tactics including use of physical punishment. The reciprocal nature of this interaction is illustrated by the ongoing development of a "coercive family process" in which a child's initial and subsequent noncompliance with parental demands may be met by more and more "extreme" measures to achieve compliance. As the child's resistance to such measures increases, there is a tendency on the part of parents to use even more coercive, aggressive strategies in an effort to gain compliance or, alternatively, to give in to the child's noncompliance. In either case, the child perceives aggression as an effective tactic for controlling others and reducing aversive events. At the same time, there is less opportunity for learning and practicing more prosocial and adaptive problem-solving skills.

Social learning theory has a long and established history in fostering research on children's aggression. From Bandura's (1973) early work on the influence of live models on aggressive expression to more contemporary approaches emphasizing multiple and reciprocal learning pathways, social learning theory continues to exert a powerful influence on our understanding of aggressive behavior. Recent research suggests that much of children's antisocial behavior can be accounted for by family process variables such as communication and discipline styles (Haapasalo & Tremblay, 1994; Hawkins, Herrenkohl, Farrington, Brewer, Catalano, & Harachi, 1998). These findings are consistent with Patterson's coercive family process model in which harsh parental discipline is reported to be the single best predictor of aggressive behavior in children (Patterson et al., 1992). From a social learning perspective, parents' modeling of aggressive behavior serves to encourage and legitimize similar behaviors in their children, which are then further reinforced by positive social outcomes (Bear, Webster-Stratton, Furlong, & Rhee, 2000).

Parents are not the only source, however, by which the potential advantages of aggressive behavior may be demonstrated to children. Social learning theory also serves to explain the powerful influence of media violence upon children's behavior. Both laboratory and naturalistic studies conducted over the past quarter of a century support the proposition that children's viewing of aggressive models on television leads to increases in the child's own level of aggression (Paik & Comstock, 1994; Wood, Wong, & Chachere, 1991). In addition, a recent review of the effects of media violence exposure on youth aggression shows that the strength of this relationship is nearly as strong as the link between tobacco smoking and lung cancer (Bushman & Anderson, 2001).

Effects of television violence upon aggressive behavior in children is mediated by a number of factors including the salience and status of the televised model, the consequences of the modeled aggression, and the context in which the modeling is viewed (Federman, 1998). Viewing violence in mass media sources can have multiple effects depending on the traits of the viewer and the perpetrator and victims (Furlong, Pavelski, Klein, Elliott, & Ko, 1999). Research has shown that youth with aggressive tendencies are more likely than their peers to watch shows with violence and that this viewing is more likely to prime them for aggression.

Information Processing

The information processing model places primary emphasis on the role of social-cognitive factors in the development of children's aggressive behavior. Based primarily on the work of Crick and Dodge (1994), aggressive behavior is seen to result from systematic biases in the processing and understanding of social cues and behaviors. At an interpretive level, chronically aggressive children are often thought to misperceive the intentions of others in social situations. This may take the form of hostile attributional biases in which others' neutral social behaviors are viewed as intentionally harmful. On the basis of such perceptions, protective or retaliatory aggressive behavior is therefore justifiable. Aggression is thus viewed as an appropriate response to the harmful intentions of others.

In addition to cognitive distortions and misperceptions, aggressive children are also subject to other types of information processing deficits that limit their ability to handle interpersonal situations in socially constructive ways. For example, aggressive children as a group tend to be limited in their ability to generate alternative solutions to interpersonal conflicts (Shure & Spivack, 1982). Aggression is viewed as a quick and simple solution to perceived challenges and this strategy is often reinforced by positive outcomes, including compliance by others. Finally, aggressive children are also less likely to consider the needs and feelings of others in social interactions. Moral reasoning among aggressive children tends to be highly hedonistic in perspective, focusing on immediate self-serving gains, rather than on the needs of others or on long-term consequences for the self (Goldstein, Glick, & Gibbs, 1998).

Research in support of social-cognitive deficits in children's processing of interpersonal events leading to aggression has focused on three interrelated processes. These include empathy, cognitive attributions, and interpersonal problem solving.

Empathy is defined as the ability to understand the feelings of others. Young children are notoriously egocentric in their ability to take the perspectives of others, which extends to understanding feelings. As children develop cognitively and socially, most acquire a heightened awareness of others' perceptions, thoughts, and feelings across a range of social situations. A growing body of research suggests that aggressive children are less proficient in understanding the perspectives of others than their nonaggressive peers (Chandler, 1973; Hudley, 1994). Children who tend to be highly empathic, on the other hand, engage in more altruistic and prosocial behaviors in school and other naturalistic settings. There is also evidence to suggest that children can acquire perspective-taking skills through direct training and instruction, and acquisition of such skills may result in less aggressive behavior toward peers (McGinnis & Goldstein, 1997).

Attributions are causal inferences that occur spontaneously in the course of understanding interpersonal events. Attributions with regard to the behavior of others are based upon selective encoding of a variety of situational and behavioral cues. Aggressive children, as a group, are more likely than their nonaggressive peers to attribute hostile intent to others in ambiguous social situations. For example, when asked to imagine themselves as the victim of an ambiguous provocation (e.g., a peer spills water on you), aggressive children are more likely to interpret the act as intentionally malicious. These interpretations serve to justify aggressive retaliation. Hostile attributional biases have been found to characterize the perceptions of a wide range of aggressive children differing in age, ethnicity, and severity of aggressive behavior (Hudley, Britsch, Wakefield, Smith, Demorat, & Cho, 1998).

The third area of social cognition, *interpersonal problem-solving*, has also stimulated considerable research comparing aggressive and nonaggressive children (Shure & Spivack, 1982). When faced with social problems, challenges, and conflicts, aggressive children tend to be limited in the number of solutions they can generate for solving these problems. Not only are these children deficient in the range of alternatives available for resolving conflicts, the types of solutions endorsed appear to be inferior to those of nonaggressive peers. For the most part, aggressive children tend to endorse atypical and maladaptive tactics for resolving conflicts with others. Not surprisingly, aggressive children value aggression, viewing it as an appropriate response and one usually supported by positive outcomes.

Cognitive–Neoassociationist

The cognitive–neoassociationist view of anger and aggression, based primarily on the work of Berkowitz (1993), places emphasis on patterns of association between previously experienced negative emotions such as anger and frustration and specific hostile thoughts and aggressive reactions. According to this model, emotions are the primary determinant of one's aggressive behavior, although certain cognitive processes such as self-regulation and control may mediate this relationship. Although sharing some common themes with social-cognitive models of aggressive behavior, the cognitive–neoassociationist view is important in its implications for understanding links between children's aggression and such variables as hormone levels, prior exposure to violence, and noxious environmental conditions such as overcrowding and high temperatures.

Research based on a cognitive–neoassociationist perspective of children's aggression has focused primarily on the construct of impulse control and particularly the role of anger in aggressive behavior. There is considerable research supporting the relationship between anger and aggression in child, adolescent, and adult samples (Furlong & Smith, 1994). Anger has also been related to a variety of other negative outcomes including poor school performance, rejection by peers, mental health problems, and alcohol and substance abuse (Cautin, Overholser, & Goetz, 2001; Grunbaum, Vernon, & Clasen, 1997; Musante & Treiber, 2000; Musante, Treiber, Davis, Waller, & Thompson, 1999). High levels of anger may signify emotional reactivity (e.g., "hot-headed") that frequently translates into reactive aggression. Impulsivity and reflectivity are opposite poles of what many would consider a personality style or trait. A reflective style is manifested in a logical, systematic, and "mindful" approach to problem solving. Rapid, inconsistent, and unorganized thinking and behavior, on the other hand, characterize impulsivity. Both impulsivity and hyperactivity are significant predictors of antisocial behavior in childhood (Hawkins et al., 1998).

STRATEGIES: OVERVIEW

Aggressive behavior in early childhood assumes many different forms and takes place in multiple contexts. Likewise, causal factors can be varied and multiplicative reflecting the complexity of understanding individual differences in the expression of aggression. Given these considerations, the distinction between prevention and early intervention of aggressive behavior is often unclear. Thus, for those children who might already be involved in teasing peers at school, a specific intervention might be designed to reduce the frequency of that particular behavior while at the same time preventing the escalation of teasing into more serious forms of aggression such as threats or physical harm.

STRATEGIES THAT WORK

Given the multiple pathways through which aggressive behavior develops in youth and the many factors that contribute both to its inhibition and disinhibition, effective prevention and intervention must necessarily be comprehensive, broadly applied, and developmentally focused. Programs meeting these criteria tend to include multiple treatment components such as individual skill building, family training, and environmental reorganization delivered across multiple contexts including home, school, and community. In this section, we begin with a brief overview of two examples of such programs followed by a more detailed analysis of specific program components that have been evaluated independently as contributing to prevention or reduction of aggressive behaviors.

Multifaceted Comprehensive Programs: Families and Schools Together

FAST Track (Bierman, Greenberg, & Conduct Problems Prevention Research (CPPR) Group, 1996) is a comprehensive, multicomponent primary prevention and early intervention program targeting students in grades 1–5 who are at-risk for development of aggressive behavior. The school-based portion of the program focuses on teaching students effective conflict resolution/interpersonal problem-solving skills, emotional competence (including empathy, communication), and prosocial skills. This is supplemented by teacher training in classroom management, remedial academic instruction for students, and consultation involving counselors, psychologists, and other mental health professionals. The home-based portion of the program includes parent education and modeling and training of appropriate interpersonal skills for both students and their families.

Evaluation of the FAST Track program with a large sample of first-grade students enrolled at multiple sites across the United States indicated decreases in peer ratings of aggressive behavior as well as observed improvements in overall classroom environment as a result of participation in the program (CPPR Group, 1999a). A separate study examining the effects of FAST Track on a sample of high-risk students already exhibiting behavioral problems at school (CPPR Group, 1999b) concluded that the program was effective in improving interpersonal cognitive skills (e.g., problem-solving, emotional regulation) and reducing aggressive–disruptive behaviors. As a result, relationships with both parents and peers improved based on multiple outcome measures.

Another comprehensive program aimed at preventing/reducing childhood aggression is the *Second Step Program* (Committee for Children, 1991) designated by the Safe, Disciplined, and Drug-Free Schools Expert Panel (US Department of Education, 2000) as one of nine exemplary violence-prevention curriculums. Second Step provides a schoolwide curriculum for elementary and middle school students focusing on developing skills related to empathy, impulse control, social problem-solving, assertiveness, and anger management. Independent controlled studies of Second Step (Grossman et al., 1997) indicate significant reductions in aggressive behaviors among children participating in the program.

Although both FAST Track and Second Step are comprehensive, multicomponent programs, each includes key components that have been independently evaluated as effective in prevention and reduction of aggressive behavior in children. These are (a) parent/family-based interventions and (b) cognitive–behavioral skills training.

Parent- and Family-Based Interventions

These approaches focus on helping parents develop better communication and conflict resolution skills and also educate parents about child development and factors that may contribute to aggressive behavior (US Department of Education, 2000). Research indicates that the earlier these family-based interventions begin, the more effective they are in reducing aggression (Webster-Stratton & Hancock, 1998). Successful, family-based interventions are individualized, culturally sensitive, home-based, and involve parents directly in planning goals and establishing an intervention plan. These strategies are designed to increase parents' sense of self-control and feelings of efficacy (Webster-Stratton & Hancock, 1998).

The program developed by Patterson et al. (1992) teaches parents prosocial behaviors, alternatives to aggression as a discipline strategy, and problem-solving skills. In addition, parents are taught to nurture and communicate effectively with children, to establish and negotiate family rules and consequences, and to reward prosocial behavior. The model has been shown to be effective in reducing family conflict and increasing a sense of family unity.

Cognitive–Behavioral Skills Training

Cognitive–behavioral skills training focuses on helping children analyze and respond to challenging social situations. Two major focal points of these efforts have been on impulse control and social problem solving.

Kendall and his associates have conducted extensive research on the role of impulsivity in children's aggressive behavior (Kendall, 1991; Kendall & Braswell, 1993). As a group, aggressive children tend not to think through the consequences of their behavior prior to acting. Based on these findings, Kendall and colleagues designed a series of activities to teach children self-control through verbal self-instruction (e.g., "what am I supposed to do?" and "how am I doing?"). These efforts are geared toward helping children restrain the tendency to respond without reflecting on the

situation at hand. Evaluation of this and similar programs suggest that impulse control is an acquired skill and can be an important deterrent to aggression.

Nowhere is the link between impulsivity and aggressive behavior more evident than in the experience and expression of anger. School- and clinic-based anger management programs for children have proliferated in recent years. Because anger is conceptualized as a multidimensional construct including affective, cognitive, and behavioral dimensions, most of these programs include multiple prevention and treatment components. In a review of anger management programs for youth, Smith, Larson, DeBaryshe, and Salzman (2000) found that the most successful programs included emotion-focused strategies such as relaxation, increased self-awareness and awareness of the feelings of others; cognitive strategies such as problem-solving and self-regulation; and behavioral strategies such as developing specific skills in communication and assertiveness. Slightly more than half of the anger management programs reviewed included elements designed to enhance maintenance and generalization of trained skills such as written homework assignments. As a group, school- and clinic-based anger management programs for youth appear to exert a strong influence on the control and regulation of aggressive behavior.

Social problem-solving training is designed to help students recognize interpersonal conflict situations, increase their repertoire of problem-solving strategies, analyze and evaluate the consequences of various actions, and select and implement socially appropriate solutions (Goldstein, 1999). Most programs utilize modeling, role-playing, and didactic instructional methods to teach problem-solving skills. The goal of such programs is to build positive peer relations by helping children learn to avoid interpersonal conflict and to handle those conflicts that are unavoidable in nonviolent, socially appropriate ways. One of the best known social problem-solving programs for young children is *I Can Problem Solve: An Interpersonal Cognitive Problem-Solving Program* (Shure, 1992; Spivack & Shure, 1974). A related program based on an information processing model is the *BrainPower* program (Hudley, 1994), which is designed to change hostile attributional biases among aggressive children. Evaluation of the program indicated increased self-control and fewer judgments of hostile intent in a sample of 3rd–6th grade boys (Hudley et al., 1998).

STRATEGIES THAT MIGHT WORK

Social and Emotional Skill Building

In a comprehensive review of prevention strategies designed to enhance social and emotional competence,

Weissberg and Greenberg (1998) discuss a range of competence-enhancement strategies for elementary age students. The major goal of such programs is "to teach children to make use of both personal and environmental resources to achieve prosocial goals" (p. 890). Because aggression is viewed primarily as a learned behavior, it can be unlearned and thus prevented by acquisition of more prosocial and positive behaviors. Hawkins, Catalano, Kosterman, Abbot, & Hill (1999) suggest that healthy bonding of children to adults, peers, and institutions that promotes healthy beliefs and prosocial attitudes is likely to result in adoption of similar views. There is growing national support for comprehensive, kindergarten through grade 12 health education that (a) emphasizes personal and social skills training; (b) promotes positive social values and health attitudes; and (c) provides honest, relevant information about health issues including violence. To date, there have been no controlled, longitudinal field experiments to evaluate the long-term effects of K to 12 social competence and health-promotion programs.

Structural/Ecological Approaches

These approaches seek to prevent aggressive behavior by establishing a school climate fostering respect for the rights of others, positive social relationships, and peaceful resolution of interpersonal conflict. By establishing school norms supporting prosocial actions toward others, the goal is to reduce the occurrence of aggressive behavior running contrary to these norms. The *Resolving Conflict Creatively Program* (DeJong, 1999) is one example of such an ecological approach that incorporates a classroom and schoolwide-value system of nonviolence. Another example is the *Peacemakers Program* (Johnson & Johnson, 2000) for students in grades 4–8 that incorporates a violence prevention curriculum in the classroom and seeks to infuse a nonviolence ethic into the entire school culture. Evaluation of this program with 1,400 students in Cleveland indicated significant decreases in aggressive incidents and subsequent disciplinary actions. More work is needed to determine the long-term effects of such ecological interventions and their applicability to students from varying backgrounds, cultures, and ethnic groups.

SYNTHESIS

Longitudinal research clearly indicates that, left undeterred, aggressive behavior in early childhood often continues unabated into later stages of childhood, adolescence, and beyond. Even if such children are not arrested for a violent crime, the quality of their interpersonal relationships

may suffer. The more serious the form of early aggression, the more likely is this pattern to occur. What then can be done to prevent the formation of early patterns of aggressive behavior in childhood? Our review of research in this area suggests a number of principles that should be considered "best practices" for prevention of aggressive behavior during childhood.

First, and most importantly, prevention efforts must begin early and include multiple components delivered across multiple settings (minimally the home and school). In the home setting, early intervention means implementing programs that engage parents in their child's education at as early a date as possible. These programs provide the context in which to disseminate effective parenting skills to all and to focus attention on parents who may be locked in a cycle of coercive child disciplinary practices. At the school level, early intervention means targeting low levels of aggressive behavior such as teasing and bullying and simultaneously establishing a school climate that reinforces positive social behaviors. Given the multiple pathways through which aggressive behavior develops in young children, it is imperative that successful prevention and intervention efforts target both individual and contextual components and that these efforts take place in the home, school, and larger community, whenever possible.

And what are the recommended strategies for preventing aggressive behavior in young children? At the individual level, available data suggest that cognitive–behavioral strategies offer the most promise with specific training in impulse control and interpersonal problem solving receiving the most empirical support. Anger management appears to be a particularly fruitful intervention direction within the broader context of cognitive–behavioral treatment. These programs seek to prevent and/or reduce the occurrence of aggressive behavior by teaching children to recognize and utilize internal cues, develop a more reflective problem-solving style, and promote usage of alternatives to aggression. Given the pervasiveness of aggression in the typical school, comprehensive aggression management programs should be a key component of all student support services plans.

At the family level, parent education and training focused on improving communication skills and fostering authoritative parenting styles appear to offer considerable promise. Gottman and DeClaire (1997) have written about the prospect of training parents as "emotional coaches" in an effort to provide more nurturing and supportive family relationships. Emotional coaches are empathetic and accepting of their children's negative emotions but guide the child in generating and choosing positive response strategies while setting limits for acceptable behavior. Programs that involve parents and help them to initiate authoritative, not authoritarian discipline practices at home have the greatest potential to reinforce the long-term reduction of a child's aggressive behaviors.

Finally, successful prevention of children's aggression means not only seeking to reduce negative affect and behaviors but also fostering higher levels of social and emotional competence. All programs need to attend to the fundamental issue of providing a positive reason for NOT being aggressive. Encouragement of prosocial behavior such as cooperation and respect, self-awareness, and empathy is the foundation for pursuing the ultimate objective of raising competent, caring, and compassionate human beings.

Also see: Anger Regulation: Childhood; Bullying: Childhood; Family Strengthening: Childhood; Peer Relationships: Childhood; Violence Prevention: Childhood; Delinquency: Childhood.

References

APBnews.com (2000, March 6). *Counselors ease fears over first-grade shooting.* [Online]. Available: www.apbnews.com/safetycenter/family/2000/03/06/kidshoot0306pm_01/html.

Bandura, A. (1973). *Aggression: A social learning analysis.* Englewood Cliffs, NJ: Prentice-Hall.

Bear, G.G, Webster-Stratton, C., Furlong, M.J., & Rhee, S. (2000). Preventing aggression and violence. In K. Minke & G. Bear (Eds.), *Preventing school problems—Promoting school success* (pp. 1–69). Bethesda, MD: National Association of School Psychologists.

Berkowitz, L. (1993). *Aggression: Its causes, consequences, and control.* New York: McGraw-Hill.

Bierman, K.L., Greenberg, M.T., & Conduct Problems Prevention Research Group. (1996). Social skills training in the FAST Track Program. In R. DeVPeters & R.J. McMahon (Eds.), *Preventing childhood disorders, substance abuse, and delinquency* (pp. 65–89). Thousand Oaks, CA: Sage.

Bushman, B.J., & Anderson, C.A. (2001). Media violence and the American public: Scientific facts versus media misinformation. *American Psychologist, 56,* 477–489.

Cautin, R.L., Overholser, J.C., & Goetz, P. (2001). Assessment of mode of anger expression in adolescent psychiatric inpatients. *Adolescence, 36,* 163–170.

Chandler, M. (1973). Egocentrism and anti-social behavior: The assessment and training of social perspective-taking skills. *Developmental Psychology, 9,* 326–332.

Coie, J.D., & Dodge, K.A. (1998). Aggression and antisocial behavior. In N. Eisenberg (Ed.), *Handbook of Child Psychology* (Vol. 3, pp. 779–862). New York: John Wiley.

Committee for Children. (1991). *Second Step: A violence prevention curriculum.* Seattle, WA: Author.

Conduct Problems Prevention Research Group. (1999a). Initial impact of the FAST Track prevention trial for conduct problems: II. Classroom effects. *Journal of Consulting and Clinical Psychology, 67,* 648–657.

Conduct Problems Prevention Research Group. (1999b). Initial impact of the FAST Track prevention trial for conduct problems: I. The high-risk sample. *Journal of Consulting and Clinical Psychology, 67,* 631–647.

Crick, N.R., & Dodge, K.A. (1994). A review and reformulation of social-information-processing mechanisms in children's social adjustment. *Psychological Bulletin, 115,* 74–101.

Crick, N.R., & Grotpeter, J.K. (1995). Relational aggression, gender, and social-psychological adjustment. *Child Development, 66,* 710–722.

DeJong, W. (1999). *Building the peace: The Resolving Conflict Creatively Program.* Washington, DC: National Institute of Justice.

Dodge, K.A., & Coie, J.D. (1987). Social-information-processing factors in reactive and proactive aggression in children's peer groups. Special Issue: Integrating personality and social psychology. *Journal of Personality and Social Psychology, 53,* 1146–1158.

Dwyer, K., Osher, D., & Warger, C. (1998). *Early warning, timely response: A guide to safe schools.* Washington, DC: US Department of Education.

Farrington, D.P. (1994). Childhood, adolescent, and adult features of violent males. In L.R. Huesman (Ed.), *Aggressive behavior: Current perspectives* (pp. 215–240). New York: Plenum.

Federman, J. (1998). *National Television Violence Study* (Vol. 3). Thousand Oaks, CA: Sage.

Furlong, M.J., Pavelski, R., Klein, J., Elliott, K., & Ko, S. (1999). The effects of media violence on children and adolescents. *Journal of Children's Legal Rights, 19,* 33–42.

Furlong, M.J., & Smith, D.C. (Eds.). (1994). *Anger, hostility, and aggression in youth: Assessment, prevention, and intervention strategies for youth.* New York: John Wiley.

Goldstein, A.P. (1999). Aggression reduction strategies: Effective and ineffective. *School Psychology Quarterly, 14,* 40–58.

Goldstein, A.P., Glick, B., & Gibbs, J.C. (1998). *Aggression Replacement Training: A comprehensive intervention for aggressive youth* (Rev. ed.). Champaign, IL: Research Press.

Gottman, J., & DeClaire, J. (1997). *The heart of parenting: Raising an emotionally intelligent child.* New York: Simon & Schuster.

Grossman, D.C., Neckerman, H.J., Koepsell, T.D., Liu, P.-Y., Asher, K.N., Beland, K., Frey, K., & Rivara, F.P. (1997). *Journal of the American Medical Association, 277,* 1605–1611.

Grunbaum, J.A., Vernon, S.W., & Clasen, C.M. (1997). The association between anger and hostility and risk factors for coronary heart disease in children and adolescents: A review. *Annals of Behavioral Medicine, 19,* 179–189.

Haapasalo, J., & Tremblay, R.E. (1994). Physically aggressive boys from age 6 to 12: Family background, parenting behavior, and prediction of delinquency. *Journal of Consulting and Clinical Psychology, 62,* 1044–1052.

Hawkins, J.D., Catalano, R.F., Kosterman, R., Abbot, R., & Hill, K.G. (1999). Preventing adolescent health-risk behaviors by strengthening protection during childhood. *Archives of Pediatrics and Adolescent Medicine, 153,* 225–234.

Hawkins, J.D., Herrenkohl, T., Farrington, D.P., Brewer, D., Catalano, R.F., & Harachi, T.W. (1998). A review of predictors of youth violence. In R. Loeber & D.P. Hawkins (Eds.), *Serious & violence juvenile offenders: Risk factors and successful interventions* (pp. 106–146). Thousand Oaks, CA: Sage.

Hudley, C.A. (1994). The reduction of childhood aggression using the BrainPower Program. In M. Furlong & D. Smith (Eds.), *Anger, hostility, and aggression: Assessment, prevention, and intervention strategies for youth.* New York: John Wiley.

Hudley, C.A., Britsch, B., Wakefield, W.D., Smith, T., Demorat, M., & Cho, S. (1998). An attribution retraining program to reduce aggression in elementary school students. *Psychology in the School, 35,* 271–282.

Johnson, D.W., & Johnson, R.T. (2000). *Teaching students to be Peacemakers: Results of twelve years of research* [Online]. Available: http://www.clcrc.com/pages/peace-meta.html.

Juvonen, J., & Graham, S. (2001). *Peer harassment at school: The plight of the vulnerable and victimized.* Thousand Oaks, CA: Sage.

Kendall, P.C. (1991). Guiding theory and therapy for children and adolescents. In P. Kendall (Ed.), *Child and adolescent therapy: Cognitive behavioral procedures* (pp. 3–22). New York: Guilford Press.

Kendall, P.C., & Braswell, L. (1993). *Cognitive-behavioral therapy for impulsive children* (2nd ed.). New York: Guilford Press.

Loeber, R., & Stouthamer-Loeber, M. (1998). Development of juvenile aggression and violence: Some common misconceptions and controversies. *American Psychologist, 53,* 242–259.

McGinnis, E., & Goldstein, A.P. (1997). *Skillstreaming the elementary school child: New strategies and perspectives for teaching social skills.* Champaign, IL: Research Press.

Musante, L., & Treiber, F.A. (2000). The relationship between anger-coping styles and lifestyle behaviors in teenagers. *Journal of Adolescent Health, 27,* 63–68.

Musante, L., Treiber, F.A., Davis, H.C., Waller, J.L., & Thompson, W.O. (1999). Assessment of self-reported anger expression in youth. *Assessment, 6,* 225–234.

Olweus, D. (1979). Stability of aggressive reaction patterns in males: A review. *Psychological Bulletin, 86,* 852–857.

Paik, H., & Comstock, G. (1994). The effects of television violence on antisocial behavior: A meta-analysis. *Communication Research, 21,* 516–546.

Patterson, G.R., Reid, J.B., & Dishion, T.J. (1992). *A social interactional approach IV: Antisocial boys.* Eugene, OR: Castalia.

Pellegrini, A.D., Bartini, M., & Brooks, F. (1999). School bullies, victims, and aggressive victims: Factors relating to group affiliation and victimization in early adolescence. *Journal of Educational Psychology, 91,* 216–224.

Shure, M.B. (1992). *I Can Problem Solve: An interpersonal cognitive problem-solving program.* Champagne, IL: Research Press.

Shure, M.B., & Spivack, G. (1982). Interpersonal cognitive problem solving in young children: A cognitive approach to prevention. *American Journal of Community Psychology, 10,* 341–356.

Smith, D.C., Larson, J., DeBaryshe, B., & Salzman, M. (2000). Anger management for youth: What works and for whom? In D.S. Sandhu & C. Aspy (Eds.), *Violence in American schools: A practical guide for counselors* (pp. 217–230). Reston, VA: American Counseling Association.

Spivack, G., & Shure, M.B. (1974). *Social adjustment of young children: A cognitive approach to solving real life problems.* San Francisco: Jossey-Bass.

US Department of Education. (2000). *The expert panel on safe, disciplined and drug-free schools searching for best programs.* Washington, DC: Safe & Drug-Free Schools Program [Online]. Available: http://www.ed.gov/offices/OESE/SDFS/programs.html

US Departments of Education and Justice. (2000). *2000 annual report on school safety.* Washington, DC: Authors.

Webster-Stratton, C., & Hancock, L. (1998). Training for parents of young children with conduct problems: Content, methods, and therapeutic processes. In J. Briesmeister & C.E. Schaefer (Eds.), *Handbook of parent training: Parents as co-therapists for children's behavior problems* (pp. 98–152). New York: John Wiley.

Weissberg, R.P., & Greenberg, M.T. (1998). School and community competence-enhancement and prevention programs. In I.E. Sigel & K.A. Renninger (Eds.), *Handbook of child psychology* (Vol. 4, pp. 877–954). New York: John Wiley.

Wood, W., Wong, F.Y., & Chachere, J.G. (1991). Effects of media violence on viewers' aggression in unconstrained social interaction. *Psychological Bulletin, 109,* 371–383.

Aggressive Behavior, Adolescence

Melinda G. Schmidt, Carrie S. Fried, and N. Dickon Reppucci

INTRODUCTION

According to the US Department of Justice, the juvenile arrest rate for violent crimes has fallen 36 percent since its peak in 1994, and the juvenile murder rate is at its lowest level since the 1960s (Snyder, 2000). However, efforts to combat adolescent aggression and violence are just now beginning to realize their potential. Research focusing on the identification and confirmation of risk factors for aggression and violence has been the basis for a number of prevention programs (Bliesener & Loesel, 1992). Few studies have explored potential protective factors, however, thus limiting the scope of prevention efforts (Bliesener & Loesel, 1992; Farrington, 1998). This is no small oversight; according to Farrington (1998), "protective factors may have more implications than risk factors for prevention and treatment" (p. 451).

This entry begins by highlighting important definitional issues and outlining the theories that underlie risk- and protective-based prevention programs. Following this, it reviews risk and potential protective factors for aggression and violence and describes promising prevention programs that successfully capitalize on protective factors to buffer risks for aggression and violence. The entry concludes with a synthesis of ideas for future research directions and prevention efforts.

DEFINITIONS

Prevention programs are often designed to simultaneously target both aggression and violence. Although the terms are often used interchangeably, *aggression* refers to the intent to hurt or gain advantage over others, without necessarily involving physical attack, whereas *violence* involves the use of physical force against another individual (Megargee, 1982). Researchers modeling developmental pathways toward violent behavior have deemed early aggression as one of the leading predictors for later violence (Loeber & Hay, 1994).

A number of researchers have identified factors that put youth at increased risk for exhibiting aggressive or violent behavior. However, ambiguity surrounding the definition of protective factors has complicated their identification.

Although researchers continue to disagree about the best way to define a protective factor for study, three general definitions have been established (Farrington, 1998). The first is that a protective factor is merely the opposite of a risk factor; thus, if low intelligence is a risk factor, high intelligence is a protective factor. The second is that protective factors may be free-standing, having no corresponding risk factor; thus, while the presence of such a factor would serve a protective benefit, its absence would not constitute a risk. Third, protective factors may be variables that interact with (buffer) risk factors to minimize their negative effects.

THEORIES

An accumulation of individual risk factors is presumed to increase the likelihood of eliciting violence or aggression, especially when coupled with multiple cultural, societal, and immediate systems level risk factors. Other factors may protect or buffer against these risks, although little research has explored potential protective factors for aggression, delinquency, and violence. Only in the last 20 years has the potential power of protective factors begun to entice researchers. This is largely due to the groundbreaking work of Garmezy and Neuchterlein (1972) and Werner and Smith (1982), whose early studies of children at risk uncovered small groups of children who grew up to be resilient adults despite their disadvantaged upbringings. Studies of these resilient children resulted in the identification of three general types of protective factors: (a) a positive disposition or likeable temperament; (b) a warm, emotionally supportive family; and (c) a source of external support (e.g., a teacher or neighbor) who rewards the child's competencies and determination (Garmezy, 1993). Risk and protective factors can be characterized under the same headings: (a) individual; (b) immediate systems; and (c) societal level factors.

RESEARCH

Individual-Level Risk Factors

At the individual level, biological, cognitive, and emotional factors contribute to the development of violence and aggression. Because the focus of this entry is on the prevention of aggression in adolescence, only those factors that are malleable in adolescence are discussed.

Cognitive precursors to aggression and violence include low IQ, reading problems, attention deficits, and hyperactivity (Farrington, 1989; Loeber, 1988). Although IQ is not in itself a very malleable factor, its associated risks may be more amenable to change. For example, Lynam, Moffitt, and Stouthamer-Loeber (1993) found that low IQ contributes to delinquency through its effect on school performance; so, youth with cognitive deficits experience school failure, which in turn contributes to delinquency. Poor school performance is also linked to high truancy rates and a high number of school transitions between the ages of 12 and 16, both of which are predictive of self-reported violence in late adolescence and early adulthood (Hawkins, Herrenkohl, Farrington, Brewer, Catalano, & Harachi, 1998).

Research indicates that aggressive adolescents have more social cognitive deficiencies (Crick & Dodge, 1994), lower moral reasoning maturity (Arbuthnot, Gordon, & Jurkovic, 1987), and poorer abstract reasoning and problem-solving skills (Seguin, Pihl, Harden, Tremblay, & Boulerice, 1995) than non-aggressive youth. An individual's cognitive appraisal of an event is a major factor in determining the subsequent behavioral response. Crick and Dodge (1994) found that aggressive children selectively attend to aggressive cues, are more likely to attribute hostile intent to others, generate fewer solutions to problems and select action-oriented rather than reflective solutions.

Immediate Systems-Level Risk Factors

The immediate systems-level factors with which the individual has direct contact that are associated with adolescent aggression and violence include neighborhood, school, peer group, and family.

Although not all poor neighborhoods experience high rates of violence, many do. Economically stressed neighborhoods share other characteristics such as transient populations and disorganization that make violence and aggression more prevalent (Hawkins et al., 1998). High levels of mobility make it more difficult for residents to develop support networks and feel a sense of attachment to the community (American Psychological Association Commission on Violence, 1993). In violent neighborhoods, children witness high levels of shootings, stabbings, and killings (Jenkins & Bell, 1994), which has an effect on the development of aggression in children (Widom, 1989).

Some consider the family to be the most powerful single influence on development of aggression and violence (McGuire, 1997). The influence of child-rearing practices on the development of an array of problem behaviors, including aggression, has received considerable attention. Coercive interactions (Capaldi & Patterson, 1996), lax and ineffective parental discipline (Weiss, Dodge, Bates, & Pettit, 1992), poor parental monitoring (Gorman-Smith, Tolan, Zelli, & Huesmann, 1996), physical punishment (Eron, Huesmann, & Zelli, 1991), and child physical abuse (Manly, Cicchetti, & Barnett, 1994) are all associated with higher rates of aggression and violence among adolescents.

However, it is unclear whether parenting practices cause aggressive behavior, or whether aggressive behaviors lead to harsh and ineffective parenting styles. The effects of parenting strategies appear to be mediated through the quality of the parent–child relationship. Lack of maternal warmth (Booth, Rose-Krasnor, McKinnon, & Rubin, 1994), insecure attachment (Erickson, Sroufe, & Egeland, 1985), and parental indifference and rejection (Farrington, 1991) have all been associated with increased levels of aggression in adolescence. Adolescents who grow up in homes characterized by high levels of family conflict and family violence are at increased risk for becoming aggressive. Exposure to parents' marital conflict is predictive of self-reported violence in adolescence (Elliott, 1994).

Unlike adults, juveniles commit most violent and serious delinquent acts in the company of peers rather than alone (Zimring, 1998). The process of association with aggressive and antisocial peers begins at a young age with rejection by prosocial peers (Coie, Dodge, & Kupersmidt, 1990). Lack of strong social ties or low satisfaction with peer group membership have been shown to be predictive of aggressiveness and delinquency in adolescence (Bender & Loesel, 1997; Lipsey & Derzon, 1998). Peer rejection leads to increased aggression and antisocial activity, and promotes association with antisocial peers (Dishion, Patterson, Stoolmiller, & Skinner, 1991). Deviant, rejected children gravitate toward each other and form their own "coercive cliques" (Cairns, Cairns, Neckerman, Gest, & Gariepy, 1988), in which aggression is valued and deviant behaviors are promoted. Other non-deviant adolescents may be attracted to the glamour of these delinquent peer groups, which may contribute to the late onset of aggression in adolescents with no prior history of delinquency or aggression (Moffitt, 1993). Several longitudinal studies have found strong positive correlations between association with delinquent peers in early adolescence and self-reported violence in late adolescence or early adulthood (Farrington, 1989).

Although violence in schools is a reflection of the community where the school is located, relations between school characteristics and aggressive behaviors exist even after controlling for neighborhood crime rates. Aggressive and violent behaviors are more likely to occur in schools with greater percentages of students who do not place a high value on good grades and do not think their school experience will have a positive influence on their lives (National Research Council, 1993). Low student attendance, high student–teacher ratios, instability in the school population, and poor academic quality of the school also characterize schools with higher rates of aggression and violence (Hellman & Beaton, 1986). Aggressive and violent behavior is more likely to occur in schools with lax enforcement of rules and undisciplined classrooms (National Research Council, 1993). It is unclear whether high rates of school violence and aggression cause or are caused by the discipline practices of the school.

Societal- and Cultural-Level Risk Factors

The high rates of adolescent aggression and violence in the United States compared to other industrialized nations make it difficult to ignore the societal and cultural factors that have contributed to the problem. These include poverty, violence in the media, accessibility of firearms, and societal abuse of drugs and alcohol. Reducing the impact of these factors would probably decrease adolescent aggression and violence, and these risks should be incorporated into multifaceted prevention programs as much as possible; however, identifying successful prevention programs that address each of these factors individually is beyond the scope of this entry.

This brief overview of risk factors associated with adolescent aggression and violence only skims the surface as there is an abundance of research available. However, what is not known is what combinations and weights of factors produce the greatest probability of increasing the likelihood of aggressive and violent behavior.

Individual-Level Protective Factors

Several potentially malleable individual-level protective factors have been identified which may be amenable to use in prevention strategies. For example, cognitive social problem-solving skills have been shown to have protective effects in the face of risk (Parker, Cowen, Work, & Wyman, 1990). In addition, resilient adolescents appear to have greater self-control, more compassion, greater attachment to others (Born, Chevalier, & Humblet, 1997), and better coping skills and higher self-esteem than their deviant peers (Bliesener & Loesel, 1992). According to Feshbach (1997), empathy may also serve as a protective factor, functioning as a coping skill in reaction to stress and inhibiting aggressive behavior.

Jessor, VanDenBos, Vanderryn, Costa, and Turbin (1995) found that intolerant attitudes toward deviant behavior, positive orientation to school, perceived regulatory controls, and perceptions of friends' modeling of prosocial behaviors had a moderating protective effect on the relationship between risk factors and adolescent problem behaviors (including delinquency). High self-efficacy (Rutter, 1985) and positive motivation (Loeber, Stouthamer-Loeber, VanKammen, & Farrington, 1991) also appear to have protective effects.

Immediate Systems-Level Protective Factors

The family, peer group, and school environments have the potential to offer protective effects. Although a limited number of studies have examined protective effects of the family environment, these studies clearly support positive family relations as mitigators of the negative effects of deviant peers (Borduin & Schaeffer, 1998). Findings from the National Longitudinal Study on Adolescent Health (Resnick et al., 1997) demonstrated that parent/family connectedness protected adolescents against a variety of risk behaviors, including violence. Similarly, using data from the Seattle Social Development Project (SSDP), Williams (1994) found that positive parent–child communication and high parental involvement during adolescence served to protect against violent behavior in later adolescence. Even more clearly, Poole and Rigoli (1979) found that if conditions of low family support existed, then involvement with delinquent peers was strongly predictive of antisocial behavior, but under conditions of high family support, such involvement with delinquent peers was only slightly predictive.

In addition to warm, supportive relationships, parenting skills such as discipline and monitoring offer protective effects. Dishion et al. (1991) found that high levels of parental discipline skill and monitoring buffered the negative effects of child involvement with deviant peers. Bliesener and Loesel (1992) found that resilient children reported having been raised in a less conflictual, more autonomous environment. Finally, Rutter (1985) highlighted positive parental modeling and child-rearing behavior as one of five general protective factors for establishing resilience.

Factors outside the family, such as peer relationships, become increasingly salient as both predictors of and protectors from aggressive and problem behaviors during adolescence. Getting along well with others, having a larger network of social support, possessing the ability to utilize social support systems, and experiencing greater satisfaction with support received have all been found to demonstrate protective effects against behavioral problems and delinquency in adolescence (Bender & Loesel, 1997; Bliesener & Loesel, 1992).

Elliott (1994) found that associating with peers who are non-approving of delinquent behavior protects against serious delinquency in adolescence. Similarly, perceptions of friends' modeling of prosocial behavior was found to protect against problem behaviors in adolescence (Jessor et al., 1995). According to Quinton, Pickles, Maughan, and Rutter (1993), good peer relationships may even mitigate the negative effects of poor family relationships if peers offer social support and model positive behaviors.

Finally, having a positive orientation to school, feeling connected to school, and being a good student have all been linked to the protection of adolescents from engaging in risk behaviors such as violence (Jessor et al., 1995; Resnick et al., 1997).

Societal-Level Protective Factors

Although societal-level protective factors per se have yet to be delineated, the importance of collective efficacy and full community involvement in reinforcing individual- and immediate-systems level protective factors cannot be overemphasized. In order to capitalize most effectively on the protective effects of individual, family, peer, and school factors in preventing negative outcomes in adolescence, a multitude of agencies, institutions, and persons must work together at the community level.

STRATEGIES THAT WORK

Although a number of prevention programs for adolescent aggression, delinquency, and violence have been initiated in recent years, relatively little emphasis has been placed on evaluation and identification of effective strategies. Moreover, many of these programs are targeted to elementary rather than middle or high school age youths. Among the most promising prevention programs for adolescents are those that take a comprehensive public health approach in enhancing protective factors and targeting multiple risk factors across a variety of settings (Loeber & Farrington, 1997). Other features of effective programs include individualized attention, community-wide multi-agency collaboration, location of programs both within and outside of schools, and engagement of peers and involvement of parents (Lerner & Galambos, 1998). Furthermore, Rutter (1985) has suggested that the potential for protection against aggressive and problem behavior lies in prevention programs that help youths develop interpersonal qualities that foster positive and adaptive interactions with others, and Howell and Hawkins (1998) have noted that programs that promote school functioning may also reduce behavioral problems in adolescence. A few promising prevention programs in several arenas are highlighted here.

Conflict Resolution and Social Skills Training

Prevention programs focusing on *conflict resolution strategies* have demonstrated reductions in aggression and violence as well as chronic school absence, suspension, and vandalism (Crawford & Bodine, 1996). Conflict resolution exists as a stand-alone prevention program or as the cornerstone piece of broader, multifaceted prevention programs targeting aggression and problem behaviors in adolescence, and may be approached as a city-wide, school-wide, classroom-focused, or distinct (outside or inside school) curriculum. Research suggests that to be effective in reducing aggressive behaviors, conflict resolution programs must be based on proven negotiation theory translated into easy-to-use instructional curricula (Crawford & Bodine, 1996). Skills enhanced by conflict resolution programs include a number of protective factors: empathy, respect for self and others, self-control, anger management, effective communication of emotions, and problem solving.

Created in the 1960s, Teaching Students to be Peacemakers is one example of a successful conflict resolution program which has grown and developed through the interaction of theory, research, and practice (Johnson & Johnson, 1996). The Peacemakers Program encourages constructive resolution of conflicts through implementation in grades 1–12 of a school-wide, age-based, guided curriculum focusing on cooperation, understanding, problem solving, negotiation, peer mediation, and continuous reinforcement of conflict resolution skills. Extensive evaluation of the program has shown that following implementation, participants knew and were able to apply conflict resolution techniques both within and outside of school. In addition, the number of discipline problems requiring teacher involvement decreased significantly. Moreover, students who received the training in the context of an English literature unit (in which negotiation and mediation strategies were applied to the dynamics of characters in a novel) showed increased academic achievement compared to a control group who read the novel without the integration of conflict resolution training (Johnson & Johnson, 1996). Thus, the protective effect of school achievement was also reinforced.

A similar curriculum implemented in grades 6–8 in Orange County, North Carolina, involving a combination of conflict resolution and peer mediation training was equally successful. During three 50-minute classroom periods, a trainer from the county's Dispute Settlement Center taught 391 middle-school students about components of conflict resolution including individuality, power, anger, self-control, and fighting fair. In addition, nine teachers were trained in conflict resolution theory. Twenty-six student mediators chosen by their peers were also trained in peer mediation during the course of four, 4-hr trainings that emphasized listening, communication, and questioning skills through the use of games, role-playing, and videos. The program was especially successful with sixth-grade students, resulting in an 82 percent drop in disciplinary referrals to the principal's office, a 42 percent drop in in-school suspensions, and 97 percent drop in out-of-school suspensions (Powell, Muir-McClain, & Halasyamani, 1995).

Other conflict resolution programs which have been evaluated with positive results include School Mediator Alternative Resolution Team (S.M.A.R.T.), and a cooperative learning and conflict resolution program initiated by the Columbia Teachers College. The S.M.A.R.T. program

resulted in a 45–70 percent reduction in suspensions for fighting during its first year within five of the six New York City high schools in which it was implemented (Lam, 1989). In the Columbia Teacher's College program, students trained by researchers in conflict resolution in an alternative high school in New York City demonstrated greater ability to manage conflict, experienced greater social support, less victimization, increased self-esteem and feelings of personal control, and improved academic achievement, all protective factors for aggressive behavior (Deutsch et al., 1992).

Related to conflict resolution programs, *social skills training* (SST) programs aim to prevent aggression and violence through training in problem solving, awareness-building, and prosocial interpersonal skills. SST programs have been successful in reducing aggressive behaviors and increasing self-esteem in boys identified as socially aggressive (Lochman, Curry, Burch, & Lampron, 1994). Moreover, culturally sensitive SST programs such as Positive Adolescents Choices Training (PACT; Yung & Hammond, 1998), targeted at African American adolescents aged 12–16, have also shown promise. PACT is a cognitive–behavioral training program designed to enhance African-American adolescents' skills in problem identification, problem solving and negotiation, and anger reduction using culturally relevant videotapes about provocative situations. Evaluation of the PACT curriculum demonstrated its success at improving in-school behavior as well as decreasing involvement with the juvenile court. Compared to youths referred on similar criteria who did not receive the training, youths receiving the PACT curriculum demonstrated a significant reduction in physically aggressive incidents at school both during the course of training and beyond the point at which the curriculum had been completed. Moreover, aggressive behavior in the control group typically remained the same or worsened (Yung & Hammond, 1998). Postintervention, youths receiving the PACT curriculum had lower levels of involvement with the juvenile court, fewer violence-related charges, and fewer arrests than the untrained youth even after 2 years. A 3-year follow-up indicated that middle-school students randomly assigned to 20 hr of PACT training had a significantly lower juvenile court referral rate than did the control group (18 vs. 49 percent) (Yung & Hammond, 1998).

Although they may be efficacious as independent curricula, conflict resolution and social skills training programs are likely to be most useful when embedded within well-funded, comprehensive, community-based programs. Moreover, even greater gains may be achieved by combining these programs with elements of prevention programs which successfully address other risk and protective factors for aggression and violence.

STRATEGIES THAT MIGHT WORK

Violence and Delinquency Prevention

A number of broad-based violence and delinquency prevention programs have been initiated in schools and communities across the United States, the elements of which have produced varying levels of success. Self-Enhancement, Inc. (SEI; Gabriel, Hopson, Haskins, & Powell, 1996) is a Portland, Oregon, community-service organization that focuses on adolescents in high-risk communities. The SEI program has several components, including: (a) classroom education, focusing on anger management, conflict resolution, and problem solving; (b) exposure education, consisting of visits to agencies and organizations that deal with the causes and consequences of violence in the community; and (c) proactive education, involving the production of newsletters, assemblies and conferences, and radio and television public service announcements that communicate antiviolence messages. The model is based on the premise that building resilience in youth from disadvantaged backgrounds will help them progress to healthy and productive lives. SEI focuses on three critical protective factors in building resiliency: (a) fostering relationships with a caring, supportive adult; (b) providing adolescents with opportunities for involvement in meaningful activities and decision-making; and (c) having high expectations for the behavior of the youth in the program. Participants included 102 African American students who were referred by teachers, based on poor attendance, academic, or behavior problems. After one year of participation in the program, participants demonstrated decreases in self-reports of fighting and carrying a weapon, whereas control youths did not demonstrate changes in either behavior.

Given the popularity of video games and electronic media among adolescents, Bosworth, Espelage, DuBay, Daytner, and Karageorge (2000) highlighted the potential for widespread impact of computer-based interventions to prevent aggression and violence. They evaluated SMART Talk, a multimedia violence prevention program for adolescents consisting of three components: (a) anger management, (b) perspective taking, and (c) dispute resolution. Results indicated that the multimedia program increased middle-school students' intentions to use nonviolent strategies and decreased their beliefs supportive of violence, although no significant changes in the frequency of aggressive behavior over time were found.

Use of mass media is another violence prevention strategy. Results from the Violence Prevention Project (VPP; Hausman, Spivak, & Prothrow-Stith, 1995), a multifaceted program initiated in two Boston neighborhoods, demonstrated that exposure to a mass media campaign against violence was the most efficacious program component, increasing adolescents' knowledge and attitudes about violence after one year.

Although broad-based violence and delinquency prevention curricula aimed at adolescents appear to have potential for success in schools and communities, there remains a relative dearth of outcome data other than self-report and attitudes. Evaluations of behavioral changes are necessary before the efficacy of such programs can truly be known.

Mentoring

Mentoring programs have produced contradictory results. Building on the protective capacity of social support, a number of mentoring programs have been established across the country in the last decade; unfortunately, most evaluations suggest that they are largely unsuccessful at accomplishing long-term positive effects on adolescent behavior problems. Rhodes' (1994) explanation for this lack of success is that the answers to questions such as what makes a good mentor, what a mentoring relationship should be like, and what outcomes may reasonably be expected from mentoring lack thorough theoretical development. Darling, Hamilton, and Niego (1994) also underscore the difficulty of both implementation and evaluation of mentoring programs. Despite these obvious weaknesses, the Office of Juvenile Justice and Delinquency Prevention's 1998 Report to Congress on juvenile mentoring (Bilchik, 1998) demonstrated that youths involved in mentoring programs were less likely to be aggressive, experiment with drugs, or skip school. Further examination of the potential of mentoring programs in preventing aggression is warranted.

Volunteerism

Primary prevention programs that include a volunteerism component have been shown to have a positive effect on adolescent behavior. Theoretically, volunteering enhances competencies in adolescents, which may increase their resistance to such behaviors as aggression and violence (Allen, Philliber, & Hoggson, 1990). In addition, adolescents are able to try new roles and take on adult-like responsibilities. According to Moffitt (1993), the lack of adult roles and responsibilities may be responsible for attracting adolescents to the glamor of delinquent behavior. Through their interactions with adult supervisors, adolescent volunteers may be more likely to identify with more prosocial values (Allen, Leadbeater, & Aber, 1990) and establish relationships with adult role models.

Two well-designed evaluations of school-based volunteerism programs, the Teen Outreach Program and the Valued Youth Program, provide the best evidence that volunteerism may be the most promising aggression prevention intervention available in adolescence (Moore & Allen, 1996). The Teen Outreach Program provides volunteer opportunities for junior high and high-school students, along with classroom-based discussions of age-appropriate issues and an opportunity to reflect on the volunteer experience. An eight-year longitudinal evaluation of the Teen Outreach Program in several states demonstrated that participating students, relative to comparison students, had an 8 percent lower rate of school suspension, a 33 percent lower rate of pregnancy, and a 50 percent lower rate of school dropout (Moore & Allen, 1996). The Valued Youth Program provided middle-school students with the opportunity to serve as tutors to younger children in the community. Results from a 2-year evaluation indicate that, compared with a control group of non-tutors, the tutors were less likely to drop out of school (1 percent of the tutors vs. 12 percent of the control group) (Cardenas, Harris, del Refugio Robledo, & Supik, 1991). Because the Teen Outreach and Valued Youth programs were designed to prevent pregnancy and/or school dropout, measures of aggression were not collected. However, remaining in school is a protective factor for involvement in aggressive and violent activities, so even if the programs did not have a direct effect on aggression, they may have an indirect effect through their effect on school dropout.

STRATEGIES THAT DO NOT WORK

The search for successful strategies for the prevention of aggression and violence in adolescence has also uncovered several ineffective approaches. Kellerman, Fuqua-Whitley, Rivara, and Mercy (1998) noted that peer group counseling, in which at-risk youths are brought together and encouraged to examine their own behavior, produced no positive effects and had the potential to be counterproductive. Furthermore, supervised after-school programs and vocational training and employment may show promise initially, but demonstrate no persistent positive effects in reducing juvenile offending rates (Kellerman et al., 1998). Finally, despite the overwhelming public support for curfew laws, empirical research has demonstrated that curfews are ineffective in reducing juvenile crime and victimization (Fried, 2001).

SYNTHESIS

According to Weissberg and Greenberg (1998), the most successful primary prevention programs are those that focus not only on improving the adolescent's skills but also on creating positive changes in the environment. Thus, the success of school-based programs such as The Peacemakers Program, S.M.A.R.T., and SMART Talk, might be further enhanced by their integration with community-based interventions such as mass media strategies, mentoring, and volunteer programs. Certainly there remains little doubt that a multifaceted community-based approach to prevention that aims to reinforce protective factors while also targeting risks is likely to be most successful; however, in order to know this with certainty, the evaluation of such broad-based programs is a necessary, albeit challenging, next step (Loeber & Farrington, 1997).

In order to continue the recent downward trend in juvenile aggression and violence, researchers should maintain their efforts to define populations at risk and to identify malleable protective factors on which to capitalize in the development of primary prevention programs. Beyond the identification of such factors, it is also necessary to begin to understand which algorithms of risk and protective factors result in successful prevention. Stated another way, the answer to why some prevention programs work and others don't may lie in the number, combination, and respective weights of risk and protective factors carried by the adolescents targeted for prevention. In order to understand these algorithms, program evaluations should incorporate a pretest/posttest approach. Knowledge of the risk and protective factors held by adolescents at the outset of a prevention program will aid in determining which youths, having which combination of risk and protective factors, benefit most from the program. Moreover, such an approach will offer insights into the mechanisms by which successful programs decrease adolescent aggression and violence. Finally, evaluations must be designed to assess not only whether youths with a particular algorithm of risk and protective factors respond positively to the program, but also whether the individual's protective factors per se are enhanced by the program. Increased knowledge about and enhancement of protective factors will be the key to continued success in the prevention of adolescent aggression and violence.

Also see: Anger Regulation: Adolescence; Delinquency: Adolescence; Family Strengthening: Adolescence; Homicide: Adolescence; Identity Promotion: Adolescence; Life Skills: Adolescence; Peer Relationships: Adolescence; Risk Taking: Adolescence.

References

Allen, J.P., Leadbeater, B.J., & Aber, J.L. (1990). The relationship of adolescents' expectations and values to delinquency, hard drug use, and unprotected sexual intercourse. *Development and Psychopathology, 2*, 85–98.

Allen, J.P., Philliber, S., & Hoggson, N. (1990). School-based prevention of teenage pregnancy and school dropout: Process evaluation of the national replication of the Teen Outreach Program. *American Journal of Community Psychology, 18*, 505–524.

American Psychological Association Commission on Violence. (1993). *Violence and youth: Psychology's response, Vol. 1*. Washington, DC: American Psychological Association.

Arbuthnot, J., Gordon, D.A., & Jurkovic, G.J. (1987). Personality. In H.C. Quay (Ed.), *Handbook of juvenile delinquency* (pp. 139–183). New York, NY: John Wiley.

Bender, D., & Loesel, F. (1997). Protective and risk effects of peer relations and social support on antisocial behaviour in adolescents from multi-problem mileus. *Journal of Adolescence, 20*, 661–678.

Bilchik, S. (1998). *Juvenile mentoring program: 1998 report to congress*. Washington, DC: Office of Juvenile Justice and Delinquency Prevention, US Department of Justice.

Bliesener, T., & Loesel, F. (1992). Resilience in juveniles with high risk of delinquency. In F. Loesel, D. Bender et al. (Eds.), *Psychology and law: International perspectives* (pp. 62–75). Berlin, Germany: Walter De Gruyter.

Booth, C.L., Rose-Krasnor, L., McKinnon, J., & Rubin, K.H. (1994). Predicting social adjustment in middle childhood: The role of preschool attachment security and maternal style. From family to peer group: Relations between relationship systems [Special issue]. *Social Development, 3*, 189–204.

Borduin, C.M., & Schaeffer, C.M. (1998). Violent offending in adolescence: Epidemiology, correlates, outcomes, and treatment. In T.P. Gullotta, G.R. Adams, & R. Montemayor (Eds.), *Delinquent violent youth: Theory and interventions* (pp. 144–174). Thousand Oaks, CA: Sage.

Born, M., Chevalier, V., & Humblet, I. (1997). Resilience, desistance and delinquent career of adolescent offenders. *Journal of Adolescence, 20*, 679–694.

Bosworth, K., Espelage, D., DuBay, T., Daytner, G., & Karageorge, K. (2000). Preliminary evaluation of a multimedia violence prevention program for adolescents. *American Journal of Health Behavior, 24*, 268–280.

Cairns, R.B., Cairns, B.D., Neckerman, H.J., Gest, S.D., & Gariepy, J.L. (1988). Social networks and aggressive behavior: Peer support or peer rejection? *Developmental Psychology, 24*, 815–823.

Capaldi, D.M., & Patterson, G.R. (1996). Can violent offenders be distinguished from frequent offenders?: Prediction from childhood to adolescence. *Journal of Research in Crime and Delinquency, 33*, 206–231.

Cardenas, J.A., Harris, R., del Refugio Robledo, M., & Supik, J.D. (1991, April). Valued Youth Program: Dropout prevention strategies for at-risk students. Paper Presented at the American Educational Research Association Meeting, Chicago, IL.

Coie, J.D., Dodge, K.A., & Kupersmidt, J. (1990). Peer group behavior and social status. In S.R. Asher & J.D. Coie (Eds.), *Peer rejection in childhood* (pp. 17–59). New York, NY: Cambridge University Press.

Crawford, D., & Bodine, R. (1996). Conflict resolution education: A guide to implementing programs in schools, youth-serving organizations, and community and juvenile justice settings. Program report. Washington, DC: Office of Juvenile Justice and Delinquency Prevention, US Department of Justice.

Crick, N.R., & Dodge, K.A. (1994). A review and reformulation of social information processing mechanisms in children's social adjustment. *Psychological Bulletin, 115*, 74–101.

Darling, N., Hamilton, S.F., & Niego, S. (1994). Adolescents' relations with adults outside the family. In R. Montemayor, G.R. Adams, & T.P. Gullotta (Eds.), *Personal relationships during adolescence* (pp. 216–235). Thousand Oaks: Sage.

Deutsch, M., Mitchell, V., Zhang, Q., Khattri, N., Tepavac, L., Weitzman, E.A., & Lynch, R. (1992). *The effects of training in cooperative learning and conflict resolution in an alternative high school*. New York, NY: Columbia University.

Dishion, T.J., Patterson, G.R., Stoolmiller, M., & Skinner, M.L. (1991). Family, school, and behavioral antecedents to early adolescent involvement with antisocial peers. *Developmental Psychology, 27*, 172–180.

Elliott, D.S. (1994). Serious violent offenders: Onset, developmental course, and termination: The American Society of Criminology 1993 presidential address. *Criminology, 32*, 1–21.

Erickson, M.F., Sroufe, L.A., & Egeland, B. (1985). The relationship between quality of attachment and behavior problems in preschool in a high-risk sample. *Monographs of the Society for Research in Child Development, 50*, 147–186.

Eron, L.D., Huesmann, L.R., & Zelli, A. (1991). The role of parental variables in the learning of aggression. In D.J. Pepler & K.H. Rubin (Eds.), *The development and treatment of childhood aggression* (pp. 169–189). Hillsdale, NJ: Erlbaum.

Farrington, D.P. (1989). Early predictors of adolescent aggression and adult violence. *Violence and Victims, 4*, 79–100.

Farrington, D.P. (1991). Childhood aggression and adult violence: Early precursors and later-life outcomes. In D.J. Pepler & K.H. Rubin (Eds.), *The development and treatment of childhood aggression* (pp. 5–29). Hillsdale, NJ: Lawrence Erlbaum.

Farrington, D.P. (1998). Predictors, causes, and correlates of male youth violence. In M. Tonry & M.H. Moore (Eds.), *Crime and justice: A review of research: Vol. 24. Youth violence* (pp. 421–476). Chicago: University of Chicago Press.

Feshbach, N.D. (1997). Empathy: The formative years. Implications for clinical practice. In A.C. Bohart & L.S. Greenberg (Eds.), *Empathy reconsidered: New directions in psychotherapy*. Washington, DC: American Psychological Association.

Fried, C.S. (2001). Juvenile curfews: Are they an effective and constitutional means of combating juvenile violence? *Behavioral Sciences and the Law, 19*, 127–141.

Gabriel, R.M., Hopson, T., Haskins, M., & Powell, K.E. (1996). Building relationships and resilience in the prevention of youth violence. *American Journal of Preventive Medicine, 12*(Suppl. 5), 48–55.

Garmezy, N. (1993). Children in poverty: Resilience despite risk. *Psychiatry, 56*, 127–136.

Garmezy, N., & Neuchterlein, K. (1972). Invulnerable children: The fact and fiction of competence and disadvantage. *American Journal of Orthopsychiatry, 42*, 328–329.

Gorman-Smith, D., Tolan, P.H., Zelli, A., & Huesmann, L.R. (1996). The relation of family functioning to violence among inner-city minority youth. *Journal of Family Psychology, 10*, 115–129.

Hausman, A.J., Spivak, H., & Prothrow-Stith, D. (1995). Evaluation of a community-based youth violence prevention project. *Journal of Adolescent Health, 17*, 353–359.

Hawkins, J.D., Herrenkohl, T., Farrington, D.P., Brewer, D., Catalano, R.F., & Harachi, T.F. (1998). A review of predictors of youth violence. In R. Loeber & D.P. Farrington (Eds.), *Serious & violent juvenile offenders: Risk factors and successful interventions* (pp. 106–146). Thousand Oaks, CA: Sage.

Hellman, D.A., & Beaton, S. (1986). The pattern of violence in urban public schools: The influence of school and community. *Journal of Research in Crime and Delinquency, 23*, 102–127.

Howell, J.C., & Hawkins, J.D. (1998). Prevention of youth violence. In M. Tonry & M.H. Moore (Eds.), *Crime and justice: A review of research: Vol. 24. Youth violence* (pp. 263–315). Chicago: University of Chicago Press.

Jenkins, E.J., & Bell, C.C. (1994). Violence exposure, psychological distress, and high risk behaviors among inner-city high school students. In S. Friedman (Ed.), *Anxiety disorders in African-Americans* (pp. 76–88). New York, NY: Springer.

Jessor, R., VanDenBos, J., Vanderryn, J., Costa, F.M., & Turbin, M.S. (1995). Protective factors in adolescent problem behavior: Moderator effects and developmental change. *Developmental Psychology, 31*, 923–933.

Johnson, D.W., & Johnson, R.T. (1996). Teaching all students how to manage conflicts constructively: The peacemakers program. *Journal of Negro Education, 65*, 322–335.

Kellerman, A.L., Fuqua-Whitley, D.S., Rivara, F.P., & Mercy, J. (1998). Preventing youth violence: What works? *Annual Review of Public Health, 19*, 271–292.

Lam, J. (1989). *The impact of conflict resolution programs on schools: A review and synthesis of the evidence* (2nd ed.). Amherst, MA: National Association for Mediation in Education.

Lerner, R.M., & Galambos, N.L. (1998). Adolescent development: Challenges and opportunities for research, programs, and policies. *Annual Review of Psychology, 49*, 413–446.

Lipsey, M.W., & Derzon, J.H. (1998). Predictors of violent or serious delinquency in adolescence and early childhood: A synthesis of longitudinal research. In R. Loeber & D.P. Farrington (Eds.), *Serious & violent juvenile offenders: Risk factors and successful interventions* (pp. 86–105). Thousand Oaks, CA: Sage.

Lochman, J., Curry, J., Burch, P., & Lampron, L. (1994). Treatment and generalization effects of cognitive-behavioral and goal-setting interventions with aggressive boys. *Journal of Counseling and Clinical Psychology, 52*, 915–916.

Loeber, R. (1988). Behavioral precursors and accelerators of delinquency. In W. Buikhuisen & S.A. Mednick (Eds.), *Explaining delinquency* (pp. 51–67). Leiden, Holland: Brill.

Loeber, R., & Farrington, D.P. (1997). Never too early, never too late: Risk factors and successful interventions for serious and violent juvenile offenders. *Studies on Crime and Crime Prevention, 7*, 7–30.

Loeber, R., & Hay, D. (1994). Developmental approaches to aggression and conduct problems. In M. Rutter & D.F. Hay (Eds.), *Development through life: A handbook for clinicians* (pp. 488–515). Oxford: Blackwell Scientific.

Loeber, R., Stouthamer-Loeber, M., VanKammen, W.B., & Farrington, D.P. (1991). Initiation, escalation and desistance in juvenile offending and their correlates. *Journal of Criminal Law and Criminology, 82*, 36–82.

Lynam, D.R., Moffitt, T.E., & Stouthamer-Loeber, M. (1993). Explaining the relation between IQ and delinquency: Class, race, test motivation, school failure, or self-control? *Journal of Abnormal Psychology, 102*, 187–196.

Manly, J.T., Cicchetti, D., & Barnett, D. (1994). The impact of subtype, frequency, chronicity, and severity of child maltreatment on social competence and behavior problems. *Developmental Psychology, 7*, 121–143.

McGuire, J. (1997). Psychosocial approaches to the understanding and reduction of violence in young people. In V. Varma (Ed.), *Violence in children and adolescents* (pp. 65–83). Bristol, PA: Jessica Kingsley.

Megargee, E.I. (1982). Psychological determinants and correlates of criminal violence. In M.E. Wolfgang & N.A. Weiner (Eds.), *Criminal violence*. Beverly Hills, CA: Sage.

Moffitt, T.E. (1993). Adolescence-limited and life-course persistent antisocial behavior: A developmental taxonomy. *Psychological Review, 100*, 674–701.

Moore, C.W., & Allen, J.P. (1996). The effects of volunteering on the young volunteer. *The Journal of Primary Prevention, 17*, 231–258.

National Research Council. (1993). *Losing generations: Adolescents in high-risk settings*. Washington, DC: National Academy Press.

Parker, G.R., Cowen, E.L., Work, W.C., & Wyman, P.A. (1990). Test correlates of stress affected and stress resilient outcomes among urban children. *Journal of Primary Prevention, 11*, 19–35.

Poole, E.D., & Rigoli, R.M. (1979). Parental support, delinquent friends, and delinquency: A test of interaction effects. *Journal of Criminal Law and Criminology, 70*, 188–193.

Powell, K.M., Muir-McClain, L., & Halasyamani, L. (1995). A review of selected school-based conflict resolution and peer mediation projects. *Journal of School Health, 65*, 426–431.

Quinton, D., Pickles, A., Maughan, B., & Rutter, M. (1993). Partners, peers, and pathways: Assortative pairing and continuities in conduct disorder. *Development and Psychopathology, 5*, 763–783.

Resnick, M.D., Bearman, P.S., Blum, R.W., Bauman, K.E., Harris, K.M., Jones, J., Tabor, J., Beuhring, T., Sieving, R.E., Shew, M., Ireland, M., Bearinger, L.H., & Udry, J.R. (1997). Protecting adolescents from harm: Findings from the National Longitudinal Study on Adolescent Health. *Journal of the American Medical Association, 278*, 823–832.

Rhodes, J.E. (1994). Older and wiser: Mentoring relationships in childhood and adolescence. *The Journal of Primary Prevention, 14*, 187–196.

Rutter, M. (1985). Resilience in the face of adversity: Protective factors and resistance to psychiatric disorder. *British Journal of Psychiatry, 147*, 598–611.

Seguin, J.R., Pihl, R.O., Harden, P.W., Tremblay, R.E., & Boulerice, B. (1995). Cognitive and neuropsychological characteristics of physically aggressive boys. *Journal of Abnormal Psychology, 104*, 614–624.

Snyder, H.N. (2000). *Juvenile arrests 1999*. Washington, DC: Office of Juvenile Justice and Delinquency Prevention, US Department of Justice.

Weiss, B., Dodge, K.A., Bates, J.E., & Pettit, G.S. (1992). Some consequences of early harsh discipline: Child aggression and a maladaptive social information processing style. *Child Development, 63*, 1321–1335.

Weissberg, R.P., & Greenberg, M.T. (1998). School and community competence-enhancement and prevention programs. In W. Damon (Series Ed.), I.E. Sigel, & K.A. Renninger (Vol. Eds.), *Handbook of child psychology: Vol. 4. Child psychology in practice* (5th ed., pp. 877–954). New York: John Wiley & Sons.

Werner, E.E., & Smith, R.S. (1982). *Vulnerable but invincible: A study of resilient children*. New York: McGraw Hill.

Widom, C.S. (1989). Does violence beget violence? A critical review of the literature. *Psychological Bulletin, 106*, 3–28.

Williams, J.H. (1994). Understanding substance abuse, delinquency involvement, and juvenile justice system involvement among African-American and European-American adolescents. Unpublished dissertation, University of Washington, Seattle.

Yung, B.R., & Hammond, W.R. (1998). Breaking the cycle: A culturally sensitive violence prevention program for African-American children and adolescents. In J.K. Lutzger (Ed.), *Handbook of child abuse research and treatment* (pp. 319–340). New York: Plenum.

Zimring, F.E. (1998). *American youth violence*. New York, NY: Oxford University Press.

Anger Regulation, Childhood

Ephrem Fernandez

INTRODUCTION

This entry introduces some general concepts in the study of anger and then focuses on the child's experience of anger. A cognitive–developmental perspective is adopted in the portrayal of this experience. Both prevention and preparation are discussed and the particular role of parents is considered. Behavioral techniques are given primacy by virtue of their usability before the very onset of anger and the minimal abstraction they demand of children at this stage of cognitive development.

It is between the ages of 4 and 6 months that infants display the first signs of anger (Stenberg, Campos, & Emde, 1983). At this stage, anger manifests itself in the form of facial and motor acts as if the child is trying to remove or overcome an obstacle. In other words, the anger is essentially a reaction to frustration from goals and is made possible by the child's understanding of basic means–ends relationships. Further into childhood, means–end struggles abound in interpersonal relations the child has with parents, siblings, and peers. This is when patterns of hostility may emerge and become compounded into diagnosable conditions such as oppositional-defiant disorder or conduct disorder.

DEFINITIONS AND SCOPE

Most scholars in the field of affect science categorize *anger* as a subjective emotion, and as such, it is episodic and often precipitated by a discernible event—unlike *moods* that tend to be enduring and vaguely linked to precipitating stimuli. As with all discrete emotions, there are unique cognitive-motivational properties of anger plus some associated physiological correlates. Cognitively, anger is an emotion that emerges from the attribution of wrongdoing (e.g., Ortony, Clore, & Collins, 1988), motivationally it involves a tendency to undo that perceived wrongdoing (e.g., Frijda, 1986), and physiologically, it is associated with sympathetic nervous system arousal such as elevated blood pressure and heart rate.

However, in children, the cognitive antecedent of anger is often a perceived frustration from a concrete goal rather than a perceived grievance. The consequence of anger is often *aggression* (motor or vocal behavior designed to hurt) or coercive behavior (designed to restrain). Alternatively, anger may be followed by passive responses such as noncooperation or inaction. Another term often employed in the literature is *hostility*. This is not an emotion or a behavior as such but a disposition to act or feel in a particular way. It is characterized by recurrent anger that suggests a proneness to this emotion. Hence, the term hostility is often equated to trait anger, as contrasted with state anger.

Adverse Effects of Anger in Children

Oppositional and conduct disorders are among the most common of childhood disorders; the core emotion in both cases is anger. Both these conditions are characterized by marked interpersonal conflict that undermines compliance with rules at home or school. There is also a component of aggression (especially in the case of conduct disorder) that may be directed at people, animals, or property. Understandably, the destructive potential of these anger-related problems is a serious concern to parents, teachers, and the community at large.

Yet, many children experience anger without getting aggressive. This too may be cause for concern because anger in such instances may be turned inward and experienced as depression. Second, unexpressed or internalized anger may, in the long run, lead to cardiovascular deterioration. Research has shown that the Type A personality is vulnerable to coronary heart disease because of a toxic core of inhibited anger and cynical hostility (Matthews, 1988; Williams & Williams, 1993). Such attributes have been found to produce greater cardiovascular reactivity in children too. For example, in a sample of 3–6-year-old boys, greater heart rate and blood pressure changes occurred among those classified as Type A than those who were Type B in response to either physically or emotionally challenging games (Lundberg, 1983).

THEORIES AND RESEARCH

Common Sources of Anger in Children

The cognitive capacities of children allow them to perceive means–end relationships far more than the complex betrayals and affronts at which adults take offense. This difference may be accentuated by issues of linguistic competence that limit the child's interpretation of various sources of anger in the adult world. Thus, we often witness bewilderment in a child when s/he observes a parent reproaching her spouse for forgetting their wedding anniversary, for disclosing a family secret to the neighbor, or for laughing at news of the downfall of a public figure. Anger in these instances is dependent on a complex understanding of the social world and the expectations, intentionality, and psychological hurt that go with it. Instead, children are more likely to get angry at tangible frustrations in their physical environment. These include aversive stimuli such as pain, extreme heat or cold, and loud noise that may well be hardwired to trigger anger in humans (Berkowitz, 1990). This may also be true of the frustration and deprivation that result from maltreatment and neglect at the hands of parents and others.

Child maltreatment (e.g., sexual abuse, physical abuse) has long been suspected as producing childhood anger (Egeland, 1991), transforming it into violence and antisocial behavior only later in life. Early evidence for intergenerational transmission of anger and violence arose out of anecdotal clinical reports, single case studies, nomothetic studies without control groups, or retrospective data from select samples of maltreated individuals. However, a recent review by Kotch, Muller, and Blakely (1999) shows that the evidence for this transmission weakens as research methodology improves. When focusing on more methodologically rigorous research, the rate of intergenerational transmission ranges from 18 to 70 percent (Kaufman & Zigler, 1989). In fact, abused children who develop supportive relationships later in life may circumvent the so-called cycle of abuse. Still, that leaves a significant minority who do perpetuate the angry, abusive behaviors that were performed on them, and a further subgroup who may not act out their anger but harbor long-term unresolved anger from the original abuse.

To the extent that it contributes to family adversity, poverty may lead to neglect, and may also be a factor in the precipitation of anger. So can other types of adversity such as criminality (Offord, 1982), social insularity (Dumas, 1986), and marital discord (Rutter & Giller, 1983). In addition to the neglect that ensues from such adversity, stress and conflict are intrinsically aversive to children who may respond with anger simply as a means of communication or coping. The cumulative effect of these stressors on emotional disturbance such as anger is multiplicative rather than additive (Dubow, Roecker, & D'Imperio, 1997).

The pervasive problem of bullying among school children may be an underlying correlate of much childhood anger. Not only do the victims tend to feel anger (Borg, 1998), but the bullies themselves often act aggressively in response to their own anger (Bosworth, Espelage, & Simon, 1999). Ultimately, a hierarchical system may evolve in which most children are recipients as well as purveyors of aggression due to anger.

STRATEGIES THAT WORK

The prevention of anger-related problems entails some sort of separation in advance of the person from the imminent problem. Thus, screening is a form of primary prevention in that the aim is to detect a risk rather than solve an existing problem. Parent training is preventive inasmuch as it targets an agent between the child and the problem. On the other hand, social skills training of children is a preparatory strategy designed to equip the child to deal with the actual prospect of anger. Put another way, primary prevention strictly applies to anger that is (in principle) avoidable, but preparation is the key when some encounter is expected between person and problem.

Screening

Children with anger-related difficulties are rarely self-referred and by the time they come to the attention of a helping professional, there may already be a problem that is overdue for intervention. Therefore, preventive approaches start early and go in search of those with a likelihood of developing such problems. One way of achieving this is through screening. This can range from mass screening to selective screening. As reviewed by Prinz and Connell (1997), screening requires the identification of marker variables, a choice of informants (e.g., teachers and peers), and administration of appropriate screening tools. The authors recommend a multiple gating procedure in which a broad and inexpensive screening determines the first level of risk followed by more detailed assessments of higher levels of risk. The evidence shows that the accuracy of predicting conduct problems in children is increased by such a multi-gate screening procedure (Lochman & the Conduct Problems Prevention Research Group, 1995).

Social Skills Training

The terms social skills, social competence, and social intelligence have been used interchangeably. Deficits in any of these are likely to put an individual at odds with social norms. Such deficits may originate from poor role models, poor peer relations, or inadequate socialization. Social skills training (SST) programs aim to rectify such deficits with a view to improving emotional adjustment. Research has been generally supportive of the efficacy of these programs.

Most SST programs for anger control use a psychoeducational approach consisting of modeling, rehearsal, performance feedback, and transfer of training (Cartledge & Milburn, 1980; Goldstein & Keller, 1989). This makes the program an exercise in coaching instead of mere instruction. Given that frustration and provocation are not always avoidable, coaching becomes a way to prepare the individual to face such challenges.

A key element in SST is modeling. This can be via video or live demonstration. The model should be someone the trainee identifies with or aspires to become. The situation should be relevant to the trainee's real-life circumstances. Target behaviors are to be presented in steps from the simple to the complex. The trainee has to mentally rehearse the target behaviors and then behaviorally emulate them in a role-play situation. Feedback is given and the behaviors are shaped by psychological rewards such as approval and praise. Finally, application to real-life situations is strongly encouraged. The outcome of such application is then jointly reviewed by trainee and trainer, and the appropriate behaviors are further reinforced.

Morrison and Sandowicz (1994) have reviewed several successful SST programs designed to prevent anger and aggression in children, such as the Lions' Quest Skills for Growing (Quest International, 1990). Here, elementary school children are trained in broad-based skills such as effective communication, resolving conflict, and cooperation—against a backdrop of self-discipline, responsibility, harmony with others, and commitment to family, school, peers, and community. Another example is the Social Decision Making Skills program (Elias & Clabby, 1989) that teaches general life skills to elementary school children.

Also worthy of mention are programs that target children at risk of anger-related problems. Stephens (1978), for instance, designed such a program for mildly disabled elementary school students. In their *Skillstreaming the elementary school child*, McGinnis and Goldstein (1984) propose a program for small groups of five to seven children with notable deficiencies in anger expression. New skills such as removing communication blocks, negotiation, reciprocating, and acknowledging subjectivity are then added to the child's repertoire for stemming the anger in its germinal stage. A spinoff of this program is the Earlscourt Social Skills Group Program (Pepler, King, & Byrd, 1991) to promote self-control in 6–12-year-olds with noncompliance or oppositional behavior.

Two premises about anger control that are rarely contested are: (a) that prevention should precede intervention and (b) that the timing of prevention is better in childhood than in adolescence or adulthood. However, peculiarities of cognitive development restrict the range of techniques that can be used to deal with anger in children. For example, children are less capable of abstraction and perspective-taking than those farther along the life span. Therefore, a developmentally appropriate prevention of anger-related problems in children might rely mainly on concrete techniques and imitative learning as often delivered through behavior therapy. Fernandez (1999) has grouped together three behavior modification techniques that are particularly effective in this regard: behavioral contract, stimulus control, and behavioral rehearsal. The last of these has already found extensive application within SST programs outlined earlier; here, there is an emphasis on observation and action-oriented practice. Stimulus control is implicit in a few SST programs but seldom conceptualized as such. Basically, the probability of occurrence of anger may be governed by certain situational cues such as place or person, in which case, the participant learns such discriminative cues and then averts those situations that invariably lead to anger. This is particularly valuable when past efforts at intervention have repeatedly failed, leaving little option but to evade the anger-provoking situation. Behavioral contracting has rarely been used here but can be used to formalize the effort against anger from the very outset. Though not a legal document, the contract fosters commitment and accountability in addition to built-in contingencies that reduce the likelihood of the undesired behavior (Fernandez & Beck, 2001). Not only are these three techniques preventive in that they target anger before its very onset, they are also suited to children

because of their focus on observable behavior more so than abstract cognition—behavior that can be shaped by social modeling instead of didactic methods. This is not to assert that cognitive techniques have no place in the prevention of anger in children. Such techniques should merely be deferred until behavioral alternatives have been exhausted and developmental changes invite their introduction.

STRATEGIES THAT MIGHT WORK

Parent Training

The work of Patterson and colleagues has demonstrated that childhood conduct and emotional expression are shaped within the context of parent–child interactions (Patterson & Reid, 1984). Therefore, a cornerstone of most prevention programs for childhood problems is parent-training (PT) in proper child-rearing skills (Bond, 1998). This offers a promising avenue for indirectly preventing childhood anger problems too. The parent not only functions as a buffer between the child and the problem, but can also become a conduit for transfer of skills to the child.

Key components of structured PT have been outlined by Miller (1994). Even though she speaks of these as interventions, the orientation is really preventive because it attempts to forestall an anger problem in the child by indirectly working on the parent. The training components include tracking, labeling, and pinpointing of problems, emphasis on positive child behavior, learning about what is developmentally appropriate, effective discipline, clear communication, troubleshooting, and generalization. Unfortunately, the long-term effectiveness and generalization of improvements from such programs is a matter of some doubt (Kazdin, 1990). This may be due to discordant expectations between parents and trainers, noncompliance with the routine, and other ecological problems such as inconducive living conditions. Therefore, more research is needed to evaluate parent training in terms of long-term effectiveness.

STRATEGIES THAT DO NOT WORK

Social modeling as practiced in SST and PT programs depends not just on the selection of an adult or peer that the target individual identifies with; it takes *appropriate behavior* on the part of the model to produce like behavior in the client. One corollary of this is that parents who lose control of their anger when relating to each other undermine their effectiveness as role models for anger control in their children. The old adage "Do as I say, not as I do" presents a conundrum that many children are unable to resolve during their phase of cognitive development when imitative learning holds sway more than instruction. Yet, this is a common reason for setbacks in early efforts at anger control.

Another pitfall in anger control for children occurs when the anger is uncritically accepted as a signal of veridical frustration. In their constant rush to help or investigate, caregivers may be reinforcing angry displays in children. It should be remembered that expressed anger is essentially a form of social communication, and the question of what is being communicated has to be astutely considered. When the underlying message is a plea for attention or (worse still) a demand for others' submission, then the anger display amounts to a tantrum, a manipulation, that can only become habitual if repeatedly attended or submitted to.

SYNTHESIS

The efficacy of preventive and preparatory programs for anger in children has been encouraging according to most published research. However, most of the efficacy data comes from investigations by the developers of these same programs. Replications by independent investigators are needed before conclusive statements about efficacy can be made.

A further issue that arises is whether it is best to attempt prevention of anger in children, adolescents, or adults. A recent meta-analysis of cognitive–behavioral anger management studies published between 1970 and 1995 sheds peripheral light on this issue (Beck & Fernandez, 1998). Ten of the studies were on children, 21 on adolescents, and 15 on adults. The effect sizes for these subsets of studies were 0.53, 0.81, and 0.97, respectively. This indicates that the control of anger was moderately successful in children, more successful in adolescents, and most successful in adults. At first glance, this might appear to challenge the notion that the earlier the prevention, the better the effect. Further reflection raises the possibility that children had low levels of anger to begin with thus creating a "floor effect." It is also possible that by virtue of less cognitive development and psychological mindedness than the other two groups, children benefited less from the kinds of interventions commonly prescribed in these studies.

Childhood, particularly the preschool years, traditionally has been viewed as the formative years of human development. It is a time for vigilance and prevention of problems. With reference to anger, this usually entails screening for those at risk, training parents in child-rearing, and training children in social skills. The emphasis is best kept behavioral since this is developmentally appropriate: it is concrete rather than abstract, relying on social modeling much more than mere instruction. Moreover, techniques such as behavioral contracting, stimulus control, and rehearsal (that form the mainstay of many SST programs) are highly suited to prevent or prepare for the onset of anger.

If we do not invest in children, we will incur their debts for the rest of our lives. Several variations of this dictum have been articulated by social scientists and lay individuals alike. On the other hand, effective upbringing, socialization, and training of children will spare families and society considerable expense and energy in helping out with the mental and physical health problems when children are grown up.

Also see: Family Strengthening: Childhood; Violence Prevention: Childhood; Peer Relationships: Childhood.

References

Berkowitz, L. (1990). On the formation and regulation of anger and aggression: A cognitive-neoassociationistic analysis. *American Psychologist, 45*, 494–503.

Beck, R., & Fernandez, E. (1998). Cognitive-behavioral therapy in the treatment of anger: A meta-analysis. *Cognitive Therapy and Research, 22*, 63–74.

Bond, L.A. (1998). Investing in parents' development as an investment in primary prevention. *Journal of Mental Health, 7*, 493–503.

Borg, M.G. (1998). The emotional reaction of school bullies and their victims. *Educational Psychology, 18*, 433–444.

Bosworth, K., Espelage, D., & Simon, T.R. (1999). Factors associated with bullying behavior in middle school students. *Journal of Early Adolescence, 19*, 341–362.

Cartledge, G., & Milburn, J.F. (1980). *Teaching social skills to children.* New York: Pergamon Press.

Dubow, E.F., Roecker, C.E., & D'Imperio, R. (1997). Mental health. In R.T. Ammerman & M. Hersen (Eds.), *Handbook of prevention and treatment with children and adolescents: Intervention in the real world context.* New York: Wiley.

Dumas, J.E. (1986). Indirect influence of maternal social contacts on mother–child interactions: A setting-event analysis. *Journal of Abnormal Child Psychology, 14*, 205–216.

Egeland, B. (1991). A longitudinal study of high-risk families. In R.H. Starr, Jr. & D.A. Wolfe (Eds.), *The effects of abuse and neglect* (pp. 33–56). New York: Guilford.

Elias, M.J., & Clabby, J.F. (1989). *Social decision-making skills: A curriculum guide for the elementary grades.* Rockville, MD: Aspen.

Fernandez, E. (1999, November). Integrating therapeutic techniques: The case of anger. The First Mid-Atlantic Conference, Society for Psychotherapy Research, Baltimore, Maryland.

Fernandez, E., & Beck, R. (2001). Cognitive-behavioral self-intervention versus self-monitoring of anger: Effects on anger frequency, duration, and intensity. *Behavioural and Cognitive Psychotherapy, 29*, 345–356.

Frijda, N. (1986). *The emotions.* New York: Cambridge University Press.

Goldstein, A.P., & Keller, H. (1989). *Aggressive behavior: Assessment and intervention.* New York: Pergamon Press.

Kaufman, J., & Zigler, E.F. (1989). The intergenerational transmission of child abuse. In D. Cichetty & V. Carlson (Eds.), *Child maltreatment: Theory and research on the causes and consequences of child abuse and neglect* (pp. 129–150). New York: Cambridge University Press.

Kazdin, A.E. (1990). Premature termination from treatment among children referred for antisocial behavior. *Journal of Child Psychology and Psychiatry, 31*, 415–425.

Kotch, J.B., Muller, G.O., & Blakely, C.H. (1999). Understanding the origins and incidence of child maltreatment. In T.P. Gullotta & S.J. McElhany (Eds.), *Violence in homes and communities: Prevention, intervention, and treatment* (pp. 1–38). New Delhi: Sage.

Lochman, J.E., & the Conduct Problems Prevention Research Group. (1995). Screening child behavior problems for prevention program at school entry. *Journal of Consulting and Clinical Psychology, 63,* 549–559.

Lundberg, M. (1983). Note on Type A behavior and cardiovascular responses to challenge in 3–6-year-old children. *Journal of Psychosomatic Research, 27,* 39–42.

Matthews, K.A. (1988). Coronary heart disease and Type A behaviors. *Psychological Bulletin, 104,* 373–380.

McGinnis, E., & Goldstein, A.P. (1984). *Skillstreaming the elementary school child.* Champaign, IL: Research Press.

Miller, G.E. (1994). Enhancing family-based interventions for managing childhood and aggression. In M. Furlong & D. Smith (Eds.), *Anger, hostility, and aggression: Assessment, prevention, and intervention strategies for youth* (pp. 83–116). Brandon, Vermont: Clinical Psychology.

Morrison, G.M., & Sandowicz, M. (1994). Importance of social skills in the prevention and intervention of anger and aggression. In M. Furlong & D. Smith (Eds.), *Anger, hostility, and aggression: Assessment, prevention, and intervention strategies for youth* (pp. 345–392). Brandon, Vermont: Clinical Psychology.

Offord, D.R. (1982). Family backgrounds of male and female delinquents. In J. Gunn & D.P. Farrington (Eds.), *Delinquency and the criminal justice system* (pp. 129–152). New York: Wiley.

Ortony, A., Clore, G., & Collins, A. (1988). *The cognitive structure of emotions.* New York: Cambridge University Press.

Patterson, G.R., & Reid, J.B. (1984). Social interactional processes within the family: The study of the moment-by-moment family transactions in which human social development is imbedded. *Journal of Applied Developmental Psychology, 5,* 237–262.

Pepler, D.J., King, G., & Byrd, W. (1991). A social-cognitively based social skills training program for aggressive children. In D.J. Pepler & K.H. Rubin (Eds.), *The development and treatment of childhood aggression* (pp. 361–379). Hillsdale, NJ: Erlbaum.

Prinz, R.J., & Connell, C.M. (1997). Conduct disorders and antisocial behavior. In R.T. Ammerman & M. Hersen (Eds.), *Handbook of prevention and treatment with children and adolescents: Intervention in the real world context* (pp. 238–258). New York: Wiley.

Quest International (1990). *Skills for growing.* Granville, OH: Author.

Rutter, M., & Giller, H. (1983). *Juvenile delinquency: Trends and perspectives.* New York: Penguin.

Stenberg, C.R., Campos, J.J., & Emde, R.N. (1983). The facial expression of anger in seven-month-old infants. *Child Development, 54,* 178–184.

Stephens, T.M. (1978). *Social skills in the classroom.* Columbus, OH: Cedars Press.

Williams, R., & Williams, V. (1993). *Anger kills.* Toronto: Random House.

Anger Regulation, Adolescence

Ephrem Fernandez

INTRODUCTION

This entry discusses factors relevant to anger in adolescence. As far as possible, research is reported where anger is measured as a subjective experience instead of an overt behavior. This means that self-report measures are the main source of data for this review. Where behavioral observations of violence and aggression are the only available dependent measures, they will be regarded as a proxy for anger. In contrast to the behavioral emphasis of the earlier entry on anger prevention in children, the perspective here is cognitive–behavioral since it is especially compatible with the developmental advances of adolescence.

DEFINITIONS AND SCOPE

The transition from childhood to adulthood is marked by dramatic physical changes in appearance and hormonal processes as well as psychosocial change in cognitive ability and interpersonal relations. These bring with them a host of opportunities and risks. Sometimes, change becomes stressful, destabilizing the adolescent to the point of an emotional or behavioral problem. One of the most striking of such problems is the aggression and underlying anger in the youth of today. On average, juveniles have been involved in one quarter of serious violent victimizations in the United States over the last quarter of a century (Snyder & Sickmund, 1999).

The difference between violence or aggression and anger merits some clarification. Smedslund (1992) theorizes that anger is an interpretation of being wronged or mistreated by a person and the ensuing tendency to counter or redress that wrongdoing. The action tendency can lead to physical aggression. As Averill remarks, "Anger and aggression are closely related phenomena, and it is not possible to discuss one without the other. Yet, not all anger is aggressive, nor can all aggression be attributed to anger" (1982, p. vii). Other responses range from reprimands to covert ones such as noncooperation and subversion. Even in the absence of active or passive aggression, anger may continue to be harbored. These subtle or concealed forms of anger often elude the so-called "behavioral measures" of anger.

Although not necessitated by anger, violence remains one of the greatest concerns in research and treatment of anger because of its blatantly destructive quality. In the adolescent population of the United States, violence is no longer confined to gangs but has increased alarmingly in and outside schools (Gullotta & McElhaney, 1999). Where anger is the precursor of violence, the prevention of anger should take primacy over the prevention of violence, just as where illness is the precursor of death, the prevention of illness precedes the prevention of death.

THEORIES AND RESEARCH

Social Skills Training

As explained in the entry on the prevention of anger in children, inappropriate anger may be viewed as a social skills deficit arising out of undersocialization, inadequate role models, or unsatisfactory peer relations. Logically, this can be averted by social skills training (SST). In this regard, the basic approach is similar to the training used to correct deficits in other areas such as motor skills, academic skills, and a variety of behaviors.

SST programs are founded upon psycho-educational principles of modeling, rehearsal, performance feedback, and transfer of training (Cartledge & Milburn, 1980; Goldstein & Keller, 1989). Modeling is often via video or live demonstration. The model should be someone with whom the trainee might identify. For adolescents, this is typically a peer; alternatively, the model may be someone the trainee aspires to be like, such as an individual a few years senior but in the same institution or organization. The situation should be relevant to the trainee's real-life circumstances, be it a problem in the family, school, or neighborhood community. Target behaviors are to be presented clearly in steps from the simple to the complex. The trainee has to mentally rehearse the target behaviors and then behaviorally reproduce them in a role-play situation. Feedback is to be given and the behaviors are to be shaped by psychological rewards such as attention, approval, and praise. Finally, application in real-life situations is encouraged. The outcome of such application is jointly reviewed by trainee and trainer, and the appropriate behaviors are further reinforced.

Morrison and Sandowicz (1994) have reviewed various SST programs designed to prevent anger and aggression in adolescents. Some of these are broad-based such as the Affective Skills Development for Adolescents (Dembrowsky, 1983) which is designed to build a classroom atmosphere conducive to growth and positive affect. Specific skills are introduced against this backdrop: communication, responsibility, assertiveness, coping with stress, problem solving, and appropriate expression of feelings. Another example is the Fighting Invisible Tigers Program (Schmitz & Hipp, 1987) which aims to enhance adolescents' awareness of stress and the lifeskills necessary to minimize it. Students are trained to exercise, relax, be assertive, have supportive relationships, and plan their lives—as part of a general prophylactic against anger and stress. The Social Competence Promotion Program (Weissberg, Caplan, Bennetto, & Jackson, 1990) is another broad, school-based program to teach students skills that minimize anger problems and conduct disorders. Spanning 45 sessions, the program adopts a social information-processing framework to educate participants on risks and to train them in prosocial values and problem solving. A critical ingredient is practice across a variety of hypothetical and real-life situations.

The success of SST in preventing anger requires ideological congruence among several parties, including teachers and parents. The former may not have the time to devote to such a program, while the latter may resist the idea on the grounds that their children get adequate lifeskills training at home. When the program works as designed, SST improves peer relations, conflict resolution, and overall adjustment (Caplan, Weissberg, Grober, Sivo, Grady, & Jacoby, 1992; Weissberg, 2000).

For youth at high risk of becoming angry, there are programs that teach skills specific to anger prevention. One example is the PACT program (Hammond & Yung, 1991) targeting anger in African-American adolescent males. This program focuses on getting participants to "give and take" by constructive expression of disapproval as well as receiving criticism from others, and problem solving one's way out of conflict. Another example is the ACCESS program (Walker, Todis, Holmes, & Horton, 1988) designed for middle- and high-school students in special and regular classrooms.

Parent Training

Patterson and colleagues have demonstrated that childhood conduct and emotional expression are shaped in the context of parent–child interactions (Patterson & Reid, 1984). Therefore, a promising approach to prevent anger problems is parent-training (PT) or the imparting of effective child-rearing skills.

Miller (1994) has outlined the key components of structured PT in this context. Even though she refers to these as interventions, the approach is really one of prevention because it attempts to forestall an anger problem in the child by indirectly working on the parent. The training components include tracking, labeling, and pinpointing of problems, emphasis on positive child behavior, learning about what is developmentally appropriate, effective discipline, clear communication, troubleshooting, and generalization. Unfortunately, the long-term effectiveness and generalization of improvements from such programs is unclear at best and inadequate at worst (Kazdin, 1990). This may be due to discordant expectations between parents and trainers, noncompliance with the routine, and broader problems such as inhospitable living conditions.

Since anger can be "infectious" (to use a metaphor), reducing anger in parents may also reduce anger and conflict in the family. Fetsch, Schultz, and Wahler (1999) provide data from the RETHINK Method: Anger Management for Parents (Institute for Mental Health Initiatives, 1991). Parents who participated in this 6-week workshop not only showed reductions in angry attitudes and behavior, but also collectively produced significant reductions in overall conflict levels within their respective families.

Promoting an Anger-Free Environment at School

Apart from the home, the school is the next most important environment where social exchanges trigger emotions and shape long-term emotional problems. Shafii and Shafii (2001) report that 30–50 cases of school violence are reported daily, many of these being attributable to some form of anger. Training teachers not to wait to intervene on anger but to fashion a classroom atmosphere that minimizes conflict is a strategic starting point.

Teachers are in a vantage position to comprehend the power structure of a class especially as related to seniority, majority versus minority, physique, and intellect. Whatever the method of stratification, bullies emerge and, with that, the spread of provocation. While the problem of bullying in schools is now widely acknowledged, the anger and resentment that it produces remain largely unaddressed. Prevention would first of all require an authority to which all students are accountable, and that authority is most appropriately the teacher. With the authority invested in him/her, the teacher can create a milieu in which there are clearly defined codes of conduct and contingencies. Together, authority figures and a system of rules can extinguish bullying and promote equity and fairness, where mere entreaties or appeals to reason and compassion fail.

Adolescent Substance Use

To the extent that substance use (whether licit or illicit) alters consciousness, affect, impulses, and behavior, it deserves special attention in the efforts to prevent anger. Poston, Norton, and Morales (1994) have reviewed important findings on the effects of drugs that may have implications for anger and its prevention. Despite being a central nervous system depressant, alcohol may precipitate or aggravate anger and agitation by clouding judgment and exerting a disinhibitory effect. When this occurs in a situation that is permissive of physical expression (e.g., at a sporting event), individuals are likely to act on their angry impulses. Marijuana may also have a disinhibitory effect on angry feelings even though there seems to be a culture of adolescent marijuana use premised on its reduction of tension and anger. At parties and other social gatherings, it may sometimes release pent-up anger. Steroids which have become more popular among young athletes are known to produce angry outbursts (called "roid rages") in about 30 percent of users. Caffeine manipulation does not produce consistent changes in anger or aggression and neither does sugar even though the latter is often viewed as a dietary culprit when children get angry. In short, the prevention of angry behavior may incorporate a component of education about substances, especially the licit and illicit drugs that exert disinhibitory effects on individuals.

STRATEGIES: OVERVIEW

Reid (1993) estimates that well-implemented primary prevention programs can get rid of emotional adjustment difficulties in 75–85 percent of students. As to which of these programs work best, the answer awaits more systematic research on comparative treatment outcomes. There is emerging evidence that with respect to anger and aggression, adolescents do better when they are not the sole participants in these programs but are joined by parents who agree with the agenda for prevention/treatment and participate in family management. Dishion, Andrews, Kavanagh, and Soberman (1996) found that participants in teen-focused groups tended to deteriorate and exhibit more delinquent behaviors than a self-directed control group; this was attributable not only to the absence of parent involvement, but to the deviant influences of certain peers within the groups.

STRATEGIES THAT WORK

Cognitive Approaches for the Cognitively Mature

In the earlier entry on the prevention of anger in children, behavioral methods were highly recommended in large part because of their compatibility with the concrete operations of children and the tangible frustrations that often trigger anger in young children. However, the transition to adolescence opens up new sources of anger based on improved capacity, speed, and depth of information processing. This enables the introduction of cognitive techniques for dealing with anger. The cognitive approach is encouraged by the adolescent's expanding domains of knowledge, increased skill with language, enhanced social cognition, and moral development.

One rudimentary point of entry to cognitive change is the individual's schema or attitude. Attitude change may invoke moral reasoning. For example, Arbuthnot (1992) described an intervention on "behavior disordered youth" that was based on Kohlberg's levels of moral reasoning. Within small group discussions, morally-relevant incidents were analyzed and the moral reasoning about the incident was introduced that was one step in moral reasoning above where the participants were. Over time, the participants showed an increase in their level of moral reasoning, but more importantly, this translated into reduced anger and lower rates of several types of antisocial behavior.

STRATEGIES THAT MIGHT WORK

To the extent that cognitive schemata drive individual appraisals, altering a schema of hate can also reduce attributions leading to anger. For example, the adolescent who has developed an attitude of hatred toward authority figures can be engaged in logical discourse to uncover the irrationality of his/her attitude, the internal contradictions among appraisals, or the discrepancies between attitude and ideals. Over an extended period, such rational disputation could ultimately bring about the collapse of the maladaptive schema and a corresponding decline in the inappropriate anger. Little recognition of this principle of schematic change is found in the anger regulation literature, even though there is frequent mention of changing individual appraisals. Compared to the reappraisal of individual self-statements as they transpire, schematic change involves changing the fundamental premises that make up an attitude; this prevents the automatic thoughts which emerge as a corollary of the underlying schema.

Advancing from prevention to the reduction of anger requires the use of more complex cognitive interventions such as problem solving. Although too advanced for children, such an approach may be attempted during adolescence by which time the individual is more adept at lateral thinking and decision-making. Problem solving involves defining the problem (in this case, an anger-related problem), brainstorming for solutions, selecting the optimal solution, implementing the solution, reviewing the outcome, and finally, reinforcing the outcome if satisfactory and reverting to the start in a recursive process until the outcome is satisfactory. A crucial part of this exercise is generating options. This demands a consideration of the hypothetical rather than the actual in a way that typically exceeds the abilities of the child, though not the adolescent. As Flavell (1985) puts it, the elementary school child has "an earth-bound, concrete, practical-minded sort of problem-solving approach, one that persistently fixates on the perceptible and inferable reality right there in front of him .... An adolescent or adult is likelier than an elementary school child to approach problems quite the other way around .... The adolescent or adult is more apt to begin with possibility and only subsequently proceed to reality" (Flavell, 1985, p. 98). Therefore, problem solving with its emphasis on generating alternatives has found a secure place in most anger regulation programs for adolescents.

Another developmental issue that is germane to how anger is controlled in adolescence as compared to childhood is social cognition. The adolescent is no longer influenced only by parents and immediate family members but also by a multitude of peers and the mass media. Now more than ever, the social construction of anger has to be heeded in any attempt to prevent or control it. Unlike the tangible frustrations that evoke anger in children, the adolescent is more susceptible to provocation by betrayal, abandonment, power, or competition. For this reason, SST at this stage of development is more advanced than when adapted for children. Adolescent SST has to address complex issues of interpersonal relations in a manner that has credibility and implications for the evolving lifestyles of adolescents. In the context of anger, it may even demand a measure of empathy or perspective-taking, accountability, and a sense of responsibility—more than is expected of children though not as much as demanded of adults.

STRATEGIES THAT DO NOT WORK

Two contraindications already discussed in the context of childhood anger are: (a) discrepancies between the words and actions of role models, and (b) contingencies between anger and rewarding consequences like attention or submission. Yet, these are two notable reasons for failed attempts to regulate anger in adolescents: the tendency for parents and authority figures to simply lecture or preach about anger control while not practicing it in their own interpersonal relations, or the tendency to listen and yield to an individual only when the latter gets angry. Altogether ignoring anger in the hope that it will go away is also a risky choice since it is likely to escalate the anger to the point that it is neither escapable nor tolerable. Clearly, a delicate balance has to be struck between ignoring versus attending, between conceding versus resisting, if there is to be a resolution to interpersonal anger. This is particularly relevant to adolescents who are relatively new to the task of negotiating and conflict resolution.

SYNTHESIS

While anger does not necessitate aggression, the latter often implies the former. Aggression among youth in North America has reached serious proportions especially with the recent violent shootings within schools across the United States and to a lesser extent in Canada. Primary prevention of anger-related problems starts with training in a broad array of social skills, the efficacy of which is well established. Parent training is also beneficial but its long-term effects are less certain. Teen-focused groups without parental involvement are vulnerable to deterioration given the risk of adverse peer influences. In schools where bullying is rampant and homes where conflict thrives, a basic code of conduct agreed upon by all and implemented by an authority figure is essential to create an environment that minimizes angry behavior.

There is widespread substance use among adolescents and to the extent that many recreational drugs have disinhibitory or mood-altering effects, they warrant attention as cofactors in the prevention of anger. Where anger prevention fails, anger regulation techniques still remain, and here special sensitivity must be paid to developmental milestones. In particular, the new capacity, speed, and depth of information processing brought on by adolescence allows the introduction of cognitive techniques that require abstraction, lateral thinking, and complex decision-making to regulate anger. While this is an advance upon the relatively concrete behavioral techniques prescribed for children, it is only a harbinger of the even more complex cognitive and experiential techniques appropriate for adults with anger problems.

Also see: Family Strengthening: Adolescence; Violence Prevention: Adolescence; Peer Relationships: Adolescence.

References

Arbuthnot, J. (1992). Socio moral reasoning in behavior-disordered adolescents: Cognitive and behavioral change. In S. McCord & R.E. Tremblay (Eds.), *Preventing antisocial behaviors: Interventions from birth through adolescence* (pp. 283–316). New York: Guilford Press.

Averill, J.R. (1982). *Anger and aggression: An essay on emotion.* Berlin: Springer-Verlag.

Caplan, M., Weissberg, R.P., Grober, J.S., Sivo, P.J., Grady, D., & Jacoby, C. (1992). Social competence promotion with inner-city and suburban young adolescents: Effects on social adjustment and alcohol use. *Journal of Consulting and Clinical Psychology, 60,* 56–63.

Cartledge, G., & Milburn, J.F. (1980). *Teaching social skills to children.* New York: Pergamon Press.

Dembrowsky, C.H. (1983). *Affective skill development for adolescents—Teacher's manual.* Jackson, WY: Constance H. Dembrowsky.

Dishion, T.J., Andrews, D.W., Kavanagh, K., & Soberman, L.H. (1996). Preventive interventions for high-risk youth. In R.DeV. Peters & R.J. McMahon (1996). *Preventing childhood disorders, substance abuse, and delinquency.* Thousand Oaks, CA: Sage.

Fetsch, R.J., Schultz, C.J., & Wahler, J.J. (1999). A preliminary evaluation of the Colorado Rethink parenting and anger management program. *Child Abuse and Neglect, 23,* 353–360.

Flavell, J.H. (1985). *Cognitive development.* Englewood-Cliffs, NJ: Prentice-Hall.

Goldstein, A.P., & Keller, H. (1989). *Aggressive behavior: Assessment and intervention.* New York: Pergamon.

Gullotta, T.P., & McElhaney, S.J. (Eds.). (1999). *Violence in homes and communities: Prevention, intervention, and treatment.* Thousand Oaks, CA: Sage.

Hammond, W.R., & Yung, B.R. (1991). *Dealing with anger: A violence prevention program for African-American Youth.* Champaign, IL: Research Press.

Institute for Mental Health Initiatives. (1991). Anger management for parents: The RETHINK method [Videotape]. Champaign, IL: Research Press.

Kazdin, A.E. (1990). Premature termination from treatment among children referred for antisocial behavior. *Journal of Child Psychology and Psychiatry, 31,* 415–425.

Miller, G.E. (1994). Enhancing family-based interventions for managing childhood anger and aggression. In M. Furlong & D. Smith (Eds.), *Anger, hostility, and aggression: Assessment, prevention, and intervention strategies for youth* (pp. 83–116). Brandon, Vermont: Clinical Psychology.

Morrison, G.M., & Sandowicz, M. (1994). Importance of social skills in the prevention and intervention of anger and aggression. In M.J. Furlong & D.C. Smith (Eds.), *Anger, hostility, and aggression: Assessment, prevention and intervention strategies for youth* (pp. 345–392). Brandon, VT: Clinical Psychology.

Poston, W.S.C., Norton, R., & Morales, M.G. (1994). Biological influences on anger and hostility. In M. Furlong & D. Smith (Eds.), *Anger, hostility, and aggression: Assessment, prevention, and intervention strategies for youth* (pp. 59–82). Brandon, Vermont: Clinical Psychology.

Patterson, G.R., & Reid, J.B. (1984). The study of the moment-by-moment family transactions in which human social development is embedded. *Journal of Applied Developmental Psychology, 5,* 237–262.

Reid, J. (1993). Prevention of conduct disorder before and after school entry: Relating interventions to developmental findings. *Development and Psychopathology, 11,* 209–223.

Schmitz, C., & Hipp, E. (1987). *A teacher's guide to fighting invisible tigers.* Minneapolis, MN: Free Spirit.

Shafii, M., & Shafii, S.L. (2001). *School violence assessment, management, prevention.* Washington, DC: American Psychiatric Association.

Smedslund, J. (1992). How shall the concept of anger be defined? *Theory and Psychology, 3,* 5–34.

Snyder, H., & Sickmund, M. (1999). *Juvenile offenders and victims: 1999 National Report* (p. 55). Washington, DC: Office of Juvenile Justice and Delinquency Prevention.

Walker, H.M., Todis, B., Holmes, D., & Horton, G. (1988). *The Walker social skills curriculum: The ACCESS program.* Austin, TX: Pro-Ed.

Weissberg, R.P. (2000). Improving the lives of millions of school children. *American Psychologist, 55,* 1360–1372.

Weissberg, R.P., Caplan, M.Z., Bennetto, L., & Jackson, A.S. (1990). The New Haven Social Competence Promotion Program for young adolescents: Social problem-solving module. Chicago, IL: University of Illinois at Chicago.

Asthma, Childhood

Elaine Gustafson

INTRODUCTION

Asthma is the most common disease of childhood in the United States (Schwartz, 1999). The US epidemiologic data on asthma underscores its high impact on children, health care institutions, schools, industry, and the economy. Recent studies have shown that it can be associated with impaired lung growth in children and with a decline in lung function in adults (Anonymous, 2000). The fact that asthma is frequently unrecognized or undertreated, especially in low income minority populations emphasizes the need for preventive care and early intervention.

The focus of this entry is primary prevention and the factors that are associated with the development of asthma in children aged 5–12. The question of whether the disease of asthma is preventable is complex because of the multiple potential precipitating factors. This entry explores primary prevention strategies with regard to the many factors associated with the development of asthma in school-age children.

DEFINITIONS

Asthma is

> a chronic airway inflammatory disorder characterized by recurrent episodes of wheezing, breathlessness, chest tightness and coughing, particularly at night or in the early morning. These episodes are usually associated with widespread but variable airflow obstruction that is often reversible either spontaneously or with treatment. The inflammation also causes an associated increase in the existing bronchial hyperresponsiveness to a variety of stimuli. (National Asthma Education and Prevention Program (National Heart, Lung and Blood Institute). Second Expert Panel on the Management of Asthma, 1998, p. 1)

Asthma usually begins in childhood often with an inherited susceptibility to environmental allergens. The severity of episodes or *exacerbation* range from mild to life threatening. These may be triggered by exposures and conditions such as respiratory illness, presence of house dust mites or cockroaches, animal dander, mold, pollen, exposure to cold air, exercise, stress, tobacco smoke, and indoor and outdoor air pollutants (Williams et al., 1995). The frequency and severity of asthma symptoms can be decreased by the use of medications and reduced exposure to environmental pollutants. Asthma cannot be cured; it can, however, be controlled by both pharmacologic and non-pharmacologic means.

Primary prevention is a process in which the intervention precedes disease development. For example, decreasing exposure to pets at school for children at risk for asthma or reducing environmental pollutants like ozone represent primary prevention approaches. Understanding the disease process and those factors contributing to the development of disease is vital to the prevention of asthma (Becker, 2000).

Secondary prevention is defined as an attempt to prevent the development of disease in individuals with allergy-associated disease or atopic illnesses. Sporik, Holgate, Platts-Mills, and Cogswell (1990) define *atopy* as a tendency to develop allergic disorders, such as asthma, allergic dermatitis, rhinitis, and food allergies. They further indicate that atopic children are at much greater risk of developing asthma than are non-atopic children. Factors that may exacerbate asthma, also known as *triggers*, precipitate asthma symptoms by causing airway inflammation in children in whom airway sensitization has already been established. Thus, if the airway is already sensitized, re-exposure to the causal factor may bring on symptoms.

SCOPE

The prevalence and severity of asthma has increased in the United States in the last 20 years, with the greatest increase among children and young adults living in the inner cities with the highest exposure to cockroaches (Eggleston, Buckley, Breysse, Wills-Karp, Kleeberger, & Jaakkola, 1999), mold, and other potential allergens like air pollution. It is the most common chronic disease in Canada affecting 6 percent of adults and 12 percent of children (Statistics Canada. Health Statistics Division, 1995). In the United States and Canada, there was a significant rise in mortality and morbidity during the 1970s and 1980s with a decrease in mortality during the past decade. Hospitalization data indicate that the disease of asthma continues to increase in Canada (Statistics Canada. Health Statistics Division, 1995). The National Heart, Lung, and Blood Institute reports that the prevalence of asthma has been increasing since the early 1980s for all age, sex, and racial groups in the United States. In 1995, the prevalence of self-reported asthma was 56.8 per 1,000 persons. In children, the prevalence was higher among males than females. In children aged 5–14, the prevalence changed from 42.8/1,000 in 1980 to 74.4/1,000 in 1993–1994 (National Asthma Education and Prevention Program, 1998). This dramatic change among school-age children represents the most significant increase among all age groups.

The components of ethnicity, poverty, and residence need to be considered together when attempting to determine risk factors for asthma development (Eggleston et al., 1999). Asthma severity and prevalence has increased over the past decade especially among children living in inner cities in the United States. Racial and ethnic minorities who populate the urban areas are the more affected populations. Their hospitalization and morbidity rates are more than double that of the white population (Clark et al., 1999). Eggleston et al. (1999) report that the prevalence of asthma in white children 7–14 years of age was 4.8 percent and in the African American population, it was 6.7 percent. This discrepancy cannot be explained by socioeconomic status alone and is statistically significant after adjusting for confounding variables such as age, gender, and residence in the inner city (Eggleston et al., 1999). Minority children also have a higher prevalence of asthma, with mortality from asthma as much as four times that of the non-minority population (Mannino et al., 1998).

Societal Costs

The use of health services for children with asthma are significant. Healthy People 2010 Objectives (2000) indicate that in 1994 alone, in the United States, there were 169,000 hospital discharges for asthma in children less than 15 years of age and asthma was second only to accidents in emergency room department visits for children (Healthy People 2010 (Group) & United States Department of Health and Human Services, 2000). Costs associated with health care use and disability are high. In 1998, the National Heart, Lung and Blood Institute estimated that the annual cost of asthma in all age groups was $11.3 billion per year. This included $7.5 billion in direct medical expenses and $3.8 billion in indirect costs such as days missed from work or school, caregiver expenditures, travel, waiting time, and premature mortality (Services, 2001).

Individual Costs

Absence from school is a frequent consequence for children with symptoms of asthma. It is estimated that children in the United States with asthma miss over 10 million days of school annually, making asthma one of the leading causes of school absenteeism (Services, 2001). This may result in poorer school performance and diminished future potential. Also, children at risk for asthma may be discouraged from participating in physical activity. Yet, it is known that exercise is important for both physical and psychological development in children.

THEORIES AND RESEARCH

Hereditary Considerations

There is no doubt that asthma has a heritable component. A family history of asthma and allergy, especially if both parents are affected, is associated with the development of asthma (Slezak, Persky, Kviz, Ramakrishnan, & Byers, 1998). Lux, Henderson, and Pocock (2000) note that among infants, the highest incidence of early wheezing occurred if the mother herself had asthma and if the infant was preterm. This early presentation is complicated by multiple other factors, the majority of which are environmental. Therefore, the recent rise in asthma prevalence is difficult to ascribe to genetics alone (Becker, 2000). Nevertheless, in a recent study of 1085 Head Start families in 18 Chicago sites, children with asthma were six times more likely to have a family member with asthma as were those without asthma (Slezak et al., 1998). The overwhelming component of environmental considerations clouds the issue of heredity in the development of asthma.

Immunologically sensitive individuals are also at risk for asthma morbidity and mortality. The genetic background of the child is a critical factor in their susceptibility to environmental stimuli. Studies in the United States, Europe, Australia, and New Zealand have established that allergy has a significant role in the development of asthma and that immune globulin E (IgE), which mediates sensitization to indoor allergens, is a major risk factor (Clark et al., 1999). Findings of a recent US study of over 5,500 children, 6–8 years old, comparing African American (AA) with European American (EA) children, suggest that AA children may be predisposed to asthma (Joseph, Ownby, Peterson, & Johnson, 2000). Significant racial differences were found between total serum IgE and airway responsiveness and between serum IgE and asthma status leading to the hypothesis that AA children may be predisposed to asthma.

Environmental Factors

The growing use and exposure of children to some chemicals has led to concern about the possible adverse effects of the environment on children's health (Samet, 1995). Current evidence suggests that environmental exposures are one of the most important factors in the development of asthma. In fact, the strongest epidemiological association has been found between asthma morbidity and the exposure of immunologically sensitive persons with asthma to airborne allergens (Eggleston et al., 1999).

Many indoor and outdoor pollutants have been considered as possibly causing or exacerbating asthma. It has been postulated that urban pollution might contribute to an increase in asthma in the inner city. However, the presence of ambient pollutants (such as air pollution) have declined steadily in cities in recent years while the incidence of asthma has risen (Lang & Polansky, 1994). Consequently, this relationship is difficult to prove. This was especially true in a case in Connecticut, in 2000, in which concerned citizens met with legislators about a bill to reduce air pollution emissions from power plants, noting the increasing incidence of asthma among inner city children. At a public meeting, a power company representative stated that asthma rates have been increasing even as air quality has improved indicating that air pollution must not be the cause of increased asthma. In fact, this statement is generally consistent with research evidence and expert opinion that air pollution is not driving the current increase in asthma rates (Vacek, 1999). Many clean air advocates believe however, that air pollution does trigger attacks among children with asthma but does not cause asthma. Others insist that this subtlety detracts from the effectiveness of their position that air pollution does cause asthma (Dixon, 2002). In support of the contention that air pollution does precipitate asthma symptoms, a study done in Atlanta, in 1996, during the Olympic Games found that the number of asthma acute care events decreased significantly among children aged 1–16 when peak weekday morning traffic counts decreased by 22 percent. This correlated with a decrease in the peak ozone concentration for the day. Researchers concluded that these data provide support for efforts to reduce air pollution and improve health through reductions in motor vehicle traffic (Friedman, Powell, Hutwagner, Graham, & Teague, 2001, p. 62).

Samet (1995) notes that there is a need to pay attention to the areas in which children spend their time, whether it is in the home, outdoors, at school, in daycare centers, on transportation or in public places. Particle exposure has been linked to higher rates of respiratory infection and outdoor pollutants have been considered as possibly causing or exacerbating asthma. A study of 138 AA children in Los Angeles attempted to identify environmental factors to explain the increase in asthma morbidity and mortality among this population. Data were collected on respiratory symptoms and medication use for 13 weeks and was compared with data on ozone (O_3), nitrogen oxide (NO_2), particulate matter, meteorological variables, pollens, and molds. New episodes of cough were associated with exposure to particulate matter, NO_2, and molds but children with asthma were found to need more medication if exposed to O_3 and particulate matter (Ostro, Lipsett, Mann, Braxton-Owens, & White, 2001).

In one study by Dekker, Dales, Bartlett, Brunekreef, and Zwanenburg (1991) of Canadian school children ($n = 17,962$), which focused on indoor environmental factors and the risk for childhood asthma, several precipitating factors were identified. These included tobacco smoke, living in a damp environment, the use of a humidifier, and use of gas for cooking. All of these risk factors were present in children with physician-diagnosed asthma except for gas cooking, which was only present in children who wheezed without a diagnosis of asthma (Dekker et al., 1991).

Sensitization to indoor aeroallergens (airborne allergens) is more likely a factor in the development of asthma than is sensitization to outdoor aeroallergens. Indoor aeroallergens would include house dust mites, pet dander, especially cat dander and exposure to cockroaches (Becker, 2000). Cat dander appears to pose a greater problem than does house dust mites in that it is present in very small particles and is more widely distributed in the home and community than are house dust mites which settle quickly after being distributed (Rosenstreich et al., 1997). Nevertheless, house dust mites are found in all homes built in temperate climates (Jones, 1998) and evidence suggests that exposure to dust mite allergen, particularly in infants, may be an important factor in the onset of asthma (Holt, Macaubas, Prescott, & Sly, 2000). However, a systematic review of 23 studies involving 686 adults and children, on controlling house dust mites, found that

reduction in exposure to house dust mite antigen does not lead to clinical improvement in patients with asthma who are sensitive to mites (Fihe, 1999).

Environmental tobacco smoke is another important factor in the development of childhood asthma and in the worsening of asthmatic conditions in children. The earlier, longer, and greater the degree of environmental tobacco smoke, the greater the chance that a child will develop asthma (Ehrlich et al., 1996). One study of 1955 children, aged 7–9 years who presented with respiratory illnesses in an urban emergency room found that 50 percent of the children had at least one smoker in their homes. Over 38 percent had elevated cotinine (a detoxification product of nicotine, eliminated by the kidneys) levels in their urine indicative of heavy exposure to environmental tobacco smoke (Ehrlich et al., 1996). Children who were older than 18 months of age had a higher incidence of wheezing if the mother smoked during pregnancy. This result implies that exposure to tobacco smoke components or their metabolites during pregnancy and early infancy has a persistent effect on lung health during early childhood and may contribute to the high prevalence of asthma (Lux et al., 2000).

A review of 51 longitudinal and case controlled studies by Strachan and Cook (1998) revealed that the studies about incidence and prognosis suggest an association between parental smoking and early non-atopic wheezing which tends to run a mild and transient course. Whereas, ten studies of prevalence and severity suggest exposure to environmental tobacco smoke increased the risk of more severe symptoms, outpatient clinic attendance, and hospital admissions. This paradox is explained by considering tobacco exposure as a cofactor with inter-current infection as a trigger of wheezing attacks rather than as the precipitant inducing the asthmatic state. The review revealed that measures of disease severity, including frequency of wheezing episodes or the incidence of intense or life-threatening attacks, which relate to acute exacerbation of existing asthma, are associated with household exposure to tobacco smoke (Strachan & Cook, 1998).

Other environmental pollutants such as diesel particulates and noxious gases such as ozone, sulfur dioxide, and nitrogen oxides may also contribute to the development of asthma. Nitrogen oxide (NO) is an industrial pollutant generated as a byproduct of hydrocarbon combustion and is considered to be an important component of urban smog (Eggleston et al., 1999). In homes, NO is generated by gas stoves and space heaters but it is rarely found at levels that would be considered a health risk. However, the Environmental Protection Agency Air Standards (Eggleston et al., 1999) consider annual average levels of NO at 50 parts per billion (ppb) to constitute a risk for acute and chronic lung disease. In the National Cooperative Inner City Asthma study (Eggleston et al., 1999) of six cities in the United States, indoor NO was measured as high as 480 ppb, with 24 percent of families in the sample exposed to 40 ppb or more. These high levels may have been related to gas-stove use and the presence of non-functioning windows in kitchens. Thus, inner city homes frequently contain levels of NO in excess of US Environmental Protection Agency standards and could be expected to contribute to asthma morbidity (Eggleston et al., 1999).

In rural communities, children are commonly exposed to organic dusts, agricultural chemicals, animal allergens, and grain dust mites that are brought into the home on work clothing (Schwartz, 1999). In comparison studies of both urban and rural children, findings suggest that the etiology of airway disease is multi-factorial and unique exposures may contribute to the development of disease in both settings (Schwartz, 1999). Rural exposures are considered to be relevant to the development of childhood asthma if the asthma is first diagnosed following exposure to agricultural dusts, allergens or fumes (Schwartz, 1999). Alternaria, a mold spore found in agrarian, semi-arid environments is a major sensitizer and is often associated with severe asthma in children from these rural areas (Becker, 2000).

Respiratory Illnesses

Another known precipitant of asthma symptoms is respiratory infection. Respiratory syncytial virus (RSV), often precedes the onset of asthma in infants (Martinez, Wright, Taussig, Holberg, Halonen, & Morgan, 1995). Although wheezing early in life is a risk factor for future decreased lung function and may be associated with later development of asthma, this relationship is not clear. In one study of 826 infants who wheezed before age 3, it was found that the majority did not have asthma or allergies at age 6 (Martinez et al., 1995). In a more recent study by Nafstad, Magnus, and Jaakkola (2000) in Norway, of 2,531 children followed for 4 years, researchers found that children who experienced any respiratory infection in infancy had an increased rather than decreased risk of having asthma later in childhood. However, in a 7-year longitudinal study of 1,314 children in Berlin, researchers found that children with two or more runny nose episodes before age 1 were less likely to be diagnosed with asthma or have a wheeze by 7 years of age (Illi et al., 2001). The findings of these two studies did concur with respect to lower respiratory tract infections which were directly associated with wheezing by age 7. These data support the hypothesis that repeated viral episodes early in life may stimulate the immature immune system, thereby reducing the risk of asthma (Illi et al., 2001).

Psychological Stress

In addition to illnesses and environmental allergens and pollutants, there are many psychological stresses of living in poor inner city neighborhoods (Eggleston et al., 1999). In a study of 150 newborn children of asthmatic mothers in Denver, CO, the infants were considered genetically at risk for asthma. This was due to early parenting difficulties, described as excessive parental anxiety, poor coping, and lack of childcare skills. These infants entered a predictive model for the onset of asthma by age 3 (Mrazek et al., 1999). Researchers hypothesize that the stress of living in urban inner city environments that may include lack of supportive relationships, lack of community resources, violence, and economic concerns, all of which may constitute psychosocial risk factors for asthma-related problems. Whether severe negative life events increased the risk of childhood asthma exacerbation, was the subject of an 18-month prospective study of 90 children in Glasgow, Scotland (Sandberg, 2000). Findings revealed that severe negative life events coupled with chronic stresses significantly increased the likelihood of asthma exacerbation in children aged 6–13 years. In fact, researchers found a threefold likelihood of new exacerbation within 2 weeks of the negative life events. Crime, noise pollution, and limited or absence of safe transportation in inner cities may also have a negative effect on children with or at risk for asthma (Clark et al., 1999).

Other Contributing Factors

Exercise is another important contributing factor in the development of asthma in the age group from 5 to 12 years. Some children only experience symptoms when physically active. These symptoms may include coughing, wheezing, chest tightness, and shortness of breath and are the result of inflammation that makes the airway overreact. Treatments available today can successfully treat exercise-induced asthma so children can fully participate in physical activity most of the time.

Food and food additives (e.g., sulfites), certain drugs (e.g., aspirin), perfumes, or strong odors may cause asthma in some children. Some evidence suggests that changes in physical and social environment, like a move or vacation may also precipitate asthma symptoms (National Asthma Education and Prevention, 1998). Also, exposure to sudden change in temperature, especially cold exposure may precipitate asthma symptoms in some children.

Other potential contributors to asthma exacerbation are related to home and building construction. Housing with little ventilation and the use of offensive building materials that emit volatile organic chemicals and formaldehyde are considered by many as influential in triggering asthma symptoms. These are speculations and have not been empirically tested (Clark et al., 1999).

STRATEGIES THAT WORK

Asthma continues to increase in the developed nations of the world with no clear indication as to what is causing this trend. Many factors are involved in this complex health issue. To date, there is no identified means to prevent asthma and no clear understanding as to how to prevent the natural progressions of the disease (Martinez, 1999). Consequently, there are no known strategies that work well in the prevention of primary asthma.

STRATEGIES THAT MIGHT WORK

Home, School, and Neighborhood Interventions

Multi-factorial approaches in the home and at school that consider the many factors that may contribute to the development of asthma are the most likely to have an impact on prevention of the disease in children. In the school-age population, the home is the single most important environment. Sources of pollutants in the home include cockroaches, cooking gas, animals, dust mites, smoking, and dust complicated by limited ventilation with outdoor air. The finding of a strong association between cockroach allergen exposure and asthma in the inner city has important public health implications. Developing interventions for cockroach control is a challenge because the allergens are found in the insect's gastrointestinal tract, saliva, feces, and body parts. Therefore, it is necessary to clean environments of the dead cockroaches after the use of pesticides. The spaces in which cockroaches reside are not easily accessible, making this a difficult challenge. A number of effective pesticides are now available for single- and multi-family housing, which reduce the populations of cockroaches by over 90 percent for up to 3 months, thus decreasing future infestation (Eggleston & Arruda, 2001). These strategies aimed at improving inner city housing may contribute to the elimination of cockroaches and consequently decrease the incidence of asthma among susceptible children. Also, there are practical measures that are effective in clinical trials for house dust mite control. In general, measures for removing the allergens are not well tested although vacuum cleaning has been found to be effective in institutional settings (Sarpong, Hamilton, Eggleston, & Adkinson, 1996). In addition, use of air conditioning and air filters may help to decrease humidity levels thus decreasing mold formation and the amount of aeroallergens.

In a study in Barcelona, Spain, installation of filters on silos to prevent airborne dissemination of allergenic soybean dust eliminated outbreaks of asthma caused by inhalation of dust. This result supports the premise that avoidance of these airborne allergens helps prevent asthma in this rural population (Anto et al., 1999).

School is the next most important environment in which children spend on average 15 percent of their time (Klepeis, 1999). Head Start may offer an unusual opportunity for asthma prevention programs in inner cities as there is a high incidence of asthma among children in those programs (Slezak et al., 1998). Identifying and removing the sources of mold and dust from rugs or ceiling tiles may enhance the environment for children at risk. Also, providing asthma self-management education to children during school time can significantly reduce the child's symptoms, improve psychological adjustment, and enhance school performance (Clark et al., 1999).

Improving outdoor air quality is a major initiative of the US Environmental Protection Agency (EPA), including protection of children from the harmful effects of ground level ozone, particulate matter, and toxic substances. This agency sets safe limits for most prevalent air pollutants and works with states to implement those standards. The ozone emission standard was strengthened in 1997 from 120 ppb averaged over 1 hr to 80 ppb averaged over 8 hr. These new limits were proposed to protect sensitive populations, such as asthmatics and children from the effects of ozone. Standards were also set for fine airborne particles for the first time. EPA estimates that these standards will protect 35 million children from potential harmful effects (Protection, 2000).

Following the guidelines of the Air Quality Index may help parents to limit exposure of children to outdoor air pollutants. This index indicates local levels of outdoor air pollutants on a daily basis and is available in the local newspaper, radio, or TV.

Psychological Approaches

Since it is known that severe stress may precipitate an asthma attack, providing children struggling with losses, family discord, or school problems, with counseling may decrease the risk of developing asthma symptoms. In a small study of 40 middle-school age children, aged 10–14 in New Haven, CT, children with asthma were randomly assigned to an asthma education group or coping skills training (CST) group (Esteban, 2000). CST sessions included opportunities for students to deal with potential life events in a small group setting. Results revealed that children who participated in the CST had higher asthma self-efficacy scores and lower depression scores than the children who had only asthma education. These findings suggest that CST may provide children with an enhanced ability to cope with the issues that may contribute to reoccurrence of an asthma attack. Neighborhood interventions that target stressors such as crime, violence, noise pollution, and lack of community resources may assist in the control of asthma as well (Clark et al., 1999).

Control of Respiratory Illness

Immunizing children against certain respiratory illnesses may prevent lower respiratory infection and future risk for development of asthma. Becker (2000) reports that many other approaches to vaccination have been suggested including the use of BCG vaccine which showed a decreased incidence of asthma in children with increased incidence of delayed hypersensitivity to tuberculin.

In addition, parents and day care workers can contribute to the control of viral infections through frequent and thorough hand washing. Support and resources for working parents to provide care for ill children may decrease the exposure of school age children to viral infections.

STRATEGIES THAT DO NOT WORK

Since the condition of asthma is complex with many contributing factors, interventions focused on single factors have the least likelihood of having an impact on its prevention. For example, cautioning parents and their children about the effects of tobacco smoke without providing them with support and resources to quit probably serves little purpose.

SYNTHESIS

This entry has attempted to address the many issues inherent in the prevention of asthma. The focus has been primary prevention, however, children with asthma would also benefit from many of the strategies in the prevention of exacerbation.

In determining the potential of a child to develop asthma, it is important to take into consideration many factors that may predispose a school-age child to asthma. First and foremost, a family history of asthma, especially if both parents are affected, places a child at greater risk. Especially, children with a family history of asthma, living in poor inner city housing, are at greater risk to develop asthma than are their suburban counterparts. Of paramount importance also is whether the child is atopic, meaning the child has a tendency toward allergies. Early sensitization to indoor allergens, especially to pets, and atopic dermatitis are predictors of subsequent development of asthma (Reijonen, Kotaniemi-Syrjanen, Korhonen, & Korppi, 2000). Of all indoor allergens, the elimination of exposure to cigarette smoke would appear to have the greatest impact on lung health.

In reducing morbidity and mortality associated with asthma, access to quality health care must be a priority. This is true in urban communities where poverty, lack of health insurance, and inadequate transportation may be a concern and in rural areas where geographic barriers to health care and health care providers are complicating factors. Although children in the age group from 5 to 12 years are at less risk to develop primary asthma than their younger and older counterparts, they are nevertheless exposed to numerous potential triggers in their home and school environments. Modification of environmental triggers is critical to the prevention of asthma. Further study is necessary to address the effectiveness of allergen avoidance in preventing allergen sensitization and in reducing asthma prevalence in children.

Further research is needed especially in high-risk populations to determine causes of asthma. More and larger studies of factors related to asthma severity among racial groups are needed. This may help to determine reasons for racial disparities in asthma prevalence and morbidity in the United States and elsewhere.

There is a need to develop public policies to address the unique vulnerabilities of children to various types of pollutants and the effects of multiple and cumulative exposures over a lifetime. There is mounting evidence to indicate that air pollution does in fact have adverse effects on children's health and improving air quality will lead to improvement in the health of children. Political and social initiatives will be required to improve air quality in our communities. Health care professionals can provide leadership and advocacy to promote environmental health initiatives in our communities (Dixon, 2002). Making our cities safe and providing adequate schools and housing for families will contribute to decreasing the incidence of asthma in the urban population. Commitment of public officials to child health issues and to the adoption of legislation that will protect our children now and in the future are critically needed.

Also see: Child Care: Early Childhood; Chronic Disease: Adolescence; Environmental Health: Early Childhood; Environmental Health: Childhood.

References

Anonymous. (2000). Long-term effects of budesonide or nedocromil in children with asthma. The Childhood Asthma Management Program Research Group. *New England Journal of Medicine, 343*(15), 1054–1063.

Anto, J.M., Soriano, J.B., Sunyer, J., Rodrigo, M.J., Morell, F., Roca, J., Rodriguez-Roisin, R., & Swanson, M.C. (1999). Long term outcome of soybean epidemic asthma after an allergen reduction intervention. *Thorax, 54*(8), 670–674.

Becker, A.B. (2000). Is primary prevention of asthma possible? *Pediatric Pulmonology, 30*(1), 63–72.

Clark, N.M., Brown, R.W., Parker, E., Robins, T.G., Remick, D.G., Jr., Philbert, M.A., Keeler, G.J., & Israel, B.A. (1999). Childhood asthma. *Environmental Health Perspectives, 107*(Suppl. 3), 421–429.

Dekker, C., Dales, R., Bartlett, S., Brunekreef, B., & Zwanenburg, H. (1991). Childhood asthma and the indoor environment. *Chest, 100*(4), 922–926.

Dixon, J.K. (2002). "Kids need clean air": Air pollution and children's health. *Family and Community Health, 24*(4), 9–26.

Eggleston, P.A., & Arruda, L.K. (2001). Ecology and elimination of cockroaches and allergens in the home. *Journal of Allergy and Clinical Immunology, 107*(Suppl. 3), S422–429.

Eggleston, P.A., Buckley, T.J., Breysse, P.N., Wills-Karp, M., Kleeberger, S.R., & Jaakkola, J.J. (1999). The environment and asthma in US inner cities. *Environmental Health Perspectives, 107*(Suppl. 3), 439–450.

Ehrlich, R.I., Du Toit, D., Jordaan, E., Zwarenstein, M., Potter, P., Volmink, J.A., & Weinberg, E. (1996). Risk factors for childhood asthma and wheezing. Importance of maternal and household smoking. *American Journal of Respiratory and Critical Care Medicine, 154*(3 Pt. 1), 681–688.

Esteban, C. (2000). *Effects of coping skills training among adolescents with asthma in school-based health clinics.* Unpublished Master's Thesis, Yale University School of Nursing, New Haven.

Fihe, D.M. (1999). Review: Controlling house dust mites is ineffective for asthmatic patients who are sensitive to mites [Commentary on Gotzsche, P.C., Hammarquist, C., Burr, M. (1998, October 24). House dust mite control measures in the management of asthma: meta-analysis. *British Medical Journal, 317*(7166), 1105–1110 and Hammarquist, C., Burr, M.L., & Gotzsche, P.C. (1998, April 30). House dust mite control measures for asthma (Cochrane Review, latest version). *Cochrane Library. Oxford: Update Software. Evidence Based Nursing, 2*(3).

Friedman, M.S., Powell, K.E., Hutwagner, L., Graham, L.M., & Teague, W.G. (2001). Impact of changes in transportation and commuting behaviors during the 1996 Summer Olympic Games in Atlanta on air quality and childhood asthma. *JAMA, 285*(7), 897–905.

Healthy People 2010 (Group), & United States Department of Health and Human Services. (2000). *Healthy people 2010.* Washington, DC: US Department of Health and Human Services.

Holt, P.G., Macaubas, C., Prescott, S.L., & Sly, P.D. (2000). Primary sensitization to inhalant allergens. *American Journal of Respiratory and Critical Care Medicine, 162*(3 Pt. 2), S91–94.

Illi, S., von Mutius, E., Lau, S., Bergmann, R., Niggemann, B., Sommerfeld, C., & Wahn, U. (2001). Early childhood infectious diseases and the development of asthma up to school age: a birth cohort study. *British Medical Journal, 322*(7283), 390–395.

Jones, A.P. (1998). Asthma and domestic air quality. *Social Science and Medicine, 47*(6), 755–764.

Joseph, C.L., Ownby, D.R., Peterson, E.L., & Johnson, C.C. (2000). Racial differences in physiologic parameters related to asthma among middle-class children. *Chest, 117*(5), 1336–1344.

Klepeis, N.E. (1999). An introduction to the indirect exposure assessment approach: modeling human exposure using microenvironmental measurements and the recent National Human Activity Pattern Survey. *Environmental Health Perspectives, 107*(Suppl. 2), 365–374.

Lang, D.M., & Polansky, M. (1994). Patterns of asthma mortality in Philadelphia from 1969 to 1991. *New England Journal of Medicine, 331*(23), 1542–1546.

Lux, A.L., Henderson, A.J., & Pocock, S.J. (2000). Wheeze associated with prenatal tobacco smoke exposure: A prospective, longitudinal study. ALSPAC Study Team. *Archives of Disease in Childhood, 83*(4), 307–312.

Mannino, D.M., Homa, D.M., Pertowski, C.A., Ashizawa, A., Nixon, L.L., Johnson, C.A., Ball, L.B., Jack, E., & Kang, D.S. (1998). Surveillance for asthma—United States, 1960–1995. *Morbidity and Mortality Weekly Report. CDC Surveillance Summaries, 47*(1), 1–27.

Martinez, F.D. (1999). Evolution of asthma through childhood. Paper Presented at the American College of Asthma, Allergy and Immunology, Chicago, IL.

Martinez, F.D., Wright, A.L., Taussig, L.M., Holberg, C.J., Halonen, M., & Morgan, W.J. (1995). Asthma and wheezing in the first six years of life. The Group Health Medical Associates. *New England Journal of Medicine, 332*(3), 133–138.

Mrazek, D.A., Klinnert, M., Mrazek, P.J., Brower, A., McCormick, D., Rubin, B., Ikle, D., Kastner, W., Larsen, G., Harbeck, R., & Jones, J. (1999). Prediction of early-onset asthma in genetically at-risk children. *Pediatric Pulmonology, 27*(2), 85–94.

Nafstad, P., Magnus, P., & Jaakkola, J.J. (2000). Early respiratory infections and childhood asthma. *Pediatrics, 106*(3), E38.

National Asthma Education and Prevention Program (National Heart, Lung and Blood Institute). Second Expert Panel on the Management of Asthma. (1998). *Expert Panel Report 2: Guidelines for the Diagnosis and Management of Asthma* (Publication No. 98-4051). Bethesda, MD: National Institutes of Health and National Heart, Lung and Blood Institute.

Ostro, B., Lipsett, M., Mann, J., Braxton-Owens, H., & White, M. (2001). Air pollution and exacerbation of asthma in African-American children in Los Angeles. *Epidemiology, 12*(2), 200–208.

Protection, U.S.E.P.A.O.o.C.s.H. (2000, 2/12/01). *Summary of EPA activities on asthma and other health effects.* Available: http://www.epa.gov/children/whatepa/national.htm#asthma

Reijonen, T.M., Kotaniemi-Syrjanen, A., Korhonen, K., & Korppi, M. (2000). Predictors of asthma three years after hospital admission for wheezing in infancy. *Pediatrics, 106*(6), 1406–1412.

Rosenstreich, D.L., Eggleston, P., Kattan, M., Baker, D., Slavin, R.G., Gergen, P., Mitchell, H., McNiff-Mortimer, K., Lynn, H., Ownby, D., & Malveaux, F. (1997). The role of cockroach allergy and exposure to cockroach allergen in causing morbidity among inner-city children with asthma. *New England Journal of Medicine, 336*(19), 1356–1363.

Samet, J.M. (1995). Asthma and the environment: Do environmental factors affect the incidence and prognosis of asthma? *Toxicology Letters, 82–83*, 33–38.

Sandberg, S. (2000). Severe stress may exacerbate childhood asthma. *The Lancet, 356*, 982–987.

Sarpong, S.B., Hamilton, R.G., Eggleston, P.A., & Adkinson, N.F., Jr. (1996). Socioeconomic status and race as risk factors for cockroach allergen exposure and sensitization in children with asthma. *Journal of Allergy and Clinical Immunology, 97*(6), 1393–1401.

Schwartz, D.A. (1999). Etiology and pathogenesis of airway disease in children and adults from rural communities. *Environmental Health Perspectives, 107*(Suppl. 3), 393–401.

Services, U.D.o.H.a.H. (2001). *Action against asthma—A strategic plan for the Department of Health and Human Services.* US Department of Health and Human Services. Available: http://aspe.hhs.gov/sp/asthma/overview.htm#overview [2002, 7/13/01].

Slezak, J.A., Persky, V.W., Kviz, F.J., Ramakrishnan, V., & Byers, C. (1998). Asthma prevalence and risk factors in selected Head Start sites in Chicago. *Journal of Asthma, 35*(2), 203–212.

Sporik, R., Holgate, S.T., Platts-Mills, T.A., & Cogswell, J.J. (1990). Exposure to house-dust mite allergen (Der p I) and the development of asthma in childhood. A prospective study. *New England Journal of Medicine, 323*(8), 502–507.

Statistics Canada. Health Statistics Division. (1995). *National population health survey overview* (Vol. 1994). Ottawa: Statistics Canada.

Strachan, D.P., & Cook, D.G. (1998). Health effects of passive smoking. 6. Parental smoking and childhood asthma: Longitudinal and case-control studies. *Thorax, 53*(3), 204–212.

Vacek, L. (1999). Is the level of pollutants a risk factor for exercise-induced asthma prevalence? *Allergy and Asthma Proceedings, 20*(2), 87–93.

Williams, P., Worstell, M., Goldberg, E., Kaluzny-Petroff, S., Golding, J., Luna, P., Majer, L. (1995). *Asthma and physical activity in the school: Making a difference* [web document]. National Heart, Lung and Blood Institute. Available: http://www.nih.gov/health/asthma/ [2001, 6/11/01].

Attention Deficit Hyperactivity Disorder (ADHD), Childhood

Miriam Mulsow and Jeong Rim Lee

INTRODUCTION

While existing knowledge does not enable us to prevent ADHD, there is much that can be done to improve the lives of children with this disorder. These preventive interventions are directed toward modifying the environment around these children to enhance their ability to function successfully as well as to strengthen the child's ability to cope with this disorder and avoid long-term problematic outcomes.

DEFINITIONS

Attention Deficit Hyperactivity Disorder (ADHD) is the most commonly diagnosed behavioral disorder of childhood. Core symptoms include developmentally inappropriate levels of attention, hyperactivity, distractibility, and impulsivity (National Institutes of Health, 1998) that appear before age 7, persist longer than 6 months, and create problems in multiple settings (e.g., home, school, work, peer group). Not all symptoms need be present for a diagnosis. ADHD has also been called attention deficit disorder, hyperactive child syndrome, hyperkinesis, minimal brain dysfunction, hyperkinetic syndrome of childhood, and hyperkinetic disorder.

Inattention symptoms include carelessness, difficulty in sustaining concentration, reluctance and difficulty in organizing and completing work correctly, failure to follow through, tendency to lose things, excessive forgetfulness, and high distractibility. *Hyperactivity* involves excessive movement, restlessness, fidgetiness, or excessive talking. *Impulsivity*, an inability to inhibit behavior, makes it difficult to stop and think before behaving or to delay gratification. *Comorbidity* means the existence of two different conditions in the same person. ADHD is commonly comorbid with *Conduct Disorder* (CD) or *Oppositional Defiant Disorder* (ODD). These two terms are sometimes used interchangeably, although ODD may be more accurately described as an earlier, less severe disorder similar to CD.

Stimulants represent the most common form of medication prescribed for children with ADHD, although other drugs have been used with varying degrees of effectiveness. *Behavioral interventions* attempt to increase positive behaviors and decrease negative behaviors by using reinforcement. *Cognitive behavioral modification* (CMB) involves techniques such as stepwise problem solving and self-monitoring.

SCOPE

Prevalence estimates for ADHD range from 3 to 10 percent of the child population and 1 to 5 percent of the adult population (Barkley, 1997; NIH, 1998). Dulcan, Dunne, Ayers, Arnold, Benson, and associates (1997) report a prevalence of 10.1 percent of males and 3.3 percent of females aged 4–11 years in Ontario, Canada. Children with ADHD are at risk to repeat a grade, be suspended from school, exhibit conduct disorder and other behavioral problems, have delays in language development, have memory deficits, make lower grades than they seem to be capable of making, and experience social rejection, depression, anxiety, accidental injuries, risk-taking behavior, poor sense of time, and sleep problems (Barkley, 1998). Family relationships are also impaired, with families of ADHD children reporting more stress, frustration, disappointment, guilt, fatigue, marital dysfunction, divorce, and psychological disorders including ADHD and depression in parents, and family therapy (Fisher, 1990). Individuals with ADHD consume numerous resources and attention from the health care system, criminal justice system, schools, and other social service agencies (NIH, 1998). "Additional national public school expenditures on behalf of students with ADHD may have exceeded $3 billion in 1995. Moreover, ADHD, often in conjunction with coexisting conduct disorders, contributes to societal problems such as violent crime and teenage pregnancy" (NIH, 1998, p. 4).

Clinical samples of ADHD overwhelmingly consist of male subjects, leading to a gender bias in existing literature. Although the ratio of males having ADHD is three to one over females, conservative estimates indicate that over one million girls and women are affected by ADHD (Dulcan et al., 1997; NIH, 1998). ADHD in girls tends to be overlooked, not just in studies, but also in diagnosis and treatment. Although girls with ADHD are less likely to develop behaviors such as criminal behavior, they do experience increased incidence of unintended pregnancy (NIH, 1998) and depression.

Long-term problems are common among adults with a history of ADHD in childhood. Some of these are more prevalent among adults who continue to have diagnosable levels of ADHD symptoms, but some occur even in those who no longer meet diagnostic criteria (Barkley, 1998). Among problems that have been reported at elevated levels in adults who have ADHD or who have a history of ADHD in childhood are occupational underachievement, substance abuse, depression, impulsivity, isolation, low educational attainment, early, unintended pregnancy, marital disruption, inadequate financial and other resources, poor coping skills, impulsive spending, arrests, gambling, accidents, impulsive aggression/violence, delayed development, poverty, excessive driving violations, failed marriages, antisocial behavior, and substance abuse (Barkley, 1997, 1998; Mulsow, O'Neal, & Murry, 2001). For example, among the children with ADHD followed prospectively into adulthood in various studies, 28 percent experienced major depression, 75 percent reported interpersonal problems, almost 10 percent attempted suicide, 20 percent committed acts of physical aggression, 36–52 percent were arrested at least once, 30–32 percent never completed high school, only 5 percent completed a university degree, 17 percent contracted a sexually transmitted disease, and 42 percent had their licenses suspended or revoked (Barkley, 1998).

THEORIES AND RESEARCH

What is ADHD? A person with ADHD is unable to delay responses to stimuli (Barkley, 1997). The apparent lack of attention in those with ADHD may result from an inability to select important stimuli in the environment versus those that can be ignored. Barkley suggests that this inability is related to a deficiency in behavioral inhibition and that "the problem ... is not one of knowing what to do but one of doing what you know when it would be most adaptive to do so" (1997, p. 78).

What causes ADHD? Although exact causes are not known, research suggests an impairment of brain functioning, with particular emphasis on the frontal lobe area (Barkley, 1998). Twin studies support a genetic transmission of ADHD accounting for 0.73–0.76 percent of the variance in children aged 5–9 years (Gjone, Stevenson, & Sundet, 1996). However, controversy surrounds the degree to which this genetic component explains the development of the disorder and how much of a contribution is made by the environment (e.g., prenatal complications). Joseph (2000) contends that neither twin nor adoption studies of families of ADHD children are reliable indicators that there is a

genetic component to ADHD or any other psychological disorder. He does not, however, address genetic mutations that have been identified in people with ADHD (Faraone, Doyle, Mick, & Biederman, 2001). Regardless of its origin, outcomes for children with ADHD are influenced by the environment surrounding the child, including the parenting they receive, the educational interventions offered, whether the disorder is treated, and the ability of other systems in the community to respond to the child's needs.

What Causes Long-Term Problems Associated with ADHD?

Individual Stress

A child's life with ADHD is not easy. Children who live with this disorder and its associated costs carry an extra burden of stressors compared to other children. When a child is stressed or discouraged, we know that one common response is misbehavior. Sometimes these children fall into the role of the family scapegoat. Other children who become discouraged may internalize the pain, thus developing problems such as depression or anxiety. In either case, the consequences of living with the stressors and discouragement associated with having ADHD may contribute to problematic outcomes for these children as they mature.

Comorbid Disorders

Many authors attribute depression and other mood disorders commonly comorbid with ADHD to a lifetime of disappointments and frustrations (Barkley, 1998). However, there is evidence that at least some of the mood disorders associated with ADHD are independent of the ADHD (Barkley, 1998). Thus, it is possible that some of the long-term problems among people with ADHD could be linked to comorbid affective disorders rather than to the ADHD.

ADHD and precursors to antisocial personality (conduct disorder and oppositional defiant disorder) commonly coexist. There is some evidence that these conduct problems may be the factors that most strongly predict problematic outcomes such as criminality and substance abuse (Dulcan et al., 1997). Recent studies, however, suggest that even when conduct problems are controlled, ADHD-linked impulsivity is associated with problematic outcomes (Babinski, Hartsough, & Lambert, 1999).

Self-Medication

Some researchers have proposed that people with comorbid ADHD and substance abuse are attempting to self-medicate their ADHD symptoms (Wilens, Biederman,

Spencer, & Frances, 1994). The incidence of stimulant use is high among people with ADHD, and studies of substance abusers with ADHD show an increase in self-esteem with the use of substances. Others suggest that the increase in life stressors associated with ADHD (Barkley, 1998) may lead to substance abuse and other negative outcomes.

Impulsivity

The association of hyperactivity and impulsivity, but not inattention, with later criminality lend support to the idea that it is the impulsivity that may lead to some of the most devastating long-term problems associated with ADHD (Babinski et al., 1999). Barkley (1998) suggests that the key symptom in ADHD is impulsivity and that the inattentive type of ADHD may be a different, and less severe, disorder. He suggests that impulsive people with ADHD lack the ability to stop and consider the consequences before acting.

Parenting Practices

As children are stressed so too are their parents. Their difficulties in managing their child may lead them to over-reacting or extreme disciplinary behaviors. Children with ADHD are more likely to experience coercive parenting practices, more physical and non-physical punishment, and more negative communication from their parents than are children from families without ADHD. When researchers examine families of children with ADHD in which parenting styles differ, they find that those children with ADHD whose parents are more coercive (Hinshaw, Klein, & Abikoff, 1998) and less protective are more likely to develop aggressive and antisocial behaviors than those children with ADHD whose parents are less coercive and more protective.

STRATEGY OVERVIEW

One approach to handling long-term problems among children with ADHD is to treat ADHD symptoms so that they do not contribute to ADHD-linked problems such as social isolation and academic failure in childhood that lead to problematic outcomes in adulthood. This focus on the child is treatment, and it has been shown to be productive (Biederman, Wilens, Mick, Spencer, & Faraone, 1999; Greenhill, 1998; Hinshaw, Klein, & Abikoff, 1998). Another approach is to modify aspects of the child's environment (e.g., classroom and parenting practices, social support) and to teach the child self-management skills (behavioral interventions) to reduce the likelihood of emotional and

behavioral problems among children with ADHD. These preventive strategies will be discussed in the following sections. But first, it is necessary to discuss the use of medications for children with ADHD.

There are some who consider the use of the words medication and prevention in the same sentence as an invitation for a heated disagreement. In this case, medication is clearly not a solution by itself but it can be a useful adjunct for the child with ADHD. Stimulant medication has been used with many individuals with ADHD to help them better manage their symptoms. It appears helpful for approximately 80 percent of all people with ADHD as long as use of the medication is continued (Barkley, 1998).

Stimulant medication has been shown to improve child behavior with parents and problem solving in interactions with peers (Greenhill, 1998). Children exhibit better compliance to requests from their mothers. Therefore, their mothers decrease their rates of commands for compliance while increasing their levels of passive observation and nondirective interactions (Fisher, 1990). Children with hyperactivity and conduct disorder become less antisocial in both structured and unstructured situations (Greenhill, 1998). Stimulant treatment has also been shown to be useful for people with comorbid ADHD and depression. Importantly, the use of medication to treat ADHD in childhood has been shown to reduce the risk of adult substance abuse compared to children with ADHD who were not treated with medication (Biederman et al., 1999). It should be noted that while medication has been shown to be effective in treating the symptoms of ADHD, it has not been shown to improve social or academic skills after its use has been discontinued. Thus, others interventions using prevention's available technology are vitally necessary. Unfortunately, the development of this technology for this problem behavior is still in its infancy. However, three interventions can be judged effective.

STRATEGIES THAT WORK

Token Economies

Interventions that teach an individual to self-manage their behavior are an example of the prevention tool of education. Children with ADHD need immediate feedback in order to reinforce positive behaviors and discourage negative ones (Barkley, 1998; Teeter, 1998). One practical and widely used method of accomplishing this is through the use of token systems. While these systems do not reduce the core symptoms of hyperactivity, impulsivity, or inattention, they are effective for producing improvements in specific behaviors (Dulcan et al., 1997).

Parent Education

Preventionists have long understood that modifications in the environment often produce positive change. Helping parents to understand the complex nature of this disorder can help them reframe their understanding, diminish family accusations and guilt, and encourage new ways of dealing more effectively with their children (Barkley, 1998; Teeter, 1998). Although parenting does not cause ADHD, parent–child interactions can influence long-term outcome for those with ADHD (Hinshaw et al., 1998; Teeter, 1998). Danforth (1998) reported that parent training improved parenting behavior, reduced maternal stress, and reduced oppositional behavior in children with ADHD. A 6-month follow-up revealed that parenting and child behavior remained stable. Cunningham, Bremner, and Secord-Gilbert (1993) reported success in offering parenting courses for parents of children with ADHD in large, school-based settings. Parent training has been used as a successful educational tool to teach and reinforce the use of authoritative methods. Hinshaw and associates (1998) demonstrate that authoritative parenting beliefs predict more positive peer relations among children with ADHD (see Teeter (1998) for reviews of several different types of parenting education programs).

Teacher Training and Classroom Interventions

In addition to increasing knowledge among family members, it is important to educate teachers about the disorder prior to involving them in classroom interventions (Teeter, 1998). Barkley (1998) reports that "a positive teacher–student relationship, based on teacher understanding of the student and the disorder, may improve academic and social functioning" (p. 459). Both Barkley (1998) and Teeter (1998) discuss the importance of and information to be included in teacher training and support. Classroom interventions that have been shown to be effective include a structured environment that limits distractions, token economies, daily report cards, homework notebooks that are reviewed and signed daily by parents and teachers, and the allowance of increased time or modified assignments as appropriate for individual children (Dulcan et al., 1997).

STRATEGIES THAT MIGHT WORK

Social Skills Training

Alone, social skills training has not, as yet, shown promising results for children with ADHD (MTA Cooperative Group, 1999). However, when it is combined with other interventions (including medication), its effectiveness does increase.

Social Support

Parent support groups, such as Children and Adults with Attention Deficit Disorder (CHADD) assist families in dealing with the stressors of living with ADHD (Barkley, 1998). They help families to recognize and overcome unhealthy patterns of interaction that have developed in response to the stress of living with ADHD (Kendall, 1999; Teeter, 1998). Further, the beneficial effects to affected families of being both caregivers to other parents struggling with this issue and care receivers is not only empowering but self-therapeutic.

Biofeedback

Biofeedback has shown promise for helping people with ADHD to control their bodies' responses to cognitive stimuli (Nash, 2000). Future research is necessary to determine if these skills can be generalized to the real world.

Summer Camps

Many families report intensive summer programs specifically tailored for their ADHD children helpful in providing support, a sense of "fitting in" for the child, and a needed respite for the parents. Although parents, staff, and children rate these programs positively, questions remain as to the actual improvements provided by these programs, their cost-to-benefit ratio, and how long improvements seen may last (Dulcan et al., 1997).

STRATEGIES THAT DO NOT WORK

It appears that problems among children with ADHD cannot be prevented by relying on the elimination of sugar from the diet, severe discipline, or relying solely on medication (MTA Cooperative Group, 1999; NIH, 1998).

Diets

To date, the number of children who have been helped by dietary restrictions has been limited. In particular, the elimination of sugar from the diet has not resulted in significant improvement in ADHD symptoms. There are studies being conducted into more complex dietary restrictions, but results to date suggest that dietary restrictions may only be effective for a small subgroup of children who have both ADHD symptoms and food allergies or sensitivities (Dulcan et al., 1997).

Severe Discipline

Commonly, parents will initially deny the existence of a disorder in their children with ADHD and will attempt to control their children's behavior with increasingly strict discipline. Although a highly structured environment has been shown to be effective in helping children with ADHD to manage their disorder, severe discipline has not. In fact, studies indicate that severe discipline contributes to a greater probability of negative outcomes among children with ADHD (Hoza, Owens, Pelham, Swanson, Connors et al., 2000).

Medication without Any Other Intervention

Often, parents and teachers of children with ADHD are so relieved at the improvements seen in children's behavior after medication is introduced that they overlook the problems that still exist despite the use of medication (MTA Cooperative Group, 1999; NIH, 1998). Findings are clear that medication alone will not prevent long-term problems (Dulcan et al., 1997).

SYNTHESIS

Dulcan and associates (1997) have compiled a summary of findings from treatment studies that have bearing for preventionists. In this document, they state that:

> Medication should not be used as a substitute for appropriate educational curricula, student-to-teacher ratios, or other environmental accommodations .... At times, the most appropriate response to a behavioral problem is behavior modification, a change in classroom placement, or modification of the teacher's classroom management style .... Even children who respond positively to medication continue to show deficits in many areas. Specific learning disabilities, gaps in academic knowledge and skills due to inattention, and impaired organizational abilities may require educational remediation. Parent training in techniques of behavior management are often indicated. Social skills deficits and family pathology may need specific treatment. (Dulcan et al., 1997, p. 91S)

These findings and the literature reviewed in this entry suggest that the following preventive interventions should be further developed and tested in the coming decade: (1) improvements in diagnostic methods for ADHD (MTA Cooperative Group, 1999; NIH, 1998); (2) education for pediatricians and family doctors concerning prevention methods that go beyond medication; (3) efficacy and cost–benefit analysis of biofeedback; (4) treating ADHD as a family issue rather than an individual problem, and designing preventative strategies accordingly; (5) further research into the nature of genetic (e.g., specific gene mutations) and environmental (e.g., prenatal environment) involvement in the disorder so that preventative strategies can be more appropriately targeted; (6) resiliency studies of adults who had ADHD in childhood who cope successfully in adulthood; and (7) the inclusion of current, accurate information on the management of ADHD in the classroom in new teacher education and inservice programs for continuing teachers.

While we have not yet developed technologies that are capable of preventing ADHD, we are able to prevent many problems associated with this disorder. We can reduce symptoms and make environmental changes to minimize the socioemotional and behavioral contexts that contribute to long-term problems. In so doing, we create a context at home and school that is less likely to interact with the child's symptoms to increase the probability that problems will occur.

Also see: Child Care: Early Childhood; Family Strengthening: Childhood; Family Strengthening: Adolescence; Physical Health: Early Childhood.

References

Babinski, L.M., Hartsough, C.S., & Lambert, N.M. (1999). Childhood conduct problems, hyperactivity-impulsivity, and inattention as predictors of adult criminal activity. *Journal of Child Psychology and Psychiatry and Allied Disciplines, 40*, 347–355.

Barkley, R. (1997). Behavioral inhibition, sustained attention, and executive functions: Constructing a unifying theory of ADHD. *Psychological Bulletin, 121*, 65–94.

Barkley, R.A. (1998). *Attention deficit hyperactivity disorder: A handbook for diagnosis and treatment.* New York: Guilford Press.

Biederman, J., Wilens, T., Mick, E., Spencer, T., & Faraone, S.V. (1999). Pharmacotherapy of attention-deficit/hyperactivity disorder reduces risk for substance use disorder. *Pediatrics, 104*, e20.

Cunningham, C.E., Bremner, R., & Secord-Gilbert, M. (1993) Increasing the availability, accessibility, and cost efficacy of services for families of ADHD children: A school-based systems-oriented parenting course. *Canadian Journal of School Psychology, 9*, 1–15.

Danforth, J.S. (1998). The outcome of parent training using the Behavior Management Flow Chart with mothers and their children with oppositional defiant disorder and attention-deficit hyperactivity disorder. *Behavior Modification, 22*, 443–473.

Dulcan, M., Dunne, J.E., Ayers, W., Arnold, V., Benson, S., Bernet, W. et al. (1997). Practice parameters for the assessment and treatment of children, adolescents, and adults with attention-deficit/hyperactivity disorder: AACAP Official Action. *Journal of the American Academy of Child and Adolescent Psychiatry, 36*(Suppl.), 85S–121S.

Faraone, S.V., Doyle, A.E., Mick, E., & Biederman, J. (2001). Meta-analysis of the association between the 7-repeat allele of the dopamine D-sub-4 receptor gene and attention deficit hyperactivity disorder. *American Journal of Psychiatry* [Special Issue], *158*, 1052–1057.

Fisher, M. (1990). Parenting stress and the child with attention deficit hyperactivity disorder. *Journal of Clinical Psychology, 19*, 337–346.

Gjone, H., Stevenson, J., & Sundet, J.M. (1996). Genetic influence on parent-reported attention-related problems in a Norwegian general population twin sample. *Journal of the American Academy of Child and Adolescent Psychiatry, 35*, 588–596.

Greenhill, L.L. (1998). Childhood attention deficit hyperactivity disorder: Pharmacological treatments. In P.E. Nathan & J.M. Gorman (Eds.), *A guide to treatments that work*, (pp. 26–41). New York: Oxford University Press.

Hinshaw, S.P., Klein, R.G., & Abikoff, H. (1998). Childhood attention deficit hyperactivity disorder: Nonpharmacological and combination treatment. In P.E. Nathan & J.M. Gorman (Eds.), *A guide to treatments that work* (pp. 26–41). New York: Oxford University Press.

Hoza, B., Owens, J.S., Pelham, W.E, Swanson, J.M, Connors, C.K. et al. (2000). Parent cognitions as predictors of child treatment response in attention-deficit/hyperactivity disorder. *Journal of Abnormal Child Psychology* [Special Issue] *Child and family characteristics as predictors and outcomes in the Multimodal Treatment Study of ADHD (MTA Study), 28*, 569–583.

Joseph, J. (2000). Not in their genes: A critical view of the genetics of attention-deficit hyperactivity disorder. *Developmental Review, 20*, 539–567.

Kendall, J. (1999). Sibling accounts of attention deficit hyperactivity disorder (ADHD). *Family Process, 38*, 117–136.

MTA Cooperative Group. (1999). A 14-month randomized clinical trial of treatment strategies for attention deficit/hyperactivity disorder. *Archives of General Psychiatry, 56*, 1073–1086.

Mulsow, M., O'Neal, K., & Murry, V.M. (2001). Adult attention deficit hyperactivity disorder, the family, and child maltreatment. *Trauma, Violence, and Abuse: A Review Journal, 2*, 36–50.

Nash, J.K. (2000). Treatment of attention deficit hyperactivity disorder with neurotherapy. *Clinical Electroencephalography, 31*, 30–37.

National Institutes of Health (NIH) Consensus Statement Online 16 (1998, November 10) Diagnosis and treatment of attention deficit hyperactivity disorder. Accessed November 16–18, 1999, pp. 1–37. Available at: http://odp.od.nih.gov/consensus/cons/110/110_statement.htm.

Teeter, P.A. (1998). *Intervention for ADHD: Treatment in developmental context.* NY: Guilford.

Thomas, J.M. (1995). Traumatic stress disorder presents as hyperactivity and disruptive behavior: Case presentation, diagnoses, and treatment. *Infant Mental Health Journal, 16* [Special Issue] Posttraumatic stress disorder (PTSD) in infants and young children. 306–317.

Wilens, T.E., Biederman, J., Spencer, T., & Frances, R.J. (1994). Comorbidity of attention-deficit hyperactivity and psychoactive substance use disorders. *Hospital and Community Psychiatry, 45*, 421–423, 435.

B

Bereavement, Childhood

Tim S. Ayers and Irwin N. Sandler

INTRODUCTION

The impact that the death of a loved one has on the development and adaptation of a child has been of great interest to both clinicians and theoreticians for many years. It has only been in the past two decades that well-controlled studies of risk and protective factors for bereaved children have begun to emerge and even more recently that rigorous evaluations of preventive interventions for these children have been conducted. This entry reviews the work in these areas. Although some children are exposed to many types of death during childhood, including but not limited to parent, sibling, grandparents, other relatives, and peers, the focus of this entry will be on the impact of parental death since the majority of the empirical work has been done examining this type of bereavement. Although there are growing bodies of empirical work examining the impact of the death of a sibling (for review, see Davies, 1999) and to a lesser extent the death of peers or other relatives (Balk, 1996; Ringler & Hayden, 2000), they are still somewhat limited.

SCOPE

The best prevalence estimates for parental death in the United States come from the Social Security Administration, which is responsible for distributing death benefits to families where there has been the death of one or both parents. Based on data from 1997 (Social Security Administration, 2000), overall 3.5 percent of children under the age of 18 had experienced the death of their parent (73.9 percent death of a father, 25 percent death of a mother, and 1.1 percent have experienced the death of both parents). For children between the ages of 0–5, approximately 1.1 percent of the population has experienced the death of a parent (75 percent death of a father, 24.6 percent death of a mother and 0.4 percent have experienced the death of both parents). This figure nearly doubles to 2.2 percent when you consider all children between the ages of 0–11 with comparable percentages of father to mother deaths as listed above. Unfortunately, no figures are available that would provide estimates of incidence or prevalence of parental death across other demographic categories such as gender or ethnicity.

The prevalence of parental deaths in other countries varies greatly from the figures available in the United States. The Demographic and Health Surveys (DHS+ Demographic and Health Surveys, 2001) are nationally representative household surveys with sample sizes of around 5,000, which have been conducted in several countries and can offer estimates of parental deaths in various regions of the world. Because of the way the DHS are summarized, estimates for parental death can be calculated for children between the ages of 0–9. DHS that have been conducted in 17 different countries across Sub-Saharan Africa, North Africa, Asia, and Latin America since 1997, indicate that the percentage of children aged 0–9 who experienced the death of either one or both parents ranges from a low of 0.4 percent in Turkey to 5.9 percent in Guatemala.[1] The average percentage of children aged 0–9 who experienced the death of a parent across these 17 countries is approximately 3 percent which is slightly higher than the figures available for the United States or the United Kingdom. It is likely that cross-national differences in rates of parental death vary as a function of factors such as wars, famines, and epidemics as well as differences across countries in rates of poverty and the quality of the public health systems.

THEORIES AND RESEARCH

Research on the impact of bereavement during childhood has increasingly begun to take into consideration the importance of the child's developmental level of cognitive, social, and emotional functioning. As Oltjenbruns (2001) noted, a more complete understanding of the bereavement process and its impact might best be accomplished by considering the context of the cognitive-language capacities and various developmental tasks to be accomplished during these periods. While no single classification of developmental levels is sacrosanct, to facilitate the discussion of material to be reviewed in this entry, we will refer to four developmental periods; infancy (spanning from approximately 0–2 years), preschool (approximately 3–4 years), middle childhood (approximately 5–7 years), and late childhood (approximately 8–11 years) periods.

One area where developmental differences have been studied is children's understanding of the concept of death (for recent reviews, see Speece & Brent, 1984, 1996; Stambrook & Parker, 1987). It is logical to believe that cognitive-language capacities will affect children's understanding of death and thereby could influence their grief experience. Piaget's (1959) four-stage model of cognitive development was initially a popular framework to understand the development of children's concepts of death.

Recently, investigators have begun to study development of children's concepts of death by comparing different components of children's concepts with adult concepts of death on these components (Speece & Brent, 1984, 1996). In this approach the concept of death is made up of several distinct components: universality, irreversibility, nonfunctionality, and causality. Speece and Brent (1996) have chosen to carefully define each of these components in what they view as an important first step to standardizing the measurement of these aspects of the concept of death. *Universality* refers to the child's understanding that death is inevitable, that it will happen to everyone, including himself or herself. *Nonfunctionality* refers to the understanding that all life-defining functions (e.g., eating, sleeping, dreaming, thinking) cease at death. *Irreversibility* refers to the understanding that all things that die do not come back to life. Finally, *causality* refers to a child's ability to understand the objective and biological causes of death.[2] In a recent review (Speece & Brent, 1996), they suggest that attention should also be paid to children's understanding of *noncorporeal continuation*, which refers to the notion that some form of personal continuation exists after the death of the physical body (e.g., reincarnation or ascension of the soul to heaven without the body).

Investigations have typically focused on determining the sequence and age or developmental level at which mature (adult-like) concepts of death are achieved on each of these components. Although there has been a great deal of variability in the reported ages at which each of the components have been obtained (varying from 4 to 12 years of age), Speece and Brent (1996) report that the majority of the studies have found that by the age of 7 (end of middle childhood), most children understand the four key components of death.

With regard to the order in which these concepts are developed, Lazar and Torney-Purta (1991) in a short-term, longitudinal study of first and second graders found that children first understand the concepts of universality and irreversibility prior to understanding the concepts of nonfunctionality and causality. In addition, they found that although these concepts were not conditional on each other at least one of them had to be understood prior to the child understanding nonfunctionality or causality.

In the few cross-cultural comparisons of the development of death concepts in children, investigators have found both transcultural similarities (Brent, Speece, Lin, Dong, & Yang, 1996) and differences (Brent et al., 1996;

---

[1] This range of estimates comes from all Demographic and Health Surveys (DHS+) completed since 1997 (Demographic and Health Surveys, 2001). This range was calculated based on the following 16 countries with the prevalence estimates of parental death for children between the ages of 0–9 for each country and the year of the survey included within the parentheses (e.g., year of survey, estimate for 0–9); Kenya (1998, 3.6), Madagascar (1997, 3.3), Mozambique (1997, 4.3), Cameroon (1998, 3.9), Ghana (1998, 4.6), Guinea (1999, 5.3), Niger (1998, 2.5), Chad (1997, 3.9), Togo (1998, 1.4), Jordan (1997, 2.5), Yemen (1997, 1.6), Kyrgyz Republic (1997, 2.2), Turkey (1998, 0.4), Indonesia (1997, 0.8), Guatemala (1999, 5.9), Nicaragua (1997, 1.7), and Bolivia (1998, 2.6).

[2] Other investigators have used other terms for each of these concepts, for example, inevitability, cessation, and permanence for universality, nonfunctionality, and irreversibility respectively. Some examples of other components that some investigators have researched are animism (i.e., the understanding that only animate things die), disposition—understanding of what happens to the physical body after death (e.g., funerals, burial, cremation), and decomposition—understanding that the body decomposes.

Schonfeld & Smilansky, 1989). Schonfeld and Smilansky (1989) in a comparison of Israeli and American school children aged 4–12 years, found that Israeli children scored higher than their American counterparts on scales of the Smilansky Death Concept Questionnaire that assess "irreversibility" and "finality" death concepts, suggesting a more mature understanding of these concepts (for a comparison of Chinese and US children, see also Brent et al., 1996). Possible reasons for these observed differences might be due to Israeli children's awareness and understanding of death due to the political unrest and ongoing military activity in their country.

Importantly, the work of Brent and colleagues (Brent & Speece, 1993; Brent et al., 1996) has begun to question the initial assumption that there would be a linear increase in the concept of "irreversibility" reflecting a more "mature" adult concept of death. Instead, these authors have begun to believe that the development of some of these concepts of death might be characterized as a species of "fuzzy" logic that governs certain types of "fuzzy" sets (Kosko & Sartoru, 1993). As an example, adult considerations of the boundaries between life and death, that is, the irreversibility concept are seemingly more ambiguous because adults now take into account the impact of modern medical technology (e.g., resuscitation), anecdotal accounts of premorbid out-of-body experiences, and the legal and clinical definitions of death when responding to questions about this concept.

Speece and Brent (1996) in their recent review of the literature conclude that ethnicity, gender, socioeconomic status, and religion have been found to be relatively unimportant factors in influencing the development of children's concepts of death. However, in addition to the cross-cultural differences mentioned earlier, concepts of death may be influenced by death-related experiences, life-threatening illnesses, and intelligence. For example, although the research literature is not definitive, bereavement writers such as Lonetto (1980) have suggested that greater and earlier experiences with death or life-threatening illnesses may stimulate development of more mature concepts of death. As Deveau (1995, 1997) notes that the challenge for those designing preventive or clinical interventions for bereaved children is to integrate the current, yet inconclusive information within this area into their thinking about the ways in which bereaved children, particularly children in the preschool (aged 2–4), and middle childhood (aged 5–7) periods are thinking about the death of a loved one.

Four recent reviews have summarized an emerging empirical literature on the relations between parental death and mental health and adaptive functioning in childhood and adulthood (Clark, Pynoos, & Goebel, 1994; Dowdney, 2000; Lutzke, Ayers, Sandler, & Barr, 1997; Tremblay & Israel, 1998). As various authors have noted (Dowdney, 2000;

Oltjenbruns, 2001), the limited number of methodologically rigorous studies and the difficulties in finding representative samples of bereaved children has led to an often confusing array of findings related to risk status for bereaved children. Oltjenbruns (2001) also emphasizes that many studies have involved children of various developmental stages and that this broad age span is rarely taken into account when interpreting the findings of these studies. A brief and yet more selective focus on methodologically rigorous studies, which have examined the risk status of primarily parentally bereaved children, is offered below.[3]

When considering studies of bereaved children who fall in the middle to late childhood periods, four studies have included children within a 4–13-year-old age span. Felner, Stolberg, and Cowen (1975) in a study of bereaved and comparison children aged 5–10 years old, who had been identified by teachers as having early school adjustment problems found that bereaved children had significantly higher overall maladjustment and moodiness/withdrawal behaviors but did not have significantly higher scores on acting out or learning problems. In a replication study of children referred by school personnel, Felner, Ginter, Boike, and Cowen (1981) found that bereaved children were significantly more shy and anxious than controls. However, in a revised study of normal school children (who were not referred) they found no differences between the bereaved and control children on the shy-anxious measure.

Nelson (1982) compared children aged 5–13 years old who had experienced the "loss" of a father by divorce or death in the past 14–25 months and children from "intact" families. Bereaved children's self-report indicated they had poorer social emotional adjustment relative to the children from intact families. The children did not differ based on parent or teacher report of symptomatology. Sood, Weller, Weller, Fristad, and Bowes (1992) examined somatic complaints of bereaved children aged 5–12 at 3 and 12 weeks following parental death with a sample of inpatient depressed children and a sample of normal control children. Based on child report there were no significant differences in overall somatic complaints between the bereaved children and the comparison groups. Bereaved children reported very few somatic complaints. When there were symptoms, the most commonly reported were gastrointestinal problems and headaches.

Those studies with samples that had a broader age range yet in which analyses examining the interaction of current age of the sample by bereavement status in the prediction of mental health status also are useful in assessing the effects of bereavement during childhood. Van Eerdewegh, Clayton, and Van Eerdewegh (1985) split their sample of bereaved

---

[3] As an initial criterion, the inclusion of a comparison condition was necessary in order for the study to be included in this selective review.

children aged 2–17 into children aged 12 and under and those older, all of whom were assessed at 1 and 13 months since the parental death. The younger bereaved children had significantly greater bed-wetting and loss of interest in activities relative to the control children. Gersten, Beals, and Kallgren (1991) dichotomized a community sample of bereaved children into groups aged 8–11 and 12–16, although they had found that bereaved children had 7.5 times greater risk for depression than controls in the overall sample, there were no main or interaction effects for age when dichotomizing the sample in this way. Worden and Silverman (1996), in a longitudinal study of a community sample of bereaved children aged 6–18 examined parent's report of symptomatology in age by gender groupings. Preadolescent boys (aged 6–11) did not differ in their symptom levels from their matched controls at 1 or 2 years following the death. However, pre-adolescent girls (aged 6–11), although not different in symptom levels at 1 year were significantly more depressed, anxious, and aggressive than their matched controls at the 2 years following the death.

As can be seen from the selective review presented above, evidence of risk for mental health problems in parentally bereaved children (aged 0–12) might best be characterized currently as inconsistent. Recent reviews of empirical studies that included the full age range of children, are more methodologically rigorous and based on representative samples have suggested that although mild depression, sadness and despair in children is fairly common following parental death, the occurrence of clinically significant levels of disorder afflict a smaller proportion (approximately 20–30 percent) of parentally bereaved children (Dowdney, 2000; Lutzke et al., 1997). In terms of types of symptomatology following parental death, there is stronger evidence of differences between bereaved and matched control groups based on symptoms of depression, withdrawal, and acting out than on somatic symptoms or serious delinquency (Lutzke et al., 1997).

Research has begun to move beyond the issue of identifying the mental health sequelae of child bereavement to ask questions concerning processes of adaptation following bereavement. Bereavement is viewed not as a single event, but as a process, and the research question is what factors lead to better outcomes. Some research on factors that are associated with healthier adaptation have focused on the surviving family system. Several studies have found that better mental health outcomes are associated with a positive relationship with the surviving parent, including parental warmth, communication, and positive time spent with the child (Deveau, 1997; Saler & Skolnick, 1992; West, Sandler, Pillow, Baca, & Gersten, 1991). The surviving parent's own grief and depressive symptoms, as well as the ability to provide a stable family environment and effective discipline

have also been found to contribute to the mental health of their children (Lutzke et al., 1997; Worden, 1996). Research has also identified individual level characteristics of children that are associated with better outcomes for bereaved children, such as self-esteem (Haine, Ayers, Sandler, Wolchik, & Lutzke, 2001), control beliefs (Worden & Silverman, 1996), and coping efficacy (Sandler, Ayers, Tein, & Wolchik, 1999). While these studies have begun to identify factors that are associated with positive adaptation of children following parental death, it is notable that there is a paucity of empirical evidence concerning the effects of several other theoretically important factors, such as expression of grief-related feelings, social support, or children's conceptions of death.

STRATEGIES THAT WORK

Research on preventive interventions is at an early stage of development. Several articles have been written describing prevention programs for bereaved children or adolescents (Gray, Zide, & Wilker, 2000; Lohnes & Kalter, 1994; Ormond & Charbonneau, 1995; Siegel, Mesagno, & Christ, 1990; Stokes, Wyer, & Crossley, 1997; Wolfe & Senta, 1995; Zambelli, Clark, Barile, & de Jong, 1988; Zambelli & DeRosa, 1992). Yet, few experimental or quasi-experimental trials of prevention programs for bereaved children have been conducted. As Stokes, Wyer, and Crossley (1997) have pointed out, the absence of experimentally controlled research designs in the implementation and evaluation of many of the bereavement interventions must encourage clinicians and practitioners to be cautious in their conclusions based on simply their observations and or descriptions of the programs.[4]

STRATEGIES THAT MIGHT WORK

Tonkins and Lambert (1996) evaluated an 8-week group for bereaved children aged 7–11 who had experienced the death of a parent (87.5 percent) or sibling (12.5 percent) in the past year. Using a pretest/posttest within group wait-list control design they assigned six children to the wait-list control condition and ten to the intervention condition. The group intervention focused on encouraging the expression of feelings, including the discussion of anger, guilt, sadness, and fears, reviving positive memories of the deceased, discussion

---

[4] Although there are studies that have used pre–posttest designs in the evaluations of interventions for bereaved children (e.g., Ormond & Charbonneau, 1995; Schilling, Koh, Abramovitz, & Gilbert, 1992; Stokes et al., 1997; Vargas-Irwin, 1999), we have chosen to only review those studies that included a control group in their design.

of "unfinished" business, and symbolic good-bye scenarios to the deceased. The group incorporated several symbolic modes of communication (i.e., through play and art projects). Results showed that participants reported significantly greater decreases in their depression and total grief-related symptomatology relative to the wait-list controls. Parent and teacher reports indicated significantly greater reductions for the program participants in overall symptomatology relative to the wait-list control group. Limitations of this study include the small sample size and a lack of random assignment to conditions.

Huss and Ritchie (1999) used a Solomon four-group design to investigate the effects of a 6-week support group intervention for 17 bereaved children aged 10–13 who had experienced the death of a parent more than 2 years prior to the study. The peer group intervention was intended to relieve the sense of isolation, normalize the experience, and offer a forum for developing and practicing coping skills, targeting outcomes of self-esteem, depression, behavior, and self-reported coping ability. Participation in the intervention did not significantly influence the children's self-esteem, depression, behavior, or self-beliefs about their ability to cope with loss.

Several studies have evaluated preventive interventions that included both children and adolescents. Ryan (1982) used a wait-list control group design to evaluate a 5-week bereavement support group that was delivered to 23 children ranging in ages from 7 to 17. No significant treatment effects were found on measures of adjustment, guilt, and anxiety. Black and Urbanowicz (1985, 1987) used a post-only design to evaluate a six-session family counseling intervention designed to provide emotional support and problem-solving assistance, and to encourage communication surrounding death and grief. Forty-six families, with children under the age of 17, participated in the intervention. For families that participated in the intervention, the parents reported that their children had fewer behavioral, health, sleep, and learning problems at a 1-year follow-up and were reported to have spent more time crying and talking about their deceased parent than children in the control group. The surviving parents in the treatment condition also reported experiencing fewer depressive symptoms or health problems. The authors found that the increased rates of crying among the children were associated with decreased behavioral problems, and concluded that the effectiveness of the intervention was in its promoting beneficial mourning. At a 2-year follow-up (Black & Urbanowicz, 1987), no significant treatment effects remained. The significant 1-year findings must also be considered with caution due to significant methodological flaws, including unblinded experimental procedures and unequal attrition between treatment and control groups.

Christ and colleagues (Christ, 2000; Christ, Raveis, Siegel, & Karus, 2001; Christ, Siegel, Mesagno, & Langosch,

1991; Siegel et al., 1990) have carried out a program of research focused on assisting families that are dealing with the death of a parent due to cancer. Christ (2000) reports results from their qualitative analyses of their work with these children with the discussion broken into five distinct age groups (3–5, 6–8, 9–11, 12–14, and 15–17). Recently they have designed and evaluated a psycho-educational parent-guidance intervention and a telephone-monitoring comparison intervention for parentally bereaved children aged 7–17 and their families (Christ et al., 2001). The parent-guidance intervention aimed to enhance surviving parents' abilities to provide support for their children, to provide an environment in which children would feel comfortable expressing their feelings about the loss, and to provide consistency and stability in the children's environment. The telephone-monitoring comparison intervention aimed to maintain contact with the surviving parents and provide referrals to various services when requested. Both interventions began before the parent's death, allowing an anticipatory intervention to be implemented and evaluated. The authors delivered these programs to 184 families, 104 of which completed the pre- and post-evaluations. Although no significant program effects were observed, there were trends for the program children to show improved depression and anxiety scores over time, as well as trends toward greater self-esteem when compared to the children in the telephone-monitoring intervention. Children in the parent-guidance intervention perceived their parent's overall competence (comprised of measures of perception of parenting and general communication) as significantly better in follow-up waves than did children in the telephone-monitoring intervention. However, there were no differences between the two groups with respect to death-related communication.

Sandler and colleagues (Sandler et al., 1992, 2001) have conducted two randomized experimental trials of preventive interventions for children and adolescents. The programs were designed to improve factors that have been found to be associated with better adaptation of bereaved children and adolescents (Sandler et al., 1992; West et al., 1991). They referred to these factors as "putative mediators" to indicate that they were theoretically causally related to outcomes for bereaved children and that change in these factors was expected to mediate the effects of the program. In their first experimental trial, 72 families were randomly assigned to the intervention condition or a 6-month delayed control group condition. The intervention targeted the following factors; demoralization of the surviving parent, family cohesion and warmth of the parent–child relationship, positive events and negative events in the family. The intervention program had two phases, a three-session family grief workshop followed by a family advisor program where para-professionals met weekly with the family for 12 weeks and taught the family skills targeted at changing the family's functioning on the theoretical mediators. Program effects immediately following the program indicated that parents in the treatment condition reported decreased symptoms of conduct problems, overall problems, and depressive symptoms among adolescents (aged 12–17) but not for children (aged 7–11). In addition, parents in the treatment condition reported significantly greater family discussion of grief-related issues, higher feelings of social support, and greater warmth of the parent–child relationship. Importantly, the increase in warmth of relationship between parent and child was found to be a significant mediator of the positive program effects on adolescents.

In a second experimental trial, Sandler and colleagues (Sandler et al., 2001) randomized 156 families with 244 bereaved children (aged 8–16) to either an intervention condition or a bibliotherapy condition. The intervention was revised and extended from that delivered in the previous trial by switching to a psycho-educational group format, with separate groups developed for children, adolescents, and caregivers. The participants in these groups met both independently and conjointly. The intervention targeted all of the same mediators included in the first trial, but also discipline strategies of the surviving parents/caregivers as well as children's coping, coping efficacy, appraisals of stress, self-esteem, control beliefs, and inhibition of feeling expression (for description of program, see Ayers et al., 2001).

Sandler and colleagues (2001) report that at immediate posttest, program participants showed improvement on a wide range of variables including positive parenting, caregiver mental health, negative events, coping, active inhibition of feelings, and a behavioral observation rating of positive affect between the parent and child. At the 11-month follow-up, the program participants continued to show improvement on the ability to share feelings and for those children who showed poor problem-solving abilities at the start of the program there was an increase in their ability to generate problem solutions. Additionally, in families where parent and child reported poor parenting practices at the start of the program, there was a greater improvement in these behaviors at posttest for the program as compared to control groups. Children and adolescents who participated in the group intervention and who had higher internalizing problems at the start of the program showed significantly lower symptomatology than the children in the bibliotherapy program at the 11-month follow-up.

Some of the program effects Sandler and colleagues observed were conditioned by gender and age (Sandler et al., 2001). At the 11-month follow-up, there was a significant decrease in internalizing and externalizing symptoms for girls who participated in the program by both parent and child report. Based on teacher report, the younger children (aged 8–11) who had high internalizing problems at the start of the program showed significantly fewer internalizing symptoms at immediate follow-up than did the control children in the same age range. At 11-month follow-up, younger children who had more adaptive control beliefs at the start of the program improved more on these beliefs than did children in the bibliotherapy condition. The overall findings from this study across multiple outcomes indicate positive effects on the putative mediating processes as well as mental health outcomes, particularly for girls.

STRATEGIES THAT DO NOT WORK

Information is not currently available on intervention strategies for bereaved children that do not work or which have been found to have iatrogenic effects.

SYNTHESIS

As can be seen by the review of prevention programs that have been evaluated, a variety of intervention approaches have been developed, including psycho-educational and parent guidance programs, family counseling, and support groups. Other formats of interventions that have been offered include use of art in an individual or group context (Zambelli et al., 1988), play therapy (Tait & Depta, 1993; Webb, 1993) and residential weekends (Stokes & Crossley, 1995; Stokes et al., 1997). Although some initial efforts have been made to evaluate these alternative approaches (e.g., Stokes et al., 1997), further work needs to be done, both in the development of appropriate evaluation instruments and in the use of more rigorous designs.

Interventions offered to bereaved children and their families have typically provided information and education on grief, and provided opportunities for expressing and understanding feelings, remembering and/or commemorating the death, and developing family communication. Less frequently (Sandler et al., 1992, 2001), interventions have focused on developing parenting skills, including effective discipline practices and building a positive relationship between the caregiver and the child. Although not as frequently a focus of intervention activities, recent evidence points to the importance of developing parenting skills, in that these skills were found to account for the observed program effects in a preventive intervention for bereaved families (Tein, Ayers, Sandler, Wolchik, & Newton, 2001). Further program development efforts in these areas might improve the effectiveness of interventions for families with bereaved children.

Overall, findings from the few controlled evaluations of preventive interventions for bereaved children have been equivocal, both with respect to the optimal combination of format, technique, and content. To further our understanding, intervention studies need to target mediators that have been demonstrated to relate to healthy outcomes of bereaved children. Sandler and colleagues (Sandler et al., 2001) have begun this work and it is hoped that an analysis of key modifiable variables will result in increasing potency and effectiveness of intervention strategies. As noted earlier, findings also suggest that the impact of the interventions on symptomatology may vary with child's age, gender and level of individual and family resources and symptoms at the time they enter the program (Sandler et al., 1992, 2001). Further research to develop our understanding of what works and *with whom* to promote healthy outcomes is critical in the design of preventive intervention services for bereaved children. Finally, there is also a need to link what we learn in these well-controlled efficacy and effectiveness trials with the constraints and realities of the existing service delivery systems for bereaved families. Utilizing information gleaned from these trials needs to be integrated into current practices and delivery systems so that programs that have demonstrated efficacy are translated into more effective services that are delivered to the public to promote healthy adaptation for *all* family members following the death of a loved one.

Also see: Bereavement: Adolescence; Grief: Older Adulthood; Religion and Spirituality: Adolescence.

ACKNOWLEDGMENTS

Support for writing this chapter was provided by the National Institute of Mental Health Grant #P30 National Institute of Mental Health Grant #P30 M439246-15 to establish a Preventive Intervention Research Center at Arizona State University, and Grant #R01 MH49155-05 to evaluate a preventive intervention for bereaved families.

References

Ayers, T.S., Twohey, J.L., Sandler, I.N., Wolchik, S.A., Lutzke, J.R., Padgett-Jones, S., Weiss, L., Cole, E., & Kriege, G. (2001). *The Family Bereavement Program: Description of a theory-based prevention program for parentally-bereaved children and adolescents.* Manuscript in preparation, Prevention Research Center, Arizona State University, P.O. Box 876005, Tempe, AZ 85287-6005.

Balk, D.E. (1996). Models for understanding adolescent coping with bereavement. *Death Studies, 20,* 367–387.

Black, D., & Urbanowicz, M.A. (1985). Bereaved children family intervention. In J.E. Stevenson (Ed.), *Recent research in developmental psychopathology* (pp. 179–187). Oxford: Pergamon.

Black, D., & Urbanowicz, M.A. (1987). Family intervention with bereaved children. *Journal of Child Psychology and Psychiatry and Allied Disciplines, 28,* 467–476.

Brent, S.B., & Speece, M.W. (1993). "Adult" conceptualization of irreversibility: Implications for the development of the concept of death. *Death Studies, 17,* 203–224.

Brent, S.B., Speece, M.W., Lin, C., Dong, Q., & Yang, C. (1996). The development of the concept of death among Chinese and US children 3–17 years of age: From binary to "fuzzy" concepts? *Omega Journal of Death and Dying, 33,* 67–83.

Christ, G.H. (2000). *Healing children's grief: Surviving a parent's death from cancer.* New York, NY, US: Oxford University Press.

Christ, G.H., Raveis, V.H., Siegel, K., & Karus, D. (2001). *Evaluation of a preventive intervention for bereaved children.* Manuscript submitted for publication, Columbia School of Social Work, New York, NY.

Christ, G.H., Siegel, K., Mesagno, F.P., & Langosch, D. (1991). A preventive intervention program for bereaved children: Problems of implementation. *American Journal of Orthopsychiatry, 61,* 168–178.

Clark, D.C., Pynoos, R.S., & Goebel, A.E. (1994). Mechanisms and processes of adolescent bereavement. In R.J. Haggerty, L.R. Sherrod, N. Garmezy, & M. Rutter (Eds.), *Stress, risk, and resilience in children and adolescents: Processes, mechanisms, and interventions* (pp. 100–146). New York: Cambridge University Press.

Davies, B. (1999). *Shadow in the sun: The experience of sibling bereavement in childhood.* Philadelphia, PA, US: Brunner/Mazel, Inc.

Demographic and Health Surveys. (2001). *MEASURE DHS+* [Data]. Macro International, Inc. Available: www.measuedhs.com [2001, 3-10-2001].

Deveau, E.J. (1995). Perceptions of death through the eyes of children and adolescents. In D.W. Adams & E.J. Deveau (Eds.), *Beyond the innocence of childhood: Factors influencing children and adolescents' perceptions and attitudes toward death* (Vol. 1, pp. 55–92). Amityville, NY: Baywood.

Deveau, E.J. (1997). The pattern of grief in children and adolescents. In J.D. Morgan (Ed.), *Readings in thanatology* (pp. 359–389). Amityville, NY: Baywood.

Dowdney, L. (2000). Childhood bereavement following parental death. *Journal of Child Psychology and Psychiatry and Allied Disciplines, 41,* 819–830.

Felner, R., Ginter, M., Boike, M., & Cowen, E. (1981). Parental death or divorce and the school adjustment of young children. *American Journal of Community Psychology, 9,* 181–191.

Felner, R.D., Stolberg, A., & Cowen, E.L. (1975). Crisis events and school mental health referral patterns of young children. *Journal of Consulting and Clinical Psychology, 43,* 305–310.

Gersten, J.C., Beals, J., & Kallgren, C.A. (1991). Epidemiology and preventive interventions: Parental death in childhood as a case example. Special Issue: Preventive Intervention Research Centers. *American Journal of Community Psychology, 19,* 481–500.

Gray, S.W., Zide, M.R., & Wilker, H. (2000). Using the solution focused brief therapy model with bereavement groups in rural communities: Resiliency at its best. *Hospice Journal, 15,* 13–30.

Haine, R.A., Ayers, T.S., Sandler, I.N., Wolchik, S.A., & Lutzke, J.R. (2001). *Locus of control and self-esteem as mediators or moderators of the relations between negative life events and mental health problems in parentally bereaved children.* Manuscript in preparation.

Huss, S.N., & Ritchie, M. (1999). Effectiveness of a group for parentally bereaved children. *Journal for Specialists in Group Work, 24,* 186–196.

Kosko, B., & Sartoru, I. (1993). Fuzzy logic. *Scientific American, 267,* 76–81.

Lazar, A., & Torney-Purta, J. (1991). The development of the subconcepts of death in young children: A short-term longitudinal study. *Child Development, 62*(6), 1321–1333.

Lohnes, K.L., & Kalter, N. (1994). Preventive intervention groups for parentally bereaved children. *American Journal of Orthopsychiatry, 64*, 594–603.

Lonetto, R. (1980). *Children's conceptions of death*. New York: Springer.

Lutzke, J.R., Ayers, T.S., Sandler, I.N., & Barr, A. (1997). Risks and interventions for the parentally bereaved child. In S.A. Wolchik & I.N. Sandler (Eds.), *Handbook of children's coping with common life stressors: Linking theory, research and interventions* (pp. 215–243). New York: Plenum.

Nelson, G. (1982). Coping with the loss of father: Family reaction to death or divorce. *Journal of Family Issues, 3*, 41–60.

Oltjenbruns, K.A. (2001). Developmental context of childhood: Grief and regrief phenomena. In M.S. Stroebe, R.O. Hansson, W. Stroebe, H. Schut (Eds.), *Handbook of bereavement research: Consequences, coping and care* (pp. 169–197). Washington, DC: American Psychological Association.

Ormond, E., & Charbonneau, H. (1995). Grief responses and group treatment interventions for five- to eight-year-old children. In D.W. Adams & E.J. Deveau (Eds.), *Beyond the innocence of childhood: Helping children and adolescents cope with death and bereavement* (Vol. 3, pp. 181–202). Amityville, NY: Baywood.

Piaget, J. (1959). *The language and thought of the child* (3 [Rev. and Enl.] ed.). New York: Humanities Press.

Ringler, L.L., & Hayden, D.C. (2000). Adolescent bereavement and social support: Peer loss compared to other losses. *Journal of Adolescent Research, 15*, 209–230.

Ryan, S.M. (1982). Childhood bereavement: Psychological test findings of a post-death intervention program (Doctoral dissertation, University of Arizona, Tucson, 1990). *Dissertation Abstracts International, 43*(3 B), 885.

Saler, L., & Skolnick, N. (1992). Childhood parental death and depression in adulthood: Roles of surviving parent and family environment. *American Journal of Orthopsychiatry, 62*, 504–516.

Sandler, I.N., Ayers, T.S., Tein, J.-Y., & Wolchik, S.A. (1999, April). Perceived coping efficacy as a mediator of the effects of coping efforts. In I.N. Sandler & B. Compas (Chair), *Beyond simple models of coping: Advance in theory and research*. Symposium conducted at the Biennial Meeting of the Society for Research in Child Development, Albuquerque, New Mexico.

Sandler, I.N., Ayers, T.S., Wolchik, S.A., Tein, J.-Y., Kwok, O.-M., Haine, R.A., Twohey, J.L., Suter, J., Lin, K., Padgett-Jones, S., Lutzke, J.R., Cole, E., Kriege, G., & Griffin, W.A. (2001). *The Family Bereavement Program: Efficacy evaluation of a theory-based prevention program for parentally-bereaved children and adolescents*. Manuscript submitted for publication, Tempe, AZ.

Sandler, I.N., West, S.G., Baca, L., Pillow, D.R., Gersten, J., Rogosch, F., Virdin, L., Beals, J., Reynolds, K., Kallgren, C., Tein, J., Krieg, G., Cole, E., & Ramirez, R. (1992). Linking empirically based theory and evaluation: The Family Bereavement Program. *American Journal of Community Psychology, 20*, 491–521.

Schilling, R.F., Koh, N., Abramovitz, R., & Gilbert, L. (1992). Bereavement groups for inner-city children. *Research on Social Work Practice, 2*, 405–419.

Schonfeld, D.J., & Smilansky, S. (1989). A cross-cultural comparison of Israeli and American children's death concepts. *Death Studies, 13*, 593–604.

Siegel, K., Mesagno, F.P., & Christ, G. (1990). A prevention program for bereaved children. *American Journal of Orthopsychiatry, 60*, 168–175.

Social Security Administration. (2000). *Intermediate Assumptions of the 2000 Trustees Report*. Washington, DC: Office of the Chief Actuary of the Social Security Administration.

Sood, B., Weller, E.B., Weller, R.A., Fristad, M.A., & Bowes, J. (1992). Somatic complaints in grieving children. *Comprehensive Mental Health Care, 2*, 17–25.

Speece, M.W., & Brent, S.B. (1984). Children's understanding of death: A review of three components of a death concept. *Child Development, 55*, 1671–1686.

Speece, M.W., & Brent, S.B. (1996). The development of children's understanding of death. In C.A. Corr & D.M. Corr (Eds.), *Handbook of childhood death and bereavement* (pp. 29–50). New York, NY, US: Springer.

Stambrook, M., & Parker, K.C. (1987). The development of the concept of death in childhood: A review of the literature. *Merrill Palmer Quarterly, 33*, 133–157.

Stokes, J., & Crossley, D. (1995). Camp Winston: A residential intervention for bereaved children. In S.C. Smith & M. Pennells (Eds.), *Interventions with bereaved children* (pp. 172–192). Bristol, PA, US: Jessica Kingsley.

Stokes, J., Wyer, S., & Crossley, D. (1997). The challenge of evaluating a child bereavement programme. *Palliative Medicine, 11*, 179–190.

Tait, D.C., & Depta, J.-L. (1993). Play therapy group for bereaved children. In N.B. Webb (Ed.), *Helping bereaved children: A handbook for practitioners* (pp. 169–185). New York, NY: The Guilford Press.

Tein, J.-Y., Ayers, T.S., Sandler, I.N., Wolchik, S.A., & Newton, C. (2001, May). *Mediated program effects for Family Bereavement Program*. Paper Presented at the Ninth Annual Meeting of the Society for Prevention Research, Washington, DC.

Tonkins, S.A.M., & Lambert, M.J. (1996). A treatment outcome study of bereavement groups for children. *Child and Adolescent Social Work Journal, 13*, 3–21.

Tremblay, G.C., & Israel, A.C. (1998). Children's adjustment to parental death. *Clinical Psychology: Science and Practice, 5*, 424–438.

Van Eerdewegh, M.M., Clayton, P.J., & Van Eerdewegh, P. (1985). The bereaved child: Variables influencing early psychopathology. *British Journal of Psychiatry, 147*, 188–194.

Vargas Irwin, M. (1999). Evaluation of a bereavement group for children. *Dissertation Abstracts International, 60*(2B), 0846 (UMI No. 9920197).

Webb, N.B. (1993). Counseling and therapy for the bereaved child. In N.B. Webb (Ed.), *Helping bereaved children: A handbook for practitioners* (pp. 43–58). New York, NY: The Guilford Press.

West, S.G., Sandler, I.N., Pillow, D.R., Baca, L., & Gersten, J.C. (1991). The use of structural equation modeling in generative research: Toward the design of a preventive intervention for bereaved children. Special Issue: Preventive Intervention Research Centers. *American Journal of Community Psychology, 19*, 459–480.

Wolfe, B.S., & Senta, L.M. (1995). Interventions with bereaved children nine to thirteen years of age: From a medical center-based young person's grief support program. In D.W. Adams & E.J. Deveau (Eds.), *Beyond the innocence of childhood: Helping children and adolescents cope with death and bereavement* (Vol. 3, pp. 203–227). Amityville, NY: Baywood.

Worden, J.W. (1996). *Children and grief: When a parent dies*. New York: Guilford.

Worden, J.W., & Silverman, P.R. (1996). Parental death and the adjustment of school-age children. *Omega Journal of Death and Dying, 33*, 91–102.

Zambelli, G.C., Clark, E.J., Barile, L., & de Jong, A.F. (1988). An interdisciplinary approach to clinical intervention for childhood bereavement. *Death Studies, 12*, 41–50.

Zambelli, G.C., & DeRosa, A.P. (1992). Bereavement support groups for school-age children: Theory, intervention, and case example. *American Journal of Orthopsychiatry, 62*, 484–493.

Bereavement, Adolescence*

Tim S. Ayers, Cara L. Kennedy, Irwin N. Sandler, and Julie Stokes

INTRODUCTION AND DEFINITIONS

Many adolescents have been exposed to bereavement experiences during their lifetimes, including but not limited to peer, sibling, and parental deaths. The long-term impact that these experiences have on an adolescent's psychological health and well-being is believed to be dependent on a variety of factors including the type and nature of the death, the relationship with the deceased, the ongoing relationships with the survivors, the family environment, and the adolescent's own socio-emotional development and personality. While authors have pointed to the resiliency and growth displayed by some bereaved adolescents (Balk & Corr, 1996; Davies, 1991; Fleming & Balmer, 1996; Martinson, Davies, & McGlowry, 1987; Oltjenbruns, 1991), a great deal of research has found that subgroups of bereaved children are at risk for long-term negative outcomes (Dowdney, 2000; Lutzke, Ayers, Sandler, & Barr, 1997; Worden, 1996). The proportion of bereaved adolescents who are viewed as being at risk typically ranges from 20 to 50 percent depending on the measure of the outcome and nature of the death (Dowdney, 2000; Hogan & Greenfield, 1991). Identifying this subgroup of children/adolescents and/or the factors that elevate the risk for poor adjustment has become an important focus of research.

This entry examines the impact of parental death and to a lesser extent sibling death on adolescents. With a few notable exceptions (Balk, 1996; Ringler & Hayden, 2000), there has been a relative lack of attention to risk and protective factors for adjustment in adolescents who have experienced the death of a peer and thus peer bereavement is not a focus of this entry.

SCOPE

The best prevalence estimates for parental death in the United States come from the Social Security Administration, which is responsible for distributing death benefits to families where there has been the death of one or both parents. Based on data from 1997 (Social Security Administration, 2000), 6.1 percent of adolescents between the ages of 13–17, have experienced the death of a parent (73.9 percent, death of a father; 25 percent, death of a mother; and 1.1 percent have experienced the death of both parents). Unfortunately, comparable prevalence figures of sibling bereavement during the adolescent years are not available.

The prevalence of parental deaths in other countries varies greatly from those figures available in the United States. The Demographic and Health Surveys (DHS+) are nationally representative household surveys with sample sizes of around 5,000 and have been conducted in several countries throughout the world. Although DHS (Demographic and Health Surveys, 2001) do not provide prevalence information for the full age range of adolescence, for children aged 10–14, the percentage that have experienced the death of either one or both parents ranges from 4.1 percent in Jordan to 14.8 percent in Mozambique.[1] Using data from these DHS one can also examine the proportion of children who have experienced either the death of a father versus a mother and who are still living with their surviving parent. These data suggest that the average proportion of father to mother deaths is 3.3 to 1, which is slightly higher but similar to that observed in the United States and the United Kingdom.

THEORIES

The numerous theoretical models that have guided past work in understanding coping with bereavement might be grouped into five broad categories. Stroebe and colleagues (Stroebe & Schut, 2001) have suggested past theories might be broadly grouped into four groups: general life event theories, general grief-related theories, specific coping with bereavement theories and more recently integrative models such as the four-component model offered by Bonanno and Kaltman (1999) and their own dual process model of coping with bereavement (Stroebe & Schut, 1999). An additional model, which has guided some of the prevention work and is not easily incorporated into the four categories offered by Stroebe and colleagues might be characterized as a

* Support for writing this chapter was provided by the National Institute of Mental Health Grant #P30 M439246-15 to establish a Preventive Intervention Research Center at Arizona State University, and Grant #R01 MH49155-05 to evaluate a preventive intervention for bereaved families.

[1] This range of estimates comes from all DHS+ completed since 1997 (Demographic and Health Surveys, 2001). This includes the following countries with the prevalence estimates of parental death for children aged 10–14 and the year of the survey included within the parentheses (e.g., year of survey, estimate for 10–14): Kenya (1998, 10.7), Madagascar (1997, 10.7), Mozambique (1997, 14.8), Cameroon (1998, 10.4), Ghana (1998, 5.7), Guinea (1999, 8.5), Niger (1998, 6.5), Chad (1997, 7.9), Togo (1998, 9.6), Jordan (1997, 4.1), Yemen (1997, 7.2), Kyrgyz Republic (1997, 5.3), Turkey (1998, 5.3), Indonesia (1997, 6.3), Guatemala (1999, 7.0), Nicaragua (1997, 5.6), and Bolivia (1998, 6.4).

resilience resource model. This model emphasizes individual, family, and stress processes that either increase or decrease the risk for children who are bereaved (Ayers et al., 2001; Sandler et al., 1992).

As an example of a general life event theory, Balk (1996) has suggested that Moos and Schaefer's (1986) general model of coping with life crisis might be a useful framework for understanding adolescent bereavement. Moos and Schaefer (1986) argued that individuals in crisis must deploy five adaptive tasks: (a) establish the meaning of the event and comprehend its personal significance, (b) confront reality and respond to the situational requirement of the event, (c) sustain interpersonal relationships, (d) maintain emotional balance, and (e) preserve a satisfactory self-image and maintain a sense of self-efficacy. Balk (1996) offers clinical anecdotes and research findings as evidence of the importance of these adaptive tasks in an adolescent's successful adaptation to a parental or sibling death.

The tasks Moos and Schaefer (1986) outline in their general model of coping with life crises are similar to the tasks Worden (1991, 1996) has offered—a model of bereavement that is reflective of the specific coping with bereavement theories. In this model, Worden proposes four "tasks" that a bereaved child/adolescent has to perform in order to adjust to bereavement. Worden (1996) prefers conceptualizing these as "tasks" rather than stages or phases in order to indicate that they are not necessarily completed in any set order or necessarily ever complete but that "work" associated with each of these tasks should facilitate adaptation. The four tasks Worden (1996) identified, which he argues are relevant to both adult (Worden, 1991) and children's bereavement involve: (a) accepting the reality of the loss, (b) experiencing the pain of grief, (c) adjusting to an environment without the deceased, and (d) "relocating" the deceased emotionally.

As another example of the specific coping with bereavement model, some researchers and theoreticians have argued that a better understanding of the natural course of adolescent bereavement cannot be achieved unless the bereavement is placed in the overall context of the developmental tasks and transitions facing adolescents (Balk & Corr, 2001). Fleming and Adolph (1986) integrated theories of adjustment to loss with theories of adolescent ego development and proposed that adolescents need to cope behaviorally, affectively, and cognitively with five core issues. They identified these issues as: (a) trusting in the predictability of events, (b) gaining a sense of mastery and control, (c) forging relationships marked by belonging, (d) believing the world is fair and just, and (e) developing a confident self-image. These authors also identify conflicts pertinent to each of the adolescent maturational periods, for example, (a) ages 11–14; the task of emotional separation from parents, with the conflict of separation vs. reunion; (b) ages 14–17; competency/mastery/control,

with the conflict of independence vs. dependence; (c) ages 17–21; intimacy and commitment, with the conflict of closeness vs. distance. In their model, they suggest that the adjustment to the death of a significant other is in part determined by the developmental phase and the major interpersonal tasks they are facing when the death occurs.

Recently authors have begun to merge theories of bereavement, emotion, and emotion regulation into more integrative theories such as the four-component model of bereavement offered by Bonanno and Kaltman (1999) and the dual process model of coping with bereavement which has been offered by Stroebe and Schut (2001). Bonanno and Kaltman's (1999) model will be briefly discussed in order to highlight some of their recent theoretical and empirical work. The first of their four components is the context of the loss, referring to the type of death, age, gender, social support, and cultural setting in which it occurs. A second component they identify is the subjective meanings associated with the loss, which range on a continuum from appraisals of everyday matters and concerns to more existential concerns about the meaning of life and death. As a third component, these authors note that there is a changing representation of the lost relationship over time, which plays an important part in the grieving process. Finally, as a fourth component, the authors highlight the importance of the role of coping and emotion-regulation processes in heightening or minimizing the stresses of the loss.

Bonanno, Keltner, Holen, and Horowitz (1995) have used a social-functional approach to emotion and its regulation within the context of bereavement to test some of the basic assumptions within the bereavement literature. In their empirical work with adults, they have challenged one of these assumptions which suggests that completing "grief work," that is, working through the emotional significance of the event, is the only appropriate means of resolving and coming to terms with the death of a loved one (Bonanno et al., 1995). This assumption has been questioned by several authors in the past 15 years (Stroebe & Stroebe, 1987; Wortman & Silver, 1989). These authors have argued that there is a lack of conceptual clarity as to what is meant by this term (Stroebe, 1992; Stroebe & Stroebe, 1987) and a lack of solid empirical evidence suggesting that "grief work" is a "necessity" and an endpoint for all individuals in order for there to be an "uncomplicated" resolution of grief (Stroebe, 1992). Recently, Stroebe and colleagues (Stroebe, Hansson, Stroebe, & Schut, 2001) note that the investigation of "grief work" has been replaced with the investigation of more narrowly defined constructs such as "rumination," "dissociation," and "confrontation-avoidance."

Finally, the resilience resource model emphasizes stressful processes as increasing adaptation problems while family and individual resources have the potential to foster healthy adaptation of bereaved adolescents (Ayers et al.,

2001; Sandler et al., 2001). The stressful processes that follow bereavement are conceptualized as arising not only from the death, but also from the cascade of stressful events that occur following the death. Several studies have found that stressful events are a significant predictor of mental health problems in bereaved children and adolescents. Empirical evidence has also indicated several possible mediating family processes. One primary focus has been on the relationship between the child and the surviving parent indicating that parental warmth, communication, and positive time spent together influence the impact of the bereavement (Saler & Skolnick, 1992; West, Sandler, Pillow, Baca, & Gersten, 1991). Related to those findings, the surviving parent's own grief and depressive symptoms, as well as ability to provide a stable family environment and effective discipline have been found to contribute to the mental health of his/her children (Lutzke et al., 1997; Worden, 1996). Additionally, there have been significant differences observed between bereaved children and their matched controls in self-system beliefs such as locus of control or self-esteem, implicating the self-system as a possible mediating process (Worden & Silverman, 1996). Indeed, Haine, Ayers, Sandler, Wolchik, and Lutzke (2001) found that self-esteem serves as a partial mediator of stress and mental health problems in parentally bereaved children. These factors have guided some of the prevention work with parentally bereaved children, which will be discussed in more detail later.

There has been increasing interest in identifying those bereaved individuals who are most at risk for long-term negative consequences. Much of this work has been done in the adult area as reflected by efforts to define diagnostic criteria for or predictors of what has been variously referred to as abnormal, morbid, pathological, complicated, or traumatic grief (Horowitz, Siegel, Holen, & Bonanno, 1997; Prigerson & Jacobs, 2001; Stroebe, van Son, Stroebe, Kleber, Schut, & van den Bout, 2000). Many contemporary writers prefer the label of "complicated grief" in order to avoid some of the more value-laden connotations of other labels and that will be the term adopted here. Although several authors have advocated for the creation of a new diagnostic entity of complicated grief (Horowitz et al., 1997), most of the work has been with conjugally bereaved individuals and little work has been done with children or adolescents. Stroebe and colleagues (Stroebe et al., 2000) in their recent review of this area have urged caution in adopting any one of these conceptualizations or criteria due to what they view as a number of unresolved issues concerning the alternative definitions, diversity in conceptualizations, distinctions between "normal" and complicated grief and overlap of complicated grief, with other disorders.

Another approach to identifying those adolescents who are most at risk for later problems in adaptation has been broader in focus than simply the detection or diagnosis of

"complicated grief." These efforts have included attempts to consider a range of personal, familial, or environmental variables that might predict greater likelihood of poor adaptation. Worden (1996) has offered some preliminary screening criteria to select those parentally bereaved children/adolescents who are most at risk for negative outcomes. Worden identified the following screening criteria, which he believed should be assessed within the first 6 months of the parent's death. The criteria included considering the surviving parent's age, their levels of stress, coping, and depression, the number of children in the family, and the child's own level of symptomatology. Using specific cut-points for these criteria and examining clinical levels of symptomatology at one and two years post death, Worden was able to correctly predict group membership based on these variables for 81 percent of the children.[2]

Worden (1996) argues that since many bereaved children adapt to the death of a loved one without significant psychological difficulties and since mental health services for children are increasingly limited, a strategy of screening for high risk children is the most efficient and cost-effective approach to provision of services for bereaved children. However, concern about the reliance on screening measures that have not established validity and efficacy across populations or time (Payne & Relf, 1994) has led other service professionals to advocate for the development of services to all bereaved children and their families (Stokes, Pennington, Monroe, Papadatou, & Relf, 1999). Thus, similar to the work attempting to identify individuals who are at risk for experiencing "complicated bereavement," the development of screening instruments for identifying children who are at risk for mental health problems is clearly in its formative stages and more work needs to be done.

RESEARCH

Recent reviews have summarized an emerging empirical literature on the relations between parental death and mental health and adaptive functioning in childhood and adulthood (Dowdney, 2000; Lutzke et al., 1997). Since each of these reviews summarized literature that included a broad age range of children, a more selective focus on the risk status for parentally bereaved adolescents is offered below. Bereaved adolescents have been found to rate themselves as having poorer academic performance, lower educational aspirations (Ambert & Saucier, 1984), and being less optimistic about their futures (Saucier & Ambert, 1982) when compared to non-bereaved adolescents. Although some authors have also noted that parentally bereaved adolescents have lower

[2] Details of the cut points for the screening criteria can be found in Worden (1996). Of the 19 percent misses, $1/4$ were false negatives and $3/4$ were false positives.

self-esteem and higher anxiety than non-bereaved adolescents (Hetherington, 1972), other investigators have found no differences in self-esteem (Hainline & Feig, 1978; Partridge & Kotler, 1987) or anxiety (Hainline & Feig, 1978). With respect to externalizing symptomatology, Gregory (1965) reviewed police and court records of a statewide sample of ninth graders and found that children who had a father die had much higher rates of delinquency than those whose mother died.

Although many investigators have focused on risk for depression or depressive symptomatology in parentally bereaved children, many of the studies typically cited in this area have samples composed of both children and adolescents (Gersten, Beals, & Kallgren, 1991; Van Eerdewegh, Bieri, Parrilla, & Clayton, 1982; Worden & Silverman, 1996). Thus, it is difficult to discern risk for these mental health problems for the adolescents within these samples. With this acknowledged, Gersten and colleagues (1991) found in their representative sample of parentally bereaved children, aged 8–15, that 9.8 percent of the bereaved and 1.3 percent of the control children met diagnostic criteria for major depression. In this sample, about half of the children who were clinically depressed were older than 11 when the death occurred. Worden and Silverman (1996) in their longitudinal study of a community sample of parentally bereaved children found that adolescent boys (ages 12–18) were significantly more withdrawn than their matched controls at two years following the death of their parent. No significant differences were observed between matched controls and the bereaved adolescent girls (ages 12–18) at either one or two years following the death. However, Reinherz, Giaconia, Hauf, Wasserman, and Silverman (1999) in a prospective longitudinal study of a cohort of 375 children found that 13 percent of females with a diagnosis of major depression at ages 18 or 21 experienced parental death by age 9, as compared with 1 percent of the non-depressed group. There was no relation between parental death and depression for males.

Findings from empirical studies indicate that the death of a sibling in childhood or adolescence affects surviving siblings across the lifespan (Davies, 1999). Specifically, experiencing the death of a sibling is associated with increased risk of symptoms of post-traumatic stress disorder (PTSD), depression, anxiety, and behavior problems, as well as decreased academic performance and social competence (Applebaum & Burns, 1991; Birenbaum, Robinson, Phillips, Stewart, & McCown, 1989). Adolescent outcomes following the sibling death are influenced by several variables, including the nature of the death, gender, and age of the surviving adolescent, and subsequent family functioning (especially parental responses to the death and facilitation of family communication, Martinson & Campos, 1991; McCown & Pratt, 1985). Several writers have proposed that sibling death can also promote psychological and/or family growth among the surviving siblings and family, in spite of the distressing outcomes that follow sibling death (Davies, 1991; Martinson & Campos, 1991).

Because of the focus on parental and sibling bereavement in this entry, it is noteworthy that Worden, Davies and McCown (1999) have recently combined their samples of parentally bereaved and sibling bereaved children (ages 6–18) in order to compare children's responses to parent and sibling bereavement. In summary, when comparing parent's report on the Child Behavior Checklist (Achenbach & Edelbrock, 1991) there were no significant differences in the impact of the two types of bereavement on the total number of problems, syndrome scales or percentage of children at risk. When considering findings for the adolescents in these two samples, gender differences emerge. Worden and colleagues (1999) report that 27 percent of teenage boys who experienced parental death and only 8 percent of the teenage boys who experienced sibling death fell in the clinical range on the internalizing, externalizing, or total symptomatology scales of the Child Behavior Checklist. However, for teenage girls who experienced parental death and sibling death, the percentage who fell into the clinical range was 14 and 33 percent, respectively. The reasons for these patterns of findings are still unclear although Worden and colleagues (1999) hypothesize that these patterns may be due to the gender of the deceased parent or deceased sibling for whom the bereaved children were grieving.

STRATEGIES THAT WORK

While there is still limited evidence concerning which critical mediators serve to promote healthy adaptation of bereaved adolescents, there are even fewer experimentally controlled research trials that have attempted to determine the preventive strategies that are most effective in reducing the risk of complicated bereavement and/or promoting resilience among children and families following the death of a parent. Stokes, Wyer, and Crossley (1997) point to the importance of experimentally controlled research designs for implementing and evaluating bereavement interventions, noting that in the absence of such designs, researchers can draw cautious conclusions based on observations and descriptions, but cannot explain any changes or their causes.

STRATEGIES THAT MIGHT WORK

A controlled outcome study of an intervention for bereaved children conducted by Black and Urbanowicz (1985) targeted 46 families with bereaved children under age 17. The six session family counseling intervention intended to provide emotional support and problem-solving assistance, as well as encourage communication surrounding death and grief. Findings indicated that, compared with the control group, children in the treatment condition had fewer behavioral, health, sleep, and learning problems at a one-year follow-up, and were reported to have spent more time crying and talking about their deceased parent than children in the control group. Additionally, the surviving parents in the treatment condition reported experiencing fewer depressive symptoms or health problems. Black and Urbanowicz (1985) found the increased rates of crying among the children to be associated with decreased behavioral problems, and concluded that the effectiveness of the intervention was in its promoting beneficial mourning. However, these findings must be considered with caution due to significant methodological weaknesses, including use of parent report only, unblinded experimental procedures and unequal attrition between treatment and control groups (which is particularly problematic given the post-only design).

Sandler and colleagues (1992) developed a randomized controlled preventive intervention based on theoretically determined mediators expected to be critical in preventing bereavement-related problems in children aged 7–17. Hypothesized mediators included demoralization of the surviving parent, reduced family cohesion and warmth, and the combination of decreased positive events and increased negative events in the family. The intervention was delivered in individual sessions with the parent as well as group family sessions. Program effects immediately following the program indicated that parents in the treatment condition reported decreased symptoms of conduct problems, overall problems, and depressive symptoms among adolescents (aged 12–17) but not for children (aged 7–11). In addition, parents in the experimental condition as compared to the controls reported significantly greater family discussion of grief-related issues, higher feelings of social support, and greater warmth of the parent–child relationship. Importantly, the increase in warmth of relationship between parent and child was found to be a significant mediator of the positive program effects. Child reports did not indicate significant differences between experimental and control conditions.

Sandler and colleagues (Sandler et al., 2001) revised and extended the intervention and conducted a second randomized experimental trial of a theory-based prevention program for bereaved children (aged 8–16) and their families. Strengths of the program evaluation included the use of a randomized controlled experimental design, inclusion of a large community-based, heterogeneous sample of 244 participants, assessment of family and child resilience resources as well as mental health problems, use of multiple reporters and methods to assess outcomes, and inclusion of a 11-month follow-up to assess maintenance of program effects. The intervention was designed to promote the development of parent–child communication and grief discussion, and enhance problem-solving

and cognitive restructuring competencies. The program also targeted discipline strategies and mental health of the surviving parents as well as children's coping, coping efficacy, appraisals of stress, self-esteem, control beliefs, and inhibition of feeling expression (Ayers et al., 2001).

At immediate posttest, program participants showed improvement on a wide range of variables including improved parent–child relationship, improved caregiver mental health, reduced negative events, improved use of active coping, reduced inhibition of feeling expression, and a behavioral observation rating of increased positive affect in parent–adolescent interactions (Sandler et al., 2001). At the 11-month follow-up, the program participants continued to show improvement on many variables such as sharing of feelings and a behavioral observational rating of generating problem solutions. Additionally, families in which parent and child reported poor parenting practices at the start of the program showed greater improvement in these behaviors at posttest relative to the families in the bibliotherapy control program. There were few differences in symptomatology between conditions at immediate posttest. However, at 11-month follow-up there was a significant effect for parents to report fewer internalizing problems for children in the program relative to the children in the bibliotherapy program for those children who were higher on internalizing problems when they entered the program. At 11-month follow-up, there was also a pattern across parent and child reports for girls in the program to have lower internalizing and externalizing problems than those in the control group. One of these significant program effects for girls, self-report on internalizing problems, also showed that the benefits occurred for girls who were higher on internalizing problems when they entered the program. Also relevant are program findings specific to the age group considered in this entry. Additional analyses indicated that adolescents who participated in the program who had reported high threat appraisals and unknown control beliefs at the start of the program showed significant positive program effects in these areas at 11-month follow-up relative to the adolescents who received the bibliotherapy program.

Current attention has also been directed toward anticipatory intervention for children and families experiencing the terminal illness of one parent. Anticipated death affords a unique set of both stressors and benefits, resulting in inconclusive findings as to whether mental health outcomes among bereaved are more positive due to forewarning of death. Empirical research is addressing the question of whether anticipatory intervention promotes ease of adaptation to the death and prevents complicated bereavement. A randomized-controlled intervention, targeted for adolescents living with a parent in terminal stages of HIV/AIDS (Rotheram-Borus, Lee, Gwadz, & Draimin, 2001), helped parents to discuss their disease with their children, prepare the adolescent for the transition to a new caretaker, and facilitate adolescents' coping. Evaluation was conducted every 3 months over the course of 2 years. Results indicated that the intervention, relative to standard care, was associated with reductions in multiple problem behaviors and emotional distress for both the parents living with HIV and their adolescents for up to 15 months following the intervention. At the 2-year assessment, adolescents involved in the intervention also reported an improvement in self-esteem relative to controls. Fortunately, many of the parents in the trial (56 percent) survived the course of the trial, due to the advent of medications to extend their lives. Therefore, these results do not generalize fully to bereaved adolescents.

In a companion paper using a different data analytic strategy, Rotheram-Borus, Stein, and Lin (2001) report that overall adolescents whose parents died during the trial reported significantly more problem behaviors and emotional distress at the 2-year assessment relative to those adolescents whose parents had survived. In terms of intervention effects, the adolescents from families that received the intervention reported significantly fewer problems behavior and sexual partners than those receiving standard care 2 years later, although the intervention did not differentially affect the bereaved and non-bereaved adolescents. In addition, similar to other findings mentioned above, the parent's own emotional distress and physical health symptoms were associated with poorer outcomes for the adolescents 2 years later.

Christ, Raveis, Siegel, & Karus (2001) designed and evaluated a psycho-educational parent-guidance intervention and a telephone-monitoring comparison intervention for parentally bereaved children aged 7–17 in families where one parent was dying from cancer. The parent-guidance intervention aimed to enhance surviving parents' abilities to provide support for their children, to provide an environment in which children would feel comfortable expressing their feelings about the loss, and to provide consistency and stability in the children's environment. The telephone-monitoring comparison intervention aimed to maintain contact with the surviving parents and provide referrals to various services when requested. Both interventions began before the parent's death, allowing an anticipatory intervention to be implemented and evaluated. Although there were no significant program effects, there were trends for program children to show improved depression and anxiety scores over time, as well as trends toward greater self-esteem when compared to the children in the telephone-monitoring intervention. Children in the parent-guidance intervention perceived their parent's overall competence (comprised of measures of perception of parenting and general communication) as significantly better in follow-up waves than did children in the telephone-monitoring intervention. However, there were no differences between the two groups with respect to death-related communication.

Interventions targeted specifically for sibling bereaved adolescents have been less prevalent, with the majority of efforts in that area focusing on individual or family-level grief counseling or therapy (Valentine, 1996), or support groups (Tedeschi, 1996), and often including participants grieving from a variety of deaths rather than only sibling bereaved adolescents. Bereavement support groups have been hypothesized to benefit adolescents by reducing their feelings of isolation, helping them share their emotions and information and helping them develop an understanding of life and death (Tedeschi, 1996). Balk, Tyson Rawson, and Colletti Wetzel (1993) developed a mutual support group intervention for bereaved college students that focused on coping with life crises and sharing personal experiences; however, no experimental trial of this intervention has been conducted to date. Although the lack of controlled outcome studies makes it difficult to assess the effect of bereavement support groups for adolescents, the anecdotal and survey evidence indicate that they have a high level of consumer acceptance and satisfaction (Baxter, 1982; Berson, 1988; Stokes et al., 1997).

STRATEGIES THAT DO NOT WORK

Information is not currently available on intervention strategies for bereaved adolescents that do not work or which have been found to have iatrogenic effects.

SYNTHESIS

An examination of bereavement interventions reveals the complexity of factors that contribute to their efficacy. Multiple intervention strategies have been developed, including family counseling, residential weekends, individual therapy, parental guidance, anticipatory grief counseling, bibliotherapy, and parent and child group interventions in parallel. These interventions have typically encouraged sharing of information, understanding and expressing feelings, and commemorating the death and family communication (Stokes & Crossley, 2001). Additionally, these approaches have employed techniques that vary from psycho-educational to supportive to therapeutic. Findings are equivocal with respect to the optimal combination of format, technique, and content, and findings with respect to symptomatology may vary with child's age, gender, and initial status as Sandler and colleagues (Sandler, Ayers, Wolchik, Tein, & Kwok, 2000; Sandler et al., 1992, 2001) report. Black and Urbanowicz (1987) attribute their positive findings to the enhancement of grief-related emotional expression, yet it is unclear as to whether an effort to improve bereavement-related communication between children and parents affect child outcomes (Christ et al., 2001).

Further research in the development of preventive interventions with adolescents who experience parental or sibling bereavement would benefit from several recommendations. First, a greater number of interventions should be conducted and evaluated as experimentally controlled outcome studies. Some investigators (Stokes et al., 1997) have acknowledged the difficulty in carrying out well-controlled studies with the bereaved due to ethical issues related to the assignment of bereaved individuals to "no treatment" conditions. However, experimental designs with treatment as usual or appropriate competing treatments may help to identify efficacious intervention components and would eliminate several threats to validity inherent in uncontrolled designs. Additionally, there is a need to carry out a greater number of experimental trials with adolescents who are bereaved due to the impact of AIDS, war, or other disasters. Unfortunately, the prevalence of bereavement related to these types of deaths is high or climbing and factors associated with the deaths may require other types of intervention approaches or strategies than what has typically been used.

Second, intervention studies need to target mediators that have been demonstrated to relate to healthy outcomes of bereaved adolescents. Sandler and colleagues (2001) have begun this work, and an analysis of key modifiable variables will allow for increasing potency and effectiveness of intervention strategies. As an important part of this process, it is necessary to build bridges from the basic science to the intervention design when developing programs. Investigators not only need to determine what mediators should be targeted but also whether current intervention strategies can lead to change in these targeted mediators.

Third, the use of more rigorous methodology such as the inclusion of multiple measures, assessment of time since the deaths, attention to age and gender of participants, and longitudinal follow-up will enhance the ability of researchers to draw meaningful conclusions from the preventive interventions they are evaluating. Finally, there is a need to link what we learn in these experimental trials with the constraints and realities of the existing service delivery systems. Of course, demonstrated efficacy in well-controlled experimental trials does not always translate into positive results in evaluation of services delivered in natural settings nor does it mean that the current service delivery systems can easily incorporate the intervention into their range of existing services. Greater attention to these kinds of dissemination issues while conducting experimental trials will likely lead to preventive interventions that can be more easily adopted in existing settings and can ultimately be more beneficial to the adolescents and families who are affected by a death in their family.

Also see: Bereavement: Childhood; Grief: Older Adulthood; Religion and Spirituality: Adolescence.

References

Achenbach, T., & Edelbrock, C. (1991). *Manual for the child behavior checklist and revised child behavior profile.* Burlington, VT: University of Vermont.

Ambert, A.M., & Saucier, J.F. (1984). Adolescents' academic success and aspirations by parental marital status. *Canadian Review of Sociology and Anthropology, 21*, 62–74.

Applebaum, D.R., & Burns, G.L. (1991). Unexpected childhood death: Posttraumatic stress disorder in surviving siblings and parents. *Journal of Clinical Child Psychology, 20*, 114–120.

Ayers, T.S., Twohey, J.L., Sandler, I.N., Wolchik, S.A., Lutzke, J.R., Padgett-Jones, S., Weiss, L., Cole, E., & Kriege, G. (2001). *The Family Bereavement Program: Description of a theory-based prevention program for parentally-bereaved children and adolescents.* Manuscript in preparation, Prevention Research Center, Arizona State University, P.O. Box 876005, Tempe, AZ 85287-6005.

Balk, D.E. (1996). Models for understanding adolescent coping with bereavement. *Death Studies, 20*, 367–387.

Balk, D.E., & Corr, C.A. (1996). Adolescents, developmental tasks, and encounters with death and bereavement. In C.A. Corr & D.E. Balk (Eds.), *Handbook of adolescent death and bereavement* (pp. 3–24). New York, NY: Springer.

Balk, D.E., & Corr, C.A. (2001). Bereavement during adolescence: A review of research. In M.S. Stroebe, R.O. Hansson, W. Stroebe, & H. Schut (Eds.), *Handbook of bereavement research: Consequences, coping and care* (pp. 199–218). Washington, DC: American Psychological Association.

Balk, D.E., Tyson Rawson, K., & Colletti Wetzel, J. (1993). Social support as an intervention with bereaved college students. *Death Studies, 17*, 427–450.

Baxter, G.W. (1982). Bereavement support groups for secondary school students. *School Guidance Worker, 38*, 27–29.

Berson, R.J. (1988). A bereavement group for college students. *Journal of American College Health, 37*, 101–108.

Birenbaum, L.K., Robinson, M.A., Phillips, D.S., Stewart, B.J., & McCown, D.E. (1989). The response of children to the dying and death of a sibling. *Omega Journal of Death and Dying, 20*, 213–228.

Black, D., & Urbanowicz, M.A. (1985). Bereaved children family intervention. In J.E. Stevenson (Ed.), *Recent research in developmental psychopathology* (pp. 179–187). Oxford: Pergamon.

Black, D., & Urbanowicz, M.A. (1987). Family intervention with bereaved children. *Journal of Child Psychology and Psychiatry and Allied Disciplines, 28*, 467–476.

Bonanno, G.A., & Kaltman, S. (1999). Toward an integrative perspective on bereavement. *Psychological Bulletin, 125*, 760–776.

Bonanno, G.A., Keltner, D., Holen, A., & Horowitz, M.J. (1995). When avoiding unpleasant emotions might not be such a bad thing: Verbal-autonomic response dissociation and midlife conjugal bereavement. *Journal of Personality and Social Psychology, 69*, 975–989.

Christ, G.H., Raveis, V.H., Siegel, K., & Karus, D. (2001). *Evaluation of a preventive intervention for bereaved children.* Manuscript submitted for publication, Columbia School of Social Work, New York, NY.

Davies, B. (1991). Long-term outcomes of adolescent sibling bereavement. Special Issue: Death and adolescent bereavement. *Journal of Adolescent Research, 6*, 83–96.

Davies, B. (1999). *Shadow in the sun: The experience of sibling bereavement in childhood.* Philadelphia, PA, US: Brunner/Mazel, Inc.

Demographic and Health Surveys. (2001). *MEASURE DHS+* [Data]. Macro International, Inc. Available: www.measuedhs.com [2001, 3–10–2001].

Dowdney, L. (2000). Childhood bereavement following parental death. *Journal of Child Psychology and Psychiatry and Allied Disciplines, 41*, 819–830.

Fleming, S., & Balmer, L. (1996). Bereavement in adolescence. In C.A. Corr & D.E. Balk (Eds.), *Handbook of adolescent death and bereavement* (pp. 139–154). New York, NY: Springer.

Fleming, S.J., & Adolph, R. (1986). Helping bereaved adolescents: Needs and responses. In C.A. Corr & J.N. McNeil (Eds.), *Adolescence and death* (pp. 97–118). New York, NY: Springer.

Gersten, J.C., Beals, J., & Kallgren, C.A. (1991). Epidemiology and preventive interventions: Parental death in childhood as a case example. Special Issue: Preventive Intervention Research Centers. *American Journal of Community Psychology, 19,* 481–500.

Gregory, I. (1965). Anterospective data following childhood loss of a parent. *Archives of General Psychiatry, 13,* 99–109.

Haine, R.A., Ayers, T.S., Sandler, I.N., Wolchik, S.A., & Lutzke, J.R. (2001). *Locus of control and self-esteem as mediators or moderators of the relations between negative life events and mental health problems in parentally bereaved children.* Manuscript in preparation.

Hainline, L., & Feig, E. (1978). The correlates of childhood father absence in college-aged women. *Child Development, 49,* 37–42.

Hetherington, E. (1972). Effects of father absence on personality development in adolescent daughters. *Developmental Psychology, 7,* 313–326.

Hogan, N.S., & Greenfield, D.B. (1991). Adolescent sibling bereavement symptomatology in a large community sample. Special Issue: Death and adolescent bereavement. *Journal of Adolescent Research, 6,* 97–112.

Horowitz, M.J., Siegel, B., Holen, A., & Bonanno, G.A. (1997). Diagnostic criteria for complicated grief disorder. *American Journal of Psychiatry, 154,* 904–910.

Lutzke, J.R., Ayers, T.S., Sandler, I.N., & Barr, A. (1997). Risks and interventions for the parentally-bereaved child. In S.A. Wolchik & I.N. Sandler (Eds.), *Handbook of children's coping with common life stressors: Linking theory, research and interventions* (pp. 215–243). New York: Plenum.

Martinson, I.M., & Campos, R.G. (1991). Adolescent bereavement: Long-term responses to a sibling's death from cancer. Special Issue: Death and adolescent bereavement. *Journal of Adolescent Research, 6,* 54–69.

Martinson, I.M., Davies, E.B., & McGlowry, S.G. (1987). The long-term effects of sibling death on self-concept. *Journal of Pediatric Nursing, 2,* 227–235.

McCown, D.E., & Pratt, C. (1985). Impact of sibling death on children's behavior. *Death Studies, 9,* 323–335.

Moos, R.H., & Schaefer, J.A. (1986). Life transitions and crises: A conceptual overview. In R.H. Moos (Ed.), *Coping with life crises: An integrated approach* (pp. 1–28). New York: Plenum Press.

Oltjenbruns, K.A. (1991). Positive outcomes of adolescents' experience with grief. Special Issue: Death and adolescent bereavement. *Journal of Adolescent Research, 6,* 43–53.

Payne, S., & Relf, M. (1994). The assessment of need for bereavement follow-up in palliative and hospice care. *Palliative Medicine, 8(4),* 291–297.

Partridge, S., & Kotler, T. (1987). Self-esteem and adjustment in adolescents from bereaved, divorced, and intact families: Family type versus family environment. *Australian Journal of Psychology, 39,* 223–234.

Prigerson, H.G., & Jacobs, S.C. (2001). Traumatic grief as a distinct disorder: A rationale, consensus criteria, and a preliminary empirical test. In M.S. Stroebe, R.O. Hansson, W. Stroebe, & H. Schut (Eds.), *Handbook of bereavement research: Consequences, coping and care* (pp. 613–645). Washington, DC: American Psychological Association.

Reinherz, H.Z., Giaconia, R.M., Hauf, A.M.C., Wasserman, M.S., & Silverman, A.B. (1999). Major depression in the transition to adulthood: Risks and impairments. *Journal of Abnormal Psychology, 108,* 500–510.

Ringler, L.L., & Hayden, D.C. (2000). Adolescent bereavement and social support: Peer loss compared to other losses. *Journal of Adolescent Research, 15,* 209–230.

Rotheram-Borus, M.J., Lee, M.B., Gwadz, M., & Draimin, B. (2001). An intervention for parents with AIDS and their adolescent children. *American Journal of Public Health, 91,* 1294–1302.

Rotheram-Borus, M.J., Stein, J.A., & Lin, Y.-Y. (2001). Impact of parent death and intervention on the adjustment of adolescents whose parents have HIV/AIDS. *Journal of Consulting and Clinical Psychology, 69,* 763–773.

Saler, L., & Skolnick, N. (1992). Childhood parental death and depression in adulthood: Roles of surviving parent and family environment. *American Journal of Orthopsychiatry, 62,* 504–516.

Sandler, I.N., Ayers, T.S., Wolchik, S.A., Tein, J.-Y., & Kwok, O. (2000, June). Evaluation of a theory based preventive intervention for bereaved children. In D.C. Godette (Chair), *Youth depression and suicide.* Symposium conducted at the Eighth Annual Meeting of the Society for Prevention Research, Montreal, Canada.

Sandler, I.N., Ayers, T.S., Wolchik, S.A., Tein, J.-Y., Kwok, O.-M., Haine, R.A., Twohey, J.L., Suter, J., Lin, K., Padgett-Jones, S., Lutzke, J.R., Cole, E., Kriege, G., & Griffin, W.A. (2001). *The Family Bereavement Program: Efficacy evaluation of a theory-based prevention program for parentally-bereaved children and adolescents.* Manuscript submitted for publication, Arizona State University, Tempe, AZ.

Sandler, I.N., West, S.G., Baca, L., Pillow, D.R., Gersten, J., Rogosch, F., Virdin, L., Beals, J., Reynolds, K., Kallgren, C., Tein, J., Krieg, G., Cole, E., & Ramirez, R. (1992). Linking empirically based theory and evaluation: The Family Bereavement Program. *American Journal of Community Psychology, 20,* 491–521.

Saucier, J.F., & Ambert, A.M. (1982). Parental marital status and adolescents' optimism about their future. *Journal of Youth and Adolescence, 11,* 345–354.

Social Security Administration. (2000). *Intermediate Assumptions of the 2000 Trustees Report.* Washington, DC: Office of the Chief Actuary of the Social Security Administration.

Stokes, J., & Crossley, D. (2001). *A child's grief.* London: Winston's Wish.

Stokes, J., Pennington, J., Monroe, B., Papadatou, D., & Relf, M. (1999). Developing services for bereaved children: A discussion of the theoretical and practical issues involved. *Mortality, 4,* 291–307.

Stokes, J., Wyer, S., & Crossley, D. (1997). The challenge of evaluating a child bereavement programme. *Palliative Medicine, 11,* 179–190.

Stroebe, M., & Schut, H. (1999). The dual process model of coping with bereavement: Rationale and description. *Death Studies, 23,* 197–224.

Stroebe, M., van Son, M., Stroebe, W., Kleber, R., Schut, H., & van den Bout, J. (2000). On the classification and diagnosis of pathological grief. *Clinical Psychology Review, 20,* 57–75.

Stroebe, M.S. (1992). Coping with bereavement: A review of the grief work hypothesis. *Omega Journal of Death and Dying, 26,* 19–42.

Stroebe, M.S., Hansson, R.O., Stroebe, W., & Schut, H. (2001). Future directions for bereavement research. In M.S. Stroebe, R.O. Hansson, W. Stroebe, & H. Schut (Eds.), *Handbook of bereavement research: Consequences, coping and care* (pp. 741–766). Washington, DC: American Psychological Association.

Stroebe, M.S., & Schut, H. (2001). Models of coping with bereavement: A review. In M.S. Stroebe, R.O. Hansson, W. Stroebe, & H. Schut (Eds.), *Handbook of bereavement research: Consequences, coping and care* (pp. 375–403). Washington, DC: American Psychological Association.

Stroebe, W., & Stroebe, M.S. (1987). *Bereavement and health: The psychological and physical consequences of partner loss.* Cambridge, England: Cambridge University Press.

Tedeschi, R.G. (1996). Support groups for bereaved adolescents. In C.A. Corr & D.E. Balk (Eds.), *Handbook of adolescent death and bereavement* (pp. 293–311). New York, NY: Springer.

Valentine, L. (1996). Professional interventions to assist adolescents who are coping with death and bereavement. In C.A. Corr & D.E. Balk (Eds.), *Handbook of adolescent death and bereavement* (pp. 312–328). New York, NY: Springer.

Van Eerdewegh, M.M., Bieri, M.D., Parrilla, R.H., & Clayton, P.J. (1982). The bereaved child. *British Journal of Psychiatry, 140,* 23–29.

West, S.G., Sandler, I.N., Pillow, D.R., Baca, L., & Gersten, J.C. (1991). The use of structural equation modeling in generative research: Toward the design of a preventive intervention for bereaved children. Special Issue: Preventive Intervention Research Centers. *American Journal of Community Psychology, 19*, 459–480.

Worden, J.W. (1991). *Grief counseling and grief therapy: A handbook for the mental health practitioner* (2nd ed.). New York: Springer.

Worden, J.W. (1996). *Children and grief: When a parent dies.* New York: Guilford.

Worden, J.W., Davies, B., & McCown, D. (1999). Comparing parent loss with sibling loss. *Death Studies, 23*, 1–15.

Worden, J.W., & Silverman, P.R. (1996). Parental death and the adjustment of school-age children. *Omega Journal of Death and Dying, 33*, 91–102.

Wortman, C.B., & Silver, R.C. (1989). The myths of coping with loss. *Journal of Consulting and Clinical Psychology, 57*, 349–357.

Birth Defects, Early Childhood

Patricia M. Newcomb

INTRODUCTION

The prevention of birth defects is an outcome desired worldwide. Primary prevention would seem to be the ideal approach, but alleviation of the morbidity of some congenital defects and diseases is also a worthy goal.

DEFINITIONS

A *congenital defect* or anomaly is an alteration in a gene (or genes) or an injury before or during birth which results in the individual affected having a visible, measurable, clinically evident disease or nonbeneficial anatomical variation. Examples of gene alterations include holes in the heart (atrial and ventricle septal defects or ASDs and VSDs), Marfan's syndrome, Tay-Sachs disease, and polydactyly. Examples of injury include contractures and limb defects due to amniotic bands (strands of membrane or scar in the uterus), direct trauma, direct poisons, and true asphyxia. Injuries also can stem from infection, such as the "TORCH" illnesses: toxoplasmosis, "other", rubella, cytomegalovirus (CMV), and herpes.

It is becoming clear that many conditions which cause difficulty in later life have both a genetic predisposition (a problem in a gene makes it more likely for that individual to develop the condition) and an environmental component. (Some other exposure must occur to cause the individual to develop the problem.) In some cases, a tiny change in a single gene creates a global illness, as in maple sugar urine disease, which affects neurological development and the excretory system. In other cases, multiple genes must be affected to cause the problem. A heart defect where the blood vessels are reversed in position, called Tetralogy of Fallot, is an example of the latter.

In many cases of single gene defects, the gene involved is known (as in sickle cell disease). A large number of congenital defects have an unknown cause. One well-known example is cerebral palsy. Some possibly preventable conditions of the fetus are now being considered a kind of birth defect. Examples would be intrauterine growth restriction (IUGR) and preterm delivery (birth before 37 weeks of gestation).

SCOPE

Incidence—3–5 percent of live-born children in the United States (150,000–250,000 per year) have a recognizable birth defect. By later childhood the incidence becomes 6–7 percent as cognitive deficits become apparent (Williams et al., 1997). Various etiologies cause these defects. The estimated contribution of various causes follows:

• Genetic (chromosomal & single gene)	20–25%
• Infections (CMV, rubella, etc.)	3–5%
• Maternal disease (diabetes, alcohol, seizure, etc.)	4%
• Drugs and medications	<1%
• Multifactorial or unknown	65–75%

Similar numbers are seen in other developed countries.

About 10,000 of these children each year have cerebral palsy (Centers for Disease Control and Prevention [CDC], 2001). About 2,750 live-born children per year have a neural tube defect (failure of the spine to close) per year in the United States (Honein, Paulozzi, Mathews, Erickson, & Lee-Yang, 2001). One percent of all births in the United States are affected by CMV infection. About 3,000 of these suffer congenital anomalies (Morrison, 2000). Approximately 13,200 infants are born to mothers who have a seizure disorder each year (Lewis, Van Dyke, Stumbo, & Berg, 1998). Conotruncal heart defects (which include major malpositions of the great vessels, Tetralogy of Fallot, and duplication in the heart structure) affect 3,000 infants a year in the United States (Botto, Khoury, Mulinare, & Erickson, 1996).

Prevalence—Data on congenital anomalies are usually reported per birth, but with the incidence of 3–5 percent, and a vast majority surviving, even though the current existing cases out of the total population of the United States are not reported, the prevalence is probably 8–9 million/300 million.

Costs to host/society—The costs to the affected individuals vary from negligible (*polydactyly*, or extra fingers) to devastating. A cerebral palsy victim, for example, averages a lifetime cost of $503,000 in 1992 dollars (CDC, 2001). A rough estimate of the cost to the US health system for cerebral palsy alone, per year, is $53 million dollars. The annual cost of treating CMV complications alone is two billion dollars (Morrison, 2000).

THEORIES

Primary prevention is the prevention of a disease or defect before it begins or is established. Secondary prevention is the prevention of consequences or morbidities in persons with established disease. Strategies to prevent birth defects take both types of prevention into account. Preconception counseling is advising parents before they attempt pregnancy how best to optimize their outcome. Some commonsense activities apply. First, avoid disease in the mother. If disease is already established in the mother, control its effects, minimizing morbidity. (Example: congenital anomalies in the offspring are reduced if blood sugar is controlled in diabetic women prior to pregnancy.) Second, avoid vitamin or micronutrient deficiencies and toxicities. (Example: folate supplementation helps prevent neural tube defects.) Third, avoid toxins and radiation exposures in both parents. (The paternal contribution is often overlooked.) Fourth, by obtaining complete histories and, at times, genetic testing of the parents, recognize specific inherited conditions for which the couple's offspring are at elevated risk.

Technology now allows us, in the case of in vitro fertilization, to test a potential embryo for genetic defects prior to implantation into the uterus (single cell genetic screening). This is one extreme of treating the problem on an individual basis. Public health theory and practice, on the other hand, hold that population-wide efforts at education or intervention will reach more people with less cost per person. Universal free prenatal visits (as in the Netherlands), financial bonuses for early prenatal care (as in France), nationwide public information campaigns, and supplementation of food products (e.g., with iron or folate) are examples.

An important concept to understand in the prevention of birth defects is the *window of effect* during the pregnancy. Doses of a toxin or exposure might be tolerated without any effect on the fetus if occurring after a critical vulnerable time. Organogenesis (the forming of organ systems in the fetus) lasts from about the 3rd week after conception to the 9th week. This is frequently the most vulnerable time for the fetus, and the time at which exposure will cause a serious defect. For this reason, many doctors advise patients to avoid all medications in the first trimester (1st twelve weeks after last menstrual period). Other windows of vulnerability exist for other substances. The nervous system takes the longest to develop in the fetus (and continues fast development after birth), and is frequently affected by third trimester exposures.

Detection of birth defects in utero allows time for definitive action (e.g., termination in lethal defects such as Potter's disease, in which the kidneys and subsequently the lungs do not form, or anencephaly, in which the brain does not form). In nonlethal diseases, early detection clearly improves the infant's outcome, when a therapy that can be promptly initiated exists. Examples would be early detection of heart defects, which allows for planning neonatal surgery, and urethral obstruction, which allows for near normal outcomes for infants undergoing sometimes risky fetal surgery.

RESEARCH

Evidence based medicine (EBM) employs the principles of best evidence to determine the most valuable strategy in treatment or in understanding prognosis. The strongest evidence in therapeutic studies comes from randomized, blinded, placebo-controlled clinical studies. Due to a long history of infamous outcomes (such as thalidomide and diethylstilbestrol [DES]), very few new drug trials are currently being carried out in populations of pregnant women. Prognosis studies involve case matched control studies, whether prospective or retrospective. Data from very large cross sectional studies are also used.

STRATEGIES THAT WORK

The best-studied intervention to prevent a specific birth defect is the provision of folic acid to pregnant women to prevent neural tube defects. Multiple studies (with, unfortunately, different dosing regimens) were carried out in several countries in the 1980s and 1990s. Both primary (new, spontaneous neural tube defects) and secondary (prevention in mothers with an affected previous child) prevention were studied. Randomized controlled studies showed a 72 percent reduction in the rate of neural tube defects when women received at least 400 μg of folate per day. These strong results led the United States to recommend 400 μg of folate per day in an average risk pregnancy, and 4 mg/day for women at high risk (or with prior history of an affected infant.) In 1996, the US Food and Drug Administration (FDA) mandated the supplementation of cereals and grains throughout the United States with a goal of increasing by approximately 50 percent the daily intake of folate among all reproductive age women in the United States to 400 μg a day. A recent study showed a 19 percent decrease in liveborn infants with neural tube defects (Honein et al., 2001).

Surely the avoidance of substances known to cause birth defects is an obvious strategy. Yet a bewildering array of substances and exposures have been linked to congenital defects. Substance use is a highly complex behavior both more entrenched and less amenable to treatment than once previously thought. Entire volumes can be written on the risks of defects caused by medicinal and other compounds. The most frequent substances and preventable defects and diseases will be addressed.

Alcohol

Maternal alcohol intake in pregnancy causes a constellation of defects known as fetal alcohol syndrome (FAS) in the offspring involving facial and musculoskeletal defects, growth defects, and mental retardation of varying degrees. There is a strong dose response, with increasing defects with increasing alcohol intake. Cessation at any point will improve the outcome (indicating the window of risk extends through the later parts of pregnancy). At least 70 percent of Americans drink some alcohol. Some recent studies indicate that continued drinking occurs in at least 1.4 percent of pregnancies. Over the last three decades, the incidence of FAS has increased to 6 births in each 10,000. FAS is the most commonly identified specific cause of mental retardation in the United States (Cunningham et al., 1997).

Widespread education campaigns and warnings on packages have increased awareness of alcohol's deleterious effects and also the stigma of drinking while pregnant. It is hoped that specific repeated screening in each trimester of pregnancy will aid in identifying problem pregnant drinkers.

Tobacco

As many as 18 percent of pregnant women smoke (Morrison, 2000). Recent large studies have demonstrated that fetuses of smokers are at increased risk for placental abruption (early separation of the placenta, often with life-threatening hemorrhage), placenta previa (placenta covering the exit from the uterus), preterm birth, low birth weight, pre-eclampsia (hypertension caused by pregnancy), developmental delay, sudden infant death syndrome (SIDS), asthma and poor lung function, and congenital anomalies such as neural tube defect, cleft palate and lip.

While cigarettes are very addicting, more so for women, pregnancy is a window of opportunity for cessation. Often women can delay, cut down, or eliminate use with the benefit for their child as a goal. Counseling efforts should include support strategies, review of facts about quitting (such as that the vast majority of successful quitters had to quit more than once or twice), and consideration of medication. Nicotine causes withdrawal syndromes in infants (has vasoactive effects) and is contraindicated. Buproprion (Wellbutrin®, Zyban®) is an effective antidepressant which reduces craving and is acceptable in pregnancy.

Other Substances of Abuse

Many substances are abused, but few are proven, in and of themselves, to cause significant birth defects. Cocaine, for example, has been widely studied and deeply feared for potentially causing neurological and development delays. While heavy use of cocaine is associated with preterm delivery, abruption, and pre-eclampsia, no studies have yet identified a long-lasting or permanent ill effect to the infant or increased incidence of birth defects. The "shaking, withdrawing crack baby" is more frequently withdrawing from nicotine.

The true issues to address are complex biological, social, and political factors leading to an overall unhealthy environment for pregnant women. This malignant milieu includes polysubstance abuse, poor self-esteem, domestic violence, poor nutrition, limitations on access to health care and inability to control the outside environment of the pregnancy (e.g., inability to undertake work with fewer exposures, or to live further from polluted areas).

STRATEGIES THAT MIGHT WORK

Preconception anticipatory guidance counseling carries hope for preventing many birth defects. Identifying risk factors facing potential parents, and beginning prevention efforts before conception, may offer great potential for optimizing outcomes. However, there are no definitive studies to support this concept overall.

The best-supported preconception intervention (or support) is folic acid supplementation. Some evidence supports the use of multivitamin (prenatal vitamins) to help prevent defects such as cleft palate. Also, immunizations carry significant promise for preconception prevention. Many illnesses, such as rubella, can cause defects, stillbirth, or loss. Because immunization for rubella is inexpensive and can prevent severe defects, it is very cost-effective. However, since the vaccine (an attenuated live vaccine) cannot be given during pregnancy, preconception anticipatory guidance is the only option (usually, in fact, immediately after the pregnancy in which lack of immunization was noted) (Morrison, 1999).

Other significant infections such as sexually transmitted diseases (STDs), especially syphilis, which causes severe congenital defects, are tracked by state Health Departments. Adequate preconception or early pregnancy intervention is essential. Varicella zoster (chicken pox), herpes, toxoplasmosis, measles, and mumps are other examples.

Paternal

Birth defects can also stem from the paternal genetic contribution, and opportunities for prevention exist. Data are incomplete but indicate certain paternal occupation exposures may put the fetus at risk (agricultural, chemical, and heavy metal-exposed occupations), environmental, and personal history or lifestyle factors (such as a history of needing anticancer agents, paternal diabetes, or smoking).

It is easy to connect the presence of a chemical in the fetus' direct environment to a defect in the child when a clear-cut mechanism of transport across the placenta from the maternal circulation exists. It is harder to understand possible paternal mechanisms. The most obvious and easy-to-accept mechanism is direct damage to the gamete (sperm) which fertilizes the egg. This mechanism is known to transmit birth defects in the case of radiation exposure, and possibly thalidomide (thalidomide binds to sperm). The damage done can be either *genetic* (direct damage to the DNA molecule in the sperm) or *epigenetic* (alterations to the "support" atoms in the DNA, such as methylation [addition of carbon molecules] changes to sperm DNA).

Other possible mechanisms include the transfer of molecules from the male to the female in seminal fluid during intercourse. These chemicals, once inside the body, affect the fetus or mother directly. Another *indirect* source of genetic damage is substances brought into the home on the father's clothing. Heavy metals have been shown to be transported this way. When clothing is handled or washed, the mother receives an exposure. Mercury, lead, and beryllium have been transported this way (Olshan and Faustman, 1993). More studies are needed to fully identify these risks and develop strategies to prevent them.

Some chronic diseases of later life involve not only a genetic predisposition but also a long subclinical period in infancy and childhood during which environmental changes are crucial. Adequate prevention will no doubt improve length and quality of life more than current advances in medication or surgery. Pregnancy is an opportunity to create a better home environment for the child through smoking cessation, reduction of fat in the diet, and decreased alcohol consumption. Currently 80 percent of children in the United States exceed dietary recommendations for fat intake. Likewise, reducing tobacco and alcohol use in parents may reduce the prevalence of these habits in adolescents (currently one third are habitual users) (Harris, 2000).

STRATEGIES THAT DO NOT WORK

Disastrous consequences have arisen whenever the balance of risk to benefit has not been carefully considered in treating pregnant women with medication. For example, in mammals, progesterone (the major steroid of pregnancy) is essential for maintaining the pregnancy. Doctors and researchers extrapolated from this and used DES, a synthetic progesterone, to combat repetitive miscarriage in humans.

The children from these exposed pregnancies suffered deformations of the uterus and cervix, infertility, and a rare form of cancer (*clear cell adenocarcinoma of the vagina*).

In the case of thalidomide, the fallacy was presuming a drug could be devoid of risks. The medication was widely believed to lack side effects, even though studies of effects were poorly done and very incomplete. When taken during organogenesis, the medication caused shortening and absence of the limbs of the child.

It is important to remember, however, that severe consequences can result in the fetus when maternal disease is allowed to progress unchecked. Fear of exposure leads many women with severe depression or seizure disorders to stop their medications. But uncontrolled mental illness may incapacitate the mother, result in suicide (or homicide by her of her children), or simply prevent adequate mothering of the child, leading to failure of the infant to thrive. Similarly, uncontrolled seizures in pregnant women may result in prolonged oxygen deprivation of the fetus, and severe neurological and developmental problems. Each patient and each drug must be considered for the complete benefit–risk relationship before continuing or stopping medications.

SYNTHESIS

Historically, the concept of improving genetic outcomes was limited by the level of intervention possible. This led to ethically unacceptable actions such as eugenics in Germany, sterilization of nonconsenting adults in the United States, and laws concerning miscegenation elsewhere (Fineman & Walton, 2000). In response, genetic health care professionals have practiced two tenets: (1) never to attempt to influence the outcome of a pregnancy and (2) always to use nondirective guidance techniques. Meanwhile, advances in medical science have allowed options other than abortion to prevent the birth of babies with congenital defects and to significantly improve the quality of life and decrease morbidity for infants born with a genetic defect. Indeed, the public health credo mandates certain interventions such as preventing isoimmunization of future pregnancies by administering Rhogam to Rh-negative mothers in pregnancy.

The core ethical principles of autonomy (respect for a person's control over her own body), and beneficence (the health care professional's obligation to provide benefit and balance risk vs. benefit for patients) come into play in these sorts of decisions. In addition, physicians have an obligation to the health of communities and populations. There are signs that genetic health care professionals are moving to consider some of the public health care precepts and to adopt more directive counseling techniques (Fineman & Walton, 2000). Care must be taken to avoid both discrimination using advanced genetic information about individuals and failure to protect innocent potential members of society (unborn children able to live outside the uterus). The coming decades will require a discernment on these issues.

Also see: Environmental Health: Early Childhood; Bullying: Childhood; Family Strengthening: Childhood; Peer Relationships: Childhood; Violence Prevention: Childhood; Delinquency: Childhood.

References

Botto, L.D., Khoury, M.J., Mulinare, J., & Erickson, J.D. (1996). Periconceptual multivitamin use and the occurrence of conotruncal heart defects: Results from a population-based, case-control study. *Pediatrics, 98*(5), 911–917.

Centers for Disease Control and Prevention (CDC). (2001). Fact Sheet. *Cerebral palsy among children*. http://www.cdc.gov/ncbddd/fact/cpfs.htm

Cunningham, G.F., Macdonald, P.C., Leveno, K.J., Gant, Norman F., Gilstrap, L.C. Williams (1993). Obstetrics 19th ed., pp. 919–921. Stanford, CT: Appleton and Lange.

Cunningham, G.F., MacDonald, P.C., Gant, N.F., Leveno, K.J., Gilstrap III, L.C., Hankins, G.D.V., Clark, S.L., & Williams, L.C. (1997). *Obstetrics* (20th ed., pp. 895, 958–959). Stamford, CT: Appleton and Lange.

Fineman, R.M., & Walton, M.T. (2000). Should genetic health care providers attempt to influence reproductive outcome using directive counseling techniques? A public health prospective. *Women & Health, 303*(3), 39–46.

Harris, G.D. (2000). Heart disease in children. *Primary Care, 27*(3), 767–784.

Honein, M.A., Paulozzi, L.J., Mathews, T.J., Erickson, J.D., & Lee-Yang, C.W. (2001). Impact of folic acid fortification of the US food supply on the occurrence of neural tube defects. *Journal of American Medical Association, 285*(23), 2981–2986.

Lewis, D.P., Van Dyke, D.C., Stumbo, P.J., & Berg, M.J. (1998). Drug and environmental factors associated with adverse pregnancy outcomes. Part I: Antiepileptic drugs, contraceptives, smoking, and folate. *The Annals of Pharmacotherapy, 32*, 802–817.

Morrison, E.H. (2000). "Periconception care" in update in maternity care. *Primary Care 27*(1), 2–5.

Morrison, E.H. (2002). Periconception care. *Primary Care, 27*(1), 1–12.

Olshan, A.F., & Faustman, E.M. (1993). Male mediated developmental toxicity. *Annual Review of Public Health, 14*, 159–81.

Bullying, Childhood

Arthur M. Horne and Pamela Orpinas

INTRODUCTION

Aggression among children and adolescents has been common throughout history and continues to be a major problem today. Neighborhoods and communities cannot be healthy for child development, nor can schools be effective institutions of learning, if they are not first and foremost safe. Yet young people face serious problems of aggression and victimization in their lives that may result in many missed opportunities for growing up as healthy young people.

Examples of aggression among young people are name-calling, teasing, threatening, pushing in hallways, and excluding a person from groups. However, some of the more extreme situations young people encounter may result in permanent physical injuries or even death. Recent examples of school shootings in the United States have heightened the attention on the seriousness of the problem of aggression. Since 1974, over two thirds of the incidents of shootings by students against fellow students have had a common theme: acting out of anger or revenge for having been victimized by other students in the school (US Secret Service National Threat Assessment Center, 2000).

DEFINITIONS

Bullying is a subset of aggression. Bullying has been defined as occurring when a student "... is exposed, repeatedly and over time, to negative actions on the part of one or more other students" (Olweus, 1994, p. 1173). It is also defined as "... long-standing violence, physical or psychological, conducted by an individual or a group, and directed against an individual who is not able to defend himself in the actual situation" (Roland, 1989, p. 143). Newman, Horne, and Bartolomucci (2000), building upon the work of Olweus, developed the "Double I/R" criteria for teachers to determine whether bullying is occurring. The double I refers to *intentional* and *imbalanced*, and the R refers to *repeated*. Not all aggressive acts are bullying, for they may not be intentional, as could occur through the hyperactive behavior of a classmate or accidental injury from rough-and-tumble play. An aggressive act that occurs between students of equal size and ability, without an imbalance of power, also would not be bullying. An aggressive event that happens only once, though not desirable, would still not fit the definition of bullying. When working with children and adolescents, aggression in general and bullying in particular should be considered.

Bullying takes several forms. Bullying may be physical (e.g., hitting, pushing, or pulling hair), verbal (e.g., teasing, ridiculing, or threatening), relational (e.g., leaving someone out of the group, not talking to someone, or ordering someone to do something to be liked), or indirect (e.g., sending nasty notes, lying about someone, or spreading rumors) (Hawker & Boulton, 2000). Bullying in the form of sexual harassment can take any of these forms. Bullies can be aggressive or passive. The *aggressive bully*, who is the most common type of bully, is usually the one who initiates the aggression and most commonly uses physical and verbal aggression. The *passive bully* does not initiate the aggression, but is the one who follows along, joins in, or encourages others to be aggressive (Newman et al., 2000).

Targets of bullying are often referred to as *victims*, but this term is misleading. *Victimization* implies a lack of ability to protect oneself, which is sometimes inaccurate. Children targeted by aggressors are exposed, often repeatedly and over time, to aggression. The effects can be far-reaching and may have an impact long after childhood. Consequences of being the target of aggression may include depression (Hawker & Boulton, 2000), somatic complaints (Williams, Chambers, Logan, & Robinson, 1996), and low self-esteem (Olweus, 1994). The targeted students are likely to report feeling unhappy and lonely, and having few friends (Boulton & Underwood, 1992). Further, they are likely to report being excluded and isolated, as well as having their personal property damaged (Hazler, 1996).

SCOPE

While the exact number of bullying incidents in schools and communities is difficult to measure or to even estimate, a number of nationwide studies indicate the extent of youth aggression and a few studies indicate the extent of bullying. In the United States in 1999, 5 percent of high school students reported missing school because of fear, almost 7 percent carried a weapon on school property, and 14 percent engaged in a physical fight on school property (Centers for Disease Control and Prevention [CDC], 2000). Similarly, a report by the National Center for Educational Statistics of children aged 12–18 years indicated that 8 percent of students reported criminal victimization at school, including either theft or violent crime, and 15 percent reported being in a physical fight at school (Kaufman et al., 2000). In that same study, 10 percent of 6th and 7th graders reported being bullied. However, when children are asked about specific acts of aggression, the prevalence of reported bullying increases. Another national study of children in grades 3–12, for example, showed that during the year prior to the survey a majority of students had been insulted by another student (60 percent); half of the students had been pushed, shoved, grabbed, or slapped by another student (49 percent); and over one third had been threatened (37 percent) (MetLife, 1999). In a cross-national study conducted in the United States, Canada, and 26 European countries among students aged 11–15 years, students in the Slovak Republic, England, Sweden, and Ireland, reported significantly less bullying than students in the United States, while students in Portugal, Austria, Czech Republic, Switzerland, Greenland, and Germany reported more (WHO Health Behaviour in School-Aged Children Study cited in US Department of Education & US Department of Justice, 1999).

THEORIES

Understanding bullies and victims requires recognition that the problem, as well as the solution, may exist at different levels or, more likely, as a function of an interaction of different levels of influence. The *Ecological model* is a framework that can be used to understand these multiple levels of risk factors that influence students' aggression, as well as the multiple levels of interventions that can be developed. The model can be visualized as concentric circles, in which the individual is the center. The second circle represents the student's family. The third circle represents the school, including peers, teachers, administrators, and staff, as well as school policies. The next circle represents the community where the child lives, and the outermost circle is the greater society that influences cultural norms about violence (Sallis & Owen, 1997).

At the core level is the individual child, who may have characteristics that place him or her at risk for bullying or for victimization. Characteristics of the child that increase the likelihood of being the aggressor are prior antisocial or behavioral problems, low verbal ability, attention deficit hyperactivity disorder, learning disability, poor motor-skill development, prenatal and perinatal complications, and head injury (Buka & Earls, 1993). The cognitive factor most studied in the area of aggression is the aggressive attributional bias, that is, bullies over-attribute hostile intentions to the actions of other students. As a result, bullies respond defensively attempting to counteract the perceived threat. Further, bullies tend to have little empathy for victims, high self-efficacy for aggression, attitudes and beliefs that support violence as a way to solve conflicts, and low ability to solve conflicts in nonviolent ways compared to nonaggressive adolescents. Children who learn that being aggressive will lead them to more opportunities, such as greater use of playground equipment, earlier lunch, or power over others, are being reinforced for that behavior.

Physical characteristics such as size or coordination problems, as well as emotional or temperament characteristics, such as being easily angered or being very timid, may influence a child to be aggressive or to be the target of aggression. Further, learning experiences may influence aggression or victimization. A child who is small, unprotected, and alone learns to fear situations and to avoid settings that will be threatening. Targets of bullies experience fear and anxiety in threatening situations, and then take protective measures to avoid or diminish the harm they may experience in those feared settings.

The family influences the child's characteristics. Family variables that predict violence are child abuse, low parental monitoring and poor discipline skills, parental approval of aggressive behaviors, negative relationship with parents, and parental criminality (DiLalla & Gottesman, 1991; Larzelere & Patterson, 1990; Orpinas, Murray, & Kelder, 1999). Similar family variables have been shown to predict bullying. Families that endorse confrontation and violence as a mean to resolve problems model that behavior for their children; thus, they contribute to the bullying experience. Likewise, families that are withdrawn, unengaged, and non-supportive may fail to provide students with the support they need to develop positive self-confidence and social skills, thus contributing to the victimization of children. The bully at school is often a victim of aggression at home and may have caretakers who are hostile, authoritarian, inconsistent in parenting, and lacking effective problem-solving skills (Horne & Sayger, 1990). Schwartz, Dodge, Pettit, and Bates (1997) concluded that boys who were both aggressive and victims belonged to the most punitive, hostile, and abusive families, while boys who were aggressive but not victims had a strong history of exposure to adult aggression, but had not been victimized by adults. In contrast, the family environment of the passive victims did not differ from the family environment of the normative group.

Schools play a major role in influencing bullying and victimization. The interaction of the child with the classroom and the culture of the school provide an environment that may result in increased—or decreased—aggression and violence. Teachers who accommodate their teaching to the needs of students, teach and promote self-management strategies and adaptive skills, and establish positive student–teacher relationships have classrooms with less bullying and victimization (Hazler, 1996). When school personnel fail to stop the problem, bullies and victims may perceive it as approval of the behavior. As a consequence, school personnel may be reinforcing the aggression (Fried & Fried, 1996).

Community and peer group influences exert a major influence on the development of bullying. The community environment may have a significant effect on the type and style of interpersonal relationships considered acceptable. Therefore, a community's lack of interest or ability to reduce bullying in essence sanctions the behavior (Fried & Fried, 1996). The final component in the development and maintenance of bullying is the larger culture. Exposure to violence and aggression through television, music, and games, increases desensitization to the impact of the violence (Bushman & Anderson, 2001; see also Hampton & Magarian, this volume).

In summary, bullying is influenced by the characteristics of the child, the family, the school, the community, and the culture, but most likely through an interaction of these different levels of influence. Programs attempting to reduce bullying need to evaluate the extent of the influence and the impact of each of these areas.

RESEARCH

Among the wealth of prevention and early intervention procedures that have been developed, too few have been carefully evaluated. Of those that have been evaluated, only a few have demonstrated effectiveness in reducing students' aggressive behaviors, while others have shown little or no program effect (Krajewski, Rybarik, Dosch, & Gilmore, 1996; Orpinas, Kelder, Frankowski, Murray, Zhang, & McAlister, 2000) or even have shown a detrimental effect (Colyer, Thompkins, Durkin, & Barlow, 1996). Generally programs with demonstrated effectiveness have been evaluated by the same researchers who develop them, and usually replication studies have not been conducted. The focus of the research has been on students, teachers, parents, or a combination of these three groups. The question of who is the best "target" of the intervention, all students versus students at high risk versus aggressive students, is still an unresolved issue.

Probably the earliest and most comprehensive school-wide program for bully reduction was the Norwegian Campaign Against Bullying (Olweus, 1994), which was identified by the Center for the Study and Prevention of Violence as one of ten that met a very high scientific standard of program effectiveness. However, this program was implemented in the 1980s in Norway and the results may not be generalizable to countries with different cultural backgrounds or to a new generation of adolescents. Further, the success of the Norwegian study has not been replicated. In the early 1990s, a comprehensive school-wide program was evaluated in England. The program included anti-bullying policies, a curriculum, environmental changes, and individual work with bullies and victims. Results were inconsistent among participating schools and the reduction of bullying was only observed among boys. In fact, in several schools bullying among girls increased (Eslea & Smith, 1998).

In the United States, several curricula designed to prevent and reduce student aggression have been evaluated. Responding in Peaceful and Positive Ways (RIPP) was evaluated twice in a sample of mostly African-American sixth graders. Results of the first evaluation showed an overall reduction of aggression among boys but not among girls (Farrell & Meyer, 1997). Results of the second evaluation indicated an overall reduction of in-school suspensions, and this effect was maintained at a 12-month follow-up for boys but not for girls. Effects measured by self-reported prevalence of specific violent behaviors were not maintained at follow-up (Farrell, Meyer, & White, 2001).

When "Second Step: A Violence Prevention Curriculum" was evaluated among elementary school children, behavioral observations showed a significant reduction of aggression; however, no effect was observed on parent or teacher reports (Grossman et al., 1997). Two evaluations of a middle school version of the curriculum showed no lasting reduction of students' aggressive behaviors (Orpinas et al., 2000; Orpinas, Parcel, McAlister, & Frankowski, 1995). The evaluation of the Resolving Conflict Creatively Program (RCCP) in a large sample of elementary school children in New York City highlights the importance of dosage of implementation. Some intervention effect was observed among students who received more lessons of the curriculum compared to those who received few or no lessons (Aber, Jones, Brown, Chaudry, & Samples, 1998). Cooper, Lutenbacher, and Faccia (2000) reviewed two decades of publications on youth violence prevention and concluded that only 15 studies had shown some reduction of students' aggression or delinquency rates.

BullyBusters is a training program for teachers to reduce bullying and aggression among young people (Newman et al., 2000). One objective of this program is to increase teachers' awareness of the role and impact of bullying in schools. Teachers are encouraged to take active steps to reduce it by providing learning experiences in the classroom, increasing monitoring of behaviors outside of the classroom, and developing an open-door policy for students who seek help with bullying problems in the school. Teachers who participated in this program, compared to teachers who did not, developed a greater knowledge of and skill in using prevention and early intervention activities, had an increased sense of self-efficacy, and had more positive expectations for students. Further, students of teachers engaged in the BullyBusting Program had fewer disciplinary problems and had fewer office referrals for aggression than students in classrooms in which teachers did not participate in training (Howard, Horne, & Jolliff, 2001; Newman et al., 2000).

STRATEGIES THAT WORK

Several research projects and government publications have highlighted the most powerful strategies to reduce and prevent violence, as well as the lessons learned in the process of implementing these programs.

Strong Support from Administrators and Teachers

The success of violence prevention programs partially depends on the level of support at different levels within the school and the school district, as well as the community (Farrell, Meyer, & Dahlberg, 1996; Orpinas et al., 1996). Before starting a program, time and effort must be spent in this process. Increasing the awareness of the problem and involving the teachers and administrators in the planning process are key factors to gain support (Kelder, Orpinas, McAlister, Frankowski, Parcel, & Friday, 1996).

Increased Awareness

As with any change program, being aware of the problem is a critical first step. In the prevention of bullying, both teachers and students should be aware of the problem. Hoover, Oliver, and Hazler (1992) reported that students believe that teachers are not aware of the extent of bullying and that they are not equipped to handle it. Only a few students (6 percent) believed that schools handled bullying problems effectively, and two of three students thought that problems were handled poorly. Awareness of the problem may be increased through anonymous classroom or school surveys, interviews with students and parents, and school data on absenteeism and conduct problems.

As part of an awareness training, teachers can analyze the extent of students' concerns and examine their own personal beliefs that impede change (e.g., a belief that bullying is a normal condition all children experience and must learn to deal with, or a belief that the problem does not even exist). Some teachers ignore bullying because they lack the skills to intervene, while others avoid action because they fear repercussions either to themselves or to the target of the bullying. Examining teachers' beliefs that maintain bullying and developing self-efficacious approaches to addressing the problem can help motivate teachers to take action. Teachers, as well as students, are more likely to perceive verbal and physical aggression as bullying than relational aggression (Boulton, 1997); therefore, awareness training should emphasize all forms of aggression. Teachers should also examine the school policies regarding bullying. A policy of identifying aggression and bullying when it happens and then providing immediate, fair, and relevant consequences is core to effective change. The school and classroom policy should focus on not allowing bullying, and the consequences associated with action should be reasonable and related to the type and extent of the aggression.

Awareness training for students is critical. A first step is to facilitate uninvolved bystanders to support children who are the targets of bullying and to support a no tolerance position on bullying. In addition, some evidence indicates that violence prevention curricula are less likely to have a positive impact in classrooms where a majority of students believe that it is acceptable to resolve conflicts through aggression (Aber et al., 1998). A second step is to increase the awareness of students who are the targets of bullying regarding the resources available to them and the opportunities for increasing their skills. For example, a study conducted in Finland showed that victims' responses of counteraggression or helplessness were more likely to make bullying start or continue, while a nonchalant attitude by the targeted student was perceived as making bullying diminish or stop (Salmivalli, Karhunen, & Lagerspetz, 1996). Similarly, in a study of young children in the United States, fighting back was associated with maintained victimization among boys (Kochenderfer & Ladd, 1997). Finally, bullies should understand the rules and consequences for their behavior. Adults should assist bullies to increase their ability to take the perspective of others, to be empathic, and to develop appropriate social skills. A number of activities have been developed specifically to facilitate awareness, including "Walking the beat," in which students are taught to be better observers of conflict and aggression in the school, or "Framing the bully," in which all students draw their perception of bullies and share it with classmates. Students develop an increased awareness that bullies are seen as undesirable. These activities can lead to greater awareness and sensitivity on the part of students and teachers alike (Newman et al., 2000).

Code of Conduct

The development of a school-wide code of conduct provides clarity on expected behaviors within the school culture and can be a very powerful strategy for reducing bullying (Olweus, 1993). The development of the code requires input from all involved in the academic community, including students, teachers, administrators, and families. Not only does the code spell out expected and not-expected behaviors, it also details the consequences for inappropriate behavior. The school code should be fair and reasonable and should specify consequences for infractions that are appropriate for the level of the offense committed. All members of the academic community are responsible for the code and are expected to participate in the process. Participation includes reporting offenders, enforcing the consequences of inappropriate behavior, taking steps to prevent and to stop bullying, and reaching out to targets of bullying to provide support and encouragement. Students should be encouraged to report bullying and must be educated to differentiate between tattling and reporting. Tattling is done for attention or to purposefully get others in trouble, whereas reporting is done to bring about a safer community for all.

Teacher and Staff Training

Many new teachers leave the profession because they feel ill prepared to handle the classroom management issues they encounter on a daily basis. Many experienced teachers have developed patterns of responding to classroom management that may no longer be effective or that may not fit the changing environment and heterogeneity of today's schools. Training that is specific to the problems of bullies and victims has been demonstrated to be very effective in reducing bullying in the school (Hazler, 1996; Howard et al., Newman et al., 2001). In addition to developing an increased awareness of bullying, teachers should learn specific skills to prevent aggression from occurring and specific skills to handle aggressive problems when they do occur. The basis for both prevention and intervention is establishing a positive, respectful relationship with students. To achieve this goal, teachers need to take care of themselves (e.g., relax, exercise), develop a strong support network among colleagues, and establish positive communication patterns with students. Examples of specific skills for prevention include: developing clear rules and routines that are common to the grade level, being prepared for class to avoid opportunities for conflict, providing classroom opportunities to develop empathy, creating a warm classroom environment, being in tune with the students' needs, encouraging cooperative group work on assignments, and creating learning experiences that involve sharing responsibilities. Examples of specific skills for intervention include: never overlooking abusive acts; providing assistance to victims, bullies, and bystanders; developing a school-wide system for reporting aggression anonymously; and developing skills for resolving conflicts, defusing aggression, and successfully implementing the school's crisis management plan.

Training opportunities need to be available to teachers, administrators and staff, for bullying occurs not only in the classroom. In fact, bullying is more likely to occur in hallways, restrooms, buses, cafeterias, or extracurricular activities than in the classroom (Davis, Schaffer, Parault, & Pellegrini, 1999; Petersen, Pietrzak, & Speaker, 1998). In particular, bullying occurs when students are not supervised. Bus drivers, janitorial staff, and kitchen workers all need to be part of the team for reducing bullying. They should endorse the school code, understand the general procedures for bully reduction, and receive specific training relevant to their area of involvement.

Support groups for teachers and staff, which are held every other week, are necessary to maintain a commitment to the program and to facilitate the implementation of skills. Workshops often lose their power if there is no ongoing review of the application of the skills learned during the workshop. During the support group, teachers share their "prouds and sorries"—the experiences that have helped to reduce bullying and experiences that have not been as successful as they had wished. Members of the support group apply problem-solving skills to assist each member in developing a more powerful intervention, so that the "prouds" become more prevalent and the "sorries" fewer.

Student Training

Just as teachers and other school personnel need training to develop the skills for reducing bullying, so do students. A number of specific programs have been developed, and each highlights particular skills that may benefit students. Depending upon the program, bullying prevention may be taught by a teacher, a counselor, or a violence prevention specialist. Examples of skills taught by most curricula include assertiveness, empathy, problem solving, anger management, and relaxation. Children need to learn to discriminate when to avoid situations that may lead to conflict and when to try to solve the conflict, as well as when to ignore a threat and when to report it. In addition to skills training, effective programs focus on helping students become more aware of the extent of the problem of bullying within their school, the impact that bullying may have upon all students—not just on the victims of aggression—and the importance of making bullying an unacceptable behavior at school.

All the strategies described above have been tested individually or in combination. However, all these strategies are being implemented and evaluated in a large multisite project. In October 1999, the National Center for Injury Prevention and Control, from the CDC, funded the Middle School Violence Prevention Project: Guiding Responsibility and Expectations for Adolescents for Today and Tomorrow (GREAT) Schools and Families. The goal of this prevention study is to evaluate the effectiveness of a student and teacher program to reduce and prevent violence among students, and to examine the additional impact of including a family program that complements the school-based activities. A common program and evaluation procedures are being implemented in four states. The four participating universities are The University of Georgia, University of Illinois at Chicago, Virginia Commonwealth University, and Duke University (Horne, Orpinas, Meyer, & The Middle School Violence Prevention Project, 2001).

STRATEGIES THAT DO NOT WORK

Perhaps the least effective strategy is ignoring the problem, for bullies then feel empowered to continue their abusive behavior and the targets of their aggression suffer the ongoing pain of victimization. However, some strategies that may be expected to be useful are not always as helpful as they would appear. For example, Turpeau (1998) evaluated the impact of group counseling on bullies in a middle school. He found that the program was popular because the bullies were thrilled to be out of class, teachers were glad not to have the bullies in their classes, administrators could report that a program was in effect, and families were pleased the school was doing something. The only problem was that the intervention did not reduce bullying in the school. Turpeau concluded that working only with bullies in a homogeneous group was ineffective because it provided a support group for bullies, while not changing the school environment. Bullying prevention requires a long-term commitment from the school. Short-term activities, an isolated curriculum, or a brief conversation with the counselor are not likely to have a long-term effect. Schools need to keep an ongoing monitoring of bullying to evaluate whether or not their programs are working.

SYNTHESIS

Bullying is a prevalent problem in schools that should be addressed, as children who are the victims are likely to suffer severe emotional and physical consequences. In theory, a comprehensive program that involves the community, neighborhoods, families, and the school should be most effective for reducing bullying. However, most communities do not have the resources to develop such programs, and not every member of the community will support it. Schools can establish a safe haven for children by defining bullying as an unacceptable behavior and taking specific steps to curtail it: develop a strong support from the administration, establish a school-wide code of conduct, develop a crisis management plan, establish a respectful and positive school climate, increase awareness on the part of teachers and students, train school personnel and students on bullying prevention, and finally implement a system to monitor whether or not the program is working.

Also see: Aggressive Behavior: Childhood; Aggressive Behavior: Adolescence; Anger Regulation: Childhood; Anger Regulation: Adolescence; Violence Prevention: Childhood.

References

Aber, J.L., Jones, S.M., Brown, J.L., Chaudry, N., & Samples, F. (1998). Resolving conflict creatively: Evaluating the developmental effects of a school-based violence prevention program in neighborhood and classroom context. *Developmental Psychopathology, 10,* 187–213.

Boulton, M.J., & Underwood, K. (1992). Bully/victim problems among middle school children. *British Journal of Educational Psychology, 62,* 73–87.

Boulton, M.J. (1997). Teachers' views on bullying: Definitions, attitudes and ability to cope. *British Journal of Educational Psychology, 67,* 223–233.

Buka, S., & Earls, F. (1993). Early determinants of delinquency and violence. *Health Affairs, 12,* 46–64.

Bushman, B.J., & Anderson, C.A. (2001). Media violence and the American Public: Scientific facts versus media misinformation. *American Psychologist, 56,* 477–489.

Centers for Disease Control and Prevention. (2000). Youth risk behavior surveillance—United States, 1999. *Morbidity and Mortality Weekly Report, 49* [SS-5].

Colyer, E., Thompkins, T., Durkin, M., & Barlow, B. (1996). Can conflict resolution training increase aggressive behavior in young adolescents? *American Journal of Public Health, 86,* 1028–1029.

Cooper, W.O., Lutenbacher, M., & Faccia, K. (2000). Components of effective youth violence prevention programs for 7- to 14-year-olds. *Archives of Pediatric Adolescent Medicine, 154,* 1134–1139.

Davis, H., Schaffer, A., Parault, S., & Pellegrini, A. (1999). Bullying and victimization in social setting: Who's who at the middle school dance? Paper Presented at the Meeting of the American Psychological Association, Washington, DC.

DiLalla, L.F., & Gottesman, I.I. (1991). Biological and genetic contributors to violence—Widom's untold tale. *Psychological Bulletin, 109,* 435–442.

Eslea, M., & Smith, P.K. (1998). The long-term effectiveness of anti-bullying work in primary schools. *Educational Research, 40,* 203–218.

Farrell, A.D., & Meyer, A.L. (1997). The effectiveness of a school-based curriculum for reducing violence among urban sixth-grade students. *American Journal of Public Health, 87,* 979–984.

Farrell, A.D., Meyer, A.L., & Dahlberg, L.L. (1996). Richmond youth against violence: A school-based program for urban adolescents. *American Journal of Preventive Medicine, 12,* 13–21.

Farrell, A.D., Meyer, A.L., & White, K.S. (2001). Evaluation of responding in peaceful and positive ways (RIPP): A school-based prevention program for reducing violence among urban adolescents. *Journal of Child Clinical Psychology, 30,* 451–463.

Fried, S., & Fried, P. (1996). *Bullies and victims.* New York: Evans & Company.

Grossman, D.C., Neckerman, H.J., Koepsell, T.D., Liu, P.Y., Asher, K.N., Beland, K., Frey, K., & Rivara, F.P. (1997). Effectiveness of a violence prevention curriculum among children in elementary school: A randomized controlled trial. *Journal of the American Medical Association, 277,* 1605–1611.

Hawker, D.S., & Boulton, M.J. (2000). Twenty years' research on peer victimization and psychosocial maladjustment: A meta-analytic review of cross-sectional studies. *Journal of Child Psychology and Psychiatry, 41,* 441–455.

Hazler, R. (1996). *Breaking the cycle of violence: Interventions for bullying and victimization.* Washington, DC: Accelerated Dynamics.

Hoover, J., Oliver, R., & Hazler, R. (1992). Bullying: Perceptions of adolescent victims in the Midwestern USA. *School Psychology International, 13,* 5–16.

Horne, A., Orpinas, P., Meyer, A., & The Middle School Violence Prevention Project. (2001, August 24–28). Violence prevention and aggression reduction in schools: Theoretical foundations. Paper Presented on the Symposium Theoretical and Methodological Issues in a Multisite Study of Youth Violence Prevention (A. Farrell, Chair) at the 109th Annual Convention of the American Psychological Association, San Francisco.

Horne, A., & Sayger, T. (1990). *Treating conduct and oppositional defiant disorders in children.* Boston: Allyn & Bacon.

Howard, N., Horne, A., & Jolliff, D. (2001). Self-efficacy in a new training model for the prevention of bullying in schools. *Journal of Emotional Abuse, 2,* 181–191.

Kaufman, P., Chen, X., Choy, S.P., Ruddy, S.A., Miller, A.K., Chandler, K.A., Rand, M.R., Klaus, P., & Planty, M.G. (2000). *Indicators of school crime and safety, 2000* (Rep. No. NCES 2001-017/NCJ 184176). Washington, DC: US Departments of Education and Justice.

Kelder, S.H., Orpinas, P., McAlister, A., Frankowski, R., Parcel, G.S., & Friday, J. (1996). The students for peace project: A comprehensive violence-prevention program for middle school students. *American Journal of Preventive Medicine, 12,* 22–30.

Kochenderfer, B.J., & Ladd, G.W. (1997). Victimized children's responses to peers' aggression: Behaviors associated with reduced versus continued victimization. *Developmental Psychopathology, 9,* 59–73.

Krajewski, S.S., Rybarik, M.F., Dosch, M.F., & Gilmore, G.D. (1996). Results of a curriculum intervention with 7th graders regarding violence in relationships. *Journal of Family Violence, 11,* 93–112.

Larzelere, R.E., & Patterson, G.R. (1990). Parental management: Mediator of the effect of socioeconomic status on early delinquency. *Criminology, 28,* 301–323.

MetLife. (1999). *The metropolitan life survey of the American teacher, 1999.* New York, NY: Louis Harris and Associates.

Newman, D.A., & Horne, A.M. (in press). The effectiveness of a psycho-educational intervention for classroom teachers aimed at reducing bullying behavior in middle school students. *Journal of Counseling and Development.*

Newman, D.A., Horne, A.M., & Bartolomucci, C. (2000). *BullyBusters: A teacher's manual for helping bullies, victims, and bystanders.* Champaign, IL: Research Press.

Olweus, D. (1993). *Bullying at school: What we know and what we can do.* Cambridge, MA: Blackwells.

Olweus, D. (1994). Annotation—Bullying at school: Basic facts and effects of a school based intervention program. *Journal of Child Psychology and Psychiatry, 35,* 1171–1190.

Orpinas, P., Kelder, S., Frankowski, R., Murray, N., Zhang, Q., & McAlister, A. (2000). Outcome evaluation of a multi-component violence-prevention program for middle schools: The Students for Peace project. *Health Education Research, 15,* 45–58.

Orpinas, P., Kelder, S., Murray, N., Fourney, A., Conroy, J., McReynolds, L., & Peters, R.J. (1996). Critical issues in implementing a comprehensive violence prevention program for middle schools: Translating theory into practice. *Education and Urban Society, 28,* 456–472.

Orpinas, P., Murray, N., & Kelder, S. (1999). Parental influences on students' aggressive behaviors and weapon carrying. *Health Education and Behavior, 26,* 774–787.

Orpinas, P., Parcel, G.S., McAlister, A., & Frankowski, R. (1995). Violence prevention in middle schools: A pilot evaluation. *Journal of Adolescent Health, 17,* 360–371.

Peterson, G.J., Pietrzak, D., & Speaker, K.M. (1998). The enemy within: A national study on school violence and prevention. *Urban Education, 33,* 331–359.

Roland, E. (1989). A system oriented strategy against bullying. In E. Roland & E. Munthe (Eds.), *Bullying: An international perspective*. London: Professional Development Foundation.

Sallis, J.F., & Owen, N. (1997). Ecological models. In K. Glanz, F.M. Lewis, & B.K. Rimer (Eds.), *Health behavior and health education: Theory, research, and practice* (2nd ed., pp. 403–424). San Francisco: Jossey-Bass.

Salmivalli, C., Karhunen, J., & Lagerspetz, M.J. (1996). How do the victims respond to bullying? *Aggressive Behavior, 22,* 99–109.

Schwartz, D., Dodge, K.A., Pettit, G.S., & Bates, J.E. (1997). The early socialization of aggressive victims of bullying. *Child Development, 68,* 665–675.

Turpeau, A. (1998). *Effectiveness of an anti-bullying classroom curriculum intervention on an American middle school*. Unpublished doctoral dissertation, University of Georgia, Athens.

US Department of Education & US Department of Justice. (1999). *1999 annual report on school safety*. US Department of Education, Education Publications Center: Washington, DC.

US Secret Service National Threat Assessment Center, US Department of Education, & National Institute of Justice (2000). *Safe school initiative: An interim report on the prevention of targeted violence in schools*. http://www.treas.gov/usss/ntac.

Williams, K., Chamgers, M., Logan, S., & Robinson, D. (1996). Association of common health symptoms with bullying in primary school children. *British Medical Journal, 313,* 17–19.

C

Cancer, Childhood

Louis Fintor

INTRODUCTION

While great strides continue to be made in the early detection and treatment of childhood cancers, primary prevention remains a formidable challenge. Childhood cancers continue to be relatively rare when compared to those afflicting adults and research advances have led to dramatic increases in survival over the last four decades. Nevertheless, childhood cancers comprise the leading cause of death by disease among US children under the age of 15 (American Cancer Society, 2001).

Even though risk-reducing cancer prevention activities involving increased cancer awareness, reduction of exposures to carcinogens, and the alteration of risk-related behaviors have demonstrated long-term cost-effectiveness, efforts in this population are often complicated by limited knowledge of the etiology of these cancers and often long intervals between exposure and progression to disease (Altman & Sarge, 1992).

DEFINITIONS

Contrary to popular perceptions, cancer is not a single disease entity but refers to more than 100 types of tumors classified in five general categories: carcinomas, sarcomas, myelomas, lymphomas, and leukemias. Cancers are characterized by the uncontrolled growth and proliferation of abnormal cells. These cells often have the ability to invade and spread ("metastasize") to normal tissue at secondary sites. These are normally organ-specific and vary in terms of cause, histology (cell type), natural history, and prognosis. Most tumors are thought to arise from a single abnormal cell (Altman & Sarge, 1992; Marina, Bowman, Pui, & Crist, 1995).

Although they are often harmless, these mutations can destroy healthy cells or cause abnormal cell growth that results in cancer. They can also increase susceptibility to carcinogenic damage. Inherited as well as spontaneous mutations can cause cancer directly or indirectly by impairing mechanisms of cellular function such as repair and division. Mutations can also arise from exposure to chemical, physical, or viral carcinogens.

It is important to frame childhood cancer prevention activities with an understanding of the mechanisms of carcinogenesis. Chemical carcinogenesis is thought to occur in two stages: initiation and promotion. Initiation occurs when exposure to a carcinogen damages cellular DNA and produces a genetic mutation. Promotion can occur years or even decades later, when the cell is exposed to chemicals known as tumor "promoters" that do not damage DNA directly but influence the proliferation of mutated cells. Physical carcinogenesis occurs when exposure to radiation and certain dusts as well as mineral and synthetic fibers (e.g., asbestos) results in mutated DNA. Finally, viral carcinogenesis describes impaired cell growth and regulation or alterations resulting from the introduction of viral material. At present, only a few classes of viruses have been identified that are associated with cancer.

Often, because these processes can involve relatively long time intervals, cancer remains largely a disease of adulthood. However, apart from early exposures to chemical and environmental cancer risks, it is important to acknowledge the role of heredity in predisposing individuals in this population to disease early in life. By identifying these genetic factors and developing novel interventions, scientists hope to expand the scope of prevention activities.

It is important to note that childhood cancers are not thought to arise from a single factor such as exposure, heredity, or behavior. Cancer is a disease of *multifactorial etiology* attributable to genetic, environmental, and physiologic factors and their interaction with biological, social, and environmental elements. In addition to chemical, physical, environmental, viral, and genetic factors, cancer is believed to result from a complicated interaction of such variables as hormones, immune status, and diet, as well as socioeconomic and lifestyle factors (Plon & Peterson, 1997).

SCOPE

While cancer prevention efforts have traditionally focused on adult and adolescent populations, public health interventions are increasingly targeting those under the age of 15 for a number of reasons. These include the increasing prevalence of tobacco use at younger ages, rising rates of melanoma and other skins cancers, an epidemic of poor nutrition contributing to obesity in the United States, and growing evidence that a pattern of long-term healthy behavior must be established early in life. However, while these early interventions have the potential to successfully prevent adult cancers over the long term, they appear to have little impact on the incidence of cancer in childhood itself.

Unlike many lifestyle-related adult cancers, those affecting children tend to occur soon after birth and are most often associated with genetic factors or exposures to ionizing radiation and chemical carcinogens. The most common risk factors for developing cancers such as smoking and years of tobacco use, excessive sun exposure, lack of exercise, poor nutrition, and alcohol use have not been recognized as critical factors among young children. In addition, the etiology of many pediatric cancers remains unknown or at best poorly understood thus hindering the development of successful primary prevention interventions in this population (Plon & Peterson, 1997).

Moreover, clinical markers are not well defined—if present at all—in the early stages of many childhood cancers. This, coupled with the relatively rare occurrence of these cancers made the potential for mass screening programs in this population unfeasible and not generally cost-effective. However, recent advances in genetic testing and familial risk assessment are prompting intense research interest in both developing new biomedical approaches to both prevention and early detection.

This may be especially valuable in understanding the mechanism of primary tumors since those diagnosed with cancer during childhood or adolescence and successfully treated may have an excess cancer mortality risk up to 25 years after their initial diagnosis.

In addition, public health advocates in the United States and abroad are beginning to shift attention from prevention of childhood cancers by minimizing in utero environmental exposures to behavioral interventions given a growing body of research validating the short- and long-term efficacy of these interventions, the potential overall health benefits they accrue, and their cost-effectiveness.

Incidence and Prevalence

When comparing worldwide rates of incidence, mortality, and survival, childhood cancer remains largely a disease phenomenon of the industrialized world. Even though children in the developing world appear to be at greater risk of death from infectious disease, malnutrition, and other conditions, it is important to note that the worldwide incidence of childhood cancer can be highly variable both between and within countries as well as by cancer type, age, socioeconomic status, race, and ethnicity.

For example, in the United States, leukemia will account for about one third of the estimated 8,600 new childhood cancer cases in 2001 while in Africa more than half of all childhood cancer diagnoses involve Burkitt's lymphomas and leukemia remains relatively rare. Caucasian United States, Canadian, Western European, and Japanese children have a peak incidence of leukemia at about four years of age while African American children have rates that are relatively static (American Cancer Society, 2001; Parkin, Pisani, & Ferlay, 1999).

The annual incidence rates per 100,000 for all childhood cancers combined in industrialized nations is relatively small and has increased only incrementally. For example, in the United States, rates for those under the age of 15 have increased just 0.7 percent from 1973 to 1997 with increases registering in the early years of this period but relatively unchanged during the last 13 years (Parkin et al., 1999; Ries et al., 1999).

In fact, recent data suggest that pediatric cancer sex- and age-specific incidence rates for children aged 14 and under tend to be relatively similar among the world's industrialized nations. For example, US rates for all cancers except skin in this age cohort are 11.02 for females and 15.14 for males while in Canada incidence is 13.57 for females and 15.31 for male children. In the United Kingdom, the rates are 11.81 for females and 13.92 for males (American Cancer Society, 2001; National Cancer Institute of Canada, & Health Canada, 2001; Ries et al., 1999).

The two most commonly diagnosed cancers in all three nations are leukemias followed by brain and central nervous system (CNS) cancers. Leukemia rates for US female children are 2.93 and 4.91 for males, while in Canada rates are 4.35 for females and 4.96 for males. Leukemia incidence among British children is 3.88 for females and 4.76 for males. Brain and nervous system rates are 2.96 for US females and 3.37 for males; 2.92 for Canadian females and 3.39 for males; and 2.51 for British females and 2.78 for males (American Cancer Society, 2001; National Cancer Institute of Canada, & Health Canada, 2001; National Cancer Intelligence Centre, 2001; Ries et al., 1999).

Since the early 1970s, biomedical treatment breakthroughs have resulted in pediatric cancer mortality rates declining by more than 50 percent for many cancers. In 2001, even though an estimated 1,500 US children will die of cancer, 5-year-survival rates have increased to almost 70 percent—up from 30 percent during the1960s. In the year 2001, even though an estimated 8,600 US children under the age of 15 are expected to be diagnosed with cancer, approximately 75 percent of all children with cancer are expected to survive five years or more (Linet, Ries, Smith, Tarone, & Devesa, 1999; Ries et al., 1999).

Overall childhood cancer mortality rates per 100,000 for all cancers except skin among US females is 4.08 and 5.04 for US males; 4.06 for Canadian females and 4.68 for males; 4.24 for British females and 4.83 for males. Leukemia has the highest mortality of all childhood cancers at 0.96 for US females and 1.26 for males; 0.95 for Canadian females and 1.37 for males; and 1.19 for British females and 1.55 for males. This is followed by brain and other CNS cancers at 0.83 for US females and 0.88 for males; 0.86 for Canadian females and 1.04 for males; and 0.92 for British females and 1.02 for males (American Cancer Society, 2001; National Cancer Institute of Canada, & Health Canada, 2001; National Cancer Intelligence Centre, 2001; Pisani, Parkin, Bray, & Ferlay, 1999; Ries et al., 1999).

In the United States, Canada, and the United Kingdom, sympathetic and allied nervous system cancers are most often diagnosed during the first year of life. Of these, neuroblastomas are most often diagnosed during the first 30 days after birth. In general, overall childhood cancer incidence rates appear to be highest among infants and then gradually decline till the age of 9 before beginning to increase. Childhood cancer appears to be higher among males than females and in 5-year age groups tends to be highest among those from birth to 4 years of age and lowest among those aged 5–9. This, however, varies by cancer site. Caucasian children appear to have the highest rates of childhood cancers followed by Latinos, Asian/Pacific Islanders, and African Americans; these cancers appear to be lowest among American Indians and Alaskan Natives (American Cancer Society, 2001; Ries et al., 1999).

Costs

The economic burden of childhood cancers on families has been relatively well studied. Many researchers have reported that indirect (nonmedical) costs far outweighed direct costs incurred by families during virtually all stages of the disease. Nonmedical costs have been estimated to consume up to 44 percent or more of family weekly budgets compared with about 5.8 percent in direct medical costs. Average weekly nonmedical expenditures have been estimated at $100. This includes $62 in out-of-pocket nonmedical expenditures and $38 in lost wages. Monthly treatment charges, about half of which accrue during the diagnostic and terminal stages of the disease, ranged from $100 to $1,800 depending on diagnosis. Meanwhile, total aggregate charges ranged from $8,000 to $53,000 with a mean of $34,558 (Brown & Fintor, 1994; Lansky, Black, & Cairns, 1983).

Since at least one parent is likely to become a primary caregiver during their peak earning years, the potential for lost income is staggering. In addition, families often carry large long-term medical debt burdens well after the recovery or death of the child (Brown & Fintor, 1994; Lansky et al., 1983).

Moreover, the psychosocial cost to children and their families is thought to be even more profound. Disability, isolation, pain, anxiety, grief, economic dependence, lost employment opportunities, relocation, and other "quality-of-life" issues for children and their families, friends, and caregivers are often extensive. In addition, there are secondary but related consequences for families such as divorce, alcoholism, and depression. Since monetary costs are only one component of the overall burden of childhood cancer, many researchers have called for studies that take a social accounting of these along with monetary costs in assessing the true burden of disease. Work in this area continues to build momentum (Brown & Fintor, 1994).

Given the enormous economic effect resulting from years of productive life lost to illness, successful prevention would benefit children diagnosed and successfully treated at the earliest possible age. Even more important, the potential long-term benefits of early cancer prevention activities targeting this population would likely yield additional and more substantial decreases in cancer morbidity and mortality later in life.

THEORIES

Even though the focus of cancer activities in this population has traditionally been largely on treatment, expanded knowledge of childhood cancer-related risks as well as the potential for sustained positive behavioral change has led to growing interest in adapting existing theoretical models to efforts at primary prevention that yields immediate and/or long-term benefits.

Among the approaches generating serious interest are *cognitive–behavioral* models acknowledging the mediation of behavior by attitudes and knowledge in conjunction with the existing social environment and perceptions of risk, motivation to change behavior, and the skills available to initiate and sustain these changes.

At the individual and intrapersonal level, three basic models have been found valuable in designing successful cancer preventive interventions involving childhood cancers. These models include Stages of Change, Health Belief, and Consumer Information Processing (Bettman, 1979; Prochaska, DiClemete, & Norcross, 1992; Rosenstock, Strecher, & Becker, 1988).

Stages of Change models used successfully in adult interventions such as smoking cessation and healthy diet promotion have been adapted for children. These models are characterized by five distinct "stages" (pre-contemplation, contemplation, decision/determination, action, and maintenance) that influence changes in health behavior (Prochaska et al., 1992).

Health Belief Models are among the oldest and perhaps most widely used conceptual frameworks in the arsenal of the primary prevention of cancer. These approaches assume that individuals weigh the risks of disease against the benefits of altering behavior and make rational choices based on those assessments. This includes perceived susceptibility, perceived severity, perceived benefits, perceived barriers, cues to action, and self-efficacy. These models have been most successfully applied in cancer-related mass media interventions, health promotional materials, and individual counseling (Rosenstock et al., 1988).

The third approach, *Consumer Information Processing*, is based on the idea that individuals have a limited capacity for grasping and using the volume of information to which they are exposed. This prompts them to selectively choose and process messages based on the *availability* of information, its perceived *usefulness*, and how *easy* the information is to adapt and use (Bettman, 1979).

With these models, successful cancer preventive interventions involving children have been designed by utilizing existing theories of interpersonal behavior that acknowledge a dynamic relationship between individual and the environment through exchanges with significant groups and individuals. Perhaps the most successful of these efforts has involved Bandura's (1986) *Social Learning Theory* or *Social Cognitive Theory*. Social learning theoretical approaches assume a three-way dynamic interaction among individual factors, the environment, and behavior. This relationship has three components: *cognition, behavior,* and *environment*; and six key concepts: *reciprocal determinism* (dynamic, but alterable relationships between the individual and the environment), *behavioral capability* (knowledge and skill), *expectations* (beliefs about the consequences of actions), *self-efficacy* (the perception that one is able to perform a specific behavior successfully), *observational learning*, and *reinforcement* (Bandura, 1986).

These last two, *observational learning* and *reinforcement*, are key elements in designing cancer preventive interventions involving children. For example, children observing parents and other role models who abstain from tobacco, engage in good dietary habits, and exercise are more likely to adopt and sustain these behaviors over time themselves. Since this population, unlike adolescents and adults, has the potential to establish baseline healthy behaviors, prevention efforts that include reinforcement rewards such as praise and encouragement have been especially important.

RESEARCH

Unlike many primary prevention efforts involving cancer in adults and adolescents, interventions designed to prevent cancer in children have been relatively limited in scope. Although the long-term economic benefits of primary prevention stand to be quite substantial, risk assessment in this population has been problematic due to obscure or unknown disease etiologies as well as the often lengthy intervals between exposure and the development of disease. Thus, the design, implementation, and evaluation of preventive interventions have often been limited by existing knowledge. Nevertheless, some attempts have used known factors associated with elevated cancer risk in children to design effective interventions with both immediate and long-term benefits. These risks fall into four major categories: genetic factors, prenatal exposures, postnatal exposures, and factors which are currently under investigation.

Genetic risk factors immediately predisposing children to cancers most often include rare chromosomal abnormalities and disease syndromes such as Down's syndrome, Li–Fraumeni syndrome, and Bloom's syndrome. Children with Fanconi's anemia, ataxia–telangiectasia, and neurofibromatosis also appear to be at higher immediate risk. Hereditary genetic mutations not related to the clinical syndromes mentioned have also been associated with Wilms' tumor and neuroblastoma (Chow, Linet, Liff, & Greenberg, 1996).

Prenatal factors include associations between childhood leukemia and in utero exposure to diagnostic ionizing radiation as well as clear-cell adenocarcinoma of the vagina in offspring and exposure to pharmaceuticals such as diethylstilbestrol (DES) and other drugs. Less often, direct placental transmission of maternal melanoma, lymphoma, and bronchogenic carcinoma has been reported (Chow et al., 1996; Robison, 1997).

Postnatal exposures involving ionizing radiation associated with the development of leukemia and solid tumors have provided some of the strongest cause-and-effect evidence to date. Japanese children exposed to radioactive fallout in 1945 developed these cancers as early as 3 years later. US children treated with radiation for enlargement of the thymus gland or ringworm during the 1940s and 1950s have a substantially increased risk for leukemia and solid head and neck tumors as adults. In addition, viral vectors such as Epstein-Barr Virus have been associated with elevated risk for nasopharyngeal cancer and certain lymphomas.

Ironically, the diagnosis and treatment of childhood cancers are sometimes associated with additional elevated risk for developing cancer later in life. It is estimated that up to 9 percent of childhood cancer patients diagnosed and treated with radiation or chemotherapy risk developing a second cancer within the first 20 years following treatment (Gurney, Davis, Severson, Fang, Ross, & Robison, 1996; Gurney, Davis, Severson, & Robison, 1994).

Finally, it is important to note that a number of factors investigated for potential association with childhood cancers have yielded inconsistent or inconclusive results. These include in utero exposures to ionizing radiation, antinausea medications, barbiturates, antibiotics, marijuana, alcohol, and nitrosamines. Meanwhile, limited associations have been reported between childhood cancer and environmental factors such as motor vehicle exhaust, pesticides, and electromagnetic fields. These deserve further investigation.

STRATEGIES: OVERVIEW

Public health advocates have persuasively argued that prevention activities should not only begin in early childhood but should take place on the individual level (clinical approach) as well as involve communities (public health approach). These interventions should be comprehensive, integrated approaches to promoting a variety of healthy behaviors. Using this approach, several pilot studies involving smoking, nutrition, and sun exposure have been designed and implemented over the last two decades which have aimed to cost-effectively reduce or eliminate risks of cancer as well as other diseases among children.

In the areas of nutrition and physical exercise, childhood cancer awareness interventions have promoted good nutritional habits. Some of the projects have stressed adequate vitamin A intake (believed to have a chemoprotective effect on cancer) in an effort to not only reduce morbidity and mortality but also promote a desirable body weight and appropriate calcium intake. This in turn has the potential to possibly reduce the downstream risk of not only developing cancer but also conditions such as diabetes and adult osteoporosis.

STRATEGIES THAT WORK

An early childhood cancer prevention and awareness intervention involved the "Know Your Body" program described by Williams (1980). This comprehensive program demonstrated that the onset of cigarette smoking could be successfully prevented and nutritional habits improved in children between the ages of 12 and 14 through an intervention using peer group interaction along with behavior modification activities.

In 1996, the Centers for Disease Control launched a similar effort to develop healthy eating patterns in early childhood by advocating school-based interventions stressing skills, social support, and environmental reinforcement. Using information guidelines on nutrition as part of a comprehensive school health program involving nutritionists, parents, teachers, and food service staff to promote healthy eating could lead to adopting and sustaining this pattern through adolescence and adulthood. This integrated approach relied on a "healthy eating" educational curriculum as well as school policy mandating the availability of healthy and nutritional foods, and family and community involvement (Kimm & Kwiterovich, 1995; Centers for Disease Control and Prevention, 1996).

Another successful cancer prevention effort involved reducing the incidence of melanoma as well as basal and squamous cell skin cancers after a Colorado study of 159 child care providers with responsibility for 13,490 infants and children under the age of 6 found that 44 percent lacked adequate sun protection policies. Only about half (54 percent) of the providers reported encouraging the regular use of sunscreen and less than 17 percent had policies requiring children to have adequate protective clothing (Crane, Marcus, & Pike, 1983).

These findings were in turn used to design comprehensive interventions in collaboration with the American Academy of Dermatology and the American Cancer Society. One of these efforts, the Arizona *Sun Awareness Project* targeted preschools and childcare facilities in developing puppet shows and other activities stressing the importance of sunscreens and protective clothing in preventing skin cancers among kindergarten and first grade students. The experimental preschool curriculum successfully raised levels of knowledge, attitudes, and behavior regarding sun exposure risk while the elementary school pilot curriculum used school nurses and teachers to conduct interactive workshops with units on skin anatomy and physiology, the nature of sunlight and skin exposure, the physical process of tanning and skin cancer, and prevention strategies (Laughlin-Richard, 2000).

The success of these interventions coupled with the potential long-term changes in cancer awareness and behavior change led Colorado public health officials to develop integrated programs of educational seminars, policy workshops, and other activities for child care workers and facilities, parents, and children (Crane et al., 1993).

STRATEGIES THAT MIGHT WORK

Although some cancer prevention strategies involving children have been relatively effective, the impact of others in both identifying risk and designing appropriate interventions have been less successful. Perhaps most significant among the obstacles to implementing effective behavioral interventions in this population is engendering an early appreciation for the association between risky behaviors and unhealthy lifestyles with long-term health consequences.

For example, the use of tobacco products among increasingly younger children, especially among young women, as well as the overall deleterious health effects of secondhand cigarette smoke has become an urgent focus for a growing number of cancer prevention efforts. Several studies have investigated parental smoking and childhood brain tumors as well as maternal exposure to passive smoke before and during pregnancy with mixed results. While no significant elevation in risk was found among women who smoked before or during pregnancy, several studies found an association between paternal smoking and maternal exposure to passive tobacco smoke during pregnancy (Norman, Holly, & Prestoin-Martin, 1996).

Investigators have identified several major predictors of tobacco use that includes peer pressure, familial use, socioeconomic status, weight control, and identification with tobacco and role models in professional sports, acting, and other arenas. However, behavioral studies have found that despite concerted efforts to reduce tobacco use among children and adolescents, a high rate of prevalence continues to persist in this population.

Recognizing the need to address this public health problem, National Cancer Institute investigators in conjunction with the American Academy of Pediatrics designed a comprehensive strategy for physicians to prevent the use of tobacco among both children and adolescents. This program relies on the "4 As": (1) Anticipate (provide continued guidance from prenatal care through adolescence); (2) Ask (assess tobacco use at each encounter with caregivers and patients); (3) Advise (reinforce positive behavior and discourage tobacco use), and (4) Assist (support efforts to discontinue tobacco use). Prenatal counseling and the use of smoking cessation and other promotional materials are encouraged throughout the intervention (Epps & Manley, 1993).

Finally, despite efforts to promote better nutrition, healthy eating, and exercise, the rate of obesity among children in the United States continues to rise.

Although there have been marked short- and medium-term successes in cancer prevention efforts involving behavioral risk reduction among children, the overall long-term impact of these strategies remains to be seen.

STRATEGIES THAT DO NOT WORK

Large-scale media educational campaigns, long thought to be the most effective way of reducing tobacco consumption, have been of limited value in preventing the use of tobacco products in younger age groups. This in turn has prompted new interventions that favor more integrated models involving the media, parents, schools, and community groups, and physicians and other health care providers in discouraging the use of tobacco (Botvin & Dusenbury, 1989; Riggs, 1992).

SYNTHESIS

As the body of evidence for the efficacy of primary prevention involving children grows, it is likely that there will be new efforts to target this group with cancer risk reduction activities. In this regard, it is important to point out that there are two distinct approaches to cancer prevention in this population. The first category involves strategic interventions that prevent the development of cancer *during* childhood while the second involves those activities, largely focused on behavior change, that are designed to engender healthy behaviors that will be sustained over time and thus prevent the development of cancer *later in life*.

The first stream largely relies on reducing environmental exposure to carcinogens both in utero and during early childhood as well as screening for genetic factors that might predispose this population to cancer. These often must necessarily involve target adult parents or caregivers instead of the children themselves.

Advances in genetic testing and immunology are not only expanding the ability to identify familial risk earlier, but to repair damaged DNA and institute treatment at even earlier stages—in some cases in utero. As these approaches are refined, it is likely that genetic screening and molecular interventions might someday be feasible. However, at the same time there are a variety of ethical, legal, and economic questions surrounding mass genetic screening and intervention which will no doubt first have to be addressed and resolved. On the other hand, ongoing cost-effective public health initiatives that encourage passive intervention—such as hepatitis A and B vaccinations among children—are likely to result in lower long-term cancer risk associated with viral vectors in this population. Similarly, active interventions involving adult parents and caregivers that are designed to prevent childhood environmental exposures to carcinogens are also likely to be more successful. As the body of knowledge regarding cancer-related risk grows, it will need to be widely and successfully disseminated.

The second category of interventions, those involving the promotion of risk-reducing behaviors designed to diminish the long-term risk of developing cancer later in life, is likely to be the most promising and cost-effective. Successful cancer preventive interventions among children will require comprehensive, integrated, interactive approaches. As already demonstrated, they must encompass children and their families, peers and public role models, health care providers and public health advocates. In addition, community involvement is crucial in providing a social support through the enlistment of schools, community organizations and religious groups, and other entities.

As McLeroy and colleagues point out, because health-related behaviors are influenced by multiple levels of interaction, incorporating behavioral change relies on several levels of influence including: (1) intrapersonal or individual factors; (2) interpersonal factors; (3) institutional or organizational factors; (4) community factors; and (5) public policy factors (McLeroy, Bibeau, Steckler, & Glanz, 1988).

On the intrapersonal and interpersonal levels, formulating peer and positive role model strategies will be critical to designing successful interventions while mass media messaging campaigns will likely be more useful with the advent of new technologies increasingly popular among children.

These will no doubt include emerging multimedia interactive modalities such as health kiosks and other computer-based approaches that are gaining momentum among children. Although the long-term success of these novel devices in primary prevention is still unknown, preliminary studies among children and adolescents are encouraging (Fintor, 1998).

Finally, multilevel models relying on an ecological perspective that addresses education, advocacy, policy, the environment, and economics will be required. To this end, public and private support for health behavior intervention involving children will be even more crucial. Childhood cancer advocacy groups, many of which were in the forefront of the earliest cancer advocacy efforts, will also continue to play a critical role in influencing public policy and helping to maintain a vigorous research agenda.

Also see: Chronic Disease: Adolescence; Environmental Health: Childhood; Family Strengthening: Childhood; Perceived Personal Control; Resilience: Childhood.

References

Altman, A., & Sarge, M.J. (1992). *The cancer dictionary*. New York: Facts on File.

American Cancer Society. (2001). *Cancer facts & figures 2001*. Atlanta: American Cancer Society.

Bandura, A. (1986). *Social foundations of thought and action*. Englewood Cliffs, New Jersey: Prentice-Hall.

Bettman, J.R. (1979). *An information processing theory of consumer choice*. Reading, MA: Addison-Wesley.

Botvin, G.J., & Dusenbury, L. (1989). Substance abuse prevention and the promotion of competence. In L.A. Bond & B.E. Compass (Eds.), *Primary prevention and promotion in the schools*. Newbury Park, CA: Sage.

Brown, M., & Fintor, L. (1994). The economic burden of cancer. In P. Greenwald, B. Kramer, & D. Weed (Eds.), *The science and practice of cancer prevention and control* (pp. 69–81). New York: Marcel Dekker.

Centers for Disease Control and Prevention. (1996). Guidelines for school programs to promote lifelong healthy eating. *Morbidity and Mortality Weekly Report, 45*, 1–41.

Chow, W., Linet, M.S., Liff, J.M., & Greenberg, R.S. (1996). Cancers in children. In D. Schottenfeld & J.F. Fraumeni, Jr. (Eds.), *Cancer epidemiology and prevention* (pp. 1331–1369). Oxford, MA: Oxford University Press.

Crane, L.A., Marcus, A.C., & Pike, D.K. (1993) Skin cancer prevention in preschools and daycare centers. *Journal of School Health, 63*, 232–234.

Epps, R.P., & Manley, M.W. (1993). Prevention of tobacco use during childhood and adolescence: Five steps to prevent the onset of smoking. *Cancer, 72*, 1002–1004.

Fintor, L. (1998). The Michigan health kiosk: Cancer info on the go. *Journal of the National Cancer Institute, 90*, 809–810.

Gurney, J.G., Davis, S., Severson, R.K., & Robison, L.L. (1994). The influence of subsequent neoplasms on incidence trends in childhood cancer. *Cancer Epidemiology, Biomarkers, and Prevention, 3*, 349–351.

Gurney, J.G., Davis, S., Severson, R.K., Fang, J.Y., Ross, J.A., & Robison, L.L. (1996). Trends in cancer incidence among children in the US. *Cancer, 78*, 532–541.

Kimm, S., & Kwiterovich, P.O. (1995). Childhood prevention of adult chronic diseases: Rationale and strategies. In L. Cheung & J.B. Richmond (Eds.), *Child Health, Nutrition, and Physical Activity* (pp. 249–273). Champaign, IL: Human Kinetics.

Lansky, S.B., Black, J.L., Cairns, N.U. (1983). Childhood cancer, medical costs. *Cancer, 52*, 762–766.

Laughlin-Richard, N. (2000). Sun exposure and skin cancer prevention in children and adolescents. *Journal of School Nursing, 16*, 20–26.

Linet, M.S., Ries, L.A., Smith, M.A., Tarone, R.E., & Devesa, S.S. (1999). Cancer surveillance series: Recent trends in childhood cancer incidence and mortality in the United States. *Journal of the National Cancer Institute, 91*, 1051–1058.

Marina, N.M., Bowman, L.C., Pui, C., & Crist, W.M. (1995). Pediatric solid tumors. In G.P. Murphy, W.L. Lawrence, & R.E. Lenhard, Jr. (Eds.), *American Cancer Society Textbook of Clinical Oncology* (pp. 524–551). Atlanta: American Cancer Society.

McLeroy, K.R., Bibeau, D., Steckler, A., & Glanz, K. (1988). An ecological perspective on health promotion programs. *Health Education Quarterly, 15*, 351–377.

National Cancer Intelligence Centre (2001). Cancer: Rates per 100,000, 1997. *Cancer registrations in England, 1995–1997.* London: Office for National Statistics.

National Cancer Institute of Canada, & Health Canada (2001). *Canadian cancer statistics 2001.* Ottawa: Health Canada.

Norman, M.A., Holly, E.A., & Preston-Martin, S. (1996). Childhood brain tumors and exposure to tobacco smoke. *Cancer Epidemiology, Biomarkers and Prevention, 5,* 85–91.

Parkin, D.M., Pisani, P., & Ferlay, J. (1999). Estimates of the worldwide incidence of 25 major cancers in 1990. *International Journal of Cancer, 80,* 827–841.

Pisani, P., Parkin, D.M., Bray, F., & Ferlay, J. (1999). Estimates of the worldwide mortality from 25 cancers in 1990. *International Journal of Cancer, 83,* 18–29.

Plon, S.E., & Peterson, L.E. (1997). Childhood cancer, heredity, and the environment. In P.A. Pizzo & Poplack (Eds.), *Principles and Practice of Pediatric Oncology* (pp. 11–36). Philadelphia: Lippincott-Raven.

Prochaska, J.O., DiClemente, C.C., & Norcross, J.C. (1992). In search of how people change: Applications to addictive behaviors. *American Psychologist, 47,* 1102–1114.

Ries, L.A.G., Smith, M.A., Gurney, J.G., Linet, M., Tamra, T., Young, J.L., & Bunin, G.R. (Eds.). (1999) *Cancer incidence and survival among children and adolescents: United States SEER Program 1975–1995* (NIH Publication No. 99-4649). Bethesda: National Cancer Institute, SEER Program.

Riggs, S. (1992). Smoking prevention and cessation in children and adolescents. *Current Opinions in Pediatrics, 4,* 590–593.

Robison, L.L. (1997). General principles of the epidemiology of childhood cancer. In P.A. Pizzo & Poplack (Eds.), *Principles and practice of pediatric oncology* (pp. 1–10). Philadelphia: Lippincott-Raven.

Rosenstock, I.M., Strecher, V.J., Becker, M.H. (1988) Social learning theory and the health belief model. *Health Education Quarterly, 15,* 175–183.

Williams, C.L. (1980). Primary prevention of cancer beginning in childhood. *Preventive Medicine, 9,* 275–280.

Cancer, Adolescence

Louis Fintor

INTRODUCTION

With lifelong behavioral patterns involving unhealthy lifestyles often initiated during adolescence, this population offers the best opportunity for successful cancer prevention activities. Even though rates of cancer incidence, prevalence, and mortality are low in this population, the long-term consequences of sustained risk-related behaviors such as smoking and poor nutrition make interventions in this group cost-effective public health social investments.

Unlike adult populations that have engaged in a lifetime of risk-related behaviors or among children who may have difficulty understanding risk-related behaviors and concepts of disease, cancer prevention and health promotion activities involving adolescents have emerged as challenging but viable public health priorities.

DEFINITIONS

Cancer is defined as more than 100 types of tumors classified in five general categories: carcinomas, sarcomas, myelomas, lymphomas, and leukemias. Cancer is characterized by the uncontrolled growth and proliferation of abnormal cells. These cells are distinguished by their ability to invade and spread ("metastasize") in normal tissue as well as travel to secondary sites. Normally organ-specific cancers vary in terms of cause, histology (cell type), natural history, and prognosis although most tumors are believed to arise from a single abnormal cell (Altman & Sarge, 1992).

Sometimes harmless, mutations can not only destroy healthy cells but can also cause abnormal cell growth resulting in cancer. In addition, they can increase susceptibility to carcinogenic damage. Mutations can be inherited and/or spontaneous and cause cancer directly or indirectly by impairing various cellular functions such as repair and division. Exposure to chemical, physical, or viral carcinogens is also a source of cellular mutations.

The long-term effects of early exposure can be illustrated through the process of *carcinogenesis*. Chemical carcinogenesis is believed to occur in two stages: initiation and promotion. During *initiation*, exposure to a carcinogen causes cellular DNA damage resulting in genetic mutation. *Promotion* on the other hand, can occur years or even decades later when the cell is exposed to chemical "promoters" which influence the proliferation of mutated cells without directly damaging DNA. Physical carcinogenesis can occur via exposure to radiation, certain dusts, and mineral and synthetic fibers (e.g., asbestos) that prompt DNA mutations. Viral carcinogenesis is impaired cell growth and regulation or cellular changes arising from exposure to certain viral materials. While only a few classes of viruses have been associated with cancer, viral agents such a human papilloma virus (linked to cervical cancer) is sexually transmitted and as such may be particularly relevant to cancer prevention efforts in adolescent populations (Altman & Sarge, 1992).

Heredity also plays an important role in predisposing individuals to cancer. Research to identify these genetic factors and to develop novel interventions have gained momentum in recent years as advances are made in molecular biology and genetics. Eventually, these discoveries are expected to result in new screening tools and interventions that will expand the scope of prevention activities.

Cancer prevention activities in adolescence are especially important because the process of carcinogenesis often requires long time intervals. Thus, exposure may occur during childhood and adolescence even though the disease will not be detectable until adulthood. In addition, prevention and early detection are important for adolescent cancer survivors who appear to be at greater risk for developing cancer later in life.

Finally, it is unlikely that a single factor such as exposure, heredity, or behavior accounts for the development of cancer among adolescents. In fact, it is thought that cancer is a disease of *multifactorial etiology* attributable to genetic, environmental, and physiologic factors and their interaction with biological, social, and environmental elements. In addition to chemical, physical, environmental, viral, and genetic factors, cancer is believed to arise from a complex interaction of hormones, immune status, diet, occupation, socioeconomic, and other lifestyle factors.

SCOPE

Because adolescent cancers result from genetic and environmental factors, prevention efforts have targeted lifestyle-related factors responsible for causing the disease later in life. These include smoking, excessive sun exposure, lack of exercise, poor nutrition, and alcohol use.

Among the known risk factors, the most significant risk factor for this group is smoking and tobacco use. Given the staggering harmful effects of adolescent smoking, this area has received the greatest public health attention. The risk of developing adult lung cancer and other diseases increases substantially with regular smoking during adolescence. It has been estimated that about one third of all adolescents who regularly smoke, or about 5 million adolescents, will eventually die of smoking-related causes (Centers for Disease Control and Prevention [CDC], 1996; 1998; Hegmann et al., 1993).

Experimentation with smoking in the United States peaks between the ages of 11 and 12. More than 33 percent of adolescents who experiment with smoking become regular, habitual smokers before leaving high school. Studies indicate that 18 percent of US high school sophomores in 1998 were regular daily smokers and that 25 percent of 1998 high school seniors were regular daily smokers. Tobacco use for those not completing high school was even higher (Grunbaum et al., 1999; University of Michigan Institute for Social Research, 1999).

Researchers estimate that every day more than 6,000 adolescents try cigarette smoking for the first time, while another 3,000 become new habitual smokers. At present, more than 90 percent of adult smokers begin smoking regularly before leaving high school (Centers for Disease Control and Prevention, 1998; United States Department of Health and Human Services, 1994).

The symptoms of tobacco addiction appear shortly after occasional smoking begins. This explains why 75 percent of US high school smokers fail at smoking cessation and that less than one in seven can stop smoking for more than 30 days. It is not surprising then that while 3 percent of adolescent smokers believe they will continue to smoke 5 years later, more than 60 percent continue to smoke up to 9 years later (Centers for Disease Control and Prevention, 1998; University of Michigan Institute for Social Research, 1999).

Epidemiology: Incidence, Mortality, and Prevalence

As with both childhood and adult cancers, US incidence rates vary among adolescents by cancer type, age, socioeconomic status, race, and ethnicity. Although cancer rates are fairly similar among industrialized nations, caution should be exercised when comparing cancer incidence and mortality rates between countries. Often, there are differences between countries in data collection and reporting in addition to methodological technicalities.

According to recent US data, cancer incidence rate for youths aged 15–19 is 20.3 per 100,000 (1993–1997) with 1,745 new cases reported during this time period. Incidence rates for the most common cancers in this age group are Hodgkin's disease (3.4); testicular cancer (3.0); ovarian cancer (2.3); leukemias (2.3); brain and other central nervous system (CNS) tumors (1.9); and non-Hodgkin's lymphoma or NHL (1.8). Childhood cancers such as neuroblastomas, retinoblastoma, and others are relatively rare among US adolescents (Ries et al., 2000).

Although there have been increases in the rates of some adolescent cancers, there have also been dramatic improvements in survival. Not only have overall 5-year US adolescent survival rates improved from 69 percent (1975–1984) to 77 percent (1985–1994), but for some common cancers 5-year survival has increased to 90 percent or more (Ries et al., 1999).

Incidence rates and the site distribution of cancers in Canada and other industrialized nations are comparable with those in the United States. According to Health Canada, consolidated (male and female) incidence rates per 100,000 for the most common adolescent cancers among those aged 15–19 are Hodgkin's disease (4.17); leukemia (2.47); brain and CNS tumors (2.10); NHL (1.67); bone cancer (1.56); and thyroid cancer (1.45). In addition, rates for testicular cancer are 2.61 (National Cancer Institute of Canada [NCIC], & Health Canada, 2000).

In England, recent data on incidence rates per 100,000 for the most common cancers among males aged 15–19 are testicular (3.2); leukemia (3.1); NHL (1.8); brain (1.1); melanoma (0.9); and lip, mouth, and pharynx (0.5). For English females, they are in situ cervical cancer (20.2); leukemia (1.9); melanoma (1); brain (1); ovary and other female sites (0.8); NHL (0.6); and colorectal cancer (0.2) (National Cancer Intelligence Centre, 2001a,b).

Cancer mortality patterns among US adolescents are comparable to those reported in other industrialized nations. According to the most recent data (1993–1997), the US cancer mortality rates per 100,000 in this age group are 3.9 with 3,522 deaths recorded during this period. Rates for the most common cancer site-specific causes of death in this group are: leukemias (1.2); brain and other CNS cancers (0.6); bone and joint cancers (0.5); NHL (0.3); and other cancers (0.1 or less) (Ries et al., 2000).

In Canada mortality rates for youths aged 15–19 peak at 4.26 per 100,000 with a trend toward declining mortality attributable to earlier diagnosis and better treatment. Recent data for England and Wales report mortality rates for all cancers except nonmelanoma skin cancers to be 4.6 for males and 2.7 for females (National Cancer Intelligence Centre, 2000, 2001a,b).

COSTS INVOLVED

As with adult and childhood cancers, direct out-of-pocket medical costs with adolescent cancers are less than indirect costs. Most of these costs accrue from foregone earnings attributable to premature death and from indirect costs to families who are primary caregivers. Still, the economic burden of adolescent cancers is significant. For childhood cancers, nonmedical costs have been estimated to consume 44 percent or more of family weekly budget. In comparison, direct medical costs average 5.8 percent with a dollar range from $8,000 to $53,000 with a mean of $34,558 (Brown & Fintor, 1994; Lansky, Black, & Cairns, 1983). Further, these parents often function as a primary caregiver to the adolescent during their peak earning years and carry large long-term medical debt after the recovery or death of their child (Brown & Fintor, 1994; Lansky et al., 1983).

Moreover, nonmonetary cancer-related psychosocial costs often accrue from pain, disability, isolation, anxiety, grief, economic dependence, lost employment opportunities, and relocation. These costs have not been well studied but should be taken into consideration when calculating the overall burden of disease on individuals and their families (Brown & Fintor, 1994).

Given these social, economic, and public health costs, it is not surprising that preventive activities with young people are cost-effective. For example, a 1997 study estimated the costs of fielding a nationwide 4-year media intervention campaign involving 209 US media markets at $8 per adolescent exposed and $162 per adolescent in whom smoking was prevented (Secker-Walker, Worden, Holland, Flynn, & Detsky, 1997).

THEORIES AND RESEARCH

Adolescent cancer prevention activities have drawn upon from a variety of theoretical approaches to construct targeted messages for different regional, age, race, sex, and SES groups. Evidence suggests that adolescents are influenced by mass marketing approaches, peer pressure, and media messages.

Less successful approaches have relied on *Fear-Appeal* models in which adverse behaviors are modified as individuals recognize a linkage between their adverse behaviors and the development of disease (Witte, 1994). These flawed models emerged from learning theory in the early 1950s. They assumed that persuasive messages would prompt individuals to fear cancer-related risks and would initiate action to reduce those threats. As negative behaviors are avoided and the perception of risk decreases, these behaviors themselves form a habitual response (McGuire, 1969). This approach does not work well with adolescents who view themselves as less vulnerable to death and disease.

Other fear-based approaches have had limited utility with adolescents. Among these are the fear-appeal *Parallel Process Model*. This approach uses messages that describe threats and efficacy in ways to resolve these threats. Adolescents often attempt to control threats through protective attitudes, intentions, and behaviors or controlling the fear itself through avoidance or denial. In cases where the perception of a threat is low, there is little or no response (Janis, 1967).

Because fear-based messages have had limited success with adolescent populations, public health professionals have turned to other social and behavioral models to achieve their health promotion objectives. These *ecological* approaches have been more successful because they involve multidimensional, multilevel prevention strategies. Using this comprehensive design, fear-based approaches are coupled with public policy, advocacy, economic support, organizational and environmental change, as well as with secondary and tertiary preventive approaches (McLeroy, Bibeau, Steckler, & Glanz, 1988).

A second approach utilizes *cognitive–behavioral* strategies. These strategies mediate behavior by taking into account perceptions of risk, motivation to change behavior, and the skills available to initiate and sustain these changes over time. In this approach, multiple factors are acknowledged to influence behavior including those that are intrapersonal/individual, interpersonal, institutional/organizational, community, and public policy-oriented. These strategies often involve families, peers, and public role models, health care providers and public health advocates. Schools, religious groups, and other community institutions provide both support and reinforcement.

Other approaches have involved cognitive–behavioral models such as *Stages of Change*, *Health Belief*, and *Consumer Information Processing*. In general, these models maintain that while individual behavior is influenced by knowledge, knowledge alone is not sufficient to change behavior (Bettman, 1979; Prochaska, DiClemete, & Norcross, 1992; Rosenstock, Strecher, & Becker, 1988).

Of the three, *Consumer Information Processing* (CIP) models have been the most successful with adolescents. CIP assumes that adolescent cancer prevention messages compete for attention and priority with other risk-related messages that youths receive. The sheer volume of information forces the adolescent to develop coping strategies for assessing the personal value of each message based on information *availability*, perceived *usefulness*, and the *ease* with which it can be adapted and used (Bettman, 1979).

A third theoretical school of interpersonal theories have also provided models for designing effective interventions involving adolescents. These models include *Social Learning Theory* and *Community-Level Models*.

Social Learning Theory describes dynamic interactions among individual cognitive factors, the environment, and behavior. These components in turn involve *reciprocal determinism* (dynamic, but alterable relationships between the individual and the environment), *behavioral capability* (knowledge and skill), *expectations* (beliefs about the consequences of actions), *self-efficacy* (belief in one's ability to initiate and sustain changes in specific behavior), *observational learning*, and *reinforcement* (Bandura, 1986).

Observational learning and *reinforcement* rely on the role played by influential individuals in modeling behaviors. In smoking, physical activity, and dietary interventions, adolescent role models who have successfully stopped smoking or lost weight motivate others. Whether the desired changes in behavior can be sustained in the short term depends on *reinforcements* such as praise, encouragement, and other "rewards." In smoking cessation and weight management examples include rewards such as refundable participation fees. Whether these behaviors can be sustained over time, however, is thought to be determined both by self-efficacy and by using strategies such as monitoring, contracting, and goal-setting.

Community-Level Models are used in smoking prevention and cessation campaigns involving children, adolescents, and adults. They are comprehensive, multilevel interventions that involve schools, religious and community groups, local governments, the media, worksites, health insurers, volunteer organizations, and others. These programs can be less cost-intensive on a per-person basis (Rothman & Tropman, 1987).

STRATEGIES THAT WORK

Successful, cost-effective, adolescent cancer prevention programs using a comprehensive, integrated approach to promoting a variety of healthy behaviors have been described in the literature. The majority of these studies have involved reducing the use of tobacco products. However, studies involving nutrition, exercise, and reducing exposure to cancer-associated viral agents have also been successful.

Interventions targeting tobacco use have been especially well-reported. For example, a comprehensive smoking education program that involved teaching adolescents a variety of self-esteem and coping skills designed to diffuse peer pressures resulted in reducing short-term smoking prevalence by up to 80 percent with sustained reductions between 20 and 25 percent over time (Botvin, Baker, Dusenbury, Botvin, & Diaz, 1995).

Another study found that identification with nonsmoking peers could lead to a 50 percent reduction in regular smoking for more than 4 years, while others have reported that media programs involving family members reduced identification with peer approval of smoking and altered knowledge, awareness, attitudes, and smoking behavior among adolescents (Flay, 1987; Murray, Pirie, Leupker, & Pallonen, 1989).

Many interventions have used the media to reinforce negative associations with smoking in an integrated approach that appears more successful than school-based interventions alone. This group of studies has combined comprehensive media public education with school-based programs and public policy efforts aimed at enforcing restrictions on tobacco advertising and sales to adolescents. These programs have resulted in reductions in rates of smoking prevalence among adolescents by up to 40 percent (Flynn et al., 1994).

In addition, a number of states have developed and initiated comprehensive adolescent public education programs in combination with overall public health smoking cessation and prevention programs. Preliminary data suggests that they have been more successful in reducing tobacco consumption among adolescents than states without these programs.

Other efforts have been designed to combat the marketing of tobacco through the media. For example, one study reported that antitobacco media education campaigns resulted in significant improvements in life-years gained—making them among the most cost-effective methods (Secker-Walker et al., 1997). Similarly, a California study found that adolescent smoking programs involving the media not only reduced the prevalence of smoking but also positively correlated higher levels of funding with higher reductions (Hu, Sung, & Keeler, 1995a).

Longitudinal studies in Sweden have reported that reductions in tobacco use could be sustained over a period of 15 years using media interventions involving schools and community groups. Investigators reported that overall cigarette consumption dropped by 22 percent among adolescents who participated in these programs. Investigators have also reported that media interventions combined with prevention's other technologies (natural caregiving and competency enhancement) using school-based health education curriculums resulted in dramatically lower rates of smoking. They found that only 14.6 percent of high school seniors who had participated in the program smoked weekly compared to 24.1 percent of adolescents in communities that did not have these programs (Perry, Kelder, Murray, & Klepp, 1992; Vartiainen, Paavola, McAlister, & Puska, 1988).

In terms of public policy, studies have demonstrated that a 3-year antismoking intervention at the end of the 1960s reduced per capita cigarette consumption by more than 5 percent while the prevalence of smoking among adolescents was reduced by 3 percent. Antismoking advertising has been demonstrated to be almost 60 percent more effective at preventing or reducing smoking than tobacco advertising (USDHHS, 1989, 1994).

Underscoring the power of comprehensive approaches, states implementing multifaceted programs have reported declines in long-term smoking of between 10 and 13 percent, while one fifth (or 2 percent) of these reductions have been reported using media only campaigns. In California, cigarette sales were reduced by 232 million packs between the third quarter of 1990 and the fourth quarter of 1992. In Massachusetts, antitobacco education efforts have been effective in preventing smoking among adolescents, substantially reducing smoking among those who already started, and encouraging smoking cessation among their parents. An evaluation of this program revealed that tobacco consumption had been reduced by 31 percent from 1992 to 1997 (Abt Associates, Inc., 1997; Hu, Sung, & Keeler, 1995; Hu, Sung, & Keeler, 1995).

While smoking and tobacco-related interventions comprise the largest single focus of primary prevention efforts in this population, nutrition, exercise and physical activity, and reducing environmental exposures are likewise important. Smoking, diet, infectious diseases, and other environmental factors are believed to be responsible for more than 75 percent of all US cancers. In addition to tobacco use, voluntary behavioral risks such as poor nutrition, physical inactivity, and obesity comprise a significantly greater proportion of individual cancer-related risk than industrial pollutants, chemicals, radiation, drug therapies, and other exposures combined.

Currently, one third of US cancer-related deaths are attributable to diet, obesity, and alcohol risk factors that are linked to cancers of the colon, rectum, stomach, breast, lung, liver, and other sites. The US prevalence of obesity alone has increased dramatically since 1976 with poor nutritional habits among US children and adolescents expected to result in even greater increases in adult obesity rates over the next few decades (Flegal, Carroll, Kuczmarski, & Johnson, 1998).

School-based interventions have targeted nutritional choice and balancing caloric intake with increased physical activity among adolescents. Among those factors that have been incorporated into these prevention activities are reducing alcohol use, emphasizing increased fruit, vegetable, and fiber intake, and reducing portion sizes. Similarly, regular physical activity has been promoted to lower the cancer risks associated with obesity.

Nutrition educators have long stressed that efforts to improve dietary habits must be targeted toward *groups* as well as *individuals*. Because the nutritional knowledge of one family member is often a good predictor of dietary behavior of the others, many interventions have targeted women since they often make household nutritional and dietary decisions (Yarbrough, 1981).

Adolescent diet is largely influenced through various media (advertising) and interpersonal interactions (peers). However, information obtained through these sources is often mediated by schools and in the home. Thus, schools have become an important resource for nutrition education. For this reason, there have been growing concerns among parents and community groups regarding the availability of low-nutritional yield snack foods and soft drinks as well as the vending of high-fat convenience foods in school cafeterias.

Nutrition educators have relied largely on diffusion models in designing interventions. Researchers have demonstrated that food choices and preferences are established early in life and are drawn from religious, ethnic, and regional influences. Hence, many educators have tried education involving substitution rather than elimination. For example, some schools have substituted high-calorie soft drinks with a selection of bottled waters and iced teas. Others have reduced serving sizes or substituted healthier ingredients. Nevertheless, many food choices appear to be *affectual*, or based on appearance and taste. Another potential problem encountered by nutrition educators involves *overadoption* such as the overuse of vitamin and mineral supplements or the adoption of nonrational choices such as "fad" diets.

Finally, some behavioral and lifestyle interventions are directed towards reducing the risks from excessive sun exposure (use sun screens and limit exposure to sunlight) which can lead to melanoma and other skin cancers. For example, the most lethal form of skin cancer, malignant melanoma, is associated with intense ultraviolet radiation exposures of relatively short duration that result in sunburn. Meanwhile, two other skin cancers, basal cell carcinomas and squamous cell carcinomas, have been linked to long-term sun exposure. A number of pilot studies have targeted children and adolescents to both reduce sun exposure and promote the use of sunscreens. These interventions have been largely school-based programs with a focus on changing knowledge, attitudes, and behaviors. One such program involved using school nurses to develop an age-appropriate curriculum for children and adolescents that integrated a series of interactive modules addressing the anatomy and physiology of skin, the physical properties of sunlight, and strategies to minimize sun exposure (e.g., protective clothing and adequate skin protection factor sunscreens) and skin damage (Laughlin-Richard, 2000).

Still other interventions have attempted to reduce the incidence of cancer-associated viral pathogens such as the sexually-acquired human papilloma virus (HPV) and hepatitis B (know your sexual partner and use latex condoms). Many of these have been undertaken by state health departments and more cost-effectively linked to AIDS education and prevention campaigns.

STRATEGIES THAT MIGHT WORK

Despite successes reported in antitobacco efforts, overall prevalence of smoking among adolescents continues to rise while the age at which smoking is first initiated continues to drop. Unfortunately, many prevention efforts are poorly funded or funded for short time intervals making long-term behavioral change both difficult to maintain and evaluate.

For example, school-based programs have long been credited with accounting for up to 60 percent in sustained reductions in smoking prevalence between 1 and 4 years. Smoking prevalence among adolescents in schools without smoking intervention programs was found to be 1.5 times higher. Even in tobacco-producing regions, the social influences that lead to smoking showed that school-based interventions could result in lower smoking rates (Noland, Kryscio, Riggs, Linville, Ford, & Tucker, 1998; USDHHS, 1994).

But more recently, a University of Washington evaluation of school-based smoking prevention in that state's 40 school districts involving more than 8,000 students over a period of 15 years (1984–1999) concluded that curriculum-based approaches alone were ineffective. In the randomized trial, investigators found that social-influences approaches which increase awareness about the social factors that lead to smoking did not improve smoking prevalence rates when compared to usual school-based health promotion and school prevention activities involving tobacco (Peterson, Kealey, Mann, Marek, & Sarason, 2000). This has generated

controversy in the public health community and led to calls for additional evaluation studies involving these approaches.

Similarly, despite individual successes in the area of diet and exercise, obesity rates among Americans continues to rise. Some studies have noted that positive change in one area such as knowledge of healthy dietary habits or substitution of health ingredients often leads to a negative change in other areas such as portion size. This phenomenon continues to be investigated.

Meanwhile, promising new efforts utilizing computer-based interactive technologies to deliver prevention messages for this population are in development. In addition, more comprehensive theory-based health communication approaches are evolving. The efficacy of these newer approaches, however, remains to be seen (Fintor, 1998).

Among these strategies are health kiosks, web-based educational sites, fax-back services, telephone support lines, computer games, and other innovations. These have been credited with the potential to become convenient, educational, and engaging ways to promote healthy behaviors as well as reach larger audiences.

However, many of these modalities require technological literacy and access, depend on substantial and expensive infrastructure, provide few incentives for behavioral change, and have not yet been demonstrated as effective.

STRATEGIES THAT DO NOT WORK

As noted earlier in this entry and elsewhere in this volume, large group interventions depending solely on education do not work. Similarly, those interventions involving only passive prevention such as altering school cafeteria menus or mandating that fast food outlets and convenience stores are zoned away from school areas likewise do not work alone.

Efforts must be both age-appropriate and culturally sensitive since the "one-size-fits-all" efforts have consistently failed in this population. It is especially important to note the difficulties in constructing "fear-based" messages that are peculiar to this population. While adolescents, like adults, have the intellectual capacity to process health risk knowledge, their time horizon and perception of personal risk differs considerably from those of adults. Thus, strategies based solely on fear have made little or no headway in this population.

In fact, many researchers have noted that educational interventions stressing the consequences of risk-taking behaviors have had the opposite effect among adolescents—in many cases generating additional appeal or creating cognitive saturation such that the risk is ignored. Likewise, those interventions involving identification with parental or other authority figures or using repetitive messaging that requires long periods of attention have similarly met with little success.

SYNTHESIS

Adolescent populations present special challenges to those designing prevention programs. Because adolescents often do not associate behavioral risks such as smoking, improper diet, and inadequate exercise with developing cancer later in life, they have difficulty grasping the concept of prevention.

On the other hand, while presenting some of the most significant challenges they also have the potential to demonstrate the most profound long-term successes.

It is clear that this population requires highly tailored interventions that involve age-appropriate, multidimensional approaches targeted at individual, family, and community level. These approaches must be culturally sensitive, engaging, timely campaigns using a combination of education, passive regulatory intervention, peer, role model, and social group identification, and positive reinforcement.

Large-scale campaigns must provide for enough flexibility to take into consideration individual and group differences. This is no doubt difficult to accomplish in a cost-effective way. However, one approach would be to "piggy back" cancer prevention messages with other health risks and benefits. For example, links between diet, exercise, and obesity. However, care must be taken such that the sheer number of messages does not overwhelm the intended audience and also that overadoption does not result in unintended negative consequences such as increased risk-taking.

The use of new computer technologies has become especially popular among many adolescents and as such has become a popular means of message delivery. However it is likewise important to determine whether the target groups at highest risk have access to these technologies and are technologically literate.

Despite modest short-term successes with cancer prevention among adolescents, much remains to be done. With adult cancers continuing to extract a heavy social and economic toll, cost-effective cancer prevention activities for adolescents will continue to grow in importance.

Also see: Chronic Disease, Adolescence; Environmental Health: Childhood; Family Strengthening: Adolescence; Perceived Personal Control; Resilience: Childhood.

References

Abt Associates, Inc. (1997). *An independent evaluation of the Massachusetts Tobacco Control Program; Fourth Annual Report: Summary; January 1994 to June 1997.*

Altman, A., & Sarge, M.J. (1992). *The cancer dictionary.* New York: Facts on File.

Bandura, A. (1986). *Social foundations of thought and action.* Englewood Cliffs, New Jersey: Prentice-Hall.

Bettman, J.R. (1979). *An information processing theory of consumer choice.* Reading, MA: Addison-Wesley.

Botvin, G.J., Baker E., Dusenbury, L., Botvin, E.M., & Diaz, T. (1995). Long-term follow-up results of a randomized drug abuse prevention trial in a white middle-class population. *Journal of the American Medical Association, 14*, 1106–1112.

Brown, M., & Fintor, L. (1994). The Economic Burden of Cancer. In P. Greenwald, B. Kramer, & D. Weed (Eds.), *The science and practice of cancer prevention and control* (pp. 69–81). New York: Marcel Dekker.

Centers for Disease Control and Prevention. (1998, May 22). Selected cigarette smoking initiation and quitting behaviors among high school students—United States, 1997. *Morbidity and Mortality Weekly Report.*

Centers for Disease Control and Prevention. (1998, October 9). Incidence of initiation of cigarette smoking—United States 1965–1996. *Morbidity and Mortality Weekly Report, 47*(19), 386–389.

Centers for Disease Control and Prevention. (1996, November 8). Projected smoking-related deaths among youths—United States. *Morbidity and Mortality Weekly Report, 45.*

Fintor, L. (1998). The Michigan health kiosk: Cancer info on the go. *Journal of the National Cancer Institute, 90*, 809–810.

Flay, B. (1987). Mass media and smoking cessation: A critical review. *American Journal of Public Health, 77*, 153–160.

Flegal, K.M., Carroll, M.D., Kuczmarski, R.J., & Johnson, C.L. (1998). Overweight and obesity in the United States: Prevalence and trends, 1960–1994. *International Journal of Obesity, 22*, 39–47.

Flynn, B.S., Worden, J.K., Secker-Walker, R.H., Pirie, P.L., Badger, G.J., Carpenter, J.H., & Geller, B.M. (1994). Mass media and school interventions for cigarette smoking prevention: Effects 2 years after completion. *American Journal of Public Health, 84*, 1148–1150.

Grunbaum, J.A., Kann, L., Kinchen, S.A., Ross, J.G., Gowda, V.R., Collins, J.L., & Kolbe, L.J. (1999). Youth risk behavior surveillance—National Alternative High School Youth Risk Behavior Survey, United States—1998. (1999) *Morbidity and Mortality Weekly Report CDC Surveillance Summary, 48*, 1–44.

Hegmann, K.T., Fraser, A.M., Keaney, R.P., Moser, S.E., Nilasena, D.S., Sedlars, M., Higham-Gren, L., & Lyon, J.L. (1993). The effect of age at smoking initiation on lung cancer risk. *Epidemiology, 4*, 444–448.

Hu, T., Sung, H.Y., & Keeler, T.E. (1995a). Reducing cigarette consumption in California: Tobacco taxes vs an anti-smoking media campaign. *American Journal of Public Health, 85*, 1218–1222.

Hu, T.W., Sung, H.Y., & Keeler, T.E. (1995b). The impact of California anti-smoking legislation on cigarette sales, consumption, and prices. *Tobacco Control, 4*(Suppl. 1), S34–S38.

Janis, I.L. (1967). Effects of fear arousal on attitude change: Recent developments in theory and experimental research. In L. Berkowitz (Ed.), *Advances in experimental social psychology* (Vol. 3, pp. 166–225). New York: Academic Press.

Lansky, S.B., Black, J.L., & Cairns, N.U. (1983). Childhood cancer, medical costs. *Cancer, 52*, 762–766.

Laughlin-Richard, N. (2000). Sun exposure and skin cancer prevention in children and adolescents. *Journal of School Nursing, 16*, 20–26.

McGuire, W.J. (1969). The nature of attitudes and attitude change. In G. Lindzey & E. Aronson (Eds.), *The handbook of social psychology* (Vol. 3, pp. 136–314). Reading, MA: Addison-Wesley.

McLeroy, K.R., Bibeau, D., Steckler, A., & Glanz, K. (1988). An ecological perspective on health promotion programs. *Health Education Quarterly, 15*, 351–377.

Murray, D.M., Pirie, P., Leupker, R.V., & Pallonen, U. (1989). Five and six year follow-up results from four seventh-grade smoking prevention strategies. *Journal of Behavioural Medicine, 12*, 207–218.

National Cancer Institute of Canada (NCIC) and Health Canada. (2000). *Canadian cancer statistics 2000.* Ottawa: Health Canada.

National Cancer Intelligence Centre. (2001a). Cancer: Rates per 100,000, 1997. *Cancer registrations in England, 1995–1997*. London: Office for National Statistics.

National Cancer Intelligence Centre. (2001b). Cancer trends appendix C2B: Mortality per 1000,000 females, England and Wales, 1999. *Cancer trends in England and Wales 1950–1999*. London: Office for National Statistics.

Noland, M.P., Kryscio, R.J., Riggs, R.S., Linville, L.H., Ford, V.Y., & Tucker, T.C. (1998). The effectiveness of a tobacco prevention program with adolescents living in a tobacco-producing region. *American Journal of Public Health, 88*, 1862–1865.

Perry, C.L., Kelder, S.H., Murray, D.M., & Klepp, KI. (1992). Communitywide smoking prevention: Long-term outcomes of the Minnesota Heart Health program and the Class of 1989 study. *American Journal of Public Health, 82*, 1210–1216.

Peterson, A.V., Kealey, K.A., Mann, S.L., Marek, P.M., & Sarason, I.G. (2000). Hutchinson Smoking Prevention Project: Long-term randomized trial in school-based tobacco use prevention. Results on smoking. *Journal of the National Cancer Institute, 92*, 1979–1991.

Prochaska, J.O., DiClemete, C.C., & Norcross, J.C. (1992). In search of how people change: Applications to addictive behaviors. *American Psychologist, 47*, 1102–1114.

Ries, L.A.G., Smith, M.A., Gurney, J.G., Linet, M., Tamra, T., Young, J.L., & Bunin, G.R. (Eds). (1999). *Cancer incidence and survival among children and adolescents: United States SEER Program 1975–1995* (NIH Publication No. 99-4649). Bethesda: National Cancer Institute, SEER Program.

Ries, L.A.G., Eisner, M.P., Kosary, C.L., Hankey, B.F., Miller, B.A., Clegg, L., & Edwards, B.K. (Eds). (2000). *SEER cancer statistics review 1973–1997* (pp. 458–478). Bethesda: National Cancer Institute, SEER Program.

Rosenstock, I.M., Strecher, V.J., & Becker, M.H. (1988). Social learning theory and the health belief model. *Health Education Quarterly, 15*, 175–183.

Rothman, J., & Tropman, J.E. (1987). Models of community organization and macro practice: Their mixing and phasing. In F.M. Cox, J.L. Ehrlich, J. Rothman, & J.E. Tropman (Eds.), *Strategies of community organization*. Itasca, Illinois: Peacock.

Secker-Walker, R.H., Worden, J.K., Holland, R.R., Flynn, B.S., & Detsky, A.S. (1997). A mass media programme to prevent smoking among adolescents: Costs and cost effectiveness. *Tobacco Control, 6*, 207–212.

United States Department of Health and Human Services. (1989). *Reducing the health consequences of smoking: 25 years of progress. A report of the Surgeon General*. Rockville, MD: Author, Public Health Service, Centers for Disease Control, Center for Chronic Disease Prevention and Health Promotion, Office of Smoking and Health.

United States Department of Health and Human Services. (1994). *Preventing tobacco use among young people: A report of the Surgeon General*. Rockville: Author, Public Health Service, Centers for Disease Control, Center for Chronic Disease Prevention and Health Promotion, Office of Smoking and Health.

University of Michigan Institute for Social Research. (1999). *Monitoring the Future Study, 1999*. Ann Arbor, Michigan.

Vartiainen, E., Paavola, M., McAlister, A., & Puska, P. (1998). Fifteen-year follow-up of smoking prevention effects in the North Karelia youth project. *American Journal of Public Health, 88*, 81–85.

Witte, K. (1994). Generating effective risk messages: How scary should your risk communication be? *Communication Yearbook, 18*, 229–254.

Yarbrough, P. (1981). Communication theory and nutrition education research. *Journal of Nutrition Education, 13*, S16–S25.

Cancer, Adulthood

Louis Fintor

INTRODUCTION

Primary cancer prevention and health promotion activities in adult populations encompass a constellation of diverse activities designed to increase cancer awareness, reduce exposures to carcinogens, and alter risk-related behaviors.

DEFINITIONS

The general term *cancer* describes more than 100 tumors which are characterized by the uncontrolled growth and proliferation of abnormal cells. Cancers can be diagnosed in many different parts of the body ("sites") and often have the ability to invade and spread ("metastasize") to normal tissue at secondary sites. Although the earliest known written descriptions of cancer are found in Egypt and thought to date from 2500 B.C.E., physical evidence of the disease has been documented even in prehistoric animal skeletal remains (Altman & Sarge, 1992). Modern researchers have developed five general categories to classify cancers. These include:

1. *Carcinoma*, the most common form of cancer comprising more than 80 percent of all diagnoses which are characterized by tumors found on epithelial tissues that line various organs such as the liver, colon, breast, lungs, and skin.
2. *Sarcoma*, which arises in connective tissues such as cartilage, bone, and muscle as well as fat.
3. *Myeloma*, which is found in bone marrow cells.
4. *Lymphoma*, a tumor of the lymphatic system.
5. *Leukemia*, a cancer of blood-forming cells.

These categories are then further subdivided to describe cancers in even greater detail. For example, acute leukemias (lymphoblastic or nonlymphoblastic) are further differentiated from chronic forms of the disease (lymphocytic or myelocytic).

Cancer can act on normal tissue in a variety of ways often depending on type. These include starving normal tissue by preferentially siphoning cellular nutrients, destroying and replacing normal tissue via the growth of a tumor mass, and by spreading and invading tissues in other parts of the body through the circulatory and lymphatic systems.

The symptoms of cancer likewise vary considerably. In general, these can include detection of a persistent abnormal growth (lump or mass), unusual bleeding, discharge, or difficulty in healing, unusual changes in bowel and bladder habits or moles, and chronic coughs, hoarseness, or difficulty in swallowing.

Today, cancer treatment has evolved to include four different approaches that can be used separately or in combination. These include, surgery (physically removing the tumor), radiation therapy (the use of radioactive agents to destroy cancer cells and shrink tumors), chemotherapy (the use of chemical agents to selectively target rapidly proliferating cells), and, more recently, biological or immunotherapies (substances that stimulate the body's own immune defenses).

Since early detection of cancer is critical to successful treatment, a variety of personal—breast cancer and testicular cancer self-examinations—and diagnostic screening interventions have been developed and continue to evolve. In addition to standard tissue biopsies, these include noninvasive radiographic diagnostic tests such as mammography used to detect breast cancer, ultrasound, and magnetic resonance imaging. In addition, new approaches such as thermography (locating tumors via changes in tissue temperature), biological markers (detecting substances associated with the presence or growth of tumors), and genetic mutations (predisposing individuals to developing cancer) continue to be investigated.

SCOPE

Although cancer prevention activities involving adult populations tend to be more numerous, varied, and well-funded than those involving children and adolescents, significant work remains to be done. Cancer continues to be a source of significant worldwide adult morbidity, mortality, and economic cost. Despite advances in early detection and treatment, prevention remains the single most effective means of cancer control. As researchers move closer to understanding the etiology of cancer, factors such as environmental exposure to carcinogens, nutrition, and genetics will play key roles in making prevention efforts an even bigger priority.

While great strides in prevention, early detection, and treatment of adult cancers over the last century are now beginning to yield measurable reductions in incidence and mortality, these are largely the result of successful interventions developed and implemented long ago. Many of these efforts have focused on behavioral changes that are measurable over time in areas such as smoking, nutrition, exercise and physical activity, and reducing environmental exposures to environmental and workplace carcinogens. This has translated into site-specific mortality rates among adults in industrialized countries beginning to show some promising signs of decline. However, at the same time an estimated 70 percent of new cases are projected in developing nations during the first two decades of this century. By the year 2020, researchers estimate 20 million cases of cancer will be diagnosed and that more than 70 percent of these will occur in countries that have less than 5 percent of the world's cancer control resources. In the absence of a cure, more than half of these patients are expected to die (American Cancer Society, 2000; Parkin, Pisani, & Ferlay 1999; Pisani, Parkin, Bray, & Ferlay 1999).

Epidemiology: Incidence and Mortality

According to the United States National Cancer Institute (NCI), incidence rates from 1990–1997 for all US cancers combined were 398.1/100,000. The four most commonly diagnosed US adult cancers are lung, colon and rectum, prostate and breast, and these comprise slightly more than half of all newly diagnosed cases. Incidence rates for lung and bronchus (55.2/100,000), colon and rectum (43.9/100,000), prostate cancer in men (149.7/100,000), and female breast cancers (109.7/100,000) remain unacceptably high. Moreover, when analyzed by race and ethnicity, African Americans currently have higher incidence and death rates than other racial and ethnic populations for all cancers except breast (American Cancer Society, 2000).

However, it is important to acknowledge that cancer rates vary widely between countries based on a variety of factors including geography, race, and the ability to reliably collect and tabulate data. In some cases, countries do not collect national incidence rates or collect them only for specific regions or groups. Overall US cancer incidence and mortality rates have declined by an average of 0.8 percent annually from 1990 to 1997 with the greatest decline in incidence (1.3 percent) occurring after 1992. This reverses a trend toward increasing incidence rates from 1972 to 1992 (American Cancer Society, 2000).

Cancer incidence and mortality rates are relatively similar among industrialized countries such as Canada, the United Kingdom, and the United States. For example, the most current (1995) overall age-adjusted Canadian cancer incidence rate is 391.98/100,000 with the four most commonly diagnosed cancers being lung (62.03/100,000), colon and rectum (50.91/100,000), female breast (49.46/100,000), and prostate in men (109.73/100,000), comprising over half of all newly diagnosed cancers in that country. As in the United States men are more often diagnosed with cancer than women and lung cancers are the leading cause of cancer-related death among both genders (National Cancer Institute of Canada, 2000). In the United Kingdom where cancer is responsible for 25 percent of all deaths, cancers of the lung, breast, large bowel (colon) and the prostate likewise account for half of all new cancer diagnoses. In addition, 23 percent of all cancer-related deaths are attributable to lung cancer with another almost 20 percent of all cancer-related deaths comprising colon and rectum cancer, female breast cancer, and prostate cancer in men (Parkin et al., 1999; Pisani et al., 1999).

Prevalence

The worldwide scope of cancer is alarming. In the United States alone, more than six million people living today have a history of cancer and of these it is estimated that more than four million were diagnosed five or more years ago. Of about one million Americans diagnosed annually with cancer, it is estimated that about half will be alive one year following diagnosis and treatment (American Cancer Society, 2000; Wingo et al., 1999). At the turn of this century, cancer is surpassed only by heart disease as the leading cause of death among American adults; one in four deaths is attributable to the disease. Since 1990, at least 13 million new cases of cancer have been diagnosed while in the year 2000 more than 1.2 million new cases of the disease were projected. It has been estimated that approximately 552,200 Americans—more than 1,500 daily—died of cancer in 2000 (American Cancer Society, 2000; Wingo et al., 1999).

Meanwhile, although there have been recently reported declines in US cancer incidence and mortality rates from 1990–1997, the mortality rate for all cancers combined was 169.9/100,000. The top four killers among Caucasians as well as all racial and ethnic groups were lung and bronchus (49.5/100,000), female breast (25.6/100,000), male prostate (25.4/100,000), and colon and rectum (17.6/100,000). In addition, mortality rates for African Americans were higher than for Caucasians, Asian and Pacific Islanders, American Indians/Alaska Natives, or Latinos (American Cancer Society, 2000).

Overall, Canadian mortality rate for the most recent year available (1997) is 188.95/100,000 with the most common causes of cancer-related death being lung (51.07/100,000), colon and rectum (23.62/100,000), female breast (27.41/100,000), and the prostate among men (28.34/100,000) (National Cancer Institute of Canada, 2000).

Economic Costs

In the United States, cancer-related economic costs are estimated to be at least $107 billion annually. Of these,

$37 billion reflects direct medical care costs (half for the treatment of lung, breast, and prostate cancers), $11 billion in indirect morbidity costs attributable to lost wages and related costs, and $59 billion in indirect mortality costs due to premature death. In a study involving outpatient chemotherapy patients, out-of-pocket indirect expenses were greater than 25 percent of weekly income for more than half of all families. Thus far, other indirect costs to family members and caregivers including those involving quality-of-life and psychological issues have not been comprehensively evaluated but are likely substantial (Brown & Fintor, 1994; Gold, Siegel, Russell, & Weinstein, 1996).

THEORIES

Primary prevention of adult cancer has drawn from a variety of theoretical approaches. Because risk varies with age, race, sex, socioeconomic status, occupation, and geography, these efforts are often tailored to specific target audiences. As such, depending on population characteristics, risk factors, and other variables, some theoretical models have been better suited than others to the task at hand and have had varying degrees of success. Some of the earliest interventions were based on changing behaviors using *Fear-Appeal* models in which adverse behaviors are modified as individuals recognize a linkage between their adverse behaviors and the development of disease.

The *Non-Monotonic* model extended this approach by arguing that fear can act either as a drive to motivate accepting desired behavior or as a *cue* to prompt habitual responses that in turn interfere with accepting behavioral messages. Thus, the optimal changes in behavior occur when there is a moderate amount of fear arousal (McGuire, 1969).

Another model, *Parallel Process*, describes two different responses (cognitive and emotional) resulting from exposure to fear stimuli. Risk-reducing behaviors then derive from attempts to mitigate the actual risk rather than the fear (Janis, 1967).

As investigators expanded their knowledge of cancer-related behavioral risks during the early 1970s, refined theories of fear appeal began to emerge and were adapted for primary prevention. *Protection-Motivation Theory* described three different factors of fear appeal messages as perceptions involving the severity of disease consequence, the likelihood that it would occur, and the efficacy of behavioral response. These factors coupled with cognitive mediators then multiply to motivate behavior change termed "protection motivation" with the magnitude of this motivation proportional to desired changes in attitudes, intent, and behavior change. This theory was later expanded to include self-efficacy as a fourth factor of fear appeal and postulated that these factors interact to prompt an individual to either appraise threats or cope with them. Threats are appraised by weighing the perceived benefits from engaging in risk-related behaviors versus the perceived degree of risk (susceptibility and severity). Coping appraisals involve behavioral adaptations which function as the response costs of a given behavior subtracted from perceived responses and self-efficacy. In both the early and later versions of this approach, fear affects the acceptance of risk reduction messages based on "severity of appraisal" (Rogers, 1975, 1983).

In the early 1980s, *Subjective–Expected Utility Model* (SEU) emerged with a comprehensive treatment of the interactions among fear-intentions and behaviors, fear-response efficacy, instructions, recommendations, and communication and recipient factors. This approach postulates that fear itself does not have a causal relationship with behavioral change, but rather results from cognitive acknowledgment of a perceived threat. In this model, individuals assess a variety of alternative behaviors before choosing those that will maximize SEU. In this respect, SEU is itself a product of subjective values and utilities relative to the potential outcomes of the alternatives. The individual assesses the subjective probabilities that the alternative behaviors will actually result in a given disease outcome (Sutton, 1982).

Leventhal (1970) described the *Parallel Process Model* in an effort to explain the process by which messages embodying threats and efficacy are perceived and processed. According to this model, perceived threats are controlled through protective attitudes, intentions, and behaviors. In addition, fear itself is also controlled by avoidance or denial. Fear arousal is initiated by perceived threats and may have a reciprocal relationship in perceptions of threats. Threats and associated fears motivate a response that is determined by efficacy such that the response will be to perceive actual danger or to control fear. In cases where the perception of a threat is low, there is little or no response. When the perception of a threat is high, low perceptions of efficacy lead to fear which is then mitigated through fear control actions. When perceptions of efficacy are high under these circumstances, the result is danger control. Danger control actions are driven by cognition of the threat and efficacy while fear is driven by fear control actions. This model has been revisited and expanded by incorporating various elements of many previously mentioned models.

RESEARCH

Smoking, diet, infectious diseases, and other environmental factors are estimated to be responsible for more than 75 percent of all US cancers diagnosed. Voluntary behavioral risks such as smoking as well as poor diet, physical inactivity, and obesity comprise significantly more individual cancer-related risk than industrial pollutants, chemicals, radiation, drug therapies, and other exposures combined. Still, it is important to acknowledge that risk from carcinogens is determined by the length of exposure as well as the concentration and intensity of exposure (Harvard Center for Cancer Prevention, 1996).

Research in the primary prevention of adult cancers has focused on behavioral and lifestyle factors as well as risk reduction and prevention of exposure to environmental and viral carcinogens. Behavioral and lifestyle interventions have largely targeted smoking, nutrition, and physical activity, while other efforts have concentrated on exposure to ultraviolet and other types of radiation as well as reducing risks of cancer-associated viral pathogens and promoting workplace safety. These efforts have often been multifaceted and frequently involved public policy interventions as well as screening (Wingo et al., 1999).

Perhaps the most concentrated efforts have been in the area of tobacco control. The United States currently has among the world's highest smoking-related death rates with at least 87 percent of lung cancer deaths and about 30 percent of all cancer deaths the result of smoking. Smoking and the use of smokeless tobacco products has been associated with cancers of the lung and bronchus, the esophagus, oral cavities, as well as other sites. Even though there have been steady declines in overall smoking prevalence among US adults since the early 1960s, 48 million adults currently smoke with recent trends indicating that Americans now begin smoking at earlier ages (American Cancer Society, 2000; Centers for Disease Control and Prevention, 1993; Wingo et al., 1999). Interventions which have been given the highest priorities include individual and community-based smoking cessation programs, tobacco awareness efforts targeting children, and tobacco control regulation and legislation in areas such as taxation, sales, and advertising (Wingo et al., 1999).

Diet and nutrition has been another area of intense primary prevention interest. Currently, at least one third of all US cancer-related deaths annually are attributable to adult diet, obesity, and alcohol. These have been linked to cancers of the colon and rectum, stomach, breast, lung, liver, and other sites. According to the *Third National Health and Nutritional Examination Survey* (NHANES), the prevalence of obesity has increased dramatically since 1976 among both men and women while increases in obesity observed among US children are expected to result in even greater increases in rates of adult obesity (Enns, Goldman, & Cook, 1997; Flegal, Carroll, Kuczmarski, & Johnson, 1998).

Public health advocates have especially targeted nonsmoking adults for interventions aimed at better nutritional choice and balancing caloric intake with increased physical activity. Among those factors that have been incorporated into these primary prevention activities is reducing alcohol use, increasing the variety and choice of foods, low-fat preparation methods, and reducing portion sizes. Emphasis has been placed on reducing cancer risk by increasing fruits, vegetables, grains, and beans while limiting meat and dairy products and restricting high-fat foods (Harvard Center for Cancer Prevention, 1996; United States Department of Health and Human Services, 1996).

Diets high in fiber, fruits, and vegetables but low in fat coupled with regular physical activity has been heavily promoted to lower the cancer risks associated with obesity. Elevated risk for postmenopausal breast cancers as well as cancers of the uterus, ovary, and gallbladder have all been associated with obesity. In addition, women who are 35 percent or more above their ideal body weight are 1.5 times more likely to develop these cancers. For men, increased risk of colon and prostate cancers have been associated with obesity while those more than 35 percent above their ideal body weight are thought to be 1.4 times more likely to develop these cancers (Harvard Center for Cancer Prevention, 1996; United States Department of Health and Human Services, 1996).

In addition to smoking, diet, and exercise, primary prevention interventions have also begun targeting hormonal, viral, and other environmental risks. Breast cancer prevention trials are currently underway to evaluate the value of chemopreventive agents such as hormone suppressors and phytoestrogenic compounds. Other interventions involve the use of vaccines for hepatitis B (HBV)—a known risk factor for liver cancer—as well as developing vaccine aimed at preventing infection with human papilloma virus (HPV) associated with cervical cancer as well as gastric *H. pylori* that has been linked with stomach cancer. In addition, a number of efforts have been launched to reduce excessive sun exposure associated with melanoma and other skin cancers. In many developing nations, the prevention of hepatitis C (HCV) exposure and aflatoxin B1 contamination have become priorities in reducing the risk of liver cancer (American Cancer Society, 2000; Keesling & Friedman, 1995; Parkin et al., 1999; Peto, Lopez, Boreham, Thun, & Health, 1994).

STRATEGIES THAT WORK

Smoking prevention and cessation interventions are among the most varied and comprehensive cancer prevention and control activities. These behavioral approaches often rely on three separate cognitive–behavioral theoretical models: *Stages of Change* (SOC), *Health Belief Model* (HBM), and *Consumer Information Processing* (CIP). These models share the idea that individual behavior is influenced by knowledge but that knowledge alone is not sufficient to change behavior.

SOC models have been used successfully in adult smoking cessation interventions and more recently in promoting better nutrition. SOC-derived interventions attempt to reach individuals at varying stages of their motivation to change adverse behaviors. SOC models are characterized by five distinct "stages" (precontemplation, contemplation, decision/determination, action, and maintenance) of changing health behaviors. Thus, an individual attempting to stop smoking might be at any one of these motivational stages and interventions can be tailored to reach those at each stage (Prochaska, DiClemete, & Norcross, 1992).

The second category of theoretical models is the most widely used conceptual framework in adult cancer prevention. HBMs rely on cognitive messages (such as those in fear-appeal) that assume individuals will balance risk against behavioral change and make appropriate choices. With a heavy reliance on the role of risk messaging, this model is useful in cancer awareness campaigns that are part of mass media interventions, the development of health promotional materials, and individual counseling. This theory describes the key factors in determining whether individuals change their behaviors as perceived susceptibility, perceived severity, perceived benefits, perceived barriers, cue to action, and self-efficacy (Rosenstock, Strecher, & Becker, 1988).

The third general category of cancer-related interventions involves CIP models. This approach assumes that cancer prevention messages compete for attention and priority among many other risk-related messages that individuals receive. The sheer volume of information forces the receiver to develop coping strategies for assessing the personal value of each message based on information *availability*, perceived *usefulness*, and the *ease* with which it can be adapted and used (Bettman, 1979).

The three categories provide the foundation for a series of interpersonal theories used to explain and modify individual behaviors. These include *Social Learning Theory* or *Social Cognitive* approaches and *Community-Level Models*.

Albert Bandura's *Social Learning Theory* or *Social Cognitive Theory*, describes dynamic interactions among individual factors, the environment, and behavior. These have three components: *cognition*, *behavior*, and *emotion*. These components in turn involve *reciprocal determinism* (dynamic, but alterable relationships between the individual and the environment), *behavioral capability* (knowledge and skill), *expectations* (beliefs about the consequences of actions), *self-efficacy* (the belief that the individual will be successful in performing a certain action), *observational learning*, and *reinforcement* (Bandura, 1986).

Observational learning and *reinforcement* rely on the role played by influential individuals in modeling behaviors. In smoking, physical activity, and dietary interventions, role models who have successfully stopped smoking or lost weight often motivates others. Whether the desired changes in behavior can be sustained in the short term often depends on *reinforcements* such as praise, encouragement, and other "rewards." In smoking cessation and weight management examples include gifts and refundable participation fees. Whether these behaviors can be sustained over time, however, is determined both by self-efficacy and by using strategies such as monitoring, contracting, and goal-setting.

Community-Level Models are often used in smoking prevention and cessation campaigns. They are comprehensive, multilevel interventions that often involve schools, religious and community groups, local governments, the local media and information systems, public health agencies, work sites, health insurers, professional societies, volunteer organizations and other groups. These programs can be less cost intensive on a per-person basis since they reach larger audiences, however, at the same time they often sacrifice the flexibility of more tailored individual interventions. Still, these models are particularly useful for integrating a variety of approaches involving public policy and organizational change (Rothman & Tropman, 1987).

STRATEGIES THAT MIGHT WORK

Despite several intense national campaigns, the results of dietary changes for primary prevention purposes have been mixed. Although more than two thirds of American adults believe it is important to consume more fruits and vegetables, there have been only small increases in actual consumption. At the same time, while less than one third of all Americans believe that consuming more grain products is important, there has been a 40 percent increase in consumption of bread, cereal, rice, and pasta during the same period. However, even though dietary fat consumption decreased from 40 percent in the late 1970s to 33 percent in the mid 1990s, only one third of adults currently meet guidelines of 30 percent or less (Enns et al., 1997; United States Department of Agriculture, 1999).

Meanwhile, interventions aimed at increasing physical activity and exercise have been less successful. According to recent survey data, less than 16 percent of Americans engage in regular light-to-moderate or vigorous physical activity in their leisure time and almost one quarter lead sedentary lifestyles. Researchers note that one in five American men and one in four women are not physically active outside their workplace (United States Department of Health and Human Services, 1998).

While the construction of fear-based messages has demonstrated utility, there has been concern over their ability to sustain behavioral change over time. Thus, contemporary interventions often rely on a broader array of social and behavioral models in which these messaging approaches can be incorporated (Witte, 1994).

Efforts derived from the *Theory of Reasoned Action* (TRA) that have involved altering attitudes and behaviors among those at high risk for skin cancers through sun exposure have also been mixed. Some researchers have noted that knowledge—not fear—is a significant predictor of attitudes, intentions, and behaviors; others have concluded that successful interventions will increasingly have to rely on intensive, targeted, individual efforts rather than large media campaigns involving fear appeal. In addition, tailoring these programs to racial and ethnic population subgroups continues to present a significant challenge (Griffin, Neuwirth, & Dunwoody, 1995).

Use of the *HBM, TRA/Theory of Planned Behavior* (TPB), and *Transtheoretical Model* (TTM) in designing intervention for minorities has been limited by social and cultural factors specific to these groups. For example, the *HBM* may not adequately address economic and social concerns that influence attitudes and beliefs about cancer risk among African Americans and other groups. Similarly, TRA/TPB models assume that behavioral intent will result in behavioral change while the TTM assumes that individuals can change behaviors based on information. Critics have argued that these models are inadequate for African Americans and other minorities because they do not address social and cultural factors such as interconnectedness, religiosity, and health system barriers (United States Department of Health and Human Services, 1998).

STRATEGIES THAT DO NOT WORK

It is difficult to say what strategies do not work. Rather, I have tried to state above what works less well. The etiology of cancer in adults remains poorly understood, and we have all-too-often witnessed a "yo-yo" effect in the literature—especially the popular press—where some preventive action was announced, and then soon thereafter, retracted. The jury is still out on many of these approaches.

SYNTHESIS

The heavy burden of cancer-related morbidity, mortality, and economic cost has made primary prevention efforts a national priority. Despite a better understanding of cancer risk and human behavior, existing theoretical applications have not provided a panacea. Smoking cessation interventions have been successful in the short term but preventing relapses has proven problematic. This has lead public health advocates to increasingly design intervention aimed at preventing tobacco use among adolescents and children.

Thus, an ecological intervention perspective has emerged in which multidimensional, multilevel prevention activities are undertaken. In addition to interventions which stress individual behavioral change, consideration is also given to public policy, advocacy, organizational and environmental change, economic support, and often a linkage to secondary and tertiary preventive interventions (McLeroy, Bibeau, Steckler, & Glanz, 1988).

Among the approaches generating serious interest are *cognitive–behavioral models*. These acknowledge the mediation of behavior through attitudes and knowledge in conjunction with existing social environment and perceptions of risk, motivation to change behavior, and the skills available to initiate and sustain these changes. This reflects an appreciation of multiple factors that affect behavior including those that are intrapersonal/individual, interpersonal, institutional/organizational, community, and public policy-oriented. In addition, they incorporate individuals as well as their communities by involving families, peers and public role models, health care providers, and public health advocates. At another level, schools, community organizations and religious groups, and other institutions provide a forum for support and reinforcement. In this context, the concept of *reciprocal causation* is key to understanding that the individual both *influences* and is *influenced by* the social environment.

More recent efforts have used emerging technologies for interactive health communication in primary cancer prevention efforts. These have included modalities such as health kiosks and electronic mail reminders. The short- and long-term efficacy of these approaches, however, remains to be seen (Fintor, 1998).

It is apparent that successful primary prevention efforts for cancer must not only integrate existing theoretical approaches but must also be multidimensional; they must be comprehensive yet flexible enough to address the social, cultural, and economic factors specific to target populations. As the complex relationships between risk and behavior is better understood, cost-effective primary prevention efforts will no doubt lead to significant reductions in the heavy burden of cancer incidence, mortality, and related costs in the coming decades.

Also see: Chronic Disease: Adulthood; Perceived Personal Control; Physical Fitness: Adulthood.

References

Altman, A., & Sarge, M.J. (1992). *The cancer dictionary*. New York: Facts on File.

American Cancer Society. (2000). *Cancer facts & figures 2000*. Atlanta: Author.

Bandura, A. (1986). *Social foundations of thought and action*. Englewood Cliffs, NJ: Prentice-Hall.

Bettman, J.R. (1979). *An information processing theory of consumer choice*. Reading, MA: Addison-Wesley.

Brown, M., & Fintor, L. (1994). The economic burden of cancer. In P. Greenwald, B. Kramer, & D. Weed (Eds.), *The science and practice of cancer prevention and control* (pp. 69–81). New York: Marcel Dekker.

Centers for Disease Control and Prevention. (1993). Cigarette smoking-attributable mortality and years of potential life lost—United States, 1990. *Morbidity & Mortality Weekly Report, 42*, 645–649.

Enns, C.W., Goldman, J.D., & Cook, A. (1997). Trends in food and nutrient intakes by adults: NFS 1977–78, CSFII 1989–91, and CSFII 1994–95. *Family Economics and Nutrition Review, 10*, 3.

Fintor, L. (1998). The Michigan health kiosk: Cancer info on the go. *Journal of the National Cancer Institute, 90*, 809–810.

Flegal, K.M., Carroll M.D., Kuczmarski, R.J., & Johnson, C.L. (1998). Overweight and obesity in the United States: Prevalence and trends, 1960–1994. *International Journal of Obesity, 22*(1), 39–47.

Gold, M.R., Siegel, J.E., Russell, L.B., & Weinstein, M.C. (1996). *Cost-effectiveness in health and medicine*. New York: Oxford University Press.

Griffin, R.J., Neuwirth, K., & Dunwoody, S. (1995). Using the theory of reasoned action to examine the health impact of risk messages. *Communication Yearbook, 18*, 201–228.

Harvard Center for Cancer Prevention. (1996). Harvard report on cancer prevention. *Cancer Causes & Control, 7*(Suppl. 1), S10–S55.

Janis, I.L. (1967). Effects of fear arousal on attitude change: Recent developments in theory and experimental research. In L. Berkowitz (Ed.), *Advances in experimental social psychology* (Vol. 3, pp. 166–225). New York: Academic Press.

Keesling, B., & Friedman, H.S. (1995). Interventions to prevent skin cancer: Experimental evaluation of informational and fear appeals. *Psychology and Health, 10*, 477–490.

Leventhal, H. (1970). Findings and theory in the study of fear communications. In L. Berkowitz (Ed.), *Advances in experimental social psychology* (Vol. 5, pp. 119–186). New York: Academic Press.

McGuire, W.J. (1969). The nature of attitudes and attitude change. In G. Lindzey & E. Aronson (Eds.), *The handbook of social psychology* (Vol. 3, pp. 136–314). Reading, MA: Addison-Wesley.

McLeroy, K.R., Bibeau, D., Steckler, A., & Glanz, K. (1988). An ecological perspective on health promotion programs. *Health Education Quarterly, 15*, 351–377.

National Cancer Institute of Canada. (2000). *Canadian cancer statistics 2000*. Toronto: Author.

Parkin, D.M., Pisani, P., & Ferlay, J. (1999). Estimates of the worldwide incidence of 25 major cancers in 1990. *International Journal of Cancer, 80*, 827–841.

Peto, R., Lopez, A.D., Boreham, J., Thun, M., & Health, C. (1994). *Mortality from smoking in developed countries, 1950–2000: Indirect estimates from national vital statistics*. New York: Oxford University Press.

Pisani, P., Parkin, D.M., Bray, F., & Ferlay, J. (1999). Estimates of the worldwide mortality from 25 cancers in 1990. *International Journal of Cancer, 83*, 18–29.

Prochaska, J.O., DiClemente, C.C., & Norcross, J.C. (1992). In search of how people change: Applications to addictive behaviors. *American Psychologist, 47*, 1102–1114.

Rogers, R.W. (1975). A Protection Motivation Theory of fear appeals and attitude change. *Journal of Psychology, 91*, 93–114.

Rogers, R.W. (1983). Cognitive and physiological processes in fear appeals and attitude change: A revised theory of protection motivation. In J. Cacioppo & R. Petty (Eds.), *Social Psychophysiology* (pp. 153–176). New York: Guilford.

Rosenstock, I.M., Strecher, V.J., Becker, M.H. (1988). Social learning theory and the health belief model. *Health Education Quarterly, 15*, 175–183.

Rothman, J., & Tropman, J.E. (1987) Models of community organization and macro practice: Their mixing and phasing. In F.M. Cox, J.L. Ehrlich, J. Rothman, & J.E. Tropman (Eds.), *Strategies of community organization.* Itasca. Illinois: Peacock.

Sutton, S.R. (1982). Fear-arousing communications: A critical examination of theory and research. In J.R. Eiser (Ed.), *Social psychology and behavioral medicine* (pp. 303–337). London: Wiley.

United States Department of Agriculture. (1999). *Results from the 1994–96 continuing survey of food intakes by individuals.* Agricultural Research Service. Beltsville Human Nutrition Research Center, Food Surveys Research Group, Beltsville, Maryland. It is available from the National Technical Information Service, Springfield, VA, accession number PB2000-500027.

United States Department of Health and Human Services. (1996). *Physical activity and health: A report of the Surgeon General.* Atlanta: Author, Centers for Disease Control and Prevention, National Center for Chronic Disease Prevention and Health Promotion.

United States Department of Health and Human Services. (1998). *Tobacco use among US racial/ethnic minority groups—African Americans, American Indians and Alaska Natives, Asian Americans and Pacific Islanders, and Hispanics: A report of the Surgeon General.* Atlanta: Author, Centers for Disease Control and Prevention, National Center for Chronic Disease Prevention and Health Promotion, Office on Smoking and Health.

Wingo, P.A. et al. (1999). Annual Report to the nation on the status of cancer, 1973–1996, with a special report on lung cancer and tobacco smoking. *Journal of the National Cancer Institute, 91,* 675–690.

Witte, K. (1994). Generating effective risk messages: How scary should your risk communication be? *Communication Yearbook, 18,* 229–254.

Cancer, Older Adulthood

Elizabeth M. Bertera

INTRODUCTION

This entry discusses the importance of non-medical approaches to preventing cancer in older adults, which is a major cause of death in this age group. Advances in medicine and public health have made it possible for people to live longer. If certain types of cancer are diagnosed in the early stages, high survival rates can be attained. Moreover, if cancer can be prevented, health care costs to the individual and to society can be minimized.

DEFINITIONS AND SCOPE

The major causes of death throughout history have been natural disasters, infant mortality, and a variety of infectious diseases. In developed nations with technological advances in public health and medicine, infectious diseases

have basically been eliminated as a cause of premature death. Mortality rates are down extending years of life. The reduction in mortality rates has led to an enormous and historically unique increase in the older population. Replacing infectious diseases has been a dramatic rise in the incidence and prevalence of lifestyle-related and stress-related chronic degenerative diseases. Among the most common causes of death today are heart disease, cancer, stroke, and diabetes. These chronic degenerative diseases, which count for a relatively long period of infirmity toward the end of life, represent the greatest health problems for the elderly. Although there is little hope for cure of these diseases through traditional medical means, their onset can be postponed through modification of risk factors (Sperry & Prosen, 1996).

One of the adopted resolutions of the 1995 White Conference on Aging made specific recommendations for education and training in social work in the area of Health Promotion and Disease Prevention (Saltz, 1997). *Health promotion* has been described by Green and Kreuter (1991) as "any combination of health education and related organizational, political, and economic changes conducive to health." Health promotion and disease prevention targeted to older persons should be designed to maximize length of life, but as important and more so, should focus on improving and maintaining good quality of life. *Disease prevention* consists of efforts to prevent disease (e.g., education, immunizations, and chemoprophylaxis).

Adults aged 65 and older represent an important growing segment of the US population. Cancer is an important cause of death in this group. Thus, the greatest risk for developing cancer is age, yet little is known about the cancer-related knowledge, attitudes and beliefs of the older adult (Fitch, Greenberg, Levstein, Muir, Plante, & King, 1997). Furthermore, much less is known about designing health promotion and early detection programs responsive to the learning needs of older adults (Muir, Greenberg, Plante, Fitch, Levstein, & King, 1997).

Approximately 16,000 new cases of invasive cancer are diagnosed each year and about 5,000 women die of this disease annually; 40 percent are aged 65 and older. The incidence of breast cancer rises with age and does not level off until age 85 or later. Colorectal cancer increases in incidence throughout old age. It was estimated that in 1996, approximately 317,000 men in the United States would receive a new diagnosis of prostate cancer and that of these 41,400 would die of it. Prostate cancer is the most common cancer diagnosed in men in the United States and the second most common cause of cancer death. Nonmelanoma skin cancers are the most common malignancies found in older adults. The incidence of basal and squamous cell carcinoma increases with age (Gallo, Busby-Whtehead, Rabins, Silliman, Murphy, & Reichel, 1999). According to the American Cancer Society

(ACS) estimates, 1,228,600 Americans were diagnosed with cancer in 1998 and approximately 568,800 people die of cancer during the year. The ACS estimates are based on an increase in the number of older Americans, who are at higher risk for developing cancer—one half of the cases occur in persons aged 65 and over. The top four causes of cancer death in the United States during 1990–1995 for all racial and ethnic groups were the same for sites as for incidence: More than 50 percent of all cancer deaths involved the lung, female breast, prostate, or colon/rectum. Persons 65 years and older bear the major burden of these malignancies. The percentages of deaths for this age group are lung (68.6 percent), female breast (58.5 percent), prostate (91.8 percent), and colon/rectum (77.0 percent).

Examination of cancer death rates for each of these sites by gender, race, and ethnicity revealed (with the exception of female lung cancer) that African Americans had higher cancer deaths rates than Whites, Asians and Pacific Islanders, or Latinos. African Americans have a vastly different cancer experience from Whites. Statistics show that African Americans have higher age-adjusted incidence and mortality rates for many cancers and lower survival rates than do Whites for all but 6 of the 25 primary cancer sites. Among the top 10 sites that were common to all four racial and ethnic groups were cancers of the pancreas, stomach, and ovary. Otherwise, the causes of cancer death among the top 10 leading sites varied by racial and ethnic group. Deaths due to cancer of the brain and central nervous system were among the top 10 mortality sites only in Whites; death due to cancer of the esophagus, cervix, and multiple myeloma were among the top 10 sites only in African Americans; and liver cancer deaths were among the top 10 sites only in Asians and Pacific Islanders and Latinos. Overall, 70 percent of cancer deaths occur in the age group 65 years and older.

The Latino cancer experience also differs from that of the White population, with Latinos having higher rates of cervical, esophageal, gallbladder, and stomach cancers. For the vast majority of cancers, including melanomas, lymphomas, and cancers of the colon, rectum, breast, and lung, Latinos are afflicted at a rate that is either the same as or lower than that of European Whites. However, among the Latino population alone, Valdez, Delgado, Cervantes, and Bowler (1993) have found the highest incidence rates for cancers of the stomach, esophagus, gallbladder, and liver.

Most common among men are cancers of the prostate, lung, and colon; most common among women are cancer of the breast, colon, and cervix (Molina & Aguirre-Molina, 1994). About 30 percent of all cancer deaths (over 175,000 deaths per year) are related to smoking. Lung cancer mortality rates for women continue to exceed the mortality rates for breast cancer. Many cancers related to dietary factors also can be prevented. Scientific evidence suggests that approximately one third of the cancer deaths that will occur this year is related to diet. In addition, many of the skin and lip cancers diagnosed this year could be prevented by limiting exposure to the sun and by wearing protective clothing and using sunscreens (Satcher, 1998).

In addition to the human toll of cancer, the financial costs of cancer are enormous. The National Cancer Institute (NCI) estimates that the overall costs for cancer are $107 billion, with $37 billion for direct medical costs, $11 billion for morbidity costs, and $59 billion for mortality costs. Treatment for lung, breast, and prostate cancers account for more than half of the direct medical costs. Although elderly Americans represent one eighth of the population, they account for more than one third of the total health care expenditures (Satcher, 1998). In view of the serious health problems many aged persons face, it is not surprising that they make heavy use of a range of health care services. If past patterns continue, as the elderly population grows, major increases can be expected in the use of hospitals and other health care services by the aged.

THEORIES AND RESEARCH

The *ecological perspective* has gained respectability in the social sciences and health promotion. Health promotion is relatively young, but ecology is not. One finds several streams of thought and action from which ecological perspectives have influenced health promotion. In the recent past, ecology influenced public health education and before that, public health. These disciplines converged with various social and behavioral sciences and other professional perspectives to form the ecological and behavioral foundation of health promotion (Poland, Green, & Rootman, 2000). The ecological perspective has become a popular framework for social work practice as a leading exemplar of nonmedical approaches, and is derived from earlier ecological theories that were popular in the fields of anthropology, sociology, and psychology. First introduced to social work by Germain (1973), the ecological perspective has been proposed as a unifying paradigm that can apply to the numerous and diverse models of social work practice. A basic assumption here is that people strive for a goodness of fit with their environments because of their interdependence between them, and in doing so, people and their environments constantly change and shape one another. This adaptation process, which involves biological, psychological, social, and cultural elements, is both reciprocal and continuous (Germain, 1973; Germain & Bloom, 1999). Unlike psychoanalytic theory, which assumes psychic determinism, or behavior theory which assumes environmental determinism, the ecological perspective views humans as purposive and goal seeking. As such, people make choices and decisions and are seen as being relatively free from deterministic forces outside their control. Given this perspective, the focus is on growth, development, and potentialities. The environment, which is physical and social, can either support or fail to support the adaptive achievements of autonomy, competence, identity formation, and relatedness to others.

The earliest formulations and applications of public health employed ecological concepts. The 19th century development of biological, especially Darwinian concepts of the "web of life" and the role of the environment and adaptation influenced public health science which first sought to ensure the survival of the human species by controlling the physical environment. Epidemiologists remained almost exclusively preoccupied with the physical, chemical, and biological environments until the 1960s. The refocusing of epidemiology on chronic diseases in the 1960s added a growing concern with behavioral determinants of health, accelerated in the 1980s with the advent of HIV and AIDS as the newest epidemic. As the behavioral emphasis narrowed the focus and the methodologies of epidemiology, health promotion sought to widen the focus to include social, economic, organizational, and political environments as determinants of health and points of interventions.

Learning theory has always given prominence to the interaction of learner and environment. These have been elaborated in *Social Learning Theory* (now *Social Cognitive Theory*) and its core concept of reciprocal determinism between person and environment (Poland et al., 2000). The ecological view of behavior holds that the organism's functioning is mediated by behavior–environment interaction. This has two implications for behavioral and social change:

1. Environment largely controls or sets limits on the behavior that occurs in it.
2. People can change environmental variables, resulting in the modification of behavior.

These two points lead to the inexorable recognition that health promotion can achieve its best results by exercising whatever control or influence it can over the environment. But the reciprocal side of this perspective also holds that the behavior of individuals, groups, and organizations also influences their environments. Hence, health promotion seeks to empower people by giving them control over the determinants of their health, whether these be behavioral or environmental (Poland et al., 2000).

STRATEGIES THAT WORK

Research on preventing diseases or limiting disabilities in older populations has been illuminating. Studies of lifestyle behaviors such as fitness, diet, smoking, and alcohol use suggest that a healthy lifestyle can lead to greater health and longevity (Fallcreek & Mettler, 1984; Guralnik, Fried, Simonsick, Kasper, & Laferty, 1995; La Croix, Newton, Leveille, & Wallace, 1997).

Disease prevention through dietary management is a cost-effective approach to promoting healthy aging. Fats, cholesterol, soluble fiber, and the trace elements copper and chromium affect the morbidity and mortality of coronary heart disease. Decreasing sodium and increasing potassium intake improves control of hypertension. Calcium and magnesium may also have a role in controlling hypertension. The antioxidant vitamins A and beta-carotene, vitamin C, vitamin E, and the trace mineral selenium may protect against some types of cancer. A decrease in simple carbohydrates and an increase in soluble dietary fiber may normalize moderately elevated blood glucose levels. Deficiencies of zinc or iron diminish immune function. Adequate levels of calcium and vitamin D can help prevent senile osteoporosis in older men and women (Johnson & Kligman, 1992). The Healthy People National Health Promotion and Disease Prevention Cancer Objectives for the year 2000 include decreasing dietary fat intake to an average of 30 percent of calories or less and average saturated fat intake to less than 10 percent of calories among people aged 2 and older (Horwath, 1989).

LaCroix and Omenn (1992) studied the benefits of smoking cessation in older adults. Older smokers who quit have a reduced risk of death compared with current smokers within 1–2 years after quitting. Their overall risk of death approaches that of those who never smoked after 15–20 years of abstinence. Smoking cessation in older adults markedly reduces the risks of coronary events and of cardiac death within 1 year of quitting, and risk continues to decline more gradually for many years. This is true for older adults both with and without a previous history of coronary disease and symptoms. Quitting reduces risks of dying from several smoking-related cancers. Although the decline in risk may be more gradual for older than middle-aged adults, the benefits of cessation are apparent within 5–10 years of quitting. Continued smoking in late life is associated with the development and progression of several major chronic conditions, loss of mobility, and poorer physical function. Former smokers appear to have higher levels of physical function and better quality of life than continuing smokers. They concluded the prospects are excellent that smoking cessation after age 65 will extend both the number of years of life and the quality of life.

Older adults are an important audience for smoking cessation programs. Over 4.5 million older adults (older than 65) continue to smoke, and the majority are long-term, heavy smokers. Rimer and Orleans (1994) point to evidence that smoking cessation programs tailored to older smokers can be effective, such as the ACS materials and programs. They reviewed the rationale for tailoring programs to older adults. Rimer and Orleans (1994) also describe the Clear Horizons program as an example of a tailored program which resulted in significantly higher rates of quitting—20 percent of Clear Horizons participants reported not smoking at 12 months compared with 15 percent for the generic guide—a general guide not tailored to older adults. They concluded that older smokers were responsive to a tailored program.

Salive, Cornoni-Huntley, LaCroix, Ostfeld, Wallace, and Hennekens (1992) examined longitudinal changes in smoking behavior among older adults in three community cohorts of the Established Populations for Epidemiologic Studies of the Elderly. Smoking prevalence declined from 15 percent at baseline to 9 percent during 6 years of follow-up. Annual smoking cessation and relapse rates were 10 percent and less than 1 percent, respectively. Interval diagnosis of myocardial infarction, stroke, or cancer increased subsequent smoking cessation but not relapse. Although smoking cessation occurred in the presence of an untoward diagnosis, primary prevention could yield greater benefits.

Goldberg and Chavin (1997) reviewed issues and studies relating to preventive medicine and screening in older adults and concluded that the goal of preventive medicine in older people should be not only reduction of premature morbidity and mortality but also the preservation of function and quality of life. Emphasis should be on offering the best proven and most effective interventions to the individuals at highest risk of important problems such as cardiovascular diseases, malignancies, infectious and endocrine diseases, and other important threats to function in older people. Breast cancer screening, smoking cessation, hypertension treatment, and vaccination for infectious diseases are thus far among the most firmly proven and well accepted specific preventive measures, with physical exercise also being particularly promising.

STRATEGIES THAT MIGHT WORK

Screening for cancer can be an important part in reducing cancer mortality. Walsh (1992) reviews and addresses screening for breast, cervical, prostate, lung, colorectal, and ovarian cancer in older Americans. Decisions about screening for cancer must consider the effects of screening, diagnostic evaluations, and treatments on the quality of life of each person (Walsh, 1992). Wardle et al. (2000) reported their randomized controlled trial of the efficacy of flexible sigmoidoscopy—examination of the intestines—for the prevention of bowel cancer. The aim of the study was to establish the predictive power of the Health Belief Model (HBM) and to evaluate the contribution of HBM elements in mediating the effect of other demographic and health variables, which have been found to be associated with screening interest and participation. A total of 5,099 participants were sent a postal questionnaire, which examined cancer worry, bowel symptoms, health status, state anxiety, and optimism. The response rate was 72 percent. The results showed that threat, barriers, and benefits explained 47 percent of the variance in interest. By addressing these points, the decision processes for participating in cancer screening, we might be able to increase the level of participation in community samples (Wardle et al., 2000).

Weinrich, Weinrich, Boyd, Atwood, and Cervenka (1994) in their ecologically oriented research on "teaching older adults by adapting for aging changes," used a quasi-experimental pretest–posttest design to measure their Adaptation for Aging Changes (ACC) Method on fecal occult blood screening (FOBS) at meals sites for the elderly in the South. The average age of participants was 72 years; average educational level was 8th grade, over half of the sample was African American; and half of the participants had incomes below the poverty level. Results suggested increase in participation in FOBS in participants taught by the ACC Method (χ^2 (1, $n = 56$) = 6.34, $p = 0.02$: odds ratio = 6.2). This research provides support for teaching that makes adaptation for aging changes, especially adaptations to participant characteristics and actual practice of the procedure.

Bertera (1999) examined the perceived health promotion needs and interest of low-income older women and men attending four senior centers and two nutrition sites. The health topics of greatest interest to older women were exercise (57.6 percent), making friends (50.9 percent), nutrition (37.5 percent), losing weight (33.6 percent), and home safety (34.6 percent). Compared with women, men were significantly more interested in exercise and its effect on mood (4.3 vs. 24.0 percent) and love and sex after 60 (44.8 vs. 18.2 percent) and significantly less interested in nutrition (17.2 vs. 37.5 percent). The fitness activities of greatest interest to women were walking (63.1 percent), back exercises (37.5 percent), toning to music (22.1 percent), and self-defense (18.2 percent) none of which was significantly different from the men in the sample. Barriers to participation most often cited were transportation, scheduling, and cost factors. These kinds of health interests offer many possibilities to address the prevention of cancer among the elderly.

Muir et al. (1997) developed a collaborative project with the intent of designing appropriate health promotion programs for early detection of cancer in older adults. The initial work included a community needs assessment using focus groups, one-on-one interviews, and self-report surveys. The use of key community contacts was effective in locating older adults through pre-established linkages with agencies. Various ethno-cultural groups, low-income communities and isolated individuals, as well as other pre-established groups, were included in this study. The needs assessment found that age is not perceived as a cancer risk factor; transportation is a barrier to screening; fear inhibits people from being screened; physicians are viewed as both the main source of expert cancer knowledge and as the gatekeepers to screening; family and peers are the main source of support, ethno-specific groups have different information needs; and that lifestyle suggestions can reduce the risk of cancer. The findings indicated that promising community health promotion programs for older adults would require multiple approaches with a combination of strategies in order to meet their learning needs.

STRATEGIES THAT DO NOT WORK

Rubenstein (1994) looked for strategies to overcome barriers to early detection of cancer among older adults and found that if health professionals wish to help increase the number of older adults who get screened regularly to detect cancer at an early stage, they must first understand the barriers to screening that older people experience (Rubenstein, 1994). For example, sigmoidoscopy, an expensive and more invasive procedure that is generally recommended as an effective cancer screening tool, was reported less likely to be practiced than prostate cancer screening, a cheaper and less invasive procedure without such recommendation. Of the types of screening about which Fried, Rosenberg, and Lipsitz (1995) asked (cholesterol, rectal exam, influenza vaccination, sigmoidoscopy, mammography, prostate cancer screening, organ donation, autopsy, health care proxy, and advance directives), age was associated only with less frequent practice of mammography. Thus, there is a need to develop strategies to emphasize the importance of cancer screening procedures that, although invasive and relatively costly, are key to early detection of cancer in older adults.

SYNTHESIS

A report on the "Healthy Older Adult" prepared by the US Department of Health and Human Services, Office of Disease Prevention and Health Promotion in 1990 affirmed that some of the conditions commonly assumed to be part of the aging process could be prevented. A key message from that report is that progress in health status cannot be made unless we do better at preventing disease and premature death. Choices about diet, exercise, smoking, and other behavioral risk factors can make the difference not only in reducing premature mortality, but also in reducing acute and chronic disability (McGinnis, 1990).

Cancer remains a major health problem in the United States and most industrialized countries. However, there is evidence that many types of cancer can be prevented and that the prospects for surviving cancer continue to improve. It is estimated that as much as 50 percent or more of cancer incidence can be prevented through smoking cessation and improved dietary habits such as reducing fat consumption and increasing fruit and vegetable consumption.

Thus, preventing cancer in older persons should emphasize research and practice on smoking cessation. Over 4.5 million older adults continue to smoke. There is evidence that smoking cessation tailored to older smokers can be effective.

Breast cancer is the most common cancer among women in the United States and older women are at higher risk. There is evidence to suggest that screening with regard to older women can save lives. Mammography is the most effective method for detecting early malignancies.

Education about dietary and lifestyle changes are also important ways to preventing cancer in older persons. According to nutrition research collated for Healthy People 2010 objectives, persons over 60 fail to meet many recommended dietary guidelines. Women older than 60 years fare worse than men on several items including having at least five servings of vegetables and fruits (39 vs. 52 percent), being over optimum weight (26 percent vs. 21 percent), having at least six servings of grains per day (28 vs. 54 percent), and meeting minimum dietary recommendations for calcium (34 vs. 33 percent) (Satcher, 1998).

Health promotion activities can be designed to address specific diseases or problems that are common to a particular population group. The ecological perspective suggests that a "goodness of fit" between people and their environment enables people and their environment to adapt to one another. Moreover, health promotion with older persons requires translating general health recommendations into personally relevant actions. The literature suggests that older adults perceive health promotion as beneficial. The need is to make such programs accessible, personally rewarding, and sustaining for older adults, so as to improve and maintain quality of life.

Also see: Chronic Disease: Older Adulthood; Perceived Personal Control; Health Promotion: Older Adulthood; Caregiver Stress: Older Adulthood.

References

Bertera, E.M. (1999). Assessing perceived health promotion needs and interests of low-income older women. *Journal of Women's Health & Gender-Based Medicine, 8*(10), 1323–1335.

Fallcreek, S., & Mettler, M. (1984). *Heathy old age: A sourcebook on health promotion with older adults.* New York: Hayworth Press.

Fitch, M.I., Greenberg, M., Levstein, L., Muir, M., Plante, S., & King, E. (1997). Health promotion and early detection of cancer in older adults: Needs assessment for program development. *Cancer and Nursing, 20*(6), 381–388.

Fried, T.R., Rosenberg, R.R., & Lipsitz, L.A. (1995). Older community-dwelling adults' attitudes toward and practices of health promotion and advance planning activities. *Journal of the American Geriatric Society, 43*(6), 645–649.

Gallo, J.G., Busby-Whtehead, J., Rabins, P.V., Silliman, R.A., Murphy, J.B., & Reichel, W. (1999). *Reichel's care of the elderly: Clinical aspects of aging*. Baltimore, MD: Lippincott Williams & Wilkins.

Germain, C.B. (1973). An ecological perspective in casework practice. *Social Casework, 54*, 323–330.

Germain, C.B., & Bloom, M. (1999). Human behavior in the social environment: An ecological view (2nd ed.). New York: Columbia University Press.

Green, L., & Kruter, M. (1991). *Health promotion planning: An educational and environmental approach*. Mountain View, CA: Mayfield.

Goldberg, T.H., & Chavin, S.I. (1997). Preventive medicine and screening in older adults [see comments]. *Journal of the American Geriatric Society, 45*(3), 344–354.

Guralnik, J., Fried, L., Simonsick, E., Kasper, J., & Laferty, M. (1995). *The women's health and aging study: Health and social characteristics of older women* (95-4009). Bethesda, MD: National Institute of Health.

Horwath, C. (1989). Dietary intake studies in elderly people. *World Review of Nutrition and Dietetics, 59*, 1–70.

Johnson, K., & Kligman, E.W. (1992). Preventive nutrition: Disease-specific dietary interventions for older adults. *Geriatrics, 47*(11), 39–40, 45–49.

La Croix, A., Newton, K., Leveille, S., & Wallace, J. (1997). Healthy aging, a women's issue. *Western Journal of Medicine, 4*, 220.

LaCroix, A.Z., & Omenn, G.S. (1992). Older adults and smoking. *Clinical Geriatric Medicine, 8*(1), 69–87.

McGinnis, J. (1990). *Healthy older people: The report of a national health promotion program*. Washington, DC: Office of Disease Prevention and Health Promotion, US Department of Health and Human Services.

Molina, C.W., & Aguirre-Molina, M. (1994). *Latino health in the US: A growing challenge*. Washington, DC: American Public Health Association.

Muir, M., Greenberg, M., Plante, S., Fitch, M., Levstein, L., & King, E. (1997). Health promotion and early detection of cancer in older adults: A practical approach. *Journal of the Canadian Oncology Nursing, 7*(2), 82–89.

Poland, B.D., Green, L.W., & Rootman, I. (2000). *Settings for health promotion*. Thousand Oaks, CA: Sage.

Rimer, B.K., & Orleans, C.T. (1994). Tailoring smoking cessation for older adults. *Cancer, 74*(Suppl. 7), 2051–2054.

Rubenstein, L. (1994). Strategies to overcome barriers to early detection of cancer among older adults. *Cancer, 74*(Suppl. 7), 2190–2193.

Salive, M.E., Cornoni-Huntley, J., LaCroix, A.Z., Ostfeld, A.M., Wallace, R.B., & Hennekens, C.H. (1992). Predictors of smoking cessation and relapse in older adults [published erratum appears in *American Journal of Public Health* [1992, Nov.], *82*(11), 1489]. *American Journal of Public Health, 82*(9), 1268–1271.

Saltz, C. (1997). *Social work response to the White House conference on aging*. New York: The Haworth Press.

Satcher, D. (1998). *Healthy People 2010 Objectives* (Government report ISBN 0-16-049722-1). Washington, DC: Department of Health and Human Services, Office of Disease Prevention and Health Promotion.

Sperry, L., & Prosen, H. (1996). *Aging in the twenty-first century*. New York: Garland.

Valdez, R.B., Delgado, D.J., Cervantes, R.C., & Bowler, S. (1993). *Cancer in Latino communities: An exploratory review*. Santa Monica, CA: RAND.

Walsh, J.M. (1992). Cancer screening in older adults [see comments]. *Western Journal of Medicine, 156*(5), 495–500.

Wardle, J., Sutton, S., Williamson, S., Taylor, T., McCaffery, K., Cuzick, J., Hart, A., & Atkin, W. (2000). Psychosocial influences on older adults' interest in participating in bowel cancer screening [In Process Citation]. *Preventive Medicine, 31*(4), 323–334.

Weinrich, S.P., Weinrich, M.C., Boyd, M.D., Atwood, J., & Cervenka, B. (1994). Teaching older adults by adapting for aging changes. *Cancer and Nursing, 17*(6), 494–500.

Caregiver Stress, Older Adulthood

Nancy R. Hooyman

INTRODUCTION

This entry addresses strategies to prevent stress among caregivers who are providing long-term care to older relatives. Because stress can negatively affect health, income, and general well-being, developing and testing prevention strategies is important for both older adults and caregivers. The entry assesses the effectiveness of three types of preventive strategies: (1) services, (2) education, individual counseling, and support groups, and (3) a multimodel that seeks change at both the individual and policy/organizational levels.

DEFINITIONS

Primary prevention in the context of caregivers for older persons refers to coordinated interventions in the early stages of the caregiving process (1) to prevent predictable primary and secondary stress, (2) to protect the caregiver's mental and physical well-being, and (3) to promote effective care that benefits both the caregiver and care recipient (Bloom, 1996). *Primary stress* includes both caregivers' acts of caring (e.g., *objective burden* or *caring for* that results from variables such as the amount of contact, care recipient's health, disruptions in income and social life) and their subjective response or *caring about* (e.g., *subjective burden* refers to caregivers' feelings, such as worry, sadness, guilt, and resentment). *Secondary stress* occurs when these primary burdens spill over into other aspects of the caregiver's life (e.g., family, work, and financial strains). In such instances, *primary and secondary stress* can lead to physical and mental health problems. Thus, preventive interventions with caregivers are important not only to their ability to care, but also to the physical and mental health of both the caregiver and older relative (Zarit, 1996).

Long-term care refers to a range of supportive assistance and services (both informal and formal) to older adults who, because of chronic illness or frailty, are unable to function independently on a daily basis.

SCOPE

Families provide nearly 80 percent of in-home long-term care. Approximately 75 percent of those aged 65 and over require some degree of home health care or personal assistance (Stone, 2000). Among these, 80 percent live in their own homes or community settings, and over 50 percent rely exclusively on family and friends for such care (National Academy on an Aging Society, 2000). These patterns are similar in most industrialized societies, although many Western European countries have more formal supports (e.g., attendant allowance and subsidized services). In Asian countries, norms of filial support are weakening, but daughters-in-law are still expected to try to provide care (Akiyama, Antonucci, & Campbell, 1990; Velkoff & Lawson, 1998).

The primary forms of family care are *emotional support*, *instrumental activities* (e.g., transportation, meal preparation, shopping), *personal care* (e.g., bathing, feeding, dressing), and *mediating with agencies for services*. The type of family care is largely determined by the older adult's functional status, intensity of needed care, co-residence, and the caregiver's gender, with over 70 percent of care provided by women (National Academy on an Aging Society, 2000). While family caregivers may save society up to $7,000 per patient annually (Peak, Toseland, & Banks, 1995), they nevertheless may experience costs in three primary areas:

Physical health includes headaches, depression, sleep disorders, stomach disturbances, weight changes, inappropriate use of prescription drugs, and self-neglect (National Academy on an Aging Society, 2000; Strang, Haughey, Gerdner, & Teel, 1999).

Financial areas relate to direct costs of medical care, adaptive equipment or hired help and indirect opportunity costs of lost income, missed promotions, or unemployment. More than 50 percent of caregiving employees have made changes at work to accommodate caregiving (National Alliance for Caregiving and AARP, 1997). Nevertheless, families are more likely to provide services directly than to purchase them, which suggests that financial demands tend to be the least burdensome (Tennstedt, 1999).

Emotional areas relate to worry, feeling alone and isolated; giving up time for oneself and family; "erosion of self" or the feeling of becoming trapped so that one's identity is completely submerged in the caregiving role; depression and other mental health problems (Aneshensel, Pearlin, Mullan, Zarit, & Whitlatch, 1995). These tend to increase with difficult levels of care and feelings of lack of control, and are experienced by women more than men (Ory, Hoffman, Yee, Tennstedt, & Schultz, 1999).

Despite these costs or burdens, most families are willing to assume care. They tend to experience more gains (closeness to relative, satisfaction) than costs when they possess effective problem-solving coping strategies, have social supports, and are in good physical health (Almberg, Grafstroem, & Winblad, 2000). Both benefits and costs vary over time, especially at points of entry and exit from the role (Seltzer & Li, 2000).

THEORIES

The most useful and widely tested theoretical model for identifying sources of stress and their possible reduction is *the stress process model* (Pearlin, Mullan, Semple, & Skaff, 1996). This model is congruent with a *person in environment or ecological model*, in which interventions aim to increase caregiver's resistance to stress (enhance their competence, self-esteem, and confidence in relation to environmental press or demands) or to decrease environmental demands (e.g., through services and social supports) (Lawton & Nahemow, 1973). Caregivers' physiological, psychological, and social responses to stress—and their interaction—are affected by two clusters of factors: *contextual* (e.g., level of care, care recipient's behavior and symptoms, quality of relationship with care recipient) and *dynamic* (e.g., social support and other resources) (McDonald, Poertner, & Pierpoint, 1999). Caregivers' *coping* refers to their internal cognitive and emotional processes as well as their ability to access social resources. The concept of *coping efficacy* encompasses the effectiveness of a copy strategy, that is, how well it results in alleviating or managing the primary/secondary stress and beliefs about one's capability in performing behaviors that lead to desired outcomes (e.g., reduced stress and enhanced quality of care).

Cognitive appraisal, especially how caregivers define the situation and their role, explains, in part, why what is difficult for one caregiver (e.g., behaviors of care recipient and severity of symptoms) may not be so for another (Walker, Pomeroy, McNeil, & Franklin, 1994; Zarit, 1996). The caregiver's subjective appraisal of the situation (feeling guilt, constantly in demand, out of control, overwhelmed) appears to be more salient than objective burden (Tennstedt, 1999; Yates, Tennstedt, & Chang, 1999). The distinction between *caring for* (e.g., the tangible tasks associated with personal assistance) and *caring about* (e.g., feelings of love, worry, and concern) also helps explain why caregivers in similar situations react in highly different ways, and why women tend to experience more stress than men (Bengtson, Rosenthal, & Burton, 1996). In other words, women more often feel responsible for their relative's psychological well-being and to perceive greater interference between caregiving and their personal and social lives (DeVries, Hamilton, Lovett, & Gallagher-Thompson, 1997).

Within this model, the goal of prevention is to reduce *stress proliferation* (e.g., effects of stress spilling over into relationships with family, friends, and work) and to enhance *stress containment*. These refer to the process by which internal (sense of efficacy) and external (social support, finances, and services) resources for caregivers reduce the impact of primary and secondary stressors.

Prevention thus encompasses different coping strategies. For example, use of respite care and adult day health are *coping by avoidance*, for example, getting away from the source of stress, even if for short periods of time. Education, support, and counseling seek to increase *coping efficacy*: the caregiver's personal care resources, such as knowledge, problem-solving skills and sense of mastery, confidence, and beliefs in one's abilities in relation to care demands. Family counseling and support seek to increase caregiving *resources* (e.g., the organization of the rest of the family to support the carer) (Ostwald, Hepburn, Caron, Burns, & Mantrell, 1999).

The extent of burden or stress also varies with the interaction among characteristics of the care recipient, the caregiver. In addition to cognitive appraisal, the extent to which caregiving has a negative effect is *mediated* by:

1. the nature of the relationship between caregiver and recipient (e.g., recipient unappreciative, making unreasonable demands, adopting manipulative behavior);
2. family support or disharmony; co-residence or geographic distance; financial resources;
3. the salience and timing in the caregiver's life course;
4. gender (women experience caregiving as more stressful than male counterparts providing similar levels of care); and
5. race and ethnicity (e.g., African Americans often turn to the church and prayer, infrequently use services, and tend to experience less caregiving stress) (Tennstedt, 1999).

Neither disability status nor the amount and type of care provided are important in explaining caregiver stress. On the other hand, a good relationship prior to caregiving minimizes stress, even in the face of heavy demands (Wolf, 1998).

The stress coping model does not include the need for changes in the larger environment; especially long-term care policies to address the needs of both the caregiver and care receiver. A feminist perspective articulates these structural changes, and is included under the proposed model given below.

STRATEGIES: OVERVIEW

The goals of preventive strategies with family caregivers can be classified as:

- reduce caregiver stress;
- ensure quality long-term care to older adults; and
- maintain the older adult at home and reduce institutionalization.

Preventive strategies tend to be two pronged, providing resources: (1) to caregivers to take better care of themselves and thereby the care recipient; and (2) to the older person and thereby to minimize their need for family care. Most interventions are brief. However, long-term support is important since caregiving is a fluid situation, shifting with care recipients' needs and caregivers' responsibilities. A preventive orientation has rarely been explicitly articulated, with many interventions often occurring too late in the caregiving cycle after stress has already spilled over into other aspects of the caregivers' lives (Whitlach, Zarit, Goodwin, & von Eye, 1995).

Early studies on the outcomes of preventive strategies used either pre-post designs with a single intervention condition or quasi-experimental designs without random assignment conditions, and focused on assessing the impact on the caregiver's well-being (Toseland & Rossiter, 1989). Later studies have involved larger and more carefully targeted randomized control groups and have examined variables other than well-being, such as use of health care and cost effectiveness (Fredriksen-Goldsen & Scharlach, 2001; Peak et al., 1995).

The primary preventive strategies evaluated here are: *formal services* (respite care, home care, adult day care); *individual and group education; individual and family counseling; and support groups.*

STRATEGIES THAT WORK

Preventive strategies that take multiple (individual, group, and family interventions) rather than single approaches are most successful in reducing nursing home placement, especially among individuals with Alzheimer's disease and subjective burden and emotional problems, such as depression (Mittelman et al., 1995). Multicomponent strategies are most effective when samples are targeted, based on an explicit assessment of caregivers' needs, and of greater intensity and duration (long-term support) than the standard 8–12-week programs characteristic of most caregiver strategies (Whitlatch et al., 1995).

Long-term preventive strategies are especially important when the goal is to prevent or postpone institutionalization for at least a year. The decision to seek nursing home placement is frequently precipitated by the family caregiver's illness or death, or by severe family strain (Seltzer & Li, 2000). Placement is thus often the result of a breakdown in the balance between the older person's care needs and self-care abilities; the primary caregiver's internal and external resources, and the larger support network (Whitlatch et al., 1995). For example, the characteristics of the caregiving context, especially perceived burden, negative family relationships, and low confidence in care, are better predictors of whether an Alzheimer's patient will be institutionalized than are the illness characteristics or symptoms of the care receiver (Fisher & Lieberman, 1999; Tennstedt, 1999). This suggests the need for multicomponent long-term models to assess and, over time, change all three contextual and mediating factors in reducing stress.

STRATEGIES THAT MIGHT WORK

Individual and group education encompass information about the older person's disease and appropriate support resources along with behavior management training and other problem-solving care skills to enhance caregivers' sense of mastery. They also frequently include self-care techniques or "taking care of the caregiver." Educational modalities are most effective when tailored to a particular caregiver situation or to specific patient behaviors (e.g., Alzheimer's supports and education group) rather than a more general approach (Ostwald et al., 1999). Education groups also increase the social supports for caregivers, with some members contacting each other after the group has ended (Toseland & McCallion, 1997).

Caregivers turn to individual counseling more than family modalities. This pattern may reflect the fact that most primary caregivers receive little regular assistance from other family members (Pearlin et al., 1996). Individual counseling is found to positively affect psychological well-being (e.g., reduce emotional stress), oftentimes by providing ways for the caregiver to identify ways to change his/her behavior and the situation (Toseland & McCallion, 1997). Barriers to participation in either counseling or education include transportation, finding someone to care for the older relative, costs of such assistance, and time. To address time and geographic barriers, telephone-based assistance is sometimes utilized; it appears to be most effective when a standardized protocol is used. Interviewers receive training on symptoms of various

illness, and caregivers are recruited via personal contact prior to the initiation of the phone intervention (Davis, 1998).

The Internet and websites also provide caregivers with information on community resources and an opportunity to connect with other caregivers on a 24-hour basis. Some corporations provide elder care information, referral, education, and adult care through employee assistance programs. However, research on the effectiveness of these computer or workplace resources is limited (Fredriksen-Goldsen & Scharlach, 2001). Nor are these strategies generally *systematic or targeted* on early caregiving, but randomly used across the caregiving career. Accordingly, the efficacy of such workplace and Internet resources vary, depending on the caregiver's subjective appraisal of need (Tennstedt, 1999).

Although findings are mixed, support groups generally appear to be more effective in preventing caregiver stress than either education or counseling alone. For example, posttest measures of a psychoeducational support group for early stage caregivers indicated a significant increase in preparedness for the caregiving role, competence, and use of positive coping strategies, and a decrease in their levels of perceived strain (subjective burden). This suggests that during the early phase of their caring, families can promote their wellness and enhance their ability to face challenges through increased emotional strength and coping skills (Cummings, Long, Peterson-Hazan, & Harrison, 1998). Support group participation is also found to be associated with decreased depression and increased morale (Mittleman et al., 1995); lower rates of institutionalization (Mittelman et al., 1995; Whitlatch et al., 1995); greater knowledge of illness and resources; and increased social support (Cummings et al., 1998). In contrast to these benefits, some studies identify support groups to be less effective than individual counseling for reducing strain and improving psychological well-being (Toseland, Rossiter, Peak, & Smith, 1990). Although support groups can provide much needed emotional assistance, they do not necessarily lower the level of caregiver stress.

Another limitation is that individual and group strategies implicitly place most responsibility for care on the family caregiver, generally a woman. From a feminist theoretical perspective, an implicit message to caregivers may be that if they were only to become more competent and efficient at caregiving, their stress will be reduced. If their stress increases, feelings of failure may surface. The focus of the intervention is on the individual, rather than on societal or structural factors. This suggests the importance of education and training to empower caregivers to advocate for policy and system-level changes. Examples of such changes are: a public long-term care policy that funds a wider array of services and values the work of family caregiving, rather than keeping it relatively invisible; economic supports for caregivers, including changes in Social

Security, especially for women who often disrupt their employment to provide care as a daughter, daughter-in-law, or wife; and assistance with economic expenditures such as household alterations, supplies, and high tech equipment.

STRATEGIES THAT DO NOT WORK

Provision of services in themselves does not improve caregivers' well-being. Most families do not use services, or do so selectively to supplement informal care for limited time periods (National Alliance for Caregiving and AARP, 1997; Tennstedt, 1999). This pattern may persist because families and their older relatives are unaware of services, unwilling to accept them, or lack the time and resources to access them (Davis, 1998). For example, for adult day care/respite to be an effective strategy, it must be flexible and accessible, and the older person must be ambulatory, in relatively stable health, able to communicate, and have someone to care for them when adult day care is unavailable (Hooyman & Gonyea, 1995). Gender and cultural differences in service utilization exist, with women and caregivers of color the least likely to turn to formal services (Dilworth-Anderson, Williams, & Cooper, 1999; National Alliance for Caregiving and AARP, 1997).

Overall, however, even when formal services are used, they have minimal effects on caregiver's well-being (Tennstedt, 1999; Worcester & Hedrick, 1997). This pattern may result because services may prolong the duration of caregiving, but not necessarily reduce the caregivers' subjective burden. Or services may be provided after problems have become too difficult to solve through short-term interventions (Given, Given, Stommel, & Azzoua, 1999). Another limiting factor is that most services are targeted to the older individual, not to reducing the structural factors underlying the burden and costs of family care. Accordingly, many services are oriented toward crisis intervention, short-term support, and long-term residential care, rather than toward personal care and in-home maintenance over the long haul needed by family caregivers (Osterbusch, Keigher, Miller, & Linsk, 1987). In many cases, families may be too poor to purchase private pay services, but not poor enough to be eligible for Medicaid-reimbursed services. And some families may experience services as discriminatory and not sensitive to cultural differences.

In addition, prevention strategies for caregivers are compromised by the limited attention given to programs delivered to and received by culturally diverse groups. Caregivers of color are less likely to use services including counseling, education, and support groups, because of economic, religious, insurance, and other barriers. In some cases, they feel like unwelcome outsiders in the locations offering services (Toseland & McCallion, 1997). Accordingly, they are more likely to turn to extended family, non-kin as family, and the church.

SYNTHESIS

Proposed Model of Interventions

A broad-based multidimensional model, which addresses both structural and individual change, would build caregivers' sense of political mastery and include advocacy for policy changes to ensure caregiver and care recipient's health and mental well-being. It would include the following components that address many of the limitations of current strategies noted previously.

1. The value and importance of family caregiving within long-term care would be *articulated explicitly* with services targeted to reducing caregiver burden. Accordingly, consistent with a feminist theoretical perspective, family members, typically women would not be assumed to be both willing and able to provide care. An ideal model would thus provide opportunities for families to learn about other care options and services to supplement and buttress the informal care network, such as respite and personal home care (Noelker & Bass, 1994). Accessible affordable respite, adult day care, and personal care are especially important, given that some research has found these services prevent institutionalization (Whitlatch et al., 1995).

2. Culturally sensitive services and multimodal interventions would address participation barriers by an array of services tailored to fit the needs of particular caregivers in accessible locations, such as churches, schools, primary care clinics, the workplace, and senior and community centers. In other words, preventive strategies would enhance the interface between family caregiving and caregivers' other community and employment roles. In evaluating strategies, the focus should not be on caregiver satisfaction, but rather which programs work best under what conditions and for whom (Fredriksen-Goldson & Scharlach, 2001).

3. Cultural beliefs and values about caregiving and service use would be assessed prior to developing preventive strategies. Outcomes evaluations would take account of the needs and experiences of diverse caregivers, including the cultural, societal, and personal factors that influence the nature of the caregiving situation (e.g., variations in filial norms and behaviors, socialization, appraisal, kinship networks, and styles of coping) (Fredriksen-Goldson & Scharlach, 2001).

4. Program targeting would occur early in the caregiving cycle or before it begins. Preventive targeting could help caregivers plan before they may be abruptly

thrust into a burdensome role. Unfortunately, it is human nature that most people do not seek out information and assistance until they need it. General information sessions about services and supports are typically not well attended. An effective early preventive strategy would engage the caregiver in planning shortly after experiencing the first acute incident or receiving the diagnosis of a fatal or chronic disease. This approach may increase receptivity to new information, which could be aimed specifically at the condition and caregiver characteristics (Tennstedt, 1999).

5. More sophisticated outcomes would identify research on controlled interventions that allow random assignment to caregivers to treatment and control conditions (both costs and benefits, including unintended and mutual ones), yet such research must also address the ethical challenges of such randomization. Qualitative research methods are needed to understand the subjective burden of caregiving and attitudes about the provision of care, including the prominence of caregiving roles, the meaning they provide and the extent to which they are perceived as under one's control.

6. A longitudinal, life course approach would take account of changes over time in responsibilities and outcomes (Fredriksen-Goldson & Scharlach, 2001).

7. Enlarging the unit of analysis to include system, not just individual, change is necessary. Although the stress coping model has typically focused on increasing the individual caregivers' skills for caring, new models, such as a feminist one, must consider the structural changes needed to support caregivers as well as to provide alternative service options.

In summary, societal changes are essential to accord greater public support to caregivers and their older relatives. Individual, group and family strategies to date are of relatively limited effectiveness. They need to be combined with political change strategies, including an intergenerational caregiver alliance, to ensure that caregiving is a shared responsibility between informal and formal supports and that preventive strategies have great impact on both systems (Hooyman, 2001; Hooyman & Gonyea, 1995).

Also see: Crises Intervention: Older Adulthood; Death with Dignity: Older Adulthood; Health Promotion: Older Adulthood; Life Challenges: Older Adulthood.

References

Akiyama, H., Antonucci, T.C., & Campbell, R. (1990). Exchange and reciprocity among two generations of Japanese and American women. In J. Sokolovsky (Ed.), *The cultural context of aging*. New York: Bergin and Garvey.

Almberg, B., Grafstroem, M., & Winblad, B. (2000). Caregivers of relatives with dementia. Experiences encompassing social support and bereavement. *Aging and Mental Health, 4*(1), 82–89.

Aneshensel, C.S., Pearlin, L.I., Mullan, J.T., Zarit, S., & Whitlatch, C.J. (1995). *Profiles in caregiving: The unexpected career*. San Diego: Academic Press.

Bengtson, V.C., Rosenthal, C.J., & Burton, C. (1996). Paradoxes of families and aging. In R.H. Binstock & C.K. George (Eds.), *Handbook of aging and the social sciences* (4th ed.). San Diego: Academic Press.

Bloom, M. (1996). *Primary prevention practices*. Thousand Oaks, CA: Sage.

Cummings, S.M., Long, J.K., Peterson-Hazan, S., & Harrison, J. (1998). The efficacy of a group treatment model in helping spouses meet the emotional and practical challenges of early stage caregiving. *Clinical Gerontologists, 20*(1), 29–45.

Davis, L.L. (1998). Telephone-based interventions with family caregivers: A feasibility study. *Journal of Family Nursing, 4*(3), 255–270.

Dilworth-Anderson, P., Williams, S.W., & Cooper, T. (1999). Family caregiving to elderly African Americans: Caregiver types and structures. *Journals of Gerontology, 54B*(4), S237–S241.

DeVries, H.M., Hamilton, D.W., Lovett, S., & Gallagher-Thompson, D. (1997). Patterns of coping preferences for male and female caregivers of frail older adults. *Psychology and Aging, 12*(2), 263–267.

Ekerdt, David, J. (ed.) (2002). *Encyclopedia of Aging*. New York: Macmillan Reference USA, an Imprint of the Gale Group.

Fisher, L., & Lieberman, M.A. (1999). A longitudinal study of predictors of nursing home placement for patients with dementia: The contribution of family characteristics. *The Gerontologist, 29*(6), 677–686.

Fredriksen-Goldsen, K., & Scharlach, A.E. (2001). *Families and work: New directions in the 21st century*. New York: Oxford University Press.

Given, C.W., Given, B.A., Stommel, M., & Azzouz, F. (1999). The impact of new demands for assistance on caregiver depression: Tests using an inception cohort. *The Gerontologist, 39*(1), 76–85.

Hooyman, N.R., & Gonyea, J. (1995). *Feminists perspectives on family care: Policies for gender justice*. Thousand Oaks, CA: Sage.

Lawton, M.P., & Nahemow, L. (1973). Ecology and the aging process. In C. Eisdorfer & M.P. Lawton (Eds.), *Psychology of adult development and aging*. Washington, DC: American Psychological Association.

McDonald, T.P., Poertner, J., & Pierpoint, J., (1999) Predicting caregiver stress: An ecological perspective. *American Journal of Orthopsychiatry, 69*(1), 100–109.

Mittelman, M., Ferris, S., Shulman, E., Steinberg, G., Ambinder, A., Mackell, J., & Cohen, J. (1995). A comprehensive support program: Effect on depression in spouse caregivers of AD patients. *The Gerontologist, 35*, 792–802.

National Academy on an Aging Society. (2000, May). *Helping the elderly with activity limitation (Caregiving, #7)*. Washington, DC: Author.

National Alliance for Caregiving and American Association for Retired Persons. (1997, June). *Family caregiving in the US: Findings from a national survey*. Washington, DC: Author.

Noelker, L., & Bass, D. (1994). Relationships between the frail elderly and informal and formal helpers. In E. Kahana, D. Biegel, and M. Wykle (Eds.) *Family caregiving across the lifespan*. Thousand Oaks, CA: Sage.

Osterbusch, S., Keigher, S., Miller, B., & Linsk, N. (1987). Community care policies and gender justice. *International Journal of Health Services, 17*, 217–232.

Ostwald, S.K., Hepburn, K.W., Caron, W., Burns, T., & Mantrell, R. (1999). Reducing caregiver burden: A randomized psychoeducational intervention for caregivers of persons with dementia. *The Gerontologist, 39*(3), 299–309.

Ory, M.G., Hoffman, R.R., Yee, J.L., Tennstedt, S., & Schultz, R. (1999). Prevalence and impact of caregiving: A detailed comparison between dementia and non-dementia caregivers. *The Gerontologist, 39*(2), 177–185.

Peak, T., Toseland, R., & Banks, S. (1995). The impact of a spouse–caregiver support group on care recipient health care costs. *Journal of Aging and Health, 7,* 427–449.

Pearlin, L., Mullan, J., Semple, J., & Skaff, M. (1996). Caregiving and the stress process: An overview of concepts and their measures. *The Gerontologist, 30,* 583–594.

Seltzer, M., & Li, L.W. (2000). The dynamics of caregiving: Transitions during a three-year prospective study. *The Gerontologist, 40*(2), 165–177.

Stone, R. (2000). *Long-term care for the elderly with disabilities: Current policy, emerging trends and implications for the 21st century.* New York: The Milbank Memorial Fund.

Strang, V.R., Haughey, M., Gerdner, A., & Teel, C.S. (1999). Respite—a coping strategy for family caregivers/commentaries/author's response. *Western Journal of Nursing Research, 21*(4), 450–471.

Tennstedt, S. (1999). Family caregiving in an aging society. *Administration on Aging.* Symposium on caregiving.

Toseland, R., & McCallion, P. (1997). Trends in caregiving intervention research. *Social Work Research, 21*(3), 154–164.

Toseland, R., & Rossiter, C. (1989). Group interventions to support caregivers: A review and analysis. *The Gerontologist, 29,* 438–448.

Toseland, R., Rossiter, C., Peak, T., & Smith, G. (1990). The comparative effectiveness of individual and group interventions to support family caregivers. *Social Work, 35,* 256–263.

Velkoff, V.A., & Lawon, V.A. (1998). *Caregiving: International brief on gender and aging.* Bureau of the Census; IB/98-3, 2–7.

Walker, R.J., Pomeroy, E.C., McNeil, J.S., & Franklin, C. (1994). A psychoeducational model for caregivers of patients with Alzheimer's disease. *Journal of Gerontological Social Work, 22*(1/2), 75–91.

Whitlatch, C.J., Zarit, S.H., Goodwin, P.E., & von Eye, A. (1995). Influence of the success of psychoeducational interventions on the course of family care. *Clinical Gerontologist, 16*(1), 17–30.

Wolf, R. (1998, March/April). Caregiver stress, Alzheimer's disease, and elder abuse. *American Journal of Alzheimer's Disease,* 81–83.

Worcester, M., & Hedrick, S. (1997). Dilemmas in using respite for family caregivers of frail elders. *Family and Community Health, 19,* 31–48.

Yates, M.E., Tennstedt, S., & Chang, B.H. (1999). Contributors to and mediators of psychological well-being for informal caregivers. *Journal of Gerontology Psychological Sciences, 54B*(1), 12–22.

Zarit, S. (1996). Interventions with family caregivers. In S. Zarit & B.G. Knight (Eds.), *A guide to psychotherapy and aging* (pp. 139–159). Washington, DC: American Psychological Association.

Child Care, Early Childhood

Angela A. Crowley and
Grace-Ann C. Whitney

INTRODUCTION AND DEFINITIONS

This entry addresses the preventive capacity of early care and education programs. *Early care and education* encompasses a variety of program types providing early childhood services, including child care, Head Start, and pre-kindergarten. It includes both center-based care and family child care. This entry discusses programs serving infants and toddlers as well as those for preschool-aged children. It will not cover school-age care for children once they enter kindergarten. However, many of the issues relevant for early care and education has relevance for early elementary school-aged populations too. This entry addresses growth and development primarily from a health perspective, while acknowledging that physical and mental development are interdependent. Cognitive issues are mentioned, but this entry does not elaborate on the variety of curricular aspects of quality early care. Finally, the World Health Organization's definition of health, "a state of complete physical, mental, and social well-being and not merely the absence of infirmity" (Tempkin, 1953, p. 21) is used.

SCOPE

The importance of understanding the preventive capacity of early care and education for healthy growth and development of young children cannot be underestimated. Today in the United States, 61 percent of mothers with children under the age of 6 years are employed, an increase of 42 percent since 1960 (US Department of Health and Human Services [USDHHS], 1999). More than 40 percent of these children are cared for outside of their homes by nonrelatives. Friedman, Haywood, and colleagues have described this phenomenon as a "watershed event.... For the first time in history, the majority of infants living in the US (are) receiving a significant amount of their care from someone other than their mothers" (NICHD Early Child Care Research Network, 1994, p. 376). With the rapid increase in child care participation, professionals have become increasingly concerned about the potential for chronic health problems, injuries, inadequate attachment, and transmission of infectious diseases (Hayes, Palmer, & Zaslow, 1990; Thacker, Addiss, Goodman, Holloway, & Spencer, 1992). Compounding the problem, in the absence of national child care policies to ensure developmentally appropriate, healthy, and safe care for young children, state child care regulations range from minimal to adequate. In a four-state study of child care centers, only 8 percent of the infant–toddler rooms met the good-quality level, that is, health and safety needs were fully met. At the same time, 40 percent were rated less than minimal (Helburn, 1995). In contrast, children in regulated child care have experienced several positive outcomes, including higher rates of immunizations and current physical examinations (Cocchi, 1994; Sterne, Hinman, & Schmid, 1986). Through daily contact with children and families, child care participation offers a unique opportunity to promote health and development.

Quality of early child care varies greatly in the United States. While most programs have basic health and safety requirements, especially if they are center-based, the United States has not set national standards. Standards and procedures for monitoring compliance with standards vary from state to state. Uniformity of quality across early care settings is achieved primarily through the work of accreditation systems, such as those of the National Association for the Education of Young Children (NAEYC), and monitoring systems, such as the federal monitoring of Head Start. These elective and compulsory systems insure the implementation of best practices. There are also models of best practice that have yet to be incorporated into formal review systems, such as *Stepping Stones*, the national model of health and safety standards developed under the auspices of the Maternal Child Health Bureau (MCHB) of USDHHS (1997). As of yet, no states have regulatory systems that require programs, whether center- or home-based, to meet such ideals.

With respect to healthy development, the extent to which early care programs are connected to the broader array of resources that bring preventive health to young children varies greatly. Most early care programs are not connected to formal health systems or providers. Other than health examinations that are required upon entry, there is no ongoing effort to monitor children's health or developmental status in order to detect problems at an early stage. In the United States, Head Start and Early Head Start, through federally established program performance standards, require ancillary staffing to monitor the health and development of participating children and ensure that family needs for social services are addressed (Zigler, Piotrowski, & Collins, 1994). While prekindergarten programs that are housed in public schools have the support of school health and social work professionals, the majority of early child care programs nationwide are not located in public school facilities and rarely have the ancillary staff to provide such preventive care. The importance of comprehensive services such as health, nutrition, mental health, special education, and family supports that connect with educational services is just beginning to be recognized for young children in early child care. This is demonstrated by a recent initiative in the state of Rhode Island to support networks of ancillary service professionals to enhance publicly funded child care programs (Rhode Island Department of Human Services, 2000). However, for early care and education provided in the vast majority of child care centers and family child care homes, service systems are fragmented, and the availability of comprehensive professional supports is rare. High quality early child care must include connections with health resources to fulfill its preventive potential.

THEORIES

The most relevant theories for the present discussion include ecological theories and transactional models of development as well as Pender's Revised Health Promotion Model (1996). Bronfenbrenner's (1979) *ecological perspective* recognizes the interrelationships among the settings that children and parents engage in and the systems outside their immediate environment that influence the quality of their experiences in those settings. Bronfenbrenner's ecological theory can provide a useful framework for understanding the importance of multiple influences on the health and development of a young child. Bronfenbrenner identifies the variety of settings in which children grow and states that, to the extent that these various systems are supportive and connected, the development of a child is enhanced. For example, when child care and health providers are closely aligned for the health of the child, there is less likelihood that health problems will go untreated and prevent full participation in learning. Specific examples include hearing and vision problems and uncontrolled asthma. Similarly, those systems outside the child's immediate environment, such as parental work policies and federal and state programs and policies supportive of families, exert a strong influence on children's healthy development. The accessibility of family medical leave allows parents to care for their sick children. Thus the child is in an optimal setting for healing, developmental needs are met, and there is less likelihood of exposing other children to disease transmission. The availability of federal programs that support quality child care, such as Head Start, the Child Care Development Block Grant funding to states, and the MCHB's Health Systems Development in Child Care/Community Integrated Services System grants, provide opportunities for creating healthy and developmentally appropriate settings for young children.

Likewise, the *transactional model* can help in understanding that a preventive capacity must persist as long as risks can occur (Sameroff, 1993). Having a requirement for immunization compliance or developmental assessment at entry into a program may be sufficient for one moment in time. However, young children must continue to receive immunizations over the course of their first five years, and developmental assessments over time tell much more about the developmental needs of a child than one snapshot ever can. Without some way of connecting health care and early care over time, important points of prevention and early intervention cannot be taken advantage of.

Pender's *Revised Health Promotion Model* (1996) provides a framework for understanding variables that influence the implementation of health promoting behaviors. The model includes three major categories: individual characteristics and experiences, behavior-specific cognitions and affect, and behavioral outcome. The extent to which variables that positively influence healthy behaviors are augmented and those that pose barriers are modified increases the likelihood that a health promoting behavior is adopted. Applying the model to child care settings, the individual characteristics and experiences of programs influence their adoption of health promotion activities. Positive past or current experiences influence the probability of future healthy behaviors. A successful hand washing initiative that reduces illness among staff and children reinforces the behavior.

Similarly, perceived benefits, barriers, self-efficacy, activity-related affect, and interpersonal and situational influences all contribute to committing to a plan of action. For example, regulations and standards with sufficient resources for implementation that are understood as positive influences on health are more likely to be fully embraced by child care programs. Finally, immediate competing demands and preferences influence the adoption of health promoting behaviors. Strategies that prioritize the health of children, staff, and families within child care settings by reinforcing positive experiences and by reducing barriers and competing demands increase the likelihood of the adoption of health promotion behaviors in child care settings.

RESEARCH

For more than three decades, health professionals and developmentalists have studied the effect of child care participation on children's health and development. Developmentalists have focused on attachment, cognitive development, and socialization skills of children in child care. Hayes et al. (1990) reported three waves of research examining the effect of child care on children's development. In the first wave, the literature focused on the influence of place, that is, comparisons of home-reared children versus those who participated in out-of-home settings. The majority of studies concluded that intellectual development appeared to be comparable across groups, although the out-of-home care children from economically disadvantaged backgrounds demonstrated greater gains in this domain as compared to children from more economically advantageous circumstances, particularly if families received parent training. However, children participating in child care had somewhat increased rates of insecure attachment. Children demonstrated more sophisticated social competence in child care settings, which may explain the additional finding that they were more oriented to peer rather than adult relationships. Major limitations of this wave of research include the type of programs studied, that is, primarily centers and model programs; measurement issues, such as almost exclusive use of the Ainsworth "Strange Situation" (Ainsworth,

Blehar, Walters, & Wall, 1978) to examine attachment; and lack of longitudinal studies. In the second wave of research, more attention was focused on variations in child care settings and how center characteristics influence development. While this phase furthered previous findings, limitations included measurement issues related to quality indicators and omission of the influence of family characteristics on developmental outcome. Finally, the third wave of research focused greater attention on child care quality and family variables.

Despite the progressive complexity of conceptual underpinnings and methodologies, most studies offered only a snap shot of child care effects on child development. Thus, in 1991 the National Institute of Child Health and Human Development (NICHD) launched a comprehensive, longitudinal study, The NICHD Study of Early Child Care (USDHHS, 1998a). This prospective study enrolled over 1,300 children and their families representative of the racial, socioeconomic, and family variations in American society. Conducted at 10 locations by university-based researchers, this study is the most comprehensive examination of the first seven years of life to date. Published scientific papers have focused on the first three years, and analysis is ongoing. A comprehensive description of the findings is beyond the scope of this entry. However, key points include the following: (1) high quality care as compared to low quality care was associated with stronger mother–child relationships, less likelihood of insecure attachment in infants of mothers with low sensitivity, fewer reports of behavior problems, higher levels of cognitive performance, language ability, and school readiness, and (2) more hours in care was associated with higher probability of insecure attachments in infants of mothers with low sensitivity, more reported child behavior problems at age two, and weaker infant–mother relationships. *High quality child care* was defined as care in which there are frequent and positive interactions between caregivers and children, smaller group size, higher staff–child ratios, and clean, safe, and stimulating environments. In addition, teachers in high quality centers have formal education, specialized training and experience in the field, as well as a philosophy of care supportive of healthy development. This study is providing ongoing evidence of the association between child care and development in addition to recommendations for optimizing the child care experience.

Recent interest in the impact of early care experiences on development has also been spurred by the concern that young children should be equipped with sufficient readiness skills to be successful upon entering school. Evidence has accumulated to show that preschool children are more capable learners than earlier thought, and that good educational experiences in the early years can have a positive impact on school learning, particularly for children from low-income families (Barnett, 1992; Helburn, 1995). Although we know that both maternal education and family income are strong correlates to school success, national statistics (Federal Interagency Forum on Child and Family Statistics, 1997) indicate that children whose mothers have attended college are nearly twice as likely to attend center-based early childhood programs as are children whose mothers have less than a high school education. Furthermore, children living in poverty are less likely to attend such programs than children whose families have higher incomes.

Lack of uniform health regulations for child care programs across states and the growing participation of children in early care settings led health professionals more than two decades ago to actively investigate children's health outcomes. Numerous studies in several countries have focused on rates of infectious disease, acute and chronic health problems, and injuries. Findings suggest that children, families, and staff are at increased risk for infectious diseases and acute and chronic health problems (Denny, Collier, & Henderson, 1987; Goodman, Churchill, Sacks, Addiss, & Osterholm, 1994; Hardy & Fowler, 1993; Thacker et al., 1992). In addition, a recent study (Moon, Patel, & Shaefer, 2000) reported that a high proportion of Sudden Infant Death Syndrome cases occurred in child care settings.

There is an extensive body of literature documenting the prevalence of gastrointestinal and respiratory infectious diseases in child care settings. Researchers have also reported increased rates of otitis media (Hardy & Fowler, 1993) and asthma (Nystad, Skronda, & Magnus, 1999), both of which may be associated with early and frequent respiratory illness among children in child care settings. Holmes, Morrow, and Pickering (1996) suggest that the increased rates of infectious diseases in child care programs contribute to greater use of antibiotics and may be associated with the emergence of antibiotic resistant organisms. Disease transmission is not limited to children. Cordell, Waterman, Chang, Saruwatari, Brown, and Solomon (1999) also demonstrated a link between provider illnesses and children's absences due to illness. Specific characteristics of such settings: non-toilet trained children, a group setting, mixing of children, immune status, hygiene practices, and exclusion policies all contribute to disease rates (Barros, Ross, Fonseca, Williams, & Moreira-Filho, 1999; St. Sauver, Khurana, Kao, & Foxman, 1998).

Multiple studies have examined injury prevalence in child care settings. Although there is a higher rate of minor unintentional injuries among children in child care settings as compared to home, the frequency of serious unintentional injuries is equivalent or less frequent (Kotch et al., 1997; Thacker et al., 1992). The most common location of injury is the playground, the most common cause is falls from climbing equipment, and the anatomical site most frequently injured is the head (Sacks, Smith, Kaplan, Lambert, & Sykes, 1989). Leland, Garrard, and Smith (1994) also reported higher rates of injury among children with disabilities as opposed to those without disabilities. This finding may be related to the lack of safe, developmentally appropriate equipment. Disabling injuries to child care providers is another aspect of injury prevalence in child care settings. Brown and Gerberich (1993) reported a high rate of injuries, particularly back injuries, among child care teachers. Addressing factors that contribute to infectious disease transmission and injuries will reduce morbidity in child care settings.

STRATEGIES THAT WORK

United States: Head Start Model

Initiated 35 years ago as a program of the War on Poverty, Head Start provides the most significant large-scale model of prevention through early care and education in the United States (Zigler & Valentine, 1979). Head Start, which serves 3- and 4-year-olds, and Early Head Start, which was established in 1994 to serve pregnant women and children up to age 3, are federally supported comprehensive child-development programs for families whose income is at or below the federal poverty line. Since its creation in 1965, Head Start has served more than 18 million children with the goal of enhancing the social competency, or school readiness, of children from poor families. Head Start and child care are not synonymous. Head Start has traditionally been part day. Not until welfare reform did programs expand to become full day, year-round programs to meet the changing demands of families. Head Start and Early Head Start programs often partner with child care programs to meet this full-time need. This results in child care that has the increased benefit of comprehensive supports that include individualized educational and child development services; physical, oral, and mental health; nutrition services; and parent involvement. Programs are locally controlled so there is a wide variation in the ways in which services are provided. However, uniform standards guide the provision of services, and compliance is monitored through centralized data-gathering and triennial on-site program reviews. Many states have recognized the value of the Head Start model of comprehensive child development services and have instituted state-financed early childhood programs that utilize Head Start Performance Standards (USDHHS, 1996) and monitoring system. Thus, greater numbers of children receive its benefits.

Early studies of the effectiveness of Head Start were conducted within the context of demonstration projects and were focused on particular policy questions. In 1985, a synthesis of 72 studies using meta-analysis methods was published by the USDHHS (McKay, Condelli, Ganson, et al., 1985, cited in Devaney, Ellwood, & Love, 1997). At the end of the Head Start year, they found a sizeable and educationally meaningful effect on children's cognitive development and beneficial effects on socioemotional development, in particular, in achievement, motivation, and social behavior. In another study (Apt Associates, Inc., 1984, cited in Devaney, Ellwood, & Love, 1997), Head Start children were more likely than controls to have received health services, enjoyed better health care services, experienced improved health status, eaten meals significantly higher in nutritional quality, and exhibited better motor control and development. Those Head Start children who experienced pediatric problems upon entry were less likely to have the same problems one year later. Zigler et al. (1994) reported that children in Head Start were more likely than their counterparts to receive immunizations, well child services, screenings, and dental care. Head Start children had fewer health problems and experienced health levels similar to those of more advantaged children.

The first national study of Head Start was begun in 1997. Although this is a longitudinal study still in progress, preliminary findings have been published (USDHHS, 1998b). With respect to the quality of Head Start programs, it was found that the average Head Start classroom is of good quality, and unlike other early care programs where quality varies from excellent to poor, no Head Start programs were found to score below the minimal quality range. Children in Head Start were performing above the levels that would be expected for children from low-income families attending center-based programs. Children in higher quality classrooms had higher performance on assessment measures, as did children who had participated in Head Start for two years rather than one.

International Models

Perhaps the best support for the concept of child care being utilized as a prevention strategy has come from what we know about early care systems operating in Europe. Three countries frequently referenced in discussions of high quality child care are France, Italy, and Denmark.

The strong pronatalist sentiment in France has created an environment for a high quality, integrated, universal, early care system that is the envy of many. Over the years France has drastically reduced rates of infant mortality and childhood disease and increased rates of immunizations and preventive health care exams. This has been done through a rigorous program of home visits to families in the early years as well as a close integration of health care and child care, so important as the rates of maternal employment and use of child care have steadily increased. One aspect of

health and child care integration has been to increase the capacity of early care to include children with congenital disorders, physical disabilities, and behavioral problems. Another aspect of system integration is the joint assurance by both health and child care systems of setting quality through licensing, monitoring, consultation, and training. A third aspect of health and child care integration involves the active participation of health personnel in outreach to early care settings to insure referrals of children for health services and to arrange for necessary health examinations.

Health and early care integration is achieved through *Protection Maternaelle et Infantile* (PMI) (Richardson & Marx, 1989). Before 1992 PMI agencies served as sources of health consultation mainly around health and safety and individual child referrals. In 1992, PMI agencies became legislatively mandated to conduct preventive health exams for all preschool children and to accomplish these exams in the child care setting for children who were not obtaining exams through the health care system. This action was taken after a survey revealed that children who were examined and appropriately referred for diagnosis and treatment at age 4 had markedly fewer medical, visual, hearing, and behavioral problems when they entered elementary school than did children who had no preschool exam (Richardson, 1994). In Cote-d'Or, where the survey was done, 4-year-old exams were universal by 1994. Parents provide permission for exams and are present whenever possible.

This same public health model is utilized in Denmark. Like early care in France, child care centers and family child care homes are linked with health professionals. In Denmark, systems of early care are supported and connected by persons whose role might be characterized as that of a team leader or supervisor (Corsini, 1998). In addition to monitoring the health and safety of settings and providing or linking providers with health and developmental training, these individuals connect early care providers, families, and children with the full range of services that exist in their communities. They may provide periodic developmental screening of children, but they serve in a more supportive way overall, having responsibility for a caseload of families to insure that regular health surveillance and health services are received and that family support services and any special services for children are accessed. This model does not place as much emphasis on providing health care *in* the child care setting and is similar to the Head Start model and others like it in the United States. However, because of the universal access to health care and family support services in Denmark, the system is much more reflective of an early care infrastructure rather than a targeted service only accessed after eligibility criteria have been met.

In Italy, the integration of early childhood programs into the broader community presents yet another model of health care and child care integration. Italy, too, has a system of universal health care access, and child care in Italy emphasizes close links among early childhood settings, family support programs, and health and social services (Kamerman & Kahn, 1995). Early childhood programs are linked to one another and to primary schools. Spaces are designed to integrate classrooms with each other and to their surrounding communities. The early care system in the municipality of Reggio Emilia, Italy, is a particularly well known example of the way in which pedagogy and the collaborative efforts of parents, teachers, and community resources can be connected to create early care experiences for children that promote their optimal growth. In this model, young children are highly valued and their healthy development involves the participation of persons beyond those in the education and health care systems. Through the process of nurturing healthy children, the whole community thrives.

These three models from Europe can provide suggestions for child care in many other nations. While having different approaches to supporting and connecting child care and health care, they nonetheless have achieved both a high level of quality in early care settings and an integration of early care into the broader realm of child and family services and supports. All three countries have universal programs for health and family support. Child care in Denmark is under the auspices of social services with greater similarity to a social work model. All three reflect the cultural variations of their communities in comparison to one another but share the strong similarity of emphasis on quality of child care and assurance of comprehensive services for all.

STRATEGIES THAT MIGHT WORK

USA: Child Care Interventions

As child care services and programs have rapidly expanded, a number of efforts have been made to mobilize strategies believed to enhance the quality and comprehensiveness of child care to benefit the health and development of children. The tremendous increase in programs for accreditation of early childhood settings is one example. Center accreditation systems have expanded their capacity to review programs, and new accreditation systems have emerged to accommodate family child care and school-age care. Efforts to promote professionalization of early care providers have resulted in the development of systematic professional development lattices in the states and initiatives to improve both the wages and benefits of early care providers. Quality initiatives also include the vast number of training and public information initiatives that have educated providers, parents, and communities about the importance of the early years

and the provision of quality programs for optimal developmental outcomes. Rediscoveries and new discoveries in the area of brain development have provided impetus for many of these activities (Committee on Integrating the Science of Early Childhood Development, Shonkoff, & Phillips, 2000). Government-sponsored initiatives such as the Healthy Child Care America campaign for health and safety on the national level and school readiness initiatives in the form of state-level legislation and programming have provided opportunities for implementing interventions believed to have the most beneficial effects for children. While some efforts have been successful, others have not. Lacking a clear national blueprint and a plan for financial support, the early care system in the United States is growing with considerable local variation. Problems include large gaps in universal utilization of best practices and piecemeal implementation of an integrated and comprehensive early care system.

Despite more than two decades of concern about health and safety risks in child care settings, few rigorous studies have examined morbidity reduction. Even fewer have explored the potential for promoting wellness in child care programs. To date, the focus of interventions includes increase in health knowledge, the relationship between health knowledge and outcomes, and the effect of providing health services on children's access to care. Colegrove (1992) and Bapat and Goclowski (1989) reported that a child care health promotion curriculum increased the health knowledge of parents and staff; however, the influence on children's health was not demonstrated. Both Kotch et al. (1994) and Ulione (1997) found improvements in hygiene practices and a reduction in illness rates among staff who participated in a health education program. Furthermore, Aronson (1993), Bapat and Goclowski (1989), and Gaines (1991) reported that access to a nurse consultant improved health outcomes through ongoing access to health information or through on-site services.

In contrast, interventions that do not provide resources such as funding or continuous access to information, to support health promotion, are clearly less effective strategies. Sacks, Brantley, Holmgreen, and Rochat (1992) found that identifying potential risk factors in child care settings without offering ongoing resources had no effect on change in practice. Similarly, while regulations may improve compliance to health standards, Crowley (1998) reported that child care directors who disagreed with child care regulations requiring health consultation visits made little use of that on-site service.

Comprehensive Services Model

The comprehensive services model is best exemplified by Head Start in the United States and the European models presented from France, Italy, and Denmark. High quality child care in the United States that has many of the characteristics of the comprehensive model also has shown strong positive developmental effects for children. The comprehensive model of early care integrates supports for children and families and increases the likelihood that families will receive the supports they need. Although Head Start began as an antipoverty program and attempted to assure the full range of services often not received by poor families and children, the comprehensive model in European countries is available for all children and families regardless of income. Evidence such as the impact of early screenings in France suggests benefits not only for children at risk due to poverty but for all children. The preventive capacity of child care seems to be inextricably linked to the provision of a range of services that can assure the quality of early care settings as well as the additional resources as needed by individual children and families. The comprehensive services model sees the child as a whole child and recognizes that when ancillary services are fragmented, often those services are never received. This prevents early detection and intervention and can lead to more serious problems for the child.

Child Care Health Consultation

The role of the child care health consultant has emerged as the embodiment of the linkage between health and child care at the program level. Head Start Health Coordinators have a long history of promoting children's health by facilitating access to services both on-site and in the community. Western European early childhood models have incorporated health consultation universally, an example being the French PMI system mentioned previously. An examination of the impact of the developing role of the child care health consultant on child and family outcomes is critical. For approximately two decades, the USDHHS, MCHB has had a sustaining interest in promoting children's health in out-of-home care settings through the linkage of child care and health professionals. Demonstration projects funded through the MCHB Special Projects of Regional and National Significance and conducted by Aronson (1993), Bapat and Goclowski (1989), and Gaines (1991) found an association between access to a health consultant and improvements in child care provider health knowledge, compliance in health practices, and health status of children in child care settings.

Additional MCHB initiatives include: The National Health and Safety Performance Standards for Out-of-Home Care (American Public Health Association [APHA] & American Academy of Pediatrics [AAP], 1992); development of the National Resource Center for Health and Safety in Child Care; launching the Healthy Child Care America Campaign with the Child Care Bureau and the AAP; state grants to build health systems in child care; and the National Training Institute for Child Care Health Consultants (AAP, 1999). Through this systemic effort, each of these initiatives contributes to child care health and safety. Present efforts are underway to investigate further the association between children's health in child care settings and access to a health consultant. Five states have required on-site health consultation for some time. Crowley (2000) found that 85 percent of 131 surveyed child care directors reported that a health consultant, who visited weekly and was required by regulation, was important or very important for the operation of their centers. As the role of the child care health consultant develops, systematic and rigorous examination of the impact of this intervention on the health and development of children and families in child care settings is essential.

STRATEGIES THAT DO NOT WORK

Approaches that are education only, that are didactic, and do not permit rehearsal and practice have not been effective.

SYNTHESIS

The child care experience presents the potential for risks or improved outcomes for children and families depending on the quality of the child care system (Helburn, 1995; NICHD Early Child Care Research Network, 1997). Models in the United States and Western Europe demonstrate that investments in systems of high quality out-of-home care promote children's health and development. These models exemplify the themes and tenets of the theories presented earlier in that they are ecological in perspective, ongoing in commitment, and focus on strategies that reduce barriers and promote healthy behaviors. Successful strategies include multisystem integration at the child, family, community and policy levels. Interventions at each of these levels foster children's well-being when they establish health and development as a priority and provide the resources to eliminate barriers. Finally, efforts are most effective when they are consistent and continuous.

From the findings shared, a discussion of promoting health and development through child care can be summarized on two levels. First, the importance of the quality of the early childhood setting itself is of great importance. At the very least, for child care to be beneficial for children it must be of good quality. This means that settings are healthy and safe, adults have appropriate training and expertise, activities and opportunities for children are developmentally appropriate and culturally sensitive, and ratios and group sizes meet accepted standards for the child's age. Dissemination of best practice standards and systems of monitoring and accreditation can help to achieve quality child care especially when resources are available from the community to insure availability of professional development programs, responsive monitoring and review systems, and programmatic consultation to meet established quality standards.

Second, the importance of the integration of child care into the wider community of child services and family supports is equally important to promote health and development through child care but perhaps more difficult to attain. Comprehensive models in the United States and Western Europe demonstrate, clearly, that when quality child care settings are integrated into resource rich and responsive communities, the overall effect on the whole child is achieved. Targeted models, such as Head Start, show evidence of success for children served by the program. Universal availability of supports in Western European models demonstrate more convincing evidence throughout whole communities and nations. High quality early childhood programs in resource-rich communities result in early detection of health and developmental problems, early intervention and treatment of identified problems, and prevention of additional problems that result from poor quality settings and communities. The same is true for the detection and prevention of disease and injury.

Building solid connections between early care settings and health services, best accomplished through quality systems of child care health consultation, has enormous potential for children in early care settings in the United States. As in Western European nations, if the bountiful resources of the United States were soon redirected to insure health consultation to all early care settings, a more solid integration of health and child care would benefit the millions of children growing up in child care today.

Also see: Abuse: Early Childhood; Environmental Health: Early Childhood; Injuries, Unintentional: Early Childhood; Nutrition: Early Childhood; Parenting: Early Childhood; Physical Health: Early Childhood; Prosocial Behavior: Early Childhood.

References

Ainsworth, M., Blehar, M., Walters, E., & Wall, S. (1978). *Patterns of attachment.* Hillsdale, NJ: Erlbaum.

American Academy of Pediatrics. (1999). The national program to train child care health consultants. *Healthy Child Care America, 3*(1), 12.

American Public Health Association, & American Academy of Pediatrics. (1992). *Caring for Our Children: National Health and Safety Performance Standards—Guidelines for Out-of-Home Child Care Programs.* Washington, DC and Elk Grove Village, IL: Authors.

Aronson, S. (1993). *Early childhood education linkage system* (Maternal Child Health Bureau Project MCJ-426025). Arlington, VA: National Center for Education in Maternal and Child Health.

Bapat, V., & Goclowski, J. (1989). *Promoting health care to infants and toddlers in child day care* (Maternal Child Health Bureau Project MCJ-093741-02-0). Arlington, VA: National Center for Education in Maternal and Child Health.

Barnett, S.W. (1992). Benefits of compensatory preschool education. *Journal of Human Resources, 27,* 279–312.

Barros, A.J., Ross, D.A., Fonseca, W.V., Williams, L.A., & Moreira-Filho, D.C. (1999). Preventing acute respiratory infections and diarrhoea in child care centers. *Acta Paediatrica, 88*(10), 1113–1118.

Bronfenbrenner, U. (1979). *The ecology of human development: Experiments by nature and design.* Cambridge, MA: Harvard University Press.

Brown, M.Z., & Gerberich, S.G. (1993). Disabling injuries to child care workers in Minnesota, 1985–1990: An analysis of risk factors. *Journal of Occupational Medicine, 35*(12), 1236–1243.

Cocchi, S.L. (1994). Overview of policies affecting vaccine use in child day care. *Reviews of Infectious Diseases, 94*(Suppl. 2), 994–996.

Colegrove, J. (1992). *New Mexico child care health promotion project* (Maternal Child Health Bureau Project MCJ-356021). Arlington, VA: National Center for Education in Maternal and Child Health.

Committee on Integrating the Science of Early Childhood Development, Shonkoff, J.P., & Phillips, D.A. (Eds.). (2000). *From neurons to neighborhoods: The science of early childhood development.* Washington, DC: National Academy Press.

Cordell, R.L., Waterman, S.H., Chang, A., Saruwatari, M., Brown, M., & Solomon, S.L. (1999). Provider-reported illness and absence due to illness among children attending child care homes and centers in San Diego, CA. *Archives of Pediatrics and Adolescent Medicine, 153*(3), 275–280.

Corsini, D.A. (1998). *Family day care in Denmark: A model to be emulated.* (ERIC Document No. 33/620).

Crowley, A.A. (1998). *Linking families, child care and health: An exploratory study of child care directors and health professionals' perceptions of consultation and collaboration.* Unpublished dissertation, University of Connecticut, Storrs, CT.

Crowley, A.A. (2000). Child care health consultation: The Connecticut experience. *Maternal and Child Health Journal, 4*(1), 67–75.

Denny, F., Collier, A., & Henderson, F. (1987). Acute respiratory infections in day care. *Reviews of Infectious Diseases, 8,* L527–L532.

Devaney, B.L., Ellwood, M.R., & Love, J.M. (1997). Programs that mitigate the effects of poverty on children. *The Future of Children, 7*(2), 88–112.

Federal Interagency Forum on Child and Family Statistics. (1997). *America's children: Key national indicators of well-being.* Washington, DC: Office of Management and Budget.

Gaines, S.K. (1991). *Health promotion in a group child care setting* (Maternal Child Health Bureau Project MCJ-133711-03). Arlington, VA: National Center for Education in Maternal and Child Health.

Goodman, R.A., Churchill, R.E., Sacks, J.J., Addiss, D.G., & Osterholm, M.G. (1994). Proceedings of the international conference on child day care health: Science, prevention, and practice. *Pediatrics, 84*(Suppl. 6), 987–1121.

Hardy, A.M., & Fowler, M.G. (1993). Child care arrangements and repeated ear infections in young children. *American Journal of Public Health, 83,* 1321–1325.

Hayes, C.D., Palmer, J.L., & Zaslow, M.J. (Eds.). (1990). *Who cares for America's children?: Child care policy for the 1990's.* Washington, DC: National Academy Press.

Helburn, S.W. (Ed.). (1995). *Cost, quality and child outcomes in child care centers: Technical report.* Denver, CO: Department of Economics, Center for Research in Economic and Social Policy, University of Colorado at Denver.

Holmes, S.J., Morrow, A.L., & Pickering, L.K. (1996). Child care practices: Effects of social change on the epidemiology of infectious diseases and antibiotic resistance. *Epidemiologic Review, 18*(1), 10–28.

Kamerman, S.B., & Kahn, A.J. (1995). Innovations in toddler day care and family support services: An international perspective. *Child Welfare, 74*(6), 1281–1300.

Kotch, J.B., Dufort, V.M., Stewart, P., Fieberg, J., McMurray, M., O'Brien, S., Ngui, E.M., & Brennan, M. (1997). Injuries among children in home and out-of-home care. *Injury Prevention, 3*(4), 267–271.

Kotch, J.B., Weigle, K.A., Weber, D.J., et al. (1994). Evaluation of an Hygienic Intervention in Child Day Care Centers. *Pediatrics, 94*(Suppl.), 991–994.

Leland, N.L., Garrard, J., & Smith, D.K. (1994). Comparison of injuries to children with and without disabilities in day care centers. *Journal of Developmental and Behavioral Pediatrics, 15*(6), 402–408.

Moon, R.Y., Patel, K.M., & Shaefer, S.J. (2000). Sudden infant death syndrome in child care settings. *Pediatrics, 106*(2 Pt. 1), 295–300.

NICHD Early Child Care Research Network. (1994). Child care and child development: The NICHD study of early child care. In S.L. Friedman & H.C. Haywood (Eds.), *Developmental follow-up: Concepts, domains and methods* (pp. 377–396). New York: Academic Press.

NICHD Early Child Care Research Network. (1997). The effects of infant child care on infant–mother attachment security: Results of the NICHD Study of early child care. *Child Development, 68*(5), 860–879.

Nystad, W., Skronda, A., & Magnus, P. (1999). Day care attendance, recurrent respiratory tract infections and asthma. *International Journal of Epidemiology, 28*(5), 882–887.

Pender, N.J. (1996). *Health promotion in nursing practice* (3rd ed.). Stamford, CT: Appleton & Lange.

Rhode Island Department of Human Services. (2000). *Starting Right.* Providence, RI: Rhode Island Department of Human Services.

Richardson, G.A. (1994). *A welcome for every child—How France protects maternal and child health—A new frame of reference for the United States.* New York: The French-American Foundation.

Richardson, G.A., & Marx, E. (1989). *A welcome for every child—How France achieves quality in child care: Practical ideas for the United States.* New York: The French-American Foundation.

Sacks, J.J., Brantley, M.D., Holmgreen, P., & Rochat, R.W. (1992). Evaluation of an intervention to reduce playground hazards in Atlanta child care centers. *American Journal of Public Health, 82*, 429–431.

Sacks, J.J., Smith, J.D., Kaplan, K.M., Lambert, D.S., & Sykes, R.K. (1989). The epidemiology of injuries in Atlanta day care centers. *Journal of the American Medical Association, 262*, 1641–1645.

Sameroff, A.J. (1993). Models of development and developmental risk. In C.H. Zeanah, Jr. (Ed.), *Handbook of infant mental health* (pp. 1–13). New York: Guilford.

St. Sauver, J., Khurana, M., Kao, A., & Foxman, B. (1998). Hygienic practices and acute respiratory illness in family and group day care homes. *Public Health Reports, 113*(6), 544–551.

Sterne, G.G., Hinman, A., & Schmid, S. (1986). Potential health benefits of child day care attendance. *Reviews of Infectious Diseases, 8*, 573–583.

Tempkin, O. (1953). What is health? Looking back and ahead. In I. Gladston (Ed.), *Epidemiology of health.* New York: New York Academy of Medicine, Health Education Council.

Thacker, S.B., Addiss, D.G., Goodman, R.A., Holloway, B.R., & Spencer, H.C. (1992). Infectious diseases and injuries in child day care: Opportunities for healthier children. *Journal of the American Medical Association, 268*, 1720–1726.

Ulione, M.S. (1997). Health promotion and injury prevention in a child development center. *Journal of Pediatric Nursing, 12*, 148–154.

US Department of Health and Human Services. (1996). *Program performance standards.* Washington, DC: Head Start Bureau.

US Department of Health and Human Services. (1998a). *The NICHD Study of Early Child Care* (NIH Publication No. 98-4318). Public Health Service, National Institute of Child Health and Human Development.

US Department of Health and Human Services. (1998b). *Head Start research: Head Start performance measures, second progress report.* Washington, DC: Head Start Bureau.

US Department of Health and Human Services. (1999). *Child Health USA 1999.* Washington, DC: Superintendent of Documents, US Government Printing Office.

US Department of Health and Human Services, Maternal Child Health Bureau. (1997). *Stepping stones to using: Caring for our children: National health and safety performance standards: Guidelines for out-of-home child care programs—Protecting children from harm.* Rockville, MD: Public Health Service, Health Resources and Services Administration.

Zigler, E., Piotrowski, C.S., & Collins, R. (1994). Health services in Head Start. *Annual Review of Public Health, 15*, 511–534.

Zigler, E., & Valentine, J. (Eds.). (1979). *Project Head Start: A legacy of the War on Poverty.* New York: The Free Press.

Children, Parents with Mental Illness, Childhood[*]

Daphna Oyserman and Carol Thiessen Mowbray

INTRODUCTION

This entry deals with promoting the mental health of young children living at home with parents with a mental illness. Therefore, we focus on programs that promote well-being of the young child directly or indirectly by promoting the well-being of the caregiver (typically the mother). The reason for this broadened focus is that improving the caregiver's well-being will have important positive consequences for the well-being of the young child.

DEFINITION AND SCOPE

According to a number of sources, at least 10 percent of women suffer a significant episode of postnatal depression meeting Research Diagnostic Criteria (RDC) for major

*Funding came from NIMH grant numbers R01 MH54321 and R01 MH57495. Kirsten Firminger, Crystal Espinoza, Mari Hashimoto, and Ben Saunders helped find references, and prepare the tables and bibliography.

depressive illness, and between 3–5 percent of women meet criteria for moderate to severe depressive illness. If not treated, a third of women with postnatal depression have episodes lasting for at least the first year of the infant's life (for a review see Oates, 2000). Perhaps due to community-based care, the fertility of individuals with schizophrenia may be rising (Stocky & Lynch, 2000) and does not differ from that of the population as a whole (Oates, 2000). In fact, women are more likely to have a major psychiatric disorder and more likely to be referred for treatment after childbirth than at other times (Nicholls & Cox, 1999). Those with preexisting severe affective disorder or schizophrenia may be at risk of relapse following child birth (Stocky & Lynch, 2000); having had one episode of puerperal psychosis increases risk of psychiatric illness in a subsequent pregnancy to as high as 60–80 percent (Stocky & Lynch, 2000). All told, about 2 percent of women are referred to psychiatric services following childbirth (Oates, 2000).

Children whose parents have a mental illness are at increased risk of having a mental health problem themselves due to complex interactions between the child and features of his or her environment (US Department of Health and Human Services [USDHHS]—US Surgeon General's Mental Health Report, 1999). Environmental features—including relationships with parents, siblings, other family, peers, neighborhood, school, and the sociocultural context within which they live—interact with and shape child characteristics (biological, psychological, and genetic) over time. Previous experiences influence children's subsequent risk for mental health problems, in part, because children attempt to adapt to their context in whatever way they can. Parenting and the caregiving environment are critical as resources as well as potential risk factors for these children. As will be outlined below, inadequate parenting can result in a child's impaired sense of self-efficacy and negative attribution style, increasing his/her risk of depression and other disorders in childhood.

Mental health problems are relatively common in childhood. The most recent US Surgeon General's Mental Health Report (USDHHS, 1999) estimates that 4 million children have serious mental health problems at any given point in time. Parental mental illness increases risk of child mental health problems, especially since maternal mental illness is associated with additional risk factors (single parenthood, family or marital discord, separation from parent due to maternal hospitalization, lack of social support, family and neighborhood poverty) that themselves can potentiate genetic and biological risks—US Surgeon General's Mental Health Report (USDHHS, 1999). Thirty-two to 56 percent of children of parents with a serious mental illness (schizophrenia or affective disorder) will themselves have a DSM diagnosable disorder (Amminger et al., 1999;

Rieder, 1973; Waters & Marchenko-Bouer, 1980). Heritability estimates vary from 75 (schizophrenia) or 80 percent (bipolar disorder) to lows of 34–48 percent (depression) (Rutter, Silberg, O'Connor, & Simonoff, 1999).

Heritability and Biological Factors

Biological factors exert especially profound influences on some mental health problems, including early-onset schizophrenia (McClellan & Werry, in press) and, according to the US Surgeon General's Mental Health Report (USDHHS, 1999), biological factors are likely to play a large part in the etiology of social phobia and obsessive-compulsive disorders. Biological factors are not necessarily genetic or heritable factors but can include abnormalities of the central nervous system due to injury, toxins, poor nutrition, or infection. According to the National Institute of Mental Health's Genetics and Mental Disorders Report (1998), autism, bipolar disorder, schizophrenia, and attention-deficit/hyperactivity disorders are likely to have genetic components, based on research with adults. Biologically based disorders can also be the result of family problems that preclude appropriate parenting, putting the fetus or infant at risk of pre- or postnatal developmental delays or deficits. Indeed disentangling family environment, biology, and genetic risk is a difficult task. For example, 20–50 percent of depressed children have a history of family depression. Children of depressed parents are three times as likely to become depressed as their peers, and also more likely to experience anxiety, conduct and substance abuse disorders, especially if both parents have a depressive illness or if depressive episodes occurred when the child was young or were recurrent (Downey & Coyne, 1990; Wickramaratne & Weissman, 1998).

Mental Illness and Parenting

Maternal depression is a common mental health problem in mothers of infants and young children, with 10–15 percent of these mothers estimated to meet DSM-IV criteria for depression severe enough to interfere with daily functioning, including parenting (O'Hara, 1997). The interplay between parenting and parental mental illness diagnoses other than depression has been the focus of less research attention (Oyserman, Mowbray, Allen-Meares, & Firminger, 2000). Even less research has focused on fathers, perhaps because men with a serious mental illness are less likely to have children or be involved in parenting. Current evidence suggests that maternal functioning and symptoms are at least as important as diagnosis itself, if not more so, in understanding current child outcomes. Though not well studied, the interface between course of maternal mental illness and child's developmental phases is also likely to be important.

Diagnosis, Functioning, and Symptoms

Particular diagnosis (e.g., unipolar depression versus schizophrenia) may matter less than the specific nature of the symptoms the mother is experiencing and the extent that her mental illness impairs parenting (see Oyserman et al., 2000).

THEORIES AND RESEARCH

Course of Mental Illness and Parenting

The parent–child relationship is critical for early child development. Infants form close bonds with their primary caregiver—usually the mother—and this early relationship is the basis for later social relationships. From the parent's perspective, these bonds often starts during pregnancy when the mother feels fetal movement, but bonding may be delayed or not occur at all when mothers have a mental illness such as depression (Kumar, 1997). Children can overcome early neglect or inadequate development of the parent–child bond if the mother becomes able to provide a sensitive and stable relationship (Downey & Coyne, 1990). When mothers are unable to provide adequately sensitive care, developmentally appropriate stimulation and model reasonable coping, risk for children increases.

This means that the timing of maternal episodes of mental illness compared to infant and child developmental phases may be critical, with children being more vulnerable to problems when their mother has an episode of mental illness that lasts longer, covers more developmental phases, and is more severe.

Cultural and Cross-Cultural Issues

Field's (1992, 1998) research over the past few decades has documented the negative effects of maternal depression on early mother–infant interactions, increasing risk for child developmental, mental health and behavioral problems. Although early mother–child interactions differ cross-culturally, most research has focused on the effect of maternal depression on interactions without regard to possible interactive influences of race–ethnicity or SES; it is thus possible that maternal depression has different effects on mother–child interactions in different cultures (Field, 1999). Mothers from different racial–ethnic subgroups may have different models of parenting, which themselves may result in differences in child responses. Cross-cultural differences in parenting goals can produce mismatches between in-group and larger societal socialization goals. These mismatches may exacerbate the negative effect of

maternal depression on parenting. Moreover, culture is likely to play a major role in how mental illness develops and the meaning it has (Field, Greenwald, Morrow, & Healy, 1992).

Concomitant Contextual Risks

Research on the process by which maternal mental illness affects child development and risk for mental health problems indicates four interlocking pathways by which risk is increased for children of mothers with a serious mental illness. (1) Mothers may pass on genetic traits, including fussy temperament. (2) Maternal mental illness can be associated with other family stresses such as family and marital conflict and problems. (3) Maternal mental illness can relate to chronic and acute psychosocial stress generally, including negative life events and daily hassles. (4) Maternal mental illness may decrease mothers' sense of competence and efficacy and increase use of punitive parenting styles (Oyserman et al., 2002; Oyserman, Bybee, Mowbray, & MacFarlane, in press).

Maternal mental illness is a risk factor for poorer parenting quality and is likely to co-occur with other stressors that may independently dampen parenting quality. These commonly co-occurring stressors include low income (Miller, 1990; Rudolph, Larson, Sweeny, Hough, & Arorian, 1990), larger than average family size (Ritsher, Coursey, & Farrell, 1997), lack of social support (Belle, 1990), increased incidence of other negative life events (Downey & Coyne, 1990), and the experience of social stigma and discrimination due to mental illness (Miller & Finnerty, 1996; Ritsher et al., 1997).

Parenting Skills and Deficits

Maternal psychopathology alone does not make a parent incapable of providing sufficient or "good enough" parenting and parents with a mental illness may feel competent as parents and function adequately at home even if they are highly anxious and have difficulties in out-of-home situations such as school or the workplace (Hall, 1996; Jacobsen, Miller, & Kirkwood, 1997). However, depressed parents may be withdrawn and lack energy and, consequently, pay little attention to or provide inadequate supervision of their children. Alternatively, these parents may be overly irritable, critical and intrusive, demoralizing and distancing toward their children (Field, Healy, Goldstein, & Guthertz, 1990). Depressed mothers often feel less competent generally and their distress can make children anxious (Downey & Coyne, 1990). Depressed parents may not model effective coping strategies and social skills (Garber & Hilsman, 1992). At each developmental phase, parenting deficiencies can reduce the child's likelihood of successfully attaining their developmental goal—resulting in impaired relationships, trust, and communication skills emerging in infancy, reduced sense of efficacy and competence in toddlerhood, and dampened cognitive–intellectual attainments in the early school years (Cicchetti & Toth, 1998).

Early parenting requires providing adequate stimulation and appropriate modulation of arousal as well as adequate physical care. In infancy, withdrawn, unresponsive, or depressed mothers can increase infant distress while intrusive, hostile mothers can "teach" infants to avoid looking at or communicating with the mother (Cohn, Tronick, & Lyons-Ruth, 1986). In the toddler stage, when mothers are depressed, they may be less adept at structuring or modifying the child's behavior, resulting in both briefer interchanges and more out-of-control child behavior (Zahn-Waxler, Iannotti, Cummings, & Denham, 1990). As these examples of parenting deficits illustrate, children of mothers with serious mental illness are at risk of both lags in socioemotional development and impaired acquirement of social and relational skills, and reduced sense of competency, worth, and efficacy (Hammen, 1997). Because mothers with a serious mental illness may require hospitalization, their children are also at risk of physical separation, acerbating the emotional withdrawal described above.

Supports and Stresses for Parents

Parental mental illness is often associated with marital discord, poverty, and social isolation—all of which are likely to have negative effects on parents and their ability to parent. Economic hardship stresses parents, reduces their ability to be warm, nurturing, and appropriately structured and these poor parenting practices increase risks for children (Zahn-Waxler et al., 1990). When children experience such unstable parenting environments, they are at risk of poor academic performance and poor social skills, further stressing parental ability to provide appropriate caregiving and family functioning. Stressful life events, such as loss of a partner through death or divorce, both stress parents and increase risk of depression in early childhood especially if they lead to permanent negative changes in the child's circumstances and the family environment (Birmaher et al., 1996).

Mental Health and Temperament

Temperament difficulties in early childhood are associated with increased risk of mental health problems while positive temperament—including long attention span, goal orientation, lack of distractibility, and curiosity—are buffering factors. Difficult temperament and quality of parenting interact—high quality parenting and a sound relationship with the primary caregiver can buffer children from the negative effects of difficult temperament, including high

reactivity. However, highly reactive, anxious, and behaviorally inhibited infants and toddlers are also more difficult to parent, increasing maternal stress. In infants and toddlers, insecure attachment, irritability, and less adaptive coping have all been associated with maternal depression (NICHD Early Child Care Research Network, 1999). In addition, risk of depression, anxiety, conduct, and attention-deficit disorders increase dramatically for children of depressed mothers (Hammen, Burge, Burney, & Adrian, 1990). Wickramaratne and Weissman (1998) found substantially increased risk of childhood depression in children of mothers with depression (15.5 vs 1.7 percent in the general population). In infancy, children of depressed mothers display less mastery motivation, a marker of efficacy (Jennings, 1991).

Socioemotional, Social, and Relational Skills

Infants of mothers with mental illness are at risk for problems in developing secure attachments to their mothers and for other more subtle relationship problems. Relational skill deficits are important because, to be healthy, children must form relationships not only with their parents but also with siblings and with peers. Children's abilities to form close relationships with peers constitutes a developmental resource, buffering other risks, as well being as a normal part of development. Children with better social skills are better able to form these relationships. Social skills are verbal and nonverbal. Verbal skills include the ability to appropriately articulate wishes or ideas as well as the ability to listen to other children's ideas and forge an appropriate compromise. Nonverbal skills include the ability to interpret and understand other children's nonverbal cues (body language, voice pitch) as well as provide appropriate nonverbal cues such as eye contact and nonintrusive touching. These skills are useful to entering already formed groups as well as maintaining one's place in the peer group (Kagen, Snidman, & Arcus, 1998). Low skill children are at risk of active rejection as well as simple neglect by their peers, both of which increase risk for mental health problems.

Cognitive Development and School-Related Problems

Children of mothers with depression are also at increased risk of behavior problems in school, attention-deficit disorder, hyperactivity, and lower intelligence scores (Downey & Coyne, 1990; Hay, 1997).

Social Stigma and Social Acceptability

We did not find empirical literature on social stigma for young children of mothers with a serious mental illness.

However, the positive psychology and resiliency literature suggests that children who have better temperaments, are more socially skilled, and physically attractive are likely to elicit more positive and supportive responses from others. Risk for problematic temperament and dampened social skills are documented. Further, since in infancy and early childhood, children rely on their mother's care for hygiene and grooming, children of depressed mothers may be generally less physically appealing, especially when mental illness combines with poverty, making access to routine medical care less likely. A fussy infant in soiled clothing with a runny nose and chaffed skin is less likely to obtain positive responses from others compared to a happy, attractively clothed, and healthy infant. More subtly, other potential caregivers may view the infant of a depressed mother more negatively simply because of the stigma of her illness.

STRATEGIES: OVERVIEW

The literature suggests that child risks emerge early and that mothers with serious mental illnesses have multiple problems that increase risks for children. Therefore, appropriate preventive interventions need to take into account the pervasiveness of risk—including poverty, unemployment and low educational attainment, lack of social support, single parenthood, or marital discord. Preventive interventions dealing with these general risk factors have also been suggested as ways to reduce risk for other problems such as substance abuse (Hawkins, Kosterman, Maguin, Catalano, & Arthur, 1997) particularly when parental alcoholism is a risk factor (Chassin, Barrera, & Montgomery, 1997). Preventive interventions must also take into account the sequential nature of risk when parents have a serious mental illness—fussy infants make attachment more difficult, difficulties in attachment set the stage for difficulties with development of self-efficacy, mastery motivation and self-competence, which in turn heighten risk of retarded cognitive development and more negative cognitive style.

STRATEGIES THAT WORK

Clear evidence of effectiveness is not yet available.

STRATEGIES THAT MIGHT WORK

Through literature reviews, searches of conference presentations, and networking with other researchers, we were able to identify ten programs that provide community-based services to infants and young children living in families with a mentally ill parent.[1] Table 1 summarizes the identified programs, their locations, and descriptions. To our knowledge, none of these has been systematically evaluated. In an earlier review, we also located literature on home visitation and mother and child hospitalization programs in England (Oyserman et al., 1994). These earlier programs focused effort on alleviating stress due to mother–child separation and deterioration of maternal mental health in the highly stressing early months of parenting. We include these in the *Encyclopedia* believing that these services act as preventive interventions for their children. We updated this review and found information on three models of care for women with puerperal mental disorder in the United Kingdom (Nicholls & Cox, 1999). Labeled as community-based, parent and baby day-units, and mother and baby units, these programs are in the table; however, their published description lacked specific details and did not provide information about program effectiveness. According to a review by Stocky and Lynch (2000), mother–baby admission principally exists in the United Kingdom, Australia, Canada, and New Zealand, has not been well evaluated, in part because randomized trials are viewed as unethical, and is based on theories of attachment and mother–child bonding. In her review, Oates (2000) calls for all psychiatric admissions of women to include their infants within specialized mother–infant psychiatric units to prevent future negative developmental outcomes for the child due to disruption in the mother–child bond; however, she does not report evaluations of this care. She suggests that provision of preventive mental health services for mothers can improve outcomes for their children, recommending regional 6-bed mother–infant units for areas including 11,000 births annually and dense populations, and more community-based supports in less dense and rural areas. We also found a brief report on a psychiatric clinic at a Dublin maternity hospital (Gannon, Barry, & Turner, 1998), suggesting that far fewer women are referred or accepted into treatment than would be predicted based on the Nicholls and Cox projects. Thus, in spite of clearly documented service needs, services do not appear to be provided in sufficient quantity—and perhaps not at all (i.e., see Nicholls & Cox, 1999, for a critique focused on services in the United Kingdom).

As can be seen from Table 1, programs vary widely in services, with some focused more on parenting skills and mother–child bonding and others providing more general services. Programs vary in location: some are residential;

---

[1] Primary sources of information were Drs. Judith Cook at the National Rehabilitation and Training Center in Chicago and Joanne Nicholson at University of Massachusetts Medical School—Center for Mental Health Services Research, who are both funded to identify and document the operations of model programs serving mothers with mental illness and their children.

Table 1. Programs for Mentally Ill Parents and their Young Children

Program	Program type, focus/goals	Children	Parents	Services/methods
Community-based care, United Kingdom developed by Oates, Nottingham, England (Oates, 2000; reviewed in Oyserman et al., 1994).	Provide in-home support for mothers with serious mental illness in the months after childbirth.	Infants		Parents must live within 20 minutes of the hospital and have a responsible adult living with them. Duration of care begins with 8 hours daily and is reduced to visits on alternate days by community-based nurses.
Parent and baby day-units, Charles Street Parent and Baby Day Unit, Stoke-on-Trent, developed by Cox (Nicholls & Cox, 1999).				Link parents to primary care and health visitors. Medication, 5-days a week day treatment during normal working hours, require good public transport and densely populated catchment areas.
Mother and baby units (Nicholls & Cox, 1999; Oates, 2000; Oyserman et al., 1994; Stocky & Lynch, 2000).	Joint admission of psychiatrically ill mothers and their babies. Either a specialized in-patient unit or a mother–child bed in a general psychiatric unit. Have existed in the UK since the 1950s.	Infants		Allow mothers to maintain as much routine care as possible for infants while psychiatrically hospitalized. In 1991 a total of 133 such beds were available in England and Wales (Nichols & Cox, 2000). Oates (2000): (1) about 10 specialist mother–baby units with 6 or more beds exist in Great Britain; (2) concern for infant safety and financial difficulties led to closure of some other general psychiatric ward mother–infant admissions; (3) although Great Britain is a world leader in mother–infant admissions, fewer than half of the health authorities have such programs.
Coombs Women's Hospital psychiatric outpatient service, Dublin, Ireland.	Liaison psychiatry outpatient service within a Dublin women's hospital. Goal is to identify and treat psychiatric disorders arising during pregnancy or the puerperium, as well as assess and monitor antenatal women with established psychiatric conditions through pregnancies and postpartum.	Infants	Expected 194–322 women, given assumed 3–5% rate of all women delivering have a severe enough disorder to warrant referral. However, only 73 women referred, 56 attended (1994).	Medication, otherwise unclear.
The Thresholds Mothers' Project, Chicago, Illinois.	Psychosocial rehabilitation facility-based program with home-visiting outreach component. Goals: stabilize and normalize familial unit; provide social network for family members; improve quality of life via independent living and parenting skills; empower parents to effectively raise children.	0 to 5 years of age	Women ages 17 and above who have custody of at least one child. Current enrollment (1997): 64% African American; 28% White; 8% Latino.	Mothers and children participate in a 5-day per week program. Children participate in activities designed to enhance motor, cognitive, social, and emotional development. Other services include: independent living skills; children's nursery/preschool and child development group; education—basic skills, GED, college prep, vocational and job training; health care referrals; psychiatric referrals; individual counseling; home visits; substance abuse support group; crisis intervention.

Program	Description	Ages	Population	Services
The Peanut Butter and Jelly Preschool, Albuquerque, New Mexico.	Private not for profit agency. Stabilize family's functioning; "graduate" children into appropriate placement; offer stabilization, reunification, and general improvement to families in conflict.	Infant to preschool aged	High-risk families living in poverty and experiencing problems such as substance abuse, family violence, developmental delays, or parental incarceration. Current enrollment (1997): 70% Latino, 20% White, 8% Native American, 2% African American.	Preschool includes parent training and education in conjunction with therapeutic early intervention for infants and preschoolers. Supported housing program. Program for parents leaving prison. Case management available to entire family, 24 hours per day, 7 days a week; staff includes teachers, other helping professionals and consultants.
LAMB Program: Loving Attachments for Mothers and Babies, Detroit, Michigan.	Voluntary prevention program connected with community mental health. Offers support to mothers with mental illness of all types and severities.	0 to 3 years of age	Primary caregivers ages 17 and above who are not active substance abusers, preference to pregnant women or mothers of newborns. Current enrollment (1997): 90% African American, 10% White.	Day-treatment format. Meet 4 days per week, with optional Parent–Toddler play, Effective Positive Parenting groups and a weekly home visiting components. Children attend developmental therapeutic nursery. Activities enhance child's language, cognitive, motor social, self-care and feeding development. Nursery can accommodate up to 16 children. Group sessions conducted by parent–infant specialists, focusing on parenting skills, stress management, daily living skills, nutrition, and information about child development. Other services include transportation, case management, psychiatric evaluations, and medication management.
Ashbury House of the Progress Foundation, San Francisco, California.	Residential treatment program. Helps families develop skills and the support system needed for independent living in the community. Family preservation/reunification program for mothers at risk of losing custody of their children.	0 to 7 years of age	Women with history of hospitalization; especially single parents. Current enrollment (1997): White, African American, and Latino (no specific breakdown).	Referrals from mental health, CPS, and temporary shelter providers. Approximately one-year stay. Services include: mental health rehabilitation; vocational and parenting instruction; "wrap-around" services; cooperative child care program; child development support group. 8 to 10 families served at a time.
The Parent and Child Education (PACE) Family Treatment Center, New York City, New York.	Community-based outpatient services. Basic tenets are to increase mutual support networks and utilize an empowerment model of mental health.	Infants to 5 year olds	Experiencing poor education, lack of marketable skills, substandard housing, inadequate medical care, and insufficient money to feed and clothe their children.	Creates with its staff a "surrogate family" for its clientele; enrichment/daycare/preschool program is critical part of service system both for benefit of children and as training site for increased parental competence.
Project CHILD Providence, Rhode Island.	Model demonstration program. Focus of project includes parent/child bonding and parenting skills. Two primary goals: to improve parenting skills and to remedy developmental delays in children	0 to 5 years of age	Most are mothers in their 30s with a first-born child or with a young second child and a much older (elementary school age or adolescent) first born. Most are welfare recipients,	Activities to foster healthy mother–child relationships and stimulate age-appropriate development in the children. Mothers seen by psychiatrist or psychiatric nurse who provides supportive therapy and medication. Services include: home visits, mother–baby school, a lunch program, social club for adults, stimulation groups for toddlers and preschoolers; transportation and community

Table 1. Continued

Program	Program type, focus/goals	Children	Parents	Services/methods
	particularly in language, attention, attachment, and ability to separate.		live alone with children in poor, urban areas and have poor social networks.	liaison. Staff include child psychiatrist, developmental psychologist, clinical MSW, special educators, clinical receptionist. Staff serve about 25 families and 35 to 40 children at any given time.
CAPT Center, Children and Parents Together, Huntington, New York.	For mothers: prevent rehospitalizations, reduce isolation, promote socialization, foster rehabilitation and normalization, enable fulfillment of parental role. For children: promote healthy growth and development; prevent or remediate developmental delays, physical or emotional problems; prevent unnecessary foster care.	0 to 5 years of age	Pregnant mothers or mothers with at least one child under 5. Current enrollment (1997): Mostly White, few African American or Latino.	Mothers' services: group counseling and support, parent education, education in community living skills, case management and crisis intervention; peer social network and activities that offer self-help and mutual support. Children's services: preschool socialization and education, age appropriate child care, early identification of developmental delays and physical or emotional problems, early intervention for these difficulties at CAPT or by referral to specialized services.
The Parent–Infant Development Program, Madison, Wisconsin.	Outpatient program; meets needs of infants and young children by providing evaluation and therapeutic services to families experiencing difficulties in early parent–child relationships or emotional/behavioral problems of infancy/early childhood.	0 to 6 years of age, exhibiting sleeping/feeding regulation difficulties; irritable, depressed mood; aggressive or withdrawn behavior; hypersensitivity to touch or sound	Mothers from urban and rural communities. Current enrollment (1997): 70% White, 20% African American, 10% Latino.	Offer diagnostic assessment and evaluation, parent–infant dyadic therapy, parent psychotherapy, play therapy; marital–family therapy, therapeutic groups, consultation and evaluation. Also coordinates with other programs the mother and child are involved in—for example, respite and family support programs, public health services, the legal system, and social services. Staff include licensed psychologists and psychiatrists with expertise in the areas of infant development and mental health as well as early family relationships. Serves 30 families.
The IMPACT Program, Dayton, Virginia.	Comprehensive adult education facility. Satisfies goals for "welfare to work" clients; court, social services, and self-referrals; young mothers wishing to complete high school.	Preschool to "older" children	Serves a wide variety of high-risk parents.	Services offered 4 days per week. Services for parents include parent training (budgeting, parenting concerns, cooking classes, etc.) and adult education (GED completion, ESL classes, vocational training, etc.). Services for children include early childhood education and child care. Serves about 40 families each year; 8–10 families at a time.

others are outreach; some focus on generally at-risk women and others target only women with mental health problems. Clearly, given the large scope of need of these mothers and children, interventions should be ongoing and family focused; provide a mix of services aimed at preventing, treating, rehabilitating, and supporting families; and be sensitive to the stigma of mental illness and the importance of custody concerns. Prevention for children thus requires interagency collaboration in treatment, support, and rehabilitation for parents.

What Can Be Learned from Interventions That Work with Other At-Risk Children?

Because the programs just described target general concerns about parenting as well as concerns specific to mental illness, we turn to interventions with other high-risk children—children growing up in poverty, at risk of abuse or neglect, and children growing up in families where the main caregiver is socially isolated and stressed. While not the focus of this entry, these issues are relevant, when children are abused or neglected, they are more at risk of depression, impaired social skill development, and insecure attachment (Kazdin, Moser, Colbus, & Bell, 1985). Similarly, risk factors like large family size, poverty, and low education can combine to produce measurable problems, such as academic lags, deficits in social skills, and conduct and affective disorders. A number of prevention programs targeting young children and their parents highlight the need for long-term, intensive interventions that include parent education and support components. In addition, when these programs are effective, it is often because they have helped structure contexts within which both parent and child can be supported and flourish, teaching social and relational as well as cognitive and other skills.

Project Head Start

Project Head Start is a nationally distributed, targeted prevention program aimed at improving the social competence and cognitive–logical capacities of preschool children at risk due to parental poverty. Although lacking a randomized trial, a number of evaluations show positive academic impact. Head Start children are more likely to graduate high school and less likely to be enrolled in special education than their peers (Barnett, 1995). That this occurs in spite of the fact that improved cognitive test scores require follow-up intervention to be maintained during elementary school (Lee, Brooks-Gunn, Schnur, & Liaw, 1990), suggests that Head Start's positive effect on graduation and reduction in special education placement may be due to its impact on children's ability to function appropriately in the social

context of school. Available research cannot clarify the extent that the parent education components of Head Start are responsible for these effects or the extent that children's learning comes from their direct involvement in the program. However, programs like this one that help children and mothers in the context of school can alleviate risk due to gaps in social skills relevant to both peer and adult–child interactions. While school-based models may not work for older children, who are more likely to feel stigmatized by their parent's mental illness, daycare and preschool-based programs that include multiply at-risk children and their mothers are likely to be helpful for infants and young children of mentally ill mothers.

Preventive Interventions for Children at Risk Due to Parental Poverty, Low Education and Other Stressors

Federal funding to develop and evaluate preventive interventions has resulted in a number of model programs. As with Head Start, these programs were not designed specifically to deal with the needs of young children of mothers with a serious mental illness. However, they provide a model for the kinds of intensive, wrap around services that are needed for families with multiple risks and the added risk of parental mental illness.

Carolina Abecedarian Project

A rigorously tested preventive daycare program for children from infancy through age 5 who are at risk of school failure due to parental poverty and other factors, identifies children at birth and continues service through an at-home component until age 8. Infants and toddlers attend 8-hour daily, 50-week yearly; their parents receive educational and supportive activities. From kindergarten on, children were visited 15 times a year at home for 3 years by a teacher with a special home curriculum to supplement the school curriculum. The intervention produced positive intellectual and academic outcomes and maintained them at age 12, four years after the intervention (Campbell & Ramey, 1994).

Infant Health and Development Program

McCarton, Brooks-Gunn, Wallace, and Bauer (1997) enrolled low-birth-weight and premature infants at birth and provided pediatric care, home visits, parent group meetings, and center-based schooling 5 days a week for children aged 1–3 years. Like the other projects, it targeted and attained positive academic and cognitive outcomes, with the additional benefit of reduced behavioral problems in enrollees compared to control children.

Elmira Prenatal/Early Infancy Project

Olds et al. (1998) targeted women pregnant with a first child at risk due to maternal youth, single parent status, and poverty. A 15-year follow-up to the study that randomly assigned mothers to four levels of intervention, showed positive results for mothers and children who received the highest level of intervention. These mothers were given developmental screening, transportation to health care, and nurse home visits every two weeks during pregnancy with regular home visits the first two years of the child's life. At age 13, their children had fewer behavioral problems and the mothers were less likely to be on welfare, use substances, or have been reported for child abuse/neglect.

STRATEGIES THAT DO NOT WORK

Given that preventive interventions to promote health and well-being of young children of parents with a serious mental illness have not benefited from empirical evaluation efforts, it is not possible to point to strategies proven not to work. We surmise that it is unlikely that strategies focused only on children that do not also support mother's well-being and ability to parent will be effective.

SYNTHESIS

Even young children of parents with serious mental illness are at risk of developmental disruptions and problems in well-being. This risk to child healthy development is likely due to the interplay between parental mental illness and the associated increased risks—of problems in parenting, of family poverty, family instability, disrupted family support networks, and high parental stress among other family context risks. While current literature does not provide an effectiveness evaluation of programs focused specifically on the young children of parents with a serious mental illness, a number of programs that work for infants and young children at risk due to the poverty, young age, and low educational attainments of their mothers were located.

Each of these latter programs is both structured and intensive, underscoring the need for sustained and intensive efforts to support the parenting of mothers with serious mental illness. As prevention researchers, we should expect that these young children experience chronic stress due to the interaction between maternal mental illness and other concurrent environmental factors. Therefore, we speculate that effective preventive interventions for this population need to provide long-term and encompassing supportive services for mothers/caregivers and stabilize the normative transitions of

childhood so that young children of parents with a serious mental illness will be able to successfully negotiate developmental milestones and their families will be able to provide adequate buffering and support.

We propose that effective preventive programs for children of parents with mental illness will need structures similar to those for other at-risk children but will need to include additional components specifically targeted to the additional needs of this group. That is, preventive interventions will need to include (a) long-term contact, (b) services for both the caregiver parents and their infants/young children, (c) comprehensive services (including social and cognitive developmental domains for children and parenting and other domains of daily living for parents), (d) services targeting the ramifications of mental illness. These latter service components include helping mothers to plan for alternative caregivers when psychiatric hospitalization is needed to minimize disruption in child/infant care and reduce risk of custody loss, educating family members about mental illness, and providing them with support so that they will not be overburdened with child care demands. Clearly targeted and well-designed evaluation of programs including these service components is a necessary part of the next decade of prevention research.

Following a prevention framework, these to-be-developed and empirically evaluated interventions must minimize risks and maximize protective factors—this means minimizing family dysfunction and stresses and maximizing family functioning, supports, and child and parent competencies. While it may seem simpler to focus only on the young child as a target of service, we believe that preventive program efforts must be multiply focused (on parents, family, and children) if they are to promote the well-being of children growing up with parents with a serious mental illness. Briefly, preventive focus on parents should be twofold: bolstering, supporting, and maintaining the parent's mental health and everyday functioning in light of their mental illness as well as concentrating on parenting itself, including support for carrying out positive, nurturing parenting and providing appropriate supervision and direction to children.

Preventive focus on family members is also necessary since these family members are likely to be turned to for support in caring for children when a parent is mentally ill. Child rearing cannot simply be displaced onto other family members. Preventive intervention for family members should be two-fold: providing information and education about mental illness generally (and what they can expect given the situation of their mentally ill relative) and helping families develop a workable plan to provide care for the young children of this family member, including setting up routines that structure and support normal development for young children. Lastly, preventive focus must also be on the young children themselves, including infant care and preschool services that can support children's social, emotional, and cognitive development and provide young children with a setting in which they can thrive independently.

To develop and empirically validate these programs, prevention researchers can begin with programs that are currently working with generally at-risk young children. These programs typically provide support for parents, structured outreach to develop parenting and daily living skills, and structured care for young children in the form of infant and child care and play groups. By adding structured outreach work to help parents develop family supports and working with mental health and rehabilitative service providers, prevention researchers can develop and evaluate plausible wrap around services for this population in need.

Also see: Families with Parental Mental Illness: Adolescence; Family Strengthening: Childhood; Self-Esteem: Childhood; Social and Emotional Learning: Childhood.

References

Amminger, G.P., Pape, S., Rock, D., Roberts, S.A., Ott, S.L., Squires-Wheeler, E., Kestenbaum, C., & Erlenmeyer-Kimling, L. (1999). Relationship between childhood behavioral disturbance and later schizophrenia in the New York high-risk project. *American Journal of Psychiatry, 156*(4), 525–530.

Barnett, W.S. (1995). Long-term effects of early childhood programs on cognitive and school outcomes. *Future of Children, 5*(3), 25–50.

Belle, D. (1990). Poverty and women's mental health. *American Psychologist, 45*(3), 385–389.

Birmaher, B., Ryan, N.D., Williamson, D.E., Brent, D.A., et al. (1996). Childhood and adolescent depression: A review of the past 10 years, Part I. *Journal of the American Academy of Child & Adolescent Psychiatry, 35*(11), 1427–1439.

Campbell, F.A., & Ramey, C.T. (1994). Effects of early intervention on intellectual and academic achievement: A follow-up study of children from low-income families. [Special issue] Children and poverty. *Child Development, 65*(2), 684–698.

Chassin, L., Barrera, M., & Montgomery, H. (1997). Parental alcoholism as a risk factor. In S.A. Wolchik & I.N. Sandler (Eds.), *Handbook of children's coping: Linking theory and intervention* (pp. 101–129). New York, NY: Plenum Press.

Cicchetti, D., & Toth, S. (1998). The development of depression in children and adolescents. *American Psychologist, 53*, 221–241.

Cohn, J.F., Tronick, E.Z., & Lyons-Ruth, K. (1986). Face-to-face interactions of depressed mothers and their infants. *New Directions for Child Development, 34*, 31–45.

Downey, G., & Coyne, J. (1990). Children of depressed parents: An integrative review. *Psychological Bulletin, 108*, 50–76.

Field, T. (1992). Mother–infant interactions of Haitian immigrants and Southern American Blacks living in Miami. In J.L. Roopnarine & D. Carter (Eds.), *Parent–child socialization in diverse cultural settings.* Norwood, NJ: Ablex.

Field, T. (1998). Maternal depression effects on infants and early intervention. *Preventive Medicine, 27*, 200–203.

Field, T. (1999). Preschoolers in America are touched less and are more aggressive than preschoolers in France. *Early Child Development and Care, 151*, 11–17.

Field, T., Greenwald, P., Morrow, C., & Healy, B. (1992). Behavior-state matching during interactions of preadolescent friends versus acquaintances. *Developmental Psychology, 28*(2), 242–250.

Field, T., Healy, B., Goldstein, S., & Guthertz, M. (1990). Behavior-state matching and synchrony in mother–infant interactions of non-depressed versus depressed dads. *Developmental Psychology, 26*, 7–14.

Gannon, M., Barry, S., & Turner, M. (1998). Audit of the first year of a psychiatric clinic at a Dublin Maternity Hospital. *Irish Journal of Psychological Medicine, 15*(4), 142–144.

Garber, J., & Hilsman, R. (1992). Cognition, stress, and depression in children and adolescents: A follow-up study. *Journal of the American Academy of Child and Adolescent Psychiatry, 1*, 129–167.

Hall, A. (1996). Parental psychiatric disorder and the developing child. In M. Goepfert, J. Webster, & M.V. Seeman (Eds.), *Parental psychiatric disorder: Distressed parents and their families* (pp. 17–41). Cambridge, MA: Cambridge University Press.

Hammen, C. (1997). Children of depressed parents: The stress context. In S.A. Wolchik & I.N. Sandler (Eds.), *Handbook of children's coping: Linking theory and intervention* (pp. 131–157). New York, NY: Plenum Press.

Hammen, C., Burge, D., Burney, E., & Adrian, C. (1990). Longitudinal study of diagnoses in children of women with unipolar and bipolar affective disorder. *Archives of General Psychiatry, 47*, 1112–1117.

Hawkins, J.D., Kosterman, R., Maguin, E., Catalano, R.F., & Arthur, M.W. (1997). Substance use and abuse. In R.T. Ammerman & M. Hersen (Eds.), *Handbook of prevention and treatment with children and adolescents: Intervention in the real world context* (pp. 203–237). New York, NY: John Wiley & Sons.

Hay, D. (1997). Postpartum depression and cognitive development. In L. Murray & P. Cooper (Eds.), *Postpartum depression and child development* (pp. 85–110). New York, NY: Guilford.

Jacobsen, T., Miller, L.J., & Kirkwood, K.P. (1997). Assessing parenting competency in individuals with severe mental illness: A comprehensive service. *Journal of Mental Health Administration, 24*(2), 189–199.

Jennings, K. (1991). Early development of mastery motivation and its relationship to the self-concept. *Contributions to Human Development, 22*, 1–13.

Kagen, J., Snidman, N., & Arcus, D. (1998). Childhood derivatives of high and low reactivity in infancy. *Child Development, 69*, 1483–1493.

Kazdin, A.E., Moser, J., Colbus, D., & Bell, R. (1985). Depressive symptoms among physically abused and psychiatrically disturbed children. *Journal of Abnormal Psychology, 94*(3), 298–307.

Kumar, R. (1997). "Anybody's child": Severe disorders of mother-to-infant bonding. *British Journal of Psychiatry, 171*, 175–181.

Lee, V.E., Brooks-Gunn, J., Schnur, E., & Liaw, F. (1990). Are Head Start effects sustained? [Special Issue] Minority children. *Child Development, 61*(2), 495–507.

McCarton, C.M., Brooks-Gunn, J., Wallace, I.F., & Bauer, C.R. (1997). Results at age 8 years of early intervention for low-birth-weight premature infants: The infant health and development program. *Journal of the American Medical Association, 277*(2), 126–132.

McClellan, J., & Werry, J. (1994). Practice parameters for the assessment and treatment of children and adolescents with schizophrenia. *Journal of the American Academy of Child and Adolescent Psychiatry, 33*(5), 616–635.

Miller, L.J. (1990). Psychotic denial of pregnancy: Phenomenology and clinical management. *Hospital and Community Psychiatry, 41*(11), 1233–1237.

Miller, L.J., & Finnerty, M. (1996). Sexuality, pregnancy, and childrearing among women with schizophrenia-spectrum disorders. *Psychiatric Services, 47*(5), 502–506.

National Institute of Mental Health. (1998). Genetics and mental disorders: Report of the National Institute of Mental Health's genetics workgroup (NIH publication No. 98-4268). Rockville, MD: Author.

NICHD Early Child Care Research Network. (1999). Chronicity of maternal depressive symptoms, maternal sensitivity, and child functioning at 36 months. *Developmental Psychology, 35*, 1297–1310.

Nicholls, K.R., & Cox, J.L. (1999). The provision of care for women with postnatal mental disorder in the United Kingdom: An overview. *Hong Kong Medical Jounal, 5*(1), 43–47.

Oates, M. (2000). *Perinatal maternal mental health services*. London: Royal College of Psychiatrists.

O'Hara, M. (1997). The nature of postpartum depressive disorders. In L. Murray & P. Cooper (Eds.), *Postpartum depression and child development* (pp. 3–31). New York, NY: Guilford.

Olds, D., Henderson, C.R., Cole, R., Eckenrode, J., Kitzman, H., Luckey, D., Pettitt, L., Sidora, K., Morris, P., & Powers, J. (1998). Long-term effects of nurse home visitation on children's criminal and antisocial behavior—15-year follow-up of a randomized controlled trial. *Journal of the American Medical Association, 280*(14), 1238–1244.

Oyserman, D., Bybee, D., Mowbray, C.T., & MacFarlane, P. (in press). Support helps: Effects of community functioning and social support on parenting of African American mothers with a serious mental illness. *Journal of Marriage and the Family*.

Oyserman, D., Mowbray, C.T., Allen-Meares, P., & Firminger, K. (2000). Parenting among mothers with a mental illness. *American Journal of Orthopsychiatry, 70*(3), 296–315.

Oyserman, D., Mowbray, C.T., & Zemencuk, J.K. (1994). Resources and supports for mothers with severe mental-illness. *Health & Social Work, 19*(2), 132–142.

Rieder, R.O. (1973). Offspring of schizophrenic parents—review. *Journal of Nervous and Mental Disease, 157*(3), 179–190.

Ritsher J.E.B., Coursey, R.D., & Farrell, E.W. (1997). A survey on issues in the lives of women with severe mental illness. *Psychiatric Services, 48*(10), 1273–1282.

Rudolph, B., Larson, G.L., Sweeny, S., Hough, E.E., & Arorian, K. (1990). Hospitalized pregnant psychotic women—characteristics and treatment issues. *Hospital and Community Psychiatry, 41*(2), 159–163.

Rutter, M., Silberg, J., O'Connor, T., & Simonoff, E. (1999). Genetics and child psychiatry: II. Empirical research findings. *Journal of Child Psychology & Psychiatry & Allied Disciplines, 40*(1), 19–55.

Stocky, A., & Lynch, J. (2000). Acute psychiatric disturbance in pregnancy and the puerperium. *Best Practice & Research in Clinical Obstetrics & Gynaecology, 14*(1), 73–87.

US Department of Health and Human Services (USDHHS). (1999). Mental health: A report of the Surgeon General. Rockville, MD: USDHHS, Substance Abuse and Mental Health Services Administration, Center for Mental Health Services, National Institutes of Health, National Institute of Mental Health.

Waters, B.G., & Marchenko-Bouer, I. (1980). Psychiatric illness in the adult offspring of bipolar manic-depressives. *Journal of Affective Disorders, 2*(2), 119–126.

Wickramaratne, P., & Weissman, M. (1998). Onset of psychopathology in offspring by developmental phase and parental depression. *Journal of the American Academy of Child and Adolescent Psychiatry, 37*, 933–942.

Zahn-Waxler, C., Iannotti, R.J., Cummings, E.M., & Denham, S. (1990). Antecedents of problem behaviors in children of depressed mothers. *Development and Psychopathology, 2*, 271–291.

Chronic Disease, Adolescence

Gary W. Harper and Sybil G. Hosek

INTRODUCTION AND DEFINITIONS

This entry discusses promoting the healthy development of youth living with a chronic illness. *Chronic illness* has been defined as a condition that often appears at birth or early childhood, interferes with daily functioning, causes hospitalizations, and involves symptoms that can often be adequately managed but not cured (Pless & Pinkerton, 1975; Wallander & Thompson, 1995). Traditionally, chronic illness has been differentiated from terminal illness in that chronic illnesses are not typically fatal. However, advances in medicine have enabled previously fatal illnesses to become chronic. Diseases most often classified as chronic among adolescents include asthma, cancer, cerebral palsy, congenital heart disease, cystic fibrosis, insulin-dependent diabetes mellitus (IDDM), hemophilia, human immunodeficiency virus (HIV), juvenile rheumatoid arthritis, leukemia, renal disease, sickle cell anemia, epilepsy, and spina bifida.

One consistency across illnesses is the importance of adherence to treatment regimens, which include medications, medical appointments, and disease-monitoring techniques. Broadly defined, *adherence*, or *compliance*, is the extent to which the patient follows the prescriptions or recommendations of health care providers (Pidgeon, 1989). The most recent nomenclature uses the term adherence, which is seen as less pejorative and more client-centered than compliance (Mehta, Moore, & Graham, 1997).

SCOPE

Worldwide, over 33 million children and adolescents died in 1999 due to chronic diseases such as cancer, diabetes, asthma, and cardiovascular disease (World Health Organization, 2000). In the United States, severe chronic conditions affect approximately 1–2 children and adolescents out of 100 (Wallander & Thompson, 1995). Asthma, which affects approximately 4–9 percent of children worldwide, is the most common chronic illness among youth (Geller, 1996). Annual estimates of asthma in the United States indicate that about 4 million children and adolescents are affected and the number of asthma-related deaths is increasing (Bender, 1996; Mannino et al., 1998). About 1 in 600 US children and adolescents have IDDM, which is comparable to European countries but much higher than Asian countries (Johnson, 1995). Sickle cell disease appears predominantly in African Americans at a rate of approximately 1 in 400, yet is also prevalent in descendants from Italy, Greece, India, and other Mediterranean countries (Lemanek, Buckloh, Woods, & Butler, 1995). Cystic fibrosis, one of the most common hereditary diseases among Caucasians, is seen in approximately 1 in 2,500 live births in the United States (Stark, Jelalian, & Miller, 1995). In the United States, the cumulative total of diagnosed AIDS cases among 13–24-year-olds as of June 2000 is 30,383 (Centers for Disease Control and Prevention [CDC], 2001).

The cost of these illnesses to society can be tremendous. For example, direct medical costs for asthma in the United States total more than $9.8 billion while the value of reduced productivity due to loss of school days is approaching $1 billion (American Lung Association, 1998). Nonadherence to medical treatment can increase medical and insurance costs by leading to unnecessary hospitalizations and diagnostic tests (Van Sciver, D'Angelo, Rappaport, & Woolf, 1995). Patients who are adherent to medical regimens incur significantly lower inpatient hospital costs, community care costs, and medical costs than patients who are non-adherent or not taking medications (Gebo, Chaisson, Folkemer, Bartlett, & Moore, 1999).

THEORIES

The majority of models that have been developed specifically to understand the impact of chronic illness on adolescents, and to guide prevention efforts for this population, are grounded in a *stress and coping paradigm* (Lazarus & Folkman, 1984). This approach proposes that the young person's individual perception and cognitive appraisal of events and situations are essential factors in predicting the youth's adaptation to the stressor (i.e., chronic illness). One of the most researched models related to the health and functioning of adolescents living with chronic illness is Wallander and Varni's (1992) *Disability-stress-coping model of adjustment*, which is based in a risk and resistance framework. This framework proposes that risk and resistance factors interact to affect an adolescent's adaptation to his/her chronic illness and/or disability. In this model, risk factors include disease/disability parameters, functional independence, and psychosocial stress. Resistance factors fall into three categories: (a) intrapersonal (e.g., competence), (b) socioecological (e.g., family environment), and (c) stress-processing (e.g., coping strategies). This model suggests that as modifiable risk and resistance factors are identified in empirical studies, they provide heuristic guidance for new

preventive interventions for adolescents living with chronic illnesses and disability.

Two related stress and coping models also have been proposed to better understand the adjustment of adolescents and children living with chronic illness. Thompson, Gustafson, Hamlett, and Spock (1992) have proposed a *Transactional ecological systems* model that focuses on the adaptational processes of the young person with a chronic illness and the mother. The illness is viewed as the primary stressor to which the chronically ill individual and his/her family system must adapt, and this adaptational process is viewed as a function of biomedical, developmental, and psychosocial processes. Garmezy, Masten, and Tellegen (1984) also have proposed an extension of traditional stress and coping models that relates stress, personal attributes, and competence to maladjustment. This approach differs from traditional stress and coping approaches by using the concept of *resiliency*, which is viewed as the adolescent's ability to maintain adaptive behavior despite experiencing a stressful situation such as a chronic illness (Garmezy, 1991).

Family systems models are another category of models that have been used to explore the impact of chronic illness on adolescents for use in preventive efforts. The *Biobehavioral family model* is a type of structural family therapy model that promotes the integration of individual, family, and social levels using a developmental biopsychosocial approach to assessment and intervention. This model addresses the reciprocal influences between interactional patterns within the family and physiological functioning of the adolescent living with a chronic illness (Wood, 1994).

Although a range of cognitively based outcome expectancy models and theories have been used to predict medical adherence behaviors for adults with chronic illness (e.g., Health belief model, Protection motivation theory, Theory of reasoned action and planned behavior), only the *Health belief model* has been specifically examined with regard to adolescents and children living with chronic illness (Riekert & Drotar, 2000).

Social cognitive theory (Bandura, 1986) is a synthesis of a number of the cognitively based outcome expectancy models that retains some of the behavioral capacity and expectancy elements, but adds the key concepts of reciprocal determinism and self-efficacy. The principle of reciprocal determinism moves this theory beyond the individual level as it represents the dynamic interaction among personal determinants, environmental influences, and behavior. Self-efficacy, which is the confidence that a person feels with regard to performing a specific behavior, is an element that has been added in various forms to other existing theories of health behaviors such as the Health belief model. This theory has been used as the basis for the development of successful multifocused interventions for adolescents living with chronic illness, such as the Cystic Fibrosis Family Education Program which has been shown to increase knowledge and general self-management scores for adolescents and their caregivers, decrease adolescent behavior problems, increase parent coping, and improve pulmonary functioning (Bartholomew et al., 1997). One criticism of the Social cognitive theory with regard to its utility in the development of health behavior change interventions and its testability as a theory is that it is so vague and broad that it does not provide direct guidance for intervention development and is difficult to empirically falsify (Baranowski, Perry, & Parcel, 1997).

RESEARCH

Youth who are living with a chronic illness must juggle the traditional developmental demands that accompany the adolescent years, in addition to illness-related burdens such as persistent physical pain and discomfort, varied medical procedures, reliance on family members for treatment assistance, and threats of sustained disability or death. This combination of stressors can have a negative impact on the healthy functioning and development of adolescents living with a chronic illness. In order to develop effective prevention programs to protect the health and healthy functioning of youth living with a chronic illness, it is important to first examine the impact that living with a chronic illness has on the developing adolescent. The vast majority of research in this area has focused on the impact of chronic illness on adolescents' developmental tasks, psychological health, and medical adherence.

Impact on Developmental Tasks

Research exploring various chronic illnesses has consistently shown negative effects on developmental issues during adolescence. Gavaghan and Roach (1987) investigated ego identity development in adolescents with cancer. When compared to a control group of healthy adolescents, adolescents with cancer were rated at significantly lower developmental levels. Sayer, Hauser, Jacobson, Willett, and Cole (1995) found that diabetic youth expressed consistently lower levels of ego identity development as compared to healthy controls. Also, in comparison to healthy controls, diabetic youth showed a significant decline in their developmental pace during late adolescence. Sayer and colleagues (1995) suggest that these between-group differences may be a reflection of the "anti-adolescent demands" that having a chronic illness places on youth. For example, dietary restrictions and medication regimes run contrary to an adolescent's desire for autonomy and close peer relationships.

Impact on Psychological Health

Research exploring various chronic illnesses during adolescence has consistently shown negative effects on psychosocial health. Wallander and Varni (1995) report that adolescents with chronic physical conditions display more behavior and social problems than the general population. In comparison to adolescents without a chronic physical condition, Varni and Setoguchi (1991) found lower levels of perceived physical appearance in adolescents living with a physical condition. In a study of adolescents with cystic fibrosis and sickle cell disease, Thompson et al. (1995) reported that over half of the participants scored poorly on measures of psychological adjustment. Also, half of the participants in this study reported levels of psychological distress that met the diagnostic criteria for a psychological disorder, primarily anxiety, and phobic disorders. Thompson and colleagues (1995) also found a high frequency of oppositional disorders in their sample of adolescents with cystic fibrosis or sickle cell disease.

Impact on Medical Adherence

While advances in medical technology have increased the effectiveness of treatment for chronic illnesses, these advances have often heightened the importance of adherence to these treatments. Studies of adherence among adolescents with diabetes and cancer have shown rates of medication adherence ranging from 20 to 60 percent (Litt & Cuskey, 1980; Pidgeon, 1989; Tebbi, 1993). Furthermore, recent research has shown that adherence to more complex treatments such as dietary changes and glucose monitoring is even lower than adherence to medication (Rapoff, 1999).

The presence of psychological or developmental difficulties is often a significant predictor of non-adherence among youth living with chronic illness. Negative affect, for example, has been associated with non-adherence in a range of illnesses, including cancer, diabetes, and epilepsy (Dunbar-Jacob, Burke, & Puczynski, 1998). Pidgeon (1989) reports that anxiety is related to non-compliance among adolescent girls living with diabetes and cancer.

STRATEGIES THAT WORK

There has been a general paucity of controlled studies examining either the efficacy or effectiveness of prevention and health promotion efforts aimed at improving the health and healthy functioning of youth living with a chronic illness or disability (Roberts, 1992).

Interventions in the general field of pediatric psychology have been categorized into four broad realms of health and functioning: (a) psychosocial and developmental factors related to disease/illness treatment and management; (b) behavioral and emotional concomitants of disease/illness; (c) promotion of health and health-related behaviors; and (d) prevention of illness and injury (La Greca & Varni, 1993). The vast majority of evidence-based prevention and health promotion strategies for youth living with chronic illness have been those related to the first two domains, but with a more specific focus on the following three areas: (a) symptom management (e.g., pain, discomfort, nausea, vomiting), (b) adherence to medical regimens and general disease management, and (c) psychological adjustment to the illness. Although some programs have a singular focus on one of these areas, interventions are increasingly incorporating a focus on multiple areas of functioning in the same program.

In order to bring about significant improvements in the health and functioning of youth, these programs typically include a combination of intervention approaches, the majority of which are based in cognitive–behavioral or behavioral modalities. A meta-analytic review of 42 studies on the effectiveness of psychological interventions for children and adolescents with chronic medical illnesses (aged 3–18) revealed that behavioral and cognitive–behavioral treatments were the most commonly used treatment techniques, and that these approaches were equally effective for affecting disease management, procedural distress, and psychosocial adjustment problems (Kibby, Tyc, & Mulhern, 1998).

Symptom Management

A variety of methods have been used to assist youth living with chronic illness in coping with a wide array of aversive symptoms, including those that are experienced during painful medical procedures (e.g., venipuncture and bone marrow aspirations), as a result of the disease process (e.g., sickle cell vaso-occlusive episodes), and/or as a side effect of medical treatments (e.g., chemotherapy). Some of these procedures are psychoeducational in nature and provide information to the adolescent prior to experiencing the symptoms to assist with pain management (e.g., anticipatory guidance), whereas others are more directly focused on teaching the adolescent skills and behavioral strategies to decrease the pain and discomfort (e.g., biofeedback, relaxation, hypnosis).

A range of health-promoting behavioral techniques have been used quite effectively with adolescents who experience nausea, vomiting, and other side effects secondary to cancer treatments (Koocher, 1996), and training in the use of a developmentally appropriate form of self-hypnosis has been shown to be effective at decreasing pain and discomfort associated with such chronic illnesses as end-stage renal disease, cancer, and HIV disease among adolescents

(Harper, 1999). The use of other behavioral and cognitive–behavioral techniques such as pain-behavior contracting, thermal biofeedback relaxation, behavioral counseling, progressive muscle relaxation, guided imagery, and meditative breathing have been shown to help adolescents manage the persistent pain associated with a range of illnesses including sickle cell disease, hemophilia, and juvenile rheumatoid arthritis; especially when parents receive education and training in these techniques, and when these strategies are combined in a comprehensive program (Lemanek et al., 1995; Walco, Varni, & Ilowite, 1992).

Adherence to Medical Regimens and General Disease Management

The majority of research in the area of adherence to medical regimens among adolescents has been conducted on the predictors of adherence, with much less focus on the systematic investigation of interventions to improve adherence. Since adolescents often report lower rates of adherence to medical regimens than both children and adults, it is critical that more interventions be thoroughly evaluated.

A variety of more recent family-focused prevention and health promotion programs to improve adherence have included nurses or other professionals from the youth's health care delivery site into the intervention. Rapoff (2000) implemented a successful intervention with children and adolescents living with juvenile rheumatoid arthritis and their families that included a parent-managed token reinforcement program, whereby youth and parents received verbal, written, and audiovisual information from a nurse about several adherence improvement strategies including visual reminders, prompting, monitoring (e.g., diary logs), positive reinforcement, and discipline. Anderson, Brackett, Ho, & Laffel (2000) implemented an office-based intervention for early adolescents living with IDDM and their families that emphasized the importance of parent–adolescent teamwork in diabetes management. This successful prevention program included a focus on strategies to avoid conflicts that would damage this teamwork, and involved the adolescents and parents working collaboratively to create a family teamwork plan which was reviewed, reinforced, and/or renegotiated at each office visit with their health care professional.

Psychological Adjustment to the Illness

Adolescents who are living with a chronic illness may experience a range of psychological consequences that may vary as a function of factors such as the visibility of their condition, severity of symptoms, threat of mortality, invasiveness of treatment procedures, level of dependence on caretakers, and limitations to independent mobility. Psychological reactions to a chronic illness may manifest in the form of more traditional psychological disturbances such as depression or anxiety, or may result in exacerbated or new physical symptoms. Another issue that is of particular note in this area is that some medications do cause behavioral side effects (e.g., attentional difficulties, impulsivity, mood swings), and it may be difficult to differentiate those behavioral and psychological changes that occur as a direct result of the medical treatment and those that have developed as a result of other factors, since the reasons for such changes are typically multifaceted.

Cognitive–behavioral interventions have been shown to be effective in helping adolescents cope with their chronic illness and to manage the negative psychological sequelae often experienced by these youth. Typically these programs include a range of psychoeducational and skills training activities related to both illness/symptom management and more general stress management. For example, Hains, Davies, Behrens, & Biller (1997) demonstrated that a cognitive–behavioral intervention was effective in reducing anxiety, decreasing disease-related maladaptive coping efforts, and increasing disease-related positive coping among adolescents living with cystic fibrosis. Rotheram-Borus and colleagues (2001) recently reported on the efficacy of a prevention program for youth living with HIV disease that involved 23 sessions of small group activities, and was focused on improving quality of life and on decreasing participation in health risk behaviors. Summer camps also have been found to be effective at improving social skills, self-esteem, and general psychosocial functioning of adolescents living with chronic illnesses such as juvenile rheumatoid arthritis and diabetes (Kaplan, Chadwick, & Schimmel, 1985; Stefl, Shear, & Levinson, 1989).

STRATEGIES THAT MIGHT WORK

Future research efforts will need to focus on identifying additional modifiable risk and resiliency factors that influence the health and functioning of youth living with chronic illness. In addition, investigators need to focus on revealing the various factors that mediate the relationship between the stressors associated with having a chronic illness and the psychological adjustment to the condition. This has exciting implications for future prevention and health promotion efforts for youth living with a range of chronic health problems.

One example of the importance of focusing prevention efforts on mediating factors is illustrated in Varni and Setoguchi's (1996) study which revealed that the effects of perceived physical appearance of adolescents with congenital/acquired limb deficiencies on psychological distress is mediated by general self-esteem, thus suggesting that interventions that focus on enhancing self-esteem may be the most effective in improving the well-being of these adolescents. Varni, La Greca, and Spirito (2000) suggest that as research uncovers additional mediating factors among chronically ill youth, creative cognitive–behavioral approaches will be developed to impact these mediating factors.

La Greca (1990) suggests that future interventions should pay greater attention to those aspects of the treatment and disease process that negatively affect social functioning, and focus more attention on the role of peers in the adolescent's management of symptoms and medication demands, as well as his/her adaptation to the disease. One innovative way to increase social support for adolescents living with a chronic illness is the use of electronic support groups through the Internet. Johnson, Ravert, and Everton (2001) report on the usefulness of a web-based, highly interactive, electronic support group developed for adolescents living with cystic fibrosis. They found that over one half of the eighteen adolescents who participated in this program e-mailed each other at least once a week, and that at the end of the study, the youth believed that they had more friends who could relate to their condition than before the study. Although no pretest/posttest changes occurred on other study outcomes, the authors noted that the youth who used the support group made increased references to peers and expressed a desire to get together with other youth in the program (Johnson et al., 2001). This may be a promising intervention for adolescents given their exposure to and use of Internet resources, especially for those youth who reside in isolated areas.

Another alternative and inexpensive method for improving adherence to treatment regimens among adolescents living with chronic illness that is congruent with current youth culture, and thus may be viewed as more acceptable, is the use of text-messaging pagers. Erickson, Ascione, Kirking, and Johnson (1998) have provided preliminary data demonstrating the utility of pagers that provide multiple daily asthma-related reminders and messages for improving adherence among adolescents with asthma. Lieberman (2001) also has utilized health education and disease management video games with youth living with diabetes to improve self-care and decrease emergency room visits, and has shown support for the use of such games in increasing self-management of asthma as well. Given the proliferation of video games in current society and the comfort with which many adolescents use such games, this is a promising new method for delivering health promotion and prevention messages in a youth-sensitive manner.

School-based approaches to addressing the health concerns of adolescents living with chronic illnesses is a promising avenue for prevention and health promotion. School-linked and school-based health centers offer enormous opportunity to reach all youth who attend schools with accessible high-quality health care, since they have the potential to link youth to needed medical services, and address both the acute and chronic health care needs of young people (American Academy of Pediatrics Committee on School Health, 2001), in an environment that is virtually stigma free, confidential, and adolescent friendly. Santelli, Kouzis, and Newcomer (1996) compared health care utilization rates of high school students in schools with and without school-based health centers and found that although students in both types of schools reported similar rates of chronic health conditions, those in schools with health centers reported increased use of primary care, reduced use of emergency rooms, and fewer hospitalizations.

STRATEGIES THAT DO NOT WORK

Given the complexity of chronic illness among youth, and the multiple systemic influences of the illness on various aspects of the adolescents' development and functioning, prevention and health promotion programs that focus on a single outcome, intervene with only the adolescent, and use simplistic methods such as basic education are generally not as effective as more multifaceted programs. Although education regarding an adolescent's chronic illness is a necessary component of most multidisciplinary prevention and health promotion programs, it must be combined with other psychologically based approaches in order to bring about significant improvements in the health and functioning of youth living with chronic illnesses (Bender, 1996). This was illustrated in a meta-analysis of randomized clinical trial studies of education-based self-management programs for pediatric asthma, which showed that such teaching programs did not reduce asthma morbidity outcomes including hospitalizations and emergency room visits (Bernard-Bonnin, Stachenko, Bonin, Charette, & Rousseau, 1995).

Since family-based interventions are becoming more the norm in preventive interventions for adolescents living with chronic illness, it is important to be observant of the theoretical approach or model on which the intervention is based, as well as the developmental level of the adolescent who is living with the chronic illness. For example, in a study by Wysocki, Greco, Harris, and White (2000), Behavioral family systems therapy was not shown to improve adherence, diabetic control, or health care utilization among a group of adolescents living with IDDM. The authors suggest that this type of intervention may be more appropriate as a preventive measure for younger adolescents, as opposed to a focused intervention for older adolescents who have been living with IDDM (see also Meijer & Oppenheimer, 1995).

Although self-help groups have been shown to be an effective intervention for adults living with a range of chronic illnesses, it appears that the formation of face-to-face self-help groups may not have the same impact with adolescents. Hinrichsen, Revenson, and Shinn (1985) compared adolescents with scoliosis who attended self-help groups to those who did not attend self-help groups and found that although the majority of those who attended reported that they enjoyed the groups, they did not evidence any significant differences on measures of psychosocial adjustment from those youth who did not attend. It may be that the adolescents' developmental concerns regarding heightened self-consciousness, especially when the illness results in physical alterations or impairments in mobility, discourage youth from traveling to and physically attending a self-help group, but when the group is in the form of a supportive Internet chat room that can be accessed comfortably and confidentially from the youth's home, it is a more acceptable form of intervention (Johnson et al., 2001).

SYNTHESIS

There is a need for prevention programs that are informed by theoretically sound conceptual models related to adolescents living with chronic illness. Many researchers and clinicians agree that there is currently a gap between the conceptual models that are being developed to explain factors that are related to health and functioning among chronically ill adolescents and the clinical interventions that are being implemented by practitioners (Drotar, Riekert, Burgess, Levi, Nobile, Kaugars, & Walders, 2000). When programs are based in well-researched conceptual models, the interventionist has a greater degree of certainty that s/he is targeting key individuals (e.g., adolescent, family, peers, health care providers) with the most effectives forms of intervention. Prevention programs that are not guided by such models may be putting valuable resources into activities and interventions that do not result in the most advantageous outcomes for adolescents living with a chronic illness and their families and friends.

Bronfenbrenner's (1992) Ecological systems theory of human development offers a theoretical framework for examining the impact of chronic illness on the lives of adolescents and can provide guidance in developing preventive interventions that expand beyond the scope of more individualistic models. Bronfenbrenner (1992) suggests that adolescents are influenced by four nested interdependent levels of environmental influences, with the most basic unit being the microsystem, which includes a pattern of roles, activities, and interpersonal relationships that are experienced in the adolescent's face-to-face daily interactions. For most adolescents, the microsystem includes arenas such as the family, school, and peer group; and for adolescents living with chronic illness, the hospital or medical facility where they receive treatments would also be included. The other three systems include interactions between various microsystems (i.e., mesosystem), the structure of the larger community and its organizations (i.e., exosystem), and overarching cultural and societal values, norms, and policies (i.e., macrosystem). The creation of interventions for adolescents should take into account the specific developmental issues that confront adolescents, and practitioners must be cognizant of these issues during the implementation of their interventions. Melamed, Kaplan, and Fogel (2001) recommend that prior to implementing interventions with youth living with a chronic illness and their families, the clinician should first examine the situation within the framework of what developmental tasks need to be accomplished during the next 5 years of the youth's life.

Cognitive development during adolescence offers young people an increased range of capabilities, as is evidenced by increases in the amount of information they can process, the speed with which they process information, and the level of abstraction and hypothetical thought that they can comprehend. Adolescents' advanced cognitive development enables them to have a more sophisticated understanding of illness than children, often leading to feelings that their life and physical integrity are threatened when confronted with medical illness and procedures. Thus, prevention efforts must attend to this increased awareness of morbidity and mortality. These advanced abilities do allow health care providers the opportunity to implement interventions with adolescents that are cognitively more complex than those used with children, and to include elements that require abstract thought and reasoning.

Another feature of adolescent cognitive development is the emergence of adolescent egocentrism and the concomitant "personal fable" beliefs, which lead the adolescent to believe in his/her own personal uniqueness, invulnerability, and indestructibility (Elkind, 1978). For some youth living with chronic illness, their thoughts of mortality may increase internal conflict and confusion, as they are in direct opposition to these "personal fable" beliefs of invulnerability. Other adolescents may feel that the intervention messages do not apply to them because they feel that other people are the ones at risk and that they are invulnerable to negative health outcomes. Therefore, preventionists may need to find creative ways to personalize risk, and to examine the individual personal susceptibility of each adolescent.

Adolescence is marked by increased exploration of occupational, sexual, and ideological roles as the adolescent attempts to form a unique and mature personal identity (Adams, Gullotta, & Montemayor, 1992; Erikson, 1968). In addition, the adolescent strives to gain independence and autonomy from parents and other adults (Havighurst, 1972). If practitioners working with adolescents living with a chronic illness are not sensitive to these independence concerns when creating and implementing interventions, resistance may develop. The adolescent must be made to feel that s/he plays an integral role in the intervention and that his/her independent decisions regarding the various components of the program are considered. This can be accomplished by working collaboratively with the adolescent during the development and implementation of the intervention so that the plan fits into his/her lifestyle, as such an interactive format may increase the adolescent's felt interest and involvement in the intervention, resulting in a heightened sense of control and independence (Harper, 1999).

Drotar et al. (2000) offer a set of recommendations for future adherence intervention efforts. These recommendations include a focus on helping to normalize less than perfect adherence, setbacks, and changes in the course of the illness; developing individualized and flexible treatment recommendations that include a collaborative problem-solving approach; reinforcing adolescents for successful adherence behaviors as well as for improvements in adherence; and using assessment data and technology to provide positive feedback to adolescents and their families and to reinforce a sense of control over the regime.

Future preventive efforts to improve the health and functioning of youth living with chronic illnesses should include increasing the frequency of contact between the adolescent and his/her various health care providers and improving provider–client communication and relationship; altering the treatment experience in an attempt to decrease negative associations and increase positive experiences; modifying aspects of the treatment regimen to be more compatable with the adolescent's lifestyle and daily routine; providing preventive, chronic, and acute care services in health care settings that are convenient and developmentally appropriate so that the adolescent can obtain services without the assistance of parents; altering the adolescent's environment to decrease the presence of triggers that may result in negative health reactions and teaching the adolescent to recognize and avoid such triggers when possible; and providing culturally appropriate services that take into account the adolescent's cultural beliefs, customs, and traditions. It is only through multifaceted programs that are sensitive to the developmental and cultural needs of the adolescent that practitioners will be able to significantly improve the health and functioning of youth living with chronic illness.

Also see: Cancer: Adolescence; Depression: Adolescence; Family Strengthening: Adolescence; Nutrition and Physical Activity: Adolescence.

References

Adams, G.R., Gullotta, T.P., & Montemayor, R. (1992). *Adolescent identity formation.* Newbury Park, CA: Sage.

American Academy of Pediatric Committee on School Health (2001). School health centers and other integrated school health services: Committee on School Health. *Pediatrics, 107*(1), 198–201.

American Lung Association. (1998). *Trends in asthma morbidity and mortality.* Washington, DC: Author.

Anderson, B.J., Brackett, J., Ho, J., & Laffel, L.M.B. (2000). An intervention to promote family teamwork in diabetes management tasks: Relationships among parental involvement, adherence to blood glucose monitoring, and glycemic control in young adolescents with type 1 diabetes. In D. Drotar (Ed.), *Promoting adherence to medical treatment in chronic childhood illness: Concepts, methods, and interventions* (pp. 347–365). Mahwah, NJ: Lawrence Erlbaum Associates.

Bandura, A. (1986). *Social foundations of thought and action: A social cognitive theory.* Englewood Cliffs, NJ: Prentice-Hall.

Baranowski, T., Perry, C.L., & Parcel. G.S. (1997). How individuals, environments, and health behavior interact: Social cognitive theory. In K. Glanz, F.M. Lewis, & B.K. Rimer (Eds.), *Health behavior and health education: Theory, research, and practice* (2nd ed., pp. 153–179). San Francisco: Jossey-Bass.

Bartholomew, L.K., Czyzewski, D.I., Parcel, G.S., Swank, P.R., Sockrider, M.M., Mariotto, M.J., Schidlow, D.V., Fink, R.J., & Seilheimer, D.K. (1997). Self-management of cystic fibrosis: Short-term outcomes of the Cystic Fibrosis Family Education Program. *Health Education and Behavior, 24*(5), 652–666.

Bender, B.G. (1996). Establishing a role for psychology in respiratory medicine. In R.J. Resnick & R.H. Rozensky (Eds.), *Health psychology through the lifespan: Practice and research opportunities* (pp. 227–238). Washington, DC: American Psychological Association.

Bernard-Bonnin, A., Stachenko, S., Bonin, D., Charette, C., & Rousseau, E. (1995). Self-management teaching programs and morbidity of pediatric asthma: A meta-analysis. *Journal of Allergy and Clinical Immunology, 95*, 34–41.

Bronfenbrenner, U. (1992). Ecological systems theory. In R. Vasta (Ed.), *Six theories of child development: Revised formulations and current issues* (pp. 187–249). Bristol, PA: Jessica Kingsley.

Centers for Disease Control and Prevention (2001). *HIV/AIDS surveillance report.* Atlanta: Author.

Dunbar-Jacob, J., Burke, L.E., & Puczynski, S. (1998). Clinical assessment and management of adherence to medical regimens. In P.M. Nicassio and T.W. Smith (Eds.), *Managing chronic illness.* Washington, DC: American Psychological Association.

Drotar, D., Riekert, K.A., Burgess, E., Levi, R., Nobile, C., Kaugars, A.S., & Walders, N. (2000). Treatment adherence in childhood chronic illness: Issues and recommendations to enhance practice, research, and training. In D. Drotar (Ed.), *Promoting adherence to medical treatment in chronic childhood illness: Concepts, methods, and interventions* (pp. 367–381). Mahwah, NJ: Lawrence Erlbaum Associates.

Elkind, D. (1978). Understanding the young adolescent. *Adolescence, 13*, 127–134.

Erickson, S.R., Ascione, F.J., Kirking, D.M., & Johnson, C.E. (1998). Use of a paging system to improve medication self-management in patients with asthma. *Journal of the American Pharmaceutical Association, 38*, 767–769.

Erikson, E.H. (1968). *Identity: Youth and crisis.* New York: Norton.

Garmezy, N. (1991). Resilience in children's adaptation to negative life events and stressed environments. *Pediatric Annals, 20*, 460–466.

Garmezy, N., Masten, A.S., & Tellegen, A. (1984). The study of stress and competence in children: A building block for developmental psychopathology. *Child Development, 55*, 97–111.

Gavaghan, M.P., & Roach, J.E. (1987). Ego identity development of adolescents with cancer. *Journal of Pediatric Psychology, 12*(2), 203–213.

Gebo, K.A., Chaisson, R.E., Folkemer, J.G., Bartlett, J.G., & Moore, R.D. (1999). Costs of HIV medical care in the era of highly active antiretroviral therapy. *AIDS, 13*, 963–969.

Geller, M. (1996). Acute management of severe childhood asthma. *AACN Clinical Issues, 7*, 519–528.

Hains, A.A., Davies, W.H., Behrens, D., & Biller, J.A. (1997). Cognitive behavioral interventions for adolescents with cystic fibrosis. *Journal of Pediatric Psychology, 22*(5), 669–687.

Harper, G.W. (1999). A developmentally sensitive approach to clinical hypnosis for chronically and terminally ill adolescents. *American Journal of Clinical Hypnosis, 42*, 50–60.

Havighurst, R.J. (1972). *Developmental tasks and education* (3rd ed.). New York: McKay.

Hinrichsen, G.A., Revenson, T.A., & Shinn, M. (1985). Does self-help help? An empirical investigation of scoliosis peer support groups. *Journal of Social Issues, 41*(1), 65–87.

Johnson, K.B., Ravert, R.D., & Everton, A. (2001). Hopkins Teen Central: Assessment of an internet-based support system for children with cystic fibrosis. *Pediatrics, 107*(2), E24.

Johnson, S.B. (1995). Insulin-dependent diabetes mellitus in childhood. In M.C. Roberts (Ed.), *Handbook of pediatric psychology* (2nd ed.). New York: Guilford Press.

Kaplan, R.M., Chadwick, M.W., & Schimmel, L.E. (1985). Social learning intervention to promote metabolic control in type I diabetes mellitus: Pilot experiment results. *Diabetes Care, 8*, 152–155.

Kibby, M.Y., Tyc, V.L., & Mulhern, R.K. (1998). Effectiveness of psychological intervention for children and adolescents with chronic medical illness: A meta-analysis. *Clinical Psychology Review, 18*(1), 103–117.

Koocher, G.P. (1996). Pediatric oncology: Medical crisis intervention. In R.J. Resnick & R.H. Rozensky (Eds.), *Health psychology through the lifespan: Practice and research opportunities* (pp. 227–238). Washington, DC: American Psychological Association.

La Greca, A.M. (1990). Social consequences of pediatric conditions: Fertile area for future investigation and intervention? *Journal of Pediatric Psychology, 15*, 285–307.

La Greca, A.M., & Varni, J.W. (1993). Editorial: Interventions in pediatric psychology: A look toward the future. *Journal of Pediatric Psychology, 18*(6), 667–679.

Lazarus, R.S., & Folkman, S. (1984). *Stress, appraisal, and coping.* New York: Springer.

Lieberman, D.A. (2001). Management of chronic pediatric diseases with interactive health games: Theory and research findings. *Journal of Ambulatory Care Management, 24*(1), 26–38.

Lemanek, K.L., Buckloh, L.M., Woods, G., & Butler, R. (1995). Diseases of the circulatory system: Sickle cell disease and hemophilia. In M.C. Roberts (Ed.), *Handbook of pediatric psychology* (2nd ed.). New York: Guilford Press.

Litt, I.F., & Cuskey, W.R. (1980). Compliance with medical regimens during adolescence. *Pediatric Clinics of North America, 27*, 1–15.

Mannino, D.M., Homa, D.M., Pertowski, C.A., Ashizawa, A., Nixon, L.L., Johnson, C.A., Ball, L.B., Jack, E., Kang, D.S. (1998, April 24). Surveillance for asthma—United States, 1960–1995. In CDC Surveillance Summaries. *Morbidity and Mortality Weekly Report, 47*(SS-1), 1–28.

Mehta, S., Moore, R.D., & Graham, N.M. (1997). Potential factors affecting adherence with HIV therapy. *AIDS, 11*, 1665–1670.

Meijer, A.M., & Oppenheimer, L. (1995). The excitation-adaptation model of pediatric chronic illness. *Family Process, 34*, 441–454.

Melamed, B.G., Kaplan, B., & Fogel, J. (2001). Childhood health issues across the life span. In A. Baum, T.A. Revenson, & J.E. Singer (Eds.), *Handbook of health psychology* (pp. 449–457). Mahwah, NJ: Lawrence Erlbaum Associates.

Pidgeon, V. (1989). Compliance with chronic illness regimens: School-aged children and adolescents. *Journal of Pediatric Nursing, 4*(1), 36–47.

Pless, I.B., & Pinkerton, P. (1975). *Chronic childhood disorders: Promoting patterns of adjustment.* Chicago: Year Book Medical.

Rapoff, M.A. (1999). *Adherence to pediatric medical regimens.* New York: Kluwer Academic/Plenum.

Rapoff, M.A. (2000). Facilitating adherence to medical regimens for pediatric rheumatic diseases: Primary, secondary, and tertiary prevention. In D. Drotar (Ed.), *Promoting adherence to medical treatment in chronic childhood illness* (pp. 329–345). Mahwah, NJ: Lawrence Erlbaum Associates.

Riekert, K.A., & Drotar, D. (2000). Adherence to medical treatment in pediatric chronic illness: Critical issues and answered questions. In D. Drotar (Ed.), *Promoting adherence to medical treatment in chronic childhood illness* (pp. 3–32). Mahwah, NJ: Lawrence Erlbaum Associates.

Roberts, M.C. (1992). Vale dictum: An editor's view of the field of pediatric psychology. *Journal of Pediatric Psychology, 13*, 329–347.

Rotheram-Borus, M.J., Lee, M.B., Murphy, D.A., Futterman, D., Duan, N., Birnbaum, J.M., & Lightfoot, M. (2001). Teens linked to care consortium. Efficacy of preventive intervention for youths living with HIV. *American Journal of Public Health, 91*(3), 400–405.

Santelli, J., Kouzis, A., & Newcomer, S. (1996). School-based health centers and adolescent use of primary care and hospital care. *Journal of Adolescent Health, 19*(4), 267–275.

Sayer, A.G., Hauser, S.T., Jacobson, A.M., Willett, J.B., & Cole, C.F. (1995). Developmental influences on adolescent health. In J.L. Wallander & L.J. Siegel (Eds.), *Adolescent Health Problems.* New York: Guilford Press.

Stark, L.J., Jelalian, E., & Miller, D.L. (1995). Cystic fibrosis. In M.C. Roberts (Ed.), *Handbook of pediatric psychology* (2nd ed.). New York: Guilford Press.

Stefl, M.E., Shear, E.S., & Levinson, J.E. (1989). Summer camps for juveniles with rheumatic disease: Do they make a difference? *Arthritis Care and Research, 2*(1), 10–15.

Tebbi, C.K. (1993). Treatment compliance in childhood and adolescence. *Cancer, 71*(10), 3441–3449.

Thompson, R.J., Gustafson, K.E., & Gil, K.G. (1995). Psychological adjustment of adolescents with cystic fibrosis or sickle cell disease and their mothers (pp. 232–247). In J.L. Wallander & L.J. Siegel (Eds.), *Adolescent Health Problems.* New York: Guilford Press.

Thompson, R.J., Jr., Gustafson, K.E., Hamlett, K.W., & Spock, A. (1992). Psychological adjustment of children with cystic fibrosis: The role of child cognitive processes and maternal adjustment. *Journal of Pediatric Psychology, 17*, 741–755.

Van Sciver, M.M., D'Angelo, E.J., Rappaport, L., & Woolf, A.D. (1995). Pediatric compliance and the roles of distinct treatment characteristics, treatment attitudes, and family stress: A preliminary report. *Developmental and Behavioral Pediatrics, 16*(5), 350–358.

Varni, J.W., La Greca, A.M., & Spirito, A. (2000). Cognitive–behavioral interventions for children with chronic health conditions. In P.C. Kendall (Ed.), *Child & adolescent therapy: Cognitive–behavioral procedures* (2nd ed., pp. 291–333). New York, NY: Guilford Press.

Varni, J.W., & Setoguchi, Y. (1991). Correlates of perceived physical appearance in children with congenital/acquired limb deficiencies. *Journal of Developmental and Behavioral Pediatrics, 12*, 171–176.

Varni, J.W., & Setoguchi, Y. (1996). Perceived physical appearance and adjustment of adolescents with congenital/acquired limb deficiencies: A path-analytic model. *Journal of Clinical Child Psychology, 25*(2), 201–208.

Walco, G.A., Varni, J.W., & Ilowite, N.T. (1992). Cognitive–behavioral pain management in children with juvenile rheumatoid arthritis. *Pediatrics, 89*(6), 1075–1079.

Wallander, J.L., & Thompson, R.J., Jr. (1995). Psychosocial adjustment of children with chronic physical conditions. In M.C. Roberts (Ed.), *Handbook of pediatric psychology* (2nd ed.). New York: Guilford Press.

Wallander, J.L., & Varni, J.W. (1992). Adjust in children with chronic physical disorders: Programmatic research on a disability-stress-coping model. In A.M. La Greca, L.J. Siegel, J.L. Wallander, & C.E. Walker (Eds.), *Stress and coping in child health* (pp. 279–298). New York: Guilford Press.

Wallander, J.L., & Varni, J.W. (1995). Appraisal, coping, and adjustment in adolescents with a physical disability. In J.L. Wallander & L.J. Siegel (Eds.), *Adolescent health problems.* New York: Guilford Press.

Wood, B.L. (1994). One articulation of the structural family therapy model: A biobehavioral family model of chronic illness in children. *Journal of Family Therapy, 16*(1), 53–72.

World Health Organization. (2000). *World Health Report 2000.* Geneva, Switzerland: Author.

Wysocki, T., Greco, P., Harris, M.A., & White, N.H. (2000). Behavioral family systems therapy for adolescents with diabetes. In D. Drotar (Ed.), *Promoting adherence to medical treatment in chronic childhood illness: Concepts, methods, and interventions* (pp. 367–381). Mahwah, NJ: Lawrence Erlbaum Associates.

Chronic Disease, Adulthood

Joshua Fogel

INTRODUCTION

Chronic diseases affect everyone regardless of race, ethnicity, or socioeconomic status. There are many types of chronic diseases. Some afflict many with pain or inconvenience but allow individuals many years of life; examples are diabetes, asthma, epilepsy, and arthritis. Other chronic diseases are life threatening and often cause death; examples are cardiovascular disease, cancer, and AIDS. This entry discusses cardiovascular disease as representative of chronic disease. It presents an overview of the evidence-based interventions that work, might work, and do not work in the primary prevention of cardiovascular disease.

DEFINITIONS

Chronic disease is a disease lasting a long time and showing a slow progression of change in the condition.

Cardiovascular disease refers to disease pertaining to the heart and blood vessels. Risk factors include high levels of triglycerides, LDL cholesterol ("bad" cholesterol), and blood pressure in the body. Cigarette use, eating a diet high in saturated fat, and obesity are behavioral risk factors. Atherosclerosis (plaque deposited in the arteries) can result from these risk factors and cause cardiovascular disease.

Ischemic heart disease is a type of cardiovascular disease where there is inadequate blood flow to the heart leading to angina pectoris (severe heart pain) and if untreated, to myocardial infarction (heart attack). *Congestive heart failure* is a condition marked by weakness, edema, abdominal discomfort, and shortness of breath due to this inadequate blood flow. Individuals with congestive heart failure can live for many years with this condition.

SCOPE

Each region has different rates of incidence and prevalence. The World Bank and World Health Organization commissioned the Global Burden of Disease Study to examine over 200 health conditions worldwide (Murray & Lopez, 1996). One of the conditions studied was ischemic heart disease, a type of cardiovascular disease. Table 1 shows the effect of congestive heart failure in established market economies (e.g., United States, Canada, Western Europe), sub-Saharan Africa, and worldwide. As can be seen, in a traditional environment such as sub-Saharan Africa, the incidence, prevalence, and average duration are approximately

Table 1. Congestive Heart Failure Rates in Selected Regions

Region	Age[a]	Incidence[b]		Prevalence[b]		Average duration[a]	
		Men	Women	Men	Women	Men	Women
Established market economy	15–44	4.9	1.4	28.6	7.7	6.9	6.8
	45–59	63.8	17.3	292.2	68.9	5.0	4.2
Sub-Saharan Africa	15–44	4.7	4.2	23.0	23.0	5.7	6.6
	45–59	29.6	23.0	121.0	98.0	4.2	4.1
Worldwide	15–44	4.7	3.1	25.5	18.7	6.7	7.5
	45–59	59.0	24.4	262.7	111.1	4.9	4.7

Notes: Based upon the Global Burden of Disease Study conducted by the World Bank and World Health Organization.
[a] In years.
[b] Per 100,000 individuals.

similar for men and women. On the other hand, established market economies are similar to the worldwide statistics where women have lower incidence and prevalence than men. Surprisingly, this does not affect the average duration of disease, where men and women have approximately the same average duration of disease.

The costs involved to society are great. Individuals are unable to work in certain labor-intensive occupations due to fear of exacerbating their disease. In the United States, coronary heart disease is the leading cause of work-related disability among men over age 50. As many as 15 percent of these individuals are unable to return to work. Cardiovascular disease is the most common reason for physician visits and was responsible for over 6 million hospitalizations in 1991. The total financial burden for treatment of cardiovascular disease was over $108 billion (Foreyt & Carlos-Poston, 1996). In the United States in 1993, 14 percent of health-care expenditures were for cardiovascular disease (Darnay, 1998).

THEORIES

Behavioral and psychological factors can influence heath-related behavior. Some of the significant theories and examples demonstrating the theory's relevance to primary prevention are discussed below.

Behavior modification relies on the successful application of principles of learning theory to change unwanted behavior (Sarafino, 2001). This can involve respondent (classical) or operant conditioning. Respondent (classical) conditioning involves learning an association by means of the pairing of a stimulus and a response. For example, due to the paired association of feeling good by eating foods high in cholesterol and sodium at your favorite restaurant, your mouth begins salivating when you pass the restaurant. This can lead to your eating foods that may not be healthy and prevent your successful attempts to lose weight.

Operant conditioning involves behavior change due to consequences. There are three important principles of consequences. The reinforcement principle suggests that behavior followed by satisfying consequences is more likely to be repeated. The punishment principle suggests that behavior followed by unpleasant consequences will be less likely to be repeated. The extinction principle suggests that the removal of all consequences that maintain an undesired behavior will likely lead to the eventual extinction of that behavior. Different combinations of the reinforcement, punishment, and extinction principles can occur. For example, the punishment principle applies in the attempt to stop smoking. After stopping, your body has physical withdrawal feelings that make you feel uncomfortable. You stop your behavior of cigarette avoidance and use cigarettes again.

Your good behavior, which led to unpleasant consequences related to withdrawal, now stops. A way to avoid this situation would be to provide yourself with positive reinforcers for avoidance of cigarettes (e.g., talking with a friend about your accomplishments of avoidance of cigarette use). As you appreciate the support from your friend, you continue your behavior of cigarette avoidance.

Another important learning principle is *modeling* (Bandura, 1986), which relies on observational learning. People can learn new thoughts or behaviors by their exposure to the complex behavior of significant others. For example, influential community leaders in an area discuss with other community members how much they enjoy their newly undertaken healthy behaviors like taking a walk during lunch hour, which contributes to the prevention of future disease. These community members might model this lunchtime walking behavior because they see the positive outcomes and enjoyment of walking by the influential community leaders.

Individual beliefs are important for preventive action. The *health belief model* (e.g., Curry & Emmons, 1994) suggests that motivation for health-related actions or behaviors is a decision-making process that relies on three factors: (1) the perceived susceptibility to disease, (2) the perceived seriousness of the disease, and (3) the belief that certain behaviors will reduce the perceived threat of disease and that taking action is better than ignoring the perceived threat. For example, you routinely weigh yourself because this awareness will help you continue your healthy diet and exercise regime that were undertaken to maintain your appropriate weight as a protective factor against cardiovascular disease.

The *theory of reasoned action* (Montano & Taplin, 1991) suggests that the most important determinant of behavior is an individual's intention. Intentions are influenced by both an individual's attitudes regarding the behavior and by the perceived social normative influence of significant people in that individual's life. For example, you routinely weigh because you believe that this is important for weight reduction and you know that your spouse thinks it is a good idea.

Self-efficacy (Bandura, 1986) involves the belief that one has the ability to deal with a specific challenging event in life. Individuals judge their capability to organize and execute actions necessary to achieve certain goals, which involves existing knowledge, skills, or motivation, and the judgment that one can use them to achieve a given objective. For example, you participate in a rigorous exercise program to lose weight. You do this since you judge that you are able to use these learned exercise skills to lower cardiovascular risk and help prevent cardiovascular disease.

The concept of *locus of control* (Rotter, Chance, & Phares, 1972) reflects the perceived control one has over one's own behavior that ranges from high internal (self-control) to high external (control by others). The theory suggests that individuals with high internal locus of control take responsibility for their own actions and view themselves as being able to control their destiny while individuals with high external locus of control believe that they cannot control events and attribute actions to outside forces. One can have a high internal locus of control but a low self-efficacy. For example, you can believe that risk factor reduction is dependent on your lifestyle and not on external events. However, you do not believe in your ability to successfully participate in an exercise program that will lower your cardiovascular risk. As a result, you will likely not attempt to exercise in an effort to lose weight.

Motivation affects the way people make decisions and change. The *transtheoretical model* (Prochaska, Norcross, & DiClimente, 1994) describes five stages of change. These stages are precontemplation, contemplation, preparation, action, and maintenance. Successful interventions work when they are compatible with an individual's stage. For example, you may smoke cigarettes. If you attend a smoking cessation treatment session because your spouse coerced you into attending, you are probably in the stage of precontemplation or contemplation. An active treatment approach involving directives to stop smoking most likely will not benefit you, as you are not motivated to actively change smoking behavior. You need treatment based on information about cigarette use and its harmful effects on cardiovascular disease. You may then progress into the preparation stage where you will be more agreeable to adhere to an active treatment regimen of stopping smoking.

RESEARCH

Primary prevention of cardiovascular disease has had excellent results in public health population interventions. Two styles exist. One targets high-risk populations through population screening for specific risk factors. The other targets the whole community.

Many advantages exist for the community primary prevention strategy (Shea & Basch, 1990a). First, health-related behaviors often involve family, social, and cultural contexts. Interventions that target the individual plus the individual's environment are more likely to be effective. Second, many risk factors have high prevalence that can best change by targeting the whole population (e.g., cigarette use, a sedentary lifestyle, LDL cholesterol—the "bad cholesterol"). Third, all of the population is at risk for poor heath-related behaviors related to diet and physical activity. These behaviors develop at a very young age, are quite difficult to change, and often lead to atherosclerosis. Most atherosclerosis occurs decades before symptomatic disease. Fourth, the initial risk-factor level does not predict those who are most likely to reduce risk factors to healthy levels. Those who are not at high risk may have a better outcome for risk reduction. Fifth, screening for high-risk populations is costly due to the expense of the screening program and the involvement of medical personnel.

Some examples of a community intervention approach involve studies in Finland and the United States (Shea & Basch, 1990b). The North Karelia Project (Puska et al., 1985) is a multi-factorial intervention that focused on serum lipids, diet, cigarette use, and hypertension but not on obesity and a sedentary lifestyle since they were not prevalent in the Finnish population. The intervention was based on the principles of modeling to encourage individuals to modify behavior (e.g., through health-education programs shown on television). Mass media messages on television indicating that these messages were endorsed by the World Health Organization also influenced individual beliefs (which would follow from the theory of reasoned action). Researchers used cultural sensitivity by working together with community leaders who helped spread the information through their social networks. Likewise, the study involved community organizations that were involved in trying to change the harmful behaviors. Healthful results were reported.

In the United States, the Stanford Three Community Study, the Stanford Five City Project, the Minnesota Heart Health Program, and the Pawtucket Heart Health Program (Ketola, Sipila, & Makela, 2000; Shea & Basch, 1990a) all used a community intervention approach. The Stanford Three Community Study (Farquhar, 1991; Farquhar et al., 1994) emphasized the mass exposure to a health-oriented media campaign delivered to two relatively isolated small communities, and not to a third (control) community. Media messages involved using television, radio, newspapers, newsletters, booklets, and self-help kits. Increased healthful results were reported.

The Stanford Five City Project extended the research findings from the Stanford Three Community Study. It focused on smoking, diet, high blood pressure, exercise, and obesity. Interventions were delivered through mass media as well as with some targeted interventions. During the 6-year intervention period, each adult in the participating communities received approximately 26 hr of exposure. Principles of modeling and involving community organizations helped modify behavior.

The study used a social marketing model. The concept behind this approach was to determine the product, promote it, find the best places to distribute it, and make the price of trying the product affordable to those who could benefit from it. The product in this situation was lifestyle modification. The results showed reduction in blood pressure, cigarette use, "bad" cholesterol, and improved physical activity for the experimental communities as compared to the control community.

Psychological factors such as social isolation, psychological stress, hostility, and depression have all been shown to contribute to cardiovascular disease (Fogel, 2000). Further primary prevention research is necessary to consider effective interventions regarding these factors.

STRATEGIES THAT WORK

The key to strategies that work is that they are comprehensive lifestyle approaches that saturate individuals and their environments. Some of these successful strategies can be performed on an individual level. Others require the resources of a comprehensive public health community intervention.

Individual Approaches

Some studies demonstrate interventions that individual primary-care practitioners can perform, often with the involvement of spouses and family members. This is consistent with the often-cited importance of social support in offering protection from cardiovascular disease (Bruhn, 1996).

In Norway, a study by Knutsen and Knutsen (1991), involved a physician making two home visits to counsel the complete family. Emphasis was placed on dietary factors, but smoking and exercise were discussed too. Follow-up was done with quarterly newsletters and with two individual phone calls only to the adult men. The results showed that men had better dietary habits, reduced triglycerides, and a reduced coronary risk score. However, the intervention did not show any positive change for body mass index, blood pressure, or cigarette use.

In the United Kingdom, Pyke, Wood, Kinmonth, and Thompson (1997) presented a study in which a nurse gave an average of two health educational sessions to participants, with a spouse attending one of those sessions. After one year, both target men and women had reduced body mass index, blood pressure, cholesterol, and cigarette use.

Community-Level Approaches

Other studies are more comprehensive and require involvement beyond that of one or two practitioners in the intervention. In Finland (Puska, 1996), the North Karelia study used a similar approach and many of the principles used in the Stanford studies. This intervention used the communication–behavior change model, massed exposure to the media, and focused on community organizations. The goal was to use a diffusion model where the early adapters would influence many others. Organizations targeted included traditional community organizations, special interest groups, and worksites. There was also collaboration with the food industry and supermarkets. The results showed that men in the experimental group compared to the control group had lower blood pressure, cigarette use, harmful cholesterol, and improved dietary habits. The areas targeted had a 46 percent decrease in coronary heart disease.

In Germany (Hoffmeister et al., 1996), a public health intervention used the media, held classes, and focused on community institutions. This intervention included public events; there were several hundred health expositions and activities held in each participating region. As compared to the control group of a national representative sample, participants had reduced blood pressure, cholesterol, and cigarette use, but no changes in body mass index.

STRATEGIES THAT MIGHT WORK

Individual Approaches

In the United Kingdom, a series of primary prevention studies were done in general-practitioner settings with patients not considered at high risk. These strategies show promise, but their results are not conclusive enough to state that they are always effective. One study by Muir, Mant, Jones, and Yudkin (1994), involved nurses performing various health checks. They measured the patient's blood pressure and weight, and gave individualized advice on smoking and cardiovascular risk factors. The results showed reduced cholesterol, blood pressure, and body mass index but no change in cigarette use. Although these results are promising, the authors of this study note that similar studies show no benefits of health checks for cholesterol levels.

Baron, Gleason, Crowe, and Mann (1990) conducted a study in which nurses advised patients individually or in groups on optimal body weight and diet. Booklets were given on diet, recipes, and local restaurants that served healthy food options. At 1- and 3-month follow-up, men had reduced cholesterol, while no change was observed for women. At 1-year, no differences were observed. This suggests that the effects remain only while being actively encouraged.

Wood et al. (1994) studied how to involve both members of a couple in their mutual health. Nurses screened a couple, and discussed their cardiovascular risk status, and where appropriate, gave them informational pamphlets. Booklets were also provided that allowed the couple to record changes in smoking, weight, diet, alcohol consumption, and exercise. The results at 1-year later showed a reduced cardiovascular risk score. However, the cholesterol and blood pressure were only minimally lower. Many who did not return were more likely to smoke cigarettes and be overweight. Family interventions appear to be successful only when they are more intensive and not just a one-session intervention.

In the United States, Dunn et al. (1997) encouraged healthy individuals to perform physical exercise. In addition, one group learned psychological strategies to enhance their exercise compliance. Although the traditional exercise group and the intervention group both had reduced cardiovascular risk factors, this self-motivational intervention may be a useful additional approach for those who are not as motivated to exercise.

In Finland (Miettinen et al., 1985), high-risk individuals were given oral and written dietary instructions. They were included in a physical activity program. Advice was given individually to stop smoking. If blood pressure was above target levels after 4 months, medication was given. This program had many follow-up sessions. Although the results were promising in that participants had reduced triglycerides, cholesterol, weight, blood pressure, and cigarette use, results usually suggesting a successful outcome, the intervention did not reduce rates of coronary morbidity and mortality. The non-intervention group had significantly less of these adverse outcomes. The authors of this study suggest that these events were due to possible adverse drug effects from the anti-hypertensive medication.

Community-Level Approaches

Community intervention approaches that have had some success usually incorporated medication for hypertension. In the United States (MRFIT, 1982), a comprehensive treatment plan included many measures found to be effective in successful primary prevention. Physicians educated participants individually. Spouses and friends had the option of attending a series of 10 lectures discussing risk factors of smoking, hypertension, and cholesterol. A multidisciplinary team included behavioral scientists, nutritionists, nurses, and physicians in the education of participants. Special smoking-cessation programs included behavior modification approaches and hypnosis. Hypertension was treated with medication. Participants were seen every 4 months. The results showed a decline in risk factors but no differences between the intervention and control group.

STRATEGIES THAT DO NOT WORK

Individual Approaches

In a Norwegian study by Meland, Laerum, and Ulvik (1997), participants received an intervention where they were given various health options. Physicians were encouraged to support their choice of option in an advisory manner. Participants were given self-help material based on psychological principles of cognitive-behavior modification.

They also were given an audiotape on stress reduction that contained relaxation and self-coping information. The results showed that their risk factors did not differ as compared to a traditional approach of a physician discussing risk factors and supplying informative handouts.

Lindholm, Ekbom, Dash, Eriksson, Tibblin, and Schersten, (1995), conducted a study in Sweden in which participants were given regular care by a physician and also shown videos on cardiovascular risk factors for six sessions. A physician or nurse discussed these videos with the group who watched them. The results showed no difference in the intervention group as compared to the control group of regular care. The authors of this study suggest that customized messages are necessary for successful intervention. Video watching does not offer that option.

Community-Level Approaches

Glasgow, Terborg, Hollis, Severson, and Boles (1995), conducted a worksite-wellness program in the United States using the transtheoretical stages of change model to reduce cardiovascular risk factors. Approaches included motivational, educational, and environmental strategies. The results showed no differences in dietary intake, cholesterol, and cigarette use. The authors of this study suggest that the program may not have been clearly structured in regard to a participant's current preventive stage, since it allowed for a lot of choice among the participants.

SYNTHESIS

Primary prevention can occur in many ways. The key to any successful cost-effective approach is to provide the least amount of intervention with the most potential benefits. Lessons learned from various primary prevention trials are applicable in traditional general-practitioner settings.

Physicians in coordination with nurses, nutritionists, and mental health professionals can offer brief interventions to reduce cardiovascular disease. This can be performed at low cost and with only a few sessions. This intervention should involve the significant others of the individual being treated. This social support can enhance treatment compliance and motivate individuals to continue their lifestyle modification.

Education by this multidisciplinary team can offer the specialized training and the unique perspective of each discipline. Nutritionists together with the individual, can plan a proper diet. Physicians and nurses can offer preventive medical advice, while mental health professionals can offer their unique perspective of applying psychological principles to motivate healthly behaviors.

Socioeconomic factors should be considered in any intervention, whether done on the individual or community level. In the United States and Western Europe, often those in the lower classes have more cardiovascular disease (Terris, 1999). Involvement of community organizations whose clientele is made up of these often-neglected groups can make a large contribution to primary prevention by combining their practice experiences with strategies used in preventing problems and promoting desired goals.

Cultural practices should be emphasized. In the United States, different lifestyles exist for different groups. For example, in the United States, African Americans have a decline in leisure-time activities at middle age (James, 1999). They may not be interested in participating in an exercise program due to cultural practices. Implementation of focus groups should help decide what methods are best for a particular cultural group. Primary prevention programmers should consider the possibility of varied cultural practices that are compatible with both health goals and acceptable cultural practices.

A community able to afford a large-scale intervention has many effective options. It is important to involve as many organizations as possible that will constantly promote the objectives of the intervention program. The media should be used to expose individuals to the messages of lifestyle change. This community approach in combination with general-medical treatment and public health outreach can enhance primary prevention of cardiovascular disease.

Also see: Cancer: Adulthood; Depression: Adulthood; Physical Fitness: Adulthood.

References

Bandura, A. (1986). *Social foundations of thought and action: A social cognitive theory*. Englewood Cliffs, NJ: Prentice-Hall.

Baron, J.A., Gleason, R., Crowe, B., & Mann, J.I. (1990). Preliminary trial of the effect of general practice based nutritional advice. *British Journal of General Practice, 40*, 137–141.

Bruhn, J.G. (1996). Social support and heart disease. In G.L. Cooper (Ed.), *Handbook of stress, medicine, and health* (pp. 253–268). Boca Raton, FL: CRC Press.

Curray, S.J., & Emmons, K.M. (1994). Theoretical models for predicting and improving compliance with breast cancer screening. *Annals of Behavioral Medicine, 16*(4), 302–316.

Darnay, A.J. (1998). *Statistical record of health & medicine* (2nd ed.). New York: Gale.

Dunn, A.L., Marcus, B.H., Kampert, J.B., Garcia, M.E., Kohl, H.W., III, & Blair, S.N. (1997). Reduction in cardiovascular disease risk factors: 6-month results from Project Active. *Preventive Medicine, 26*, 883–892.

Farquhar, J.W. (1991). The Stanford cardiovascular disease prevention programs. *Annals of the New York Academy of Sciences, 623*, 327–331.

Farquhar, J.W., Maccoby, N., Wood, P.W., Alexander, J.K., Breitrose, H., Brown, B.W., Jr., Haskell, W.L., McAlister, A.L., Meyer, A.J., Nash, J.D., & Stern, M.P. (1994). Community education for cardiovascular disease. In A. Steptoe & J. Wardle (Eds.), *Psychosocial processes and health: A reader* (pp. 316–324). New York: Cambridge University Press.

Fogel, J. (2000). Psychosocial factors affecting atherosclerotic coronary artery disease. *Einstein Quarterly Journal of Biology and Medicine, 17,* 91–97.

Foreyt, J.P., & Carlos-Poston, W.S., II. (1996). Reducing risk for cardiovascular disease. *Psychotherapy, 33,* 576–586.

Glasgow, R.E., Terborg, J.R., Hollis, J.F., Severson, H.H., & Boles, S.M. (1995). Take heart: Results from the initial phase of a work-site wellness program. *American Journal of Public Health, 85*(2), 209–216.

Hoffmeister, H., Mensink, G.B.M., Stolzenberg, H., Hoeltz, J., Kreuter, H., Laaser, U., Nussel, E., Hullemann, K.D., & van Troschke, J. (1996). Reduction of coronary heart disease risk factors in the German cardiovascular prevention study. *Preventive Medicine, 25,* 135–145.

James, S.A., (1999). Primordial prevention of cardiovascular disease among African-Americans: A social epidemiological perspective. *Preventive Medicine, 29,* S84-S89.

Ketola, E., Sipila, R., & Makela, M. (2000). Effectiveness of individual lifestyle interventions in reducing cardiovascular disease and risk factors. *Annals of Medicine, 32,* 239–251.

Knutsen, S.F., & Knutsen, R. (1991). The Tromso survey: The family intervention study—the effect of intervention on some coronary risk factors and dietary habits, a 6-year follow-up. *Preventive Medicine, 20,* 197–212.

Lindholm, L.H., Ekbom, T., Dash, C., Eriksson, M., Tibblin, G., & Schersten, B. (1995). The impact of health care advice given in primary care on cardiovascular risk. *British Medical Journal, 310,* 1105–1109.

Meland, E., Laerum, E., & Ulvik, R.J. (1997). Effectiveness of two preventive interventions for coronary heart disease in primary care. *Scandinavian Journal of Primary Health Care, 15,* 57–64.

Miettinen, T.A., Huttunen, J.K., Naukkarinen, V., Strandberg, T., Mattila, S., Kumlin, T., & Sarna, S. (1985). Multifactorial primary prevention of cardiovascular disease in middle-aged men. *JAMA, 254,* 2097–2102.

Montano, D.E., & Taplin, S.H. (1991). A test of an expanded theory of reasoned action to predict mammography participation. *Social Science and Medicine, 32*(6), 733–741.

MRFIT (1982). Multiple risk factor intervention trial: Risk factor changes and mortality results. *JAMA, 248,* 1465–1477.

Muir, J., Mant, D., Jones, L., & Yudkin, P. (1994). Effectiveness of health checks conducted by nurses in primary care: Results of the OXCHECK study after one year. *British Medical Journal, 308,* 308–312.

Murray, C.J.L., & Lopez, A.D. (1996). *Global health statistics.* Boston: Harvard.

Prochaska, J.O., Norcross, J.C., & DiClemente, C.C. (1994). *Changing for good.* New York: Avon.

Puska, P. (1996). Community interventions in cardiovascular disease prevention. In K. Orth-Gomer & N. Schneiderman (Eds.), *Behavioral medicine approaches to cardiovsacular disease prevention* (pp. 237–262). Mahwah, NJ: Erlbaum.

Puska, P., Nissinen, A., Tuomilehto, J., Salonen, J.T., Koskela, K., McAlister, A., Kottke, T.E., Maccoby, N., & Farquhar, J.W. (1985). The community-based strategy to prevent coronary heart disease: Conclusions from the ten years of the North Karelia project. *Annual Review of Public Health, 6,* 147–193.

Pyke, S.D.M., Wood, D.A., Kinmonth, A.-L., Thompson, S.G. (1997). Change in coronary risk and coronary risk factor levels in couples following lifestyle intervention. *Archives of Family Medicine, 6,* 354–360.

Rotter, J.B., Chance, J.E., & Phares, E.J. (1972). *Applications of a social learning theory of personality.* New York: Holt, Rinehart, & Winston.

Sarafino, E.P. (2001). *Behavior modification: Understanding principles of behavior change* (2nd ed.). Mountain View, CA: Mayfield.

Shea, S., & Basch, C.E. (1990a). A review of five major community-based cardiovascular disease prevention programs. Part I: Rationale, design, and theoretical framework. *American Journal of Health Promotion, 4*(3), 203–213.

Shea, S., & Basch, C.E. (1990b). A review of five major community-based cardiovascular disease prevention programs. Part II: Intervention strategies, evaluation methods, and results. *American Journal of Health Promotion, 4*(4), 279–287.

Terris, M. (1999). The development and prevention of cardiovascular disease risk factors: Socioenvironmental influences. *Preventive Medicine, 29,* S11–S17.

Wood, D.A., Kinmonth, A.L., Davies, G.A., Yarwood, J., Thompson, S.G., Pyke, S.D.M., Kok, Y., Cramb, R., Le Guen, C., Marteau, T.M., & Durrington, P.N. (1994). Randomised controlled trial evaluating cardiovascular screening and intervention in general practice: Principal results of the British family heart study. *British Medical Journal, 308,* 313–320.

Chronic Disease and Caregivers, Adulthood

Carlos Vallbona

INTRODUCTION

This entry focuses on health promotion activities for family members who assume the role of caregivers for the chronically ill/invalid with the intention of increasing healthy development for all involved persons to the extent possible.

DEFINITIONS

Caregivers are individuals who provide assistance to elderly or chronically ill persons with mental or physical problems which interfere with their activities of daily living. There are five overlapping categories of caregiving roles: anticipatory, preventive, supervisory, instrumental, and protective. They can be assumed by direct or indirect caregivers. *Direct caregivers* are persons who provide appropriate personal and health care to a family member or significant other (Swanson, Jenses, Specht, Johnson, Maas, and Saylor, 1997). These caregivers may be "formal", professionally trained or "informal", usually untrained family members or friends. *Indirect caregivers* are persons who make arrangements for a family member or significant other to receive the services of a paid or a voluntary family care provider (Swanson et al., 1997).

SCOPE

Caregiving has grown considerably in industrialized nations because of the growing percentage of the elderly population as well as the number of younger persons who have contracted a chronic illness or survived disabling episodes (such as a myocardial infarction or a cerebrovascular accident). Of major interest is the Alzheimer's disease which may lead to severe dependency. In the USA it has been estimated that there are four million persons with diagnosed Alzheimer's, and 3.7 million in Europe (Alzheimer's Brief, 2001). Worldwide, the estimate of persons with this disease is 15 million. The prevalence increases with age: it occurs in 1–3 percent of the population, 65–74 years old, and in 25–50 percent of persons over 85. The sufferers of Alzheimer's require almost constant attention by caregivers who must pay attention to their own health lest their ability to care for the patient becomes seriously compromised.

Caregiver characteristics: The US Special Committee on Aging (Administration on Aging Elder Action, 2001) reports that over 70 percent of caregivers are women who are providing services for at least a year. Of those, 80 percent are involved in caregiving seven days a week. It also reported that caregivers are most often women in their late 40s, married, with children at home and active in the workforce. In the words of Wood (1987), the term caregiver may be a euphemism for an unpaid female relative. According to Schulz and Quittner (1998), the number of caregivers in the United States is conservatively estimated at 15 million. The estimate is based on the fact that four percent of the non-institutionalized persons under 55, present health-related mobility and self-care limitations. The prevalence increases with age to the point that over 50 percent of the population after 85 has serious limitations. Results reported after the 1997's National Survey of Caregivers indicated that 22.4 million households met the broad criteria for home caregiving in the past 12 months (National Alliance for Caregiving, & the American Association of Retired Persons, 1997). The range of intensity and type of care is rather wide. Some caregivers may provide intermittent service a few hours a week while others do it for more than 40 hrs per week and may be on call 24 hrs per day. The issue of caregiving has assumed worldwide proportions. For example, several studies reported by Herrman et al. (1993) reveal a growing number of caregivers in Australia.

The economic cost of caregivers has not been adequately quantified. Even the total cost of funded home health services in the United States of $32.2 billion in 1997 is only part of the story. Unpaid informal caregivers add a large amount to the costs to the nation (Caregivers At Risk, 1999).

THEORIES

Bull, Maruyamama, and Luo (1995, 1997) tested a model of the impact of posthospitalized elder behavior on the health of their caregivers. The model is based on Lazarus and Folkman's (1984) *Transactional Stress Theory*. According to this theory, four concepts are critical to analyze the response to a stressful situation: (1) assessment of the stressor or the stressful situation, (2) appraising whether the situation is irrelevant, stressful, or benign, (3) evaluation of what might be done to manage the situation, and (4) production of a stress reaction or response. This reaction is considered to be a "burden," and may lead to deterioration in the caregivers' health. The ability to cope, and the extent of available social support are potential mediators of the stress response. This model could help in the establishment of strategies to minimize the physical or mental impact of caregiving, and preserve a reasonable quality of life for the individuals who are recipients of care.

Traditional *stress coping models* (Schulz & Quittner, 1998) have been utilized to assess the physical or mental impact of caregiving. The literature shows a direct relationship between the level of patient disability and psychological distress of the caregiver. Several mediating factors may include: economic and social support resources, gender, personality attributes (optimism, self-esteem, self-mastering), coping strategies used, and the quality of the relationship between caregiver and care recipient.

Swanson et al. (1997) emphasize the importance of developing a standardized language for outcomes. They suggest a set of categories which are based in part on the medical outcome study (MOS) of Tarlov, Ware, Greenfield, Nelson, Perrin, and Zubkoff (1989) and other outcomes identified in the nursing literature. These categories are: psychological and cognitive status; social role status; physical functional status; safety status; family caregiver status; health attitudes/knowledge/behavior; and perceived well-being. I want to emphasize that these categories consider the well-being of both caregiver and care receiver, as components of a common social system.

Regardless of the model used to analyze the caregiving performance, it is clear that the caregiver must receive adequate information on the nature of the physiological or psychological problems presented by the person being card for. This highlights the role that health professionals must assume in facilitating access to, and understanding of, such information. Transmission of information can be most effective through three channels: (a) oral, (b) visual through written messages, photographs, drawings, etc., and (c) kinesthetic which involves the transmission of sensations that help the caregiver understand the nature of the problem presented by the patient. The kinesthetic channel has been successfully tested in hypertensive patients. While the blood pressure is measured, the patient is invited to equate the discomfort produced by an inflated arm cuff (at the level of the current systolic or diastolic pressure) to the work that the heart must do. By deflating the cuff to the desired level of blood pressure control, the patient realizes the beneficial decreased load to the heart (Scherwitz, Priddy, & Vallbona, 1983).

The *health belief model* proposed by Becker, Drachman, and Firscht (1974) analyzes several factors that prompt individuals to undertake any preventive action. The perceived threat and severity of any illness are obvious determinants, but personal characteristics also influence the level of perceived threat. With reference to the caretaker situation, whatever action the caregiver undertakes, it is a combined function of his or her own characteristics and strengths, as well as the limitations and strengths of the care recipient. This combined recognition may lead a caregiver to get needed assistance even though the recipient's condition alone is not that burdensome.

RESEARCH

There is an abundant literature on the level of physical or psychological burden on caregivers as identified by Given and Given (1998), but the number of articles dealing with health promotion in caregivers is small. The psychological health status of caregivers has been reviewed by Schulz and Quittner (1998). Several papers deal with the problems of caregivers of dementia patients, mostly high rates of clinical depression, and anxiety. Often these problems are related to uncertainties of income and the caregiver's perceived barriers to undertaking preventive measures may be overwhelming.

Killeen (1989) conducted a study of primary caregivers for elderly at home. Most were women with at least a high-school education and were Caucasian. Perceptions of health were negatively associated with the amount of care rendered by the caregivers, but not with the length of time in the care-giving role. By utilizing the Current Health Scale Index (Ware & Karmos, 1976), Killeen identified the caregivers' perception of their own health. Most prevalent physical problems with caregivers were high blood pressure, and increase in the frequency of episodic illnesses. Perception of health was negatively correlated with the percent of care provided. However, by using a Personal Life Style Questionnaire (Muhlenkamp et al., 1983), Killeen found a positive relationship between free time and health promotion activities. Healthy activities related to abstinence of tobacco and moderate or no alcohol ingestion were most frequently reported while activities related to the physical exercise ranked the lowest.

Contradictory results were obtained by different studies on the physical health consequences of caregiving. Neundorfer (1991) concluded that most caregivers of spouses with dementia can manage their roles without significant health deterioration. However, Haley, Levine, Brown, Berry, and Hughes (1987), and Jutras and Lavoie (1995) reported alterations in the physical health status of caregivers as measured by health ratings, the number of reported chronic illnesses, health care utilization, or use of prescribed medications. In an interesting study, Bergman-Evans (1994) compared spousal caregivers of Alzheimer patients living at home and living at a nursing home. They did not find any significant differences between the two groups. O'Brien (1993) reported an inverse relationship between the health promotion behavior of caregivers and the severity of dependence of their recipients of care. Wives of multiple sclerosis patients reported higher health promoting activities than husbands of similar patients but scored lower on exercise. Similar findings were reported by Fuller-Jonap and Haley (1995) in a study of health habits of male spouses of women with Alzheimer's disease.

Pruchno and Potashnik's (1989) research led them to conclude that fewer caregivers were reported to have excellent health than the general population, but they actually spent less time sick in bed and reported less health care utilization. Ethnicity did not appear to be a confounding factor in a study conducted by Haley et al. (1995).

Given and Given (1998) reported only three studies that specifically examine health promotion behaviors (Connell, Davis, Gallant, & Sharpe, 1994; Fuller-Jonap & Haley, 1995; O'Brien, 1993), but the methodologies and the instruments employed by these investigators were different and no clear conclusions could be established. Given and Given (1998) summarized that there are always differences between the physical health of caregivers and noncaregivers, but they suggested that the caregiving process does not have a substantial effect on physical health, that caregivers adapt reasonably well, and that in spite of the considerable stress imposed by entering into a caregiving role, physical health remains uncompromised. Assuming that this summarizes a contradictory situation, the question remains: Would it be possible to promote a healthier quality of life for caregivers and indirectly for care recipients?

STRATEGIES THAT WORK

Despite an abundant literature on caregiver mental and physical health, much of the literature on the impact of health promoting strategies oriented to family members is limited. Therefore, I will review various strategies that show promise of being effective, but need further research and development.

STRATEGIES THAT MIGHT WORK

As discussed previously, Killeen (1989) conducted a study to assess adherence to health promotion activities in a group of 120 primary caregivers for a disabled elder at home. Killeen reported that participation in health promotion activities was associated with a positive assessment of the caregiver's health. An interesting finding was that half of those interviewed responded that they did not have time to be concerned about their own health, and were unable to specify activities that they could do to maintain and promote health. Most of these persons were daughters of the elderly. In contrast, spouses seemed to be more amenable to undertake health promotion activities such as exercise, eating nutritious meals, resting, permitting time for themselves, setting limits on the amount of caregiving and following physician's orders regarding prescribed medications. They also participated in psychological activities such as practicing a positive mental attitude, patience, finding enjoyment in relating to grandchildren, and communicating with others. Caregivers with high levels of dedication were older, and had been caregivers longer with greater participation on health promotion activities than younger caregivers who were mostly daughters, less likely to participate in health promotion activities, more likely to be in the workforce, and had their own child care responsibilities. Clearly, these younger persons had many competing tasks to carry out, less time to devote to caregiving and less time to think about their own preventive health practices.

Montgomery and Borgata (1989), in the United States, carried out a longitudinal study of caregivers and found that those who were randomized to receive a 12 month-training on coping with the stress of caring for patients with dementia, reported lower levels of subjective burden than those assigned to other strategies which did not include such training.

Seltzer, Litchfield, Lowy, and Levin (1989) conducted a longitudinal study to assess the effectiveness of a trained program in case management for families caring for elderly relatives. Those who participated in the program performed significantly more preventive management tasks than those individuals in the control group. After two years these control family members achieved the same level of case management activity as the intervention group. What is promising is the possibility of achieving desired goals two years earlier that seems to occur naturally.

In summary, the following points might be made about programs that might promote the healthy development when a family member is chronically ill. The first point is to achieve an acceptable degree of satisfaction in the part of caregiver (Worchester & Quaghagen, 1983). The second point is that caregiving and receiving is a mutual enterprise, and that only if the caregiver is healthy can the care given be health producing. This provides impetus to programs that promote the health of the caregiver as well as the care receiver. Third, this joint caregiving/receiving goal should mobilize health professionals to give active advice and training on how to make the task optimally satisfying and healthful to both parties. This advice and training should be given as a continuum including the period when the patient is at home, intermittently hospitalized, or admitted to a hospice before the end of life (Lynn, 2000, 2001).

STRATEGIES THAT DO NOT WORK

There is no specific research on what does not promote healthy development in families with a chronically ill or invalid person.

SYNTHESIS

In view of the caregiving tasks, the health problems presented by chronically ill or fragile elderly persons, and the need to ensure community support for health promotion activities, I believe that multifactorial strategies that take into consideration the interaction among the caregiver, the patient, and the community should be emphasized.

From a systems perspective, promoting the health of the caregiver will influence the health of the recipient. Therefore, health care personnel should set realistic health goals for the recipient living in the community that include health-promoting objectives for the caregiver. Moreover, as the recipient will likely need treatment services over a period of time, so, too, should health care personnel take these opportunities to encourage preventive thinking and action by the family caregiver on a regular basis. This may include forms of respite care, or even Hospice, as needed. These supportive services should be viewed as primary prevention for the caregiver, while they serve treatment functions for the recipient. Or there may be other forms of community service, such as support groups that bring together caregivers facing common problems so that effective solutions might be shared as well as emotional support provided. Fortunately, there are increasing numbers of such support groups being formed. A list of Internet web sites is provided in the References for this entry. Finally, I want to emphasize the importance of community infrastructure resources such as transportation, recreation, and religious groups. These resources are critical to connect the caregiver to the rest of the community, and to feel supported in their often-isolated tasks.

Health promotion of the families of chronically ill/disabled takes on extraordinary importance in keeping with Breslow's (1999) ideas which emphasize the active role that individuals must play in achieving their maximum health potential at all stages in their life. To this must be added the systems perspective that all components of the system are involved in the health and healthy development, even when one member of that system has a chronic condition.

ACKNOWLEDGMENT

The author of this chapter acknowledges the helpful assistance of Ms. Patricia Parra-Arévalo in the preparation of this manuscript.

Also see: Cancer, Adulthood; Depression: Adulthood; Physical Fitness: Adulthood; Chronic Disease: Older Adulthood.

References

Administration on Aging Elder Action. (2001). Action ideas for Older persons and Their Families. Retrieved October 11, 2001, from http://www.aoa.dhhs.gov/aoa/eldractn/caregive.html

Alzheimer's Brief August 2001. (2001). Retrieved October 11, 2001, from http://www.biopharmafund.nl/NewsMainBody5.htm

Becker, M.H., Drachman, R.H., & Firsctl, J.P. (1974). A new approach to explaining sick-role behavior in low-income populations. *American Journal of Public Health, 64,* 205–216.

Bergman-Evans, B. (1994). A health profile of spousal Alzheimer's patients. *Journal of Psychosocial Nursing, 32,* 25–30.

Breslow, D. (1999). From disease prevention to health promotion. *Journal of the American Medical Association, 281*(11), 1030–1033.

Bull, M.J., Maruyamama, G., & Luo, D. (1995). Testing a model for hospital transition of family care givers for elderly persons. *Nursing Research, 44*(3), 132–138.

Bull, M., Maruyama, G., & Luo, D. (1997). Testing a model of family caregivers' perceptions of elder behavior two weeks posthospitalization on caregiver response and health. *Scholarly Inquiry for Nursing Practice: An International Journal, 11*(3), 231–248.

Caregivers At Risk. (1999). Retrieved October 11, 2001, from http://www.caregiver.org/stat_riskC.html

Connell, C.M., Davis, W.K., Gallant, M.P., & Sharpe, P.A. (1994). Impact of social support, social cognitive variables, and perceived threat on depression among adults with diabetes. *Health Psychology, 13,* 263–273.

Fuller-Jonap, F., & Haley, W.E. (1995). Mental and physical health of male caregivers of a spouse with Alzheimer's disease. *Journal of Aging and Health, 7,* 99–118.

Given, B.A., & Given, C.W. (1998). Health promotion for family caregivers of chronically ill elders. *Annual Review of Nursing Research, 16,* 197–217.

Haley, W.E., Levine, E.G., Brown, S.L., Berry, J.W., & Hughes, G.H. (1987). Psychological, social and health consequences of caring for a relative with senile dementia. *Journal of American Geriatric Society, 35*(5), 405–411.

Haley, W.E., West, C.A.C., Wadley, V.G., Ford, G.R., White, F.A., Barrett, J.J., Harrell, L.E., & Roth, D.L. (1995). Psychological, social and health impact of caregiving: A comparison of Black and White dementia family caregivers and noncaregivers. *Psychology of Aging, 10,* 540–552.

Herrman, H., Singh, B., Schofield, H., Eastwood, R., Burgess, P., Lewis, V., & Scotton, R. (1993). The health and wellbeing of informal caregivers: A review and study program. *Australian Journal of Public Health, 17*(3), 261–266.

Internet Addresses:

American Association of Retired Persons (AARP), http://www.aarp.org

American Cancer Society (ACS), http://www.cancer.org

American Diabetes Association (ADA), http://www.diabetes.org

American Geriatrics Society (AGS), http://www.americangeriatrics.org

American Lung Association (ALA), http://www.lungusa.org

Arthritis Foundation, http://www.arthritis.org

National Kidney Foundation, http://kidney.org

National Mental Health Association, http://www.nmha.org

National Stroke Association, http://www.stroke.org

National Health Information Center, http://www.health.gov/nhic

Jutras, S., & Lavoie, J. (1995). Living with an impaired elderly person: The informal caregiver's physical and mental health. *Journal of Aging and Health, 7,* 46–73.

Killeen, M. (1989). Health promotion practices of family caregivers. *Health Values, 13*(4), 3–10.

Lazarus, R., & Folkman, S. (1984). Stress, appraisal, and coping. New York: Springer.

Lynn, J. (2000). Learning to care for people with chronic illness facing the end of life. *Journal of the American Medical Association, 284*(19), 2508–2511.

Lynn, J. (2001). Serving patients who may die soon and their families. *Journal of the American Medical Association, 285*(7), 925–932.

Montgomery, T.J.V., & Borgata E.F. (1989). The effects of alternative support strategies on family caregivers. *Gerontologist, 29,* 457–464.

Muhlenkamp, A., Brown, N., Fox, L., et al. (1983). The relationship between health beliefs, health values and health promotion activities. *Western Journal of Nursing Research, 5,* 155–163.

National Alliance for Caregiving, & the American Association of Retired Persons. (1997). *Family caregivers in the US findings from a national survey. Final report.* Bethesda, MD: National Alliance for Caregiving.

Neundorfer, M.M. (1991). Coping and health outcomes in spouse caregivers of persons with dementia. *Nursing Research, 40,* 260–265.

O'Brien, M.T. (1993). Multiple sclerosis: Stressors and coping strategies in spousal caregivers. *Journal of Community Health Nursing, 10,* 123–135.

Pruchno, R.A., & Potashnik, S.L. (1989). Caregiving spouses: Physical and mental health in perspective. *Journal of the American Geriatrics Society, 37,* 697–705.

Scherwitz, L., Priddy, D., & Vallbona, C. (1983). A three-dimensional model for teaching hypertension. *Health Values, 7,* 25–27.

Schulz, R., & Quittner, A. (1998). Caregiving for children and adults with chronic conditions: Introduction to the special issue. *Health Psychology, 17*(2), 107–111.

Seltzer, M.M., Litchfield, L.C., Lowy, L., & Levin, R.J. (1989). Families as case managers: A longitudinal study. *Family Relations, 38,* 332–336.

Swanson, E.A., Jenses, D.P., Specht, J., Johnson, M.L., Maas, M., & Saylor, D. (1997). Caregiving: Concept analysis and outcomes. *Scholarly Inquiry for Nursing Practice: An International Journal, 11,* 65–76.

Tarlov, A.R., Ware, J.E., Greenfield, S., Nelson, E.C., Perrin, E., & Zubkoff, M. (1989). The medical outcomes study: An application of methods for monitoring the results of medical care. *Journal of the American Medical Association, 262,* 925–930.

Ware, J., & Karmos, A. (1976). *Development & validation of scales to measure perceived health & patient role prosperity* (Vol. II) (Publication No 288–331). Springfield, VA: National Technical Information Services.

Wood, J. (1987). Labors of love. *Modern Maturity, 30*(4), 28–34, 90, 92–94.

Worchester, M., & Quaghagen, M. (1983). Correlates of caregiver satisfaction: Prerequisites to elder home care. *Research in Nursing and Health, 6,* 61–67.

Chronic Disease, Older Adulthood

Colette V. Browne

INTRODUCTION

This entry describes a number of strategies and interventions that may prevent chronic diseases and conditions in the aged, or minimize their effects. Examples of interventions are reviewed, along with findings of studies testing their impact. This entry concludes with a synthesis together with research and practice recommendations aimed at maximizing the potential for a healthy old age.

DEFINITIONS

In this entry, the term *older adult* refers to those individuals who are 65 years of age and over. *Chronic conditions* are defined as persistent or recurring health illnesses or impairments that cannot be cured and that last for years. Some of the most prevalent chronic conditions, such as sinusitis, are generally not disabling; however, others such as heart disease and arthritis, can result in serious limitations in people's abilities to perform daily activities. *Impairments* refer to dysfunction once the chronic condition has entered the clinical stage, and may or may not require assistance from others. A more serious term is *disability*, which, according to the World Health Organization, refers to impairments in the ability to complete multiple daily tasks. Disability affects one's *functional health*, often referred to as either *Activities of Daily Living (ADL)* or *Instrumental Activities of Daily Living (IADL)*. ADLs are those activities one needs to perform in order to maintain independent living such as eating, dressing, bathing, and grooming. IADLs are those complex activities that further support one's independence, such as shopping for food and home management tasks. *Health promotion* is a model of care that emphasizes individual responsibility for and control of one's health and that includes health education and other social and economic changes aimed at improving health. *Long-term care* is used here to refer to the wide array of familial and professional supports provided to individuals who suffer or are at-risk from chronic conditions or disability that places limits on their ability to live well and independently. In addition to medical services, people with chronic conditions often need personal, social or *preventive care* for a long period of time to prevent disease from turning into disability or at least prevent further deterioration. *Rehabilitative care* refers to restoration of the person to the highest level of functioning possible after treatment of the problem.

SCOPE

Chronic conditions and diseases are the major causes of illness, disability, and death in the United States (National Academy on an Aging Society, 1999). All age groups suffer from chronic conditions, and while distinct gender, age, and racial variations exist in types of chronic conditions, no one is immune from them. Nearly 100 million Americans have chronic conditions, and projections indicate that the number will increase to nearly 160 million by 2040. The cost of medical care for Americans with chronic conditions is startling $470 billion in 1995, with estimated costs jumping to nearly $864 billion by 2040 (National Center for Health Statistics [NCH], 2000).

The prevalence of chronic diseases varies with age. Some diseases, such as asthma, are more common in children, but conditions that are more disabling and more difficult and costly to treat are those found among the aged (National Academy on an Aging Society, 1999). Although old age may not be synonymous with chronic conditions and disability, the risk for disability does increase with age. The population most at-risk is the "oldest-old"—those 85 years of age and over—the fastest growing age group within the aged population (Moody, 2000). Chronic conditions can be mildly or severely disabling, affecting a person's life in different degrees and at different times in one's life. Far from having influence on only the person suffering from the condition, others affected include family members and friends, work associates, the work environment, and the society at large.

Although the normal aging process is marked by progressive changes that ultimately increase the risk of morbidity and mortality, recent research informs us that older Americans are living longer and reporting generally good health in their old age. Indeed, in self-reports, the vast majority identifies their health as good or excellent (NCH, 2000). Nonetheless, chronic disease, memory impairment, and depressive symptoms affect on the aged, and the risk of such problems often increases with age. The most common types of chronic conditions affecting the aged are hypertension, heart disease, cancer, diabetes, and stroke. Increases in memory impairment and depressive symptoms occur with advancing age; one third or more of men and women over the age of 85 and old have moderate or severe memory impairment and 23 percent of this group experience severe depressive symptoms (NCH, 2000).

Recent data reported by the Federal Interagency Forum on Aging Related Statistics (NCH, 2000) suggest that the overall prevalence of illness or chronic conditions among the aged may be improving. Comparing the most recent data collected in 1999 to that from 1982, the proportion of Medicare beneficiaries who are 65 years of age and over with a chronic disability was 21 percent, a decease from 24 percent in 1982. Although the older population grew dramatically in this time period, the number of older people estimated to have functional limitations increased by 600,000. Although not inconsequential, this is a more conservative number compared to earlier projections. Not all individuals with chronic conditions are disabled; most continue to have contributory and active and fulfilling lives. Nonetheless, some do experience significant challenges to independent living due to their chronic conditions. Of the nearly 100 million people with chronic conditions, approximately 40 million are limited in their ADLs by their condition (Robert Wood Johnson Foundation, 1996). In 2000, approximately 8 million persons 65 years of age and over needed some assistance in order to remain in the community with numbers increasing with the person' age. Projections estimate that these figures will increase to 12 million by 2020, and 17 million by 2040. Of those disabled, about 20 percent will have severe limitations. While numbers who are severely limited appear small, their numbers have huge consequences to the health and long-term care systems, and to their families. And, as previously stated, chronic conditions are costly. In part, this is due to higher rates of hospitalization among those with chronic conditions—specifically those with hypertension and arthritis (National Academy of an Aging Society, 2000).

In addition to age, other influences on the prevalence and incidence of chronic conditions are gender, race, and socioeconomic status (SES). Men and women suffer from the same five chronic conditions—arthritis, hearing, heart disease, cataracts, and hypertension (National Academy of an Aging Society, 1999). However, gender variations exist in their prevalence, as women over the age of 75 years are more likely to report a diagnosis of arthritis, hypertension, sinusitis, or cataracts, whereas men in the same age group report heart disease, hearing impairment, tinnitus, and visual impairment (NCH, 1995). Some of the major effects of such diseases and conditions are decreased mobility and other ADLs. Higher dependency increases the likelihood that one may end up in a nursing home or other resident care facility. Gender patterns are here as well: 75 percent of nursing home residents are females (Hooyman & Kiyak, 1999).

The prevalence of chronic conditions also varies by race and ethnicity. While there exist overall commonalities (the five most common chronic conditions are the same for Black and White Americans), diabetes is more common among Blacks. Although Whites are more likely to develop coronary heart disease than other races, Blacks are more likely to die of heart disease, with the gaps in the heart disease death rate between Blacks and Whites widening since the 1980s (Centers for Disease Control and Prevention, 2000a). Moreover, Blacks, Latinos, and Native Americans are more apt to be disabled at younger ages and to have more limitation in ADLs compared to Whites (John, 1994; NCH, 2000). Among the Asian and Pacific Islander population, itself a diverse group, hypertension and cancer rates are higher compared to Whites (Wykle & Kaskel, 1994). Finally, SES matters, as those with lower education and lower income are more at risk for chronic conditions (NCH, 2000).

THEORIES

There are generally four theoretical frameworks that guide gerontological services. These are health promotion/behavioral, the biomedical perspective, the ecological perspective, and public health approaches.

Health Promotion

The theories and frameworks that underlie health promotion efforts—the *health belief model* and individual change—are based on individual psychology and are aimed at behavioral change (Bandura, 1977). While some have argued that health promotion can be described in terms of the interrelationships between individual behavior and the physical and social environments (Minkler, Schauffler, & Clements-Nolle, 2000), health promotion strategies have clearly taken an individualistic/lifestyle approach to the prevention of chronic conditions and disability (Wallace, 2000). Primary preventive strategies emphasize that an individual's risk factors for chronic conditions and disability can be modified with the right lifestyle choices. Indeed, choices about diet, exercise, smoking, and other behavioral risk factors have been found to reduce premature mortality and reduce chronic disability (McGinnis, 1990). According to the National Academy on an Aging Society (2000), the five modifiable risk factors associated with chronic conditions are: being overweight (defined as having a body mass index above 25), not exercising, smoking cigarettes, having high cholesterol, and consuming more than two alcoholic drinks per day.

Exactly how do older adults fare regarding their health behaviors? The majority of adults approaching their later years have risk factors for chronic conditions that may be due to their health-related behaviors, and are associated with five chronic conditions—hypertension, heart disease, diabetes, cancer, and stroke. Two thirds of the older adult population are overweight, and more than one third of those who are overweight are obese. Nearly 50 percent do not participate in light physical activity three or more times per week, and estimates identify between 2 and 10 percent of older adults to be alcoholic (NCH, 2000; Osgood, Wood, & Parham, 1995). Overall, 25 percent of persons with hypertension, heart disease, diabetes, or stroke have three or more risk factors (National Academy on an Aging Society, 2000). For a variety of reasons, ethnic minority aged have generally poorer health behavior profiles compared to Whites (Meyers, Kagawa-Singer, Kumanyhika, Lex, & Markides, 1995). In addition to this focus on health promotion and risk factors, the range of primary preventive services also include immunizations, diabetes education, and osteoporosis prevention.

The Genetic/Biomedical Perspective

Not all risk factors are modifiable: age, gender, and genetic predisposition influence risks for chronic conditions and disability. An overall mechanism that results in decreased functional capacity in older adults has yet to be identified (Moody, 2000). Increasingly, researchers are focusing on how the aging process may be controlled by DNA, the basis for heredity in living cells. Interventions into the genetic causes of longevity may help to identify ways to reduce disabilities and dysfunctions of old age. In other words, altering the genetic code could delay the onset of age-dependent illnesses, many of which are chronic (Moody, 2000).

Biomedical perspectives also examine the individual's immune system to chronic disease. Humans come equipped with an immune system which prevents diseases that may be caused by pathogens (fungi, parasites, viruses, bacteria) or cancerous cells. A damaged system can allow pathogens to overwhelm defenses, leading to illness. The immune system can also attack its host, causing major damage of a different kind, known as autoimmune diseases. Insulin-dependent diabetes and rheumatoid arthritis are examples. Accordingly, epidemiologists, environmentalists, and other scientists are paying increased attention to the ways in which air, water, and food pollution may disrupt the immune system. Common agents and environmental contaminants known to harm the immune system include Dioxin and PBS, a class of industrialized chemicals not outlawed but still present in the environment, and a wide array of pesticides, asbestos, and other work sites hazardous chemicals. Subsequently, this approach often teams up with public health interventions to prevent pollution and other environmental concerns.

The Ecological Perspective

In contrast to health promotion's focus on changing individual behaviors or the biomedical focus on pharmacologic or gene therapies, the focus of this perspective is on the conditions that shape people's behaviors—in other words, the social and environmental conditions that are seen as more determinative of health than behaviors (Cockerham, 2000). Rather than viewing aging and chronic diseases as developed and controlled by lifestyle behaviors or genes, the ecological model examines the person in his or her environment, and develops interventions that are often interdisciplinary, require prevention strategies, and demonstrate the importance of and interrelationships among psychological, structural, cultural, and economic factors.

The environment and the person's location in his or her environment provide varying advantages and disadvantages throughout the life course that culminate in a more or less stressful old age. One possible outcome is the documented existence of persistent racial and ethnic disparities in health status (Brach & Fraser, 2000). For example, the recent challenge set by *Healthy People 2000*—whereby 60 percent of older Americans received vaccinations—was only true for non-Latino Whites. Among older women, rates for mammograms increased between 1998 and 1987 (55 percent compared to 23 percent in 1987) but not all ethnic groups benefited equally (NCH, 2000). Influenza morbidity rates are higher among African Americans and American Indians/Native Alaskans compared to White Americans (Brach & Fraser, 2000). Subsequently, this perspective emphasizes that attention must be paid to the older adults' response—ability or capacity for effectively responding to their own needs and the challenges in the environment (Minkler, 1989). In other words, placing responsibility on only the individual seems akin to victim blaming; instead, the society has a responsibility in promoting the health of its citizens.

Accordingly, the ecological perspective's emphasis on health strategies takes into account inequality in income, education, and access to health care. As poverty is recognized as a main predictor of poor health, and contributor to other health problems (Holden, 2001; World Health Organization, 1999), ecological interventions are concerned with its eradication. To understand the difference between the health promotion and ecological focus, consider this example. Although exercise may be a goal and strategy for both the health promotion and ecological perspectives, the former focuses on individual behavioral change while the latter focuses on ways that the context—society, structural factors, and the environment—can provide more conditions to improve exercise (Wallace, 2000).

Public Health

Whereas health promotion has generally taken a more clinical approach to healthy aging, prevention from the public health approach examines population health. Avoiding or eliminating germ vectors, building host resistance through immunizations, improving sanitation, promoting decent and safe housing, advocating for more stringent antipollution legislation to prevent contaminated water and the use of chemicals in food, and developing and arguing for more inclusive health care policies that include attention to prevention have been the primary strategies for understanding and treating risk factors. Public health approaches include: (1) assessment of the health status of individuals, and their community, (2) the identification of key community health problems, and (3) outreach, screening, and action to ensure that individuals needing health care are identified and receive appropriate services (Schmidt, 1994).

STRATEGIES THAT WORK

Regardless of the theoretical framework used, each approach hopes to keep people away from disease and toward full health. A comprehensive review of the intervention literature is beyond the scope of this entry. Instead, I will attempt to summarize some of the more recent primary preventive strategies and services of each perspective and highlight those that have been demonstrated by scientific criteria to be effective with older adults.

Health Promotion

A basic belief within health promotion strategies is that the choices one makes with regard to social and behavioral aspects of life throughout the life course make a difference in the promotion of health and well-being. In other words, aging is viewed as a cumulative experience that is influenced by the choices and situations from earlier years. Accordingly, while it is never too late to start eating a healthy diet, begin an exercise program, minimize contact with the sun, or to stop smoking, the life course perspective examines those interventions that begin in childhood and the teenage years.

Recent evidence suggests that health promotion strategies that have focused on individual health behaviors have a positive impact on well-being. One behavior often analyzed is smoking due to its association with the development of several chronic conditions such as heart disease and stroke, loss of mobility, and overall poor physical function. More than 4.5 million older adults continue to smoke and the majority are long-term smokers. Studies have reported on smoking cessation programs (LaCroix & Omenn, 1992;

Rimer & Orleans, 1994), with results indicating that older adults who participate in these programs having a reduced rate of death compared with current smokers within 1–6 years after quitting (Hermanson, 1988; LaCroix & Omenn, 1992). Programs tailored to meet the needs of older Americans had higher rates of quitting smoking compared to those who received a generic guide (Rimer & Orleans, 1994).

Diet programs have also been studied as to their effect on heart disease and other chronic conditions. High fat and sugar diets are associated with chronic conditions such as heart disease and diabetes. While a poor diet can be associated with many factors, including poor financial status, research suggests that even a moderate reduction in fat consumption can be beneficial in reducing the risk for heart disease (Knopp et al., 1997). Increased amounts of regular exercise have also been found to be associated with maintained cardiovascular and respiratory functioning (Clark, 1996; Jette, Harris, Sleeper, Lachman, Heislein, & Georgetti, 1996). These activities appear to be the most successful when the older adult is an active participant along with their health care provider in the development of a personal health promotion plan.

A health promotion program that appears to be successful is one recently reported by the Prevention Research Center at the University of Washington, one of 11 prevention centers funded by the Center for Disease Control (2000b). Results to date have shown that a combination of prevention strategies, targeting such factors as physical inactivity, alcohol use, home hazards, medication use, social isolation, and sensory impairment among older adults can reduce hospital bed days by as much as 70 percent and the number of days of restricted activity by 25 percent. Study results have also found that regular walking reduces the risk for heart disease, and exercise classes as well as home-based exercise programs among older adults can reduce falls by as much as 30 percent in one year.

Another positive impact on the health of older adults associated with participation in a health promotion program was recently found in the analysis of data from 103 Health Enhancement Programs (HEP) enrollees at 1 of 9 senior centers in western Washington for whom 12-month follow-up information was available (Phelan, Williams, Snyder, Simmons, Wagner, & LoGerfo, 2000). The HEP reaches seniors at risk for functional decline and consists of education and monitoring of health information on diet, smoking, exercise, and other behaviors. The study examined participant characteristics and program impact on health and functional status and health care use. Participants were primarily females, had a mean age of 74 years, and reported an average of three chronic conditions each. At follow-up, 84 percent rated their health the same or better than a year prior to program attendance. Twenty-seven percent reported hospitalization in the year before enrollment and 18 percent were hospitalized while participating in the program. Depression scores improved from baseline to follow-up for participants and physical activity improved for those who chose to address exercise.

Still another study used a prospective, randomized design to evaluate the effectiveness of individualized assessment and counseling together with the addition of a written health care plan on client adherence to health-behavior recommendations established by a statewide health promotion program (Fox, Breuer, & Wright, 1997). The sample consisted of 237 ethnically diverse low-income older adults 60 years of age and over who were participating for the first time in an established health promotion program. Use of logistic regression and controlling for socioeconomic and demographic variables found that the treatment group that had received a personal health plan and counseling completed significantly more preventive referrals and health behavior changes. Data suggest that a client-centered planning process, together with supportive counseling and heath care plans provided to clients, can increase prevention measures taken by the older adult. Collectively taken together, results from these and other health promotion studies provide some evidence of the positive impact of health promotion strategies on health outcomes. Successful program characteristics target the elder as active participant, and use a didactic educational focus, offer a supervised and group exercise program, have a family focus, use peer counselors, and provide literature geared to older adults (Knopp et al., 1997).

Biomedical/Pharmacologic

Biomedical and pharmacologic interventions can also help prevent chronic conditions and disability. For example, although a diet of an increased calcium intake is important in the prevention of osteoporosis, equally important may be the biomedical and pharmacologic treatments. Research has identified hormone replacement therapy (HRT) as a positive strategy for some; however, data are controversial as other studies suggest a link between HRT and certain kinds of cancer in women (Colditz et al., 1995). Biomedical technologies can replace body parts with increasing frequency—hip replacements are common operations and researchers are investigating the use of artificial heart valves and laboratory-grown cartilage to replace worn out ones (Moody, 2000).

Rehabilitative services also play a role in the prevention of disability. The Well-Elderly study is an example of a randomized clinical trial study that was conducted from 1994 to 1998 to evaluate the efficacy of preventive occupational therapy (OT) interventions to reduce health-related declines among a sample of urban, multiethnic independent-living older adults. Significant improvement in health, functional

status, and quality of life resulted in the experimental group from the 9-month OT intervention (Clark et al., 1997). A follow-up study whereby participants were followed for 6 months without further intervention and then reevaluated found that approximately 90 percent of participants had kept gains in their ADLs.

Ecological

Communities have varying attitudes and beliefs about health and disease. Programs that appear to be effective tailor the development and introduction of prevention strategies to the targeted community. The Reach 2010 program, part of the Department of Health and Human Services (DHHS) response to the President' Race Initiative and Goal for 2010, aims to eliminate disparities in health status experienced by racial and ethic minority populations. Grants are provided to community coalitions to design, implement, and evaluate community-driven strategies to eliminate health disparities. One example is a community-based chronic disease management program that is attempting to intervene in the health status of African Americans with diabetes and hypertension (Nine, Lakies, & Jarrett, 2000). Program outcomes provide evidence of improvement produced in diabetes-related outcomes with preventive measures offered in a community-based structured environment. Seeking community support, the researchers sought the advice of the community's Black Pastor's Association to allow for trust to develop between program staff with possible participants. A successful program of interventions that promoted healthier eating, exercise, and a supportive environment was then implemented. Initial data show improvement in blood pressure, cholesterol, and quality of life. The emphasis is on developing strategies for building successful community partnerships that, in turn, can eliminate health disparities.

Public Health

Public health interventions include those that monitor and provide education and services to assure prevention of infectious and chronic diseases, monitor the safety of air, water, and food supplies, work with community constituents in community organizing, advocate for improved and affordable service delivery and policies, and conduct preventive research to better understand the causal pathways for better health. Examples of the wide array of public health strategies aimed at smoking cessation have included banning the advertisement of tobacco products, raising taxes on cigarettes, prohibiting smoking in public places, and restricting access to cigarettes by minors (McLeroy and Crump, 1994), as well as working with attorneys in litigation against tobacco manufacturers.

Prevention research is a major public health strategy. Public health intervention studies have taken two general research strategies over the last 25 years. The first is high-risk approaches, such as the Multiple Risk Factor Intervention Trial (MRAFIT) and the CDC-funded studies described previously. The second is community-based approaches such as the Stanford Three-Community Study (Flora, Maibach, & Maccoby, 1985) and the North Karelia Project (Puska et al., 1985). Results to-date find the community-based approaches producing more positive results in morbidity and mortality reductions than the high-risk approaches (McLeroy & Crump, 1994). Strategies that lead to changes in health behaviors and risk factors have included educational programs, community organization, service development, and policy change. Results from both of the community-based interventions provide positive results for reductions in negative health-related behaviors, and significant declines were observed in heart disease mortality (McLeroy & Crump, 1994).

Policies

Improved health policies seek to provide citizens with the health care they need, increase efforts to fund comprehensive interdisciplinary research on prevention interventions, and offer health promotion strategies. In the long run, these may be the most effective strategies to prevent chronic conditions and disability. Because more than 80 percent of older adults have a chronic condition, a broadening of the definition of prevention to include all levels of intervention should be considered (Quarterlyn, 1994). Long-term care can be viewed as prevention strategy if the services can prevent unnecessary disability and decline before a problem emerges, as in the prevention of injuries from falling. Unfortunately, the present long-term care system remains fragmented with no national or universal funding base. Stone (2000) suggests that the following should be essential design features of such a system. Services must be tailored to people with varying degrees of mental and physical impairment, sensitive to the needs of the family and the older adult, flexible to address the social, chronic, and non-medical and acute needs of the long-term care client, and public and private funds would follow the client, not the provider, as individuals and families make choices that reflect preferences and values. Even among the disabled, the right mix of care—prevention, treatment, and rehabilitative services—can be very beneficial.

A major problem with long-term care in the United States is the absence of a national long-term care policy that pays for services. At this point in that nation's history, long-term care is paid for primarily for individual resources, private insurance, and Medicaid. Other nations are turning to more of a health insurance model. To deal with their own long-term care problem, the Japanese government instituted the *kaigo hoken* (nursing care insurance) in April 2000; payment will be provided for both community/home care and institutional care via the charging of premiums to Japanese workers 40 years of age and over. Unlike in the United States, this new system was planned to provide everyone with services as long as they meet the service eligibility criteria. Although too new to evaluate its effectiveness, initial data suggest a number of issues must be reworked; for example, quality of care through patient choice of services, and the reconsideration of cash benefits to families (Japan Echo, 2000).

STRATEGIES THAT MIGHT WORK

Health Promotion

The theory that older adults will use more health promotion services—aimed at changing behaviors, if available at no cost—was the rationale for a series of demonstration projects funded by the Health Care Financing Administration (HCFA) that examined the implications of extending coverage for disease prevention/health promotion services to Medicare beneficiaries. Individuals enrolled in one such demonstration project were eligible for specific health promotions, including nutrition, smoking cessation, alcohol counseling, and dementia/depression evaluations, to be covered by Medicare (Lave, Ives, Traven, & Kuller, 1995). Participation improved only among those with higher education, and rural beneficiaries were more likely to use preventive services when recommended by their physician compared to a hospital-based program. Data suggest that affordability may be only one reason for the adoption of health promotion behaviors. Whether or not this or other health promotion programs work has been difficult to answer due to two research design problems. The first is the sole attention to the effects of single-factor population-based intervention studies directed at reducing obesity, physical inactivity, stress, or cholesterol as opposed to multiple risk factor intervention studies. The second is the lack of longitudinal data that tracks outcomes over time to evaluate the sustained benefits of program participation (McLeroy & Crump, 1994).

Biomedical

Another strategy that might work is gene therapy—the elimination or replacement of defective genes with normal genes. While this belongs to the future, it is within the realm of possibility that gene therapy may result in the slowing down of the aging process and a decrease in chronic conditions. The Human Genome Project, a project of the US government, has uncovered the map of the entire sequence of genes on the human chromosome. In the near future, it is possible that gene therapy may result in cures for such age-related chronic conditions diseases as Parkinson's, Alzheimer's, and cancer. New developments in cell biology and genetic engineering may ultimately lengthen life and result in a healthier one (Smith-Sonneborn, 1990).

Cultural Competence

Women, ethnic minorities, and those without access to health care will be at high risk for a slow decline for chronic conditions (Kiyak and Hooyman, 2000). Elimination of health disparities and increasing the quality of years of healthy living is a major goal of the Healthy People 2010 project. Increasingly, professionals are referring to the use and importance of cultural competence in interventions for ethnic and minority populations. A typical definition of *cultural competence* involves some set of common behaviors, attitudes, and policies that an agency and its practitioners use to work effectively in cross-cultural situations (Cross, Bazron, Kennis, & Isaacs, 1989). Theory and logic would suggest that this is an appropriate strategy for a nation that is struggling to become more sensitive to a changing citizenry. The question is: Do they work?

In a recent review article that examined the cultural competency literature, rigorous research was found to be lacking in the impact evaluation of particular cultural competency techniques to health outcomes and to strategies that may reduce health disparities (Brach & Fraser, 2000). Examples of specific techniques include interpreter services, training of staff, coordinating with traditional helpers, use of community health workers, and culturally competent health promotion. There is evidence that using natural helpers has increased the use of the cancer screening test to Latina women (Navarro, Senn, McNicholas, Kaplan, Roppe, & Campo, 1998). Literature on dementia care translated into different languages may increase knowledge by older diverse adults and family members (Braun, Takamura, Forman, Sasaki, & Meinenger, 1995). More rigorous research will enable health professionals to test theoretical premises and provide them with information about effective techniques to promote health and well-being.

Assisted Technology

A number of factors may reduce chronic conditions and disability in the future years—increasing health, new forms of service delivery, and the growth of assisted technology (Longino, 1999). For example, the Georgia Tech Center for Rehabilitation Technology has created *Rehabilitation Assistivetech.net*, an online information resource providing up-to-date information on assistive technologies, adaptive

environments and community resources for people with disabilities, including their families, service providers, and their communities. Low technology items such as adapting writing and eating implements are described as well as high technology tools such as voice-activated computers. Assistive and information technology provides support for people in doing their daily tasks at home or at work, and is especially good for the homebound and disabled.

STRATEGIES THAT DO NOT WORK

Not following a healthy lifestyle, living in areas with high levels of air and water pollution, and not following a medical regimen recommended by one's physician can result in poor health. Poverty, little or no access to quality health care, and the lack of social supports can also have negative effects on health (Holden, 2001). Furthermore, numerous alternative strategies offer the consumer little if any real evidence that they prevent or cure diseases. For example, many health food products advertise the prevention and cure of a number of chronic conditions, but provide minimal empirical support to such claims. While we may find that some have value, the average citizen should proceed with caution about using some alternative treatments.

SYNTHESIS

Chronic conditions are serious problems for millions of Americans. As the nation's populace grows increasingly older, more Americans will live with chronic conditions. A number of different interventions have been profiled in this entry. These include health promotion/behavioral, biomedical, ecological, and public health. Research has primarily focused on examining how changing older adults' health-behaviors can improve their health and decrease the propensity for chronic conditions. Results to-date show that the health status of older adult is in fact improving, and data suggest that personal health care behaviors have improved (although racial and ethnic disparities continue to exist in health behaviors). Older adults who follow a sensible diet, do not smoke, exercise, and check blood pressure regularly reported less hospital admissions and had lower Medicare reimbursements than others surveyed in the National Survey of Self Care and Aging (Stearns, Bernard, Konrad, Schwartz, & Defriese, 1997). Programs that seem to work well with older adults have the following characteristics: the older adult is an active participant in the plan, and the program used a didactic-education format, easy and large print, and multiple methods (e.g., supervised exercise, peer exchange, and family support). Clearly, it is never too late to learn new healthy habits. Additionally, older adults must be trained to be better consumers and primary care providers must be trained to work with older adults in their health education. To be effective, health promotion services must be universally based and must extend beyond the confinements of any individual health care provider or facility (Schmidt, 1994).

Medical technology and biomedical advances will change our prevention efforts in ways we may not at this time be able to imagine. Medical attention to chronic conditions is making progress, notably in osteoporosis. Although much will depend on future research with Alzheimer's Disease, Parkinson's Disease, and other chronic conditions, we also know that the overall social environment must be revamped to foster healthy living. Clearly, the prevention of pollution-related illnesses and conditions is less expensive than treatment and warrants the nation's leadership. Moreover, we can look to ecological models that uncover the relationships among poverty, discrimination, and poor health. A history of inadequate or nonexistent access to health care, poor nutrition, and poor health status in the younger years leads to poor health status in later life. All of this speaks to a much needed broader perspective which suggests that interventions at the policy level are necessary to improve health care access and that also address the challenging issues of long-term care. Accordingly, policy makers must understand the special needs of all older adults but especially older women, the very frail and old, and ethnic minorities, many of whom find health care inaccessible, unaffordable and not community-based. Moreover, definitions of prevention in the elderly must be broadened to include all levels of interventions as nearly 80 percent have at least one chronic condition. Interventions that may minimize the effects of chronic conditions turning into disabilities is worthy of policy change. The important role of preventive research is critical in increasing our understanding of ways to prevent chronic conditions from turning into disabilities. More rigorous longitudinal designs are needed that will allow for more informative data on program evaluation as well as a better understanding of the relationship between chronic disease and disability. Developing and implementing the best health care system to deal with chronic conditions—from prevention to treatment—will require a commitment to a healthy citizenry by both government and private funding options. Regardless of intervention, the aim is to postpone chronic conditions and loss of functional status disability indefinitely or at least until very late in life.

Also see: Cancer: Older Adulthood; Caregiver Stress: Older Adulthood; Crises Intervention: Older Adulthood; Death with Dignity: Older Adulthood; Depression: Older Adulthood; Health Promotion: Older Adulthood.

References

Bandura, A. (1977). Self efficacy: Toward a unifying theory of behavioral change. *Psychological Review, 84*, 191–215.

Brach, C., & Fraser, I. (2000). Can cultural competency reduce racial and ethnic health disparities? A review and conceptual model. *Medicare Care Research and Review, 57*(Suppl. 1), 181–217.

Braun, K., Takamura, J., Forman, S., Sasaki, P., & Meinenger, L. (1995). Developing and testing outreach materials on Alzheimer's Disease for Asian and Pacific Islanders. *Gerontologist, 35*(1), 122–126.

Centers for Disease Control and Prevention. (2000a). Trends in ischemic heart disease death rates for blacks and whites—United States 1981–1995. *Mortality and Morbidity Weekly Report, 47*(44), 945–949.

Center for Disease Control, & Prevention Research Center. (2000b). Improving health care for older adults Available: www.cdc.gov/pre/glance/html

Clark, D.O. (1996). The effect of walking on body disability in blacks and whites. *American Journal of Public Health, 86*, 57–61.

Clark, F., Azen, S.P., Zemke, R., Jackson, J., Carlson, M., Mandel, D., Hay, J., Josephson, K., Cherry, B., Hessel, C., Palmer, J., & Lipson, L. (1997). *JAMA, 278*(16), 1321–1326.

Cockerham, W.C. (2000). The sociology of health behavior and health life styles. In C.E. Bird, C.P. Conrad, & A.M. Fremont (Eds.), *Handbook of medical sociology* (5th ed.). Upper Saddle Road, New Jersey: Prentice-Hall.

Colditz, G., Hankinson, S., Hunger, D., Willett, W., Manslon, J., Stampfer, M., Hennekens, C., & Speizer, F. (1995). The use of estrogen and progestin and the risk of breast cancer in postmenopausal women. *New England Journal of Medicine, 332*, 1589–1593.

Cross, T.L., Bazron, B.J., Kennis, K.W., & Isaacs, M.R. (1989). *Towards a culturally competent system of care: A monograph for effective services for minority children who are severely emotionally disturbed.* Washington, DC: CASSP Technical Assistance Center, Georgetown University Child Development Center.

Flora, J.A., Maibach, E.W., & Maccoby, N. (1985). The role of media across four levels of health promotion intervention. *Annual Review of Public Health, 10*, 281–307. Palo Alto, CA, Annual Review.

Fox, P.J., Breuer, W., & Wright, J.A. (1997). Effects of a health promotion program on sustaining health behaviors in older adults. *American Journal of Preventive Medicine, 13*(4), 257–264.

Hermanson, B. (1988). Beneficial six year outcome of smoking cessation in older men and women with coronary artery disease: Results from the CAS registry. *New England Journal of Medicine, 320*, 1365–1369.

Holden, K. (2001). Chronic and disability conditions: The economic costs to individuals and families. *The Public Policy and Aging Report, 11*(2), 1–6.

Hooyman, N., & Kiyak, A. (2000). *Social gerontology* (5th ed.). Boston: Allyn and Bacon.

Japan Echo. (2000, June 3). The launch of long term care insurance, 27.

Jette, A.M., Harris, B.A., Sleeper, L., Lachman, M.E., Heislein, D., & Georgetti, M. (1996). A home based exercise program for nondisabled older adults. *Journal of the American Geriatrics Society, 44*, 644–649.

John, R. (1994). The state of research on American Indian elder's health, income security, and social support network. In *Minority elders: Five goals toward building a public policy base* (2nd ed.). Washington, DC: The Gerontological Society of America.

Kiyak, A., & Hooyman, N. (1999). Aging in the 21st century. *Hallyn International Journal of Aging, 1*(1), 56–66.

Knopp, R.H., Walden, C.E., Rfetzlaff, B.M., McCann, B.S., Dowdy, A.A., Albers, J.J., Gey, G.O., & Cooper, M.N. (1997). Long term cholesterol-lowering effects of fat restricted diets in hyper cholesterolemic and combined hyperlipidemic men. The dietary alternatives study. *Journal of the American Medical Association, 278*, 1509–1515.

LaCroix, A.Z., & Omenn, G.S. (1992). Older adults and smoking. *Clinical Geriatric Medicine, 8*(1), 69–87.

Lave, J.R., Ives, D.G., Traven, N.D., & Kuller, L.H. (1995). Participation in health promotion programs by the rural elderly. *American Journal of Preventive Medicine, 11*(1), 46–53.

Longino, C. (1999). The future population aging in the USA and Pacific Rim countries. *Hallym International Journal of Aging, 1*(1), 33–42.

McGinnis, J. (1990). *Healthy older people: The report of a national health promotion program*. Washington, DC: Office of Disease Prevention and Health Promotion, DHHS.

McLeroy, K., & Crump, C. (1994). Health promotion and disease prevention: A historical perspective. *Generations, 18*(1), 9–15.

Meyers, H., Kagawa-Singer, M., Kumanyhika, S., Lex, B., & Markides, K. (1995). Behavioral risk factors related to chronic diseases in ethnic minorities. *Health Psychology, 14*(7), 613–621.

Minkler, M. (1989). Health education, health promotion, and the open society. A historian perspective. *Health Education Quarterly, 16*(1), 17–30.

Minkler, M., Schauffler, J., & Clements-Nolle, K. (2000). Health promotion for older Americans in the 21st century. *American Journal of Health Promotion, 14*(5), 371–379.

Moody, H. (2000). *Concepts and controversies in aging* (2nd ed.). Thousand Oaks: Pine Forge Press.

Navarro, A.M., Senn, K.L., McNicholas, L.J., Kaplan, R.M., Roppe, B., & Campo, M.C. (1998). Por La Vida model intervention enhances use of cancer screening tests among Latinas. *American Journal of Preventive Medicine, 15*(1), 32–41.

National Academy on an Aging Society. (1999). *Chronic conditions: A challenge in the 21st century*. Washington, DC: The Gerontological Society of America.

National Academy on an Aging Society. (2000). *At risk: Developing chronic conditions later in life*. Washington, DC: The Gerontological Society of America.

National Center for Health Statistics. (2000). *Older Americans 2000: Key indicators of well-being*. Washington, DC: Author.

National Center for Health Statistics. (1995). Washington, DC: Author.

Nine, S., Lakies, C., & Jarrett, H. (2000, November 29–December 1). Development and early outcomes of a chronic disease management program in an African American community. Paper Presented at the 15th National Conference on Chronic Disease Prevention and Control.

Phelan, E., Williams, B., Snyder, Simmons, L., Wagner, E., & LoGerfo, J. (2000, November 29–December 1). Outcomes of a community based replication of the senior health Enhancement Program. Paper Presented at the 15th National Conference on Chronic Disease Prevention and Control.

Puska, P., Nissinen, A., Tuomilehto, J., Salonen, J., Koskela, K., McAlister, A., Kottke, T., Maccoby, N., & Farquhar, J. (1990). The community-based strategy to prevent coronary heart disease: Conclusions from the ten years of the North Karelia Project. In L. Breslow, J. Fielding, & Lave, L. (Eds.) (1985). *Annual Review of Public Health, 6*, 147–193. Palo Alto, CA: Annual Reviews.

Quarterlyn, P.S. (1994). The meaning of prevention for older people: Changing common perceptions. *Generation, 18*(1), 28–32.

Osgood, N.J., Wood, H.E., & Parham, I. (1995). *Alcoholism and aging: An annotated bibliography and review*. Westport, CT: Greenwood.

Rimer, B.K., & Orleans, C.T. (1994). Tailoring smoking cessation for older adults. *Cancer, 74*(Suppl. 7), 2051–2054.

Robert Wood Johnson Foundation. (1996). *Chronic care in America: A 21st century challenge*. Princeton, New Jersey.

Schmidt, R.M. (1994). Preventive health care for older adults: Societal and individual services. *Generations, 18*(1), 33–38.

Smith-Sonneborn, J. (1990). How we age. In R. Butler, M. Oberlink, & M. Schecter (Eds.), *The promise of productive aging* (pp. 7–11). New York: Springer.

Stearns, S.C., Bernard, S.L., Konrad, T.R., Schwartz, R.J., & Defriese, G.H. (1997). Medicare use and costs in relation to self-care practices. Poster Presented at the Annual Meeting of the Association for Health Services Research.

Stone, R. (2000). *Long term care for the elderly with disabilities: Current policy, emerging trends, and implications for the twenty-first century*. New York: Millbank Memorial Fund.

Wallace, S.P. (2000). American health promotion: Where individualism rules. *The Gerontologist, 40*(3), 373–377.

World Health Organization. (1999). *Health 21: The health for all policy framework for the WHO European Region* (*European Health for All Series, No. 6*). Copenhagen, Denmark: Author, Regional Office for Europe.

Wykle, M., & Kaskel, B. (1994). Increasing the longevity of older adults through improved health status. Minority elders: Five goals toward building a public policy base (2nd ed.). Washington, DC: The Gerontological Society of America.

Community Capacity

Jay A. Mancini, James A. Martin, and Gary L. Bowen

INTRODUCTION

Dimensions of social organization are significant in the health and well-being of individuals and their families. *Social organization* is a term that describes the collection of values, norms, processes, and behavior patterns within a community that organize, facilitate, and constrain the interactions among community members. This entry highlights key aspects of social organization, community capacity, and social support with regard to primary prevention activities.

Our discussion weaves together several important everyday life strands of human development and the community that reflect social organization. The social organization of a community has a direct bearing on its well-being and community capacity represents an important dimension of that social organization. We believe health promotion and illness prevention can be substantially influenced by the willingness and ability of community members to assume shared responsibility for one another, and by corresponding behavioral evidence of their collective competence in reducing risks and promoting assets associated with health and health promotion.

We begin by discussing the various ways in which community can be conceptualized. Our model of community capacity is presented as an organizing schema for understanding the relationship between community and health. This model includes community capacity itself, community results, formal and informal networks, and levels of effects. With the exception of community results, which are products of social organization, each component of the model is an aspect of social organization. We next review the research literature on health, well-being, social support, and community; social support is also a dimension of social organization, as well as an indicator of community capacity at a microlevel. Our discussion concludes by positing the implications of the model for enhancing overall community health and well-being.

The Significance of Community Networks

The role of community networks in promoting the physical, psychological, social, and spiritual well-being of community members is receiving increasing attention from scientists, public leaders, and government officials, as well as community members. These formal and informal community linkages are linchpins in how well individuals and families experience everyday life. The community is a composite of individual and social life, and as such has become an important force in intervening between life circumstances and the various effects of those circumstances on individuals and families (Bowen, Richman, & Bowen, 2000; Garbarino & Kostelny, 1992; Sampson, Raudenbush, & Earls, 1997).

The Community as a Protective Factor

Discussions around community often center on social problems and associated risk factors, and risk behaviors. However, more is transpiring in communities aside from risk factors and risk behaviors. As the work of Garbarino and Kostelny (1992) on child maltreatment, and of Sampson and colleagues (1997) on violent crime demonstrate, communities with similar risk factors vary in health-related outcomes. These findings are significant for our discussion on the role of community as it pertains to health. Intervention and prevention planning depend on identifying community-level processes that account for community variation in health-related outcomes in the context of similar levels of risk.

We propose the concept of *community capacity* as a key protective factor that allows communities to achieve better health-related outcomes, especially when risk factors are substantial. As a feature of social organization in a community, "community capacity is the degree to which people in a community demonstrate a sense of *shared responsibility* for the general welfare of the community and its individual members, and also demonstrate *collective competence* by

taking advantage of opportunities for addressing community needs and confronting situations that threaten the safety and well-being of community members" (Bowen, Martin, Mancini, & Nelson, 2000, p. 7). Our approach emphasizes a resilience and protective factor perspective (Richman & Fraser, 2001) and we believe that communities vary in their level of adaptation at any single point in time, which reflects the status of the population within a defined area on multiple community results, including health-related results (Coulton, 1995). *Community resilience* is the ability of a community to maintain, regain, or establish favorable community results over time even when there is adversity or when there are positive challenges (e.g., there may be situations that a community faces that are opportunities for positive change, which require that people join together in order to advance community life). The community is resilient in part because it possesses various protective factors, one of which is community capacity, that provide it with resources to deal with difficult situations.

Community Influences and Health

The capacity of a community to influence matters of health, including illness and wellness, can be substantial if a community possesses the sentiment that places a high value on mutual support, and also demonstrates that it is actually able to provide support to its members. A core reflection of this sentiment of shared responsibility is represented by a sense of community and community altruism. People who have a strong *sense of community* indicate that they feel a part of their community, and they believe their community will support them when necessary. People who are *altruistic* feel it is important to do supportive things for others, even when it is not clear what benefits might be coming back to them. Both of these concepts represent individual level characteristics of community members. We believe that the power associated with a sense of shared responsibility and with collective competence allows community members individually and collectively to make a difference in people's health. While individuals make a difference on their own, improving the quality of life in a community is largely up to the collective force of the community itself, since it requires consensus about how well the community is doing and what community results *should be* addressed. An assumption of our approach is that the community as a collective is what determines the overall health and well-being because it represents the talents and positive sentiments of community members across the breadth of the community.

The aggregate health and well-being of its members may be the most telling indicator of how well a community is functioning. Using Maslow's heuristic description of the human condition and motivations for taking action, the health and well-being of community members are at the core of community health (Maslow, 1954). Community members can be expected to place greater effort into other higher order aspects of community life (such as the arts, beautification projects, etc.) when essential matters of health and well-being are adequately addressed (whether they be access to basic health care or knowing that the streets are safe).

Caveats and Considerations

Several caveats are required in any discussion of research and theory about community and health. First, definitions of what comprises a community vary across studies. As we discuss in a later section, community is defined in numerous ways, and each definition gives a different understanding of the community. Second, terms such as social support, social network, and interpersonal relationships are often used interchangeably in the social science literature (Cohen, 1988). Consequently, it is more difficult to compare studies and their results. Third, measuring aspects of community and of social support are challenging (Cohen, Gottlieb, & Underwood, 2000; Coulton, 1995). A community level indicator of well-being is not simply the addition of individual level indicators. Fourth, as we note in a later section, some community studies are confounded by the ecological fallacy, that is, generalizing from aggregated information to the situation of a particular person in the community. Knowing about community indicators does not mean that you can explain the situation of any one person in that community (Macintyre & Ellaway, 2000). As a result of these constraints, conceptualizing and researching community collectively, in addition to an individual or a dyadic level, is not well-refined. Even with these limitations, the consideration of the role of community has merit. We believe that it represents a more powerful way to think about prevention and intervention.

The Nature of a Community

The word "community" is defined and applied in differing ways. We speak of being a part of a community (identity and membership), of experiencing community with others (interaction and closeness), and of being concerned about our community (commitment and corresponding opportunities for community involvement). While the word community can be used and applied in any number of ways, it is important from a research perspective to denote some precision about how this term is actually being used. This is especially so when constructing prevention and intervention strategies because understanding the specific meaning of the term community provides an opportunity to establish clearer and more specific goals and desired outcomes.

"Community" is both a social and a geographic unit (Coulton, 1995). In all cases, when we specify a community we are discussing boundaries, some geographical and spatial and others interpersonal and psychosocial. Coulton (1995) has discussed four types of boundaries, including phenomenological, interactional, statistical, and political. Phenomenological boundaries are those agreed upon by most people living in contiguity to each other; simply most people agree their neighborhood exists in an area bounded by certain geographic coordinates. This consensus may change over time since this type of boundary is not concrete, nor is it simply comprised of particular objects. Interactional boundaries are based on people sharing a spatial area and spending time together in interaction and transaction. One might focus on patterns of friendship and activities of daily living in order to define this kind of community boundary. Statistically based boundaries involve information from sources such as the US Census, where tract information may be used to establish community boundaries. A final approach discussed by Coulton is based on political or governmental units such as wards, districts in a city, or towns.

Furstenberg and Hughes (1997) have pointed out aspects of community that help expand and explain this notion of people and institutions within a defined space. They discuss community with regard to physical infrastructure, social and demographic infrastructure, institutional resources, and social organization. Each reflects a critical aspect of the total community picture. Physical features include streets, buildings, parks and their juxtaposition; social and demographic features include descriptions of people in the community along economic, racial, ethnic, and age lines; institutional resource features include agencies and organizations supporting community members' needs (schools, hospitals, etc.); social organization features include what happens between people in the community, that is, how people interrelate, cooperate, and provide support to each other. Social organization also includes networks of people, the exchange and reciprocity that transpire in relationships, accepted standards (norms) of social support, and social controls that regulate behavior and interaction. Our discussion of community capacity is anchored by the social organization part of Furstenberg and Hughes' (1997) discussion of community.

"Neighborhood" is often used interchangeably with community, and the neighborhood may be the place where prevention and intervention activities actually occur. Sampson et al. (1997, p. 919) define a *neighborhood* as "a collection of people and institutions occupying a subsection of a larger community." Defining community from a neighborhood perspective has a great deal of appeal since the concept of a neighborhood is more easily visualized and therefore easier to understand and describe than some other definitions of community. For most of us the term neighborhood suggests both a land area (including streets and buildings) and a sense of something shared between and among the people residing in that physical space.

How a community is defined is important when considering matters of health and well-being. For example, if there is a campaign to immunize 100 percent of children at risk in a neighborhood or community, then the community boundaries must be clearly understood so that the actual number of targeted children can be determined. Or if an important community result deals with improving the safety of youth during after-school hours, then the community where that improvement needs to occur should be identified so that specific actions can be undertaken where these youth are actually located. Or if insuring that access to health care is adequate and efficient for certain community residents, then community boundaries need to be well understood with particular attention to the juxtaposition of people and health care institutions. Without this specificity it is difficult to develop and evaluate prevention and intervention efforts. It is also difficult to assess and monitor associated community results. If a community is to be mobilized and if its capacity to improve itself is to be strengthened, then the parameters of that community must be known.

Without regard to how it is defined, community is a context that has a bearing on many aspects of everyday life and therefore requires inclusion in discussions of how to improve the lives of individuals and families who live and work in contiguity to one another. Various aspects of a community make a difference in matters related to health, especially as they relate to social organization.

The Community Capacity Model and Social Organization

We have noted that social organization is a key element in enhancing community health and well-being. The following model of community capacity builds on a social organization framework, and captures the interaction, cooperation, and support that occur among people in a community (Furstenberg & Hughes, 1997). Our community capacity model contains three main parts: community capacity, community results, and formal and informal networks of social care. In addition, we discuss effect levels as they relate to how formal and informal networks interact. We also discuss social capital as part of community capacity. Our empirical work has partially examined this model. It shows that the sense of community is informed by an individual's level of participation in community activities, the ease in connecting with others in the community, and by the extent of shared responsibility and collective competence among community members (Bowen, Martin, Mancini, & Nelson, 2001).

The literature cited in a later section on community and health demonstrates that the informal network is a powerful ally in prevention and intervention.

Theoretical History and Context of our Model

The community capacity model presented in this review is informed by the work of numerous other social and behavioral scientists (Coleman, 1988; Putnam, 2000; Sampson, 2001; Sampson et al., 1997). The concepts and the findings from this body of research have been beneficial to our specification of community capacity, community results, formal and informal networks, and effect levels.

In the late 1980s, Coleman (1988) discussed several kinds of capital, including *social capital*. He viewed social capital as a force that enables certain outcomes to occur that otherwise would not be attainable in a community. From this perspective, social capital can occur in various kinds of human relationships, including those between family members, between work associates, and even between strangers. These many sources of social capital are significant in our framework because we contend that, for communities to do well, social capital must have the contributions of many rather than of a few. Certainly for community health to be improved, the collective efforts of individuals, families, and neighborhoods all play an important role.

Coleman (1988) discussed obligations and expectations, information channels, and social norms as forms of social capital. Obligations and expectations pertain to the exchanges that occur between people, that is, the back and forth support that typifies both interpersonal and group relationships. For this process to effectively occur there must be a certain level of trust and cooperation, factors that underlie the process of successfully connecting with others. Information and the vehicles that provide it are important to Coleman's view of social capital because it is through information that particular needs and goals are realized. In the modern society, information is a highly valued source of capital. The informed community is one that can more effectively address its problems and achieve its goals because the information that it possesses is a powerful and effective resource. Coleman also discusses *social norms*, that is, those socio-community guidelines that encourage prosocial behavior and discourage antisocial behavior. Consequently there are norms that pertain to altruism, that promote interacting with others, and that move people to behave in collective, supportive ways. Our own model benefits from Coleman's work in that we incorporate his focus on collective processes that bring people to pool their sentiments and their actions.

Our work is also informed by Sampson (2001) and by Sampson et al. (1997). These researchers have focused on collective efficacy, a process that adds an important dimension to the understanding of community capacity. *Collective efficacy* goes beyond social capital in that it involves people feeling connected and being willing to act on behalf of themselves and their neighbors (Sampson et al., 1997). Sampson (2001, p. 10) has recently stated that collective efficacy "is meant to signify an emphasis on shared beliefs in a neighborhood's conjoint capability for action to achieve an intended effect, and hence an active sense of engagement on the part of residents." Our definition of community capacity parallels the thinking of those who have discussed collective efficacy because we place high value on the action complement of social capital. For us, the sentiment to act is insufficient unless the action itself is also evident.

Robert Putnam (1995, 2000) captured the attention of numerous social scientists when he used the phrase "bowling alone" to describe his view of the current status of community. In short, Putnam was struck that while more people were bowling, there were fewer bowling leagues—individuals are not connected to one another by their everyday activities. Putnam has discussed social capital as including two key terms, reciprocity and trust. He also ascribes cohesive and lubricating characteristics to social capital. In the former sense, social capital is a force in bringing people together, and in the later it is a force for enhancing human relationships. Putnam notes that social capital belongs to the collective rather than to an individual, that it allows the community to achieve results otherwise not achievable, and that it increases the more that it is used (also an action element of social capital).

Our community capacity model has benefited from the work of these scholars and throughout the following discussion you will read elements of these earlier works. In addition to these primary social capital and collective efficacy concepts, we enhance the discussion of supporting people and their communities by examining the nature of community results, by differentiating informal and formal networks, and by discussing effect levels that emerge from these networks.

Community Capacity

Community capacity is the central concept in this model. As stated earlier, "Community capacity is the degree to which people in a community demonstrate a sense of *shared responsibility* for the general welfare of the community and its individual members, and also demonstrate *collective competence* by taking advantage of opportunities for addressing community needs and confronting situations that threaten the safety and well-being of community members" (Bowen et al., 2000, p. 7). "Demonstrate" is a key word in our definition of community capacity. Community capacity

is more than a willingness to think or feel in a particular way; it is seen in observable results. We believe that community capacity mediates what transpires between the social capital that is generated by formal and informal networks, and achieving community results.

Social capital supports the development of community capacity and provides its "fuel." *Social capital* is the sum of resources (information, opportunities, and practical support) that develop from reciprocal relationships that are embodied in the social networks among people in both formal and informal settings. Putnam (2000, p. 326), who has been the most recent articulator of social capital thinking draws the following conclusion: "Of all the domains in which I have traced the consequences of social capital, in none is the importance of social connectedness so well established as in the case of health and well-being."

Our definition of social capital is consistent with Putnam, as well as with several other social scientists who have been studying the relationships between social capital and health (Kawachi & Berkman, 2000; Kawachi, Kennedy, Lochner, & Prothrow-Stith, 1997). Social capital involves reciprocity and trust among people. It is seen in civic engagement, that is, the involvement of community members themselves in the community through activities in civic associations and religious groups, in various groups via official membership, and in community initiatives. One study that warrants discussion has reported on the relationship between social capital and health (Kawachi, 1999). This investigator examined self-reported health and found that people residing in states with low social capital (as measured by levels of interpersonal trust, norms of reciprocity, and associational membership) were more likely to indicate poorer self-rated health levels. While there is very little research that tries to connect social capital with health, this report does suggest that aspects of community in a collective sense have some relevance to health.

It is community capacity that is active and that ultimately leads toward achieving community results. By this we mean that community capacity is not just sentiment about doing good for the community and its members. It is the actual demonstration of shared responsibility and of collective competence.

Community Results

Matters of health are at the core of community well-being. Oftentimes when people speak about their community or about people in their community or about themselves, the conversation contains an element of health and well-being. For example, we hear discussions about which communities are the healthiest, which are the best places to raise children, which are the best for retirement, and so on. Health and well-being issues can include just about anything and everything across a biopsychosocial spectrum. They represent both the macro aspects of community well-being and the micro aspects of individual well-being, from safety to disease, from crime to pregnancy rates among teenagers, from family financial success and unemployment rates to smoking behaviors in an area or a neighborhood. In our model of community capacity, we have spoken about community results, which are broad-based and which reflect the consensus of the community. Community results reflect the aspirations that community members might have collectively. Community results, to the extent they are recognized and discussed, provide guidance to a community on how it could use its resources to improve the lives and life chances of its members. It is important to recognize community results, otherwise to what end is community capacity operating?

Social epidemiologists and other health-oriented professionals examine a range of health and well-being issues that can be discussed in terms of community results. At a collective level, rates would be established that reflect each of these issues (e.g., rates of a particular event, disease, or circumstance per 1,000 people in a circumscribed community). These issues include living free from violence and intimidation on the streets and at home, avoidance of preventable accidents and illnesses, being able to have adequate care when ill, being risk-free from sexually transmitted diseases, and exhibiting positive health behaviors (including moderation in alcohol use, abstinence with regard to smoking and non-prescribed drug use, and the appropriate use of safety devices like child car restraints). Many community results that are health-oriented can be seen with regard to the human and family life cycle. As examples, a community result pertinent to young families might involve insuring that infants and young children have adequate nutrition; one that is more applicable to adolescents might involve insuring that teenagers have adequate supervision in the after school hours; one that is particular to older adults might involve insuring that people at this life cycle stage are provided every opportunity to maintain their independence.

Formal and Informal Networks of Social Care

Two important vehicles in our conceptualization of community capacity are the formal and informal networks. Formal networks are based on role and position, and often reflect obligation or duty. Informal networks include relationships with work associates, friends, neighbors, voluntary associations, and other collective relationships that are entered into and maintained voluntarily. The notion of network is consistent with the social capital perspective and reflects the long history of work in the social sciences that

has addressed interaction patterns. The term "social care" suggests that networks function to provide support for individuals and for families. "Social" is a key term in that it suggests that the products of being in a network, such as interaction and transaction, emanate from connecting with others. The term social care suggests that humans, individually and in groups, have needs for association in order to live healthy lives.

In our model of community capacity, the focus is on informal networks because we believe that informal networks continue to be a relatively untapped source in building healthy communities. This is not to say that the recognition of the significance of informal networks is anything new. It does reflect that for the most part communities have not been sufficiently intentional in building these networks. We believe that supporting informal networks is a primary responsibility of the formal network, which includes agencies, organizations, and generally people and structures that function out of obligation. We believe that the formal network can more readily achieve its objectives by mobilizing and empowering the informal community.

Community capacity comes alive to the extent that the informal network is strong and to the extent the formal network supports it, rather than taking on responsibilities that should be addressed by people and their connections. Formal and informal networks are interrelated, in that each informs the other and potentially strengthens the other. For example, a formal network organization dealing with health information is far more effective when the informal networks in a community are supportive of it, and are talking about that organization's public awareness campaign; additionally, it may well be that change will occur only if the informal network takes what the formal network provides, endorses it, and shapes the community members' health behaviors accordingly.

Levels of Effects

In our community capacity model, as formal and informal networks operate, several kinds of effects and associations occur. These effects in turn contribute to the building of community capacity. Our conceptualization of effect levels is based on the work of Small and Supple (2001). First-level effects pertain to what transpires within a homogeneous network, whether it is formal or informal. For example, if we focus on a formal community support organization such as a mental health agency, we could examine their contribution to community capacity as evidenced by the willingness of its staff to deal with sensitive health-related issues such as depression and suicide. If we were to focus on the informal network, we might look at the degree to which residents in a particular neighborhood share information about safety on the streets. In this instance community capacity is enhanced by activities that have been described by Putnam (2000) by the term "bonding." These kinds of activities occur within a group and produce cohesion, trust, and positive regard.

Second-level effects involve what transpires between similar networks. If we extend our first level effects examples, we would be interested in how staff from various community agencies deal with sensitive health-related issues and how they collectively address those issues (in this case depression and suicide). And with regard to the informal network, we would focus on how various adjoining neighborhoods in a community share information about safety on the streets, including safest paths for walking and reports of crime.

Third-level effects involve interactions between dissimilar network types that contribute to community capacity. These may involve, for example, neighborhoods collaborating with community service agencies around such issues as improving safety on the streets, or around preventing suicide among youth. In the case of third-level effects there is crossover between formal and informal networks of social care. We believe that as this crossover occurs, there is potential for building the capacity of a community to deal with internal and external threats (respond to crises), and with enhancing the quality of community life (proactively addressing desired community results, aside from crisis situations). In Putnam's (2000) schema, these kinds of effects involve activities that have a "bridging" function, that is, those that involve ties among people across groups. Bridging activities, as well as bonding activities, become forces behind the development of community capacity.

Research on Health, Well-Being, and Social Support

To this point we have discussed the ways community can be defined. We have also discussed our model of community capacity, which reflects the social organization within a community from a macro perspective. In this section, we highlight the health-related literature demonstrating the role of social organization, and providing the rationale for our focus on community capacity. This literature includes analyses of social networks, interpersonal relationships, and social support (which represent microlevel perspectives), as well as analyses of more global aspects of the community (Berkman & Glass, 2000; Cohen et al., 2000; Kawachi, 1999; Patrick & Wickizer, 1995). Our own review is based on the summaries of these resources.

Our approach to the understanding of community, as well as our approach to how to build community capacity, is dependent on interpersonal connections. As a consequence, we focus mainly on these aspects of community in our discussion. The net result of this part of our discussion is our

contention that relational aspects of community can make a great difference in the health and well-being of community members. However, as is noted by Brissette, Cohen and Seeman (2000), social networks can also be hostile to good health and well-being since interpersonal relationships themselves can be laced with negative emotions, conflictual communication, competition, and stress. In these instances, the benefits for health associated with social support will be tempered. We mention this because all too often the social network is over identified with positive outcomes, and recognition is not given to the possibility of negative outcomes.

Microlevel Research Perspectives

Social epidemiologists and other social scientists have been studying the many ways that aspects of community and health interrelate. There is a growing number of research studies on social support in areas related to arthritis, cancer, cardiovascular disease, diabetes, HIV/AIDS, kidney disease, multiple sclerosis, and pregnancy (Wills & Shiner, 2000). We are limiting our discussion to a few main dimensions of health as examples of how aspects of community social organization come into play. Most of these studies employ a microlevel perspective, with the individual or family as the unit of analysis.

Recently, Berkman and Glass (2000) summarized the research that connects health with social integration, social networks, and social support. Berkman and Glass review this work with regard to all-cause mortality, and to cardiovascular, disease, stroke, and to infectious diseases. In their analysis of all-cause mortality, they conclude that "virtually all of these studies find that people who are socially isolated or disconnected to others have between two and five times the risk of dying from all causes compared to those who maintain strong ties to friends, family, and community" (Berkman & Glass, 2000, p. 160). In short, people who are isolated are at increased risk of dying "before their time." What is interesting to note is that the studies they report on were conducted across a number of countries in North America, Europe, and Asia.

In a research reviewed by Berkman and Glass (2000) involving a sample of Californians, those with fewer social ties were at higher risk of dying from ischemic heart disease, cerebrovascular and circulatory disease, cancer, and from other causes of death related to the respiratory and gastrointestinal systems. These researchers found that the association between these diseases and social networks was not directly related to health behaviors such as smoking and drinking, a further indication of the power of social support. In a Michigan study, there were similar findings for men but they did not hold for women. Additional research conducted in North Carolina, and in Georgia also demonstrate the social network and health relationship, that is, being connected with others has a positive impact on mortality. Outside of the United States, the findings are similar (Berkman & Glass, 2000). In Sweden, it was found that people more socially isolated were at higher risk for dying without regard to their age and physical risk factors. In Finland, the results are similar but again more so for men than for women when controlling for other risk factors. Finally, research in Denmark and in Japan also indicates that social support lessens overall mortality risk.

In their summary of research specifically focused on cardiovascular disease, Berkman and Glass (2000) note that the onset of this disease must be distinguished from prognosis and survival when examining the impact of social support. On average social support appears to influence post-heart attack well-being rather than preventing the onset of heart disease. The authors note that the emotional support that emanates from connections with others has a role in heart patients' recovery. In other research cited by these social epidemiologists, being married or having a close confidant had a positive influence on survival among people with serious heart disease. Other aspects of social support also have a positive correlation with heart disease survival, including involvement in civic and religious organizations, and religious beliefs.

Somewhat parallel to the findings concerning cardiovascular disease, Berkman and Glass (2000) report that social network factors are more important for recovering from stroke than for preventing stroke. They cite numerous study results that suggest that emotional support after a stroke influences positively how well a person functions physically and how well they adjust psychologically (such as having fewer suicidal thoughts). It appears that social support is a strong intervention in quality of life post-stroke, including fewer hospitalized days and more positive conditions at discharge.

A final general category discussed by Berkman and Glass (2000) is infectious disease, namely HIV/AIDS and the common cold. Social mixing becomes a context and a vehicle whereby both good and bad results can occur, and the latter is certainly the case with injection drug abuse. For example, these authors cite research that found that drug injectors with a non-injecting spouse or other intimate non-injecting partner were not injecting as frequently. Other research has reported parallel findings that support the protection that positive relationships have on destructive behavior such as drug use. There is also increasing evidence that aspects of social support have some bearing on the immune system itself. For example, Berkman and Glass (2000) discuss a study conducted in Sweden among HIV-infected men that found that immune system levels were lower among those who reported fewer available close relationships. At the opposite end of the serious infection spectrum is the common cold. Research indicates that people who have a wider and more diverse social network are less susceptible to common colds, and when they have a cold suffer fewer symptoms (Cohen, Doyle, Skoner, Rabin, & Gwaltney, 1997).

Theoretical Models

Cohen et al. (2000) have discussed three models that help explain the association between social relationships and health, and that reflect social organization. Their discussion helps inform our community capacity model. The *"main effect"* model covers the paths that show direct effects between social relationships and associated psychological and physical health. As examples, they suggest that a social network can provide a generally positive outlook on life that mitigates despair, can be a source of information about health that keeps people more aware of healthy habits of daily living or keeps them better informed about community services, and can provide practical assistance such as food and clothing.

The *"stress buffering"* model is more particular to when people are in stressful situations. In this model the social network and social support help by keeping people away from making poor responses to stressful events (social network and social support operate as protective factors and counteract the influence of stressors or risk factors on health-related outcomes). Social network members may provide useful advice in response to stress or may provide respite during a stressful time (an example that comes to mind is in the case where an elderly person is providing constant care to her/his spouse). In the absence of specific stressors or risk factors, social network and social support may have few demonstrable effects.

A third model is called *"threshold or gradient"* model and has to do with how incremental increases or decreases in social support affect an individual or a family. It may be that once a certain level of support is reached, then additional levels of support do not provide additional benefits. On the other hand, once protective factors, like social support, decline past a certain level, the individual or family has no immunity against stressors or risk factors and may become very vulnerable. This discussion by Cohen and his colleagues provides an understanding of why social support (an important part of this community concept) makes a difference.

Macrolevel Research Perspectives

Patrick and Wickizer (1995) and Macintyre and Ellaway (2000) have summarized various studies related to health and community but with more of a focus on community-level interventions than on social networks and social support per se. Kawachi (1999) has examined social capital and its relationship to community and health. Patrick and Wickizer (1995) discuss a conceptual model that includes components of cultural systems, political and policy systems, economics systems and prosperity, the community social environment (including poverty, gender, social cohesion, and social norms), community physical environment (including pollution, population density, and climate), community responses (activation and social support), and community outcomes (social behaviors, community health, and quality of life). Patrick and Wickizer (1995) state:

> As a determinant of health, community interacts with broader determinants, notably the social and physical environment. Communities contain the social environment, including worksites, schools, families, friends, and a range of organizations and institutions. These social units are sources of reciprocal social influence that affect the health and well-being of individuals. Individuals and groups are both agents and recipients of social influence. Community also incorporates the physical environment, and for this reason alone its definition must include a geographic component: the physical environment of a locale, influenced by the larger global environment, affects the health of its residents. (pp. 52–53)

Patrick and Wickizer (1995) and Macintyre and Ellaway (2000) discuss the problems of generalizing from aggregated information to the situation of a specific individual in the community (called the ecological fallacy). In short, knowing about community indicators does not mean that you can explain the situation of any one person in that community. Patrick and Wickizer use the example of the hung jury. As a group, the jury is indecisive but on an individual level each juror is quite decisive, which is why the jury as a whole is indecisive. Consequently, in trying to understand the influence of aspects of the community generally on people at the individual level, great care must be exercised.

While our main interest involves social organization as it is embodied in the sentiments and actions of people and groups, we briefly note that there are those who examine the effects that community has on everyday life from a much broader perspective. Macintyre and Ellaway (2000) discuss at length the process of studying "area effects" on people's health (whether it be health behavior, health status, health risks, or mortality). They make an important distinction between compositional and contextual explanations. The former refers to the fact that some places (or areas) are composed of people with very similar characteristics, whereas the latter refers to the fact that some physical or geographic places have particular features or characteristics, like differing levels of community capacity, that influence the health of those who live there, including any number of environmental features.

If these two types of explanations are confused, then conclusions about community and health can be very different and consequently very wrong. For example, effects attributed to an area may be only due to the characteristics associated with the homogeneity of the people who live there. It appears to us that current research designs rarely uncover contextual explanations, including those relating to collective characteristics of community members. Macintyre and Ellaway's review of the literature leads us to believe that the available evidence is now on the side of compositional explanations. These authors cite various studies from the United States and from Europe that find it difficult to attach a close relationship between "area" and health. For example, a Dutch study of mental illness found that rates were more attributable to people who resided in a place as opposed to the place itself. However, they cite other studies that suggest that people characteristics cannot fully explain health status and health behaviors in a particular area. Our own take on these studies is that overall the verdict is still out on the influence of place on health, when place (contextual effects rather than environmental contamination effects) is separated from the people (compositional effects) in that place. Even though our main interest around community capacity and social organization is process focused, it is important to be aware of possible influences of place on what happens within a community.

In this section, we have summarized comprehensive examinations of aspects of health and their relationships to aspects of community, more particularly the social network and the support that it provides. We have discussed these studies of social support as examples of social organization in a community. We have used these as examples of the significance that community can have in people's lives. The degree to which people are "connected" to other people (including the practical aid that this represents, as well as the emotional benefits of these social relationships) makes a difference in their health, and helps determine how well they respond to disease conditions. In general, social aspects of the community do affect health—those aspects that are about people and connections rather than solely about geography. Such connections are significant for our conceptualization of community capacity.

Conclusions: Community Capacity, Social Organization, and Health

Gottlieb (2000) has noted that effective support interventions must attend to the needs of people and to the nature of the social environment. He observes that little has been done "on ways of altering the structure and policies of organizations and institutions in order to enhance their occupants' access to or actual receipt of support" (Gottlieb, 2000, p. 196). A key piece of our thinking about community capacity and pathways to build it is that the juxtaposition of formal (organizations and institutions) and informal networks of support is significant. Our suggestion about altering the structure and the functions of organizations and institutions is that these formal networks can be more intentional about what happens within their organization, how they relate to other formal networks around key community health issues, and how they relate to informal networks in their community. The first response really has to do with whether a single organization is geared to addressing key health issues, the second has to do with whether organizations that are concerned about similar health issues are effectively collaborating, and the third has to do with whether organizations are working with informal network members. This third response is what we discussed in our model earlier and involves formal networks of social care being intentional about working with informal networks of social care in partnership rather than as professional to client (the latter being a hierarchical approach which keeps the informal community network dependent and ineffective). This third response assumes that the informal network is powerful, resourceful and asset-rich, rather than unskilled and deficit-laden. The research that we have cited that connects social networks with health outcomes shows the power of the informal network at a dyadic and family level. What remains to be seen is how collectively this power can be directed to achieving desired community health results.

In his discussion on strategically thinking about society and health, Miller (1995) speaks of the relational dimensions of a community, including the "social fabric" of everyday life (he notes that building a successful community is not only a matter of economic improvement). He rightly points out that social relations are the foundation of community and social support. Miller goes on to discuss the importance of promoting social interactions and of developing ways of connecting people. Community connections are important vehicles for enhancing the everyday life of community members, for building a sense of shared responsibility, and for building the collective competence of community members, which are the elements of community capacity. As formal networks of social care rethink their partnerships with the informal community, an important consideration is how these formal networks can foster and enrich connections among people and groups in the informal network. Through their normal activities formal networks can provide those connecting opportunities, which in turn contribute to the building of community (Bowen et al., 2001).

Miller (1995) calls for thinking broadly about health care reform, and notes that the discussion seems to be mainly about financing rather than about care per se. The financing-oriented discussion focuses on remedial matters and not so much on prevention matters. Building community capacity is about structuring communities in which prevention is supported by community members feeling responsible for other community members and by community members collectively accomplishing results that otherwise would be unattainable.

We are struck by a comment made by Glass (2000) in his review of psychosocial interventions as they involve health. He notes that certain interventions must arrive at a particular point in a health crisis for there to be a maximum helpful effect, and then cites a study which reports that the intervention started too late. A community capacity approach is not only oriented to unanticipated crises but is mostly oriented to normative everyday life situations. A community can have the capacity to meet desired community results on a daily basis, so that people are supported in their everyday life activities and supported in those times when crises occur as well. The connections that typify the informal network become a web that can respond to a variety of health-related demands, whether they are informing neighborhoods about childhood infectious disease outbreaks or whether they are supporting families with relatives that are hospitalized.

Emmons (2000) has recently reviewed the literature on health behavior change research. She notes in her analysis that theoretical models in this area are limited because too little attention is given to community, organizational, or system factors that affect health. In her social ecological model, five intervention levels are described: intrapersonal, interpersonal, organizational/environmental, community, and policy. When Emmons speaks of the community as a target of intervention, she includes these suggestions (p. 252): develop strategies that involve one's family, friends, and community; provide cues for health behavior throughout the community; connect participants with community organizations; train key community leaders to deliver important prevention messages; develop interventions that enhance the fit between people and their surroundings; and imbed interventions into ongoing community programs and activities. These suggestions are consonant with the notion of building community capacity because they are multilayered, because they are partnership based, and because they are likely vehicles for supporting the sentiment of shared responsibility and for contributing to the collective competence that community members possess.

Community capacity is a social organization generic framework of prevention and intervention that argues for developing partnerships between formal and informal networks of social care. The framework highlights community results because a focus on results provides direction to those trying to make positive differences in a community. It assumes that social capital provides the resources that support the development of community capacity. Communities high in capacity demonstrate a sense of *shared responsibility* for the general welfare of the community and its individual members, and also demonstrate *collective competence* by taking advantage of opportunities for addressing community needs and confronting situations that threaten the safety and well-being of community members. The application of the community capacity model to the promotion of health and the prevention of illness appears to have great promise in that health is a significant issue at the individual, family, organizational, and community levels. Since optimum health is not just a matter of treating diseases by the medical profession, the role of the larger community itself in health and well-being is significant. This larger community includes people in neighborhoods, work associates, and human and health services professionals. The community that has high capacity for addressing health issues on a normative basis and during times of crises is effective because there is a sense of shared responsibility (an altruistic sentiment to support all community members) and because the community takes collective action that corresponds to that sentiment. As a framework of social organization, the community capacity model incorporates multiple levels of community life, including processes that occur among community members in informal ways as well as processes that occur between community members and the formal organizations that they rely upon. The model is a natural context for understanding the relationships between the community and the health of its members, and for continuing a dialogue in particular on how collective aspects of community life affect the promotion of health and the prevention of illness.

Also see: Culture, Society, and Social Class: Foundation; Politics and Systems Change: Foundation; Parenting: Early Childhood; Substances: Adolescence (Roona).

References

Berkman, L.F., & Glass, T. (2000). Social integration, social networks, social support, and health. In L.F. Berkman & I. Kawachi (Eds.), *Social epidemiology* (pp. 137–173). New York: Oxford University Press.

Bowen, G.L., Richman, J.M., & Bowen, N.K. (2000). Families in the context of communities across time. In S.J. Price, P.C. McKenry, & M.J. Murphy (Eds.), *Families across time: A life course perspective* (pp. 117–128). Los Angeles, CA: Roxbury.

Bowen, G.L., Martin, J.A., Mancini, J.A., & Nelson, J.P. (2000). Community capacity: Antecedents and consequences. *Journal of Community Practice, 8*, 1–21.

Bowen, G.L., Martin, J.A., Mancini, J.A., & Nelson, J.P. (in press). Civic engagement and sense of community in the military. *Journal of Community Practice, 9*(2), 71–93.

Brissette, I., Cohen, S., & Seeman, T.E. (2000). Measuring social integration and social networks. In S. Cohen, L.G. Underwood, & B.H. Gottlieb (Eds.), *Social support measurement and intervention: A guide for health and social scientists* (pp. 53–85). New York: Oxford University Press.

Cohen, S. (1988). Psychosocial models of the role of social support in the etiology of physical disease. *Health Psychology, 7*, 269–297.

Cohen, S., Doyle, W.J., Skoner, D.P., Rabin, B.S., & Gwaltney, J.M. (1997). Social ties and susceptibility to the common cold. *Journal of the American Medical Association, 277*, 1941–1944.

Cohen, S., Gottlieb, B.H., & Underwood, L.G. (2000). Social relationships and health. In S. Cohen, L.G. Underwood, & B.H. Gottlieb (Eds.), *Social support measurement and intervention: A guide for health and social scientists* (pp. 3–25). New York: Oxford University Press.

Coleman, J. (1988). Social capital in the creation of human capital. *American Sociological Review, 94*, 95–120.

Coulton, C.J. (1995). Using community-level indicators of children's well-being in comprehensive community initiatives. In J.P. Connell, A.C. Kubisch, L.B. Schorr, B., & C.H. Weiss (Eds.), *New approaches to evaluating community initiatives: Concepts, methods, and contexts* (pp. 173–199). Washington, DC: The Aspen Institute.

Emmons, K.M. (2000). Health behaviors in a social context. In L.F. Berkman & I. Kawachi (Eds.), *Social epidemiology* (pp. 242–266). New York: Oxford University Press.

Furstenberg, F.F., & Hughes, M.E. (1997). The influence of neighborhoods on children's development: A theoretical perspective and research agenda. In J. Brooks-Gunn, G.J. Duncan, & J.L. Abner (Eds.), *Neighborhood poverty: Vol. 2. Policy implications in studying neighborhoods* (pp. 23–47). New York: Russell Sage Foundation.

Garbarino, J., & Kostelny, K. (1992). Child maltreatment as a community problem. *Child Abuse and Neglect, 16*, 455–464.

Glass, T.A. (2000). Psychosocial intervention. In L.F. Berkman & I. Kawachi (Eds.), *Social epidemiology* (pp. 267–305). New York: Oxford University Press.

Gottlieb, B.H. (2000). Selecting and planning support interventions. In S. Cohen, L.G. Underwood, & B.H. Gottlieb (Eds.), *Social support measurement and intervention: A guide for health and social scientists* (pp. 195–220). New York: Oxford University Press.

Kawachi, I. (1999). Social capital and community effects on population and individual health. *Annals of the New York Academy of Sciences, 896*, 120–130.

Kawachi, I., Kennedy, B.P., Lochner, K., & Prothrow-Stith, D. (1997). Social capital, income inequality, and mortality. *American Journal of Public Health, 87*, 1491–1498.

Kawachi, I., & Berkman, L.F. (2000). Social cohesion, social capital, and health. In L.F. Berkman & I. Kawachi (Eds.), *Social epidemiology* (pp. 174–190). New York: Oxford University Press.

Macintyre, S., & Ellaway, A. (2000). Ecological approaches: Rediscovering the role of the physical and social environment. In L.F. Berkman & I. Kawachi (Eds.), *Social epidemiology* (pp. 332–348). New York: Oxford University Press.

Maslow, A. (1954). *Motivation and personality*. New York: Harper.

Miller, S.M. (1995). Thinking strategically about society and health. In B.C. Amick, S. Levine, A.R. Tarlov, & D.C. Walsh (Eds.), *Society and health* (pp. 342–358). New York: Oxford University Press.

Patrick, D.L., & Wickizer, T.M. (1995). Community and health. In B.C. Amick, S. Levine, A.R. Tarlov, & D.C. Walsh (Eds.), *Society and health* (pp. 46–73). New York: Oxford University Press.

Putnam, R.D. (1995). Bowling alone: America's declining social capital. *Journal of Democracy, 6*, 65–78.

Putnam, R.D. (2000). *Bowling alone: The collapse and revival of American community*. New York: Simon & Schuster.

Richman, J.M., & Fraser, M.W. (2001). Resilience in childhood: The role of risk and protection. In J.M. Richman & M.W. Fraser (Eds.), *The context of youth violence: Resilience, risk, and protection* (pp. 1–12). Westport, CT: Praeger.

Sampson, R.J. (2001). How do communities undergird or undermine human development? Relevant contexts and social mechanisms. In A. Booth & A.C. Crouter (Eds.), *Does it take a village? Community effects on children, adolescents, and families* (pp. 3–30). New York: Lawrence Erlbaum.

Sampson, R.J., Raudenbush, S.W., & Earls, F. (1997). Neighborhoods and violent crime: A multilevel study of collective efficacy. *Science, 277,* 918–924.

Small, S., & Supple, A. (2001). Communities as systems: Is a community more than the sum of its parts? In A. Booth & A.C. Crouter (Eds.), *Does it take a village? Community effects on children, adolescents, and families* (pp. 161–174). New York: Lawrence Erlbaum.

Wills, T.A., & Shiner, O. (2000). Measuring perceived and received social support. In S. Cohen, L.G. Underwood, & B.H. Gottlieb (Eds.), *Social support measurement and intervention: A guide for health and social scientists* (pp. 86–135). New York: Oxford University Press.

Cost Benefit Analysis

Carrie Yodanis and Alberto Godenzi

INTRODUCTION

Measures of cost efficiency, including cost/benefit and cost-effectiveness estimates, are important for evaluating prevention programs. Since the 1990s, cost/benefit analyses of a wide assortment of negative social conditions have become very popular in countries worldwide. In this entry, we rely on examples of studies related to family issues, breastfeeding, work/family policies, and violence against women, in order to highlight a trend in the use of cost/benefit analysis. Over the past decade, cost/benefit studies have often been used as claims-making activities in the construction of social problems and to build a rationale for preventive action.

DEFINITIONS

According to Rossi and Freeman (1990), there are three general modes of decision-making, which can result from evaluation research. These include: Go or No Go decisions, Legitimation and accountability, and Developing a rationale for action. Cost/benefit analysis is commonly done to legitimize and account for the money given for certain programs. With cost/benefit data, it is possible to demonstrate the significant advances made with the money provided. In addition cost efficiency data are often helpful in deciding whether or not to take action and if so, which action to take. It can be shown that the amount saved through a prevention program outweighs the costs of the program and thus makes economical sense to adopt the program. The choice between two possible programs can also be made based on which saves the most per dollar spent. Yet since the 1990s, cost/benefit studies have taken a new tone in relation to social problems.

The studies are being used with the goal of building a rationale for action. The goal is not to decide if a certain action or program is best or to decide between programs. Rather, the researchers aim to convince those who are in a decision-making position to take the action for which they are calling. This approach is rooted in the theoretical framework of the social construction of social problems.

Spector and Kitsuse (1987) define social problems not as objective facts, measured in terms of number of people affected or seriousness of results, but as *claims-making* activities, actions intended to produce the definition of a given condition as a problem in need of solving. These activities, and therefore what are and are not social problems, varies across time and place. They outline four specific stages in the social construction of social problems. In the first stage, "Group(s) attempt to assert the existence of some condition, define it as offensive, harmful, or otherwise undesirable, publicize their assertions, stimulate controversy, and create public or political issues over the matter" (p. 142). In Stage 2, the group(s) and their actions are legitimized by the recognition of established organizations, agencies, and institutions. Stage 3 involves a re-emergence of claims by the original groups against the organizations that handle the problem. This results from dissatisfaction with the ways or extent to which the organizations have dealt with the complaints. In Stage 4, the group(s) reject the established organizations, institutions, and agencies and act to create new, alternative institutions to meet their needs.

In this entry, we discuss how cost/benefit studies can be viewed as claims-making activities used by groups in the social construction of social problems. Cost/benefit language is a tool used to increase acceptance that particular negative social conditions are indeed social problems which need to be addressed, or more ideally, prevented. Thus, cost/benefit analyses are now used not only for the evaluation of, but in the argument for, the very existence of prevention programs.

SCOPE

Becker (1981) was one of the first to use cost/benefit analysis to understand the institution of the family. Becker argues that people, acting to maximize utility, marry, divide the household labor, and have children when benefits are higher than the costs. Taking this theoretical perspective a step further, a number of recent studies have tried to calculate the costs of such actions as having children. The costs vary by region, income levels, family composition but are always quite expensive. In their annual report, the US Department of Agriculture (2000) estimates that a wife and husband who have a child in the year 2000 will spend between US$171,500 and $340,000 on housing, food, transportation, clothing, health care, child care and education, and other miscellaneous goods and services to raise the child to the age of 18. A Swiss National Science Foundation study estimates the costs of one child to total about US$30,000 in direct and indirect costs each year (Spycher, Bauer, & Baumann, 1995). Another Swiss study found the direct and indirect costs for two parents to raise one child for the first 20 years of life to be approximately US$500,000 (Bauer, 1998). These studies are intended to bring attention to the need for better social policies to help parents manage the currently high costs of raising children and to discourage teen pregnancy.

THEORY AND RESEARCH

These studies capture the new direction of cost/benefit studies for social problem in the 1990s. Over the past 20 years, states, businesses, and other institutions have made decisions regarding where to cut expenses when faced with pressure from recession to globalization (Jenson & Sineau, 2000). In this environment, cost/benefit arguments become increasingly important (Yodanis, Godenzi, & Stanko, 2000). They are now political tools for taking action to prevent the negative condition. The beneficiaries and benefits are defined in terms of those people who are in the positions to enforce or contribute to the change. The topics of these studies are wide and varied. Many focus on health issues, such as environmental health hazards, smoking, and drug and alcohol abuse, and traffic accidents (Alfaro, Chapuis, & Fabre/European Commission, 1994; Hutton/World Health Organization, 2001; National Institute of Drug Abuse & National Institute on Alcohol Abuse and Alcoholism, 1992; Physicians for a Smoke-Free Canada, 1998). Others focus on crime, including murder, robbery, drunk driving, and arson (Travis/National Institute of Justice, 1996). Still others focus on problems of inequality and injustice (United Nations Population Fund, 2000). Below we discuss three examples from the family to provide empirical depth to this argument.

PREVENTING PROBLEMS IN FAMILIES: COST/BENEFIT ANALYSES

Breastfeeding

Medical studies have found that breastfeeding can prevent a wide array of health problems in infants and mothers.

For infants, there is evidence that breastfeeding prevents childhood diabetes and cancers as well as heart disease, stroke, and autoimmune diseases later in adulthood. It can also improve intelligence and visual development in children. For mothers, breastfeeding can aid in the recovery from childbirth, reduce the risk of breast and ovarian cancers, multiple sclerosis, and osteoporosis (see studies cited in Galtry, 1997; Wight, 1997). While there was a decrease between 1980 and 1990 in the number of US mothers who breastfed, over the last decade, the rates of breastfeeding have increased between 17 and 100 percent, depending on ethnic group. Today about 68 percent of white, 66 percent of Latinos, and 45 percent of Black mothers in the United States breastfeed (Labbok, 2001).

Labbok (2001) computed the cost/benefit ratios of breastfeeding. Under the costs of breastfeeding were included maternity leave from work and "lactation consultant" support. Health benefits included the wide range of health problems in children which have been shown to be reduced by breastfeeding, such as infectious diseases, gastrointestinal problems, and diabetes. Health system and household savings, including the cost of formula and additional visits to health care providers, were also estimated. The models show the potential cost savings of breastfeeding to be over $4 billion for the health care system and at least $2 billion in household savings. The cost/benefit ratios reveal that for every dollar spent to enable breastfeeding, the savings to the country as a whole are between $1.11 and $1.73. Public and private insurers and HMOs nationwide, themselves, would save $1.55 for every dollar spent.

Other studies have focused on the benefits, or cost savings, to government, social services, and health care and insurance providers resulting from breastfeeding. Zeretzke (1997) summarizes the total annual cost in the United States of not breastfeeding to be between $1.186 and $1.3 billion. Montgomery and Splett (1997) defined benefits as savings to Women, Infant and Children (WIC) and Medicaid program and found that breastfeeding is associated with a cost savings of $478 per infant in the first six months of life. Similarly, Tuttle and Dewey (1996) estimate that breastfeeding would result in a savings to public assistance programs of between $450 and $800 per enrolled family. In addition to estimating the cost of health problems associated with not breastfeeding, Riordan (1997) concludes that the federal government must spend an additional $2.67 million for the WIC program each year to pay for infant formula. In Australia, Drane (1997) estimates that breastfeeding could save US$6 million annually.

Work–Family Policies

Labor force participation of women, particularly mothers of infants, is growing in countries worldwide. The traditional nuclear family comprising a mother working at home and a father working for pay in the labor force is becoming rare. Rather, families now largely consist of an employed mother and father (Drew, Emerek, & Mahon, 1998; Moen, 1992). The problems experienced by dual earner families are well documented. Stress, guilt, lack of sleep, and lack of time with family all result from parents' efforts to juggle both long hours in the workplace and the high demands of unpaid work in the family (Garey, 1999; Hochschild, 1997). Until recently, this balancing act was considered to be an employed woman's problem to solve. However, policies, programs, and services are being suggested and increasingly implemented in workplaces which better allow both women and men to manage both their careers and families. These include flexible hours, part-time work, job sharing, telecommuting, homework, family leave, financial support for child and elder care, onsite day care, and lactation rooms for breastfeeding mothers.

Models, which businesses can use to calculate cost/benefit analysis of their work–family policies, have been developed from a number of sources, including the Families and Work Institute, the Oregon and Washington State Child Care Resource and Referral Networks, and Work/Family Directions, Inc. (WFD). The costs for the programs include developing and operating services such as resource, counseling, and referral services, child care services, and flexible work and leave policies. The benefits include increased employee retention, saved employee time, decreased absenteeism, increased productivity, and stress and health care cost reduction. The US Department of Education's (1997) *A business guide to support employee and family involvement in education* reports the findings from various companies when they applied the WFD model. A food company with 2,400 employees with average salaries of $24,700 spent $42,638 on their work–family programs. Based on the calculations, this company saved an estimated $3.59 for every dollar spent. A delivery company with 90,000 employees who have average salaries of $32,000 spent over $1 million on programs and saved $2.73 for every dollar spent. The cost/benefit ratios of the work–family policies in a law firm was $5.52 : 1, for an entertainment firm, $4.11 : 1, and for a bank, $3.01 : 1.

Also commonly cited are reports of companies' estimated savings from various work/family policies. Families and Work Institute, the Women's Bureau of the US Department of Labour, *Working Woman* and *Working Mother* magazines, and the *National Report on Work & Family* as well as consulting agencies and business magazines either collaborate in cost/benefit studies with companies or report company data which shows the benefits of family/work policies. These include a large insurance company's estimated annual savings of $1 million as a result of maternity leave, with a flexible return to work; a bank's estimated profits of $106 million resulting from the implementation, marketing, and manager training related to flexible work hours and a wide assortment of family–work programs; and a law firm's $800,000 annual savings from providing back-up child care for employees (Hammonds, 1996; Johnson, 1995; Martinez, 1997).

An Institute for Women's Policy Research Report, "Unnecessary Losses" also considers the costs to taxpayers when a national family and medical leave policy is not enacted. The costs, related to the increased need for unemployment compensation, welfare payments, and other social support, are estimated as $1.2 billion for childbirth or adoption, $108 million for lack of parental leave, $7.5 billion for absence of illness, and $4.3 billion for lack of temporary medical leave (Spalter-Roth & Hartmann, 1990).

Stopping Violence against Women

Violence against women exists in multiple forms in every culture of the world. Decades of research confirm the far-reaching negative consequences of violence, including physical, verbal, sexual, and psychological. Women who are victims of violence are more likely to experience poor physical and mental health, drug and alcohol addiction, lower economic status, and a lower quality of life due to fear and suffering (Stark & Flitcraft, 1996). Societies, as a result of violence against women, also suffer in terms of life quality and economic well-being (Heise, 1994). A wide range of programs and policies have been suggested and adopted for reducing violence against women. Many of these are reactive strategies aimed at minimizing the possibility of further damage and repeat offenses. These include mandatory arrest policies, hotlines, shelters, and counseling for men. Prevention efforts are often focused on efforts at education, consciousness-raising, and zero tolerance (Godenzi & De Puy, 2001). There are also calls for macrolevel efforts for greater gender equality and the elimination of pervasive cultures of violence, which research shows is related to the prevalence of violence against women (Dobash & Dobash, 1992; Yodanis, 2001).

In their cost/benefit analysis of services provided by an Arizona domestic violence shelter, Chanley, Chanley, and Campbell (2001) estimate the cost of shelter services to range between $250,000 and $440,000. When including the cost of public assistance as well, the total social costs are estimated to be between $654,655 and $960,110. Social benefits include assaults and injuries averted and benefits to mental health and range from $4.5 to $17.7 million. Using these figures, the net benefits of shelter services are estimated to be between $3.8 and $16.7 million. The benefit/cost ratio is estimated to be between $6.80 and $18.40 saved for every $1 spent, with an absolute minimum benefit/cost ratio of $4.6 : 1.

Most other studies examining violence against women from a cost perspective have focused primarily on the benefits of reducing the violence, that is, the costs of having the violence continue. Potential savings are computed not only for individuals but health care, criminal justice, and social service institutions as well as businesses. In Australia, the annual costs of violence to government, employers, third parties, and individuals in New South Wales is estimated at US$1 billion, in Queensland, US$407 million, and in the Northern Territory, US$5.8 million (Blumel, Gibb, Innis, Justo, & Wilson, 1993; NSW Women's Coordination Unit, 1991; Office of Women's Policy, 1996). In New Zealand, the costs are estimated to be between $625 million and $2.75 billion (Snively, 1994). In Canada, health care costs are estimated at over $1 billion per year and total costs are $2.8–260 billion in British Columbia alone (Day, 1995; Greaves, Hankivsky, Kingston-Riechers, 1995; Kerr & McLean, 1996). In Europe, costs in the Netherlands are estimated at $160 million, $290 million in Switzerland, $8.3 million in one UK borough, and $46 million in Finland (Korf, Meulenbeek, Mot, & van den Brandt, 1997; Piispa & Heiskanen, 2001; Stanko, Crisp, Hale, & Lucraft, 1997; Yodanis & Godenzi, 1999a). While it is not possible to compare these studies as a result of varying methodologies and cost equations, all studies reveal strikingly high costs associated with violence against women and thus high potential benefits for reducing violence.

STRATEGIES: OVERVIEW

These examples are just three of many which can be used to highlight the trend of using cost/benefit arguments to build a rationale for action and in the construction of social problems. In this section, we consider the characteristics of these studies.

First, the studies tend to be conducted in the context of a particular social movement or by agents of social change. The studies of violence against women are done by feminist researchers and organizations that fight against family violence, such as the Family Violence Unit of the New Zealand Department of Social Welfare or the Ministry of Women's Equality of British Columbia. Some of the cost/benefit analyses of breastfeeding were originally computed for, presented at, and continue to be cited by organizations which are formed around the advocacy of breastfeeding, including La Leche League International and International Lactation Consultant Association (Labbok, 1994). Likewise, the studies of work and family policies are often conducted or used by organizations that have as their goal improving the quality of life

for women and children. These include *Working Women* magazine, Work and Families Institute, the Institute for Women's Policy Research, and the US Department of Education. Exceptions are consulting businesses, which aim to advise companies on profit-making and employee relations strategies. In sum, the authors are often not neutral researchers seeking to provide neutral data. Rather, the authors and the organizations they work for come to the research as actors of social change and social improvement (Nelson, 1993).

A second characteristic is that one specific prevention program is often not the focus of the analysis. Rather, the studies tend to analyze a general behavioral change, such as breastfeeding, a whole category of programs, such as work–family policies, or no specific program at all, such as ending domestic violence (Rappaport & Holden, 1981). Even if a specific program is used in the analysis, such as Chanley, Chanley, and Campbell's cost/benefit analysis of a domestic violence shelter, the results are often not intended specifically for those who are involved with the particular program. Rather, the results are intended for a wider audience of individuals, organizations, and institutions who could potentially adopt the program. This makes sense when the focus is on calling for social change—making breastfeeding popular, making it possible for women and men to have both careers and families, and ending violence against women.

A third and related characteristic of these studies is the greater reliance on analyzing benefits than a ratio of benefits to costs. When the evaluation of the efficiency of a certain prevention program is not the focus of the analysis, then it is not possible to estimate the costs. Beyond methodological reasons, the focus on benefits can also be politically strategic. Reporting the exorbitant costs of the continuation of the problem is an act in the construction of social problems. It is a clear way of demonstrating that what was previously considered a private family matter is now a public matter affecting us all, at least monetarily. In this process, a resulting cost figure of $1 billion is likely to receive more media attention than reporting a cost/benefit ratio of $1.53 savings for every $1 spent. The focus on benefits can also take the emphasis away from the costs associated with the actors' actions.

Finally in these studies, the conceptualization and operationalization of benefits and beneficiaries are targeted to meet the goal of social change. Benefits are defined in terms of those in power who are being targeted to contribute to the social change. Therefore, the benefits of breastfeeding are defined largely in terms of savings for HMOs, insurance companies, and public assistance from government. The benefits of work–family policies are defined in terms of savings for business, rather than benefits in mothers, fathers, and children. Reducing violence against women is defined as benefiting states, social service agencies, business, and other various "third parties." In addition, tax payers are often included as those who would benefit as a result of a reduction in the problems. The authors and organizations who conduct the studies are not as concerned about business profits and tax savings as improving the lives of women, children, and working families. Still, they use this information in their arguments to encourage individuals and organizations with political leverage for change, who may have other interests, to join them in acting for change. Through social marketing, public opinion is swayed to care about these problems (Kotler & Andreasen, 1991; Kotler & Roberto, 1989). It is a way to turn what was previously defined as negative family matters into opportunities for social benefits, both financial and social improvement.

SYNTHESIS

In evaluation research, including cost/benefit studies, one has to weigh methodological rigor, practicality, and ethical issues (Rossi & Freeman, 1990). Within each of these three areas, it is possible to see the value and sense of using cost/benefit analysis, or at times only benefit analysis, as claims-making activities.

Methodologically, cost/benefit studies are estimates, at best. Measures of costs and benefits always contain error (Yodanis & Godenzi, 1999b). This is particularly problematic when considering highly complicated, multifaceted issues such as violence against women, balancing work and family, and breastfeeding. With these issues, it is often not possible to establish solid causal relationships between causes or prevention efforts and the extent of certain outcomes. It is then even more difficult to cost all of the many monetary and nonmonetary, direct and indirect, variable and fixed costs and benefits associated with the problem and any program to prevent it (Chambers, Wedel, & Rodwell, 1992). It may make sense, given these methodological difficulties, to reduce the assumed precision and complication of the equation. Therefore, a large, yet conservative, underestimate of some of the total benefits definitely to be gained by preventing a problem may be the most realistic goal.

Similarly, there are practical reasons for this approach. In terms of preventive efforts, building evidence to encourage others to take action may be more *cost efficient*, given the limited time and resources available, than doing individual cost/benefit analysis for individual prevention programs. Furthermore, it is widely known that evaluation research occurs within political social contexts (Rossi & Freeman, 1990). Therefore, it seems quite practical that those working within these contexts use and shape the analysis to meet their needs.

Finally, there are ethical reasons for this approach. Cost/benefit analysis is based on the assumption that if the costs for action outweigh the benefits, then action should not be taken. The results may not justify the costs. But this new trend in cost/benefit analysis starts with the assumption that prevention is essential, whether or not it is cost efficient. Within the context of these problems, emphasizing the benefits over the costs makes ethical sense.

In sum, the use of cost/benefit analysis as claims-making activities in the construction of social problems and to build a rationale for preventative action can be quite powerful in the current climate of streamlining costs and downsizing government and business. While different from traditional approaches to cost/benefit analysis, it is a way to build a clear, convincing, and far-reaching argument for the need for prevention efforts.

Also see: Financing: Foundation; Evaluation: Foundation; Environment: Foundation; Politics and Systems Change: Foundation.

References

Alfaro, J.L., Chapuis, M., & Fabre, F. (1994). *Volkswirtschaftliche Kosten der Strassenverkehrsunfälle (Economic costs of traffic accidents)*. Brussels: European Commission.

Bauer, T. (1998). *Kinder, Zeit und Geld (Children, time, and money)*. Bern: Swiss Federal Office of Social Insurance.

Becker, G. (1981). *A treatise on the family*. Cambridge: Harvard University.

Blumel, D.K., Gibb, G.L., Innis, B.N., Justo, D.L., & Wilson, D.V. (1993). *Who pays? The economic costs of violence against women*. Queensland: Women's Policy Unit, Office of the Cabinet.

Chambers, D.E., Wedel, K., & Rodwell, M. (1992). *Evaluating social programs*. Boston: Allyn and Bacon.

Chanley, S.A., Chanley, J.J., & Campbell, H.A. (2001). Providing refuge: The value of domestic violence shelter services. *American Review of Public Administration, 31*.

Day, T. (1995). *The health-related costs of violence against women in Canada: The tip of the iceberg*. London, Ontario: Centre for Research on Violence Against Women and Children.

Dobash, R.E., & Dobash, R.P. (1992). *Women, violence, and social change*. London: Routledge.

Drane, D. (1997). Breastfeeding and formula feeding: A preliminary economic analysis. *Breastfeeding Review, 5*, 7–15.

Drew, E., Emerek, R., & Mahon, E. (Eds.). (1998). *Women, work, and the family in Europe*. London: Routledge.

Galtry, J. (1997). Suckling and silence in the USA: The costs and benefits of breastfeeding. *Feminist Economics, 3*, 1–24.

Garey, A.I. (1999). *Weaving work and motherhood*. Philadelphia: Temple.

Godenzi, A., & De Puy, J. (2001). Overcoming boundaries: A cross-cultural inventory of primary prevention programs against wife abuse and child abuse. *Journal of Primary Prevention, 21*, 455–475.

Greaves, L., Hankivsky, O., & Kingston-Riechers, J. (1995). *Selected estimates of the costs of violence against women*. London, Ontario: Centre for Research on Violence Against Women and Children.

Hammonds, K.H. (1996, September 19). Balancing work and family: Big returns for companies willing to give family strategies a chance. *Business Week*, 74–80.

Heise, L. (1994). *Violence against women: The hidden health burden* (Discussion Paper No. 255). Washington DC: The World Bank.

Hochschild, A.R. (1997). *The time bind: When work becomes home and home becomes work.* New York: Metropolitan Books.

Hutton, G. (2000). *Considerations in evaluating the cost effectiveness of environmental health interventions.* Geneva: World Health Organization.

Jenson, J., & Sineau, M. (2000). *Who cares?: Women's work, childcare, and welfare state redesign.* Toronto: University of Toronto Press.

Johnson, A.A. (1995, August). The business case for work–family programs. *Journal of Accountancy*, 53–58.

Kerr, R., & McLean, J. (1996). *Paying for violence: Some of the costs of violence against women in B.C.* British Columbia: Ministry of Women's Equality.

Kotler, P., & Andreasen, A. (1991). *Strategic marketing for nonprofit organizations.* Englewood Cliffs: Prentice-Hall.

Kotler, P., & Roberto, E. (1989). *Social marketing: Strategies for changing behavior.* New York: Free Press.

Korf, D.J., Meulenbeek, H., Mot, E., & van den Brandt, T. (1997). *Economic costs of domestic violence against women.* Utrecht, Netherlands: Dutch Foundation of Women's Shelters.

Labbok, M.H. (1994). Breastfeeding as a women's issue: Conclusions, consensus, complementary concerns, and next actions. *International Journal of Gynecology and Obstetrics, 47*, S55–S61.

Labbok, M.H. (2001). Cost benefit analysis for breastfeeding in the United States: Is supporting exclusive breastfeeding worth the costs? In D.Michels (Ed.), *Breastfeeding Annual International.* Washington DC: Platypus Media Press.

Martinez, M.N. (1997). Work-life programs reap business benefits. *HRMagazine, 42*, 110–114.

Moen, P. (1992). *Women's two roles: A contemporary dilemma.* New York: Auburn House.

Montgomery, D., & Splett, P.L. (1997). Economic benefit of breast-feeding infants enrolled in WIC. *Journal of the American Dietetic Association, 97*, 379–385.

National Institute on Drug Abuse, & National Institute on Alcohol Abuse and Alcoholism. (1992). *The economic costs of alcohol and drug abuse in the United States.* Washington, DC: National Institute on Drug Abuse.

Nelson, J. (1993). Persuasion and economic efficiency. *Economics and Philosophy, 9*, 229–252.

NSW Women's Coordination Unit. (1991). *Costs of domestic violence.* Haymarket, NSW: Author.

Office of Women's Policy. (1996). *The financial and economic costs of domestic violence in the Northern Territory.* Northern Territory: KPMG.

Physicians for a Smoke-Free Canada. (1998). *The cost of smoking.* Ottawa: Author.

Piispa, M., & Heiskanen, M. (2001). *The price of violence: The costs of men's violence against women in Finland.* Helsinki: Statistics Finland.

Rappaport, J., & Holden, K. (1981). Prevention of violence: The case for a nonspecific social policy. In J.R. Hays et al. (Eds.), *Violence and the violent individual* (pp. 409–440). New York: Spectrum.

Riordan, J.M. (1997). The cost of not breastfeeding: A commentary. *Journal of Human Lactation, 13*, 93–97.

Rossi, P.H., & Freeman, H.E. (1990). *Evaluation: A systematic approach.* London: Sage.

Snively, S. (1994). *The New Zealand economic costs of family violence.* Auckland: Coopers and Lybrand.

Spalter-Roth, R., & Hartmann, H. (1990). *Unnecessary losses: Costs to Americans of the lack of family and medical leave.* Washington, DC: Institute for Women's Policy Research.

Spector, M., & Kitsuse, J.I. (1987). *Constructing social problems.* New York: Aldine De Gruyter.

Spycher, S., Bauer, T., & Baumann, B. (1995). *Kinder Kosten und Kinderkosten-Ausgleich in der Schweiz (The costs of children and child cost assistance in Switzerland).* Bern: Swiss National Science Foundation.

Stanko, E.A., Crisp, D., Hale, C., & Lucraft, H. (1997). *Counting the costs: Estimating the impact of domestic violence in the London borough of Hackney.* Middlesex, UK: Brunel University.

Stark, E., & Flitcraft, A. (1996). Women at risk: Domestic violence and women's health. Thousand Oaks: Sage.

Travis, J. (1996). *The extent and costs of crime victimization: A new look.* Washington, DC: National Institute of Justice.

Tuttle, C.R., & Dewey, K.G. (1996). Potential cost savings for Medi-Cal, AFDC, Food Stamps, and WIC programs associated with increasing breast-feeding among low-income Hmong women in California. *Journal of the American Dietetic Association, 96*, 885–890.

United Nations Population Fund. (2000). Counting the costs of gender inequality. In UNFPA (Ed.), *The state of the world population 2000.* New York: United Nations.

US Department of Agriculture. (2000). *Expenditures on children by families, 2000 annual report.* Washington, DC: Author.

US Department of Education. (1997). *A business guide to support employee and family involvement in education.* Washington, DC: Author.

Wight, N.E. (1997). *The benefits of breastfeeding.* San Diego: San Diego County Breastfeeding Coalition.

Yodanis, C., & Godenzi, A. (1999a). *Report on the economic costs of violence against women.* Fribourg: University of Fribourg.

Yodanis, C., & Godenzi, A. (1999b, October 7–8). *Male violence: The economic costs—A methodological review.* Proceedings of the Council of Europe seminar "Men and Violence against Women". Strasbourg: Council of Europe Press.

Yodanis, C., Godenzi, A., & Stanko, E.A. (2000). The benefits of studying costs: A review and agenda for studies on the economic costs of violence against women. *Policy Studies, 21*, 264–276.

Yodanis, C. (2001, June). *Gender inequality and violence against women in European countries.* Paper Presented at the International Crime Victimization Workshop, Leiden, The Netherlands.

Zeretzke, K.M. (1997). *Cost benefits of breastfeeding.* Illinois: La Leche League.

Creativity, Early Childhood

Charlotte Doyle

INTRODUCTION

Are young children "naturally" creative? Can the creative episode in young children be compared to the process by which the major creators in a society produce their works? The answers to these questions suggest possibilities for how parents and teachers might promote creativity in young children.

WHAT IS CREATIVITY?

Young children often delight observers with their exuberant curiosity, their spontaneity, their emotional expressiveness, and their free imaginations. These qualities have led some observers to say that all young children are creative. Various psychologists have theorized about the cognitive and affective processes that underlie these characteristics.

Freud (1959) saw young children as dominated by *primary process* thought and described it in both cognitive and affective terms. Cognitively, primary process implies a free flow of thought, one in which many different kinds of associations can link one idea to the next. Modern psychologists have done systematic studies of the cognitive aspects of primary process by devising *divergent thinking* tests, which ask children questions which don't have single answers but which ask for a variety of possible answers. "Think of uses for a brick" is a classic example. (Guilford, 1959; Torrance, 1988; Wallach and Kogan, 1965). According to Freud, primary process thinking is infused with affect; in fact its direction is determined by feeling and desire. Russ (1996) has studied this aspect of primary process in young children by observing access to emotion and affect-laden fantasies in children's play.

Werner also theorized that young children are dominated by different cognitive modes than adults. He put forth the concept of *physiognomic perception*, a mode in which seeing and feeling are merged in contrast to the geometrical–technical perception of adults. Schachtel (1959) emphasized curiosity and a desire to explore the world as a basic motivation of young children, an idea that has been supported by many studies (e.g., see Ainsworth, 1973; Mahler, Pine, & Bergman, 1975).

Freud, Werner, and Schachtel all saw the process of growing up as involving the internalization of conceptual and linguistic categories leading to the suppression of primitive modes of thought and/or of spontaneous, uncensored encounters with the world. Now instead of spontaneity, there is intention and planned action; instead of freedom, there is careful reflection and self-evaluation; instead of easy access to emotion and feeling, there is self-consciousness, self-judgment, and conscious control over thinking; instead of free imagination, thought follows culturally prescribed directions. Most people lose the childlike qualities which underlie creativity, according to these theorists, and only a few creative adults retain the capacity to return to childlike modes of thought.

Other theorists take a completely different view of the meaning of being creative. A creative person is someone who has contributed something genuinely new to his or her culture, they say. These theorists study outstanding people such as Virginia Woolf and Charles Darwin (Gardner, 1993; Gruber, 1981) as a starting point for defining and studying creativity. They notice that such creativity always draws on an already established cultural domain such as literature or biology, and that someone who is creative in one domain is not necessarily creative in another. The creative contributors did a long apprenticeship in learning the skills and heuristics of their medium including expertise in using a symbol system. They understand the history of their domains. They intentionally structure their time and activity in order to make creative work possible, and critical evaluation of their work in progress is part of the process. These theorists question the idea that primitive modes of thought are the essence of creativity, question whether its cognitive aspects can be captured by the use of short item tests. No matter how delightful the traits of young children according to this view, no young child can be truly creative.

A middle view distinguishes two kinds of creativity: cultural and personal. People show personal creativity if they discover or create ideas or products original to themselves if not to the culture. Curious, imaginative young children can be creative in this sense. Theorists do not agree on how to relate personal creativity to the creativity of major innovators whose works contribute to and modify a cultural domain (Boden, 1996; Csikszentmihalyi, 1996).

One way out of these definitional dilemmas has been to take a look at the creative process itself. Then questions can be raised about whether, amid obvious differences, some common features emerge in the creative process as it is manifested in a variety of contexts including early childhood. A convenient unit of analysis is the *creative episode*—the period between the initial impulse to begin work on a project to the point at which the final product feels complete, and something new has been created or discovered.

RESEARCH ON THE CREATIVE EPISODE

Studies of the creative episode have been primarily associated with interview studies of the creative episode in adults who are culturally recognized as creative (Csikszentmihalyi, 1996; Doyle, 1976; Franklin, 1989). But developmental researchers, in the course of empirical studies of children's art (Smith, 1993), pretend play (Franklin, 1983; Garvey, 1990), and children's story-telling (Doyle, 2001; Dyson and Genishi, 1994; Engel, 1995) have described creative episodes in young children, and, surprisingly, many of the features of the adult creative episode appear in many childhood episodes as well. A close look at the episode, its phases, and its features, provides a framework for thinking about facilitating the creative episode in young children.

Phases of the Creative Episode: Beginnings

Adult creators, when they are asked, how does the creative process begin, sometimes speak of a specific event that triggered the sense that this was a beginning that could be developed. But some speak of a general intention to write, or paint or work in clay and speak of playing around until something takes shape (Doyle, 1998; Franklin, 1989). In either case, they begin with an intention, with something pulling at their minds strongly enough so that they give themselves the time and the opportunity to let the creative process take place. Far from the studio or office or laboratory, in a preschool, we see a young child's equivalent as a child takes a piece of paper off a shelf, picks up a magic marker, and begins to draw or as one child says to another "Let's play house."

Initial Reflections

Before the creative work begins to flow, creators sometimes reflect on how they are going to go about the project—writers make notes on possible characters or some themes the work should embody, for example. Young children sometimes also make explicit statements about how they are going to go about their creative projects (Franklin, 1983; Smith, 1993). "I am going to draw a very big man," says the young artist. "I'll be the doctor and you'll be sick," says a young child to another in a nursery school pretend area. "I don't want to be sick," says the other, "I'll be the Mommy and my baby is sick."

Thinking in the Medium: Entering an Imaginary World

In the creative episode, the reflective, planful, self-conscious mode of thought gives way to another way of thinking. For the writer, it is entering into an imagined reality, listening to what the characters say and do (Doyle, 1998); for the musician it involves being immersed in a world of sound and thinking in sounds alone (Berliner, 1997; Sessions, 1952). In the preschool, the young builder now thinks directly in blocks; the young painter is engaged with brush and paint. And in the pretend play of children, in this phase the young players are no longer planning their drama, they become their characters and freely and spontaneously improvise (Franklin, 1983). This full engagement in an ongoing project has been called the flow (Csikszentmihalyi, 1996) and centration (Doyle, 1976), and both children and adults find it deeply satisfying. No longer self-conscious or judgmental, everything the creator knows, feels, is puzzled by, and hopes for can flow into the developing creation without self-consciousness or censorship. This phase is experienced as a time of great freedom and spontaneity. The medium and the imaginary world created by it allow the creator both to express and get perspective on material that is moving, puzzling, or overwhelming, and the process itself can lead to new discoveries.

Interruptions

The flow typically does not always move to completion unblocked. At times, the non-reflective, unself-conscious thinking in the medium ends abruptly. In the case of adult creators, the sense that something is wrong may throw them out of their imaginary world recurrently and usher in another phase of reflection. They think about what is wrong in terms of craft, and try to solve the problem that blocked the flow. At times their reflections take a harsher turn and take the form of severe self-criticism, questioning their own capacities to do what they set out to do (Steinbeck, 1989). Though young children are typically less self-critical than adults, we see this on a small scale in the young children as well. A 4-year-old boy crosses out the sketch he just made (M. Franklin, personal communication, 2000). A 3-year-old, unable to make a vertical block stand on its side, knocks down the building she is working on and says sadly, "I can't do it." A 5-year-old girl who has been dictating a story, stops and says, "I don't know what to say next" (Doyle, 1989). Contrary to some models, even young children sometimes reflect on and judge their small-scale creations-in-progress as well as their own capacities as creators.

A Sense of Completion

There are times when the creative episode ends here, without completion. But frequently the creators, young and old, find ways to re-enter the imaginary worlds of their own creation and to bring their work to fruition. The little boy who crossed out his first sketch made several more and finally made one that satisfied him (M. Franklin, personal communication, 2000). The story-teller found a way to finish her story (Doyle, 1989). Both adults and young creators have a sense of satisfaction when their project has fulfilled their developing intentions.

Sharing

There is typically one more phase in many creative episodes. Creators, both young and old, typically seek to share what they have done with others. In young children, this takes the form of showing what they have made to a teacher, a classmate, or a parent. The boy who made the many sketches until one satisfied him found his mother, pointed to his satisfying sketch and said, "flower" (M. Franklin, personal communication, 2000). The story-teller smiled shyly as her completed story was read to her classmates (Doyle, 1989). Sharing the work can be a time of vulnerability and self-consciousness for the adult creator and the young child alike. But it is also an opportunity to win that special satisfaction that comes when others recognize and truly understand something meaningful you have said and done. (Benjamin, 1988; Rogers, 1959).

Thus, even in young children, the creative episode draws on intentions, reflective planning, the ability to use a medium, the capacity to deal with frustrations and blocks, and the impulse to share (features noted by those who research creativity find in cultural innovators). At the same time, the creative episode also draws on traits more typically associated with young children: curiosity and a sense of adventure, the freedom to allow thinking to flow directly and spontaneously, the willingness to follow unexpected paths without censorship. During the moments of non-reflective flow in an imaginary world, children as well as adult creators allow what they know and as well as what intrigues, puzzles, overwhelms, or disturbs them to shape their creations as they use the symbolic forms of a medium. Thus the process as it unfolds over time embodies both planful intention *and* spontaneity, knowledge of cultural ways of doing and thinking *and* imaginative and affective freedom, frustration, perhaps self-criticism *and* unself-conscious exuberance. And, in children and adults alike, such creating is meaning-making, and has the potential to lead to discovery.

So, the creative episode engages different, apparently contradictory, aspects of a child or an adult. Because of this, facilitating the creative process is an amazing way to accomplish many goals at the same time. Promoting the creative process in young children has the potential for supporting intellectual, emotional, and social development simultaneously.

STRATEGIES

Promoting Creative Episodes in Young Children

Since the definition of creativity itself is still in flux, it would be presumptuous to state categorically that some strategies definitely work and some definitely do not. However, there are studies and demonstrations that suggest ways in which the various phases of the creative episode may be facilitated in young children.

First, it should be noted that in contemporary discussions of educating young children at home and in preschool, fostering creativity is not usually mentioned as a major goal. Instead, the emphasis today is on training in academic skills. The current rhetoric speaks of high standards, behavioral goals, and measuring the extent to which children meet those standards and goals with objective tests. Many parents and teachers hope to train children from age 2 to meet those standards using materials such as flash cards and arithmetic cards or their more technological versions, computer phonics, and arithmetic programs. Creativity is usually far from

the minds of those who plan such activities; nevertheless such activities do support one aspect of the creative episode: They introduce children to the cultural symbol systems which are also the media for creation. As long as the training is in the context of games that children enjoy and as long as children have other opportunities to engage in creative episodes of their own making, the training may prove helpful to some children. Still, it is also important to remember that the learning of symbol systems is not an end in itself. Symbol systems are ways of making meaning (Smith, 1993; Wells, 1986), and children need to be introduced to those systems as more than a collection of rote associations.

There are less decontextualized ways of introducing various media to children. Sharing and pointing at the words and pictures in books, playing music, taking children to dance performances and plays, going on nature walks and talking together about what has been seen are all ways to introduce children to our culture's ways of representing and understanding experience symbolically. These introductions can embody what is too often left out in rote training sessions—the excitement and the joy of using those symbol systems to reveal and convey meaning. In fact, for a small number of children, such an introduction to a medium can become life changing, as they become passionately engaged in learning and using a particular medium. These are the so-called gifted children who become passionate about learning and creating in art, music, words, or numbers, and now choose to spend many hours learning and working in their medium (Winner, 1996).

Some parents who value the creative arts pay for structured lessons in music or dance. Again these are ways of introducing young children to the media in which creative episodes take place. Lessons can be useful for some children as long as the lessons do not sap the children of self-confidence and joy in the activity and as long as there are opportunities for other kinds of activities as well.

The current emphasis on academic training for young children is a relatively new way of thinking about preschool children. Most societies began explicit systematic training in the skills of their culture at around the age of 6, the age at which children enter primary school. Nursery school and kindergarten were given other goals in the past, a tradition that is still maintained in some progressive educational traditions such as the developmental–interactionist approach (Nager & Shapiro, 2000). Preschool classrooms organized according to this tradition support many aspects of the creative process directly, and the principles that emerge from those classrooms can be applied in other contexts as well.

Preschools following the developmental–interactionist approach are sometimes described by saying that the children do "nothing but play." This description was belied by systematic observations in such a school (Doyle, 2001).

Such classrooms also put children in touch with the many media in which creative work goes on. Teachers read stories and poems. They played music. They had conversations with children about scientific topics like where rain comes from and why popcorn pops. They introduced number concepts and mathematical notation in ways that had meaning to the children, such as a graph which showed the number of teeth each child lost (Doyle, 2001).

Researchers have assembled evidence that play itself facilitates various outcome measures that some theorists relate to creativity. A period of play enhances divergent thinking scores (Dansky, 1980; Feitelstein & Ross, 1973; Hughes, 1987). Play also facilitates subsequent flexibility in social problem solving (Pelligrini, 1992) and insight (Vandenberg, 1988). Russ (1996) makes the argument that play itself embodies the cognitive and affective processes that underlie creativity. Similarly, Franklin (1994) points out that play, along with art-making and story-telling are examples of the creative process in the sense that each of these activities involves the creation of imaginary worlds.

In the developmental–interactionist classroom, the structures and routines of the classroom invite children's participation in such activities and support various phases of the creative episode that emerge.

Opportunities to Explore Various Media

Progressive classrooms have areas that invite making: a pretend corner for creating a drama, a painting area for creating visual representations, a place for block building, occasional opportunities to shape play dough or try woodworking. There are chances to explore the "I wonder" world of science: by noting the growth of plants and the behavior of animals, by inviting discoveries with use of mirrors and magnifying glasses and magnets. The creative process takes root in a cultural and social context, one in which various media are available and which gives children opportunities to try them out. These everyday setups and activities provide the preconditions of the creative process.

Time for Nonreflective Engagement

Soon after the free play periods begins, creative episodes begin to unfold all over the classroom: children painting at easels or drawing with magic markers, miniature architects creating buildings, young scientists studying their own fingers under magnifying glasses, young improvisers creating characters and stories in a pretend corner. The children tend to be intently concentrated, deeply engaged in what they are doing, engrossed in worlds different from the pragmatic world of everyday life (Doyle, 2001).

Learning

As with adults, young children's creative episodes involve using and developing skills of observation and representation, using the symbol systems of various media. Children learn the tricks of their media by watching and listening to teachers and to each other and by their own discoveries. Various observers reported that children discovered how to mix paints (Gwathmey & Mott, 2000), that words rhyme (Doyle, 1989), that a stick can serve as a vacuum cleaner (Franklin, 1983), that a large block on top of a small block can be unsteady, and how to draw a particular kind of thing such as an ant (Doyle, 2001).

Allowing Autonomy, Listening to an Inner Voice

In reviews of the literature, Rejskind (1982) and Amabile (2001) concluded that autonomy tends to enhance creativity. Allowing such freedom was a feature of the "free play" periods. At these times, teachers respected the children as active agents with intentions and invited the children to allow their own intentions to structure what they did. Very occasionally, a child found the freedom of free play daunting, and then the teachers gave the children support, suggestions, and encouragement, but even then the activities themselves were self-chosen (Doyle, 2001).

Children sometimes short-circuit their own autonomy by asking an adult to do something for them instead of experimenting on their own. For example, children sometimes ask an adult to draw something for them, such as a giraffe (Smith, 1993). An adult can dazzle children with a drawing, but, if the adult's drawing takes the place of their own creative attempts, it saps children of their sense of competence and agency. Smith suggests that the adult help the children to generate their own drawings.

Accepting the Unusual

Some theorists tie creativity to divergent thinking such as imagining unusual uses. In the progressive classroom, teachers accepted and supported the unorthodox uses of materials. One day a child discovered that magic markers could be lined up end to end like a train. She built a long magic marker train. The markers, which were sometimes put on the table for use in art project, on this day had been on a shelf, not intended for use that day. The teacher did not say, "We're not using markers today," or "Markers are for drawing." She was genuinely impressed with the child's inventive construction (Doyle, 2001).

Encouraging Exploration and New Paths

A given activity, even if it is in an artistic domain can sometimes become routinized and unimaginative, as when a child draws the same picture over and over again. Teachers can show children the variety of ways that a medium can be used to encourage new creative episodes. Smith (1993) suggests putting out paint brushes and papers of different sizes and shapes on different days. She also begins art periods by having discussions of specific topics such as "what is your favorite toy?" and suggesting that a picture could tell people about it. For children who have been painting the same sun, flowers, and a house day after day, this can give new focus and allow a fuller creative episode to take place. Smith also demonstrated that young children who have representational intentions but have fallen into undifferentiated and stereotyped images can be encouraged to look closely as they draw, resulting in a deeper process and a more satisfying product. In the realm of pretend play, unusual props and clothes can elicit completely new episodes.

Respect: Helping Children to Reflect on Their Own Creations and Discoveries

Part of respect is taking the children's creations seriously. This can take place in conversation, with the child's work as the focus of the conversation. Smith (1993) suggests that a teacher or parent can ask a child to tell about a painting. Then the adult can notice distinctive features of the child's work and give children a vocabulary for talking about their own work. For example, a teacher can say, "The way you made a big shape here and a lot of little shapes here makes my eyes go all over your painting." In a very different context, a little girl found a worm under the sliding board and wanted to take it home. The teacher admired her discovery and asked her to tell where she found the worm and what it felt like to pick it up—helping her to find words to describe the worm and the conditions that help worms thrive (Doyle, 2001)

Scaffolding Creative Activities That Children Cannot Carry Out on Their Own

Adults can encourage creative activities which cannot take place without their assistance. An example is writing stories. Young children cannot write stories on their own, and yet, with the help of an adult willing to take dictation, children around the age of 3 can become young authors of little books (Doyle, 1989). In a sense, the adult becomes the child's instrument in such creative episodes, and, in order for the child to feel the autonomy of creativity, the adult allows the child to be the sole determiner of the words that are written. Once the children understand this, they are willing to go to great lengths to make sure that the adult has written their words correctly. One teacher kept hearing a child dictate, "Once upon a time there were lots." The child kept correcting

the teacher's read-back by repeating the same sentence. Finally the child took the teacher by the hand, led her out the door and pointed at the rocks on the playground (Doyle, 1989).

Hints and Helps in the Face of Discouragement

There were times when children could not solve a problem that emerged in the course of the creative episode, and like the adult creators, became discouraged and deflated. Here, the teachers found ways to help children do what they wanted to do with hints and helps. They sometimes framed the situation so that the child could learn a heuristic, a trick of craft that would enable a child to carry out his or her own intention. A boy started out to draw something very large. One piece of paper could not contain his monumental creation. "It's no good," the boy told the teacher, "There's no room for the legs." "What could you do to make more room?" the teacher asked. The boy thought and then brightened and said, "Get another piece of paper." He did, but the papers kept slipping in relation to one another. The teacher brought out some tape. The boy found it and used it. A little girl was building a building and was becoming increasingly frustrated at the inability of a block to stay vertical. She became so angry she was about to knock down the rest of the building, as she had done several times before. The teacher guided her in buttressing the vertical block with supporting blocks on each side. A young story-teller faltered mid-story and said, "I don't know what comes next." The teacher told him to shut his eyes and listen as she read what she had so far. If that didn't stimulate a flow, she asked questions related to the story already written such as, "What did the boy do when he saw the monster?" (Doyle, 2001).

Allowing Time for Transitions

When a child is engaged in a creative episode, being abruptly routed from the created world can be a difficult moment. One way teachers supported the creative process was by how they dealt with those transitions—with respect and understanding. Three children invented a jumping game as the group was moving from free play to meeting time. Instead of saying, "You can't" or "You shouldn't", the teacher said, "Three more jumps and then it will be meeting time." The project was acknowledged and respected even though the teacher needed for it to stop (Doyle, 2001).

Opportunities for Sharing

Young children's creative endeavors do not always have a clear beginning, middle, and end. Dramatic play, typically co-constructed by several children drifting in and out of it, often trails off into another activity. But frequently children have a clear sense of project and know when they completed it. Now they seek to show others what they had done. The progressive classrooms were full of occasions that allowed children to share their creations. Children often first showed their work to their teachers. As Smith suggested, teachers did not offer empty praise, did not say, "I like your painting or I think your block building is great." Instead, they gave recognition to interesting features of the children's creation. "Wow. You drew different all the parts of the ants" or "I like the way the polar bear is walking on the high plank so he can talk to the giraffe." Children also had opportunities to share with each other, not only the classic show-and-tell, but talking to classmates about buildings they built, worms they found, discoveries they made by playing with mirrors. Children's stories were given an honored place in the classroom either by reading them at meeting time or using them as little plays for the others to act out. One child, then another, experienced the special pleasure that comes from sharing and finding recognition for what was created (Doyle, 2001).

Creation and Discovery as Part of the Culture of the Classroom

Homes and classrooms that honor children's creative activities make these kinds of activities part of the children's sense of their own capacities and possibilities. The classroom that honors creativity also conveys that these are activities that are enjoyed by many children. With a creative culture in the classroom, children learn about possibilities from their classmates as well as from exposure from adult versions. In some classrooms, story-telling becomes part of the shared culture (Dyson & Genishi, 1994). Doyle (2001) found that one humorous story inspired several others. In the same classroom, story-telling began as primarily a girls' activity, until one shy boy told a story about a heroic knight, a story that began a tradition of boys also telling stories, often about heroes of various sorts. Such a culture can also recognize quiet children who otherwise rarely call attention to themselves. In another "story-telling" classroom, a little girl, one who otherwise seemed unexceptional and in fact seemed less verbally gifted than other children in terms of phonics and printing letters, became known to the others as an exceptionally humorous and imaginative story-teller (Doyle, 2001).

SYNTHESIS

The preschool years are times of tremendous development and change in many realms: in thinking and language,

in social and emotional life, in the sense of self. Creative episodes facilitate positive development in many of these realms simultaneously. Fostering them involves supporting each of the episode's phases as it unfolds over time. Adults can help by introducing symbol systems, by providing opportunities for children to choose creative activities, become completely engaged in them, then bring them to completion, by respecting the work through allowing transitions and helping children to reflect on their own creations, by scaffolding activities children cannot carry out on their own, by encouraging the explorations of new paths, by providing support and help during times of discouragement, by offering opportunities for sharing and recognition of the completed work—in effect, establishing a culture of creativity. Putting these principles into practice allows the curiosity, spontaneity, emotional expressiveness, and imagination so typical of young children to find pathways for discovery via episodes of creative meaning-making.

Also see: Creativity: Childhood; Creativity: Adolescence; Creativity: Adulthood; Creativity: Older Adulthood; Culture, Society, and Social Class: Foundation.

References

Ainsworth, M.D.S. (1973). The development of infant–mother attachment. In B.M. Caldwell & H.N. Ricciuti (Eds.), *Review of child development research* (Vol. 3, pp. 1–94). Chicago: University of Chicago Press.

Amabile, T.M. (2001). Beyond talent: John Irving and the passionate craft of creativity. *American Psychologist, 56*(4), 333–336.

Benjamin, J. (1988). *The bonds of love*. New York: Pantheon.

Berliner, P. (1997). Give and take: The collective conversation of jazz performance. In R.K. Sawyer (Ed.), *Creativity in performance* (pp. 9–41). Greenwich, CT: Ablex.

Boden, M.A. (1996). Computer models of creativity. In R.J. Sternberg (Ed.), *Handbook of creativity* (pp. 251–273). New York: Cambridge University Press.

Csikszentmihalyi, M. (1996). *Creativity: Flow and the psychology of discovery and invention*. New York: HarperCollins.

Dansky, J. (1980) Make-believe: A mediator of the relationship between play and associative fluency. *Child Development, 51*, 576–579.

Doyle, C. (1976). The creative process: A study in paradox. In C. Winsor (Ed.), *The creative process*. New York: Bank Street College.

Doyle, C. (1989, August). Young children as authors: The creative process in first stories. Paper Presented at the American Psychological Association Meetings in New Orleans.

Doyle, C. (1998). The writer tells: The creative process in the writing of literary fiction. *Creativity Research Journal, 11*(1), 29–36.

Doyle, C. (2001). "I'm too busy": The creative paradox and the young child. In M. Bloom & T.P. Gullotta (Eds.), *Promoting creativity across the lifespan* (pp. 45–82). New London, CT: CWLA Press.

Dyson, A.H., & Genishi, C. (1994). Introduction: The need for story. In A.H. Dyson & C. Genishi (Eds.), *The need for story* (pp. 1–7). Urbana, IL: National Council of Teachers of English.

Engel, S. (1995). *The stories children tell*. New York: W.H. Freeman.

Feitelstein, D., & Ross, G. (1973). The neglected factor—play. *Human Development, 16*, 202–223.

Franklin, M.B. (1983) Play as the creation of imaginary situations: The role of language. In S. Wapner & B. Kaplan (Eds.), *Toward a holistic developmental psychology*. Hillsdale, NJ: Erlbaum.

Franklin, M. (1989). A convergence of streams: Dramatic change in the artistic work of Melissa Zink. In D.B. Wallace and H.E. Gruber (Eds.), *Creative people at work* (pp. 255–277). New York: Oxford University Press.

Franklin, M. (1994). Art, play, and symbolization in childhood and beyond: Reconsidering connections. *Teacher's College Record, 95*(4), 526–541.

Freud, S. (1959). *Collected papers*. (J. Riviere Trans.). London: Hogarth.

Garvey, C. (1990) *Play*. Cambridge, MA: Harvard University Press.

Gardner, H. (1993). *Creating minds*. New York: Basic Books.

Gruber, H.E. (1981). *Darwin on man: A psychological study of scientific creativity*. Chicago: University of Chicago Press.

Guilford, J.P. (1959). The three faces of intellect. *American Psychologist, 14*, 469–479.

Gwathmey, E., & Mott, A. (2000). Visualizing experience. In N. Nager & E.K. Shapiro (Eds.), *Revisiting a progressive pedagogy: The developmental interaction approach* (pp. 139–160). Albany, NY: SUNY.

Hughes, M. (1987). The relationship between symbolic and manipulative (object) play. In D. Gorelitz & J. Wohwill (Eds.), *Curiosity, imagination, and play* (pp. 247–257). Hillsdale, NJ: Erlbaum.

Mahler, M.S., Pine, F., & Bergman, A. (1975). *The psychological birth of the human infant: Symbiosis and individuation*, New York: Basic Books.

Nager, N., & Shapiro, E.K (Eds.). (2000). *Revisiting a progressive pedagogy: The developmental interaction approach*. Albany, NY: SUNY.

Pelligrini, A. (1992). Rough and tumble play and social problem solving flexibility. *Creativity Research Journal, 5*, 13–26.

Rejskind, F.G.(1982). Autonomy and creativity in children. *Journal of Creative Behavior, 16*(1), 58–67.

Rogers, C. (1959). A theory of therapy, personality, and interpersonal relationships, as developed in the client-centered framework. In S. Koch (Ed.), *Psychology: A study of a science* (Vol. 3, pp. 184–256). New York: McGraw-Hill.

Russ, S.W. (1996). Development of creative processes in children. In M. Runco (Ed.), *Creativity from childhood through adulthood: The developmental issues*. New York: Wiley.

Schachtel, E.G. (1959). *Metamorphosis*. New York: Basic Books.

Sessions, R. (1952). The composer and his message. In B. Ghiselm (Ed.), *The creative process* (pp. 45–49). Berkeley, CA: University of California Press.

Smith, N.R. (1993) *Experience and art: Teaching children to paint* (2nd ed.). New York: Teachers College Press.

Steinbeck, J. (1989) *Working days: The journals of the grapes of wrath*. R. DeMott. Ed.. New York: Viking.

Torrance, E.P. (1988). The nature of creativity as manifest in its testing. In R.J. Sternberg (Ed.). *The nature of creativity: Contemporary psychological perspectives* (pp. 43–75). New York: Cambridge University Press.

Vandenberg, B. (1988) The realities of play. In D. Morrison (Ed.), *Organizing early experience: Imagination and cognition in childhood*. Amityville, NY: Baywood.

Wallach, M.A., & Kogan, N. (1965) *Modes of thinking in young children: A study of the creativity-intelligence distinction*. New York: Holt, Rinehart, Winston.

Wells, C.G. (1986) *The meaning makers: Children learning language and using language to learn*. Portsmouth, NH: Heinemann.

Winner, E. (1996). *Gifted children: Myths and realities*. New York: Basic Books.

Creativity, Childhood

Charlotte Doyle

INTRODUCTION

An article in preparation for a magazine for parents plans to ask in its title, "Oh no. Where did all the creativity go?" (Hoyt, in preparation). Young children seem full of curiosity, spontaneity, imagination, and expressiveness. But during the school years these qualities seem to decline, according to the article. Psychological researchers who study creativity also have pointed to a decline. Although there is no single, generally agreed-on measure of creativity in children, investigators from different traditions using different ways of measuring creativity seem to agree that during the school years, creativity scores tend to fall. This entry explores this apparent drop in creativity first by looking at definitions of creativity and attempts to measure it in children. Next, the issue is examined in developmental and cultural context. Finally, descriptions of the phases of the creative process provide a basis for suggesting strategies to promote creativity in school children.

DEFINITIONS AND SCOPE

One aspect of creativity, according to many visions, is the capacity for psychic freedom, originality, and fluency of thought. In Freud's vision of primary process (Freud, 1959), thought bounces freely from one idea to another unhampered by the learned ways of categorizing and thinking that children learn from their cultures. Without drawing on all of psychoanalytic theory, this notion of free, *divergent thinking* became the basis of attempting to differentiate intelligence from creativity through the psychological tests (Wallach & Kogan, 1965). Intelligence tests, according to this view, tend to measure convergent thinking, that is, the ability to come up with a single correct answer such as, "If Tim is older than Dan and younger than Carl, who is the oldest?" In contrast, divergent thinking tests ask children to think of as many different answers as possible to a single question such as "Think of uses for a brick." The greater the number, variety, and originality of the answers, the higher the divergent thinking test score. Researchers report a "fourth grade slump" in divergent thinking test scores, a dip that they interpret as a drop in creativity (Runco, 1999).

Some psychologists have questioned whether such test items meaningfully measure creativity. They even question whether it is appropriate to try to measure a general trait, creativity. From Guilford (1959) to Gardner (1983, 1993), psychologists have challenged the notion that intelligence and creativity are broad general abilities. Instead, they suggest that each domain involves different operations and symbol systems, and that each domain has independent biological roots. Thus, it is more appropriate to ask about the extent to which a child is verbally creative or creative in the visual arts or music or mathematics than to ask whether or not a child is creative. Creativity in one domain does not say anything about creativity in another, according to this view. Furthermore, Gardner and Winner (1991) argue that a child's actual creative works in a domain are better indicators of creativity than short items on a test. Nevertheless, within domains, they found evidence of a drop in creativity during the school years. Gardner and Winner report that adult artists rate the drawings of school children as less aesthetic, replete, and expressive than those of preschool children. In the verbal realm, they note that school children produce fewer spontaneous metaphors than they did when they were younger. Even with this very different approach to what creativity consists of and how it should be observed, researchers report a dip during the school years.

This apparent drop needs to be examined in two contexts: the context of psychological development and the context of the contemporary American and European culture with particular emphasis on the schools. Such exploration also suggests directions for promoting creativity during the primary school years.

THEORIES AND RESEARCH

The Primary School Years in Developmental and Cultural Context

In most cultures, at around the ages of 6 or 7, children begin to be trained in the skills needed by adults in order to take their places in their societies. Developmental theories suggest why this age may so often be chosen to begin such training. Children of this age have longer attention spans and can take on longer and more complex projects. In addition, Piaget and Inhelder (1969) place the 6–7-year-old child at the beginning of the concrete operational period, when children become more capable of thinking systematically about the world around them—to arrange, to classify, to use mental processes to imagine reversing present and past, self and other. It is also a time when children are ready to learn the rules that underlie the concrete world that they live in, whether it be the rules of games, the rules of social

life, or scientific laws underlying the physical and biological worlds in which they live. In the aesthetic realm, they are ready to study the rules of various domains: how to deal with viewpoint in two-dimensional visual art, various chords structures in the domain of music, spelling, and grammar in the domain of language. The close attention to learning the rules may inhibit the expressiveness of the preschool years. Interestingly, a few studies fail to find the middle years dip. Wohwill (1985) found no dip in the realm of visual arts when children were asked to generate non-representational designs using a computer. One explanation is that the children were freed of the demand of realism and the need to attend to the complex rules of perspective.

Cognitive development implies changes in social development as well. The increase in skill in arranging from most to least and the ability to reverse the position of self and peer lead to an increase in what social psychologists have called social comparison—getting a perspective on self by comparing self with others and, at times, judging one's accomplishments, in part, by the reactions of significant others, be they adults or peers. Self-judgment can be a spur to greater accomplishment, but it can have negative effects as well (Dweck, 1999).

These changes are also inextricably intertwined with emotional developments. Freud referred to the elementary school years as latency, a time when biological urges have been tamed and their energies channeled into aims that are socially acceptable and useful. Erikson (1950) developed and broadened Freud's view and called the period a time when the central emotional issue pits the desire for industry with fear of inferiority. Experimental psychologists have brought these ideas into systematic studies showing that some children enjoy challenges, while many others fear failure and tend to attribute any and all failure to lacks within themselves (Dweck, 1999).

These theories evolved in Europe and North America, and discussion continues about the extent to which various concepts speak to human universals or are culturally specific. As mentioned, earlier, however, most cultures seem to emphasize skill training at around the age of 7 years. At least this aspect represents cultures building on the developing capacities of children in comparable ways.

Contemporary North American and European cultures provide a specific context in which those developments take place. Current educational practice in the United States emphasizes the learning of specific material and skills, objective assessments, the ranking of students on various scales of achievement, threats for failing and rewards for the few who outdo the many. For children who desire to do what the culture asks, the message is to learn what is required, and even the hint of a failure to do so may cost a child a loss of status among adults and peers and damage to self-esteem.

These cognitive, social, and emotional developments, particularly as they are played out in our contemporary culture, might explain the apparent dip in creativity in the elementary school years. Though the requirements and incentives children discern may facilitate some aspects of the creative process, they inhibit others. These helps and hindrances can be seen most clearly by considering the creative episode as it unfolds over time (Doyle, 1976) and in research that studies the contexts that make the creative process likely (Amabile, 1996).

Phases of the Creative Process and the Challenges They Bring

(1) The Beginning: Problem Finding

The creative episode begins when a person senses that the creative process has begun. This may sound as if this is a tautology, but phenomenologically it is not. Something pulls at the mind strongly enough so that the person decides to spend time and energy in carrying out a creative task. That something may be a specific intriguing idea or problem. But sometimes, there is only a general sense of wanting to work in the medium. In this case, playing around, exploring different possibilities may result in the emergence of a compelling idea (Stokes, 2001). In either case, discovering a problem that pulls at the mind is the threshold to creative work (Csikszentmihalyi & Getzels, 1988). The challenge for those who want to facilitate creativity is to encourage children to explore possibilities and to help them to find an engaging project.

During the elementary school years, children are rarely encouraged to find their own problems. Instead, the culture provides a set curriculum with demands for learning specific contents. And even if a school demand is to find a problem within a general framework, such as "Write an essay about your summer vacation," the decision to give time and energy to making something in a medium is the teacher's and not the child's. Amabile (1996) has suggested that, in general, projects are likely to be carried out in a more creative way when the motivation to do so is intrinsic rather than extrinsic. (*Extrinsic motivation* derives from external incentives such as the reward of good grades in contrast with *intrinsic motivation* that comes from within the child.) For those who want to promote creativity, the challenge is to find a way to help children find projects that are so meaningful personally that the children find intrinsic as well as extrinsic reasons for carrying them out.

(2) Learning the Skills and Possibilities of a Medium

Once there is a sense of direction—to do something in words or paints or think about the natural world, for example—creative people report thinking in the medium. The physicist thinks in forces and movement, the composer in melodies and harmonies, the playwright in dialogue and action. Thinking in a medium requires skill in using the medium, facility in manipulating symbol systems to create meanings. The more proficient a child is in using a symbol system, the greater the possibilities for meaning-making with it.

The challenge here is to introduce and give the possibility of acquiring ever increasing skill in the uses of the medium without losing the idea that the reason for learning these symbols systems is their potential for meaning-making. In fact, showing children the different ways symbol systems can be used to make different kinds of meanings—representational versus non-representational painting, differences in the language used for letters, poems, essays, stories— increases the children's sense of possibility of what their own work can comprise.

Each medium, as it develops in a particular cultural context, develops its own heuristics, that is, tricks of the trade that guide the creator toward realization of creative goals. For example, realistic fiction writers, once they imagine a character in a scene, learn to ask themselves questions about the character such as who is the character, how did the character come to be in this scene, what is the character wearing and why. The challenge is to allow children to learn heuristics that will help develop projects without these guides becoming mechanically applied rules that inhibit rather than move the creative process ahead.

(3) Reflective and Non-Reflective Thinking

Working on a creative project often involves a dialectic between two modes of thought called variously reflective versus non-reflective thinking (Sartre, 1975) or living and knowing (Merleau-Ponty, 1962). Reflective thinking about a project includes planning, thinking explicitly about what should be accomplished, remembering heuristics, and evaluating what has been accomplished so far. In non-reflective thinking, the creator does not think *about* the project. Instead, the project takes over consciousness, and the representations of a particular medium flow without self-consciousness. Nothing pulls at the mind other than the puzzles and pushes and pulls that derive from the project itself and from other lived concerns of the creator. There is no explicit thinking about aims or goals or rewards—only the world of the project itself engages the mind. These periods have been called *task-centered thinking* (Wertheimer, 1959), *flow* (Csikszentmihalyi, 1996), and *centration* (Doyle, 1976). The challenge for facilitating creativity in children is to allow the time and opportunity for this kind of full engagement in the work.

These unreflective "flow" periods alternate with reflective thinking—thinking about the project in evaluative terms such as what has been accomplished so far, what needs to be changed, and where the project needs to go and ways to get there. These reflective phases sometimes include self-evaluation, including harsh destructive criticism of ones' own ability to carry out the project. The challenge here is to guide children to reflect on what they have already done in ways that propel them back into those flow periods of full unreflective engagement and to give support and guidance in the face of discouragement and sensed helplessness.

Young children typically take on projects that can be completed in minutes. Older children have longer attention spans and attempt projects that require more time, often intermittently time over a period of days. It is also a challenge to give children the time and the support as the unfolding reflective and non-reflective periods share the days with other tasks.

(4) Sharing the Work

Completing a project brings its own intrinsic satisfactions, but we are social human beings, and child and adult alike seek to share what they have done with others. Something personally meaningful needs to have a meaningful place in the social world as well (Csikszentmihalyi, 1996). The challenge here is to provide opportunities that allow children to see that their projects are recognized, appreciated, and understood by others.

STRATEGIES FOR PROMOTING CREATIVITY IN SCHOOL CHILDREN: OVERVIEW

The dominant educational practices in our contemporary culture do not support most of the phases of the creative episode during the elementary school years. They do allow for learning certain symbol systems, and evaluation of products is emphasized. But allowing the child to become an active agent in choosing a personally meaningful project from a wide range of possibilities is not commonly a part of educational practice. Nor is there help in how to find such a project or the time to carry it out during periods of full personal private engagement. And the sense of constantly being evaluated and ranked with respect to fellow students increases the tendency for critical personal self-evaluation. So it is not surprising that just at the time when a child is set to discern the rules and practices of our culture, is motivated to meet its work demands, is expected to take on more complex projects, and is self-consciously aware of one's status with respect to peers, psychologists report a dip in creativity, be it measured by a tiny timed sample of the free flow of thought or by aesthetic judgment of art work.

The irony is that our culture honors creativity at least in its rhetoric and sees the inventiveness of its people as one of the factors that have led to cultural progress. In China, art education does not take creativity as one of the goals to which school-aged children should aspire. Instead, young Chinese art students are encouraged to learn by copying the masters. Skill in carrying out this task is what is aspired to and honored. In China, no one bewails the drop in creativity in the school years, because creativity in the Western sense is not even an aim in aesthetic domains until much later in life. Learning to make accurate copies is the child's age-appropriate task in that culture (Gardner & Winner, 1991). Another question is whether the dip has any implications for the future creative productions of gifted individuals. Pariser (1985) found the creative dip in the artworks of great artists such as Picasso and Klee. Perhaps the school-aged years should be devoted to learning the rules of the medium, leaving creative projects for later times in development.

Interestingly, it is in the United States that this dip in creativity has been a concern, and this concern dovetails with critiques of the dominant trends in contemporary education (e.g., see Nager & Shapiro, 2000). Those critiques question whether demands for rote learning and objective assessment are the most efficient ways of teaching students the skills needed for our culture, a culture that emphasizes inventiveness, individual initiative, and citizen empowerment in the face of change. Furthermore, these critics see meaningful engagement as a sine qua non, not only of high quality education as preparation for the future, but as part of a generative, fulfilling way to live during all the periods of development. Promoting creativity, according to this view, not only prepares for future creativity but also brings special and important kinds of cognitive, social, and emotional fulfillment to the life of a child in the middle years.

STRATEGIES THAT WORK

The definition of creativity and empirical ways of assessing it are still in flux, so it is premature to state categorically that the effectiveness of a particular strategy has been clearly proved or disproved.

STRATEGIES THAT MIGHT WORK

The general cultural trend not withstanding, gifted teachers and parents have put together intriguing programs to nourish the creative potential of children in the elementary school years in a variety of domains. The following are some examples.

Facilitating Creativity in Writing: The Teacher's College Writing Project

The Teacher's College Writing Workshop (Caulkins, 1991) has developed methods for facilitating many of the phases of the creative process in children in the school context. Instead of the demand to write on a specific topic, the invitation is to find something meaningful to write about. Most children do not know how to do this. So the first task is to help children discover their subjects, finding the ones that pull at the children's mind for intrinsic reasons as well as address the external demand to do a piece of writing. One way of doing this, the Workshop suggests, is to teach the heuristic of keeping notebooks in which children record observations, questions, reactions to books, feelings, and thoughts. After a while, the child and teacher talk about the notebook, with the idea of finding a meaningful project. Sometimes the conversation begins by asking the child which entry mattered most. For example, one child said, "When I had to let my hamster go in the park, because then I have no one to come home to." The teacher asked whether any other entries related to that. The child found an entry about her grandmother who used to be at home before she died. This led to the child's writing a story of losing her grandmother, coming home to a hamster, and having to let the hamster loose in the park.

Once a child decides to write on a specific topic, there is discussion about how an idea might be developed. Some heuristics that may guide project development are studying published work that deals with a similar topic or getting more information about an incident through interviews or making more entries on a specific topic. Ten-year-old Chris discovered that many of his entries had to do with moving away from his mother to live with his father; he articulated three intentions: to write more entries explicitly on that topic, to write something that had the feel of literature, and to begin with one specific entry. Another child, a class comedian, decided to write a list of funny rules regarding how to request permission to use the bathroom. Part of the planning is the understanding that there are many different ways to use writing—for poems, stories, autobiographies, picture books, letters, even signs that can be posted.

The Workshop recommends a period of reflection and talk about writing and then, what Caulkins calls a silent space: a quiet time in the classroom, a period, that can allow the children to engage in their projects non-reflectively. Thereafter, the teacher is available to help children reflect on what they have written and to help plan what to do next. Caulkins also notes that it is very important not to do and say too much, not to rob the child of the sense of ownership of his or her own work.

The children read their completed work to one another. But the children are also encouraged to understand that their words can affect audiences outside of the classroom. A boy who was upset about not being invited to be part of his brother's wedding actually drafted a letter to him. A child who lived in a homeless shelter wrote an extensive report of conditions and sent it to the governor. A girl who wrote about the death of her brother made it into a picture book and read it to younger children. Thus, the Workshop methods support problem finding, developing intentions, opportunities to study various uses of a medium, heuristics as guides to further planning, periods of reflective thinking and non-reflective engagement, and, at the completion, ways of giving the project a respected place in the social world.

Promoting Creativity in Other Domains

Other teachers and parents have invented procedures that promote creative episodes in other domains. The physicist Feynman (1988) wrote appreciatively about how his father introduced him to the realm of science. In particular he remembered their nature walks. His father helped him to find mysteries in what they saw. He scoffed at simply naming birds or plants and instead asked his son questions something like, "What do you see the bird doing?" "Why do you think the bird does that?" "Can you think of a way of testing that guess?" Feynman also remembers himself noticing that a marble in the middle of his wagon rolled to the back when he pulled on it. When he told his father, his father suggested that the boy look closely from the side as the wagon is pulled to see what moves and what stands still. The boy, completely engaged in the problem, stared as his father pulled the wagon slowly several times and discovered that the wagon, not the marble, was doing most of the moving. Finding problems, inventing hypotheses, learning how to derive specific questions from hypotheses that observations can answer, using the skills of observation and thought to solve them—all these shared experiences introduced the boy to the pleasures of creative thinking in science.

The late Viola Farber (personal communication, 1998), a dancer and choreographer, used to visit schools with groups of her Sarah Lawrence College students. First, the students put on a little show. It began with a single dancer saying, "This is the right way to dance." Soon a second dancer, moving very differently entered and said, "No, this is the right way to dance." By the end, eight dancers each moving in very different ways were on the stage. The children—now aware of many possibilities, the idea there is no one right way to dance, and the sense that criticism can be ignored—were then invited to move. Then they were divided into groups, each led by a college student, and their movements adapted and integrated into a group dance that they then showed to each other. Dance became a medium with a variety of possibilities, a medium in which there is no single set of rules to follow and in which the individual creations become part of a larger performance piece. Similarly, in an after-school program, in conjunction with deciding how to paint scenery for a play, teacher Jim Doyle (2001) took his fourth and fifth graders on an art history tour, showing them the many possible ways artists used paint to represent.

Teacher Bill McKeon (personal communication, 2000) invited each of his fourth- or fifth-grade students to learn the skills of research and presentation by investigating a topic of special interest. As in the writing workshops, McKeon helped each student to find a topic. A child captivated by basketball or special effects in movies could choose it as a topic. A child fascinated by horses or fashion could choose that topic. The mission was to learn more about the topic, to find ways to organize it, and then to present it to the other children. In the process, the children read, visited the library, used the Internet, wrote, and drew. They shared their projects at several points during the semester as works in progress and listened to questions from other children about the project. At the end, each child made a final presentation. Again, the child had ownership of the topic, was invited to develop it in a variety of ways, acquired the sense that a project needs to be developed over time, learned heuristics for doing so, had opportunity for non-self-conscious engagement and for reflection, and came at the end to share the completed work with others.

Art educator Nancy Smith (1993) has worked with elementary school children and teachers in the realm of painting. She, too, noticed that children's paintings often become rather stereotyped in these years. To avoid this she begins art periods with questions that both stimulate topics and sensitize children to issues of craft. During one period in which she wanted children to think about how emotion can be reflected visually, she asked questions such as: how can you tell what an animal is feeling by how the animal moves? When you feel dreamy, how do you stand or sit; what do you think about? What happened that made you feel frightened or brave? As part of the discussion, she elicited specific details such as what kinds of plants grew in their gardens, thus helping children avoid stereotypic forms. Smith (1993) also teaches the heuristics of planning by asking questions such as "if you want to show the crowd watching the skater, where will you place them on the page." She suggests that children assume body positions that may be difficult to depict. Once children are engaged and committed to a particular project, she is careful not to tromp on their intentions with comments. But when they come to her with difficulties, she again uses question to guide the children to solve the problems themselves. A child puzzled about how to draw a table can be guided by questions such as: "What shape is the table? Do you want to draw it from the top or from the side? How does it fit into the rest of the painting?" When a child brings a finished painting to her, she does not simply say she likes it. Instead, she acknowledges what she sees in the painting explicitly, making comments that show that she recognizes what the child has done in terms of color, form, composition, representation, and expression. These evaluations recognize what the child has accomplished, communicate it in a detailed way, and, at the same time, give the child a language through which to think about craft.

STRATEGIES THAT DO NOT WORK

Given the variety in definition and assessment of creativity, it is not appropriate to label any procedure as proven to be ineffective.

SYNTHESIS

All the examples of strategies that might work suggest that the way to promote creativity in school children is to give children opportunities to participate in extended creative episodes. For children of this age, it is not enough to "have an art period" or to be asked to write in a journal. Children, primed to learn the right way to do things, need to understand that there are many right ways to be creative. They can learn this by seeing different, varying examples of using various media and by experiencing encouragement and acceptance for exploring a variety of approaches. Children intent on doing what is expected need help in realizing that what they really care about can become a project that is respected in the context of school. They may need guidance in becoming explicit about what is meaningful to them; probing, supportive conversations, and the use of notebooks can help here. Children who are old enough to design and evaluate complex projects but are intimidated by the prospect of carrying them out need to learn the heuristics that will enable the development of a project they care about over time. This can involve explicit instruction in the techniques for using symbol systems, teaching strategies for working in a particular genre, asking guiding questions, and/or exploring works related to what the child is trying to accomplish. Children used to the clamor of demands need silent times and spaces so that they can become deeply engaged. This suggests designating special work places and work times in which children can do things quietly and privately. Children expecting to be evaluated need to feel respect and recognition without being ranked. Serious conversations about the project and the ways in which intentions were realized help children feel that respect. So does the opportunity for sharing the accomplishment with adults and peers—giving the project a place in the social world.

Many of these suggestions put the adult in the role of a helper, someone who finds ways to allow the projects to go on. Vygotsky (1973) teaches that interpersonal experiences such as dialogues with others in the context of a task later become an inner dialogue, an intrapersonal experience. When parents and teachers ask guiding questions at various phases of a project, they are teaching children heuristics for how to guide themselves in the future. The emphasis here is not on an adult's evaluation of the child, but on what this project needs to develop it further—on intrinsic rather than extrinsic aspects. And the children's creations become objects of respect from others, with specific recognition of what has been accomplished. Though the adult may participate as a helper, the children need to feel the projects to be theirs: They find a project that has meaning for them and they are the shapers of its development.

Do these ways of promoting creativity eliminate the primary school dip to which researchers pointed? Perhaps, but the research has not been done. This kind of evaluation, based on one or another creativity measure, may not be the issue, however. Participating in creative episodes allows children to learn contents and skills in the context of activities that matter to them. Such participation brings a sense of agency and competence, of recognition and respect. Creative episodes allow children to get perspective on what fascinates, puzzles, confuses, or overwhelms them. To mentor children as they engage in developmentally appropriate creative episodes is to nurture cognitive, social, and emotional growth in ways that children find deeply fulfilling.

Also see: Creativity: Early Childhood; Creativity: Adolescence; Creativity: Adulthood; Creativity: Older Adulthood; Culture, Society, and Social Class: Foundation.

References

Amabile, T.M. (1996). *Update to the social psychology of creativity.* Booker, CO: Westview.

Caulkins, L.M. (1991). *Living between the lines.* Portsmouth, NH: Heinemann.

Csikszentmihalyi, M. (1996). *Creativity: Flow and the psychology of discovery and invention.* New York: HarperCollins.

Csikszentmihalyi, M., & Getzels, J.W. (1988). Creativity and problem finding. In F.G. Farley (Ed.), *The foundations of aesthetics, art, and art education* (pp. 91–106). New York: Praeger.

Doyle, C. (1976). The creative process: A study in paradox. In C. Winsor (Ed.), *The creative process* (pp. 6–15). New York: Bank Street College.

Doyle, J. (2001). *The college bound class: A differentiated curriculum for the enrichment of the motivated students.* Unpublished master's thesis, LaVerne University, LaVerne, CA.

Dweck, C.S. (1999). *Self-theories: Their role in motivation, personality, and development.* Philadelphia, PA: Psychology Press/Taylor & Francis.

Erikson, E. (1950). *Childhood & society.* New York: Norton.

Feynman, R. (1988). *What do you care what other people think.* New York: Norton.

Freud, S. (1959). *Collected papers* (J. Riviere, Trans.). London: Hogarth.

Guilford, J.P. (1959). The three faces of intellect. *American Psychologist, 14,* 469–479.

Gardner, H. (1983). *Frames of mind.* New York: Basic Books.

Gardner, H. (1993). *Creating minds.* New York: Basic Books.

Gardner, H., & Winner, E. (1991). The course of creative growth: A tribute to Joachim Wohwill. In R.M. Downs, L.S. Liben et al. (Eds.), *Visions of aesthetics, the environment, and development: The legacy of Joachim Wohwill* (pp. 23–43). Hillsdale, NJ: Lawrence Erlbaum.

Hoyt, C. (in preparation). Oh no. Where did the creativity go? *Sesame Street Parent Magazine,*

Merleau-Ponty, M. (1962). *Phenomenology of perception* (C. Smith, Trans.). New York: Humanities Press.

Nager, N., & Shapiro, E.K. (Eds.). (2000). *Revisiting a progressive pedagogy: The developmental interaction approach.* Albany, NY: SUNY.

Pariser, D. (1985, November). *The juvenalia of Klee, Toulouse-Lautrec, and Picasso.* Paper Presented at Conference on the History of Education, Pennsylvania State University, College Park, PA.

Piaget, J., & Inhelder, B. (1969). *The psychology of the child* (H. Weaver, Trans.). New York: Basic Books.

Runco, M. (1999). Fourth grade slump. In M.A. Runco & S. Pritzker (Eds.), *Encyclopedia of creativity* (pp. 743–744). San Diego, CA: Academic Press.

Sartre, J.P. (1975). *The emotions: Outline of a theory.* New York: Citadel Press.

Smith, N.R. (1993). *Experience and art: Teaching children to paint* (2nd ed.). New York: Teachers College Press.

Stokes, P. (2001) Variability, constraints, and creativity: Shedding light on Claude Monet. *American Psychologist, 56*(4), 355–359.

Vygotsky, L. (1973). *Mind in society* (M. Cole et al., Trans. and Eds.), Cambridge, MA: Harvard University Press.

Wallach, M.A., & Kogan, N. (1965). *Modes of thinking in young children: A study of the creativity-intelligence distinction.* New York: Holt, Rinehart, & Winston.

Wertheimer, M. (1959). *Productive thinking.* New York: Harper & Row.

Wohwill, J. (1985). The Gardner–Winner view of children's visual-artistic development: Overview, assessment, and critique. *Visual Arts Research, 11,* 1–22.

Creativity, Adolescence

Sally M. Reis and Joseph S. Renzulli

INTRODUCTION

This entry highlights some of the major issues associated with promoting high levels of creative potential and achievement in talented adolescents. It summarizes recent research about the environmental factors, and school and home programs, that are more likely to result in the realization of creative talent.

DEFINITIONS

Schoolhouse giftedness and talent refers to test-taking, lesson-learning, or academic giftedness or talents. Individuals who fall into this category generally score well on more traditional intellectual or cognitive assessments and perform well in school.

Creative/productive giftedness and talent, on the other hand, is reflected in individuals who tend to be or have the potential to become producers (rather than consumers) of original knowledge, materials, or products and who employ thought processes that tend to be inductive, integrated, and problem oriented.

SCOPE

We have no way of estimating the number of talented young people with high creative potential who currently fail to develop this potential in American schools; nor do we have a way to estimate how many adolescents and children have creative potential. Nationally, approximately 5–10 percent of students are identified as gifted or talented, but not all of these young people demonstrate high creative potential, and indeed, many of these talented students underachieve in school (Reis & McCoach, 2000).

THEORIES

Gardner's (1983) theory of multiple intelligences (MI) and Renzulli's (1978) "three ring" definition of gifted behavior serve as examples of multifaceted and well-researched conceptualizations of intelligence and giftedness. Gardner's definition of *intelligence* is the ability to solve problems, or create products, that are valued within one or more cultural settings (Gardner, 1993). Within his MI theory, he articulates eight specific intelligences: linguistic, musical, logical-mathematical, spatial, bodily-kinesthetic, interpersonal, intrapersonal, and naturalistic. Gardner believes that people are more comfortable using the term "talents" and that "intelligence" is generally reserved to describe linguistic or logical "smartness"; however, he does not believe that certain human abilities should arbitrarily qualify as "intelligence" over others (e.g., language as an intelligence vs. dance as a talent) (Gardner, 1993).

Renzulli's (1978) theory examines gifted behaviors, rather than gifted individuals: Gifted behavior consists of behaviors that reflect an interaction among three basic clusters of human traits—above average ability, high levels of task commitment, and high levels of creativity. Individuals capable of developing gifted behavior are those possessing or capable of developing this composite set of traits and applying them to any potentially valuable area of human performance. Persons who manifest or are capable of developing an interaction among the three clusters require a wide variety of educational opportunities and services that are not ordinarily provided through regular instructional programs (Renzulli & Reis, 1997). These three basic clusters of human traits contain the following characteristics:

Above average ability, viewed as a general ability, includes: (1) high levels of abstract thought, (2) adaptation to novel situations, and (3) rapid and accurate retrieval of information. Viewed as a specific ability, it includes (1) application of general abilities to a specific area of knowledge, (2) the capacity to sort out relevant from irrelevant information, and (3) the capacity to acquire and use advanced knowledge and strategies while pursuing a problem.

Task commitment includes: (1) a capacity for high levels of interest and enthusiasm, (2) a capacity for hard work and determination in a particular area, (3) self-confidence and drive to achieve, (4) the ability to identify significant problems within an area of study, and (5) setting high standards for one's work.

Creativity includes: (1) fluency, flexibility, and originality of thought, (2) being open to new experiences and ideas, (3) being curious, (4) being willing to take risks, and (5) being sensitive to aesthetic characteristics (adapted from Renzulli & Reis, 1997, p. 9).

RESEARCH

A discussion of "high intellectual ability or potential" and "high creative ability or potential" must be presented separately because existing research and discussion often identify the existence of two broad categories, which Renzulli (1986) referred to as either "schoolhouse giftedness" and/or "creative/productive giftedness."

Many research studies support a general approach that develops the creative potential of adolescents in school (Renzulli & Reis, 1994). Results of several recent longitudinal studies (Delcourt, 1994; Hébert, 1993; Perleth, Sierwald, & Heller, 1993) provide research support for Renzulli's distinction between schoolhouse giftedness and creative/productive giftedness. Perleth et al. (1993), in their Munich Longitudinal Study of Giftedness (1985–1989) focusing on a large number of secondary students, found clear differences between students who demonstrated creative/productive as opposed to schoolhouse giftedness. Renzulli believes that both schoolhouse giftedness and creative productive giftedness should be developed in adolescents and that an interaction logically exists between them (Renzulli & Reis, 1985, 1997).

Many authors have described the personality traits, social environment, and thinking and learning styles of creatively gifted adults (Davis, 1992, 1999; Rothenberg, 1990; Walberg & Stariha, 1992; Walberg & Zeiser, 1997). However, few studies have examined similarly talented adolescents who may have the potential for high levels of creative productive work (Bloom, 1985; Csikszentmihalyi, Rathunde, & Whalen, 1993; Winner, 1996; Winner & Martino, 1993). A consistent finding from the adolescent studies is that several characteristics, personality traits, and environmental factors facilitate the development of high levels of creativity and creative productive giftedness in young people and adolescents (Czikszentmihalyi, 1998; Gardner, 1983; Reis, 1998; Renzulli, 1986; Sternberg & Lubart, 1993).

Personality Traits and Characteristics of Highly Creative Persons

Much of the work on personality factors associated with high creative achievement suggests that there is a consistent psychological profile of creative persons, though there is considerable variety from one person to the next (Barron, 1988; Bloom, 1985; Csikszentmihalyi, 1996; Csikszentmihalyi et al., 1993; Renzulli, 1978, 1986; Runco, 1992; Simonton, 1988; Torrance, 1978, 1995). This cluster of personality traits distinguishes more creative individuals from those with lower levels of creative potential. Creative persons are generally considered to be open to new experience, persevering, nonconforming, and intellectually and emotionally independent. They may be impulsive yet self-confident, and often have good insight into their abilities. They may be less group-oriented, more introverted, seeking more time alone than do average people.

Other characteristics that researchers and theorists have associated with creative giftedness include awareness of one's own creativity (Daniels, 1997) and emotional maturity, including the courage to actualize one's abilities (Sternberg & Lubart, 1993). Creative achievers may withdraw more often, and seek solitude for some creative tasks require long stretches of concentration without interruption. Creatively gifted individuals also tend to be much less motivated by external rewards like grades and public recognition, and more driven by a love for creative work (Kirshenbaum & Reis, 1997). More recent work has also concluded that youngsters who are exceptionally creative engage in fantasy, and can openly express emotion (Russ, Robins, & Christano, 1999). The same study also found that their emotional expression was relatively stable over time; young people who expressed more emotion in their early years also did so later in their childhood.

Davis (1992, 1999) reviewed over 200 personality characteristics compiled by researchers of creative persons and categorized them into 16 positive characteristics of individuals with high creative ability or potential, as well as 12 negative traits. The positive traits include: awareness of creativeness, independent, energetic, thorough, sense of humor, original, risk taking, capacity for fantasy, curious, attracted to complexity and ambiguity, artistic, need for time alone, emotional, open-minded, perceptive, and ethical.

The negative traits include: questioning rules and authority, stubbornness, low interest in details, forgetfulness, careless and disorganized, egotistical, indifference to common conventions, rebellious and argumentative, tendency to be emotional, absentminded, neurotic, and impulsive or hyperactive.

These negative traits tend to upset the parents and educators, as well as some of the peers, of creative children, since they lead to behaviors not considered appropriate in traditional classrooms. A challenge exists for educators and parents to identify these characteristics of creativity in children and to channel creative energy into constructive outlets (Renzulli & Reis, 1985, 1997) by encouraging playfulness, flexibility, and the production of wild and unusual ideas (Torrance, 1962), as well as opportunities to pursue real problems (Renzulli & Reis, 1985, 1997).

In summary, creatively talented children may exhibit different characteristics than academically gifted children. Those with high academic abilities may have the potential to develop creative gifts and talents, yet many creatively talented students do not necessarily display high academic performance in school.

Environmental Factors

Several researchers also suggest that certain environments can help to nurture high levels of creative potential (Amabile, 1989; Csikszentmihalyi, 1990; Torrance, 1978). For instance, families with moderate levels of stress may promote creativity in children because children learn to tolerate tension, ambiguity, and are less pressured to conform (Torrance, 1978). Yet, the creative person also needs support. For example, MacKinnon (1978) concluded that creative talent requires a need for understanding from others to convey confidence in abilities. This reinforcement and affirmation seems to address the anxieties that may be associated with creative ideas, but it does not belittle the intensity nor dismiss the reality of the creative ideas. Runco (1992) also found that creativity requires an environment that nurtures and then actively supports independence of judgment. Runco also found that creative individuals tend to be self-evaluative by nature, but this self-evaluation cannot be sustained without external support systems, and when support is unavailable, frustration may develop.

Torrance (1978, 1988) determined that the creative personality requires a variety of social and emotional support mechanisms and that denial of those needs would likely result in both physiological and psychological illnesses. These needs include parental support and understanding of frustration as it develops and the need for reinforcing experimentation. In other words, the creatively gifted individual is more likely to thrive in environments where risk taking is valued and promoted, and where there is less pressure to conform to prescribed conventions (Wildauer, 1984). These needs do not end with adolescence, but continue throughout life (Willings, 1983).

In studies of talented adolescents, Bloom (1985) points to the important influence of gifted peers who match or surpass a student's abilities, and share the motivation needed for persistent effort over a prolonged period. Access to a peer group of students with similar passions and abilities prepares creatively gifted adolescents to cope with the realities of the intense competition and stardom that characterizes some creative careers later in life.

Csikszentmihalyi's (1996) research on creative adolescents suggests that the pursuit of high creative achievement among this group is likely to result in reduced popularity and perhaps increased marginalization or alienation from peers. Creatively gifted persons may appear particularly odd to peers when they have interests and passions that differ from the mainstream, and a proclivity for unique thinking and self-expression. Development of creative talent often necessitates more time spent alone than for average teens, and the amount of time allocated to mental play appears to inhibit sexual awareness and independence.

STRATEGIES: OVERVIEW

Several instructional strategies, programs, and models can be used to develop and nurture creativity in adolescents. A brief summary of some of these is provided as well as a thorough description of one model designed to develop creative productivity in students. The Schoolwide Enrichment Model (SEM) (Renzulli, 1977; Renzulli & Reis, 1985, 1997) is one of the mostly widely used enrichment models in the United States. It is based on an enrichment programming model called the Enrichment Triad Model (Renzulli, 1977), developed in the mid-1970s.

STRATEGIES THAT WORK

In the SEM, a talent pool of 15–20 percent of above average ability, creative, high potential students is identified through a variety of measures including: achievement tests, teacher nominations, assessment of potential for creativity and task commitment, as well as alternative pathways of entrance (self-nomination, parent nomination, etc.). High achievement and IQ test scores automatically include a student in the talent pool, enabling those creative students who are underachieving in their academic schoolwork to be included.

Once students are identified for the talent pool, they are eligible for three services. First, interest and learning styles assessments are used with talent pool students. Many schools use this process for all students. Informal and formal methods are used to create or identify students' interests and to encourage students to further develop and pursue these interests in various ways. Learning style preferences which are assessed include: projects, independent study, teaching games, simulations, peer teaching, programmed instruction, lecture, drill and recitation, and discussion. This information, which focuses on strengths rather than deficits, is compiled into a Total Talent Portfolio used to make decisions about talent development opportunities, either for students in the talent pool or for all students. This approach is also consistent with the more flexible conception of *developing* creative gifts and talents that has been a cornerstone of this approach promoting more equity in enrichment or gifted programs.

Second, curriculum compacting is provided to all eligible students for whom the regular curriculum is modified by eliminating portions of previously mastered content. This streamlining of curriculum enables above-average students to avoid repetition of previously mastered work and guarantees mastery while simultaneously finding time for more creative and appropriately challenging activities (Reis, Burns, & Renzulli, 1992). A form, entitled the Compactor (Renzulli & Smith, 1978), is used to document which content areas have been compacted and what alternative work has been substituted.

Third, three types of enrichment experiences are offered, based on the theoretical approach underlying the SEM, the Enrichment Triad. The goal is to encourage creative productivity on the part of young people by exposing them to various topics, areas of interest, and fields of study; and to further train them to *apply* advanced content, process-training skills, and methodology training to self-selected areas of interest. In the SEM, Type I (exposure to new topics, areas, and issues), Type II (thinking skills, problem solving, and methods training within content areas, such as historical, scientific, etc.), and Type III Enrichment (small group or individual self-selected studies in academic or artistic areas) are offered to all students; however, Type III enrichment is usually more appropriate for students with higher levels of ability, interest, and task commitment.

Evidence that the SEM approach works is supported by numerous studies (Renzulli & Reis, 1994). Delcourt (1988) and Starko (1986) investigated student creative productivity in the SEM. Delcourt (1988) investigated characteristics related to creative/productive behavior in 18 adolescents who consistently engaged in first-hand research of self-selected topics both in or out of school, finding that: (1) targeted students do exhibit characteristics similar to those of creative/productive adults; (2) these students can be producers of information as well as consumers; and (3) the learning processes of these students merit closer attention if their abilities are to be better understood by themselves, their parents, and their teachers. Delcourt (1994) also conducted longitudinal research using the same subjects and focusing on their interests, educational and professional experiences, career plans, and projects. Results indicated that students maintained similar or identical career goals to their plans in high school and remained in major fields of study in colleges. Based upon each student's level of involvement with his or her investigations and the quality of the projects, Delcourt's study supports the concept that adolescents can continue to become creative young adults.

Starko (1986) examined the effects of SEM participation on student creative productivity. Students who participated in SEM programs for at least four years were compared with students who qualified for such programs but received no services. Data were analyzed by hierarchical multiple regression, as well as qualitative analysis of open-ended questionnaire items. Results indicated that students who became involved in independent study projects in the SEM more often initiated their own creative products both *in and outside of school* than did students in the comparison group. A total of 103 students, 58 program students and 45 non-program students of similar ability, participated in the study. The group in the enrichment program reported more than twice as many creative projects per student (3.37) as the comparison group (1.4). The group that participated in the enrichment program also reported doing more than twice as many creative products outside of school on their own time (1.03) than the comparison group (0.50).

In a longitudinal study of SEM program participants, Hébert (1993) examined the educational experiences of nine senior high school students ten years after their involvement in the program. The students selected for the study were chosen because of the number and quality of the Type III products they completed during their elementary TAG program experience. He found that: (1) Type III interests of students affect post-secondary plans, (2) creative outlets are needed in high school, (3) a decrease in creative Type III productivity occurs during the junior high experience (perhaps due to increasing demands of more teachers and peer pressure not to pursue additional academic work), and (4) the Type III process serves as an important training for later productivity. Baum, Renzulli, and Hébert (1995) found that Type III studies can work to reverse underachievement in talented students, as well.

In a comprehensive examination of widespread efforts to teach creativity, Torrance (1987) analyzed over 150 different studies and reported that he had found "massive evidence" of positive results. Some of the programs studied by Torrance included those discussed in this section that have been implemented to nurture creativity in talented students. National programs such as Future Problem Solving, conceived by Torrance, have taught hundreds of thousands of students to apply creative problem-solving techniques to the real problems of our society. Although not developed solely for talented students, Future Problem Solving is widely used in programs for academically talented students because of the curricular freedom associated with these programs.

The Future Problem Solving Program is a year-long program in which teams of four students use a six-step problem solving process to solve complex scientific and social problems of the future such as the overcrowding of prisons or the greenhouse effect. At regular intervals throughout the year, the teams mail their work to evaluators, who review it and return it with their suggestions for improvement. As the year progresses, the teams become increasingly more proficient at problem solving. The Future Problem Solving Program takes students beyond memorization. The program challenges students to apply information they have learned to some of the most complex issues facing society. They are asked to *think*, to make decisions, and, in some instances, to carry out their solutions. Little research has been conducted on this program, however. Other articles have described the success of the program in general (Chapman, 1991; Torrance, 1984), as well as success using Future Problem Solving with underachieving students (Rimm & Olenchak, 1991).

Eleven states have created separate schools for talented students in math and science such as The North Carolina School for Math and Science, and several of these stress creative products and self-selected research. Some large school districts have established magnet schools to serve the needs of talented students. In New York City, for example, the Bronx High School of Science has helped to nurture and develop mathematical and scientific talent for decades, producing internationally known scientists and Nobel laureates. In other states, Governor's Schools provide advanced, intensive summer programs in a variety of content areas. It is clear, however, that these opportunities touch a small percentage of creatively gifted adolescents who could benefit from them.

STRATEGIES THAT MIGHT WORK

Within schools that have gifted or enrichment programs, some options for the development of creativity exist through the use of resource room programs in which a student leaves his/her regular classroom and spends time doing creative projects or independent study. Some students also become involved in advanced research on topics that they select in a resource room or in a classroom. Some classroom teachers provide opportunities for creativity training or creative work or even independent study projects that provide students with opportunities to engage in pursuing both individual interests and creative work. Many districts have created innovative mentorship programs that pair students with older students or adults who have similar interests.

In addition to Future Problem Solving, programs such as Odyssey of the Mind, a national program in which teams of students use creative problem solving to design structures, vehicles, and solutions to problems such as designing a vehicle which uses a mousetrap as its primary power source. Many talented students have the opportunity to participate in History Day in which students work individually or in small groups to research an historical event, person from the past, or invention related to a theme that is determined each year. Using primary source data including diaries or other sources gathered in libraries, museums, and interviews, students prepare research papers, projects, media presentations, or performances as entries. These entries are judged by local historians, educators, and other professionals and state finalists compete with winners from other states each June. Additional research is needed concerning the overall effectiveness of this program.

STRATEGIES THAT DO NOT WORK

It is difficult to identify what does not work to develop creativity as researchers usually focus on what can increase creativity, rather than diminish it. It seems clear that some classroom environments seem to constrict creative thoughts and productivity. Too much rigidity, too few opportunities for freedom of choice and enjoyment exist in the learning process and too few teachers today concentrate on trying to develop creativity. Instead, they seem to focus on how to increase achievement test scores. The most common manner in which the underachievement of talented students is described involves identifying a discrepancy between ability and achievement described in detail by Reis and McCoach (2000) who review the issues surrounding the definition and identification of underachievement in the gifted.

The absence of creative opportunities for work is widely mentioned as one reason that creatively talented students underachieve. Many talented underachievers are bored or unstimulated in school (Pirozzo, 1982; Reis, Hébert, Diaz, Maxfield, & Ratley, 1995). Whitmore (1980) specifically found that the creativity of talented underachieving students is stifled in the typical classroom situation that focuses on achieving the "one right answer." Whitmore (1980) further argued that the instructional strategies of classroom teachers, curricula, and the typical classroom climate are unsuitable for high ability students. Teachers may judge students only on the basis of their performance or apply unreasonable pressure for achievement and conduct strict, autocratic classes emphasizing rote, repetitive learning that may stifle creativity in talented learners.

SYNTHESIS

The ultimate goal of education for adolescents should be engagement in current learning that inspires adolescents to continue learning and working to develop their academic and creative potential. This potential is best developed in a systematic approach that targets the benefits of the development of creative productivity, such as the three types of enrichment that are a part of the SEM approach. Type I enrichment is designed to expose students to a wide variety of disciplines, topics, occupations, hobbies, persons, places, and events that would not ordinarily be covered in the regular curriculum. In schools that use this model, an enrichment team consisting of parents, teachers, and students often organizes and plans Type I experiences by contacting speakers, arranging mini-courses, demonstrations, or performances, or by ordering and distributing films, slides, videotapes, or other print or non-print media.

Type II enrichment consists of materials and methods designed to promote the development of thinking and feeling processes. Some Type II enrichment is general, consisting of training in areas such as creative thinking and problem solving, learning how to learn skills such as classifying and analyzing data, and advanced reference and communication skills. Other Type II enrichment is specific, as it cannot be planned in advance and usually involves advanced instruction in an interest area selected by the student.

Type III enrichment occurs when students become interested in pursuing a self-selected area and are willing to commit the time necessary for advanced content acquisition and process training in which they assume the role of a first-hand inquirer. The goals of Type III enrichment include: providing opportunities for applying interests, knowledge, creative ideas and task commitment to a self-selected problem or area of study; acquiring advanced level understanding of the knowledge (content) and methodology (process) used within particular disciplines, artistic areas of expression, and interdisciplinary studies; developing authentic products primarily directed toward bringing about a desired impact upon a specified audience; developing self-directed learning skills in the areas of planning, organization, resource utilization, time management, decision making and self-evaluation; developing task commitment, self-confidence, and feelings of creative accomplishment.

Today, many educators and politicians seem to be more interested in raising achievement scores, rather than in developing creativity in their students. This may be very shortsighted from an historical and societal perspective. By using some of the strategies developed in the programs that nurture creativity, we can help some students develop their creativity, as well as their academic potential, as part of their overall school experiences. It may very well be that these creative opportunities matter much more in students' futures, and in society as well.

Also see: Creativity: Early Childhood; Creativity: Childhood; Creativity: Adulthood; Creativity: Older Adulthood; Culture, Society, and Social Class: Foundation.

References

Amabile, T. (1989). *Growing up creative: Nurturing a lifetime of creativity.* New York: Crown.

Barron, F. (1988). Putting creativity to work. In R.J. Sternberg (Ed.), *The nature of creativity.* New York: Cambridge University Press.

Baum, S., Renzulli, J.S., & Hébert, T.P. (1995). *The prism metaphor: A new paradigm for reversing underachievement* (Collaborative Research Study 95310). Storrs, CT: The National Research Center on the Gifted and Talented.

Bloom, B. (Ed.). (1985). *Developing talent in young people.* New York: Ballantine Books.

Chapman, S.M. (1991). Introducing young children to real problems of today and tomorrow. *Gifted Child Today, 14*(2), 14–18.

Csikszentmihalyi, M. (1990). *Flow: The psychology of optimal experience.* New York: Harper and Row.

Csikszentmihalyi, M. (1996). *Creativity: Flow and the psychology of discovery and invention.* New York: HarperCollins.

Csikszentmihalyi, M. (1998). Creativity and genius: A systems perspective. In A. Steptoe (Ed.), *Genius and the mind: Studies of creativity and temperament.* New York: Oxford University Press.

Csikszentmihalyi, M., Rathunde, K., & Whalen, S. (1993). *Talented teenagers: The roots of success and failure.* New York: Cambridge University Press.

Daniels, S. (1997). Creativity in the classroom: Characteristics, climate, and curriculum. In N. Colangelo & G.A. Davis (Eds.), *Handbook of gifted education* (2nd ed.). Boston: Allyn & Bacon.

Davis, G.A. (1992). *Creativity is forever.* Dubuque, IA: Kendall/Hunt.

Davis, G.A. (1999). *Creativity is forever* (4th ed.). Dubuque, IA: Kendall/Hunt.

Delcourt, M.A.B. (1988). *Characteristics related to high levels of creative/productive behavior in secondary school students: A multi-case study.* Unpublished doctoral dissertation, The University of Connecticut, Storrs.

Delcourt, M.A.B. (1994). Characteristics of high level creative productivity: A longitudinal study of students identified by Renzulli's three-ring conception of giftedness. In R.F. Subotnik & K.D. Arnold (Eds.), *Beyond Terman* (pp. 401–436). Norwood, NJ: Ablex.

Gardner, H. (1983). *Frames of mind: The theory of multiple intelligences.* New York: Basic Books.

Gardner, H. (1993). *Creating minds.* New York: Basic Books.

Hébert, T.P. (1993). A developmental examination of young creative producers. *Roeper Review: A Journal on Gifted Education, 16,* 22–28.

Kirschenbaum, R.J., & Reis, S.M. (1997). Conflicts in creativity: Talented female artists. *Creativity Research Journal, 10*(2&3), 251–263.

MacKinnon, D.W. (1978). *In search of human effectiveness.* Buffalo, NY: Creative Education Foundation.

Perleth, C., Sierwald, W., & Heller, K.A. (1993). Selected results of the Munich longitudinal study of giftedness: The multidimensional/typological giftedness model. *Roeper Review, 15*(3), 149–155.

Pirozzo, R. (1982). Gifted underachievers. *Roeper Review, 4,* 18–21.

Reis, S.M. (1998). *Work left undone: Compromises and challenges of talented females.* Mansfield Center, CT: Creative Learning Press.

Reis, S.M., Burns, D.E., & Renzulli, J.S. (1992). *Curriculum compacting: The complete guide to modifying the regular curriculum for high ability students.* Mansfield Center, CT: Creative Learning Press.

Reis, S.M., Hébert, T.P., Diaz, E.P., Maxfield, L.R., & Ratley, M.E. (1995). *Case studies of talented students who achieve and underachieve in an urban high school* [Research Monograph 95120]. Storrs, CT: National Research Center for the Gifted and Talented.

Reis, S.M., & McCoach, D.B. (2000). The underachievement of gifted students: What do we know and where do we go? *Gifted Child Quarterly, 44,* 152–170.

Renzulli, J.S. (1977). *The enrichment triad model: A guide for developing defensible programs for the gifted and talented.* Mansfield Center, CT: Creative Learning Press.

Renzulli, J.S. (1978). What makes giftedness? Reexamining a definition. *Phi Delta Kappan, 60,* 180–184, 261.

Renzulli, J.S. (1986). The three ring conception of giftedness: A developmental model for creative productivity. In R.J. Sternberg & J.E. Davidson (Eds.), *Conceptions of giftedness* (pp. 53–92). New York: Cambridge University Press.

Renzulli, J.S., & Reis, S.M. (1985). *The schoolwide enrichment model: A comprehensive plan for educational excellence.* Mansfield Center, CT: Creative Learning Press.

Renzulli, J.S., & Reis, S.M. (1994). Research related to the Schoolwide Enrichment Model. *Gifted Child Quarterly, 38,* 2–14.

Renzulli, J.S., & Reis, S.M. (1997). *The schoolwide enrichment model: A how-to guide for educational excellence.* Mansfield Center, CT: Creative Learning Press.

Renzulli, J.S., & Smith, L.H. (1978). *The compactor.* Mansfield Center, CT: Creative Learning Press.

Rimm, S.B., & Olenchak, F.R. (1991). How FPS helps underachieving gifted students. *Gifted Child Today, 14*(2), 19–22.

Rothenberg, A. (1990). *Creativity and madness: New findings and old stereotypes.* Baltimore: Johns Hopkins University Press.

Runco, M.A. (1992). The evaluative, valuative, and divergent thinking of children. *Journal of Creative Behavior, 25,* 311–319.

Russ, S., Robins, A., & Christano, B. (1999). Imaginative youngsters become creative problem solvers. *Creativity Research Journal, 12,* 129–139.

Simonton, D.K. (1988). *Scientific genius: A psychology of science.* Cambridge, England: Cambridge University Press.

Starko, A.J. (1986). *The effects of the revolving door identification model on creative productivity and self-efficacy.* Unpublished doctoral dissertation, The University of Connecticut, Storrs.

Sternberg, R.J., & Lubart, T. (1993). Creative giftedness: A multivariate investment approach. *Gifted Child Quarterly, 37*(1), 7–15.

Torrance, E.P. (1962). *Guiding creative talent.* Englewood Cliffs, NJ: Prentice-Hall.

Torrance, E.P. (1978). Healing qualities of creative behavior. *Creative Child and Adult Quarterly, 3*(3), 146–158.

Torrance, E.P. (1984). Some products of twenty-five years of creativity research. *Educational perspectives, 22*(3), 3–8.

Torrance, E.P. (1987). Teaching for creativity. In S.G. Isaksen (Ed.), *Frontiers of creativity research: Beyond the basics* (pp. 189–215). Buffalo, NY: Bearly Limited.

Torrance, E.P. (1988). The nature of creativity as manifest in its testing. In R.W. Sternberg (Ed.), *The nature of creativity*. New York: Cambridge University Press.

Torrance, E.P. (1995). *Why fly? A philosophy of creativity*. Norwood, NJ: Ablex.

Walberg, H.J., & Stariha (1992). Productive human capital: Learning, creativity, and eminence. *Creativity Research Journal, 5*, 323–340.

Walberg, H.J., & Zeiser, S. (1997). Productivity, accomplishment, and eminence. In N. Colangelo & G.A. Davis (Eds.), *Handbook of gifted education* (2nd ed.). Boston: Allyn & Bacon.

Whitmore, J.R. (1980). *Giftedness, conflict, and underachievement*. Boston: Allen & Bacon.

Wildauer, C.A. (1984). *Identification and nurturance of the intellectually gifted young child within the regular classroom: Case histories*. Washington, DC: US Department of Education, Educational Information Center (ERIC Document No. ED254041).

Willings, D. (1983). *The gifted child grows up*. Washington, DC: US Department of Education, Educational Information Center (ERIC Document No. ED252038).

Winner, E. (1996). *Gifted children: Myths and realities*. New York: Basic Books.

Winner, E., & Martino, G. (1993). Giftedness in the visual arts and music. In K.A. Heller, F.J. Monks, & A.H. Passow (Eds.), *International handbook of research and development of giftedness and talent* (pp. 253–281). New York: Pergamon Press.

Creativity, Adulthood

Sally M. Reis

INTRODUCTION

This entry discusses the major theories associated with the development of creativity in talented adults. Significant theories associated with creativity are reviewed, as are gender differences and blocks to creativity that may emerge in the creative process. The entry concludes with suggestions for promoting creativity in adulthood.

DEFINITIONS

Creativity is often defined in one of four categories of definitions: the creative person, process, product, or environment.

The Creative Person. Some theorists believe that some persons have higher innate levels of creative potential, even though this is expressed in creative products through environmental support.

The Creative Process. Several researchers have discussed a process that persons undertake in creative work, described by Wallas (1926) as including four steps: preparation, incubation, illumination, and verification.

The Creative Product. The creative product is usually discussed in terms of attributes such as originality, elaboration, novelty, but also social value. For example, Barron (1988) defines a creative product as something new that has been brought into existence purposefully.

The Creative Environment. Theorists discuss the environment, either social or psychological, as a necessary component to the development of creativity because some environments may support creative works, while others may repress them.

A *talented adult* is a person with the potential and motivation to create new and original work that will have a significant impact on a field or area of work.

SCOPE

It is impossible to identify the incidence of creativity in talented adults. Even indicators like the number of patents merely skims the surface of creative acts, large and small. However, almost everything of value in society is likely to have been the product of a creative act.

THEORIES

Near the beginning of the 20th century, Freud hypothesized that creativity focused on the motivation to create as a sublimation of the libido of the Id into a redirection of energy into more acceptable forms of creative work. By the middle of that century, Maslow described 15 characteristics of self-actualized persons; most relevant here, Maslow suggested that a person actively uses his/her potential in becoming whatever he/she is capable of becoming. In more recent years, other theories of creativity have tried to identify components of that potential.

Sternberg and Lubart's Investment Theory

Sternberg (1988) offered a three-facet model of creativity, defining it as an intersection among intelligence, cognitive style, and personality/motivation. Sternberg and Lubart (1993) viewed creativity as a type of giftedness, rather than as a dimension of intelligence. They propose that a person's "resources" for creativity enable a process of creative production to occur. Because they believe that six separate resources combine to interactively yield creativity, they find creative giftedness to be a rare occurrence. Sternberg and Lubart's six "resources" succinctly describe many of the traits of creative individuals:

1. *Intellectual Processes.* Creatively gifted people excel in problem definition, using insight (selective encoding, selective comparison, selective combination, and divergent thought) to solve problems. These intellectual processes of creatively gifted learners are not measurable by traditional IQ tests.

2. *Knowledge.* Knowledge of the domain allows for one to identify areas where new and novel work is needed. To some extent knowledge may serve as a hindrance to creativity, as too much of it can limit the ability to have fresh ideas.

3. *Intellectual (Cognitive) Styles.* Creatively gifted people tend to prefer a legislative style (creating, formulating, and planning) and a global mode of processing information (thinking abstractly, generalizing, and extrapolating).

4. *Personality.* Five key personality attributes are important to creative giftedness: tolerance of ambiguity, moderate risk-taking, willingness to surmount obstacles and persevere, willingness to grow, and belief in self and ideas.

5. *Motivation.* A task-focused orientation (drive or goal that leads a person to work on a task, as opposed to a goal-focused orientation (extrinsic motivators, rewards, or recognition which lead people to see a task as a means to an end), often exists in creatively gifted individuals. (See also Renzulli, 1978, 1986.)

6. *Environmental Context.* Environmental resources play into creativity as well. Implications for primary prevention include providing surroundings that promote creativity, a reward system for creative ideas, and an evaluation of creative products by appropriate audiences in both children and adults.

Csikszentmihalyi's Concept of Flow

Csikszentmihalyi (1988) defines creativity as the product of a talented person who experiences a period of training; this person is adventurous, and perhaps even insubordinate; there is an encouraging domain or discipline within which the individual works; and there is an audience that decides the quality of the creations. In his more recent work, Csikszentmihalyi (1990) discusses *flow* as the complete involvement in an activity to such an extent that nothing else seems to matter and the experience is totally enjoyable.

Gardner's Theory

Gardner's (1993) conception of a creative individual is one who "*regularly* solves problems or fashions products in

a *domain*, and whose work is considered both novel and acceptable by knowledgeable members of a field" (p. xvii). Creativity should not be regarded as a construct in the mind or personality of an individual; rather it is something that emerges from the interactions of intelligence (personal profile of competencies), domain (disciplines or crafts within a culture), and field (people and institutions that judge quality within a domain).

Renzulli's Theory of Creative Productivity

Renzulli's (1978, 1986) theory identifies three clusters that contribute to the creative productiveness of an individual. He identifies the interaction among above-average ability, task commitment, and creativity as the necessary components for "gifted behavior" that results in creative productivity. He later identified "a host of other factors (personality and environmental) that must be taken into account in our efforts to explain what causes some persons to display gifted behaviors at certain times and under certain circumstances" (Renzulli & Reis, 1997, p. 8). These factors can be studied in the lives of creative people.

Renzulli also discusses the differences between "high intellectual ability or potential" and "high creative ability or potential" as two broad categories. In school-aged youngsters, Renzulli (1986) referred to these as "schoolhouse giftedness" and "creative/productive giftedness." Schoolhouse giftedness refers to test-taking, lesson-learning, or academic giftedness. Individuals who fall into this category generally score well on more traditional intellectual or cognitive assessments, and also perform well in school. Creative/productive giftedness, on the other hand, is reflected in individuals who tend to be producers (rather than consumers) of original knowledge, materials, or products, and who employ thought processes that tend to be inductive, integrated, and problem-oriented.

Runco's Theory

Runco (1991) suggested that two broad personality and cognitive "transformations" occur in the development of high levels of creativity in persons of high ability. The first is the development of outstanding creative ability during the first two decades of life and the second begins in adolescence and entails the transformation of creative abilities into an integrated set of cognitive skills, career-focused interests and values, specific creative personality dispositions, and moderately high ambitions. Runco (1990) also discussed the viability of an implicit theory of creativity as a specific conception of creativity that exists in one's mind, and that can serve a prototype of creativity used by persons within a field to decide if either a product or a person is creative.

MacKinnon's Threshold Concept

MacKinnon's (1978) controversial concept of the threshold suggests that individuals with high intelligence may or may not have high creative ability or potential as well (Davis & Rimm, 1988; Renzulli & Reis, 1997). There is evidence, however, to suggest that a relationship exists between creativity and intelligence. MacKinnon's threshold concept describes a base level (an IQ of about 120) of intelligence as essential for creative productivity. Beyond that threshold, no relationship exists between creativity and intelligence as measured by IQ tests (Davis & Rimm, 1988; Sternberg, 1988).

Reis' Diversification of Creativity Theory

Reis discusses how gender differences influence creative accomplishment in talented women. She suggests that women tend to diversify their creative efforts or be obliged to diversify their efforts into several different areas including relationships, work-related to family and home, personal interests, aesthetic sensitivities, and appearance (Reis, 1987, 1991, 1995, 1996, 1998). The effect of this diversification is that women's creative efforts take many forms, which reduces the possibility of focusing on any one specific area, such as high culture art or laboratory science. This diversification of creativity is eloquently illustrated by one participant in a study of older creative women (Reis, 1995). When asked about the periods of creative productivity in her life (as one of the first female producers on Broadway), she expressed the key idea of the diversity model:

> Women spend their lives moving from one creative act to another and they find satisfaction from their creative expression in many different outlets. I have found that men, on the other hand, see an end goal and move directly toward the pursuit of that creative goal. That is why men are able to achieve goals and fame more quickly than women, but I think that women have a richer creative journey, find joy in the diversity of their creative acts, and in the end, enjoy the creative process so much more. (As reported in Reis, 2001, p. 251)

Systems Approach

Another approach to the organization of studying creativity evolved in the late 1980s—the systems model. This perspective emerged in the creativity literature from Gruber's work focusing on the life of Charles Darwin, and his attempt to put that life into the context of the social milieu in which Darwin lived. The study of eminent adults was found to be an appropriate way to look at the development of the person, process, product, and situation in which the person's life existed. Gruber called this *the evolving systems theory* (Piirto, 1999).

RESEARCH

The study of creativity has intrigued thinkers for centuries with the Greeks attributing it to the Muses and different generations of humanity extolling it as either a gift from God or a curse. Theorists have speculated regarding how education, parenting, mentoring, motivation, life experiences, environment, and even chance contributes to the development of creativity in those with innate talents and gifts (Albert & Runco, 1990; Simonton, 1988; Tannenbaum, 1990). Creativity and the creative process of talented persons have been studied by examining the lives of adults who have achieved high levels of recognition in their fields (Albert, 1996; Gardner, 1993; Goertzel, Goertzel, & Goertzel, 1978; Wallace & Gruber, 1989) and analyzing common factors during the developmental years (Goertzel & Goertzel, 1962; Simonton, 1987). Definitions of creativity often focus on the original product and its uniqueness as determined by society (Albert & Runco, 1990; Csikszentmihalyi, 1988). I will focus this discussion of research on the four components of creativity.

The Creative Individual

For many years, the study of creativity focused on the individual and the identification of personality traits of talented, creative people (MacKinnon, 1978; Torrance, 1962) with the implication that creativity was essentially innate. Is a very talented person born with the potential to be more creative than a person with fewer obvious talents, or does a person who becomes recognized as having creative talents simply have the opportunities, resources, and encouragement (Renzulli & Reis, 1997)? Researchers have begun to study the traits that distinguish creatively talented persons from those who are not creative. For example, distinctive characteristics of creative and talented artists can include openness to experience, imagination, impulsivity, anxiety, emotional sensitivity, ambition, non-conformity, and independence (Davis, 1999).

The Creative Process

Over the years, ways to describe different creative processes have evolved. One way has been to examine the stages or processes that a creative person goes through. Most models generally describe a combination of seemingly unrelated thoughts that form a new idea. The first published stage model delineated four steps: preparation (looking for the "real" problem), incubation (preconscious thinking during an unrelated activity), illumination (a sudden change in perception—an "Aha!"), and verification (checking the solution) (Wallas, 1926). The Creative Problem Solving Model (CPS), includes six steps and emphasizes problem finding, fact finding, and solution finding (Osborn, 1963).

This process has also been described as a change in perception or mental transformation (Guilford, 1986). Perceptual change or transformation is characterized by examining the elements of creative inspiration or insight often in Gestalt psychology. How this process works is not well understood, yet observation reveals that it is somewhat involuntary or unconscious (Davidson, 1986).

The Creative Product

The third major area of study in creativity focuses the development of creative products. Some people create a product that a knowledgeable audience recognizes as unique and distinctive, while others make products that are sellable without being unique. The characteristics of a creative product have been long debated and include adjectives such as: innovativeness, originality, style and uniqueness. However, it is difficult to define these terms satisfactorily.

The Creative Environment

Researchers have also studied the environments that support or block creative expression. Many believe that creative work blossoms in some receptive work, home, and learning environments and is stifled in other non-receptive ones. Blocks to creative expression have been studied by a number of researchers and are discussed in a later section.

Research on Gender Differences in the Creativity in Talented Persons

Ajzenberg-Selove (1994) and Bateson (1990) have observed that male professors publish more than female professors. Callahan (1979) and Reis (1987, 1998) note that men earn more degrees in professional fields then females. Even in areas such as literature men are more productive than women. Also, more men than women have been recipients of grants from the National Endowment Fellowships in Literature.

The majority of research on creativity and productivity in adult life has concentrated on men (Cattell, 1903; Diamond, 1986; Lindauer, 1992; McLeish, 1976; Schneidman, 1989; Sears, 1977; Simonton, 1977, 1984, 1989). However, this emphasis has been questioned, and recent research is now studying creativity in women as well (Ochse, 1991; Piirto, 1991). For example, Nichol and Long (1996) have studied creativity, stress, and female musicians. Reis (1995) found that the reason some talented women who have children cannot pursue creative professional endeavors is the absence of large blocks of time to devote to their work. Walberg and Stariha (1992) suggested that achieving recognition in a given field may require 70 hours per week of disciplined effort over a decade or more, a time commitment which is nearly impossible for women who are raising children.

Helson (1996) studied the creative personality in women, finding that self-reports of imaginative and artistic interests correlate with occupational creativity, and that creative vitality was associated with being in an encouraging environment. Helson compared a sample of highly creative women mathematicians with a sample of other female mathematicians. The two groups differed only slightly on measures of intelligence, cognition, and masculine traits, but creative subjects engaged in more research activity, were highly flexible and original, and rejected outside influence. Half of the creative women were foreign born, and most had professional men as fathers. As compared with creative male mathematicians, the creative women had less assurance, published less, and occupied less prestigious positions. Helson also found differences between creative and comparison subjects in background and personality. The traits most characteristic of the creative women seemed to be (a) rebellious independence, introversion, and a rejection of outside influence; (b) strong symbolic interests and a marked ability to find self-expression and self-gratification in directed research activity; and (c) flexibility, both in general attitudes and in mathematical work. Helson attributed differences in creative productivity between men and women after graduate school to social roles and institutional arrangements.

Foley (1986) studied 15 artists who were mothers and found that these women experienced guilt and conflict between their roles as mothers and artists. The extent to which female artists have uninterrupted time to work on their art, and the manner in which they find time to produce art, remains largely ignored in the research literature and was the subject of this study. The age at which women artists create art and find uninterrupted time for their work was also investigated in this study. Reis (1995) suggested that some talented women's peak age for creative productivity and eminence may occur at a later age. Kirschenbaum and Reis (1997) used a comparative case study approach to investigate the development of artistic talent among female artists who also had children. Intensive interviews with 10 female artists revealed that their priority in life was their family but that their art was also essential for creative self-expression. Artistic productivity was dependent upon a number of factors, including self-discipline, financial support and security, spousal encouragement and support, childrearing responsibilities, job demands, access to artistic materials/ equipment, and workspace availability. The female artists in this study reported that they often faced difficult choices related to their art, their relationships with their husbands, and with their children who often diverted their attention from their art. However, they all persevered and continued with their art. Ironically, the obstacles that they encountered, such as the absence of support from spouses and parents, financial difficulties and time necessary to raise their children were perceived by these women as contributing in some ways to their creative process and the development of their identities as artists.

STRATEGIES THAT WORK

There is no available information about a program to promote creativity in adults that has received rigorous documentation. We do have a great deal of information about *creative persons* (Barron, 1988; MacKinnon, 1978); *processes* (Gardner, 1993), and *environments* (Davis, 1999; Sternberg, 1988; Sternberg & Lubart, 1993) that are associated with creative products, but no one has turned this information into a program to promote creativity in talented adults.

STRATEGIES THAT MIGHT WORK

Gardner (1993) studied creative and talented persons across several domains, finding that creativity is a dynamic process that occurs as an ongoing dialectic among talented individuals, domains of expertise, and fields charged with judging the quality of creations. According to Gardner (1993), this dynamic process can be characterized by various kinds of tensions and asynchronies that, if not overwhelming, can prove conducive to the fostering of creative individuals, processes, and products. Gardner also summarizes a portrait of the Exemplary Creator (EC), generalizing from his research on highly talented creators, such as Einstein, Gandhi, Stravinsky, and Martha Graham.

The basic question is how to use these and other pieces of information about known creative persons, processes, and environments, in order to promote creativity in other talented adults, while being sensitive to such issues as gender, culture, and other circumstances. We are only at the beginning of this process.

STRATEGIES THAT DO NOT WORK

Blocks to Creativity in Talented Adults   Davis (1999) discusses some of the most common blocks to creative thinking and productivity as: habit and learning, rules and traditions, perceptual blocks, cultural blocks, emotional blocks, and resource blocks. Habit and learning blocks occur because of our well-learned responses and customary ways of thinking and responding. Rules and traditions that seem necessary for life may restrict creative thought or processes. Perceptual blocks occur because humans are accustomed to perceiving things in familiar ways and it is difficult to see new meanings in occurrences that we encounter regularly. Perceptual blocks may prevent us from identifying problems or from understanding the world around us.

Cultural blocks may also affect creative potential in talented individuals and involve social norms and expectations as well as pressures to conform. Torrance (1977, 1979) found that creativity in children drops when they enter kindergarten and then slumps again when they reach fourth grade, perhaps due to the conformity expected in school. There may be equivalent cultural blocks when people reach adulthood and become part of the fabric of society.

Davis (1999) also discusses emotional blocks to creativity that may include anger, fear, hate, or even love. Van Gundy (1987) noted that emotional barriers such as a fear of taking risks and of being viewed as uncertain or different may have an impact on the ability to work creatively. Van Gundy also discussed resource barriers to the development of high levels of creativity such as the lack of time, money, materials, or information that may impair one's ability to do creative work.

SYNTHESIS

New Directions for Developing Creative Potential in Talented Adults   Too few talented people have opportunities as adults to engage in sustained creative work; the routines of conventional society are very strong and necessary. However, there is also a great need to innovate, to discover new questions as well as new solutions, if society is to progress. What can be suggested to promote creativity in adulthood?

Creative Adults

There are many adults who have the potential to make creative contributions to society. We know what they are like: independent-minded, non-conformists, and energetic (Barron, 1988). We know what they need: encouragement to make use of their skills, a place in which to do them, and rewards for beginning efforts. Schools and colleges, businesses, and non-profit corporations might set up structures to encourage creative efforts—from scholarships, to "think tanks" that provide the space, resources, and security to exercise these talents, to support groups for innovative thinking. The critical issue is to have people believe in themselves as having creative talents, and to offer encouragement as broad-based as possible to nurture these talents.

Creative Processes

Most of these creative processes seem to involve ordinary problem solving set at a higher complexity of effort. Adults can be given education and encouragement for considering divergent ideas in combinations, or breaking out of the box of conventional solutions, of seeking new ways of seeing old problems. In short, it is possible to teach techniques for creative thinking. It is an empirical question as to whether people who use these techniques will actually create new products, but it is fairly certain that if they do not use them, there is little likelihood of their being creative.

Creative Products

It is difficult to know the unknown, but one fruitful method is to work backward from what one wants to attain, to find the possible stepping stones by which to attain it. The first task is to imagine what products would be desirable, and then to figure out ways of moving toward them.

Creative Environments

The role of the audience is critical in artistic, commercial, and scientific products. In these cases, we can encourage these audiences to be receptive to new ideas and to give approval to those efforts that are innovative and have social value.

We have to imagine a world without its Einsteins, Gandhis, O'Keefes, and Curies, in order to understand that we may have already lost their equivalents by lack of support for promoting creativity. This is not to say that we should abandon all of the other worthy educational programs across the human spectrum, while favoring only the talented. Rather, it is that we have to recognize the value of creativity as the foundation for an optimal life for all of us.

Also see: Creativity: Early Childhood; Creativity: Childhood; Creativity: Adolescence; Creativity: Older Adulthood; Culture, Society, and Social Class: Foundation.

References

Ajzenberg-Selove, F. (1994). *A matter of choices: Memoirs of a female physicist*. Brunswick, NJ: Rutgers University Press.

Albert, R.S. (1996). What the study of eminence can teach us. *Creativity Research Journal, 9*(4), 307–315.

Albert, R.S., & Runco, M.A. (1990). The achievement of eminence: A model based on a longitudinal study of exceptionally gifted boys and their families. In R.J. Sternberg & J.E. Davidson (Eds.), *Conceptions of giftedness* (pp. 332–357). Cambridge, MA: Cambridge University Press.

Barron, F. (1988). Putting creativity to work. In R.J. Sternberg (Ed.), *The nature of creativity* (pp. 76–98). New York: Cambridge University Press.

Bateson, M.C. (1990). *Composing a life*. New York: Plume, The Penguin Group.

Callahan, C.M. (1979). The gifted and talented woman. In A.H. Passow (Ed.), *The gifted and talented* (pp. 401–423). Chicago: National Society for the Study of Education.

Cattell, J.M. (1903). A statistical study of eminent men. *Popular Science Monthly, 62*, 359–377.

Csikszentmihalyi, M. (1988). Society, culture and person: A systems view of creativity. In R.J. Sternberg (Ed.), *The nature of creativity* (pp. 325–339). Cambridge, MA: Cambridge Press.

Csikszentmihalyi, M. (1990). *Flow: The psychology of optimal experience*. New York: Harper & Row.

Davidson, J.E. (1986). Insight and giftedness. In R.J. Sternberg & J.E. Davidson (Eds.), *Conceptions of giftedness* (pp. 201–222). Cambridge, MA: Cambridge University Press.

Davis, G.A. (1999). *Creativity is forever* (4th ed.). Dubuque, IA: Kendall/Hunt Publishing Company.

Davis, G.A., & Rimm, S. (1988). *Education of the gifted and talented* (4th ed.). Boston: Allyn & Bacon.

Diamond, A.M. (1986). The life-cycle research productivity of mathematicians and scientists. *Journal of Gerontology, 41*, 520–525.

Foley, P. (1986). *The dual role of experience of artistic mothers*. Unpublished dissertation, Northwestern University, Chicago.

Gardner, H. (1993). *Creating minds*. New York: Basic Books.

Goertzel, M.G., Goertzel, V., & Goertzel, T.G. (1978). *Three hundred eminent personalities*. San Francisco: Jossey-Bass Publishers.

Goertzel, V., & Goertzel, M.G. (1962). *Cradles of eminence*. Boston: Little, Brown.

Guilford, J.P. (1986). *Creative talents: Their nature, uses and development*. Buffalo, NY: Bearly Limited.

Helson, R. (1996). In search of the creative personality. *Creativity Research Journal, 9*(4), 295–306.

Kirschenbaum, R.J., & Reis, S.M. (1997). Conflicts in creativity: Talented female artists. *Creativity Research Journal, 10*(2,3), 251–263.

Lindauer, M.S. (1992). Creativity in aging artists: Contributions from the humanities to the psychology of old age. *Creativity Research Journal, 5*, 211–231.

MacKinnon, D.W. (1978). *In search of human effectiveness: Identifying and developing creativity*. Buffalo, NY: The Creative Education Foundation, Inc.

McLeish, J.A.B. (1976). *The Ulyssean adult: Creativity in the middle and later years*. New York: McGraw-Hill/Ryerson.

Nichol, J.J., & Long, B.C. (1996). Creativity and perceived stress of female music therapists and hobbyists. *Creativity Research Journal, 9*(1), 1–10.

Ochse, R. (1991). Why there were relatively few eminent women creators. *Journal of Creative Behavior, 25*(4), 334–343.

Osborn, A.F. (1963). *Applied imagination* (3rd ed.). New York: Scribners.

Piirto, J. (1991). Why are there so few? (Creative women: Visual artists, mathematicians, musicians). *Roeper Review, 13*(3), 142–147.

Piirto, J. (1999). A survey of psychological studies in creativity. In A.S. Fishkin, B. Cramond, & P. Olszewski-Kubilius (Eds.), *Investigating creativity in youth: Research & methods* (pp. 27–48). Creskill, NJ: Hampton Press, Inc.

Reis, S.M. (1987). We can't change what we don't recognize: Understanding the special needs of gifted females. *Gifted Child Quarterly, 31*(2), 83–89.

Reis, S.M. (1991). The need for clarification in research designed to examine gender differences in achievement and accomplishment. *Roeper Review, 13*(4), 193–198.

Reis, S.M. (1995). Talent ignored, talent diverted: The cultural context underlying giftedness in females. *Gifted Child Quarterly, 39*(3), 162–170.

Reis, S.M. (1996). Older women's reflections on eminence: Obstacles and opportunities. In K.D. Arnold, K.D. Noble, & R.F. Subotnik (Eds.), *Remarkable women: Perspectives on female talent development* (pp. 149–168). Cresskill, NJ: Hampton Press, Inc.

Reis, S.M. (1998). *Work left undone: Compromises and challenges of talented females*. Mansfield Center, CT: Creative Learning Press.

Reis, S.M. (2001). Toward a theory of creativity in diverse creative women. In M. Bloom & T. Gullotta (Eds.), *Promoting creativity across the life span* (pp. 231–275). Washington, DC: CWLA Press.

Renzulli, J.S. (1978). What makes giftedness?: Reexamining a definition. *Phi Delta Kappan, 60*, 180–184.

Renzulli, J.S. (1986). The three-rings conception of giftedness: A developmental model for creative productivity. In R.J. Sternberg & J.E. Davidson (Eds.), *Conceptions of giftedness* (pp. 53–92). New York: Cambridge University Press.

Renzulli, J.S., & Reis S.M. (1997). *The schoolwide enrichment model: A how-to guide for educational excellence*. Mansfield Center, CT: Creative Learning Press.

Runco, M.A. (1990). Implicit theories and ideational creativity. In M.A. Runco & R.S. Albert (Eds.), *Theories of creativity* (pp. 234–252). Newbury Park, CA: Sage.

Runco, M.A. (1991). The evaluative, valuative, and divergent thinking of children. *Journal of Creative Behavior, 25*(4), 311–319.

Schneidman, E. (1989). The Indian summer of life: A preliminary study of septuagenarians. *American Psychologist, 44*, 684–694.

Sears, R. (1977). Sources of satisfaction of Terman's gifted men. *American Psychologist, 32*, 719–728.

Simonton, D.K. (1977). Creative productivity, age, and stress: A biographical time-series analysis of 10 classical composers. *Journal of Personality and Social Psychology, 35*, 791–804.

Simonton, D.K. (1984). *Genius, creativity, and leadership*. Cambridge, MA: Harvard University Press.

Simonton, D.K. (1987). Developmental antecedents of achieved eminence. *Annals of Child Development, 5*, 131–169.

Simonton, D.K. (1988). Creativity, leadership, and chance. In R.J. Sternberg (Ed.), *The nature of creativity* (pp. 386–426). New York: Cambridge University Press.

Simonton, D.K. (1989). *Scientific genius*. New York: Cambridge University Press.

Sternberg, R.J. (1988). A three-faceted model of creativity. In R.J. Sternberg (Ed.), *The nature of creativity* (pp. 125–147). Cambridge: Cambridge Press University.

Sternberg, R.J., & Lubart, T.I. (1993). Creative giftedness: A multivariate investment approach. *Gifted Child Quarterly, 37*(1), 7–15.

Tannenbaum, A.J. (1990). Giftedness: A psychosocial approach. In R.J. Sternberg & J. E. Davidson (Eds.), *Conceptions of giftedness* (pp. 21–52). Cambridge, MA: Cambridge University Press.

Torrance, E.P. (1962). *Guiding creative talent*. Englewood Cliffs, NJ: Prentice-Hall.

Torrance, E.P. (1977). *Creativity in the classroom*. Washington, DC: National Education Association.

Torrance, E.P. (1979). *The search for satori and creativity*. Buffalo, NY: Creative Education Foundation.

Van Gundy, A.B. (1987). Organizational creativity and innovation. In S.G. Isaksen (Ed.), *Frontiers of creativity research: Beyond the basics* (pp. 358–379). Buffalo, NY: Bearly Limited.

Walberg, H.J., & Stariha, W.E. (1992). Productive human capital: Learning, creativity, and eminence. *Creativity Research Journal, 5*, 323–340.

Wallace, D.B., & Gruber, H.E. (1989). *Creative people at work*. New York: Oxford University Press.

Wallas, G. (1926). *The art of thought*. New York: Harcourt, Brace, Jovanovich.

Creativity, Older Adulthood

Martin Bloom

INTRODUCTION

This entry will discuss the promotion of creativity in older persons, a topic on which little is known, and less studied empirically. Yet, fascination with creative people has tantalized observers throughout history. It may be fruitful to speculate from what is known about creativity in general, and about the "new" older person in the 21st century, to consider what might be possible in promoting creativity in older persons.

DEFINITIONS

The term creativity has been defined in several ways. First, creativity refers to the generating of an idea, a process, or product that is new to the individual and is accepted by others as original and socially useful (Fasko, 1999; Simonton, 2000). The research literature generally uses this national reputation sense in studies of "creative people." However, there is a second sense used within a developmental or personal context because the creation of a child or some adults or older persons may be qualitatively different. The child's creation may be new and innovative, even if it never gets beyond posting on the refrigerator door. An adult or older person who undertakes some enterprise new to him or her, which pushes beyond where he or she has ever gone, may be said to be creative to that person, even if no other audience defines it as socially useful. It serves its purpose for the creator alone. A third or local sense of creativity would involve a person pursuing his or her creative interests, whose work comes to the attention of a local community audience, and gains a local reputation—even though this person may never enter the national scene.

These three definitions—let me distinguish the national/international sense as creativity, the local sense as creativity, and the personal sense as creativity—may, on occasion, blur, as when a Grandma Moses, originally painting for her own amusement, finds that her neighbors also enjoy her paintings, and then by good luck becomes a commercial success on a national level. This entry focuses on the promotion of personal creativity, because this is where the overwhelming numbers of older people are in terms of their experiences in creative efforts. The other levels of creative production are probably self-initiated and self-sustained. However, seeking ways to promote creativity at the personal level does not mean promoting trivial pursuits. Rather, personal creativity may be linked with finding important meanings and self-satisfaction in life, beyond whatever products emerge.

Gerontologists make the distinction among the young old (roughly age 65–74), the middle old (75–84), and the old old (85 and over) because each has differences that are developmentally important (Hooyman & Kiyak, 1996). The elderly in general, but the young old in particular, are very different from older persons of a generation or two ago. They tend to be better educated, healthier, and wealthier, and by virtue of these factors, in the context of retirement, they are involved in their extended family, the community, and the world like no other generation before them (Klein & Bloom, 1997). The middle old and the old old benefit from advances in social security, nutrition, medicine, and education so that more of these older persons are living longer and in better circumstances than any group of older persons in past times. This means that more people will have more time and resources to be actively engaged in the community, and to do more for themselves and others than ever before, even though many have various chronic conditions that are impediments to creative activities. A whole new ball game exists with regard to being old in the 21st century, at least in developed nations. However, this is not to say that the picture for older persons is perfect, for all people will die and most will sustain some period of difficulty, disease, and/or disability before death.

SCOPE

There are approximately 6 billion creative people on this planet, albeit varying by degree, assuming that creativity is normally distributed among persons in a society (Nicholls, 1972; Simonton, 2000). Theoretically, we should expect to find creative ideas, processes, and products evenly distributed across the life span and between the genders. However, this is not the case. Simonton (1988, p. 252) described the observed patterns this way:

> One empirical generalization appears to be fairly secure. If one plots creative output as a function of age, productivity tends to rise fairly rapidly to a definite peak and thereafter declines gradually until output is about half the rate at the peak .... This cross-cultural and transhistorical invariance strongly suggests that the age curves reflect underlying psychological universals rather than sociocultural determinants ....

Perhaps Simonton is correct, but these empirical findings may also reflect near universal patterns of pervasive discrimination and differential access to resources and support for some types of individuals, which could equally well account for Simonton's curve. Men, and mostly young to middle-aged men, are predominant among the lists of recognized creative artists and scientists. Although there are exceptions like Grandma Moses and the elderly Michelangelo, what is important in the context of this entry is the paucity of older persons among the highest levels of creativity in any domain. There are many barriers and facilitators for different groups of persons at different stages of life. The fundamental question for this entry is whether personal creativity itself diminishes or is eliminated in older persons. If not, then how can it be promoted in older persons?

THEORIES AND RESEARCH

Many theories of creativity involve developmental considerations. Levy and Langer (1999) present a *peak and decline model* in which creativity is supposed to peak in a person's 30s and decline thereafter. This model receives some empirical support from the listings of the age at which artists' and scientists' most effective creations were produced. Lehman's (1953) classic investigation indicated that effective productivity was a function of age, but different forms of creative efforts had different peaks and declines: poetry and mathematics peaked early; longer and more complex novels or plays were generally produced later in life. These developmental models reflect a common bias against older persons. Even Freud suggested that psychoanalysis should not be conducted with persons over 50 because they lacked personal insight and the ability to make meaningful changes. Dennis (1956) challenged Lehman's work on grounds that total productivity did not vary by age, and by the obvious fact that many well-known artists and scientists (including Freud) made important contributions in their later years.

Levy and Langer (1999) describe a second type of theory of creativity in older persons, a *life span developmental model*, which views creativity as the result of one's underlying cognitive processes that change with one's life stage, as well as with one's social and cultural experiences. This perspective may help to explain why there are differential rates of recognized creative productivity between men and women, younger and older adults, and among the various cultural groups, because of the differential life experiences each group faced. This position also permits multiple creative careers, in which a person finds some way to relaunch him or herself by undertaking new challenges, using new media, or in new disciplines.

The Freudian model of the artist hypothesizes a psychological regression into the unconscious in order to experience the raw materials of creativity, and then a return to reality to rework these materials into some public form (Vaillant, 2000). A behavioral model of creativity would involve combining things that are only remotely associated in conventional life into something unique and socially useful (Fasko, 1999). A social learning model (Bandura, 1986) would seek to identify what knowledge, skills, and motivation, and what perceived self-efficacy a person possessed in order to engage in creative activities. Neither the Freudian, the behavioral, or the social learning approaches has led to any notable research in creative production, although many writers use the terms to describe ex post facto what must have been the case to generate some given artistic product.

As Atchley (2000) points out, there are physical, sensory, and motoric losses in old age, but many of these losses may be coped with, compensated for, and overcome in the pursuit of some creative effort. Indeed, the very pursuit of creativity may be a factor in adapting successfully with the changes that occur during old age, including the middle old and the old old. Levy and Langer (1999) discuss how creativity can influence aging, indeed how creative acts may contribute to life itself. Great artists, they point out, live longer than the general population (cf. Vaillant & Vaillant, 1990). In general, the stimulation of the creative process appears to bring "life to years," as well as "years to life." This is a provocative hypothesis.

In a different context, Pelz and Andrews (1966) and Pelz (1972) discuss creativity in organizational settings, contrasting what is characteristic of highly successful organizations with less successful ones. What they describe is a complex view of the interaction of both persons and environments. Essentially, they suggest that creative productivity in scientific organizations is a combined function of a high degree of challenge and a high degree of support that moves through a process leading to a high probability of a creative product. (There is no inevitability in being successful, but as Pasteur commented, "nature favors the prepared mind.") By challenge, Pelz means some demand made by a legitimate authority for the person (or team) to achieve some goal. This is pressure; this generates anxiety during the work process. By support, Pelz means the provision of time, space, resources, the climate that this appropriately educated and trained individual (or team) can do it, and ultimately the rewarding feedback of informed peers. Thus, by inference, to promote creativity in older persons, we have to provide the range of support and the individual has to accept the (social or personal) challenge. However, this is exactly what society does not do for older persons, and others (women, minorities in particular).

We have some general theoretical ideas about creativity, in the individual and between the individual and his or her environment. The question is how to use this body of theory and research to provide strategies to promote personal creativity in older persons. How and where can we invite creativity in older persons?

There are numerous studies of art programs in nursing homes, institutional settings, and in continuing education courses where creativity is invited. These reports are often intriguing, although not yet of compelling scientific design. For example, Doric-Henry (1997) used an intervention involving an 8-session pottery class with 20 nursing home residents (ages 50–95 years) and compared their psychological well-being, self-esteem, and levels of depression and anxiety with 20 non-participating elderly nursing home residents. Qualitative evaluations showed that participants improved in measures of self-esteem and in reduced depression and anxiety. Wikstroem, Ekvall, and Sandstroem (1994) reported their controlled intervention with 40 elderly institutionalized females who were randomly assigned to an intervention or control group. The intervention consisted of nondirected use of pictures of art as a way of stimulating creativity. Results showed the intervention group more open

and flexible, with increased imagination and freedom in their own drawings, than the controls, a finding that continued after a 4-month follow-up. Wikstroem, Theorell, and Sandstroem (1993) report that these women (aged 70–97) also improved their well-being, as indicated by positive mood indicators such as happiness and peacefulness; improvements were also reported in their medical health status.

Callanan (1994) described art therapy with frail older persons as a means of accessing personal experiences and dealing with them. Although this involves working with conflicted individuals, the author makes the point that art work reinforces the autonomy of the older person when other losses make such autonomy limited—in a therapy or a non-therapy context. Likewise, qualitative data in Wilkinson, Srikumar, Shaw, and Orrell's (1998) study support the hypothesis that drama and movement therapy improved social interactions in everyday life. However, the cautions that Marshall and Hutchinson (2001) offer on the use of activities with persons with Alzheimer's disease should be considered in this entire discussion of the promotion of creativity in older persons: There are, as yet, many theoretical and methodological limitations in these studies that lead to limited findings and unclarity as to important questions of gender, ethnic, and cultural differences. More rigorous theory and research are needed, adapted to capture the distinctive features of older persons in everyday life.

It is important to add that creativity has a dark side (Kastenbaum, 2001) because to create often means to destroy what had been accepted as right, true, or beautiful before. Creativity as the creation of new and socially useful products may be socially useful to evil leaders—how to build a better bomb. Like fire, creativity may burn brightly, but remember that it may also burn.

STRATEGIES: OVERVIEW

The search for strategies to promote personal creativity in older persons involves providing opportunities for older persons in their homes, in senior centers or other places where older persons may congregate, and in institutions where necessary. Opportunities will likely involve challenges and resources (Pelz), as appropriate to the setting and to the participants. The challenges may include positive opportunities as well as negative barriers regarding creative experiences. The resources will include internal traits, as well as what social and cultural resources are available. Programs should be conceptually clear (in terms of a theory guiding practice), empirically rigorous, with replications involving persons and environments in different contexts. Has any program in promoting personal creativity in older persons fulfilled these criteria?

STRATEGIES THAT WORK

A search of the literature revealed no empirically based, theoretically guided programs that fulfill the high standard described above.

STRATEGIES THAT MIGHT WORK

Promising strategies probably follow the Pelz model, of creating challenges appropriate to the situation, and providing opportunities that are relevant. We certainly prime the pump with preschoolers in high quality Head Start programs, offering them many types of tools and setting up time for creative endeavors. We may prime the pump as well in high quality senior centers or places for assisted living. Unfortunately, none of these situations have been studied to see what effect challenge and opportunity have on the person's creative effort. Nor do we have adequate theory to guide that practice.

Creativity in old age, especially the middle old and the old old, may reflect a fear of death and the now-or-never motivational component, something like the swan song as Simonton (1989) describes it, but in every form of creative production. On the other hand, personal creativity in old age may reflect engagement with life, the integrity that Erikson (1968) describes, the putting together of the strands of one's life in some new and personally meaningful form. If it is also socially useful, society is the beneficiary. Journal writing offers one approach to coming to terms with one's life, and in so doing, leaving the record of a life to one's posterity (Berman, 1991). It may have a therapeutic effect, as in Butler's (1963) notion of life review. But it can also serve a healthy function, a positive life review, as described by Klein and Bloom (1997, pp. 87–93). Perhaps, the first-time creative explorations into drawing, or story-telling, or being a foster grandparent, may also represent a new expanded or integrated sense of self, as a meaningful contributor to humanity.

STRATEGIES THAT DO NOT WORK

We cannot order (force) creativity; it must be invited, provided for, facilitated. We cannot lecture about creativity; we must involve people in interactive, or hands-on ventures. Any strategy may eventually meet unmovable obstacles in the serious illness and decline of the older person, but short of this, almost every other condition, from poverty to isolation, may find adaptations that help to fulfill a person's creative urge and possibly make contributions to self and society.

SYNTHESIS

Csikszentmihalyi (1996) and Reis (2001) describe what may be the best set of proposals for enhancing personal creativity. I will adapt these suggestions to the promotion of personal creativity in older persons as a source of their mental health and, where the stars are properly aligned, for the social good as well.

1. *Engage one's energies for creative purposes.* As people retire, they generally restrict their social interactions to what is more essential to them. This may include a full range of beginnings or continuations of what they had been doing throughout their lives, from consummate volunteer community service or consummate fishing, to the fine arts or fine conversations with friends. In the older years, they may begin to devote major and undivided attention to these endeavors, rather than spending their time on the formerly necessary tasks of making a living or making someone else's living more agreeable. To begin these new endeavors requires support of family and friends, and the availability of resources in the community.

2. *Curiosity and interest should be cultivated, an independence of mind and self-permission for artistic risk taking.* For one long experienced with everyday events and objects, it will require effort to move beyond the familiar, to see things in a new way, even when energy and sensory equipment may be diminished. But adaptive measures abound. Memory always serves us, as Mark Twain once remarked, whether the event happened or not. Many stimulating books on tape and CDs are available for persons whose vision is becoming limited. Reis (personal communication, 1995) described an older creative woman on her death bed who was working her way through a stack of classic books on tape. She remarked to her interviewer: "So many books to hear, so little time." Curiosity can be cultivated to last a lifetime. Drawing by computer opens up new possibilities for persons of any age. Senior centers are available in local areas, and elderhostel-type organizations make travel to distant areas more available. Curiosity probably comes easily to an older person long accustomed to be creative; it may require pump priming for the ordinary older person regarding the knowledge, skills, motivation, and sense of self-efficacy to achieve a particular goal (Bandura, 1986).

3. *Cultivate the flow of creativity in everyday life.* Csikszentmihalyi suggests that one wake up in the morning with a specific goal to look forward to, especially what one does well and enjoys. To keep enjoying something, one must become increasingly aware of its nature, simple or complex. This suggestion is especially important for older persons whose external world may not provide the structure that it once did.

4. *Keep awakened creative energy active.* Many writers advise that we should stop distracting ourselves (Csikszentmihalyi, 1996). This would involve making better channels for one's creative energy to flow by taking charge of one's time schedule and making sure one leaves time for reflection and relaxation. This principle would also suggest that people shape their living/working spaces to make them serve the creative tasks. A room of one's own, as Virginia Woolf said, and an adequate income to provide the time to be creative in that room. This may be difficult for some older persons relocating to smaller accommodations. Prioritize: One should do more of what one wants to do, and less of what one doesn't want to do.

5. *Accentuate one's strengths.* We know a lot about general factors that are related to creativity, but whether some set of such factors will in fact lead to creative products is unknown. Csikszentmihalyi suggests developing what you lack; this may not always be possible for older persons who may become dependent on the services of others. He also suggests shifting from openness to closure as a part of living the sometimes contradictory life of a creative person in a conforming society. Again, older persons may not have an option to do this, especially as they grow much older. However, a final suggestion is quite possible: to aim at careful examination of the target of one's creativity and to observe the complexity of it. Here is where the wisdom of older persons, the innumerable life experiences that provide perspective and nuance on the human condition, may enable the older person to accentuate his/her strengths.

6. *Extend one's self beyond the envelope of everyday motions.* Reis (2001) suggests that problem finding—look for questions and not only the answers—is important in the creative life. This may involve finding a way to express oneself that moves one to see something in a new way. Look at the problems or challenges from as many viewpoints as possible, as ways to consider divergent viewpoints. Creativity is never a finished business, but a process in process.

Also see: Creativity: Early Childhood; Creativity: Childhood; Creativity: Adolescence; Creativity: Adulthood; Culture, Society, and Social Class: Foundation.

References

Atchley, R.C. (2000). *Social forces and aging: An introduction to social gerontology* (9th edition). Belmont, CA: Wadsworth Thomson Learning.

Bandura, A. (1986). *Social foundations of thought and action: A social cognitive theory*. Englewood Cliffs, NJ: Prentice-Hall.

Berman, J.J. (1991, Spring). For the pages of my life. *Generations*, 33–40.

Butler, R.N. (1963). The life review: An interpretation of reminiscence in the aged. *Psychiatry, 26*, 65–76.

Callanan, B.O. (1994). Art therapy with the frail elderly. *Journal of Long Term Home Health Care, 13*(2), 20–23.

Csikszentmihalyi, M. (1996). *Creativity: Flow and the psychology of discovery and invention*. New York: HarperCollins.

Davis, G.A. (1999). Barriers to creativity and creative attitude. In M.A. Runco & S.R. Pritzker (Eds.), *Encyclopedia of creativity* (pp. 165–174). San Diego, CA: Academic Press.

Dennis, W. (1956). Age and achievement: A critque. *Journal of Gerontology, 11*, 331–333.

Doric-Henry, L. (1997). Pottery as art therapy with elderly nursing home residents. *Art Therapy, 14*(3), 163–171.

Erikson, E.H. (1968). Life cycle. In D.L. Sills (Ed.), *The international encyclopedia of the social sciences*. New York: Crowell, Collier, & Macmillan.

Fasko, D. (1999). Associative theory. In M.A. Runco & S.R. Pritzker (Eds.), *Encyclopedia of creativity* (pp. 135–139). San Diego, CA: Academic Press.

Hooyman, N., & Kiyak, A. (1996). *Social Gerontology*. Needham Heights, MA: Allyn & Bacon.

Kastenbaum, R. (2001). Riding the tiger: The challenge of the creative renewal in the later adult years. In M. Bloom & T.P. Gullotta (Eds.), *Promoting creativity across the life span* (pp. 277–310). Washington, DC: CWLA Press.

Klein, W.C., & Bloom, M. (1997). Successful aging: Strategies for healthy living. New York: Plenum.

Lehman, H.C. (1953). *Age and achievement*. Princeton, NJ: Princeton University Press.

Levy, B., & Langer, E. (1999). Life span development model. In M.A. Runco & S.R. Pritzker (Eds.), *Encyclopedia of creativity* (pp. 45–52). San Diego, CA: Academic Press.

Marshall, M.J., & Hutchinson, S.A. (2001). A critique of research on the use of activities with persons with Alzheimer's disease: A systematic literature review. *Journal of Advanced Nursing, 35*(4), 488–496.

Nicholls, J.G. (1972). Creativity in the person who will never produce anything original and useful: The concept of creativity as a normally distributed trait. *American Psychologist, 27*(8), 717–727.

Pelz, D.C. (1972). Environments for creative performance within universities. Paper Presented at the Conference on Cognitive Styles and Creativity in Higher Education, Montreal.

Pelz, D.C., & Andrews, F.M. (1966). *Scientists in organizations: Productive climates for research and development*. New York: Wiley.

Reis, S.M. (1995). Older women's reflections on eminence: Obstacles and opportunities. *Roeper Review, 18*(1), 66–72.

Reis, S.M. (2001). Toward a theory of creativity in diverse creative women. In M. Bloom & T.P. Gullotta (Eds.), *Promoting creativity across the life span* (pp. 231–275). Washington, DC: CWLA Press.

Simonton, D.K. (1988). Age and outstanding achievement: What do we know after a century of research? *Psychological Bulletin, 10*(2), 251–267.

Simonton, D.K. (1989). The swan-song phenomenon: Last works effects for 172 classical composers. *Psychology and Aging, 4*(1), 42–47.

Simonton, D.K. (2000). Creativity: Cognitive, personal, developmental, and social aspects. *American Psychologist, 55*(1), 151–158.

Vaillant, G.E. (2000). Adaptive mental mechanisms: Their role in a positive psychology. *American Psychologist, 55*(1), 89–98.

Vaillant, G.E., & Vaillant, C.O. (1990). Determinants and consequences of creativity in a cohort of gifted women. *Psychology of Women Quarterly, 14*, 607–616.

Wikstroem, B., Ekvall, B., & Sandstroem, S. (1994). Stimulating the creativity of elderly institutionalized women through works of art. *Creativity Research Journal, 7*(2), 171–182.

Wikstroem, B., Theorell, T., & Sandstroem, S. (1993). Medical health and emotional effects of art stimulation in old age: A controlled intervention study concerning the effects of visual stimulation provided in the form of pictures. *Psychotherapy and Psychosomatics, 60*(3–4), 195–206.

Criminal Behavior, Adulthood

Mark B. Borg, Jr. and Emily Garrod

INTRODUCTION

Theoretical approaches to the prevention of adult criminal behavior range from those that focus on the individual and the community to those that target specific crimes and their prevention in specific areas. With the exception of strategies that target specific crimes in specific areas, there appear to be few direct links between primary prevention and adult criminal behavior. Public health approaches to crime prevention claim to implement primary prevention strategies, but these approaches do not target adults (Tonry & Farrington, 1995). The highly controversial, and historically political nature of defining criminals and criminal behavior may contribute to the paucity of primary prevention strategies in this area (Foucault, 1975). While the link between primary prevention and adult criminal behavior is often tenuous, we can address theories and approaches that have attempted to locate and influence people who are naturally exposed to the conditions that foster crime.

DEFINITIONS

Felner and Lorion (1989) state that "a preventative intervention involves the systematic alteration and modification of processes related to the development of adaptation and well-being or disorder, with the goals of increasing or decreasing, respectively, the rate or level with which these occur in the [target] population" (p. 93). Developmental studies have shown that common antecedents, such as family resources and interaction patterns, economic and social deprivation, life stresses, powerlessness, and a number of non-specific resiliency factors (e.g., social support, self-efficacy, hope), all influence the probability that members of a population will develop patterns of disordered behavior (Felner, Felner, & Silverman, 2000). We must also consider the possibility that target (criminal) behaviors may reflect adaptive solutions to disordered contextual conditions (Moynihan, 1986). Primary prevention of criminal behavior is, therefore, defined as the modification of criminogenic conditions in the physical and social environment at large.

The definition of criminal and criminality is a highly controversial process that ranges in perspective from political to psychiatric. Political definitions of criminality which include aspects of racial identity and/or political ideology, such as those implemented in Nazi Germany, South Africa's Apartheid, and a multitude of dictatorial regimes serve as potent examples of the potential for definitions of criminality to be used in ways that oppress and terrorize, rather than protect, targeted segments of the population.

From an historic psychiatric perspective, the "typical criminal" has had a history that, if monitored and diagnosed, began in childhood or adolescence with Oppositional Defiant Disorder, which was, at some point, reassessed as Conduct Disorder and finally led to Antisocial Personality Disorder. According to the DSM-IV (APA, 1994) "The essential feature of Antisocial Personality Disorder is a pervasive pattern of disregard for, and violation of, the rights of others that begins in early childhood or early adolescence and continues into adulthood" (p. 645). Deceit and manipulation, failure to conform to social norms regarding lawful behavior, impulsivity, irritability, aggressiveness, lack of remorse and repetitive patterns of illegal actions are among the criteria for this disorder. Traditionally this disorder is associated with low socio-economic status and urban settings, and questions have been raised regarding misapplication of this diagnosis to individuals in settings in which such behaviors may be part of protective survival strategies (Sadock & Kaplan, 1998). In contexts of both political oppression and severe socio-economic deprivation behaviors defined as criminal by those outside the immediate community may be viewed by community members as necessary survival strategies (Skogan, 1994; Sperry, 1995). Therefore, in the definition of adult criminal behavior we must be aware of relevant community norms and values.

SCOPE

According to *Crime state rankings 2000* (Morgan & Morgan, 2000), the most recent findings on the number of victims of all types of crimes (including "personal crimes," "property crimes," but not including murder) was 31,307,000 in 1998.[1] In the case of murder, the reported national arrest rate for 1998 was 6.5 percent reported arrests per 100,000 in

---

[1] The most comprehensive and objective assessment of overall national crime rates was completed 12/29/99 by the US Bureau of the Census (Morgan & Morgan, 2000, p. A-2).

the US population (p. 8). Nationally, there were 5,563 reported arrests per 100,000, resulting in a 4.4 percent increase in the number of state prisoners from 1997 to 1998 (p. 48); 6.4 percent of state prisoners are female (p. 55).[2] The expense of state and local government judicial and legal payroll in 1998 was $13,750,837,716 (p. 179).[3] This figure accounts only for the legal expenses associated with court proceedings regarding adult criminal behavior and does not reflect the huge expense of housing and managing inmate populations. In general, studies have shown that for every dollar spent on prevention, cost savings of between $3 and $10 may be realized in reduced demand for after-the-fact service (Felner et al., 2000). However, as the incidence, prevalence, and reported costs of adult criminal behavior is greatly under-reported, and existing statistics do not adequately represent the broad range of crimes, criminals, and expenditures, the accuracy of this equation is difficult to assess.

THEORIES

There are two broad approaches to crime prevention: the public health approach and the criminal justice approach. The public health perspective views crime or, more specifically, violence as emerging from complex causal systems, not only offenders' intentions, motivations and characters. Favored interventions take place at the level of primary prevention—the prevention of harms before they occur (Moore, 1995). Criminal justice approaches generally intervene at the secondary or tertiary levels, when the signs of crime have been identified or when rehabilitation after adjudication has begun. Moore (1995) states that,

> Advocates of the criminal justice approach view arresting, prosecuting and jailing offenders as preventing crime through four mechanisms: (1) general deterrence (i.e., the effect that comes from threatening everyone in the population with criminal prosecution if they violate laws); (2) specific deterrence (i.e., the effect on an individual criminal offender that comes from punishing him for a specific offense); (3) incapacitation (i.e., the effect that comes from holding an offender under such close supervision that it is impossible for him to commit offenses); and (4) rehabilitation. (p. 249)

[2] The national arrest rates noted by Morgan and Morgan (2000) are based on arrest numbers reported by the FBI and are only from those law enforcement agencies that submitted complete arrest reports for 12 months in 1998. The editors stated that these numbers were, therefore, subject to underestimating the actual incidence and prevalence rates of crime in the United States and should be interpreted with caution.

[3] This includes court and court-related activities (except probation and parole), activities of sheriff's offices, prosecuting attorneys' and public defenders' offices, legal departments and attorneys providing government-wide legal services.

The public health approach to prevention also has a number of strategies: (1) preventing first offenses (i.e., developmental crime prevention); (2) technological manipulations of the environment (i.e., physically changing the environment to reduce its vulnerability to crime); (3) cultural approaches (i.e., addressing risk factors such as violence on TV); and (4) education. In trying to shape attitudes and behavior, the public health approach often prefers educational to legal strategies. Public health efforts to prevent adult criminal behavior generally target violent behaviors, focus interventions on children and adolescents, and redirect attention and resources to victims. This approach encourages an assessment of the causes of crime, which influence, rather than begin with, the offender.

The criminal justice system, while a key deterrent and a necessary component in crime prevention, is not sufficient. For every 100 offenses committed, 49 are reported to the police, 30 are reported by them, seven are cleared up, and two result in a conviction (Laycock & Tilley, 1995). The main problem with crime prevention strategies that focus solely on the use of the criminal justice system is that, given the high degree of effort, they are increasingly understood to have only modest effects on rates or patterns of crime (Glensor, Correia, & Peak, 2000). The public health approach, in contrast, may neglect the law as an instrument for education as well as a device for authorizing state intervention. Both approaches, singularly, appear limited and inadequate to address the severity and variability of adult criminal behavior. The public health perspective views the criminal justice system as being reactive and overly reliant on traditional police tactics (i.e., arrest and incarceration), while the criminal justice approach views the public health approach as being overly optimistic in its view of the mutability of human behavior (Clarke, 1997). The public health perspective potentially complements that of criminal justice by focusing on crime as a threat to both community health and community order, both victims and offenders, and on crime between intimates as well as strangers.

STRATEGIES: OVERVIEW

An assessment of crime and criminals, as well as the recorded differences between Antisocial Personality Disorder prevalence rates and general crime statistics, suggests an immense diversity of crimes and criminals (Duff, 1995). A variety of offenders commit a variety of crimes for a variety of reasons, and prevention strategies need to take account of those differences. The following strategies approach prevention of adult criminal behavior from a wide variety of perspectives and intervention techniques.

STRATEGIES THAT WORK

It appears that the most effective potential strategy would be a blend of public health and criminal justice approaches, which included situational crime prevention techniques, specific policing tactics, and communitarian concepts; all within the larger context of community building as crime prevention. For example, increasing natural surveillance through street-lighting (a situational technique) and traditional policing tactics, such as crackdowns on known drug-retailing sites are likely to be maximally effective when they are viewed by members of the community they effect as collaboratively derived solutions by community members to community problems (a communitarian ideal). Community building projects maximize the effectiveness of crime prevention when specific strategies are viewed as only one aspect in a larger, integrative effort to empower community residents to articulate and solve their own problems. The complex, integrative community building approach to adult crime prevention is a primary prevention strategy that directly reduces targeted criminal behaviors while also addressing the larger context in which they occur.

Community Building as Crime Prevention

The National Crime Prevention Council (1994) states that, "Crime prevention is defined as patterns of attitudes and behaviors directed at reducing the threat of crime and enhancing the sense of safety and security, to positively influence the quality of life in our society and to help build environments where crime cannot flourish" (p. 107). This definition clarifies the importance of community as a base for prevention. It also recognizes that there is a dual task: reducing crime's threat to the community and developing communities that discourage crime.

The US Department of Housing and Urban Development (HUD) has developed a Healthy and Safe Communities initiative, which is an approach to comprehensive community revitalization that identifies crime prevention as a primary goal. Previous program interventions share the common goal of stabilizing and transforming communities through coordinated and broad-based efforts that engage community members in restoring the social fabric of their respective communities. Primary interventions tend to cluster around specific issues: (1) community organizing and broadening of participation; (2) strengthening local collaborations and linkages (with special attention paid to the role of community policing); (3) improving access to education, skills, training and jobs; (4) enhancing the quality of school life, and creating better youth motivational programs; (5) improving social and other services; (6) developing

a base of economic prosperity for the community; and (7) enhancing the physical quality of life (Borg, 1997). The community building approach assumes that crime is part of an ecological picture that includes other community variables, not only economic ones, but cultural, moral, symbolic and perhaps even spiritual (DeLeon-Granados, 1999). According to this model, the community and the police (as well as representatives from within both the public health and criminal justice system) co-produce safety. Indigenous solutions—specific to a time and place and developed from within the community's own agenda—are derived collaboratively. The overriding assumption is that people stop crime, specifically people who form cohesive, interdependent communities. The key to this community-based collaborative approach is sustained involvement, not temporary mobilization to address specific threats.

A four-year comprehensive community revitalization pilot program run in collaboration with the US Department of Housing and Urban Development's Safe and Healthy Communities initiative in the South Bronx, evidenced a 54 percent reduction in crime (Mills, 1996). A four-year community revitalization program that was modeled after the South Bronx intervention was implemented in 1993 in South Central Los Angeles in the immediate aftermath of the "civil unrest" (e.g., riots) and showed equally promising results (Borg, 1997; Borg, Garrod, & Dalla, 2001). Similar programs are now being conducted nationally and are considered exemplars of community crime prevention.

STRATEGIES THAT MIGHT WORK

Situational, community policing, and communitarian approaches may work as primary prevention strategies on a limited basis. It is when we begin to address long-term implications that these specific approaches, in isolation, are likely to be lacking in efficiency and, in certain instances, may be detrimental. Short-term effectiveness must be weighed, on a case by case basis, against negative long-term effects (e.g., increased community apathy and alienation from law enforcement personnel) through increasing awareness of specific community issues, values and norms.

Situational Prevention

Situational prevention theories support strategies that are designed to prevent the occurrence of crimes by reducing opportunities and increasing risks, based on the premise that much crime is contextual and opportunistic. Situational crime prevention, according to Clarke (1997), is defined as:

> Comprising measures directed at highly specific forms of crime that involved the management, design, or manipulation

of the immediate environment in as systemic and permanent a way as possible so as to reduce the opportunities of crime and increase its risks as perceived by a wide range of offenders. (p. 91)

Situational prevention techniques include: (1) increasing perceived efforts (e.g., through target hardening by electronic tagging of merchandise and increasing access control through parking lot barriers), to reduce opportunities by making crimes more difficult to commit; (2) increasing perceived risks (e.g., through formal surveillance by closed-circuit TV and increased entry/exit screening); and (3) reducing anticipated rewards (e.g., through removing inducements by putting smaller, more valuable items behind the counter and identifying property to prevent resale); among others. Studies suggest that situational crime prevention strategies are highly effective. Clarke (2000) cites evidence from 23 successful case studies of situational crime prevention programs conducted in the United States and Britain, where the most effective reductions in crime were evidenced at 50 percent, although the author adds that "situational measures usually ameliorate, rather than eliminate problems" (p. 202). Other critics of this approach have stated that it displaces crime, rather than genuinely preventing it by addressing underlying causes and situational factors such as unemployment, socioeconomic status, family constellation and make up, lack of education and career training (Tonry & Farrington, 1995).

Community Crime Prevention

Community crime prevention targets the community but does not directly link police and community members. Interventions are designed to change the social conditions that influence offending in residential communities. Whether individuals commit crimes, in this model, is probabilistically related to where they live. Community crime prevention is based on the premise that changing the community may change the behavior of the people who live there. It has included efforts to control crime by altering building and neighborhood design to increase natural surveillance and guardianship, improving the physical appearance of areas, organizing community residents to take preventive actions and to solicit additional political and material resources, and organizing self-conscious community crime prevention strategies (Felson, 1994).

The effectiveness of the community approach appears to depend, in part, on how broadly one defines community. Residential groups, who attempt to stem crime without the support of local institutions, groups, and/or agencies, feel such approaches generally cannot sustain a unified program for the area as a whole (Foster & Hope, 1993). Efforts to reshape contextual cues to prevent crime, such as citizens banding together to change the look of their neighborhoods or

to provide neighborhood watch groups, often fall short along class lines as poorer communities seldom independently start, carry through, or maintain collective efforts because of their transient populations (Skogan, 1990). Therefore, community action occurs less often among those who need it the most—the disadvantaged (Verba, Schlozman, Brady, & Nie, 1993). The empirical evidence for the effectiveness of community crime prevention, in the absence of other community development approaches, is lacking (Carter & Sapp, 2000; Hope, 1995). While communities that have implemented these strategies have shown significant reductions in the incidence of specific crimes, these interventions have coincided with other community development projects and, therefore, their specific contribution to crime reduction is unknown (Forrester, Chatterton, & Pease, 1988; Henggeler, Schoenwald, Borduin, Rowland, & Cunningham, 1998).

Communitarianism

Communitarianism is founded on the belief that neighborhood crime problems can be solved primarily through self-help efforts of residents, and that "laws communicate and symbolize those values that the community holds dear" (Etzioni, 1993, p. 133). Braithwaite (1989) describes Communitarian society as:

> A dense network of individual interdependencies with strong cultural commitments to mutuality of obligation.... Interdependence and mutual obligation together provide the resource for social control; not only are members of such a community likely to be subject to shame or exclusion if they individually transgress, but also each individual feels confident to enlist the support of others to act on deviants and maintain the norms of the community. (pp. 85–86)

This is a strategy of social avoidance where in-group members strictly control outside influence. Ultimately, in the Communitarian ideal, community members would either have to enforce a segmented order, based on a consensus on agreed-upon (by the in-group) laws of the moral majority, or strive to integrate offenders into their communities. There have been no empirical studies of the Communitarian approach. Media strategies to prevent minor offenses, such as littering, suggest that appeals to common ideals of citizenship may, at times, be effective. Critics of Communitarianism view it as tending toward discrimination and insularity through its narrow emphasis on conventional or normative values and behavior (DeLeon-Granados, 1999).

Community Policing

The practice of community policing is based on the assumption that police interventions are severely hampered without the full cooperation of community members and resources. Community policing views police acting as catalysts for local change by helping community members to exploit their own informal social control abilities. Some important characteristics of community policing are: (1) decentralization (to encourage officer initiative and the effective use of local knowledge); (2) geographically defined rather than functionally defined subordinate units (to encourage the development of local knowledge); and (3) close interactions with local communities (Peak & Glensor, 2000).

Community-Oriented Policing and Problem Solving (COPPS) is a specific approach to community policing that has been developed from Goldstein's (1979) identification of the concept of problem-oriented policing to the present time. COPPS is a proactive philosophy that involves identifying, analyzing, and addressing crime and other community problems at their source. The COPPS philosophy emphasizes the need to redefine who is responsible for public safety and the roles and relationships between the police and the community. Police and community members work cooperatively to identify problems and develop long-term, proactive community-wide solutions. COPPS requires shared ownership, decision making, accountability, and sustained commitment from both the police and the community. To be effective, this approach requires a police management style, which includes diverse public feedback into the decision making process and the establishment of new public expectations of, and measurement standards for, police effectiveness (Community Policing Consortium, 1994; Glensor et al., 2000). Empirical evidence for the effectiveness of community policing is mixed (Eck & Maguire, 2000; Sherman, 1997). There is little empirical evidence to support the effectiveness of increasing the number of police officers in a given area. However, directed patrols in hot spots, firearms enforcement, and retail drug market enforcement have shown reasonably strong quasi-experimental support for their effects (Blumstein & Wallman, 2000). It is not clear, however, whether these effects are based on specific implementation strategies, targeting repeat offenders, or other trends effecting drug markets and crime (Eck & Maguire, 2000). Critics of community policing argue that its reliance on arrest and conviction statistics is likely to negate latent problem-solving skills indigenous to the community. The net effect can result in a crime-control model that disturbs the community ecology more than it stabilizes it, one in which officers fail to exploit fully cohesive, resourceful community networks, in favor of surveillance, crackdowns, sweeps, arrests, and problem obliteration (DeLeon-Granados, 1999).

STRATEGIES THAT DO NOT WORK

Strategies that do not work as primary prevention techniques are those which have either negligible immediate

effectiveness or whose short-term effectiveness is outweighed by severe long-term negative effects. For instance, increasing the number of police officers in a given area without any effort to integrate them into the community has been found to be ineffective (Blumstein & Wallman, 2000). On the other hand, zero-tolerance strategies may have short-term effectiveness in reducing crime; however, their long-term consequences of alienating and criminalizing community members are likely to outweigh short-term effectiveness.

Zero-Tolerance Policing

In contrast to community police measures, which attempt to produce order and reduce crime through cooperation with community members, zero-tolerance policing attempts to impose control through strict law enforcement (Cordner, 1998). This approach tends toward invasive measures and has been labeled "harassment policing" (Panzarella, 1998). A component of this approach is to "crackdown" on misdemeanors and minor violations, hence increasing the visibility of the police. Critics allege that minorities bear the brunt of this strategy, as minority members have been frequently and disproportionately subjected to arrest, stop-and-frisk searches, disrespect, and brutality (Human Rights Watch, 1998; Yardley, 1999). While such strategies claim to have significantly reduced crime, in New York City for example, significant concerns have been expressed about their inherent potential for abuse, discrimination, and violation of civil liberties (Eck & Maguire, 2000; Greene, 1999; Hassell, Peyton, Zhao, & Maguire, 1999). There is little evidence to support the effectiveness of zero-tolerance policing. Evidence on the effectiveness of related generic order-maintenance strategies on reducing violent crime are mixed (Reiss, 1985; Sherman, 1990). Critics of these strategies believe they increase criminality by leading offenders (or potential offenders) to become more angry and defiant, or by labeling minor offenders as criminals, thereby increasing their potential to commit future crimes (Buerger, 1994; Cordner, 1998).

Strategy Assessment

Clearly, there is need for assessment techniques that accurately measure the outcomes of crime prevention strategies. Empirical evidence for strategy effectiveness, at this time, is generally in the form of case studies, action research or, at best, quasi-experimental. Crime statistics, arrest, and indictment records are generally utilized to validate quasi-experimental evaluations of crime prevention programs (Glensor & Peak, 2000). Often, the objective of empirical evaluations in the area of crime prevention is not to document the precise value of particular interventions observed under particular circumstances, but to build a detailed understanding of the principles of effective crime reducing strategies. This more qualitative approach is based upon the assumption that crime prevention practitioners are called upon to provide tailor-made solutions for new problems arising in fresh circumstances and, therefore, quantitative measures of effectiveness are of limited generalizability (Clarke, 1997, 2000; Glensor et al., 2000).

The interlocking patterns (individual, social, environmental) that influence criminal behavior suggests that we must address larger issues, such as parenting and role-modeling, and the presence or lack of educational and financial opportunities in a given community in order to adequately account for the diverse nature of crimes and criminals. Considering the paucity of direct links between the prevention of adult criminal behavior and primary prevention strategies, we might do well to, as Albee (1981) has suggested, "look to the dynamics of the larger societal context as we attempt to formulate primary prevention programs" (p. 26).

SYNTHESIS

Generally, current crime prevention strategies remain rooted in: (1) a public health system that attempts only indirectly to prevent adult criminal behavior by targeting circumscribed age groups (children and adolescents) and specific (violent) behaviors; or, (2) a punitive, arrest- and indictment-driven criminal justice system. Neither system addresses the existing diversity of crime, criminal, and context. As DeLeon-Granados (1999) states,

> The community project is pursued with the best of intentions, and people are working hard to build community and respond to crime. But even if such a project is given every opportunity to work, there is still a disturbing tension underlying it. It is a tension about division between race and class, about using community to oil the cogs of a punitive criminal justice system and about locking people away rather than forging new relations with one another as the most important problem-solving strategy. (p. 149)

Strategies, which derive from and for specific communities, seem the most promising. A community building approach that empowers community members to address patterns and perceptions of isolation, inequality, and stagnation provides the best context for crime prevention. Crime may, after all, be viewed as a symptom of a society that is not adequately addressing the immediate and long-term developmental needs of all of its members. Therefore, the search for crime prevention must go beyond the symptom toward an awareness of crime as, in part, a reflection of the way a culture represents itself. New multidisciplinary paradigms must reflect the vast diversity of crimes, criminals, victims, and the contexts within which these three elements interact.

Also see: Culture, Society, and Social Class: Foundations; Delinquency: Childhood; Delinquency: Adolescence; Intimate Partner Violence: Adulthood; Homicide: Adolescence.

References

Albee, G.W. (1981). The prevention of sexism. *Professional Psychology, 12*, 20–28.

American Psychiatric Association (APA). (1994). *Diagnostic and statistical manual of mental disorder—fourth edition (DSM-IV)*. Washington, DC: Author.

Blumstein, A., & Wallman, J. (2000). *The crime drop in America*. New York: Cambridge University Press.

Borg, M.B. (1997). *The impact of health realization training on affective states of psychological distress and well-being*. Ann Arbor, MI: UMI.

Borg, M.B., Garrod, E., & Dalla, M. (2001). Intersecting "real worlds": Community psychology and psychoanalysis. *The Community Psychologist, 34*(2), 16–19.

Braithwaite, J. (1989). *Crime, shame and reintegration*. Cambridge: Cambridge University Press.

Buerger, M. (1994). The problems of problem-solving. *American Journal of Police, 13*, 1–36.

Carter, D., & Sapp, A.D. (2000). Community policing evaluation. In R.W. Glensor, M.E. Correia, & K.J. Peak (Eds.), *Policing communities: Understanding crime and solving problems*. Los Angeles: Roxbury.

Clarke, R.V. (1997). *Situational crime prevention: Successful case studies*. Albany, NY: Harrow and Heston.

Clarke, R.V. (2000). Situational crime prevention: Successful studies. In R.W. Glensor, M.E. Correia, & K.J. Peak (Eds.), *Policing communities: Understanding crime and solving problems*. Los Angeles: Roxbury.

Community Policing Consortium. (1994). *Understanding community policing: A framework for action*. Washington, DC: US Bureau of Justice Assistance.

Cordner, G.W. (1998). Problem-oriented policing vs. zero tolerance. In T.O. Shelley & A.C. Grant (Eds.), *Problem-oriented policing*. Washington, DC: Police Executive Research Forum.

DeLeon-Granados, W. (1999). *Travels through crime and place: Community building as crime control*. Boston: Northeastern University Press.

Duff, A. (1995). Penal communications and the philosophy of punishment. In M. Tonry (Ed.), *Crime and justice: A review of research*. Chicago: University of Chicago Press.

Eck, J.E., & Maguire, E.R. (2000). Have changes in policing reduced violent crime? In A. Blumstein & J. Wallman (Eds.), *The crime drop in America*. New York: Cambridge University Press.

Etzioni, A. (1993). *The spirit of community: Rights, responsibilities, and the communitarian agenda*. New York: Crown.

Felner, R.D., Felner, T.Y., & Silverman, M.M. (2000). Prevention in mental health and social intervention: Conceptual and methodological issues in the evolution of the science and practice of prevention. In J. Rappaport & E. Seidman (Eds.), *Handbook of community psychology*. New York: Kluwer Academic/Plenum.

Felner, R.D., & Lorion, R.P. (1989). Clinical child psychology and prevention: Toward a workable and satisfying marriage. *Proceedings: National Conference on Clinical Child Psychologists*, 41–95.

Felson, M. (1994). *Crime and everyday life*. Thousand Oaks, CA: Pine Forge Press.

Forrester, D., Chatterton, M., & Pease, K. (1988). *The Kirkholt burglary prevention project: Roachdale*. London: Home Office.

Foster, J., & Hope, T. (1993). *Housing, community and crime: The impact of the priority estates project*. London: H.M. Stationary Office.

Foucault, M. (1975). *Discipline and punish: The birth of the prison*. New York: Vintage Books.

Glensor, R.W., & Peak, K.J. (2000). Implementing change: Community-oriented policing and problem solving. In R.W. Glensor, M.E. Correia, & K.J. Peak (Eds.), *Policing communities: Understanding crime and solving problems*. Los Angeles: Roxbury.

Glensor, R.W., Correia, M.E., & Peak, K.J. (2000). *Policing communities: Understanding crime and solving problems*. Los Angeles: Roxbury.

Goldstein, H. (1979). Improving policing: A problem-oriented approach. *Crime and delinquency, 25*, 236–258.

Greene, J.A. (1999). Zero tolerance: A case study of police policies and practices in New York City. *Crime and Delinquency, 45*, 171–187.

Hassell, K., Peyton, J., Zhao, J., & Maguire, E.R. (1999). *Structural change in large municipal police organizations*. Orlando, FL: Academy of Criminal Justice Sciences.

Henggeler, S.W., Schoenwald, S.K., Borduin, C.M., Rowland, M.D., & Cunningham, P.B. (1998). *Multisystemic treatment of antisocial behavior in children and adolescents*. New York: Guilford.

Hope, T. (1995). Community crime prevention. In M. Tonry & D.P. Farrington (Eds.), *Building a safer society: Strategic approaches to crime prevention*. Chicago: University of Chicago Press.

Human Rights Watch. (1998). *Shielded from justice: Police brutality and accountability in the United States*. New York: Human Rights Watch.

Laycock, G., & Tilley, N. (1995). Implementing crime prevention. In M. Tonry & D.P. Farrington (Eds.), *Building a safer society: Strategic approaches to crime prevention*. Chicago: University of Chicago Press.

Mills, R.C. (1996). *Psychology of mind-health realization: Summary of clinical, prevention, and community empowerment applications—Documented outcomes*. Los Angeles: California School of Professional Psychology.

Moore, M.H. (1995). Public health and criminal justice approaches to prevention. In M. Tonry & D.P. Farrington (Eds.), *Building a safer society: Strategic approaches to crime prevention*. Chicago: University of Chicago Press.

Morgan, K.O., & Morgan, S. (2000). *Crime state rankings 2000*. Lawrence, KS: Morgan Quitno Press.

Moynihan, D.P. (1986). *Family and nation*. Orlando: FL: Harcourt Brace Javonovich.

National Crime Prevention Council. (1994). *Uniting communities through crime prevention*. Washington, DC: Crime Prevention Coalition.

Panzarella, R. (1998). Bratton reinvests "harassment model" of policing. *Law Enforcement News, June 15*, 13–15.

Peak, K.J., & Glensor, R.W. (2000). *Community policing and problem solving: Strategies and practices*. Upper Saddle River, NJ: Prentice-Hall.

Reiss, A.J. (1985). Policing a city's central district: The Oakland story. *National institute of justice research report*. Washington, DC: US Government Printing Office.

Sadock, B.J., & Kaplan, H.I. (1998). *Synopsis of psychiatry: Behavioral sciences, clinical psychiatry*. Baltimore, MD: Williams & Wilkins.

Sherman, L.W. (1990). Police crackdowns: Initial and residual deterrents. In M. Tonry and N. Morris (Eds.), *Crime and justice: A review of research*. Chicago: University of Chicago Press.

Sherman, L.W. (1997). Policing for crime prevention. In *Preventing crime: What works, what doesn't work, what's promising—A report to the Attorney General of the United States*. Washington, DC: US Department of Justice.

Skogan, W.G. (1990). *Disorder and decline*. Berkeley, CA: University of California Press.

Skogan, W.G. (1994). The impact of community policing on community residents: A cross-sites analysis. In D.P. Rosenbaum (Ed.), *The challenge of community policing*. Thousand Oaks, CA: Sage.

Sperry, L. (1995). *Handbook of diagnosis and treatment of the DSM-IV Personality Disorders*. Levittown, PA: Brunner/Mazel.

Tonry, M., & Farrington, D.P. (1995). *Building a safer society: Strategic approaches to crime prevention*. Chicago: University of Chicago Press.

Verba, S., Schlozman, K.L., Brady, H., & Nie, N.H. (1993). Citizen activity: Who participates? *American Political Science Review, 87*, 303–318.

Yardley, J. (1999). In two minority neighborhoods, residents see a pattern of hostile street searches. *The New York Times, March 29*, B-3.

Crisis Intervention, Older Adulthood

Ira Iscoe and Michael Duffy

INTRODUCTION

At the beginning of the new millennium, the life expectancy in the United States, was about 74 years, a truly remarkable increase from the previous century, where, at its beginning, life expectancy was about 55 years. Improving working and living conditions, enforced public health practices, advances in preventive medicine, and health education have all contributed to this increase, to mention some of the more prominent ones. At the same time the increase in longevity presents enormous problems and challenges to the behavioral and health sciences as well as public policy practices and formulations.

Currently about 14 percent of the American population is 65 years or older, and the prediction is that this will increase to about 20 percent in the next 15–20 years as the baby boomers enter the so-called third age. The fastest growing segment of the 65 plus age group is referred to as the "old old", that is, 80 years and above. There are changing perceptions of the aging population. No longer is it rare for octenagarians to actively participate in foot and bicycle races, go through successful hip and knee replacements, and to celebrate 50th and 60th wedding anniversaries. The political power of the third age population is considerable and understandably major debates center around the extent of funding for social security and the provision of health services. How can the diverse needs of an increasingly aging population be best accommodated within the framework of our society? What types of financial health and social support systems should be implemented? As the autumn of life moves into winter, what transition can be facilitated and what difficulties prevented or ameliorated? These are complex, value-laden issues that involve not only the individuals but also their spouses, families, the community at large, and many cultural and religious factors. Developmental psychology is concerned with changes in abilities as a function of increasing age. It is an appropriate starting point to a consideration of the concept of crisis, with special emphasis on aging populations.

In contrast to infancy, childhood, adolescence, and adulthood, where there is a progression in the development of various physical and mental capacities leading to an increased repertoire of competencies, the later years of life bring on gradual or sometimes sudden diminution of mental and physical functions, sometimes separately, sometimes combined. Inevitably, however, there is a decrease or impairment of activities that could be performed in earlier years. There is a saying that old age brings on increase in some functions and decreases in others. A major concern is health. There is a Chinese custom of not wishing a person long life without wishing good health also. The increase in longevity has also brought on a crisis in the science of developmental psychology. Never in history has it had to confront increased aging in large numbers of people. There is a recognition that there is a transition from autonomy to some degree of dependency, and sometimes to complete dependency. The decrease in the nuclear family has led to increased reliance on extrafamilial resources, and it is predicted that this type of reliance will increase in the future, leading to the ultimate so-called nursing or long-term arrangements, where independence is traded for security and safety, moving people from an environment they can no longer cope with, increasing their dependence on family members and other support systems.

How are these progressions to be measured? The extent of diminution of functions is frequently assessed by the Activities of Daily Living scale (ADL). This measure is designed to gauge how well a person can get along without assistance or, in reverse, what type of activities does the person need for "assisted living." The ability to get out of bed without assistance, walking without assistance, mounting steps, bathing oneself, attending to toilet needs, level of vision and hearing, short- and long-term memory functioning are some examples of assessing current ability to function independently. The number of functions that a person needs assistance with is equated to the amount of independent functions the person has. There is no full agreement as to the absence of how many functions results in the need for assisted living or that with the inability to perform most of these functions there is a need for long-term care or a change in treatment or other support areas.

In an encyclopedia devoted to prevention and health maintenance, the concept of crisis has an important part to play in helping the reader to understand the complexities

facing older persons and their families to accommodate to changes, keeping in mind that it is usually difficult for older persons to accommodate to changes in behaviors and routines that they have performed for a good part of their lives. As will be explained, crisis theory basically dictates that the individual recognizes and accepts the fact that some activities that worked in the past cannot work in the present situation. *Competent coping* is defined as recognizing the need for change and taking those actions that lead to an adjustment, to the situation that is confronted. The term adjustment does not mean acceptance. It does infer the examination of options and the acceptance of interventions designed to improve an individual's coping capacity.

Besides activities of daily living, there are changes that range from changes of living quarters, loss of loved ones, diminution of family support, financial inadequacies, and failing health. The reduction in financial resources is, as always, an important ingredient and usually increases with advancing age. The repertoire of options open to older persons is significantly less than that of younger persons, and the time available to deal with such changing situations is usually more limited. It is all the more important, therefore, that older persons are prepared for, or at least made aware of, potential changes in their daily functions, be they physical or mental. In what follows, the essentials of crisis theory are presented and descriptive examples are given of its application. An understanding of the essential basis of crisis resolution, or of the avoidance of crises, can be of material aid to older persons as well as those who play a part in helping them cope with crisis such as state and municipal agencies as well as extended families.

DEFINITION

The term crisis has many meanings in lay persons' language as well as in professional health services, all of which are pertinent in our understanding the occurrence of crises in older adults (65 plus in this context). The various concepts of crisis range from the initial and classical work within community psychiatry and community psychology (Bloom, 1984; Caplan, 1964; Lindemann, 1944; Miller & Iscoe, 1963), through application in crisis and emergency services and hotlines (Losee, Parham, Auerbach, & Teileman, 1988; Slaikeu, 1990) through the development and concept of Acute Stress Disorder (ASD) and Post-Traumatic Stress Disorder (PTSD) (Green, Wilson, & Lindy, 1985). Definitions therefore range from the popular notion of equating crisis with the stressful event itself, to the classical concept of the inner psychological destabilization that such an event may engender in some persons, to the pattern of stress-related symptoms that might follow either or both of the above situations. It should be noted that these concepts, while not synonymous, do follow a coherent trajectory from the event to the experience to the effect. Each of these aspects will be included in this entry. While work on crisis theory and intervention is not specific to any age group, it certainly is relevant to older adults (DeVries & Gallagher-Thompson, 2000; Duffy & Iscoe, 1990). Duffy (1999) deals with many of the problems of living presented by older adults and the role that counseling and therapy in the resolution.

SCOPE

Determining the prevalence and incidence of crises among older persons is complicated by several factors. First, crises are not classified as disorders and do not appear in the Diagnostic Statistical Manual of the American Psychiatric Association (1994) classification system as a basis for enumeration. Second, by definition, the classical concept of crisis involves an internal state which generally is not amenable to identification. Finally, where external symptoms can be used to estimate prevalence of crisis, these figures do not reliably apply to older cohorts. For example, PTSD is estimated to have a prevalence of 1–14 percent for the general community and 3–58 percent for high-risk groups such as crime victims, but we know of no quantifiable reliable estimates of crises among older adults. Even using symptom patterns as a basis for estimation, there is a further complication based on definitional range mentioned earlier, the presence of acute post-traumatic symptoms while clearly an indicator of an experienced stressful event do not necessarily imply a crisis in the sense of internal psychological destabilization. A person can experience stress and be traumatized without the immobilization of an internal crisis.

The consensus of clinical opinion, therefore, continues to be a useful guide to understanding the presence and proportion of crisis among older adults. There is some evidence that older adults may be more resilient than younger adults in weathering some stressful situations. However, there are also high-risk groups among the elderly, for example, those in the process of institutionalization in a nursing home (Duffy & Iscoe, 1990).

THEORIES

The classical *theory of crisis* mentioned above is composed of four elements. There is the occurrence of a *stressful event*. This may be external and situational such as a natural disaster, the experience of violent crime, or sexual violence or abuse. Alternatively, the stressful event may be internal or developmental in nature, as may be encountered in very difficult life transitions such as the stress of retirement or chronic age-related physical decline in later life. For older adults, stressful events may be hidden. For example, change of location of living, loss of the ability to drive, loss of a loved one. The insidious nature of these hidden losses can precipitate a crisis in a previously resilient older person. A nursing home example will illustrate another feature of crisis in late life. Stressful events are often multiple, simultaneous, and interacting (Duffy & Iscoe, 1990). Within a 24-hr period an older person entering a nursing home without a well-formulated orientation and adjustment period will experience these many changes simultaneously. The Geriatric Social Readjustment Scale (Amster & Krauss, 1974) identifies a series of stressful events that frequently coexist for older adults and test their coping capabilities as well as those of their concerned families.

The second element in crisis theory is the relative *internal perception* of the stressful event by the person. Most persons would experience the above events as highly stressful and even be traumatized by them, as captured in the concept of ASD and PTSD. While one person may experience such stress and still be able to function (albeit with difficulty), another might find such experiences beyond "customary methods of problem solving" (Slaikeu, 1990). Depending on previous life experience and level of resilience, a person might not only be stressed but be temporarily immobilized by the experience. The lack of previously learned strategies for this (or psychological equivalent) experience leads to an impasse. It is important to note that this concept of the crisis experience does not involve the presence of pathology. It is an essentially normal and naturalistic concept, although the presence of "premorbid psychological disorder" increases vulnerability to this type of impasse.

The third element of the crisis experience is the *symptomatic expression* of the psychological impasse, or *immobilization*. Predictably, this experience results in acute anxiety or panic symptoms or the presence of disassociative symptoms. Understandably, such an experience can alternatively be expressed as a frantic speeding up or closing down of the organism. The presence of these symptoms will be familiar to emergency care workers at disaster sites but less obvious to "quiet" crises such as complicated bereavements. The recognition of the presence of a genuine crisis is vitally important in the diagnosis and treatment of stress symptoms. ASD or PTSD may or may not involve the presence of a crisis experience as we have defined it. Similarly, "crisis hotlines" are frequently dealing with "emergencies" rather than true crises and the difference is clinically important in intervening effectively.

The fourth and final element in the crisis experience is the *resolution phase*. In naturalistic terms, the arousal of crisis will inevitably subdue over time. The key issue during this final phase is whether the person will chose an effective or ineffective solution to the situation. "Effectiveness" is defined in functional rather than ideal terms. An effective response is one that teaches a new coping skill so that a person may more successfully weather future similar or stressful events. This is the basis for the suggestion that older adults in general may have superior skills in coping with crisis. Navigating and mastering life stresses has taught them much, but at the same time they may be faced with situations in which previous coping capacities and strategies are not effective in reducing the tension and leading to constructive activities.

The theory of intervention parallels the various phases of the crisis experience. Predictable stressful events invite a preventive approach such as providing an anticipatory psychoeducational program for new nursing home residents and their families. During the resolution phase of the crisis trajectory, problem solving and solution finding will be appropriate. The timing of these interventions is important. A person who is in the highly symptomatic affective phase will most likely be "intolerant and resistant" of the kind of logical and cognitive interventions that will be timely and effective in the problem solving phases (DeVries & Gallagher-Thompson, 2000). Either the person involved will eventually decide upon a course of action that is most attractive and anxiety reducing or, as frequently happens, a decision will be made by those responsible or closely associated with the person.

In the best of all circumstances, persons can profit by anticipatory guidance (more to be discussed later) and taking stock of their resources and options, and making a declaration of preferred procedures should they become incapacitated and unable to act on their own. Failing to record these activities, decisions may be made contrary to the best wishes of the person or in recognition of the depletion of options available to the person.

The high point of crisis and crisis intervention theory was in the 1960s and 1970s, where early research shows its treatment effectiveness (Auerbach & Kilmann, 1977). Due to the medicalization (e.g., managed care of psychology) in the 1980s and 1990s and the relative demise of community psychology and psychiatry, there was a clear neglect of the contributions of positive mental health concepts of an illness model of disorder that fit the narrowing reimbursement systems. Understandably, research followed suit, with decreasing amounts of attention devoted to community mental health and the study of effective crisis interventions. The recent renewed interest of crisis intervention and critical incidence of stress management has been researched with both individual and metaanalytic studies which mostly have demonstrated the effectiveness of intervention and debriefing techniques (Everly, Flannery, & Mitchell, 1999). The ambiguity and range in the precise meaning of crisis complicates research in this area. There is a rather limited number of studies of crisis intervention among older adults, which will be reviewed in the next section under various headings.

RESEARCH

Kahana, Redmond, Hill, and Kercher (1995) studied the effects of a series of stressors in a sample of 397 elderly, ages 65 plus, as well as the possible moderating effects of subjects' satisfaction with key domains such as activities, relationships, health, and income. The stressors studied were recent negative events, cumulative life crises, living with illnesses with a relative, and isolation. The results indicated that levels of satisfaction in major life domains did affect well-being. Stressors are buffered when other resources are present. This finding is consistent with clinical data from other sources. The absence of resources is a crucial factor in well-being and as yet little research has dealt with the withdrawal or absence of resources. The results fit the concept that mental health is closely related to the availability of options. The decrease in options is a key factor in mental health and positive coping.

Much clinical and research attention has been devoted to suicide among older adults. As part of an evaluation of a suicide hotline service, Morrow-Howell, Becker-Kemppainen, and Judy (1998) conducted a quasi-experimental study on the effects of crisis intervention aimed at depression, isolation, and unmet needs. They found a reduction of depressive symptomatology at four months, with some diminution of this effect at eight months. It is clear that suicide is a significant problem in later life, especially with older White males. Suicide in later life tends to be more determined and planful, although with less violent methods (Conwell et al., 1998). The relatively modest success of suicide prevention at this age group strongly suggests that suicide in older adults may at times be phenomenologically different than in younger persons. In later life, suicide may not always derive from depression. Older persons may at times choose death as a rational solution to their life situation. This concept of "elective death" can explain the early result suggesting a more planful, less crisis-related meaning for late life suicide. It may be asserted that while suicide is often an emergency, it is not always the product of a true inner crisis. Indeed, suicide in late life is not always an emergency except, perhaps, to the helpers and family members. It is frequently a clear choice on the part of an older person; men, more socially isolated in old age than women, may have less resilience and be more suicide vulnerable. Also, when trait anxiety decreases with age, late life may herald a vulnerability and loss of control in situational events that increase state anxiety.

Anticipatory Guidance and Interventions

The purpose of *anticipatory guidance* is to prepare persons to meet situations in which they most likely have not had any previous experience. The great bulk of research and planning for the future of older persons is tied into retirement, and while there is increasing attention being paid to the problems being faced and yet to be faced as persons age, anticipatory guidance has yet to take its place as a strong ingredient in counseling and programmatic changes for older persons. From the point of view of crisis theory, decisions can be made taking into account available options and resources, or neglected, leaving the responsibility to family members or, in the last resort, to the courts or government agencies. This neglect is mirrored in the fact that the great majority of persons with some means die without a written will and frequently leave the disposition of their assets to their survivors or, failing them, to the courts. An increase in educational procedures stressing anticipatory guidance is clearly called for in terms of public policy and in programs dealing with older persons. Although life expectancy has been extended, this does not guarantee that the person will live to an older age nor that they will have the good fortune of not experiencing a variety of physical and mental conditions which are debilitating and definitely limit their coping capacities.

There are a number of preventive activities that public health policy and programs for aging persons could stress and indeed should be stressed. While they may seem inconsequential, they can be of enormous importance. The need for continuing physical activity commensurate with a person's health should be a dictum for the elderly. Such activities should include practice and training in maintaining and improving balance, walking, and stretching. Knowledge about the availability and instruction in the use of various devices designed to assist mobility and decrease the possibility of falling or injuries is likewise necessary in any progressive program.

The decision of when and how to intervene is one complicated by many value systems. Crises can be avoided or ameliorated by instigating preventive activities. Preparation would appear to be the key factor. It is not easy to recognize that at some time in the future the end of life will occur. How it will occur and when it will occur and how it can be faced with the least amount of pain, suffering, and loss of dignity is a major problem for society to face now and with increasing frequency in the future.

There are a number of potentially difficult areas and stress for older persons and their families which have to be faced. These can be done either at the preventive, symptom management, or problem solving phases. Most suggestions have not been systematically researched but represent the accumulated experience by practitioners working with adults. It is arguable that these intensive case histories more closely represent the phenomenon of crises than more extensive or remote surveys and statistical approaches.

It is beyond the scope of this entry to deal with the myriad of conditions leading to crises in older persons. The authors attempt a brief description and suggestions for what appear to be some of the main factors. Depression is one of the most common conditions prevalent in older populations. The symptomatology of depression might better be viewed as an ineffective response to crisis rather than a crisis itself. It is understandable that in a review of one's life there are many regrets and wishes that early activities and energies had taken different paths. Depression can be best dealt with in a combination of cognitive therapy and medication, although it should be stated that there are limitations to the medication of negative mood conditions. Closely linked to depression is the overuse of alcohol and over-the-counter drugs by elderly populations. Not all depressives become alcoholics nor do all persons abusing alcohol become depressives. This is a continuing area of concern not only for older populations but also for adult populations as a whole.

It is generally agreed that given current incidence figures, entering a nursing facility will be encountered at some point by about 25 percent of older adults. Nursing facilities vary greatly in the quality of care, depending upon the financial status of the recipient and local and state regulations. Even the most adequate and caring location can be traumatic for a number of reasons. There is a sudden loss of many freedoms and this is more impactful emotionally because a person has lost many subtle and hidden freedoms that were not recognized and therefore not prepared for. This situation is clearly suggestive of the need for primary anticipatory guidance and preventive programs which should include familiarization with the new setting, the ability to take along a few treasured objects, and generally to allow the person to become better oriented to the new environment. Perspective residents and family members need preparation for the many painful and surprising emotions encountered. The challenge of such programming is all the more difficult because adult children frequently utilize denial for admission and avoid dealing with issues until the situation is pressured. When a crisis has emerged, then aggressive crisis intervention is necessary for all concerned. Ongoing family councils can provide a setting where experienced family members may be able to mentor adult children of new residents (Duffy, 1987; Duffy & Shuttlesworth, 1987).

With increases in longevity and increasing neurological conditions such as dementias, highlighted by Alzheimer's Disease, society is faced with the decision of where and how to best care for individuals who may be in good physical health but whose mental capacity is sadly diminished, causing enormous sorrow and confusion to the remaining family and friends. The loss of cognitive acuity can be truly frightening and is the type of experience that has no precursor in adaptive and coping skills. The fear of Alzheimer's Disease can certainly evoke a sense of panic and call for timely interventions designed to correctly evaluate the situation, reduce anxiety, and consider alternatives. An enlightened public health and policy approach can do much to avoid a crisis and encourage a recognition that the steps that are taken are those that in the end are most beneficial both for the person and the family.

SYNTHESIS

Crisis theory has a long history. While it reached an early significance within the community mental health movement of the 1960s, awareness and training in anticipatory guidance in crisis intervention saw a decline in the 1970s as community psychology and psychiatry lost visibility with an increasing medical model of mental health services. The systematic and natural philosophy of health promotion and prevention at the individual and community level has much to offer in the present. It is best represented in multidisciplinary health care settings such as high quality health maintenance organizations with their emphasis on prevention and health.

An effective crisis avoidance and successful intervention are best supported by an enlightened public health policy designed to deal with inevitable mental and physical limitations that face older people, who are an increasing percentage of the population. Public policy that provided for hearing and dental care under Medicare would certainly be a first step.

Also see: Caregiver Stress: Older Adulthood; Grief: Older Adulthood; Health Promotion: Older Adulthood; HIV/AIDS: Older Adulthood; Life Challenges: Older Adulthood; Suicide: Older Adulthood.

References

American Psychiatric Association. (1994). *Diagnostic and statistical manual of mental disorders* (4th ed.). Washington, DC: Author.

Amster, L.E., & Krauss, H.H. (1974). The relationship between life crises and mental deterioration in old age. *International Journal of Aging and Human Development, 5*(1), 51–55.

Auerbach, S., & Kilmann, P. (1977). Crisis intervention: A review of outcome research. *Psychological Bulletin, 84*, 1189–1217.

Bloom, B.L. (1984). *Community mental health: A general introduction.* Belmont, CA: Wadsworth.

Caplan, G. (1964). *Principles of preventive psychiatry.* New York: Basic Books.

Conwell, Y. et al. (1998). Differences in behaviors leading to completed suicide. *American Journal of Geriatric Psychiatry, 6*(2), 28–46.

DeVries, H.M., & Gallagher-Thompson. (2000). Assessment and crisis intervention with older adults. In F.M. Dattilio & A. Freeman (Eds.), *Cognitive–behavioral strategies in crisis intervention.* New York: The Guilford Press.

Duffy, M. (1987). The techniques and contexts of multigenerational family therapy. *Clinical Gerontologist, 5*(3–4), 347–362.

Duffy, M., & Iscoe, I. (1990). Crisis theory and management: The case of the older person. *Journal of Mental Health Counseling, 12*(3), 303–313.

Duffy, M., & Shuttlesworth, G.E. (1987). The residents family: Adversary or advocate in longterm care. *Journal of Long Term Care Administration, 15*(3), 9–11.

Duffy, M. (1999). *Handbook of counseling and psychotherapy with older adults.* New York: Wiley and Sons.

Everly, G.S., Flannery, R.B., & Mitchell, J.T. (1999). *Aggression and Violent Behavior, 5*(1), 23–40.

Green, B.L., Wilson, J.P., & Lindy, J.D. (1985). Conceptualizing PTSD: A psychological framework. In C.R. Figley (Ed.), *Trauma and its wake.* New York: Bruner Mazel.

Kahana, E., Redmond, C., Hill, G., & Kercher, K. (1995). The effects of stress, vulnerability, and appraisals on the psychological well-being of the elderly. *Research in Aging, 17*(4), 459–489.

Lindemann, E . (1944). Symptomatology and management of acute grief. *American Journal of Psychiatry, 101*, 141–148.

Losee, N., Parham, I., Auerbach, S., & Teileman. (1988). *Crisis intervention with the elderly: Theory, practical issues and training procedures.* Springfield, IL: C.C. Thomas.

Miller, K., & Iscoe, I. (1963). The concept of crisis: Current status and mental health implications. *Human Organization, 22*(3).

Morrow-Howell, N., Becker-Kemppainen, S., & Judy, L. (1998). Evaluating an intervention for the elderly at increased risk of suicide. *Research in Social Work Practice, 8*(1), 28–46.

Slaikeu, K.A. (1990). *Crisis intervention* (2nd ed.). Boston: Allyn & Bacon.

D

Death with Dignity, Older Adulthood

Kathryn L. Braun

INTRODUCTION

This entry defines a "good death" and presents evidence that suggests that few older Americans are able to achieve this goal. Interventions to improve end-of-life care target change at the intrapersonal, interpersonal, community, and policy levels. Examples of these interventions are reviewed, along with findings of studies testing their impact. The entry concludes with recommendations for actions necessary to increase the number of older adults who achieve a good death.

DEFINITIONS

Although the definition of a *good death* may vary across individuals and cultures, North American research suggests that a good death has the following characteristics: pain and symptoms are managed; inappropriate prolongation of dying is avoided; decisions are clear; wishes are respected; the situation is not burdensome; the surroundings are familiar; loved ones are present; the dignity of the patient and caregiver are respected; relationships are strengthened;

and a sense of meaning and completion are achieved (Cassel & Foley, 1999; Lawton, 2000; Singer, Martin, & Kelner, 1999; Steinhauser, Clipp, McNeilly, Christakis, McIntyre, & Tulsky, 2000).

Therapy that is of no value to the patient, and only serves to prolong the dying process, is called *futile care.* Policies and documents that can help people to avoid a long, painful, burdensome dying process (and to terminate care that proves futile) are based on the individual's fundamental right to control decisions relating to his/her own medical care, including the decision to have life-prolonging treatments provided, continued, withheld, or withdrawn. For example, laws related to *informed consent* require health care providers to disclose the risks and benefits of recommended treatment, no treatment, and alternatives to recommended treatment. *Advance directives* (AD) are documents that allow competent individuals to provide treatment instructions in case of future incapacitation (through a *living will*) or to designate a proxy or surrogate to make future treatment decisions for them (through a *healthcare power of attorney*). The *Patient Self Determination Act* (PSDA) of 1990 requires health care facilities and agencies, upon a patient's admission, to provide information about patient's rights and AD and to place a copy of the patient's AD (if one exists) in the medical record (Braun, Pietsch, & Blanchette, 2000).

Others feel that death can be improved through legalization of assisted-death options, including *physician-assisted suicide* (PAS), in which a doctor provides a competent, dying patient who requests it access to a lethal dose of medicine for the patient to use with the primary intention of ending his/her own life, and *voluntary active euthanasia* (VAE), in which a doctor gives a competent dying patient who requests it a lethal injection with the primary intention of ending the patient's life. Others emphasize the need to embrace and better finance *palliative care* (therapies provided to ease distress and increase comfort, rather than to cure) for people at the end of life. *Hospice*, which can be provided in home and institutional settings, provides palliative care services and also attends to the non-medical needs of dying patients and their family members (Field & Cassel, 1997; Lawton, 2000).

SCOPE

Everyone will die and, at least in developed countries, the majority of deaths occur in older adulthood and are accompanied by chronic illnesses and physical and mental impairments. Findings from the Study to Understand Prognoses and Preferences for Outcomes and Risks of Treatment (SUPPORT), a landmark investigation involving 9,105 dying patients across five hospitals, suggested that physicians often misunderstand patient preferences, dying patients often are over-treated (receiving more life-extending care than desired), orders to withdraw or withhold life-extending care are not written until the last minute, and perhaps 50 percent of conscious patients die in pain (SUPPORT Principal Investigators, 1995). Although most healthy Americans report wanting to die at home, statistics suggest that only 20 percent of US deaths occur in the home, whereas the majority occur in institutions, primarily hospitals. For patients in the last month of life, hospice is thought to be the best care option and may generate cost savings of 25–40 percent. At present, hospice services are covered by Medicare and some other insurers, but only for individuals expected to survive another 6 months or less, and many eligible patients are referred very late in their illnesses, if at all. Thus, it is not surprising that only about 17 percent of US deaths are attended by hospice (Field & Cassel, 1997; Lawton, 2000).

A hospital death is not necessarily a bad death. However, in the United States, hospitals are built, staffed, and reimbursed to provide curative care. They are equipped with technology that saves lives, as in the case of the heart attack victim who receives emergency bypass surgery and goes on to live another 20 years. For individuals who are dying, however, hospitals may not be equipped or reimbursed to provide palliative care. Kaufman (1998) described four components of the hospital as it influences death and dying: (1) medicine (rather than ethnic culture, religion, or family) is the dominant framework for understanding old age and death; (2) technology is allowed to determine end-of-life events; (3) players are unclear about and often have competing goals for end-of-life care; and (4) few people are knowledgeable about the available technology and the implications for technology-related decisions in hospitals, nor are they prepared for the level of participation in decision making that is demanded of them.

End-of-life practices in the United States have been compared with those of the Netherlands. The values of autonomy and individual freedom are prized highly in both countries, and medical technology is similarly advanced. A significant difference, however, is in health care access. Over 95 percent of Holland's residents have comprehensive health insurance that covers their primary, acute, palliative, and long-term care needs. (In contrast, an estimated 40 million Americans, about 13 percent, are uninsured, and those with insurance rarely enjoy comprehensive coverage.) Dutch citizens can enjoy life-long relationships with their family physicians, who refer patients to a variety of home and community (as well as institutional) services to meet their changing needs. Palliative care and hospice services are available, and Dutch patients may access PAS and VAE if specified criteria are met, for example, unacceptable suffering, a well-considered and durable request, and a concurring second opinion (Keizer, 1997; Quill & Kimsma, 1997). Within the United States, many states have launched efforts to improve end-of-life care, but Oregon stands out as the state with the lowest in-hospital death rates and for its legalization of PAS (Emanuel, Fairclough, & Emanuel, 2000; Tolle, Rosenfeld, Tilden, & Park, 1999).

Theory for Improving End-of-Life Care

Interventions to improve end-of-life care in the United States target change at the intrapersonal, interpersonal, community, and policy levels.

Intrapersonal

At the intrapersonal (or individual) level, most Americans have witnessed or heard about someone whose death was unnecessarily prolonged, painful, and burdensome. Many Americans want to take steps personally to avoid this for themselves, and thus support autonomy and self-determination in health care. These values are reflected in the PSDA, which encourages individuals to document their wishes for future care. Calls to legalize a patient's right to end his/her own life are based in the same values (autonomy and self-determination), that is, "if I'm dying anyway, and want to minimize the time I spend in a painful, burdensome state, I should be able to direct a physician to assist me in dying."

Interpersonal

Although the concepts of autonomy and self-determination resonate with most Americans, the process of dying is rarely a solitary, individual event. It is preceded, in most cases (and especially in older adulthood), by a crisis or a disease process that brings the individual in contact with the health care system and involves the elder's significant others in caregiving and decision making. Communication patterns, especially about death, are influenced by family, cultural, and religious norms, so it is not uncommon for end-of-life conflict to arise among family members, between the family and the physician, and between the patient and the health care system (Braun et al., 2000). Thus, simply documenting and filing one's wishes may not be enough to improve one's chances for a good death. Interventions on the interpersonal level strive to improve communications by encouraging dialogue about death, teaching active listening skills, and increasing the cultural competence of health care professionals and facilities.

Community

Having a good death may depend on availability of community resources. For example, which health services exist in the dying person's community? Are family and friends able and willing to provide care that is not available or covered? Do churches and other spiritual groups provide outreach to the dying and bereaved, assist families in resolving conflict, or help dying people achieve a sense of completion and acceptance at life's end?

Policy

End-of-life care can be improved through changes in policy as well. Professional societies establish and promulgate standards of care. Health care review agencies establish standards and impose sanctions on facilities that do not meet them. Government and private insurers can expand coverage of palliative care and limit reimbursement for futile care. Legislators can be asked to change laws related to end-of-life care, for example, by legislating fines against providers who do not honor a patient's documented wishes or by legalizing assisted-death options.

STRATEGIES

Interventions have been proposed and tried at each of the four levels—intrapersonal, interpersonal, community, and policy. These are reviewed here, along with findings from studies testing their impact. In general, no single strategy has been shown to work best. In this section, information is provided on the benefits and limitations of each approach.

Intrapersonal Interventions: Advance Directives

All 50 states have passed legislation on AD, and surveys have shown that Americans are in favor of such legislation. Studies suggest, however, that only 15–25 percent of

the general public have completed AD, although percentages increase among the aged, people in hospitals and nursing homes, persons with terminal diagnoses, and individuals with higher-than-average education and income (Miles, Koepp, & Weber, 1996). Several studies of adults affiliated with specific programs or clinics have looked at ethnicity, and most have found lower AD completion rates for African and Latino Americans than non-Latino whites (Braun et al., 2000).

Interventions to increase AD completion include anticipatory guidance efforts and mailed materials. Face-to-face interventions work best, and response is higher among individuals already aged and/or under medical care for chronic conditions. Research suggests, however, that a completed AD may never appear in the medical record; an AD may be misplaced as a patient moves across settings (e.g., outpatient, acute, rehabilitation, long-term care); an AD influences hospital care for only 25 percent of patients who have them; and no differences are seen when comparing outcomes of ill patients with and without AD. Thus, interventions that simply increase rates of AD completion appear to have minimal effect on improving the quality of end-of-life care (Lawton, 2000; Miles et al., 1996).

An exception has been seen in Oregon, where a dying patient's wishes are recorded as medical orders on a form called the Physician Orders for Life-Sustaining Treatment (POLST), a document that accompanies the patient across health care settings (and even into the ambulance). This intervention has helped many dying patients avoid that last, futile admission to a hospital, resulting in a very low in-hospital death rate for Oregon (Tolle et al., 1999).

Intrapersonal Interventions: Assisted-Death Options

A great number of surveys have been conducted to ascertain support for assisted-death options among members of the public, patients, and physicians. Among members of the North American public, opinion-poll data suggest that 53–69 percent support the legalization of VAE and that 52–66 percent support the legalization of PAS for terminally or hopelessly ill patients. For both VAE and PAS, support varies among respondents, with generally less support among the elderly, minorities, and individuals with strong religious beliefs (Braun, Kayashima, Somogyi-Zalud, & Sakai, 2001).

Among terminally ill patients, support ranges from 52–67 percent for legalizing PAS and 65–73 percent for legalizing VAE (Braun et al., 2001). Research suggests, however that patients who consider VAE or PAS are likely to be depressed, to have moderate to severe pain, and to have substantial care needs, suggesting that improvements to pain control, mental health interventions, insurance coverage, and caregiver support may reduce consumer desire for the legalization of assisted-death options (Emanuel et al., 2000; Foley, 1997). Investigators and practitioners also have found that many patients who initially request PAS or VAE change their minds about it later on, either on their own or following reassurance that they will not be left alone or in unbearable pain (Emanuel et al., 2000; Keizer, 1997; Quill & Kimsma, 1997).

Among physicians, support for legalizing PAS and VAE generally is lower than among patient and public samples, and varies by ethnicity (minority physicians generally are less supportive than white physicians), religion (those reporting "no religion" are more supportive than those with strong religious beliefs), medical specialty (psychiatrists are more supportive than oncologists), and residence (with relatively high levels of support in Oregon and Washington and lower levels of support in east-coast samples). These findings, coupled with an inequitable health care system, have led a number of physicians and ethicists to speak against legalizing PAS/VAE in the United States, warning of possible abuses of vulnerable patient groups (Braun et al., 2001; Foley, 1997; Meier, Emmons, Wallenstein, Quill, Morrison, & Cassel, 1998; Quill & Kimsma, 1997).

It is interesting to note that few dying individuals have actually availed themselves of VAE and PAS. In a prospective, cohort study of 988 terminally ill patients across the United States, 60 percent supported VAE or PAS in a hypothetical situation. However, only 11 percent considered it for themselves, less than 4 percent hoarded drugs for PAS or discussed either assisted-death option with a physician, and only 1 out of the 256 patients who died during the study period actually died by VAE or PAS (Emanuel et al., 2000). In the first 2 years that PAS was legal in Oregon, only 43 (0.09 percent) deaths were so assisted, and assisted-death rates in the Netherlands are estimated at only 3.4 percent (Emanuel et al., 2000). Thus, "euthanasia and PAS may not be particularly pivotal interventions, since for more than 95% of deaths they do not contribute to a good death" (Emanuel et al., 2000, p. 2466).

Interpersonal Interventions

If an AD document in itself will not improve one's chances of a good death, would it help if individuals discussed their wishes with their family, health care providers (especially their physicians), lawyer, and perhaps clergy? Research suggests that individuals want their doctors to initiate discussions about advance planning, and that these discussions should occur after their physician–patient relationship is established but while the patient is still well (Miles et al., 1996). Conversations should address values and expectations related to life prolongation, proxy decision-making, preference of place of death, potential benefits of hospice,

and so forth. This is especially important where patients and physicians are from different cultures. These conversations take time, and providers and insurers must develop mechanisms that encourage these conversations (Braun et al., 2000; Doukas & McCullough, 1991; Field & Cassel, 1997).

In a 2-year controlled trial, the SUPPORT Investigators (1995) tested a hospital-based intervention to improve end-of-life outcomes through communication, but results suggested that the intervention was ineffective. Specifically, 2,652 patients were assigned to an intervention group, in which their physicians "received estimates of the likelihood of 6-month survival for every day up to 6 months, outcomes of cardiopulmonary resuscitation, and functional disability at 2 months ... [while] a specially trained nurse made multiple contacts with the patient, family, physician, and hospital staff to elicit preferences, improve understanding of outcomes, encourage attention to pain control, and facilitate advance care planning and patient–physician communication" (p. 1591). Unfortunately, this hospital-based intervention did not increase patient–physician communication or physician knowledge of patient preferences. Nor did it reduce the number of ICU days, use of hospital resources, levels of pain for dying patients, or number of patients on ventilators or comatose before death.

In Oregon, however, efforts to encourage discussions and to honor end-of-life wishes have resulted in a high rate of patient–family–physician agreement on the withholding and withdrawing of life-sustaining treatment for dying patients. Oregon's success is attributable, in part, to its health care system's support of dying patients who want to avoid admission to the hospital or want to be discharged from the hospital to a home or community setting when death appears imminent (Tolle et al., 1999).

Community Interventions

End-of-life care is influenced by the availability (or lack) of resources in one's community. For example, a study of Medicare death records from 1992 and 1993 revealed great variation across the country in the percent of hospital-based deaths, from 23 percent in Portland to 54 percent in Newark. Variance was associated strongly with availability and use of hospital beds, that is, residents are more likely to die in a hospital if their community has a lot of hospital beds and the hospital occupancy rates are high. The same association was found in an analysis of SUPPORT deaths (Lawton, 2000; Pritchard et al., 1998).

Additional evidence of the impact of a community's resource base on the dying experience comes from Oregon. This state has a relatively high level of hospice penetration, and about 30 percent of deaths in 1997 were attended by hospice (compared to about 17 percent nationally). Oregon also has developed an extensive network of services to support dying patients (and their families) who wish to die at home. Dying patients without families may receive hospice care in an adult foster home. Nursing home facilities and staff also are comfortable with caring for patients through the dying process (Tolle et al., 1999). The Netherlands, as well, has an array of insurance-covered health and community-based services that are distributed evenly throughout the country and increase the likelihood of a good death outside of the hospital (Quill & Kimsma, 1997).

In 1999, the Robert Wood Johnson Foundation (RWJF) funded a number of Community–State Partnerships to Improve End-of-Life Care. Several of these coalitions have established programs to increase community awareness about death and dying and to stimulate community-wide changes in professional education, local policy, and church involvement. Hawaii's Partnership, for example, leveraged RWJF funds to expand palliative care resources; to increase access to and financing for hospice; to engage churches in outreach to the dying and the bereaved; to educate the public about AD and one's right to a good death; and to strengthen health practitioners' abilities to assess and treat pain, give bad news, ask directly about patients' wishes, and respect requests to withhold or withdraw treatment. As a result, the state boasts high rates of AD completion (68 percent among residents 65 and older in 2000) and has seen increasing demands for and referrals to hospice care.

Policy Interventions

Even when community resources are available, an AD is in place, and discussions have occurred, an individual still may encounter barriers to a good death. A review of the SUPPORT findings suggests that patient preferences change as patients confront new situations and are re-asked about their wishes in light of new developments. For hospital-based patients, players (patients, families, and physicians) tend to go along with "the program" rather than advocate for less aggressive care, and families tend to feel guilty if they do not ask for everything to be done for the dying person. Rather than depend on patients and families to recognize a short dying trajectory and to reject care that is likely to have little effect, Lynn and colleagues (2000) proposed changes to the standards of care for advanced diseases so that standards specify procedures that most people would want (e.g., good pain control for metastatic cancer) and contraindicate procedures, like CPR, that would be unlikely to improve the quality of the patient's life or death. Individuals could use an AD to document a desire for CPR, but the standard of care would not require it.

Because the US health care environment encourages heroic and aggressive treatment for all patients, perhaps

drastic improvements in end-of-life care may only occur with changes to the structure and financing of care. Tolle and colleagues (1999) certainly believe that policy decisions in Oregon, which expanded funding to hospice and community-based care options and allowed the institutionalization of the POLST document, have helped shape a health care environment that is supportive of a good death.

SYNTHESIS

What should be done to improve end-of-life care in the United States? Returning to our definition, a good death requires a dying process in which pain and symptoms are managed, inappropriate prolongation of dying is avoided, decisions are clear, wishes are respected, the situation is not burdensome, the surroundings are familiar, loved ones are present, dignity is respected, relationships are strengthened, and a sense of meaning and completion are achieved (Lawton, 2000; Singer et al., 1999; Steinhauser et al., 2000). This is a tall order, and the solution will involve action on several fronts.

1. *Early Discussion and Documentation of Preferences.* Improvements to end-of-life care begin with increased patient–family–physician dialogue about preferences, and these discussions should start before a patient has a health crisis. Preferences should be documented, and documents should accompany patients across settings. Training of physicians and other health care providers must emphasize communication skills, including active listening, cultural sensitivity, and the ability to give bad news. Because most patients lack knowledge about the realities of dying and the limitations (as well as the abilities) of technology, physicians need to be able to tell patients when they are on a short death trajectory and which care options are futile. The early sharing of values and the establishment of trust can help reduce misunderstandings and facilitate meaningful communication as the patient goes through the process of his/her dying (Braun et al., 2000; Field & Cassel, 1997; Foley, 1997; Kaufman, 1998; Lawton, 2000).

2. *Changes in Professional Standards and Training.* Clinical policy for care at the end of life has been advanced through the development and promulgation of Core Principles for End-of-Life Care, shown in Table 1 (Cassel & Foley, 1999). By 1999, these principles had been adopted in full or part by the American Medical Association, 13 subspecialty medical societies, and the Joint Commission for the Accreditation of Healthcare Organizations (JCAHO).

Table 1. Core Principles for End-of-Life Care
(Cassel & Foley, 1999)

Clinical policy of care at the end of life and the professional practice it
guides should:
   1. Respect the dignity of both patient and caregivers;
   2. Be sensitive to and respectful of the patient's and family's wishes;
   3. Use the most appropriate measures that are consistent with patient
      choices;
   4. Encompass alleviation of pain and other physical symptoms;
   5. Assess and manage psychological, social, and spiritual/religious
      problems;
   6. Offer continuity (the patient should be able to continue to be cared
      for, if so desired, by his/her primary care and specialist providers);
   7. Provide access to any therapy which may realistically be expected to
      improve the patient's quality of life, including alternative or non-
      traditional treatments;
   8. Provide access to palliative care and hospice care;
   9. Respect the right to refuse treatment;
  10. Respect the physician's professional responsibility to discontinue
      some treatments when appropriate, with consideration for both
      patient and family preferences;
  11. Promote clinical and evidence-based research on providing care at the
      end of life.

Standards for the assessment and management of
pain have evolved as well and, in 2000, JCAHO
began penalizing health care facilities that ignored
such standards. These developments, along with
research findings that indicate a lack of provider
training in death and dying (Foley, 1997), require
that end-of-life care be incorporated into professional education. This includes additions to the
didactic program, along with the development of
end-of-life scenarios for use in problem-based
learning and by standardized patients and families.
Professional schools also should require students to
train and function as hospice volunteers prior to
graduation. Physicians already in practice should
enroll in offerings of a curriculum developed by the
American Medical Association called Educating
Physicians in End-of-Life Care (EPEC). US physicians' practices are influenced by litigation, and it is
likely that a few well-publicized lawsuits (e.g., for
inadequately controlling pain or for ignoring a
patient's wishes) may increase physician attention
to palliative care principles.
   3. *Changes to Federal Policy.*   As in any country, the
      US health care system is shaped by the availability
      of funding, and funding streams are often a matter of
      federal policy. The largest impact on the quality of
      end-of-life care for Americans, especially for the esti-
      mated 40 million without health insurance, would be
      the establishment of a universal health care system
      that includes preventive, primary, acute, long-term,

and palliative care. Efforts to do so have not met with
much success, or even enthusiasm. Barring this type
of policy change, the next best recommendation is for
expanded development of and coverage for palliative
care services across settings, including hospital,
nursing home, and home-based settings.
   4. *Community Awareness and Resources.*   Policies
      that encourage the development and financing of
      home and community-based palliative care will lead
      to increased availability of and access to such serv-
      ices. Support for family caregivers, and access to
      home-like residential care for dying people without
      families, are equally crucial. A good death, however,
      involves more than just good health care. For most, a
      good death also requires the strengthening of rela-
      tionships and the realization of meaning and com-
      pletion. Although hospice providers and volunteers
      can facilitate progress toward these goals, there is a
      clear role in this arena for faith communities to help
      congregants prepare for death, both spiritually and
      practically, and to facilitate the resolution of conflict
      and forgiveness.
   5. *Research and Measurement.*   As academic disci-
      plines, thanatology and palliative care are relative
      newcomers. The science of measuring the problems
      associated with death and dying, and gauging
      progress in their resolution, is still in its infancy.
      Researchers evaluating specific interventions to
      improve end-of-life care (e.g., new or expanded
      services, new standards of care, new reimbursement
      rules) will gain insights from the evolving work
      of Teno and colleagues, who have proposed ways
      to measure several important components of good
      end-of-life care. These include communication
      and shared decision-making, effective symptom
      management, and family perceptions of the coordi-
      nation and continuity of the health care system
      (Lawton, 2000). Other researchers need to test inter-
      ventions designed to increase the usefulness of AD,
      to reduce inappropriate prolongation of dying, to
      allow individuals to die in familiar surroundings,
      to strengthen relationships, to support caregivers, to
      validate life's meaning, and to give a sense of
      completion.

In this age of increasing life expectancy and advanced
medical technology, too many Americans die in pain and in
situations that are neither familiar nor comforting. To
improve end-of-life care and help assure that each older
adult will have a good death, individuals and groups must
work together to affect change at the intrapersonal, interpersonal, community, and policy levels.

Also see: Suicide: Childhood; Suicide: Adolescence; Suicide: Adulthood; Suicide: Older Adulthood; Ethics: Foundation; Depression: Older Adulthood.

References

Braun, K.L., Kayashima, R., Somogyi-Zalud, E., & Sakai, D. (2001, November). *Physician, public, and patient support of assisted suicide and euthanasia: Why the large variance?* Paper presented at the annual meeting of the Gerontological Society of America, Chicago, IL.

Braun, K.L., Pietsch, J.H., & Blanchette, P.L. (2000). *Cultural issues in end-of-life decision making.* Thousand Oaks, CA: Sage

Cassel, C.K., & Foley, K.M. (1999). *Principles for care of patients at the end of life: An emerging consensus among the specialties of medicine.* New York, NY: Milbank Memorial Fund.

Doukas, D.J., & McCullough, L.B. (1991). The values history: The evaluation of the patient's values and advance directives. *Journal of Family Practice, 32*, 145–153.

Emanuel, E.J., Fairclough, D.L., & Emanuel, L.L. (2000). Attitudes and desires related to euthanasia and physician-assisted suicide among terminally ill patients and their caregivers. *Journal of the American Medical Association, 284*, 2460–2468.

Field, M.J., & Cassel, C.K. (1997). *Approaching death: Improving care at the end of life.* Washington, DC: National Academy Press.

Foley, K.M. (1997). Competent care for the dying instead of physician-assisted suicide. *New England Journal of Medicine, 336*, 54–57.

Kaufman, S.R. (1998). Intensive care, old age, and the problem of death in America. *The Gerontologist, 38*, 715–725.

Keizer, B. (1997). *Dancing with Mister D: Notes on life and death.* New York: Doubleday.

Lawton, M.P. (2000). *Annual review of gerontology and geriatrics, volume 20. Focus on the end of life: Scientific and social issues.* New York, NY: Springer.

Lynn, J., Arkes, H.R., Stevens, M., Cohn, F., Koenig, B., Fox, E., Dawson, N.V., Phillips, R.S., Hamel, M.B., & Tsevat, J. (2000). Rethinking fundamental assumptions: SUPPORT's implications for future reform. *Journal of the American Geriatrics Society, 48*, S214–S221.

Meier, D.E., Emmons, C., Wallenstein, S., Quill, T., Morrison, R.S., & Cassel, C. (1998). A national survey of physician-assisted suicide and euthanasia in the United States. *New England Journal of Medicine, 338*, 193–201.

Miles, S.H., Koepp, R., & Weber, E.P. (1996). Advance end-of-life treatment planning: A research review. *Archives of Internal Medicine, 156*, 1062–1068.

Pritchard, R.S., Fisher, E.S., Teno, J.M., Sharp, S.M., Reding, D.J., Knaus, W.A., Wennberg, J.E., & Lynn, J. (1998). Influence of patient preferences and local health system characteristics on the place of death. *Journal of the American Geriatrics Society, 46*, 1242–1250.

Quill, T.E., & Kimsma, G. (1997). End-of-life care in the Netherlands and the United States: A comparison of values, justifications, and practices. *Cambridge Quarterly of Healthcare Ethics, 6*, 189–204.

Singer, P.A., Martin, D.K., & Kelner, M. (1999). Quality end-of-life care: Patients' perspectives. *Journal of the American Medical Association, 281*, 163–168.

Steinhauser, K.E., Clipp, E.C., McNeilly, M., Christakis, N.A., McIntyre, L., & Tulsky, J.A. (2000). In search of a good death: Observations of patients, families, and providers. *Annals of Internal Medicine, 132*(10), 825–832.

SUPPORT Principal Investigators. (1995). A controlled trial to improve care for seriously ill hospitalized patients. *Journal of the American Medical Association, 274*, 1591–1598.

Tolle, S.W., Rosenfeld, A.G., Tilden, V.P., & Park, Y. (1999). Oregon's low in-hospital death rates: What determines where people die and satisfaction with decisions on place of death? *Annals of Internal Medicine, 130*, 681–685.

Delinquency, Childhood

Brandon C. Welsh and David P. Farrington

INTRODUCTION, DEFINITIONS, AND SCOPE

Juvenile delinquency is a serious problem. In 1997, there were about 30 million juveniles aged 10–17 in the United States. About 123,000 were arrested for serious violent crimes (murder, rape, robbery, or aggravated assault) and 702,000 were arrested for serious property crimes (burglary, theft, vehicle theft, or arson). The juvenile arrest rate for serious violence stayed constant from 1975–1988 at about 3 per 1,000 population, but then suddenly increased by two thirds to over 5 per 1,000 in 1994 before deceasing somewhat (Snyder & Sickmund, 1999). In contrast, the juvenile arrest rate for serious property offenses stayed constant over this whole time period, at about 25 per 1,000 population each year.

The cumulative prevalence of delinquency is much higher than the annual prevalence, of course. For example, one third of boys and 14 percent of girls born in Philadelphia in 1958 were arrested for nontraffic offenses as juveniles, and 18 percent of boys and 4 percent of girls were arrested for one of the eight serious offenses (Tracy, Wolfgang, & Figlio, 1985). There was a considerable racial differential; 26 percent of African American boys were arrested for serious offenses, compared with 9 percent of Caucasian boys.

This entry is concerned with the primary prevention of juvenile delinquency through programs that are initiated in the childhood years. In this sense, primary prevention is focused on preventing delinquency and later offending before offenses actually occur. Essentially, it aims positively to influence the early risk factors or "root causes" of delinquency and later offending, typically through broad-based strategies. Some of the major causes or risk factors include: growing up in poverty, living in poor housing, inadequate parental supervision and harsh or inconsistent discipline, parental conflict and separation, low intelligence and poor school performance, and a high level of impulsiveness and hyperactivity.

We review leading early childhood delinquency prevention programs that have been implemented in the four most important settings: home (home visitation), day care, preschool, and elementary school. Only programs including outcome measures of delinquency, antisocial behavior, or disruptive child behavior are included; programs were excluded if they only had outcome measures of risk factors such as low IQ or poor parenting. Some of the programs did not have a direct measure of delinquency, because that would have required a long-term follow-up. However, there is considerable continuity between disruptive child behavior and juvenile delinquency (Farrington, 1998). Therefore, programs that have immediate effects on disruptive child behavior are likely to have long-term effects on delinquency and later offending. We also look at the monetary costs and benefits of preventing juvenile delinquency, for those programs that have carried out a benefit–cost analysis.

STRATEGIES

Most early prevention programs have not been evaluated adequately. Rather than attempt to review a large number of programs (e.g., in a meta-analysis; see Lipsey & Wilson, 1998), we have chosen to focus on the best: those evaluated in randomized experiments with relatively large samples (see Farrington & Coid, 2002; Farrington & Welsh, 1999). This entry is organized around the four most important types of programs: home visitation, day care, preschool, and school-based.

Home Visiting Programs

Teenage mothers can be helped, child abuse and neglect can be reduced, and problems in pregnancy and infancy can be alleviated by intensive home visiting programs. The Elmira (New York) Prenatal/Early Infancy Project (PEIP) was designed with three broad objectives: "(1) to improve the outcomes of pregnancy; (2) to improve the quality of care that parents provide to their children (and their children's subsequent health and development); and (3) to improve the women's own personal life-course development (completing their education, finding work, and planning future pregnancies)" (Olds, Henderson, Phelps, Kitzman, & Hanks, 1993, p. 158). The program enrolled 400 at-risk women prior to their 30th week of pregnancy. The mothers were randomly assigned to receive home visits from nurses during pregnancy, to receive visits both during pregnancy and during the first two years of life, or to a control group who received no visits. Each visit lasted about one and one quarter hours, and the mothers were visited on average every two weeks. The home visitors gave advice about prenatal and postnatal care of the child, about infant development, and about the importance of proper nutrition and avoiding smoking and drinking during pregnancy.

The results of the experiment showed that home visits during pregnancy led to teenage mothers having heavier babies. Also, women who had previously smoked decreased their smoking and had fewer preterm deliveries. In addition, the postnatal home visits caused a decrease in recorded child physical abuse and neglect during the first two years of life, especially by poor, unmarried teenage mothers; 4 percent of visited versus 19 percent of nonvisited mothers of this type were guilty of child abuse or neglect. This last result is important because of the common observation that being physically abused or neglected as a child predicts later violent offending.

This experiment had a 15-year follow-up, and the main focus in the follow-up was on the higher risk sample of disadvantaged unmarried mothers. Among these mothers, those who received prenatal and postnatal home visits had fewer arrests than those who received prenatal visits or no visits (Olds et al., 1997). Also, children of these mothers who received prenatal and/or postnatal home visits had less than half as many arrests as children of mothers who received no visits (Olds et al., 1998).

Benefit–cost analyses of PEIP carried out at 2 and 13 years after the completion of the program showed that it produced value for money (for the government), but only for the higher risk sample (Greenwood et al., 2001; Olds et al., 1993). For the higher risk sample, program benefits surpassed costs, for benefit–cost ratios of 1.1 (2-year follow-up) and 4.1 (13-year follow-up); for the lower risk sample, benefit–cost ratios for the 2- and 13-year follow-ups were 0.5 and 0.6, respectively.

The first benefit–cost analysis revealed that, of government savings to the higher risk sample ($3,313 per family, in 1980 US dollars), the largest portion (56 percent) was attributed to reductions in Aid for Dependent Children (AFDC) payments. Reductions in Food Stamps accounted for 26 percent of the savings; Medicaid, 11 percent; and increases in tax revenue, 5 percent. Fewer cases of child abuse and neglect among the program group compared to the control group accounted for only 3 percent of the government savings (to Child Protective Services), or approximately $100 per family. The second benefit–cost analysis also showed that the majority of government savings were due to similar noncrime benefits.

In Memphis, Tennessee, Kitzman and her colleagues (1997) carried out a replication of the Elmira intervention program. In this, 1,139 African American mothers (primarily poor and unmarried) were randomly assigned to receive home visits from nurses during pregnancy, to receive visits both during pregnancy and during the first two years of life, or to a control group who received no visits. As before, the home visitors gave the mothers advice about child care and avoiding substance use. The initial results showed that the nurse-visited children suffered fewer injuries during the first two years of life.

Around the same time that the Elmira PEIP began, a similar home visitation program had been started in Montreal, Canada, by Larson (1980). Mothers from disadvantaged neighborhoods were the focus of the program. One hundred and fifteen mothers were assigned to one of the three conditions: home visits both before and after the child's birth, home visits only after the child's birth, or no home visits. The home visitors (child psychologists) provided advice about taking care of the infant and about infant development. The home visits produced beneficial effects, since the children of visited mothers sustained significantly fewer injuries in the first year of life. The children of mothers visited both before and after birth had only half as many injuries as the children of the nonvisited mothers. Also, the mothers visited both prenatally and postnatally were rated by observers as the most skilled in taking care of the child.

Another home visitation program, carried out in Miami, Florida, by Stone, Bendell, and Field (1988), randomly assigned 131 disadvantaged teenage mothers either to receive parent education during the first year of their child's lives or to a control group. The parent education focused on infant care, developmental milestones, and age-appropriate infant stimulation exercises. Two years after the intervention, the mothers in the treatment group, compared to their control group counterparts, had fewer repeat pregnancies and a higher rate of return to work or school. However, a later follow-up, when the children were between the ages of 5 and 8, found that the children who received the treatment were not significantly different in rated behavior problems from those who did not receive the treatment. The loss of a large number of the original subjects (53 percent), however, limits the confidence in this finding.

Trying to isolate the key features that make some home visitation programs successful in preventing child aggression and later antisocial behavior problems is no easy task. This is because these programs are invariably multidimensional; that is, there is a combination of interventions which are in operation either simultaneously or consecutively. It may be that the success of programs lies not in one particular programmatic feature, but rather in the interaction between the package of measures and the targeted population. In each one of the four programs reviewed here the targeted mothers had some preexisting disadvantage (e.g., low socioeconomic status [SES]), which can further exacerbate the difficult situation of raising a newborn. By providing generic services (e.g., links to community resources) to help mothers improve their life course development, and providing them with basic information on parenting, some of the hardships can be alleviated. This may translate into improved care and attention for the child, both at a physical and socioemotional level.

Child Care Programs

Child care, available to children as young as six weeks old in the United States and other industrialized countries (Michel, 1999), is another setting that has been used to stimulate socioemotional functioning and address child and family risk factors for aggression and later delinquency. Three high quality child care programs deserve mention.

One of the very few prevention experiments beginning in pregnancy and collecting outcome data on delinquency was the Syracuse (New York) Family Development Research Program (Lally, Mangione, & Honig, 1988). The researchers began with a sample of pregnant women—mostly poor, single mothers—and gave them weekly help with child-rearing, health, nutrition, and other issues. In addition, their children received free full-time day care, designed to develop their intellectual abilities, up to age 5. This was not a randomized experiment, but a matched control group was chosen when the children were aged 3. The children receiving the program had significantly higher intelligence than the controls at age 3, but were not significantly different at age 5. Ten years later, 119 children in the treatment and control groups were followed-up to about age 15. Significantly fewer of the treatment group children (2 vs. 17 percent) had been referred to the juvenile court for delinquency offenses.

A benefit–cost analysis of the Syracuse program by Aos, Phipps, Barnoski, and Lieb (2001) found that it provided poor financial value (to the government and crime victims), for a benefit–cost ratio of 0.4. There are two main reasons for the program's poor economic showing: first, it was very costly, at more than $45,000 per participant (in 1998 US dollars); and, second, only effects on crime (i.e., crimes avoided) were monetized, thus leaving out many of the social or noncrime benefits.

Another high quality child care program was that of the Houston (Texas) Parent–Child Development Center (Johnson & Walker, 1987), which randomly allocated 458 poor families of Mexican American heritage with one-year-old children to experimental or control groups. The experimental mothers received home visits for one year and attended a child development center with their child during the second year. The program focused on advising the mother about child development and parenting skills, helping her develop an affectionate relationship with her child, and fostering the cognitive skills of the child. At the end of the program when the children were aged 3, the experimental mothers were rated as more affectionate, as using more praise and less criticism, and as providing a more stimulating home environment; however, attrition rates for both the experimental and control groups was high. An 8-year follow-up of the Houston program, when the children were aged 8–11, found that experimental children were less involved in fights and less impulsive than controls according to their teachers.

The largest child care program was the Infant Health and Development Program (IHDP), involving 985 low-birth-weight infants in eight sites across the United States. Children were selected at birth and randomly allocated to experimental or control groups. The program included home visits, parent group meetings, and attendance at specially designed child development centers. Home visits occurred weekly in the first year and biweekly in the second and third years. Parent group meetings were held four times per year. The day care was for an average of 267 full days per year, and the average program cost was more than $15,000 per child per year, although about one third of this was for transportation to the child development centers. The program had immediate beneficial effects, with the experimental infants demonstrating higher intelligence and fewer behavior problems at ages 2 and 3. However, at age 8, the experimental and control children were not significantly different in behavior problems, according to parent ratings on the Child Behavior Checklist (McCarton et al., 1997).

Mostly encouraging messages can be drawn from the findings of these three child care programs. Importantly, each produced a desirable effect on outcomes of interest (e.g., behavior problems) at some follow-up. On the other hand, the passage of time resulted in the decay of beneficial effects for the largest of the programs. Again, the multidimensional nature of these programs makes it difficult to say with any certainty what the key elements are that make a program successful or unsuccessful.

Preschool Programs

Preschool is another important setting for delivering programs to improve school readiness and address early risk factors for problem behaviors and delinquency in later childhood years. Provided to children typically aged 3–5—the formative years of brain development according to theorists—a number of preschool programs, particularly those of a high quality nature, have demonstrated numerous benefits for participants.

The most important is the Perry Preschool program started in 1962 in Ypsilanti, Michigan, which is perhaps the best known longitudinal study in the Western world that has rigorously charted the effects of an early childhood primary prevention program. The principal hypothesis of the program was that "good preschool programs can help children in poverty make a better start in their transition from home to community and thereby set more of them on paths to becoming economically self-sufficient, socially responsible adults" (Schweinhart, Barnes, & Weikart, 1993, p. 3).

Prior to the start of the program, 123 children aged 3–4 years were randomly assigned to either an experimental group that received the preschool programming or a control group that did not. Families were recruited if they had low SES and their children showed low intellectual performance. The main approach involved high quality, active learning preschool programming administered by professional teachers for two years. Preschool sessions were one-half day long and were provided five days a week for the duration of the 30-week school year. The educational approach focused on supporting the development of the children's cognitive and social skills through individualized teaching and learning. Weekly home visits were also carried out by the teachers to provide parents with educational information and to enable them to take an active role in their child's early education. The sample was most recently assessed at the age of 27, or 22 years after the program ended. Sample attrition was exceedingly low at this follow-up stage, at under 5 percent.

At age 27, compared to the control group, experimental group participants showed a number of benefits across a range of prosocial functioning indicators. They had statistically significantly fewer police arrests, with the mean number of lifetime arrests being only half as many for experimental group participants compared to controls (2.3 vs. 4.6). Also, fewer experimental group members were judged to be chronic offenders (5 or more arrests) compared to controls (7 vs. 35 percent).

A comprehensive benefit–cost analysis of the Perry program found that the program's effects translated into substantial savings for the program group participants, government (or taxpayers), and crime victims. Benefits were estimated at $88,433 (in 1992 US dollars) for each program group participant. The greatest benefits were from savings to the justice system ($12,796) and crime victims ($57,585). Savings to the justice system alone covered program costs ($12,356). The other benefits received by the public for each preschool participant included: higher educational output and reduced schooling costs, $6,287; revenue generated from taxes on increased earnings, $8,847; and reduced reliance on welfare, $2,918. Dividing total financial benefits per participant ($88,433) by total financial costs per participant ($12,356) produced a highly desirable benefit–cost ratio of 7.2. In other words, the public received $7.2 for every dollar invested in the program.

Pagani, Tremblay, Vitaro, & Parent (1998) used a subset of boys involved in the Montreal longitudinal experimental study (described in the next section) to investigate the effect of attending preschool programs. Of 404 boys attending 28 schools at age 6 which had publicly funded preschool programs, 117 had attended the preschool at ages 4–5 and 287 had not. The two groups were not equivalent, but Pagani and her colleagues carried out regression analyses which controlled for preexisting differences in maternal age, education, and social class. The main aim of the preschool programs were to develop skills in oral and written expression, social and personal skills, and problem-solving skills. In addition, teachers worked with parents to promote child development, and parents attended parent-effectiveness workshops on positive child-rearing practices.

Self-reported delinquency measures were obtained at age 12. Pagani and her colleagues found that the results depended on whether children had perinatal complications. For those without complications, the prevalence of extreme delinquency was about half in the preschool group compared with the control group, but there was no significant difference for those who had experienced complications.

The third preschool program took place in Seattle, Washington. Webster-Stratton (1998) randomly assigned 64 classes in nine Head Start centers to experimental or control conditions; 426 children (average age 4.7) completed baseline assessments, in most cases drawn from families on social assistance with single mothers. The main approach in the experimental group was weekly parent training for 8–9 weeks, covering such topics as playing with your child, helping your child learn, using praise and encouragement to bring out the best in your child, effective setting of limits, and handling of misbehavior.

An evaluation of the program at its completion showed that experimental mothers became more consistent and less harsh compared with control mothers. Home observations showed a decrease in child misbehavior by experimental children, but there were no effects on rated externalizing (aggressive or impulsive) behavior according to mothers and teachers. A 1-year follow-up showed that experimental mothers maintained their decreases in harsh discipline and experimental children maintained their decreases in observed misbehavior.

Taken together, these three studies show that preschool programs including parenting interventions can lead to decreases in childhood antisocial behavior and delinquency.

School-Based Programs

Schools are a critical social context for delinquency and crime prevention efforts, even for the early grades. Two of the school-based programs we review here—one in Montreal (Tremblay, Pagani-Kurtz, Mâsse, Vitaro, & Pihl, 1995) and the other in Seattle (Hawkins et al., 1999)—are among the highest quality and most successful early delinquency prevention programs.

The Montreal longitudinal experimental study targeted disruptive (aggressive/hyperactive) boys from low SES neighborhoods. From an original sample of 1,161 boys, Tremblay and his colleagues (1995) identified 366 disruptive boys at age 6 and randomly allocated 319 of these to experimental or control conditions. The program lasted for 2 years and had 2 components: school-based social skills training and home-based parent training. Social skills training for the children was focused predominantly on improving child–peer interaction. The parent training component was based in social learning principles and involved training parents on how to provide positive reinforcement for desirable behavior, use nonpunitive and consistent discipline practices, and develop family crisis management techniques. At the latest follow-up, six years after the completion of the program, experimentals, in contrast to the controls, showed many desirable effects, including lower rates of self-reported delinquency.

The Seattle Social Development Project (SSDP), by Hawkins, Catalano, Kosterman, Abbott, and Hill (1999), involved about 500 first grade children (aged 6) in 21 classes in 8 schools, who were randomly assigned to be in experimental or control classes. The program included modified classroom teaching practices, parent training, and child social skills training. The parents were trained to notice and reinforce their children's socially desirable behavior in a program called "Catch them being good." At the end of the intervention period, treatment effects on delinquency and academic achievement varied by gender; no effect on delinquency was found for girls, but a desirable effect was found for boys. At the 6-year follow-up period, the full intervention group reported less violence, less alcohol abuse, and fewer sexual partners than the controls.

An external benefit–cost analysis of SSDP by Aos and his colleagues (2001) found that the program was economically efficient, with a benefit–cost ratio of 1.8. There was just about an equal split in the contribution of criminal justice system and crime victim benefits to the program's overall economic worth.

The largest school-based delinquency prevention study reported here, the Metropolitan Area Child Study (MACS) (Eron et al., 2000), which took place in Chicago and Aurora, Illinois, assessed the effectiveness of three different types of prevention programs: (1) general enhancement classroom intervention (GECI); (2) GECI plus small group peer-skills training (SGPST); and (3) GECI plus SGPST plus family intervention (FI), compared to a no-treatment control group. The study involved almost 2,200 children and randomly allocated 16 schools to the four different conditions. The program found varied effects as a function of the time of intervention and school resource level. Just focusing on the comparison between the most intensive intervention (GECI plus SGPST plus FI) and the control group, in the early grades (2–3) and early plus late grades (2–3 and 5–6, respectively) intervention cohorts, aggression was found to be lower for the experimental group, while for the late intervention cohort, the program showed no effect on aggression. In addition to these largely beneficial results, Eron and his colleagues (2000, p. 2) reported that, "Iatrogenic [harmful] effects on aggression were noted for younger children in low resource schools receiving the most intensive intervention as well as for older children receiving classroom plus small group training regardless of school resource level."

In the State of Oregon, Reid, Eddy, Fetrow, & Stoolmiller (1999) randomly allocated 12 elementary schools to experimental or control conditions. First and fifth grade children (aged about 7 and 11) in experimental schools received skills training in the classroom, backed up by parent training. The immediate impact of the intervention was successful, since the observed physical aggression of children in the playground decreased significantly for the experimental children.

Another important school-based prevention experiment was carried out by Kolvin, Garside, Nicol, MacMillan, Wolstenholme, & Leitch (1981) in Newcastle-upon-Tyne, England. They randomly allocated 270 junior school children (ages 7–8) and 322 senior school children (ages 11–12) to experimental or control groups. All children had been identified as showing some kind of social or psychiatric disturbance or learning problems (according to teacher and peer ratings). There were three types of experimental programs: (1) behavior modification—reinforcement with the seniors, "nurture work" teaching healthy interactions with the juniors; (2) parent counseling—teacher consultation with both; and (3) group therapy with the seniors, play groups with the juniors.

The programs were evaluated after 18 months and after 3 years using clinical ratings of conduct disturbance. Generally, the experimental and control groups were not significantly different for the juniors, although there was some tendency for the nurture work and play group conditions to be superior to the controls at the 3-year follow-up. For the seniors, those who received group therapy showed significantly less conduct disturbance at both follow-ups, and there was some tendency for the other two programs also to be effective at the 3-year follow-up.

Overall, these five school-based programs were of very high quality conceptually, methodologically, and in delivery. It is more than likely that their success has a great deal to do with these qualities. Indeed, the provision of child training in the school environment in a nonstigmatizing manner, combined with high quality parent training, were special features of these programs.

SYNTHESIS

This entry reviewed leading primary prevention programs implemented in the childhood years to address juvenile delinquency. Four different types of programs were examined: home visitation, child care, preschool, and school-based. Many of the programs in these different settings produced substantial benefits in the form of reductions in current acting-out behaviors such as aggression towards parents, teachers, and other children, and conduct problems, lower rates of delinquency in later childhood and adolescence, and improvements in the children's life course development. This entry also showed that some of these programs produced financial benefits that exceeded the costs of the program, and these benefits translated into cost savings to government and taxpayers, crime victims, and the program participants themselves.

Advancing knowledge about the benefits of early primary prevention programs to reduce antisocial behavior and later delinquency needs to begin with a program of research dedicated to replicating—particularly in high crime and high needs areas—more of those programs that have been shown to work and are promising, and ending funding for those programs that have been shown not to work or, more importantly, cause harm. This calls for greater use of experimental research designs, particularly randomized experiments, to assess program effects, because the more rigorous the evaluation design the more confidence that can be placed in the findings. There is also a great need for translating scientific research on what works and is promising into public policy and local practice. An evidence-based approach to the development of early delinquency prevention programs and policy has many advantages over current practice (Sherman, Farrington, Welsh, & MacKenzie, 2002).

It would also be desirable to know more about the long-term effects of many of these different types of early delinquency prevention programs. Long-term follow-up occurred in only a handful of the programs reviewed here, and few programs assess outcomes beyond the first year. Whether the benefits of programs persist beyond short-term time horizons is an important issue for policy development in this area.

Research is also needed to identify the active ingredients of successful (and promising) early delinquency prevention programs. Most programs are multidimensional, making it difficult to isolate the independent effects of the different components. Future experiments are needed which attempt to disentangle the effects of different elements of the most successful programs, such as the home visiting program of Olds and the school-based program of Hawkins. Nevertheless, there is generally good news: many early prevention programs are effective.

Also see: Delinquency: Adolescence; Peer Relationships: Childhood; School Absenteeism: Childhood; Self-Esteem: Childhood; Violence Prevention: Childhood.

References

Aos, S., Phipps, P., Barnoski, R., & Lieb, R. (2001). The comparative costs and benefits of programs to reduce crime: A review of research findings with implications for Washington State. In B.C. Welsh, D.P. Farrington, & L.W. Sherman (Eds.), *Costs and benefits of preventing crime* (pp. 149–75). Boulder, CO: Westview Press.

Eron, L.D., Guerra, N.G., Henry, D., Huesmann, L.R., Spindler, A., Tolan, P.H., & Van Acker, R. (2000). *A cognitive–ecological approach to preventing aggression in urban settings: Initial outcomes for high-risk children*. Manuscript under review.

Farrington, D.P. (1998). Youth crime and antisocial behaviour. In A. Campbell & S. Muncer (Eds.), *The social child* (pp. 353–392). Hove, East Sussex, England: Psychology Press.

Farrington, D.P., & Coid, J.W. (Eds.). (2002). *Early prevention of adult antisocial behaviour*. Cambridge, England: Cambridge University Press.

Farrington, D.P., & Welsh, B.C. (1999). Delinquency prevention using family-based interventions. *Children and Society, 13*, 287–303.

Greenwood, P.W., Karoly, L.A., Everingham, S.S., Houbé, J., Kilburn, M.R., Rydell, C.P., Sanders, M., & Chiesa, J. (2001). Estimating the costs and benefits of early childhood interventions: Nurse home visits and the Perry Preschool. In B.C. Welsh, D.P. Farrington, & L.W. Sherman (Eds.), *Costs and benefits of preventing crime* (pp. 112–148). Boulder, CO: Westview Press.

Hawkins, J.D., Catalano, R.F., Kosterman, R., Abbott, R., & Hill, K.G. (1999). Preventing adolescent health-risk behaviors by strengthening protection during childhood. *Archives of Pediatrics and Adolescent Medicine, 153*, 226–234.

Johnson, D.L., & Walker, T. (1987). Primary prevention of behavior problems in Mexican-American children. *American Journal of Community Psychology, 15*, 375–385.

Kitzman, H., Olds, D.L., Henderson, C.R., Hanks, C., Cole, R., Tatelbaum, R., McConnochie, K.M., Sidora, K., Luckey, D.W., Shaver, D., Engelhardt, K., James, D., & Barnard, K. (1997). Effect of prenatal and infancy home visitation by nurses on pregnancy outcomes, childhood injuries, and repeated childbearing: A randomized controlled trial. *Journal of the American Medical Association, 278*, 644–652.

Kolvin, I., Garside, R.F., Nicol, A.R., MacMillan, A., Wolstenholme, F., & Leitch, I.M. (1981). *Help starts here: The maladjusted child in the ordinary school*. London, England: Tavistock.

Lally, J.R., Mangione, P.L., & Honig, A.S. (1988). The Syracuse University Family Development Research Program: Long-range impact of an early intervention with low-income children and their families. In D.R. Powell (Ed.), *Parent education as early childhood intervention: emerging directions in theory, research and practice* (pp. 79–104). Norwood, NJ: Ablex.

Larson, C.P. (1980). Efficacy of prenatal and postpartum home visits on child health and development. *Pediatrics, 66*, 191–197.

Lipsey, M.W., & Wilson, D.B. (1998). Effective intervention for serious juvenile offenders: A synthesis of research. In R. Loeber & D.P. Farrington (Eds.), *Serious and violent juvenile offenders: Risk factors and successful interventions* (pp. 313–345). Thousand Oaks, CA: Sage.

McCarton, C.M., Brooks-Gunn, J., Wallace, I.F., Bauer, C.R., Bennett, F.C., Bernbaum, J.C., Broyles, R.S., Casey, P.H., McCormick, M.C., Scott, D.T., Tyson, J., Tonascia, J., & Meinert, C.L. (1997). Results at age 8 years of early intervention for low-birth-weight premature infants: The Infant Health and Development Program. *Journal of the American Medical Association, 277*, 126–132.

Michel, S. ((1999). *Children's interests/mother's rights: The shaping of America's child care policy*. New Haven, CT: Yale University Press.

Olds, D.L., Eckenrode, J., Henderson, C.R., Kitzman, H., Powers, J., Cole, R., Sidora, K., Morris, P., Pettitt, L.M., & Luckey, D. (1997). Long-term effects of home visitation on maternal life course and child abuse and neglect: Fifteen-year follow-up of a randomized trial. *Journal of the American Medical Association, 278*, 637–643.

Olds, D.L., Henderson, C.R., Cole, R., Eckenrode, J., Kitzman, H., Luckey, D., Pettitt, L., Sidora, K., Morris, P., & Powers, J. (1998). Long-term effects of nurse home visitation on children's criminal and antisocial behavior: 15-year follow-up of a randomized controlled trial. *Journal of the American Medical Association, 280*, 1238–1244.

Olds, D.L., Henderson, C.R., Phelps, C., Kitzman, H., & Hanks, C. (1993). Effects of prenatal and infancy home visitation on government spending. *Medical Care, 31*, 155–174.

Pagani, I., Tremblay, R.E., Vitaro, F., & Parent, S. (1998). Does preschool help prevent delinquency in boys with a history of perinatal complications? *Criminology, 36*, 297–313.

Reid, J.B., Eddy, J.M., Fetrow, R.A., & Stoolmiller, M. (1999). Description and immediate impacts of a preventive intervention for conduct problems. *American Journal of Community Psychology, 27*, 483–517.

Schweinhart, L.J., Barnes, H.V., & Weikart, D.P. (1993). *Significant benefits: The High/Scope Perry preschool study through age 27*. Ypsilanti, MI: High/Scope Press.

Sherman, L.W., Farrington, D.P., Welsh, B.C., & MacKenzie, D.L. (Eds.). (2002). *Evidence-Based Crime Prevention*. New York: Routledge.

Snyder, H.N., & Sickmund, M. (1999). *Juvenile offenders and victims: 1999 national report*. Washington, DC: Office of Juvenile Justice and Delinquency Prevention, US Department of Justice.

Stone, W.L., Bendell, R.D., & Field, T.M. (1988). The impact of socioeconomic status on teenage mothers and children who received early intervention. *Journal of Applied Developmental Psychology, 9*, 391–408.

Tracy, P.E., Wolfgang, M.E., & Figlio, R.M. (1985). *Delinquency in two birth cohorts*. Washington, DC: Office of Juvenile Justice and Delinquency Prevention, US Department of Justice.

Tremblay, R.E., Pagani-Kurtz, L., Mâsse, L.C., Vitaro, F., & Pihl, R.O. (1995). A bimodal preventive intervention for disruptive kindergarten boys: Its impact through mid-adolescence. *Journal of Consulting and Clinical Psychology, 63*, 560–568.

Webster-Stratton, C. (1998). Preventing conduct problems in Head Start children: Strengthening parenting competencies. *Journal of Consulting and Clinical Psychology, 66*, 715–730.

Delinquency, Adolescence

Brandon C. Welsh and
David P. Farrington

INTRODUCTION, DEFINITION, AND SCOPE

Juvenile delinquency is a serious problem. In 1997, there were about 30 million juveniles aged 10–17 in the United States. About 123,000 were arrested for *serious violent crimes* (murder, rape, robbery, or aggravated assault) and 702,000 were arrested for *serious property crimes* (burglary, theft, vehicle theft, or arson). The juvenile arrest rate for serious violence stayed constant from 1975 to 1988 at about 3 per 1,000 population, but then suddenly increased by two thirds to over 5 per 1,000 in 1994 before deceasing somewhat (Snyder & Sickmund, 1999). In contrast, the juvenile arrest rate for serious property offenses stayed constant over this whole time period, at about 25 per 1,000 population each year.

The cumulative prevalence of delinquency is much higher than the annual prevalence, of course. For example, one third of boys and 14 percent of girls born in Philadelphia in 1958 were arrested for nontraffic offenses as juveniles, and 18 percent of boys and 4 percent of girls were arrested for one of the eight serious index offenses (Tracy, Wolfgang, & Figlio, 1985). There was a considerable racial differential; 26 percent of African American boys were arrested for serious offenses, compared with 9 percent of Caucasian boys.

This entry is concerned with the primary prevention of juvenile delinquency through programs that are initiated in the adolescent years. We review leading adolescent delinquency prevention programs organized by the four most important approaches: school-based, mentoring, after-school recreation, and community-based. Only programs including outcome measures of delinquency or antisocial behavior are included. We also look at the monetary costs and benefits of preventing juvenile delinquency, for those programs that carried out a benefit–cost analysis.

Like early childhood delinquency prevention programs, most delinquency prevention programs implemented in the teenage years have not been evaluated adequately. Rather than attempt to review a large number of programs (e.g., in a meta-analysis; see Lipsey & Wilson, 1998), we have chosen to focus on the best: those evaluated in randomized experiments or quasi-experiments (i.e., comparing experimental and control conditions with before and after measures), with relatively large samples (for more extensive information on the prevention of delinquency in the teenage years, see Loeber & Farrington, 1998).

THEORY, RESEARCH, AND STRATEGIES

School-Based Programs

Schools are an important social context for juvenile delinquency and crime prevention efforts, and evaluation studies of school-based programs number in the hundreds. We review two important programs here, but interested readers should consult Gottfredson's (2000) excellent book on schools and delinquency.

Several school-based programs have been designed to decrease bullying, which is known to predict later delinquency. The most famous of these was implemented by Olweus (1994) in Norway. It aimed to increase awareness and knowledge of teachers, parents, and children about bullying and to dispel myths about it. A 30-page booklet was distributed to all schools in Norway describing what was known about bullying and recommending what steps schools and teachers could take to reduce it. Also, a 25-min video about bullying was made available to schools. Simultaneously, the schools distributed to all parents a four-page folder containing information and advice about bullying. In addition, anonymous self-report questionnaires about bullying were completed by all children.

The program was evaluated in Bergen. Each of the 42 participating schools received feedback information from the questionnaire, about the prevalence of bullies and victims, in a specially arranged school conference day. Also, teachers were encouraged to develop explicit rules about bullying (e.g., do not bully, tell someone when bullying happens, bullying will not be tolerated, try to help victims, try to include children who are being left out) and to discuss bullying in class, using the video and role-playing exercises. Also, teachers were encouraged to improve monitoring and supervision of children, especially in the playground. The program was successful in reducing the prevalence of bullying by half.

A similar program was implemented in 23 Sheffield (England) schools by Smith and Sharp (1994). The core program involved establishing a "whole-school" anti-bullying policy, raising awareness of bullying, and clearly defining roles and responsibilities of teachers and students, so that everyone knew what bullying was and what they should do about it. In addition, there were optional interventions tailored to particular schools: curriculum work (e.g., reading books, watching videos), direct work with students (e.g., assertiveness training for those who were bullied), and playground work (e.g., training lunch-time supervisors). This program was successful in reducing bullying in primary schools, but had a relatively small effect in secondary schools. (For reviews of anti-bullying programs in many different countries, see Smith, Morita, Junger-Tas, Olweus, Catalano, & Slee, 1999.)

Mentoring Programs

Mentoring programs typically involve nonprofessional volunteers spending time with young individuals in a "supportive, nonjudgmental manner while acting as role models" (Howell, 1995, p. 90). The Office of Juvenile Justice and Delinquency Prevention has supported mentoring for many years across the United States, most substantially through the Juvenile Mentoring Program (JUMP), which offers "one-to-one mentoring for youth at risk of delinquency, gang involvement, educational failure, or dropping out of school" (Novotney, Mertinko, Lange, & Baker, 2000, p. 1).

Two of the earliest mentoring programs that were experimentally evaluated for their effects on delinquency were conducted in the early 1970s in Hawaii by Fo and O'Donnell (1974, 1975). Called the "Buddy System," these two experimental mentoring programs were provided to at-risk youth between ages 11 and 17 years; mentors were between 17 and 65 years. The first Buddy System program (Fo & O'Donnell, 1974) lasted 12 weeks and consisted of two six-week interventions. Forty-two children with behavior management problems were randomly assigned to three treatment groups and one control group. In all three experimental groups, mentors received $10 to spend on each mentee per month. While the "relationship" and "social approval" treatment groups spent the money in a non-contingent way on the mentee, the "social/material reinforcement" treatment group provided social approval and money contingent on appropriate behaviors of the youngsters.

Fo and O'Donnell's assessment of program effectiveness focused on the truancy rate, academic achievement, and behavior problems (e.g., fighting) of the children. Results after the first six weeks showed a substantial reduction in truancy for those mentees who received the social approval and social/material reinforcement treatment but not for those in the relationship treatment group or no-treatment control group. After "stabilization" of the target behavior, all mentees were switched to the social/material reinforcement condition for the second intervention period. Results from the second six weeks of intervention showed lower truancy rates for all treatment groups compared to the control group. Child problem behaviors were also reduced through the social/material reinforcement treatment. These findings indicate that the use of behavioral contingency procedures may be highly effective. However, the small sample size and short intervention periods limit the strength of these findings.

Fo and O'Donnell (1975) evaluated a second, much larger and longer Buddy System program. This program lasted one year and included a sample of 442 children and youth, ages 10–17 years. Much less complex than the first program, comparisons were made only between those who received mentoring and those who did not. The results of this program were rather interesting: while the Buddy System seemed to be effective for youngsters with prior offenses, it was ineffective (harmful) for those without any criminal history. One explanation for this outcome could be that mentees with no prior offenses formed relationships with delinquent youngsters. The authors noted that, "The results raise the spectre of possible iatrogenic treatment effects of the Buddy System approach with youngsters with no record of prior major offenses" (Fo & O'Donnell, 1975, p. 524).

A more recent mentoring program known as the Quantum Opportunities Program (QOP; Hahn, 1999) found desirable effects on criminal activity. QOP was started in 1989 in five sites across the United States: Philadelphia, Oklahoma City, San Antonio, Saginaw, and Milwaukee. The program aimed to improve the life course opportunities of disadvantaged, at-risk youth during the high school years.

The sample consisted of 250 youths who were in the ninth grade of school. Youths were randomly assigned to the program or to the control group. The sample sizes in each of the five sites were identical ($N = 50$), with an equal number in both the program and control groups, and the program and control groups were similar in their level of disadvantage. The program ran for four years or up to grade 12, and was designed around the provision of three "quantum opportunities": (1) educational activities (e.g., peer tutoring, computer-based instruction, homework assistance); (2) service activities (e.g., volunteering with community projects); and (3) development activities (e.g., curricula focused on life and family skills, and college and career planning) (Hahn, 1994). Each of these opportunities was guaranteed for up to 250 hr each year for the duration of the program. Cash and scholarship incentives were also offered to students for work carried out in the three program areas—education, service, and development—to provide short-run motivation for school completion and future academic and social achievement. Staff received cash incentives and bonuses for keeping youths involved in the program.

Six months after the program ended a number of significant effects were observed. Compared to the control group, QOP group members were: more likely to have graduated from high school (63 vs. 42 percent); more likely to be enrolled in some form of post-secondary education (42 vs. 16 percent); less likely to have dropped out of high school (23 vs. 50 percent); and less likely to have been arrested (17 vs. 58 percent).

A benefit–cost analysis of the program revealed substantial benefits for both participating QOP members and taxpayers. Total costs of the program were estimated at $10,600 per program group member; benefits were estimated at $39,037 per program group member. Dividing benefits by costs produced a desirable benefit–cost ratio of 3.7, meaning that for each dollar spent on the program almost four dollars were saved.

Other mentoring programs have also been successful. For example, Baker, Pollack, and Kohn (1995) evaluated an after-school mentoring program in a Baltimore youth center, and found that the delinquency and drug use of experimental youth decreased relative to control youth. However, this evaluation was hindered by high attrition of youth between pretest and posttest questionnaires.

Mixed messages can be drawn from the findings of these four juvenile mentoring programs. On the one hand, the graduation incentives mentoring program of Hahn, the first experiment on the Buddy System, and the Baltimore youth center program showed desirable and in some cases significant results; on the other hand, the second experiment on the Buddy System produced harmful results for one group who received the intervention. This latter finding is perhaps deserving of special attention.

Afterschool Recreation

Recreation programs are based on the belief that providing prosocial opportunities for young people in the afterschool hours can reduce their involvement in delinquent behavior in the community. Afterschool programs seek to target a range of risk factors for delinquency and later criminal behavior, including alienation and association with delinquent and violent peers. Two high quality programs, one in Canada and one in the United States, are reviewed.

The Canadian program (Jones & Offord, 1989), implemented in 1980 in a public housing complex in the city of Ottawa, recruited low-income children (ages 5–15) to participate in afterschool activities aimed at improving skills in sports, music, dance, scouting, and other nonsport areas. Known as the Participate and Learn Skills (PALS) program, it lasted for 32 months and sought to advance children toward higher skill levels and to integrate children from the housing complex into activities in the wider community. It was also assumed that this skill-development program could affect other areas of a child's life (e.g., prosocial attitudes and behaviors). The housing project was matched with a control public housing complex, which did not receive this specialized treatment.

At the end of the program, children in the experimental housing site fared better than their control counterparts on a range of measures. The strongest program effect was found for juvenile delinquency. During the 32 months of the program, the monthly average of juveniles charged by the police was 80 percent less at the experimental site compared to the control site. This effect was diminished somewhat in the 16 months after the program ended. Possibly, the effects of the program were wearing off. Substantial gains were also observed in skill acquisition, as measured by the number of levels advanced in an activity, and in integration in the wider community, among experimental site children compared with the controls. Spill-over effects on participating children included an increase in self-esteem, but no change in behavior at school or home was observed.

A benefit–cost analysis of the program produced a desirable benefit–cost ratio of 2.6. Over the course of the 48 months (intervention and follow-up periods), program

costs totaled $258,694 (in 1983 Canadian dollars) and benefits were estimated at $659,058. The calculation of monetary benefits was limited to only those areas where significant differences were observed between the experimental and control complexes: fewer police charges against juveniles, reduced private security reports, and reduced calls for fire department service. The city housing authority reaped the largest share of the benefits (84 percent). These benefits were due to the reduced demand for private security services in the experimental housing complex relative to the control complex.

Schinke and his colleagues (1992) analyzed the impact of the Boys and Girls Clubs in a number of public housing sites across the United States. The study's goal was to compare "substance abuse and other problem behavior rates between youth who lived in public housing developments and youth who do and do not have access to Boys and Girls Clubs" (Schinke, Orlandi, & Cole, 1992, p. 120). The evaluation design used three groups of five housing project sites: ten treatment sites and five control sites. Five sites had a traditional Boys and Girls Club (BGC) program, five sites received the BGC program in combination with a substance abuse prevention program called Self-Management and Resistance Training (SMART Moves), and five sites had no intervention (control groups). Evaluation results showed that housing projects with BGC, with and without SMART Moves, had fewer damaged units and less criminal activity than housing projects without clubs. There was also an overall reduction in substance abuse, drug trafficking, and other drug-related criminal activity.

Taken together, these two studies show that afterschool recreation interventions can lead to decreases in juvenile delinquency and make improvements in other important life course outcomes.

Community-Based Programs

These programs sometimes incorporate numerous interventions targeted at an array of risk factors for juvenile delinquency and are typically implemented in high crime neighborhoods. The three programs we review below are among the most well known and are of the highest quality methodologically.

In the famous Cambridge-Somerville youth study, 650 Boston boys (median age 10) who were rated as difficult or average in behavior were randomly allocated to experimental or control conditions. The experimental boys received regular friendly attention from counselors for an average of five years, and whatever medical and educational services were needed. The counselors talked to the boys, took them on trips and to recreational activities, tutored them in reading and arithmetic, played games with them at the project's center, encouraged them to attend church, and visited their families to give advice and general support (McCord & McCord, 1959). Family problems were the focus of attention for approximately one third of the experimental group.

The men in both groups were followed up to age 45, 30 years after the program had ended. Unfortunately, the results were disappointing. Generally, there was little difference between the experimental and control groups in recorded crimes, but significantly more of the experimental group had committed two or more crimes. Similarly, there was little difference between the groups in the prevalence of mental illness, but significantly more of the experimental group showed signs of alcoholism and more had died early. Nevertheless, two thirds of the experimental men thought that the program had helped them. McCord (1978) speculated that the negative results could have been caused by the program generating high expectations which may later have been dashed when the program was terminated.

Feldman, Caplinger, and Wodarski (1983) in St. Louis evaluated a program based on the influence of prosocial (well-behaved) friends. Over 400 boys (aged about 11) who were referred because of their antisocial behavior were randomly assigned to two types of activity groups, each comprising about 10–12 adolescents. The groups consisted either totally of referred youths or of one or two referred youths and about 10 non-referred (prosocial) peers. The focus was on group-level behavior modification. On the basis of systematic observation, self-reports by the youths, and ratings by group leaders, it was concluded that the antisocial behavior of referred youths who were interacting with prosocial peers decreased relative to that of referred youths in homogeneously antisocial groups. Similarly, experiments using high-status conventional peers to teach adolescents ways of reducing peer pressure have been effective in reducing drug use (Tobler, Lessard, Marshall, Ochshorn, & Roona, 1999).

More recently, the large-scale Children At Risk (CAR) program targeted high risk youths (average age 12.4) in poor neighborhoods of five cities across the United States (Harrell, Cavanagh, & Sridharan, 1999). Eligible youths were identified in schools and randomly assigned to experimental or control groups. The program was a comprehensive community-based prevention strategy targeting risk factors for delinquency, including case management and family counseling, family skills training, tutoring, mentoring, afterschool activities, and community policing. The program was different in each neighborhood.

The initial results were disappointing, but a one-year follow-up showed that (according to self-reports) experimental youths were less likely to have committed violent crimes and used or sold drugs. The process evaluation showed that the greatest change was in peer risk factors. Experimental youths associated less often with delinquent peers, felt less peer pressure to engage in delinquency, and

had more positive peer support. In contrast, there were few changes in individual, family, or community risk factors, possibly linked to the low participation of parents in parent training and of youths in mentoring and tutoring. The implementation problems of the program were related to the serious and multiple needs and problems of the families.

SYNTHESIS

This entry reviewed leading primary prevention programs implemented in the adolescent years to address juvenile delinquency. Four different types of programs were examined: school-based, mentoring, afterschool recreation, and community-based. Decreases in delinquency were achieved by programs in each of these four different program categories. This entry also showed that a couple of these programs produced financial benefits that exceeded the costs of the program, and these benefits translated into cost savings to government and taxpayers, crime victims, and the program participants themselves.

Our recommended program of research to advance knowledge about the benefits of primary prevention programs in the teenage years to reduce juvenile delinquency is very similar to the one we described for delinquency prevention programs in the childhood years. First, there needs to be a commitment to replicating—particularly in high crime and high need areas—more of those programs that have been shown to work and are promising, and ending funding for those programs that have been shown not to work or, more importantly, cause harm. This calls for greater use of experimental research designs, particularly randomized experiments, to assess program effects, because the more rigorous the evaluation design the more confidence that can be placed in the findings. Second, there is a need for translating scientific research on what works and is promising into public policy and local practice, as an evidence-based approach to the development of juvenile delinquency prevention programs and policy has many advantages over current practice (Sherman, Farrington, Welsh, & MacKenzie, 2002).

Third, attention should be given to understanding more about the long-term effects of many of these different types of juvenile delinquency prevention programs. Few programs assess outcomes beyond the first year, and long-term follow-up occurred in only a handful of the programs reviewed here. Whether the benefits of programs persist beyond short-term time horizons is an important issue for policy development in this area, just as it is for early childhood delinquency prevention programs.

Lastly, we need to learn more about harmful effects caused by programs designed to "do good" and how these harmful effects can be avoided in the future. This is a particularly important issue facing social interventions of all kinds and for all ages, but seems to be of particular concern for programs, which are targeted on antisocial adolescents (see Dishion, McCord, & Poulin, 1999). It is logical to target peer influences in attempting to prevent adolescent offending, but there is always the danger that peer influences are bad. Preventing harmful effects and putting more of what works into practice should be the main goals of efforts to prevent juvenile delinquency.

Also see: Homicide: Adolescence; Life Skills: Adolescence; Peer Relationships: Adolescence; Risk-Taking: Adolescence; School Violence: Adolescence; Self-Esteem: Adolescence; Sexual Assault: Adolescence.

References

Baker, K., Pollack, M., & Kohn, I. (1995). Violence prevention through informal socialization: An evaluation of the South Baltimore Youth Center. *Studies on Crime and Crime Prevention, 4,* 61–85.

Dishion, T.J., McCord, J., & Poulin, F. (1999). When intervention harms: Peer groups and problem behavior. *American Psychologist, 54,* 755–764.

Feldman, R.A., Caplinger, T.E., & Wodarski, J.S. (1983). *The St. Louis conundrum.* Englewood Cliffs, NJ: Prentice-Hall.

Fo, W.S.O., & O'Donnell, C.R. (1974). The buddy system: Relationship and contingency conditioning in a community intervention program for youth with nonprofessionals as behavior change agents. *Journal of Consulting and Clinical Psychology, 42,* 163–169.

Fo, W.S.O., & O'Donnell, C.R. (1975). The buddy system: Effect of community intervention on delinquent offenses. *Behavior Therapy, 6,* 522–524.

Gottfredson, D.C. (2000). *Schools and delinquency.* New York: Cambridge University Press.

Hahn, A. (1994). *Evaluation of the Quantum Opportunities Program (QOP): Did the program work?* Waltham, MA: Brandeis University.

Hahn, A. (1999). Extending the time of learning. In D.J. Besharov (Ed.), *America's disconnected youth: Toward a preventive strategy* (pp. 233–265). Washington, DC: Child Welfare League of America Press.

Harrell, A.V., Cavanagh, S.E., & Sridharan, S. (1999, November). Evaluation of the Children At Risk Program: Results 1 year after the end of the program. *Research in brief.* Washington, DC: National Institute of Justice, US Department of Justice.

Howell, J.C. (Ed.). (1995). *Guide for implementing the comprehensive strategy for serious, violent, and chronic juvenile offenders.* Washington, DC: Office of Juvenile Justice and Delinquency Prevention, US Department of Justice.

Jones, M.B., & Offord, D.R. (1989). Reduction of anti-social behaviour in poor children by nonschool skill development. *Journal of Child Psychology and Psychiatry, 30,* 737–750.

Lipsey, M.W., & Wilson, D.B. (1998). Effective intervention for serious juvenile offenders: A synthesis of research. In R. Loeber & D.P. Farrington (Eds.), *Serious and violent juvenile offenders: Risk factors and successful interventions* (pp. 313–345). Thousand Oaks, CA: Sage.

Loeber, R., & Farrington, D.P. (Eds.). (1998). *Serious and violent juvenile offenders: Risk factors and successful interventions.* Thousand Oaks, CA: Sage.

McCord, J. (1978). A thirty-year follow-up of treatment effects. *American Psychologist, 33,* 284–289.

McCord, J., & McCord, W. (1959). A follow-up report on the Cambridge-Somerville Youth Study. *Annals of the American Academy of Political and Social Science, 322,* 89–96.

Novotney, L.C., Mertinko, E., Lange, J., & Baker, T.K. (2000, September). Juvenile mentoring program: A progress review. *OJJDP Juvenile Justice Bulletin.* Washington, DC: Office of Juvenile Justice and Delinquency Prevention, US Department of Justice.

Olweus, D. (1994). Bullying at school: Basic facts and effects of a school based intervention program. *Journal of Child Psychology and Psychiatry, 35,* 1171–1190.

Schinke, S.P., Orlandi, M.A., & Cole, K.C. (1992). Boys & Girls Clubs in public housing developments: Prevention services for youth at risk [OSAP Special Issue]. *Journal of Community Psychology,* 118–128.

Sherman, L.W., Farrington, D.P., Welsh, B.C., & MacKenzie, D.L. (Eds.). (2002). *Evidence-based crime prevention.* New York: Routledge.

Smith, P.K., Morita, Y., Junger-Tas, J., Olweus, D., Catalano, R., & Slee, P. (1999). *The nature of school bullying: A cross-national perspective.* London, UK: Routledge.

Smith, P.K., & Sharp, S. (1994). *School bullying.* London, UK: Routledge.

Snyder, H.N., & Sickmund, M. (1999). *Juvenile offenders and victims: 1999 national report.* Washington, DC: Office of Juvenile Justice and Delinquency Prevention, US Department of Justice.

Tobler, N.S., Lessard, T., Marshall, D., Ochshorn, P., & Roona, M. (1999). Effectiveness of school-based drug prevention programs for marijuana use. *School Psychology International, 20,* 105–37.

Tracy, P.E., Wolfgang, M.E., & Figlio, R.M. (1985). *Delinquency in two birth cohorts.* Washington, DC: Office of Juvenile Justice and Delinquency Prevention, US Department of Justice.

Depression, Childhood

Clare Roberts and Brian Bishop

INTRODUCTION

Children with depression report symptoms such as sadness, irritability, social withdrawal, somatic complaints, and a lack of interest in usual activities. Their suffering leads to impairments in home, school, and interpersonal contexts. While not a common childhood mental health problem, incidence in childhood is a strong predictor for adolescent and adult depression (Kovacs, 1996). Furthermore, depression is showing increasing incidence in cohorts born in the later part of this century (Roberts, 1999). These factors make childhood depression an important target for preventive efforts.

DEFINITIONS

Depression is a generic term used to describe a number of phenomena, measured by a variety of approaches.

Depressed mood, commonly measured by self-report, is defined as an unhappy or sad mood. While not necessarily evidence of a clinical disorder, severely depressed mood predicts future depressive disorders in children (Cicchetti & Toth, 1998). *Depressive syndrome* is defined as a sad mood accompanied by a constellation of other emotional symptoms, for example, anhedonia, low self-esteem, worry, pessimism, guilt, and loneliness. It is measured by questionnaire; information is often sought from more than one source; and clinical cut-offs based on empirically validated levels of symptom clusters are used. *Depressive disorders* are defined by clinically derived standard diagnostic criteria involving specific profiles of emotional, behavioral, cognitive, and somatic symptoms. Assessment is usually based upon structured clinical interviews. *Major depressive disorder* (MDD), which is episodic and often recurrent, and *dysthymic disorder* (DD) involving more chronic mood disturbance will be addressed in this entry. Bipolar disorder has different phenomenology and aetiology and will not be discussed.

SCOPE

No studies of the incidence of depression in children were found. However, studies from the United States (Cohen et al., 1993), Spain (Polaino-Lorente & Domenech, 1993), and New Zealand (Anderson, Williams, McGee, & Silva, 1987) have found 0.4–2.5 percent of youngsters under 12 years experience MDD at any point in time. Also, less than one percent of pre-schoolers experienced MDD. DD is rarer than MDD, with point prevalence rates of 0.6–1.7 percent in US and New Zealand studies, and 6.4 percent in Spain (Birmaher et al., 1996).

Studies of depressive syndrome revealed similar rates. In Australia, 3 percent, of 4–11-year-olds evidenced clinically significant levels of anxious and depressed symptoms, rated by their parents and teachers on the Child Behavior Checklist (Zubrick et al., 1995). In Canada, Flemming, Offord, and Boyle (1989) found rates of 5.5 percent using the same instrument, in a population sample of 4–16-year-olds. Where depressive mood has been measured, rates are higher, with 13 percent of 10–11-year-olds in the Isle of Wight study reporting depressive feelings (Rutter, Izard, & Read, 1986). Girls and boys have approximately equal prevalence rates for depressive disorders and symptoms below 13–14 years (Cohen et al., 1993).

The median episode length for childhood MDD is 9 months, and 3.9 years for DD. Further, children with DD frequently develop MDD within 2–3 years. Significant comorbidity with other psychological disorders is also a feature. Anxiety disorders (30–75 percent) and conduct disorders (21–83 percent) are common. Comorbidity increases the risk of recurrent episodes and functional impairments, and reduces the response to treatment (Kovacs, 1996).

THEORIES AND RESEARCH

A number of models of depression have been proposed: genetic, biological, cognitive, behavioral and interpersonal, environmental stress, and family theories. Unlike adult models, models of childhood depression need to take developmental and transactional perspectives that consider the impact of development on depression and the impact of depression upon emerging developmental processes.

Genetic Theories

Depression runs in families. While twin studies indicate a genetic component for depressive symptoms, the impact of genetic factors is not clear in children. A higher incidence of affective disorders has been found in the adult relatives and cousins of children with depressive disorders compared to normal controls. However, when offspring studies of affective and anxiety disorders in children have been reviewed, a lack of specificity for depression has been found in offspring (Todd & Heath, 1996). Research from adoption studies of depressive symptoms in childhood suggests that heritability is negligible, the effects of shared environment are modest, and non-shared environmental effects are more substantial (Eley, Deater-Deckard, Fombonne, Fulker, & Plomin, 1998). Hence, while genetic vulnerability may be a factor in childhood depressive disorders, the effect may neither be specific to depressive disorders nor as relevant for depressive symptoms, and the effects may vary with age.

Biological Theories

Research into biological markers of childhood depression has been disappointing. There is some support for neuroendocrine system dysfunction, particularly in relation to hypothalamic–pituitary–adrenal axis abnormalities and dysregulation of the sleep-onset mechanism in depressed adolescents, but findings are less consistent in pre-pubertal children (Birmaher et al., 1996). Researchers have found some evidence that biochemical differences in depressed children involve increased sensitivity to stress or environmental challenge, rather than the chronic dysregulation or hyperarousal found in depressed adults (Birmaher et al., 1996). Hammen and Rudolph (1996) report on research that has found an association between rises in neuroendocrine activation immediately following a psychosocial stressor, and anxiety and social inhibition in outpatient children. These rises also predicted anxiety and depression 6 months later. Further, Birmaher et al. (1996) reviewed research that has found abnormal variations in growth hormone, prolactin secretion, and serotonergic functioning in response to psycho-pharmacological stressors in depressed children. They suggest that changes in growth hormone secretion and serotonergic regulation may be associated with earlier onset of depressive disorders. These findings suggest a developmental sequence in which repeated neuroendocrine activation following environmental stress increases children's susceptibility to internalizing problems.

Cognitive Theories

A number of cognitive theories of depression have been investigated in children, cognitive errors/schema (Beck, Rush, Shaw, & Emery, 1979), attributional style (Peterson & Seligman, 1984), personal control (Weisz, Rudolph, Granger, & Sweeney, 1992), and self-control theory (Rehm, 1977). These theories all represent diathesis-stress models in proposing that a child's perception and processing of adverse events leads to depression rather than aversive events alone.

Beck's theory proposes that depressed children make systematic errors in their interpretation of negative events leading to negative self-talk. Depression is associated with stable, internal belief systems that structure memory, guide information processing, and stimulate self-critical beliefs, resulting in a "negative cognitive triad" of the self, the world, and the future. Negative schema and self-talk leave the individual vulnerable to depression in the face of external stressors.

General population studies have linked depressive symptoms to lowered self-esteem, irrational beliefs, dysfunctional attitudes, negative automatic thoughts, and pessimism in children (Roberts, 1999). Also, clinical studies have distinguished depressed, from anxious and normal, children by less positive views the self, others, and the future, and more negative automatic thoughts. Clinically depressed children have more negative styles of processing self-evaluative information, more distorted self-perceptions, and they judge themselves more harshly than non-depressed children (Compas, Connor, & Wadsworth, 1997). In addition, depressive symptoms in children have been predicted by the interaction of negative cognitions and self-perceptions, and aversive events in longitudinal studies (Roberts, 1999). However, cognitive bias has been found to mediate the relationship between negative peer evaluations and depressive symptoms in early adolescence, but not in younger children (Cole & Jordan, 1995).

Peterson and Seligman (1984) proposed that a pessimistic attributional style, that is, attributing negative outcomes to internal, global and stable, causes and positive outcomes to external, specific and temporary, causes leads to helplessness, hopelessness, and ultimately depression in the face of negative life events. The related locus of control theory presented by Weisz et al. (1992) implicates a link between low perceived competence, external locus of control and depression. Further, Bandura's self-efficacy theory proposed that belief in one's ability to regulate functioning and to control events that affect your life are strongly related to depression (Bandura, Pastorelli, Barbaranelli, & Caprara, 1999).

Gladstone and Kaslow's (1995) meta-analyses found moderate to large effect sizes for associations between children's pessimistic attributional style and depressive symptoms. However, the proposed diathesis-stress effect has been found in older children just beginning adolescence, but not younger children. Nolan-Hoeksema, Girgus, and Seligman (1992) found that negative events predicted depressive symptoms in early childhood, but pessimistic attributional style predicted depressive symptoms alone and in interaction with negative events by late childhood. Pessimism worsened during depressive episodes and persisted following recovery from episodes supporting the theory of learned helplessness.

Compas, Banez, Malcarne, and Worsham (1991) indicated that children's perceptions of contingency, competence, and control are not well developed until 11 years of age. In support, Weisz, Sweeney, Proffitt, and Carr (1993) found positive associations between depressive symptoms and perceived competence and contingency beliefs in late childhood. Also, low levels of perceived social and academic efficacy have been found to contribute to concurrent and subsequent depression in children, both directly and via an impact upon actual academic achievement and behavior. Perceived social inefficacy appears to be more important for girls than boys (Bandura et al., 1999).

Rehm's self-control theory proposed that impairments in processes such as self-monitoring, setting standards, and rewarding successes, result in vulnerability to depression. The research on cognitive factors reviewed by Roberts (1999) supports deficits in self-monitoring and self-evaluation, including memory impairments related to recall of success, setting harsh standards, and confirmation of negative self-cognitions, in depressed children from clinical and community samples. In addition, positive self-evaluations in just one domain can have a compensatory effect.

The research reviewed supports a developmental sequence whereby negative cognitive processes are developed in response to repeated environmental stressors, and these processes become habitual by late childhood to early adolescence and act as vulnerability factors in interaction with life stress. Indeed these vulnerabilities may be evolving from an early age, in that pre-school children of depressed mothers have been found to display negative affective tone in their causal attributions and self-statements to their mothers (Cicchetti & Toth, 1998).

Behavioral and Interpersonal Theories

Negative cognitions do not preclude behavioral or interpersonal deficits also being related to the development and maintenance of childhood depression. Lewinsohn (1974) conceptualized depression as the consequence of skills deficits that are associated with low rates of response contingent positive reinforcement. Three areas of skills are important here, social competence skills, social problem-solving skills, and coping skills.

Social competence difficulties have been associated with depression in children, including lower levels of peer acceptance, negative peer nominations, friendship difficulties, and poor social skills, such as less assertion, more submissiveness, and more angry impulsive behavior. These results have been found in studies using ratings from teachers, peers, and self-reports, both concurrently and over time. In addition, the effects of negative social behavior appear to be mediated in part by peer rejection and self-perceptions of rejection in children (Roberts, 1999). Cole, Martin, and Powers (1997) demonstrated interactions between interpersonal and cognitive risk factors and depressive symptoms over time. Competency ratings by peers, teachers, and parents predicted changes in self-evaluations of competency over time, in girls, and these changes were associated with increased depression over time in both genders.

Nezu, Nezu, and Perri (1989) proposed that depression is directly influenced by how people cope with major and minor daily stressors, and how well they solve social problems. In support, Hammen and Rudolph (1996) review research indicating that the effectiveness of children's solutions to peer conflict problems, not the number of solutions, moderates the relationship between negative life stress and depressive symptoms. Further, depressed youngsters have been found to be more hostile than anxious youngsters, and their problem-solving efforts resulted in more peer conflict, less collaboration, and less joint problem solving. Depressed children evoked negative affect and peer rejection in their problem-solving partners. Hence, the negative self-perceptions of depressed children may be realistic. Compas et al. (1997) presented evidence that problem-focused coping skills emerge in childhood, but emotion-focused coping skills develop more rapidly in the late childhood and early adolescence. They also reported that the coping skills repertoire of depressed children are often deficient in active problem-focused strategies and over supplied with emotion-focused, passive, avoidant, and ruminative coping strategies.

Hence, depression in children is associated with lower levels of social competence, and more limited social problem-solving and coping skills. These lower levels of competence and problem-solving skills also lead to more negative interpersonal relationships and depression. Indeed infants of depressed mothers show more frequent expressions of sadness, fewer expressions of interest, and more gaze and head aversion in mother–child interaction, than other infants of well mothers (Cicchetti & Toth, 1998).

Environmental Stress Theories

Stress models of depression have been alluded to in the review of cognitive and interpersonal diathesis-stress theories of depression. These theories include stress-reactive models and stress-generation models. Research reviewed previously indicates some support for stress-reactive models or an interaction between attributional style and life stress, at least in late childhood (Gladstone & Kaslow, 1995). There is also support for interactions between stress and interpersonal factors. Moderation effects relating stress in specific life domains that are valued by children, particularly the interpersonal domain, to depressive symptoms have been found in older but not younger children. In addition, researchers have proposed mediation models, where individual cognitive and interpersonal risk factors are caused by stress, then predispose younger children to depression (Roberts, 1999). Rudolph, Hammen, Burge, Lindberg, Herzberg, and Daley (2000) presented evidence that depressed children generate stressful circumstances particularly in the interpersonal domain, which in turn result in more depression. Hence, environmental stress is related to depression in children. It is implicated in the development of cognitive and interpersonal vulnerabilities for depression in younger children and these vulnerabilities moderate the impact of stress as children reach late childhood and early adolescence, by providing a buffering effect or by creating additional interpersonal stress (Roberts, 1999).

Family Theories

Family theories propose that vulnerabilities for childhood depression arise in the context of insecure infant attachments that then contribute to the development of internal models of the self and others, and influence on the development of cognition, affect regulation, and behavior (Cicchetti & Toth, 1998). Further, social learning occurs through the day-to-day parent–child interactions (Rapee, 1997). Family variables that have been investigated include parental affective disorders, parent–child interactions and childrearing practices, marital conflict, general family functioning and attachment (Dadds & Barrett, 1996).

Impaired attachment processes have been implicated in the development of childhood depression. However, little specificity for particular clinical problems has been found in studies of children (Main, 1996). Main's review found five attachment difficulties associated with psychological problems in children: failure to form attachment between 6 months and 3 years, disorganized insecure attachments, separations and loss of attachment figures, and disorganized attachments as a result of maltreatment or parental trauma. These difficulties have been associated with emotional delay, affect regulation disturbances, later attachment problems, behavior problems, and depression in later childhood.

Downey and Coyne's (1990) review and analysis indicated that depression was the only disorder for which children of depressed parents showed a heightened risk. In addition, Hammen and her colleagues have consistently found that children of depressed mothers experience depressive episodes in close proximity to maternal episodes, and that such families experience more stressful episodes and chronic daily stress than other families (Hammen & Rudolph, 1996). Some of this stress is created by the interactions of the depressed parent, for example, marital conflict and more parent–child conflict. Downey and Coyne (1990) suggested that by creating and supporting parental depression, marital discord indirectly increased the risk for depression in children. Indeed when marital discord has been measured by children's perceptions, strong relationships with depression have been found (Nolen-Hoeksema et al., 1992). Depressed mothers have been found to give more attention to children's failures, reward their children at much lower rates than mothers of other clinic-referred or normal children, are more restricted in their emotional expression and behavior, and less engaged in interactions with their children (Dadds & Barrett, 1996). They respond more slowly to their children, less consistently, and when they do respond it is less positive, than non-depressed mothers. Also, Rapee (1997) found that rejection and excessive control in childrearing were positively associated with depression and anxiety in children, with rejection more closely related to depression.

Conclusions

Implications for the prevention of depression include the developmental timing of interventions, contexts to target interventions, and intervention content. The impact of parental depression and insecure attachments is already obvious in infancy. To prevent childhood depression, it is important to intervene with postnatal depression in particular and parental depression in general. Late childhood is another important development period for intervention, as indicated by genetic, cognitive, coping, and competency-based theories. Studies of family theories suggest that children of depressed parents should be routinely targeted for intervention. Furthermore, children who experience multiple stressful life events may benefit from targeted interventions.

The need to include both cognitive and interpersonal strategies in depression prevention programs aimed at children has been clearly indicated. These programs should target cognitive errors, pessimistic attributions, self-esteem and self-perceptions, social and friendship skills, interpersonal problem-solving, personal competencies, and coping skills. The research on family models also emphasizes the importance of focusing on attachment, parent–child interaction and childrearing, in addition to child characteristics.

STRATEGIES THAT WORK

The prevention strategies described below aim to reduce depressive mood, symptoms and syndrome, and ultimately to reduce the incidence of depressive disorders in children. However, depressive disorders are relatively rare in childhood. Hence, none of the programs have measured depressive disorders, assessing instead more proximal outcomes such as depressive symptoms, syndrome and risk factors, for example, attributional style, coping skills, and other behavioral and interpersonal factors. Efforts have focused mainly on children with known risk factors or elevated levels of depressive symptoms, rather than primary prevention programs for all children. Some strategies are child-centered, school-based strategies targeting cognitive and interpersonal factors. Others are environment-centered focusing on the family context in which children of depressed parents live. School-based strategies are reviewed first.

The Penn Prevention Program targeted 10–13-year-olds who were at risk for depression by way of sub-clinical levels of depressive symptoms and/or high levels of perceived parental conflict (Jaycox, Reivich, Gillham, & Seligman, 1994). The program focused on skills to reduce cognitive errors and promote optimistic attributional styles, and enhance social problem-solving and coping skills. Compared to the control group, significant improvements in depressive symptoms and classroom behavior were found for the intervention group at posttest. Prevention of depressive symptoms was maintained at a 6-month follow-up and parents of intervention group children reported fewer externalizing problems compared to controls. Prevention effects were maintained at a 2-year follow-up (Gillham, Reivich, Jaycox, & Seligman, 1995), but were no longer significant at a 3-year follow-up (Gillham & Reivich, 1999). Also, the intervention group made fewer pessimistic attributions for negative events compared to the control group at posttest and all follow-ups indicating effective reduction of this risk factor.

Working with elementary school children with mild to moderate depressive symptoms, Weisz, Thurber, Sweeney, Proffitt, and LeGagnoux (1997) implemented an 8-session intervention program aimed at enhancing primary control (changing the situation) and secondary control (changing one's interpretations). The program was conducted in small groups in schools. Children who received the intervention showed significantly greater reductions in depressive symptoms at posttest and 9-month follow-up than control group children. Also, intervention group children were more likely than control group children to move into the non-clinical range on depression measures.

Beardslee and his colleagues (1993) focused their efforts on family factors, using cognitive therapy and psycho-educational approaches aimed at children whose parents have affective disorders. The 6–10 session family intervention helps families to develop a shared perspective of the depressive illness and to change parent's behavior toward their children. The development of resilience in children was promoted by providing information about the parent's illness, ways of coping, and encouraging supportive relationships outside the home. Following the intervention, parents reported significantly more changes in behavior and attitudes to their illness, compared to families that received an information-based intervention only (Beardslee et al., 1993). These effects were sustained at an 18-month follow-up, with the family-based intervention associated with more positive parent-reported and assessor-rated changes (Beardslee, Salt, Veersage, Gladstone, Wright, & Rothberg, 1997). Family risk factors for childhood depression were reduced and prevented over time; however, no measures of child functioning have been reported to determine if depression was prevented in the offspring of depressed parents.

The development of depression prevention strategies in childhood is still in its infancy. Primary prevention programs for children as young as fourth graders, with elevated risk factors have been effective in the short term. Programs targeting the late childhood to early adolescent period have also demonstrated efficacy in the longer term. These programs have been largely child-centered and school-based. The only family-based program currently published has shown efficacy in modifying the home environments of children at high risk, in the medium term. These studies indicate the efficacy of prevention strategies based upon cognitive, interpersonal, and family models of childhood depression.

STRATEGIES THAT MIGHT WORK

Strategies that might prevent depression in children include interventions that have shown, as yet, only short-term effects and primary prevention strategies for disorders that have high comorbidity with depression, for example, anxiety. In addition, a number of primary prevention strategies target variables associated with depression and the theoretical models presented above, for example, social competence and social skills (see Durlak & Wells, 1997 for a meta-analysis). While research on these strategies has not

measured depressive symptoms or disorders, many have shown promising outcomes with proximal factors that place children at risk for depression or alternatively protect children from the impact of aversive life events. These strategies are presented elsewhere in this encyclopedia and are not reviewed in this entry.

Strategies targeting risk factors such as, low social competence and poor academic achievement in the early and middle childhood years show promise. However, as yet no long-term intervention effects have been established. King and Kirschenbaum (1990) used a 9-session social skills and social problem-solving intervention, plus a parent and teacher consultation service for fourth grade children who were at risk for depression because of poor social competence. The program was modeled on the Primary Mental Health Project (Cowen, Hightower, Pedro-Carroll, Work, Wyman, & Haffey, 1996). The combined service program showed decreased depressive symptoms compared to the parent/teacher consultation service only, and a control group at posttest, with social competencies improving for all groups.

Kellam, Bebok, Mayer, Ialongo, and Kalodner (1994) proposed that pessimistic attributional style in association with poor academic mastery, was important in the development and maintenance of childhood depression. They implemented a universal school-based prevention strategy designed to enhance mastery of academic skills in first grade children. It included an enriched reading curriculum and flexible, individualized correction procedures, implemented by teachers throughout the first year of school. They found that intervention group boys with high initial levels of depressive symptoms and good gains in reading achievement, reported lower levels of symptoms at the end of their first school year. However, girls with high initial levels of depressive symptoms who made gains in reading achievement, reported lower levels of symptoms regardless of whether they attended intervention or control group classes. While these two interventions target different mechanisms in the development of childhood depression, they show some promise as prevention strategies, by way of reducing depressive symptoms in younger children.

Other strategies show promise by way of reducing comorbid mental health problems. The Primary Mental Health Project (Cowen et al., 1996) involves the screening and identification of young children with early school adjustment problems. It then provides prompt and effective intervention services for high-risk youngsters. The program has been evaluated in numerous sites throughout the United States. For example, one evaluation in California, where 50,000 children from 750 schools were involved, found effect sizes of between 0.37 and 0.49 for improvements in adjustment variables such as acting out, shyness, and anxiety. In addition Dadds, Holland, Spence, Laurens, Mullins, and Barrett (1999) found that a 10-week anxiety prevention program for 7–14-year-olds who were at high risk for anxiety disorders resulted in reductions in the rate of anxiety disorders and the prevention of onset of new anxiety disorders at 6-month and 24-month follow-up, compared to a no-treatment control group.

STRATEGIES THAT DO NOT WORK

There is no published research on unsuccessful depression prevention strategies specific to childhood. However, there are studies on related areas that suggest that interpersonal problem-solving strategies are not effective in reducing mental health problems when implemented universally, although they are effective in increasing competence (Durlak & Wells, 1997). Brief classroom-based programs are not as effective as longer multiyear programs in producing stable effects on children's knowledge, attitudes, and behavior in social competence. Also, school-based programs that are focused only on the child or the environment are less effective than strategies that focus on both simultaneously (Durlak, 2000).

SYNTHESIS

Empirically supported theories suggest that depressive symptoms and disorders in childhood develop in the context of individual genetic and biological vulnerabilities, insecure early attachments, impaired parent–child interactions, and high levels of environmental stress. These early factors result in decreased behavioral and interpersonal skills, and impairments in internal cognitive schema, and information processing mechanisms. These deficits may result in additional negative feedback from peers, teachers, and family members. Hence, when aversive life events are encountered, children are vulnerable to depression. Vulnerability may come from a number of distinct or combined pathways, for example, few coping skills or processes for accessing coping skills, cognitive distortions that promote helplessness, overly high standards or negative self-evaluations, or few supportive relationships; this vulnerability may subsequently lead to depression.

Research on the prevention of depression in children indicates that both school-based and family-based interventions targeted at children with known risk factors, such as elevated depressive symptoms, poor social competence, and parental affective disorder, result in reductions in risk factors for depression, reductions in depressive symptoms, and changes to family contexts. Prevention effects have been maintained for up to 2 years. These interventions have been based upon cognitive, interpersonal, and family models of depression, and have largely used cognitive–behavioral strategies to facilitate the process of change. The mechanisms of change have been investigated for only one school-based intervention program, which found that depression prevention effects were mediated by changes in attributional style for negative events.

Other promising strategies with sound theoretical underpinnings and some empirical support include school-based interventions targeting social skills in children with low levels of social competence, environment-centered strategies such as parent and teacher consultations, and enriched curriculum materials that promote academic mastery. Strategies that are yet to be tested include universal interventions for all children regardless of risk, multiyear interventions and those that integrate child- and family-centered strategies. In addition, interventions early in children's lives, which promote attachment, reduce the impact of maternal depression, promote positive parenting, and build social competencies and school readiness, are likely to have important impacts upon child and family adjustment overall, thereby reducing vulnerability to depression.

This field is still in its infancy and there is much work to be done. There have been few randomized controlled efficacy trials, no replications trials, and no effectiveness studies to determine what strategies work when incorporated into regular service delivery conditions. In addition, there have been no component analyses of the available programs. Hence, it is unclear which strategies are the active ingredients in preventing childhood depression. In addition, there has been only one trial of a strategy offered to all children regardless of risk status, and only one study that attempted to integrate child-centered and environment-centered approaches. These are all important areas for future research.

Also see: Depression: Adolescence; Depression: Adulthood; Depression: Older Adulthood; Bereavement: Childhood; Children, Parents with Mental Illness: Childhood; Family Strengthening: Childhood.

References

Anderson, J., Williams, S., McGee, R., & Silva, P. (1987). DSM-III disorders in pre-adolescent children. *Archives of General Psychiatry, 44,* 69–76.

Bandura, A., Pastorelli, C., Barbaranelli, C., & Caprara, G.V. (1999). Self-efficacy pathways to childhood depression. *Journal of Personality and Social Psychology, 76,* 258–269.

Beardslee, W.R., Salt, P., Porterfield, K., Rothberg, P.C., van der Velde, P., Swatling, S., Hoke, L., Moilanen, D.L., & Wheelock, I. (1993). Comparison of preventative interventions for families with parental affective disorder. *Journal of the American Academy of Child and Adolescent Psychiatry, 32,* 254–263.

Beardslee, W.R., Salt, P., Veersage, M.A., Gladstone, T.R.G., Wright, E.J., & Rothberg, P.C. (1997). Sustained change in parents receiving preventive interventions for families with depression. *American Journal of Psychiatry, 154,* 510–515.

Beck, A.T., Rush, A.J., Shaw, B.F., & Emery, G. (1979). *Cognitive theory of depression.* New York: Guilford Press.

Birmaher, B., Ryan, N.D., Williamson, D.E., Brent, D.A., Kaufman, J., Dahl, R.E., Perel, J., & Nelson, B. (1996). Childhood and adolescent depression: A review of the past 10 years. Part 1. *Journal of the American Academy of Child and Adolescent Psychiatry, 35,* 1427–1439.

Cicchetti, D., & Toth, S.L. (1998). The development of depression in children and adolescents. *American Psychologist, 53,* 221–241.

Cohen, P., Cohen, J., Kasen, S., Velez, C.N., Hartmark, C., Johnson, J., Rojas, M., Brook, J., & Streuning, E.L. (1993). An epidemiological study of disorders in late childhood and adolescence—I. Age- and gender-specific prevalence. *Journal of Child Psychology and Psychiatry and Allied Disciplines, 34,* 857–867.

Cole, D.A., & Jordan, A.E. (1995). Competence and memory: Integrating psychosocial and cognitive correlates of child depression. *Child Development, 66,* 459–473.

Cole, D.A., Martin, J.M., & Powers, B. (1997). A competency-based model of child depression: A longitudinal study of peer, parent, teacher and self-evaluations. *Journal of Child Psychology and Psychiatry, 38,* 505–514.

Compas, B.E., Banez, G.A., Malcarne, V.L., & Worsham, N.L. (1991). *Perceived control, coping with stress, and depressive symptoms in school-aged children.* Burlington, VT: University of Vermont.

Compas, B.E., Connor, J., & Wadsworth, M. (1997). Prevention of depression. In P.P. Weissberg, T.P. Gullota, R.L. Hampton, B.A. Ryan, & G.R. Adams (Eds.), *Enhancing children's wellness. Healthy children 2010. Issues in children's and families' lives* (Vol. 8, pp. 129–174). Thousand Oaks, CA: Sage.

Cowen, E.L., Hightower, A.D., Pedro-Carroll, J.L., Work, W.C., Wyman, P.A., & Haffey, W.G. (1996). *School-based prevention for children at risk. The Primary Mental Health Project.* Washington, DC: American Psychological Association.

Dadds, M.R., & Barrett, P.M. (1996). Family processes in child and adolescent anxiety and depression. *Behavior Change, 13,* 231–239.

Dadds, M.R., Holland, D.E., Spence, S.H., Laurens, K.R., Mullins, M., & Barrett, P.M. (1999). Early intervention and prevention of anxiety disorders in children: Results at 2-year follow-up. *Journal of Consulting and Clinical Psychology, 67,* 145–150.

Downey, G., & Coyne, J.C. (1990). Children of depressed parents: An integrative review. *Psychological Bulletin, 108,* 50–76.

Durlak, J.A. (2000). Health promotion as a strategy in primary prevention. In D. Cicchetti, J. Rappaport, I. Sandler, & R.P. Weissberg (Eds.), *The promotion of wellness in children and adolescents* (pp. 221–242). Washington, DC: CWLA Press.

Durlak, J.A., & Wells, A.M. (1997). Primary prevention mental health programs for children and adolescents: A meta-analytic review. *American Journal of Community Psychology, 25,* 115–152.

Eley, T.C., Deater-Deckard, K., Fombonne, E., Fulker, D.W., & Plomin, R. (1998). An adoption study of depressive symptoms in middle childhood. *Journal of Child Psychology and Psychiatry, 39,* 337–345.

Flemming, J.E., Offord, D.R., & Boyle, M.H. (1989). Prevalence of childhood and adolescent depression in the community: Ontario Child Health Study. *British Journal of Psychiatry, 155,* 647–654.

Gillham, J.E., Reivich, K.J., Jaycox, L.H., & Seligman, M.E. (1995). Prevention of depressive symptoms in school children: Two-year follow-up. *Psychological Science, 6*(6), 343–350.

Gillham, J.E., & Reivich, K. (1999). Prevention of depressive symptoms in school children: A research update. *Psychological Science, 10,* 461–463.

Gladstone, T.R.G., & Kaslow, N.J. (1995). Depression and attributions in children and adolescents: A meta-analytic review. *Journal of Abnormal Child Psychology, 23,* 597–606.

Hammen, C., & Rudolph, K.D. (1996). Childhood depression. In E.J. Mash & R.A. Barkley (Eds.), *Child psychopathology.* New York: Guilford.

Jaycox, L.H., Reivich, K.J., Gillham, J., & Seligman, M.E.P. (1994). Prevention of depressive symptoms in school children. *Behavior Research and Therapy, 32*(8), 801–816.

Kellam, S.G., Bebok, G.W., Mayer, L.S., Ialongo, N., & Kalodner, C.R. (1994). Depressive symptoms over first grade and their response to a developmental epidemiologically based prevention trial aimed at improving achievement. *Development and Psychopathology, 6,* 473–481.

King, C.A., & Kirschenbaum, D.S. (1990). An experimental evaluation of a school-based program for children at risk: Wisconsin early intervention. *Journal of Community Psychology, 18,* 167–177.

Kovacs, M. (1996). Presentation and course of major depressive disorder during childhood and later years of the life span. *Journal of the American Academy of Child and Adolescent Psychiatry, 35,* 705–715.

Lewinsohn, P.M. (1974). A behavioral approach to depression. In R. Friedman & M. Katz (Eds.), *The psychology of depression: Contemporary theory and research* (pp. 157–185). Washington, DC: Winston-Wiley.

Main, M. (1996). Overview of the field of attachment. *Journal of Consulting and Clinical Psychology, 64,* 237–243.

Nezu, A.M., Nezu, C.M., & Perri, M.G. (1989). *Problem solving therapy for depression.* New York: John Wiley & Sons.

Nolen-Hoeksema, S., Girus, J., & Seligman, M. (1992). Predictors and consequences of childhood depressive symptoms: A 5-year longitudinal study. *Journal of Abnormal Psychology, 101,* 405–422.

Peterson, C., & Seligman, M.E.P. (1984). Causal explanations as a risk factor for depression: Theory and evidence. *Psychological Review, 91,* 347–374.

Polaino-Lorente, A., & Domenech, E. (1993). Prevalence of childhood depression: Results of the first study in Spain. *Journal of Child Psychology and Psychiatry, 34,* 1007–1017.

Rapee, R.M. (1997). Potential role of childrearing practices in the development of anxiety and depression. *Clinical Psychology Review, 17,* 47–67.

Rehm, L.P. (1977). A self-control model of depression. *Behavior Therapy, 8,* 787–804.

Roberts, C. (1999). The prevention of depression in children and adolescents. *Australian Psychologist, 34,* 49–57.

Rudolph, K.D., Hammen, C., Burge, D., Lindberg, N., Herzberg, D., & Daley, S.E. (2000). Toward an interpersonal life-stress model of depression: The developmental context of stress generation. *Development and Psychopathology, 12,* 215–234.

Rutter, M., Izard, C., & Read, P. (1986). *Depression in young people: Issues and Perspectives.* New York: Guildford Press:

Todd, R.D., & Heath, A. (1996). The genetic architecture of depression and anxiety in youth. *Current Opinion in Psychiatry, 9,* 257–261.

Weisz, J.R., Rudolph, K.D., Granger, D.A., & Sweeney, L. (1992). Cognition, competence, and coping in child and adolescent depression: Research findings, developmental concerns, and therapeutic implications. *Developmental Psychopathology, 4,* 627–653.

Weisz, J.R., Thurber, Sweeney, L., Proffitt, V., & LeGagnoux (1997). Brief treatment of mild to moderate child depression using primary and secondary control enhancement training. *Journal of Consulting and Clinical Psychology, 65,* 703–707.

Weisz, J.R., Sweeney, L., Proffitt, V., & Carr, T. (1993). Control-beliefs and self-reported depressive symptoms in late childhood. *Journal of Abnormal Psychology, 102,* 411–418.

Zubrick, S.R., Silburn, S.R., Garton, A., Burton, P., Dalby, R., Shepard, C., & Lawrence, D. (1995). *Western Australian Child Health Survey: Developing health and well-being in the nineties.* Perth, Western Australia: Australian Bureau of Statistics and the Institute for Child Health Research.

Depression, Adolescence

Clare Roberts and Brian Bishop

INTRODUCTION

Adolescent depression is a set of psychological phenomena characterized by mood, thoughts, and behaviors that range from a mild reactive despondency or sadness to more extreme feelings of dysphoria, hopeless thoughts, and withdrawn or irritable behavior. This entry discusses theories, research, and strategies related to preventing depression in adolescence. The burden of depression on those young people suffering from it, their families and careers, and the community at large is considerable. The financial burden of depression has been estimated to be $43 billion in the United States alone in the mid-1990s, in terms of treatment, absenteeism, loss of production, and early death (Cicchetti & Toth, 1998). These costs will only increase if, as described in an earlier entry in this volume, depression becomes more prevalent and the age of first onset continues to decline.

DEFINITIONS

Depressive symptomology for children and adolescents is similar, other than increased hypersomnia and slightly more weight loss apparent in depressed adolescents. Differences between depression in adolescents and adults include increased anhedonia and psychomotor retardation with age, and more depressed appearance, somatic complaints, and poor self-esteem occurring at younger ages (Roberts, Lewinsohn, & Seeley, 1995). Despite these minor differences, diagnostic systems such as the DSM-IV use the same criteria to diagnose depressive disorders in children, adolescents, and adults.

Depressed mood, depressive syndromes, and depressive disorders (DD) are categories of adolescent depression used in the literature (Petersen, Compas, Brooks-Gunn, Stemmler, Ey, & Grant, 1993). Definitions of these phenomena and their measurement are provided in an earlier entry.

SCOPE

Studies of the prevalence of adolescent DD have been conducted in a variety of countries including the United States (Lewinsohn, Hops, Roberts, Seeley, & Andrews, 1993), New Zealand (McGee, Feehan, Williams, Partridge, Silva, & Kelly, 1990), and Ireland (Donnelly, 1995). Estimates of the point prevalence of Manic Depressive Disorder (MDD) in adolescence, range from 0.4 percent to 8.3 percent (Birmaher et al., 1996), while lifetime prevalence rates across adolescence have been estimated at 15–20 percent (Cicchetti & Toth, 1998). Point prevalence rates for DD range from 1.6 to 8.0 percent (Cicchetti & Toth, 1998), with a small proportion of youngsters having both disorders. These rates are nearly twice those of childhood and are comparable to adult prevalence rates by late adolescence. Studies of depressive syndromes as measured by instruments such as the Child Behavior Checklist, have found a similar doubling of rates in adolescence. Zubrick et al. (1995) found 4.8 percent of 12–16-year-old Western Australians were rated by their parents and teachers as having clinically significant levels of anxious and depressed symptoms.

Studies of depressive mood in adolescence indicate even higher rates. There is strong evidence that subclinical and clinical levels of depressive symptoms increase the risk for depressive disorders in adolescence (Lewinsohn, Clarke, Seeley, & Rohde, 1994). Roberts et al. (1995) found 29.5 percent of adolescents reported depressive symptoms and 2.6 percent were diagnosable with clinical depression. Estimates of the 6-month prevalence of depressed mood in adolescents vary from 20 to 35 percent in boys and 25 to 40 percent in girls (Petersen et al., 1993). In early adolescence, depressive mood becomes more common in females (Wichstrom, 1999). By late adolescence, the prevalence rates for depressive mood and disorders are two to three times greater for females than males (Hankin, Abramson, Moffitt, Silva, McGee, & Angell, 1998). Differential hormonal changes at puberty do not predict gender differences when age is controlled. Rather, adolescent girls' greater socialization and more ruminating coping style disadvantages them compared to boys, when they are faced with the stresses and changes in adolescence (Nolen-Hoeksema & Girgus, 1994).

Incidence data is less commonly reported. Lewinsohn et al. (1993) defined *first incidence* as the percentage of people who developed an episode for the first time in their lives compared to those who never had an episode prior to the research. They reported a first incidence rate of 6.32 percent for females and 4.25 percent for males in adolescence. The breakdown for MDD and DD were 7.14 and 0.13 percent, respectively, for females and 4.35 and 0.00 percent, for males. Further, New Zealand data shows an increased rate of first incidence of depressive disorders throughout adolescence, particularly for females. Incidence at age 11 was 1.79 percent for males and 0.31 percent for females compared to 0.56 percent for males and 4.39 percent for females at age 15, and 9.58 percent for males and 20.69 percent for females at age 18 (Hankin et al., 1998).

Depressive symptoms and disorders in adolescence are associated with a range of other problems. The most common comorbid conditions are anxiety and behavior problems such as conduct disorder. However, other common comorbid problems in adolescence include attention-deficit disorders, substance abuse and eating disorders, early school dropout for females and discontinuity of employment in males, social adjustment difficulties, and increased risk of suicide and suicidal behavior (Harrington & Clark, 1998).

THEORIES AND RESEARCH

Adolescence is a period of considerable change. There are biological changes associated with puberty, the relative influence of the family is reduced, and peers become more important. In many countries, schooling changes from having a single teacher in primary school to having a variety of teachers in middle or high school. This change is often accompanied by location and cohort changes that mean establishing a new sense of place and new friendships. All these factors make adolescence a period of considerable challenge. Theories of adolescent depression need to incorporate these developmental and environmental considerations.

Genetic Theories

An earlier entry in this book showed that depression runs in families. However, these findings can be related to both genetic and social explanations, and the evidence for direct genetic effects in adolescence is modest. Twin studies have suggested a genetic vulnerability for depressive symptomology that may begin to take effect in adolescence rather than childhood (Thaper & McGuffin, 1994). However, adoption studies and offspring studies attest to the importance of both shared and non-shared environmental effects on the offspring of depressed parents (Eley, Deater-Deckard, Fombonne, Fulker, & Plomin, 1998; Todd & Heath, 1996). In a study of genetic and environmental influences on depressive symptomology in adolescents, Rende, Plomin, Reiss, and Hetherington (1993) found a strong genetic influence (34 percent) and minimal environmental influence for the full range of depressive symptoms. However, for adolescents with clinical levels of symptoms, shared environment accounted for 23 percent of the variance, while genetic influences were negligible. Hence, it is evident that depressed

adolescents inherit both environmental and genetic risk factors from their depressed parents.

Biological Theories

The evidence for biological markers in adolescents is not as well developed as that for adults. Growth hormone has been investigated and there is some evidence that stressful events may lead to elevated nocturnal growth hormone secretion in adolescents (Birmaher et al., 1996). Studies of abnormalities in hypothalamic–pituitary–adrenal (HPA) axis suggest that depression in adolescents is more closely linked to dysfunction in this area and sleep disturbance, than it is in pre-pubertal children (Hammen & Rudolph, 1996). In addition, studies that have included inpatient and suicidal adolescent samples have found more evidence for biological impairment in these extreme groups (Hammen & Rudolph, 1996). Although sleep disturbance is a common complaint among depressed adolescents, research has not demonstrated the same relationships between sleep changes and depression in adults (Birmaher et al., 1996). Hence, biological markers in depressed adolescents more closely resemble those found in adults than children, but there are still differences. Markers such as HPA dysfunctions are more evident in severe inpatient cases and adolescents who are suicidal. More research with children and adolescents is necessary to identify biological mechanisms involved in early onset depression and the developmental sequence of effect.

Cognitive Theories

Cognitive errors such as over generalizations and personalization are common in depressed adolescents and negative experiences are often magnified while positive experiences are minimized, in comparison to non-depressed adolescents (Hammen & Rudolph, 1996). Lewinsohn, Roberts et al.'s (1994) community-based study of adolescents supports this interpretation, in that low self-esteem and to a lesser extent self-consciousness were both predictive of, and concurrently associated with, depressive symptoms over a 12-month period. Pessimistic attributional style was a significant risk factor for depressive symptoms, prospectively. Turner and Cole (1994) found support for both Beck (Beck, Rush, Shaw, & Emery, 1979) and Seligman's (Peterson & Seligman, 1984) theories of depression in young adolescents. In their study, pessimistic attributional style and negative cognitive errors moderated the relationship between negative life events (in specific valued domains) and depression, in young adolescents, but not younger children. Recently, Schwartz, Kaslow, Seeley, and Lewinsohn (2000) found that maladaptive attributions were associated with increased depressive symptoms and suicidal ideation, plus impaired self-esteem, coping skills and interpersonal functioning both concurrently and prospectively. Hence, by early adolescence, cognitive styles such as schema and attributions have become more stable. Rehm's (1977) self-control theory of depression has found relatively consistent support in adolescent studies (Hammen & Rudolph, 1996). For example, Jackson and Frick (1998) found that social support and internal perceptions of control moderated the effect of negative life events on internalizing symptoms particularly in girls in early adolescence.

The research on applications of cognitive theories to adolescent depression support a developmental sequence whereby negative cognitions are developed in response to repeated environmental stressors. These cognitive processes become habitual by early adolescence, take a moderator role and act as filters for the interpretation of important life events, interacting with negative events to produce depression in adolescence and adulthood (Cicchetti & Toth, 1998).

Behavioral and Interpersonal Theories

Social competence problems, such as relationship difficulties, poor social skills, social problem solving, and coping skills have been found to be associated with depression in adolescents (Lewinsohn, Rohde, & Seeley, 1998). Lewinsohn, Roberts et al. (1994) found that self-rated social competence in adolescents was associated with depression, but not predictive of future episodes. However, Schwartz et al. (2000) found that maladaptive attributions were associated with impaired coping skills and interpersonal functioning both concurrently and prospectively, suggesting interactions between cognitive and interpersonal models in the development and maintenance of depression in adolescents. In support of this transactional theory, Cole, Martin, and Powers (1997) found that competency ratings by peers, teachers, and parents predicted changes in self-evaluations of competency over time, in girls but not boys, and these changes were associated with changes in depression over time in both genders as they reached adolescence.

Relationship difficulties are also important factors at this time of change from reliance upon family to more identification with peers. Puskar, Tusaie-Mumford, Sereika, and Lamb (1999) found significant relationships between depressive symptomology and losing a close friend, arguments with parents, and trouble with classmates, in rural adolescents in the United States. Goodyer and Altham (1991) found that friendship difficulties exerted a direct effect of similar magnitude to aversive life events, on the probability of depressive and anxiety disorders in 7–16-year-olds. Compas, Banez, Malcarne, and Worsham (1991) suggested that the ability to cope with the emotional impact and loss of

reinforcement caused by interpersonal difficulties is more evident in adolescence. Such abilities may protect youngsters from depression. However, Rudolph, Hammen, Burge, Lindberg, Herzberg, and Daley (2000) indicated that high levels of interpersonal stress often overwhelmed young people's coping resources and contributed to a sense of helplessness.

More longitudinal research is needed to determine whether deficits in social and interpersonal functioning place the adolescent at risk for depression or whether heightened depressive symptoms lead to decreased social performance and further depression. Lewinsohn, Roberts et al.'s (1994) research suggests that in adolescence, the relationship is a concurrent one. However, Cole et al.'s (1997) work suggests that both pathways to depression hold true for boys but that only the first pathway is significant for girls.

Family Theories

Beardslee, Versage, and Gladstone (1998) found that episodes of major depression in adolescents and young adults whose parents had a diagnosable depressive disorder were more frequent, longer in duration, had an earlier onset, and were more likely to have comorbid diagnoses than the offspring of healthy parents. Genetic and attachment theories, dysfunctional parent–adolescent interaction patterns, marital conflict, and general family functioning have been used to explain the increased likelihood of depression in the offspring of depressed parents (Roberts, 1999). The evidence for these influences varies.

Rosenstein and Horowitz (1996) found that anxious/ambiguous attachment styles were associated with internalizing problems such as anxiety and depression while avoidant/dismissive attachments were associated more with conduct problems in adolescent inpatients. These attachment problems may be exhibited in parent–adolescent interaction styles. Ge, Best, Conger, and Simons (1996) found that parents of tenth graders with depressive or conduct problems, or the co-occurrence of both, were more hostile and demonstrated lower levels of warmth and effective parenting skills when their children were in seventh, eighth, and ninth grades, but parents of depressed adolescents were less hostile than parents of adolescents with conduct problems. Also, Lewinsohn, Roberts et al. (1994) found that adolescent conflict with parents predicted future depression. These studies suggest that the parenting behavior of depressed and nondepressed parents may play a role in both the development and the maintenance of depressive symptoms of their offspring.

Parental divorce and marital conflict have a negative effect on adolescent rates of depression. Puig-Antich et al. (1993) found the depressed adolescents reported more severe marital difficulties in their parents. In their review,

Petersen et al. (1993) claimed that a good relationship with parents was a protective factor against depressive symptoms. Indeed Reinherz, Giaconia, Pakiz, Silverman, Frost, and Lefkowitz's (1993) longitudinal study found that family cohesiveness and satisfactory social support from peers and family mediated the effects of negative life events on depressive symptoms. In contrast, poor family adjustment is associated with more negative life events, daily hassles, and less access to family support (Puskar et al., 1999). Hence attachment difficulties, negative parental interactions, and marital conflict have been implicated as mechanisms in adolescent depression, while family cohesiveness and family support have been found to act as protective factors.

Environmental Stress Theories

Compas, Orosan, and Grant (1993) have proposed a model of the role of environmental stress and coping in the development of depression and other psychological problems in adolescence. These researchers have proposed that biological and environmental changes associated with puberty and adolescence interact with interpersonal stress to result in depressed mood. The way adolescents cope with depressed mood can then result in the development of depressive disorders or in successful adaptation to life challenges. They posit that the development of emotion-focused coping in early adolescence and the common usage of these strategies by females may explain the differential gender prevalence rates for male and female adolescents. This model is supported by Nolen-Hoeksema and Girgus (1994) who found that adolescent girls reported more ruminating coping styles compared to boys. Also, research reviewed by Petersen, Leffert, Graham, Alwin, and Ding (1997) showed that adolescents with positive adjustment used more approach-oriented coping strategies and less avoidant coping strategies, than youths with poor adjustment.

Overall, studies suggest that multiple stressors, either major events or daily hassles are strongly related to depressive symptoms in adolescents (Lewinsohn, Roberts et al., 1994). Further, Rudolph et al.'s (2000) research found that both episodic and chronic interpersonal stress was associated with depression in young people, but that depressed youngsters also create stressful events and circumstances, leading to self-perpetuating cycles. Therefore, negative life events and daily hassles have a place to play in a model of depression, but may not be specific to depression, as major negative life events and chronic daily stress have been implicated as risk factors for a number of childhood disorders: depression, anxiety, and phobic disorders (Compas et al., 1993). The effect of environmental stress occurs in interaction with other vulnerabilities, be they biological, cognitive, interpersonal, or family-based. Also, depressed adolescents cause additional stress in their own lives resulting in an interactive process which influences emergent developmental processes.

Conclusions

Most of the theoretical models outlined above have come from the adult literature. The adolescent domain has not been as fully researched and theories need to be developed and evaluated with this population. The diversity of theory has also led to the call for integrated bio-psychosocial models. Hammen and Rudolph (1996) and Cicchetti and Toth (1998) have provided integrated models suggesting that a single depression theory is unlikely to account for all depressive episodes. Depression occurs in the context of a variety of factors and the need for an integrative model is based on the assumption that a broader contextual approach is required.

STRATEGIES THAT WORK

School-based prevention and health promotion programs for depression has been strongly advocated and have shown some efficacy (Roberts, 1999). However, there have not been many programs developed to date and these are based primarily on cognitive–behavioral strategies. The prevention programs reviewed here tend to be selectively applied to adolescents with known risk factors, or adolescents showing early depressive symptoms. One trial has been conducted in which the intervention was given to a non-selected group of adolescents. The merits of non-targeted or universal interventions for adolescents have been debated (Harrington & Clark, 1998; Roberts, 1999). Such approaches have advantages in terms of higher recruitment and retention rates. Universal school-based interventions also avoid the risk of labeling that can come when students are removed from class or are treated separately from their peers. In addition, school-based programs for all students offer that opportunity for modeling from competent peers and significant adult figures such as teachers.

A disadvantage of universal programs is that they can be more costly as they provide the intervention to those at risk and those not at risk indiscriminately. Targeting those at risk, such as adolescents with depressed parents or those with elevated, but sub-diagnostic, symptom levels can increase the cost-effectiveness of interventions (Harrington & Clark, 1998). Harrington and Clark (1998) argued that it is possible that universal prevention programs may create indirect harmful effects, for example, universal suicide prevention programs that may do little good to those not at risk, and may do harm by upsetting some adolescents or even normalizing suicidal behavior.

Trials of strategies for children (Jaycox, Reivich, Gillham, & Seligman, 1994) and adolescents (Clarke, Hawkins, Murphy, Sheeber, Lewinson, & Seeley, 1995) at risk, aim to reduce the incidence of depression in the adolescent years. In the first reported randomized controlled study on the prevention of MDD and DD in high-risk adolescents, Clarke et al. identified adolescents who were "demoralized" on the basis of elevated self-reports of depressed mood. The "Coping with Stress Course" consisted of 15, 45-minute sessions and involved techniques to identify and challenge negative thoughts, social skills training, activity scheduling, problem solving, and education about feelings and interpersonal behavior. Survival analysis revealed that those in the intervention group were less likely to develop a depressive disorder (14.5 percent) compared to the control group (25.7 percent) at a 12-month follow-up.

Jaycox et al. (1994) developed the Penn Prevention Program based on a cognitive–behavioral models, and evaluated its implementation with groups of 10–13-year-olds who reported elevated levels of depressive symptoms and parental conflict. The content of this intervention and the results of the evaluation trial have been reviewed in a previous entry. Although this intervention was conducted after school, for children of average age 11 years, the results of follow-up studies indicated that it was successful in decreasing and preventing depressive symptoms as the children made their transition to early and middle adolescence (Gilham, Reivich, Jaycox, & Seligman, 1995). In addition, the intervention group maintained more optimistic attributional styles, compared to the control group, 3 years after completing the program (Gillham & Reivich, 1999).

Hence, programs targeting young adolescents with elevated risk factors of depression have been successful in reducing and preventing depressive symptoms and disorders. Further, their effects have been maintained up to 2 years. However, neither of the above-mentioned programs have been integrated into the school curriculum, which reduces access for many adolescents. Universal school approaches where prevention strategies are offered to all adolescents regardless of risk level are described below.

Shochet et al. (2001) have developed a universal school-based prevention program for young adolescents regardless of their level of risk. The Resourceful Adolescent Program (RAP) is an 11-week cognitive–behavioral program oriented toward resilience and skill building. The program content includes cognitive and interpersonal strategies, and an adjunctive 3-session family program is available. In a controlled trial with 12–15-year-olds, Shochet et al. implemented the 40–50-minute weekly sessions during school hours with graduate level psychologists as facilitators. Intervention and usual care control groups included sequential cohorts of students from one high school in Brisbane,

Australia. The results indicated that depression and hopelessness symptoms were lower in the RAP group than the controls at posttest. This difference was maintained at a 10-month follow-up and the number of adolescents with clinically significant levels of depressive symptoms was significantly reduced in the intervention group. This prevention program was easily integrated into the school curriculum, and by offering it to all adolescents, problems of labeling were reduced.

STRATEGIES THAT MIGHT WORK

A promising environment-centered intervention that is based upon cognitive and interpersonal theories of adolescent depression has been described in the literature. Glover, Burns, Butler, and Patton (1998) described a universal mental health promotion program, the Gatehouse Project currently being studied in Victoria, Australia. This intervention is designed for young adolescents (13–14-year-olds) and aims to build capacity in the school system by promoting a more supportive school environment with greater safety, less bullying, and increasing social connectedness and positive regard. While no outcome data are available for this project, early results indicate associations between a sense of security, social connectedness and positive regard, as provided in a supportive school environment and emotional well-being in young adolescents, not just who at high risk levels.

There are a number of programs that are based on competence enhancement, which may have benefits of reducing depression. Weissberg, Barton, and Shriver (1997) have focused on harm reduction using an extensive program aimed at enhancing self-efficacy skills in dealing with the environment and positive self-perceptions. The school-based program involves 45 sessions, designed to enhance adolescent's social problem-solving skills and their application of these skills to the development of healthy lifestyles and limitation of high-risk activities, such as substance abuse and risky sexual behavior. Controlled outcome studies indicate that this program results in improved social problem-solving skills, better peer relationships, and better behavioral adjustment (Weissberg et al., 1997). Furthermore, intervention group adolescents implemented more adaptive stress management strategies when faced with challenging negative life situations. Weissberg et al. argued that programs such as these must be integrated into comprehensive and coordinated interventions throughout the school years.

Danish (1997) also developed a life skills program designed to build transferable problem-solving skills in adolescents, the GOAL program. Danish's approach is integrated at a number of levels in the school, and includes the use of high school student leaders to facilitate program workshops. The program teaches young adolescents to identify and plan for positive life goals, to identify barriers to goal achievement, and to seek and create social support to help achieve goals. The program makes use of 10, one-hr workshops. The use of student leaders provides peer support, but also reflects a whole of school approach, and the importance of locating the school in the community. While evaluations of this program have not been strong methodologically, research indicates that participants were able to achieve the goals that they set themselves, and they had better school attendance than a control group. Further, boys who attended these workshops displayed fewer health compromising behaviors, such as smoking and drinking, and showed less violence and behavior problems than control group boys. This approach extends the preventive intervention into sectors of the school and community that are not typically included. While this program was not designed to prevent depression per se, its focus on social competence could be valuable.

STRATEGIES THAT DO NOT WORK

There is some information on depression prevention strategies for adolescents that do not work. Clarke, Hawkins, Murphy, and Sheeber (1993) looked at two low-intensity interventions, that were incorporated into mandatory health classes for ninth or tenth grade students. In the first study, teachers administered a 3-session intervention based on a behavioral theory of depression, designed to encourage adolescents to increase their rates of pleasant activities. The results of a randomized controlled trial indicated no effect on depression for girls, a short-term effect for boys at posttest, but no effects at a 12-week follow-up. The second study involved a 5-session skills development program targeting pleasant events and irrational thinking styles. The results indicated that the program was ineffective in the short term and at a 12-week follow-up. The authors suggested that the programs were too brief and that more intensive universal programs may not be cost effective.

Rice and Meyer's (1994) universal 16-session psychoeducational program was based upon stress and coping skills models of adolescent depression. The intervention resulted in better coping in both girls and boys and reductions in depressive symptoms in girls in the short term, compared to the control group. However, depressive symptoms were increased in the intervention group boys. Follow-up assessments 12 months later indicated that the intervention effects did not persist over time (Petersen et al., 1997). The authors argued that the intervention was effective in assisting adolescents to cope better with the challenges and transitions of early adolescence, but that it was too brief to have strong long-term effects.

Finally, Hains and Ellmann (1994) reported a trial of a stress inoculation program based in high schools and designed for adolescents with high levels of arousal. The program involved a variety of cognitive–behavioral strategies such as cognitive restructuring, problem solving, and anxiety management training. They found reductions in depression, anxiety, and anger symptoms. These gains were maintained at follow-up, conducted at the end of the fourth quarter of the school year. However, the wait-list control group showed similar gains. These studies indicate that strategies that are brief, whether targeted at adolescents at risk or universal, are unlikely to have lasting preventive effects. Further, brief interventions that are based on stress and coping models have not demonstrated maintenance over time.

In summary, brief classroom-based programs have been less effective than longer multiyear programs; school-based programs that focus only on the child or their environment are likely to be less effective than strategies that focus on both simultaneously, and inadequate organizational support for program delivery can result in diminished program effects. These features may be more important for high schools that traditionally involve students being taught by multiple teachers in different classrooms with different mixes of peer groups.

SYNTHESIS

While the theory and research on the prevention of depression in adolescence is still developing, there are already a number of effective strategies available. Controlled trials of school-based intervention strategies for young adolescents with elevated risk factors have resulted in the prevention of depressive symptoms, and reduction in the incidence of clinical depression. These effects have been maintained 1–2 years after intervention. Also, one nontargeted school-based intervention provided to all ninth grade adolescents has been effective in preventing depressive symptoms in the medium term. These interventions were all based upon cognitive and interpersonal models of adolescent depression, and used cognitive–behavioral and interpersonal approaches to impart skills and competencies to students. Although, replication studies with more rigorous methodology are required, this research provides a sound foundation on which to build.

There is evidence that universal competence-enhancement interventions have positive outcomes on factors that have been implicated in the development and maintenance of adolescent depression, for example, social problem solving, self-efficacy, positive self-perceptions, and connectedness to school (Danish, 1997; Weissberg et al., 1997). Hence, strategies that focus upon the promotion of competence as well as models of depression may be even more effective in preventing depression. The results of Shochet et al.'s (in press) trial of a universal depression prevention program supports this argument. Furthermore, both Weissberg et al. and Danish recommend integration of strategies at a variety of levels within the school and the community, providing more environment-centered strategies rather than focusing on individual risk and protective factors.

We can conclude that brief school-based interventions do not work, and that interventions based on stress and coping models of adolescent depression may not be effective in the long term. However, little is known about the best time to target interventions developmentally. Jaycox et al. (1994) achieved long-term success with depressive symptoms by targeting their interventions during a period of change, from primary school to high school, while Clarke et al.'s (1995) successful intervention achieved reductions in the incidence of depressive disorders, by intervening during middle adolescence. This is an important area for future research. In addition, the issue of whether programs targeted at adolescents who are at risk are better than universal programs is yet to be investigated. Dissemination of strategies on a broader scale will depend on the issue of comparative efficacy of these approaches and the cost effectiveness. If preventive programs are to be truly effective, they need to be broadly applied (Weissberg et al., 1997). Effective prevention programs need to be disseminated and implemented widely under usual service delivery conditions. Strategies of doing this, while maintaining program integrity will be a challenge for the future.

As the science of prevention improves, we need to look at the issues of broad social change, evaluate the positive and negative aspects of that change, and address the negative psychological implications through effective preventive and promotive programs that are sensitive to the social ecology.

Also see: Depression: Childhood; Depression: Adulthood; Depression: Older Adulthood; Bereavement: Adolescence; Chronic Disease: Adolescence; Family Strengthening: Adolescence.

References

Beardslee, W.R., Versage, E.M., & Gladstone, T.R.G. (1998). Children of affectively ill parents: A review of the past 10 years. *Journal of the American Academy of Child and Adolescent Psychiatry, 37,* 1134–1144.

Beck, A.T., Rush, A.J., Shaw, B.F., & Emery, G. (1979). *Cognitive theory of depression.* New York: Guilford Press.

Birmaher, B., Ryan, N.D., Williamson, D.E., Brent, D.A., Kaufman, J., Dahl, R.E., Perel, J., & Nelson, B. (1996). Childhood and adolescent depression: A review of the past 10 years. Part 1. *Journal of the American Academy of Child and Adolescent Psychiatry, 35,* 1427–1439.

Cicchetti, D., & Toth, S.L. (1998). The development of depression in children and adolescents. *American Psychologist, 53,* 221–241.

Clarke, G.N., Hawkins, W., Murphy, M., & Sheeber, L. (1993). School-based primary prevention of depressive symptomology in adolescents: Findings from two studies. *Journal of Adolescent Research, 8,* 183–204.

Clarke, G.N., Hawkins, W., Murphy, M., Sheeber, L.B., Lewinson, P.M., & Seeley, J.R. (1995). Targeted prevention of unipolar depressive disorder in an at-risk sample of high school adolescents: A randomized trial of a group cognitive intervention. *Journal of the American Academy of Child Adolescent Psychiatry, 34,* 312–321.

Cole, D.A., Martin, J.M., & Powers, B. (1997). A competency-based model of child depression: A longitudinal study of peer, parent, teacher and self-evaluations. *Journal of Child Psychology and Psychiatry, 38,* 505–514.

Compas, B.E., Banez, G.A., Malcarne, V.L., & Worsham, N.L. (1991). *Perceived control, coping with stress, and depressive symptoms in school-aged children.* Burlington, VT: University of Vermont.

Compas, B.E., Orosan, P.G., & Grant, K.E. (1993). Adolescent stress and coping: Implications for psychopathology during adolescence. *Journal of Adolescence, 16,* 331–349.

Danish, S.J. (1997). Going for the goal: A life skills program for adolescents. In G.W. Albee & T.P. Gullotta (Eds.), *Primary prevention works* (pp. 291–312). Thousand Oaks, CA: Sage.

Donnelly, M. (1995). Depression among adolescents in Northern Ireland. *Adolescence, 30,* 339–350.

Eley, T.C., Deater-Deckard, K., Fombonne, E., Fulker, D.W., & Plomin, R. (1998). An adoption study of depressive symptoms in middle childhood. *Journal of Child Psychology and Psychiatry, 39,* 337–345.

Ge, X., Best, K.M., Conger, R.D., & Simons, R.L. (1996). Parenting behaviours and the occurrence and co-occurrence of adolescent depressive symptoms and conduct problems. *Developmental Psychology, 32,* 717–731.

Gillham, J.E., & Reivich, K. (1999). Prevention of depressive symptoms in school children: A research update. *Psychological Science, 10,* 461–463.

Gillham, J.E., Reivich, K.J., Jaycox, L.H., & Seligman, M.E. (1995). Prevention of depressive symptoms in school children: Two year follow-up. *Psychological Science, 6,* 343–350.

Glover, A., Burns, J., Butler, H., & Patton, G. (1998). Social environments and the emotional wellbeing of young people. *Family Matters, 49,* 11–16.

Goodyer, I.M., & Altham, P.M. (1991). Lifetime exit events and recent social and family adversities in anxious and depressed school-age children and adolescents: II. *Journal of Affective Disorders, 21,* 229–238.

Hains, A.A., & Ellmann, S.W. (1994). Stress inoculation training as a preventative intervention for high school youths. *Journal of Cognitive Psychotherapy, 8,* 219–232.

Hammen, C., & Rudolph, K.D. (1996). Childhood depression. In E.J. Mash & R.A. Barkley (Eds.), *Child psychopathology.* New York: Guilford.

Hankin, B.L., Abramson, L.Y., Moffitt, T.E., Silva, P.A., McGee, R., & Angell, K.E. (1998). Development of depression from pre-adolescence to young adulthood: Emerging gender differences in a 10-year longitudinal study. *Journal of Abnormal Psychology, 107,* 128–140.

Harrington, R., & Clark, A. (1998). Prevention and early intervention for depression in adolescence and early adult life. *European Archives of Psychiatry and Clinical Neuroscience, 248,* 32–45.

Jackson Y., & Frick, P.J. (1998). Negative life events and the adjustment of school-age-children: Testing protective models. *Journal of Clinical Child Psychology, 27,* 370–380.

Jaycox, L.H., Reivich, K.J., Gillham, J., & Seligman, M.E.P. (1994). Prevention of depressive symptoms in school children. *Behavior Research and Therapy, 32*(8), 801–816.

Lewinsohn, P.M., Clarke, G.N., Seeley, J.R., & Rohde, P. (1994). Major depression in community adolescents: Age at onset, episode duration, and time to recurrence. *Journal of the American Academy of Child and Adolescent Psychiatry, 33,* 714–722.

Lewinsohn, P.M., Hops, H., Roberts, R.E., Seeley, J.R., & Andrews, J.A. (1993). Adolescent psychopathology: I. Prevalence and incidence of depression and other DSM-III-R disorders in high school students. *Journal of Abnormal Psychology, 102,* 133–144.

Lewinsohn, P.M., Roberts, R.E., Seeley, J.R., Rohde, P., Gotlib, I.H., & Hops, H. (1994). Adolescent psychopathology: II. Psychosocial risk factors for depression. *Journal of Abnormal Psychology, 103,* 302–315.

Lewinsohn, P.M., Rohde, P., & Seeley, J.R. (1998). Major depressive disorder in older adolescents: Prevalence, risk factors, and clinical implications. *Clinical Psychology Review, 18,* 765–794.

McGee, R., Feehan, M., Williams, S., Partridge, F., Silva, P.A., & Kelly, J. (1990). DSM-III disorders in a large sample of adolescents. *Journal of the American Academy of Child and Adolescent Psychiatry, 29,* 611–619.

Nolen-Hoeksema, S., & Girgus, J.S. (1994). The emergence of gender differences in depression in adolescence. *Psychological Bulletin, 115,* 424–443.

Petersen, A.C., Compas, B.E., Brooks-Gunn, J., Stemmler, M., Ey, S., & Grant, K.E. (1993). Depression in adolescence. *American Psychologist, 48,* 155–168.

Petersen, A.C., Leffert, N., Graham, B., Alwin, J., & Ding, S. (1997). Promoting mental health during the transition into adolescence. In J. Schulenberg, J.L. Maggs, & K. Hurrelmann (Eds.), *Health risks and developmental transitions during adolescence* (pp. 471–497). Cambridge: Cambridge University Press.

Peterson, C., & Seligman, M.E.P. (1984). Causal explanations as a risk factor for depression: Theory and evidence. *Psychological Review, 91,* 347–374.

Puig-Antich, J., Kaufman, J., Ryan, N.D., Williamson, D.E., Dahl, R.E., Lukens, E., Todak, G., Ambrosini, P., Rabinovich, H., & Nelson, B. (1993). The psychosocial functioning and family environment of depressed adolescents. *Journal of the American Academy of Child and Adolescent Psychiatry, 32,* 244–253.

Puskar, K.R., Tusaie-Mumford, K., Sereika, S.M., & Lamb, J. (1999). Screening and predicting adolescent depressive symptoms in rural settings. *Archives of Psychiatric Nursing, 13,* 3–11.

Rehm, L.P. (1977). A self control measure of depression. *Behavior Therapy, 8,* 787–804.

Reinherz, H.Z., Giaconia, R.M., Pakiz, B., Silverman, A.B., Frost, A.K., & Lefkowitz, E.S. (1993). Psychosocial risks for major depression in late adolescence: A longitudinal community sample. *Journal of the American Academy of Child and Adolescent Psychiatry, 32,* 1159–1164.

Rende, R., Plomin, R., Reiss, D., & Hetherington, M. (1993). Genetic and environmental influences on depressive symptomatology in adolescents: Individual differences and extreme scores. *Journal of Child Psychology and Psychiatry, 34,* 1387–1398.

Rice, K.G., & Meyer, A.L. (1994). Preventing depression among young adolescents: Preliminary process results of a psycho-educational intervention program. *Journal of Counseling and Development, 73,* 145–152.

Roberts, C. (1999). The prevention of depression in children and adolescents. *Australian Psychologist, 34,* 49–57.

Roberts, R.E., Lewinsohn, P.M., & Seeley, J.R. (1995). Symptoms of DSM-III-R major depression in adolescence: Evidence from an epidemiological survey. *Journal of the American Academy of Child Adolescent Psychiatry, 34,* 1608–1617.

Rosenstein, D.S., & Horowitz, H.A. (1996). Adolescent attachment and psychopathology. *Journal of Consulting and Clinical Psychology, 64,* 244–253.

Rudolph, K.D., Hammen, C., Burge, D., Lindberg, N., Herzberg, D., & Daley, S.E. (2000). Toward an interpersonal life-stress model of depression: The developmental context of stress generation. *Development and Psychopathology, 12,* 215–234.

Shochet, I.M., Dadds, M.R., Holland, D., Whitefield, K., Harnett, P.H., & Osgarby, S.M. (2001). The efficacy of a universal school-based program to prevent adolescent depression. *Journal of Clinical Psychology, 30,* 303–315.

Schwartz, J.A., Kaslow, N.J., Seeley, J., & Lewinsohn, P. (2000). Psychological, cognitive and interpersonal correlates of attributional change in adolescents. *Journal of Clinical Child Psychology, 29,* 188–198.

Thaper, A., & McGuffin, P. (1994). A twin study of depressive symptoms in childhood. *British Journal of Psychiatry, 65,* 259–265.

Todd, R.D., & Heath, A. (1995). The genetic architecture of depression and anxiety in youth. *Current Opinion in Psychiatry, 9,* 257–261.

Turner, J.E., & Cole, D.A. (1994). Developmental differences in cognitive diatheses for child depression. *Journal of Abnormal Child Psychology, 22,* 15–32.

Weissberg, R.P., Barton, H.A., & Shriver, T.P. (1997). The social-competence promotion program for young adolescents. In G.W. Albee & T.P. Gullotta (Eds.), *Primary prevention works* (pp. 291–312). Thousand Oaks, CA: Sage.

Wichstrom, L. (1999). The emergence of gender difference in depressed mood during adolescence: The role of intensified gender socialization. *Developmental Psychology, 35,* 232–245.

Zubrick, S.R., Silburn, S.R., Garton, A., Burton, P., Dalby, R., Shepard, C., & Lawrence, D. (1995). *Western Australian Child Health Survey: Developing health and well-being in the nineties.* Perth, Western Australia: Australian Bureau of Statistics and the Institute for Child Health Research.

Depression, Adulthood

Jane E. Gillham, Derek R. Freres, and Andrew J. Shatté

INTRODUCTION

Depression is one of the most prevalent psychological disorders, affecting most of us, either directly, or through its impact on friends or family members. Depression exacts an emotional and monetary toll in the form of emotional suffering, decrease in achievement and productivity, impairments in important interpersonal relationships, and in the worst cases, suicide. For more than half of the depressed population, the depressive profile is one of recurrent episodes throughout the lifespan.

Over the past 20 years, researchers have learned a great deal about risk factors for depression and efficacious approaches to treatment. More recent research has attempted to apply this knowledge to the prevention of depression. This entry discusses several possible strategies for the prevention of depression and reviews empirical research on programs designed to prevent depression in adulthood.

DEFINITIONS

Depression. This entry focuses on the prevention of depressive symptoms and the two main types of unipolar depressive disorders: major depression and dysthymia. An episode of *major depression* is characterized by a variety of symptoms, including sad mood, anhedonia (or loss of interest or pleasure), fatigue, psychomotor retardation or agitation, significant changes in weight or appetite, sleep difficulties, difficulty concentrating, feelings of worthlessness or excessive guilt, and suicidal ideation. At least five of these symptoms (including sad mood and/or anhedonia) must be present throughout two or more weeks in order to meet diagnostic criteria. Major depressive episodes typically last for more than four months, but endure for more than two years in approximately 5–10 percent of individuals (American Psychiatric Association, 1994).

Dysthymia, a milder but more chronic form of unipolar depression, is characterized by the presence of four or more of these symptoms over a two-year period or longer (or a one-year period in children) (American Psychiatric Association, 1994). In this entry, we focus on the prevention of major depression, dysthymia, and symptoms of these two disorders.

There is debate as to whether depression is a discrete phenomenon, or whether depression is best conceptualized as symptoms on a continuum, with the clinical threshold determined by the number of symptoms and their frequency, intensity, and duration. Individuals who report high but subclinical levels of depressive symptoms are at a substantially increased risk for depressive disorders (Clarke, Hawkins, Murphy, Sheeber, Lewinsohn, & Seeley, 1995; Muñoz, 1993). Therefore, an intervention that prevents or reduces high levels of depressive symptoms may prevent depressive disorders.

SCOPE

Unipolar depression is one of the most common psychological disorders. In the United States, approximately 3–6 percent of the population will suffer from a depressive episode in a given year (American Psychiatric Association, 1994; Greenberg, Stiglin, Finkelstein, & Berndt, 1993). Between 7 and 20 percent of adults in the United States will experience an episode of depression in their lifetimes

(American Psychiatric Association, 1994). Epidemiological studies indicate that the incidence of depression in the United States increased dramatically during the past century, with some estimates suggesting a tenfold rise (Klerman et al., 1985). The high incidence of depression is a common Western phenomenon. In Switzerland, for example, approximately 18 percent of individuals will experience a major depressive episode during their lifetimes. Approximately 35 percent will experience major depression or dysthymia (Angst, 1995). Recent research indicates that between 4 and 11 percent of Canadians become depressed each year (Parikh, Wasylenki, Goering, & Wong, 1996; Patten, 2000), and approximately 8 percent of Italians may become depressed in a 6-month period (Dubini, Mannheimer, & Pancheri, 2001). The lifetime prevalence of depressive disorders appears to be much lower outside the West. In Ethiopia, for example, only about 3 percent of the population will experience major depression in their lifetimes (Kebede & Alem, 1999).

Depression is associated with other problems, including substance abuse, decreased work productivity, physical health problems, mortality and increased risk of suicide (American Psychiatric Association, 1994; Greenberg et al., 1993). Depression also appears to impair interpersonal relationships, including marital and parent–child relationships (American Psychiatric Association, 1994; Downey & Coyne, 1990). Maternal depression substantially increases the risk of depression in offspring (Downey & Coyne, 1990). For at least 60 percent of those affected, depression will be a recurrent disorder, with each recurrence further increasing the likelihood of future episodes (American Psychiatric Association, 1994).

The financial cost of depression is enormous. Recent estimates put the economic consequences of major depression and dysthymia (in terms of healthcare expenses and lost productivity) at $30 billion per year (Gillham, Shatté, & Freres, 2000; Greenberg et al., 1993). In a study of the global mortality and disability associated with 107 disorders and risk factors, unipolar depression ranked fourth, only falling below lower respiratory infections, diarrheal diseases and perinatal disorders on the measure of disease burden. Depression ranked above many disorders considered to be significant public health problems such as ischemic heart disease, tuberculosis, measles, traffic accidents, and HIV (Murray & Lopez, 1997).

THEORIES AND RESEARCH

Researchers have identified numerous *risk factors* for depression including negative cognitive styles (Robins & Hayes, 1995), maladaptive interpersonal styles (Joiner, Metalsky, Katz, & Beach, 1999), stressful life events

(Jenaway & Paykel, 1998), chronic medical problems (American Psychiatric Association, 1994) and poverty (Bruce, Takeuchi, & Leaf, 1991). In most Western cultures, women are twice as likely to suffer from depression as men. Although the sex difference has not been completely accounted for, possible explanations include differences in societal roles, differences in coping responses, and biological differences (Nolen-Hoeksema, 1990). Depression may be prevented by targeting these risk factors or by increasing *protective factors* such as coping skills and social support.

There are now several efficacious *treatments* for adult depression including cognitive–behavioral therapy, interpersonal therapy, and pharmacotherapy (e.g., Elkin et al., 1989). It is possible that cognitive–behavioral or interpersonal therapy techniques could be used to *prevent* depression from occurring in the first place. Although pharmacotherapy is more controversial as a preventive intervention, it may be useful for individuals with very high levels of symptoms who have a strong family history of the disorder.

The prevention of depression is a relatively new field. Consequently, only a few approaches to prevention have been evaluated. Existing studies have not yet provided strong support for the prevention of depressive disorders, and there is still little evidence for the prevention of high levels of symptoms. In the review that follows, we examine those approaches to the prevention of depression that (1) compare an intervention to a control condition and (2) assess depressive symptoms and/or depressive disorders as outcomes.

STRATEGIES: OVERVIEW

Prevention programs that have been empirically evaluated tend to target cognitive–behavioral risk and protective factors or assist individuals with difficult life circumstances or transitions. Interventions often overlap in the specific techniques or strategies they employ. For example, many of the interventions reviewed attempt to provide participants with social support and many interventions that target life transitions include cognitive–behavioral skills.

STRATEGIES THAT WORK

Treatment outcome researchers have recommended reserving the term "efficacious" for those interventions that have yielded successful outcomes in well-designed and well-controlled studies, and whose effects have been replicated (ideally by independent research teams) (e.g., Chambless & Hollon, 1998). Successful programs for preventing depression will prevent depressive disorders (major depression and/or dysthymia) and/or increases in depressive symptoms over time. Using these criteria, none of the programs designed to prevent adult depression can be classified as efficacious. Several interventions have yielded promising findings, and these are reviewed in the next section.

STRATEGIES THAT MIGHT WORK

Cognitive–Behavioral Programs Designed to Prevent Depression

The majority of programs for the prevention of depression that have been evaluated in the literature are based on cognitive–behavioral theories of depression. These theories link depression to negative cognitive styles, negative assumptions about the self and the world, biased information processing, maladaptive coping styles, and/or engagement in few pleasurable events. There is a great deal of research linking depressive symptoms and depressive disorders to these variables. For example, compared with nondepressed individuals, individuals with depressive disorders and depressive symptoms are more pessimistic in their explanations for events (Robins & Hayes, 1995), endorse more unrealistic stringent standards for success, and interpret information in a more negative manner (Gotlib & Krasnoperova, 1998). While these cognitive variables are almost certainly correlated with depression, the evidence that they are causes of depression is mixed (see Gotlib & Krasnoperova, 1998; Robins & Hayes, 1995). Abramson and colleagues recently found that negative cognitive styles preceded and predicted the onset of depressive episodes in young adults (Abramson et al., 2000).

Cognitive–behavioral therapy (CBT), an efficacious treatment for adult depression, targets depressotypic cognitions and teaches problem-solving skills. In CBT, clients are taught to recognize their negative assumptions and interpretive styles, to consider alternative interpretations for events, and to evaluate evidence for and against negative beliefs. Clients are typically taught a variety of behavioral skills including relaxation and assertiveness techniques, as well as how to divide large tasks into manageable components.

CBT is a validated treatment for depression and several studies have found that clients treated with CBT are less likely to relapse than those treated with pharmacotherapy (Evans et al., 1992). One reason for this may be that CBT provides patients with skills that can be used to effectively handle problems and painful emotions long after therapy ends. This raises the possibility that, if administered earlier, CBT techniques may be useful in preventing depression from developing.

A handful of studies have evaluated the effects of cognitive–behavioral interventions in preventing depression in adults. Studies with the strongest methodological designs (control or comparison groups, follow-up beyond the end of the intervention phase) are reviewed below (for a more detailed review of research on cognitive–behavioral prevention of depression, see Gillham et al., 2000).

One of the earliest investigations of cognitive–behavioral prevention programs was conducted by Vega and colleagues (Vega & Murphy, 1990). They evaluated two cognitive–behavioral interventions with low-income Mexican American women between the ages of 35 and 55. This particular sample was targeted because epidemiological research indicates that low-income minority women may be at especially high risk for depression. Participants were randomly assigned to one of two interventions or to a no intervention control. In the first intervention condition, participants received one-on-one counseling. In the second condition, a group format was used. Both interventions met once a week for approximately 12 weeks and provided social support, taught coping skills (including assertiveness), and attempted to build self-esteem by encouraging participants to think about difficult experiences they had surmounted. Depressive symptoms were assessed through self-report questionnaires prior to the intervention and 6 months after the intervention ended. When results were analyzed for all participants, no significant intervention effect was found. However, a significant preventive effect was found among participants who initially reported low levels of depressive symptoms. There were no differences in effects for the two interventions.

Muñoz and colleagues conducted the first study investigating the prevention of depressive disorders in adults (Muñoz et al., 1995). Non-depressed medical outpatients (ages 18–69) from a predominantly low-income minority community were randomly assigned to the intervention or control condition. The intervention consisted of eight 2-hr group meetings that focused on identifying and changing negative thoughts, increasing pleasant events, relaxation, and goal setting. Depressive symptoms and depressive disorders were assessed prior to the intervention and through one year of follow-up. No significant effect was found for depressive disorders. However, the incidence of depressive disorders was low (affecting less than 5 percent of the sample) and results were in the expected direction. Results for depressive symptoms differed for the two self-report measures used. Prevention group participants reported greater reductions in symptoms than controls on the Beck Depression Inventory (BDI), but no effect was found on the Center for Epidemiological Studies Depression Scale (CES-D).

Seligman and colleagues also conducted a randomized study of the prevention of depressive disorders (Seligman, Schulman, DeRubeis, & Hollon, 1999). This intervention was conducted with non-depressed university freshmen identified as at risk for depression based on their scores on a measure of explanatory style. Participants were randomly assigned to the intervention or a no-intervention control. The intervention consisted of eight 2-hr sessions that included cognitive restructuring and problem-solving techniques. Depressive disorders, depressive symptoms, anxiety disorders, anxiety symptoms, and measures of physical illness were assessed through three years of follow-up. Findings revealed no significant effect for definite depressive episodes. However, a significant prevention effect was found for moderate depression. Over the three-year follow-up period, the incidence of moderate depression was 31 percent in the control group and only 19 percent in the prevention group. A significant effect was found for self-reported depressive symptoms (on the BDI), with prevention group participants reporting fewer symptoms throughout the follow-up period. However, no effect was found for clinician reported symptoms on the Hamilton Depression Rating Scale. Prevention participants experienced fewer moderate episodes of Generalized Anxiety Disorder and reported fewer symptoms of anxiety on self-report measures. Prevention participants also reported fewer symptoms of physical illness and made fewer illness-related visits to the student health center (Buchanan, Gardenswartz, & Seligman, 1999).

Cognitive–behavioral interventions provide one promising route toward the prevention of adult depression. The interventions evaluated by Muñoz and Seligman and their colleagues reduced depressive symptoms and improved cognitions that are related to depression (Muñoz et al., 1995; Seligman et al., 1999). These findings are encouraging since depressive symptoms and depressotypic cognitions are risk factors for depressive disorders. However, we classify cognitive–behavioral interventions as strategies that *might* work since there is much less evidence that these interventions *prevent* depressive disorders or high levels of depressive symptoms in adults. Although Seligman and colleagues found significant prevention of moderate depressive symptomatology, neither study that assessed definite depressive disorders found a significant intervention effect.

Research on the prevention of depression in adolescents has yielded stronger findings. For example, Clarke and colleagues conducted a study of a group cognitive–behavioral intervention for high school students who reported high but subclinical levels of depression. A significant prevention effect was found for depressive disorders through one year of follow-up (Clarke et al., 1995). In a recent study, Clarke and colleagues recruited adolescents with high but subclinical levels of depression who had a parent affected by depression. These adolescents were randomly assigned to a group cognitive–behavioral intervention or a usual care condition. A significant prevention effect was found for depressive disorders through the 15-month follow-up period (Clarke et al., 1999). These findings indicate that cognitive–behavioral prevention programs are applicable to adolescent depression. Indeed, one path to the prevention of depression in adults may be through teaching cognitive–behavioral skills to individuals during childhood or adolescence. Longitudinal studies are needed to determine whether effects of these interventions can endure into adulthood.

The discrepancy in findings for cognitive–behavioral prevention in adults and adolescents is intriguing. There are several possible explanations. It could be that the intervention developed by Clarke and colleagues is more powerful than the interventions used in other research. All of the interventions described (including the intervention used by Clarke and colleagues) derive from CBT for adult depression. Although there is considerable overlap in the concepts and techniques covered, there is also a fair amount of variability in the actual cognitive–behavioral techniques included and in the ways concepts and skills are presented and practiced. Clarke and colleagues' intervention may provide more emphasis on the behavioral skills, including more focus on interpersonal skills and increasing pleasant events.

Another important difference between the studies by Clarke and colleagues and the studies of cognitive–behavioral programs for adult depression is in the level of symptoms displayed by participants. Clarke and colleagues recruited participants with high (but subclinical) levels of symptoms. In contrast, participants in the other studies were selected on the basis of other risk factors (demographic characteristics, pessimistic explanatory style) that are more distal to depression. On average, these participants displayed dramatically lower levels of depressive symptoms. It is possible that cognitive–behavioral and, perhaps, other preventive interventions are most relevant and useful for participants with very high levels of depressive symptoms. One finding that seems to contradict this hypothesis is the stronger effect for low symptom participants in the study by Vega and colleagues.

Finally, selecting participants with very high levels of symptoms increases the probability that participants will develop depressive disorders over the follow-up period. This increases the likelihood of finding an intervention effect since intervention effects for categorical outcomes (e.g., depressive disorder) are easier to detect when the incidence of the condition is high in the control group (Gillham et al., 2000; Muñoz, 1993). It will be important for future studies to examine whether cognitive–behavioral programs can prevent depressive disorders in adults with very high (but subclinical) levels of symptoms.

Coping with Difficult Life Transitions and Circumstances

Another approach to the prevention of depression involves administering interventions that help individuals cope with specific stressors or life transitions that are linked to depression. These interventions typically employ a variety of strategies including providing social support, teaching cognitive–behavioral skills, and teaching other skills relevant to particular stressors or circumstances. The research on these types of interventions is sparse. Only a few studies have attempted to prevent depressive symptoms and no studies have explored the prevention of depressive disorders.

An Intervention Targeting Job Searching Skills in Unemployed Adults

Price, Van Ryn, and Vinokur (1992), Vinokur, Price, and Caplan (1991), and Vinokur, Price, and Schul (1995), have developed an intervention for unemployed adults. This is an important risk factor to target since job loss, unemployment and poverty are linked to depression in adults (American Psychiatric Association, 1994; Kebede & Alem, 1999). It has been estimated that poverty accounts for as much as 10 percent of new episodes of major depression (Bruce et al., 1991).

The intervention developed by Vinokur and colleagues consisted of eight 3-hr group sessions held over a 2-week period. The sessions provided social support, taught problem-solving and decision making techniques, and covered a variety of skills related to job seeking such as identifying work related skills, using social networks to obtain job leads, contacting potential employers, preparing applications and resumes, and preparing for job interviews (Price et al., 1992; Vinokur et al., 1991, 1995).

Two studies have evaluated the effects of the intervention on depressive symptoms. Intervention participants were compared with participants in a control condition who received a brief booklet describing job seeking tips. A variety of outcomes were assessed including employment status, quality of work, and monthly earnings. Although the major goal of this intervention was to help participants find employment, the researchers also investigated the effects of the intervention on depressive symptoms.

In the first study, adults were randomly assigned to the intervention or control conditions and were followed for $2^1/_2$ years after the intervention ended. Intervention participants achieved significantly higher levels of reemployment than did controls (Vinokur et al., 1991). Among participants identified at high risk for depression (based on self-reports of financial strain, depressive symptoms, and social assertiveness), those in the intervention group reported lower levels of depressive symptoms than controls through the follow-up period. About 51 percent of high risk controls reported moderate to severe levels of depressive symptoms during one or more of the follow-up assessments, compared with 39 percent of high risk participants in the experimental group (Price et al., 1992).

In the second study, participants were randomly assigned to the intervention or control condition and followed for 6 months after the intervention ended. Results differed by participants' levels of risk. Among low risk participants, no intervention effect was found for reemployment status or depressive symptoms at the 6-month follow-up. Among high risk participants, significant intervention effects were found. Intervention participants were more likely to be reemployed and reported greater reductions in depressive symptoms than controls at the 6-month follow-up (Vinokur et al., 1995).

A Stress Management Program for Low-Income Women

Tableman and her colleagues conducted several studies investigating the effects of a stress management program for low-income women (Tableman, 1987, 1989; Tableman, Marciniak, Johnson, & Rodgers, 1982). Their group intervention consisted of 10 weekly meetings. The program included many cognitive and behavioral techniques including goal setting, decision making, relaxation training, and identifying signs of stress. Other topics included developing positive attitudes about women's roles, exploring interpersonal relationships, and positive approaches to child rearing. Depressive symptoms was one of several outcomes assessed. Two studies were conducted with women on public assistance (one with a predominantly Caucasian sample and another with a predominantly African American sample). Participants who attended the intervention reported greater reductions in depressive symptoms than controls who received no training.

The research of Tableman and her colleagues have produced promising results. Low-income women are a particularly important population to target since they experience considerable day-to-day stress and are at increased risk for depressive symptomatology. Women in general are at twice the risk for depression as men, and there is evidence that low-income women may be particularly vulnerable (American Psychiatric Association, 1994).

Like the intervention developed by Vinokur, Price and their colleagues, this intervention is classified as an intervention that *might* work because: (1) the effects of the intervention on depressive disorders was not assessed, (2) it is not clear whether the intervention *prevented* or simply reduced depressive symptoms, and (3) findings have not yet been replicated by other research groups.

Many other stressors and life transitions could be targeted by programs that aim to prevent depression. Interventions that assist individuals in coping with divorce, the death of a loved one, or the postpartum period may prevent sadness and dysphoria from becoming a clinical depression. It is estimated that 10–20 percent of new mothers experience depression during the postpartum period, yet preventive interventions have not been empirically evaluated for this group (Locicero, Weiss, & Issokson, 1997; Spinelli, 1999).

STRATEGIES THAT DO NOT WORK

In the published literature on interventions designed to prevent depression, there is a virtual lack of negative findings. This may be due in part to a bias to publish studies with positive results. But, research on the prevention of depression is in its early stages and many strategies remain to be evaluated. It is too early to draw conclusions about strategies that lack efficacy.

One study that yielded negative findings evaluated the efficacy of the anti-depressant mianserin in preventing depression in stroke victims (Palomäki et al., 1999). In this study, patients who had recently suffered a stroke were randomly assigned to mianserin treatment or to a usual care condition. No overall effect of mianserin was found on depressive symptoms or depressive disorders. The researchers noted, however, that the prevalence of depression was quite low in their sample. Only 16 percent of patients became depressed during the 18 month follow-up period. Thus, there was little depression to prevent. Future studies may find mianserin and other anti-depressants are efficacious in preventing depression in higher risk samples.

SYNTHESIS

The emerging field of preventing depression in adults has employed several approaches, including cognitive–behavioral interventions and interventions that help individuals adjust to and cope with life transitions and chronic stressors. Several of these interventions use similar strategies such as providing social support, targeting cognitive styles linked to depression, and teaching problem solving.

Although many of these interventions reduce depressive symptoms, there is not yet convincing evidence that depressive disorders and dysthymia can be prevented. Few interventions have prevented increases in depressive symptoms and no intervention has prevented definite depressive disorders in adults.

There are several possible explanations for this failure to find strong prevention effects. Existing prevention programs may not be powerful enough or may not have effects that endure over time. More successful programs might increase the duration of the intervention, include booster sessions, increase the amount of time participants spend practicing specific skills, increase the amount of feedback participants receive, or target additional risk and protective factors. Interventions that combine approaches (e.g., cognitive–behavioral approaches that also focus on improving interpersonal relationships) may prove particularly powerful.

The prevention of depression may also be achieved through other pathways that have not yet been empirically evaluated. For example, although there is evidence that women with little social support are particularly vulnerable to postpartum depression, interventions that attempt to increase social support at this time have not yet been evaluated. Although CBT, interpersonal psychotherapy, and pharmacotherapy are all efficacious treatments for depression, only CBT has received much attention as a preventive intervention.

The majority of interventions that have been evaluated target individual risk factors for depression. The prevention of depression may be achieved through targeting societal risk factors. Such interventions could provide individuals with skills to change negative circumstances in their own lives and/or take a broader approach by directly targeting relevant societal and cultural institutions and policies relevant to depression (Muñoz et al., 1995; Offord, 1996). Bruce and colleagues estimate that poverty accounts for 10 percent of new episodes of major depression (Bruce et al., 1991). Thus, depression may be prevented by teaching skills and creating policies that enhance the ability of individuals to support themselves and their families.

Stronger effects may also be found by targeting interventions to participants who are at extremely high risk for depression. Significant prevention of depression has been found in adolescents when investigators selected participants with very high (but subclinical) levels of symptoms (Clarke et al., 1995, 1999). It will also be important, however, to develop and evaluate interventions with individuals with lower levels of depressive symptoms as it may be possible to prevent high levels of symptoms, and ultimately depressive disorders from developing in these participants as well. The prevention of high levels of depressive symptoms is an important goal in itself since these symptoms are associated with many of the same problems (e.g., academic difficulties, decreased productivity, impaired relationships) as depressive disorders.

Depression may be prevented more effectively by providing interventions before individuals reach adulthood, perhaps even at multiple points in development. Recent research indicates that rates of depression in childhood and adolescence have risen dramatically. Individuals who experience depression during adolescence are at an increased risk for depression as adults. Thus, it is possible that the preventive effects of successful interventions delivered during childhood or adolescence endure as participants grow older and enter adulthood.

In conclusion, research on the prevention of depression has progressed considerably in the past decade. Several interventions have been developed and evaluated with promising results. Currently, there is no convincing evidence that depressive disorders can be prevented in adults. However, we believe that evidence for prevention will emerge as researchers expand their interventions, target additional risk factors, and investigate new approaches. Given the tremendous personal and societal costs of depression, the development of efficacious and effective prevention programs is a high priority for future research.

Also see: Depression: Childhood; Depression: Adolescence; Depression: Older Adulthood; Chronic Disease: Adulthood.

References

Abramson, L.Y., Alloy, L.B., Hankin, B.L., Clements, C.M., Zhu, L., Hogan, M.E., & Whitehouse, W.G. (2000). Optimistic cognitive styles and invulnerability to depression. In J.E. Gillham (Ed.), *The science of optimism and hope: Research essays in honor of Martin E.P. Seligman.* Radnor, PA: Templeton Foundation Press.

American Psychiatric Association. (1994). *Diagnostic and statistical manual of mental disorders* (4th ed.). Washington, DC: Author.

Angst, J. (1995). The epidemiology of depressive disorders. *European Neuropsychopharmacology, 5* (Suppl.), 95–98.

Bruce, M.L., Takeuchi, D.T., & Leaf, P.J. (1991). Poverty and psychiatric status: Longitudinal evidence from the New Haven epidemiologic catchment area study. *Archives of General Psychiatry, 48,* 470–474.

Buchanan, G., Gardenswartz, C.A.R., & Seligman, M.E.P. (1999). Physical health following a cognitive–behavioral intervention. *Prevention and Treatment, 2.*

Chambless, D.L., & Hollon, S.D. (1998). Defining empirically supported therapies. *Journal of Consulting and Clinical Psychology, 66,* 7–18.

Clarke, G.N., Hawkins, W., Murphy, M., Sheeber, L.B., Lewinsohn, P.M., & Seeley, J.R. (1995). Targeted prevention of unipolar depressive disorder in an at-risk sample of high school adolescents: A randomized trial of a group cognitive intervention. *Journal of the American Academy of Child and Adolescent Psychiatry, 34,* 312–321.

Clarke, G., Hornbrook, M., Lynch, F., Polen, M., Gale, J., O'Connor, E., & Haworth, L. (1999, March). *Prevention of depression in at-risk offspring of depressed HMO members.* Paper presented at the HMO Research Network annual conference, Hawaii.

Downey, G., & Coyne, J.C. (1990). Children of depressed parents: An integrative review. *Psychological Bulletin, 108,* 50–76.

Dubini, A., Mannheimer, R., & Pancheri, P. (2001). Depression in the community: Results of the first Italian survey. *International Clinical Psychopharmacololgy, 16,* 49–53.

Elkin, I., Shea, M.T., Watkins, J.T., Imber, S.D., Sotsky, S.M., Collins, J.F., Glass, D.R., Pilkonis, P.A., Leber, W.R., Docherty, J.P, Fiester, S.J., & Parloff, M.B. (1989). NIMH treatment of depression collaborative research program: General effectiveness of treatments. *Archives of General Psychiatry, 46,* 971–982.

Evans, M.D., Hollon, S.D., DeRubeis, R.J., Piasecki, J.M., Grove, W.M., Garvey, M.J., & Tuason, V.B. (1992). Differential relapse following cognitive therapy and pharmacotherapy for depression. *Archives of General Psychiatry, 49,* 802–808.

Gillham, J.E., Shatté, A.J., & Freres, D.R. (2000). Depression prevention: A review of cognitive–behavioral and family interventions. *Applied & Preventive Psychology, 9*, 63–88.

Gotlib, I.H., & Krasnoperova, E. (1998). Biased information processing as a vulnerability factor for depression. *Behavior Therapy, 29*, 603–617.

Greenberg, P.E., Stiglin, L.E., Finkelstein, S.N., & Brendt, E.R. (1993). The economic burden of depression in 1990. *Journal of Clinical Psychiatry, 54*, 405–426.

Jenaway, A., & Paykel, E.S. (1988). Life events and depression. In A. Honig & H.M. van Praag (Eds.), *Depression: Neurobiological, psychopathological and therapeutic advances* (pp. 279–295). New York: Wiley & Sons.

Joiner, T.E., Metalsky, G.I., Katz, J., & Beach, S.R.H. (1999). Depression and excessive reassurance-seeking. *Psychological Inquiry, 10*, 269–278.

Kebede, D., & Alem, A. (1999). Major mental disorders in Addis Ababa, Ethiopia. II: Affective disorders. *Acta Psychiatrica Scandinavica, 100* (Suppl. 397), 18–23.

Klerman, G.L., Lavori, P.W., Rice, J., Reich, T., Endicott, J., Andreasen, N.C., Keller, M., & Hirschfeld, R.M.A. (1985). Birth cohort trends in rates of major depressive disorder: A study of relatives of patients with affective disorder. *Archives of General Psychiatry, 42*, 689–693.

Locicero, A.K., Weiss, D.M., & Issokson, D. (1997). Postpartum depression: Proposal for prevention through an integrated care and support network. *Applied and Preventive Psychology, 6*, 169–178.

Muñoz, R.F. (1993). The prevention of depression: Current research and practice. *Applied and Preventive Psychology, 2*, 21–33.

Muñoz, R.F., Ying, Y., Bernal, G., Perez-Stable, E.J., Sorensen, J.L., Hargreaves, W.A., Miranda, J., & Miller, L.S. (1995). Prevention of depression with primary care patients: A randomized controlled trial. *American Journal of Community Psychology, 23*, 199–222.

Murray, C.J.L., & Lopez, A.D. (1997). Global mortality, disability, and the contribution of risk factors: Global burden of disease study. *Lancet, 349*, 1436–1442.

Nolen-Hoeksema, S. (1990). *Sex differences in depression.* Stanford, CA: Stanford University Press.

Offord, D.R. (1996). The state of prevention and early intervention. In R.D. Peters & R.J. McMahon (Eds.), *Preventing childhood disorders, substance abuse, and delinquency* (pp. 329–344). Thousand Oaks, CA: Sage.

Palomäki, H., Kaste, M., Berg, A., Löennqvist, R., Löennqvist, J., Lehtihalmes, M., & Hares, J. (1999). Prevention of poststroke depression: 1 year randomised placebo controlled double blind trial of mianserin with 6 month follow-up after therapy. *Journal of Neurology Neurosurgery, and Psychiatry, 66*, 490–494.

Parikh, S.V., Wasylenki, D., Goering, P., & Wong, J. (1996). Mood disorders: Rural/urban differences in prevalence, health care utilization, and disability in Ontario. *Journal of Affective Disorders, 38*, 57–65.

Patten, S.B. (2000). Major depression prevalence in Calgary. *Canadian Journal of Psychiatry, 45*, 923–926.

Price, R.H., Van Ryn, M., & Vinokur, A.D. (1992). Impact of a preventive job search intervention on the likelihood of depression among the unemployed. *Journal of Health and Social Behavior, 33*, 158–167.

Robins, C.J., & Hayes, A.M. (1995). The role of causal attributions in the prediction of depression. In G.M. Buchanan & M.E.P. Seligman (Eds.), *Explanatory style* (pp. 71–98). Hillsdale, NJ: Lawrence Erlbaum Associates.

Seligman, M.E.P., Schulman, P., DeRubeis, R.J., & Hollon, S.D. (1999). The prevention of depression and anxiety. *Prevention and Treatment, 2*, article 8. Available on www:http:journals.apa.org/prevention/volume2/pre0020008a.html

Spinelli, M.G. (1999). Prevention of postpartum mood disorders. In L.J. Miller (Ed.), *Postpartum mood disorders* (pp. 217–235). Washington, DC: American Psychiatric Press.

Tableman, B. (1987). Stress management training: An approach to the prevention of depression in low-income populations. In R.F. Muñoz (Ed.), *Depression prevention: Research directions* (pp. 171–184). Washington, DC: Hemisphere.

Tableman, B. (1989). Stress management training for low income women. *Prevention in Human Services, 6*, 259–284.

Tableman, B., Marciniak, D., Johnson, D., & Rodgers, R. (1982). Stress management training for women on public assistance. *American Journal of Community Psychology, 10*, 357–367.

Vega, W.A., & Murphy, J.W. (1990). *Culture and the restructuring of community mental health.* New York: Greewood Press.

Vinokur, A.D., Price, R.H., & Caplan, R.D. (1991). From field experiments to program implementation: Assessing potential outcomes of an experimental intervention program for unemployed persons. *American Journal of Community Psychology, 19*(1), 543–562.

Vinokur, A.D., Price, R.H., & Schul, Y. (1995). Impact of the JOBS intervention on unemployed workers varying in risk for depression. *American Journal of Community Psychology, 23*, 39–73.

Depression, Older Adulthood

Velma A. Kameoka, Elaine M. Heiby, and Judy H. Lee

INTRODUCTION

This entry presents a definition of major depression and the prevalence of this mood disorder among older adults. While dozens of theories of depression have been proposed over the past century, the two most significant ones in terms of generating research, treatment, and prevention approaches will be noted: an organic theory and a psychosocial theory. Probable risk factors, such as disability, and potential preventive techniques, such as learning new social skills, will be addressed. Finally, a synthesis suggesting a multidisciplinary approach to the prevention of depression will be offered.

DEFINITIONS

The term depression has been used in different ways in the literature to refer to a clinical syndrome, a cluster of depressive symptoms, or a mood state. The fourth edition of the Diagnostic and Statistical Manual of Mental Disorders (DSM-IV) defines two clinical syndromes of depression (also termed "unipolar depression")—*major depression* and *dysthymia*. Diagnostic criteria for *major depression* include at least one episode of at least five of the following symptoms that together interfere with daily functioning during a two-week period: depressed mood, loss of pleasure, significant weight loss, insomnia or hypersomnia, psychomotor retardation or agitation, loss of energy, feelings of worthlessness or excessive guilt, diminished ability to think, concentrate, or make decisions, and suicidal ideation. *Dysthsmia*, in contrast, is a chronic disorder characterized by less severe depressive symptoms lasting most of the time over two years. Although clinical syndromes of depression are clearly defined by the DSM-IV, symptom manifestations of depression unique to the population of older adults are not adequately defined and not easily recognized (Mulsant & Ganguli, 1999; NIH, 1991; Pachana, Gallagher-Thompson, & Thompson, 1994).

SCOPE

In many countries, depression among adults over the age of 65 is a common problem that is underrecognized, underdiagnosed, and undertreated. Although cross-national prevalence estimates for major depressive disorder is relatively low (1–3 percent), prevalence estimates for depressive symptoms that do not meet diagnostic criteria for major depression is quite high (15 percent) among older adults living in the community (Beekman, Copeland, & Prince, 1999; Mulsant & Ganguli, 1999). Prevalence and incidence estimates for depression vary widely across studies due to differences in the definition of depression, criteria for diagnosing depression, characteristics of the population sampled, and method of assessment.

Epidemiological data indicate that rates for depression increase dramatically as health and functional status of elders deteriorate. For example, rates for major depressive disorders and depressive symptoms range from 5–20 percent in primary care clinics, 10–25 percent in hospital settings, and 12–40 percent in nursing homes (Cole, Bellavance, & Mansour, 1999; Mulsant & Ganguli, 1999). In the United States, one-year incidence of major depression among nursing home residents is 13 percent and an additional 18 percent develop new symptoms of depression over the one-year period (NIH, 1991). These cross-national estimates are striking and suggest that depression is a serious public health problem that exacts significant costs from society. Untreated, depressive symptoms increase risk for major depression and suicide, exacerbate co-occurring medical disorders, increase use of health care services, and increase health care costs by contributing to poorer prognosis for depression and comorbid medical disorders. Less than 20 percent of depressed elders in community and primary care settings, however, are diagnosed or receive treatment (Cole et al., 1999).

THEORIES

The most significant theories of depression focus on either organic or psychosocial determinants. *Organic theories* (Paykel, 1992) suggest depression at any age is due to brain dysfunctions in neurotransmitter systems. The dysfunction may be due to genetics or environmental trauma that affect hypothalamic–pituitary–adrenal regulation. Particular neurotransmitters that contribute to mood are inferred from animal models and the effects of antidepressant medications. No gene that causes depression has been identified. The hypothesized brain dysfunctions include catecholamine and indoleamine receptor dysregulation. As people age, the amount of environmental stress accumulates and may impair neuroendocrine responses to current stressors, rendering older people at greater risk for catecholamine and indoleamine receptor dysregulation. This dysregulation would impair an older person's ability to deal with both daily hassles and major life changes such as the death of a spouse, physical illness, and reduced functional ability. Therefore, the preventive implication of the organic theories includes strategies that enhance the ability to cope with stressful life events.

Psychosocial theories (Craighead, Craighead, & Ilardi, 1998) postulate numerous behavioral and cognitive competencies that facilitate coping with stressful life events and thus prevent depression at any age. These theories also postulate that environmental engineering that reduces the number of negative events and increases the number of positive events may prevent depression.

Hypothesized behavioral competencies include social and recreational skills. Social skills include the ability to be assertive about one's needs and preferences. As people age, they may need to learn to make new friends and ask for assistance with daily tasks. Recreational skills may include developing new interests and pastimes following retirement and changes in functional ability. Hypothesized cognitive competencies include self-reinforcement, attributional style, and perceived control. *Self-reinforcement* refers to rewarding oneself overtly or covertly for one's accomplishments and assets rather than depending upon other people to do so. Older adults often lose sources of recognition, such as from friends and co-workers who have died. *Attributional style* refers to how one interprets response-outcome contingencies. Depression is more likely to follow a negative life event if one attributes the cause of the event to oneself and expects the negative event to occur in a wide range of current and future situations. For example, it would be depressogenic to attribute reduced visual acuity to one's teenage junk food diet rather than a natural aging process. *Perceived control* is sometimes called *self-efficacy*. Perceived control refers to one's sense of ability to accomplish a specific goal.

For example, an older adult who wants to continue to play tennis and believes it is possible to do so is more likely to retain this recreational pastime, perhaps by playing doubles or a less competitive game.

Environmental engineering to increase positive events can take several forms. The physical environment can be changed, such as providing hand rails in the bathroom so basic self-care skills can be maintained. The social environment can also be changed to enhance informational, material, and emotional social support, such as by joining senior centers or moving into a retirement community.

RESEARCH

A major challenge for prevention research is the identification of factors that lead an older adult to be at increased risk for depression. The identification of risk factors requires prospective studies on the etiology and course of depression. Although such longitudinal studies have not been conducted, the organic and psychosocial theories discussed above have generated a vast body of empirical studies on biological, socio-environmental, and psychological variables associated with greater vulnerability to depression among older adults.

Research findings indicate that biological factors play a more prominent role in precipitating depression later rather than earlier in life. Biological factors that have been found to increase risk for depression among older adults include comorbid medical illness, neurobiological changes, and drug reactions (Karel, 1997). Studies show that depression co-occurs with stroke, cardiovascular disease, cancer, diabetes, Parkinson's disease, Alzheimer's disease, and chronic pain. Studies also show that depression, in turn, can exacerbate the course of these illnesses (Karel, 1997; Mulsant & Ganguli, 1999; NIH, 1991). Neurobiological correlates of depression that have received most attention include decreased serotonin concentrations in the brain and impaired hypothalamic–pituitary–adrenal activity, changes that are commonly associated with aging itself (Schneider, 1996). The importance of these neurobiological factors, in comparison to medical and psychosocial risk factors, in accounting for increased risk for depression is unclear. In contrast, studies have shown that various medications are clearly associated with increased risk for depression among older adults including those prescribed for cardiovascular problems, hypertension, and Parkinson's disease, chemotherapy drugs, and steroids (Karel, 1997).

The vast body of research on socio-environmental risk factors suggests that stressful life events and lack of social support are associated with greater risk for depression. Stressful life events that have been shown to be particularly salient in rendering an older adult to be at increased risk for depression include illness, disability, interpersonal loss, bereavement, and associated deficits in social support (Karel, 1997). Not all older adults, however, who experience socio-environmental changes, report depression. The evidence suggests that the effects of these life stresses on depression depend on an individual's psychological predispositions or ability to cope with stressful socio-environmental conditions.

Evidence pertaining to psychological risk factors support the importance of behavioral and cognitive competencies, or "coping resources," posited by theory as discussed earlier. Among the behavioral risk factors, studies of late life depression suggest that poor social skills and recreational inactivity, as characterized by lack of assertiveness, social withdrawal, and inertia, may predispose an elder to depression (Dubanoski, Heiby, Kameoka, & Wong, 1996). Studies of cognitive competencies have shown that perceived control and self-reinforcement skills are associated with decreased risk for depression throughout adulthood and among older adults (Karel, 1997). The results suggest that an elder's perception of his or her ability to influence environmental contingencies and, also, to accommodate to environmental events that are beyond the individual's control, may render the elder less vulnerable to depression. Also, studies have shown that the ability to monitor and evaluate the positive aspects of one's behavior and to self-administer positive reinforcement for those behaviors decrease risk for depression among older adults and in samples of Asian and Caucasian elders (Wong, Heiby, Kameoka, & Dubanoski, 1999).

STRATEGIES THAT WORK

The longitudinal studies needed to demonstrate prevention of depression in later life have not been conducted. There are, however, numerous studies of the various methods for treating depression in the aged (Cole et al., 1999; Craighead et al., 1998; Duffy, 1999; Karel & Hinrichsen, 2000; Salzman, 1999). We will generate some possible preventive strategies from these treatment methods.

STRATEGIES THAT MIGHT WORK

All of the following suggestions will require further research, but theoretically they hold promise for the prevention of depression in older persons. Health education and pre-retirement planning that include the development of positive expectations of a new life phase, new interests, and more social support, might be helpful to prevent depression in the older age group. Training in problem-solving also might be useful in managing specific daily life stressors.

Reminiscence or life review therapies have been shown to enhance life satisfaction, a salient variable for this age group shown to be negatively associated with depression (Dubanoski et al., 1996), although some research presents conflicting results, when the intervention addresses painful life events from the elder's past (Karel & Hinrichsen, 2000). Being a part of groups that have planned social and leisure activities might be promising in preventing depression (cf. Salzman, 1999). Cognitive and behavioral bibliotherapy (reading books on behavioral or cognitive therapy for depression) also have shown to alleviate mild depressive symptoms (Karel & Hinrichsen, 2000).

Given the treatment outcome support for cognitive–behavioral therapy (CBT) and interpersonal therapy (IPT), primary prevention programming may be guided by the behaviors targeted in these forms of treatments. For example, providing instruction on the relations among thoughts, feelings, and behaviors and how one can control these experiences may be useful in preventing depression among elders. CBT includes challenging the negative triad, suggesting prevention strategies that would include attention to how one interprets negative events, their causes, and their probability of recurrence (Beck, Rush, Shaw, & Emery, 1979). CBT also includes exposure to pleasant events, which suggests a preventive approach in which older persons might benefit from recreational skills training and acceptance that new interests may be necessary in later life. IPT involves social skills training, from which we might derive the idea of developing communication and assertiveness skills relevant to the transitions in one's social support network and personal needs.

There are a number of psychosocial interventions for depression that have been shown to be effective with young and middle age adults, but have not yet been systematically evaluated for older adults (Craighead et al., 1998). Behavior and cognitive therapy that focuses on enhancing frequency of self-reinforcement and perceived control have been shown to be effective and could be adapted for the elderly.

Research on correlates of depression among community-dwelling elders (Dubanoski et al., 1996) also suggests prevention strategies may need to be tailored according to an elder's ethnic identity. It has been shown that correlates differ for elders of Asian, Caucasian, and Hawaiian ancestry. Asian American elders were more likely to exhibit depressive symptoms if they also exhibited deficits in assertiveness, self-reinforcement, perceived control, and functional ability. Caucasian American elders were more likely to exhibit depressive symptoms if they also reported high stressful life events and exhibited deficits in emotional social support, reciprocal social support, recreational activity, assertiveness, self-reinforcement, perceived control, perceived health, functional ability, and objective health. Hawaiian American elders were more likely to exhibit depressive symptoms if they also reported high stressful life events and exhibited deficits in reciprocal social support, assertiveness, self-reinforcement, perceived control, perceived health, functional ability, and objective health. Therefore, generic community-based prevention strategies may not be indicated for each vulnerability factor. For example, it has been suggested that increasing social support may prevent depression among older adults (Duffy, 1999), but these findings may not be relevant to elders whose cultural environment includes strong communal values. On the other hand, some vulnerability factors may be universal. Deficits in assertiveness, self-reinforcement, and functional ability may render an elder at risk for depression regardless of cultural differences. Perhaps the aging process inherently requires one to learn to ask for help, evaluate oneself and life experiences in a positive way, and be able to conduct the basic tasks of daily living in order to avoid depression.

STRATEGIES THAT DO NOT WORK

One implication of organic theories of depression is that medication be applied at the earliest signs of depression, but this may be ineffective as a prevention strategy due to potential serious negative side effects of antidepressant medication among older adults. Approximately 20 percent of older adults have serious health problems that can be exacerbated by antidepressant medications, including increased risk of hip fractures and elevated blood pressure (Karel & Hinrichsen, 2000).

Psychosocial risk factors vary across cultural groups (Dubanoski et al., 1996). Therefore, psychosocial, competency-based prevention strategies may not be effective unless preventive interventions are tailored to address cultural variations in behavioral and cognitive repertoires. In addition, training in psychosocial skills may need to be adjusted for cognitive and physical deficits (Montano, 1999).

Difficulties in assessing depression among older adults, however, present challenges for evaluating the efficacy of prevention strategies. There are numerous mitigating factors that render it difficult to identify elders who are at risk for depression. Assessment of depression and risk factors depends on the accuracy of reports by self, caregivers, health professionals, and family members (Pachana et al., 1994). Older adults and their loved ones may feel stigmatized by admitting depressive symptoms (Montano, 1999). Primary care physicians underdiagnose depression in all age groups, have less reimbursement incentives to treat depression, and may lack comprehensive knowledge in treating subclinical depressive symptoms (e.g., Mulsant & Ganguli, 1999; Pearson & Brown, 2000). In addition, the expression of depression is heterogeneous and confounded with bereavement, natural aging processes, and other disorders that affect mood, appetite, and sleep (Beekman et al., 1999). Therefore, in order to identify prevention strategies that do and do not work, it is critical to develop accurate methods of assessment of depression among elders.

SYNTHESIS

The organic and psychosocial theories of depression have been integrated in a psychological behaviorism theory proposed by Heiby and Staats (1990). The theory posits that three types of organic factors can render an individual at risk for depression. These organic factors include genetic conditions that interfere with the learning of mood regulation skills, physical conditions that impair the use of mood regulation skills (e.g., loss of visual acuity), and physical conditions that directly elicit dysphoria (e.g., hypoglycemia). The theory also posits that early learning conditions can impair the acquisition of mood regulating skills and that current learning conditions may fail to reinforce the expression of these skills. The mood-regulating skills posited in the theory are classified as including language-cognitive skills (e.g., attributional style), emotional-motivational skills (e.g., recreational interests), and sensory-motor instrumental skills (e.g., assertiveness). The theory includes those skills involved in CBT and IPT, as well as the factors studied by Dubanoski et al. (1996).

According to this theory, the prevention of depression must be multifaceted. Medical strategies to facilitate the use of mood-regulating skills could include the use of assistive devices, such as a cane or hearing aide, as well as treatment for physical diseases. Environmental strategies could include engineering more reinforcement for adaptive behavior, such as social acceptance upon joining a senior center. Psychoeducational strategies would include training in recreational activities, assertiveness, self-reinforcement, and perceived control. Health facilities and senior centers could provide assessment of risk factors for depression, and training in the use of medical, situational, and mood regulating skills. Because primary care physicians are often the first contact with an older adult at risk for depression, it would be useful to educate physicians on risk factors and referrals for prevention training.

The psychological behaviorism theory suggests prevention of depression among older adults would involve a multidisciplinary approach, which is consistent with recommendations from reviews of the elder depression literature (Karel & Hinrichsen, 2000; Montano, 1999). In addition, to avoid further medical risks and complications, the first line of prevention for depression should be nonpharmacologic (Salzman, 1999). Instead, primary prevention strategies should involve psychoeducational outreach programs (Hogstel, 1995; Kennedy, 1996) and changing the way primary care addresses detection of depressive symptoms. The Elder Life Adjustment Interview Schedule (ELAIS) developed by Dubanoski et al. (1996) is designed to assess depressive symptoms, life satisfaction, and the organic conditions, socio-environmental conditions, and behavioral and cognitive competencies associated with risk for depression. Therefore, the ELAIS is consistent with psychological behaviorism theory and the elder depression literature and may prove to be useful in identifying persons at risk for depression in later life.

Also see: Depression: Childhood; Depression: Adolescence; Depression: Adulthood; Chronic Disease: Older Adulthood; Crises Intervention: Older Adulthood; Death with Dignity: Older Adulthood; Grief: Older Adulthood; Health Promotion: Older Adulthood; Life Challenges: Older Adulthood.

References

Beck, A.T., Rush, A.J., Shaw, B.R., & Emery, G. (1979). *Cognitive therapy of depression.* New York: The Guilford Press.

Beekman, A.T.F., Copeland, J.R.M., & Prince, M.J. (1999). Review of community prevalence of depression in later life. *British Journal of Psychiatry, 174,* 307–311.

Cole, M.G., Bellavance, F., & Mansour, A. (1999). Prognosis of depression in elderly community and primary care populations: A systematic review and meta-analysis. *American Journal of Psychiatry, 156,* 1182–1189.

Craighead, W.E., Craighead, L.W., & Ilardi, S.S. (1998). Psychosocial treatments for major depressive disorder. In P.E. Nathan & J.M. Gorman (Eds.), *A guide to treatments that work.* New York: Oxford University Press.

Dubanoksi, J.P., Heiby, E.M., Kameoka, V.A., & Wong, E. (1996). A cross-ethnic psychometric evaluation of the elder life adjustment interview schedule. *Journal of Clinical Geropsychology, 2,* 247–262.

Duffy, M. (1999). *Handbook of counseling and psychotherapy with older adults.* New York: John Wiley & Sons.

Heiby, E.M., & Staats, A. (1990). Depression and its classification. In G. Eifert & I. Evans (Eds.), *Unifying behavior therapy: Contributions of paradigmatic behaviorism.* New York: Springer.

Hogstel, M.O. (Ed.). (1995). *Geropsychiatric nursing* (2nd ed.). St. Louis, MO: Mosby-Year.

Karel, M.J. (1997). Aging and depression: Vulnerability and stress across adulthood. *Clinical Psychology Review, 8,* 847–879.

Karel, M.J., & Hinrichsen, G. (2000). Treatment of depression in late life: Psychotherapeutic interventions. *Clinical Psychology Review, 20,* 707–729.

Kennedy, G.J. (1996). The epidemiology of late-life depression. In G.J. Kennedy (Ed.), *Suicide and depression in late life: Critical issues in treatment, research, and public policy* (pp. 23–33). New York: Wiley & Sons.

Montano, C.B. (1999). Primary care issues related to the treatment of depression in elderly patients. *Journal of Clinical Psychiatry, 60*(Suppl. 20), 45–51.

Mulsant, B.H., & Ganguli, M. (1999). Epidemiology and diagnosis of depression in late life. *Journal of Clinical Psychiatry, 60*(Suppl. 20), 9–15.

National Institutes of Health (NIH). (1991, November). *Diagnosis and treatment of depression in late life: NIH consensus statement, 9*(3), 1–27.

Pachana, N.A., Gallagher-Thompson, D., & Thompson, L.W. (1994). Assessment of depression. In M.P. Lawton (Series Ed.) & M.P. Lawton & J.A. Teresi (Vol. Eds.), *Annual review of gerontology and geriatrics: Vol. 14. Focus on assessment techniques* (pp. 234–256). New York: Springer.

Paykel, E.S. (1992). *Handbook of affective disorders*. New York: The Guilford Press.

Pearson, J.L., & Brown, G.K. (2000). Suicide prevention in late life: Directions for science and practice. *Clinical Psychology Review, 20,* 685–705.

Salzman, C. (1999). Practical considerations for the treatment of depression in elderly and very elderly long-term care patients. *Journal of Clinical Psychiatry, 60*(Suppl. 20), 30–33.

Schneider, L.S. (1996). Biological commonalities among aging, depression, and suicidal behavior. In G.J. Kennedy (Ed.), *Suicide and depression in late life: Critical issues in treatment, research, and public policy* (pp. 39–50). New York: Wiley & Sons.

Wong, S.S., Heiby, E.M., Kameoka, V.A., & Dubanoski, J.P. (1999). Perceived control, self-reinforcement, and depression among Asian American and Caucasian American elders. *The Journal of Applied Gerontology, 18,* 48–64.

Disordered Eating Behavior, Adolescence

Michael P. Levine, Niva Piran, and Lori M. Irving*

INTRODUCTION AND DEFINITIONS

Eating disorders are part of a spectrum of *disordered eating behavior* (DEB). This spectrum encompasses varying combinations and degrees of negative body image, binge-eating, and unhealthy forms of weight management such as restrictive dieting, self-induced vomiting after eating, and abuse of laxatives, diuretics, diet pills, and exercise as well as excessive eating that contributes to obesity. At the extreme end of the spectrum are the prototypical syndromes of anorexia nervosa, bulimia nervosa, and binge-eating disorder. *Anorexia nervosa* is characterized by rigid refusal to eat adequate amounts, resulting in fierce maintenance of body weight at a very low, sometimes deadly level. *Bulimia nervosa* involves cycles of binge eating, purging (e.g., use of self-induced vomiting, laxatives, diuretics, etc.), and restrictive dieting. *Binge- eating disorder* is similar to bulimia nervosa but without compensatory purging. The DEB spectrum involves various combinations, at varying levels of intensity, of body

dissatisfaction, disordered eating patterns, low self-esteem, and negative emotions such as shame, social anxiety, and depression. At least part of the negative emotion reflects self-deprecation about the disordered eating. In many instances, but not always, the body dissatisfaction results from the idealization of slenderness, irrational fear of fat, and belief in weight and shape as central determinants of one's identity. A minority of obese adolescents have problems with binge-eating and/or use a variety of unhealthy weight loss strategies (e.g., diet pills).

SCOPE

Prevalence

The point prevalence of bulimia nervosa and anorexia nervosa among middle and high school girls is 1–2 and 0.2–0.5 percent, respectively (Van Hoeken, Lucas, & Hoek, 1998). The prevalence of binge-eating disorder among adolescents is unknown. The prevalence of DEB that produces significant physical, psychological, and social problems, but does not meet the full anorexia nervosa or bulimia nervosa criteria is, conservatively, 8 percent (Austin, 2000; Shisslak, Crago, & Estes, 1995). Thus, the DEB spectrum affects at least 10 percent of adolescent girls. The prevalence of anorexia nervosa and bulimia nervosa among adolescent males is estimated at 0.5–1 percent, indicating 8 : 1 as a conservative estimate of the ratio of females to males for the more severe syndromes. If one applies the female-to-male ratio observed in adults to adolescents, it is likely that this gender difference is far less extreme in the case of binge-eating disorder; in adults, the ratio of females to males with binge-eating disorder is 1.5 : 1. The prevalence of DEB among adolescent males may be underestimated, because many boys suffer from obsessive anxieties about becoming more muscular and less fat (Pope, Phillips, & Olivardia, 2000).

Framing the DEB spectrum are cultural values extolling the glories of thinness, the horrors of fat, the primacy of "image," and the body as life-long project to be managed as a consumer or investor would a commodity. These values have led many adolescents to be dissatisfied with their bodies and to engage in eating and weight-management practices that form the initial portion of the DEB spectrum (Thompson, Heinberg, Altabe, & Tantleff-Dunn, 1999). This is especially true for girls. On any given day, approximately 40–45 percent of US girls and 15–20 percent of US boys ages 12–18 are trying to lose weight, and about 15–20 percent of adolescent girls report dieting five or more times in the past year (French, Story, Neumark-Sztainer, Downes, Resnick, & Blum, 1997). Weight and shape concerns frequently emerge or intensify during puberty. Field et al. (1999) found that 15–19 percent of a very large sample of girls ages 12–14 were "overweight" according to body mass, while 17 percent of those who were not objectively over-weight thought that they were. Moreover, in this sample the prevalence of girls trying to lose weight increased from 35 to 40 to 44 percent for ages 12, 13, and 14, respectively. The comparable data for boys from this study reflects the gendered nature of weight and shape concerns. Approximately 22–27 percent of the boys were overweight, 5–6 percent perceived themselves to be overweight when they were not, and 20 percent were trying to lose weight, a figure that declined from ages 12 to 14.

Incidence

The number of new cases of anorexia nervosa and bulimia nervosa among males does not appear to be increasing, but the overall incidence of anorexia nervosa in many countries increased during the 1970s and into the 1980s, particularly for females ages 10–24. The incidence of bulimia nervosa in females also rose dramatically in the 1970s and early 1980s. The incidence of both bulimia nervosa and anorexia nervosa appears to have leveled off in the last decade of the 20th century (Gordon, 2000).

Costs

Anorexia nervosa and bulimia nervosa seriously impair physical and social functioning while undermining self-confidence and effectiveness in fulfilling individual responsibilities at school and at work. They cause substantial misery and dysfunction for sufferers, families, friends, treatment providers, and many societies around the world (Gordon, 2000). The more severe forms of DEB often deteriorate into chronic, debilitating, and even fatal conditions (Herzog, Nussbaum, & Marmor, 1996). Treatment for eating disorders is difficult and expensive, and the most effective treatments produce recovery in less than half of patients (Johnson, Tsoh, & Varnado, 1996). The mortality rate for anorexia nervosa is 12 times higher than it is for young women in the general population (Becker, Grinspoon, Klibanski, & Herzog, 1999). Less severe manifestations of DEB are associated with poor nutrition, social anxiety, restricted physical and social activity, low self-esteem, and abuse of tobacco. Overall, the costs to society of DEB—in terms of health care, productivity, and wasted human potential—are enormous.

THEORIES

Disease-Specific Social Cognition (DISC) Model

The DISC approach to prevention (Perry, 1999) focuses on eliminating risk factors seen as specific to a disorder.

Applied to DEB the general objectives of the DISC approach are: (1) increased resistance to internalization of the slender beauty ideal and to calorie-restrictive dieting, binge-eating in response to stress, and unhealthy weight management techniques; (2) improved body image; (3) healthy resolution of developmental challenges such as the clash between normal pubertal weight gain and a culture that vilifies fat; and (4) increased awareness of the nature and dangers of the DEB spectrum itself. Prevention programs that follow a DISC model use various agents of social influence (psychologists, teachers, peers, video) to transmit information, teach skills for positive behavioral changes (e.g., self-monitoring, goal-setting, decision-making), teach skills for resisting negative social influences, and increase incentives for learning healthier attitudes and behaviors toward weight and shape. Curricular material such as lesson plans are seen as critical elements for preventive change.

Non-Specific Vulnerability-Stressor (NOVS) Model

According to the NOVS perspective, there is a *nonspecific* relationship between psychological problems (including DEB) and life stress, lack of coping skills and other behavioral competencies, and lack of social support (Cowen, 2000). Therefore, prevention need not wait for specification of risk factors for DEB because adolescents will benefit in numerous ways from opportunities to develop general "life skills" for stress management, decision-making, and communication. Self-acceptance and self-esteem are also critical for health promotion. The DISC model incorporates environmental change within assumptions about behavior being reciprocally determined by environmental and personal factors (Neumark-Sztainer, 1996; Perry, 1999). The NOVS model, however, emphasizes directly the need for social change to make the environments of adolescents less stressful and more supportive of positive, nurturing relationships with peers and adults.

Participatory-Empowerment-Ecological-Relational (PEER) Model

The PEER model (Piran, 1999; Piran, Levine, & Steiner-Adair, 1999; see also Friedman, 2000) shares important features with the other paradigms, for example, concern about the unhealthy tension between the natural diversity and beauty of human shapes versus idealized images of thin white women. The PEER model departs radically from the DISC perspective, however, in locating the specific targets and mechanisms for change in the "lived experience," "knowledge," and "authority" of adolescents themselves. The fundamental mechanism of change, therefore, is not assimilation of knowledge and skills emanating from didactic lessons presented by an authority. Rather, prevention is facilitated by the *process* of empowering girls—and boys—to clarify, critique, and change or (re-)create themselves and their environments.

To do so, adult women foster respectful dialogue with the adolescents and between the adolescents themselves. Expressing and listening to the adolescents' own concerns, knowledge, and anxieties invariably raise sociocultural issues that underlie DEB and weight and shape preoccupation (i.e., harassment, racism, objectification, and power imbalance), but are missing (silenced) from DISC prevention curricula. The knowledge that is constructed in dialogues among adolescents with adult mentors is then used to transform the social environment, including peer norms, school policies, curricula, and administrative structures. A new set of personal and social experiences is therefore created through: (1) development of a critical social perspective about body image, weight, and eating; and (2) actual transformation of the social environment. In summary, the PEER approach differs from the other two models, not only in its emphasis on the authority of adolescents, but also in its multi-layered blend of disease-specific and non-specific factors, in its insistence on centrality of social change, and in the fact that it works with boys and girls in similar ways.

These models specify proximal goals associated with decreases in certain risk factors and increases in particular forms of resilience (e.g., coping skills). A "prevention effect" would be demonstrated by evidence, from valid measures, of: (1) careful implementation of the complete program; (2) the hypothesized changes in risk and resilience; (3) reduced incidence or delayed onset of DEB during the protracted period of risk, relative to a comparable group of non-participants; and (4) a meaningfully low rate of new cases of DEB. To date, no study has fulfilled these requirements.

Research

Several excellent reviews of DEB prevention research are available (Austin, 2000; Franko & Orosan-Weine, 1998). As of January 2001, we have obtained 42 published and unpublished studies of youth ages 8–18. Most are classroom-based didactic programs (mean time = 6 hr), delivered without tailoring to individuals with different levels of risk or symptomatology. Sixty-four percent of the 42 studies had ≥3 elements of the DISC model, 48 percent had ≥2 elements of the NOVS model, and 19 percent had ≥2 elements of the PEER model.

Some experts (Stice, Mazotti, Weibel, & Agras, 2000) on DEB argue that primary-universal prevention programs, most of which are based on the DISC and NOVS models, are less effective in producing positive results than are secondary-targeted programs. However, 90 percent of the studies reviewed had a positive effect on knowledge, 65 percent had at least one positive effect on attitudes (e.g., idealization of slenderness), and 38 percent had one or more positive effects on behavior. As important, comparable figures for the 15 controlled outcome studies with a follow-up (ranging from 1 month to 2 years) are 91 percent, 62 percent, and 21 percent. Prevention programs definitely can have a positive *short-term* effect on knowledge, body image, the glorification of thinness, and eating behaviors. However, achievement (maintenance) of long-term behavioral changes and demonstration of full prevention effects remain elusive goals.

STRATEGIES THAT WORK

Thus far, no prevention program is a clear standard for what works.

STRATEGIES THAT MIGHT WORK

Here, in chronological order, are five programs that merit further attention and research because they have produced promising results (see Levine & Piran, 2001).

Neumark-Sztainer, Butler, and Palti (1995) presented a 10-hr curriculum to several hundred Israeli girls ages 15–16. Based explicitly on the DISC model, the lessons used presentations, discussions, and assignments to teach girls about nutrition, exercise, physical and psychological development in adolescence, and ways to understand, resist, and actively change sociocultural factors at school and at home. Teachers were trained to speak constructively with the girls about weight concerns and to support activism. At the 6-month follow-up girls participating in the program had more regular eating patterns, exercised more frequently, and were less likely to initiate unhealthy dieting and binge-eating. There was a similar, non-significant trend at the 2-year follow-up.

Santonastaso, Zanetti, Ferrara, Olivetto, Magnavita, and Favaro (1999) engaged 10 groups of 16-year-old Italian girls ($N = 154$) in four 2-hr presentations and group discussions. Topics reflected a combination of DISC and NOVS elements: pubertal changes, including weight gain; body image; the nature and epidemiology of DEB; sociocultural aspects of eating and of the idealization of slenderness; and general challenges in coping with adolescence. At the 1-year follow-up the program had a significant preventive effect on body dissatisfaction and bulimic behavior of "low risk" participants. There was no prevention effect for high risk participants and no effect for either risk group with respect to drive for thinness.

During the period 1987–1996, Piran (1999) evaluated a sustained application of the PEER model to prevention within an elite residential ballet school for students ages 10–18. Serving as a consultant to the staff and students in this high risk setting, Piran helped participants to explore factors that adversely affected their body image, and to pursue constructive changes in their peer norms and the school's policies, norms, and staff. Piran found that, compared to students of the same age in the 1987 cohort (the prior to program implementation), ballet students in the 1991 and 1996 cohorts ate more regularly, engaged in significantly less disordered eating (e.g., restriction, bingeing, and purging), and reported greater body satisfaction.

In a study by O'Dea and Abraham (2000) Australian boys and girls ages 11–14 participated in a nine-part program called *Everybody's Different*. Consistent with some aspects of the PEER and NOVS models, this curriculum eschews didactic lessons in favor of group-oriented, cooperative, "student-centered learning." The program "included absolutely nothing about food, weight, exercise, healthy eating, eating disorders, dieting, etc." (J. O'Dea, personal communication, February 6, 2000). Instead, activities were designed to improve self-esteem by reinforcing the message that everyone is unique and valuable, to promote life skills, and to increase positive feedback from significant others. The program was developed in conjunction with school personnel, but there was no explicit emphasis on changing adult behavior or school policies.

The pattern of O'Dea and Abraham's (2000) results illuminates the challenges facing prevention. At posttest and relative to the control group, body satisfaction increased and weight loss efforts decreased for program participants. The program also successfully produced long-term reductions in concerns about physical appearance and social acceptance. However, there were no significant changes in the drive for thinness, and the relative improvement in body satisfaction dissipated at the 12-month follow-up. More troubling, there was a significant pretest to follow-up increase of 9 percent in the number of girls in the intervention group trying to lose weight, versus a nonsignificant increase in the control group of 6 percent.

Smolak and Levine (2001) conducted a longitudinal evaluation of a 10-lesson curriculum for children ages 8–11. Based primarily on the DISC model, lessons promoted healthy eating and exercising; tolerance of and appreciation for diversity in weight and shape, including avoidance of shape-related teasing; and critiques of dieting and of cultural messages insisting on a thin standard of beauty. Parents of children receiving the curriculum were sent nine newsletters paralleling the lessons. Two years later experimental and control participants (ages 11–13) were assessed, along with a new control group who had attended schools not included in the original study. Compared to this new control group, program participants were more knowledgeable, had higher body esteem, and used fewer unhealthy weight management techniques. Scores of the original control group were intermediate, suggesting that the original curriculum's emphasis on new norms and values may have "spilled over" to influence control participants within the same elementary schools.

The themes found in these heterogeneous projects are consistent with effective components of programs to prevent cigarette smoking and AIDS (Raczynski & DiClemente, 1999). First, these programs include a critique of cultural messages that encourage DEB and provide information and behavioral training in regard to healthy alternatives. Second, explicit attempts are made to create healthier, more flexible values and norms about weight, shape, and beauty. And, third, there is general support for developing a positive sense of self—as unique, competent, and connected to others—in a culture that promotes unhealthy attitudes about gender, adolescence, and identity.

Several other promising programs are worth describing, especially because: (1) the target audiences are children who have not yet entered adolescence, the period of greatest risk for DEB; (2) the programs are based on experiential learning, not just didactic presentations; and (3) there is clear matching of program content with the audience's developmental stage.

Kater, Rohwer, and Levine (2000; see Smolak & Levine, 2001) conducted an uncontrolled, pre-to-post evaluation of a 10-lesson program for children ages 9–12. The curriculum, written by Kater, combines the DISC and NOVS models. One category of lessons addresses what children *cannot and should not try to control*, such as the developmental changes of puberty and genetic effects on size and shape. A second set of lessons concerns *what children can control*, for example, development of a multifaceted identity, and selection of realistic but inspiring role models. The final set of lessons develops resistance to unhealthy sociocultural messages about thinness and weight management, with a focus on critical thinking about media and about the history of cultural attitudes concerning body image. This program produced very positive short-term improvements in body esteem, acceptance of diversity in shape and weight, and rejection of the thin beauty standard. A controlled evaluation of this program with 390 boys and girls ages 9–11 has recently been completed, and the preliminary results are equally promising (Kater, personal communication, September 28, 1999).

A growing number of DEB prevention programs have adopted "media literacy" strategies. Media literacy helps participants analyze positive, negative, and ambiguous effects of mass media on body image, gender roles, eating patterns, etc. (Berel & Irving, 1998; Piran et al., 1999).

As explicated by the PEER model, groups of girls research, discuss, and clarify links between mass media (operating as business, entertainment, and advertising) and how girls feel about their bodies and themselves. This analysis leads to activism for changes in mass media and to media-based advocacy for cultural changes.

Neumark-Sztainer, Sherwood, Coller, and Hannan (2000) designed a media literacy program for American girl scouts ages 10–12. At the 3-month follow-up, participants in the six 90-min lessons were less likely to read *Seventeen* magazine, which promotes the slender beauty ideal and feminine identity based primarily on appearance. In addition, internalization of the slender ideal was reduced and belief in one's ability to affect weight-related social norms was increased. However, there was no effect on dieting, and the modest pre-to-posttest improvement in body size acceptance was not maintained at follow-up. Recently, similar results emerged from an evaluation of GO GIRLS!™ (Giving Our Girls Inspiration and Resources for Lasting Self-Esteem!), a 12-lesson program for girls ages 14–18 (National Eating Disorders Association; see www.edap.org). The girls' personal statements and their activism projects strongly suggest that media literacy helped them to critically evaluate sociocultural determinants of body image, to learn life skills, and to feel empowered as citizens capable of challenging unhealthy cultural factors.

STRATEGIES THAT DO NOT WORK

These promising programs need to be interpreted cautiously. Several notable failures have employed very similar lesson plans and strong methodology, and many programs work well in the short run, only to see absolute or comparative improvements dissipate at follow-up (see Levine & Piran, 2001; Levine & Smolak, 2001). It is fair to say that even well designed cognitive–behavioral programs using didactic lessons and various exercises to improve body image, prevent dieting behaviors, and increase healthy eating and weight regulation have only a 50–50 chance of producing significant, lasting effects in groups of adolescents ages 12–14 (see Killen et al., 1993; Stewart, Carter, Drinkwater, Hainsworth, & Fairburn, 2001). Based on anecdotal evidence and research in other areas of health promotion (see Perry, 1999), we can state with much more confidence that "one shot" presentations emphasizing the lurid details and dangers of disordered eating are not only ineffective, they may also transmit unhealthy practices such as purging to control weight. We believe that the probability of an ineffective prevention program will be reduced to the extent that the program helps students and adults to develop a critical perspective toward the sociocultural bases of DEB

while fostering meaningful relationships with peers, active learning opportunities, and environmental changes that continue beyond a clearly demarcated set of lessons (Perry, 1999; Piran, 1999).

SYNTHESIS

Principles and Assumptions

Prevention benefits from a clear sense of the program's underlying principles and assumptions. The following examples constitute a starting point for discussion:

1. The targets of prevention are not just clinical syndromes, but the DEB spectrum of body image problems and disordered eating.
2. The DEB spectrum is not "just a female issue," it is a community issue affecting and affected by males as well as females.
3. Prevention involves more than education based on scientific research regarding predictive factors. It also requires political activism toward social justice. Specifically, prevention must address broad factors that influence the health and well-being of women from diverse ethnocultural and socioeconomic groups. These factors include the culture's fear of women's desires and hungers, the problems of sexual harassment and sexual abuse, limitations in women's avenues for success apart from beauty and sexuality, and the impact of multiple systems of prejudice.
4. Prevention should draw from all three models to promote the "4 *C*'s": *C*onsciousness-raising, *C*ompetencies (life skills), *C*onnections with others, and *C*hange in community norms and values.
5. Prevention research is an important part of risk factor research. A successful outcome in a program that seeks to eliminate or minimize a risk factor strongly suggests that this factor plays a causal role in the disorder(s) targeted for prevention.

PROPOSED STRATEGIES

Classroom Lessons

Knowledge is insufficient for long-term preventive change, but it is undoubtedly necessary. Educators and adolescents should be taught, in multiple classes (e.g., biology, health, social studies, art) about: (1) mass media effects on shifting beauty ideals in industrialized cultures; (2) the genetics of diversity in shape and weight; (3) biopsychosocial costs of dieting and the dieting mentality; (4) the nature and unacceptability of prejudice, including prejudice against fat people; (5) the value of healthy eating, healthy exercise, and self-respect, rather than worrying about Body Mass Index; and (6) the history of women's and men's struggles for equality and justice, featuring strong, caring, and accomplished people of both genders and all sizes and shapes.

Modes of Learning and Action

The PEER model's success (Piran, 1999) demonstrates that classroom lessons delivered by teachers, psychologists, or other authorities should not be the sole or even the major mechanism for prevention. Adolescents in general, and adolescent girls in particular, need safe and respectful opportunities to discuss, wrestle with, research, and clarify the complex determinants of body image, weight management, and eating (Friedman, 2000). Adolescents also need support for finding and constructing the power to change their social environment (Piran, 1999). Working with peers to construct personally meaningful knowledge and to take action to improve one's world constitute are a clear embodiment of the "4 C's."

Health-Promoting Communities

By definition, primary prevention emphasizes health promotion and reduction of illness risk through changes in groups, institutions, and communities (Cowen, 2000). All three prevention models support a multidimensional, ecological approach (Austin, 2000; Levine & Piran, 2001). Specialists in preventing adolescent problems such as substance use, cardiovascular risks, and AIDS have for some time been designing programs to change the behavior of teachers, parents, and other influential adults, and to create healthier policies, values, and norms within multiple, interlocking systems such as schools, communities, and mass media (Perry, 1999; Raczynski & DiClemente, 1999). Therefore, it is troubling that there is such a broad gap between this rich tradition and the classroom/individual student focus of nearly all of the evaluated DEB prevention research reviewed here.

According to the PEER model, activism is most effective when directed by the specific, contextualized concerns of adolescent and adult stakeholders, but prevention facilitators can advocate general environmental targets for change. Objectives in developing a "health-promoting school" (Neumark-Sztainer, 1996; O'Dea & Maloney, 2000; Piran, 1999) should include teacher modeling of positive body image; system-wide reduction in gender-related teasing; removal of weightist practices (e.g., weight/shape requirements for cheerleading; posters making fun of fat people), and enhanced presence of books, posters, and guest speakers that emphasize people of character and accomplishment at varying sizes.

Facing Some Tough Issues

The potential for sweeping cultural transformations is reinforced by revolutions such as mass participation of females in athletics and the decline of cigarette smoking and imperious tobacco companies. However, to advance prevention of the DEB spectrum four very challenging issues need to be addressed. *First*, sociocultural perspectives and universal prevention strategies are difficult to promote in the current environment of reverence and massive funding for the psychobiology of narrowly defined "mental disorders." To the extent that biomedical psychiatry embraces prevention at all, its seeks to identify and "treat" high-risk or proto-symptomatic individuals, not to proactively transform cultural contexts. *Second*, all three prevention models agree there is no single set of "sociocultural" determinants needing to be changed. Prevention programs must be sensitive to the fact that body image, weight management, and eating patterns are influenced by many sociocultural factors that include, but are not limited to, ethnicity, sexual orientation, social class, and regional variation in norms and values.

Third, prevention of DEB is an interdisciplinary endeavor requiring involvement of (among others) psychology, anthropology, public health, and medical science. Therefore, prevention programs must coordinate, integrate, and/or choose carefully from different interventions, research designs, and quantitative and qualitative methodologies.

Finally, prevention specialists in the fields of eating disorders and obesity need to acknowledge and expand upon their common ground: A concern about the well-being of adolescents that is shaped by a critical, multifaceted, and evolving understanding of how eating, fitness, and health in general are defined and influenced by the complex intersection of biology, psychology, and culture.

Also see: Nutrition: Early Childhood; Nutrition: Childhood; Nutrition: Adulthood; Nutrition: Older Adulthood; Nutrition and Physical Activity: Adolescence; Obesity: Adolescence; Self-Esteem: Adolescence.

References

Austin, S.B. (2000). Prevention research in eating disorders: Theory and new directions. *Psychological Medicine, 30,* 1249–1262.

Becker, A.E., Grinspoon, S.K., Klibanski, A., & Herzog, D.B. (1999). Eating disorders. *New England Journal of Medicine, 340,* 1092–1098.

Berel, S., & Irving, L. (1998). Media and disturbed eating: An analysis of media influence and implications for prevention. *Journal of Primary Prevention, 18,* 415–430.

Cowen, E.L. (2000). Psychological wellness: Some hopes for the future. In D. Cicchetti, J. Rappaport, I. Sandler, & R.P. Weissberg (Eds.), *The promotion of wellness in children and adolescents* (pp. 477–503). Washington, DC: Child Welfare League of America.

Field, A.E., Camargo, C.A., Jr., Taylor, C.B., Berkey, C., Frazier, A.L., Gillman, M.W., & Colditz, G.A. (1999). Overweight, weight concerns, and bulimic behaviors among girls and boys. *Journal of the American Academy of Child and Adolescent Psychiatry, 38,* 754–760.

Franko, D.L., & Orosan-Weine, P. (1998). The prevention of eating disorders: Empirical, methodological and conceptual considerations. *Clinical Psychology: Science and Practice, 5,* 459–477.

French, S.A., Story, M., Neumark-Sztainer, D., Downes, B., Resnick, M., & Blum, R. (1997). Ethnic differences in psychosocial and health behavior correlates of dieting, purging, and binge eating in a population-based sample of adolescents. *International Journal of Eating Disorders, 22,* 315–322.

Friedman, S.S. (2000). *Nurturing GirlPower: Integrating eating disorder prevention/intervention skills into your practice.* Salal Books. Available from Salal Communications, Ltd., 101–1184 Denman St. #309, Vancouver, BC V6G 2M9 Canada (604-689-8399).

Gordon, R.A. (2000). *Eating disorders: Anatomy of a social epidemic* (2nd ed.). Malden, MA: Basil Blackwell.

Herzog, D.B., Nussbaum, K.M., & Marmor, A.K. (1996). Comorbidity and outcome in eating disorders. *The Psychiatric Clinics of North America, 19,* 843–859.

Johnson, W.G., Tsoh, J.Y., & Varnado, P.J. (1996). Eating disorders: Efficacy of pharmacological and psychological interventions. *Clinical Psychology Review, 16,* 457–478.

Kater, K.J., Rohwer, J., & Levine, M.P. (2000). An elementary school project for developing healthy body image and reducing risk factros for unhealthy and disordered eating. *Eating Disorders: The Journal of Treatment & Prevention, 8,* 3–16.

Killen, J.D., Taylor, C.B., Hammer, L., Litt, I., Wilson, D.M., Rich, T., Simmonds, B., Kraemer, H., & Varady, A. (1993). An attempt to modify unhealthful eating attitudes and weight regulation practices of young adolescent girls. *International Journal of Eating Disorders, 13,* 369–384.

Levine, M.P., & Piran, N. (2001). The prevention of eating disorders: Towards a participatory ecology of knowledge, action, and advocacy. In R. Striegel-Moore & L. Smolak (Eds.), *Eating disorders: New directions for research and practice* (pp. 233–253). Washington, DC: American Psychological Association.

Levine, M.P., & Smolak, L. (2001). Primary prevention of body image disturbances and disordered eating in childhood and early adolescence. In J.K. Thompson & L. Smolak (Eds.), *Body image, eating disorders, and obesity in childhood and adolescence* (pp. 237–260). Washington, DC: American Psychological Association.

Neumark-Sztainer, D. (1996). School-based programs for preventing eating disturbances. *Journal of School Health, 66*(2), 64–71.

Neumark-Sztainer, D., Butler, R., & Palti, H. (1995). Eating disturbances among adolescent girls: Evaluation of a school-based primary prevention program. *Journal of Nutrition Education, 27,* 24–30.

Neumark-Sztainer D., Sherwood N., Coller T., & Hannan, P.J. (2000). Primary prevention of disordered eating among pre-adolescent girls: Feasibility and short-term impact of a community-based intervention. *Journal of the American Dietetic Association, 100,* 1466–1473.

O'Dea, J., & Abraham, S. (2000). Improving the body image, eating attitudes and behaviors of young and behaviors of young male and female adolescents: A new educational approach which focuses on self esteem. *International Journal of Eating Disorders, 28,* 43–57.

O'Dea, J., & Maloney, D. (2000). Preventing eating and body image problems in children and adolescents using the Health Promoting Schools Framework. *Journal of School Health, 70,* 18–21.

Perry, C.L. (1999). *Creating health behavior change: How to develop community-wide programs for youth.* Thousand Oaks, CA: Sage.

Piran, N. (1999). Eating disorders: A trial of prevention in a high risk school setting. *Journal of Primary Prevention, 20,* 75–90.

Piran, N., Levine, M.P., & Steiner-Adair, C. (Eds.). (1999). *Preventing eating disorders: A handbook of interventions and special challenges.* Philadelphia: Brunner/Mazel.

Pope, H.G., Jr., Phillips, K.A., & Olivardia, R. (2000). *The Adonis complex: The secret crisis of male body obsession.* New York: Free Press.

Raczynski, J.M., & DiClemente, R.J. (Eds.). (1999). *Handbook of health promotion and disease prevention.* New York: Kluwer Academic/ Plenum.

Santonastaso, P., Zanetti, T., Ferrara, S., Olivetto, M.C., Magnavita, N., & Favaro, A. (1999). A preventive intervention program in adolescent school girls: A longitudinal study. *Psychotherapy and Psychosomatics, 68,* 46–50.

Shisslak, C.M., Crago, M., & Estes, L. (1995). The spectrum of eating disturbances. *International Journal of Eating Disorders, 18,* 209–219.

Smolak, L., & Levine, M.P. (2001). A two-year follow-up of a primary prevention program for negative body image and unhealthy weight regulation. *Eating Disorders: The Journal of Treatment & Prevention, 9,* 313–325.

Stewart, D.A., Carter, J.C., Drinkwater, J., Hainsworth, J., & Fairburn, C.G. (2001). Modification of eating attitudes and behavior in adolescent girls: A controlled study. *International Journal of Eating Disorders, 29,* 107–118.

Stice, E., Mazotti, L., Weibel, D., & Agras, S. (2000). Dissonance prevention program decreases thin-ideal internalization, body dissatisfaction, dieting, negative affect, and bulimic symptoms: A preliminary experiment. *International Journal of Eating Disorders, 27,* 206–217.

Thompson, J.K., Heinberg, L.J., Altabe, M., & Tantleff-Dunn, S. (1999). *Exacting beauty: Theory, assessment, and treatment of body image disturbance.* Washington, DC: American Psychological Association.

Van Hoeken, D., Lucas, A.R., & Hoek, H.W. (1998). Epidemiology. In H.W. Hoek, J.L. Treasure, & M.A. Kaztman (Eds.), *Neurobiology in the treatment of eating disorders* (pp. 97–126). London: John Wiley & Sons.

Disordered Eating Behavior, Adulthood

Lori M. Irving,* Michael P. Levine, and Niva Piran

INTRODUCTION

This entry focuses on eating disorders in adults, and what we know about preventing these conditions.

DEFINITIONS AND SCOPE

Prevalence and Implications for Prevention with Adults

Currently, we lack solid epidemiological data about the prevalence and incidence of "diagnosable" eating disorders (see earlier entries for definitions). In addition, the database for current estimates makes it impossible to distinguish

* Deceased

between statistics for adolescents and adults. Judicious estimates suggest that about 0.5–1 percent of adolescent girls meet the diagnostic criteria for anorexia nervosa (AN), 1–3 percent of adolescent and young adult women meet the criteria for bulimia (BN), and 0.7–4 percent of community samples meet the criteria for binge eating disorder (BED) (American Psychiatric Association, 1994; Van Hoeken, Lucas, & Hoek, 1998). The ratio of females to males with AN and BN is at least 8 : 1, while the ratio of females to males with BED is 1.5 : 1.

A substantial proportion of adult women experience eating problems that occur along the spectrum of disordered eating behavior (DEB). The proportion of college women with potentially serious sub-clinical eating problems is estimated to range from 10 (Drenowski, Yee, Kurth, & Krahn, 1994) to 30 percent (Hesse-Biber, 1991). Among college women (in samples typically encompassing ages 18–25), various forms of DEB may be the rule rather than exception. Mintz and Betz (1988) reported that only 33 percent of their sample of college women could be characterized as "normal" eaters (i.e., eating when hungry, stopping when full), and that 61 percent engaged in some form of disordered eating (e.g., chronic dieting, binge-eating, purging). By age 18, most women exhibit attitudes and behaviors considered precursors to or part of the DEB spectrum, including internalization of a thin white ideal of female beauty, irrational concerns about dietary and bodily fat, weight and shape preoccupation, and repeated attempts at weight loss through dieting. Thus, although prevention of the DEB spectrum in childhood and early adolescence often involves prevention with asymptomatic populations by early adulthood, prevention programs must acknowledge the need to intervene with individuals who already demonstrate attitudes and behaviors along the DEB spectrum.

Costs and Correlates

Those behaviors have serious consequences for women. Psychological problems associated with DEB range from low self-esteem, excessive self-consciousness, and difficulty in coping with stress to depression, anxiety disorders, and substance abuse. More extreme forms of DEB can have medical consequences that include osteoporosis and reproductive, gastrointestinal, and cardiovascular problems (Pike & Striegel-Moore, 1997). Further, without intervention, less severe forms of DEB may evolve into full-blown eating disorders. In a prospective study of college women, Drenowski et al. (1994) reported that, at baseline, 31 and 10 percent of their sample could be classified as "intensive dieters" and "dieters at risk," respectively. By the following semester, 4 percent of "intensive dieters"

and 15 percent of "dieters at risk" were diagnosed with BN. Early intervention for less extreme forms of DEB is probably much more cost-effective than treating a full-blown eating disorder. The "most effective" treatments for eating disorders produce recovery in less than half of patients, and inpatient treatment for AN is similar in cost to that for schizophrenia (Striegel-Moore, Leslie, Petrill, Garvin, & Rosenheck, 2000).

Late Adolescence/Early Adulthood as a Period of Heightened Risk

For young women, the transition from late adolescence to early adulthood poses unique challenges that can contribute to the development of DEB (Smolak, Levine, & Striegel-Moore, 1996). Young women at this developmental stage are engaged in the process of identity formation, separation from families, and coping with expectations for more adult-like sexual behavior and career decisions. As such, they may be particularly vulnerable to a combination of insecurities, loss of confidence, and receiving and/or creating peer pressure to engage in high risk behaviors, including DEB. In the context of these developmental tasks, the college environment may inadvertently contribute to DEB by: (1) introducing academic, financial, and interpersonal stressors; (2) encouraging participation in activities or groups that promote unhealthy eating (e.g., competitive athletics, sorority membership); (3) confronting students with radically altered food choices and access (e.g., restricted access to cafeteria; an abundance of high carbohydrate, high fat foods); and (4) offering a social "scene" that intensifies and confuses issues of autonomy, control, and status in regard to sexuality and substance use.

THEORY AND RESEARCH

Theoretical perspectives, such as the social cognition model, the vulnerability-stressor model, and the empowerment-ecological model, are covered in other entries and will be mentioned again in connection with research to be discussed below.

Several extensive reviews of DEB prevention research are available (Franko & Orosan-Weine, 1998; Levine & Piran, 2001). As of January 2001, we have obtained 21 published and unpublished DEB prevention studies of adults (i.e., >18 years). Most programs (n = 19) targeted college students, and all but two targeted women exclusively. Eighteen (86 percent) of the studies reviewed had a positive effect on one or more outcome variables of interest. We discuss the details of some of these studies in the strategies sections to follow.

STRATEGIES THAT WORK

Several programs stand out in their ability to affect multiple risk and protective factors. These programs are characterized by: (1) a "fit" between program content and characteristics of the target population; (2) multiple sessions rather than a "one-shot" intervention; (3) a multidimensional approach that addresses personal, interpersonal, and sociocultural factors; (4) an interactive, rather than exclusively didactic, style of presentation; and (5) a well-controlled research design. These programs are reviewed below.

Kaminski and McNamara (1996) administered measures of self- and body-esteem, beliefs about attractiveness, and eating disordered attitudes and behaviors to 315 women enrolled in an introductory psychology course at a US university. There were 29 (9.2 percent) women who were not bulimic but were considered "at risk" for a serious eating disorder because they had high scores on measures of negative body image or eating disordered attitudes and behaviors. These women were randomly assigned to a no-treatment control or a cognitive–behavioral program incorporating elements of the Disease-Specific Social Cognition (DISC) and the Non-Specific Vulnerability-Stressor (NOVS) models (Levine & Piran, 2001).

Kaminski and McNamara (1996) arranged for eight weekly 90-min group sessions led by two female graduate students in counseling psychology. Participants learned about healthy weight management, the negative effects of yo-yo dieting, and techniques for challenging both cultural pressures for thinness and individual negative thoughts about weight and shape. Participants also learned more effective techniques for coping with stress and meeting their emotional needs. At 1-month follow-up the intervention group demonstrated significant improvements in weight management behavior, body satisfaction, self-esteem, and fear of negative evaluation.

In two controlled studies Stice and colleagues (Stice, Chase, Stormer, & Appel, 2001; Stice, Mazotti, Weibel, & Agras, 2000) found evidence for the ability of a "dissonance-based" prevention program to reduce DEB risk factors and symptoms in college women with "elevated body image concerns." In the first study, students participated in either an intervention or a no-intervention control group; assignment was not random. In the second study, participants were randomly assigned to an intervention or healthy weight management control condition. The experimental intervention consisted of three 1-hr sessions in which participants were invited to create a "body acceptance program" for high school females. This "cognitive dissonance manipulation" encouraged participants to act contrary to their previously held attitudes by articulating a respect for diverse body weight and shapes despite their own preoccupation with weight and shape. Guided by a doctoral or masters level psychologist and an undergraduate student, participants discussed ways that adolescents can avoid internalizing the thin ideal of beauty. Based on the DISC model, topics included origins of the thin ideal, how it is perpetuated, the impact of the ideal, and who benefits from the thin ideal. Participants also completed a counter-attitudinal role-play and counter-attitudinal essay in which they provided reasons for challenging the thin ideal. In the first study, compared to the no-intervention control, the intervention was successful at one-month follow-up in reducing thin-ideal internalization, body dissatisfaction, and bulimic symptoms. In the second study, both interventions produced significant reductions in thin-ideal internalization, body dissatisfaction, negative affect, dieting, and bulimic symptoms at 1-month follow-up. However, compared to the weight management program, the dissonance prevention program more immediately reduced thin-ideal internalization and body dissatisfaction, factors that are specific to DEB.

In a series of randomized, controlled studies, Stanford University researchers (Taylor, Winzelberg, & Celio, 2001) demonstrated the ability of a computer-based psychoeducational prevention program to reduce DEB risk factors in college women. The interactive program, called *Student Bodies*, is based on the DISC model. It offers multimedia education about the development and consequences of eating disorders, cultural determinants of beauty, and healthy nutrition and exercise. Accompanying this information are a moderated on-line discussion and cognitive–behavioral exercises (Cash, 1996) to improve body image. Two studies found that *Student Bodies* was most effective for college women with high levels of body dissatisfaction when it was combined with a set of readings about women, culture, body image, and dieting, and with three face-to-face discussion sessions.

Together, the three sets of studies reviewed suggest that interventions for adult women at risk for DEB or with moderately severe forms of DEB can be effective. This proposition is supported further by prevention studies designed to benefit young adult women who are clearly at risk for eating disorders. For example, Chase (2000) identified a group of women at a large US university who "exhibited elevated levels of preoccupation with body weight and shape and unhealthful dieting behaviors and did not meet diagnostic criteria for an eating disorder" (p. 48). The intervention, delivered in three 45-min group sessions over a 2-week period, was a modification of Kaminski and McNamara's (1996) program. Individual activities, group discussions, and homework assignments were used to teach general information about eating disorders and healthy weight management. Participants were also taught specific cognitive–behavioral techniques for challenging sociocultural pressures and for correcting negative thoughts and feelings in regard to body image and weight/shape preoccupation. Compared to a placebo-group control, participants in Chase's (2000) program demonstrated (at 1-month follow-up) increased knowledge about program components and reductions in dieting behavior, body dissatisfaction and weight concerns, and anxiety.

The results of these studies are promising and impressive. They are also consistent with a body of literature that demonstrates the effectiveness of cognitive–behavioral techniques for helping college women with negative body image (Cash, 1996). However, the relevance of this research to (more heterogeneous) community samples of adult women is unclear. In the only randomized controlled study to utilize a community sample, Higgins and Gray (1998) evaluated Freedom From Dieting (FFD). This program explicitly reflects the concern that dieting can be a precursor to DEB, but it includes NOVS components as well as DISC elements. The 82 adult women (*M* age = 44.4, range 24–67 years) who participated were recruited from the community via mass media. FFD is delivered in six 2-hr sessions consisting of content and activities to: (1) replace feelings of self-worth based on weight with self-worth based on meeting all of one's basic needs; (2) reinterpret feelings about stressful situations; and (3) replace chronic dieting with "natural eating"—being aware of and responding to the body's naturally occurring signals of hunger and satiety (as opposed to eating in response to emotional or situational triggers). The program relied on group participation and discussion. Positive modeling was provided by former chronic dieters who had become successful "natural eaters." At posttest, compared to a control condition, FFD produced reductions in restrained eating and in eating triggered by emotions and external factors, reductions in body shape concern, and increased self-esteem. Reductions in body shape concerns were maintained at 6- and 12-month follow-up. Moreover, further reductions in unhealthy eating attitudes and increases in self-esteem were observed at 6- and 12-month follow-up.

STRATEGIES THAT MIGHT WORK

We now turn our attention to programs that are promising but have not been evaluated rigorously in terms of random assignment to groups, careful attention to valid assessment, or follow-up evaluation. College campuses are a logical setting for prevention programs, so various forms of education are attractive possibilities for reaching fairly large target audiences. One type of educational program is an Eating Disorders course. The Stanford University group (Springer, Winzelberg, Perkins, & Taylor, 1999) developed a 10-week course called *Body Traps*. The components of the seminar, emphasized in readings, reaction papers, and discussions, combined *content* from the DISC model and the

Participatory-Empowerment-Ecological-Relational Model (PEER; Piran, 1999, 2001). That is, there were "lessons" on, for example, media and body image; culture, gender, and beliefs about fat; and facts about the biopsychosocial determinants of weight, shape, obesity, and eating disorders. Springer et al. (1999) found that a non-randomized control group demonstrated little change from the beginning to the end of the course, whereas the course participants reported improved body satisfaction, fewer bulimic symptoms, a lower drive for thinness, and reduced weight and shape concerns.

Stice and Ragan (2001) offered an eating disorders seminar, which they describe as an "intensive psychoeducational intervention." This course was advertised and conducted as a university class, not as a prevention or intervention, but, not surprisingly, those who signed up had moderate levels of DEB. Didactic presentations and group discussion were used to cover the nature, epidemiology, and etiology of disordered eating, as well a topics pertaining to obesity, nutrition, and healthy weight management. Consistent with the work of Springer et al. (1999), Stice and Ragan found that, compared to matched control participants from other university psychology courses, the eating disorders class significantly reduced internalization of the thin beauty ideal, body dissatisfaction, dieting, and eating disorder symptoms.

A second type of educational approach to prevention on college campuses is media literacy. Proponents of this approach argue that critical viewing skills reduce the degree to which women internalize social beauty standards and, consequently, may prevent development of body dissatisfaction and disordered eating (Berel & Irving, 1998). Media literacy programs have proven successful at reducing intentions to use alcohol and increasing skepticism about violent media in children. In a 1995 study and a 1998 replication (Thompson, Heinberg, Altabe, & Tantleff-Dunn, 1999), Stormer and Thompson assigned college women to either: (1) a 30-min psychoeducational program and discussion concerning how media manipulate women's bodies in order to present "perfect" images, and how to challenge the negative impact of the media by reminding oneself of their deceptive methods; (2) a 30-min control condition that provided information on nutrition, exercise, stress management, and dental hygiene; or (3) no-intervention. Participants completed surveys immediately before and after the program. In both studies, compared to the control conditions, women receiving this brief psychoeducational media education program reported decreases in appearance- and weight-related anxiety and reduced internalization of the sociocultural ideal of beauty. This 30 min of media literacy may not seem like much, but Posavac, Posavac, and Weigel (2001) found that just 8 min of a psychoeducational presentation designed to contrast media constructions of artificial beauty with the genetic realities of diversity in weight and shape mitigated the negative effect of slides of slender models from fashion magazines.

A third type of promising program has been developed by Phelps, Sapia, Nathanson, and Nelson (2000). The lessons are noteworthy for their unique combination of DISC and NOVS elements. As is the case for most prevention programs, this one explores sociocultural determinants of negative body image and disordered eating, as well as the negative effects of dieting. However, Phelps and colleagues also teach participants how to emphasize: (1) positive aspects of one's appearance; (2) the importance of self-efficacy and an internal locus of control in regard to one's health and fitness; and (3) the advantages of physical strength and stamina attained from healthy eating and exercising. Working in the high-risk setting of a sorority, a quasi-experimental pilot study found that four 75-min sessions, including a question and answer period with a woman who has recovered from an eating disorder, reduced current use of unhealthy weight management techniques, decreased body dissatisfaction, and increased physical self-esteem.

STRATEGIES THAT DO NOT WORK

Our review of effective programs also illustrates strategies that have not been effective. The following characteristics are associated with the absence of a prevention effect: (1) lack of "fit" between the program and program participants (e.g., trying to prevent the development of unhealthy attitudes who already have high levels of DEB); (2) "one-shot" interventions; (3) a unidimensional focus (e.g., an emphasis on clinical eating disorders without attention to the multidimensional factors that underlie DEB); and (4) an exclusively didactic presentational style. This type of program can be illustrated by single session college intervention programs that have as a goal both prevention and identification and referral of severe DEB. Not only can such programs be ineffective, they may do harm by providing knowledge about disordered eating strategies (e.g., purging behaviors) without addressing and challenging personal, interpersonal, and sociocultural factors that motivate the development of DEB (Mann, Nolen-Hoeksema, Huang, Burgard, Wright, & Hanson, 1997).

SYNTHESIS

Eating disorders prevention is a relatively young field within the broader area of prevention. DEB typically develops during adolescence, so most prevention research has been conducted with adolescents. Further research is needed to examine the onset of DEB among college students and other adult groups and to assess the effectiveness of prevention with adult samples. The following recommendations arise from our review of prevention programs for adults.

The Status of Prevention on College Campuses

Studies of prevention with high-risk college students suggest that varied short-term interventions subsumed under the broad "psychoeducational" model produce significant changes in attitudes and behaviors that are sustained during short-term follow-up. Longer follow-up assessments are needed. These prevention programs overlap to a large degree with the cognitive–behavioral approaches that have been successful in the treatment of negative body image in eating disordered and non-eating disordered, but weight dissatisfied women (Cash, 1996). In contrast, little is known about prevention of eating disorders with late adolescent or young adult women who come to college with low levels of unhealthy weight-shape concerns. Although, some research has identified the transition from high school to college as a time of increased vulnerability to DEB (Smolak et al., 1996), no studies have assessed the ability of a specific program to prevent this pattern on a particular university campus.

The Need for Integrated, Multidimensional Programs on College Campuses

University counseling center staff are the most vocal proponents for integrated, multidimensional programs to address the full spectrum of DEB (Hotelling, 1999; Schwitzer, Bergholz, Dore, & Salimi, 1998; Sigall, 1999). As part of their mission to protect the campus' mental health, counseling center staff are called upon to intervene at every point along the DEB spectrum by: (1) providing education for the general student body about healthy body image and weight management, as well as how to help a friend with severe DEB; (2) offering specialized interventions for "high risk" groups such as student athletes and sororities; (3) consulting with dining hall staff, coaching personnel, faculty, residence hall staff, and other relevant individuals or groups; and (4) providing individual and group therapy for individuals with an identified eating disorder (Hotelling, 1999).

The overall goal of these programs is to create a college campus where staffs are informed about DEB and about ways to enhance resilience and reduce risk for eating disorders among students. This will help expose students to constructive messages about the natural and beautiful diversity of body shapes. An educated and engaged staff will also work with students to foster critical discussions and to support them as they challenge adverse cultural messages, and as they participate in the process of identification, treatment referral, and support for students with eating disorders. Hotelling (1999) has established a multi-disciplinary campus task force comprised of health and mental health professionals, teachers, and administrative staff to provide a continuum of services for students displaying DEB. Sigall (1999) has developed a program for college sororities, as they are high-risk groups on campus. Unique aspects of Sigall's program involve making preventive activities an ongoing part of the fabric of life in all campus sororities. These programs are important initial developments, but as yet no research has closed the gap between calls for multilevel college-wide interventions (Hotelling, 1999) and evaluation research focused on relatively small, targeted groups of high-risk individuals displaying some level of DEB (Chase, 2000). Research is needed to assess, not only individual-level change, but also institutional change in response to programs addressing environmental risk factors.

The Need for Programming with High-Risk Groups on College Campuses

In designing prevention programs for college students, the need for specific interventions among high risk student groups should be emphasized. Goldberg et al. (1996) have developed successful programs for male and female high school athletes to prevent use of anabolic steroids, alcohol, or other illicit drugs, as well to enhance healthy forms of eating and strength development. Their program, which includes interactive classroom and exercise training sessions given by peer educators, coaches, and trainers, has been found to be effective in inducing long-term attitudinal and behavioral changes. Similar prevention programs that use the DISC model to form a combination of psychoeducational and cognitive–behavioral approaches are being developed for high risk adolescents (e.g., those with Type I diabetes; Colton, Rodin, Olmsted, & Daneman, 1999). This type of program could be applied on campus for students with diabetes or other health problems in which the illness or the drug treatments affect weight gain, body image, and eating behavior. Another group that may benefit from carefully designed programs of this sort are male or female students who are at high risk for negative body image and DEB because they are obese. Such prevention work must carefully balance concern about the health risks of obesity with the need for obese adults to avoid unhealthy dieting and to have the opportunity to eat reasonably, to exercise regularly, and to learn to effectively manage various forms of stress, including cultural prejudices about fat.

Beyond the College Campus: A Social Ecological Perspective

As is the case for most significant health problems, negative body image and DEB are definitely rooted in complex social values and factors operating at multiple levels

of the physical and social environment (Maton, 2000; Perry, 1999; Piran, 2001; Thompson et al., 1999). For example, pressures stemming from gender inequality in power and status have made women much more susceptible to appearance-related messages and to the practice of various unhealthy behaviors such as dieting and cigarette smoking. Similarly, ethnocultural, class-based, and acculturation pressures may put particular individuals at risk. The prominence of mass marketing and "virtual reality" in modern life introduces the blurring of boundaries between "real" and constructed images (including the representation of the biological body) and between what can and cannot be safely changed through "technology." These larger scale social forces, in turn, interact with and affect social communities and systems, including schools, neighborhoods, families, peers groups, etc.

In other words, all relational experiences embedded within these multiple communities will therefore be informed and shaped by larger social values, prejudices, and structures. With regard to negative body image and DEB, both qualitative and quantitative research have indeed documented these complex interactions between larger social variables, social systems, and individuals' experiences of their body, eating, and self-esteem (Piran, 2001; Thompson, 1994; Thompson et al., 1999). As these relational contexts provide the breeding grounds for disruptions in body- and self-image, prevention of DEB and concomitant problems (e.g., depression and substance abuse) in adults must necessarily involve larger social scale changes.

Community-based prevention has been applied with promising results to a variety of problems, including cardiovascular health and substance abuse (Perry, 1999). To date there has been little progress in the development and evaluation of multidimensional community programs for preventing DEB. Working with psychological and nursing professionals living on an Israeli kibbutz, Latzer and Shatz (1999) arranged for programs to: (1) educate adolescents and adults; (2) train professionals in identification and referral of eating disorders; and (3) provide skilled counseling, treatment and support services for eating disordered individuals and their families. The entire effort integrated programs with a wide scope (e.g., raising community awareness of how sociocultural factors contribute to many challenges faced by adolescent girls), a moderate scope (e.g., helping families with teenage girls understand the impact of the pubertal transition on body image), and a narrow focus (e.g., helping girls evincing the warning signs of disordered eating). Preliminary evidence indicated an increase in public awareness about the nature and causes of eating disorders, an increase in early identification of disordered eating, and a possible reduction in the incidence of serious eating disorders.

Transforming communities, which themselves are internally heterogeneous and externally embedded in larger social contexts, is a daunting task. Yet, given the recent developments in such diverse areas as women's athletics and seat-belt use, there is reason to be optimistic about health promotion through social change. In order to move from possibility to practice, eating disorder prevention specialists will need to draw from theoretical developments and practical experience in community psychology and in other disciplines such as applied anthropology.

Maton (2000) and Piran (1999, 2001) offer compatible theoretical frameworks that could prove useful in community-based prevention via social transformation. In general, these theories focus on relational community-building, development of group empowerment and of individual skills within a group setting, and critical analysis and actions toward unhealthy sociocultural influences. Specifically, these theorists advocate that mental health professionals, parents, educators, adolescents, and other stakeholders convene to discuss and eventually assess their community's concerns and needs. In these dialogues emphasis would be on patient, respectful construction of a shared understanding of beliefs, needs, concerns, fears, etc., concerning the core issues associated with DEB. Some of these issues would likely be very specific. Examples include negative body image in adolescent girls, obesity and poor nutrition, and the influence of mass media's glorification of slenderness. Other issues raised will probably be much more general, for example, ethnic prejudice or inequitable gender roles. Psychologists, social workers, or other social activists may have a role in creating forums to facilitate the type of intensive and critical group dialogues required for social change. However, it is critically important that community members assume leadership and power in the process of communal change(s). Similarly, the initial dialogues and efforts toward program development should work toward supportive relationships, social cohesion, and respect for diversity. Regardless of their socioeconomic status, communities characterized by disenfranchisement, demoralization, and disengagement are likely to be fertile soil for a large number of health problems, including DEB. Critical understanding derived from the experience of different communities can, in turn, inform and transform larger scale social forces.

Patient construction of this communal process sets the stage for clarification of specific sociocultural factors that operate within a community to either increase the probability of DEB (risk factors that increase vulnerability) or work against emergence of DEB (protective factors that contribute to resilience). As these contextualized factors are identified, plans will emerge to challenge and change them on multiple levels. For example, consider a community whose stakeholders are concerned about mass media's manipulative portrayals of women and girls as slender sex objects and of men as muscular, unfeeling "hunks." At the community

level, adults could engage in a coordinated campaign to protest publicly these images, to meet with and educate media and business leaders, and to develop healthier images of individual style and beauty. Efforts to raise awareness about the topic and to educate the public could incorporate displays at public libraries, billboards, and newspaper articles. At the family level, stakeholders could work with the schools, supermarkets, medical professionals, and churches to educate parents and grandparents about, for example: (1) normative bodily and psychological changes during puberty and late adolescence; and (2) how to encourage youth to appreciate and enjoy mass media while being critical consumers. At the school level, stakeholders could work with teachers and students to develop media literacy, including involvement in active construction of media that promotes healthy attitudes and behaviors in regard body image, nutrition, and exercise. This type of critical education can be reinforced in many settings, such as girl scouts. If done carefully, media literacy (and cultural literacy in general) connects youth and the adults who teach and mentor them to overarching prevention principles of relational dialogue, group empowerment, and constructive action to improve culture and one's self simultaneously (Maton, 2000; Levine & Piran, 2001; Piran, 1999, 2001).

Also see: Nutrition: Early Childhood; Nutrition: Childhood; Nutrition: Adolescence; Nutrition: Older Adulthood; Obesity: Adolescence.

References

American Psychiatric Association. (1994). *Diagnostic and statistical manual of mental disorders* (4th ed.). Washington, DC: Author.

Berel, S., & Irving, L. (1998). Media and disturbed eating: An analysis of media influence and implications for prevention. *Journal of Primary Prevention, 18*, 415–430.

Cash, T.F. (1996). The treatment of body image disturbances. In J.K. Thompson (Ed.), *Body image, eating disorders, and obesity: An integrative guide for assessment and treatment* (pp. 83–107). Washington, DC: American Psychological Association.

Chase, A.C. (2000). *Eating disorder prevention: An intervention for "at-risk" college women*. Doctoral Dissertation, University of Texas at Austin.

Colton, P.A., Rodin, G.M., Olmsted, M.P., & Daneman, D. (1999). Preventing eating disorders in young women with diabetes. In N. Piran, M.P. Levine, & C. Steiner-Adair (Eds.), *Preventing eating disorders: A handbook of interventions and special challenges* (pp. 270–284). Philadelphia: Brunner/Mazel.

Drenowski, A., Yee, D.K., Kurth, C.L., & Krahn, D.D. (1994). Eating pathology and DSM-III-R bulimia nervosa: A continuum of behavior. *American Journal of Psychiatry, 151*, 1217–1219.

Franko, D.L., & Orosan-Weine, P. (1998). The prevention of eating disorders: Empirical, methodological and conceptual considerations. *Clinical Psychology: Science and Practice, 5*, 459–477.

Goldberg, L., Elliot, D., Clarke, G.N., MacKinnon, D.P., Moe, E., Zoref, L., Green, C., Wolf, S.L., Greffrath, E., Miller, D.J., & Lapin, A. (1996). Effects of a multidimensional anabolic steroid prevention intervention.

The adolescents training and learning to avoid steroids (ATLAS) program. *Journal of the American Medical Association, 276,* 1555–1562.

Hesse-Biber, S. (1991). Women, weight, and eating disorders: A sociocultural and political-economic analysis. *Women's Studies International Forum, 14,* 173–191.

Higgins, L.C., & Gray, W. (1998). Changing the body image concern and eating behaviour of chronic dieters: The effects of a psychoeducational intervention. *Psychology and Health, 13,* 1045–1060.

Hotelling, K. (1999). An integrated prevention/intervention program for the university setting. In N. Piran, M.P. Levine, & C. Steiner-Adair (Eds.), *Preventing eating disorders: A handbook of interventions and special challenges* (pp. 208–221). Philadelphia: Brunner/Mazel.

Kaminski, P.L., & McNamara, K. (1996). A treatment for college women at risk for bulimia: A controlled evaluation. *Journal of Counseling & Development, 74,* 288–294.

Latzer, Y., & Shatz, S. (1999). Comprehensive community prevention of disturbed attitudes to weight control: A three-level intervention program. *Eating Disorders: The Journal of Treatment & Prevention, 7,* 3–31.

Levine, M.P., & Piran, N. (2001). The prevention of eating disorders: Towards a participatory ecology of knowledge, action, and advocacy. In R. Striegel-Moore & L. Smolak (Eds.), *Eating disorders: Innovative directions in research and practice* (pp. 233–253). Washington, DC: American Psychological Association.

Mann, T., Nolen-Hoeksema, S., Huang, K., Burgard, D., Wright, A., & Hanson, K. (1997). Are two interventions worse than none? Joint primary and secondary prevention of eating disorders in college females. *Health Psychology, 16,* 215–225.

Maton, K.I. (2000). Making a difference: The social ecology of social transformation. *American Journal of Community Psychology, 28,* 25–57.

Mintz, L., & Betz, N. (1988). Prevalence and correlates of eating disordered behaviors among undergraduate women. *Journal of Counseling Psychology, 35,* 463–471.

Perry, C.L. (1999). *Creating health behavior change: How to develop community-wide programs for youth.* Thousand Oaks, CA: Sage.

Phelps, L., Sapia, J., Nathanson, D., & Nelson, L. (2000). An empirically supported eating disorder prevention program. *Psychology in the Schools, 37,* 443–452.

Pike, K.M., & Striegel-Moore, R.H. (1997). Disordered eating and eating disorders. In S.J. Gallant, G.P. Keita, & R. Royak-Schaler (Eds.), *Health care for women: Psychological, social, and behavioral influence* (pp. 97–114). Washington, DC: American Psychological Association.

Piran, N. (1999). The reduction of preoccupation with body weight and shape in schools: A feminist approach. In N. Piran, M.P. Levine, & C. Steiner-Adair (Eds.), *Preventing eating disorders: A handbook of interventions and special challenges* (pp. 148–159). Philadelphia: Brunner/Mazel.

Piran, N. (2001). Re-inhabiting the body from the inside out: Girls transform their school environment. In D.L. Tolman & M. Brydon-Miller (Eds.), *From subjects to subjectivities: A handbook of interpretative and participatory methods* (pp. 218–238) New York: NYU Press.

Posavac, H.D., Posavac, S.S., & Weigel, R.G. (2001). Reducing the impact of media images on women at risk for body image disturbance: Three targeted interventions. *Journal of Social and Clinical Psychology, 20,* 324–340.

Schwitzer, A.M., Bergholz, K., Dore, T., & Salimi, L. (1998). Eating disorders among college women: Prevention, education, and treatment responses. *Journal of American College Health, 46,* 199–207.

Sigall, B. (1999). The Panhellenic task force on eating disorders: A program of primary and secondary prevention for sororities. In N. Piran, M.P. Levine, & C. Steiner-Adair (Eds.), *Preventing eating disorders: A handbook of interventions and special challenges* (pp. 222–237). Philadelphia: Brunner/Mazel.

Smolak, L., Levine, M.P., & Striegel-Moore, R.H. (Eds.). (1996). *The developmental psychopathology of eating disorders: Implications for research, prevention, and treatment.* Mahwah, NJ: Lawrence Erlbaum.

Springer, E.A., Winzelberg, A.J., Perkins, R., & Taylor, C.B. (1999). Effects of a body image curriculum for college students on improved body image. *International Journal of Eating Disorders, 26,* 13–20.

Stice, E., Chase, A., Stormer, S., & Appel, A. (2001). A randomized trial of a dissonance-based eating disorder prevention program. *International Journal of Eating Disorders, 29,* 247–262.

Stice, E., Mazotti, L., Weibel, D., & Agras, S. (2000). Dissonance prevention program decreases thin-ideal internalization, body dissatisfaction, dieting, negative affect, and bulimic symptoms: A preliminary experiment. *International Journal of Eating Disorders, 27,* 206–217.

Stice, E., & Ragan, J. (in press). A preliminary controlled evaluation of an eating disturbance psychoeducational intervention for college students. *International Journal of Eating Disorders, 31,* 159–171.

Striegel-Moore, R.H., Leslie D., Petrill S.A., Garvin V., & Rosenheck, R.A. (2000). One-year use and cost of inpatient and outpatient services among female and male patients with an eating disorder: evidence from a national database of health insurance claims. *International Journal of Eating Disorders, 27,* 381–389.

Taylor, C.B., Winzelberg, A.J., & Celio, A.A. (2001). The use of interactive media to prevent eating disorders. In R. Striegel-Moore & L. Smolak (Eds.), *Eating disorders: Innovative directions in research and practice* (pp. 255–269). Washington, DC: American Psychological Association.

Thompson, B. (1994). Food, bodies, and growing up female: Childhood lessons about culture, race, and class. In P. Fallon, M. Katzman, & S.C. Wooley (Eds.), *Feminist perspectives on eating disorders* (pp. 355–378). New York: Guilford Press.

Thompson, J.K., Heinberg, L., Altabe, M., & Tantleff-Dunn, S. (1999). *Exacting beauty: Theory, assessment, and treatment of body image disturbance.* Washington, DC: American Psychological Association.

Van Hoeken, D.V., Lucas, A.R., & Hoek, H.W. (1998). Epidemiology. In H.W. Hoek, J.L. Treasure, & M.A. Katzman (Eds.), *Neurobiology in the treatment of eating disorders* (pp. 97–126). Chichester, UK: John Wiley.

Divorce, Childhood

Mark A. Fine

INTRODUCTION

Approximately 50 percent of children in the United States will experience the divorce of their parents before they reach the age of 18 years. The adjustment of these children has been a source of concern for both practitioners and researchers and, indeed, the adjustment of children who have experienced parental divorce tends to be somewhat poorer than that of children whose parents remain married. Nevertheless, the differences in adjustment are relatively small, and parents can enhance their children's adaptation by reducing their levels of spousal conflict, communicating directly with each other, and keeping the children out of their disputes. Accordingly, interventions have been developed to help parents facilitate their children's adaptation. Some promising interventions have also been developed for children themselves.

DEFINITIONS

Divorce is the legal termination of a marriage. *Legal custody* refers to who has the legal authority to make decisions regarding the child's welfare. Legal custody can be *sole*, in which case one parent has legal responsibility for the child (the other parent is referred to as the *noncustodial parent*), or *joint*, in which case both parents have legal responsibility. *Physical custody* refers to where the child physically resides, regardless of who has legal custody of the child. If one parent lives with the child for a majority of the time, that parent is considered the *residential parent*, whereas the other parent is called the *nonresidential parent*. *Visitation* refers to time spent between the child and the noncustodial and/or the nonresidential parent. *Child support* refers to the funds provided by one parent (usually the nonresidential or noncustodial parent) to the other parent to use to raise the child. A *parenting plan* is a document that reflects agreements reached between the parents regarding matters pertaining to raising the child, such as custody, visitation, financial support, which parent will spend which holidays with the child, how special expenses such as music lessons or college will be managed, and how the parents will communicate with each other. A *motion to modify decree* reflects a legal attempt to change the terms of the original divorce settlement, which may occur many years after the divorce itself.

SCOPE

By all indicators, both the incidence and prevalence of divorce have increased considerably over the last several hundred years in the United States. Whereas only an estimated 5 percent of first marriages in the middle of the 19th century ended in divorce, approximately 50 percent of current marriages will end in divorce (Amato, 2000). The greatest increase in divorce rates occurred between 1960 and 1980, with rates increasing only slightly since 1980 (Teachman, Tedrow, & Crowder, 2000). Further, about one-half of all divorces involve children under the age of 18 years; as a result, over one million children in the United States experience parental divorce each year and approximately 40 percent of all children born in the 1990s will experience the divorce of their parents before they turn 18 years (Amato, 2000). There are racial/ethnic group differences in the prevalence of divorce, with African Americans having higher rates than Whites, who, in turn, have higher rates than Latinos (Teachman et al., 2000).

Several trends noted in the United States have also been noted in other Western and Eastern countries. Divorce rates in Western European countries increased substantially in the second half of the 20th century, although they stabilized during the last decade, and most countries have moved toward "no-fault" grounds for divorce (i.e., based on the notions that marriages may be irreversibly damaged through no fault of either spouse and/or that post-divorce adjustment is facilitated when spouses do not have to establish that one or the other spouse is responsible for the breakdown of the marriage) (Fine & Fine, 1994). Countries that are predominantly Catholic, such as Italy, Spain, France, and Ireland, tend to have lower divorce rates and more restrictive divorce laws. Similarly, in many Eastern countries, divorce rates have increased dramatically in recent years, although they remain considerably lower than in Western countries (Goode, 1993). For example, the divorce rate in Taiwan, which has the highest rate in Asian countries, is approximately one half of the rate in the United States (National Center for Health Statistics, 1998; *Taiwan Executive Yuan*, 1998).

THEORIES

A wide array of theories have been used to understand divorce and its effects on family members. The *social exchange perspective* suggests that individuals decide whether to continue their relationships on the basis of their assessment of costs and benefits, relative to alternative relationships that they could be involved in, and that they end relationships when the cost/benefit ratio exceeds what they believe that they could obtain in an alternative relationship. The *symbolic interaction perspective* suggests that individuals attach meaning to their experience and that this meaning influences their behavior. With respect to divorce, this perspective leads us to acknowledge that individuals actively attempt to "make sense" of their experience in ways that help them cope with difficult circumstances and that individuals may attach very different meanings to the same divorce-related events. Finally, the *social learning perspective* emphasizes that children learn from observing how their parents respond to various circumstances and events. With respect to divorce, this perspective has been used to explain why children whose parents divorce are themselves more likely to divorce and why boys seem to experience more negative consequences from divorce than girls (i.e., boys "lose" their same-sex role model when their fathers spend less time with them). This perspective also forms much of the basis for the content of parenting education programs for divorcing parents, which emphasizes that parents should not argue in the presence of children, should model positive problem-solving strategies, and communicate directly with one another.

RESEARCH

Children from divorced families fare more poorly than children from first-marriage families on virtually all outcome dimensions that have been studied, including academic performance, behavior problems, social competence, self-esteem, psychological adjustment, and health (Amato, 2000). In a series of meta-analyses, Amato found that the mean effect sizes describing the difference between children from divorced and first-marriage families on conduct problems and psychological adjustment were −0.19 and −0.17, respectively, for studies conducted in the 1990s. Those in the divorced group, on average, performed approximately two tenths of a standard deviation below children from first-marriage families.

One of the critiques levied against much of the literature that has compared children's adjustment in different types of families is that causal inferences (e.g., divorce causes adjustment problems) are inappropriately drawn from correlational research designs. To address this issue, several longitudinal studies have been conducted. In general, these studies have found that children whose parents later divorce are also more poorly adjusted before the divorce, suggesting that divorce itself is not the sole cause of later adjustment difficulties (Baydar, 1988; Block, Block, & Gjerde, 1986; Cherlin et al., 1991).

If divorce is not the sole cause of some children's adjustment difficulties, what other factors are influential? Research has suggested that a variety of factors that have been referred to as "family processes" have important effects on children. Such processes include parenting behaviors, with parents showing simultaneously high levels of parental supervision and warmth fostering the most positive child outcomes; conflict, with children faring best when they are exposed to little conflict between the ex-spouses; and family interactions, with children adjusting most effectively when their family environments, including siblings as well as parents, are ordered, supportive, supervised, and relatively free of conflict (Fine, 2000).

Parents' adjustment is also important to consider because it strongly affects children's well-being. With that in mind, divorced parents, on average, experience more mental health problems than parents from first-marriage families. For example, Demo and Acock (1996) found that divorced and never-married mothers had lower levels of well-being than did mothers in first-marriage families. Nevertheless, divorced parents' level of adjustment improves over time (Hetherington, Bridges, & Insabella, 1998) and, as is the case for children, a variety of other factors, besides the divorce itself, strongly affect parents' well-being. For example, parents' adjustment is facilitated to the extent that they are relatively free of depression, have a supportive social network, and establish new, mutually satisfying romantic partnerships.

STRATEGIES THAT WORK

Mediation

Mediation has grown as an alternative to contested divorces. When successful, mediation allows the divorcing parents to maintain control of decisions pertaining to their children, such as child support, how parents will spend time with their child, and financial settlements. Often, these agreements are recorded in written parenting plans. Although considerably more research on the effects of mediation needs to be conducted, evidence (see Emery, 1998; Demo, Fine, & Ganong, 2000) suggests that: (a) compliance with mediated agreements is greater than compliance with adjudicated agreements; (b) mediation may be less costly than litigation; (c) mediation may take less time than litigation; (d) couples with mediated agreements are less likely to return to court to file motion to modify decrees than are couples with other types of agreements; and (e) in medicated cases, parents are more likely to remain in contact with children, child support is more likely to be paid, and parents are more satisfied with postdivorce arrangements. Couples who mediate tend to be more satisfied with decisions surrounding the divorce and with the divorce process itself (Emery, Matthews, & Wyer, 1991; Kelly, 1991), although men are generally more satisfied than women.

Despite this supportive evidence, mediation is not without its critics. One criticism levied against mediation is that mediators, in their attempts to be neutral and unbiased, tend to ignore or minimize the power inequities (i.e., men's greater financial resources, risk of physical violence by men) that place women at a negotiating disadvantage and that culminate in solutions that they perceive as unfair to them. In addition, mediation is not indicated for all couples, as some may not be able to engage in the necessary negotiation and compromise because of personality or relational problems.

Programs for Children

There are a number of programs developed for children whose parents are divorced or divorcing (Grych & Fincham, 1992). Most use a structured group format, consist of 8–14 sessions, and are provided in schools. The groups tend to have both educational and therapeutic elements, focusing on such goals as helping children to: (a) gain a clearer understanding of difficult divorce-related issues and situations; (b) adjust to stressful issues stemming from the divorce; (c) improve parent–child communication; (d) learn new coping skills; and (e) improve their self-image (Grych & Fincham, 1997).

The child-focused program that has most thoroughly been evaluated is the Children of Divorce Intervention Project (CODIP; Alpert-Gillis, Pedro-Carroll, & Cowen, 1989;

Pedro-Carroll, Alpert-Gillis, & Cowen, 1992). This program helps children gain a clearer understanding of the divorce, and assists them in learning new coping skills and improving their self-esteem. According to Grych and Fincham (1997), evidence suggests that the program is effective with children from a variety of racial and ethnic backgrounds. For example, the CODIP program has been modified for a racially mixed urban population by placing greater emphasis on the extended family and by recognizing the acceptability of a variety of types of families. In one study, compared to children from first-marriage families and children whose parents divorced but did not participate in the program, children who participated in the modified CODIP reported feeling more positively about themselves, their parents reported that the children were better adjusted, and their teachers rated the children as more assertive, task-oriented, and better able to tolerate frustration (Alpert-Gillis et al., 1989).

STRATEGIES THAT MIGHT WORK

Parent Education for Divorcing Parents

Among the most common and fastest growing interventions for families experiencing a divorce is parent education for divorcing parents (Arbuthnot & Gordon, 1997; Blaisure & Geasler, 1996). Such programs now can be found in almost one half of the counties in the United States (Geasler & Blaisure, 1999), as well as in most Canadian provinces, Israel, New Zealand, People's Republic of China, Australia, Puerto Rico, and South Africa (Arbuthnot & Gordon, 1997). The primary assumption underlying the proliferation of these programs is that the process of divorce for children can be made much less stressful and harmful by educating parents concerning how to help their children navigate through this difficult experience. Thus, the focus of the sessions is on children and not the parents, although some attention is obviously given to parents' well-being because it so strongly influences children's adjustment. Not surprisingly, given the focus on children's adjustment to divorce, topics that are usually covered in these programs include: (a) the typical reactions of children and parents to divorce; (b) children's developmental needs at different ages; (c) the benefits of ex-spouses being able to cooperatively parent following divorce; and (d) the benefits of keeping children out of the "middle" of their parents' disputes (Braver, Salem, Pearson, & DeLuse, 1996).

Most evaluations of these programs, when they are even conducted, consist primarily of "consumer satisfaction" questionnaires that are administered to participants immediately after the completion of the program (Blaisure & Geasler, 1996). These questionnaires typically show that participants are very satisfied with the programs (Blaisure & Geasler, 1996; Feng & Fine, 2000; Fine et al., 1999; Kramer & Washo, 1993) and that they report that the program was helpful to them, even after 12-month follow-ups (cf. Frieman, Garon, & Garon, 2000). These positive evaluations are not surprising given that clients usually report having positive experiences with a wide range of interventions.

Although it is promising that participants report being so pleased with these programs, such reports do not necessarily mean that the programs are successfully changing parents' behavior and helping children cope with divorce. Unfortunately, there have only been a few studies that have assessed the short- and long-term effectiveness of these parenting education programs. The few studies that have been done have suggested that these programs may have limited positive effects on participants. For example, Kramer and Washo (1993) found that parents with initially high levels of parental conflict reported a significant decline (over 3 years) in their ex-spouse's triangulating childrearing behaviors (e.g., blaming the other parent for the divorce in front of the child) at follow-up. However, with respect to parents' reports of childrearing behaviors or parent–child relationship quality, there were no program effects. Further, children in both the educational and comparison groups were reported as being better adjusted at the follow-up than they were at the time of the program. Arbuthnot and Gordon (1997) found that, over a 6-month follow-up period, parents learned useful parenting and communication skills and that children were exposed to less parental conflict. However, there were few differences between the parent education and comparison groups in child adjustment.

Because these educational programs have political and intuitive appeal, it is likely that the absence of evaluation data will not deter their continued widespread implementation. However, as Braver et al. (1996) noted, without sound evaluation findings, courts and legislatures will find it increasingly difficult to justify mandating such programs. Thus, evaluations of these programs that extend beyond consumer satisfaction are much needed.

Programs for Parents

Wolchik, Sandler, Braver, and Fogas (1993) designed a group for residential divorced mothers that targeted the quality of mother–child relationships, discipline, interparental conflict, contact with fathers, and support from adults other than the child's parents. The group intervention was intensive, requiring 10 group sessions and 2 individual sessions for residential mothers. The results were somewhat mixed. There were positive changes in the quality of mother–child relationships in the program group, but there were no differences between the program and control group participants in interparental conflict, contact with fathers, or discipline. In addition, contrary to expectation, children in the program group reported *less* support from other adults than did those in the control group. With respect to child outcomes, children in the program group fared better than their control counterparts on some dimensions (e.g., lower levels of aggression), but not on others (e.g., self-reported anxiety). Clearly, programs such as this one have considerable potential in effecting positive outcomes among children and parents following divorce. Balanced against the benefits of this strong potential, however, is the limited evaluation support of this (and other) programs targeted to parents and the potential difficulties in engaging parents to participate in such an intensive (and possibly costly) intervention.

Programs for Children

There is a wide array of programs for children that have not received as much evaluation support as has the CODIP program (Grych & Fincham, 1992). According to Grych and Fincham (1997), some of these programs have reported positive outcomes on some adjustment dimensions, but they have yet to show consistent and broad-based positive effects on children who participate. For example, Bornstein, Bornstein, and Walters (1988) reported mixed results from a group treatment program for children who have experienced divorce and Kalter, Schaefer, Lesowitz, Alpern, and Pickar (1988) found some support for the utility of a school-based support group for children experiencing divorce. The lack of clear, general, and consistent positive effects from these programs may be partially due to the presence of serious methodological flaws in the evaluation designs (Grych & Fincham, 1997). In addition, it should also be noted that there are many programs and/or support groups for children who have experienced parental divorce that have not been presented in the scholarly literature and the effectiveness of these programs is unknown.

Newsletters for Divorced Parents

There is some limited evidence that newsletters for divorced parents can be an effective intervention strategy. Hughes, Clark, Schaefer-Hernan, and Good (1994) evaluated the effectiveness of a series of 14 newsletters (containing information on a number of divorce-related issues) that were sent to 142 divorced mothers identified from public court records. Hughes et al. found that 86 percent of the divorced mothers indicated that they read the newsletters at least some of the time, that they were satisfied with the newsletter intervention, and that the information contained in the newsletters was helpful to them. However, those receiving the newsletters did not improve in the areas of

coping skills, psychological well-being, and parenting to a greater extent than did those mothers in the comparison group. These results suggest that divorced mothers are likely to feel positively about a newsletter intervention, but that the newsletters are unlikely to have significant long-term positive effects in terms of behavior change and psychological functioning. Hughes et al. suggest that the newsletter intervention might not be intensive enough to effect change among individuals as highly stressed as recently divorced parents.

STRATEGIES THAT DO NOT WORK

Voluntary Parenting Education Programs

As noted earlier, most parent education programs for divorcing parents are mandatory. By contrast, some have attempted to offer voluntary classes to the same audience. However, these have met with less than optimal success. Arbuthnot and Gordon (1997) reported that their efforts in offering free, voluntary classes were "disappointing" (p. 351), as very few parents registered to attend the classes and even fewer still actually attended the class. This lack of involvement may be one reason why courts have required divorcing parents to attend such programs, although others have claimed that a lack of interest and participation in voluntary classes are not adequate justifications for mandating that parents attend these classes.

One Session Classes/Programs

Given that there is only relatively weak evidence that existing single session mandatory parent education classes for divorcing parents actually change parent behavior and improve child outcomes, it may be unrealistic to expect that any single session program consisting of only a few hours would have a lasting impact on behavior and child well-being. Thus, while research has suggested that one session educational programs are likely to lead to positive attitudinal change (Feng & Fine, 2000; Fine et al., 1999) and can serve as a catalyst for subsequent changes if additional intervention strategies are employed (Kramer & Washo, 1993), future research is sorely needed to test whether the programs have long-term (more than 3 years) behavioral impacts that extend beyond satisfaction with the program and attitudinal change. To date, this research has yet to be conducted.

SYNTHESIS

Who is likely to benefit from which preventive interventions under which conditions and at which stages of the divorce process? The literature reviewed in this entry suggests that some preliminary answers to this question can be advanced. Available evidence suggests that some brief interventions, such as parenting education sessions for divorcing parents and possibly newsletters, may provide some assistance to parents, and subsequently to their children, following divorce. Parenting education programs for divorcing parents are typically offered just before the actual legal divorce, which may fall at any one of a number of different time periods during the process of marital breakdown. Although no research has yet been conducted on the optimal timing of this intervention, it is plausible to hypothesize that parents who have only recently decided to end their relationship may benefit more from these educational sessions than will parents who have been separated for an extended period of time before filing for divorce. Further, because educational programs are often more readily received by individuals from higher socioeconomic levels, it is likely that middle and upper socioeconomic status parents are likely to be more receptive to these interventions than those with more limited financial resources and less previous education. However, investigators have yet to empirically test this hypothesis. Similarly, it is plausible to expect that a newsletter intervention would be most effective for parents who have recently initiated the divorce process and who have higher levels of socioeconomic status; however, again, until the requisite research is undertaken, these possibilities will remain hypotheses.

However, even if subsequent research shows that parenting education programs and newsletters are effective, the brief nature of these interventions suggests that their impact is necessarily limited and that more intensive interventions are likely to be needed to effect lasting change. Toward this end, a number of intensive programs have been developed, most of which occur in a group milieu; a few of these have received empirical support from well-conducted evaluations, whereas others have received less support and mixed results. In most cases, these programs have been developed for white, middle-class parents and children, but a few (e.g., the CODIP program) have been successfully modified for ethnically and racially diverse participants.

Given these considerations, it is likely that the ease with which brief interventions can be delivered (e.g., only one session or only one mailing) must be balanced against their only limited potential impact. By contrast, the likelihood of longer lasting positive impacts from the more intensive programs must be weighed against their greater cost, greater time investment required, and limited availability for some parents. With these balances in mind, the current literature justifies the conclusion that a multifaceted intervention, with differing degrees of intensity, which targets multiple family members is likely to provide the greatest benefit to children and families who have experienced divorce. Perhaps the greatest impact can be achieved by combining some (possibly mandated) brief interventions targeted to parents (no known brief interventions directly target children), with some choices available to family members from a menu of programs (including mediation) for either parents, children, or both. Programs that target both children and parents are understandably few in number, given the logistical problems involved in intervening with multiple family members, but show some promise (Stolberg & Mahler, 1994).

As an alternative to developing programs for divorced children and parents, another route toward the desired end of preventing negative consequences following divorce lies in the area of public policy. Public policy reforms have the potential to facilitate the difficult adjustment process following divorce. As has been noted by several scholars (e.g., Mason, 2000), children are likely to benefit from policy changes that lead to less adversarial divorce proceedings (e.g., through mediation and other alternative-dispute resolution approaches), that increase the financial resources available to the child (via child support), that increase the children's involvement with their nonresidential parent, and that foster clearer agreements between parents regarding childrearing (i.e., parenting plans). These legal and policy reforms hold great promise, at least partly because they can affect the experiences of many more people than can parent- and child-targeted interventions.

Also see: Divorce: Adolescence; Bereavement: Childhood; Single-Parent Families: Childhood.

References

Alpert-Gillis, L.J., Pedro-Carroll, J.L., & Cowen, E.L. (1989). The children of divorce intervention program: Development, implementation, and evaluation of a program for young urban children. *Journal of Consulting and Clinical Psychology, 57*, 583–589.

Amato, P.R. (2000). The consequences of divorce for adults and children. *Journal of Marriage and the Family, 62*, 1269–1287.

Arbuthnot, J., & Gordon, D.A. (1997). Divorce education for parents and children. In L. VandeCreek, S. Knapp, & T.J. Jackson (Eds.), *Innovations in clinical practice* (Vol. 15, pp. 341–364). Sarasota, FL: Professional Resource Press.

Baydar, N. (1988). Effects of parental separation and reentry into union on the emotional well-being of children. *Journal of Marriage and the Family, 50*, 967–981.

Blaisure, K.R., & Geasler, M.J. (1996). Results of a survey of court-connected parent education programs in US counties. *Family and Conciliation Courts Review, 34*, 23–40.

Block, J.H., Block, J., & Gjerde, P.F. (1986). The personality of children prior to divorce: A prospective study. *Child Development, 57*, 827–840.

Bornstein, M.T., Bornstein, P.H., & Walters, H.A. (1988). Children of divorce: Empirical evaluation of a group-treatment program. *Journal of Clinical Child Psychology, 17*, 248–254.

Braver, S.L., Salem, P., Pearson, J., & DeLuse, S.R. (1996). The content of divorce education programs: Results of a survey. *Family and Conciliation Courts Review, 34*, 41–59.

Cherlin, A.J., Furstenberg, F.F., Jr., Chase-Lansdale, L.P., Kiernan, K.E., Robins, P.K., Morrison, D.R., & Teitler, J.O. (1991). Longitudinal effects of divorce in Great Britain and the United States. *Science, 252,* 1386–1389.

Demo, D.H., & Acock, A.C. (1996). Singlehood, marriage, and remarriage: The effects of family structure and family relationships on mothers' well-being. *Journal of Family Issues, 17,* 388–407.

Demo, D.H., Fine, M.A., & Ganong, L.H. (2000). Divorce as a family stressor. In P.C. McKenry & S.J. Price (Eds.), *Families and change: Coping with stressful events* (2nd ed., pp. 279–302). Newbury Park, CA: Sage.

Emery, R. (1998). *Marriage, divorce, and children's adjustment* (2nd ed.). Thousand Oaks, CA: Sage.

Emery, R., Matthews, S.G., & Wyer, M.M. (1991). Child custody mediation and litigation: Further evidence on the differing views of mothers and fathers. *Journal of Consulting and Clinical Psychology, 59,* 410–418.

Feng, P., & Fine, M.A. (2000). Evaluation of a research-based parenting education program for divorcing parents: The Focus on Kids program. *Journal of Divorce and Remarriage, 34,* 1–23.

Fine, M.A. (2000). Divorce and single parenting. In C. Hendrick & S.S. Hendrick (Eds.), *Sourcebook of close relationships* (pp. 139–152). Newbury Park, CA: Sage.

Fine, M.A., Coleman, M., Gable, S., Ganong, L.H., Ispa, J., Morrison, J., & Thornburg, K.R. (1999). Research-based parenting education for divorcing parents: A university-community collaboration. In T.R. Chibocos & R.M. Lerner (Eds.), *Serving children and families through community-university partnerships: Success stories* (pp. 251–258). Norwell, MA: Kluwer.

Fine, M.A., & Fine, D.R. (1994). An examination and evaluation of recent changes in divorce laws in five Western countries: The critical role of values. *Journal of Marriage and the Family, 56,* 249–263.

Frieman, B.B., Garon, H.M., & Garon, R.J. (2000). Parenting seminars for divorcing parents: One year later. *Journal of Divorce and Remarriage, 33,* 129–143.

Geasler, M.J., & Blaisure, K.R. (1999). 1998 nationwide survey of court-connected divorce education programs. *Family and Conciliation Courts Review, 37,* 36–63.

Goode, W.J. (1993). *World changes in divorce patterns.* New Haven, CT: Yale University Press.

Grych, J.H., & Fincham, F. (1992). Interventions for children of divorce: Toward greater integration of research and action. *Psychological Bulletin, 111,* 434–454.

Grych, J.H., & Fincham, F. (1997). Children's adaptation to divorce: From description to explanation. In S. Wolchik & I. Sandler (Eds.), *Handbook of children's coping: Linking theory and explanation* (pp. 159–193). New York: Plenum Press.

Hetherington, E.M., Bridges, M., & Insabella, G.M. (1998). What matters? What does not? Five perspectives on the association between marital transitions and children's adjustment. *American Psychologist, 53,* 167–184.

Hughes, R., Jr., Clark, C.D., Schaefer-Hernan, & Good, E.S. (1994). An evaluation of a for divorced mothers. *Family Relations, 43,* 298–304.

Kalter, N., Schaefer, M., Lesowitz, M., Alpern, D., & Pickar, J. (1988). School-based support groups for children of divorce. In B.H. Gottlieb (Ed.), *Martialing social support: Formats, processes, and effects* (pp. 165–185). Newbury Park, CA: Sage.

Kelly, J.B. (1991). Parent interaction after divorce: Comparison of mediated and adversarial divorce processes. *Behavioral Science and the Law, 9,* 387–398.

Kramer, L., & Washo, C.A. (1993). Evaluation of a court-mandated prevention program for divorcing parents. *Family Relations, 42,* 179–186.

Mason, M.A. (2000). *The custody wars: Why children are losing the legal battle and what we can do about it.* New York: Basic Books.

National Center for Health Statistics (1998). Divorce. *Monthly vital statistics report, 47*(21) http://www.cdc.gov/nchs/fastats/divorce.htm

Pedro-Carroll, J.L., Alpert-Gillis, L.J., & Cowen, E.L. (1992). An evaluation of the efficacy of a preventive intervention for 4th–6th grade urban children of divorce. *Journal of Primary Prevention, 13,* 115–130.

Stolberg, A.L., & Mahler, J. (1994). Enhancing treatment gains in a school-based intervention for children of divorce through skill training, parental involvement, and transfer procedures. *Journal of Consulting and Clinical Psychology, 62,* 147–156.

Taiwan Executive Yuan (1998). *Social indicators of Taiwan area 7.*

Teachman, J.D., Tedrow, L.M., & Crowder, K.D. (2000). The changing demography of America's families. *Journal of Marriage and the Family, 62,* 1234–1246.

Wolchik, S.A., Sandler, I.N., Braver, S.L., & Fogas, B. (1993). Events of parental divorce: Stressfulness ratings by children, parents, and clinicians. *American Journal of Community Psychology, 14,* 59–74.

Divorce, Adolescence

Spring R. Dawson-McClure, Irwin N. Sandler, and Sharlene A. Wolchik

INTRODUCTION

The large number of adolescents who experience parental divorce each year and the well-documented association between parental divorce and adjustment problems clearly indicate the importance of programs that facilitate postdivorce adjustment. The development of such programs requires an understanding of the factors that increase risk of maladjustment and those that promote adaptation. Theory-guided prevention programs of multiple modalities have been shown to be effective in improving adolescents' postdivorce adjustment.

SCOPE

Incidence and Prevalence

In 1998, 1,135,000 divorces occurred in the United States, and over 3 million adolescents (aged 12–17) were living with a divorced parent. It is predicted that 40 percent of American children will reside with a divorced parent prior to age 16. The divorce rate is markedly higher in the United States than in other developed countries; for example, compared to 20.7 divorces per year per 1,000 married women in the United States, there were 12.9 in Canada, 12.3 in the United Kingdom, and 5.4 in Japan.

Costs to Host and Society

In comparison to adolescents in two-parent homes, those with divorced parents exhibit higher levels of teen pregnancy, school drop out, delinquent behavior, substance use, greater externalizing and internalizing problems and reduced academic and social competence (Hetherington et al., 1992; Amato & Keith, 1991a). Adolescents of divorced parents are more likely to display a cluster of "norm-breaking" behaviors, which includes cheating, stealing, and truancy, than are those from nondivorced families. Furthermore, following parental divorce, adolescents are two to three times as likely to receive psychological help than adolescents whose parents are not divorced (Zill, Morrison, & Coiro, 1993). Although divorce is associated with approximately a twofold increase in rates of adjustment problems in multiple domains, most adolescents from divorced homes adapt well.

The effects of parental divorce persist over time for some adolescents. Studies with representative samples in the United States, Britain, and Finland have demonstrated long-term effects on mental health problems, substance use, and educational attainment (Aro & Palosaari, 1992; Chase-Lansdale, Cherlin, & Kiernan, 1995; Zill et al., 1993). Similarly, a meta-analysis on the impact of parental divorce on adult adjustment reveals negative effects on psychological well-being, interpersonal relationships, educational and occupational success, and physical health (Amato & Keith, 1991b). Finally, it has been demonstrated that the life spans of people who experienced parental divorce prior to age 21 were more than 4 years shorter than their counterparts from intact homes.

THEORIES

There are two main theoretical perspectives for understanding the higher levels of adjustment problems among those who have experienced parental divorce. One focuses on the genetic transmission of personality traits and asserts that the link between parental divorce and adolescent adjustment problems is explained by a common genetic pathway. The other suggests that the constellation of stressful events associated with divorce adversely affects children's adjustment.

The *genetic self-selection hypothesis* suggests that personality traits of parents (e.g., antisocial traits) contribute to both divorce and child adjustment problems. According to this view, parents' personality traits increase the risk of family conflict and divorce, so that some people are more genetically vulnerable to marital dissolution. Twin studies indicate that genetic factors strongly influence personality characteristics that increase the likelihood of divorce (Jockin, McGue, & Lykken, 1996). According to these authors, personality characteristics may relate to children's adjustment problems

through an association with poor parenting, and also be genetically transmitted, thus directly increasing children's vulnerability to adjustment problems. While there is some support for this perspective, it appears that rather than genetically-transmitted traits wholly accounting for postdivorce adjustment problems, both genetic and environmental influences play important roles (O'Connor, Caspi, DeFries, & Plomin, 2000).

An alternative perspective, the *transitional-events model*, focuses on the process of multiple stressful changes and disruptions that occur in the family's social and physical environment before and after parental separation (Felner, Farber, & Primavera, 1983), such as interparental conflict, maternal depression, reduced contact with the non-residential parent, and financial distress. These stressors influences adjustment to the extent that they are mediated or moderated by intrapersonal factors, such as appraisals and coping strategies, and interpersonal factors (primarily within the family), such as parent–adolescent relationship and discipline. For example, interparental conflict may weaken adolescents' beliefs that they will be cared for, which in turn may lead to increased internalizing and externalizing problems. In this case, the beliefs that they will not be cared for mediate, or explain, the relations between conflict and problems. A warm parent–adolescent relationship may lessen the negative effects of divorce-related stressful events on adolescent problems. In this case, parental warmth would moderate, or reduce the strength of, the relation between stressors and problems.

Intra- and interpersonal factors that are causally linked to adolescent adjustment are potential targets for preventive interventions. If interventions can effectively modify these factors, then program-induced changes should prevent adjustment problems. Thus, research, that identifies potentially modifiable mediators and moderators can guide the development of effective interventions.

RESEARCH

We discuss the potentially modifiable intra- and interpersonal factors that have been most consistently associated with adjustment. Most evidence comes from cross-sectional studies; where they exist, prospective studies will be highlighted, as they provide more rigorous support for causal relations. When relations have been found consistently across multiple domains, we refer generally to adjustment; when the associations are more limited, we specify the particular outcome.

Stressful Divorce-Related Events

Consistent with the transitional events model, researchers have developed measures of the stressful events that occur following parental divorce. Inventories include both positive and negative events, such as "Mom and Dad argue in front of you" and "You do fun things with Dad." Stable positive events are associated with higher levels of adjustment, while increases in negative events are related to more adjustment problems (Sandler, Wolchik, Braver, & Fogas, 1991). The occurrence of life change events, such as moving, changing schools, or mother beginning work, are also related to adolescents' postdivorce adjustment problems (Stolberg, Camplair, Currier, & Wells, 1987). In addition, multiple transitions surrounding parents' partners living in the household are associated with higher levels of adjustment problems.

Accumulated research indicates that interparental conflict is one of the most damaging stressors associated with divorce (Amato & Keith, 1991a). Interparental conflict is related to conflict in the mother–adolescent relationship, and the detrimental impact of interparental conflict on adjustment may operate in part by creating feelings of being caught between parents and reducing the effectiveness of parenting. High levels of conflict are also associated with disengagement from the family, which in combination with antisocial peers, can lead to early sexual activity, drug use, and deviant behavior.

Interpersonal Factors

Mother–adolescent relationships that are characterized by warmth, supportiveness, effective problem-solving skills, positive communication, and low levels of conflict and negativity are associated with successful adolescent adaptation (Hetherington et al., 1992; Simons, 1996). Discipline that is consistent and appropriate also facilitates adolescent adjustment. In addition, high quality mother–adolescent relationships reduce the negative impact of divorce-related stressors on adjustment, and predict delinquent behavior in young adulthood.

Parental monitoring and family decision-making are additional aspects of parenting that are especially relevant to adolescent adjustment given the normative increases in independence, affiliation with peer groups, and the importance of educational and occupational goals. High levels of parental monitoring and joint decision-making are associated with low levels of externalizing, substance use, and academic difficulties (Buchanan, Maccoby, & Dornbusch, 1996).

Increases in maternal adjustment problems following divorce are not uncommon. Adjustment problems may reduce maternal warmth and place strains on the mother–adolescent relationship. This diminished parenting competence is related to higher adjustment problems in adolescents (Forgatch, Patterson, & Ray, 1996).

Father–Adolescent Relationship

The father–adolescent relationship has been relatively understudied. Although studies of the amount of contact have yielded mixed results, there is support for an association between relationship quality and adolescent adjustment. Non-custodial fathers' authoritative parenting is associated with lower levels of adjustment problems (Amato & Gilbreth, 1999). Further, some research suggests that a positive father–adolescent relationship mitigates the effect of interparental conflict on internalizing problems and predicts educational attainment and psychological adjustment in young adulthood (Forehand et al., 1991).

Intrapersonal Factors

Based on stress and coping theory assertions that the impact of stressful events is mediated through appraisals of them and that coping efforts are mobilized on the basis of these appraisals, researchers have examined the relations between appraisals, coping, and postdivorce adjustment. Threat appraisals, or the understanding of the personal significance of negative events, relate to internalizing problems cross-sectionally and longitudinally, and explain additional variance in adjustment above and beyond negative events (Sheets, Sandler, & West, 1996). Negatively biased appraisals about divorce events and attributions for the divorce itself are also related to adjustment. Researchers have demonstrated that *avoidant coping strategies* are associated with increased adjustment problems; while *active coping strategies* relate concurrently to lower antisocial behavior and substance use, and predict lower depression over time (Sandler, Tein, & West, 1994). Furthermore, coping efficacy, a global belief that one can deal with the demands made and the emotions aroused by a situation, is related to lower internalizing problems over time.

Summary

Researchers have demonstrated that divorce stressors, parenting, appraisals, and coping are consistently related to adolescents' postdivorce adjustment. However, it is important to note that these studies have focused almost exclusively on late childhood and early adolescence. Similarly, while the interventions reviewed in the following section have been evaluated in samples that include early adolescents, they were not specifically designed to foster adolescent adaptation to divorce. Although the findings may apply to mid- to late adolescence, research that specifically examines this developmental period is needed. In particular, longitudinal studies are necessary to elucidate the impact of divorce on adolescent developmental tasks and to identify risk and protective factors that are especially salient at this stage.

STRATEGIES: OVERVIEW

The transitional events model and empirical evidence supporting relations between intra- and interpersonal factors and postdivorce adjustment create a framework for the development of theory-based preventive interventions. Within this framework, the correlates of adjustment problems are viewed as putative mediators that are targeted for change. Carefully designed intervention trials, which include random assignment to condition, comparison of the intervention condition to a control group, and assessment of program effects on mediators as well as outcomes, evaluate the effectiveness of the intervention and provide an experimental test of the relations between putative mediators and adjustment problems. Preventive interventions to facilitate children's postdivorce adjustment have taken three forms: child-focused, parent-focused, and combined parent and child programs.

STRATEGIES THAT WORK

The interventions reviewed in this section have been evaluated in two experimental or quasi-experimental trials and have demonstrated program effects on adjustment problems. Some have also been shown to influence the putative mediators specified by the theory underlying the program.

Child/Adolescent-Focused Programs

These programs target intrapersonal factors, such as coping, problem-solving skills, and beliefs, and interpersonal factors over which children have some control (e.g., parent–child relationship). A key component is the group format, which is intended to provide social support and reduce the isolation and stigmatization that may follow parental divorce.

The Children's Support Group (CSG; Stolberg et al., 1987) and the Children of Divorce Intervention Program (CODIP; Pedro-Carroll, Alpert-Gillis, & Cowen, 1992; Pedro-Carroll, Sutton, & Black, 1993) are highly-similar school-based programs that teach specific cognitive–behavioral coping skills (i.e., anger control, problem-solving, relaxation), and foster the identification and expression of emotions. Both focus on distinguishing between problems that are within and beyond children's control, and practicing solving, or disengaging from problems. Unique to CODIP are its emphasis on processing of divorce-related feelings and experiences, and its aim to promote self-esteem and positive perceptions of one's family through discussions of the diversity of family structures. These programs consist of 10–12 sessions, and utilize techniques to facilitate emotional processing and maintain a high level of involvement (e.g., role plays, games).

These two programs have been evaluated with samples ranging from late childhood to early adolescence in multiple experimental and quasi-experimental trials. Program effects were assessed in terms of multiple measures of child adjustment, and in the case of CODIP, also on mediators of adjustment (e.g., divorce-related beliefs, problem-solving skills). Maintenance of effects over one year has also been evaluated. The strongest evaluation, conducted by Stolberg and Mahler (1994), demonstrated that participants (ages 8–12) in the CSG improved more on internalizing and externalizing problems at posttest and 1-year follow-up than did those in the randomly-assigned control group. In addition, compared to the control group, the CSG resulted in greater reductions in clinically significant levels of symptomatology. Three other evaluations provide further support for the effectiveness of these programs. Specifically, Stolberg and Garrison (1985) reported improvements in children's self-concept that were maintained at a 5-month follow-up, while Pedro-Carroll and her colleagues demonstrated program effects on teacher and group leader report of problem behavior and competence and child report of anxiety relative to a randomly-assigned control group (Pedro-Carroll & Cowen, 1985). In addition, the evaluations of CODIP provide some support for positive effects on children's cognitions (e.g., divorce-related misconceptions) and have demonstrated program effects in low-income populations (Pedro-Carroll et al., 1992).

Residential Parent-Focused Programs

These programs are designed to improve parenting practices and other interpersonal factors that parents may be able to influence (e.g., interparental conflict, non-residential parent visitation). Wolchik and her colleagues (1993) developed an intervention to change the following empirically supported mediators: mother–child relationship quality, effective discipline, father–child contact, and interparental conflict. The program consisted of 11 group and two individual sessions, which were used to tailor the program skills to individual family's needs.

The initial evaluation indicated positive program effects on mediators (i.e., mother–child relationship quality, effective discipline, maternal attitudes toward father's parenting, and willingness to change scheduled visits) as well as outcomes (i.e., child report of aggression and mother report of total behavior problems), relative to a randomly assigned control group (Wolchik et al., 1993). Mediational analyses indicated that mother–child relationship quality accounted for the program effect on children's adjustment. In general, the program effects were stronger for families functioning more poorly prior to participation in the program. A more recent evaluation of the program provides a replication of its beneficial effects with a larger sample (Wolchik et al., 2000). In comparison to a randomly assigned self-study condition, the program resulted in improved mother–child relationship quality, effective discipline, and maternal attitudes toward the father–child relationship. As with the first evaluation, there were no program effects on father–child contact or interparental conflict. At posttest, the children whose mothers participated in the program displayed lower levels of internalizing and externalizing problems than those in the self-study condition. At 6-month follow-up, the program effect on externalizing problems was maintained, and an effect on teacher report of acting out behavior emerged. Mother–child relationship and effective discipline mediated the effect of the program on child adjustment. Consistent with the first evaluation, program effects were stronger for families in which adjustment problems were higher and parenting was poorer prior to participation.

Summary

Carefully conducted evaluations provide an opportunity to determine which of the targeted intra- and interpersonal factors produce program effects, and thus increase understanding of the processes underlying postdivorce adjustment. Evaluations of residential parent-focused programs indicate that program-induced changes in parenting accounted for improvements in adjustment. Mediational analyses have not been conducted for the child/adolescent-focused programs. Thus, it is not clear which cognitive-behavioral coping skills or aspects of emotional processing account for program effects on adjustment.

STRATEGIES THAT MIGHT WORK

The programs reviewed in this section are diverse in intervention design and strength of evaluation. Some have demonstrated program effects on adjustment but evaluation design was weak; others have shown effects on empirically supported correlates of adjustment, but not on adjustment, and may also have been poorly evaluated. Future work that includes more rigorous methodology, refinements in program content, or both may indicate that these strategies reduce adjustment problems.

Adolescent-Focused Programs

While previously reviewed studies with children and early adolescents have demonstrated positive effects on adjustment, only two programs have been specifically designed to foster adolescent adjustment. However, these programs have not been evaluated using strong research designs (randomized experiments or strong quasi-experimental designs) and additional evidence of program effects is needed.

Pedro-Carroll et al. (1993) modified CODIP for seventh and eighth graders by incorporating material that is especially relevant to adolescent developmental tasks (e.g., trust in interpersonal relationships, hopes and goals for the future), and using techniques that are developmentally appropriate and interesting to adolescents (e.g., creative dramatics, charting significant life events, discussion of popular song lyrics). The results of a small pilot without a control group indicated that program participants reported improvements in anger control, as well as communication skills, trust, and more positive expectations for the future.

Short (1998) evaluated a 12-session school-based program designed specifically to reduce substance use given that children of divorce are at increased risk of developing such problems. This modification of the Stress Management and Alcohol Awareness Program (SMAAP), developed for children of alcoholics, targets the following potential mediators: coping, self-esteem, assertiveness, and alcohol expectancies. Participants in SMAAP (ages 10–13) reported improvements on mediators (i.e., self-esteem and problem-focused coping), as well as outcomes (i.e., anxiety, aggression, and alcohol use) in comparison to demographically matched adolescents whose parents were married.

Parent-Focused Programs

Several programs have shown encouraging effects to change empirically validated correlates of adjustment, but have not been shown to influence adolescent adjustment itself. One such program, the Single Parents' Support Group (SPSG), is a 12-session program for residential mothers that aims to facilitate children's adjustment primarily by improving mothers' adjustment (Stolberg & Garrison, 1985). The program was designed to provide social support, focus on aspects of identity development, and address parenting issues. Although the adjustment of mothers in the SPSG was marginally better than that of mothers in the control group at posttest, the program did not affect parenting skills or children's adjustment. These findings are surprising given that the link between maternal adjustment and child adjustment is well established. It appears that further work is needed to integrate programs that improve parents' adjustment with effective programs that improve parenting skills.

A second promising approach involves working with non-residential parents, such as Devlin and colleagues' Parenting for Divorced Fathers program. This 6-session program focuses on normalizing the experience of fatherhood following divorce and improving the father–child and co-parent relationships. A posttest evaluation indicated that fathers reported improvements on communication skills with children, as assessed by two items, relative to a waitlist control group (Devlin, Brown, Beebe, & Parulis, 1992). Child adjustment measures were not included.

Another approach is the parent education program that provides information in a brief, often didactic framework. These programs emphasize children's needs and the detrimental effects of interparental conflict, and are typically one session. The number of programs affiliated with the court system has almost tripled since 1994, with mandatory attendance to two thirds of them.

Three evaluations of parent education programs have shown some positive effects on interparental conflict. Shifflett and Cummings' (1999) evaluation demonstrated that relative to parents who attended a general parenting class, program participants reported a decrease in their own conflict behaviors. Participants in a program based on the "Children in the Middle" video reported putting their children in the middle of conflict less frequently at 6-month follow-up than a comparison group of parents who had filed for divorce before institution of the program (Arbuthnot & Gordon, 1996). Finally, an evaluation of the Children First program showed that compared to a group of divorcing parents from a county without a mandated program, parents who were more conflictual prior to participation reported declines on a measure that included conflict behaviors (Kramer & Washo, 1993). While Shifflett and Cummings did not assess child adjustment, the other two evaluations included single item measures and did not find program effects. Although the possibility of reducing conflict is promising, non-random assignment and inadequate measurement limit the interpretability of these findings. The preventive impact of such programs may involve an increased likelihood of obtaining more comprehensive services to facilitate postdivorce adjustment (Kramer & Washo, 1993).

A fourth strategy, divorce mediation, provides a dispute resolution alternative to the adversarial litigation process. Mediation has been successful in producing settlements more quickly and with which parents are more satisfied, and in reducing the likelihood of proceeding to court hearings. However, improvements in family functioning are limited and there is no evidence for program effects on child adjustment. A 12-year follow-up conducted by Emery and his colleagues provides a strong test of the effects of mediation as families were randomly offered mediation or litigation (Emery, Laumann-Billings, Waldron, Sbarra, & Dillon, 2001). Non-residential parents who mediated had more frequent contact with their children and were more involved in parenting (e.g., disciplining, discussing problems) relative to non-residential parents who litigated.

Combined Parent and Child/Adolescent Programs

A final promising, but as yet unproven, approach is to combine programs that involve both parents and children in an effort to produce additive effects over child-focused or parent-focused programs alone. Two models of combined programs have been evaluated. In one model, mothers and children attend separate, but concurrent groups. Stolberg and Garrison (1985) combined their CSG and SPSG programs; Wolchik and colleagues (2000) combined their residential mother-focused program and a child-focused program that targeted active and avoidant coping, negative appraisals of divorce stressors, and quality of mother–child relationship. An alternative model involves the addition of a transfer component to a child-focused program. Stolberg and Mahler (1994) developed a home workbook and a series of four parent workshops to facilitate the transfer of therapeutic gains to the home environment and increase parental support.

Three evaluations of combined programs have not demonstrated additive effects. Although Wolchik et al.'s (2000) combined program produced additive effects on threat appraisals and knowledge of appropriate coping strategies, no additive effects occurred for child adjustment at posttest or 6-month follow-up. The authors propose that also targeting coping efficacy may be necessary to impact adjustment. Stolberg and Garrison (1985) did not find additive effects, and moreover, the program effects demonstrated on children and mother's adjustment by the CSG and SPSG alone were not obtained in the combined condition. It is important to note that non-random assignment resulted in pre-intervention differences across conditions (e.g., lower employment status, longer time since separation). Finally, improvements in symptomatology in Stolberg and Mahler's (1994) combined and child-focused conditions were comparable. The authors suggest that the lack of additive effects may be due to problems surrounding sharing of the workbook, or alternatively, increased involvement by distressed parents may have had adverse effects on children's adjustment.

STRATEGIES THAT DO NOT WORK

The determination that strategies do not work depends on methodologically rigorous evaluations that include random assignment to condition, sufficient sample size to detect program effects, and measurement strategies with acceptable psychometric properties. To date, the paucity of such evaluations does not allow the identification of programs that do not affect adolescent adjustment. Careful evaluation of the promising programs reviewed above is a critical direction for the field. Such work, along with research that compares the effects of the few empirically supported programs, is needed to identify the programs that have the greatest potential to prevent mental health problems and to inform policy decisions about funding and mandating of programs.

SYNTHESIS

The evaluations reviewed provide support for the effectiveness of both child-focused and residential mother-focused interventions in facilitating adolescents' postdivorce adjustment. The findings demonstrate that both types of programs improved adjustment relative to randomly assigned control groups, and that these gains were maintained at short-term follow-ups. Moreover, these results support the effectiveness of targeting empirically supported correlates of adjustment. With regard to mother-focused programs, changes in parenting account for improved adolescent adjustment. Because the child-focused programs teach multiple skills and mediational analyses have not been conducted, it is not possible to determine which program components (e.g., self-disclosure, supportive feedback, problem-solving, anger management) contribute to changes in adjustment.

Efforts to develop programs that combine the effective child-focused and parent-focused interventions have been disappointing; the evaluations have demonstrated that the simple combination of programs is not sufficient. The lack of additive effects is surprising given that a wider array of putative mediators can be affected by involving both parents and adolescents. Greater integration of the parent and child programs, such as practicing skills together in session, discussing barriers to change, and developing family-related program goals, may lead to additive effects.

Future efforts to develop integrated approaches should focus not only on empirically supported correlates of postdivorce adjustment, but also on the ways in which divorce influences the developmental challenges of adolescence. For example, witnessing the disruption of marriage, and high levels of conflict in particular, may influence one's views of intimacy, trust, and commitment, and in turn make it more difficult to form stable, intimate relationships. Also, the detrimental impact of poor parenting often associated with divorce may be especially pronounced during adolescence. If parents are less available to provide support, help problem-solve, or monitor activities, adolescents may be at greater risk of affiliating with deviant peers and experiencing serious outcomes, such as substance abuse, arrests, or pregnancy. In addition, evidence that divorce may exacerbate adolescent developmental tasks is provided by the occurrence of a "sleeper" effect in which problems reemerge after desisting during childhood or develop for the first time during adolescence. For example, a longitudinal study of children of divorce found marked improvements in adjustment 2 years following divorce, but by mid-adolescence there were again elevations in adjustment problems compared to adolescents from nondivorced families.

Barber (1995) has proposed a framework for developing preventive interventions to improve adolescents' postdivorce adjustment based on an integration of empirically supported mediators and adolescent developmental tasks. She argues that targeting the parent–adolescent relationship, discipline, family decision-making, and maternal expectations in parallel programs for adolescents and residential mothers is the most effective and appropriate method given that family influences remain important in spite of increasing autonomy needs and reliance on peer networks. Such programs could incorporate interactive components that focus on developmentally appropriate tasks, such as renegotiation of the parent–adolescent relationship and conflict resolution skills. Rigorous evaluations are needed to determine if integrated programs for divorced families produce additive effects on adolescent outcomes. It is especially important for evaluations to assess program effects through the developmental transitions into late adolescence and adulthood when rates of serious problems, such as mental disorder and substance abuse, normatively increase.

Also see: Divorce: Childhood; Bereavement: Adolescence; Single-Parent Families: Childhood.

References

Amato, P.R., & Gilbreth, J. (1999). Nonresident fathers and children's well-being: A meta-analysis. *Journal of Marriage and the Family, 61,* 557–573.

Amato, P.R., & Keith, B. (1991a). Parental divorce and the well-being of children: A meta-analysis. *Psychological Bulletin, 110,* 26–46.

Amato, P.R., & Keith, B. (1991b). Parental divorce and adult well-being: A meta-analysis. *Journal of Marriage and the Family, 53,* 43–58.

Arbuthnot, J., & Gordon, D.A. (1996). Does mandatory divorce education for parents work? A six-month outcome evaluation. *Family and Conciliation Courts Review, 34,* 60–81.

Aro, H.M., & Palosaari, U.K. (1992). Parental divorce, adolescence, and transition to young adulthood: A follow-up study. *American Journal of Orthopsychiatry, 62,* 421–429.

Barber, B.L. (1995). Preventive intervention with adolescents and divorced mothers: A conceptual framework for program design and evaluation. *Journal of Applied Developmental Psychology, 16,* 481–503.

Buchanan, C.M., Maccoby, E.E., & Dornbusch, S.M. (1996). *Adolescents after divorce.* Cambridge, MA: Harvard University Press.

Chase-Lansdale, L.P., Cherlin, A.J., & Kiernan, K.E. (1995). The long term effects of parental divorce on the mental health of young adults: A developmental perspective. *Child Development, 66,* 1614–1634.

Devlin, A.S., Brown, E.H., Beebe, J., & Parulis, E. (1992). Parent education for divorced fathers. *Family Relations, 41,* 290–296.

Emery, R.E., Laumann-Billings, L., Waldron, M.C., Sbarra, D.A., & Dillon, P. (2001). Child custody mediation and litigation: Custody, contact, and coparenting 12 years after initial dispute resolution. *Journal of Consulting and Clinical Psychology, 69*, 323–332.

Felner, R.D., Farber, S.S., & Primavera, J. (1983). Transitions and stressful life events: A model for primary prevention. In R.D. Felner, L.A. Jason, J.N. Mortisugu, & S.S. Farber (Eds.), *Preventive psychology: Theory, research and practice* (pp. 81–108). New York: Pergamon Press.

Forehand, R., Wierson, M., McCombs Thomas, A., Fauber, R., Armistead, L., Kemptom, T., & Long, N. (1991). A short-term longitudinal examination of young adolescent functioning following divorce: The role of family factors. *Journal of Abnormal Child Psychology, 19*, 97–111.

Forgatch, M.S., Patterson, G.R., & Ray, J.A. (1996). Divorce and boys' adjustment problems: Two paths with a single model. In E.M. Hetherington & E.A. Blechman (Eds.), *Stress, coping, and resiliency in children and families*. Mahwah, NJ: L. Erlbaum Associates.

Hetherington, E.M., Clingmpeel, W.G., Anderson, E.R., Deal, J.E., Stanley Hagan, M., Hollier, E.A., & Linder, M.S. (1992). Coping with marital transitions: A family systems perspective. *Monographs of the Society for Research in Child Development, 57* (2–3, Serial No. 227).

Jockin, V., McGue, M., & Lykken, D.T. (1996). Personality and divorce: A genetic analysis. *Journal of Personality and Social Psychology, 71*, 288–244.

Kramer, L., & Washo, C.A. (1993). Evaluation of a court-mandated prevention program for divorcing parent: The Children First program. *Family Relations, 42*, 179–186.

O'Connor, T.G., Caspi, A., DeFries, J.C., & Plomin, R. (2000). Are associations between parental divorce and children's adjustment genetically mediated? An adoption study. *Developmental Psychology, 36*, 429–437.

Pedro-Carroll, J.L., Alpert-Gillis, L.J., & Cowen, E.L. (1992). An evaluation of the efficacy of a preventive intervention for 4th–6th grade urban children of divorce. *The Journal of Primary Prevention, 13*, 115–129.

Pedro-Carroll, J.L., & Cowen, E.L. (1985). The children of divorce intervention program: An investigation of the efficacy of a school-based prevention program. *Journal of Consulting and Clinical Psychology, 53*, 603–611.

Pedro-Carroll, J.L., Sutton, J.L., & Black, A.E. (1993). *The children of divorce intervention program: Preventive outreach to early adolescents* (Final report). Rochester, NY: Rochester Mental Health Association.

Sandler, I.N., Tein, J.Y., & West, S.G. (1994). Coping, stress, and the psychological symptoms of children of divorce: A cross-sectional and longitudinal study. *Child Develoment, 65*, 1744–1763.

Sandler, I., Wolchik, S., Braver, S., & Fogas, B. (1991). Stability and quality of life events and psychological symptomatology in children of divorce. *American Journal of Community Psychology, 19*, 501–520.

Sheets, V., Sandler, I.N., & West, S.G. (1996). Appraisals of negative events by preadolescent children of divorce. *Child Development, 67*, 2166–2182.

Shifflett, K., & Cummings, E.M. (1999). A program for educating parents about the effects of divorce and conflict on children: An initial evaluation. *Family Relations, 48*, 79–89.

Short, J.L. (1998). Evaluation of a substance abuse prevention and mental health promotion program for children of divorce. *Journal of Divorce and Remarriage, 28*, 139–155.

Simons, R.L. (1996). *Understanding differences between divorced and intact families: Stress, interaction, and child outcome.* Thousand Oaks, CA: Sage.

Stolberg, A.L., Camplair, C., Currier, K., & Wells, M.J. (1987). Individual, familial and environmental determinants of children's post-divorce adjustment and maladjustment. *Journal of Divorce, 11*, 51–70.

Stolberg, A.L., & Garrison, K.M. (1985). Evaluating a primary prevention program for children of divorce. *American Journal of Community Psychology, 13*, 111–124.

Stolberg, A.L., & Mahler, J. (1994). Enhancing treatment gains in a school-based intervention for children of divorce through skill training, parental involvement, and transfer procedures. *Journal of Consulting and Clinical Psychology, 62*, 147–156.

Wolchik, S.A., West, S.G., Sandler, I.N., Tein, J.Y., Coatsworth, D., Lengua, L., Weiss, L., Anderson, E.R., Greene, S.M., & Griffin, W.A. (2000). An experimental evaluation of theory-based mother and mother-child programs for children of divorce. *Journal of Consulting and Clinical Psychology, 68*, 843–856.

Wolchik, S.A., West, S.G., Westover, S., Sandler, I.N., Martin, A., Lustig, J., Tein, J.Y., & Fisher, J. (1993). The children of divorce parenting intervention: Outcome evaluation of an empirically-based program. *American Journal of Community Psychology, 21*, 293–331.

Zill, N., Morrison, D.R., & Coiro, M.J. (1993). Long term effects of parental divorce on parent–child relationships, adjustment, and achivement in young adulthood. *Journal of Family Psychology, 7*, 91–103.

E

Elder Abuse

Jane E. Fisher, Deborah Henderson, and Jeffrey Buchanan

INTRODUCTION

Elder abuse is often invisible. There are many reasons for this, including potential legal consequences for both the victim and the perpetrator which may affect their motivation to report the problem. Elderly persons competent to report their victimization are often ashamed or fearful of other potential consequences, including recrimination and the potential negative consequences for the perpetrator, who is typically a family member. The private setting in which abuse occurs further limits its detection. In recent years, a few widely publicized cases occurring in nursing homes have alerted and alarmed the public to this problem. While these accounts have served to raise interest in elder abuse, recent evidence suggests that abuse occurs etc. more frequently in private homes than in institutions. In this entry, we will describe dominant theoretical explanations for elder abuse. We will then summarize findings regarding risk factors associated with abuse. Drawing from the limited empirical literature we will then describe potentially effective primary prevention strategies for physical and psychological mistreatment.

DEFINITIONS

Research on elder abuse has been hindered by a lack of consensus on the definition of abuse. This lack of consensus has impeded advances in explanation and prevention, and limited a comparison of findings across studies. In addition, research reports rarely employ any theoretical framework, further limiting advances in explanation, and prevention.

While definitions vary, *elder abuse* is characterized by the following forms of maltreatment: physical abuse, psychological or verbal abuse, financial abuse or exploitation, and neglect. *Physical abuse* of an elderly person includes striking, pushing, or otherwise causing physical harm; *psychological abuse* includes threats, humiliation, enforced isolation, or repeated name calling; *financial abuse* or *exploitation* includes misusing money or taking control of possessions or property without permission or legal rights to do so; *neglect* includes refusing medical assistance, food or required medications, failure to provide adequate care such as bathing, or (in the case of self-neglect) failing to perform adequate daily care activities such as grooming or eating (Penhale, 1993; Wolf, 1996).

SCOPE

It is estimated that between 4 and 10 percent of the elderly population has been or is being abused (Ansello, 1996). While the majority of abuse occurs in private homes, abuse within nursing homes is common. In a survey of nursing home aides, 10 percent reported committing a physically abusive act, either using excessive restraint or hitting, punching or shoving a resident; 41 percent admitted committing psychological abuse during the past year; and 9 percent admitted that they had sworn at or insulted a resident under their care (Bitzan & Kruzich, 1990). Unfortunately, there are no data available with regard to the costs associated with elder abuse.

THEORIES

Few theories address elder abuse per se but instead have been developed to explain violence in other populations and then extended to the victimization of the elderly.

Social Exchange Theory

Social exchange theory assumes that social interactions involve the exchange of rewards and costs (Finkelhor, 1983; Phillips, 1989). According to this theory, rewards include resources (e.g., money, support), services or positive sentiments while costs includes negative sentiments or the withdrawal or loss of resources. When the exchange of rewards and costs is unbalanced in a relationship for which there is little likelihood of future reciprocity (e.g., when one person always gives more rewards than he or she receives in return), then that person may become frustrated, and this frustration might lead to aggression, including abuse. This theory has received support from the descriptive literature which shows that dependency of the abuser on the victim is a risk factor for elder abuse (Wolf, Strugnell, & Godkin, 1982).

Stress Theory and its Variations

Social exchange theory is one type of stress model, where an exhausted caregiver has such stress as to behave in an abusive manner (Curry & Stone, 1995). Other forms of this model include the external stress theory, which suggests that when individuals face intense stress not directly related to caregiving (such as from job stress, marital stress, financial pressures), then their care recipients are at greater risk of abuse. Prevention efforts derived from stress theories involve relieving caregiving stress through provision of respite, emotional support such as through support groups and helplines (Eastman, 1984; Grafstrom, Nordberg, & Winblad, 1992) and through instrumental support services like Meals on Wheels, and home care services.

Transgenerational Violence

The theory of transgenerational violence holds that abuse is a learned behavior. Victims of child abuse are considered to be at greater risk for becoming abusers than are individuals who were not child abuse victims (Kosberg, 1988; Janz, 1990). This pattern has been called the "cycle of violence." According to this theory, perpetrators are likely to have a learning history in which aggression was negatively reinforced by consequences such as a reduction in frustration or physiological arousal. This theory has been empirically tested with other types of perpetrators (e.g., spouse abusers, Hotaling and Sugarman, 1990; and child abusers, Straus, Gelles, & Steinmetz, 1980), but there have been no empirical reports describing the validity of transgenerational violence theory for elder abuse (Biggs, Kingston, & Phillipson, 1995).

Ageism

Ageism is a form of prejudice that involves devaluing elderly individuals based on their chronological age (Palmore, 1990). Prejudicial attitudes may lead to abusive behavior if the needs or rights of the elderly are seen as less important than the needs or rights of other people, particularly the caregiver (Fulmer, 1989). This theory would lead to predictions of higher rates of elder abuse in cultures where old age is associated with negative stereotypes involving dependency and incompetence (e.g., in industrialized western culture) than in cultures where old age is associated with desirable attributes such as knowledge or wisdom. Caregiving of an elderly relative in an ageist culture may be viewed more with resentment than with privilege, thus increasing the risk of abuse.

RESEARCH

Risk Factors Associated with Elder Abuse

For ethical reasons research on the etiology of elder abuse is correlational, focusing on identifying risk rather than causal factors. *Risk factors* are characteristics of the victim, the perpetrator, or the environment that increase the probability that elder abuse will occur. Identifying risk factors is critical if prevention is to be initiated (Henderson, Buchanan, & Fisher, 2002).

Victim Characteristics
Gender

Historically, it has been assumed that most victims of elder abuse were women (O'Malley, 1987; Wolf et al., 1982). This assumption was based on the greater proportion of elderly women in the population, and perceptions of women as physically weaker and more passive—characteristics believed to increase their vulnerability to physical mistreatment. However, empirical accounts indicate that there in fact are more male than female victims of elder abuse (Tatara, 1993). Explanations for this finding have included retribution by women against men for past abuse and the greater likelihood of caregivers being women.

Age/Impairment

As elderly people age, the probability that they will be abused increases (Whittaker, 1993). Age is associated with more health problems and therefore greater impairment, which may make the elderly person more reliant upon and therefore more vulnerable to the abuser (who may be experiencing excessive stress). Block and Sinnot (1979) have documented that the risk of abuse increases with physical or mental impairment. This is especially the case when we consider individuals with a diagnosis of dementia, who can exhibit aggressive behaviors during caregiving tasks (O'Malley, Everitt, O'Malley, & Campion, 1983). Caregivers may not understand this aggressive behavior as being a consequence of a medical condition and instead view the behavior as uncooperativeness or retaliatory in nature (Garcia & Kosberg, 1993; Kosberg & Cairl, 1986). Alternatively, some caregivers state that even though they do understand that the elderly person's behavior is due to an impairment and not intentional, they justify their abusive behavior as resulting from anger toward the elderly person's behavior (Garcia & Kosberg, 1993).

Psychological Problems

Depression, anxiety, and substance abuse are problems that have been found to increase the risk of abuse. Elderly individuals with these problems have been found to be more likely to deny abuse, make internal attributions for the abuse, fail to take action to protect oneself from abuse, and/or experience social isolation which is another risk factor for abuse (Grafstrom et al., 1992). For substance abusing elderly individuals, the risk may be an unstable living situation or the likelihood of the elderly person experiencing impaired judgment placing them in jeopardy (Kosberg, 1988). Further, a substance-abusing individual may behave in erratic, insensitive, or otherwise ineffective ways that provoke confrontation. Aggressive behavior directed toward a caregiver may function to increase the probability of abusive behavior (Henderson et al., in press).

Perpetrator Characteristics

Gender

Perpetrators of elder abuse tend to be young or middle-aged caregiving adults living with or close to the elderly victim (Quinn & Tomita, 1986). Women are more likely to be caregivers and hence to perpetrate elder abuse.

Psychological Problems

Psychopathology has been identified as a risk factor for engaging in elder abuse. Substance abuse has been identified as a particular risk factor. Substance abuse may reduce a caregiver's ability to regulate his/her emotions and behavior during stressful caregiving situations thereby increasing the risk of abuse (Fulmer, 1989; Godkin, Wolf, & Pillemer, 1989; O'Malley, Segel, & Perez, 1979; Pillemer & Wolf, 1989). In addition, substance abuse may impair a caregiver's judgment regarding the care receiver's needs.

Caregiving Skills

Caregivers of elderly individuals are usually family members who lack formal training in caregiving skills. Skills deficits are problematic when the care recipient is physically frail, cognitively impaired, and/or exhibits challenging behaviors such as aggression or agitation. In these circumstances, caregiver aggression may be used to gain control. It is also common for untrained caregivers to personalize a cognitively impaired care receiver's challenging behavior or to interpret it as voluntary rather than as the result of a dementing illness.

Stress

Extensive research over the past 20 years has documented that providing care for an elderly person can be extremely stressful (Lawton & Rubenstein, 2000; Schulz, 2000). When the stress of caregiving, in addition to everyday life stressors, exceeds the emotional and instrumental resources of the caregiver, caregivers are at greater risk for engaging in abusive behavior (Hudson, 1986). To illustrate, Wolf and Pillemer (1989) found that 34 percent of a sample of caregivers in abuse cases reported long-term financial problems while 24 percent reported a recent financial difficulty; 32 percent reported a recent change in living arrangements; 26 percent reported a long-term medical complaint; 24 percent reported a recent medical complaint; and 15 percent reported a recent divorce.

Dependence

Dependence of the caregiver on the care recipient, typically financial, has been associated with an increased probability of physical and psychological abuse (Pillemer, 1985; Wolf & Pillemer, 1989). It has been generally assumed that it is the dependency of the victim, not the abuser, that determines the vulnerability of the older person to abuse. However, it appears that this is more often true in cases of neglect, where caregiving is seen as an unwanted obligation. When caregivers depend upon the elderly care recipient for financial or emotional support, they tend to report more feelings of anger, impotence, and frustration (Curry & Stone, 1995). These feelings may lead to an increased probability of abuse.

Contextual Risk Factors

Environmental factors may increase the probability of elder abuse. These include financial difficulties, a history of family violence or family conflict, and inadequate social support.

Financial Difficulties

Caregiving often results in financial burden for families. Expenses associated with medication, medical equipment, and the need for 24 hr care coupled with a loss of wages for an employed caregiver may contribute to feelings of frustration, anxiety, depression, and/or hopelessness in both the caregiver and care receiver. When the demands of caregiving occur against a background of financial pressure, the risk of provocative and/or abusive behavior is increased.

Inadequate Social Support

Research has consistently demonstrated the importance of social support for decreasing the burden of caregiving (Schulz, 2000). Social support assists both the caregiver and the care recipient. Socially isolated caregivers experience low rates of pleasant activities, increased stress, increased risk of depression, anger, and related symptoms. Socially isolated care recipients are at risk for depression and increased health problems leading to an increased demand on the caregiver (Gottlieb, 1991).

STRATEGIES THAT WORK

Unfortunately, the nature of elder abuse—including the covert nature of abuse and the stigma associated with it and attendant methodological issues—prevents researchers from establishing with certainty that any particular approach to prevention is effective in the prevention of elder abuse. However, there are some promising interventions being implemented that could be effective.

STRATEGIES THAT MIGHT WORK

Educational Programs

Prevention strategies reduce the probability that elder abuse will occur by addressing the risk factors that are associated with abuse. The most common primary prevention programs focus on education (Wiehe, 1998), which may be directed toward the general public, health care personnel and other professionals, caregivers, family members, or the potential elderly victim. Public service announcements, advertisements, workshops, published research findings, and other types of awareness enhancing strategies provide individuals with information on the definition and prevalence of abuse, the risk factors for elder abuse, and how to report potentially abusive situations (Weiner, 1991).

Public education programs function to normalize the stress of caregiving by informing caregivers that their experience is not unique and that it is not unusual for people in their position to feel overwhelmed. Normalizing caregiver stress may reduce the stigma associated with common emotional responses, resulting in increased utilization of available resources and a decrease in the number and/or severity of risk factors (Henderson et al., in press). Educational programs should avoid tactics that punish the caregiver by blaming him or her for ineffective behavior, a strategy that typically results in increasing feelings of guilt and defensiveness. Programs that evoke such negative affect in a caregiver will likely reduce willingness to self-report and to address problematic behaviors.

Providing potential victims with information about elder abuse and resources available to prevent abuse may increase assistance-seeking behavior. It is important that education programs validate the elderly person's fears and target irrational views involving shame, self-blame, and the consequences of reporting abuse.

Primary care physicians, in particular, are on the front lines in the prevention of elder abuse. Educating physicians about risk factors associated with elder abuse and informing them that it is critically important that they directly assess for abuse is an inexpensive and potentially far-reaching approach to prevention given the extensive contact elderly individuals have with their primary care physicians. If elder abuse is suspected, the physician (or other health care professional) must conduct a more directed assessment that is designed to obtain specific information about what kind of abuse may be occurring. Several protocols are available to assist physicians in conducting more thorough investigations of elder abuse, including the American Medical Association's diagnostic and treatment guidelines (1992). This said, it must be emphasized that education alone is insufficient to reduce elder abuse. It is when education is combined with the next intervention that positive results might occur.

Caregiver Services

In addition to education, important prevention strategies include providing services which decrease the dependency of the caregiver on the potential victim—and vice versa—and providing services that directly address the risk factors for elder abuse, such as substance abuse, stress, or inadequate caregiving skills (see Biegel & Schulz, 1999) for reviews of caregiver interventions). Services that may decrease the dependency of the caregiver on the elderly care recipient include job training skills or child care services and psychological treatment targeted at increasing social support, interpersonal skills or other relevant domains that are interfering with normal adult functioning. Services that target the dependency of the elderly person on the caregiver include respite programs such as adult day care services, programs such as Meals on Wheels, home health care services, assistance with personal finances and other household tasks such as shopping and housecleaning, and psychological treatment to address problems (e.g., depression, social isolation) that may make it more difficult for the elderly person to engage in self-care or to find support from someone other than the caregiver.

Alternative services that address risk factors for elder abuse include stress and anger management workshops, caregiver skills training, and social support. Gallagher-Thompson (1994) describes two interventions for reducing caregiver stress, *Coping With the Blues* and *Coping With Frustration*. Both programs are designed for a group format, maximizing cost-effectiveness and efficiency while at the same time providing social interaction/support opportunities for caregivers. The *Coping With the Blues* workshop focuses on integrating pleasant events into caregivers' daily routines, with an emphasis on developing plans to overcome barriers to engaging in these activities. The *Coping With Frustration* workshop is designed to teach caregivers relaxation skills, coping skills to use when angry, assertiveness skills, and appropriate ways to express anger and frustration.

STRATEGIES THAT DO NOT WORK

For the same reasons that we cannot determine which strategies are clearly effective for the prevention of elder abuse, we cannot say with certainty which strategies are not effective. However, it can be inferred that strategies which focus only on the "immorality" of abuse, and ignore the factors involved in initiating and maintaining abusive behaviors will not be effective in eliminating abuse. It can be further inferred that strategies which ignore the perpetrator will be of limited effectiveness.

SYNTHESIS

A consequence of the graying of America is that the problem of elder abuse is likely to increase. The need for research on the effectiveness of primary prevention programs is clear. While programs are in place, problems of detection limit the ability to determine if they are effective and, if so, with whom. Consensus regarding the definition of elder abuse would increase meaningful comparisons across prevention programs and enhance efforts to understand the possible causes of elder abuse. In particular, we would suggest that successful strategies for the prevention of elder abuse would be aimed at both at-risk elders and potential perpetrators. These strategies should be systematically interconnected: educational programs for frontline helping professionals, as well as for elders and family members or other caregivers, in order to make them aware of the concern and that there are preventive solutions for it. Caregiver services like anger management workshops, respite care, and support groups, in order to help caregivers manage their tasks more effectively and with less personal stress. These few strategies serve to highlight the important fact that we have only begun to consider the ways to prevent elder abuse.

Also see: Age Bias: Older Adulthood; Caregiver Strees: Older Adulthood; Life Challenges: Older Adulthood.

References

Ansello, E.F. (1996). Causes and theories. In L.A. Baumhover & S.C. Beall (Eds.), *Abuse, neglect and exploitation of older persons* (pp. 9–29). Baltimore, MD: Health Professions Press.

Biegel, D.E., & Schulz, R. (1999). Caregiving and caregiver interventions in aging and mental illness. *Family relations: Interdisciplinary Journal of Applied Family Studies, 48*, 345–354.

Biggs, S., Kingston, P.A., & Phillipson, C. (1995). *Elder abuse perspectives*. Buckingham: Open University Press.

Bitzan, J.E., & Kruzich, J.M. (1990). Interpersonal relationships of nursing home residents. *Gerontologist, 30*, 385–390.

Block, M.R., & Sinnot, J.D. (1979). *The battered elder syndrome: An exploratory study*. College Park: University of Maryland Centre on Ageing.

Curry, L.C., & Stone, J.G. (1995). Understanding elder abuse: The social problem of the 1990s. *Journal of Clinical Geropsychology, 1*(2), 147–156.

Eastman, M. (1984). At worst just picking up the pieces. *Community Care, 20*(1), 20–22.

Finkelhor, D. (1983). Common features of family abuse. In D. Finkelhor, R. Gelles, G. Hotaling, & M. Strauss (Eds.), *The dark side of families: Current family violence research*. Beverly Hills: Sage.

Fulmer, T.T. (1989). Mistreatment of elders: Assessment, diagnosis, and intervention. *Nursing Clinics of North America, 23*(3), 707–716.

Gallagher-Thompson, D. (1994). Clinical intervention strategies for distressed caregivers: Rationale and development of psychoeducational approaches. In E. Light, G. Niederehe, & B.D. Lebowitz (Eds.), *Stress effects on family caregivers of Alzheimer's patients: Research and interventions* (pp. 260–277). New York: Springer.

Garcia, J.L., & Kosberg, J.I. (1993). Understanding anger: Implications for formal and informal caregivers. *Journal of Elder Abuse and Neglect, 4*(4), 87–99.

Gottlieb, B.H. (1991). Social support and family care of the elderly. *Canadian Journal on Aging, 10*(4), 359–375.

Grafstrom, M., Nordberg, A., & Winblad, B. (1992). Abuse is in the eye of the beholder. *Scandinavian Journal of Social Medicine, 21*(4), 247–255.

Henderson, D., Buchanan, J.A., & Fisher, J.E. (in press). Prevention of elder abuse. In P. Schewe (Ed.), *Developmentally appropriate approaches to the prevention of intimate partner violence.* Washington, DC: American Psychological Association.

Hotaling, G.T., & Sugarman, D.B. (1990). Prevention of wife assault. In R.T. Ammerman & M. Hersen (Eds.), *Treatment of family violence.* New York: John Wiley & Sons.

Hudson, M.F. (1986). Elder mistreatment: Current research. In K.A. Pillemer & R.S. Wolf (Eds.), *Elder abuse: Conflict in the family* (pp.125–166). Dover, MA: Auburn House.

Janz, M. (1990, September–October). Clues to elder abuse. *Geriatric Nursing,* 220–222.

Kosberg, J.I. (1988). Preventing elder abuse: Identification of high risk factors prior to placement decisions. *Gerontologist, 28*(1), 43–50.

Kosberg, J.I., & Cairl, R.E. (1986). The cost of care index: A case management tool for screening informal care providers. *Gerontologist, 26,* 273–278.

Lawton, M.P., & Rubenstein, R.L. (2000). *Interventions in dementia care: Towards improving quality of life.* New York, NY: Springer.

O'Malley, T.A. (1987). Abuse and neglect of the elderly: The wrong issue? *Pride Institute Journal of Long Term Health Care, 5,* 25–28.

O'Malley, T.A., Everitt, D.E., O'Malley, H.C., & Campion, E.W. (1983). Identifying and preventing family-mediated abuse and neglect of elderly persons. *Annals of Internal Medicine, 98,* 998–1005.

Palmore, E.B. (1990). *Ageism: Negative and positive.* NY: Springer.

Penhale, B.(1993). The abuse of elderly people: Considerations for practice. *British Journal of Social Work, 23,* 95–112.

Phillips, L.R. (1989). Issues involved in identifying and intervening in elder abuse. In R. Finlinson & S. Ingman (Eds.), *Elder abuse: Practice and policy* (pp. 197–217). New York: Human Sciences Press.

Pillemer, K.A. (1985). The dangers of dependency: New findings on domestic violence of the elderly. *Social Problems, 33,* 146–158.

Quinn, M.J., & Tomita, S.K. (1986). *Elder abuse and neglect: Causes, diagnoses, and intervention strategies.* New York: Springer.

Schulz, R. (Ed.) (2000). *Handbook on dementia caregiving: Evidence-based interventions for family caregivers.* New York, NY: Springer.

Strauss, M., Gelles, R., & Steinmetz, S. (1980). *Behind closed doors: Violence in the American family.* New York: Doubleday.

Tatara, T. (1993). *Summaries of the statistical data on elder abuse in domestic settings for FY90 and FY91: A final report.* Washington, DC: National Aging Resource Center on Elder Abuse.

Weiner, A. (1991). A community-based education model for identification and prevention of elder abuse. *Journal of Gerontological Social Work, 16,* 107–119.

Whittaker, T. (1993). Rethinking elder abuse: Towards an age and gender integrated theory of elder abuse. In P. Decalmer & F. Glendenning (Eds.), *The mistreatment of elderly people* (pp. 116–128). London: Sage.

Wiehe, V.R. (1998). *Understanding family violence: Treating and preventing partner, child, sibling, and elder abuse.* London: Sage.

Wolf, R.S. (1996). Elder abuse and family violence: Testimony presented before the Senate Special Committee on Aging. *Journal of Elder Abuse & Neglect, 8*(1), 81–96.

Wolf, R.S., & Pillemer, K. (1989). *Helping elder victims: The reality of elder abuse.* New York: Columbia University Press.

Wolf, R.S., Strugnell, E.P., & Godkin, M.A. (1982). *Preliminary findings from the model projects on elderly abuse.* Worcester, MA: University of Massachusetts Center on Aging.

Environmental Health, Early Childhood

Maureen T. Mulroy and Joan Bothell

INTRODUCTION AND DEFINITIONS

Environmental health, according to the World Health Organization (WHO, 1997b), "comprises those aspects of human health, disease, and injury that are determined or influenced by factors in the environment. This includes the direct pathological effects of various chemical, physical and biological agents, as well as the effects on health of the broad physical and social environment, which includes housing, urban development, land-use and transportation, industry, and agriculture." WHO (2000) divides environmental threats into two categories—"traditional" hazards and "modern" hazards—each of which has associated health risks.

Traditional environmental hazards are those associated with poverty and lack of economic or technical development. They include lack of access to safe drinking water, inadequate basic household and community sanitation, food contaminated with pathogens, indoor air pollution from cooking and heating using coal or biomass fuel, inadequate solid waste disposal, occupational injury hazards in agriculture and cottage industries, and natural disasters, including floods, droughts, and earthquakes (WHO, 2000). Today, the children who suffer most from traditional hazards are poor children—especially those under five years old—who live in the poorest countries. Among the most serious problems are unsafe drinking water and contaminated foods, which cause illness and death through diarrhea and other infections, both because the children are exposed to infectious organisms and because their immune systems may be suppressed by contaminants and malnutrition. Street children in Cambodia, for example, scavenge food from a city dump, where they are exposed not only to contaminated food and water, but also to disease-carrying mosquitoes, rats, and other pests and contaminants. Moreover, these children and their families lack access to immunizations, quality health care, and knowledge necessary to avoid illness (Carpenter et al., 2000, p. 989).

In the developed world, many traditional hazards have been addressed through vaccines and antibiotics and through technical improvements in sanitation, heating, and ventilation. As less developed countries modernize, the environmental hazards they face are changing from the traditional to the modern. *Modern environmental hazards* are those related to development that is not sustainable (i.e., development that exhausts or degrades finite natural resources) and that lacks health and environmental safeguards.

Worldwide, modern hazards include water pollution from populated areas, industry, and intensive agriculture; urban air pollution from automobiles, coal-powered energy generators, and industry; solid and hazardous waste accumulation; chemical and radiation hazards stemming from industrial and agricultural technologies; emerging and re-emerging infectious disease hazards; deforestation, land degradation, and major ecological changes; and climate change, stratospheric ozone depletion, and transboundary pollution (WHO, 2000). New aspects of environmental hazards are emerging. For example, in the next decade, hundreds of millions of computers, most of them containing significant amounts of lead and other hazardous materials, will become obsolete and may end up in landfills.

More than 75,000 chemicals are manufactured in the United States (Roe, Pease, Florini, & Silbergeld, 1997). US industries put at least 2.4 billion pounds of chemicals into the air every year. Yet little is known about the health effects on children of most of these chemicals. Some are known or suspected of causing cancer, while others affect the nervous system or disrupt the endocrine (hormonal) system.

Primary prevention efforts in the United States increasingly emphasizes chronic conditions, which include asthma, learning disabilities, birth defects, and childhood cancers, all of which may have some environmental causes or triggers. Today, chronic conditions comprise the number one cause of death in the United States.

Worldwide, acute exposures caused by environmental disasters are yet another concern. Some of the worst examples have been widely reported. From 1956 to 1967, residents of Minamata, Japan, ate fish contaminated with methyl mercury that was discharged from a local chemical factory. The children of women who had eaten the fish showed an elevated incidence of cerebral palsy, mental retardation, severe birth defects, sight and hearing loss, paralysis, and death. In 1976, an explosion at a chemical factory in Seveso, Italy, released dioxin and other chemicals into the atmosphere, contaminating people, animals, plants, and soil around the factory. In 1978, when an investigation of health problems revealed that the Love Canal neighborhood in Niagara Falls, New York, had been built on a former chemical waste dump, the area had to be evacuated. In 1984, a toxic gas leak from a US chemical plant in Bhopal, India, killed thousands of people and injured hundreds of thousands. In 1986, a nuclear reactor accident in Chernobyl, Ukraine, contaminated a large area of Ukraine, Belarus, and Russia, requiring the evacuation of some 200,000 people. Radiation from the accident spread over most of Europe. This nuclear disaster is believed to be the cause of genetic mutations and a substantial increase in the incidence of thyroid cancer in children living around Chernobyl.

SCOPE

According to the WHO (2000), "poor environmental quality is responsible for around 25 percent of all preventable ill-health in the world today." In Asia, millions of children die each year from diarrhea, often the result of drinking contaminated water. In Bangladesh, children are at risk of developing cancer from drinking well water that is contaminated with naturally occurring arsenic. In the Philippines, they are at risk of poisoning from eating fish contaminated with mercury, cadmium, and lead from mining waste dumped into the offshore ocean. In Vietnam, where millions of gallons of the defoliant Agent Orange were sprayed during the Vietnam War, stillbirths, spontaneous abortions, and birth defects have increased (Carpenter et al., 2000). Elsewhere, children have been poisoned—sometimes killed—by exposures to lead from leaded gasoline and mining operations, fungicides in seed grain, pesticides in agricultural fields, PCBs in cooking oil, and rat-killing chemicals in tortillas. Moreover, children are often exposed to multiple toxins, which may greatly increase their risks.

In the United States, according to the Pew Environmental Health Commission (2000, p. 2), chronic health problems with known or suspected links to environmental causes affect more than 100 million Americans a year, at a cost of $325 billion in healthcare and lost productivity. Children are the most susceptible members of the population.

Respiratory ailments related to environmental conditions illustrate the problem. According to the US Environmental Protection Agency (EPA), more than 25 percent of US children live in areas that do not meet national air quality standards. Asthma, a disease that is believed to have both environmental and genetic causes, is the most prevalent chronic disease among children. Nearly 5 million US children under 18 years of age have asthma. About 150,000 of these children are hospitalized each year, and 600 die from the disease (USEPA, 1998, p. 7). Treatment costs in 1990 were estimated at $6.2 billion. Projected costs for the year 2000 were $14.5 billion, with the increase attributed to higher incidence and greater medical costs.

Exposure to environmental tobacco smoke (ETS) may account for 150,000–300,000 cases of lung infections, such as bronchitis and pneumonia, in infants and toddlers each year. Of these, 7,500–15,000 young children are hospitalized. It is estimated that children exposed to ETS in their homes miss 7 million more school days each year than do other children because of respiratory illnesses (USEPA, 1998, pp. 8–9).

Developmental disorders in children are another important area of concern. The National Academy of Sciences (NAS) estimates that 25 percent of such disorders may be caused by a combination of genes and environmental factors. The academy warned that at least 60,000 infants each year could be at risk for lower intelligence and learning disabilities because their mothers had eaten mercury-contaminated fish and seafood (NAS, 2000). Some 890,000 US children under the age of 6 suffer from lead poisoning, which permanently lowers their intelligence, decreases attention span, causes hyperactivity, and impairs growth.

The USEPA (1998, p. 36) estimates that 4 million US children live within one mile of a hazardous waste site, that is, a site that contains substances that are known to be carcinogenic or corrosive, present the danger of fire or explosion, or otherwise represent a serious health hazard.

Environmental factors are believed to play a role in many birth defects, which are the leading cause of infant mortality in the United States and result in some 6,500 deaths each year (Pew Environmental Health Commission, 2000, p. 5).

THEORY AND RESEARCH

Children's Special Vulnerabilities

Like adults, children are exposed to toxic substances by eating and drinking them (ingestion), breathing them (inhalation), and coming into skin (dermal) contact with them. But physiologically, metabolically, psychologically, and behaviorally, children are not "little" adults. They are at greater risk than adults for exposure to environmental hazards and are more susceptible to illnesses from those hazards. Nonetheless, current environmental health standards are based on exposures of healthy adult males, not developing fetuses, infants, children, and adolescents. According to the world's economic leaders, "evidence is growing that pollution at levels or concentrations below existing alert thresholds can cause or contribute to human health problems and our countries' present levels of protection may not, in some cases, provide children with adequate protection" (WHO, 1997a). Among the most important environmental health threats to children worldwide are persistent organic pollutants, pesticides, hazardous chemicals and hazardous waste, lead, microbiologically contaminated drinking water, air pollution, ETS, and endocrine-disrupting chemicals (EDCs).

There are several reasons for children's special vulnerability to environmental hazards.

Children Are Exposed to More Environmental Threats Than Are Adults

In comparison to adults, children eat proportionately more food, drink more fluids, and breathe more air per pound of body weight. Their diets are usually less varied, and they generally eat more fruit, vegetables, and dairy products than do adults. Children therefore have substantially heavier exposures pound for pound than adults to any toxins that are present in water, food, or air (Landrigan et al., 1998, p. 788).

Children Are More Susceptible to Environmental Threats

Children's metabolic and physiological processes are different from those of adults. Their immune systems are developing, and they may be less able than healthy adults to recover rapidly from illnesses and stressors. Very young children may not metabolize, detoxify, and excrete certain toxins as effectively as adults. For example, children absorb up to 50 percent of the lead they ingest, while adults absorb only about 10 percent. Their smaller body size may make them more vulnerable. For example, their smaller airways are more susceptible to breathing problems caused by air pollution.

Children Are Undergoing Rapid Growth and Development, and the Developmental Processes Are Easily Disrupted

Cells are most susceptible to damage from environmental toxins when they are actively growing. From conception through early childhood, children's immune, respiratory, and nervous systems undergo rapid growth and development. If the growth and development of the critical structures and pathways are adversely influenced at this time, the chances of attaining a healthy adulthood are dramatically decreased. For this reason, the timing of exposure with respect to a child's development, as well as the degree of exposure, may have important health consequences (Chai & Bearer, 1999). Each of the following developmental stages has characteristic sources of exposure and health effects (Chai & Bearer, 1999).

Preconception. Parental environmental exposures even before a child is conceived can damage the fetus, because toxins can damage the maternal or paternal reproductive organs or can be stored in the body and mobilized during pregnancy, when they may affect the developing fetus. For example, a woman's exposure to lead or PCBs, even before she becomes pregnant, may damage an infant conceived later.

Fetus. Fetal cells are growing very rapidly and are especially susceptible to damage. Toxic substances that are known to cross the placenta and reach the fetus include lead, mercury, carbon monoxide (CO), ETS, PCBs, and dioxin. Many of these substances are neurotoxic, that is, they may alter the normal processes of cell growth and the development of the brain and nervous system.

Newborn. Newborns may be exposed to toxic substances through ingestion, inhalation, and dermal contact. Breast milk may contain smoking byproducts, lead, or PCBs, and formula, especially if it is made with contaminated water, may contain various toxins. A newborn's gastrointestinal system more readily absorbs lead, PCBs, and dioxin compounds. Babies can also be harmed by inhaling lead dust or ETS, and their skin can readily absorb some toxic substances, such as some pesticides.

Infant/toddler. Children in this stage are particularly vulnerable to inhaled and ingested toxins. Because they have higher respiration rates than do adults, infants/toddlers exposed to ETS absorb more toxicants per kilogram than adults. Normal behavior also places infants and toddlers at risk. They may chew on lead-painted windowsills or on objects contaminated with pesticides. Crawling on the floor exposes them to pesticides, radon, formaldehyde from new synthetic carpeting, and particles from ETS.

Preschool and School-Age Child. Childcare facilities, schools, and playgrounds may present environmental hazards. Dangers can include lead-based paint, lead-contaminated water, asbestos in playground sand or in building components, poor indoor or outdoor air quality (from sources such as art or janitorial supplies, or exhaust from school buses), toxic residues from prior use of the site, pesticides, and the use of toxic preservatives like arsenic on wooden playground equipment.

Children's Normal Behavior Exposes Them to Different Environmental Hazards

Normal behaviors, such as hand-to-mouth activities, curiosity, exploration, crawling, and playing on the floor and outside, increase children's exposures to environmental toxins. When children put objects in their mouths, they can ingest toxins (such as lead from lead-based paint) found in dust or soil. When they crawl or play close to the ground, they are exposed to toxins in dust, soil, and carpets. When they explore their world, they may be exposed to household chemicals and other hazardous substances. When they play actively outdoors, they may breathe in more air pollutants. Young children are also unable to protect themselves from health risks that adults can easily avoid.

Children Have More Time to Develop Chronic Disease That May Be Triggered by Early Environmental Exposures

Some diseases that are triggered by toxic exposures in childhood require years or even decades to develop. Examples include mesothelioma caused by exposure to asbestos, leukemia caused by benzene, breast cancer that may be caused by DDT, and possibly some chronic neurological diseases such as Parkinson's disease, which may be caused by exposures to environmental neurotoxins. Many of these diseases are now thought to be the products of multistage processes that require years to develop (Landrigan et al., 1998, p. 788).

STRATEGIES AND SYNTHESIS

In 1997, an international body of the world's leading democracies affirmed that "prevention of exposure is the single most effective means of protecting children against environmental threats" (WHO, 1997a). Strategies for preventing exposure can be divided into individual or family responses and community or regional responses.

Individual/Familial Strategies

To promote environmental health at the individual/familial level, adults must educate themselves about ways to protect children from known and addressable environmental threats in their homes and neighborhoods; remain alert to changing environmental conditions, such as levels of outdoor air pollution, by monitoring local news sources; and keep themselves informed as new knowledge about emerging environmental hazards becomes available.

At this level, immediate and often inexpensive steps can be taken to reduce children's exposure to some common environmental hazards. Strategies include modifying the child's environment (e.g., putting dangerous chemicals out of the child's reach); modifying the child's behavior (e.g., using good personal hygiene, such as hand washing); and modifying the adult's behavior (e.g., quitting smoking or washing fruits and vegetables thoroughly). The following are specific strategies for some of the most common environmental health hazards for children.

Asbestos

Long used in construction materials, such as insulation, flooring, and roofing, and in appliances, asbestos is found in residences, schools, and other public buildings. Old, crumbly asbestos that flakes into a fine dust is the most dangerous.

When inhaled, asbestos fibers can cause lung cancer and mesothelioma, diseases that often take a long time to develop. If testing shows that asbestos is present, the material must be sprayed with a sealant, enclosed with newly constructed walls or ceilings, or removed by trained, qualified, and properly equipped workers. Asbestos remediation is *not* a do-it-yourself project.

Carbon Monoxide (CO)

A colorless, odorless gas, CO is produced from the incomplete burning of almost any combustible substance, such as natural gas, oil, kerosene, coal, and wood. Poorly ventilated or poorly maintained combustion appliances, attached garages, and tobacco smoking are common sources of CO indoors. Inhaling CO, which blocks the blood's ability to carry oxygen, can cause fatigue, headache, nausea and vomiting, confusion, brain damage, and death. If pregnant women are exposed to low levels of CO over long periods, the fetus may be injured. Prevention strategies include annual professional checkups of fuel-burning appliances, installation of CO detectors, and elimination of smoking, especially around young children. Gas ranges should not be used for heating a living space, and charcoal grills should never be used indoors. Automobiles, snow blowers, lawnmowers, and other internal combustion engines should never be run in enclosed spaces, such as garages.

Dioxin

A group of toxic compounds that comes from both natural and industrial sources, such as waste incineration and paper production, dioxin enters the food chain when animals eat contaminated plants. Most human exposures come from eating meat, fish, and dairy products, where dioxin tends to accumulate in fat. Mothers can pass dioxin to their children through the umbilical cord and breast milk. Fetuses and newborns are particularly vulnerable to dioxin, which is associated with developmental defects, diabetes, and cancer. To reduce exposure, children's diets should be carefully monitored for fat intake. Providing a balanced diet can help to avoid excessive exposure from a single source.

Endocrine-Disrupting Chemicals (EDCs)

By interfering with the role of natural hormones in the body, such substances are suspected of causing birth defects; alterations of normal growth and development; reproductive cancers; infertility; and impaired mental, immune, and thyroid function in developing children. Endocrine disruptors (also known as hormonally active agents) are found in thousands of products, ranging from pesticides to plastics.

The USEPA is currently screening 15,000 chemicals, each of which is produced in annual volume exceeding 10,000 pounds, for their endocrine-disrupting potential.

Environmental Tobacco Smoke (ETS) or Secondhand Smoke

The smoke from the burning end of a cigarette and the smoker's exhalation contains more than 4,000 chemicals, including several that are known to be carcinogenic or respiratory irritants. Some 43 percent of all children between the ages of 2 months and 11 years live in a home with a smoker (USEPA, 1998, p. 8). Children who are exposed to ETS suffer more bronchitis, pneumonia, respiratory infections, middle ear infections, and asthma attacks than do other children. The most effective strategy is for adults to cease smoking; if they cannot or will not do so, they should not smoke in the house or anywhere near young children.

Lead

A toxic metal, lead is especially dangerous to children under the age of 6, whose developing nervous systems are most vulnerable and whose normal behavior exposes them to lead-contaminated dust and soil. The US Centers for Disease Control and Prevention recommend assessing children's risk of exposure and screening, at ages 12 and 24 months, for blood lead levels for all children at high risk. Even at relatively low levels, lead can reduce children's IQ, produce significant learning and behavioral problems, and harm hearing and growth. At high levels, lead can cause coma, convulsions, and death.

The most common source of childhood lead poisoning in the United States today is deteriorating lead-based paint. Though banned for residential use in 1978, such paint remains in millions of homes, where it can contaminate dust and soil. Unless testing shows otherwise, caregivers should assume that any house built before 1978 contains lead-based paint. Adults should clean frequently, using a vacuum with a high efficiency particulate air (HEPA) filter and wet methods to reduce the spread of lead dust. Children should be encouraged to wash their hands after they play and before they eat to remove any lead dust. Children should be fed frequently (empty stomachs absorb more lead); their diets should include adequate amounts of calcium and iron and limited amounts of fat, which seems to encourage the absorption of lead. In pre-1978 homes, repairs and remodeling should be conducted using lead-safe procedures. Improper removal of lead-based paint can *increase*, rather than decrease, lead hazards.

In older homes, where lead may enter the drinking water from pipes, water should be run until it is cold; hot water directly from the tap should never be used to cook, drink, or make infant formula. Lead may also be found in some imported ceramics and miniblinds, leaded crystal, some hobby supplies (e.g., fishing sinkers and bullets), some folk remedies, and some ethnic cosmetics. Adults who work in lead-related industries must be careful to avoid bringing home lead dust and exposing their children.

Mercury

Used in thermometers, thermostats, barometers, fluorescent lights, some switches, and some medical equipment, liquid mercury is a toxic metal. Symptoms of mercury poisoning include muscle cramps or tremors, headache, rapid heart rate, intermittent fever, personality change, and neurological problems. Where possible, products that do not contain mercury (e.g., digital thermometers) can be substituted for mercury-containing ones. Even small mercury spills (e.g., from a broken thermometer) should be cleaned up in a way that will not spread or disperse the mercury. Because debris or products containing mercury may be considered hazardous waste, all cleanup materials should be disposed of in accordance with state regulations.

Methyl mercury, a highly toxic organic form of mercury, is released into the air by incinerators and fossil-fuel power plants and is then deposited on land and in water, where it may accumulate in predatory fish, shellfish, and marine mammals. Exposure to high levels of methyl mercury *in utero* or early infancy may damage a child's brain and nervous system, leading to mental retardation, cerebral palsy, deafness, blindness, and speech problems. Chronic, low-dose exposure from maternal consumption of contaminated food may also damage a child's developing nervous, cardiovascular, and immune systems. Pregnant women and children's caretakers must therefore pay attention to local fish advisories that recommend restricted consumption of certain fish species.

Outdoor Air Pollutants

Including ozone (the principal component of smog), CO, nitrogen oxides, and particulate matter (e.g., pollen, soot, and dust), outdoor air pollutants are thought to contribute to asthma attacks and other respiratory problems. Sources of outdoor air pollution include automobile and truck exhaust and emissions from industrial plants. Diesel exhaust alone contains more than 40 chemicals considered toxic air contaminants, known or probable human carcinogens, reproductive toxicants, or endocrine disruptors. If possible, children's outdoor activities should be conducted away from areas with heavy traffic. When air pollution is high (the air quality index is 100 or above), children should not play outdoors. On smoggy days, especially in summer,

children should play outdoors in the early morning, when smog levels are usually lowest.

Persistent Organic Pollutants (POPs)

A variety of highly stable chemicals that endure in the environment for very long periods before breaking down, POPs are widespread and are particularly dangerous because they concentrate in living organisms through the process of bioaccumulation. Organisms at the top of the food chain, like humans, absorb the greatest concentrations. POPs include PCBs, dioxins, and furans (both of which are byproducts of combustion and industrial processes), and other chemicals that have been linked to cancer, birth defects, allergies and hypersensitivity, damage to the nervous system, reproductive disorders, and disruption of the immune system. Avoiding foods that have high fat content, where POPs tend to accumulate, may help to reduce exposure.

Pesticides

A variety of chemicals used to control insects, rodents, weeds, molds, bacteria, and other pests, both indoors and outdoors, pesticides include some highly toxic materials. Children may be exposed through foods they eat (including milk, breast milk, fruits, and vegetables), contaminated drinking water, and air and dermal contact at home or in school. Exposure to some pesticides in utero and early childhood may cause cancer, respiratory problems, and damage to the central nervous, reproductive, endocrine, and immune systems (USEPA, 1998, pp. 83–86).

Although pesticides must be federally registered for use in the United States, registration does not ensure that the chemicals have been fully tested to determine their effects on fetuses, infants, and children. The USEPA is currently reviewing more than 9,000 old pesticides to ensure children's safety with respect to the residue limits in or on foods, aggregate exposures to pesticides from all sources (such as lawn treatments, household uses, and drinking water, as well as food), and cumulative or combined effects from groups of pesticides that may act on the body in similar ways (US General Accounting Office [GAO], 2000).

To reduce children's risks, the use of toxic pesticides in the home and the garden should be minimized. An alternative method, integrated pest management, uses chemical-free strategies first and pesticides only as a last resort. For example, indoor pest infestations may be prevented by blocking pest entries, and outdoor pests may be controlled through beneficial predators. If a pesticide must be used, the least toxic possible agent should be selected and the smallest effective amount used. Label directions about use and disposal should be followed carefully. Children, toys, and pets should always be removed from areas (homes, childcare facilities, and schools) where pesticides are to be applied, and the chemicals should always be stored (in their original, labeled containers) in locked areas, well out of reach of children. Buildings should be aired out thoroughly after the application.

Organic produce, grown without pesticides, can be purchased. If organic foods are not an option, produce should be scrubbed thoroughly with water or very diluted dishwashing detergent before eating or cooking. Running water removes more residues than soaking does. Fruits and vegetables should be peeled when possible, and the outer leaves of leafy vegetables should be discarded. (It must be noted, however, that some pesticides permeate produce and cannot be washed off.) Because some pesticide residues concentrate in animal fats, fat should be trimmed from meat and poultry, and skin from fish.

Phthalates

Industrial chemicals, often used to soften polyvinyl chloride (PVC), phthalates have been used in products ranging from infant teething devices and soft plastic toys to personal care and medical products, building products, detergents, and solvents. Phthalates can be ingested, inhaled, or absorbed through the skin. Some may pass to a fetus from the mother. Some phthalates may cause birth defects and disrupt hormone functions. In the United States and Europe, they have been removed from new chewable teething and other toys because of concern that the phthalates could leach out. Adults should allow children to use only products that are phthalate-free.

Polychlorinated Biphenyls (PCBs)

A variety of chemicals formerly used in many industrial and commercial applications, PCBs were banned in 1976. PCBs may cause cancer, as well as skin, nose, and lung irritations, and they may affect the immune, nervous, endocrine, and reproductive systems. Children whose mothers were exposed to PCBs during pregnancy may suffer from learning disabilities and delayed development. Children may be exposed to PCBs by inhaling contaminated air, touching PCBs in soil or other media, and ingesting contaminated water or food (including breast milk and predatory fish, such as tuna, shark, and swordfish). Monitoring the diet to avoid potentially contaminated foods and monitoring intake of fat, where PCBs concentrate, may reduce risk of exposure.

Radon

A colorless, odorless, tasteless radioactive gas, radon occurs naturally in soil, rocks, water, and some building materials. Radon gas usually enters homes, schools, and workplaces through cracks or holes in the foundation. It may also enter through well water. A known carcinogen, it is considered the most significant cause of lung cancer among nonsmokers in the United States. An individual's risk depends on the level of radon, the duration of exposure, and smoking habits (smoking greatly increases the risk of dying from lung cancer caused by radon). Professional services and inexpensive do-it-yourself kits (federal- or state-certified) that measure radon levels are readily available. If radon is present, home repairs, such as sealing cracks in foundations, can reduce exposure.

Volatile Organic Compounds (VOCs)

Found in cleaning products, adhesives, paints, drycleaning fluids, aerosol sprays, and wood preservatives, VOCs may irritate the eyes, nose, and lungs; may cause rashes, headaches, nausea, vomiting, and asthma; and may damage the liver, kidney, and nervous system. Some VOCs, such as formaldehyde and benzene, may cause cancer. To reduce exposure, household products should be used according to manufacturer's directions, and good ventilation should be provided when these products are used. Only limited quantities—as much as will be needed in a short period—should be purchased. Stored chemicals should be kept in well-ventilated areas and out of reach of children. Partly empty containers of old or unneeded chemicals should be disposed of safely.

Community/Regional Strategies

Although individuals can help to mitigate children's exposure to some environmental toxins, governmental and international efforts are essential to deal with many environmental health concerns. Collecting information on chronic diseases that may have environmental causes may be a first step in reducing them. At the international level, WHO (2000) notes that "existing health statistics do not reflect the real morbidity and mortality rate due to acute and chronic exposures to chemicals." WHO places high priority on collecting sound data and demonstrating cost-effective intervention strategies.

In the United States, the Pew Environmental Health Commission (2000) urged the federal government to establish a systematic, comprehensive, nationwide health tracking network that could document possible links between environmental hazards (including POPs, heavy metals, pesticides, air contaminants, and drinking water contaminants) and chronic diseases (including asthma and other chronic respiratory diseases, birth defects, developmental disabilities, neurological diseases, and cancers, especially childhood cancers).

Tracking information could be used to guide other community strategies. It would serve to identify populations at risk; formulate responses to outbreaks, disease clusters, and emerging threats; establish relationships between environmental hazards and diseases; guide intervention and prevention strategies; identify, reduce, and prevent harmful environmental risks; improve the public health basis for policymaking; implement the public's right to know about health and the environment; and track progress toward achieving better environmental health.

The Children's Environmental Health Network has proposed a national agenda that includes prevention-oriented research, a child-centered paradigm for health risk assessment and policymaking, and education to persuade the public, health professionals, and policymakers that environmental disease is preventable (Landrigan et al., 1998, p. 787).

Other community strategies include the prevention of environmental contamination through regulation and legislation (e.g., the US Clean Air Act), the cleanup of contaminated sites (e.g., lead and asbestos abatement), and the education of residents and public officials about environmental hazards (e.g., antismoking campaigns). These strategies can be highly successful. Since US governmental measures to eliminate lead in gasoline, in paint for residential use, and in solder in food cans have been put into effect, mean blood lead levels in children have declined by 80 percent, and the number of children with elevated blood lead levels has decreased by 90 percent (Ryan, Levy, Pollack, & Walker, 1999). Some community strategies, however, may be slow, technically difficult, extremely expensive, or subject to industry resistance or political controversy.

It must be noted that not all communities are equally subject to environmental hazards. Throughout the world, poor and minority children are at greatest risk from environmental threats. In the United States, for example, African American and low-income children are at five to eight times higher risk for lead poisoning than other children (Ryan et al., 1999). The United Nations, USEPA, state agencies, and community organizations have implemented programs in environmental justice, or environmental equity, to reduce disparities.

Current laws and regulations may not be adequate to protect children. For example, the EPA requires that chemical manufacturers prove that their products do not cause cancer or birth defects, but it does not require them to prove that the products do not cause neurological damage. Moreover, the test standards are for hazards to adults, not children. US legislation specifically designed to protect children's environmental health had been proposed but had not yet been passed by the end of the millennium.

In less developed countries, lack of understanding of environmental risks, education, and enforcement of environmental laws, as well as lack of resources and facilities, all contribute to environmental risks to children. Many sources of environmental contaminants that are regulated in developed nations are not controlled elsewhere. For example, leaded gasoline, no longer used for automobiles in the United States or Japan, is still used in 150 other nations (Ryan et al., 1999). In addition, cultural features may increase risk. In parts of Asia, for example, families commonly live where the father works, so that children as well as adults suffer from occupational exposures. Environmental standards may be viewed as Western concerns rather than indigenous ones, and attitudes toward risk may be different from Western attitudes (Carpenter et al., 2000, p. 989).

Nonetheless, some progress is being made. In 1995, the USEPA announced a national policy to "consistently and explicitly take into account health risks to children and infants from environmental hazards when conducting assessments of environmental risks." A 1997 executive order made it a federal priority "to identify and assess environmental health risks and safety risks that may disproportionately affect children" and to ensure that policies and programs addressed these risks.

At year-end 2000, the United Nations announced that 122 nations had agreed on a treaty that will ban or reduce the use or production of twelve highly toxic POPs, including eight pesticides, two industrial chemicals, and two byproducts of combustion and industrial processes. Exemptions to the immediate ban, however, illustrate some of the complexities of improving environmental health. DDT is still needed to control malaria-carrying mosquitoes in some countries and cannot be eliminated until cost-effective and more environmentally friendly replacements are available. PCBs, though no longer produced, are still used in hundreds of thousands of tons of electrical transformers and other equipment, and their replacement will take decades.

Also see: Culture, Society, and Social Class: Foundation; Child Care: Early Childhood; Nutrition: Early Childhood; Parenting: Early Childhood; Physical Health: Early Childhood.

References

Carpenter, D.O., Chew, F.T., Danstra, T., Lam, L.H., Landrigan, P.J., Makalinao, I., Peralta, G.L., & Suk, W. (2000). Environmental threats to the health of children: The Asian perspective. *Environmental Health Perspectives, 198*(10), 989–992.

Chai, S., & Bearer, C. (1999, June). A developmental approach to pediatric environmental health. In *Training manual on pediatric environmental health: Putting it into practice* (pp. 57–68). Children's Environmental Health Network.

Landrigan, P., Carlson, J., Bearer, C., Cranmer, J., Bullard, R., Etzel, R., Groopman, J., McLachlan, J., Perera, F., Reigart, J., Robison, L., Schell, L., & Suk, W. (1998, June). Children's health and the environment: A new agenda for prevention research. *Environmental Health Perspectives, 106*(Suppl. 3), 787–794.

National Academy of Sciences (NAS), & National Research Council. (2000). *Toxicological effects of methylmercury.* Committee on the Toxicological Effects of Methylmercury, Board on Environmental Studies and Toxicology, Commission on Life Sciences, National Research Council. Washington, DC: National Academy Press.

Pew Environmental Health Commission. (2000, September). *America's environmental health gap: Why the country needs a nationwide health tracking network.* Environmental Health Tracking Project Team, Johns Hopkins School of Hygiene and Public Health, Department of Health Policy and Management. http://pewenvirohealth.jhsph.edu

Roe, D., Pease, W., Florini, K., & Silbergeld, E. (1997, Summer). *Toxic ignorance.* Washington, DC: Environmental Defense Fund.

Ryan, D., Levy, B., Pollack, S., & Walker, B. (1999, June). Protecting children from lead poisoning and building healthy communities. *American Journal of Public Health.* Editorial. American Public Health Association. http://www.apha.org/journal/editorials/edryan.htm

US Environmental Protection Agency (EPA). (1998). Office of Children's Health Protection. *The EPA's children's environmental health yearbook.* EPA 100-R-98-100. Washington, DC: Author

US General Accounting Office (GAO). (2000, September). *Children and pesticides: New approach to considering risk is partly in place.* United States General Accounting Office, Report to Congressional Requesters. GAO/HEHS-00-175.

World Health Organization (WHO). (1997a). Declaration of the environment leaders of the eight on children's environmental health. http://www.who.int/peh/child/1997declaraton.htm (retrieved 9/8/00).

World Health Organization (WHO). (1997b). Indicators for policy and decision making in environmental health (draft). Geneva, Switzerland: Author.

World Health Organization (WHO). (2000). Sustainable development and healthy environments: Protection of the human environment: Environmental toxic exposures and poisoning in children. http://www.who.int/peh/child/toxexpo.htm (retrieved 9/8/00).

Environmental Health, Childhood

Shelley Hearne

INTRODUCTION

Preadolescent children interact with a diverse array of physical, chemical, biological, and social factors in the environment that can pose a threat to their health. These can be naturally occurring risks such as bacterial contaminants in water, or pollutants, such as tobacco smoke, chemicals, and heavy metals. The potential for harmful effects from different environmental hazards depends on many factors including the intensity of the exposure, the toxicity of the substance, the duration of exposure, and route of contact. Most environmental threats pose a risk to the entire population, though children are usually more vulnerable.

In general, the most effective means of reducing these risks is through population-based strategies to prevent or reduce the use and/or release of harmful substances into the environment. For naturally occurring materials, control options are available to help avoid exposure.

DEFINITIONS

Combustion products are hazardous materials such as carbon monoxide, nitrogen oxide and small inhalable particles that are released into both indoor and outdoor air when burning fuel or other materials.

Environmental tobacco smoke (ETS) is a complex mixture of more than 4,000 chemicals, including carbon monoxide, nicotine, tars, formaldehyde, and hydrogen cyanide, many of which are known as human carcinogens or respiratory irritants. Also known as "second hand smoke" or "passive smoking," ETS is released into the air from burning tobacco products.

Heavy metals are naturally found elements with high atomic weights (e.g., mercury, chromium, cadmium, arsenic, and lead) that can damage living organisms at low concentrations and can bioaccumulate in human and animal food chains.

Pesticides are any substance intended to destroy, prevent, or repel pests such as insects, weeds, fungi, and rodents. The term pesticide includes numerous types of substances designed for different purposes. For instance, herbicides kill unwanted plants, fungicides kill fungi, rodenticides kill rodents, and disinfectants kill microorganisms.

Volatile Organic Compounds (VOCs) are compounds that vaporize at room temperature. Housekeeping and maintenance products and building and furnishing materials are common sources of VOC emissions.

SCOPE

Preadolescent children are exposed on a daily basis to a wide array of environmental hazards found in air, water, soil, and consumer products. Each environmental contaminant has its own risks, exposures, and costs. Despite significant measures by the US federal government to control environmental threats over the past 30 years, children continue to be exposed to environmental hazards. Research and policy efforts are just beginning to address the unique susceptibilities of children in order to prevent or reduce their exposure to environmental threats.

Lead is a primary example of an environmental hazard associated with adverse acute and chronic health outcomes that disproportionately affects children. Children can be exposed to lead via multiple routes, including hand-to-mouth behavior, playing close to the ground, and breathing leaded gasoline.

Evidence indicates that children more readily absorb the heavy metal and are physically more susceptible to its ill effects. Research has shown that children absorb about 50 percent of lead ingested, while almost all the lead passes through adults when ingested (Royce, 2000). Once the lead gets into a child's body, this heavy metal can inhibit proper neurologic development. Numerous studies have found associations between elevated blood lead levels and reduced IQ, behavioral problems, and learning disabilities (NRC, 1993a). The CDC has determined that lead levels above 10 μg/dL (micrograms/deciliter) in the blood stream pose an unacceptable risk. A CDC cost-benefit analysis showed that an elevated blood lead level (>10 μg/dL) resulted in avoidable medical and special education costs of $1300 and $3331 per child, respectively (CDC, 1991).

The prevalence of children with unacceptable lead levels varies significantly in the United States, Canada, and other parts of the world, depending on how lead is used locally. For example, India still uses leaded gasoline, though this fuel additive is scheduled to be removed. There are estimates that over 40–50 percent of Indian children aged 1–12 in medium-sized and larger cities have blood lead levels greater than 10 μg/dL (George Foundation, 1999). One study found that lead levels were significantly higher among children aged eight and over than among younger children. Mean blood lead levels for children aged 8–11 were 32 μg/dL and for children under age seven, 19 μg/dL (Kumar & Kesaree, 1999). This directly contrasts with the United States and Canada, which no longer use leaded gasoline, though exposures in these countries occur from old paint and other limited sources. Lead contamination profiles indicate that school-aged children have the lowest blood lead levels of all age groups. The percentage of US children with elevated blood lead levels has dropped from 88.2 percent in the 1970s to 4.4 percent in the early 1990s. In the United States, prevention measures and health promotion have substantially reduced lead poisoning cases, but lead exposure remains a threat for children who live in older housing, near mining and industrial sites, or who participate in hobbies or activities involving lead.

THEORIES

While environmental hazards pose a risk to all members of society, preadolescent children are highly vulnerable due to their unique exposures and physical characteristics. In order to take appropriate preventive action and health promotion, it is critical to understand that children are not "little adults" and, pound for pound of body weight, are more susceptible to environmental toxicants than adults. In addition, children often are limited by their inability to take action to avoid certain hazards. Unfortunately, many environmental laws and standards do not take into account children's unique vulnerabilities.

Different Exposures to Environmental Hazards. Preadolescent children's exposures to environmental hazards vary depending on location, body weight ratios, and behavioral factors.

Physical Location. Preadolescents spend a significant amount of time in school, homes, and playing areas, which may lead to a variety of environmental exposures, ranging from lead, VOCs, and pesticides to air pollution and ventilation problems.

Breathing and Consumption Differences. Children have smaller body mass than adults (i.e., weight range for children aged 5–12 is 40–90 pounds vs. the average adult male at 154 pounds). As a result, children breathe more air, consume more food, and drink more water as a percentage of their body weight than adults. In relative terms, children receive higher doses of contaminants that are present in any of these sources.

Behavioral. Childhood activities, such as playing on the ground, outdoors, or with increased exertion, can cause greater exposures to pollutants than in adults. Children playing on the ground will be exposed to toxic substances that have been applied to or accumulate at ground level, such as pesticides, lead, and solvents. Preadolescent children are not as prone to exposures from hand to mouth activity, which is a significant source of toxic exposure in younger children, unless they are developmentally delayed.

Greater Physiological Susceptibility to Environmental Hazards. Children aged 5–12 are still involved in significant growth and maturation of their organs, which may be affected by toxicants. The two key organs developing during this age are the lungs and nervous systems. The myelination of the brain, which creates a protective barrier from toxicants, is not completed until adolescence. Similarly, the lung's alveoli—the terminal sacs that increase blood oxygen exchange—are not fully formed until adolescence. This lengthy development period leaves preadolescent children particularly vulnerable to toxic substances, which could impede proper development or increase susceptibility to cancer (Bearer, 1995).

Though most kidney and liver functions have matured by preadolescence, these children still may absorb, distribute, metabolize, and excrete toxic substances differently than adults. This has the potential to make chemicals either more or less hazardous, depending on their chemical properties and the body's metabolic development.

RESEARCH

Air Pollution

Air pollution has a wide variety of health impacts on children, including increased duration of infectious disease, increased aggravation of asthma, decreased lung function, and even death in severe cases. School-age children may have relatively high outdoor pollutant exposures because of physical outdoor activities and because leaving school in the afternoon correlates with highest ozone levels (Bates, 1995).

Indoor

In the United States, children spend the majority of their day indoors (Schwab, 1992). Research indicates that indoor air pollution in homes and schools poses a threat to children's health. Poor ventilation, lack of upkeep, leaky roofs, and indoor contaminants such as allergens, combustion materials, pesticides, volatile organic compounds, and tobacco smoke can contribute to poor indoor air quality. Allergens and biological agents in indoor air, including animal dander, insect materials, mold spores, and bacteria, may induce adverse respiratory and asthmatic responses (AAP, 1999). Combustion products have a range of effects. Exposure to particulate materials and various oxides may result in irritation and inflammation of the upper and lower respiratory tract (Pope & Ransom, 1992). The health effects of carbon monoxide (CO), another combustion product, range from flu-like symptoms to coma and death from prolonged or intense exposures. Hundreds of deaths in children occur annually from unintentional CO poisonings (AAP, 1999).

VOCs may result in skin and/or respiratory irritation, depending on the route and level of exposure. Other signs and symptoms include nasal congestion, rash, headaches, and nausea (AAP, 1999). Long-term exposures to high levels of some VOCs, such as benzene, have been shown to cause cancer, but health effects from low-level exposures to VOCs are generally unknown. Studies conducted by the US Environmental Protection Agency have shown that the levels of VOCs inside homes are often two to five times higher than they are outside (EPA, 2000a).

In developing nations, respiratory disease is the primary cause of death in children and indoor pollution from improperly ventilated burning fuel may play a significant role (Smith, Samet, Romieu, & Bruce, 2000).

Outdoor

Almost 25 percent of US children live in counties that exceed national air quality standards for one or more leading air pollutants (ozone, carbon monoxide, nitrogen dioxide, sulfur dioxide, particulate matter (soot), and lead) (EPA, 2000b). Research indicates that particulate matter, ground level ozone, and sulfur dioxide have harmful effects on lung function and the upper respiratory tract (Bates, 2000; Clark, 1999; Pope, & Ransom, 1992; Samet, Dominici, Currier, Coursac, & Zeger, 2000). Children are particularly sensitive. Elevated levels of air pollutants correspond with a rise in lost school days (Gilliland et al., 2001), higher numbers of medical visits (Ostro, Eskeland, Sanchez, & Feyzioglu, 1999), more cases of restricted activity, and increases in children with reduced lung function (Chen, Chan, Lai, Hwang, Yang, & Wang, 1999; Jedrychowski, Flak, & Mroz, 1999). Recent studies have found a significant adverse effect of air pollution upon preadolescent children's proper lung development (Jedrychowski et al., 1999; Peters et al., 1999).

Asthma Exacerbaters

Pediatric asthma rates have increased substantially, and growing evidence indicates an environmental role. While the cause of asthma remains unknown, research has identified many environmental factors that may trigger children's asthma attacks. These include inhalant allergens (dust mites, cockroach feces, animal dander, and other animal allergens, indoor fungi, outdoor mold spores, and pollens) and irritants (ETS, ozone, particulate matter, sulfur dioxide, nitrogen dioxides and certain chemicals) (Clark, 1999).

Environmental Tobacco Smoke

The CDC reports that 43 percent of preadolescent children in the United States live in a home with at least one smoker. Children exposed to ETS have higher rates of bronchitis, pneumonia, respiratory infections, otitis media (fluid in the middle ear), and asthma symptoms (Clark, 1999; Eggleston, Breysse, Buckley, Wills-Karp, Kleeberger, & Jaakkola, 1999; EPA, 1990; Gold, 2000). Studies suggest that decreasing children's ETS exposure could prevent asthmatic attacks (Gold, 2000).

Water Pollution

Children can be exposed to water contaminants by swimming in polluted lakes and streams, consuming contaminated fish, and drinking contaminated water supplies. Drinking water contamination is one of the top public health risks posed by environmental problems. In the United States, approximately 8 percent of children live in areas served by public water systems that exceed a drinking water standard or violate treatment requirements (EPA, 2000b). Experts estimate that up to 900,000 people per year in the United States become ill from drinking contaminated water and as many as 900 die from waterborne infectious diseases (ASM, 1999). These estimates are considered low, in part, because the country lacks an active nationwide surveillance of water-based illness. In developing countries without sanitation and drinking water systems, contaminated water supplies can be the leading cause of death. Drinking water can be contaminated by chemicals or microbial pathogens like bacteria, viruses, or protozoa (parasites). Disease causing organisms in sewage-contaminated water can result in hepatitis, dysentery, gastrointestinal illness, fever, ear infections, and other health problems. Common microbiological contaminants, such as Cryptosporidium, Giardia, and Norwalk virus, can cause immediate health threats in local conditions. Water can also be contaminated with toxic substances such as heavy metals, PCBs, disinfectant byproducts, and organic chemicals, which are associated with a wide range of serious health problems, including cancer, birth defects and skin irritations. Many of these contaminants cannot be destroyed by conventional water treatment.

Pesticides

Children are exposed to pesticides through household and school use, consuming produce and drinking water with pesticide residues, and exposures associated with parents working with pesticides. Whether there will be any effect and, if so, the type of effect, depends not only on the particular pesticide and the amount taken into the body, but also on the frequency and duration of the contact. Since children consume substantially more fruits and vegetables and play on the ground where pesticides are applied and persist, they can receive higher doses of these pesticides than adults.

Some symptoms associated with high, short-term exposures to pesticides include headaches, blurred vision, salivation, dizziness, nausea and vomiting, abdominal cramps, slow pulse and even death. The long-term health effects of pesticides on children are not well studied, but the National Academy of Sciences reports that some pesticides may interfere with physiological processes of children, including their immune, respiratory, and neurological systems (NRC, 1993b). Studies have found an increased risk of developing leukemia and non-Hodgkin's lymphoma among children whose parents use pesticides occupationally or at home (Buckley, 2000; Lowengart, 1987).

Heavy Metals

Heavy metals are found in a variety of products ranging from fossil fuels to consumer goods. Heavy metals pose a particular risk to children because of their ability to cause neurological damage while the nervous system is developing. Some symptoms associated with high mercury and lead exposures are tremors, memory problems, and changes in vision. Low level, long-term exposures can decrease mental ability or reduce growth. A National Academy of Sciences' report indicated that mercury contributes to learning disabilities, and that in the United States approximately 60,000 newborns annually may be at risk of adverse neurological damage due to in-utero exposure to methylmercury (NRC, 2000).

Children can be exposed to cadmium from cigarette smoke or eating cadmium-contaminated food, which can damage the lungs, cause kidney disease, and may irritate the digestive tract. Inorganic arsenic can increase the risk of certain cancers and abnormal heart rhythms, damage blood cells, and cause skin disorders and nausea. Exposures can occur from natural sources, hazardous waste sites, and treated wood products.

STRATEGIES THAT WORK

Reducing Indoor Air Pollution

To date, the federal government does not regulate indoor air quality. Most measures to reduce indoor pollutants in buildings frequented by children are voluntary, except for prohibitions on tobacco smoking. The following strategies offer effective reductions for specific indoor air pollutants.

Combustion Products

Prevention methods to reduce children's exposures to combustion products include the following measures: (1) routine professional inspection and maintenance of furnaces, gas water heaters, gas stoves and clothes dryers, all of which should be properly vented outdoors; (2) regular cleaning and inspection of fireplaces and wood stoves; (3) restricting use of cooking grills to outdoors; and (4) leaving idling cars and building garages away from the building's air intake system. Carbon monoxide (CO) warning units can also alert residents to fatally high levels of CO in homes using gas-based equipment.

Volatile Organic Compounds

Indoor VOC concentrations and resulting exposures may vary significantly depending on the level of ventilation in buildings and activities such as smoking, remodeling, or painting. To prevent exposure to VOCs, consumer products and building materials containing these substances should be avoided or substituted for low VOC-containing products. To minimize exposures, building ventilation can be increased and VOC-containing materials (such as paints, solvents, and furniture lacquers) should not be stored in homes or left open.

If formaldehyde is suspected, many sources can be removed, including carpeting or urea–formaldehyde insulation or paneling. If it is not possible to remove them, these materials could be coated with a nontoxic sealant, and building ventilation could be increased (AAP, 1999). Children should avoid vehicle exhaust and gasoline vapors during refueling.

Asthma Exacerbaters

Prevention includes interventions to reduce and eliminate dust mites, ETS, and mold in buildings occupied by children. Smoking bans in public places frequented by children are effective measures to reduce asthmatic symptoms. To reduce mold, measures need to be taken to improve ventilation and repair leaking roofs and other water sources. The most effective measures to decrease mite infestation in the home is to cover bed mattresses with plastic covers, wash bedding in very hot water (over 55°C) and control indoor humidity in buildings (Clark, 1999; Etzel, 1995).

Outdoor Air Pollutants

Due to the wide range of sources, prevention of outdoor air pollutants requires government action or voluntary initiatives in limiting the levels of pollutants emitted by industry, transportation and energy utility operations.

Reducing Exposure to Harmful Heavy Metals

Prevention encourages reduced use of heavy metals that may produce childhood exposures. As proven in the United States and other countries, heavy metal fuel additives should be avoided since their use produces widespread and extensive exposures to vast populations.

Reducing Exposure to Lead

Lead poisoning is a disease that is not highly treatable, and therefore, prevention efforts offer the most effective solution. In developing countries that still use lead in gasoline or paints, the most effective prevention strategy for lead poisoning is to eliminate these significant lead uses. Since the phase out of lead in gasoline, there has been a 70 percent reduction in lead levels in US children aged 6–19 years (Pirkle, 1994). Overall, children of this age now have the lowest geometric mean blood lead for the entire population. Similar reductions have occurred in Canada. In the United States and Canada, lead-based paints in home remain the most significant source of potential lead exposure. The CDC has determined that removing lead-based paint from homes provides long-term benefits that significantly outweigh short-term financial costs. The costs for abating the average

Table 1. American Academy of Pediatrics Recommended Prevention Strategies for Lead Risks

Risk factor	Prevention strategy
Paint	Identify if lead contaminated and abate
Dust	Wet mop, frequent hand washing
Soil	Restrict play in area, ground cover, frequent hand washing
Drinking water	Flush water faucet for 2 min in the morning; use of cold water for cooking and drinking
Folk remedies	Avoid use
Old ceramic or pewter cookware	Avoid use
Some imported cosmetics, toys, crayons	Avoid use
Parental occupations associated with lead	Remove work clothing at work
Hobbies involving lead-based materials	Proper use, storage and ventilation
Home renovation	Proper containment, ventilation
Buying or renting a new home	Inquire about lead hazards

pre-1950 home with lead-based paint is approximately $2,225 and would yield cost saving of $4,323 over the lifetime of the home (CDC, 1999) considering, for example, medical and special education costs of lead poisoning.

The top priority for reducing lead contamination in US children today is to reduce lead-based exposures to old paints, dusts, and soil and consider other possible exposures including leaded pipes, hobby materials, and certain folk remedies. Depending on the source of lead exposure, different prevention strategies can be applied. Table 1 summarizes the recommended prevention techniques for different risk factors (AAP, 1999).

Reducing Exposure to Mercury

Preadolescent children's exposure to mercury is most likely via ambient air sources or consumption of mercury contaminated food products, such as fish. Acute mercury exposure can occur in limited events, such as thermometer breakage or leaking electric meter devices. In such an event, the beaded mercury should be rolled onto paper and then placed in an airtight jar for appropriate disposal. Mercury should not be vacuumed as this may cause vaporization and increase exposure risks (AAP, 1999).

Reducing Exposure to Contaminated Water

The most effective prevention strategy for water-borne illness is to eliminate contamination at the source. The federal and state governments require municipal and commercial water suppliers serving more than 25 people to meet the Safe Drinking Water Act standards. National drinking water standards—known as Maximum Contaminant Levels (MCLs)—have been established for more than 80 microbial, chemical and radionuclide contaminants (EPA, 2000b). For public water systems, health-based violations of drinking water standards have decreased from 19 percent in 1993 to 8 percent in 1998 (EPA, 2000b).

Another method of prevention includes water testing. Parents can have water tested for contamination to determine if corrective steps are necessary. Local water companies are now required under the US law to provide consumers with a report on contamination of their water supply.

Reducing Exposure to Pesticides

Integrated Pest Management (IPM) is a problem-solving approach that emphasizes preventing and reducing the source of the pest problems rather than treating the symptoms with routine pesticide spraying (Chase, 1995). Its objective is to suppress pest populations below the level that causes economic, aesthetic, or medical injury using a minimal level of pesticides.

IPM consists of a five-step process: (1) inspect and gather information about the pest's lifecycle and habits; (2) monitor to determine the seriousness of the problem; (3) establish the threshold level to determine at what point to take action; (4) determine treatment using least toxic methods first and timing for efficacy; and (5) evaluate IPM program's successfulness (Chase, 1995). Under IPM, rather than implement routine pesticide spraying, treatments are only used when regular monitoring indicates a problem. Management tactics include physical (caulking cracks), mechanical (vacuuming pests), cultural (appropriate plantings), biological (beneficial insects), and educational (cleaning up food wastes) approaches (AAP, 1999).

There is evidence that IPM can be more cost-effective than chemical-based pest control programs and have been used successfully in US schools, government agencies, and farms (AAP, 1999; Chase, 1995).

STRATEGIES THAT MIGHT WORK

Air Pollution: Indoor Air Pollution

It is recognized that the most effective means of reducing indoor air contamination is avoiding the use of toxic substances and materials. Home air cleaners can also be used, and generally can remove certain air contaminants. However, most cannot remove a broad spectrum of pollutants and can sometimes create health hazards (Manuel, 1999). Studies indicate that portable air cleaner units are more effective at reducing solid matter, such as

dust, smoke, and pollen, than gaseous-phase contaminants such as VOCs, carbon monoxide, and nitrogen oxide. The cleaners that work via filtration have the greatest efficiency for particles, though this decreases over time unless the filters are routinely cleaned. The ionizing and ozone generating units are least efficient. For gaseous pollutants, no unit has been able to remove more than 49 percent of any pollutant, and many have shown no effect at all (Manuel, 1999).

Asthma Inducers

The prevention of the development of asthma is not well understood. There is limited evidence that in-utero exposure to tobacco-smoke products is an important determinant of wheezing in the first year, though no studies have been conducted on whether asthma incidence can be reduced by decreasing smoking during pregnancy (Etzel, 1995).

Prevention of asthmatic attacks may be achieved by reducing children's exposures to asthma exacerbaters, such as tobacco smoke and indoor allergens. Despite research associating environmental tobacco smoke with childhood asthma, the efficacy of asthma reduction initiatives that reduce ETS have not been adequately evaluated (Clark, 1999; Etzel, 1995). One study indicated that parents who limited children's exposure to ETS reported less severe asthmatic symptoms, but the study could not document actual ETS levels or diagnosed symptoms (Etzel, 1995). Research is being conducted to determine the effectiveness of measures to control children's activity patterns and community-based interventions for reducing environmental asthma excaberators (Clark, 1999).

Reducing Exposure to Contaminated Water

Increasing numbers of homes are installing water filter and treatment systems that remove lead, chlorine by-products, organic compounds, and bacteria. This measure can be applied for precautionary purposes and to improve overall taste and odor. Researchers have estimated that 35 percent of these control systems are used at the end of the tap or water faucet in homes or schools and have limited health benefits. Additionally, they are not highly cost effective for the following reasons: (1) most drinking water supplies already meet federal and state standards; (2) many systems are not highly effective in removing trace substances; and (3) if not properly maintained, filters using activated carbon can become reservoirs for growing bacteria (AAP, 1999). If a water contamination problem has been identified, it is more effective for water suppliers to correct the problem, as required by law.

STRATEGIES THAT DO NOT WORK

Reducing Exposure to Air Pollution: Indoor Air

All portable air cleaning units have limited, if any, ability to remove gaseous pollutants (Manuel, 1999). None of these machines can effectively remove carbon monoxide. Some portable air cleaning units are based on a mechanism of generating ozone and negative ions that claims to kill undesirable organisms and clean particles from indoor air. Advertisements state that these units can reduce dust, odors, allergens, mold, mildew, secondhand smoke, bacteria, and/or pollen. Research has shown that these units are the least efficient at reducing particulate matter and are marginally effective (7–15 percent) for gaseous pollutants. Some federal and state agencies have issued warnings against ozone generating air cleaners. Ozone is also a lung irritant and is associated with decreased lung function over the long-term (Manuel, 1999).

Reducing Asthma Excaberators

While many environmental factors have been identified as asthma triggers, not all measures will be effective in reducing asthma symptoms for every child due to the individualistic response of the condition. Certain common remedial activities, such as vacuuming with a standard vacuum cleaner, can increase allergen-containing particles in the air and induce adverse respiratory conditions for children with specific allergic reactions (Clark, 1999).

SYNTHESIS

School-Based Initiatives

Children are rarely exposed to only one environmental hazard, so it is critical that prevention programs are integrated to address multiple potential exposures. Children aged 5–12 spend 35–50 hr per week in and around school buildings where they can come into contact with many environmental hazards that may be in building materials, cleaning products, ventilation systems, and even arts and crafts. A properly engineered building that considers environment in its original design and that is maintained properly is the ideal prevention strategy. A comprehensive school program aimed at identifying, eliminating and minimizing pesticides, air pollution and other toxic substances can substantially reduce children's risks.

Pesticides are frequently used in and around schools to control rodents, insects, and weeds. Recognizing the potential health risks posed to children, several school systems have adopted IPM programs. The US federal legislation recently passed a bill requiring the EPA to develop IPM guidelines for schools.

Indoor air quality problems are frequently found in school buildings and can range from a wide variety of hazards—from VOCs to molds and allergens to particulate matter. Five basic prevention strategies can be employed to reduce indoor air pollution (AAP, 1999):

1. Educate school staff about: (a) sources and effects of toxic substances that they can control; and (b) proper operation and maintenance of the school's ventilation system, which can result in reduction of multiple exposures.
2. Manage the sources of toxic substances through removal, substitution, or encapsulation. The preferred management approach is prevention whereby a pollutant is never introduced to the school. This includes preventing buses from idling near ventilation air intakes and prohibiting smoking in building areas. Substitution involves replacing those substances with less toxic materials, such as safer art supplies or pest controls. Encapsulation involves erecting an impervious barrier around the source so that less toxic materials are released into the school environment.
3. Ensure that specific sources are exhausted outdoors, such as science laboratories, kitchens, bathrooms, vocational areas, housekeeping storage rooms and printing/duplicating areas.
4. Frequent and effective circulation with outside air throughout the building to ensure cleaner indoor air.
5. Administrative control over activities involving toxic substances, such as painting, pest control and intensive solvent use when students are away for substantial time (i.e., holidays or Friday afternoons).

The USEPA has developed a school-based initiative for improving an existing school's indoor air quality through cost-effective prevention tactics (EPA, 2000a).

Environmental Laws, Health Tracking and Pollution Prevention

Most countries have established extensive environmental laws that regulate pollution in air, water, and land. Many of these laws have provisions to set pollution standards based on public health and technology goals. In the US, environmental regulation is embodied in eight primary environmental laws:

- The Clean Air Act (CAA)
- The Safe Drinking Water Act (SDWA)
- The Federal Water Pollution Control Act or Clean Water Act (CWA)

- The Toxic Substances Control Act (TSCA)
- The Federal Insecticide, Fungicide and Rodenticide Act (FIFRA)
- The National Environmental Policy Act (NEPA)
- The Resource Conservation and Recovery Act (RCRA)
- The Comprehensive Environmental Response, Compensation, and Liability Act (CERCLA or Superfund)

Although it is difficult to generalize, these laws seek to protect the environment and public health by establishing policies, regulations and enforcement mechanisms that encourage or force behavior changes in the way that society uses environmental resources such as the land, air, and water. They also seek to control the introduction into commerce of new chemical compounds and industrial processes. This population-based approach is critical for reducing environmental risks, as individuals cannot effectively prevent or control ambient exposures (Pew Commission, 2001).

Conceptually, the goal of environmental health is to prevent harm at the source rather than assess risk afterwards. In order for environmental regulations to better prevent environmental health risks and promote children's health, three measures are needed:

1. *Revise Environmental Standards to Consider Children's Risks.* Environmental standards are designed to limit dangerous levels of pollution. The US government recognized in 1997 that children are uniquely vulnerable to environmental hazards and has mandated that all existing and future regulatory actions adequately consider children's health. For example, drinking water standards are currently based on the consumption patterns of an adult and should be reevaluated based on children's higher exposures and physiological vulnerabilities.

2. *Promote Pollution Prevention and Holistic Regulation.* While environmental laws have been successful by many measures, in general the laws have promoted treating pollution rather than more efficiently preventing its generation at the source. Pollution prevention is any practice that reduces the use or generation of hazardous substances prior to recycling, storage, treatment, or control. Several laws or strategies have been effective in promoting toxics use reduction at the source, including right-to-know laws that publicly report on pollution releases, drinking water contamination-product labeling requirements for hazardous ingredients and pollution prevention planning laws for industrial facilities (Hearne, 1996).

3. *Track Human Health Information to Take Preventive Action and Better Inform Environmental Decision-Making.* The success of environmental laws has been measured largely by charting reductions in ambient pollution, except for blood lead programs to reduce lead exposure. Little, if any, effort has gone into evaluating whether reduction in pollution levels are linked to improved health outcomes, such as fewer new cases of cancer, reduced severity of asthma attacks, or fewer birth defects. In cases where data about human disease or exposure is available, it should be incorporated into environmental decision-making. Disease surveillance systems need to be improved to track chronic disease and the associated environmental factors so that the public, health and environmental officials, and researchers can identify health promotion and disease prevention opportunities (Pew Commission, 2001).

Also see: Culture, Society, and Social Class: Foundation; Child Care: Early Childhood; Nutrition: Childhood.

References

American Academy of Pediatrics (AAP). (1999). *Handbook of pediatric environmental health.* Author.

American Society for Microbiology (ASM). (1999). *Microbial pollutants in our nation's water.* Washington, DC: Author.

Bates, D. (1995). The effects of air pollution on children. *Environmental Health Perspectives, 103*(Suppl. 6), 49–53.

Bates, D. (2000, February). Lines that connect: Assessing the causality inference in the case of particulate pollution. *Environmental Health Perspectives, 108*, 91–92.

Bearer, C.F. (1995). How are children different from adults? *Environmental Health Perspective Supplements, 103*(Suppl. 6), 7–12.

Buckley, J.D. (2000). Pesticide exposures in children with non-Hodgkin Lymphoma. *Cancer, 89*(11), 2315–2321.

Centers for Disease Control and Prevention (CDC). (1991). *Strategic plan for the elimination of childhood lead poisoning.* Atlanta: Department of Health and Human Services.

Centers for Disease Control and Prevention (CDC). (1999). *An ounce of prevention … What are the Returns?* (2nd ed.). Atlanta: US DHHS.

Chase, J. (1995). *Blueprint for a green school.* New York: Scholastic.

Chen, P.C., Chan, C.C., Lai, Y.M., Hwang, J.S., Yang, C.Y., & Wang, J.D. (1999, November). Short-term effect of ozone on the pulmonary function of children in primary school. *Environmental Health Perspectives, 107*, 921–925.

Clark, N. (1999, June). Childhood asthma. *Environmental Health Perspectives, 107*(Suppl. 3), 421–429.

Eggleston, P.A., Breysse, P.N., Buckley, T.J., Wills-Karp, M., Kleeberger, S.R., & Jaakkola, J.J. (1999, June). The environment and asthma in US inner cities. *Environmental Health Perspectives, 107*, 439–450.

Environmental Protection Agency (EPA). (1990). *Respiratory health effects of passive smoking: Lung, cancer and other disorders* (EPA 600-6-90-006F). Washington, DC.

Environmental Protection Agency (EPA). (2000a). *The Indoor Air Quality (IAQ) tools for schools* kit (EPA 402-C-00-002). Washington, DC.

Environmental Protection Agency (EPA). (2000b). *America's children and the environment: A first view of available measures* (EPA 240-R-00-006). Washington, DC.

Etzel, R.A. (1995). Indoor air-pollution and childhood asthma—effective environmental interventions. *Environmental Health Perspectives, 103* (Suppl. 6), 55–58.

George Foundation. (1999). *Project Lead-Free: A study of lead poisoning in major Indian cities.* Bangalore, India: The George Foundation.

Gilliland, F.D., Herhane, K., Rappaport, E.B., Thomas, D.C., Avol, E., Gauderman, W.J., et al. (2001). The effects of ambient air pollution on school absenteeism due to respiratory illnesses. *Epidemiology, 12*(1), 43–54.

Gold, D. (2000, August). Environmental tobacco smoke, indoor allergens and childhood asthma. *Environmental Health Perspectives, 109*(Supp. 4), 643–651.

Hearne, S. (1996). Tracking toxics: Chemical use and the public's "right-to-know." *Environment 38*, 4–34.

Jedrychowski, W., Flak, E., & Mroz, E. (1999, August). The adverse effect of low levels of ambient air pollutants on lung function growth in preadolescent children. *Environmental Health Perspectives, 107*, 669–674.

Kumar, R.K., & Kesaree, N. (1999). Blood lead levels in urban and rural Indian children. *Indian Pediatrics, 36*(3), 303–306.

Lowengart, R.A. (1987). Childhood leukemia and parents occupation and home exposures. *Journal of National Cancer Institute, 79*, 39–46.

Manuel, J. (1999, July). A healthy home environment? *Environmental Health Perspectives*, 107–117.

National Research Council (NRC). (1993a). *Measuring lead exposure in infants, children and other sensitive populations.* Washington, DC: National Academy Press.

National Research Council (NRC). (1993b). *Pesticides in the diet of infants and children.* Washington, DC: National Academy Press.

National Research Council (NRC). (2000). *Toxicological effects of Methylmercury.* Washington, DC: National Academy Press.

Ostro, B., Eskeland, G., Sanchez, J., & Feyzioglu, T. (1999). Air pollution and health effects: A study of medical visits among children in Santiago, Chile. *Environmental Health Perspectives, 107*(1), 69–73.

Peters, J., Avol, E., Gauderman, W.J., Linn, W.S., Navidi, W., London, S.J., Margolis, H., Rappaport, E., Vora, H., Gong, H., Jr., & Thomas, D.C. (1999). A study of twelve Southern California communities with differing levels and types of air pollution. *American Journal of Respiratory and Critical Care Medicine, 159*(3), 768–775.

Pew Environmental Health Commission. (2001). *Strengthening our public health defense against environmental threats.* Baltimore: Johns Hopkins School of Public Health.

Pirkle, J.L. (1994). The decline in blood lead levels in the United States— The National Health and Nutrition Examination Surveys. *Journal of the American Medical Association, 272*(4), 284–291.

Pope, C., & Ransom, M. (1992, August). Elementary school absences and PM10 pollution in Utah Valley. *Environmental Research, 58*, 204–219.

Royce, S. (2000). *Case studies in environmental medicine: Lead toxicity.* Atlanta, GA: Agency for Toxic Substances and Disease Registry.

Samet, M., Dominici, F., Currier, F., Coursac, I., & Zeger, S. (2000, December). Fine particulate air pollution and mortality in 20 US cities, 1987–1994. *New England Journal of Medicine, 343*, 1742–1749.

Schwab, M. (1992). Using longitudinal data to understand children's activity patterns in an exposure context: Data from the Kanawha County health study. *Environmental Health Perspectives, 18*, 173–189.

Smith, K., Samet, J., Romieu, I., & Bruce, N. (2000). Indoor air pollution in developing countries and acute lower respiratory infections in children. *Thorax, 55*, 518–532.

F

Families with Parental Mental Illness, Adolescence[*]

Carol Thiessen Mowbray and
Daphna Oyserman

INTRODUCTION

The offspring of parents with mental illness have long been a focus of research and a concern for practitioners. During childhood and adolescence, this population is considered at risk for problematic behavioral, academic, and social outcomes. In adulthood, their likelihood of having a diagnosable mental illness is significantly elevated. Vulnerability emanates from a combination of biological and environmental sources, including genetic factors (US DHHS, 1999, pp. 129, 237, 251, 254, 276), problematic parenting, and parental separations, as well as from social/contextual factors such as poverty, social isolation, stigma, and discrimination (Oyserman, Mowbray, Allen-Meares, & Firminger, 2000). This entry focuses on how interventions with school age and adolescent offspring of parents with mental illness may be planned and conducted to prevent predictable problems, protect their healthy functioning, and promote desired goals.

[*] Funding came from NIMH grant numbers R01 MH54321 and R01 MH57495. Crystal Espinoza and Mari Hashimoto helped prepare the tables and references.

DEFINITIONS

For the purposes of this entry, we have defined *mental illness* to be any disorder that fits the diagnostic criteria of DSM IV and is evidenced in more than one acute episode. We define *serious mental illness* additionally as a diagnosed disorder with duration more than 12 months and which seriously affects functioning in one or more major life areas.

SCOPE

A large body of literature exists concerning children of mentally ill parents, including some research outside the United States. The effects on children of parental psychiatric diagnosis or symptoms has been studied with individuals in Canada (Boyle & Pickles, 1997), New Zealand (Fergusson & Lynskey, 1993), London (Rutter & Quinton, 1984), Australia (Cowling, 1999), and Sweden (Persson-Blennow, Naeslund, McNeil, & Kaij, 1986). Changes in the likelihood of parenting and in the efficacy of psychotropic treatment for adults with mental illness make continued attention to this topic critical. That is, because of the deinstitutionalization movement begun in the 1950s in the United States, which has become a worldwide phenomenon, adults with a serious mental illness are now likely to remain in their communities and participate in more of the normal experiences of adulthood, such as having children and parenting. Available research indicates that most women with mental illness do marry, have normal fertility rates, are likely to be sexually active, and bear an above average number of children (Mowbray, Oyserman, & Zemencuk, 1995). Thus, many are likely to be mothers (59 percent according to McGrath, Hearle, Plant, Drummond, & Baskle, 1999). Further, in the last decade, there have been substantial improvements in psychiatric rehabilitation treatments and psychotherapeutic

471

medications, positively affecting the community functioning of adults with serious mental illness and thus their abilities to parent successfully. Based on several sources, we estimate that about one third of women with serious mental illnesses in community treatment have minor children and are carrying out childcare responsibilities (Mowbray, Oyserman, Bybee, MacFarlane, & Rueda-Riedle, in press).

Numerous studies have identified problematic outcomes for the offspring of parents with mental illness; most have studied infants and preschool children (Oyserman & Mowbray, see Children, Parents with Mental Illness: Childhood). For school age children and adolescents, maternal depressive mood correlates consistently with behavior problems and lower levels of social competence (Thomas, Forehand, & Neighbors, 1995; mean age of children, 13.1 years). Concerning academic and cognitive outcomes, results are more complex. Arbelle et al. (1997) found offspring (median age 16–17) of parents with schizophrenia performed significantly worse on a cognitive battery than children of parents with other mental illnesses or having no mental illness. But other studies find either no significant impairments for children of parents with mental illness or mediating relationships; for example, in one study, the relationship between maternal mental illness and self-perception of scholastic ability in children (mean age 10.11 years) was mediated by children's perceptions of emotional distress in their mothers (Scherer, Melloh, Buyck, Anderson, & Foster, 1996). Where gender differences do occur, they favor male children; that is, girls are more often adversely affected by having a mother with a mental illness than are boys (Oyserman et al., 2000), although results are inconsistent and not examined often enough.

It might be expected that families with a parent with a serious mental illness would have access to services necessary for identified and emergent needs. Unfortunately, this seems not to be the case. According to our own research and that of others, few mental health treatment programs or practitioners address the parenting needs of their clients. Few state information services collect data about whether clients have children; clinical records of mental health agencies often fail to even note the existence of children for adult clients; and only a minority of mothers identify their therapist or case manager as someone who could give advice or support about being a mother (Mowbray, Schwartz, Bybee, Spang, Rueda-Riedle, & Oyserman, 2000).

THEORIES

This review adopts a bio-psychosocial perspective as most helpful in understanding the situation of children with a mentally ill parent. The biological aspect of this perspective is well established; multiple research methods have documented

that for many mental illness diagnoses "heredity—that is, genes—plays a role in the transmission of vulnerability... from generation to generation" (US DHHS, 1999, p. 53). However, multiple environmental factors affect the extent to which genetic predispositions are expressed. In this regard, ecological theory seems most applicable to conducting comprehensive research on outcomes for children with mentally ill parents (Dulmus & Rapp-Paglicci, 2000). Bronfenbrenner (1979) conceptualized environmental influences on development as emanating from four domains: micro-, meso-, exo-, and macro-systems. Outcomes reflect the influences of these domains, as well as interactions between characteristics of the individual and of each domain. Thus, concerning children with mentally ill parents, research has focused most attention on the microsystem of parent–child interactions being influenced (negatively) by parental mental illness, the particular mechanisms through which this occurs, and, to a limited extent, the ways in which child characteristics (such as age or gender) may affect (moderate) this impact. Some research has also identified factors in the meso- and exo-systems that are relevant (such as marital discord or family functioning; Beardslee & Wheelock, 1994). Case studies have discussed how negative community and societal attitudes towards mental illness may affect children's adaptation and social integration (Marsh & Dickens, 1997). However, comprehensive research studies have not addressed these influences overall, nor studied their differential impact. The question we would like answered is: what characteristics of children and their contexts, including parents, families, peer interactions, community and societal influences, are the most prominent risk factors for negative outcomes?

RESEARCH

Biological Risk Factors

According to the recent report on mental health from the Surgeon General (US DHHS, 1999), biological factors (including genetics as well as early-onset abnormalities of the central nervous system) play a large part in the etiology of schizophrenia, bipolar disorder, social phobia, obsessive compulsive disorder, and Tourette's disorder (US DHHS, 1999, p. 129). However, heritability indices[1] vary from estimates

---

[1] Heritability indices reflect the estimated proportion of the phenotypic variance that is genetically determined. However, this is the estimate of genetic contribution in the population, not in each individual; and the partitioning of variance is specific to the particular trait, population, and environment. Further, heritability does not indicate what proportion of the trait is genetic, only what proportion of the variation in the trait is genetic. Finally, a trait can be genetically transmitted in a population but this does not necessarily mean that group differences in the trait are genetic in origin (Cann, 2001; Schelonka, 1999).

of 80 percent for bipolar disorder, 75 percent for schizophrenia, to 34–48 percent for depression (Rutter, Silberg, O'Connor, & Siminoff, 1999). As summarized by Downey and Coyne (1990), research studies on parents referred for depression indicate that their children are six times more likely to receive a diagnosis of major affective disorder than are children without an affectively ill parent. For these and other mental illness diagnoses, the likelihood of the identified patient's first-degree relatives also having a diagnosis reflects genetic contributions, but environmental circumstances are necessary to trigger genetic vulnerabilities. A number of epidemiological studies have found high rates of diagnosis in children of mentally ill parents, but the diagnoses are not necessarily the same as their parents'. For example, schizophrenia has a high concordance rate, but schizoaffective and bipolar diagnoses do not (Erlenmeyer-Kimling et al., 1997). Rutter and Quinton (1984) concluded that the association between parental and child mental disorders is environmentally mediated rather than genetically determined.

Parenting Problems

This summary of what is known about parenting problems draws from a more extensive literature review on parenting among mothers with a serious mental illness (Oyserman et al., 2000). That review covered parents of children from infancy to adolescence, and examined results from small clinical studies, as well as from larger and more diverse field studies. Unfortunately, a minority of published studies involves school age or adolescent children. Nevertheless, the studies available did show that, in comparison to non-mentally ill parents, mothers with schizophrenia or other psychotic disorders and mothers with unipolar depression have less encouraging parenting behaviors (Scherer et al., 1996), are less positive and more critical, and show less task-oriented behavior (Gordon, Burge, Hammen, & Adrian, 1989). Existing literature does not provide an adequate basis to determine differential effects of specific diagnoses. Studies do indicate that the current community functioning and symptomatology of mothers with mental illness have significant effects on parenting variables, such as the quality of the mother–child relationship, affective problems in family interactions, and children's task persistence (Hammen, Adrian, Gordon, & Jaenicke, 1987). Children's self-reports, gathered through qualitative research, indicate that their mothers are often inconsistent and unpredictable (Cowling, 1999).

A few qualitative studies have identified the parenting strengths of women with severe mental illness, presenting evidence that parenting can have positive and motivating effects upon the mothers. In these studies, mothers with serious mental illness articulated the significance of having children, its positive contribution to recovery, and their struggles to maintain custody (Nicholson, Sweeney, & Geller, 1998).

Contextual Factors

While studies have clearly established parenting difficulties among mothers with mental illness, research has not determined the separate effects of common confounding risk factors. For example, marital discord and social isolation are common for seriously mentally ill mothers and their children, as are conflicts with extended family. Some research indicates that adults with depression tend to marry spouses with psychiatric illness, a history of psychopathology, and/or substance abuse. Mothers with a mental illness are also likely to have more stressful lives, including past experiences of physical and sexual abuse. Multiple hospitalizations and the chronicity of mental health problems affect mothers' relationships with children and contribute to marital break-ups. Furthermore, all these factors are likely to interact and exacerbate overall family functioning; thus, marital discord contributes to negative interactions with children for depressed mothers, child behavior disturbances relate to mothers' more distant and withdrawn behaviors, and children with externalizing disorders have fewer and less positive interactions with mentally ill mothers (Oyserman et al., 2000).

Narratives from now-adult children of mentally ill parents describe other risk factors. Risks for children include role reversals (children taking care of parents) and heightened anxieties about whether they will inherit their parents' mental illness. More generally, risks may be due to a decrease in family social life and loss of "normal" family activities (e.g., outings and fun things to do), with concomitant instability, chaos, crises, and household disarray. Also periods of neglect, either relative or statutorily defined, and inconsistent parenting caused by separations when mothers are hospitalized (Barankin & Greenberg, 1996) have been cited. These strains deplete family energies, leaving caretakers less able to help children with tasks that they must accomplish developmentally, and less capable of providing love, guidance, or supervision (Marsh & Dickens, 1997). Children may respond by feeling resentful and rejecting, increasing the likelihood of family burnout (Hatfield, 1996).

Economic factors are also likely to significantly affect families; nearly all individuals with a serious mental illness, especially women, are living in poverty and at risk for chronic economic hardships. Lack of social support is another risk factor because adults with serious mental illness consistently have smaller social networks than the general population (Mowbray, Schwartz et al., 2000). Culture can interact with mental illness symptoms to affect labeling and treatment. For example, gender and race/ethnicity influence the reliability and stability of diagnoses (Nathan & Langenbucher, 1999; Prudo & Blum, 1987); in particular, African Americans with affective disorders are significantly more likely than Caucasians to be mis-diagnosed with schizophrenia-spectrum disorders, especially paranoia (Whaley, 1998).

Although not systematically examined in research, studies on risk factors, stigma and discrimination experienced from neighbors and others in the community, as well as rejection and abandonment by extended family and family friends are frequently reported by adults who grew up with a mentally ill parent (Marsh & Dickens, 1997). These adult children report losing friends, being afraid or ashamed to bring friends home, feeling different, and feeling that they came from a "defective" family. School age and adolescence are particularly critical, as children report that it is the time when they realize that their family is different (Cowling, 1999).

Thus correlations between maternal mental illness, parenting, and children's outcomes, may be due to a direct effect of mental illness, but are also likely to be due, in part, to the many other social and economic hardships associated with mental illness—hardships that can interfere with important developmental opportunities. These effects seem particularly significant for school age children and adolescents, as they establish their own identity, sense of competence, networks of social support, and autonomy in their communities.

Unfortunately, very little research has attempted to disentangle the direct effects of maternal psychiatric variables, such as diagnosis, symptom severity, duration and chronicity of mental illness, or community functioning, from social/contextual variables that negatively affect mothers and their children, such as poverty, single parenting, social support. Mowbray, Oyserman, Bybee, and MacFarlane (2000) found that controlling for demographic variables, mothers' diagnosis made independent, but small contributions to explaining variability in parenting; mothers' symptomatology and community functioning had much stronger effects. Some research has begun to investigate the pathways through which maternal diagnoses or symptoms affect child and adolescent outcomes. For example, Davies and Windle (1997), found that family discord was a strong mediator of the relationship between maternal depressive symptoms and children's conduct disturbances and depressive symptoms, at least for girls.

STRATEGIES: OVERVIEW

There is a disturbing lack of research addressing the needs of school aged and adolescent children of mentally ill parents. This gap is surprising given the long history of attributing children's mental disturbances to parental influences (e.g., the "schizophrenogenic" mother) and the

acknowledged potency of parental psychopathology as a risk factor for child/adolescent mental illness. Most existing research has focused on epidemiology, but additional research of that type is likely to provide diminishing returns. More helpful to the development of effective prevention interventions would be studies addressing: "What is the best way to intervene with these children and their families?" Answers to this question would assist in developing and testing the effectiveness of alternative approaches, including early preventive interventions with children, parents, families, and broader support systems, as well as in identifying the critical components of these interventions.

Pertaining to such research, some prevention approaches for school age and adolescent offspring of mentally ill parents have still been developed. Through literature reviews, searches of conference presentations, and networking with other researchers, we were able to identify seven programs that provide services to the target group.[2]

STRATEGIES THAT WORK

Only one of the identified programs has undergone any rigorous evaluation: "Preventive Intervention for Families with Depression." For this program, Beardslee, Salt, Versage, Gladstone, Wright, and Rothberg (1997) utilized an experimental design, with random assignment to a clinician-facilitated (active treatment) or lecture-based intervention (quasi-control condition). Eligible families, recruited from a large health maintenance organization, included at least one parent who experienced an episode of affective disorder and one child between ages 8 and 15 who had never been treated for affective disorder. The purpose of the intervention was to decrease the effect of family and marital risk factors, encourage the promotion of resiliency in children through enhanced parental and family functioning, and prevent the onset of depression and other mental health problems. The clinician-facilitated (active) condition involved 6–10 sessions, starting with an assessment of all family members. It included individual sessions with parents, an individual session with each child and one or two family meetings, along with an information packet about depression. The program had a strong cognitive orientation, with a goal of increasing all family members' understanding of the illness experience, increasing adults' understanding of their children's perspective, and helping parents to promote children's ability to cope with

---

[2] Primary sources of information were Drs. Judith Cook at the National Rehabilitation and Training Center in Chicago and Joanne Nicholson at University of Massachusetts Medical School-Center for Mental Health Services Research, both of whom have been funded to identify and document the operations of model programs serving mothers with mental illness and their children.

the illness and to move on with their lives. In the lecture condition, families received the same packet of information and attended two 1-hr lectures, followed by brief question and answer periods.

Beardslee, Salt, Versage, Gladstone, Wright, and Rothberg (1997) reported the follow-up results for 37 families served, 18 months after the initial intervention. Independent raters documented significant improvements for all families in number of positive changes in behaviors and attitudes, global benefits, self-understanding, and the family's focus on their children. Additionally, families in the clinician-facilitated (vs. lecture) condition reported significantly more satisfaction and more benefits from the intervention. However, no data were reported on differential outcomes for children.

STRATEGIES THAT MIGHT WORK

Table 1 summarizes information for all the relevant programs identified in the literature, their locations and descriptions. Listed programs are located all over the United States, Canada, Australia and Israel, suggesting recognition of this problem in diverse societies. Interestingly, we identified urban programs serving mothers with serious mental illness and their infants and/or young children, but programs for families with older children are primarily located in rural or suburban areas. Possibly, urban services put less emphasis on mental health and more on behavioral problems: Mrazek and Haggerty (1994) found no prevention programs for adolescents focused on preventing depression or schizophrenia. All the programs for adolescents they identified involve preventing substance abuse or conduct disorder.

The programs described in Table 1 are extremely heterogeneous. Some are add-ons to existing services provided to the parent with a mental illness, offering parenting support and/or training, such as Beardslee et al. (1997) or Lifequest. Some are comprehensive, offering services that the parents' mental health agency should provide, at least for a limited period of time, such as crisis intervention, coordination of needed services, housing availability, family reunification services (FSS in Iowa City and the Invisible Children's Program in Goshen, New York). Several of the programs were for children only, utilizing a group support model (Group intervention—Tel Aviv; Kids Link—Vancouver, Champs and Kids with Confidence—Victoria, Australia).

STRATEGIES THAT DO NOT WORK

The lack of comprehensive research on intervention models and their components precludes a definitive answer to this question. However, some research reviews have offered some speculation. While the specifics vary, the overall answer is that a "one size fits all" prevention approach for families with a mentally ill parent should be avoided. Thus, Downey and Coyne (1990), presenting an integrative review of research on children of depressed parents, concluded "adequate explanatory models must incorporate considerable complexity" (p. 68). They note the importance of reciprocal influences between mothers and children and the significance of the family context. Obviously, race/ethnicity, class, and culture need attention in all family treatment and prevention programs (Corcoran, 2000)—but perhaps even more so where mental illness is involved, since its labeling, acceptance, treatment, and recovery definitions are extremely culture-bound.

At a minimum, these considerations imply first, that the target of prevention efforts should be the entire family—not just children and not just parents. Second, interventions should be individualized, or alternative models should be available. Thus, while some parents may need parent training, others have this knowledge and would find such services boring, irrelevant, or insulting. However, these families may need assistance in budgeting or in accessing additional resources, so they can do the best job they can with what they have available. Finally, although one would hope that this would not need to be said, based on our accumulated research knowledge, interventions must avoid blaming mothers with mental illness for their children's problems. Downey and Coyne (1990) remarked that they found "a distinct and consistent, even if unintentional, 'mother-bashing' quality to much of this body of work" (p. 72). From a prevention perspective, capitalizing on family strengths not just weaknesses should enhance willingness to stay involved in services.

SYNTHESIS

Despite the heterogeneity of available models, program descriptions and summative reviews (Cook & Steigman, 2000) present some common, important ingredients for interventions that are successful in preventing mental health and other problems in school age and adolescent children of parents with mental illness. Following a prevention framework, interventions must minimize risks and maximize protective factors; this means minimizing family dysfunction and maximizing the child's support system and his/her own competencies. Whether the program provides direct services or coordinates and links with other services, prevention activities must have a multiple focus on parents, family, and children. With regard to parents, prevention efforts need to ensure that the parent with a mental illness remains as healthy as possible, minimizing negative effects on parenting. Family members need support and education about

Table 1. Programs for Parents with Mental Illness and/or Their School Age/Adolescent Children

Program	Focus/goals	Children	Parents	Services/methods
Preventive interventions for families with depression (Beardslee et al., 1997)	Project aims to decrease impact of parental illness on family functioning and promote changes in parental behavior and attitudes that would result in fostering resiliency in children	Ages 8–15 ($X = 12$)	Mean age = 42.9 $N = 37$ families. 29 dual-parent families; 8 single parents. All single parents were mothers White middle-class	A clinician-facilitated group intervention was designed to prevent childhood depression and related problems through decreasing the impact of related risk factors and encouraging resiliency-promoting behaviors and attitudes
Short-term group therapy for children of mentally ill parents (Finzi & Stange, 1997)	Group therapy intervention aimed at creating support systems for improving children's coping mechanisms and adjustment via positive peer experiences, and assisting in rehabilitation of damaged interpersonal skills and self-concept.	Ages 9–12 15 boys and girls	11 families referred by local general practitioners	Traditional aspects of activity group therapy with special activities and dramatic games through which children could express inner world fantasies and fears and real world distress, become aware of and learn new coping strategies in a safe, accepting atmosphere
The family support services program, Iowa City, Iowa (J. Cook, personal communication, 2000)	Reduce hospitalizations by coordination of treatment services; reduce out-of-home placements of children; bridge gap between mental health and child welfare	Ages 0–18 Many diagnosed as oppositional, ADHD, or developmentally delayed	Most are single-parent and impoverished, with little or no family support 95% White, 2% African American, 2% Latino, 1% Native American (1997)	Crisis intervention 24 hr/day, 7 days/week teaching decision-making, problem-solving skills, and helping with child management. Teaching children about parent's mental illness and assisting in preparations for hospitalization. Families engage in self-assessment, strengths identification, family goal-setting, and establishment of formal/informal supports
The invisible children's program Goshen, NY (J. Nicholson, personal communication, 2000)	First priority is to empower parent to be a role model. Provide guidance to help develop quality way of life; support to avoid separation of parent(s) and child; prevent child(ren) from repeated foster care; preservation of family	Ages 0–12	Voluntary, self-referred clients 60% White, 40% African American (1997)	Quality housing to keep families together; 17 apartments and 24 hr case management provided. Respite care, job training, and safety planning. Art therapy for children. Children educated about their parents' disorders
Lifequest Wasilla, Alaska (J. Cook, personal communication, 2000)	Large, diverse, community-oriented mental health services agency	Ages 0–18	Mothers w/parental role impairment, homeless. Mostly White, small percentage Native American, African American (1997)	Clinical, emergency, rehabilitation, medical, residential, and prevention/early intervention/community education services, including supported housing and home-based services
Kids in control Vancouver, British Columbia, Canada (J. Cook, personal communication, 2000)	Psycho-educational support group program for children/adolescents. Promotes children's development of healthy coping skills	Young children to early adolescents	Adults with serious mental illness	Group runs once/year in four BC communities, and consists of 1.5 hr sessions once/week for 4 weeks. Group members given opportunity to work with and develop weekly themes through use of different arts, crafts, and interactive game activities
Southern partnership project—"Listen to the Children" Victoria, Australia (Cowling, 1999)	Develop 4 inter-agency networks to more effectively meet the needs of families. Facilitate collaborative and cooperative links among service providers to ensure children are identified and receive support and parents feel entitled to ask for help in caring for children; develop prevention and early intervention programs for children	Dependent children, all ages	Adults with serious mental illness	Regional level: questionnaire for service providers; reference group initiatives— identified shortcomings of Dept of Human Services data collection forms re service provision to families. Network level: lobbying; workshops on understanding effects of MI on parents and parenting; service development— a planned support program for parents

mental illness. Children need their own sources of support and advocacy, and help understanding their parent's mental illness and their own independence from it.

Minimizing Risks

1. *Keeping the Parent with Mental Illness Healthy.* The identified consumer in the family must receive appropriate, state of the art mental health and rehabilitation services. This usually means psychiatric diagnostic assessments and medication, rehabilitative assistance through recovery counseling, and psycho-education targeted on consumers' understanding their disorder and making necessary lifestyle changes to maximize functioning. Usually case management services are necessary to assure that services are coordinated, available, accessible, and acceptable. This may require making funding arrangements, identifying programs to meet special needs (e.g., for those with English as a second language, or with a physical disability), finding programs acceptable to the individual's cultural values, or accessing services provided through other agencies, like supported education or vocational rehabilitation. Case management is often necessary to help families meet basic needs such as housing that is affordable, safe, and appropriate for children, and funds for food, clothing, and children's developmental needs. Programs should build on the newly found recognition that child rearing is a significant role for parents with mental illness and one that often can serve as the foundation for a parent's recovery (Cook & Steigman, 2000).

2. *Maintaining a Functioning Family System.* As parents are working on their own recovery, the family system needs to provide assistance and also needs help meeting needs of each individual adult family member. All family members must understand that psychiatric disorders are *real* illnesses—not disorders of character or morality. Families often need assistance in how they communicate about mental illness, because keeping this problem a family secret usually exacerbates functioning difficulties. Families also need probo feel that there is a stable back-up for their parent with mental illness. Psycho-education programs, developed primarily for families where an adult child has a mental illness, can be adapted to families in which a parent has mental illness.

3. *Minimizing Crises, Family Disruptions and Child Placements.* Mental health treatments, psychiatric rehabilitation and case management services should help minimize the likelihood of serious problems that require hospitalizations. Suicide attempts, extremely bizarre behaviors, or interpersonal violence are problems that disrupt family functioning and children's need for stability, cause parental separations that disturb parenting continuity, heighten children's anxieties and fears, and may produce trauma and other stresses. Because psychiatric disorders are illnesses with variable courses, procedures for early intervention and for immediate and sensitive crisis resolution must be in place to handle serious problems when they do arise. These procedures need to take into account the care of children when the main caregiving parent is in the hospital. Because many mothers with mental illness are not married and live alone with their children, lack of advance planning is likely to result in child welfare placement that may be difficult to reverse, even when the mother is subsequently released and stabilized. To avoid such placements, some states and advocacy groups have information available on how to establish temporary custody arrangements in advance or execute advance directives specifying childcare arrangements and the authority of the temporary care provider when the parent is unavailable.

4. *Parenting Assistance.* Many adults with mental illness were functioning successfully as parents before the onset of their disorder. However, those adults who experienced an early onset of mental illness may need considerable education and training in parenting skills. All families with a mentally ill parent should be involved in an assessment of strengths and weaknesses that gives the identified parent–patient the opportunity to voice his/her concerns and needs. Based on the assessment, parents should have available any needed education and training about child and adolescent development, group support and mentoring from other parents with mental illness (which also helps with problem-solving and communication issues), and parent skill training (which can be provided through in-home services or by role-modeling of other parent support group members). Mental health and rehabilitation staff and/or client case managers will need to involve themselves in parenting issues by including parenting goals in individual treatment plans. Parents will often need assistance and advocacy support to deal with other agencies, such as child welfare services with regard to TANF payments or abuse/neglect allegations, schools regarding children's academic or behavior problems, and children's health providers.

Maximizing Protective Factors

1. *Supportive Adults in the Child/Adolescent's Life.* Research literature and self-reports of children with a mentally ill parent confirm the importance of the child having alternative caretakers or other supportive adults that they trust and feel they can rely on. Supportive adults can provide consistent, warm, and affectionate relationships and a source for building the child's self esteem and his/her sense of independence and accomplishment (Cowling, 1999). If the child does not have rapport with adults in the family system, prevention programs should help build such connections (e.g., with a coach, teacher, religious or youth group leader, a neighbor, etc.) and this adult support person should be invited to attend family support activities so that he/she has an understanding of mental illness and of the family situation.

2. *Peer Support for Children/Adolescents.* A number of programs include peer support groups for children, composed of a small group whose parents all have a mental illness. Peer groups serve the significant function of helping children believe (rather than just hearing or being told) that their problems are not unique. This experience can help decrease stigma and shame experienced, increase social connectedness, provide opportunities to help others, and give some children opportunities to practice interpersonal skills that may be under-developed because of social isolation and discrimination.

3. *Child/Adolescent Understanding and Competence.* Many self-reports from adult children who experienced parental mental illness emphasize the importance of their understanding and believing that they are not responsible for parental behavior and outcomes and therefore do not need to compensate—by being "good" or filling adult roles—and that their own outcomes are separate from their parents'. Thus, children/adolescents individually or through group support need to hear these messages clearly and repeatedly. Their own competence and autonomy need to be enhanced and promoted to reduce guilt, anxiety, and fear and the stress these produce, especially because these stresses, themselves, can increase risk of mental and emotional problems.

4. *Early Identification of Child Problems and Ready Access to Child and Family Mental Health Services.* Even if all the above critical ingredients are available to a family, child/adolescent problems may develop as a result of genetic, constitutional, or other biological bases of mental illness as well as psychosocial factors such as maternal prenatal stress, poverty, or exposure to external toxins experienced in urban areas (accidents, crime, and the like). Parents, family members, and the child's adult support/advocate need education and awareness for early identification of such problems. Case managers, mental health staff and rehabilitation workers all need to be tuned in and responsive to early warning signs of child disorders. Barankin and Greenberg (1996) recommend that all children of parents with serious mental illnesses be given annual "check-ups," much as is the case when parents have other chronic disorders with a genetic basis (e.g., diabetes). We now know that many serious mental illnesses have a long prodromal period, and that early interventions can markedly decrease the likelihood of relapse and disability throughout life. Agency procedures must facilitate rapid response and integrated treatments for parent and child.

Thus, prevention programs targeting children/adolescents of mentally ill parents need to have many components and work effectively with other services utilized or needed by families, in a wrap-around fashion, where meeting family needs is more important than the administrative procedures of various funding sources. It would seem that most often, child/adolescent prevention services should be associated with the parent's mental health or rehabilitation provider. This contrasts with many traditional school-based child/adolescent prevention programs that target at-risk groups such as children of divorce, and children coping with grief and mourning. Because creating an understanding and a supportive context is central to prevention with school age and adolescent children of parents with mental illness, school-based services would be inappropriate because of the stigma of being the child of a mentally ill parent and the discrimination likely directed at group members. An exception might be Student Assistance Programs (SAP), which operate much like Employee Assistance Programs in industry; that is, schools provide information to help students realize that they may have a problem and then self-refer or obtain referral for confidential treatment and assessment. It is up to the SAP to identify the risk factors contributing to problems and to address them (Dupont, 1997). A similar approach is used with children from families with addictions and could potentially be applied to other family-based problems like parental mental illness, since family dysfunction is often similar under both sets of risk factors.

Also see: Family Strengthening: Childhood; Family Strengthening: Adolescence; Self-Esteem: Early Childhood; Self-Esteem: Childhood; Self-Esteem: Adolescence; Social and Emotional Learning: Early Childhood; Social and Emotional Learning: Childhood; Social and Emotional Learning: Adolescence.

References

Arbelle, S., Magharious, W., Auerbach, J.G., Hans, S.L., Marcus, J., Baruch, S., & Caplan, R. (1997). Formal thought disorder in offspring of schizophrenic parents. *Israel Journal of Psychiatry & Related Sciences, 34*(3), 210–221. Israel: Gefen.

Barankin, T., & Greenberg, M. (1996). The impact of parental affective disorders on families. In B. Abosh & A. Collins (Eds.), *Mental illness in the family* (pp. 105–119). Toronto: University of Toronto Press.

Beardslee, W.R., Salt, P., Versage, E.M., Gladstone, T.R.G., Wright, E.J., & Rothberg, P.C. (1997). Sustained change in parents receiving preventive interventions for families with depression. *American Journal of Psychiatry, 154*(4), 510–515.

Beardslee, W., & Wheelock, I. (1994). Children of parents with affective disorders. In W. Reynolds, & H. Johnston (Eds.), *Handbook of depression in children and adolescents*. New York: Plenum Press.

Boyle, M., & Pickles, A. (1997). Influence of maternal depressive symptoms on ratings of childhood behavior. *Journal of Abnormal Child Psychology, 25*(5), 399–412.

Bronfenbrenner, U. (1979). *The ecology of human development: Experiment by nature and design.* Cambridge, MA: Harvard University Press.

Cann, R. (2001). *Genetics* [On-line]. Available: http://www.hawaii.edu/genetics/week_16_Thursday.htm

Cook, J., & Steigman, P. (2000). Experiences of parents with mental illnesses and their service needs. *The Journal of NAMI California, 11*(2), 21–23.

Corcoran, J. (2000). Family treatment of preschool behavior problems. *Research on Social Work Practice, 10*(5), 547–588.

Cowling, V. (Ed.) (1999). *Children of parents with mental illness.* Melbourne, Victoria: The Australian Council for Educational Research.

Davies, P.T., & Windle, M. (1997). Gender-specific pathways between maternal depressive symptoms, family discord, and adolescent adjustment. *Developmental Psychology, 33*(4), 657–668.

Downey, G., & Coyne, J.C. (1990). Children of depressed parents—An integrative review. *Psychological Bulletin, 108*(1), 50–76.

Dulmus, C.N., & Rapp-Paglicci, L.A. (2000). The prevention of mental disorders in children and adolescents: Future research and public-policy recommendations. *Families in Society, 81*(3), 294–303.

Dupont, R.L. (1997). *The selfish brain: Learning from addiction.* Washington, DC: American Psychiatric Press.

Erlenmeyer-Kimling, L., Adamo, U., Rock, D., Roberts, S., Bassett, A., Squires-Wheeler, E., Cornblatt, B., Endicott, J., Pape, S., & Gottesman, I. (1997). The New York high-risk project: Prevalence and comorbidity of Axis I disorders in offspring of schizophrenic parents at 25 year follow-up. *Archives of General Psychiatry, 54*(12), 1096–1102.

Fergusson, D., & Lynskey, M. (1993). The effects of maternal depression on child conduct disorder and attention deficit behaviours. *Social Psychiatry & Psychiatric Epidemiology, 28*, 116–123.

Finzi, R., & Stange, D. (1997). Short term group intervention as a means of improving the adjustment of children of mentally ill parents. *Social Work with Groups, 20*(4), 69–80.

Gordon, D., Burge, D., Hammen, C., & Adrian, C. (1989). Observations of interactions of depressed women with their children. *American Journal of Psychiatry, 146*(1), 50–55.

Hammen, C., Adrian, C., Gordon, D., & Jaenicke, C. (1987). Children of depressed mothers: Maternal strain and symptom predictors of dysfunction. *Journal of Abnormal Psychology, 96*(3), 190–198.

Hatfield, A. (1996). Out of the ashes of mental illness. In B. Abosh & A. Collins (Eds.), *Mental illness in the family* (pp. 58–66). Toronto: University of Toronto Press.

Marsh, D.T., & Dickens, R.M. (1997). *Troubled journey.* New York: Penguin Putnam.

McGrath, J.J., Hearle, J., Plant, K., Drummond, A., & Barkla, J.M. (1999). The fertility and fecundity of patients with psychoses. *Acta Psychiatrica Sandinavica, 99*, 441–446.

Mowbray, C.T., Oyserman, D., Bybee, D., & MacFarlane, P. (2000). Parenting of mothers with a serious mental illness: Differential effects of diagnosis, clinical history and other mental health variables. Unpublished manuscript. University of Michigan, Ann Arbor, MI.

Mowbray, C.T., Oyserman, D., Bybee, D., MacFarlane, P., & Rueda-Riedle, A. (2000). Life circumstances of mothers with serious mental illness. *Psychiatric Rehabilitation Journal, 25*(2), 114–123.

Mowbray, C.T., Oyserman, D., & Zemencuk, J. (1995). Motherhood for women with serious mental illness: Pregnancy, childbirth and the postpartum period. *American Journal of Orthopsychiatry, 65*(1), 21–38.

Mowbray, C.T., Schwartz, S., Bybee, D., Spang, J., Rueda-Riedle, A., & Oyserman, D. (2000). Mothers with mental illness: Stressors and resources for parenting and living. *Families & Society, 81*(2), 118–129.

Mrazek, P.J., & Haggerty, R.P. (1994). *Reducing risks for mental disorders: Frontiers for preventative intervention research.* Washington, DC: National Academy Press.

Nathan, P.E., & Langenbucher, J.W. (1999). Psychopathology: Description and classification. *Annual Review of Psychology, 50*, 79–107.

Nicholson, J., Sweeney, E.M., & Geller, J.L. (1998). Mothers with mental illness: I. The competing demands of parenting and living with mental illness. *Psychiatric Services, 49*(5), 635–642.

Oyserman, D., Mowbray, C.T., Allen-Meares, P., & Firminger, K. (2000). Parenting among mothers with a mental illness. *American Journal of Orthopsychiatry, 70*(3), 296–315.

Persson-Blennow, I., Naeslund, B., McNeil, T.F., & Kaij, L. (1986). Offspring of women with nonorganic psychosis: Mother–infant interaction at one year of age. *Acta Psychiatrica Scandinavia, 73*, 207–213.

Prudo, R., & Blum, M. (1987). Five-year outcome and prognosis in schizophrenia: A report from the London Field Research Centre of the international pilot study of schizophrenia. *British Journal of Psychiatry, 150*, 345–354.

Rutter, M., & Quinton, D. (1984). Parental psychiatric disorder: Effects on children. *Psychological Medicine, 14*(4), 853–880.

Rutter, M., Silberg, J., O'Connor, T., & Siminoff, E. (1999). Genetics and child psychiatry: II. Empirical research findings. *Journal of Child Psychology & Psychiatry & Allied Disciplines, 40*(1), 19–55.

Scherer, D.G., Melloh, T., Buyck, D., Anderson, C., & Foster, A. (1996). Relation between children's perceptions of maternal mental illness and children's psychological adjustment. *Journal of Clinical Child Psychology, 25*(2), 156–169.

Schelonka, E.P. (1999). Applications of genetics in sports medicine. *Medicine, 50*(2) [On-line]. Available: http://www.dcmsonline.org/jax-medicine/february99/index.htm

Thomas, A.M, Forehand, R., & Neighbors, B. (1995). Change in maternal depressive mood: Unique contributions to adolescent functioning over time. *Adolescence, 30*(117), 43–52.

US Department of Health and Human Services (US DHHS). (1999). *Mental health: A report of the Surgeon General.* Rockville, MD: US DHHS, Substance Abuse and Mental Health Services Administration, Center for Mental Health Services, National Institutes of Health, National Institute of Mental Health.

Whaley, A.L. (1998). Cross-cultural perspective on paranoia: A focus on the Black American experience. *Psychiatric Quarterly, 69*(4), 325–343.

Family Strengthening, Childhood

Larry E. Dumka

INTRODUCTION

This entry focuses on empirically based family strengthening interventions aimed at improving aspects of family members' interactions with children aged 5–12, and that have been shown to prevent or ameliorate negative developmental outcomes in children (e.g., conduct problems, academic failure, substance abuse, and high risk sex) and to promote positive ones. This focus includes interventions that target parents or adult caretakers only, typically termed "parenting" programs, and interventions that involve both parents and children and interactions between them, called "family" approaches (Kumpfer, 1999).

DEFINITIONS

Across cultures, the healthy development of children appears to be fostered by three key functions of families: the provision of adequate resources for sustenance (food, shelter, medical care), training for economic viability (adequate education), and socialization into the local standards of virtuous behavior (LeVine, 1974). For the purposes of this article, *family* is defined as the system of adults and siblings that perform these key functions for children (Kumpfer, 1999). In the broadest sense, *family strengthening* can involve activities that contribute to family members' ability to perform and manage any of the key functions mentioned (e.g., income, employment, and tax assistance, improving schools, character education).

SCOPE

Early problems with children strongly predict more serious problems later in adolescence (Patterson & Joerger, 1993). Troubling signs in the United States, include the highest rates of violent crime and pregnancy among teenagers in developed countries as well as very high rates of substance abuse, sexually transmitted diseases, and academic failure (e.g., failure to graduate from high school). In addition, these problems appear to be interconnected, with young people who engage in one of the problem behaviors being more likely also to engage in others (Donovan, Jessor, & Costa, 1988). Moreover, there is evidence that negative developmental outcomes in children tend to be visited on the subsequent generation (Conger, Cui, Bryant, & Elder, 2000). One response to these problems has been the development of family strengthening interventions.

THEORIES

Prominent among the theoretical sources for empirically based family strengthening interventions are the *social learning models* of human behavior that have emphasized the bi-directional nature of parent–child relations and identified coercive patterns of family interaction that predict antisocial adjustment in children (Patterson & Joerger, 1993). Consequently, many intervention developers have focused on attempting to interdict these patterns and replace them with more benign and adaptive ones. Furthermore, intervention developers have relied frequently on social learning principles (e.g., modeling, guided practice, and feedback) as the basis for the change strategies employed in their interventions (Taylor & Biglan, 1998).

Another major theoretical source for empirically based family strengthening interventions has been research on *developmental risks and protective factors* that are linked to children's developmental outcomes. Risk factors are those variables that have been shown to increase the probability of children developing problems. Empirically identified risk factors within the family include parental mental illness, substance abuse, antisocial behavior, excessive family conflict or marital discord, and poor parenting practices, particularly inadequate discipline, monitoring, and supportiveness (Rutter, 1987). Moreover, the chances of children developing behavioral and mental health problems increase markedly as the number of risk factors increases. Protective factors, in contrast, are variables that have been shown to decrease the risk of children experiencing problems. Consequently, developers of empirically based family strengthening interventions have focused on trying to reduce modifiable family risk factors (e.g., family conflict) and/or increase modifiable family protective factors (e.g., effective parenting practices).

A closely related theoretical source for family-strengthening interventions is individual and *family stress process models* (McCubbin & Patterson, 1983). In these models, stress is seen as resulting when the perceived demands of a situation (e.g., the arbitrariness of a parent's behavior) appear to exceed the available resources to cope adaptively with the stressors and resolve the predicament (e.g., knowing what the parent will view as compliant behavior). The additional contribution of stress process models pertains to the coping capacities. In some family strengthening interventions, parents have been engaged to help children increase their coping capacities through teaching problem solving, help seeking, and cognitive and emotion regulation skills. More recently, intervention developers have acknowledged stressors operating on parents, both within and outside the family. When the demands of these stressors exceed parents' coping resources, parents' capacity to maintain protective family functions for children (e.g., adequate discipline, monitoring, and support) are compromised. Thus, in addition to teaching child management skills, family strengthening intervention developers have begun to address parents' personal stress management capacities (e.g., problem-solving skills, soliciting social support, and cognitive and emotion regulation skills).

A theoretical source that is increasingly influencing family strengthening interventions is *contextualism* (Lerner, Castellino, Terry, Villarruel, & McKinney, 1995). Contextualism highlights the embeddedness of human systems and seeks to explain not only how children, parents, and families influence each other but also how family members are influenced by and, in turn, influence their ecological niches. For example, certain ecological niches (e.g., violent neighborhoods) can negatively affect children's proximal environments (e.g., family relations and quality of parenting) and thus compromise protective factors (Brooks-Gunn, Duncan, Klebanov, & Sealand, 1993). Conversely, families joining together to provide mutual support and jointly monitor children can make the neighborhood a safer place for children (Furstenberg, 1993). In addition, broad systemic changes over the past 50 years, including increases in marital dissolution, mothers in the labor force, single-parent households, and child poverty, have significantly altered the developmental contexts of many children (Hernandez, 1993).

RESEARCH

Research has indicated that serious behavioral and mental health problems in teenagers and young adults are often predicted by negative patterns in childhood established as early as age five (Kazdin, 1987). These early patterns include conduct problems (e.g., aggression and coercion) interacting with child temperament conditions (e.g., impulsivity and low verbal IQ) in ways that contribute to social rejection by prosocial peers and academic underperformance. These, in turn, lead to increased association with deviant peers, which is the most proximal influence on deviant behavior (Patterson & Joerger, 1993). At the same time, research has shown that family factors such as prevalent conflict and poor parenting influence children's developmental trajectories (Grych & Fincham, 2001; Rothbaum & Weisz, 1994). Parents' family management practices have

been seen as an important pathway of the mechanism of influence, primarily because of the parents' role in structuring children's social learning environments, not just within the family, but also through parents' ability to influence peer association and school interactions and performance.

Research has consistently shown four parenting practices to be linked to children's problem behavior: (1) lack of parents' prosocial involvement with children (e.g., teaching and reinforcement of verbal skills and cooperative behavior); (2) lack of supportiveness (e.g., responsiveness to children's concerns, affirmation, enjoyable time spent together); (3) harsh and inconsistent discipline (e.g., lack of clear rules and even-tempered enforcement of appropriate consequences); and (4) lack of monitoring (i.e., knowledge of children's whereabouts and behavior at home, at school, and with peers) (Patterson & Joerger, 1993). Thus, behaviorally oriented interventions to promote children's healthy development initially tended to focus on training parents to use complementary and positive child management practices.

Furthermore, research has identified additional factors that significantly affect parents' parenting behavior. These include marital conflict, parent depression, and parent social isolation (Patterson, Reid, & Dishion, 1992). As a result, intervention developers have added components to child management training in order to increase intervention effectiveness. Examples of added components include parent self-control training (Wells, Griest, & Forehand, 1980), assistance with marital problems (Webster-Stratton & Herbert, 1994), and social problem-solving skills for isolated single parents (Pfiffner, Jouriles, Brown, Etscheidt, & Kelly, 1990). Thus, in response to research findings, family strengthening interventions have evolved from behavioral parent training, limited to training in child management skills, into what are now termed behavioral family interventions, addressing a range of factors influencing positive parenting behavior (Taylor & Biglan, 1998).

Much of the research supporting behavioral family interventions has been conducted on indicated level interventions (i.e., preventive interventions aimed at people already exhibiting some level of the problem, e.g., children with conduct disorder, hyperactivity, various medical disorders). Recent reviews of this research (Serketich & Dumas, 1996; Taylor & Biglan, 1998) conclude that behavioral family interventions have demonstrated efficacy with children at risk due to a wide variety of conditions and who live in diverse family contexts. Also, in most cases, behavioral family interventions have demonstrated effects superior to alternative treatments. They also appear to benefit parents as well as children, with participating parents reporting reduced stress and better communication with parenting partners. At the same time, there are few studies that have measured intervention effect maintenance beyond a year.

More recently some universal interventions (i.e., interventions provided to members of a population regardless of risk level) that incorporate aspects of behavioral family treatments have demonstrated efficacy in reducing risk for children developing violent behavior and substance abuse problems (Kumpfer, 1999; US Department of Health and Human Services, 2001). Additionally, involvement in these universal interventions appears to increase family members' willingness to participate in future interventions when they become necessary (Spoth & Redmond, 1996).

STRATEGIES: OVERVIEW

Fortunately, quite a number of family strengthening interventions aimed at promoting healthy development in children aged 5–12 have been tested and garnered empirical support. Furthermore, recent reviews, using rigorous criteria and multiple raters, have evaluated the strength of the empirical support for these interventions and rated them (i.e., "model" and "promising" programs, see Kumpfer, 1999; US Department of Health and Human Services, 2001). The review by Kumpfer (1999) focused specifically on family strengthening interventions and also categorized interventions according to the targeted age group and risk level. These reviews show an encouraging level of consistency in rating criteria and in ratings (see US Department of Health and Human Services, 2001 for a ratings consistency table).

Family Strengthening Strategies

Strategies refers here to processes that have been employed in various family strengthening interventions that evaluators have identified as instrumental to intervention effectiveness. Although reviews have identified a variety of strategies that have been associated with success, four appear quite consistently across reviews.

Skills Training

Interventions that target improvement in parents' child management skills (listed above), parents' personal coping and problem solving skills, and children's coping and problem solving skills have consistently demonstrated the capacity to enhance family–child interaction patterns and children's behavioral and mental health (Taylor & Biglan, 1998; US Department of Health and Human Services, 2001). For skills training to be effective, however, the intervention must allot sufficient time for skill modeling, practice, and feedback.

Addressing Multiple Contexts

Research on indicated interventions with families of conduct problem adolescents indicates that approaches that include both parent and child components may be more effective than approaches that focus on either parents or children alone (Kazdin, Siegel, & Bass, 1992). Moreover, a number of the interventions with the strongest evidence for success have targeted both family and school contexts for change as well as facilitated communication and consistency between these contexts (e.g., Eddy, Reid, & Fetrow, 2000; Webster-Stratton, 1992). The school components of the interventions have often taught adaptive coping skills to children in group settings and/or modified teachers' classroom practices to better accommodate the learning needs of at-risk children.

Sufficient Intervention Dosage

The intervention dosage or extensiveness needs to match the level of risk factors present in the targeted population. Targeted populations with high levels of risk factors require a higher dosage of intervention. Higher dosages can be obtained by addressing more contexts in the change process (e.g., the school, parents' marital relationship, peer network), using more complex or individualized intervention methods (e.g., family therapy), or extending the time of the intervention (more contact time). Some interventions have designed components of graduated intensity matched to increasing levels of risk (e.g., Sanders, 1999).

Adequate Trainer Intervention Skills and Implementation

The effectiveness of family strengthening interventions appears to be moderated by the skills level of trainers. Key skills are the ability of trainers to communicate an understanding of parents' perspectives, to establish a collaborative working relationship with family members, to present rationales for and respectful management of skills training, and to encourage continued engagement of families who vacillate in their self-efficacy and outcome expectancies (Taylor & Biglan, 1998). In addition, trainers must be able to implement interventions as the developers intended so that all active components are delivered.

STRATEGIES THAT WORK

Although an impressive number of family strengthening interventions have employed evidence-based strategies and demonstrated efficacy in decreasing risk for negative developmental outcomes in children, only a limited number can be featured here. Readers interested in more comprehensive listings and comparisons are referred to excellent recent reviews by Kumpfer (1999) and US Department of Health and Human Services (2001).

Two universal level family-based interventions have repeatedly demonstrated efficacy in enhancing child–family relationships and increasing children's avoidance of tobacco, alcohol, and drugs. "Preparing for the drug free years" (Kosterman, Hawkins, Spoth, Haggerty, & Zhu, 1997) targets parents with 8–14 year old children and consists of five (2-hr) sessions that focus on parenting skills, managing family conflict, and enhancing children's involvement in family activities. One session, focusing on peer pressure, includes and actively involves the children. The "Iowa strengthening families program" (Molgaard & Kumpfer, 1994) targets families with 10–14 year old children. This program consists of seven sessions that include separate parent and child components conducted simultaneously with a family component immediately following. Four booster sessions are conducted approximately 6 months after the initial sessions. Parent sessions deal with monitoring and discipline skills and protecting against substance abuse. Youth sessions focus on goal setting, stress management, communication, and handling peer pressure. Family sessions provide opportunities for skill reinforcement and positive parent–child involvement. Both "Preparing for the drug free years" and the "Iowa strengthening families program" include parents and children, are conducted outside of children's school hours, and make extensive use of video stimuli to reduce the need for professional leaders or extensive leader training.

Several selected level preventive interventions (i.e., those targeted at people at greater risk for problems because of some factor, e.g., poverty, parental substance abuse) with demonstrated efficacy illustrate addressing and involving multiple contexts and/or providing increased dosage for children at higher risk. One of these, "The incredible years series" (Webster-Stratton, 1992), is for families with aggressive children at risk for conduct disorder. The series has skill development components for parents (separate 11–14 week versions for children aged 2–7 and 5–12 years), teachers (36 hr of training including how to teach social and problem solving skills in the classroom), and children (22 weeks). Additional available components for parents address supporting children's academic performance and parent self-management skills. "The incredible years series" makes extensive and effective use of videotaped stimulus material and modeling which has facilitated dissemination of this intervention. The "Linking the interests of families and teachers" program (Eddy et al., 2000) includes school-based skills training for first and fifth grade students (20 1-hr sessions over 10 weeks), a peer component promoting prosocial behavior on the playground, and parent training (six sessions). The "Families and schools together—FAST track program" (Conduct Problems Prevention Group, 1992) is an even more comprehensive, multiyear intervention targeting at-risk children identified as disruptive in kindergarten. "FAST track" uses home visitation and academic tutoring in addition to parent training, social skills training, and classroom management training to prevent the development of severe conduct problems by increasing connections between home, school, and child.

At the indicated level, "Functional family therapy" (Alexander & Parsons, 1982), conducted by skilled clinicians with individual families with children aged 6–18, has admirably demonstrated efficacy in preventing delinquency recidivism over multiple replications and trial sites. This family therapy approach involves reducing intense family negativity, increasing positive communication, strengthening parental problem solving, and maintaining change through coordinating home, school, peer, and correctional system contexts.

STRATEGIES THAT MIGHT WORK

Promising interventions incorporate innovative strategies and have demonstrated an initial level of efficacy that merits additional development and evaluation efforts. Again, the reader is referred to the recent reviews for detailed descriptions and comparisons of promising interventions (Kumpfer, 1999; US Department of Health and Human Services, 2001). Two interventions with different levels of parental involvement and family interaction are highlighted here. Both access contexts beyond the family and school to promote healthy development in children.

The Midwestern Prevention Project (MPP; Pentz, Mihalic, & Grotpeter, 1998) is a multiyear, multi-component, community wide intervention aimed at preventing drug abuse, beginning when children make the transition to middle school in the United States (age 11–13). The MPP is based on a person by situation by environment theoretical model and includes five components instituted at prescribed intervals over a five-year period. The media component includes TV, radio, and print broadcasts. A school intervention component with students is conducted by trained teachers and facilitated by peer leaders (10–13 sessions). A parent component reinforces non-drug use norms, provides parent training, and organizes parental involvement. A community organization component engages community and government leaders to form a planning group that develops additional complementary services, networks with local agencies, and makes referrals. Finally, a policy change component organizes a committee of government leaders that seeks to implement community health policies that reduce drug demand and supply. Trials of the MPP have resulted in significant reductions in children's drug and alcohol use at the end of high school and beyond as well as lower parent alcohol and marijuana use, increased positive parent–child communication, and improvements in community drug policy and treatment services. Family strengthening is only one component of the MPP. However, the MPP illustrates how family strengthening can be integrated into a comprehensive intervention aimed at producing significant and enduring change in environmental factors affecting children's development.

In comparison, the "Families and schools together" program (FAST; McDonald & Sayger, 1998, not to be confused with the earlier mentioned FAST track program), centrally focuses on family strengthening. FAST is distinguished by an innovative strategy to engage multiple community agents to sustain and institutionalize the intervention. As a first step, FAST requires the establishment of an adopting community team that is culturally representative of the community and includes parents, school professionals, and members of community-based agencies (a mental health agency, a substance abuse treatment agency). This team is then trained by FAST consultants to conduct outreach to targeted families. The core of the FAST intervention is 8–10 multifamily group sessions in which whole families participate. The focus of the sessions is on activities that build relationships within the family, between parents, between children and their peers, between families and school personnel, and between families and community agencies. Specific skill training does not appear to be a central feature of FAST. After these sessions, graduating parents, with support, lead their own follow-up multifamily meetings for two years. Evaluations, primarily using non-experimental repeated measures designs, have shown immediate reductions in home and classroom behavior problems and increases in family cohesion. Assessments at 6-month follow-up have additionally revealed increases in parent involvement in school and decreases in parent isolation. No data on FAST's effects on substance abuse or delinquency appear to have been reported. The developers report several experimental field trials in progress. Although FAST is less comprehensive in scope than the MPP and has not, as yet, demonstrated long-term effects on children's risk behaviors, FAST requires fewer resources to implement than the MPP, has been much more widely disseminated, and presents a promising model for sustaining family strengthening interventions in communities.

STRATEGIES THAT DO NOT WORK

Reviewers report that a sizable proportion of family-strengthening interventions have little or no empirical support. Lack of empirical support does not necessarily mean that these interventions are ineffective. Rather, adequate comparative evaluation studies may not yet have been conducted on these interventions. However, there are features that appear to contribute to the ineffectiveness of family strengthening interventions. One is insufficient dosage. Brief parent education sessions that are limited to providing information do not appear to produce change, especially for families at higher risk. Another factor contributing to ineffectiveness is lack of training in empirically supported parenting skills. For example, the widely used "Systematic training for effective parenting program" (STEP; Dinkmeyer & McKay, 1976) that emphasizes understanding children's behavior, using encouragement, listening, and disciplining by natural consequences, does not emphasize skill training and has not demonstrated that it actually changes parent or child behavior. Lack of accommodation of participants' cultural beliefs is another factor likely to contribute to intervention ineffectiveness. For example, approaches that promote children's autonomous decision making and the use of democratic family management practices may run counter to the widely acknowledged Latino family values of interdependency and respect for generational hierarchies. Culturally incompetent interventions are likely to be dismissed by targeted participants. Research indicates that approaches that congregate conduct problem youth risk increasing problem behavior (Dishion & Andrews, 1995). Finally, lack of key skills in trainers and/or ineffective implementation can contribute to the failure of even the best empirically supported interventions.

SYNTHESIS

We are fortunate in having a critical mass of effective family strengthening technology. At the same time, we are confronted with the persistence of social problems, cited at the outset of this entry, arising from inadequately socialized and educated children. This predicament highlights perhaps the main limitation of family strengthening interventions today, the lack of widespread competent implementation of existing empirically supported interventions with a large proportion of families and children who could benefit from them. This is analogous to having developed a vaccine to prevent a contagious disease but having no effective systems in place to produce adequate amounts of the vaccine or get the vaccine to the majority of people at risk for the disease. Accordingly, some have advocated adopting a public health perspective in addressing childrearing and children's behavioral and mental health (e.g., Biglan, 1995).

Contextualist ideas have already motivated researchers to expand the design of family strengthening interventions to involve multiple socializing agents of children and to address coping with neighborhood, school, and economic stressors. Moreover, researchers have now just begun to investigate the process of disseminating effective family strengthening interventions. These investigations hopefully will lead to identifying factors and processes that are critical to mobilizing and organizing large communities to adopt and sustain family strengthening policies and practices at multiple levels over long periods. However, technological knowledge in the hands of researchers will be insufficient to meet the looming challenge. Leadership must also be developed to instigate the change processes.

Biglan (1995) has identified some possible components of a community based public health approach to inadequate child socialization including programs for families, changes in school practices, extrafamilial supervised activities for children, and structures for policy development and implementation. Under programs for families, two elements have sometimes been included in family strengthening interventions but rarely emphasized. The first is a family support component that is able to link families suffering housing, health, and financial problems to services in the community. Parent training interventions conducted in low-income neighborhoods often attend to helping families with their instrumental needs informally. The effectiveness of family interventions could be enhanced if this family support function were sufficiently developed.

The second underdeveloped element of family strengthening interventions is the treatment of marital distress. Marital distress and dissolution negatively affect children's developmental contexts in a number of ways. Chronic marital distress increases conflict and negative affect in the family, often models coercive behavior, erodes the spouse support for parenting, and reduces parenting self-efficacy and adaptive parenting practices (Grych & Fincham, 2001). Marital dissolution most often results in single parenting for some period, which makes monitoring children more difficult because there is less parenting resource available to it. Parenting resources are further reduced when single parents must take on additional work hours outside the home to compensate for decreased financial resources. These negative effects on childrearing resources point to the need for family strengthening interventions to take a more direct role in addressing and reducing marital discord. Because the family is the primary socializing for children aged 5–12, any interventions that increase marital satisfaction and stability need to be viewed as key to family strengthening.

A third underdeveloped dimension of family strengthening interventions is the provision of prosocial activities for children that are supervised by adults. The increased prevalence of two full time worker households has also significantly reduced the parenting and monitoring resources available to children. Providing supervised recreational and skill-building activities for older children, who are otherwise left alone at home for extended periods (after school, evenings, weekends, during school breaks), can compensate for the reduction in parenting resources and play a significant role in preventing antisocial behavior. Family strengthening interventions can help parents locate inexpensive, adequately supervised activities and help parents organize themselves to take advantage of them. Alternatively, programs providing supervised activities for children provide a means to engage families in skill training and supporting children's development in other ways (e.g., increasing parents' involvement in schoolwork).

The increased mobility of contemporary families has led to many parents' separation from extended family members and neighbors. It has also contributed to neighborhoods where standards for child and parent behavior are no longer upheld in common. The erosion of these traditional supports means that more and more families have to go at it alone and are increasingly vulnerable to problems. When families fail to perform their key functions, not only the child's development is compromised, the health of the whole society is compromised. Conversely, when families are strengthened to perform their key functions successfully, not only the healthy development of the child is promoted, the health of the whole society is enhanced. Family strengthening interventions hold great potential in helping families cope with raising children in a rapidly changing world.

Also see: Effective Programming: Foundation; Parenting: Early Childhood; Parenting: Adolescence; Parenting, Single Parent: Adolescence; Parenting: Adulthood.

References

Alexander, J.F., & Parsons, B.V. (1982). *Functional family therapy: Principles and procedures*. Carmel, CA: Brooks/Cole.

Biglan, A. (1995). *Changing cultural practices: A contextual framework for intervention research*. Reno, NV: Context Press.

Brooks-Gunn, J., Duncan, G.J., Klebanov, P.K., & Sealand, N. (1993). Do neighborhoods influence child and adolescent development? *American Journal of Sociology, 99*, 353–395.

Conduct Problems Prevention Group (Bierman, K., Coie, J., Dodge, K., Greenberg, M., Lochman, J., & McMahon, R.). (1992). A developmental and clinical model for the prevention of conduct disorder: The FAST track program. *Development and Psychopathology, 4*, 509–527.

Conger, R.D., Cui, M., Bryant, C.M., & Elder, G.H., Jr. (2000). Competence in early adult romantic relationships: A developmental perspective on family influences. *Journal of Personality and Social Psychology, 79*, 224–237.

Dinkmeyer, D., & McKay, G. (1976). *Systematic training for effective parenting*. Circle Pines, MN: American Guidance Service.

Dishion, T.J., & Andrews, D.W. (1995). Preventing escalation in problem behaviors with high-risk young adolescents: Immediate and 1-year outcomes. *Journal of Consulting and Clinical Psychology, 63*, 538–548.

Donovan, J.E., Jessor, R., & Costa, F.M. (1988). Syndrome of problem behavior in adolescence: A replication. *Journal of Consulting and Clinical Psychology, 56,* 762–765.

Eddy, J.M., Reid, J.B., & Fetrow, R.A. (2000). An elementary-school based prevention program targeting modifiable antecedents of youth delinquency and violence: Linking the Interests of Families and Teachers (LIFT). *Journal of Emotional and Behavioral Disorders, 8,* 165–176.

Furstenberg, F.F., Jr. (1993). How families manage risk and opportunity in dangerous neighborhoods. In W. J. Wilson (Ed.), *Sociology and the public agenda* (pp. 231–258). Newbury Park, CA: Sage.

Grych, J.H., & Fincham, F.D. (2001). *Interparental conflict and child development.* New York: Cambridge University Press.

Hernandez, D.J. (1993). *America's children: Resources from family, government, and the economy.* New York: Russell Sage Foundation.

Kazdin, A.E. (1987). Treatment of antisocial behavior in children: Current status and future directions. *Psychological Bulletin, 10,* 187–203.

Kazdin, A.E., Siegel, T.C., & Bass, D. (1992). Cognitive problem-solving skills training and parent management training in the treatment of antisocial behavior in children. *Journal of Consulting and Clinical Psychology, 60,* 733–747.

Kosterman, R., Hawkins, J.D., Spoth, R., Haggerty, K.P., & Zhu, K. (1997). Effects of preventive parent training intervention on observed family interactions: Proximal outcomes from preparing for the drug-free years. *Journal of Community Psychology, 25,* 277–292.

Kumpfer, K.L. (1999). *Strengthening America's families: Exemplary parenting and family strategies for delinquency prevention.* Washington, DC: US Department of Justice, Office of Juvenile Justice and Delinquency Prevention. Available on the World Wide Web: http://www.strengtheningfamilies.org

Lerner, R.M., Castellino, D.R., Terry, P.A., Villarruel, F.A., & McKinney, M.H. (1995). Developmental contextual perspective on parenting. In M. H. Bornstein (Ed.), *Handbook of parenting: Volume 2, biology and ecology of parenting* (pp. 285–309). Mahwah, NJ: Lawrence Erlbaum Associates.

LeVine, R.A. (1974). Parental goals: A cross-cultural view. *Teachers College Record, 76,* 226–239.

McCubbin, H.I., & Patterson, J.M. (1983). The family stress process: The double ABCX model of family adjustment and adaptation. *Marriage and Family Review, 6,* 7–37.

McDonald, L., & Sayger, T.V. (1998). Impact of a family and school based prevention program on protective factors for high risk youth. *Drugs & Society, 12,* 61–85.

Molgaard, V., & Kumpfer, K.L. (1994). *Strengthening families program II.* Ames: Iowa State University, Social and Behavioral Research Center for Rural Health.

Patterson, G.R., & Joerger, K. (1993). Developmental models for delinquent behavior. In S. Hodgins (Ed.), *Mental disorder and crime.* Newbury Park, CA: Sage.

Patterson, G.R., Reid, J.B., & Dishion, T.J. (1992). *Antisocial boys.* Eugene, OR: Castalia.

Pentz, M.A., Mihalic, S.F., & Grotpeter, J.K. (1998). *Blueprints for violence prevention, book one: The Midwestern prevention project.* Boulder, CO: Center for the Study of and Prevention of Violence. Available on the World Wide Web: http://www.colorado.edu/cspv

Pfiffner, L.J., Jouriles, E.N., Brown, M.M., Etscheidt, M.A., & Kelly, J.A. (1990). Effects of problem-solving training for single-parent families. *Child and Family Behavior Therapy, 12,* 1–11.

Rothbaum, F., & Weisz, J.R. (1994). Parental caregiving and child externalizing behavior in nonclinical samples: A meta-analysis. *Psychological Bulletin, 116,* 55–74.

Rutter, M. (1987). Continuities and discontinuities from infancy. In J. Rolf, A.S. Masten, D. Cicchetti, K.H. Neuchterlein, & S. Weintraub (Eds.), *Risk and protective factors in the development of psychopathology* (pp. 181–214). New York: Cambridge University Press.

Sanders, M.R. (1999). Triple P-positive parenting program: Towards an empirically validated multilevel parenting and family support strategy for the prevention of behavior and emotional problems in children. *Clinical Child and Family Psychology, 2,* 71–90.

Serketich, W.J., & Dumas, J.E. (1996). The effectiveness of behavioral parent training to modify antisocial behavior in children: A meta-analysis. *Behavior Therapy, 27,* 171–186.

Spoth, R., & Redmond, C. (1996). Illustrating a framework for prevention research: Project Family studies of rural family participation and outcomes. In R. Peters & R.J. McMahon (Eds.), *Childhood disorders, substance abuse, and delinquency: Prevention and early intervention approaches* (pp. 299–328). Newbury Park, CA: Sage.

Taylor, T.K., & Biglan, A. (1998). Behavioral family interventions for improving child-rearing: A review of the literature for clinicians and policy makers. *Clinical Child and Family Psychology Review, 1,* 41–60.

US Department of Health and Human Services. (2001). Youth violence: A report of the US Department of Health and Human Services. Washington, DC: Author. Available on the World Wide Web: http://www.surgeongeneral.gov/library/youthviolence

Webster-Stratton, C. (1992). *The incredible years: A trouble-shooting guide for parents of children age 3–8.* Toronto, Canada: Umbrella. Order on the World Wide Web: http://www.incredibleyears.com

Webster-Stratton, C., & Herbert, M. (1994). *Troubled families, problem children, working with parents: A collaborative process.* New York: Wiley.

Wells, K.C., Griest, D.L., & Forehand, R. (1980). The use of a self-control package to enhance temporal generality of a parent training program. *Behavioral Research and Therapy, 18,* 347–358.

Family Strengthening, Adolescence

Stephen M. Gavazzi

INTRODUCTION AND DEFINITIONS

This entry provides a review of family strengthening programs that target families containing youth between the ages of twelve and twenty-one years of age. For present purposes, family strengthening programs are asserted to be intergenerational, systems-oriented, and asset-based. As such, the criteria used to categorize a program as of the "family strengthening" type are threefold.

First, the intergenerational criterion translates into the fact that the program requires the participation of *two* generations of family members (i.e., parent and adolescent) in *shared* program activities. This condition rules out parenting programs being reviewed in this entry, as well as eliminating those programs that have parents and adolescents involved in an initiative that includes their participation only in separate activities. The second criterion, that it is system-oriented, means that the program is designed to affect the family as a whole, or at the very least a subsystem of the family (i.e., the parent–adolescent dyad). This eliminates any review of programs that target only individual-oriented phenomena. The third and final component of the present definition of a family strengthening program—the asset-based criterion—asserts that the program must target positive features of family life that are applicable to universal populations of families. Unless a given program is dedicated primarily to topic areas that are generally pertinent to all families, the present entry will not review initiatives that target either families identified as high risk (i.e., those programs known as selective prevention) or families in need of actual treatment (i.e., those programs that provide targeted interventions, therapy, etc.).

SCOPE

There are approximately 40 million youth between the ages of 12 and 20 years of age living in the United States in the year 2000. This figure represents about 15 percent of the overall population, a proportion that is expected to remain steady throughout the next 10 years (US Census Bureau, 2000).

Worldwide, there are approximately 520 million adolescents between the ages of 15 and 19 years of age. About two-thirds of these adolescents live in Africa, Asia, the Near East, Latin America, and the Caribbean, and this population is expected to increase on the order of 25 percent by the year 2020. In the remainder of the world, the adolescent population is expected to shrink by approximately 15 percent over the same time period (United Nations Population Information Network, 2000).

Family strengthening programs thus have a sizable audience for the services that they offer. Marketplace estimates for universal programs are tempered by existing evidence that supports the notion that many problem behaviors seen in adolescence are preexistent in childhood (Montemayor, Adams, & Gullotta, 1990). Hence, some families will enter this life cycle stage already in need of more selective and/or indicated services. Additionally, estimates that anywhere between 10 and 20 percent of all adolescents will experience some sort of individual and/or interpersonal difficulty requiring more intensive services than can be offered by a universally based family strengthening program further attenuates these figures (McKenry & Gavazzi, 1994).

THEORIES

A variety of approaches and labels currently exist with regard to the development and implementation of family strengthening programs. Some of these initiatives are explicitly discussed as "family strengthening" programs; other descriptors include "family enrichment," "family life education," "family skills training," "family empowerment," "family wellness," and "family support" programs.

The theoretical underpinnings of these programs are quite divergent. For instance, some of the family skills training programs were developed by professionals who were interested in outcomes related to delinquency and related antisocial behavior, and thus based their work on principles that came out of social learning theory and/or the social development model. Other professionals who developed family skills training programs were influenced by theories from the family therapy movement. In another realm, family life education programs largely were created by family scientists who utilized family development theory to guide their work. Different still are those family support programs that largely came out of an ecological theory framework.

In the present review, theoretical foundations are identified to the extent that such information is provided by the developers of each separate program. At the same time, the present entry identifies one unifying theoretical principle underlying the development of most if not all of these related efforts. To wit, these many and varied family strengthening programs are built on the basic premise that "human relationships can be taught and, therefore, can be learned" (L'Abate, 1990, p. 129).

RESEARCH

Just as there is great variety in terms of the theoretical backgrounds represented in the literature concerning family strengthening programs, so too is there a rather wide range of efforts undertaken in order to conduct an empirical evaluation of the implementation of these programs. First of all, it should be said that there are many more family strengthening programs currently being implemented than are contained in the literature that has been reviewed. Most simply put, many of the programs that are absent from this literature have lacked the empirical testing required for acceptance into many refereed journals. Those programs that have undergone such rigorous examination are oftentimes given the label "best practice." At the same time, the gathering of summative evaluation data is not an appropriate task for those developers whose programs are at the more beginning stages of development. Hence, there are some programs that have made it into the literature with formative evaluation data, often with the label "promising approach." The present review covers programs of both types, and reports the general findings of these formative and summative evaluation efforts.

STRATEGIES: OVERVIEW

This section presents information on those family strengthening programs that were identified in searches of the following bodies of literature: the Institute for Scientific Information's Web of Science Citation Database, the Office of Juvenile Justice and Delinquency Prevention's Family Strengthening Series, and the table of contents of the *Journal of Primary Prevention*. These programs are divided into sections entitled "programs that work" (following a rule that a program has been tested at least three times with successful results) or "programs that might work" (having been tested less than three times). Further, these programs are reviewed in alphabetical order, are described in summary fashion according to their main objectives, their theoretical framework, and the empirical evidence that has been generated through implementation and evaluation efforts. Due to space restrictions, only one citation concerning each program is made available in this review.

STRATEGIES THAT WORK

The families and schools together program (McDonald & Frey, 1999) is an initial 8–10-session family strengthening program (followed by two years of monthly booster sessions) that is designed to assist families of youth (up to the age of 14 years) to prevent school failure and substance use while concurrently increasing family functioning levels. Program activities include quite a variety of experiential activities (singing, game-playing, eating, drawing) that are linked to programmatic objectives. The theoretical frameworks of this program include a number of therapy literatures (psychiatry, psychology, play therapy, family therapy), as well as more generic parent, family, and communication literatures. Interestingly, this program is strongly connected to the school system as a source of referrals, a site for program implementation, and a connection point for family member involvement in community-oriented activities. This program has been evaluated through a number of studies that have gathered follow-up data from program participants, and analyses have indicated programmatic impact in terms of decreased externalizing problem behaviors and increased family functioning. Additionally, the results of one unpublished experimental design study are reported to show significant improvement in participating youth versus controls.

The preparing for the drug free years program (Haggerty, Kosterman, Catalano, & Hawkins, 1999) is a five-session family strengthening program designed to assist families of adolescents (up to 14 years of age) in reducing risk factors and increasing protective factors related to substance use and related problem behaviors. Many of the program activities are attended by parents only, and include family conflict management, education on the extent of substance use and its connection to family and peer factors, and parent communication skill building. There also is a session attended by parents and adolescents together that focuses on the development of substance use refusal skills. This program is grounded in the social development model (the program developers include some of the original theorists who created this model). Evaluation of this program has included both formative and summative data collection efforts. Formative data collected on program dissemination indicated that the program reaches its intended audience and that parents perceive their participation to have been helpful in reaching the program's stated objectives. The results of one experimental design study indicated improvement in participating adults' parenting and communication skills versus controls, as well as decreases in adolescent substance use.

The strengthening families program (Kumpfer & Tait, 2000) is a 14-week family strengthening program that is designed to assist families of adolescents (up to 14 years of age) in the deterrence of substance use and the improvement of parent–adolescent relationships. Program activities include a combination of parent skill development (anger and stress management, discipline, use of rewards, communication), adolescent skill development (social skills, coping, communication), and family skill development (problem-solving, practicing communication skills, use of family meeting times). The theoretical framework of this program is a combination of the Values-Attitudes-Stressors-Coping (VASC) and Social Ecology models of substance abuse. This program has been rigorously examined in at least 12 summative evaluation studies conducted by independent program evaluators. Reports of results include significant decreases in adolescent substance use and increased family functioning. A number of culturally specific variations of this program concurrently have been developed, and include initiatives that target African American, Hawaiian Asian/Pacific Islander, Latino, and American Indian families.

The strengthening families program: For parents and youth 10–14 (Molgaard, Spoth, & Redmond, 2000) is a seven-week family strengthening program (with four additional booster sessions) that resulted from a significant modification of the original Strengthening Families Program (SFP) described above. In essence, the program was altered in order to better fit the universal needs of rural families with adolescents (aged 10–14 years of age) such that intermediate outcomes related to improved family skills would serve the more long-term outcome of decreased adolescent problem behaviors. Each program session consists of 1 hr of separate parent and adolescent activities that cover a spectrum of skills, and a second hour that unites the family members in order to put into practice the skills just learned. While there is theoretical kinship to the original SFP initiative, conceptual linkages to a biopsychosocial vulnerability model, the resiliency literature, and attention to family processes also are emphasized. At least one study incorporating an experimental design has been conducted to date, and results are reported that indicate increases in functional parenting skills, as well as decreases in a variety of adolescent problem behaviors. Interestingly, researchers were able to document the direct and indirect effects of this program on certain parenting variables as part of this study. Finally, more recent efforts that have been undertaken to develop a videotape-based curriculum are particularly noteworthy.

STRATEGIES THAT MIGHT WORK

The Chicago HIV prevention and adolescent mental health project (Madison, McKay, Paikoff, & Bell, 2000) is a 12-week family strengthening program that is designed to help urban families of early adolescents (aged 10–12 years of age) deal with sexual activity and related behaviors that increase HIV exposure risk. Program activities include: family communication skill building; discussion of the impact of neighborhood and peer environments; the role of parental monitoring and discipline; and education about issues concerning adolescent sexuality and HIV/AIDS transmission. The program utilizes a generic set of theoretical assumptions stemming from the adolescent developmental literature that includes the impact of biological, cognitive/psychological, and social context factors on risk-taking behaviors. Data have been reported on relatively successful recruitment and retention rates, as well as preliminary outcomes that suggest programmatic impact on variables related to knowledge gain and increased parental functioning.

The families in action program (Pilgrim, Abbey, Hendrickson, & Lorenz, 1998) is a six-session family strengthening program that is designed to assist rural families of adolescents (entering junior high or middle school) increase protective factors and decrease risk factors associated with alcohol, tobacco, and other substance use. Program activities include communication skill building, focusing on positive thinking, school success, and substance use avoidance strategies. Theoretically, this program is based on the social development model. Formative data has focused on curriculum adherence and group discussion facilitation. Additionally, the results of one quasi-experimental design

study have indicated that participating adolescents were more receptive to the use of social services than were adolescent controls, while male adolescents (but not females) reported greater attachment to school and peers and more functional attitudes toward substance use. In turn, participating parents reported increased family functioning and more functional attitudes towards substance use than did parent controls.

The growing up FAST: Families with adolescents surviving and thriving program (Gavazzi, 1995) is a two-session family strengthening program that is designed to assist families of adolescents (aged 12–18 years) in meeting a variety of developmental demands through identification of family strengths and capabilities. Program activities include: the creation of a definition of what successful adulthood means to family members; identification of those behaviors family members are engaged in presently or could become engaged in that support achievement of successful adulthood status; development of needs assessment and decision-making skills; and the utilization of community resources. The theoretical framework of this program includes a blend of literatures concerning rites of passage, multicultural studies, and the solution-focused perspective. To date, empirical evidence is primarily formative. This information includes the actual use of this program to generate outputs that are consistent with its stated objectives (i.e., creating definitions of successful adulthood), as well as family member perceptions of program effectiveness.

The home and on your own program (Colan, Mague, Cohen, & Schneider, 1994) is a six-session family strengthening program designed to increase safety in homes where adolescents are alone for periods of time after school (although no age range is specified by the program developers, this program was included in the present entry due to the program's general applicability to 12–18 year-old students). Program activities include: family communication and decision-making skill building; education about safety issues in the home and neighborhood environments; and issues involving risk-taking behaviors, including substance use. The self-care literature is the primary theoretical underpinning of this program. Interestingly, this program utilizes a recruitment strategy that involves employee assistance programs. Reported evaluative data are formative, and involves participant perceptions of the program's effectiveness. Additionally, relatively high rates of retention are reported.

Larger critical reviews of family strengthening programs is to date, a comprehensive review of the entire body of family strengthening programs represented by the specific efforts examined above has yet to be undertaken. Less inclusive reviews that usually confine themselves to working to achieve a specific aim (i.e., preventing delinquency or providing family life education) have provided readers with comparisons and contrasts of the relative merits of programs that target families of adolescents. However, even these reviews tend to be long on generalities and short on specific information that identifies "best practices" and "promising approaches" based on empirical evidence.

This section begins with a brief recounting of the one review of family strengthening programs that utilizes specific research evidence to ground their assertions about "what works," at least in terms of an examination of family-based initiatives that target illegal behavior. Building on this, a somewhat larger picture of the current "state of the art" regarding family strengthening programs more generally is constructed through the additional review of studies conducted on the specific programs covered above in the previous section of this entry.

Kumpfer and Alvarado (1998) were the authors who reviewed family-based programs that sought to reduce the involvement of adolescents in delinquency and substance abuse. Borrowing from guidelines developed through the National Institute on Drug Abuse (NIDA), these reviewers called attention to a set of principles that they believed seemed to characterize effective family-focused interventions. These principles included: allowance of family members to remain involved in programming for a sufficient length of time and intensity level that would permit them to solidify changes in family dynamics; use of post-program booster sessions to counter the degradation of program gains; comprehensive attention given to skill development in such areas as family cohesiveness, interpersonal communication, and parental monitoring; attention paid to culturally specific issues in both program content and recruitment/retention efforts; program material being developmentally appropriate to adolescents and starting as early as possible in this developmental period; use of audiovisual instructional material for skill-building components of the program; and attention given to advanced training opportunities for program facilitators.

The first issue that these authors deal with concerns "dosage"; quite literally, how much programming is enough to make a difference in family functioning levels? The programs reviewed above range from 2 to 14 sessions, with seven times being the average number of contacts. Rather than making the assertion that there is some minimum number of contacts with families that will make a given program effective, instead it might be more useful to affirm the notion that more sessions would be needed for families that were at lower levels of functioning. There seems to be general consistency with that premise in terms of the programs reviewed above and the amount of sessions that are offered to families.

The dosage issue overlaps with the second principle regarding the comprehensiveness of programming. Obviously, programs that have more built-in contacts with families are able to cover material in more breadth (and

depth, for that matter). An examination of the programs reviewed above indicates that very trend; programs with more sessions seem to cover family dynamics in more detail.

Even so, it is important to note that the reality of the situation might be that the most impaired families actually are able to access the least amount of resources, and the most functional families are operating well enough to be able to choose non-participation without negative repercussions. This would leave mid-range functioning families as the ones most likely to take full advantage of programs that offer the most contact points.

The third issue discussed by Kumpfer and Alvarado (1998) concerns the specific areas of family dynamics covered by family strengthening programs. Clearly, many of these programs cover areas that directly and indirectly tap into concerns related to family cohesiveness, interpersonal communication, and parental monitoring. At the same time, these programs also aim to have an impact on other important areas of family life, including family adaptability, family problem-solving and decision-making skills, conflict management in the family, and the interplay of family and larger social systems (including most notably the school setting).

Culturally specific issues of one kind or another have been discussed in the general social sciences literature as being one of the most important yet under utilized factors related to the successful transition into adulthood (Spencer & Dornbusch, 1990). There seems to be some attention paid to these types of issues in many of the family strengthening programs reviewed above. In particular, ethnic background and/or geographical location of the families are two of the more salient issues that permeate descriptions of these programs. However, more information about how these culturally specific issues form a fundamental part of the program itself (instead of something that was thrown in at the end for reasons that might have more to do with being politically correct) would be most beneficial.

The issue of cultural specificity is linked to the effective programming principle concerning the developmental appropriateness of program content, as they both involve attention paid to the fit between the specialized needs of the target population and what the programs actually provide. The family-strengthening initiatives reviewed above all seem to take on issues that are developmentally suitable for the families of adolescents being served by these programs. Additionally, these entire programs target the lower bounds of the adolescent period (although at least one program allows for the participation of older adolescents and their families), and thus are focused more on helping families earlier than later.

Where greater criticism can be lodged against at least some of these family strengthening programs are in areas that touch on the last two principles of effective program covered by Kumpfer and Alvarado (1998): the use of audio-visual instructional material and advanced training opportunities for program facilitators. Having audiovisual material available for use by family members facilitates the transfer of learning of skills covered by program facilitators in family sessions. The availability of such material is emphasized only by a few of the programs reviewed above. Additionally, the availability of advanced training opportunities also is highlighted infrequently. Already robust in so many other principles of effective programming, the family strengthening programs reviewed above would be strengthened greatly by increased attention to these two areas.

STRATEGIES THAT DO NOT WORK

Based on Kumpfer and Alvarado's (1998) review of the literature, we can say that programs that are of shorter duration, restricted in the breadth and depth of material covered, less focused on compelling family processes, inattentive to culturally specific issues, and lacking in developmentally appropriate content all seem to become factors associated with potentially ineffective programming efforts. In addition, the use of lecture-based formats (Tobler & Stratton, 1997) and other information-only modalities of program implementation (Norman & Turner, 1993) largely have failed to generate much in the way of empirical support.

SYNTHESIS

The family strengthening programs reviewed above represent a praiseworthy collection of best practices and promising approaches to prevention-oriented work with the families of adolescents. The developers of these programs are to be commended for their attention to both theoretical and empirical rigor. At the same time, there are a number of directions that future work in this area must take.

First, greater attention must be paid to culturally specific issues in program development. While a number of current efforts have looked at the generalizability of family strengthening programs across ethnic groups, fewer have developed program content that is explicitly connected to the cultural heritage of participating families. Additionally, those culturally specific programs already in existence that either target younger children or higher risk youth and their families should be given support in order to be modified for more prevention-oriented activities with culturally diverse families of adolescents. Two examples that immediately come to mind include the "DAYS La Familia program" (Hernandez & Lucero, 1996) and the "Family effectiveness training program" (Szapocznik, Santisteban, Rio,

Perez-Vidal, Santisteban, & Kurtines, 1989), both of which are designed for use with families of high-risk Latino children and adolescents. There also has been limited attention paid to the geographical location of the families served by these programs, especially with regard to urban families. Again, effort could and should be undertaken to modify programs already in existence that currently target inner-city families of higher risk youth (Tolan & McKay, 1996).

In related fashion, greater attention must be paid in the future to the classification schemes used to categorize programs. It has been pointed out elsewhere that there are inconsistencies in the use of terminology related to primary, secondary, and tertiary prevention that lead to confusion about what a given program is supposed to accomplish and with whom those program activities should be targeted (Froom & Benbassat, 2000). In addition to future work aimed at standardizing such terminology, whatever programs end up in the prevention category must continue to advance efforts to focus on the building up of protective factors associated with the assets, strengths, and capabilities of families, not just the reduction of family-oriented risk factors.

The overall family prevention field has been portrayed as being behind in the use of the most up to date methods of empirical inquiry (Dumka, Roosa, Michaels, & Suh, 1995). One major shortfall has been the scant attention given to the standardization of family assessment devices in the family strengthening literature. Hence, there seems to be significant variation in how youth and families are classified according to their level of risk. Debate on questions surrounding the selection of measures that might be used to homogenize our understanding of family risk levels should begin immediately. Also, because program developers are interested in the family as the unit of analysis, planning of these future research efforts should be influenced by the overall family field's growing interest in the gathering and analysis of data from multiple family members (Bartle-Haring & Gavazzi, 1996).

While the family by definition is the central focus of family strengthening efforts, program developers have been urged to become more comprehensive in their focus by including components that affect multiple systems and multiple factors within those systems (Ellis, 1998). One important outcome of this call would be the expansion of parenting skills efforts to include adolescents in family-specific program activities. At the same time, recommendations to promote the development of linkages to other social organizations beyond the family might be reinforced most importantly in work with ethnically diverse families, who often rely on churches and related religious organizations to provide prevention and intervention services (Sutherland, Hale, & Harris, 1995).

Also see: Effective Programming, Parenting: Early Childhood; Parenting: Adolescence; Parenting, Single Parent: Adolescence; Parenting: Adulthood.

References

Bartle-Haring, S.E., & Gavazzi, S.M. (1996). Multiple views on family data: The sample case of adolescent, maternal, and paternal perspectives on family differentiation levels. *Family Process, 35,* 457–472.

Colan, N.B., Mague, K.C., Cohen, R.S., & Schneider, R.J. (1994). Family education in the workplace: A prevention program for working parents and school-age children. *Journal of Primary Prevention, 15,* 161–172.

Dumka, L.E., Roosa, M.W., Michaels, M.L., & Suh, K.W. (1995). Using research and theory to develop prevention programs for high risk families. *Family Relations, 44,* 78–86.

Ellis, R.A. (1998). Filling the prevention gap: Multi-factor, multi-system, multi-level intervention. *Journal of Primary Prevention, 19,* 57–71.

Froom, P., & Benbassat, J. (2000). Inconsistencies in the classification of preventative interventions. *Preventative Medicine, 31,* 153–158.

Gavazzi, S.M. (1995). The growing up FAST: Families with adolescents surviving and thriving program. *Journal of Adolescence, 18,* 31–47.

Haggerty, K., Kosterman, R., Catalano, R.F., & Hawkins, J.D. (1999). *Preparing for the drug free years.* Washington, DC: US Department of Justice, Office of Justice Programs, Office of Juvenile Justice and Delinquency Prevention.

Hernandez, L.P., & Lucero, E. (1996), DAYS La Familia community drug and alcohol prevention program: Family-centered model for working with inner-city Latino families. *Journal of Primary Prevention, 16,* 255–272.

Kumpfer, K.L., & Alvarado, R. (1998). *Effective family strengthening interventions.* Washington, DC: US Department of Justice, Office of Justice Programs, Office of Juvenile Justice and Delinquency Prevention.

Kumpfer, K.L., & Tait, C.M. (2000). *Family skills training for parents and children.* Washington, DC: US Department of Justice, Office of Justice Programs, Office of Juvenile Justice and Delinquency Prevention.

L'Abate, L. (1990). *Building family competence: Primary and secondary prevention strategies.* Newbury Park, CA: Sage.

Madison, S.M., McKay, M.M., Paikoff, R., & Bell, C.C. (2000). Basic research and community collaboration: Necessary ingredients for the development of a family-based HIV prevention program. *AIDS Education and Prevention, 12,* 281–298.

McDonald, L., & Frey, H.E. (1999). *Families and schools together: Building relationships.* Washington, DC: US Department of Justice, Office of Justice Programs, Office of Juvenile Justice and Delinquency Prevention.

McKenry, P.C., & Gavazzi, S.M. (1994). *Vision 2010: Families and Adolescents.* Minneapolis, MN: National Council on Family Relations.

Molgaard, V., Spoth, R.L., & Redmond, C. (2000). *Competency training: The strengthening families program for parents and youth 10–14.* Washington, DC: US Department of Justice, Office of Justice Programs, Office of Juvenile Justice and Delinquency Prevention.

Montemayor, R., Adams, G.R., & Gullotta, T.P. (1990). *From childhood to adolescence: A transitional period?* Newbury Park, CA: Sage.

Norman, E., & Turner, S. (1993). Adolescent substance abuse prevention programs: Theories, models, and research in the encouraging 80's. *Journal of Primary Prevention, 14,* 3–20.

Pilgrim, C., Abbey, A., Hendrickson, P., & Lorenz, S. (1998). Implementation and impact of a family-based substance abuse prevention program in rural communities. *Journal of Primary Prevention, 18,* 341–361.

Spencer, M.B., & Dornbusch, S.M. (1990). Challenges in studying minority youth. In S.S. Feldman & G.R. Elliott (Eds.), *At the threshold: The developing adolescent* (pp. 123–146). Cambridge, MA: Harvard University Press.

Sutherland, M., Hale, C.D., & Harris, G.J. (1995). Community health promotion: The church as partner. *Journal of Primary Prevention, 16,* 201–216.

Szapocznik, J., Santisteban, D., Rio, A., Perez-Vidal, A., Santiseban, D., & Kurtines, W.M. (1989). Family effectiveness training: An intervention to prevent drug abuse and problem behaviors in Latino adolescents. *Latino Journal of Behavioral Sciences, 11,* 4–27.

Tobler, N.S., & Stratton, H.H. (1997). Effectiveness of school-based prevention programs: A meta-analysis of the research. *Journal of Primary Prevention, 18,* 71–128.

Tolan, P.H., & McKay, M.M. (1996). Preventing serious antisocial behavior in inner-city children: An empirically based family prevention program. *Family Relations, 45,* 139–147.

United Nations Population Information Network. (2000). *Charting the progress of populations.* New York: Department of Economic and Social Affairs, Population Division, United Nations.

US Census Bureau. (2000). *Population projections of the United States by age, sex, race, Latino origin, and nativity: 1999 to 2100.* Washington, DC: Population Projections Program, Population Division, US Census Bureau.

Foster Care, Childhood

Chris Downs and Jason Williams

INTRODUCTION

Whether it is a local government department or a private agency that has taken on the parenting role, foster children are truly the village's children. Foster care entails a great many costs to the children themselves, the families and agencies charged with their care, and to the society at large. All too often, foster care has negative outcomes, such as educational underachievement, substance abuse, homelessness, mental illness, or crime. But there are many positive stories as well, stories of children who triumphed over maltreatment, destroyed attachments, and sadness to develop loving relationships and healthy adult lives. It is critical that the agencies charged by the village with caring for these children examine what works and what does not work in promoting positive outcomes for foster children in order to promote healthy development in children of foster care families.

DEFINITIONS

A *child living with a foster family* is typically a minor who has been judged by a state, county, or court administrator as temporarily or permanently unable to live with his or her family of origin. A *foster parent* is an adult who meets the legal requirements for providing temporary, intermediate, or long-term care for a child living in out-of-home care. Foster parents can be part of the child's larger family (or *kin*), neighborhood, tribe, or, more often, strangers who provide safe homes for the child. Foster care can be brief or long lasting, with 60 percent of children in out-of-home care remaining in care for one or more years (Tatara, 1992). The *basic goals of foster care* are to provide safety, permanence, and well-being (Altshuler & Gleeson, 1999). *Emancipation* refers to the end of foster care, particularly the process of aging out of care, which until recently generally came at age 18 or the completion of high school.

SCOPE

In 1998, there were over 520,000 children in the United States who needed a foster care placement and only 130,000 foster families available to care for them (Casey Family Programs, 2000a). In many areas of the United States, foster children come in disproportionate numbers from minority groups including African American, Latino, and Native American groups (Courtney & Barth, 1996). As of March 31, 1999, there are approximately 62,450 children in the care of provincial and territorial child welfare authorities in Canada (Human Resources Development Canada, 2000). In other countries, the number of youths living in foster care are similarly high. In the United Kingdom, there were 58,100 children in the custody of local authorities and about 65 percent of them were in foster care (Department of Health, 2000). In the Russian Federation, the foster care system is very fragile and overwhelmed. The exact numbers are elusive, but the need is so great that many potential foster youths are never placed into homes and become homeless. In fact, there are approximately 60,000 homeless children in Moscow alone primarily because of a lack of available foster homes (Hellinckx, Grietens, & Bodrova, 1997).

Most youth enter the foster care system because they have experienced neglect, abandonment, or physical, psychological, or sexual abuse (Fanshel, Finch, & Grundy, 1990), usually as a result of dysfunction in their homes of origin. Original (usually biological but sometimes early adoptive) parents of these youths tend to have high rates of substance abuse and/or mental illness (Courtney & Barth, 1996).

The costs to children who enter and remain in foster care are substantial. Maltreated or not, children who are removed from their original parent(s) and who are subsequently placed in foster care experience loss. This loss is frequently traumatic and results in physical, cognitive, emotional, identity, and social deficits.

The costs to society are very high. The basic *tangible* costs of foster care include training and paying staff members; licensing, training, and compensating foster parents; and health insurance, clothing and food expenses, and other forms of public assistance as required by the child or jurisdiction (e.g., special needs assessments, tutoring, independent living classes). In the United States, the monthly maintenance payments to resource families alone averaged about $400 per child in 1998 (Child Welfare League of America [CWLA], 2000). The combined measurable cost of the foster care system to American society easily exceeds $2.5 billion per year.

The *intangible* costs to society are also substantial. The emotional, cognitive, physical, educational and safety needs of foster children can be very high and probably exceed the support capacity of most public and private agencies. Some evidence suggests that the unmet, intangible needs of foster children may lead to higher levels of unintended pregnancy, educational underachievement, substance abuse, homelessness, mental illness, and crime (Fanshel et al., 1990; Yancey, 1998).

THEORIES

There has been very few theoretical discussion of the long-term effects of early neglect and abuse on youths who subsequently entered the foster care system. Downs and Pecora (2001) have applied Erikson's psychosocial theory to the impact of maltreatment and foster care. They argue that: (1) the timing and severity of early trauma, and (2) the quality of foster care have single and interactive predictability for eventual outcomes once a foster youth has left care (i.e., by returning home or emancipating into adulthood). Specifically, the earlier and more severe the abuse or neglect, the lower the overall probability of successful adult outcomes. The higher the quality of foster care, the greater the overall probability of successful adult outcomes. And the better the match between the types/severity of early trauma and the ameliorative quality of foster care, the greater the likelihood of an eventual positive and successful adult outcome.

Landsverk, Davis, Garland, Hough, Litrownik, & Price (1995) prepared a detailed *developmental model* of the impact of foster care as well. This conceptual model places the child in a developmental context wherein the interactive effects of birth family characteristics (e.g., age, gender, mental health, history of maltreatment of the parent[s]), the child's characteristics (e.g., age, gender, ethnicity, mental and physical health), community ecology (e.g., social and economic factors, attitudes toward abuse), and maltreatment (relationship to perpetrator, types, severity, time of onset, and duration) are considered as important pre-foster care factors before the child enters the child welfare system. Once in the system, several factors mediate the types and quality of foster care delivered. These include characteristics of the foster home, connections to the birth family, the systems of care available (e.g., availability, quality, and accessibility of services) and the ecological and community supports available for the child (e.g., supportive teachers, schools, neighbors, peers). Together, factors present before and during care mediate the eventual outcomes for the child who lives in foster care. These outcomes include mental and physical health, cognitive and social functioning, educational attainment, and employment/economic status.

RESEARCH

It is difficult to untangle the effects of pre-foster care maltreatment from foster care itself. Indeed, even in the better literature described below, it is often not clear what is the stronger predictor of eventual outcomes—the early abuse, the negative or positive quality of foster care, or an interaction of early trauma and the foster care experience.

Many studies have demonstrated the negative health and physical consequences encountered by foster children. These include physical disabilities, missed immunizations, chronic health problems, developmental delays, and motor skills deficits (Altshuler & Gleeson, 1999; Horowitz, Owens, & Simms, 2000). Speech, language, and cognitive functioning deficits have also been demonstrated (American Academy of Pediatrics [AAP], 2000) along with a predictably lower educational achievement (Altshuler & Gleeson, 1999).

Psychosocial development is often delayed (AAP, 2000; Horowitz et al., 2000) and attachment difficulties are common. Problems with attachment greatly hinder the ability to develop into a psychologically healthy adult with a sense of emotional security, identity, and social conscience (AAP, 2000; Downs & Pecora, 2001). Moreover, infants and children under chronic stress, such as that resulting from abuse, family violence, and other disruption, often turn to apathy, detachment, and withdrawal to cope with the stress, and may exhibit failure to thrive, even after being placed in very good foster homes (AAP, 2000).

Children in care who experienced trauma and/or frequent stress may also exhibit hypervigilance and exaggerated startle responses, impulsivity, hyperactivity, and mood swings (AAP, 2000). Overall, many studies have shown that children in foster care exhibit greater levels of behavioral problems, emotional disturbance, and psychopathology than children not in care (AAP, 2000; Altshuler & Gleeson, 1999).

Courtney, Piliavin, and Grogan-Kaylor (1995) found that 37 percent of their sample had been in at least one special education class, and 30 percent reported failing a grade, thus requiring at least one more year of publicly funded schooling. In her review of the literature, Yancey (1998) noted that estimates of the prevalence of emotional disturbances in foster children ranged from 35 to 85 percent, and foster children are 28 times more likely to be referred for mental health services compared with mainstream peers.

A small number of investigations have looked at the long-term, adult outcomes when youths spend a year or more of their childhoods in foster care. The outcomes include, on the average, increased levels of alcohol and drug use, criminal behavior, and homelessness, and decreased levels of educational attainment and income (Barth, 1990). Some of these adults are, of course, functioning well, with healthy social relationships, financial stability, physical health, and overall wellness. The foster care outcomes literature, however, illustrates that foster children are at an increased risk for relatively negative adult outcomes.

Problems with health and development have also been noted in other countries and groups. For example, Mosek (1993) reported that foster children in Israel exhibit difficulties in overall adjustment and particularly in social adjustment. In Denmark, Rothe (1985) reported that the large numbers of placements often encountered by foster children lead to lower intellectual performance, emotional development, and attachment. In a study of very young Vietnamese refugee foster children in the United States, Sokoloff, Carlin, and Pham (1984) found higher than average medical problems, nightmares, temper tantrums, excessive fears, and jealousy. In general, the long-term outcomes for children in foster care are relatively analogous for France, Canada, the United States, and Great Britain (Minty, 1999).

STRATEGIES: OVERVIEW

Society relies on the child welfare system to take on the task of nurturing these at-risk children. The task of this entry is to focus on primary prevention, before problems become manifested. For those children who do not have serious psychological or social problems, primary prevention regarding foster care takes the form of a consistent, nurturing, protective adult who can repair deficits in attachment, trust, emotional stability, and socialization skills, provide environmental stimulation to improve cognitive skills, help "overcome the stress and trauma of abuse and neglect" (AAP, 2000, p. 1146), and in general, provide the parental care that fosters healthy development. If not alleviated, the impact of these problems will worsen. Early crisis intervention then takes the form of mitigating or stopping the impact of earlier abuse and neglect, allowing the child to establish the cognitive, emotional, social, and physical foundation from which he or she can develop into healthy adulthood.

Foster care agencies seek to provide safe, permanent, nurturing homes for troubled children. The resulting improvements in environmental stimulation, predictability, trust and security, and mental health and other services can both repair past and prevent future problems in all aspects of development—physical, emotional, cognitive, social, and spiritual (AAP, 2000). The earlier this positive intervention, the better the child's development, particularly if the ameliorative and preventive effects occur while brain development is still in the plasticity stage of early childhood (AAP, 2000). The quality of foster care parents may control the effects of prior abuse, prevent escalation of current problems, and promote positive social and emotional development. Youth–parent matching and placement longevity become especially important factors in the success of this prevention strategy.

Unfortunately, very few foster children are able to have the experience of only one consistent caregiver. Fanshel et al. (1990) found the average number of placements to be over 10 during a multiyear stay in foster care. As the research cited above demonstrated, most foster children require additional services, such as special education and tutoring, health care, mental health, employment training, independent living skills training, and other specialized services (e.g., AAP, 2000; Courtney et al., 1995; Horowitz et al., 2000; Yancey, 1998). In terms of primary prevention, a single or consistent foster caregiver can maximize the chances of success when these services are delivered. For instance, children needing special education classes, but who are moved from one foster home to another, receive less benefit from those classes compared with children who remain in a consistent, supportive, and stable placement (e.g., Renihan & Renihan, 1995).

One of the more important aspects of foster care is the long-term (and perhaps stable and preventive) versus transient (or unstable) nature of care. When stable, long-term foster care is provided, even for youths who have previously been in large numbers of placements, they tend to show remarkable improvements on a wide array of physical, psychological, and intellectual fronts (Altshuler & Gleeson, 1999). Foster children have resilience and other strengths that are best manifested and utilized within stable, supportive environments.

The quality of the foster child's relationship to others, particularly to the foster parents, is highly important (AAP, 2000). Like all children, foster children need nurturing, warmth and affection, protection, and the stability of a permanent placement to develop trust, security, and, eventually, overall psychological health and optimal functioning in school, relationships, work, and adulthood (AAP, 2000). A foster parent must be prepared to provide unconditional love to the hurt and wary foster child, acceptance of that child's unique behaviors and reactions, consistency and flexibility, empathy, environmental stimulation, safety and security, a sense of belonging and, of course, room and board (AAP, 2000). Facilitating these qualities in foster parents is a major objective of primary prevention programs.

No foster family, however, no matter how much they meet the above ideals, can be fully effective in isolation. There must be proactive aid from the larger society. Much research has shown the importance of child welfare agency involvement (e.g., Fanshel et al., 1990; Sokoloff et al., 1984). Although foster parent training is a critical variable (Pasztor & Wynne, 1995; Sokoloff et al., 1984), the relationship between the agency and the foster family must be maintained in both directions, providing mutual feedback, respect and value, and financial, psychological, and resource support (AAP, 2000; Pasztor & Wynne, 1995).

STRATEGIES THAT WORK

Even though we believe we know what should be done to optimize the healthy growth and development in at-risk foster children, there is no available evidence that such a program has been consistently delivered and shows positive results.

STRATEGIES THAT MIGHT WORK

One controversial aspect of an agency's involvement with the foster child is how those in charge of the child's care involve the birth family. A main focus of child welfare in Western society has been to reunite the child with the biological family. Unfortunately, as seen in the news as well as in research, contact with birth parents does not always have positive effects.

Many attempts at family reunification fail to provide a permanent home for the child, resulting in reentry into the foster care system and further trauma to the child's emotions, psychological development, and attachment (AAP, 2000). Careful consideration of all aspects of child development and of the child's current attachment, *and* the current level of social and emotional functioning of the biological parents, must be part of any determination of foster care versus birth family placement (e.g., AAP, 2000; McDonald, Allen, Westerfelt, & Piliavin, 1996). Indeed, authors from both the United States and Canada have argued that connections to siblings and other significant people (e.g., neighbors, other family members, teachers) are more important to the overall adjustment in foster care than connections to birth parents (e.g., Thorpe & Swart, 1992).

There has been much discussion of who are the best candidates to provide foster care to a specific child. Partly because of the huge shortfall in available foster parents, child welfare agencies have frequently turned to kinship care, recruiting birth relatives (aunts and uncles, grandparents, etc.) to provide a home for foster children. While kinship care may provide such advantages as familiarity for the child and pre-existing relationships that will presumably result in stable caregiving (AAP, 2000), there is no conclusive research demonstrating consistent positive outcomes of placement with relatives. For example, Altshuler and Gleeson (1999) found generally positive evidence for the efficacy of kinship care in their review of foster child well-being research, but did note that some studies found inferior outcomes in certain areas for kinship care versus regular foster care.

As with kinship care, other aspects of foster parenting continue to be studied. In the interest of cultural competency, many argue that minority children should be placed with parents of the same ethnicity; however, being of the same ethnicity as the foster child does not automatically grant a parent cultural competency or the ability to help that child develop his or her cultural identity. Further research is necessary in this area; Courtney (1997) has noted that because the research is all weakened by methodological problems, no definitive study has yet shown the relative value or equivalency of transracial adoption. In addition, Downs (1998) reports initial findings of equivalence between gay, lesbian, and bisexual foster parents vis-à-vis heterosexual counterparts in providing safe, permanent homes for children in out-of-home care.

STRATEGIES THAT DO NOT WORK

Other strategies for caring for children tried over the years did not work. Among them were orphanages wherein children were warehoused until age 18 unless adopted. In other instances, children were kept in their homes of origin while services were delivered to those families despite the fact that these homes often remained dangerous. Other foster care strategies have involved forcing children to leave their foster homes at age 18 or at high school graduation (whichever came later). This strategy was common until the end of the 20th century when US states and the federal government finally recognized that these young people were not necessarily ready to live on their own as adults by that age (e.g., Casey Family Programs, 2000b). None of these strategies have shown promise in promoting positive emotional, mental, or physical development or in preventing the long-term negative effects of early abuse and neglect.

SYNTHESIS

First, it would be most beneficial if we could prevent the large numbers of children from becoming "foster" in the first place. Other entries in this Encyclopedia speak about ways to promote healthy families. However, given the reality of large numbers of children entering the foster care system with varying degrees of potential or manifest problems, this system has to take responsible actions. We are focusing on primary prevention of predictable problems and protection of existing strengths in these young people, as well as the promotion of their healthy development. What is needed most of all for these vulnerable young people are qualified, willing, and able adults who care deeply for the well-being and safety of children living in out-of-home care. There is a critical lack of available, trained, and devoted foster parents. Expansion of definitions of foster parents, to include those not traditionally considered ideal (e.g., kin adults; gay, lesbian, and bisexual adults; single adults; retirees), is a very promising practice in order to identify more devoted foster parents. More resources are necessary for initial recruitment and retention of an expanded definition of prospective foster parents.

Thorough review of foster parent recruitment and retention procedures and programs are available (Casey Family Programs, 2000a; Pasztor & Wynne, 1995). The Child Welfare League of America (Pasztor & Wynne, 1995) carefully reviewed best practices in retention and recruitment of foster homes and best practices for foster children. They emphasized the importance of elevating the role and voice of the foster parent in the child welfare system, of providing competency-based training to these parents, and of matching prospective foster children and foster parents. The latter has been an approach of some private foster care agencies and has been successful in minimizing placement disruptions. Other foster parent supports are extremely important and include respite care, recognition for accomplishments, professional development, liability insurance, increased stipends, connections with other foster families, and availability of social workers.

Foster parent training must include helping parents understand the meaning and implication of common needs and experiences of foster children (abuse and neglect, placement disruption, loss of social ties with family and friends, medical and developmental needs, etc.), necessary principles of child development, household safety, cultural competence, attachment, behavior management skills, and available community resources (e.g., AAP, 2000; Pasztor & Wynne, 1995). Foster parent training should be frequent, proactive, regular, and held at convenient times.

Foster care parents must be supported within a broader, comprehensive, integrated system of services that considers the physical health and development, attachment and social development, identity development, extended family, emotional development, adjustment and performance in school, placement stability and safety, spirituality, nutrition, and individuality of that child (and, as applicable, the foster family) (e.g., Bloom, 1998). This holistic focus must be taken both in terms of primary prevention and treatment. More resources must be made available to decrease caseloads and increase support for all facets of the child/foster parent/social worker system.

Many child welfare agencies are developing multidisciplinary wraparound service programs, as such programs have been found to be generally effective in other populations. For instance, The Oregon Social Learning Center began a multidisciplinary treatment foster care approach involving early intervention with young children diverted from juvenile justice (Fisher & Chamberlain, 2000). The Florida Mental Health Institute's Fostering Individualized Assistance Program involves strengths-based assessment and family specialists linking resource families to needed services available in the community; this program has shown promise in both the home and school behaviors of foster children (e.g., McDonald, Boyd, Clark, & Stewart, 1995).

There are many programs and specialized services proven to work in the community at large that are appropriate and needed for foster children. These include dentistry, nutrition, pediatric medicine (AAP, 2000), regular and special education services, psychological and psychiatric services, and social skills development programs (Renihan & Renihan, 1995). These programs and services should all be integrated into an individualized system of care for foster children (AAP, 2000; Bloom, 1998), focusing on reparation and prevention in all elements of childhood health and development.

Although, as discussed above, placement longevity is highly important in fostering health and positive development, sometimes it becomes necessary to remove a child from a foster placement. Promising practices include providing continuity of a child's school when a foster placement is disrupted. Specifically, using a neighborhood foster care approach, even if a child must leave a specific foster placement, the child's next placement is in the same neighborhood and school district. This minimizes disruption to the child's educational and social development.

Finally, preparation for emancipation from foster care must begin at the time the child enters the child welfare system. Foster care alumni sometimes note that they felt "coddled" or ignored during their time in care, unable to do and learn for themselves before being thrust upon the world at emancipation. Consequently, early independent living training, beginning as early as age 8, is highly desirable. This may maximize the chances of promoting competency and self-sufficiency in early adulthood (Nollan & Downs, 2001). For example, foster children, as with other children, could be given an allowance and later encouraged to establish a bank account, all in order that they might learn money management skills. This notion is consistent with another suggestion

sometimes heard from alumni—that they be directly given a portion of the foster care payment for their own use.

Foster children enter the child welfare system with many strengths, but also with many needs and negative factors associated with poor outcomes. They need stable, holistic, integrated systems of care, involving a nurturing foster parent and other community supports, in order to capitalize on their resiliency and allow them to develop into healthy adults.

Also see: Foster Care: Adolescence; Self-Esteem: Childhood.

References

Altshuler, S.J., & Gleeson, J.P. (1999). Completing the evaluation triangle for the next century: Measuring child "well-being" in family foster care. *Child Welfare, 78,* 125–147.

American Academy of Pediatrics Committee on Early Childhood, Adoption, and Dependent Care (AAP). (2000). Developmental issues for young children in foster care. *Pediatrics, 106,* 1,145–1,150.

Barth, R.P. (1990). On their own: The experience of youth after foster care. *Child and Adolescent Social work, 7,* 419–440.

Bloom, M. (1998). Primary prevention and foster care. *Children & Youth Services, 20*(8), 667–696.

Casey Family Programs. (2000a). *Lighting the way: Attracting and supporting foster families.* Seattle: Author.

Casey Family Programs. (2000b). *Frequently asked questions about the Foster Care Independent Act of 1999 and The John H. Chafee Foster Care Independent Program.* Seattle: Author.

Child Welfare League of America (CWLA). (2000, November/December). *National data analysis system.* Available: http://ndas.cwla.org

Courtney, M.E. (1997). The politics and realities of transracial adoption. *Child Welfare, 76,* 749–779.

Courtney, M.E., & Barth, R.P. (1996). Race and child welfare services: Past research and future directions. *Child Welfare, 75,* 99–137.

Courtney, M.E., Piliavin, I., & Grogan-Kaylor, A. (1995). *The Wisconsin study of youth aging out of out-of-home care: A portrait of children about to leave care.* Madison, WI: University of Wisconsin-Madison.

Department of Health. (2000). *Modern social services: Ninth report of the Chief Inspector for social services.* London: Author.

Downs, A.C. (1998, August). *Gay and lesbian foster parents.* Paper presented at the American Psychological Association, San Francisco. Available from cdowns@casey.org

Downs, A.C., & Pecora, P.J. (2001). *Application of Erikson's psychosocial development theory to foster care research.* Seattle: Casey Family Programs.

Fanshel, D., Finch, S.J., & Grundy, J.F. (1990). *Foster children in a life course perspective.* New York: Columbia University Press.

Fisher, P.A., & Chamberlain, P. (2000). Multidimensional treatment foster care: A program for intensive parenting, family support, and skill building. *Journal of Emotional & Behavioral Disorders, 8,* 155–164.

Hellinckx, W., Grietens, H., & Bodrova, V. (1997). Prevalence and correlates of problem behavior in 12-to-16-year-old adolescents in the Russian Federation. *International Journal of Child & Family Welfare, 97,* 86–112.

Horowitz, S.M., Owens, P., & Simms, M.D. (2000). Specialized assessments for children in foster care. *Pediatrics, 106,* 59–66.

Human Resources Development Canada, Social Policy, Strategic Policy Branch. (2000). *Social Security statistics, Canada and Provinces, 1974–75 to 1998–99.* Available: http://www.hrdc-drhc.gc.ca/socpol/statistics/74-75/tab437.shtml

Landsverk, J., Davis, I., Garland, A., Hough, R., Litrownik, A., & Price, J. (1995). *A developmental framework for research with victims of child maltreatment placed in foster care.* San Diego: Center for Research on Child and Adolescent Mental Health Services.

McDonald, B.A., Boyd, L.A., Clark, H.B., & Stewart, E.S. (1995). Recommended individualized wraparound strategies for foster children with emotional/behavioral disturbances and their families. *Community Alternatives: International Journal of Family Care, 7,* 63–82.

McDonald, T.P., Allen, R.I., Westerfelt, A., & Piliavin, I. (1996). *Assessing the long-term effects of foster care: A research synthesis.* Washington, DC: CWLA Press.

Minty, B. (1999). Annotation: Outcomes in long-term foster family care. *Journal of Child Psychology, Psychiatry & Allied Disciplines, 40,* 991–1000.

Mosek, A. (1993). Well-being and parental contact of foster children in Israel: A different situation from the USA? *International Social Work, 36,* 261–275.

Nollan, K.A., & Downs, A.C. (2001). *Preparing youth for long-term success. Proceedings from the Casey Family Program National Independent Living Forum.* Washington, DC: CWLA Press.

Pasztor, E.M., & Wynne, S.F. (1995). *Foster parent retention and recruitment: The state of the art in practice and policy.* Washington, DC: CWLA Press.

Renihan, F.I., & Renihan, P.J. (1995). Responsive high schools: Structuring success for the at-risk student. *High School Journal, 79,* 1–13.

Rothe, W. (1985). Some consequences of frequent changes of environment in early childhood. *International Journal of Rehabilitation Research, 8,* 196–199.

Sokoloff, B., Carlin, J., & Pham, H. (1984). Five-year follow-up of Vietnamese refugee children in the United States. *Clinical Pediatrics, 23,* 565–570.

Tatara, T. (1992). *Characteristics of children in substitute and adoptive care—A statistical summary of the VCIS national child welfare data base.* Washington: American Public Welfare Association.

Thorpe, M.B., & Swart, G.T. (1992). Risk and protective factors affecting children in foster care: A pilot study of the role of siblings. *Canadian Journal of Psychiatry, 37,* 616–622.

Yancey, A.K. (1998). Building positive self-image in adolescents in foster care: The use of role models in an interactive group approach. *Adolescence, 33,* 253–267.

Foster Care, Adolescence

Chris Downs and Kathryn Caldwell

INTRODUCTION

Many youths are unable to live with their original birth or adoptive parents and become the custody of the public welfare system. The impact of the early trauma or abuse leading to disruption from their homes of origin, and the impact of subsequent foster care are the subjects of infrequent theory and research. This entry reviews existing theory, research, and strategies that have differential effectiveness in promoting healthy development among youths living in out-of-home care.

DEFINITIONS

An adolescent living with a foster family is typically a minor who has been judged by a state, county or court administrator as temporarily or permanently unable to live with his or her family of origin. A *foster parent* is an adult who meets the legal requirements for providing temporary, immediate, respite, or long-term care for an adolescent living in out-of-home care. Foster parents can be part of the adolescent's larger family (or kin), neighborhood, tribe, or more often a stranger who provides a safe home for the youth. Foster care can be brief or long-lasting with 60 percent of youths in out-of-home care remaining in care for one or more years (Tatara, 1992). The *basic goals of foster care* are to provide safety, permanence, and well-being (Altshuler & Gleeson, 1999). *Emancipation* refers to the end of foster care, usually the process of aging out of care, which often occurs at age 18 or at the completion of high school.

SCOPE

In 1998, there were over 520,000 minors in the United States in foster care. Of these, 77,000 were adolescents between the ages of 16 and 20 (Casey Family Programs, 2000; US GAO, 1999). About 24,000 adolescents emancipate each year and many have no connection to families or other close relatives (Pizzigati, 2001). In most areas of the United States, foster youths are disproportionately African American, Latino, or Native American rather than Caucasian (Courtney & Barth, 1996; Dillon, 1994; Yancey, 1992).

In other countries, the numbers of youths living in foster care are as high or higher. In Canada, there are 62,450 youths in the care of provincial and territorial child welfare authorities (Human Resources Development Canada, 2000). In the United Kingdom, 65 percent of the 58,100 youth in the custody of local authorities are in foster care (Department of Health, 2000). In the Russian Federation, the numbers of adolescents in foster care are unknown, but with about 60,000 homeless youths in Moscow alone, the numbers are probably small in comparison to the need for such care (Hellinckx, Grietens, & Bodrova, 1997).

Most adolescents who enter the foster care system have experienced prior neglect or abuse, typically in their homes of origin. Some adolescents enter care because of their own serious behavior problems (McDonald, Allen, Westerfelt, & Piliavin, 1996).

An additional, but as yet unknown number of adolescents are known as "throwaways" (Gullotta, 1979). These are lesbian, gay, bisexual, or transgender youths who have been forced out of their homes because their parents reject their sexual orientation. Estimates of such youths range from 25 percent (in Los Angeles) to 40 percent (in Seattle) of all homeless youths are runaway or throwaway gay or lesbian youths (Kruks, 1991). Additional research has shown that many of these youths end up in the child welfare system in foster care (Mallon, 1994).

Costs towards adolescents who exit their homes of origin and then enter and remain in foster care are often elusive, but substantial. Whether or not they are the victims of child abuse or neglect, adolescents who are removed from their original parent(s) experience loss. Such losses are frequently related to later physical, cognitive, emotional, identity, and social deficits.

The *tangible* costs to society are very high. The basic costs include staff support, foster parent preparation and payment, insurance, clothing, food, and housing allowances, public assistance, and independent living supports (US GAO, 1999). The Child Welfare League of America (CWLA) has estimated that the average monthly maintenance payments to foster families are about $400 per youth (CWLA, 2000).

The *intangible* costs foster care presents to society are substantial. The emotional, cognitive, physical, educational and safety needs of foster adolescents can be very high and probably exceed the support capacity of most social welfare agencies. Some evidence suggests that the unmet, intangible needs of foster youths may lead to higher levels of unintended pregnancy, educational underachievement, substance abuse, homelessness, mental illness, and crime (Courtney, Piliavin, Grogan-Kaylor, & Nesmith, 1998; Fanshel, Finch, & Grundy, 1990).

THEORIES

There have been very few theoretical treatments of the long-term effects of neglect and abuse on adolescents who subsequently entered the foster care system. Applications of existing theories have included ecological and protective factors models (Cicchetti & Lynch, 1993), attachment theory (Goldberg, Muir, & Kerr, 1995), and risk and protective frameworks (Catalano & Hawkins, 1996).

Landsverk, Davis, Garland, Hough, Litrownik, and Price (1995) prepared one of the more detailed developmental models of the impact of foster care. This conceptual model places the adolescent in a developmental context wherein the interactive effects of birth family characteristics (e.g., age, gender, mental health, history of maltreatment),

the adolescent's own characteristics (e.g., age, gender, ethnicity, mental and physical health), community ecology (e.g., social and economic factors, attitudes toward abuse), and maltreatment (types, severity, time of onset, and duration) are all jointly considered as important pre-foster care factors before the adolescent enters the social welfare system. Once in the system, several factors mediate the types and quality of foster care delivered. These include characteristics of the foster home, connections to the birth family, the systems of care available (e.g., availability, quality, and accessibility of services) and the ecological and community supports available for the youth (e.g., supportive teachers, schools, neighbors, peers). Together, factors present before and during care mediate the eventual outcomes for the adolescent who lived in foster care. These outcomes include mental and physical health, cognitive and social functioning, educational attainment, and employment/economic status.

Downs and Pecora (2001) have applied Erikson's psychosocial theory to the impact on adolescents of maltreatment and foster care. They propose that: (1) the timing and severity of early trauma and (2) the quality of foster care have single and interactive predictability for foster care outcomes after emancipation. They predict that the earlier and more severe the abuse and neglect, the lower the overall probability of successful adult outcomes. However, the higher the quality of foster care during adolescence, the greater the overall probability of adult outcomes. They also argue that the match between the youth's prior trauma and the supportive qualities of the foster home are important in predicting successful adult outcomes.

RESEARCH

The effects of early maltreatment and of later foster care on adolescents are well documented in the empirical literature. While many adolescents who were abused or neglected and enter foster care function well later as adults, many do not (Becker et al., 1995; McDonald et al., 1996). The consequences depend on a variety of factors including the types and timing of abuse or neglect, and the quality and length of foster care.

Adolescents in care who experienced chronic stress, such as from abuse and neglect, family violence, removal from the home, and foster care placement disruptions often exhibit apathy, withdrawal, and daydreaming (AAP, 2000) as well as anxiety, depression, somatic complains, and problems with attachment (Altshuler & Gleeson, 1999). Those with a history of trauma often suffer from post-traumatic stress disorder symptomatology. When faced with current stress, such as that encountered in school or on the job, such youths may "freeze" and are sometimes labeled oppositional or defiant (AAP, 2000). Identity disturbances can also be frequent for foster adolescents, especially those from minority groups (Dillon, 1994; Ryan & Futterman, 1998).

Adolescents in foster care may experience greater sensitivity to rejection and higher rates of aggressive, delinquent, and anti-social behaviors (Feldman & Downey, 1994; Manly, Cicchetti & Barnett, 1994). For instance, adults who have spent a year or more in foster care as adolescents were more likely to have been involved in criminal activities, drug and alcohol use, depression, and homelessness (Barth, 1990; Courtney, Piliavin, & Grogan-Kaylor, 1995; Festinger, 1983). In addition, these young adults are more likely to receive public assistance (Fanshel et al., 1990).

Problems with health and development have also been noted in other countries and groups. For example, Mosek (1993) reported that foster youth in Israel exhibit difficulties in adjustment, particularly social adjustment.

In urban areas, foster children tend to be disproportionately from minority groups, particularly African American, Latino, and Native American (Dillon, 1994; Yancey, 1992). Minorities in urban centers, whether in child welfare or not, also disproportionately experience unintended pregnancies, academic underachievement and discontinuation, substance abuse, and, ultimately, homelessness (Yancey, 1992). Identity disturbances can be frequent for minorities in child welfare when the negative attitudes toward and beliefs about minority groups and other aspects of the historical and sociopolitical context are not properly confronted (Dillon, 1994; Yancey, 1992). It is also important to note the importance of within-group variability of minority groups that may become relevant in same-group placements as well as cross-group placements. The well-being of foster youth, including intellectual and spiritual development, is likely to suffer if "cultural identification, ethnicity, and social class" are not considered during placement decisions (Dillon, 1994, p. 129). Thus, while all foster youth have experienced varying levels of trauma, disruption, poor attachment, and inconsistent relationships which are likely to result in problems in identity formation (AAP, 2000), ethnicity and social class introduce other variables that may affect eventual outcomes.

In general, adolescents in foster care are likely to have experienced difficulty in school achievement, social development, and trust. They may suffer from emotional or physical disabilities. They are likely to have little contact with their biological parents, and if they do, the parent is likely not able to offer much support, financially or emotionally.

The process of emancipation often comes before optimal social, emotional, intellectual, vocational, and identity development. Imagine being forced to leave home on your 18th birthday, having been judged by the "state" as a "self-sufficient adult!" Upon emancipation, youth often face such problems as not having a driver's license or a high school diploma, having little money, and feeling unprepared for independent living (Courtney et al., 1998; Nollan & Downs, 2001). As a result, follow-up studies have shown that many young people experience inadequate income and financial stress, employment difficulties, life dissatisfaction, loneliness, psychological distress, criminal involvement, and inadequate medical and dental care (Courtney et al., 1998; Fanshel et al., 1990). For example, Fanshel and colleagues (Fanshel et al., 1990) found that approximately 10 percent of the alumni interviewed from a private child welfare agency were on public assistance as adults. Courtney and Piliavin (1998) found that 32 percent of their respondents received public assistance and 12 percent had been homeless at least once since leaving care.

STRATEGIES THAT WORK

Many of the problems described in the previous section are present when adolescents enter foster care in the first place. Assuming we have not been able to prevent the problems that led to the need of foster care, then the first intervention comes from the foster care itself—the existence of a consistent, nurturing, protective adult who can repair deficits in attachment, trust, emotional stability, and socialization skills, provide environmental stimulation to improve cognitive skills, and help "overcome the stress and trauma of abuse and neglect" (AAP, 2000, p. 1146). Unfortunately, very few foster youth are able to have the experience of only one consistent caregiver. And during that time, most foster children/youth require additional services, such as special education and tutoring, health care, mental health, employment training, independent living skills training, and other specialized services (AAP, 2000; Courtney et al., 1995; Horwitz, Owens, & Simms, 2000; US GAO, 1998; Yancey, 1998).

We rely on the child welfare system to take on this task of "fixing" our most vulnerable and harmed children. Indeed, oftentimes the best intervention for children in foster care is the foster care itself. Although research continues to attempt to demonstrate the efficacy of foster care in general and aspects of care in particular, various authors have discussed the success of foster care agencies in helping abused, neglected, and troubled young people become more functional and productive, and much of the research demonstrates positive outcomes for the majority of the youth because of high quality care (Altshuler & Gleeson, 1999; Courtney et al., 1995, 1998; Fanshel et al., 1990; Sokoloff, Cavlin, & Pham, 1984).

Foster care agencies seek to provide safe, permanent, nurturing homes for troubled children. The resulting improvements in environmental stimulation, predictability, trust and security, and mental health and other services can both repair past and prevent future problems in all aspects of development—physical, emotional, cognitive, social (AAP, 2000), and spiritual (Dillon, 1994). The earlier this positive intervention comes, the better the adolescent's development will be (AAP, 2000).

The quality of the foster adolescent's relationship to others, particularly the foster parents, is highly important (AAP, 2000; Marcus, 1991). Foster children need nurturing, warmth and affection, protection, and the stability of a permanent placement to optimally develop trust, security, and, eventually, overall psychological health and optimal functioning in school, relationships, work, and adulthood (AAP, 2000; Marcus, 1991). A foster parent must be prepared to provide unconditional love to the hurt and wary foster child, acceptance of that child's unique behaviors and reactions, consistency and flexibility, empathy, environmental stimulation, safety and security, a sense of belonging, and, of course, room and board (AAP, 2000; Marcus, 1991).

STRATEGIES THAT MIGHT WORK

Among the basic prevention strategies that would ameliorate the need for and effects of foster care are to attack the root causes of foster care in the first place. The two most important factors leading to the need for foster care are: (a) mental illness of parents and (b) substance abuse of parents. In both instances, abuse and neglect are the sequelae of problem parental behavior (Courtney & Barth, 1996). Additional root causes of foster care include family and community poverty (Courtney & Barth, 1996), and homophobia for sexual minority youths (Ryan & Futterman, 1998).

Most child welfare agencies try to provide independent living skills to increase the chances that youth can emancipate successfully. A large number of specific approaches to this training have shown promise. Bach, Downs, Friend, Patz, and Topkins (2001) report on a unique approach to preparing youth for economic self-sufficiency. Their approach is built on a team concept wherein youth help to develop their own independent living curricula, identify mentors, and evaluate experiences with jobs during adolescence. Another program at Boysville (Michigan) emphasizes a comprehensive supervised independent living program with both short- and long-term outcome goals specified (Hoge & Idalski, 2001). Other promising programs have included job development programs wherein the goal is to align summer employment with stated career interests (Rodriguez et al., 2001).

Kroner (2001) has developed what appears to be a highly effective method for developing housing options for adolescents in foster care. His agency, Lighthouse Youth Services in Cincinnati, Ohio, works with local landlords of scattered-site apartments, to provide safe, affordable housing. As of 2001, more than 600 adolescents had successfully made the difficult transition from foster care to independent living with the support of this program.

A controversial aspect of agency involvement with foster youths is how social workers connect with the original or birth family. A great deal of attention in child welfare agencies has been to unite youths with biological families. Unfortunately, birth family contact is not always in the best interests of the adolescent. Some attempts at family reunification fail to provide permanent homes, resulting in disruption and reentry into the child welfare system (AAP, 2000). McDonald et al. (1996) argue that careful consideration of all aspects of development and the youth's current attachment must be important factors in foster care versus birth family placement.

STRATEGIES THAT DO NOT WORK

During the 20th century, numerous strategies were tried in order to meet the needs of children living in out-of-home care. Some of these did not work. Among them are orphanages wherein children were warehoused until age 18 unless adopted. In other instances, children were kept in their homes of origin while services were delivered to those homes despite the fact that these homes often remained dangerous. Other foster care strategies have involved forcing children to leave their foster homes at age 18 or after high school graduation (whichever came later). This strategy was common until the end of the 20th century when US states and the federal government finally recognized that these young people were not ready to live on their own as adults by that age (Casey Family Programs, 2000).

SYNTHESIS

What is needed most of all are qualified, willing, and able adults who care deeply for the well-being and safety of adolescents living in out-of-home care. There is a critical lack of available, trained, and devoted foster parents. Thorough review of foster parent recruitment and retention procedures and programs are available to identify and retain excellent parents (Casey Family Programs, 2000; Pasztor & Wynne, 1995).

The Child Welfare League of America (Pasztor & Wynne, 1995) reviewed best practices on the retention and recruitment of foster homes and best practices for foster children. They emphasized the importance of elevating the role and voice of the foster parent in the child welfare system, of providing competency-based training to these parents, and of matching prospective foster children and foster parents. The latter has been an approach of some private foster care agencies (Casey Family Programs) and has been successful in minimizing placement disruptions. Other foster parent supports are important and include respite care, recognition for accomplishments, professional development, liability insurance and connections with other foster families.

Many social welfare agencies are developing multidisciplinary services designed to meet varying levels and types of needs for youths in care. The Florida Mental Health Institute's Fostering Individualized Assistance Program involves strengths-based assessment and family specialists linking resource families to needed services available in the community; this program has shown promise in both the home and school behaviors of foster children (McDonald, Boyd, Clark, & Stewart, 1995).

The Casey Family Programs, a large private foster care foundation based in Seattle, have encouraged the use of practice-friendly independent living assessments. The Ansell-Casey Life Skills Assessment (ACLSA) was designed for this purpose and has been shown to have excellent practice utility in preparing youths aged 8–18 to live on their own at emancipation. The ACLSA is self-administered, with a companion for caregivers, web-based, free, and provides an instant score report to the end users (i.e., the social worker, parent, and youth). The instrument is linked with curricula resources to set independent living goals for the coming period, typically six months. Instruments like the ACLSA are showing great promise for future practice and research in work with adolescents in foster care (Nollan, Horn, Downs, & Pecora, 2001).

There are many other programs and specialized services proven to work in the community at large that are appropriate and needed for foster youths. These include dentistry, nutrition, pediatric medicine (AAP, 2000), regular and special education services (Renihan & Renihan, 1995), psychological and psychiatric services (Rivera & Kutash, 1994), social skills development programs (Swetnam, Peterson, & Clark, 1982), and other interventions discussed elsewhere in this encyclopedia. These programs and services should all be integrated into an individualized system of care for foster children, focusing on reparation and prevention in all facets of adolescent health and development.

Also see: Foster Care: Childhood; Self-Esteem: Adolescence.

References

Altshuler, S.J., & Gleeson, J.P. (1999). Completing the evaluation triangle for the next century: Measuring child "well-being" in family foster care. *Child Welfare, 78*(1), 125–147.

American Academy of Pediatrics Committee on Early Childhood, Adoption, and Dependent Care (AAP). (2000). Developmental issues for young children in foster care. *Pediatrics, 106*, 1145–1150.

Bach, C., Downs, A.C., Friend, R., Patz, C.R., & Topkins, R. (2001). Preparation of youth for employment (PYE): Description and evaluation of a competency-based approach to economic independence. In K.A. Nollan & A.C. Downs (Eds.), *Preparing youth for long-term success: Proceedings from the Casey Family Program National Independent Living Forum.* Washington, DC: CWLA.

Barth, R.P. (1990). On their own: The experience of youth after foster care. *Child and Adolescent Social work, 7*(5), 419–440.

Becker, J.V., Alpert, J.L., Bigfoot, D.S., Bonner, B.L., Geddie, L.F., Henggeler, S.W., Kaufman, K.L., & Walter, C.E. (1995). Empirical research on child abuse treatment: Report by the Child Abuse and Neglect Treatment Working Groups, American Psychological Association. *Journal of Child Clinical Psychology, 24*, 23–46.

Casey Family Programs. (2000). *Lighting the way: Attracting and supporting foster families.* Seattle: Author.

Catalano, R.F., & Hawkins, J.D. (1996). The social developmental model: A theory of antisocial behavior. In J.D. Hawkins (Ed.), *Delinquency and crime: Current theories.* New York: Cambridge.

Child Welfare League of American. (2000). *National data analysis system,* ndas.cwla.org, compiled November and December, 2000.

Cicchetti, D., & Lynch, M. (1993). Toward an ecological/transactional model of community violence and child maltreatment: Consequence for children's development. *Psychiatry, 56*, 96–118.

Courtney, M.E., & Barth, R.P. (1996). Race and child welfare services: Past research and future directions. *Child Welfare, 75*(2), 99–137.

Courtney, M.E., Piliavin, I., & Grogan-Kaylor, A. (1995). *The Wisconsin Study of youth aging out of out-of-home care: A portrait of children about to leave care.* Madison, WI: University of Wisconsin-Madison.

Courtney, M.E., Piliavin, I., Grogan-Kaylor, A., & Nesmith, A. (1998). *Foster youth transitions to adulthood: Outcomes 12 to 18 months after leaving out-of-home care.* Madison, WI: University of Wisconsin-Madison.

Department of Health. (2000). *Modern social services: Ninth report of the Chief Inspector for social services.* London: Author.

Dillon, D. (1994). Understanding and assessment of intragroup dynamics in family foster care: African American families. *Child Welfare, 73*, 129–139.

Downs, A.C., & Pecora, P.J. (2001). *Application of Erikson's psychosocial development theory to foster care research.* Seattle: Casey Family Programs.

Fanshel, D., Finch, S.J., & Grundy, J.F. (1990). *Foster children in a life course perspective.* New York: Columbia University Press.

Feldman, S., & Downey, G. (1994). Rejection sensitivity as a mediator of the impact of childhood exposure to family violence on adult attachment behavior. *Development and Psychopathology, 6*, 231–247.

Festinger, T. (1983). *No one ever asked us…A postscript to foster care.* New York: Columbia University Press.

Goldberg, S., Muir, R., & Kerr, J. (Eds.). (1995). *Attachment theory: Social, developmental, and clinical perspectives.* Hillsdale, NJ: Analytic Press.

Gullotta, T.P. (1979). Leaving home: Family Relationships of the runaway. *Social Casework, 60*, 111–114.

Hellinckx, W., Grietens, H., & Bodrova, V. (1997). Prevalence and correlates of problem behavior in 12-to-16-year-old adolescents in the Russian Federation. *International Journal of Child & Family Welfare, 97*(2), 86–112.

Hoge, J., & Idalski, A. (2001). How Boysville of Michigan specified and evaluated its supervised independent living program. In K.A. Nollan & A.C. Downs (Eds.), *Preparing youth for long-term success: Proceedings from the Casey Family Program National Independent Living Forum.* Washington, DC: CWLA.

Horwitz, S.M., Owens, P., & Simms, M.D. (2000). Specialized assessments for children in foster care. *Pediatrics, 106,* 59–66.

Human Resources Development Canada, Social Policy, Strategic Policy Branch. (2000). *Social Security statistics, Canada and Provinces, 1974–75 to 1998–99* [On-line]. Available: http://www.hrdc-drhc.gc.ca/socpol/statistics/74-75tab437.shtml.

Kroner, M.J. (2001). Developing housing options for independent living preparation. In K.A. Nollan & A.C. Downs (Eds.), *Preparing youth for long-term success: Proceedings from the Casey Family Program National Independent Living Forum.* Washington, DC: CWLA.

Kruks, G.P. (1991). Gay and lesbian homeless/street youth: Special issues and concerns. *Journal of Adolescent Health, 12,* 515.

Landsverk, J., Davis, I., Garland, A., Hough, R., Litrownik, A., & Price, J. (1995). *A developmental framework for research with victims of child maltreatment placed in foster care.* San Diego: Center for Research on Child and Adolescent Mental Health Services.

Mallon, G.P. (1994). The experience of gay and lesbian adolescents in New York City's child welfare system. In A. Siskind & F. Kunreuther (Eds.), *Report and Recommendations of a Joint Task Force of New York City's Child Welfare Administration and the Council of Family and Child Caring Agencies.* New York: Author.

Manly, J.T., Cicchetti, D., & Barnett, D. (1994). The impact of subtype, frequency, chronicity, and severity of child maltreatment on social competence and behavior problems. *Development and Psychopathology, 6,* 121–143.

Marcus, R. (1991). The attachments of children in foster care. *Genetic, Social & General Psychology Monographs, 117,* 367–394.

McDonald, B.A., Boyd, L.A., Clark, H.B., & Stewart, E.S. (1995). Recommended individualized wraparound strategies for foster children with emotional/behavioral disturbances and their families. *Community Alternatives: International Journal of Family Care, 7,* 63–82.

McDonald, T.P., Allen, R.I., Westerfelt, A., & Piliavin, I. (1996). *Assessing the long-term effects of foster care: A research synthesis.* Washington, DC: CWLA.

Mosek, A. (1993). Well-being and parental contact of foster children in Israel: A different situation from the USA? *International Social Work, 36,* 261–275.

Nollan, K.A., & Downs, A.C. (2001). *Preparing youth for long-term success: Proceedings from the Casey Family Program National Independent Living Forum.* Washington, DC: CWLA.

Nollan, K.A., Horn, M., Downs, A.C., & Pecora, P.J. (2001). *Ansell-Casey Life Skills Assessment (ACLSA) and Life Skills Guidebook Manual* [On-line]. Available: www.caseylifeskills.org

Pasztor, E.M., & Wynne, S.F. (1995). *Foster parent retention and recruitment: The state of the art in practice and policy.* Washington, DC: Child Welfare League of America.

Pizzigati, K. (2001). Public policy to help youth leaving foster care achieve independence: Where are we going? How do we get there? In K.A. Nollan & A.C. Downs (Eds.), *Preparing youth for long-term success: Proceedings from the Casey Family Program National Independent Living Forum.* Washington, DC: CWLA.

Renihan, F.I., & Renihan, P.J. (1995). Responsive high schools: Structuring success for the at-risk student. *High School Journal, 79,* 1–13.

Rivera, V.R., & Kutash, K. (1994). *Components of a System of Care: What Does the Research Say?* Tampa, FL: University of South Florida, Florida Mental Health Institute, Research and Training Center for Children's Mental Health.

Rodriguez, C.B., Downs, A.C., Burns, J., Hill, R., Patz, C.R., Meyer, J., Eutsey, N., & Sherman, P. (2001). The Job Development Initiative (JDI): An intensive jobs-based approach to youth self-sufficiency. In K.A. Nollan & A.C. Downs (Eds.), *Preparing youth for long-term success: Proceedings from the Casey Family Program National Independent Living Forum.* Washington, DC: CWLA.

Ryan, C., & Futterman, D. (1998). *Lesbian & gay youth: Care & counseling.* New York: Columbia University Press.

Sokoloff, B., Carlin, J., & Pham, H. (1984). Five-year follow-up of Vietnamese refugee children in the United States. *Clinical Pediatrics, 23,* 565–570.

Swetnam, L., Peterson, C.R., & Clark, H.B. (1982). Social skills development in young children: Preventive and therapeutic approaches. *Child & Youth Services, 5,* 5–27.

Tatara, T. (1992). *Characteristics of children in substitute and adoptive care—A statistical summary of the VCIS National Child Welfare Data Base.* Washington: American Public Welfare Association.

United States General Accounting Office (US GAO). (1999). *Foster care: Effectiveness of independent living services unknown.* Washington, DC: Author.

Yancey, A.K. (1992). Identity formation and social maladaptation in foster adolescents. *Adolescence, 27,* 819–831.

Yancey, A.K. (1998). Building positive self-image in adolescents in foster care: The use of role models in an interactive group approach. *Adolescence, 33,* 253–267.

G

Gambling, Adolescence

Robert Ladouceur and Francine Ferland

INTRODUCTION AND DEFINITIONS

Gambling has always existed, but only recently has it taken on the endlessly colorful and infinitely accessible forms we know today. Legalized gambling opportunities have markedly increased in most industrialized countries and, beyond any doubt, gambling is now a widespread phenomenon. While most people gamble occasionally, some people become addicted to gambling. The accessibility and availability of gambling opportunities are in direct relation to the number of pathological gamblers in a given area. This has created a situation in which more and more people are likely to develop serious gambling problems, for which they will need to seek professional help.

Pathological gambling was officially recognized in 1980 with the publication of the DSM-III (American Psychiatric Association [APA], 1980) and was classified as an impulse control disorder. According to the DSM-IV, problem gambling is characterized by a loss of control over gambling, lies about the extent of involvement with gambling, family and job disruption, stealing money, and chasing losses (e.g., continuing to gamble in order to recuperate money lost while gambling) (APA, 1994). Essentially, gambling takes place when something valuable—usually money—is staked on the outcome of an event that is entirely unpredictable. The pivotal characteristics of gambling are that its outcomes are based on uncertainty, randomness, or chance. But from the gambler's point of view, the primary task of gambling is to use the information available to them to try to predict the outcome of an event that is in reality unpredictable.

SCOPE

Constant changes in gaming legislation have led to a substantial expansion of gambling opportunities in America, Canada, Australia, and Europe. Prevalence studies show that this has led to an increase in gambling rates among adults and, despite legal restrictions, among adolescents as well (National Research Council, 1999). A recent matter for concern has been a rise in the number of individuals identified on surveys as meeting DSM criteria for pathological gambling (APA, 1980, 1994), particularly children and adolescents. Children and adolescents are drawn to games of chance and skill, particularly the computer-based arcade and hand-held game variety; this renders them exceptionally vulnerable to the lure of similar electronic gaming devices such as video-draw poker, keno, and slot machines. The attractiveness of these games can lead young people to develop a dependency on them, and ultimately to develop serious gambling problems (Griffiths, 1995). Yet, despite legislated restrictions, survey data reveal that a majority of adolescents gamble. Although it is possible that such rates have peaked in recent years (Stinchfield, Cassuto, Winters, & Latimer, 1997), recent data nevertheless show that 24–40 percent of adolescents gamble weekly, 10–15 percent appear at-risk, and 2–9 percent meet diagnostic criteria for pathological gambling (Derevensky & Gupta, 2000; Griffiths, 1995; Ladouceur, Dubé, & Bujold, 1994). Furthermore, Shaffer, Hall, and Vander Bilt (1997) conducted a meta-analytic study of 120 North American prevalence studies to calculate a reported lifetime rate of 3.9 percent (95 percent confidence interval 2.33–5.43), and a 12-month rate of 5.8 percent (95 percent confidence interval 3.17–8.37) for adolescent disordered gambling. The estimated median prevalence rate of up to 6 percent for adolescent pathological gambling is generally three to four times greater than the median figure of 1.5 percent reported for adults.

THEORIES

The acquisition of wealth is usually assumed to be the primary motivation for gambling. Ironically, however, all legalized forms of gambling are designed so that the expected return is less than the wagered sum. Thus, if the individual's goal is to acquire wealth, the most rational course of action would be to avoid gambling. The paradox of gambling, however, is that people, in attempting to gain wealth, engage in an activity which is impoverishing by nature. *Cognitive theories* of gambling explain this paradox by assuming that gamblers believe and expect to win regardless of adverse odds.

Studies show that cognitive factors play a key role in the development and maintenance of gambling problems. More specifically, perceiving logical connections between events that are actually random appears to be a core misconception held by gamblers (Ladouceur & Walker, 1996, 1998). Gamblers employ various game strategies based on this misconception, and believe that their strategies and abilities will help them win. Many studies have shown the importance of erroneous perceptions held by individuals while they are gambling. In studies evaluating the perceptions of gamblers, participants were asked to think aloud while playing roulette, slot machines, blackjack, and video poker. Results revealed that over 75 percent of their perceptions were erroneous, and most of them deviated from the notion of randomness. This cognitive misconception plays an important role in the development and maintenance of gambling (see Ladouceur & Walker, 1996, 1998).

An interesting illustration of this phenomenon is Henslin's observational study of gamblers in the casinos of Las Vegas. He described a revealing, if not amusing, characteristic behavior displayed by some gamblers: when "craps" players wished to obtain a high number on the roll of a dice, they threw the dice rapidly and forcefully, while if they desired a low number, they threw them slowly and lightly. In this case, the illusion of control can be seen through the player's attempt to "control" which numbers come up through the use of a specific type and pattern of wrist motion when throwing the dice!

In our psychology laboratories at Laval University, we have verified that both gamblers' erroneous perceptions about randomness, and their illusions of control play a central role in the overall process of gambling. In one experiment, we invited two groups of gamblers to participate in a session of roulette. The two groups were exposed to the same conditions as those found in a casino, with one exception: a first group of "active gamblers" were allocated the responsibility of throwing a roulette ball themselves, while for a second group of "passive gamblers," the experiment's croupier performed this task. In reality, the numbered slot where the ball finally came to rest was left to chance regardless of whether the gambler or the experimental croupier threw the ball. However, the results of the experiment clearly demonstrated that participants who threw the ball themselves placed higher bets and overestimated their chances of winning far more often than did the "passive gamblers" in the second group.

In other studies conducted by our research group, we have found similar evidence of the prevalence of erroneous perceptions and illusions of control among gamblers. For example, when we asked gamblers to generate sequences of "heads and tails," we observed that more than 70–80 percent of the participants relied on the outcome of past events when trying to predict future outcomes. Yet, it is a fact that for each flip of the coin, "heads" or "tails" has, and will always have, a one in two chance of appearing. A detailed analysis indicated that the gamblers' principal error was their desire to have an equal proportion of "heads" and "tails" in a sequence, and their desire to avoid any apparent form of pattern or long sequence of the same event. In this particular study, for example, the participants tended to prefer a selection of "heads" after a run of six or seven "tails."

In summary, the core cognitive errors involved in pathological gambling, illusion of control and the belief that events are predictable, both stem from a misconception of randomness. More specifically, when involved in a gambling situation, most of us seem to forget that all events are independent, and tend to make logical connections between random events in order to increase our probability of winning. This is probably because, as intelligent beings, we like to feel that there is order and logic in the events that happen around us. We feel uncomfortable believing that chance is an accurate and plausible explanation of events. In fact, we tend to rely on the concept of chance only when confronted with unusual, unpredictable, and unexpected events such as coincidences. Thus, it is not surprising that, in general, people are not very good at tasks such as generating random sequences of numbers, because they misunderstand the respective contributions of chance and skill in determining the outcome of events.

If illusion of control and the belief that events are predictable play a key role in the development and maintenance of gambling pathology, then confronting and correcting these erroneous perceptions should reduce or eliminate gambling problems. Targeting these variables is therefore the main focus of the prevention programs that will be discussed in this entry.

RESEARCH

There is little history of empirically validated prevention programs for pathological gambling. Until very recently, only one gambling prevention study had been conducted and published in peer review journal. This study was conducted by Gaboury and Ladouceur (1993) which mostly involved delivering information about gambling in the same way a teacher would. They have conducted the only experimental study on gambling prevention that has been published to date. The prevention program used by these researchers was a universal type of implementation, which was open to all youths regardless of their gambling habits. The prevention program involved supplying the young people with information about gambling in a classroom setting. Some of the themes that were covered during the prevention included information about the gambling industry, the legal aspects of gambling, the potential consequences of gambling activities, and an explanation of automatic gambling-related behaviors and pathological gambling. Results indicated that the experimental group significantly improved in their knowledge about gambling compared to the control group, a difference which was still apparent 6 months after the intervention. In the control group, gambling behaviors and misconceptions showed no significant change.

A recent youth gambling prevention program, created by Ferland, Ladouceur, and Jacques (2000), shared some characteristics with the Gaboury and Ladouceur (1993) program in that it also used a universal mode of transmission. However, the Ferland et al. (2000) study differed in that it used an interactive learning element in addition to the provision of information in a classroom setting. Students were asked to actively participate in the learning process by testing the concepts and ideas they had been taught outside of the classroom. In addition to the theories explained and demonstrated in class, each student received a 20-page manual containing a number of take-home activities whose goal was to allow the students to experience the things they had learned firsthand.

The in-class portion of the prevention program was administered by psychologists specializing in pathological gambling, during three separate sessions. The first session was dedicated to explaining what gambling activities really are, helping the students recognize the pitfalls of gambling, and the common error of failing to understand the random nature of games of chance. The second session was devoted to explaining and putting into practice a six-step problem-solving strategy for resisting social pressure to gamble, while the last session addressed the issue of excessive gambling and its eventual consequences. Results from this study revealed that the intervention significantly improved the students' knowledge and decreased the number of misconceptions they had about gambling activities. Unfortunately, the prevention program did not succeed in improving students' ability to solve problems, even though the students reported that they used the problem-solving strategies that were taught to them. Further analyses will be conducted in order to determine whether this prevention program has effectively reduced gambling activities, and if so, whether this reduction will be sustained at a follow-up assessment. Even if we suppose that Gaboury and Ladouceur's intervention had little immediate impact on gambling behavior, it could be argued that modifying process variables such as erroneous perceptions and information should have a long-term effect, decreasing the young people's motivation to gamble by convincing them that gambling is a truly uncontrollable activity.

A third study was conducted evaluating the effectiveness of the video used in the Ferland et al. (2000) study described above to target the misconceptions and cognitive errors involved in gambling. The video lasted 20 min and had a humorous style. The two main characters were "Lucky," a sarcastic clown who had lost all his money gambling, and his assistant. In the video, these characters were invited to a school to present a show about gambling. Throughout the video, Lucky explained the differences between gambling and games of skill. Lucky also talked about the real odds of winning a game of chance, about illusion of control, randomness, good luck charms, the uselessness of winning strategies, and so on. To evaluate the effectiveness of the video, 423 participants (students in grades 7 and 8) were randomly assigned to four treatment and control conditions. Results indicated that the video was successful in modifying students' knowledge and attitudes toward gambling, as compared to participants in the control group (Ferland & Ladouceur, 2001).

In summary, although few controlled prevention studies have been conducted, results obtained so far clearly demonstrate that erroneous perceptions can be modified and that individuals can be taught to distinguish between gambling and games of skill. Targeting misconceptions toward the notion of randomness which leads to the illusion of control therefore appears to be a key factor in the treatment and prevention of pathological gambling.

STRATEGIES THAT WORK

Only one published program has been tested. It is therefore difficult to say what type of prevention program works.

STRATEGIES THAT MIGHT WORK

Prevention of problem gambling is quite a recent area of research. As previously mentioned, few published papers report the efficacy of gambling prevention programs. This may be because the gambling prevention programs that do exist are carried out on a very small scale, and their effects are not necessarily being recorded, analyzed, and published. Nevertheless, some important efforts have been made by a number of groups who create and implement gambling prevention programs. For example, the North American Training Institute (NATI) is an organization for the training of professionals involved in the field of problem gambling. The NATI has produced at least two important gambling prevention programs, one of which focuses on young people, and the other on an elderly population. In both cases, the NATI has created an intervention guide for professionals who work with these populations. Unfortunately, the NATI, as far as we know, has yet to evaluate the effectiveness of their prevention programs.

In Canada, the Addiction Foundation of Manitoba has created a gambling prevention program especially designed for secondary school students. The program is named "Keep Your Shirt On" and is taught by specialists in the field of addiction. Once again, however, the effectiveness of this prevention program has not been formally assessed. In the province of Quebec, a program called "Count Me Out" was applied to all students in the last 3 years of primary school and in the 5 years of high school. Main components included information about gambling, cognitive misconceptions, problem solving, and peer pressure. Although interesting, no studies evaluating the effectiveness of this program have been published.

Gambling prevention research may be scarce because this issue has yet to capture the interest of university researchers. In fact, as mentioned earlier, many gambling prevention programs are implemented by community groups, groups of ex-gamblers, or government organizations. It may be that pathological gambling has not produced much research interest for the simple reason that it is such a new area of study, and the creation of any prevention program requires a detailed knowledge of the variables involved. However, the few studies that have been conducted so far illustrate the type of active elements that might make up a successful prevention program.

Contributions That Can Be Made by Other Types of Prevention Research

Although the gambling prevention studies previously reviewed describe some promising strategies, it is nonetheless difficult to draw definite conclusions about effectiveness based on such a small body of research. Thus, it is difficult to know which evidence-based strategies really work. However, programs targeting the prevention of drug, alcohol, and tobacco use may, in a more general sense, provide helpful information about designing an effective prevention program for gambling.

For Botvin and Wills (1985), the main goal of a prevention program should be to decrease the individual's motivation to try the substance or perform the target behavior. For these researchers, a prevention program addressing any addiction must aim to teach students how to resist the social pressures that can lead to consumption. In a study published in 1997, Donaldson, Graham, Piccinin, and Hansen observed that prevention programs that address social pressure variables seem to be the most effective ones. Graham, Marks, and Hansen (1991) also emphasized the importance of focusing on social pressure processes when designing a prevention program. According to this group of researchers, prevention programs that target erroneous social perceptions can effectively reduce undesirable consumption behavior. One of the most widespread erroneous perceptions that youths have is that they drastically overestimate the rate at which their peers have engaged in addictive behaviors. Therefore, this inaccurate perception must be addressed in a prevention program if each youth is to normalize his or her own behavior, and realize that they are not an exception in abstaining from the behavior (Johnson, Farquhar, & Sussman, 1996). This view of prevention is consistent with that taken by Vander Pligt (1998), who recommends focusing on proximal variables that are most likely to result in behavior change, rather than on distal variables which are difficult to modify.

Both the Ferland et al. (2000) and Gaboury and Ladouceur (1993) prevention programs were based on the prevention theory reviewed at the beginning of this entry. In fact, both programs target proximal variables such as erroneous perceptions, lack of knowledge, and attitudes, and focus on the normalization of abstinence from gambling behaviors by emphasizing that while many young people have tried gambling, very few actually gamble regularly.

The gambling prevention program used by Ferland et al. (2000) emphasized the importance of teaching young people how to resist various social pressures to gamble. Even if the problem-solving strategies taught to the students did not significantly improve their problem-solving abilities, the students nonetheless reported using the strategies more frequently than before the intervention. Thus, it is possible that the students understood and assimilated the problem-solving strategies and would use them when they were needed, which may have been a week or a year after the intervention. Unfortunately, the study did not assess the students at a later period.

In summary, effective alcohol, drug, and tobacco prevention strategies focus on resistance to social pressure and the correction of erroneous cognitions. By helping youths resist social pressure and correct their erroneous perceptions toward the target behavior or substance, a prevention program should successfully alter behavior. It is important to remember that, as Botvin and Wills (1985) emphasized, a change in behavior necessitates a reduction in the motivation to engage in that behavior. Thus, a successful prevention program is one that can reduce this motivation and thereby decrease the behavior. By targeting these factors in their gambling prevention programs, Gaboury and Ladouceur (1993), Ferland and Ladouceur (2001), and Ferland et al. (2000) successfully modified the proximal variables that motivate young people's gambling behavior.

SYNTHESIS

To date, the three gambling prevention programs reviewed here are based on an empirical evaluation. They all used a universal approach, including students regardless of their gambling habits before the beginning of the program. This means that all the students received the same intervention, whether they were at a high or low risk of developing a gambling problem; this also means that subgroups (i.e., classroom groups who received the intervention) included both at-risk and not at-risk students. Dent, Sussman, Ellickson, Brown, and Richardson (1996) have argued that in addiction prevention, universal prevention programs have had positive effects on at-risk groups of individuals, but these interventions might not be the optimal approach to take with not at-risk groups. For example, young people who have gambled might interpret the prevention program differently from those who have no gambling experience. Therefore, it may be necessary to develop specific prevention programs for different categories of young people. One possibility is that the existing validated universal prevention programs could be implemented in elementary schools, as an introduction to the topic. After this general introduction, prevention programs could be implemented for specific categories of young people, and address their individual needs. The more specific prevention could then place more emphasis on factors like illusion of control, failure to understand randomness which contribute to the development of gambling problems.

Another aspect of prevention to consider is parental involvement. As gambling is a behavior that is learned within a familial context, it would make sense to offer families information about gambling, erroneous perceptions, and so on. Not only are parents in general an important influence in a young person's life, but any prevention is more likely to be effective if the young person receives the same information from the prevention program and from their parents. Hopefully, the combination of these influences will enable the young person to acquire a realistic attitude toward gambling.

Because gambling prevention is such a new topic of research, not only do few studies exist, but the studies that are published mostly focus on positive results, making it difficult to know which prevention strategies are ineffective, or even counter-productive. Once again, however, we can turn to prevention research for other types of problem behaviors to get an idea of what to avoid. According to Johnson et al. (1996), every preventive intervention with youths must include the transmission of realistic information, but caution must be exercised in the way this information is put across. Research has shown that using a fear-inspiring approach, scare tactics, or dissuasion emphasizing negative effects have limited results (Botvin & Wills, 1985; Hansen, 1992), can be ineffective (Donaldson et al., 1997; Tobler, 1992), or can even have negative effects such as increasing the target behavior one hoped to reduce (Vander Pligt, 1998). Additional research shows that prevention programs based solely on the transmission of information produce few positive effects (Botvin, Baker, Renick, Filazzola, & Botvin, 1984; Botvin & Wills, 1985; Donaldson et al., 1997; Tobler, 1992; Vander Pligt, 1998). It also appears that increasing knowledge about the legal and medical consequences of use has virtually no impact on the target behavior, or the motivation to engage in it (Botvin et al., 1984).

Given these findings from prevention research in other areas, it appears that a prevention should not only increase the young person's knowledge of the negative consequences of the target behavior, but should improve their overall understanding of the problem. For example, a gambling prevention program for young people should focus on the real probabilities of winning, the independence of events in the game, the ineffectiveness of lucky charms, and the illusion of control, rather than on the eventual drawbacks of gambling, such as becoming a pathological gambler at 50 and losing one's house or car.

Also see: Gambling: Adulthood.

References

American Psychiatric Association. (1980). *Diagnostic and statistical manual of mental disorders* (3rd ed.). Washington, DC: Author.

American Psychiatric Association. (1994). *Diagnostic and statistical manual of mental disorders* (4th ed.). Washington, DC: Author.

Botvin, G.J., Baker, E., Renick, N.L., Filazzola, A.D., & Botvin, E.M. (1984). A cognitive–behavioral approach to substance abuse prevention, *Addictive Behavior, 9*, 137–147.

Botvin, G., & Wills, J. (1985). Personal and social skill training: Cognitive–behavioral approaches to substance abuse prevention, *National Institutes of Drug Abuse Monographs, 63*, 8–49.

Dent, C.W., Sussman, S., Ellickson, P., Brown, P., & Richardson, J.L. (1996). Is current drug abuse prevention programming generalizable across ethnic groups? *American Behavioral Scientist, 39*, 911–918.

Derevensky, J.L., & Gupta, R. (2000). Prevalence estimates of adolescent gambling: A comparison of the SOGS-RA, DSM-IV-J, and the GA 20 questions. *Journal of Gambling Studies, 16*, 227–252.

Donaldson, S.I., Graham, J.W., Piccinin, A.M., & Hansen, W.B. (1997). Resistance-skills training and onset of alcohol use: Evidence for beneficial and potentially harmful effects in public schools and private catholic schools. In G.A. Marlatt & G.R. Vanden Bos (Eds.), *Addictive behaviors: Readings on etiology, prevention, and treatment* (pp. 215–238). Washington, DC: American Psychological Association.

Ferland, F., & Ladouceur, R. (2001). *Prevention of problem gambling: Modifying misconceptions and increasing knowledge*, Submitted to the Journal of Counseling and Clinical Psychology.

Ferland, F., Ladouceur, R., & Jacques, C. (2000, June). *Evaluation of a gambling prevention program for youths*. 11th International Conference on Gambling and Risk-Taking, Las Vegas, Nevada, USA.

Gaboury, A., & Ladouceur, R. (1993). Evaluation of a preventing program for pathological gambling among adolescents, *The Journal of Primary Prevention, 14*(1), 21–28.

Graham, J.W., Marks, G., & Hansen, W.B. (1991). Social influence processes affecting adolescent substance use, *Journal of Applied Psychology, 76*(2), 291–298.

Griffiths, M. (1995). *Adolescent gambling*. Routledge: London.

Hansen, W.B. (1992). School-based substance abuse prevention: A review of the state of the art in curriculum, 1980–1990. *Health Education Research, 7*(3), 403–430.

Johnson, C.A., Farquhar, J.W., & Sussman, S. (1996). Methodological and substantive issues in substance abuse prevention research: An integration, *American Behavioral Scientist, 39*(7), 935–942.

Ladouceur, R., Dubé, D., & Bujold, A. (1994). Gambling among primary school students. *Journal of Gambling Studies, 10*, 363–370.

Ladouceur, R., & Walker, M. (1996). Cognitive perspective on gambling. In P.M. Salkovskis (Ed.), *Trends in cognitive therapy* (pp. 89–120). Oxford: Wiley.

Ladouceur, R., & Walker, M. (1998). The cognitive approach to understanding and treating pathological gambling. In A.S. Bellack & M. Hersen (Eds.), *Comprehensive clinical psychology*. New York: Pergamon.

National Research Council. (1999). *Pathological gambling: A critical review*. Washington, DC: National Academy Press.

Shaffer, H.J., Hall, M.N., & Vander Bilt, J. (1997). *Estimating the prevalence of disordered gambling behavior in the United States and Canada: A meta-analysis*. Published by the Harvard Medical School: Division on Addictions, 122 pp.

Stinchfield, R., Cassuto, N., Winters, K., & Latimer, W. (1997). Prevalence of gambling among Minnesota public school students in 1992 and 1995. *Journal of Gambling Studies, 13*, 25–48.

Tobler, N.S. (1992). Drug prevention programs can work: Research findings, *Journal of Addictive Diseases, 11*(3), 1–28.

Vander Pligt, J. (1998). Perceived risk and vulnerability as predictors of precautionary behavior, *British Journal of Health Psychology, 3*, 1–14.

Gambling, Adulthood[*]

Anne-Marie Cantwell and Gerald R. Adams

INTRODUCTION

Given time and place, gambling has been considered a form of entertainment, of deviant or sinful behavior, and often considered both simultaneously. Presently across North America, gambling is widely accepted as a recreational activity. In large part this is due to the financial link that exits between legal gambling and government, which heavily taxes this enterprise (Stebbins, 1996). Gambling takes many forms such as lotteries, slots, gaming tables, and sports betting. The majority of adults (greater than 80 percent) indicate having participated in recreational gambling activities at some time (National Research Council, 1999). Of this number, only a small percentage have been identified as "problem" or "pathological" gamblers. It is only recently that the problems associated with gambling (debt, family suffering, etc.) have received public and scientific attention (Hollander, Buchalter, & DeCaria, 2000). These gambling related problems have "taken the front stage in the continuing debate over legalized gambling" (Lesieur, 1998) and led Petry and Armentano (1999) to describe gambling as the addiction of the 1990s.

DEFINITIONS

According to Devereux (1979), *gambling* involves the wagering of money or other personal belongings on activities or events of chance that involve random or uncertain outcomes. Gambling is an act whereby a person pursues monetary gain without the use of his or her skills (Brenner & Brenner, 1990). Pathological gambling was recognized as a psychiatric disorder in 1980 and listed in the *Diagnostic and Statistical Manual of Psychiatric Disorders* as an impulse control disorder not classified elsewhere (American Psychiatric Association, 1980). The criteria for diagnosis was similar to alcohol or drug dependence (Rosenthal, 1986). The majority of scholars now agree that pathological gambling may be conceptualized as a combination of factors including, psychological, biological, and social factors (Shaffer & Gambino, 1989). The terms problem, pathological, and compulsive are used to describe the problems associated with gambling.

The term *problem gambler* has been used in two ways: (1) to indicate those with less serious gambling problems than those who have been identified as pathological gamblers, and (2) as an all-encompassing term including all levels of gambling problems, both problem gamblers and pathological gamblers (Lesieur, 1998). According to Lesieur and Rosenthal (1991), *problem gambling* is a comprehensive term used to describe gambling behaviors that compromise, disrupt, or damage the individual, his/her relationship, or career. *Pathological gambling*, as defined by Rosenthal (1992), is "a progressive disorder characterized by a continuous or periodic loss of control over gambling; a preoccupation with gambling and with obtaining money with which to gamble; irrational thinking; and a continuation of the behavior despite adverse consequences" (p. 73). The term *compulsive*

[*] This paper was partially supported by a grant from the Ontario Problem Gambling Research Centre (OPGRC). Any ideas presented here are not representative of the OPGRC; but are the sole expression of the authors.

gambler is a lay term used by the general public to signify problem or pathological gambling (Lesieur, 1998).

SCOPE

Continued growth in the gambling industry increases public concern regarding the increase of problem and pathological gambling. Pathological gambling creates difficulties for afflicted individuals, their families, employers, and the wider society (Ladouceur, Sylvain, Letarte, Giroux, & Jacques, 1998). According to Politzer, Yesalis, and Hudak (1992), there are as many as 10–17 people around the gambler who are affected negatively. In Canada, the expansion of gambling institutions have routinely been made without public debate. Expansions are implemented without seeking voter approval because citizens usually reject new gambling proposals. The expansion of gaming activities in Canada has led to the formation of grass roots groups like Citizens Against Gambling Expansion in British Columbia (Smith, 1997) and the Ontario Coalition Against Gambling.

Comparing and interpreting prevalence findings can be problematic. Often studies use different screening and diagnostic instruments or varying criterion levels to measure levels of gambling problems (National Research Council, 1999). Evidence supports a logic model—with a rise in the availability of gambling opportunities, there is a parallel increase in the rates of problem and pathological gambling. Many of the prevalence studies have been conducted to determine the extent of this increase in gambling problems as well as associated individual and societal costs. For example, Canada, the United States, and Australia use prevalence surveys as part of an effort to monitor gaming initiatives. Prevalence surveys enable governments to make informed decisions regarding education, prevention, and treatment strategies (Volberg, Dickerson, Ladouceur, & Abbott, 1996).

In each of these countries, the motivating force encouraging research is the expansion of gaming opportunities, particularly casinos and lotteries. In Australia, more than 80 percent of people gamble at least once a year with between 0.25 and 1.73 percent of those scoring in the pathological gambling range (Dickerson & Hinchy, 1988). In the United States, there have been prevalence studies conducted in several states. Volberg (1993, 1996) has reported between 86 and 91 percent of people indicated that they have gambled at some point in their lives. In 17 states where studies have been undertaken, the rate of pathological gambling was between 1.7 and 7.3 percent. Canada has reported similar results with 67 percent of respondents in Ontario and 97 percent of respondents in British Columbia indicating that they have gambled in their lifetimes (National Council of Welfare, 1996). The higher rates in British Columbia and other western provinces, such as Alberta (93 percent) may reflect the fact that legalized gambling has a longer history here than in other regions of the country. Problem and pathological gambling rates for Canada were reported to be between 1.9–4.0 and 0.8–1.9 percent respectively (National Council of Welfare, 1996).

Age Differences in Gambling Behavior

The relationship between gambling and age has received little attention in the social sciences (Mok & Hraba, 1993). However with the increasing aging of the population, research in this area is required. In their review, Mok and Hraba (1993) maintain that chronological age was negatively correlated with gambling behavior, and age differences resulted in different types of gambling activity. For example, middle-aged adults (35–64) participate in gambling opportunities that are more likely to bring greater financial rewards and risks. On the other hand, older adults, are more likely to participate in games that are less competitive and provide an environment conducive to developing and maintaining social relationships (such as bingo) (Mok & Hraba, 1993).

For Mok and Hraba (1993) older adults appear to be less likely to gamble because they have less need to experiment for self-identity and to take risks for financial success. From this perspective, we would expect a linear decline in gambling behavior because older adults have more stable and positive concepts (McPherson, 1983) and therefore would be less likely to turn to gambling for self-presentation. In addition to conceptions regarding stability in self-identity among older adults, it is also important to consider cohort effects when exploring gambling behavior.

Cohorts are groups of people born within time periods of 5–10 years. Cohort effects refer to the influence of specific historical occurrences on different age groups (Riley, 1988). For example, an older cohort socialized during the Great Depression might frown on gambling because of lessons learned that stressed the need for frugality. In contrast, a cohort born during prosperous times might have a far different attitude toward activities of chance. As Mok and Hraba note, understanding age differences in relation to gambling participation can provide guidance for policies regarding gambling.

THEORIES AND RESEARCH

Shaffer and Gambino (1989) suggest there are several limitations in published gambling research. In particular, they recognize the absence of an accepted research paradigm and a lack of integration among research, theory, and practice. Since this criticism, there has been some correction of these limitations in research using the medical model and subsequent treatment (Ferris, Wynne, & Single, 1999). Although the medical model has been identified as the prevailing model in gambling research, there are competing models evident in the literature. Taber (1987) suggested that it is necessary to consider the perspectives of a variety of models because gambling is such a complex behavior.

The Medical Model

According to Ferris et al. (1999), the medical model of gambling is "the dominant one in North America at the moment" (p. 9). Within the parameters of this model, pathological gambling is identified as a disease that needs to be diagnosed and treated. From this perspective, pathological gambling is seen as either present or absent; pathological gamblers are viewed as unable to control their impulses for gaming. This qualitative difference is seen as central to the model and is often identified as some physiological factor that predisposes the individual to pathological gambling (Jacobs, 1986). Blume (1987) has differentiated the disease of pathological gambling from other gaming behavior by stating it must represent a characteristic pattern for the individual that is outside the individual's control, and is continually harmful to the individual and/or others.

While pathological gambling is believed by some to be a neurosis or psychiatric disturbance (Bergler, 1958; Moran, 1993), this view is debatable (Blume, 1994). However, there is evidence suggesting that there are parallels between pathological gambling and alcohol/drug dependence. Indeed, it is common to observe pathological gambling and chemical dependence (47–52 percent) in the same individuals (Briggs, Goodin, & Nelson, 1996; Lesieur, 2000).

In addition to the evidence of comorbidity between pathological gambling and alcohol/drug dependence, it has been suggested that there is a correlation between gambling problems and affective disorders. Blaszczynski and McConaghy (1988) found that the mean depression score of pathological gamblers was significantly higher than that of a psychiatric outpatient sample. They also reported that the pathological gamblers in their study exhibited significantly higher psychopathology than the control group. These results support a view that negative emotional states play a central role in pathological gambling.

Biological Theories

These theories view pathological gambling as the result of an interaction between a physiological pre-disposition and the environment that results in dysfunctional gambling behavior (Ferris et al., 1999). According to Blume (1987),

addictive behaviors tend to run in families. Given such family links, a genetic tendency towards addictions may be present for pathological gambling. Early evidence suggests that the biological determinants will be more important for those with a history of family addictions (Jacobs, 1987).

Within the biological school of thought, three primary models have emerged: (1) models based on EEG waves (Carlton & Goldstein, 1987; Goldstein, Manowitz, Nora, Swartsberg, & Carlton, 1985); (2) models that look at plasma endorphin levels (arousal) (Blaszczynski, Winter, & McConaghy, 1986) and (3) models which focus on other chemical imbalances in the brain (Roy, Adinoff, Roehrich, & Lamparski, 1988; Roy et al., 1988). According to Ferris et al. (1999), these three divisions are still appropriate considering the research that has occurred since that literature review.

The studies that looked at EEG waves found that the patterns in the pathological gamblers more closely resembled patterns displayed by children with attention deficit hyperactivity disorder (ADHD) than those of controls (Carlton & Goldstein, 1987; Carlton & Manowitz, 1994; Goldstein et al., 1985). In addition to the brain wave patterns observed, pathological gamblers were more likely than controls to report childhood behaviors that were indicative of attention deficits (Carlton, Manowitz, McBride, Nopra, Swartzberg, & Goldstein, 1987). Such findings offer further evidence for possible comorbidity between pathological gambling and other disorders.

When examining arousal, researchers have generally conducted laboratory experiments and then attempted to validate findings through naturalistic studies (Anderson & Brown, 1984). While some have measured arousal levels by plasma endorphins (Blaszczynski et al., 1986), others have assessed an increase in heart rate (Anderson & Brown, 1984; Leary & Dickerson, 1985). Findings indicate that gamblers who are more aroused continue playing for longer periods of time (Dickerson & Adcock, 1987). It is important to note that although there is some evidence of increased endorphin levels in gamblers, the research to date remains inconclusive (Lesieur & Rosenthal, 1991). Further, Anderson and Brown indicate that although elevated heart rates are not found in the laboratory setting, there is evidence of an increase in heart rates during a gambling experience. These findings suggest that caution should be applied when making recommendations based on the biological perspective until further work suggests otherwise.

Other work by Roy and colleagues (1988) falls into a psychobiological framework. In this research investigators measured levels of norepinephrine, monoamine metabolites, and peptides in cerebrospinal fluid, plasma, and urine. The findings indicate that pathological gamblers have higher levels of 3-methoxy-4-hydrophenylglycol and norepinephrine, suggesting that they may be suffering from an abnormality in their noradrengic system. Increased activity in this system has been linked to sensation-seeking that underlies risk-taking behavior including pathological gambling.

Psychological Theories

Psychological perspectives of pathological gambling can be found in psychodynamic theory, personality theory, and cognitive social learning theory (behavioral). Researchers working within a psychodynamic (or psycho-analytic) framework view the problems associated with gambling as within the individual's psyche that is beyond the voluntary control of the individual (Lesieur & Rosenthal, 1991; Rosenthal, 1992). According to Ferris et al. (1999), "pathological gambling occurs in response to some trigger, often an event which causes psychic pain" (p. 14). Pathological gambling is seen as an attempt to escape or self-medicate in order to avoid pain (Anderson & Brown, 1984; Jacobs, 1986).

There have been attempts to link various traits/characteristics to pathological gambling. The most common link identified in the literature is between pathological gambling and depression (Blaszczynski & McConaghy, 1988; McCormick, Russo, Ramirez, & Taber, 1984). In addition to depression, other traits include impulsivity (Blaszczynski, Steel, & McConaghy, 1997; Castellani & Rugle, 1995), low self-esteem (Rosenthal, 1993), anxiety (Blaszczynski et al., 1997), and antisocial personality or behaviors (Blaszczynski, McConaghy, & Frankova, 1989; Rosenthal, 1993). The direction of causality remains unknown. It is difficult to determine whether the trait is a cause of pathological gambling or if it is a result of gambling (Blaszczynski & McConaghy, 1988).

From a *social learning perspective*, gambling is viewed as a behavior that has been learned through imitation from a parent, other adult or peers in the child's life (Ferris et al., 1999). The amount of gambling participation is determined by opportunities available in the surrounding environment. Gambling is seen to fall on a continuum from problem-free to problem-dominated where an individual's movement along this continuum is dynamic depending on various factors including available opportunities (Brown, 1987). The distinguishing feature that identifies those who support a social learning theory is the belief that because the behavior is learned, it can also be unlearned (Lesieur & Rosenthal, 1991).

Sociological Theories

Rather than focus on those in treatment, researchers employing a sociological framework examine gamblers in varying settings and different types of gambling activities (Lesieur & Rosenthal, 1991). A primary focal point from this perspective is that of social worlds (Mok & Hraba, 1993). It has been suggested that the social rewards gained from involvement in gambling may outweigh the costs in the minds of pathological gamblers. The social rewards may include a desire to belong to a group of like-minded peers, as well as a desire to adopt their language and identity (Ashley, 1990). One often cited criticism in relation to the sociological perspective is the lack of a clinical focus (Lesieur & Rosenthal, 1991).

STRATEGIES THAT WORK

There is no available research information on the prevention of gambling in adults. The few efforts that have been undertaken in gambling prevention focuses on youth (Derevensky & Gupta, 2000; Griffiths, 1995; Gupta & Derevensky, 1997).

STRATEGIES THAT MIGHT WORK

Recognizing that our efforts are directed at minimizing the harmful effects of this *legal* behavior, we believe several activities deserve testing. Using our previous review of the literature which suggested similarities between pathological gambling and alcohol/drug addiction, these activities draw upon prevention's technology that has been successfully applied to the prevention of substance abuse. While we will address each prevention tool separately, it must be remembered that alone any one of these prevention strategies is not as powerful as when they are combined.

Natural Caregiving

Support groups might be useful in the prevention of gambling with adults where people at risk for problematic behavior provide support for others in similar circumstances to avoid the behavior. Whether social support alone at this early recognition of the problems that gambling may pose is a possible preventive measure remains to be tested. However, evidence from attempts to treat pathological gambling raises concerns.

Gamblers Anonymous (GA) is the most popular intervention for problem and pathological gambling (Lesieur, 1998); unfortunately, it does not appear to be as effective as it is popular (Petry & Armentano, 1999). GA is based on the principles of Alcoholics Anonymous employing a 12-step program based on the abstinence-disease model. The belief that pathological gambling is a disease means that it cannot be cured and as a result abstinence is the only means of coping with it. Typically a crisis precipitates entry into GA (Hollander et al., 2000; Livingston, 1974).

Although many gamblers adopt the principles set forth by GA upon entering the group, relapse rates are high with 70 to 90 percent dropping out (Brown, 1985, as cited in Petry & Armentano, 1999). Further, in a study of 232 gamblers attending GA, Stewart and Brown (1988) report that only 8 percent of GA attendees report total abstinence after 1 year, and fewer still (7 percent) after 2 years.

Would support from others prevent the pathological gambler from engaging in this dysfunctional behavior? While the GA continued participation rate is extremely modest so too are its operational costs. Thus, experiments in natural caregiving combined with other technologies might prove worthy of implementation from a cost/benefit perspective.

Education

Education increases awareness and knowledge; occasionally it affects attitudes; rarely does it alone change behavior. Still, workplace and community educational interventions using public service announcements, incorporating information into employee assistance program workplace presentations, and elsewhere could bring significant added value. These educational messages could focus on the outcomes of problem gambling ensuring that people understand the full meaning of gambling. Further, they could alert people to the warning signs of problem gambling, thus engaging natural caregivers like family members and friends to exercise their influence (to the extent that is possible) at a point before the gambling behavior becomes unmanageable.

Further, it appears that pathological gamblers have irrational beliefs about gambling and that they live with the illusion that they can "control the uncontrollable" (Rosenthal, 1993, p. 143). As a result of these illogical thoughts, one promising approach uses cognitive behavioral techniques to counteract these underlying beliefs or attitudes (Ladouceur et al., 1998). These self-managing educational strategies involve educating gamblers about the principles of probability and randomness in an effort to correct their misguided thinking (National Research Council, 1999).

Systems Intervention

The prevention technology of systems intervention is built upon the premise that our society and its institutions (in this example gambling establishments) contribute to the dysfunction behavior of its members. To have a healthier society means changing those practices that encourage illness. Again, drawing from the field of addiction studies, the concept of harm reduction (Daugherty & Leukefeld, 1998) offers several intriguing possibilities. For example, the following might be tried: limiting the operating hours of gambling establishments, limiting the daily amount of money that could be spent on this activity, and prohibiting the use of credit cards or issuing loans within gambling establishments to patrons. Imagine a smoke free casino where posters caution people about excessive wagering and at regular intervals the public address system airs a warning message not to gamble excessively. Further, we suspect that if laws were changed to prevent gambling institutions from collecting on loans to patrons (and thus preventing their bankruptcy) that the industry exercising self-interested behavior might very well reduce the incidence of pathological gambling behavior by still other methods.

Competency Promotion

To belong, to be valued, to contribute meaningfully to your community define competency. Competent people have a positive self-esteem, a positive self-concept of ability, and an internal locus of control. They can explain "meaning" in their life. The literature reviewed earlier suggests that many of these elements are lacking from the lives of pathological gamblers. From a prevention perspective, efforts should have been undertaken much earlier. Nevertheless, meaning can still be realised and lives changed by the power of a single caring person or group of people through natural caregiving.

STRATEGIES THAT DO NOT WORK

Given the paucity of work undertaken in this area, we are not able to identify strategies that do not work. That said, from the substance abuse prevention literature we can infer that didatic education only approaches are ill-advised.

SYNTHESIS

Gambling is a widespread and expanding industry. For a minority it is addictive and results in a host of problems for the individual, family and friends, and society. As noted earlier, it is challenging to determine which combination of strategies might be effective in preventing gambling problems. We believe that a harm reduction approach offers promise. To the system intervention examples offered earlier other possibilities include limiting the time spent at tables/slot machines, installing clocks and large windows in casinos, and reducing the availability of alcohol and food on the floor thus requiring individuals to take a break from their gaming activity.

It is vital that research be conducted to examine the issue of comorbidity. This is crucial if gambling problems are to be reduced. The concept of "switching addictions" suggests that we need to look beyond the gambling problem and understand the underlying features that are outwardly displayed as addictive and impulse control disorders (Blume, 1994).

By understanding the experience of the individual we can begin to make recommendations based on empirical evidence for prevention. Through the use of effective education and other prevention strategies, we may reduce the costs associated with problem and pathological gambling for both the individual and society.

Also see: Gambling: Adolescence.

References

American Psychiatric Association (APA). (1980). *Diagnostic and statistical manual of psychiatric disorders*. Washington, DC: Author.

Anderson, G., & Brown, R.I. (1984). Real and laboratory gambling, sensation seeking and arousal. *British Journal of Psychology, 75*, 401–410.

Ashley, L.R. (1990). "The words of my mouth and the meditation of my heart": The mindset of gamblers revealed in their language. *Journal of Gambling Studies, 6*, 241–261.

Bergler, E. (1958). *The psychology of gambling*. New York: International Universities Press.

Blaszczynski, A.P., & McConaghy, N. (1988). SCL-90 assessed psychopathology in pathological gamblers. *Psychological Reports, 62*, 547–552.

Blaszczynski, A.P., McConaghy, N., & Frankova, A. (1989). Crime, antisocial personality and pathological gambling. *Journal of Gambling Behavior, 5*, 137–152.

Blaszczynski, A.P., Steel, Z.P., & McConaghy, N. (1997). Implusivity in pathological gambling: The antisocial impulsivist. *Addiction, 92*, 75–87.

Blaszczynski, A.P., Winter, S.S., & McConaghy, N. (1986). Sensation seeking and pathological gambling. *Journal of Gambling Behavior, 2*, 3–14.

Blume, S.B. (1987). Compulsive gambling and the medical model. *Journal of Gambling Behavior, 3*, 237–247.

Blume, S.B. (1994). Pathological gambling and switching addictions: Report of a case. *Journal of Gambling Studies, 10*, 87–96.

Brenner, R., & Brenner, R.A. (1990). *Gambling and speculation: A theory, a history, and a future of some human decisions*. New York: Cambridge University Press.

Briggs, J.R., Goodin, B.J., & Nelson, T. (1996). Pathological gamblers and alcoholics: Do they share the same addiction? *Addictive Behaviors, 21*, 515–519.

Brown, R.I.F. (1987). Classical and operant paradigms in the management of gambling addictions. *Behavioural Psychotherapy, 15*, 111–122.

Carlton, P.L., & Goldstein, L. (1987). Physiological determinants of pathological gambling. In T. Galski (Ed.), *The handbook of pathological gambling* (pp. 111–122). Springfield, IL: Charles C. Thomas.

Carlton, P.L., & Manowitz, P. (1994). Factors determining the severity of pathological gambling in males. *Journal of Gambling Studies, 10*, 147–158.

Carlton, P.L., Manowitz, P., McBride, H., Nopra, R., Swartzberg, M., & Goldstein, L. (1987). Attention deficit disorder and pathological gambling. *Journal of Clinical Psychiatry, 48*, 487–488.

Castellani, B., & Rugle, L. (1995). A comparison of pathological gamblers to alcoholics and cocaine misusers on impulsivity, sensation seeking and craving. *International Journal of the Addictions, 30*, 275–289.

Daugherty, R.P., & Leukefeld, C. (1998). *Reducing the risks for substance abuse: A lifespan approach*. New York and London: Plenum.

Derevensky, J., & Gupta, R. (2000). Youth gambling: A clinical and research perspective. *e-Gambling: The Electronic Journal of Gambling, 2*, 1–10.

Devereux, E.C. (1979). Gambling. In *The international encyclopedia of the social sciences* (Vol. 17). New York: Macmillan.

Dickerson, M., & Adcock, S. (1987). Mood, arousals and cognitions in persistent gambling: Preliminary investigation of a theoretical model. *Journal of Gambling Behavior, 3*, 3–15.

Dickerson, M., & Hinchy, J. (1988). The prevalence of excessive and pathological gambling in Australia. *Journal of Gambling Behavior, 4*, 135–151.

Ferris, J., Wynne, H., & Single, E. (1999). *Measuring problem gambling in Canada final report: Phase I*. Canadian Centre on Substance Abuse, Ontario, Canada.

Goldstein, L., Manowitz, P., Nora, R., Swartzberg, M., & Carlton, P. (1985). Differential EEG activation and pathological gambling. *Biological Psychiatry, 20*, 1232–1234.

Griffiths, M. (1995). *Adolescent gambling*. London: Routledge.

Gupta, R., & Derevensky (1997). Familial and social influences on juvenile gambling. *Journal of Gambling Studies, 13*, 179–192.

Hollander, E., Buchalter, A.J., & DeCaria, C.M. (2000). Pathological gambling. In E. Hollander & A. Allen (Eds.), *The Psychiatric Clinics of North America, 23*, 629–642.

Jacobs, D.F. (1986). A general theory of addictions: A new theoretical mode. *Journal of Gambling Behavior, 2*, 15–31.

Jacobs, D.F. (1987). A general theory of addictions: Application to treatment and rehabilitation planning for pathological gamblers. In T. Galski (Ed.), *The handbook of pathological gambling* (pp. 169–194). Springfield, IL: Charles C. Thomas.

Ladouceur, R., Sylvain, C., Letarte, H., Giroux, I., & Jacques, C. (1998). Cognitive treatment of pathological gamblers. *Behaviour Research and Therapy, 36*, 1111–1119.

Leary, K., & Dickerson, M. (1985). Levels of arousal in high- and low-frequency gamblers. *Behaviour Research and Therapy, 23*, 635–640.

Lesieur, H.R. (1998). Costs and treatment of pathological gambling. *Annals of the American Academy of Political and Social Science, 556*, 153–171.

Lesieur, H.R. (2000). Commentary: Types, lotteries, and substance abuse among problem gamblers. *Journal of the American Academy of Psychiatry and the Law, 28*, 404–407.

Lesieur, H.R., & Rosenthal, R. (1991). Pathological gambling: A review of the literature. *Journal of Gambling Studies, 7*, 5–40.

Livingston, J. (1974). *Compulsive gamblers: Observations on action and abstinence*. New York: Harper Touchbooks.

McCormick, R.A., Russo, A.M., Ramirez, L.F., & Taber, J.I. (1984). Affective disorders among pathological gamblers seeking treatment. *American Journal of Psychiatry, 141*, 215–218.

McPherson, B.D. (1983). *Aging as a social process: An introduction to individual and population aging*. Toronto, ON: Butterworth.

Mok, W.P., & Hraba, J. (1993). Age and gambling behavior: A declining and shifting pattern of participation. In W.R. Eadington & J.A. Cornelius (Eds.), *Gambling behavior and problem gambling* (pp. 51–74). Reno, NV: University of Nevada.

Moran, E. (1993). The growing presence of pathological gambling in society: What we know now. In W.R. Eadington & J.A. Cornelius (Eds.), *Gambling behavior and problem gambling* (pp. 135–142). Reno, NV: University of Nevada.

National Council of Welfare (1996). *A guide to the proposed seniors benefit: A report*. Ottawa, ON: The Council.

National Research Council (1999). *Pathological gambling: A critical review*. Washington, DC: National Academy Press.

Petry, N.M., & Armentano, C. (1999). Prevalence, assessment, and treatment of pathological gambling: A review. *Psychiatric Services, 50,* 1021–1027.

Politzer, R., Yesalis, C., & Hudak, C., Jr. (1992). The epidemiologic model and the risks of legal gambling: Where are we headed? *Health Values, 16*(2), 20–27.

Riley, M.W. (1988). On the significance of age in sociology. In M.W. Riley (Ed.), *Social change and the life course* (Vol. 1). Newbury Park, CA: Sage.

Rosenthal, R. (1986). The pathological gambler's system for self-deception. *Journal of Gambling Behavior, 2,* 108–120.

Rosenthal, R. (1992). Pathological gambling. *Psychiatric Annals, 22*(2), 72–78.

Rosenthal, R.J. (1993). Some causes of pathological gambling. In W.R. Eadington & J.A. Cornelius (Eds.), *Gambling behavior and problem gambling* (pp. 143–148). Reno, NV: University of Nevada.

Roy, A., Adinoff, B., Roehrich, L., & Lamparski, D. (1988). Pathological gambling: A psychobiological study. *Archives of General Psychiatry, 45,* 369–373.

Roy, A., Adinoff, B., Roehrich, L., Lamparski, D., Custer, R., Lorenz, V., Barbaccia, M., Guidotti, A., Costa, E., & Linnoila, M. (1988). Extraversion in pathological gamblers. *Archives of General Psychiatry, 46,* 679–681.

Shaffer, H.J., & Gambino, B. (1989). The epistemology of "addictive disease": Gambling as a predicament. *Journal of Gambling Behavior, 5,* 211–229.

Smith, G. (1997). *Gambling and the public interest?* Calgary, AB: Canada West Foundation.

Stebbins, R. (1996). *Tolerable differences: Living with deviance.* Toronto, ON: McGraw-Hill Ryerson.

Stewart, R.M., & Brown, R.I.F. (1988). An outcome study of Gamblers Anonymous. *British Journal of Psychiatry, 152,* 284–288.

Taber, J.I. (1987). Compulsive gambling: An examination of relevant models. *Journal of Gambling Behavior, 3,* 219–223.

Volberg, R.A. (1993). Estimating the prevalence of pathological gambling in the United States. In W.R. Eadington & J.A. Cornelius (Eds.), *Gambling behavior and problem gambling* (pp. 365–378). Reno, NV: University of Nevada.

Volberg, R.A. (1996). Prevalence studies of problem gambling in the United States. *Journal of Gambling Studies, 12,* 111–128.

Volberg R.A., Dickerson, M.G., Ladouceur, R., & Abbott, M.W. (1996). Prevalence studies and the development of services for problem gamblers and their families. *Journal of Gambling Studies, 12,* 215–231.

Grief, Older Adulthood

Robert O. Hansson and
Margaret S. Stroebe

INTRODUCTION

Bereavement, particularly spousal bereavement, can be an especially disruptive experience in old age because it occurs in the context of age-related changes in health, abilities, and available support and coping resources. These issues may complicate the grief experience and undermine one's ability to continue to cope. In addition, the emotional impact of loss may interact with or exacerbate any pre-existing health or psychological problems with which an older person may be dealing. Strategies to promote normal grieving and to prevent complicated grief among older persons should be based on an understanding of the broader nature of age-related risks and potentially adaptive processes.

DEFINITIONS

Bereavement is the situation of having recently lost a loved one to death.

Normal Grief (or Grief) is the emotional response to the death of a loved one. Grief reactions involve psychological and physical distress, and the disruption of social and behavioral functioning. This is a normal response to the loss of an attachment figure, rather than a disorder, and with time, most bereaved persons are able to adapt.

Complicated Grief is a deviation from the normative grief experience, involving an absence of usual symptoms, delayed onset of symptoms, or a chronic and more intense emotional experience.

Mourning is the social expression of grief, actions, and grief rituals that reflect one's culture or social group.

SCOPE

Only a small proportion of bereaved persons in any age group suffers complicated grief. Nevertheless, bereavement is associated with distress and suffering for the majority of affected persons, and is a particular concern among the elderly, given their frailty, a likelihood of smaller support networks, increased isolation and loneliness, and experience of multiple losses. Among older persons, baseline levels of physical health and adaptive capacity are lower, and can be exacerbated by the stress associated with bereavement. This can, in turn, threaten their ability to live and function independently.

Incidence

Formal statistics are not compiled for complicated bereavement. However, field studies suggest that perhaps 25–45 percent of bereaved persons experience mild levels of depressive symptoms, and that 10–20 percent may exhibit clinically significant levels. Approximately 20 percent of bereaved persons may meet the criteria for complicated grief. Recently bereaved persons are also estimated to be at approximately 40 percent increased risk for new physical health problems, use of medical services, and prescribed medication (Gallagher-Thompson, Futterman, Farberow, Thompson, & Peterson, 1993).

Prevalence

Among the elderly, spousal bereavement is most frequent and most studied. Approximately 45 percent of women and 15 percent of men aged 65 and over in the United States are widowed.

Costs to Society

Bereavement is a life-stressor with mental and physical health consequences that may require intervention and care from family or formal sources. However, older adults exhibit a variety of health, economic, and social risk factors that make them even more likely to become dependent on others for basic needs in daily life or to require formal long-term care. For example, 36 percent of persons aged 65+ are limited by chronic health conditions, and 52 percent have at least one disability. Such factors, then, have resulted in large numbers of elderly persons needing assistance with the basic activities of daily living (e.g., washing, cooking, hygiene), and in the United States, over 50 percent of public health care expenditures tend to be devoted to elderly persons (American Association of Retired Persons, 1999). Insofar as conjugal bereavement entails the loss of a significant, supportive other, there is likely to be an increase in the need for family and formal support.

THEORIES AND RESEARCH

Grief reactions may involve a diversity of cognitive symptoms (e.g., preoccupation with the deceased, helplessness, diminished concentration); affective responses (sadness, despair, loneliness, anger); social and behavioral distress (withdrawal, crying); and stress-related physiological symptoms (e.g., modulated immune response, increased incidence of illness, need for medications, hospitalization). A number of theoretical models have been proposed to account for the grief experience, and have guided thinking about intervention. Bowlby (1980) proposed that the emotional response to the *loss of an attachment figure* would involve a sequence of four phases: (a) initially shock, numbness, and denial, (b) a time of yearning and protest as the finality of the loss becomes understood, (c) a longer period of despair, emotional upset, and withdrawal, and (d) an eventual period of recovery, in which the loss becomes more tolerable, and is accepted, and in which feelings of well-being begin to increase. Such theoretical models have been useful in conceptualizing bereavement process. However, they should not be viewed as prescriptive.

Other models consider the *tasks of grieving*. For example, Weiss (1988) argued that three processes (cognitive acceptance, emotional acceptance, and identity change) were essential to recovery. Worden (1991) proposed four tasks at the core of the grieving process: (a) accepting the loss, (b) experiencing the pain, (c) learning to live a life without the deceased, and (d) relocating the deceased within one's emotional space, allowing the bereaved person to move on with life. More recently, M. Stroebe and Schut (1999) have proposed a *dual-process model* of coping with grief. They suggest that in addition to coping emotionally with the loss, it is important to cope with "secondary stressors" associated with the death, such as re-establishing family security, rebuilding relationships, and adapting to new social or economic roles, and that bereaved persons will likely need to "oscillate" between these two domains of coping.

It is important to understand, however, that grief is a natural and normal (if harrowing) emotional response to the loss of a loved one. Most bereaved persons do adapt to their loss within a year or two (Gallagher-Thompson et al., 1993), and in the process may experience an *increased* sense of personal growth and mastery (Lund, Caserta, & Dimond, 1993). Researchers and clinicians agree, then, that bereavement itself should not automatically signal a need for formal therapeutic intervention. There is consensus, also, on two additional assumptions. *First*, that comfort and support are available from many naturally occurring sources, such as family, friends, religious and community groups, and even the Internet, and that for most bereaved persons these will be the most accessible and useful coping resources. *Second*, that bereaved individuals will vary in the nature and intensity of their grief-related distress, and in their degree of need for intervention to prevent problematic outcomes (Raphael, Minkov, & Dobson, 2001).

Intervention strategies may be grouped into (a) primary preventive interventions, intended for any older bereaved person facing bereavement, (b) primary preventive interventions for those at high risk, and (c) other than primary prevention for those having identifiable problems related to bereavement. To this end, research and theory have addressed three important questions: (a) What are the most important risk factors? (b) What are the important protective factors? (c) What kinds of preventive, treatment, and maintenance interventions work, why, and for whom?

Risk Factors

Three types of factors appear to be important: *Situational* risk factors such as mode of death (e.g., suddenness); *person* factors such as pre-death levels of emotional stability, self-esteem, sense of personal control, religious beliefs, and gender (some research has indicated that elderly widowers may be a particularly high risk group, due to their relative social isolation and less communicative ways of coping with bereavement, relative to elderly widows); and *interpersonal* risk factors such as lack of social/emotional support from family or friends (W. Stroebe & Schut, 2001). It is noteworthy, also, that entire populations may be placed at risk in the event of a natural or community disaster or in time of war. Such events, for example, expose large numbers of people to traumatic death circumstances, and to the sudden and untimely deaths of loved ones.

Protective Factors

A number of the risk factors noted above should (from another viewpoint) also be viewed as protective factors, with respect to primary prevention and promotion of adaptation to bereavement. Generally speaking, bereaved individuals are remarkably resilient; most eventually find ways to cope with the emotional side of a loss and with the practical consequences (Stein, Folkman, Trabasso, & Richards, 1997). Their natural support networks among family, friends, and community play an important protective role as well (Lopata, 1996), but also participate in the adaptive processes of sharing and sorting out of emotions and in the search for meaning in the death (Nadeau, 1998; Pennebaker, 1997). Bereavement researchers widely agree on the need to encourage these naturally occurring protective resources and to facilitate their efforts, rather than rush to more formal treatment solutions (Bonanno, 2001; Raphael & Nunn, 1988). Protective factors more relevant to the aging context will be discussed further in the Adaptive Processes section, below.

Issues in Assessing Grief—and Establishing Intervention Goals

The bereavement reaction is a process, not a disease. A broad range of cognitive, affective, and physiological reactions are likely to arise and to change across the course of the bereavement, with considerable variability across individuals and across cultures. It is therefore difficult, theoretically, to establish developmental norms for the bereavement process, per se. The impact and course of bereavement have, therefore, typically been assessed using (in addition to measures of grief symptoms) traditional measures for such outcomes as depression and physical health, for which diagnostic criteria have been established, and measures of variables such as traumatic symptomatology (e.g., intrusion/avoidance of memories), loneliness, sense of control, and social involvement. Readers should be cautioned, however, that among elderly persons, psychological symptoms of this type may be multi-determined (they can reflect a significant health event, medication interactions, dietary problems, lack

of stimulation, etc.); thus it may be difficult to isolate the causal influence of a bereavement-related reaction for any given individual (Kane & Kane, 2000).

Aging Issues in Bereavement: Age-Related Vulnerabilities

Older persons experience bereavement reactions similar to younger persons, as assessed by traditional measures of emotional and physical symptoms. However, in spousal bereavement especially there are also longer term concerns, as the issue of what is lost in the death broadens. Over time, a couple will have developed shared resources, traditions, identities, and interdependencies. The death, then, in addition to one's emotional reaction to the loss, may disrupt the important social, support, and meaning structures of a widowed person's life, fostering isolation, undermining reasons to continue to cope and maintain function, and threatening independence. In addition, the death of a spouse in old age may interact with or intensify the consequences of other stressors that tend to cluster in late-life, such as chronic illness and disability, retirement, and involuntary change of residence (Hansson & Carpenter, 1994).

Aging Issues in Bereavement: Adaptive Process

It is important to understand that older adults exhibit increasing diversity in psychological and physiological status, life experience, coping styles and competencies, and also in their reactions to bereavement. That said, older widowed persons appear to benefit from social support, and over time to increase the percentage of other widowed persons in their friendship networks (Carstensen, Gross, & Fung, 1997). Also, those who try to use the time during a spouse's lingering illness to prepare for how to deal with the practical consequences of the death (e.g., learning to drive, handle finances, and making new friends), report less emotional disruption at the death and increased success in dealing with the practical consequences of their loss. It is also of interest that the sequence of caregiving for a dying spouse, followed by the bereavement does not necessarily imply an accumulation of stressors; rather, a period of successful caregiving may broaden one's perspectives, and enhance one's sense of competency (Wells & Kendig, 1997).

Aging Issues in Bereavement: Emotion Regulation in Late-Life

Although late-life entails greater risks of disability, decline and loss, subjective reports of emotional well-being tend to increase. Such findings would seem counterintuitive. However, a number of explanations seem reasonable (Magai & McFadden, 1996). For example, older persons appear to appraise life-stressors differently, with potential implications for experienced emotion and perceived demands for coping. Older persons tend to report fewer life problems generally, compared to middle-aged counterparts, and feel less upset or challenged by problems they do encounter. Even though they more frequently experience bereavements, sense of threat or loss is not elevated, and they feel relatively confident in their ability to handle emotionally demanding events. It has been suggested that they experience a dampening of emotions, both positive and negative, and physiological assessments of emotional responsiveness are consistent with this hypothesis (Lawton, Kleban, Rajagopal, & Dean, 1992). This may reflect age-related changes in the brain's emotion systems. It may also indicate that older persons are likely to have come to terms with the many implications of aging, and that they have learned through experience how best to manage or prevent the consequences of many late-life stressors, precluding the need to constantly rise to the occasion to cope with a crisis. Finally, older adults also appear to learn to manage (regulate) their emotions in response to a stressful life-event. They may realistically lower their standards or goals for coping, compare themselves only with similar others, and re-appraise the event to find a balance of positive and negative consequences.

Issues in Psychological Intervention with Older Adults

Although grief is a normal emotional reaction to loss, and not a psychiatric disorder, it is in some cases associated with higher risks of clinical symptoms (e.g., depression and physical illness). In this connection, older adults can experience most of the psychological disorders seen in younger persons. However, a variety of contextual factors make assessment and understanding of symptoms more difficult. For example, among older persons, psychological distress may also reflect one's frustration with physical illness and chronic pain, or problems in dealing with multiple-medications. Also, the likelihood of dementia increases among elderly persons (5 percent among those over age 65, and about 30 percent of those over age 85), threatening an elderly person's ability to cope independently with life-events (APA Working Group on the Older Adult, 1998).

Most psychological interventions used with younger persons appear effective with older adults as well, although they may need to be adapted to the abilities and circumstances of the older client. It may be necessary, for example, to determine the older person's understanding of the assessment and helping process, and to provide some education about the nature and goals of service. It is also helpful to consider concurrent physical, cognitive, or social problems that could affect this process.

Older persons are found to benefit from individual and group therapy, and from cognitive–behavioral, psychodynamic, and interpersonal therapy. Given the frequent dependency of older clients on family support, it may also be useful to involve family members in the intervention. Similarly, given the interrelation of physical and psychological problems in the elderly, providers may also want to consider physical therapy, pain control, or environmental-modifications as part of treatment. Intervention protocols also may need to be modified to accommodate slower learning and problem-solving processes in the elderly. Finally, it should be understood that among elderly persons, many problems are chronic and progressive. It may therefore be necessary to adopt more flexible goals for treatment, focusing on the management of symptoms and rehabilitation or maintenance of function, rather than on recovery (APA Working Group on the Older Adult, 1998). The APA Working Group's emphasis on protecting existing strengths and resources, then, is consistent with the focus of the present volume on prevention.

Intervention research with older persons has traditionally distinguished between (a) the prevention of disabling consequences of age-related change in health or life-circumstances, (b) the identification and control of risk factors, and (c) the rehabilitation or restoration of function (Jette, 1996; Schulz & Martire, 1999). Among the elderly, however, an important issue is the target of the intervention. Most interventions directly target the aging individual, for example with medical treatment, educational or counseling strategies to enhance positive health behavior, social, and intellectual maintenance. However, because issues of dependency arise in late life, interventions often focus, as well, on strengthening the older person's social or physical environment, for example with home modifications, support for caregivers, or education for staff. Finally, some interventions are directed to society at large. These might include public health programs, Medicare policy, or preventive home health initiatives (Schulz & Martire, 1999).

STRATEGIES: OVERVIEW

We noted earlier a variety of naturally occurring processes believed to be important to successful adaptation to bereavement. These generally involved coming to terms with the loss, finding meaning and emotional acceptance, learning to live one's life without the deceased while retaining emotional bonds, and coping with the secondary stressors such as threats to family security and the need to continue to perform ongoing social or economic roles. Such processes are quite demanding, given the suffering, emotional and physical distress typical of the early phases of bereavement.

During this time, the support of friends and family can be immensely helpful. Social support can provide companionship, affection, understanding, distraction, someone with whom to compare feelings, and help with practical problems. However, older bereaved persons vary immensely in their access to competent, reliable social support networks. An important role for helping professionals, then, is in supporting or orchestrating these natural helping resources.

In uncomplicated bereavements, the goals of grief counseling are (a) to encourage natural grieving processes, (b) to provide support and comfort, and (c) to provide assistance with the secondary stresses that surround a death in the family. These efforts may complement available support from family and naturally occurring community resources. Counseling may be provided by pastors, health care professionals, or self-help groups such as "Widow to Widow" programs (involving persons who have themselves been through the bereavement process: Silverman, 1986).

Grief therapy may be indicated where the grief process is more problematic, of abnormal intensity, prolonged, or where the bereaved individual is determined to be at risk for related disorder. Its goals may include assisting the bereaved person to face the reality of the loss, to openly experience emotional reactions until they become tolerable, to adjust to life-changes associated with the death, new roles, and a changed identity.

Schut, Stroebe, van den Bout, and Terheggen (2001) recently reviewed the efficacy studies on bereavement interventions for persons of varying levels of risk. They found serious methodological shortcomings in much of this research (lack of appropriate control groups, inadequate sampling, etc). However, a number of patterns were apparent from that review, and are summarized in the sections that follow. The reader will note from this summary of findings that it is not so much which strategies work (similar strategies have been used with persons of varying risk), but for *whom* they work.

STRATEGIES THAT WORK

The natural helping network of family, neighbors, and friends, as well as members of familiar religious, social, or business groups appears to be successful in helping most bereaved people through the normal grieving process. Moreover, as we will indicate below, it may be unwise to add professional services in the case of normal grieving. In the case of complicated grieving which goes beyond the scope of primary prevention, see Stroebe, Hansson, Stroebe, and Schut (2001) for a discussion of intervention and treatment strategies.

STRATEGIES THAT MIGHT WORK

A number of interventions have targeted bereaved persons determined to be at increased risk for problematic outcome. Here, outcome studies have produced mixed, but somewhat positive results. For example, interventions that provide support and encourage expression of emotions in the months after a traumatic or sudden death appear to be associated with reduced symptoms (Raphael, 1977, 1978). Similarly, high risk bereaved persons who receive support in dealing with their grief immediately after the death appear to benefit, as indicated by lower levels of physical symptoms, depression, worrying, and use of health care services (Parkes, 1981). Those who receive practical and emotional support appear to benefit, at least in the short term, with respect to general health and anxiety.

STRATEGIES THAT DO NOT WORK

A variety of studies have focused on professional or non-family strategies for facilitating normal bereavement processes. Bereaved persons in these studies are not selected on the basis of expressed need or the existence of suspected risk factors. Interventions have included crisis teams visiting family members within hours of the loss, self-help groups with the goal of fostering friendship, programs to educate bereaved persons about the tasks of working through one's grief, cognitive-restructuring and behavioral-skills programs, treatments involving the sharing of information, emotions, and support, and brief group psychotherapy. Unfortunately, there is very little empirical support for the effectiveness of these primary preventive interventions among adults (Caserta & Lund, 1993; Lieberman & Yalom, 1992; Reich & Zautra, 1989). The rare positive effects tended to be temporary, and occasionally there were reports of negative consequences of the intervention. For most bereaved persons, the bereavement would not be expected to be complicated, and naturally occurring support resources would already be available. While at least temporary relief of suffering may be perceived as a benefit of such intervention, it seems likely that normal grief must indeed "run its course."

SYNTHESIS

Several points from the preceding discussion deserve emphasis. *First*, grief is a natural and normal process. The vast majority of bereavements are not complicated, and for most persons there are natural support resources available that appear to be successful in helping. These include family, friends, religious and community groups, the self-help literature, and the Internet. These resources may provide emotional and practical support, companionship, an opportunity to share and work through feelings, health care, housing, and so on.

Second, evidence suggests that formal intervention is generally not effective or justified for uncomplicated bereavements. That means that helping professionals are likely to be most effective by providing support to natural helpers. Helping professionals should also understand that the provision of formal outreach services, even to elderly bereaved persons, might result in the withdrawal of (most important) family and informal support.

Third, for those elderly at high risk for complicated bereavement, a variety of intervention approaches have been found to be effective, and may be useful when appropriately applied.

Finally, it is important to remember that, among older persons, the psychological distress associated with bereavement is likely to involve physical and environmental co-determinants, in addition to the expected emotional impact of the loss. Many elderly bereaved persons will be at increased risk because of previously existing chronic illness, pain, disability, limited physical or cognitive functioning. Others will be socially isolated, or unable to manage in their homes after the loss of a spouse-caregiver. Primary prevention strategies for older bereaved persons should therefore always include a response to any assessed needs with respect to such physical, family, or environmental variables.

Also see: Crisis Intervention: Older Adulthood; Depression: Adulthood; Loneliness/Isolation: Older Adulthood.

References

American Association of Retired Persons. (1999). *A profile of older Americans.* wysiwyg://37/http://www.aoa.dhhs.gov/aoa/stats/profile/

APA Working Group on the Older Adult. (1998). What practitioners should know about working with older adults. *Professional Psychology: Research and Practice, 29,* 413–427.

Bonanno, G.A. (2001). Introduction: New directions in bereavement research and theory. *American Behavioral Scientist, 44*(5), 718–725.

Bowlby, J. (1980). *Attachment and loss: Vol. 3: Loss: Sadness and depression.* London: Hogarth Press.

Carstensen, L.L., Gross, J.J., & Fung, H.H. (1997). The social context of emotional experience. *Annual Review of Gerontology and Geriatrics, 17,* 325–352.

Caserta, M.S., & Lund, D.A. (1993). Intrapersonal resources and the effectiveness of self-help groups for bereaved older adults. *The Gerontologist, 33,* 619–629.

Gallagher-Thompson, D., Futterman, A., Farberow, N., Thompson, L.W., & Peterson, J. (1993). The impact of spousal bereavement on older widows and widowers. In M.S. Stroebe, W. Stroebe, & R.O. Hansson (Eds.), *Handbook of bereavement: Theory, research, and intervention* (pp. 227–239). Cambridge: Cambridge University Press.

Hansson, R.O., & Carpenter, B.N. (1994). *Relationships in old age: Coping with the challenge of transition.* New York: Guilford.

Jette, A.M. (1996). Disability trends and transitions. In R.H. Binstock & L.K. George (Eds.), *Handbook of aging and the social sciences* (pp. 94–116). San Diego: Academic Press.

Kane, R.L., & Kane, R.A. (Eds.). (2000). *Assessing older persons: Measures, meaning, and practical applications.* Oxford: Oxford University Press.

Lawton, M.P., Kleban, M.H., Rajagopal, D., & Dean, J. (1992). Dimensions of affective experience in three age groups. *Psychology and Aging, 7,* 171–184.

Lieberman, M.A., & Yalom, I. (1992). Brief group psychotherapy for the spousally bereaved: A controlled study. *International Journal of Group Psychotherapy, 42,* 117–132.

Lopata, H.Z. (1996). *Current widowhood: Myths and realities.* Thousand Oaks, CA: Sage.

Lund, D.A., Caserta, M.S., & Dimond, M.F. (1993). The course of spousal bereavement in later life. In M.S. Stroebe, W. Stroebe, & R.O. Hansson (Eds.), *Handbook of bereavement: Theory, research, and intervention* (pp. 240–254). Cambridge: Cambridge University Press.

Magai, C., & McFadden, S.H. (Eds.). (1996). *Handbook of emotion, adult development, and aging.* San Diego: Academic Press.

Nadeau, J.W. (1998). *Families making sense of death.* Thousand Oaks, CA: Sage.

Parkes, C.M. (1981). Evaluation of a bereavement service. *Journal of Preventive Psychiatry, 1,* 179–188.

Pennebaker, J.W. (1997). *Opening up: The healing power of expressing emotions* (Rev. ed.). New York: Guilford Press.

Raphael, B. (1977). Preventive intervention with the recently bereaved. *Archives of General Psychiatry, 34,* 1450–1454.

Raphael, B. (1978). Mourning and the prevention of melancholia. *British Journal of Medical Psychology, 51,* 303–310.

Raphael, B., Minkov, C., & Dobson, M. (2001). Psychotherapeutic and pharmacological intervention for bereaved persons. In M.S. Stroebe, R.O. Hansson, W. Stroebe, & H. Schut (Eds.), *Handbook of bereavement research: Consequences, coping and care* (pp. 587–612). Washington, DC: American Psychological Association.

Raphael, B., & Nunn, K. (1988). Counseling the bereaved. *Journal of Social Issues, 44*(3), 191–206.

Reich, G.W., & Zautra, A.G. (1989). A perceived control intervention for at-risk older adults. *Psychology and Aging, 4,* 415–424.

Schulz, R., & Martire, L.M. (1999). Intervention research with older adults: Introduction, overview, and future directions. *Annual Review of Gerontology and Geriatrics, 18,* 1–16.

Schut, H., Stroebe, M., van den Bout, J., & Terheggen, M. (2001). The efficacy of bereavement interventions: Who benefits? In M.S. Stroebe, R.O. Hansson, W. Stroebe, & H. Schut (Eds.), *Handbook of bereavement research: Consequences, coping and care* (pp. 705–737). Washington, DC: American Psychological Association.

Silverman, P.R. (1986). *Widow-to-widow.* New York: Springer.

Stein, N., Folkman, S., Trabasso, T., & Richards, T.A. (1997). Appraisal and goal processes as predictors of well-being in bereaved caregivers. *Journal of Personality and Social Psychology, 72,* 872–884.

Stroebe, M.S., & Schut, H.A.W. (1999). The dual process model of coping with bereavement: Rationale and description. *Death Studies, 23,* 197–224.

Stroebe, M.S. Hansson, R.O. Stroebe, W., & Schut H. (Eds.). (2001). *Handbook of bereavement research: Consequences, coping and care.* Washington, DC: American Psychological Association.

Stroebe, W., & Schut, H.A.W. (2001). Risk factors in bereavement outcome: A methodological and empirical review. In M.S. Stroebe, R.O. Hansson, W. Stroebe, & H. Schut (Eds.), *Handbook of bereavement research: Consequences, coping and care* (pp. 349–371). Washington, DC: American Psychological Association.

Weiss, R.S. (1988). Loss and recovery. *Journal of Social Issues, 44*, 37–52.

Wells, Y.D., & Kendig, H.L. (1997). Health and well-being of spouse caregivers and the widowed. *The Gerontologist, 37*, 666–674.

Worden, J.W. (1991). *Grief counseling and grief therapy: A handbook for the mental health practitioner*. New York: Springer.

H

Health Promotion, Older Adulthood

Jasmin Tahmaseb McConatha and Lori Riley

INTRODUCTION

The difference between a successful and unsuccessful aging experience depends, to a large extent, on the ways in which people are able to successfully engage in health-promoting behaviors. The 21st century presents a formidable challenge for health care professionals concerned with promoting healthy lifestyles for an increasingly diverse older adult population in the United States. This entry focuses on the ways in which cultural values and beliefs interact with personal and social factors to influence health promotion activities for older minority adults. Cultural values and belief systems shape choices about diet, alcohol consumption, tobacco use, attitudes toward exercise, and other preventive health practices. Medical advances have enabled people to live longer, healthier, and happier lives; however, an increase in life expectancy has also contributed to greater incidence rates of chronic and debilitating illnesses among older adults. The average current life expectancy in Western societies is 76, which is a significant change from the turn of the last century when it was only 45 (Grossman, 1998).

A large percentage of the older adult population, however, has not yet been able to fully realize the benefits of improved health care and health-promoting lifestyles that enhance the quality of life in later adulthood.

DEFINITIONS

In this entry, we use several terms relating to health promotion in later adulthood. *Health promotion* is understood as a lifelong process that involves personal growth and fulfillment, physical health and well-being, and self-actualization. As such, health promotion is a holistic process that involves a person's well-being in the physical, mental, spiritual, and social realms (Campbell & Kreidler, 1994).

Health promotion activities are related to factors such as gender, ethnicity, and culture, as well as personal habits, health practices, lifestyle choices, and previous health concerns. These interact to influence an individual's overall health in late adulthood. Studies have found that if people are willing to engage in health-promoting behaviors, a large percentage of such major chronic conditions as heart disease, cancers, cerebrovascular disease, pneumonia, influenza, and diabetes can be either prevented or more effectively treated.

Wellness is an important underlying component of health promotion. Wellness focuses on an individual's self-responsibility for his or her well-being. A wellness-oriented lifestyle is based on the premise of personal responsibility and self-care. Ruffing-Rahal and Wallace (2000) proposed an ecological model of wellness. This model focuses on the advancement of health and wellness promotion within the context of everyday well-being. The model constitutes a framework for health promotion that includes activity, affirmation, and synthesis. Activity deals with meaningful pursuits that incorporate self-care and health-promoting lifestyles. Affirmation deals with hope, faith, religiosity, and life satisfaction. Synthesis is concerned with the ways that people deal with and incorporate negative life experiences.

Health promotion and wellness are related to feelings of control and competence. These can be increased by participation in activities that improve health and well-being. According to some researchers, one of the most important factors that determine an individual's reaction to health-threatening situations is her or his sense of control. The attempt to maintain a sense of control over one's life is an important challenge for people of all ages. People who believe that their personal efforts have influenced their life circumstances tend to be healthier than individuals without a sense self-control. Augmenting one's sense of personal control has also been found to lead to positive changes in health-promoting behaviors (Krause, 1990; McConatha, McConatha, Deaner, & Dermigny, 1995; Rodin, 1986; Schulz & Heckhausen, 1996).

Competence, a consequence of control, refers to a person's ability to adapt to an environment by making effective choices, plans, and controlling—as much as possible—the events and outcomes of daily life. In this entry, we suggest that an individual's ability to engage in behaviors that increase his or her health and well-being are to a large extent dependent upon his or her sense of competence. This competence can enable individuals to effectively engage in physical and psychological health-promoting behaviors. A lack of competence, on the other hand, has been associated with lower self-esteem, life satisfaction, greater use of home health care services, greater risk of hospitalization and institutionalization, and higher mortality (Diehl, 1998).

Health promotion activities, wellness, a sense of control, and competence are important factors that influence the well-being of older adults. They vary by culture and ethnicity. For example, older men and women in the United States, who are recent immigrants or belong to a minority groups, may have a history of poor access to health care, decent employment, proper nutrition, and adequate living conditions, all of which will affect their wellness.

SCOPE

In the United States, significant inequalities continue to exist in the health concerns of older men and women. Poverty, for example, has a direct bearing on health-related factors such as living conditions, diet, exercise, and preventive health care. Minority populations in the United States are more likely to have lower incomes. Thirty seven percent of Blacks and 36 percent of Latino older adults have incomes that fall below the Federal Poverty Line. Poverty

rates also increase with age and are highest among minority women (*Family Economics and Nutrition Review*, 1999).

Income levels have been related to preventive health behaviors and practices. As a consequence, mortality rates are still divergent for white Americans and African Americans. Beyond the discrepancies in life expectancy are other disparities. African American men and women suffer from more chronic conditions than do other Americans. They also have less access to preventive health care, and as a consequence, they have higher mortality rates from heart disease, stroke, cancer, diabetes, and cirrhosis of the liver than do Whites. In fact, many African Americans die from these diseases before the age of 65 (Yee & Weaver, 1994). Gender differences are also relevant. Women have a greater life expectancy than do men. By the same token, they also tend to have more limited financial means. As a consequence, they suffer more from various chronic illnesses as well as from such psychological disorders as depression.

Older adults with lower educational attainment and income have been found to have more unhealthy behaviors and lifestyles. For example, a greater number of older adults with lower educational attainment smoke cigarettes, consume alcohol, and have decreased levels of physical activity than those with higher educational attainment. High-density lipoprotein cholesterol, sickness, disability, and increased premature death rates have also been found to be related to lower education levels (Kubzansky, Berkman, Glass, & Seeman, 1998). This may devolve from poor living conditions as well as the necessity of doing physically demanding work to support themselves. Those with greater educational attainment, on the other hand, are usually in better health. They tend to be less resistant to appeals from health care professionals to adopt a more health-promoting lifestyle (Green & Ottoson, 1999).

THEORIES AND RESEARCH

Several theoretical approaches can be used in understanding the relationship between health, well-being, and minority older adult populations in the United States. The *Health Belief Model* (Becker, 1974) is particularly relevant when considering the well-being of older minority populations. This model illustrates people's perceptions of their health and illness. It incorporates subjective factors such as perceived susceptibility, perceived seriousness of a health concern, and perceived benefits of certain actions such as preventative behaviors. The model also addresses the relationship between individuals' perceptions of their health and the interaction they have with health care providers. Factors such as ethnicity and culture may influence in the type and quality of care provided. Additionally, a person's belief about the causes of illnesses may be related to her or his cultural values. These values sometimes conflict with those of a health care provider. Frequently care providers are from a white and majority background and may be ignorant or dismissive of a patient's traditional belief system.

There are many changes that occur as people grow older. The key to successful aging is to accept and adapt to age-related transformations by developing and maintaining healthy behaviors and lifestyles. The health belief model can be utilized to help health care professionals in their understanding of the health concerns of older minority adults. By understanding the ways in which cultural values and beliefs influence their understanding of health-promoting activities, professionals can assist patients in aging successfully and providing appropriate health programs to educate and foster healthy behaviors and lifestyles.

Control Theory is another approach that provides an understanding of an individual's set of beliefs concerning their health and well-being. The attempt to maintain a sense of control over one's life is an important challenge for people of all ages, but it becomes particularly important as a person ages and the possibility for health concerns and impairment increases. Feeling in control has been shown to be inversely related to positive health and well-being. Feeling out of control, by contrast, has been associated with negative psychological and physiological responses (McConatha et al., 1995; Rodin & Langer, 1980).

Self-efficacy expectations, related to *social cognitive theory*, also play an important role in overall feelings of control. Bandura (1986) has argued that self-efficacy is one of the most powerful explanatory agents in human behavior. Self-efficacy is described as a belief in one's ability to successfully perform a given behavior. Self-efficacy has an impact on health-related choices, the amount of effort invested in prevention activities, how long to persevere, and whether tasks are approached with confidence or hesitation. Positive changes in an individual's health behaviors and lifestyles can greatly decrease their risk of being inflicted with a serious debilitating illness.

Theories of Social Support have found that one of the most influential components of health and well-being in later adulthood is the availability of supportive social contact. Conceptualizations of social support vary by individual, culture, age, and ethnicity. Sarason, Levine, Basham, and Sarason (1983) define social support as "the existence or availability of people on whom we can rely, people who let us know that they care about, value, and love us" (p. 127). The social support resource theory considers people's attempts to obtain and protect their physical and psychological resources (Hobfoll, Freedy, Lane, & Geller, 1990). In times of stress and illness, these resources are perceived as buffers; they help a person feel more in control.

Additionally, social support provides a person with a sense of interpersonal connectedness, a more positive and valued sense of self, and assistance in times of need.

STRATEGIES THAT WORK

Cultures vary in their understanding of what constitutes a healthy life. Cultural values and expectations influence health promotion activities as well as the treatment of illnesses. The case of Moussa Boureima, a West African immigrant, illustrates potential problems that may arise for older minority men and women.

> Moussa Boureima, a 65 year old immigrant from West Africa, lives in New York City. He suffers from rheumatism. The condition, which makes his knees ache, his ankles swell, and his joints stiffen, is aggravated by the fact that in order to make ends meet, he sells merchandise, baseball hats, gloves, shawls, outside—in the damp chill of fall and winter as well as the stifling humidity of summer. Despite his continuous pain and discomfort, Moussa is hesitant to seek treatment.
>
> "I don't speak much English," he says, "Not enough to explain what's wrong with me. Last year I found a doctor on 72nd Street who spoke French. He gave me a shot and my pain went away, but it came back. I don't want to go to a hospital. I have no insurance and no money. I don't want any trouble."

For help and information on health-related issues, Moussa generally relies on advice from a social support network of friends and family. Moussa's situation is not atypical for immigrants to the United States. Many immigrants to the United States do not have an understanding of the health care system, have limited financial resources, and are not able to engage in health-promoting behaviors (Stoller & McConatha, 2001).

As Fred Williams's case illustrates, long-standing belief systems can also become a barrier to effective health promotion.

> It is lunchtime and two older African American men are sitting in the delivery alcove of an apartment building enjoying a fried chicken lunch. Fred Williams, is 76, he is the head super of the building. As he chews on a chicken wing he complains about the declining quality of plumbers. "They don't take pride in their work," he says to Ernest Thorpe, his assistant. Fred and Ernest are overweight. Fred has high blood pressure and high cholesterol and suffers from a bad back. Even so, he and Ernest, who is 68, continue to eat fried foods, like their noontime chicken, that are not good for their various conditions. Fred doesn't worry about his doctor's advice about diet and exercise. "If I work hard everyday, it doesn't matter what I eat or what I lift. Hard work is the best medicine. It has kept me going so far."

Various ethnic and cultural beliefs play a central role in health promotion among older ethnic minorities in the United States. For example, many African Americans believe that natural illness is caused by "thin blood," an unalterable condition that is generated by the aging process. For them, "thin blood" illnesses are not the result of an unhealthy diet or a sedentary lifestyle. Accordingly, they may not seek treatment for such asymptomatic illnesses as hypertension (Yee & Weaver, 1994).

Native Americans continue to retain many of their traditional health values and practices. Although many differences exist, one important aspect of Native American belief systems focuses on the view that health results from a sense of harmony between the person and nature. Holistic healing of the mind, body, and spirit is consistent with traditional belief systems. Healing from this perspective focuses on a restoration of harmony (Yee & Weaver, 1994). These traditional beliefs can serve as an important health-promoting factor. They may also make an older person more distrustful of modern medical techniques. They therefore may be less likely to use preventive and/or treatment methods.

Differences have also been noted in health concerns and death rates between Asian American older men and women. Asian and Asian Americans, even those from a lower socio-economic background, tend to have higher life expectancy and engage in more positive health practices than poor elderly Whites, African Americans, or Latinos. Asian American adults have reduced their rate of smoking and alcohol consumption-actions that have lowered death rates. Like the Native Americans, many older Asian Americans believe that health is derived from harmony between the person, society, and the forces of the universe. A lifelong belief in the potential benefits associated with natural healing and the use of herbs have been widely effective in helping promote health and well-being for many Asian Americans.

Little is known about the health practices of older Latino men and women. There is some evidence, however, that many older Latinos suffer a higher rate of obesity as a result of poor eating habits, lack of exercise, smoking, and alcohol abuse than do comparable minority groups. As can be seen, in order to be effective, health promotion practitioners must have some awareness of traditional values and beliefs (Brislin, 1993).

Culturally-contoured processes of interpretation variously shape both the concept of wellness and what conditions constitute illness. As in the case of Fred Williams, cultural values and norms both promote and serve as barriers to health promotion. As these cases illustrate, cultural gaps may also separate health care professionals from minority populations (Green & Ottoson, 1999). What one culture or ethnic group may consider unhealthy behavior may be socially acceptable in another culture or ethnic group. Lifelong cultural belief systems may also be in conflict with health-promoting behaviors. For example, *Gaman*, or self-control, can cause Japanese older men and women to accept pain stoically; it may make them reluctant to seek help or use services that could provide relief or alleviate the problem (Yee & Weaver, 1994). In certain religions such as Islam, adherents believe that the time of one's death is predetermined. This belief may make a person less likely to participate in difficult or painful health-promoting activities.

The fast pace of cultural and environmental changes can affect feelings of control and competence for older adults. Older adults who are unable to cope and adapt to these changes have a greater likelihood of suffering from psychological and physical illness. Gergen (1991) describes how feelings of stress, inadequacy, and self-doubt emerge from the effects of rapid change in contemporary societies.

STRATEGIES THAT WORK

Health promotion strategies and programs need to focus on increasing older minority adults' awareness that an unhealthy lifestyle can result in a loss of autonomy, desired lifestyles, and independence. One possible avenue of health promotion involves utilizing existing resources. One can, for example, rely on family or other social support. Studies have found that minority older adults often have many family ties. They would therefore be in a better position to receive positive support from their relationships. Peer and family influences may promote healthy behaviors and lifestyles more successfully than health care professionals (Kubzansky et al., 1998).

Physical fitness, good nutrition, safety, management of stress are all essential to health promotion and disease prevention activities among older minority adults (Campbell & Kreidler, 1994). Even small changes in these areas have been proven to be effective in promoting more positive health. Basic awareness of health promotion activities such as quitting smoking, increasing exercise, making changes in diet, and managing stress can make significant differences in overall well-being. For example, exercise has been identified as a major health-promoting activity in later adulthood (Fontane, 1996). Repeated studies have found that exercise tones and heals the body, influences psychological well-being and increases life expectancy. However, only one fourth to one third of older adults exercise regularly. These percentages are even lower for older minority populations (Clark, 1996). Airhihenbuwa, Kumanyika, Agurs, and Lowe (1995) stated that older adults from different cultural and ethnic backgrounds have varying attitudes toward exercise. For example, older African Americans were found to engage in less physical activity than their White counterparts, a fact that may be related to the fact that many African Americans had occupations that required them to be physically active. Accordingly, they may perceive retirement as a time of physical rest and relaxation.

Maintaining a sense of control and competence in later adulthood requires the availability of support and resources. Cultural changes and transformation such as the computerization of everyday life can serve as an important health-promoting resource for older adults. Computer technology is one such resource that has been demonstrated to improve sensorimotor, cognitive, personality, and social skills. Computers can serve as links for communication to get older adults involved in social activities, friends and relatives, as well as health-related educational programs.

Older adults with greater social and cultural resources adjust more positively to the aging process. Environmental resources can serve a buffering function. People who have access to resources such as a social support network or computer technology may have a more successful aging experience because they are able to select, optimize, and compensate for areas of decline (Baltes & Lang, 1997). Computer technology can also reduce feelings of isolation experienced by some older adults. Recent studies have found that anxiety about computer use has been diminishing and an increasing number of older men and men of all backgrounds are making use of computer technology (McConatha et al., 1995).

STRATEGIES THAT MIGHT WORK

Ginkgo biloba, St Johns' Wort, acupuncture, reflexology, massage, are some of the many terms associated with "alternative medicine." Alternative treatments constitute procedures that are based on a mind–body connection. The procedures focus on methods that include the prevention of disease as well as the treatment of illnesses. Many of these therapies are especially useful when considering health promotion for older adults. Juxtaposed to a disease causation model, most alternative therapies are based on a holistic model that focuses on a balanced integration of factors that constitute the individual. This paradigm acknowledges the presence of an intelligent life force referred to as "chi" in China and "prana" in India. Symptoms of illness are often seen as evidence that the mind, body, and spirit are attempting to correct an existing imbalance (Light, 1997). Whereas conventional medical practitioners often focus on a single cause of a health concern, alternative practitioners, by contrast, focus on the interconnectedness of the mind, body, and the environment. They also assume that individuals have the capacity to assume a degree of responsibility for their own health.

Reliance on "alternative medicine" is on the increase among both minority and mainstream Americans of all ages.

In a 1993 study, Eisenberg, Lessler, Foster, Norlock, Calkins, and Delbanco conducted a telephone survey of 1,539 adults. They found that one in three of their respondents reported having utilized "alternative" treatment methods. In another recent study of Mexican Americans and Anglo-Americans, both groups were found to rely upon what has traditionally been referred to as alternative medicines, though Mexican Americans utilized these treatment methods more frequently. Minority populations in the United States often rely upon various folk therapies for the treatment of health disorders (Keegan, 2000). For example, many Latinos with health concerns often visit a shaman, or curandero, who prescribes spiritual as well as medical treatments.

Various health promotion methods which have long been utilized in Asia are recently becoming more widely accepted in the United States. Acupuncture has been reported to be successful for alleviating pain and treating conditions such as obesity, smoking, insomnia, and nausea (Kaniegal, 1998). Massage therapy is a widely used practice that helps to expel toxins from the body and improve blood flow (Siegel-Maier, 1999). Massage therapy has been proven to be effective for a number of wide-ranging health conditions including depression and migraine headaches (O'Donnell, 1999). Certain medicinal herbs that have been widely used for various healing purposes for centuries, are now being accepted by the American Medical Association. For example, ginkgo is now accepted as an effective treatment for the symptoms of Alzheimer's Disease (Spector, 1996). Tai Chi, meditation, and Yoga are becoming widely practiced as an effective form of exercise, stress management, and health promotion for older adults.

Astin (1998) states that at times conventional western medicine may be dissatisfying because it has been ineffective, expensive, or has produced adverse side effects. Given the increasing acceptance of alternative therapies, it becomes even more necessary for health care providers to become familiar with various cultural practices. Many health care professionals tend to be skeptical of alternative therapies and indeed some have been shown to have no beneficial effects. As a consequence, individuals who rely upon alternative therapies may not feel comfortable discussing these with their health care providers. If health care providers are not aware of other treatment methods, a number of complications may arise.

STRATEGIES THAT DO NOT WORK

As noted elsewhere in this encyclopedia, didactic educational approaches alone do not work. Health care professionals cannot simply distribute brochures (often written in

English and at an educational level beyond many of their intended readers), nor provide didactic advice alone, and expect these efforts to promote the health of older persons.

SYNTHESIS

Primary prevention should consist of providing older adults with comprehensive educational opportunities that provide ample time for interaction and practice in the language and context in which these people are comfortable. They and their families should be encouraged to attend health education seminars about nutrition, ways to lower blood pressure as well as other educational programs offered at aging and health services organizations. However, information alone rarely changes behavior.

Health prevention programs should involve older adults in self-screening as far as possible, such as breast cancer checks and testicular checks. Lifestyle changes within specific cultural milieus should be fostered, such as healthy foods eaten in supportive social contexts, or group exercises in aquatic classes. The combination of individual efforts and various social and cultural supports in promoting healthy behavior among the older adult population is crucial.

The media can be utilized as an important tool in the education process. When developing a health promotion plan, it is important to examine the cultural values and beliefs, educational level, income, and other demographic characteristics of target population. Programs and advertisements can be strategically placed to maximize the impact of health-related messages. Television, in particular, may be one effective way of providing health information to minority populations. McConatha, Schnell, and McKenna's (1999) found that all groups of older adults watched television news more than reading the newspaper or engaging in other forms of recreation.

Health promotion practices can help a person achieve high levels of good health. This entry has focused on a number of interrelated factors which can influence an individual's decision to engage in health-promoting activities within culturally acceptable practices. There are many different paths to health and well-being. All of them require a blending of different practices that take into account the cultural background and belief systems of the persons, families, friends, neighborhoods, and the communities involved.

Also see: Age Bias: Older Adulthood; Caregiver Stress: Older Adulthood; Chronic Disease: Older Adulthood; Nutrition: Older Adulthood; Oral Health: Older Adulthood; Retirement Satisfaction: Older Adulthood; Sexuality: Older Adulthood.

References

Airhihenbuwa, C.O., Kumanyika, S., Agurs, T.D., & Lowe (1995). Perceptions and beliefs about exercise, rest, and health among African Americans. *American Journal of Heath Promotions, 9*, 426–429.

Astin, J.A. (1998). Why patients use alternative medicine. *Journal of the American Medical Association, 279*, 1548–1553.

Baltes, M., & Lang, F.R. (1997). Everyday functioning and successful aging: The impact of resources. *Psychology and Aging, 12*(3), 433–443.

Bandura, A. (1986). *Social foundations of thought and action: A social cognitive theory.* Englewood Cliffs, NJ: Prentice-Hall.

Becker, M.H. (1974). *The health belief model and personal health behavior.* Thorofare, NJ: Slack.

Brislin, R. (1993). *Understanding culture's influence on behavior.* Fort Worth, Philadelphia, New York, & Orlando: Harcourt Brace College Publishers.

Campbell, J., & Kreidler, M. (1994, December). Older adults' perceptions about wellness. *Journal of Holistic Nursing, 12*(4), 437–448.

Clark, D.O. (1996). Age, socioeconomic status, and exercise self-efficacy. *The Gerontologist, 36*, 157–164.

Diehl, M. (1998). Everyday competence in later life: Current status and future directions. *Gerontological Society of America, 38*(4), 422–433.

Eisenberg, D.M, Lessler, R.C., Foster, C., Norlock, F.E., Calkins, D.R., & Delbanco, T.L. (1993). Unconventional medicine in the United States: Prevalence, costs, and patterns of use. *The New England Journal of Medicine, 12*, 246–252.

Family Economics and Nutrition Review (1999, Summer). Poverty among women *11*(1), 71–74.

Fontane, P.E. (1996). Exercise, fitness, and feeling well. *American Behavioral Scientist, 39*, 288–305.

Green, L.W., & Ottoson, J.M. (1999). *Community and population health* (8th ed., p. 44). New York: McGraw-Hill.

Gergen, K.J. (1991). *The saturated self: Dilemmas of identity in contemporary life.* US: Basic Books.

Grossman, L.K. (1998). Aging viewers: The best is yet to come. *Columbia Journalism Review, 36*(5), 568–569.

Hobfoll, S.E., Freedy, J., Lane, C., & Geller, P. (1990). Conservation of social resources: Social support theory. *Journal of Social and Personal Relationships, 7*, 465–478.

Kaniegal, R. (1998). Aching for relief. *Health, 12*, 46–49.

Keegan, L. (2000). A comparison of the use of alternative therapies among Mexican Americans and Anglo-Americans in the Texas Rio Grande Valley. *Journal of Holistic Nursing, 18*, 280–295.

Krause, N. (1990). Perceived health problems, formal/informal support, and life satisfaction among older adults. *Journal of Gerontology: Social Sciences, 45*, 193–205.

Kubzansky, L.D., Berkman, L.F., Glass, T.A., & Seeman, T.E. (1998). Is educational attainment associated with shared determinants of health in the elderly? Findings from the MacArthur studies of successful aging. *American Psychosomatic Society, 60*, 578–585.

Light, K.M. (1997). Florence Nightingale and holistic philosophy. *Journal of Holistic Nursing, 15*, 25–40.

McConatha, J.T., McConatha, D., Deaner, S.L., & Dermigny, R. (1995). A computer-based intervention and therapy of institutionalized older adults. *Educational Gerontology, 21*, 141–150.

McConatha, J.T., Schnell, F., & McKenna, A. (1999). Description of older adults as depicted in magazine advertisements. *Psychological Reports, 85U*, 1051–1056.

O'Donnell, S.A. (1999). Hands-on migraine relief. *Prevention, 51*, 1.

Rodin, J. (1986). Aging and health: Effects of the sense of control. *Science, 23*, 1271–1276.

Rodin, J., & Langer, E.J. (1980) Aging labels: The decline of control and the fall of self-esteem. *Journal of Social Issues, 36,* 12–29.

Ruffing-Rahal, M.R., & Wallace, J. (2000). Successful aging in a wellness group for older women. *Health Care for Women International, 21*(4), 267–275.

Sarason, I.G., Levine, H.M., Basham, R.B., & Sarason, B.R. (1983). Assessing social support: The Social Support Questionnaire. *Journal of Personality and Social Psychology, 44*(1), 127–139.

Schulz, R., & Heckhausen, J. (1996). A life span model of successful aging. *American Psychologist, 51*(7), 702–714.

Siegel-Maier, K. (1999). Aromatherapy and massage. *Better Nutrition, 61,* 72–76.

Spector, R.E. (1996). *Cultural diversity in health and illness.* Stamford, CT: Appleton and Lange.

Stoller, P., & McConatha, J.T. (2001). City life: Community and social support among West Africans in New York. *Journal of Contemporary Ethnography, 30*(6), 651–678.

Yee, B., & Weaver, G.D. (1994, Spring). Ethnic minorities and health promotion: Developing a culturally competent agenda. *Generations, 18*(1), 39–44.

HIV/AIDS, Early Childhood

Deborah H. Cornman and
Blair T. Johnson

INTRODUCTION AND DEFINITIONS

Human immunodeficiency virus (HIV) and other sexually transmitted infections (STIs) are among the most common infectious diseases today, with well over 20 STIs having now been identified. Individuals become infected with STIs through contact with infected body fluids during sex, the sharing of injection drug equipment, breastfeeding, or pregnancy and delivery. The impact of STIs varies widely across diseases, from little or none (e.g., scabies, pubic lice) to moderate (e.g., human papillomavirus [HPV], gonorrhea) to life-threatening (e.g., HIV, syphilis). These diseases affect men and women of all backgrounds, ages, and economic levels, presenting wide-ranging challenges for public health around the world.

The STI that currently presents the greatest challenge worldwide is HIV, which causes AIDS, a disease that progressively destroys the body's ability to fight infections and certain cancers and usually results in death. Although healthy individuals rarely succumb to these "opportunistic" infections, the weakened immune systems that characterize people with AIDS render them more susceptible to infections and less able to fight them off. Concurrent infection with other STIs weakens their immune system even more and worsens their prognosis. Fortunately, the use of antiretroviral drug therapies can prevent or delay the onset of AIDS and significantly prolong the lifespan of those who are living with HIV.

Most HIV-infected people unknowingly carry the virus for years, only learning about their status when enough damage has been done to the immune system to result in AIDS. Consequently, they may infect many others with the virus during those years when they are unaware of their own infection. Because there is currently no vaccine to prevent the acquisition of HIV and no cure to eradicate the virus once it is contracted, the only effective way to prevent HIV transmission at this point is through behavior change.

Due to the seriousness of the HIV/AIDS pandemic, the current entry and the four that follow it will focus primarily on prevention of HIV/AIDS, with less attention given to other STIs. Generally, though, prevention of HIV/AIDS is similar to prevention of many of the other STIs, so HIV/AIDS prevention recommendations that appear here logically extend to other STIs. It is important to note that preventive recommendations for HIV/AIDS and other STIs vary widely across the lifespan, owing to both the different routes with which these diseases can be acquired (e.g., sharing drug injection equipment vs. perinatally vs. sexual intercourse) and the differing cognitive capacities of the targeted group (e.g., infants vs. adolescents vs. adults vs. the elderly).

SCOPE

Since the beginning of the HIV epidemic, an estimated 21.8 million people have died from AIDS worldwide, and 4.3 million of those have been children less than 15 years of age (UNAIDS, 2000). During 1999 alone, 500,000 children died from AIDS and 620,000 children became newly infected, resulting in a total of 1.3 million children living with HIV/AIDS. UNAIDS reported that 2.4 million HIV-infected women give birth annually throughout the world, and that approximately 600,000 of their children are infected with HIV through mother-to-child transmission. Thus, about 1,600 children per day become infected with HIV perinatally. Over 90 percent of these HIV-infected children are living in sub-Saharan Africa, but the rate of infection of children is growing rapidly in southeast Asia as well. If the spread of HIV is not contained in these and other developing countries, it is projected that by 2010, infant mortality will increase by 25 percent, and the mortality of children under five will increase by 100 percent (McIntyre, 1998).

Over 90 percent of HIV-infected children less than 15 years of age became infected through mother-to-child transmission (UNAIDS, 1996). These children acquired the virus either in the uterus (antepartum), at the time of labor and delivery (intrapartum), or during breastfeeding (postpartum). Most perinatal transmission is believed to occur close to or during childbirth (Mofenson, 1997). Studies have reported that 30–50 percent of infants who contract HIV do so in utero, and 50–70 percent acquire HIV during the intrapartum period (Cao et al., 1997; Mayaux, Dussaix et al., 1997a).

Prior to the US Public Health Service recommendation to use antiretroviral medications with HIV-infected pregnant women and their newborns (see below), the rates of transmission of HIV from mother to child ranged from 15 to 40 percent, with some variation across geographical areas (Connor et al., 1994; Working Group on Mother-to-Child Transmission of HIV, 1995). For example, perinatal transmission rates were reported to be 15 percent in Europe, 25 percent in the United States, and 40 percent in Africa. However, with the advent of routine antiretroviral therapy use in many developed countries, much lower transmission rates are now being reported in those countries—as low as 2 percent (Simonds et al., 1998). The transmission rates continue to remain high, however, in developing and resource-poor countries. In South Africa, for example, prevention efforts have been unable to keep up with the rate of new infection in children, which is as high as 45 percent in some areas. Pediatric wards of hospitals there are overflowing with infants and children who are dying from AIDS (Matchaba & Chapanduka, 1997).

THEORIES AND RESEARCH

Behavioral theories and supporting research will be discussed in succeeding entries. This section will focus predominantly on prevention from a medical/biological perspective.

STRATEGIES: OVERVIEW

This section will discuss three strategies that work in settings that can support them, especially developed nations. In addition, it will enumerate the various barriers that exist in many developing nations to fully implementing these strategies and the modifications that are being utilized to overcome these barriers.

Since the vast majority of HIV-infected children acquire HIV from their mothers through perinatal transmission, the primary strategy for preventing pediatric HIV infection should be the prevention of HIV infection in women of childbearing age. Because the majority of these women become infected through unprotected heterosexual intercourse, it is important to offer primary prevention programs that provide information about HIV/AIDS and its prevention, promote safer sex and the use of condoms, and provide access to facilities that can diagnose and treat other STIs that can significantly increase the risk of HIV transmission (see HIV/AIDS: Adolescence by Marsh, Johnson, & Carey). In addition, policies and programs that are aimed at improving women's status in society should also be prioritized because women's social and economic vulnerability ultimately makes them and their children susceptible to HIV as well.

STRATEGIES THAT WORK

Once a woman becomes infected, however, there are other interventions that need to be implemented to minimize the risk of transmission to her newborn. The remainder of this entry will focus on those prevention interventions— interventions that help to reduce the risk of mother-to-child transmission from women already infected with HIV. Fortunately, a great deal of progress has been made in this domain. To minimize the risk of transmission, three different preventive interventions have been demonstrated to be effective: (1) the use of antiretroviral medications during pregnancy, delivery, and following birth, (2) delivery by caesarean section, and (3) avoiding breastfeeding and using breast milk replacements after delivery. These three strategies have been found to dramatically decrease mother-to-child transmission of HIV. Although all three of these strategies have been effectively implemented in developed nations such as the United States and Europe, there are many barriers to their implementation in resource-poor areas such as South Africa.

Maternal Therapeutic Intervention as Prevention of HIV in Fetuses and Newborns: Antiretroviral Therapy

In February 1994, the Pediatric AIDS Clinical Trials Group (PACTG) reported the preliminary findings from Protocol 076, which was a randomized, double-blind, placebo-controlled study of the effectiveness of zidovudine (ZDV) in preventing mother-to-child transmission of HIV-1 (Connor et al., 1994). The risk of mother-to-child, or perinatal, HIV-1 transmission was reduced by two thirds with the use of a three-part regimen of ZDV, from 25 percent in infants of women who received the placebo to 8 percent in infants of women who received ZDV. This regimen included oral ZDV initiated at 14–34 weeks' gestation and continued for the duration of the pregnancy, followed by intravenous ZDV started at the onset of and continued throughout labor, and then oral ZDV administered to the infant for the first 6 weeks of the infant's life. None of the women in this study breastfed their infants after birth, which also protected their infants from HIV transmission. Subsequent research demonstrated that the use of ZDV can significantly reduce the risk of HIV transmission in both breastfeeding and non-breastfeeding women, as well as in women with advanced HIV disease, low CD4+ or T-cell counts (indicative of a weakened immune system), and prior ZDV therapy (Stiehm et al., 1999).

Based on these results, in the August of 1994, the United States Public Health Service (PHS) recommended that the PACTG076 ZDV regimen be "discussed with and offered" to all HIV-1 infected women for the purpose of reducing the risk of perinatal transmission (Centers for Disease Control and Prevention [CDC], 1994). A year later, the PHS also recommended universal HIV-1 prenatal counseling and voluntary HIV-1 testing for all pregnant women in the United States (CDC, 1995). Subsequent epidemiological studies in the United States and France have demonstrated that the incorporation of this PACTG 076 ZDV regimen into general clinical practice along with increased prenatal HIV-1 counseling and testing have resulted in dramatic declines in perinatal transmission rates to as low as 4–6 percent (Mayaux, Teglas et al., 1997b), with few adverse toxic or safety effects being found on a short-term basis (i.e., up to 6 years following birth) for either the recipient women or their infants (Connor et al., 1994; Culnane et al., 1999). Long-term safety for children exposed in utero to ZDV has not yet been determined, however, and long-term follow-up studies of children are needed. Based on data from rodent studies, some scholars have expressed concern about the potential long-term toxicity of ZDV, including the potential for carcinogenic effects (e.g., Ayers, Torrey, & Reynolds, 1997).

Since the PACTG 076 study in 1994, other significant advances have been made in understanding the pathogenesis of HIV-1 infection as well as in the treatment of the disease. Research has shown that the most effective way to prevent the virus from replicating, to maintain the strength of the immune system, and to minimize the chances for the virus to become resistant to the medications is to start the patient early in his/her disease on an aggressive combination of antiretroviral medications (Havlir & Richman, 1996). Combination drug therapy is now the currently recommended standard treatment for HIV-1 infected adults who are not pregnant. This therapy usually consists of a protease inhibitor used in combination with two nucleoside analogue reverse transcriptase inhibitors (Office of Public Health and Science, 1997). Combination therapy has been found to reduce or maintain the viral load, or the level of HIV virus in the blood, at very low levels.

In January 1998, the PHS Task Force new guidelines concluded that "pregnancy is not a reason to defer standard therapy" and recommended that standard antiretroviral therapy be "discussed with and offered" to all HIV-1 infected pregnant women (CDC, 1998). According to these guidelines, monotherapy, or treating a person with a single medication such as ZDV, is suboptimal for treatment (Office of Public Health and Science, 1997). Consequently, an increasing proportion of HIV-infected women in the United States and Europe are receiving combination antiretroviral therapy during pregnancy for the benefit of their own health.

Moreover, evidence now suggests that combination therapy may benefit the infant as well, with perinatal HIV transmission rates at least as low as those produced by the PACTG 076 protocol (e.g., Khoury, Kovacs, Stek, Kramer, & Homans, 1998). Specifically, research has found that women who have low or undetectable viral loads (i.e., <1,000 copies/mL) have very low rates of perinatal transmission, which suggests that there are significant benefits to the infant if the mother adheres to her antiretroviral therapy (e.g., Garcia et al., 1999). For many of these antiretroviral drugs, however, the short- and long-term effects on the fetus and newborn are unknown, which has made the decision about the use of antiretroviral medications very complex. It has become a delicate balancing act between effectively treating the mother's HIV-1 infection and reducing perinatal transmission. PHS has recommended that drug choice be individualized and based on careful consideration of the mother's health, the fetus' health, and the risks and benefits associated with the available antiretroviral drugs (CDC, 1998). When evaluating the potential harm of the drug to the fetus, many factors must be taken into account, including the dosage taken, the gestational age of the fetus when exposed to the drug, the duration of the exposure, the interaction between the drugs and other agents to which the fetus is exposed, and the genetic make-up of the mother and fetus.

The three-part zidovudine regimen has contributed to a declining perinatal HIV-1 transmission rate in North America and Western Europe, but a comparable decline has not been observed thus far in less-developed countries due to the regimen's expense and complexity of usage (Mofenson & McIntyre, 2000). As a result, several simpler and less expensive short-course antiretroviral regimens have been developed for use in resource-poor countries. Short-course therapy with ZDV, whether given from 36 weeks until delivery or from delivery until one week postpartum, appears to decrease transmission risk by approximately 40–50 percent. This reduction was observed whether or not the mother breastfed, although the reduction was smaller in breastfeeding populations (e.g., Dabis et al., 1999; Shaffer et al., 1999). Similarly, in studies of HIV-infected women who breastfed their infants, the use of a short-course combination regimen of ZDV and lamivudine (3TC) reduced the risk of perinatal transmission by 38–50 percent (Saba, 1999). Thus, both short-course oral ZDV and short-course ZDV plus 3TC appear to be successful at reducing mother-to-infant HIV transmission and are feasible for use in developing countries.

Obstetric Intervention: Caesarean Section versus Vaginal Delivery

Strong evidence has emerged that HIV-infected women with "elective" caesarean section delivery—caesarean section performed before rupture of membranes and before onset of labor—are at significantly lower risk of transmitting HIV infection to their children. More specifically, the International Perinatal Group (1999) reviewed over 8,000 births from 15 studies and found that there was a 57 percent lower risk of transmission of HIV when caesarean delivery was performed before the onset of labor and membrane rupture, and an 87 percent lower risk among the women who were also receiving the PACTG 076 ZDV regimen. Transmission rates of 2 percent or less have been consistently reported when the ZDV regimen is combined with elective caesarean delivery (European Mode of Delivery Collaboration, 1999; International Perinatal HIV Group, 1999; Women and Infants Transmission Study Investigators, 1999). Based on these and other findings, in 1999, the Committee on Obstetric Practice of The American College of Obstetricians and Gynecologists (ACOG) recommended that HIV-infected women be offered elective, or scheduled, caesarean section delivery to reduce the risk of vertical transmission of HIV. Elective caesarean section lowers transmission rates by protecting the infant from direct contact with the mother's genital tract secretions and blood, which may contain HIV. In 2000, ACOG then modified their recommendations and stated that cesarean section should only be considered for women with viral loads above 1,000 copies/mL. Because women with low or undetectable viral loads typically have low rates of transmission, it is unlikely that the addition of a scheduled cesarean delivery would reduce those rates any further (Perinatal HIV Guidelines Working Group, 2001).

Although caesarean section provides protection against mother-to-child transmission, it is accompanied by an increased risk of maternal morbidity and mortality compared with vaginal delivery, which is true whether or not the mother is HIV-infected (Nielsen & Hokegaard, 1983). The risks include maternal hemorrhage (uncontrolled bleeding), infection, and other complications. Further research is needed to determine whether HIV serostatus affects the extent to which women experience these complications. At this point, the decision about what type of delivery is best for both mother and baby remains a matter of medical opinion and personal choice. It is also a matter of availability, as elective caesarean section is not readily available in most developing countries where the HIV prevalence is very high.

Modification of Breastfeeding Practice

Although the mechanisms of HIV transmission through breast milk are not yet fully understood, the transmission of HIV through breastfeeding has been well documented (e.g., Van de Perre et al., 1991). It is estimated that 200,000 infants a year worldwide acquire HIV through breastfeeding. Breastfeeding in developing countries is particularly problematic because it is an extremely high-prevalence behavior and thus is responsible for a high proportion of mother-to-child transmissions. Specifically, UNAIDS reported that one in seven children born to HIV-positive mothers in developing countries are infected through breast milk (1997). Studies of HIV-positive women estimate that, beyond the risk of transmission that occurs during pregnancy and delivery, the added risk of transmission from the breast milk of women with "established HIV infection" is approximately 15 percent (Bertolli et al., 1996; Dunn, Newell, Ades, & Peckham, 1992). The risk of transmission from the breast milk of women with "recent infection"—HIV infection that was acquired during the postpartum period—is about 29 percent, most likely due to the increased viral load caused by new infections (Sepou et al., 1998; Dunn et al., 1992).

These findings suggest that breastfeeding can actually double the transmission rate, and it may be the main reason for the difference in transmission rates between developed and developing countries. For example, the highest rates of mother-to-child transmission have been found in women in sub-Saharan Africa; there the rates are as high as 45 percent (vs. a maximum of 15–25 percent in Europe and the United States). The fact that many women in Africa breastfeed for about 2 years could account for most of the increased rate of transmission that is found there.

On the surface, the solution to this problem seems simple: have HIV-positive mothers avoid breastfeeding altogether and feed their infants with breast milk replacements such as commercial infant formula or homemade infant formula. In developed nations, this viable option has in fact been adopted by the majority of HIV-positive mothers. In resource-poor developing countries, in contrast, the situation is much more complex. The use of breast milk replacements is often not feasible because of cost (e.g., breast milk substitutes are not affordable), practical considerations (e.g., nutritionally adequate substitutes are not consistently available, or there is no access to clean water for making the milk replacement), and cultural reasons (e.g., there is a stigma attached to not breastfeeding) (Nicoll, Newell, Van Praag, Van de Perre, & Peckham, 1995).

Overall, breastfeeding plays an important role in the health of both the mother and her child that cannot be ignored when making the decision to stop breastfeeding. Specifically, breastfeeding contributes to maternal health by prolonging the interval between births and by helping to protect the mother from developing ovarian or breast cancer. For the child, breast milk provides the nutrition that the child needs in order to thrive and grow. These nutrients can of course be supplied by acceptable milk replacements. However, milk replacements cannot replace maternal antibodies, which can protect the child against common childhood illnesses such as diarrhea, pneumonia, neonatal sepsis, acute otitis media, and other potentially fatal diseases (Golding, Emmett, & Rogers, 1997; Goldman, 1993). There is a presumption, as yet undemonstrated, that the breast milk of HIV-infected women also protects their children against these infectious diseases.

In response to the debate over HIV-infected mothers and breastfeeding, UNAIDS, WHO, and UNICEF issued a joint policy statement on HIV and breastfeeding in 1997, supporting breastfeeding but encouraging extensive counseling for pregnant women who are HIV-positive. They suggested several infant feeding options for possible use by HIV-positive mothers including (1) replacement feeding with commercial formula or homemade formula; (2) breastfeeding exclusively and stopping early when the infant is 3–6 months old; (3) conventional breastfeeding; (4) use of pasteurized, or heat-treated, expressed breast-milk; and (5) wet-nursing by an HIV-negative woman. In some countries, milk banks—places where women donate breast milk—also are an option, as long as the breast milk has been evaluated to be safe.

Research has yet to demonstrate the exact relationship between the risk of transmission and the duration of breastfeeding, but current evidence suggests that the risk of transmission increases the longer the child continues to breastfeed (Taha et al., 1998; Leroy, Newell, & Dabis, 1998). Thus, one option for reducing transmission risk is for HIV-infected women to stop breastfeeding when their infants are 3–6 months old. The child thus avoids the cumulative risk of longer breastfeeding duration, and the health hazards for the child of not consuming breast milk are fewer at this age than at birth (Leroy et al., 1998).

Other research is relevant to the manner in which the breast milk is consumed. First, breastfeeding exclusively with no other food or drink provided to the infant appears to be less likely to transmit HIV than mixed feeding, apparently because other foods can cause abrasions in the mucous linings of the infant's digestive tract, which make it easier for HIV to enter the infant's bloodstream (Coutsoudis,

Pillary, Spooner, Kuhn, & Coovadia, 1999). Second, heating breast milk that contains HIV to 62.5°C for 30 min has been found to dramatically reduce the amount of infectious virus in the milk (Orloff, Wallingford, & McDougal, 1993). Similarly, HIV appears to be inactivated when the breast milk is left at room temperature for 30 min (Orloff et al., 1993). Further research is needed to determine how these findings can be applied in real-world settings.

In their 1997 policy statement, UNAIDS, UNICEF, and WHO recommended that mothers be provided with all of the available information on the advantages and disadvantages of breastfeeding with regard to HIV infection so they can make a fully informed decision about infant feeding. The infant-feeding method chosen has significant health and financial implications for the entire family, so it is important that all of the facts are known. If an HIV-infected mother has continuous access to affordable and nutritionally adequate breast milk replacements, and if she can safely prepare the replacements and feed them to her child, then it would clearly place her child at less risk of illness and death not to be breastfed. However, if these conditions are not met, then the benefits of breast milk replacements may not outweigh the benefits of breastfeeding, especially in settings where infectious diseases and malnutrition are the primary causes of death during infancy. In these settings, artificial feeding may actually increase the child's risk of illness and death.

SYNTHESIS

The main HIV transmission mode for children younger than 15 years of age is perinatal, or mother-to-child. It is clear that the primary means of preventing HIV in children is to prevent it in their mothers. However, if these prevention efforts are not successful, then there are demonstrated effective strategies for reducing the risk of transmission from mother to child. The first of these strategies involves making voluntary HIV counseling and testing available to all pregnant women. Because research has shown that treatment with antiretrovirals during pregnancy reduces the risk of HIV transmission to the infant, it is important to be able to identify those women who are living with HIV. This does not mean, however, that testing and counseling should necessarily be mandatory, because requiring testing may make women reluctant to seek out prenatal care or treatment for their HIV, particularly in developing countries where being HIV-positive is highly stigmatizing. Thus, HIV counseling and testing must be a voluntary, confidential, free-of-charge service that women are encouraged but not mandated to use.

Recommendations for the next set of strategies vary as a function of whether the mother is from a developed country such as the United States or a resource-poor developing country such as South Africa. When it comes to mother-to-child transmission, the HIV epidemic has traveled divergent paths in developed and developing countries. In developed countries, the use of antiretroviral medications during pregnancy and delivery in conjunction with elective caesarean sections and replacement breast milk has significantly reduced the incidence of vertical transmission from 25 to 2 percent or less. Unfortunately, these successes have yet to be realized in developing nations. Significant barriers exist to the use of these strategies in these resource-poor countries, and the result has been that a comparable decrease in the incidence of mother-to-child transmission has not occurred. To the contrary, as progressively more and more women have become infected with HIV in developing nations, the number of children acquiring HIV through perinatal transmission has increased.

In these countries, where HIV prevalence is high and resources are few, UNAIDS, UNICEF, and WHO (1998) jointly recommended that a six-step intervention be used to reduce the risk of mother-to-child transmission, modifying successful strategies from developed countries to make them simpler and less costly. Besides voluntary and confidential counseling and testing, the intervention includes early access to prenatal care, a short- as opposed to a long-course of ZDV treatment given to the mother in the last weeks of pregnancy and during delivery, improved care during labor and delivery, counseling for the mother on alternative methods of infant feeding, and support for any mother who chooses not to breastfeed. This intervention is currently being evaluated for its feasibility and effectiveness.

At the present time, prevention research makes it clear that any preventive intervention to reduce the risk of mother-to-child transmission must be customized to meet the needs of the individual within her culture. Developing an intervention that is biologically sound is useless if there are social, cultural, political, financial, psychological, and practical barriers that prevent its use. Theoretically, we understand enough about mother-to-child transmission to prevent children from becoming infected with HIV. Practically, we are faced with numerous and complex challenges that make it extremely difficult to put this knowledge into practice.

Also see: HIV/AIDS: Childhood; HIV/AIDS: Adolescence; HIV/AIDS: Adulthood; HIV/AIDS: Older Adulthood.

References

American College of Obstetricians and Gynecologists (ACOG). (1999, August). *Scheduled cesarean delivery and the prevention of vertical transmission of HIV infection* (ACOG Committee Opinion Number 219). Washington, DC: Author.

American College of Obstetricians and Gynecologists (ACOG). (2000, May). *Scheduled cesarean delivery and the prevention of vertical transmission of HIV infection* (ACOG Committee Opinion Number 234). Washington, DC: Author.

Ayers, K.M., Torrey, C.E., & Reynolds, D.J. (1997). A transplacental carcinogenicity bioassay in Cd-1 mice with zidovudine. *Fundamental and Applied Toxicology, 38,* 195–198.

Bertolli, J., St. Louis, M.E., Simonds, R.J., Nieburg, P., Kamenga, M., Brown, C., Tarande, M., & Quinn, T. (1996). Estimating the timing of mother-to-child transmission of human immunodeficiency virus in a breast-feeding population in Kinshasa, Zaire. *Journal of Infectious Diseases, 174,* 722–726.

Cao, Y., Krogstad, P., Korber, B.T., Koup, R.A., Muldoon, M., Macken, C., Song, J.L., Jin, Z., & Zhao, J.Q. (1997). Maternal HIV-1 viral load and vertical transmission of infection: The Ariel Project for the prevention of HIV transmission from mother to infant. *Nature Medicine, 3,* 549–552.

Centers for Disease Control and Prevention (CDC). (1994). Recommendations of the Public Health Service Task Force on the use of zidovudine to reduce perinatal transmission of human immunodeficiency virus. *MMWR, 43*(RR-11), 1–21.

Centers for Disease Control and Prevention (CDC). (1995). Public Health Service recommendations for human immunodeficiency virus counseling and voluntary testing for pregnant women. *MMWR, 44*(RR-7), 1–14.

Centers for Disease Control and Prevention (CDC). (1998). Public Health Service Task Force recommendations for the use of antiretroviral drugs in pregnant women infected with HIV-1 for maternal health and for reducing perinatal HIV-1 transmission in the United States. *MMWR, 47*(RR-2), 1–30.

Connor, E.M., Sperling, R.S., Gelber, R., Kiselev, P., Scott, H., O'Sullivan, M.J., VanDyke, R., & Bey, M. (1994). Reduction of maternal-infant transmission of human immunodeficiency virus type I with zidovudine treatment. Pediatric AIDS Clinical Trials Group Protocol 076 Study Group. *New England Journal of Medicine, 331,* 1173–1180.

Coutsoudis, A., Pillary, K., Spooner, E., Kuhn, L., & Coovadia, H.M. (1999). Influence of infant-feeding patterns on early mother-to-child transmission of HIV-1 in Durban, South Africa: A prospective cohort study. *The Lancet, 354,* 471–476.

Culnane, M., Fowler, M., Lee, S.S., McSherry, G., Brady, M., O'Donnell, K., Mofenson, L., Gortmaker, S.L., Shapiro, D.E., Scott, G., Jimenez, E., Moore, E.C., Diaz, C., Flynn, P.M., Cunningham, B., & Oleske, J. (1999). Lack of long-term effects of in utero exposure to zidovudine among uninfected children born to HIV-infected women. *Journal of the American Medical Association, 281*(2), 151–157.

Dabis, F., Msellati, P., Meda, N., Welffens-Ekra, C., You, B., Manigart, O., Leroy, V., Simonon, A., Cartoux, M., Combe, P., Ouangre, A., Ramon, R., Ky-Zerbo, O., Montcho, C., Salamon, R., Rouzioux, C., Van-de-Perre, P., & Mandelbrot, L. (1999). 6-month efficacy, tolerance and acceptability of a short regimen of oral zidovudine to reduce vertical transmission of HIV in breastfed children in Côte d'Ivoire and Burkina Faso: A double-blind placebo-controlled multicentre trial. *The Lancet, 353,* 786–792.

Dunn, D.T., Newell, M.L., Ades, A.E., & Peckham, C.S. (1992). Risk of human immunodeficiency virus type 1 transmission through breast-feeding. *The Lancet, 340,* 585–588.

European Mode of Delivery Collaboration. (1999). Elective caesarean-section versus vaginal delivery in prevention of vertical HIV-1 transmission: A randomized clinical trial. *The Lancet, 353,* 1035–1039.

Garcia, P.M., Kalish, L.A., Pitt, J., Minkoff, H., Quinn, T.C., Burchett, S.K., Kornegay, J., Jackson, B., Moye, J., Hanson, C., Zorrilla, C., & Lew, J.F. (1999). Maternal levels of plasma human immunodeficiency virus type 1 RNA and the risk of perinatal transmission. *New England Journal of Medicine, 341*(6), 394–402.

Golding, J., Emmett, P.M., & Rogers, I.S. (1997). Breastfeeding and infant mortality. *Early Human Development, 49*(Suppl.), S143–S155.

Goldman, A. (1993). The immune system of human milk: Antimicrobial, anti-inflammatory and immunomodulating properties. *Pediatric Infectious Disease Journal, 12*, 664–671.

Havlir, D.V., & Richman, D.D. (1996). Viral dynamics of HIV: Implications for drug development and therapeutic strategies. *Annals of Internal Medicine, 124*, 984–994.

International Perinatal HIV Group. (1999). The mode of delivery and the risk of vertical transmission of human immunodeficiency virus type 1: A meta-analysis of 15 prospective cohort studies. *New England Journal of Medicine, 340*, 977–987.

Khoury, M., Kovacs, A., Stek, A., Kramer, F., & Homans, J. (1998, July). *Combination therapy with nevirapine, zidovudine and a second nucleoside analog during pregnancy.* (Abstract No. 463/12152). Paper Presented at Twelfth World AIDS Conference, Geneva, Switzerland.

Leroy, V., Newell, M.L., & Dabis, F. (1998). International multicentre pooled analysis of late postnatal mother-to-child transmission of HIV infection. *The Lancet, 352*, 597–600.

Matchaba, P.T., & Chapanduka, Z.C. (1997). Paediatric AIDS—is now not the right time to act? *South African Medical Journal, 87*, 1343–1345.

Mayaux, M.J., Dussaix, E., Isopet, J., Rekacewicz, C., Mandelbrot, L., Ciraru-Vigneron, N., & Allemon, M.C. (1997a). Maternal virus load during pregnancy and the mother-to-child transmission of human immunodeficiency virus type: The French Perinatal Cohort Studies. *Journal of Infectious Diseases, 175*, 172–175.

Mayaux, J.M., Teglas, J.P., Mandelbrot, L., Berrebi, A., Gallais, H., Matheron, S., & Ciraru-Vigneron, N. (1997b). Acceptability and impact of zidovudine for prevention of mother-to-child human immunodeficiency virus-1 transmission in France. *Journal of Pediatrics, 131*, 857–862.

McIntyre, J. (1998). *HIV in pregnancy: A review.* Geneva: World Health Organization, & Joint United Nations Programme on HIV/AIDS (UNAIDS).

Mofenson, L.M. (1997). Interaction between timing of perinatal human immunodeficiency virus infection and the design of preventive and therapeutic interventions. *Acta Paediatrics, 491*(Suppl.), 1–9.

Mofenson, L.M., & McIntyre, J.A. (2000). Advances and research directions in the prevention of mother-to-child HIV-1 transmission. *The Lancet, 355*, 2237–2244.

Nicoll, A., Newell, M.L., Van Praag, E., Van de Perre, P., & Peckham, C. (1995). Infant feeding policy and practice in the presence of HIV-1 infection. *AIDS, 9*, 107–119.

Nielsen, T.F., & Hokegaard, K.H. (1983). Postoperative cesarean section morbidity: A prospective study. *American Journal of Obstetrics and Gynecology, 146*, 911–915.

Office of Public Health and Science, Department of Health and Human Services. (1997). Guidelines for the use of antiretroviral agents in HIV-infected adults. *Federal Register, 62*, 33417–33418.

Orloff, S.L., Wallingford, J.C., & McDougal, J.S. (1993). Inactivation of human immunodeficiency virus type 1 in human milk: Effect of intrinsic factors in human milk and of pasteurization. *Journal of Human Lactation, 9*, 13–17.

Perinatal HIV Guidelines Working Group. (2001, May 4). Public Health Service Task Force recommendations for use of antiretroviral drugs in pregnant HIV-1-infected women for maternal health and interventions to reduce perinatal HIV-1 transmission in the United States. *HIV/AIDS Treatment Information Service (ATIS).* Retrieved July 5, 2001 from http://www.hivatis.org/guidelines/perinatal/May03_01/PerinatalMay04_01.pdf.

Saba, J. (1999). Interim analysis of early efficacy of three short ZDV/3TC combination regimens to prevent mother-to-child transmission of HIV-1: The PETRA trial. (Abstract No. S7). Paper Presented at 6th Conference on Retroviruses and Opportunistic Infections, Geneva, Switzerland.

Sepou, A., Becquart, P., Hocini, H., Belec, L., Matta, M., Kazatchkine, M., Barre-Sinoussi, F., Brogan, T. & Garin., B. (1998, February). *Early postnatal mother-to-child transmission of HIV-1 in Bangui, Central African Republic.* (Abstract 242). Paper Presented at 5th Conference on Retroviruses and Opportunistic Infections, Chicago, IL.

Shaffer, N., Chuachoowong, R., Mock, P.A., Bhadrakom, C., Siriwasin, W., Young, N.L., Chotpitayasunondh, T.. Chearskul, S., Roongpisuthipong, A., Chinayon, P., Karon, J., Mastro, T.D., & Simonds, R.J. (1999). Short-course zidovudine for perinatal HIV-1 transmission in Bangkok, Thailand: A randomized controlled trial. *The Lancet, 353*, 773–780.

Simonds, R.J., Steketee, R., Nesheim, S., Matheson, P., Palumbo, P., Alger, L., Abrams, E.J., Orloff, S., Lindsay, M., Bardeguez, A., Vink, P., Byers, R., & Rogers, M. (1998). Impact of zidovudine use on risk and risk factors for perinatal transmission of HIV. *AIDS, 12*(3), 301–308.

Stiehm, E.R. Lambert, J.S., Mofenson, L.M., Bethel, J., Whitehouse, J., Nugent, R., Moye, J., Glenn-Fowler, M., Mathieson, B.J., Reichelderfer, P., Nemo, G.J., Korelitz, J., Meyer, W.A., Sapan, C.V., Jimenez, E., Gandia, J., Scott, G., O'Sullivan, M.J., Kovacs, A., Stek, A., Shearer, W.T., & Hammill, H. (1999). Efficacy of zidovudine and hyperimmune HIV immunoglobulin for reducing perinatal HIV transmission from HIV-infected women with advanced disease: Results of pediatric AIDS clinical trials group protocol 185. *Journal of Infectious Diseases, 179*, 567–575.

Taha, T., Miotti, P., Markakis, D., Kumwenda, N., Van der Hoeven, H., Biggar, R., & Hoover, D. (1998, July). *HIV infection due to breastfeeding in a cohort of babies not infected at enrollment.* (Abstract 23270). Paper Presented at XII International Conference on AIDS, Geneva, Switzerland.

UNAIDS. (1996). *HIV/AIDS: The global epidemic.* (Fact Sheet). Geneva: Joint United Nations Programme on HIV/AIDS.

UNAIDS. (1998, June 29). *New initiative to reduce HIV transmission from mother to child in low-income countries.* Geneva: Joint United Nations Programme on HIV/AIDS.

UNAIDS. (2000, December). *AIDS epidemic update: December 2000.* Geneva: Joint United Nations Programme on HIV/AIDS.

UNAIDS, UNICEF, & WHO. (1997). *HIV and infant feeding. A policy statement developed collaboratively by UNAIDS, UNICEF and WHO.* Retrieved January 12, 2001, from http://www.unaids.org/publications/documents/mtct/infantpole.html

Van de Perre, P., Simonon, A., Msellati, P., Hitimana, D.G., Vaira, D., Bazubagira, A., Van Goethem, C., Stevens, A.M., Karita, E., & Sondag-Thull, D. (1991). Postnatal transmission of human immunodeficiency virus type 1 from mother to infant. A prospective cohort study in Kigali, Rwanda. *New England Journal of Medicine, 325*, 593–598.

Women and Infants Transmission Study Investigators. (1999, September). *Trends in mother-to-infant transmission of HIV in the WITS cohort: Impact of 076 and HAART therapy.* (Abstract 212). Paper Presented at 2nd Conference on Global Strategies for the Prevention of HIV Transmission from Mothers to Infants, Montreal, Canada.

Working Group on Mother-to-Child Transmission of HIV. (1995). Rates of mother-to-child transmission of HIV-1 in Africa, America and Europe: Results from 13 perinatal studies. *Journal of Acquired Immune Deficiency Syndromes and Human Retrovirology, 8*, 506–510.

HIV/AIDS, Childhood

Angela Bryan and Blair T. Johnson

INTRODUCTION AND DEFINITIONS

This entry reviews research and knowledge relating to the development and implementation of HIV/AIDS prevention programs for school-aged children. The entry reviews the scope of the problem and outlines the current recommendations for effective HIV/AIDS prevention programs for school-aged children, those between the ages of 6 and 12.

SCOPE

The HIV/AIDS pandemic has had devastating effects on the world's children (UNICEF, 2000). Organizations such as UNAIDS and UNICEF expect that in hardest-hit countries, namely Botswana, Namibia, and Zimbabwe, half of all 15-year-olds alive today will eventually die of the disease (UNAIDS, 2000). UNAIDS estimates that over 600,000 children were infected with HIV in 1999, and 1.3 million children are currently living with HIV or AIDS. Many more children are affected by the epidemic, in that they have lost their parents to the disease. To date, more than 13 million children have lost one or both parents to AIDS, and estimates suggest that before the end of the next decade this figure may bulge to 30 million.

The picture is not so bleak in the industrialized world, but HIV/AIDS among children still presents a substantial public health threat. In the United States, the number of pediatric AIDS cases has been reduced dramatically, from 945 cases reported in 1992 to only 155 reported in 1999 (CDC, 2000a). This decrease is largely due to the use of zidovudine (AZT) during pregnancy amongst HIV+ women. Despite these advances, the CDC estimates that over 5,000 children under the age of 13 are currently living with HIV or AIDS. More important from a prevention standpoint, a large percentage of HIV infections are detected in early adulthood (e.g., 21–30 years). Given the latency from infection to detection of the HIV virus, these figures suggest that patterns of risk behavior established in late childhood and early adolescence place young people at high risk for HIV infection later in life. For these reasons, UNAIDS (1997) urged that HIV prevention programs, and particularly school-based HIV prevention programs, be implemented "at the earliest possible age, and certainly before the onset of sexual activity" (p. 2). Recent reports in the United States suggest that average age of first intercourse is approximately 16 years old, and in higher risk groups, such as criminally involved adolescents, first intercourse occurs between the ages of 12 and 14. Thus, both parents and schools must undertake HIV prevention efforts, preferably before children reach the age of 12; these efforts can have the added benefit of protection from sexually transmitted diseases (STDs). The focus of this entry is the current state of HIV prevention efforts for these young people. Specifically, we review HIV prevention programs for children between the ages of 6 and 12. Given the extremely high costs associated with HIV/AIDS in both economic and personal terms, it is crucially important to start prevention programs early so as to avoid as many infections as possible.

THEORIES AND RESEARCH

Despite the importance of HIV/STD prevention for school-aged children, theories directed towards this group remain poorly developed. Moreover, the vast majority of all HIV prevention programs for young people, and particularly school-based programs, have been conducted with adolescents of high-school age. We could find only one example of a program conducted with school-aged children. Schonfeld, O'Hare, Perrin, Quackenbush, Showalter, and Cicchetti (1995) designed and implemented an AIDS education curriculum in a randomized controlled trial in one elementary school. The participants were children in grades ranging from kindergarten to sixth grade, and the program was developmentally tailored. The educational program involved discussions of general concepts of illness (e.g., germs, the immune system) followed by a specific discussion of the transmission and prevention of HIV and the progression of AIDS. This program was successful at increasing conceptual understanding of HIV transmission and prevention, and did not increase fears about HIV/AIDS among the children. Schonfeld et al. (1995) conclude that young children are indeed capable of understanding and processing factual information regarding HIV transmission and prevention.

Based on this program and those conducted with older adolescents, some conclusions regarding the development of effective HIV prevention programs for school-aged children are reasonable. First, the CDC guidelines for Effective School Health Education to Prevent the Spread of AIDS (CDC, 1988) recommend that HIV prevention interventions are most likely to be effective when they are integrated into a health education curriculum. The overall health education curriculum should emphasize the strong connection between personal behavior and health in all domains (e.g., sexual behavior, exercise, nutrition, substance use, etc.). Such an integrative approach to health education is expected to foster an early belief in the controllability of health outcomes later in life.

In a review of 20 years of school-based sexuality education, Kirby (1999a) concluded that simply imparting correct knowledge about sex, contraception, and disease prevention has been shown to be insufficient to influence risk behavior. While behaviorally relevant information regarding HIV transmission and prevention is a necessary component of an HIV prevention educational program (Fisher & Fisher, 2000), it is clear that increases in such knowledge are only weakly related to behavior. Thus, a focus on the complex set of skills necessary to manage sexual risk behavior becomes crucial. UNAIDS (1997) recommends a "life skills approach," wherein young people are given the self-confidence and ability to handle risky situations in all domains, including that of sexual behavior.

Importantly, the same findings applicable to all other populations targeted for HIV prevention appear to be true of school-aged children. Interventions that are theoretically and empirically based, and tailored to the population of interest, are mostly likely to be successful (Kirby, 1999b). Examples of theoretical underpinnings of successful HIV prevention programs for older adolescents and for adults include the *Theory of reasoned action/Planned behavior* (Fishbein & Ajzen, 1980; Ajzen & Madden, 1986), *Social cognitive theory* (Bandura, 1992), and the *Information-motivation-behavioral skills model* (Fisher & Fisher, 1992). Central to each of these theories is the notion that information alone is not enough, and that in order to engage in HIV prevention, individuals must have positive *attitudes* towards prevention, perceive *normative support* for prevention, have the perceived and actual *skills* (i.e., self-efficacy) necessary to engage in prevention, and have strong *intentions* to engage in preventive behavior.

At present, the exact content necessary to optimally promote each of these prevention components for children between the ages of 6 and 12 has not been empirically investigated. Recall that the work of Schonfeld et al. (1995) only examined the effectiveness of their program for increasing factual knowledge. But it is clear that such children should have developmentally appropriate information designed to increase positive attitudes, normative support, perceived self-efficacy, and intentions to engage in safer behavior. For example, a self-efficacy intervention component on the intricacies of negotiating condom use with a sexual partner, while crucial for teenagers, would be wholly inappropriate for a 10 year-old. Later in the entry, we review some suggestions made by developmental psychologists about what content an HIV prevention program for young children should contain.

A final theoretical perspective that is important when considering children's risk behavior is *Problem behavior theory* (Jessor & Jessor, 1977; Jessor, Turbin, & Costa 1998). Problem behavior theory asserts that there are multiple distal personality and environmental characteristics that serve as risk and protective factors, and that often these factors do not have obvious, content-related similarity to the risk behavior at focus (Jessor et al., 1998). For example, Jessor and colleagues have shown that distal personality factors such as high self-esteem and environmental factors such as community service involvement serve as protective factors that decrease risky behaviors including early and unprotected sexual behavior (Jessor et al., 1998). Thus, in addition to education specific to sexual risk reduction, it is crucial that efforts be made to strengthen distal protective factors including self-esteem, a sense of hope for the future, and community involvement.

STRATEGIES THAT WORK

Thus far, there are no large-scale research projects in the literature that adequately address the success of HIV prevention interventions among school-aged children. The research that does exist is largely descriptive, and typically compares "high-risk" children (e.g., children of HIV+ mothers, children of drug dependent parents, children in high seroprevalence areas) to age and gender-matched community controls (e.g., Armistead, Summers, Forehand, Morse, Morse, & Clark, 1999; Sigelman, Goldenberg, Siegel, & Dwyer, 1998). Generally speaking, young people directly affected by HIV disease tend to have slightly higher knowledge about the disease and its sequellae, but few differences in attitudes or behavior are observed. Schonfeld et al.'s (1995) study of a program for elementary school children demonstrated that knowledge levels regarding HIV/AIDS can be increased through classroom-based education, but this study did not target or measure crucial variables known to be more predictive of behavior (e.g., attitudes towards prevention, normative support for prevention, self-efficacy for prevention or intentions to engage in preventive behavior).

According to Healthy People 2010 (Wolff & Schoeberlein, 1999), schools have actually been moving farther away from the Healthy People 2000 goal of having age-appropriate HIV/STD curricula in grades K-12 in 95 percent of schools. This goal was apparently deemed too ambitious by the time of the final report, as the published goal was to have HIV/STD curricula in all grades in 90 percent of schools (Healthy People, 2010, US Department of Health and Human Services). One problem is the dearth of available curricula with proven effectiveness for children between the ages of 6 and 12.

According to a review by Wolff and Schoeberlein (1999), those middle schools that do implement any HIV prevention education at all tend to use locally developed programs with unproven efficacy. Although the CDC maintains a list of HIV/STD prevention "Programs that Work" (CDC, 2000b), all listed programs but one are targeted to older students (the exception being one community-based program appropriate for 9–15 year olds) and thus little formal information is available for developing curricula for students under the age of 12. Prevention education efforts are further hampered by local control and local decision-making, both of which are often unsupportive of HIV prevention efforts that include frank discussions of sexual issues with young people (Wolff & Schoeberlein, 1999).

STRATEGIES THAT MIGHT WORK

At this point, there are virtually no evidence-based guidelines for effective HIV prevention education with young people ages 6–12. Nonetheless, developmental psychologists, the work of Schonfeld (2000), and the CDC concur on the sort of program that is likely to lead to success in this age group. The following outline of an age-appropriate HIV/STD prevention curriculum is taken partially from Pozen (1995, pp. 249–251) and from Kirby (1999b, pp. 202–205), and includes suggestions from Schonfeld (2000).

The outline also includes specific sample content based on each of the components of the Theory of planned behavior (TPB; Ajzen & Madden, 1986) in order to demonstrate how a theoretical model guides intervention content. The TPB specifies that intentions to carry out a behavior are the most proximal predictor of engaging in the behavior. Intentions, in turn, may be determined by individuals' attitudes towards the behavior, perceptions of subjective normative support for the behavior, and perceptions of behavioral control (PBC) or self-efficacy with respect to the act in question. This model has been successfully applied to condom use in numerous studies (Albarracín, Johnson, Fishbein, & Muellerleile, 2001).

Kindergarten through Third Grade (ages 5–8). In early elementary school, there are two important goals for HIV/STD prevention education. The first is to reduce anxiety related to AIDS. Numerous descriptive studies of young children's views about HIV/AIDS suggest a high level of fear and misconception, and an overestimate of both the prevalence of HIV/AIDS and the ease with which one can contract the disease (Schonfeld, 2000). Thus, children should be taught that it is not possible to contract the disease via casual contact or insect bites, and that only very intimate contact between two people results in HIV transmission.

The second goal of HIV/STD prevention education is to lay the groundwork for healthy patterns of behavior that are linked to later risk reduction. For example, a basic description of viruses and bacteria and how they cause disease is important. Children should understand that usually the body can fight off these organisms, and sometimes we need medicines to help, but that there is currently no medicine available that will help a body completely "kill" HIV. At this point, it is appropriate to teach children the importance of good hygiene and of not touching others' blood or bodily fluids. An HIV prevention curriculum should include a drug abuse prevention component, and children at this age can be taught about the link between the abuse of alcohol and illicit drugs and the propensity to make bad decisions regarding one's health. Further, they can be taught that injection drug use is one way that the virus is spread, and that they should never touch discarded needles or syringes. Finally, the link between personal behavior and health should be stressed in order to increase self-efficacy. Children should be taught that it is both their right and their responsibility to be assertive in protecting their own health.

This is the goal to which TPB content can be directed. Interventions can include exercises encouraging positive attitudes towards being responsible for one's health, for example, that it is important, that it is a good thing to do. Telling children that their parents and teachers believe it is important for them to take responsibility for their health can generate normative support. Peer group discussions of ways in which individuals can protect their health also promote a strong descriptive norm for responsibility. Finally, fostering a sense of general self-respect and self-esteem is crucial in the development of a sense of behavioral control over and self-efficacy for protecting one's health. Finally students can be asked to describe their intentions to protect their health, and give specific examples of how they will accomplish this.

Fourth and Fifth Grades (ages 9–10). The goal of HIV/STD prevention in this age group is to prepare young people to make decisions with regard to their participation in sexual and alcohol/drug use activity. At this stage, it is appropriate to begin basic sex education, including anatomy and the physiology of reproduction. Some educators recommend that this introduction to sex education is most effective when boys and girls are taught separately. Once the basics of sexual intercourse are explained, children should be taught that this type of intimate sexual activity is a primary way that HIV and other sexually transmitted diseases are spread. The anxiety-reduction component can be re-introduced at this point both to reinforce earlier education and to highlight the ways in which HIV can be spread (e.g., sexual contact) versus the ways it cannot (e.g., hugging, sharing bathroom facilities).

More specific information regarding the link between alcohol and drug abuse and dangers associated with HIV transmission can be given at this age. Children should be taught not only about the transmission of HIV via certain types of drug use (e.g., sharing needles) but that the use of such substances can impede one's decision-making abilities and make them less likely to make healthy choices. An explanation of the effects of alcohol and illicit drugs on the body, and the process of addiction may also be appropriate. Primary education on the role of viruses and bacteria in the disease process can be increased. The role of the immune system can be made more concrete, and the general effects of HIV on the immune system can be elucidated. Children can also be taught about the formation of antibodies, and how HIV screening tests work via the detection of these antibodies in a person's blood. A continuing focus on assertiveness and responsibility training is also important, as these young people will soon encounter opportunities to engage in risky behaviors including alcohol and substance use.

Behavioral goals to be targeted by TPB intervention content can be more concrete at this stage, perhaps focusing on the ability to resist becoming sexually active and to resist involvement in drug and alcohol use. To encourage positive attitudes towards these behaviors, students can be told to list all the benefits of *not* being sexually active and of *not* being involved in drug use. Discussion can focus on abstinence as the most certain way of protecting oneself from HIV and STD infection. Normative support can again be generated by discussions about parents' and teachers' beliefs that it is important for young people to delay intercourse and refrain from drug and alcohol use. Perceived behavioral control can be enhanced through role-plays of ways to resist peer pressure to engage in sexual activity and drug or alcohol use. Young people can then write down or discuss their intentions to delay sexual activity and avoid substance use.

Sixth through Eighth Grades (ages 11–13). At this stage, the HIV/STD prevention education should be focused heavily on equipping young people with correct and specific information regarding HIV/STD transmission and prevention, positive attitudes towards important preventive behaviors such as delaying sexual intercourse or using condoms consistently, normative support for prevention from peers and important others, and an enhancement of their belief in their ability to negotiate risky situations and engage in safer behaviors. Kirby (1999b), in a review of school sexuality education programs, emphasized that successful programs incorporated goals that were appropriate to the age of the students. In the case of 11–13 year olds, depending on the demographic make-up of the young people, most are probably not sexually active, so an abstinence-focused program is most appropriate. However, a subset of this age group is very likely to become sexually active during this time frame (Aarons et al., 2000), so adequate information about effective condom and contraception use should also be included.

Exercises to enhance attitudes towards prevention behaviors should include the generation of benefits of abstinence and the benefits of condom use if one chooses to be sexually active. Young people should be asked to discuss why they believe abstinence or condom use are important in order to enhance descriptive normative support for prevention. While parents are still crucially important as sources of normative support, in the early teenage years the focus shifts from parents to peers, so believing one's peers think abstinence and/or condom use are important and is likely to heavily influence behavior. Research with adolescents across domains of risk behavior consistently shows a strong association between perception of peer norms and levels of risk behavior (Chassin, Presson, Sherman, & McConnell, 1995). In the case of sexual risk behavior, perceived peer norms are strongly related to both age at first intercourse (Kinsman, Romer, Furstenberg, & Schwarz, 1998) and frequency of condom use (Norris & Ford, 1998).

Particularly in the seventh and eighth grades, HIV prevention education should begin to focus more on specific information about the proper use of condoms including a condom demonstration in order to help young people begin to develop a sense of behavioral control over this activity. Young people this age are likely to be uncomfortable handling condoms themselves, but should be shown how to properly apply, remove, and dispose of a condom by a teacher/facilitator. Behavioral control also involves social skills for negotiating risky situations in a number of domains. These skills should be fostered in this age group, ideally using a variety of methods including role-play and rehearsal, written strategies for dealing with particular situations, and modeling by peers or facilitators of ways to communicate with peers and romantic partners regarding risk behavior (Kirby, 1999b). Such skill rehearsal can be focused on less sensitive areas first (e.g., a peer tries to get you to try a cigarette) and move on to more sensitive areas (e.g., a boyfriend tries to get you to have sexual intercourse) once the former are mastered. Skill rehearsal is an extremely effective method for increasing both perceived self-efficacy as well as actual ability for dealing with risky situations. Further, watching peers model risk-reduction role-plays is likely to further increase normative support for preventive behavior. Finally, young people should again be encouraged to think about their particularly behavioral goal (e.g., to remain abstinent or to use condoms consistently if they become sexually active) and how they can go about achieving it. Many programs for older adolescents use the strategy of having young people write down their behavioral goal and why they chose it in order to strengthen a sense of commitment to the goal (Kirby, Barth, Leland, & Fetro, 1991).

Aarons et al. (2000) reported on the effectiveness of an intervention to postpone sexual intercourse among junior high school students. The program took place in Washington, DC and included the use of a standard of care comparison group. Health professionals implemented the program, which included reproductive health classes, the *Postponing Sexual Involvement Curriculum* in the seventh grade year, and a variety of educational activities in the eighth grade year meant to bolster program effectiveness. There were large gender differences at baseline in terms of sexual activity; while 81 percent of girls reported being virgins at baseline, only 44 percent of boys were virgins. The intervention appeared to have some desired effects for girls, in that significantly more of the intervention girls remained virgins at the end of the eighth grade follow-up year compared to the control group girls. In addition, intervention girls who reported being sexually active were significantly more likely to have used some form of birth control during the last intercourse and all post-intervention measurements. The program appeared unsuccessful with boys, as there was no difference in intervention versus control boys' rate of virginity, attitudes regarding abstinence, or the use of birth control.

This study highlights the importance of tailoring intervention content to the age and maturity of the students with whom one is intervening (cf. Jemmott & Jemmott, 2000). For these girls, the vast majority of whom were not sexually active, a focus on postponing sexual activity, while also providing adequate information about reproductive health, condom use, and contraception, seemed a successful strategy. For boys, most of whom were already sexually active, the program should have taken a risk-reduction approach, and emphasized the effective and consistent use of condoms. These findings also highlight the potential necessity of different program focus for boys and girls of the same age. A consistent finding both in the United States and cross-culturally is that boys initiate sexual activity at a younger age than girls. Formative research on the current sexual activity level of the population at focus becomes very important in the determination of the use of an abstinence focused or condom use focused intervention strategy.

STRATEGIES THAT DO NOT WORK

While the definitive formula for an effective program has yet to be ascertained, there is some converging evidence to suggest strategies that are unlikely to be effective. It is clear that information-only strategies, while they definitely increase knowledge related to HIV transmission and prevention, have little or no effect on actual risk behavior (Kirby, 1999a). This finding is completely consistent with HIV prevention research with other populations and is by now assumed by virtually all HIV prevention researchers and practitioners.

The lack of success of a second strategy may seem somewhat counterintuitive. Although many people would consider parent–child communication about sexual issues to be an important part of an overall strategy for reducing sexual risk, studies of such interventions show that "there is no reasonably simple and robust relationship between parent–adolescent communication about sexuality and delay in the onset of intercourse" (Kirby, 1999b, p. 196). The same is true of the influence of specific parent–child discussion of contraceptive use and HIV/STDs. There appears to be no clear relationship of such discussion to higher rates of health protective behavior, and in fact some studies have shown that parents who engage in discussions of HIV and STDs have children who engage in *higher* levels of sexual risk behavior (Kirby, 1999b). The causal direction of that particular relationship is not clear, and there are serious methodological limitations involved in research on this topic. Nevertheless, both parents and adolescents believe that such discussion is important, and thus programs should endeavor to improve such communication where possible. Further, in a recent study by Blake, Simkin, Ledsky, Perkins, and Calabrese (2001), parent–child "homework" exercises were designed to reinforce school-based sexual risk reduction curricula in a middle school. Their results suggested that the classroom curriculum enhanced with parent–child homework assignments resulted in stronger effects on self-efficacy for refusing high-risk behaviors and stronger intentions to delay intercourse than did the classroom curriculum alone. These results are encouraging, but without more reliable evidence of effectiveness, the responsibility for teaching young children HIV/STD preventive behavior should not be left to parents alone. On a more positive note, and consistent with problem behavior theory, family connectedness including warmth, closeness, good parental supervision, and boundary setting, does appear to be related to the delay of sexual intercourse as well as to other health-protective behaviors.

Finally, reviews of different preventive interventions for HIV/STD conclude definitively that abstinence-only interventions—that is, those that focus explicitly on delaying intercourse (typically until marriage) and only mention condom and contraceptives in the context of their failure to completely protect against unwanted pregnancy or STDs—are wholly ineffective. The weight of the evidence is that such programs fail to delay the onset of intercourse (Kirby, 1999b). Further, since they give only passive coverage to ways to make sexual behavior safer, they also fail to increase condom and contraceptive use among those who become sexually active. It has become increasingly obvious that the inclusion of *both* abstinence and safer sex content is crucial for program success. The weight of program time devoted to a focus on abstinence versus a focus on safer sexual behavior should be determined, as has been reviewed, by the age and maturity of those who are the targets of the intervention.

SYNTHESIS

The best HIV prevention program for young children between the ages of 6 and 12 years of age is one that integrates HIV prevention into an ongoing health behavior curriculum in schools. Typically, there is not a high dropout rate in this age group, so interventions implemented in the school setting are likely to cover the broadest audience of young people. Yet, placing the burden on the shoulders of elementary educators brings up the most important barrier to the provision of HIV prevention programs (Schonfeld, 2000). Because of discomfort discussing sexual issues with children, a lack of training in human sexuality in general or HIV/STDs more specifically, and fear of reprisal from parents or administrations for explicitly answering frank questions about sex, teachers are reluctant to participate as facilitators in HIV prevention programs. Schonfeld (2000) reviews ways of helping teachers to become more comfortable addressing such sensitive topics, including in-service trainings by HIV prevention professionals. It also important that teachers are fully supported by school administrators in their efforts, and that both teachers and administrators be made aware that parents overwhelmingly support the provision of HIV/AIDS information in schools (Schonfeld, 2000).

An ideal health behavior curriculum should include an early and direct focus on individual responsibility for one's own health and on the link between personal choices about health behavior and health outcomes. Specific content with regard to drug use and sexual behavior should be included at age-appropriate intervals, and techniques to address these behaviors should be grounded in behavioral science theories (e.g., Theory of Reasoned Action/Planned Behavior and Social Cognitive Theory, used in Jemmott, Jemmott, & Fong, 1998; Protection-Motivation Theory used in Stanton, Li, Ricardo, Galbraith, Feigelman, & Kaljee, 1996; Social Learning Theory used in Kirby et al., 1991) with proven empirical success in HIV risk reduction with older adolescents.

Despite the fact that there is no evidence to suggest that they are effective, the United States spent approximately $440 million on abstinence-only programs in 1999 (Institute of Medicine, 2001). The empirical evidence suggests that this is not money well spent. It is absolutely crucial that for every age group HIV/AIDS prevention programs include comprehensive information on methods of making sexual behavior safer. Finally, key to the success of interventions meant to discourage risky sexual behavior is that they be implemented *well before young people are sexually active.* It is far easier to establish healthy patterns of behavior early on than to attempt to change risky behaviors once they have been initiated.

Also see: HIV/AIDS: Early Childhood; HIV/AIDS: Adolescence; HIV/AIDS: Adulthood; HIV/AIDS: Older Adulthood; Sexuality: Childhood.

References

Aarons, S.J., Jenkins, R.R., Raine, T.R., El-Khorazaty, M.N., Woodward, K.M., Williams, R.L., Clark, M.C., & Wingrove, B.K. (2000). Postponing sexual intercourse among urban junior high school students—A randomized controlled evaluation. *Journal of Adolescent Health, 27,* 236–247.

Ajzen, I., & Madden, T. (1986). Prediction of goal-directed behavior: Attitudes, intentions, and perceived behavioral control. *Journal of Experimental Social Psychology, 22,* 453–474.

Albarracín, D., Johnson, B.T., Fishbein, M., & Muellerleile, P.A. (2001). Theories of reasoned action and planned behavior as models of condom use: A meta-analysis. *Psychological Bulletin, 127,* 142–161.

Armistead, L., Summers, P., Forehand, R., Morse, P.S., Morse, E., & Clark, L. (1999). Understanding of HIV/AIDS among children of HIV-infected mothers: Implications for prevention, disclosure, and bereavement. *Children's Health Care, 28,* 277–295.

Bandura, A. (1992). A social cognitive approach to the exercise of control over AIDS infection. In R.J. DiClemente (Ed.), *Adolescents and AIDS: A generation in jeopardy* (pp. 89–116). Newbury Park: Sage.

Blake, S.M., Simkin, L., Ledsky, R., Perkins, C., & Calabrese, J.M. (2001). Effects of a parent–child communications intervention on young adolescents' risk for early onset of sexual intercourse. *Family Planning Perspectives, 33,* 52–61.

Centers for Disease Control and Prevention (CDC). (1988). Effective school health education to prevent the spread of AIDS. *MMWR, 37,* 1–14 [on-line]. Available: http://www.cdc.gov/epo/mmwr/preview/mmwrhtml/00001751.htm

Centers for Disease Control and Prevention (CDC). (2000a). *HIV/AIDS Surveillance Report, 12*(1) [on-line]. Available: http://www.cdc.gov/hiv/stats/hasr1201.htm

Centers for Disease Control and Prevention (CDC). (2000b). Programs that work. *HIV prevention fact sheets* [on-line]. Available: http://www.cdc.gov/nccdphp/dash/rtc/hiv-curric.htm

Chassin, L., Presson, C.C., Sherman, S.J., & McConnell, A.R. (1995). Adolescent health issues. In M. Roberts (Ed.), *Handbook of pediatric psychology* (2nd ed., pp. 723–740). New York: Guilford Press.

Fishbein, M., & Ajzen, I. (1980). *Understanding attitudes and predicting behavior.* Englewood Cliffs: Prentice-Hall.

Fisher, J.D., & Fisher, W.A. (1992). Changing AIDS-risk behavior. *Psychological Bulletin, 111,* 455–474.

Fisher, J.D., & Fisher, W.A. (2000). Theoretical approaches to individual-level change in HIV risk behavior. In J.L. Peterson & R.J. DiClemente (Eds.), *Handbook of HIV prevention* (pp. 3–55). New York, NY: Kluwer Academic/Plenum.

Healthy People. (2010). *National health promotion and disease prevention objectives* [on-line]. Washington, DC: US Department of Health and Human Services. Available: http://web.health.gov/healthypeople/document/

Institute of Medicine. (2001). *No time to lose: Getting more from HIV prevention.* Washington, DC: National Academy Press.

Jemmott, J.B., & Jemmott, L.S. (2000). HIV risk reduction behavioral interventions with heterosexual adolescents. *AIDS, 14,* S40–S52.

Jemmott, J.B., Jemmott, L.S., & Fong, G.T. (1998). Abstinence and safer sex HIV risk-reduction interventions for African American adolescents: A randomized controlled trial. *Journal of the American Medical Association, 279,* 1529–1536.

Jessor, R., & Jessor, S.L. (1977). *Problem behavior and psychosocial development: A longitudinal study of youth.* New York: Academic Press.

Jessor, R., Turbin, M.S., & Costa, F.M. (1998). Protective factors in adolescent health behavior. *Journal of Personality and Social Psychology, 75,* 788–800.

Kinsman, S.B., Romer, D., Furstenberg, F.F., & Schwarz, D.F. (1998). Early sexual initiation: the role of peer norms. *Pediatrics, 102,* 1185–1192.

Kirby, D. (1999a). Reflections on two decades of research on teen sexual behavior and pregnancy. *Journal of School Health, 69,* 89–94.

Kirby, D. (1999b). Sexuality and sex education at home and school. *Adolescent Medicine: State of the Art Reviews, 10,* 195–209.

Kirby, D., Barth, R.P., Leland, N., & Fetro, J.V. (1991). Reducing the risk: Impact of a new curriculum on sexual risk-taking. *Family Planning Perspectives, 23,* 253–263.

Norris, A.E., & Ford, K. (1998). Moderating influence of peer norms on gender differences in condom use. *Applied Developmental Science, 2,* 174–181.

Pozen, A.S. (1995). HIV/AIDS in the schools. In N. Boyd-Franklin & G.L. Steiner (Eds.), *Children, families, and HIV/AIDS: Psychosocial and therapeutic issues* (pp. 233–255). New York, NY: The Guilford Press.

Schonfeld, D.J. (2000). Teaching young children about HIV and AIDS. *Child and Adolescent Psychiatric Clinics of North America, 9,* 375–387.

Schonfeld, D.J., O'Hare, L.L., Perrin, E.C., Quackenbush, M., Showalter, D.R., & Cicchetti, D.V. (1995). A randomized, controlled trial of a school-based, multi-faceted AIDS education program in the elementary grades: The impact on comprehension, knowledge and fears. *Pediatrics, 95,* 480–486.

Sigelman, C.K., Goldenberg, J.L., Siegel, C.B., & Dwyer, K.M. (1998). Parental drug use and the socialization of AIDS knowledge and attitudes in children. *AIDS Education and Prevention, 10,* 180–192.

Stanton, B.F., Li, X., Ricardo, I., Galbraith, J., Feigelman, S., & Kaljee, L. (1996). A randomized, controlled effectiveness trial of an AIDS prevention program for low-income African-American youths. *Archives of Pediatric and Adolescent Medicine, 150,* 363–372.

UNAIDS. (1997). *Integrating HIV/STD prevention in the school setting: A position paper* [on-line]. Available: http://www.unaids.org/publications/documents/children/schools/Pos_Paper_Schools-E.doc

UNAIDS. (2000). *Report on the Global HIV/AIDS epidemic—June 2000* [on-line]. Available: http://www.unaids.org/epidemic_update/report/Epi_report.htm

UNICEF. (2000). *The state of the World's children: 2000* [on-line]. Foreword by Secretary General Kofi A. Annan. Available: http://www.unicef.org/sowc00/

Wolff, W.J., & Schoeberlein, D.R. (1999). The status of middle level HIV/STD education as assessed by state and local education agencies. *Journal of School Health, 69,* 239–242.

HIV/AIDS, Adolescence

Kerry L. Marsh, Blair T. Johnson, and Michael P. Carey

INTRODUCTION

An essential step in attacking the pandemic of HIV is changing adolescents' sexual risk behavior. Individuals become infected with the human immunodeficiency virus (HIV) through contact with infected body fluids, primarily through sexual intercourse or contact with infected blood (sharing needles in drug injection or receiving blood transfusions). Though unsafe drug injection practices render some adolescents (e.g., drug users) at high risk, *every* adolescent has potential sexual risk.

SCOPE

In areas of the world such as sub-Saharan Africa where prevalence rates of HIV are astoundingly high, heterosexual contact and limited condom use leads to prevalence rates twice as high for young females aged 15–24 as for males (UNAIDS, 2000). For example in countries such as Botswana, South Africa, and Zimbabwe, rates from 1997 to 1998 were 25 percent or higher for females aged 15–24. The implications of such rates are terrifying; in South Africa alone, the total population living with HIV or acquired immune deficiency syndrome (AIDS) was more than 4 million in 1999.

In North America, the increasing tendency for adolescents to initiate intercourse in middle adolescence (14–16 years) means that exposure to HIV also is a significant concern. In Canada, as of the end of 1999, 597 positive HIV tests had been reported for youth aged 15–19 (Bureau of HIV/AIDS, STD and TB, Health Canada, 2000). In the United States, the rates are higher. As of December 2000 (CDC, 2001), 2,412 male and 3,167 female adolescents of ages 13–19 were reportedly infected with HIV and an additional 2,366 males and 1,695 females had AIDS. In 1999, the estimated incidence of new diagnoses of AIDS in adolescents was 141 male and 155 females. Of new cases for which risk factors were identifiable, over 70 percent involved sexual contact. Although rates of infection in US adolescents are substantially lower than for older adults, for many other sexually transmitted diseases (STDs), adolescents are at especially high risk. Among women, 15- to 19-year-olds had the highest rate of gonorrhea in 1999 compared to other age categories; the third highest rates among men were in this age group (Division of STD Prevention, 2000). Rates of many STDs decreased between 1995 and 1999. For example among those 15- to 19-years-old, gonorrhea rates were 71.7 cases per 100,000 females in 1995 and 54.6 cases in 1999; rates for males of this age declined from 503.2 cases to 341.1 cases. Chlamydia rates, however, remain exceptionally high in females of this age group, with indications that chlamydia infection is widespread geographically and highly prevalent among economically disadvantaged young women. For example, the average chlamydia prevalence rates by state were 9.9 percent for female entrants into the US Army and 11.1 percent for

Job Corps in 1999 (Division of STD Prevention, 2000). Although bacterial STDs can be cured, other STDs (e.g., chlamydia) are often asymptomatic and may go undetected and therefore uncured. These facts are particularly troubling in that STDs put individuals at risk for other health problems, including sterility and increased susceptibility to HIV infection. The consequences of HIV infection are most dire. Because there currently is no cure or vaccine for HIV, all such cases must be considered as on going until death.

Adolescence is a critical time for successfully establishing behaviors that will protect individuals and their partners from exposure to HIV and other STDs throughout the course of their life. Many begin initiating sexual intercourse during adolescence; thus it is a critical time for shaping attitudes relevant to delaying initiation of sex, abstaining from sex unprotected by condoms, and choosing safer sexual behavior over higher risk ones. As young and healthy individuals, adolescents have a substantial length of time to be exposed to, and expose others to, HIV and other STDs. Providing adolescents with the appropriate information and skills to engage in self-protective behavior, and motivating them to engage in such action are the only ways available to ensure that individuals who will eventually have sex will not contract or transmit HIV in doing so.

THEORIES

From the earliest *health models* used for explaining adolescents' sexual risk behavior (Rosenstock, Strecher, & Becker, 1994), to the most current, one basic assumption is that individuals must have adequate information regarding HIV, AIDS, and STDs in order to engage in appropriately protective behavior. The failure of approaches that merely provided general education (Helweg-Larson & Collins, 1997) lies primarily on the failure to appropriately target the specific, proximal beliefs most closely linked to protective behavior. Individuals must believe that they are personally at risk of such diseases, and they must have information about what behaviors reduce this risk. Current dominant perspectives on risk behavior emphasize the necessity of increasing adolescents' perceptions of personal vulnerability in order to motivate them to remain abstinent longer and use condoms when they have sex. Even so, increasing perceptions of personal vulnerability has not been demonstrated to affect behavior that protects against HIV.

Current models of HIV prevention indicate that providing information about HIV and one's risk of contracting HIV is necessary but not sufficient for inducing protective sexual behavior. In general, three other processes that need to be considered involve attitudes, peer influence, and skills development. From the perspective of the *Theory of reasoned action* and *Theory of planned behavior* (Fishbein & Middlestadt, 1989), interventions should attempt to change adolescents' attitudes toward engaging in behaviors such as abstaining from sex or using a condom. These attitudes determine behavioral intentions that are in turn highly predictive of behavior (Albarracin, Johnson, Fishbein, & Muellerleile, 2001). Thus, interventions target individuals' beliefs about the consequences of an action, and how desirable or undesirable they personally find those consequences. For instance, interventions might address adolescents' beliefs that resisting pressure to have sex will lead to a partner's rejection, that buying condoms will be embarrassing, or that using condoms will feel unpleasant. These theories, as well as *social influence approaches* (Kelly, St. Lawrence, & Stevenson, 1992), suggest that interventions should also address the role of peer influences in determining adolescents' behavior. To the extent that an adolescent believes that remaining abstinent or using condoms is a typical and acceptable behavior to their peers, they will be more likely to intentionally engage in that behavior.

The third critical process involves skills development. Theorizing about *self-efficacy* processes (Bandura, 1994) suggests that an adolescent must learn appropriate skills in order to be able to perform a risk reduction behavior. Thus, providing adolescents with skills experiences such as practicing sexual refusal in peer role-playing has multiple benefits. It results in greater skill at refusing sex should such situations arise. It also means an adolescent will be more motivated to attempt the behavior as a consequence of both increased confidence in their skills (feelings of self-efficacy) as well as increased perception that peers support such behavior.

Several models developed specifically in response to the HIV crisis build on multiple aspects of these theories. The *AIDS risk reduction model* (ARRM; Catania, Kegeles, Coates, 1990) and *Transtheoretical model* (Prochaska & Velicer, 1997) emphasize that changing risk behavior involves shifting individuals toward stages in which they recognize the need to change their behavior, begin to contemplate and prepare to change their behavior, before committing to change and finally maintaining this change. The model that most comprehensively integrates these various processes is the *Information motivation behavioral skills model* (Fisher & Fisher, 1992, 2000). It suggests that inducing appropriate sexual behavior in adolescents would require addressing informational deficits, instantiating motivation in attitudes, normative influence, and perceived vulnerability to HIV, as well as developing behavioral skills. In particular, this model suggests careful tailoring of an intervention's content to the specific practices relevant to adolescents. For example, abstinence-based approaches that did not address sexual communication and condom use skills would be inappropriate in a sample of adolescents who were sexually active. Practice at managing one's own impulses and managing one's environment to avoid risky situations (intrapersonal skills) would be essential for adolescents whose failures to use condoms were based in poor self-management skills.

In sum, theories of HIV risk reduction suggest that changing adolescents' behavior means making progress in changing the underlying psychological constructs that move the individual toward less risky behavior. Changing behavior therefore means attending to adolescents' beliefs about the specific costs and benefits of engaging in the behavior, actual and perceived self-efficacy, peer and informational influences, and motivation to engage in less risky behavior. We consider prevention research on risky behavior into the two categories that have received investigation, sexual risk and injection drug use.

RESEARCH ON REDUCING SEXUAL RISK

While vast numbers of schools have instituted programs relevant to youth HIV-risk reduction, relatively few have rigorously evaluated these interventions. Nonetheless, an increasing number of studies have now evaluated school-based intervention programs, and other HIV-prevention programs conducted in small group community settings. The content of these varies considerably, from a focus on factual education only, focus on encouraging abstinence only, to providing information about condom use, and providing participants with skills-building experiences (e.g., role-playing or condom skills). Facilitators in these interventions are sometimes adults, peers, or a combination of adults and peers. A number of studies have evaluated small-group or individual interventions tailored to minority individuals living in areas of higher HIV incidence. Moreover, interventions have been conducted in populations at high risk such as juvenile detainees, runaway youths, and drug users. In some cases, the primary focus of relevant interventions has been STD or pregnancy prevention rather than HIV prevention specifically, but the intervention contained information about HIV risk. In many of these studies, staff in settings such as health clinics delivered one-to-one or small group interventions.

Some pregnancy prevention, abstinence-only or STD interventions had no substantive information about HIV or AIDS. Such studies are, however, relevant to assessing the effectiveness of primary prevention of HIV, AIDS, and STDs more generally if they included relevant intervention content (taught abstinence skills, or provided condom information) and assessed outcomes such as condom use or frequency of sex. Reviews of pregnancy prevention studies

(Franklin, Grant, Corcoran, Miller, & Bultman, 1997) and abstinence-only programs (Wilcox & Wyatt, 1997) provide little evidence for decreased initiation or frequency of sexual activity. For example, evidence for decreased initiation of sex was present only in weak designs (Guyatt, DiCenso, Farewell, Willan, & Griffith, 2000). It is difficult to draw clear conclusions from these reviews, however, because they typically included many studies of poor methodological quality.

The evidence discussed in this entry is limited to rigorously designed outcome evaluation studies that involve controlled delivery of an educational or psychosocial intervention designed to affect HIV risk behaviors. Thus, excluded are mass media studies and street-outreach interventions that had uncontrolled dosages or self-selection confounds. Many studies reviewed had randomized controlled trials (RCT), meaning the designs involved individuals randomly assigned to condition, but some used quasi-experimental pretest posttest designs with alternative means of control. Inferences that an intervention worked well were based on systematically assessing the relative differences between the intervention and the control conditions on their primary outcomes measures that affect contracting of HIV (e.g., reduced incidence of sex and increased condom use). Such inferences were possible for approximately 60 high quality studies with HIV-content (Johnson, Carey, Marsh, & Levin, 2001) and 30 without HIV content that produced reports between 1981 and January 1, 2001.

STRATEGIES THAT WORK

We define interventions that work as having shown at least moderate impact on critical behaviors relevant to HIV risk: condom use, abstinence from sex, frequency of sex, and number of sexual partners. Participants in these conditions, when compared to participants who did not receive the intervention or received an alternative minimal intervention (e.g., education-only), should have decreased sexual activity and increased condom use when they are sexually active. We adopted conventional standards regarding the success of interventions based on the size of the differences between the treatment and control conditions compared on a standardized scale (i.e., effect size).

Relevant research has included both interventions that have targeted HIV and those that have not. Recent reviews (Jemmott & Jemmott, 2000; Johnson et al., 2001) indicate that *HIV interventions* can lead to detectable reductions in sexual risk behavior, especially for behaviors such as condom use and acquisition. Effective HIV interventions are predominantly skills-based interventions that have particular goals of reducing sexual risk behaviors rather than more diffuse goals. In such studies, researchers typically deliver the content to small groups of 6–8 participants and use procedures that actively engage adolescents in the material. In addition to basic HIV information, effective interventions provide information about condoms. Such information, however, is relatively minimal in a few interventions with more extensive emphasis on abstinence. In other cases where interventions are effective, extensive condom information is often provided; sometimes participants are provided explicit instruction (modeling and rehearsal) of condom use. Programs that have more lasting effects are more likely to have emphasized condom use than to have focused on abstinence alone (Jemmott & Jemmott, 2000). In *all* cases of effective interventions, HIV risk is personalized through information and exercises designed to enhance perceptions of personal risk.

Moreover, interpersonal skills training is a significant component of interventions demonstrated as effective. Such training involves demonstration and discussion of how to handle communication and negotiation with a potential sexual partner, and includes role-playing by the participants themselves. In these cases, youths rehearse scenarios in which they learn how to resist pressure to engage in sex or persuade a partner to use a condom, they receive feedback and encouragement from the facilitators and the other group members, and they watch others role-play scenarios. In many interventions, youth also receive some exposure to intrapersonal skill development. Occasionally these components require active involvement much like the role-playing exercises; students discuss how to manage their own feelings in potentially sexual situations, describe their own goals and plans regarding sexual risk behavior, and develop personal plans and strategies for self-management of themselves and their risk environment. More commonly, intrapersonal skill components are either omitted or delivered with less extensive active participation, in which participants merely discussed goals and self-management issues.

The studies demonstrating effective interventions have been conducted predominantly with minority youth in community settings; some have been conducted in residential treatment centers (St. Lawrence, Brasfield, Jefferson, Alleyne, O'Bannon, & Shirley, 1995) or classroom settings (Hubbard, Giese, & Rainey, 1998). In these effective interventions, the intervention involves at least one session of 5 hr; in other community settings, interventions are delivered in at least six sessions of typically 90 min or more and have total dosages of between 9 and 14 hr. Effective classroom interventions, however, may require lengthier sessions (e.g., at least 14 sessions, Hubbard et al., 1998).

For example, one study demonstrated that an intervention can have beneficial effects on condom use, number of sexual partners, and frequency of sex, 13 weeks after the end of the intervention (Jemmott, Jemmott, & Fong, 1992). Other studies have similarly found effects on male youths' condom use at short times after the intervention, 8–13 weeks later (St. Lawrence et al., 1995). In one unpublished study, condom use was reassessed at 6 months and 1 year postintervention. Although the effects for boys had dropped somewhat at 6 months, becoming negligible by 1 year, the effects were delayed for girls, becoming moderate by the last measurement occasion. Intervention effects on condom use in other studies have typically shown only a slight decay across time (Johnson et al., 2001).

Overall, the bulk of the evidence for effectiveness has been demonstrated on condom use measures. There is no evidence, however, that increases in condom use have been associated with increased sexual activity. In fact, there is some evidence that frequency of sex can be reduced at least 8 weeks after the intervention. There is other evidence that interventions have consequences such as reduced incidence of sex under risky circumstances and reduced diagnoses of STDs (St. Lawrence, Jefferson, Alleyne, & Brasfield, 1995).

Other behavioral skills interventions have provided evidence of success on outcomes that are theorized as necessary precursors to engaging in safer sexual behavior. Such studies had interventions involving active interpersonal skills component as well as condom information (often with condom skills). Some studies demonstrated increased tendency for participants to take condoms upon leaving the study (Rickert, Gottlieb, & Jay, 1992). Other studies measured communication skill in sexual risk role-playing scenarios and found that the interventions were in fact improving such skills (Hovell et al., 1998); these effects had decayed after several months.

As with the HIV-content interventions, *non-HIV interventions* studies have demonstrated that including skills-based components does affect outcomes that theories presume are precursors to risk behavior. For example, studies have found that interpersonal skills training improves skill at sexual assertiveness (refusing sex and insisting on condom use) in role-played interactions relative to control condition participants (Gilchrist & Schinke, 1983).

In fact, non-HIV interventions that have had moderate effects on behavior all provide substantial emphasis on skills training and have some sex education component. Typically the skills training involves interpersonal skills training, often with primary focus on abstinence (e.g., adolescents practice how to refuse sex, but not how to negotiate condom use). In a few studies, the focus of skills training has been primarily intrapersonal skills (self-management). Overall, effective skills-based interventions have 10–12.5 hr of content.

For example, two classroom-based studies used early versions of the curriculum *Reducing the Risk* (RTR). Though later versions of RTR have had a significant HIV component (Hubbard et al., 1998), studies conducted with the earliest version had no substantive HIV component (Barth, Leland, Kirby, & Fetro, 1992). RTR is strongly abstinence-oriented, but treatment components also include condom information and role-played experience such as refusing sex. In addition, intrapersonal skills information is discussed in RTR, but goal setting is primarily focused on life goals (and how having sex might interfere) in the intervention-active self-management skills such as planning behaviors proximal to abstinence or sex is not a primary focus. In two studies that evaluated RTR, neither demonstrated moderate effects of the intervention on whether or not participants had sex. One study demonstrated no effectiveness of the intervention on any behavioral measures whereas the other study found that the intervention affected only those youth who had not yet initiated sex at the time of the intervention (Barth et al., 1992). These individuals had less frequent sex and more condom use 6 months after the intervention; effects had decayed by 18 months post-intervention.

Smith (1994) used a RCT to evaluate the effectiveness of an intervention that provides four sessions of intervention imbedded in a 14-session health promotion intervention. In this intervention, small groups of high school freshmen meet weekly for sessions that include two sessions of active interpersonal skills training, one session of active intrapersonal skills training, and one factual session (condoms are also provided). Evaluation of this program demonstrated that such interventions could decrease frequency of sex 18 weeks after it ends.

A study conducted in Norwegian classrooms suggests that leading an intervention as a peer educator can reduce sexual risk. Classes in the study were randomly assigned to control condition or to the intervention provided by peer educators (Kvalem, Sundet, Rivo, Eilertsen, & Bakketeig, 1996). In this intervention, peers provide active interpersonal training and some condom information. Although conducting the training had no effect on whether peer educators initiated sex, it did have some effect on condom use (assessed only in those who were already having sex at pretest). The study demonstrates that this kind of intervention can have effects up to 6 months afterwards, with effects decaying by 1 year after the intervention.

STRATEGIES THAT MIGHT WORK

Despite evidence that interventions that are effective have strong skill components as well as other theoretically important components, there is less evidence that skill-based interventions *generally* work well. In many cases, well-designed studies conducted in community settings or in large-scale school-settings have all the theoretically relevant

components and yet yield only minimal effects. In some of these cases the interventions were still viewed by the researchers as successful because of statistical significance on an individual measure or some subsample of the study, albeit not on most relevant measures or for participants taken as a whole. Other studies achieve statistical significance because they include an enormous number of participants, but the sizes of the effects are actually quite small. Extracting some general understanding of why some studies demonstrate moderate effects where others provide less evidence of effectiveness is difficult, but some trends are apparent.

It is much easier to demonstrate effectiveness on psychological variables, including knowledge, attitudes, perceptions of peer's norms for behavior, and intentions, than to influence risk-related behaviors of primary interest. Theoretically, this pattern is sensible because change in behaviors requires adequate knowledge *as well as* appropriate attitudes, norms, intentions, and skills. Moreover, with sexual risk reduction, the fact that the behaviors in question are dyadic further increases the complexity of reducing risk behaviors. For behavioral outcomes, interventions are more effective at increasing condom use than at decreasing frequency of sex and number of partners. Increasing abstinence rates may be the most difficult because one would expect decreased abstinence as adolescents approach adulthood. Moreover, how well the intervention is matched to the concerns relevant to that age and cultural group of adolescents will be important in intervention effectiveness. For instance, older adolescents are more likely to be sexually experienced and also have more risky behavior (less condom use) as evidenced by their higher rates of STDs and pregnancy (Jemmott & Jemmott, 2000). Interventions with older adolescents need to be designed with consideration of the greater risk behavior already present in such samples. Finally, it appears that interventions with smaller groups are more successful (Kirby, 1995). Kirby's review of school-based programs concluded that for larger groups (e.g., classrooms), at least 14 hr of treatment were necessary to produce a positive impact.

STRATEGIES THAT DO NOT WORK

In general, whether or not programs provide HIV content, those that lack skills training and merely provide sex education or condom information alone in a didactic manner are minimally effective at inducing safer behavior (Kirby, 1999). Nonetheless, there are a few studies in which providing sex education or condom information may have been effective. The distinguishing feature in most of these exceptions appears to be increased motivational engagement of participants. The exceptions were varied but lead to some potential conclusions. Such interventions might be effective if they either engage active individualized motivation via very brief one-to-one interventions in clinical settings or engage peer support through very lengthy involvement in a peer support group that sustains its identity over an extended period.

Providing information alone without arousing additional motivation seems especially unlikely to be effective in populations that already have received sufficient information. For example, HIV-content studies published in earlier years had significantly stronger effects on measured knowledge than in recent years. Presumably this pattern reflects the fact that, societally, adolescents know more about HIV today than they knew in the years early in the HIV crisis.

RESEARCH ON REDUCING DRUG INJECTING-RELATED RISK

Most interventions designed to reduce HIV risk in adolescents have focused on sexual risk rather than injection risk. For some teens, however, risk of HIV infection via drug injection is a serious concern. Moreover, adolescents who inject drugs have considerably greater risk of HIV infection through multiple routes. Because incidence of HIV is exceptionally high in segments of the population that inject drugs, participating actively in such subcultures means increased HIV risk. Drug-injecting teens expose themselves to HIV through using HIV-contaminated needles as well as by engaging in sex under the circumstances least likely to engage thoughtful action about the consequences of risky behavior. They may have sex while under the influence of drugs or alcohol, or the need for drugs may lead them to exchange sex for money or drugs.

STRATEGIES THAT WORK

Because of the limited research in this area of injection-related risks to adolescents, we will focus on strategies that might work.

STRATEGIES THAT MIGHT WORK

Beyond minimal information regarding transmission of HIV through unclean needles, most HIV interventions directed at youth do not include a needle risk component. However, a more substantial needle risk component is typically included for higher risk samples: those teens who are in the criminal justice system, drug treatment programs, or residential centers, or teens who are homeless or runaways. In studies evaluating interventions in such populations, teens report substantial illegal drug use but the percentage reporting that they ever injected drugs is typically much lower

about 1–2 percent. Only a few studies report substantial rates of teens injecting drugs (6–17 percent). Thus in evaluation studies with high risk youth, outcomes such as general frequency of drug use are often assessed, but rarely are outcomes reported such as drug injecting or needle bleaching. In all cases, interventions focus substantially more on sexual risk components than on drug-related risk and find less evidence of the effectiveness of injection-related content than of the effectiveness of sexual risk content. One study that did measure IV drug use and needle sharing (after a brief small group informational session) did not find evidence of effectiveness (Slonim-Nevo, Ozawa, & Auslander, 1991). In some limited cases, however, interventions with drug risk content have been associated with greater decrease in drug use than in control conditions.

Overall, evidence is insufficient regarding whether interventions can be effective at directly changing injection-related risk behaviors in adolescents. However, interventions that have been associated with decreased drug use and seem to offer the most potential for reducing HIV risk in adolescents have a substantial skills component analogous to sexual risk reduction interventions (Rotheram-Borus, Koopman, Haignere, & Davies, 1991). It appears likely that to be more successful at reducing drug-related HIV risk, an intervention should provide information about the relations among substance abuse, sexual risk, and HIV in a manner that personalizes the risk to the teen. In addition, cleaning needles with bleach should be demonstrated and rehearsed by teens. Ideally, an intervention designed for adolescents at substantial injection-related risk should also provide intrapersonal and interpersonal skills training specific to these risks. For instance, teens should learn to identify the triggers that elicit substance abuse, and practice problem solving skills to deal with the negative feelings, cravings, and urges leading to risky drug-related behaviors (Rotheram-Borus et al., 1991). Moreover, teens should practice refusing drugs and alcohol and learn how to resist pressure to engage in drug use.

SYNTHESIS

In general, the evidence regarding effectiveness of interventions for reducing HIV and STD risk in adolescents lends support to Kirby's (1999) recommendations for effective curricula. Namely, messages in the interventions should be consistent and repeatedly reinforced, not diluted by too many goals or by messages that are diffuse or ambiguous. Moreover, interventions should provide information about the risks of unprotected sex and how to reduce these risks. In addition, they should involve active learning processes rather than passive reception of information. Conveyed information needs to be closely tied to the specific facts that the adolescent needs to make choices about action rather than technical and abstract information of less relevance to specific behavioral goals. Providing information that specifically is relevant to youth's perceived barriers to safer sexual behavior has a greater likelihood at changing the appropriate attitudes toward engaging in these behaviors.

Moreover, interventions must engage the adolescents in the subject material. Effective interventions accomplish this goal through experiential techniques, using, for instance, role-playing to teach teens refusal skills and sexual communication skills as well as to enhance feelings of self-efficacy. Skills and information regarding condom use, interpersonal skills training, and in some cases, intrapersonal skill training were used. Moreover, to be effective, interventions should be tailored to the appropriate age, sexual experience, and needs of the participants (Kirby, 1999), which is a practice followed by practically all successful interventions.

As experts have concluded (Kirby, 1995), there is no evidence that any interventions in any category of content decrease levels of abstinence or increase levels of sexual behavior. This conclusion is true of even those studies that are full of "safer sex interventions," providing not just encouragement of abstinence, but extensive information and training regarding condom use and condom negotiating/ sexual assertiveness training. Interestingly, of those interventions that are heavily abstinence oriented, effectiveness is evident through increased condom use in most cases, and occasionally on sexual frequency measures. Finding that an intervention delayed initiation of sex is rare when such effects were quantified across appropriate measures and compared on a common statistical metric (effect size).

Interpersonal skills experiences are critical for increasing individual teens' skills in sexual pressure interactions. Ideally, such training should provide preparation for situations in which an adolescent does choose to have sex, because statistics demonstrate that such behavior will commonly be occurring and the evidence shows that providing such preparation does not deter abstinence. In those interventions with minimal safer sex component, but that still had strong interpersonal skills training, it may seem paradoxical to find positive effects on subsequent condom use. Skills training may be important not only for the specific skills they provide, but also because of more general skill at interpersonal negotiation surrounding sexual issues. Moreover, these and other active successful elements (personalized risk assessment, condom skills practice, intrapersonal skills development) should theoretically increase perceptions of control over sexual issues, helping increase adolescents' feelings of self-efficacy and responsibility for their sexual decisions. Moreover, the interventions that hold the most promise for reducing injection-related HIV risk have the same key components: accurate information, personalized risk, addressing specific barriers to safer behavior, and active interpersonal and intrapersonal skills components.

One final component of interventions that appears critical for effectiveness is normative support for engaging in behavior of lower risk (e.g., abstinence and protected sex). In abstinence-oriented interventions, such information is often provided explicitly, typically by adult facilitators leading a discussion of how media images promote sexual behavior, and by promoting the notion that adolescents' peers are not typically sexually active. Explicit efforts to influence adolescents' perceptions of peer support for abstinence or condom use have a danger of backfiring if the information is not believable to adolescents. A more indirect way in which changing adolescents' perceptions of peer support is through use of peer facilitators. Although there is no clear evidence that peer leaders have more or less impact than adult facilitators, in some cases peers who are in such leadership roles show improved behavior (Kvalem et al., 1996). One reason that small group interventions are generally more effective than classroom interventions (unless such interventions were much lengthier) may be because the extensive interaction among group members allows for peer influence processes and leads to changes in their perceptions of peer support for risky behavior. Nevertheless, no studies to date have taken the step of implementing natural opinion leader, peer influence interventions (Kelly et al., 1992) in adolescent populations. Such interventions involve having popular peers in natural settings conduct casual one-to-one brief attempts to persuade others to engage in appropriate behavior. Given the obvious centrality of peer influence in youth's sexual behavior, attempting such interventions seems warranted.

Overall, the evidence for primary prevention of HIV in adolescents is that some interventions with the appropriate intervention content can have modest effects on behavior, in particular on condom use. Yet the magnitude of impact is not large and many well-designed interventions with appropriate content does not yield modest effects. Without exception, however, the impact of interventions on the psychological variables that are theorized as critical precursors to behavior change is substantially larger. The task of influencing behavior in such a domain is an extremely difficult one, for which modest effects are quite laudable. Sexual behavior is a behavior in which nearly all individuals, at some point in adulthood (if not before) inevitably feel strongly impelled to engage. To affect change in a behavioral arena for which biological imperatives to act are so strong is progress indeed.

Also see: HIV/AIDS: Early Childhood; HIV/AIDS: Childhood; HIV/AIDS: Adulthood; HIV/AIDS: Older Adulthood; Sexuality: Adolescence; Sexually Transmitted Diseases: Adolescence.

References

Albarracin, D., Johnson, B.T., Fishbein, M., Muellerleile, P.A. (2001). Theories of reasoned action and planned behavior as models of condom use: A meta-analysis. *Psychological Bulletin, 127,* 142–161.

Bandura, A. (1994). Social cognitive theory and exercise of control over AIDS. In R. DiClemente & J. Peterson (Eds.), *Preventing AIDS: Theories, methods, and behavioral interventions* (pp. 25–60). New York: Plenum.

Barth, R.P., Leland, N., Kirby, D., & Fetro, J.V. (1992). Enhancing social and cognitive skills. In B.C. Miller (Ed.), *Preventing adolescent pregnancy: Model, programs, and evaluations* (pp. 53–83). Newbury Park: Sage.

Bureau of HIV/AIDS, STD and TB, Health Canada (2000, April). *HIV and AIDS among youth in Canada.* HIV/AIDS Epi Update.

Catania, J.A., Kegeles, S.M., & Coates, T.J. (1990). Towards an understanding of risk behavior: An AIDS risk reduction model (ARRM). *Health Education Quarterly, 17,* 53–72.

Centers for Disease Control and Prevention (CDC). (2001). *HIV/AIDS Surveillance Report, 2000, 12(2).*

Division of STD Prevention. (2000, September). *Sexually transmitted disease surveillance, 1999.* Department of Health and Human Services, Atlanta: Centers for Disease Control and Prevention (CDC).

Fishbein, M., & Middlestadt, S.E. (1989). Using the theory of reasoned action as a framework for understanding and changing AIDS-related behaviors. In V. Mays, G. Albee, & S. Schneider (Eds.), *Primary prevention of AIDS: Psychological approaches* (pp. 93–110). Beverly Hills: Sage.

Fisher, J.D., & Fisher, W.A. (1992). Changing AIDS-risk behavior. *Psychological Bulletin, 111,* 455–474.

Fisher, J.D., & Fisher, W.A. (2000). Theoretical approaches to individual-level change in HIV-risk behavior. In J. Peterson & R. DiClemente (Eds.), *HIV prevention handbook* (pp. 3–55). New York: Plenum.

Franklin, C., Grant, D., Corcoran, J., Miller, P.O.D., & Bultman, L. (1997). Effectiveness of prevention programs for adolescent pregnancy: A meta-analysis. *Journal of Marriage and the Family, 59,* 551–567.

Gilchrist, L.D., & Schinke, S.P. (1983). Coping with contraception: Cognitive and behavioral methods with adolescents. *Journal of Consulting and Clinical Psychology, 58,* 432–436.

Guyatt, G.H., DiCenso, A., Farewell, V., Willan, A., & Griffith, L. (2000). Randomized trials versus observational studies in adolescent pregnancy prevention. *Journal of Clinical Epidemiology, 53,* 167–174.

Helweg-Larson, M., & Collins, B.E. (1997). A social psychological perspective on the role of knowledge about AIDS in AIDS prevention. *Current Directions, 6,* 23–26.

Hovell, M., Blumberg, E., Sipan, C., Hofstetter, C.R., Burkham, S., Atkins, C., & Felice, M. (1998). Skills training for pregnancy and AIDS prevention in Anglo and Latino youth. *Journal of Adolescent Health, 23,* 139–149.

Hubbard, B.M., Giese, M.L., & Rainey, J. (1998). A replication study of Reducing the Risk: A theory-based sexuality curriculum for adolescents. *Journal of School Health, 68,* 243–247.

Jemmott, J.B., & Jemmott, L.S. (2000). HIV behavioral interventions for adolescents in community settings. In J.L. Peterson & R.J. DiClemente (Eds.), *Handbook of HIV prevention* (pp. 103–127). New York: Kluwer Academic/Plenum.

Jemmott, J.B., Jemmott, L.S., & Fong, G.T. (1992). Reductions in HIV risk-associated sexual behaviors among black male adolescents: Effects of an AIDS prevention intervention. *American Journal of Public Health, 82,* 372–377.

Johnson, B.T., Carey, M.P., Marsh, K.L., & Levin, K.D. (2001). *Interventions to prevent HIV in adolescents (1985–2000): A meta-analysis.* Unpublished manuscript.

Kelly, J.A., St. Lawrence, J.S., & Stevenson, L.Y. (1992). Community AIDS/HIV risk reduction: The effects of endorsements by popular people in three cities. *American Journal of Public Health, 82,* 1483–1489.

Kirby, D. (1995). *A review of educational programs designed to reduce sexual risk-taking behaviors among school-aged youth in the United States.* Santa Cruz, CA: ETR Associates.

Kirby, D. (1999). Sexuality and sex education at home and school. *Adolescent Medicine: State of the Art Reviews, 10,* 195–209.

Kvalem, I.L., Sundet, J.M., Rivo, K.I., Eilertsen, D.E., & Bakketeig, L.S. (1996). The effect of sex education on adolescents' use of condoms: Applying the Solomon four-group design. *Health Education Quarterly, 23,* 34–47.

Prochaska, J.O., & Velicer, W.F. (1997). The transtheoretical model of health behavior change. *American Journal of Health Promotion, 12,* 38–48.

Rickert, V.I., Gottlieb, A.A., & Jay, M.S. (1992). Is AIDS education related to condom acquisition? *Clinical Pediatrics, 31,* 205–210.

Rosenstock, M., Strecher, V., & Becker, M. (1994). The Health Belief Model and HIV risk behavior change. In R. DiClemente & J. Peterson (Eds.), *Preventing AIDS: Theories, methods, and behavioral interventions* (pp. 5–24). New York: Plenum Press.

Rotheram-Borus, M.J., Koopman, C., Haignere, C., & Davies, M. (1991). Reducing HIV_sexual risk behaviors among runaway adolescents. *Journal of the American Medical Association, 266,* 1237–1241.

Slonim-Nevo, V., Ozawa, M.N., & Auslander, W.F. (1991). Knowledge, attitudes and behaviors related to AIDS among youth in residential centers: Results from an exploratory study. *Journal of Adolescence, 14,* 17–33.

Smith, M.A.B. (1994). Teen Incentives Program: Evaluation of a health promotion model for adolescent pregnancy prevention. *Journal of Health Education, 25,* 24–29.

St. Lawrence, J., Brasfield, T., Jefferson, K.W., Alleyne, E., O'Bannon III, R.E., & Shirley, A. (1995). Cognitive-behavioral interventions to reduce African American adolescents' risk for HIV infection. *Cognitive Therapy and Research, 7,* 379–388.

St. Lawrence, J., Jefferson, K.W., Alleyne, E., & Brasfield, T. (1995). Comparison of education versus behavioral skills training interventions in lowering sexual HIV-risk behavior of substance dependent adolescents. *Journal of Consulting and Clinical Psychology, 63,* 154–157.

UNAIDS (2000, June). *Report on the global HIV/AIDS epidemic.*

Wilcox, B.L., & Wyatt, J. (1997, November). *Adolescent abstinence education programs: A meta-analysis.* Paper presented at the Joint Annual Meeting of the Society for the Scientific Study of Sexuality and the American Association of Sex Educators, Counselors, and Therapists, Arlington, VA.

HIV/AIDS, Adulthood

Blair T. Johnson, Kerry L. Marsh, and Michael P. Carey

INTRODUCTION AND DEFINITIONS

Adults become infected with the human immunodeficiency virus (HIV) and sexually transmitting diseases (STDs) through contact with infected body fluids, primarily through sexual intercourse or contact with infected blood (e.g., sharing needles in drug injection). Unfortunately, most people who acquire HIV do not learn about their status until much later, when they seek testing or develop acquired immunodeficiency syndrome (AIDS); in the meantime, these individuals may unknowingly infect others. (See other definitions in HIV/AIDS, Early childhood.) Opportunistic infections from certain bacteria, viruses, and other microbes characterize AIDS. Although healthy individuals rarely acquire these infections, the weakened immune systems of people with AIDS render them more susceptible to opportunistic infections. Such infections are often severe and can be fatal for AIDS victims.

SCOPE

The HIV/AIDS pandemic continues unabated. According to figures from the Joint United Nations Programme on HIV/AIDS (UNAIDS, 2000), 21.8 million people have died from AIDS since the beginning of the epidemic, with 3 million having died during 2000. By the end of 2000, there were 36.1 million people living with HIV, with these cases disproportionately found in Sub-Saharan Africa (70 percent) and in South and South-East Asia (16 percent); Latin America (4 percent) and North America (3 percent) have disproportionately fewer cases. Encouragingly, UNAIDS concluded that new cases of HIV have finally started to stabilize in Sub-Saharan Africa, but there is always the risk of new outbreaks in areas that have to date had low-prevalence (e.g., Nigeria). Similarly, although to date Eastern Europe has had relatively low prevalence rates to date (only 2 percent of people currently living with HIV), there is the risk of an HIV outbreak, as the incidence rate of HIV has yet to slow. For example, in 1999, the Russian Federation had only 29,000 documented cases of HIV from 1987 to 1999, yet in 2000 this number is likely to rise over 50,000 (UNAIDS, 2000). In contrast, the incidence of new HIV cases in the United States has stabilized, yet there are still a significant number of individuals who acquire HIV each year. In the 12 months through December 2000, the Centers for Disease Control and Prevention (CDC, 2000) recorded 21,704 new cases of HIV in the United States and its possessions. AIDS prevalence continues to rise, given the longer lives that antiretroviral therapies (e.g., zidovudine or AZT) have made possible.

Most people who have been diagnosed with HIV are at least 15 years of age, but this age of AIDS diagnosis is poorly descriptive as to when HIV was acquired. In fact, many individuals contract HIV as adolescents, and owing to the long latency period before actual AIDS symptoms appear, HIV infection is not diagnosed until the adult years (see HIV/AIDS: Adolescence). Historically in the United States and other industrialized countries, HIV/AIDS has been more common in men than women, reflecting the facts that HIV has been spread (1) by injection drug users (IDUs) who are more likely to be men than women, and by (2) men who have sex with men. IDUs were among the earliest victims of AIDS, with the HIV spreading rapidly through this group due primarily to sharing of needles from HIV-positive individuals. They may also engage in sex under the circumstances least likely to engage thoughtful action about the consequences of risky behavior. They may have unprotected sex while under the influence of drugs or alcohol, or the need for drugs may lead them to exchange sex for money or drugs. Thus, IDUs are more vulnerable to HIV infection through multiple routes. Because incidence of HIV is exceptionally high in segments of the population that inject drugs, participating actively in such social networks also means increased HIV risk.

Despite the early trends that mainly concerned IDUs and gay men, women have increasingly been victimized by HIV in the United States and elsewhere; in Sub-Saharan Africa, women represent the majority of cases (55 percent). Moreover, whereas HIV/AIDS was once thought relevant only to gay men, the pandemic now affects men and women, gay and straight. Individuals living in poverty are the most vulnerable, not just in Sub-Saharan Africa and in Southern and Southeastern Asia, but also in more affluent countries such as the United States.

To date, there is neither a vaccine to prevent HIV nor a cure for it, once contracted. Therefore, the current best hope for stemming the pandemic is changing the behaviors and environments that put individuals at risk for HIV. Providing individuals with the appropriate information and skills to engage in self-protective behavior (e.g., using or negotiating condom use; safe drug use), and motivating them to engage in such action are the primary means available to ensure that individuals who will eventually have sex or use drugs will not contract or transmit HIV in doing so. Finally, although HIV/AIDS receives the most contemporary attention, STDs such as chlamydia, syphilis, and gonorrhea are also an important public health problem, given their greater frequency and often-pernicious consequences. In the United States, there are approximately 10 times more STD cases identified each year than there are HIV cases (Division of STD Prevention, 2000). Similarly, there are approximately 333 million new cases of curable (i.e., bacterial) STDs each year among adults. Having even one STD makes an individual between two and five times more susceptible to HIV (Division of STD Prevention, 2000). Fortunately, there are effective medical therapies to cure most STD infections, although vaccines are less common. Moreover, in many respects, primary prevention of STDs parallels prevention of HIV.

THEORIES

Current models of HIV prevention indicate that providing information about HIV and one's risk of contracting HIV are necessary but not sufficient for inducing protective sexual behavior (Fisher & Fisher, 2000). Mere knowledge of HIV transmission and risk reduction is not enough; individuals must believe that they are personally at risk of such diseases, and they must be motivated to reduce this risk (Carey & Lewis, 1999). However, merely increasing perceptions of personal vulnerability appears not to improve HIV- and STD-risk-protective behavior (Gerrard, Gibbons, & Bushman, 1996). In general, three other processes that need to be considered involve attitudes, peer influence, and skills development. From the perspective of the *Theory of Reasoned Action* and *Theory of Planned Behavior* (Albarracín, Johnson, Fishbein, & Muellerleile, 2001), risk behaviors are predicted best by people's intentions to engage in such behavior, which are in turn influenced by an individual's attitude and perceived social norms toward the behavior. In short, if individuals have positive attitudes toward the behavior and if they are motivated to comply with their peers' acceptance of the behavior, they will intend to engage the behavior. These theories, as well as *social influence* approaches (Kelly, St. Lawrence, & Stevenson, 1992), suggest the importance that peers play in influencing behavior. To the extent to which an individual believes that remaining abstinent or using condoms is a typical and acceptable behavior to people they find important, they will be more likely to intentionally engage in that behavior.

A final critical process involves skills development. Theorizing about *self-efficacy* (Bandura, 1994) suggests that to enact a behavior, a person must have learned the appropriate skills such as how to resist pressure to engage in unwanted action, how to use a condom, or how to clean drug equipment. Skills-based experiences provide not only the necessary competencies to allow action to occur when an individual is motivated to do so, but also, by enhancing confidence in those competencies to perform some specific behaviors (feelings of self-efficacy), it increases motivation to act.

The models developed specifically in response to the HIV crisis build on multiple aspects of these theories. The *AIDS Risk Reduction Model* (ARRM; Catania, Kegeles, & Coates, 1990) and *Transtheoretical Model* (Prochaska & Velicer, 1997) emphasize that changing risk behavior involves shifting individuals toward stages in which they recognize the need to change their behavior, begin to contemplate, and prepare to change their behavior, before committing to change and finally maintaining this change. The most comprehensive model that guides HIV interventions is the *Information–Motivation–Behavioral Skills Model* (IMB; Fisher & Fisher, 2000), which posits that inducing appropriate sexual behavior requires addressing informational deficits, instantiating motivation in attitudes, normative influence, and perceived vulnerability to HIV, as well as developing behavioral skills. In particular, this model suggests that interventions should be tailored to targeted populations. For example, approaches that center on men having sex with men would be largely inappropriate for a sample of inner-city women. As another example, practice at managing one's own impulses and managing one's environment to avoid risky situations (intrapersonal skills) would be essential for people whose failures to use condoms were based in poor self-management skills.

STRATEGIES THAT WORK

From the perspective of current models of HIV risk reduction, changing risk behavior means one of two things. One strategy, a *structural* approach, is making permanent changes to the environment of people at risk, thus increasing lower-risk behaviors. When community-wide policies make condoms or clean injection drug equipment more available, at-risk behaviors decline. Alternatively, *psychological* approaches use persuasive mechanisms, education, and skills training to move individuals toward safer behavior. In this strategy, changing behavior means focusing on beliefs about the specific costs and benefits of engaging in the risk and protective behavior, feelings of self-efficacy, peer and informational influences, and motivation to act on their attitudes. Such strategies may be pursued from individual, small-group, or community-level perspectives. Structural and psychological interventions are not mutually exclusive categories (Carey, 1999). Changes to structure do result in changes in psychological underpinnings of behavior, and to some extent the reverse route is possible, also. Here we organize findings about reducing risk of HIV starting with individualized strategies leading to the most general, structural strategies. Each strategy may involve use of the other strategies, but generally individual interventions fall into only one of these categories.

Individualized Strategies to Reduce Risk of HIV (and STDs)

In the United States, the most commonly employed strategy to reduce individual's risks of receiving HIV or transmitting it is HIV counseling and testing. To date, more than one third of adult Americans have been tested, with about 2 million individuals voluntarily seeking tests each year (Anderson, 1996). (An unknown number of Americans are tested in other employment, insurance, and health care contexts.) The CDC has a large commitment to HIV testing supplemented with counseling and has recently endorsed testing for all Americans. Many states offer anonymous and/or confidential HIV tests without charge. A large number of trials have now evaluated the efficacy of HIV counseling and testing regarding sexual transmission of HIV. To date, the results show that, for individuals who test negative, negligible risk reduction occurs, but that for individuals who test positive, significant risk reduction occurs on the dimensions of unprotected intercourse, condom use, and number of sexual partners (Weinhardt, Carey, Johnson, & Bickham, 1999). Serodiscordant couples—those with one member HIV-positive and the other HIV-negative—change the most. This evidence strongly suggests that HIV counseling and testing as it has been practiced to date is a powerful secondary prevention strategy, but is not very effective for primary prevention. Unfortunately, little is known about the content of the counseling portion of such trials; it is possible that counseling and testing interventions can prove effective for primary prevention if such interventions conform to other techniques that have now been shown to be effective, such as for example including skills training for risk reduction (Kalichman, Carey, & Johnson, 1996). The evidence regarding HIV counseling and testing in IDUs has yet to be cumulated.

Traditionally STDs have been treated with antibiotics and other drugs following testing; those who test positive for a particular STD are interviewed regarding their past partners to facilitate partner notification in order that the STD will not spread more widely. But here the picture becomes more complex because, as we mentioned earlier, having an STD makes an individual two to five times more susceptible to contracting HIV. STDs often cause genital lesions in both men and women, which permits easier access for HIV into the bloodstream. Similarly, in women, STDs can increase the number of HIV target cells (CD4 cells) in cervical mucous, increasing susceptibility to HIV. Perhaps even more importantly, individuals who have both one or more STDs and HIV have greater detectable HIV in their secretions (e.g., semen). Consequently, prevention of STDs—which in many cases are treatable—has a direct added benefit of being an HIV prevention strategy.

Small-Group Strategies to Reduce Risk of HIV

Most of the available psychosocial prevention trials to reduce HIV-risk behaviors have been conducted using relatively small groups. In such studies, researchers typically deliver the content to small groups of 6–8 participants who are peers and use procedures that actively engage them in the material. In addition to extensive information about HIV, effective interventions provide information about condoms. Sometimes participants are provided explicit instruction (modeling and rehearsal) of condom use. HIV risk is

personalized through information and exercises designed to enhance perceptions of personal risk. Moreover, interpersonal skills training is often included and appears to be a significant component of effective interventions, consistent with self-efficacy theory and the IMB model. Such training often involves role-playing to enhance communication and negotiation skills with a potential sexual partner. In these cases, individuals rehearse scenarios in which they learn how to resist pressure to engage in sex or persuade a partner to use a condom; they receive feedback and encouragement from the facilitators and the other group members; and they watch others role-play scenarios. Many interventions also include intrapersonal skill development.

Occasionally these components require active involvement much like the role-playing exercises; participants discuss how to manage their own feelings in potentially sexual situations, describe their own goals and plans regarding risk behavior, and develop personal plans and strategies for managing both themselves and their risk environment. Some interventions add relapse management as an aspect of intrapersonal skills development. More commonly, intrapersonal skill components are either omitted or delivered with less extensive active participation, in which participants merely discussed goals and self-management issues.

Facilitators in these interventions are sometimes health-care professionals, paraprofessionals, peers, or some combination thereof. A number of studies have evaluated interventions tailored to minority individuals living in areas of higher HIV incidence, not limited to the United States. Moreover, interventions have been conducted in populations at high risk such as drug users and the severely mentally ill. These programs focus on reducing risky behaviors (e.g., unprotected intercourse) or increasing healthier behaviors (e.g., using clean needles).

The content of psychosocial interventions varies widely from those that focus on education only, to providing information about condom or drug use, and providing participants with skills-building experiences (e.g., role-playing or condom skills). Participants in these enriched programs, when compared to participants who did not receive the intervention or received an alternative minimal intervention (e.g., education-only), tend to have decreased risky sexual activity and increased condom use when they are sexually active, and/or decreased injection drug use or decreased unsafe drug use. An early research synthesis of small-group trials focusing on sexual risk reduction revealed that the interventions are at least modestly successful (Kalichman et al., 1996). Similarly, skill-training interventions for IDUs are effective at reducing sexual risk for HIV, although studies have had minimal success at increasing the safety of injection behaviors, as shown in a recent meta-analysis (Prendergast, Urada, & Podus, 2001). It also seems clear that the best interventions are tailored to the specific barriers and risk factors present for a given population. Because the concerns of each population differ, it is important to conduct elicitation research in order to determine the specific beliefs and behaviors that place participants at risk, or to identify barriers to risk reduction. The intervention can then target the particular beliefs and behaviors that are the most relevant or the most feasible to change. Increasingly, interventions place less concern on general HIV/AIDS education and focus on providing information that is most proximal to the risk behaviors in question.

Community-Level Strategies to Reduce Risk of HIV

Strategies at the community level have typically tried to identify individuals who are already peer leaders in the community, or who can be trained to be community advocates. The principle is that the best advocates for reducing risk behaviors are peers who already are embedded in the social network. For example, investigators might look at an area already high in HIV prevalence to identify a popular bar where men meet men and ask regulars at the bar to identify the most popular individuals, who are often called "popular opinion leaders" or "gatekeepers" because they serve as a link to at-risk individuals of the community (Kelly et al., 1992). These individuals may be recruited to help to design the intervention (e.g., to make it more sensitive to the needs of the targeted individuals). The intervention might be supplemented by small or mass media (e.g., posters about safe sex, radio ads). The popular opinion leaders are often also trained to give personal accounts on how to reduce HIV-risk behaviors to other members of the community. The studies also often make condoms more available to people in the targeted community (e.g., at popular bars). Other community-wide interventions have merely exposed residents of treatment towns to extensive clinic-based medical treatments for STDs. Results to date have suggested that communities using such strategies have reduced risk behaviors relative to matched communities without such strategies (e.g., Kelly et al., 1992).

Mass-Media Strategies to Reduce Risk of HIV

Mass media campaigns have sometimes been deployed in the public health fight against HIV infection, although their use in the United States has not been widespread (Carey & Vanable, in press). Numerous studies suggest that broad-based HIV-education campaigns that target risk-related beliefs among the general public may change knowledge and attitudes (Wolber, 1987), but many studies have shown little change of subsequent high-risk behaviors

(Abraham & Sheeran, 1993). For cost-effectiveness reasons, public health officials have generally favored more targeted media interventions at "hot spots" in epidemics rather than blanketing large regions of the country simultaneously. For example, an area with a high incidence of STDs may be targeted with public service announcements. Safer sexual behaviors can be diffused through the media. For example, a radio-broadcast HIV prevention program in the guise of a soap opera has proven effective at reducing risk behaviors in Tanzania (Rogers, 2000).

Structural Interventions to Reduce Risk of HIV

Some countries have implemented large national prevention programs, such as Thailand's *100 percent Condom Program*, targeted at sex workers. The government mandated condom use during commercial sex, with the result that unprotected sex decreased dramatically, as did the incidence of STDs and HIV infections among the sex workers and in groups that frequent them (Celentano et al., 1998). Structural interventions have also focused extensively on IDUs, trying to reduce the practice of exchanging needles, by, for example, offering methadone, free condoms, and bleach kits or needle-exchange programs for addicted adults (for a review, see Des Jarlais, Guydish, Friedman, & Hagan, 2000). Methadone treatments help heroin addicts reduce drug use, which in turn decreases injection behaviors and lowers risk because there is less sharing of needles. There may also be an indirect risk reduction in that reducing drug use often leads to a reduction in sexual risk behavior. Finally, having free, clean needles available means that addicts do not need to share needles, with the consequence that bodily fluids are also not shared. Research to date appears to show that the interventions are successful, resulting in greater use of needle disinfection, entry into drug treatment, and even reduce HIV seroincidence (Des Jarlais et al., 2000).

STRATEGIES THAT MIGHT WORK

Although the preceding section makes clear that many strategies work, the changing nature of the HIV pandemic across time urges caution. Because cultures and subcultures change, there is no single solution guaranteed to work well in every instance. For example, after a decade of lowered HIV incidence in the Castro District of San Francisco, incidence rates recently began to rise again. Prevention messages and strategies that had worked became ineffective in the face of life-prolonging medications. Any strategy that can work in one location and time must be first considered to be a strategy that *might* work in some new context. It is for these reasons that many HIV prevention scholars recommend piloting interventions and their components before proceeding full-scale.

STRATEGIES THAT DO NOT WORK

In general, prevention programs that lack skills training and merely provide information alone are minimally effective at inducing safer behavior. There are few studies in which merely providing sex education or condom information has been effective. Yet the success of relatively brief counseling and testing interventions on those who test positive for HIV suggests that behavior change can take place quickly after an individual learns about the positive test, even without all of the usual components of a successful intervention (Weinhardt et al., 1999). Such an experience engages active individualized motivation in understanding and coping with the infection.

SYNTHESIS

HIV/AIDS has had a devastating impact around the world, an impact that continues to worsen. Until such time as a preventive vaccine for HIV becomes available, which is not likely in the near future, behavioral change will continue to be an essential way to prevent HIV. Fortunately, psychosocial interventions, whether implemented on an individualized or very broad scale, have been shown to be effective in reducing risk for HIV and STD infection among adults around the world. The most successful interventions use elicitation research to determine what beliefs most need changing, provide information, enhance health-promotion skills, and improve motivation to practice safer behaviors.

It is worth drawing attention to the fact that although HIV prevention efforts have a statistically detectable impact on risk behaviors, the impact is generally small in absolute terms, smaller than what other psycho-social-educational interventions have produced in the past (cf. Lipsey & Wilson, 1993). Our view is that changing HIV-risk behaviors is more difficult than changing other health promotion behaviors for two main reasons. First, HIV-risk behaviors are almost always relational. That is, the amount of risk an individual incurs is determined not simply by that individual but also by others around him or her. For example, a woman may not ask her partner to use a condom because he has more relationship power than she does. Thus, the best risk reduction requires that both the intrapersonal *and* the interpersonal parts of the equation are addressed. Interventions that have provided not only information but also appropriate skills training have proven the most successful at reducing risk for acquiring HIV.

The second reason that HIV preventions may have a smaller-than-desirable impact is that society gives conflicting signals about the need for safe behavior. For example, norms for adolescents might support not only risk reduction but also increased levels of sexuality. Psychosocial interventions must pay close attention to the ebbs and flows of societal and cultural changes, not to mention the psychological changes that occur because of new treatments. San Francisco recently witnessed a sharp increase in new HIV infections, particularly among young gay men, perhaps because as a result of the perception that HIV is now a manageable disease rather than a fatal one. Clearly, there are broad-level risk changes that require interventions to be continual, always on the watch for reactance to the interventions. This conclusion also holds for periods when interventions seem to be working particularly well. Just because there is reduced risk is no assurance that it will last.

Other impediments to HIV prevention are structural. In all too many locales, residents are leery of needle exchange programs, it is illegal for individuals to purchase needles, drug treatments are not available on demand, and there are many blocks even to make condoms available to students who request them at school clinics. We probably need to make just as much attempt to "intervene" with public opinion than we do with those at individual risk. For example, the public can be educated about what the research data show: Condom availability does *not* reduce abstinence rates.

With growing numbers of HIV-positive individuals living normal life spans, future interventions are certain to develop secondary prevention efforts extensively, making sure that people know their HIV status and that they behave safely with regard to others. With no cure or vaccine in sight, the fact that more HIV-positive individuals will survive means that the prevention of infecting others will grow more important with time. The recent drug company decisions to make antiretroviral drug treatments more widely available in economically challenged areas has the potential to keep individuals healthy and alive longer. Yet, to the extent that individuals do not comply with the regimens of the drug treatments, new and more resistant strains of HIV emerge, making HIV prevention and management even more difficult. Thus, preventive services are crucial for ensuring that present HIV strains do not become ever more dangerous. Adhering to the drug treatment regimens can be challenging; thus, psychosocial and structural interventions to remove the barriers to adherence in HIV individuals are fast becoming essential for worldwide public health.

Also see: HIV/AIDS: Early Childhood; HIV/AIDS: Childhood; HIV/AIDS: Adolescence; HIV/AIDS: Older Adulthood; Sexually Transmitted Diseases: Adolescence.

References

Abraham, C., & Sheeran, P. (1993). In search of a psychology of safer-sex promotion: Beyond beliefs and texts. *Health Education Research, 8,* 245–254.

Albarracín, D., Johnson, B.T., Fishbein, M., & Muellerleile, P.A. (2001). Theories of reasoned action and planned behavior as models of condom use: A meta-analysis. *Psychological Bulletin, 127,* 142–161.

Anderson, J.E. (1996). CDC data systems collecting behavioral data on HIV counseling and testing. *Public Health Reports, 11,* 129–132.

Bandura, A. (1994). Social cognitive theory and exercise of control over AIDS. In R. DiClemente & J. Peterson (Eds.), *Preventing AIDS: Theories, methods, and behavioral interventions* (pp. 25–60). New York: Plenum.

Catania, J.A., Kegeles, S.M., & Coates, T.J. (1990). Towards an understanding of risk behavior: An AIDS risk reduction model (ARRM). *Health Education Quarterly, 17,* 53–72.

Carey, M.P., & Vanable, P.A. (in press). HIV/AIDS. In A.M. Nezu, C.M. Nezu, & P.A. Geller (Eds.), *Comprehensive handbook of psychology, Volume 9: Health psychology.* New York: Wiley.

Carey, M.P. (1999). Prevention of HIV infection through changes in sexual behavior. *American Journal of Health Promotion, 14,* 104–111.

Carey, M.P., & Lewis, B.P. (1999). Motivational strategies can augment HIV-risk reduction programs. *AIDS and Behavior, 3,* 269–276.

Celentano, D.D., Nelson, K.E., Lyles, C.M., Beyrer, C., Eiumtrakul, S., Go, V.F., Kuntolbutra, S., & Khamboonruang, C. (1998). Decreasing incidence of HIV and sexually transmitted diseases in young Thai men: Evidence for success of the HIV/AIDS control and prevention program. *AIDS, 12,* F29–F36.

Centers for Disease Control and Prevention (CDC). (2000). *HIV/AIDS surveillance report, 2000, 12*(1).

Des Jarlais, D.C., Guydish, J., Friedman, S.R., & Hagan, H. (2000). HIV/AIDS prevention for drug users in natural settings. In J. Peterson & R. DiClemente (Eds.), *Handbook of HIV prevention* (pp. 159–177). New York: Kluwer Academic/Plenum.

Division of STD Prevention. (2000, September). *Sexually transmitted disease surveillance, 1999.* Department of Health and Human Services, Atlanta: Centers for Disease Control and Prevention (CDC).

Fisher, J.D., & Fisher, W.A. (2000). Theoretical approaches to individual-level change in HIV risk behavior. In J. Peterson & R. DiClemente (Eds.), *Handbook of HIV prevention* (pp. 3–55). New York: Kluwer Academic/Plenum.

Gerrard, M., Gibbons, F.X., & Bushman, B.J. (1996). Relation between perceived vulnerability to HIV and precautionary sexual behavior. *Psychological Bulletin, 119,* 390–409.

Kalichman, S.C., Carey, M.P., & Johnson, B.T. (1996). Prevention of sexually transmitted HIV infection: A meta-analytic review of the behavioral outcome literature. *Annals of Behavioral Medicine, 18,* 6–15.

Kelly, J.A., St. Lawrence, J.S., & Stevenson, L.Y. (1992). Community AIDS/HIV risk reduction: The effects of endorsements by popular people in three cities. *American Journal of Public Health, 82,* 1483–1489.

Lipsey, M.W., & Wilson, D.B. (1993). The efficacy of psychological, educational, and behavioral treatment: Confirmation from meta-analysis. *American Psychologist, 48,* 1181–1209.

Prochaska, J.O., & Velicer, W.F. (1997). The transtheoretical model of health behavior change. *American Journal of Health Promotion, 12,* 38–48.

Prendergast, M.L., Urada, D., & Podus, D. (2001). Meta-analysis of HIV risk-reduction interventions within drug abuse treatment programs. *Journal of Consulting and Clinical Psychology, 69,* 389–405.

Rogers, E.M. (2000). Diffusion theory: A theoretical approach to promote community-level change. In J.L. Peterson & R.J. DiClemente (Eds.), *Handbook of HIV prevention* (pp. 57–65). New York: Kluwer Academic/Plenum.

UNAIDS (2000, December). *AIDS epidemic update: December 2000.* Geneva, Switzerland: World Health Organization.

Weinhardt, L.S., Carey, M.P., Johnson, B.T., & Bickham, N. (1999). Effects of HIV counseling and testing on sexual risk behavior: Meta-analytic review of published research, 1985–1997. *American Journal of Public Health, 89,* 1397–1405.

Wolber, J.M. (1987). *Youth and television: Some patterns of behaviour, appreciation and attitudes, particularly concerning AIDS.* London: Independent Broadcasting Authority.

HIV/AIDS, Older Adulthood

K. Rivet Amico and Blair T. Johnson

INTRODUCTION, DEFINITIONS, AND SCOPE

Infection with the human immunodeficiency virus (HIV), which causes acquired immunodeficiency syndrome (AIDS), is a serious public health threat around the world. (See other definitions in Cornman & Johnson: HIV/AIDS, Early Childhood.) In the United States, approximately 80,000 (6 percent) of known cases of HIV are 50 years of age and older and about 11 percent of all US cases of AIDS are in this age group (Centers for Disease Control and Prevention [CDC], 2000). AIDS has been identified as the 15th leading cause of death in those over 65 years of age in the United States (Hillman & Stricker, 1998) and the picture is similar in other developed countries (UNAIDS, 2000). In developing countries (e.g., sub-Saharan Africa), the HIV/AIDS has appeared in older adults less frequently than in developed countries because AIDS has killed younger adults so frequently (UNAIDS, 2000). Despite the sizable number of older individuals directly affected by HIV/AIDS, this community continues to be under-served and neglected in terms of HIV primary and secondary prevention efforts. Moreover, the number of HIV infections in older adults is almost certain to grow substantially in the coming years.

Our ability to curb the epidemic in older adults depends primarily on the ability to meet challenges unique to this population and to implement creative prevention strategies. Older adults are unique or distinguished from their younger cohorts by a number of features relevant to HIV transmission risk. Modes of HIV transmission interact with the aging processes, placing older adults at greater risk for contracting HIV. Older adults have a disease presentation that tends to delay diagnosis of HIV, which in turn delays treatment and offers a larger window of opportunity of unwitting transmission to others. There is a need for the development of intervention strategies that can better equip older adults in maintaining healthy behaviors and decreasing those behaviors that place individuals at risk. This entry discusses how HIV manifests itself in older populations and how to prevent the spread of HIV in older populations. We explore how HIV is expressed in older adults by reviewing current and anticipated prevalence rates of HIV in older populations, modes of transmission with emphasis on age-related and cultural sensitivity, the problems with delayed diagnosis in this population, and issues surrounding disease progression and treatment. Primary prevention of HIV in older adults is a newly burgeoning area of research, with a handful of localized efforts that promise to provide us with the first evaluations of what might be effective with this population. While efficacy results are still needed, we offer some possibilities for interventions that may maximize yields from past research and theory in this area.

Prevalence of HIV in Older and Elderly Adults

Although prevalence estimates indicate that the HIV/AIDS epidemic is substantial among older adults and the elderly, it is very likely that the magnitude of the epidemic in this group has been underestimated. Research shows that health care providers make delayed diagnoses of HIV/AIDS when dealing with elderly patients, despite striking clinical indications and markers (Ankrom & Greenough, 1997; Gaeta, LaPolla, & Malendez, 1996; Gordon & Thompson, 1995). Older adults may feel most acutely the stigma of an HIV/AIDS diagnosis, which may prevent them from accurately reporting risks and/or seeking medical advice (Szirony, 1999). These delays or failures to reach an appropriate HIV/AIDS diagnosis make accurate estimates of prevalence difficult but point to the all-but-certain conclusion that available prevalence rates are an underestimate. Additionally, campaigns to encourage respectful and appropriate treatment of individuals with HIV/AIDS have traditionally targeted younger populations, which may help these individuals, more than the elderly, to come forward for treatment. Consequently, an accurate HIV/AIDS diagnosis may not even be reached until after death and sometimes not even then (el Sadr & Gettler, 1995). Demographic trends indicate that the incidence of HIV/AIDS in elderly populations will increase over time. In the year 2000, those 65 and above made up one eighth of the US population. With babyboomers approaching retirement age, this population should double in the next 50 years (Lieberman, 2000). As the sheer size of the population increases, even if the percentages remain the same, the actual numbers of HIV/AIDS cases in the US population of those 50 and older can easily double. Additionally, there will be more individuals with HIV who will have the opportunity to grow older in this country due to the longevity benefits of highly active antiretroviral therapies.

Several factors create a situation in which risk of HIV transmission among elderly persons is acute. The elderly population is growing and along with this growth a larger number of HIV-positive individuals will enter this stage of life, owing to the success of antiretroviral therapies. Although age-related maladies may once have limited engagement in HIV-risk behaviors, improved health and medical remedies for erectile dysfunction such as Viagra (Hilton, 1998) make the elderly increasingly similar to middle- and younger-adults. If elders continue to show a lack of knowledge about HIV-risk behaviors and safer sexual behaviors (Linsk, 1994; Nocera, 1997; Szirony, 1999), then the incidence of HIV/AIDS cases in older adult and elderly populations may increase.

HIV/AIDS Modes of Transmission in Older and Elderly Adults

In order to identify goals for prevention strategies, one must be familiar with the common modes of transmission of HIV in the older adult population, which tends to be similar to those for younger individuals. The leading cause is homosexual transmission among men, followed by needle sharing among intravenous drug users, blood transfusion, and, finally, heterosexual transmission (Catania, Turner, Kegeles, Stall, Pollack, & Coates, 1989; Hillman & Stricker, 1998; Szirony, 1999; Whipple & Scura, 1989). Transmission via men having sex with men appears to be the leading transmission route up to the age of 70 for US men (Wallace, Paauw, & Spach, 1993), while transmission via blood transfusion has dropped since the advent of blood screening in the United States in 1985. Another mode of transmission commonly overlooked is the exchange of blood or fluids during caregiving from an older adult to his or her adult child suffering from HIV/AIDS (Brabant, 1994; Levine-Perkell, 1996; Lloyd, 1998). Unlike younger HIV-positive individuals, older adults who acquire HIV are more likely to indicate that they do not know how they contracted HIV, suggesting that prevalence rates for different modes of transmission may be very difficult to estimate (Gordon & Thompson, 1995).

Within these trends, modes of transmission appear to differ across cultures. Men having sex with men is a more prevalent risk behavior in Western society than in sub-Saharan Africa and Eastern countries, where women and children are the higher risk groups (Lee, Leo, Snodgrass, & Wang, 1997). Transmission of HIV via shared needles is more likely in US older adults compared to UK elders (Hilton, 1998). Ingstad, Brunn, and Tlou (1997) noted the increased potential for blood transmission of HIV in cultures that practice rituals that involve blood exchange and/or exposure.

Across cultures, unique changes due to hormone level decreases in older women have created growing concern about the risks of heterosexual transmission via vaginal intercourse (Hillman & Stricker, 1998). Not only vaginal dryness but also thinning of vaginal walls in post-menopausal women, which is due to decreases in progesterone, create greater potential for micro and macro tears allowing for easier exchange of the virus (Catania et al., 1989; Hillman & Stricker, 1998; Szirony, 1999). Thus, heterosexual transmission is clearly an area of increased concern for older adults. Heightening the concern is the fact that older and elderly adults tend *not* to use protective barriers such as condoms during intercourse (Chiao, Ries, & Sande, 1999; Nocera, 1997; Szirony, 1999) and frequently report sexual activity outside of a steady relationship (Nokes, 1999).

A number of reasons may underlie this avoidance of condom use. Older men may be reluctant to use a condom due to complications the condom may cause with maintaining an erection (Hilton, 1998). Post-menopausal women may not consider condom use during heterosexual intercourse because they no longer need protection from pregnancy (Szirony, 1999). There also appears to be a relative lack of knowledge in the older heterosexual population about HIV/AIDS as a sexually transmitted disease (Johnson, Haight, & Benedict, 1989; Szirony, 1999). Even in samples where there was some degree of knowledge about HIV/AIDS transmission, older adults, much like their younger counterparts, continued to engage in heterosexual and homosexual risk behaviors (Leigh, Temple, & Trocki, 1993).

THEORIES AND RESEARCH

The theories discussed in earlier entries on HIV prevention are relevant to older persons as well. The cognitive-behavioral models, which emphasize how people's beliefs about their world influence their behavior—including risky behavior—are especially pertinent for older persons.

HIV/AIDS Symptoms and Diagnosis in Older and Elderly Adults

Early detection and diagnosis of HIV infection can help to prevent further transmissions of HIV and have been identified as critical to all prevention efforts (Janssen, 2001). In reaching these prevention goals, we must increase both health care providers' and the general public's understanding of the reality of HIV as a health threat to an older population. Once it has been contracted, HIV/AIDS can be unique for the

older adult populations in terms of the disease progression, diagnosis, and course of the illness. The "window" period between contraction of the HIV virus and the development of symptoms is shorter for older adults than their younger counterparts, about 4–7 years (Catania et al., 1989), with an average of 5.5 years (Medley, Anderson, Cox, & Billard, 1987). Common symptoms in the elderly are ambiguous and non-specific (Wallace et al., 1993), including anorexia, weight loss, fatigue, decreased physical endurance, and diminished mental abilities (Wooten, 1999), which are often dismissed as artifacts of the normal aging process (Lieberman, 2000). Frequently, an older adult makes his or her first presentation to medical care providers with opportunistic infection(s) (OIs) and/or HIV/AIDS dementia complex (HADC; Hillman & Stricker, 1998; Szirony, 1999). Older adults and elderly with HIV tend to have lower numbers of helper T-cells (CD4 counts) than their younger counterparts (Adler, Baskar, Chrest, Dorsey, Winchurch, & Nagel, 1997; de Gorgolas, Bello, Gracia, Moya, Gracia, & Fernandez-Guerrero, 1999), leaving them with lowered ability to fight and overcome viral infections. HIV, through a number of mechanisms, overtakes CD4 cells rendering them incapable of attacking the virus. Although the rate of CD4 destruction is about the same for younger and older HIV positive individuals, the older individual cannot as easily replace the destroyed or mutated CD4 cells with new viable ones (Adler et al., 1997), thus placing the older HIV positive adult at considerable risk for OIs such as Pneumocystis Carinii Pneumonia (PCP) or Mycobacterium Tuberculosis (TB) (cf. Szirony, 1999; Wooten, 1999). Similar to the general symptoms of HIV for the older adult, general practitioners often do not associate these infections with possible HIV infection (Crisologo, Campbell, & Forte, 1996; Hillman & Stricker, 1998).

It is also common for the first complaints brought to medical attention to be cognitive or neurological in nature (Szirony, 1999). HDAC in the older adult can easily be misdiagnosed as Dementia of Alzheimer's type (Hilton, 1998; Wallace et al., 1993). Unique to HADC, however, patients may present with rapid onset of symptoms over a 6-month period, substantial social withdrawal, unsteady gait as a symptom developed early on, overall psychomotor slowing, and a relative absence of aphasias (Hillman & Stricker, 1998). Hilton (1998) recommends the use of speeded tests, as opposed to the standard Mini-Mental State Exam screen typically used in medical settings, as a potential tool in differential diagnosis. Quite unlike other dementias, HADC symptoms can be completely reversed with appropriate treatment (Hillman & Stricker, 1998), though many health and mental health care providers appear to be generally unaware of this course of action (Hillman, 1998).

Because the general symptoms of HIV and presentation of OIs and HDAC can have a number of different possible underlying causes, HIV in the elderly has earned the term of the "new great imitator" (Sabin, 1987). General practitioners treating geriatric patients are not generally well versed in HIV risks and manifestations, making signs and symptoms difficult to identify (Lieberman, 2000). In addition, stereotypes of elderly as asexual and non-drug abusing can impede the clinician from fully assessing HIV risk factors or giving HIV infection serious consideration with their elderly patients (Puleo, 1996), even in the face of positive STD histories (Gordon & Thompson, 1995). Such factors can interact to create long delays between presentation of HIV/AIDS symptoms and diagnosis. Reports of delayed diagnosis range from 3 (Gordon & Thompson, 1995) to 10 months (Ankrom & Greenough, 1997). These delays are particularly disturbing on the individual level given the rapid progression of HIV/AIDS and poor survival rates in the elderly (Adler et al., 1997; Chiao et al., 1999) and on an epidemic level in terms of allowing for a greater opportunity for the HIV positive person to unknowingly infect others.

HIV/AIDS Disease Progression and Treatment

Prevention strategies must make use of what is currently known about the ravaging effects of HIV on its elder hosts. HIV is a health threat to all individuals, but is particularly dramatic for elder adults. HIV has a faster disease progression rate in older and elderly individuals (Chiao et al., 1999), owing primarily to the inability to produce new CD4 cells in older adults (Adler et al., 1997). The weakened immunity allows OIs to have fatal impacts on their hosts, a progression often hastened by late medical attention. Survival rates for older individuals have been estimated to range from 3 months from diagnosis (Lee et al., 1997) to 24 months (Skiest, Rubinstien, Carely, Gioiella, & Lyons, 1996), although co-morbid conditions (such as OIs) appear to have a larger role in disease progression than age per se (Skiest et al., 1996). Our understanding of the rapid development of fatal illnesses calls for a distinctive approach to preventing HIV/AIDS in older persons, which we will describe below. It also calls for equally rapid identification, diagnosis, and treatment. With slowed identification and diagnosis, treatment of HIV is currently an unknown proposition for elderly adults. Older and elderly adults are rarely included in clinical trials of antiretroviral treatments for HIV, often because co-morbid conditions exclude them as ineligible (Szirony, 1999). Consequently, there is little information available in terms of optimal treatments for HIV in the older and elderly populations (Adler & Nagel, 1994; Szirony, 1999). What is known is that Zidovudine (AZT) can be effective in older patients with HIV (de Gorgolas et al., 1999), with survival rates similar to that of their younger counterparts at 24-month follow-ups. Because only a minority of older patients can tolerate AZT, however, applicability is severely limited. Antiretrovirals appear to be the most promising treatment for older individuals, with smaller doses required as well as frequent monitoring (Adler et al., 1997).

Since the advent of highly active antiretroviral therapy in 1996, many HIV positive patients have effectively treated their HIV, often to the point of the HIV being undetectable by our typical viral load assessment measures (Arnsten, Demas, Gourevitch, Buono, Farzadegan, & Schoenbaum, 2000; Bangsberg et al., 2000). Older and elderly HIV patients, however, have not been a large part of these advances (Szirony, 1999). The seriousness of an HIV diagnosis for an elderly individual, in terms of natural progression and limited treatment options, must be conveyed in prevention strategies in a manner that does not "scare" the recipients of such messages into inaction. A delicate balance between the reality of HIV's grave effects and the possibility of protecting oneself from HIV through a menu of actions must be achieved.

STRATEGIES THAT WORK

Just as older and elderly adults have been de-emphasized relative to younger adults in terms of diagnosis and treatment of HIV/AIDS, to date prevention studies focusing on this population are virtually non-existent. For example, less than 1 percent of HIV/AIDS research published as of the year 2000 explicitly addresses the elderly. While there is a current lack of published, scientific evaluations of educational campaigns for HIV/AIDS prevention in the older adult and elderly populations, ongoing studies should, in the near future, ameliorate this problem. Currently, the National Institute of Nursing Research is sponsoring Momentum AIDS Project's implementation and evaluation of a psychoeducational group program for older HIV positive adults in New York City, and the National Institute on Aging is sponsoring the development of an intervention program targeting coping in older HIV-positive adults. Efforts in primary prevention of HIV in older adults continue to be an area in need of exploration. To date, interventions influencing older adults tend to be directed at a younger cohort and reach elders by way of indirect (e.g., publicity campaigns) as opposed to direct (interventions developed specifically for an aged population) routes.

STRATEGIES THAT MIGHT WORK

Because there is a paucity of prevention studies targeting older adult populations, prevention strategies developed for adolescents and young adults continue to be used with the aged. Although it is tempting to translate these models, we should be cautious about such generalizations because of the discrepancy in history, cultural climate, and expression of HIV between the age groups. With these cautions in mind, we have compiled a brief list of prevention strategies that may translate well into older populations with minor modifications and note their potential misapplication. In addition, we consider the strategies of information dissemination, enlisting care provider support, and extending current behavior change theory in greater detail. Strategies likely to be effective for prevention of HIV transmission within the older and elderly adult populations include making more information available about the risks to and expression of this disease in elderly individuals. Effectiveness seems likely to increase as the message becomes more specific and relevant to the receiver and offers specific strategies for avoiding negative consequences. Information must be tailored to address the issues faced by older adults in the specific area targeted by the prevention effort (e.g., rural Kentucky vs. New York City). Messages will likely be ineffective if they are too heavily steeped in scare tactics, rely on colloquialisms irrelevant to the targeted populations, or provide no recourse for action. Programs that focus only on information dissemination are likely only to have minimal effectiveness.

Effective prevention campaigns must use more than mere information. Strategies should use a multi-pronged, tiered approach, focusing, at minimum, on information, skills necessary to perform safer behaviors, and the motivation to perform them. Past experience with prevention strategies suggests that information alone is a necessary but insufficient condition for change. Information dissemination should be one of several strategies.

Like any age group, prevention efforts should emphasize, where relevant, eliminating unsafe sexual practices (e.g., fewer partners, more condom use), eliminating drug use, or increasing safe drug-use strategies (e.g., cleaning injection drug equipment). Strategies that may be most effective are likely to take a harm-reduction approach, in which abstinence is but one of several possible goals.

Important for some elder individuals is the provision of sexual education. Alternatives to intercourse may need to be specifically identified and detailed. Behaviors such as touching and massage may not be a part of an elder individual's repertoire of sexual expression. Note that strategies may quickly be rendered ineffective when the preventive behavior is too distal and possibly inappropriate from current behaviors (e.g., advocating abstinence with a sexually active steady couple).

Prevention efforts must target *both* this population *and* its providers of service and care. Providers can work toward enhancing prevention, or can unwittingly undermine

prevention efforts. Effective prevention programs must solicit and maintain support from care providers.

While we are not yet in the position to rate intervention strategies in terms of their empirical evaluation, there are some strategies that hold promise to be more effective than others in working toward the prevention of HIV in an elderly population. Possible strategies to increase funds of accurate information in a culturally-sensitive manner, to involve care providers, and to apply behavioral change theory to preventing HIV in older populations are reviewed.

Effective Content for Prevention Messages

To meet the goal of providing accurate information, strategies and campaigns could benefit from: (a) using a nonstigmatizing manner to define HIV as the transmittable virus that causes AIDS; (b) defining known routes of transmission including sexual contacts and shared needle (whether for illicit drug use or for insulin injection or as caretakers of an adult child who is an AIDS victim) with emphasis on elevated risk factors in the elderly; (c) providing detailed strategies that can be used for protection, including male condoms, female condoms, and abstinence, emphasizing the possibility for mutually satisfying yet safer sexual relationships; (d) providing easily accessed support services for testing and information, expressly noting confidentiality (e.g., the National AIDS CDC Hotline; Welch, 1999); and (e) correcting misperceptions about HIV and AIDS.

To date, commercials and posters, as well as slogans, have mainly focused on younger persons (Nokes, 1999), unintentionally supporting the perception that HIV is not an illness that elderly individuals should consider a threat. The idea that "it can't happen to me" can easily support heuristics that one can "tell" whether his/her partner is HIV positive or that the risks are non-existent because of beliefs that HIV is quite rare in one's peer or age group. While accurate information should help to correct the misinformation, the format of delivery of the information may help to address more implicit processes (i.e., faulty heuristics). It would be helpful for campaigns to involve older individuals in their visual and audio strategies.

The content and format of prevention messages for older individuals also must differ. Unlike their younger counterparts, changes associated with menopause create conditions of greater transmission risk through sexual contact, yet knowledge of elevated risks is uncommon in older adults (Szirony, 1999). Education campaigns at the individual and community levels may help to address these deficits in knowledge by providing accurate information regarding transmission risks and by correcting inaccurate information (Hillman & Stricker, 1998; Szirony, 1999). The format for delivering information to an elderly population must be carefully constructed. Testimonials and the use of same-age models in messages can help to "normalize" and de-stigmatize HIV in older individuals. Posters, slogans, commercials, and advertisements in areas and venues where reaching an older population can be maximized should employ actors or presenters that mirror the population of interest.

Geographic regions, cultural affiliations, and cohort history can guide the development of educational/informational campaigns. While we continue to have limited research that would help to identify general information deficits, competencies, or misperceptions in elderly and older adults in specific regions in the United States, the use of local focus groups could inform prevention developers. Differences based on cohort history should also be considered. Individuals currently in their seventh and eighth decades came of age in the 1940s and 1950s, which were relatively conservative and private sexual eras (Linsk, 1994). In contrast, individuals currently in their fifth and sixth decades of life came of age in the 1960s and 1970s, a very different history with many participating in the freedoms of the sexual revolution and recreational drug use. Clearly, the manner in which information is presented to these two different groups would require sensitivity to one's comfort level in discussing issues of sex and drug use.

Caregivers as Change Agent

Another promising strategy for prevention of HIV in older populations is the enlistment of care providers in prevention efforts. Care providers are often characterized as having either undermining or neutral effects on HIV prevention in older adults. A lack of understanding about the expression of HIV in the elderly (Liebermann, 2000) or risk factors (Hillman, 1998), and stereotypes of the elderly as generally inactive sexually or unlikely to be drug abusers (Hillman & Stricker, 1998; Puleo, 1996) can interfere with a care provider's assessment of risk for HIV and the diagnosis and treatment of the disease. Because of these factors, it would be advisable for any prevention program targeting older adults to include a campaign for care provider support and education as a key component. Strategies to enlist care providers can take advantage of the resources available at the State and National levels (e.g., the National Association on HIV Over Fifty's (NAHOF) training material and information for service providers over the Internet— http://www.hivoverfifty.org).

Care providers can also be supported in efforts to include a sexual history (of perhaps the past 7 years) as a standard part of a medical evaluation for all individuals across the life-span (Hillman, 1998; Hillman & Stricker, 1998). The sexual history can be an opportunity for service or care providers to check an individual's fund of information and offer accurate information about HIV and AIDS (Linsk, 1994). On-line training (Linsk, 2000) can be used to sensitize providers to pertinent issues, though the availability of this, in itself, would not be expected to address the critical issues as sexual histories continue to be uncommon in general practice. Perhaps the growing prescription of medication to address erectile dysfunction associated with aging will offer the opportunity for discussions of sexual behavior and risk to become more common and familiar in medical and clinical care settings offering such treatments (Hilton, 1998). Prevention work with care providers, particularly medical care providers that may see their older patients quite frequently, is an area that offers tremendous promise for prevention intervention developers and evaluators.

Translating Models of Behavior Change

There is a need for translation of general models of risk behavior to HIV prevention in older adult populations. For several prominent models of HIV-risk behavior, information is a starting point for other change agents. In addition to information, the *Information Motivation Behavioral Skills (IMB) Model* (Fisher, Fisher, Williams, & Malloy, 1994), for example, identifies motivation to change behavior and behavioral skills as critical determinants of risk behavior. Included in the behavioral skills component are abilities needed for safer behavior (e.g., condom use skills; barrier-use skills in caring for AIDS patients at home; needle cleaning or exchange skills). Included in the motivational component is one's sense of social support for behavior change, one's perceived vulnerability, one's attitude towards behavior maintenance and change, and one's perceived intent to change behavior. Using community campaigns or individual care providers to deliver an intervention, in addition to increasing one's accurate information about HIV/AIDS, motivation to take precautions could be enhanced through manipulation of one's perceived vulnerability, or sense of support from peers, family, or care providers. A care provider can invite the exploration of attitudes and skills toward condom use, recognizing possible erectile difficulties and religious convictions that may support avoiding condom use. Similar to the cultural competency required in formatting informational campaigns, interventions utilizing IMB factors must be grounded in the culture of the target group, which is often informed through the use of localized focus groups.

SYNTHESIS

HIV/AIDS, a catastrophic and often fatal condition for individuals who are in their later years, affects some 80,000

US citizens over the age of 50. Despite this large number of cases, prevention efforts have focused primarily on younger individuals, unfortunately supporting misperceptions of invulnerability on the part of both older adults and their clinical and medical care providers. There is a present challenge to the scientific/research communities to adequately address the problem of HIV/AIDS in older populations.

Issues essential to understanding the scope and gravity of the HIV/AIDS problem in older adult and elderly populations include a understanding of current prevalence rates, modes of transmission and risk, and the characteristics and symptoms of HIV/AIDS in this age group, as well as diagnostic issues, disease progression, and prevention issues. While there are many theoretical models that address HIV prevention behaviors (Peterson & DiClemente, 2000), there has not yet been a model proposed or translated specific to older adults. Nonetheless, it is logical that currently used prevention strategies and behavior change models may, with some modification, generalize to this population. It is our belief that the most promising prevention strategies include: (a) targeting an increase in accurate information available about HIV in elderly persons; (b) working with care providers as change supporters and agents; and (c) providing prevention strategies are informed by the specific belief systems and cultural norms of the age cohort being targeted.

Prevention programs that appear to hold the most promise should target elder adults who are currently HIV negative, older adults who are HIV positive so as to prevent the spread of HIV, and their medical or other critical care providers. Behaviors targeted for change, based on what is known about common modes of transmission, would include risky sexual behaviors and needle sharing. Behaviors targeted for maintenance reinforcement would include safe and safer sexual behavior. Interventions for these individuals and these behaviors could be implemented via information enhancement campaigns, motivational enhancement, and imparting prevention and safer behavioral skills. These interventions may be accomplished in numerous sites (such as church groups, community recreation centers, life-long education centers, malls), so long as the information is creatively packaged. In particular, one avenue for intervention that might be particularly promising is the implementation of programs within the medical clinical care setting. This strategy may offer a two-prong effect of sensitizing clinicians to issues surrounding HIV with elderly populations and would allow prevention programs to reach a large number of seniors in a credible, respected setting. Such programs may be too large and encompassing for small organizations or groups to implement. Portions of such types of interventions, however, are underway in several States to educate older adults as well as their service care providers. Evaluation of such efforts and the development of

theory-driven prevention programs are essential components to reconciling the current disparity between the HIV/AIDS prevention efforts being provided for younger adults and what has thus far been offered to help older adults prevent HIV infection.

Also see: HIV/AIDS: Early Childhood; HIV/AIDS: Childhood; HIV/AIDS: Adolescence; HIV/AIDS: Adulthood; Sexually Transmitted Diseases: Adolescence.

References

Adler, W.H., Baskar, P.V., Chrest, F.J., Dorsey, C.B., Winchurch, R.A., & Nagel, J.E. (1997). HIV infection and aging: Mechanisms to explain the accelerated rate of progression in the older patient. *Mechanisms of Aging and Development, 96*, 137–155.

Adler, W.H., & Nagel, J.E. (1994). Acquired immunodeficiency syndrome in the elderly. *Drugs and Aging, 4*, 410–416.

Ankrom, M., & Greenough, W.B.I. (1997). Delayed diagnosis: A 78 year old man with AIDS. *Journal of the American Geriatrics Society, 45*, 1282–1283.

Arnsten, J., Demas, P., Gourevitch, M., Buono, D., Farzadegan, H., & Schoenbaum, E. (2000). Adherence and viral load in HIV-infected drug-users: Comparison of self-report and medication event monitors (MEMS). *Seventh Conference on Retroviruses and Opportunistic Infections.* San Francisco, CA.

Bangsberg, D.R., Hecht, F.M., Clague, H., Charlebois, E., Ciccarone, D., Chesney, M., & Moss, A.R. (2000). Provider estimate and structured patient report of adherence compared with unannounced pill count. *Seventh Conference on Retroviruses and Opportunistic Infections.* San Francisco, CA.

Brabant, S. (1994). An overlooked AIDS affected population: The elderly parent as caregiver. *Journal of Gerontological Social Work, 22*, 131–145.

Catania, J.A., Turner, H., Kegeles, S.M., Stall, R., Pollack, M.A., & Coates, T.J. (1989). Older Americans and AIDS: Transmission risks and primary prevention. *Gerontologist, 29*, 373–381.

Centers for Disease Control and Prevention (CDC). (2000). *HIV/AIDS surveillance report, 12* (1). Atlanta, GA.

Chiao, E.Y., Ries, K.M., & Sande, M.A. (1999). AIDS and the elderly. *Clinical Infectious Diseases, 28*, 740–745.

Crisologo, S., Campbell, M.H., & Forte, J.A. (1996). Social work, AIDS, and the elderly: Current knowledge and practice. *Journal of Gerontological Social Work, 26*, 49–69.

de Gorgolas, M., Bello, E., Garcia, V.E., Moya, M.J., Garcia, D.R., & Fernandez-Guerrero, M.L. (1999). In old age … AIDS: Is it worth it to initiate antiretroviral treatment? A review of 37 patients more than 60 years of age. *Anals de Medicina International, 16*, 273–276.

el Sadr, W., & Gettler, J. (1995). Unrecognized human immunodeficiency virus infection in the elderly. *Archives of Internal Medicine, 155*, 184–186.

Fisher, J.D., Fisher, W.A., Williams, S.S., & Malloy, T.E. (1994). Empirical tests of an Information-Motivation-Behavioral Skills model of AIDS preventative behavior. *Health Psychology, 13*, 238–250.

Gaeta, T.J., LaPolla, C., & Melendez, E. (1996). AIDS in the elderly: New York City vital statistics. *Journal of Emergency Medicine, 14*, 19–23.

Gordon, S.M., & Thompson, S. (1995). The changing epidemiology of human immunodeficiency virus infection in older persons. *Journal of the American Geriatric Society, 43*, 7–9.

Hillman, J.L. (1998). Health care providers' knowledge about HIV induced dementia among older adults. *Sexuality and Disability, 16*, 181–192.

Hillman, J.L., & Stricker, G. (1998). Some issues in the assessment of HIV among older adult patients. *Psychotherapy: Theory, Research, Practice, and Training, 35*, 483–489.

Hilton, C. (1998). General paralysis of the insane and AIDS in old age psychiatry: Epidemiology, clinical diagnosis, serology, and ethics-the way forward. *International Journal of Geriatric Psychiatry, 13*, 875–885.

Ingstad, B., Brunn, F.J., & Tlou, S. (1997). AIDS and the elderly Twasana: The concept of pollution and consequences for AIDS prevention. *Journal of Cross Cultural Gerontology, 12*(4), 357–372.

Janssen, R. (2001, February). Sereostatus approach to fighting the HIV epidemic (SAFE): A new prevention strategy to reduce transmission. *Conference Abstracts (S20): Paper presented at the 8th Conference on Retroviruses and Opportunistic Infections.* Chicago, IL.

Johnson, M., Haight, B.K., & Benedict, S. (1998). AIDS in older people: A literature review for clinical nursing research and practice. *Journal of Gerontological Nursing, 24, Journal of Gerontological Nursing, 24*, 8–13.

Lee, C.C., Leo, Y.S., Snodgrass, I., & Wong, S.Y. (1997). The demography, clinical manifestations, and natural history of human immunodeficiency virus (HIV) infection in an older population in Singapore. *Annals of the Academy of Medicine, Singapore, 26*, 731–735.

Leigh, B.C., Temple, M.T., & Trocki, K.F. (1993). The sexual behavior of US adults: Results from a national survey. *American Journal of Public Health, 83*, 1200–1208.

Levine-Perkell, J. (1996). Caregiving issues. In K.M. Nokes (Ed.), *HIV/AIDS and the older adult* (pp. 115–128). Philadelphia: Taylor & Francis.

Lieberman, R. (2000). HIV in older Americans: An epidemiological perspective. *Journal of Midwifery and Women's Health, 45*, 176–182.

Linsk, N.L. (1994). HIV and the elderly. *Families in Society, 75*, 362–372.

Linsk, N.L. (2000). HIV among older adults: Age-specific issues in prevention and treatment. *The AIDS Reader, 10*, 430–440.

Lloyd, G.A. (1989). AIDS & elders: Advocacy, activism, and coalitions. *Generations, 13*, 32–35.

Medley, G.F., Anderson, R.M., Cox, D.R., & Billard, L. (1987). Incubation period of AIDS in patients infected via blood transfusion. *Nature, 328*, 719–721.

Nocera, R. (1997). AIDS and the older person. *Topics in Geriatric Rehabilitation, 12*, 72–85.

Nokes, K.M. (1999, November). Are older persons engaging in risk behaviors associated with HIV? *Conference Abstracts: The National Association on HIV Over Fifty's Third Annual Conference.* Chicago, IL.

Peterson, J.L., & DiClemente, R.J. (2000). *Handbook of HIV prevention.* New York: Kluwer Academic/ Plenum.

Puleo, J.H. (1996). Scope of the challenge. In K.M. Nokes (Ed.), *HIV/AIDS and the older adult* (pp. 1–8). Philadelphia: Taylor & Francis.

Sabin, T.D. (1987). AIDS: The new "great imitator." *Journal of the American Geriatric Society, 35*, 467–471.

Skiest, D.J., Rubinstien, E., Carely, N., Gioiella, L., & Lyons, R. (1996). The importance of comorbidity in HIV-infected patients over 55: A retrospective case-control study, *American Journal of Medicine, 101*, 605–611.

Szirony, T.A. (1999). Infection with HIV in the elderly population. *Journal of Gerontological Nursing, 25*, 25–31.

UNAIDS: Joint United Nations Programme on HIV/AIDS World Health Organization. (2000, December). *AIDS epidemic update: December, 2000.* Geneva, Switzerland.

Wallace, J.I., Paauw, D.S., & Spach, D.H. (1993). HIV infection in older patients: When to suspect the unexpected. *Geriatrics, 48*, 61–70.

Welch, S. (1999, November). CDC National hotline: A resource for people over 50. *Conference Abstracts: The National Association on HIV Over Fifty's Third Annual Conference.* Chicago, IL.

Whipple, B., & Scura, K.W. (1989). HIV and the older adult: Taking the necessary precautions. *Journal of Gerontological Nursing, 15*, 15–19.

Wooten, B.K. (1999). HIV and AIDS in older adults. *Geriatric Nursing, 20*, 268–272.

Homelessness, Childhood

Paul A. Toro, Sylvie A. Lombardo, and Courtney J. Yapchai

INTRODUCTION

Research produced in the past 15 years (mainly conducted in the United States) has produced substantial knowledge on homelessness (Baumohl, 1996; Toro, 1998). Although most of this research has been conducted on homeless adults, research has begun to focus on homeless children and adolescents. This entry provides an overview of this recent research and then describes various interventions that show promise for the prevention of homelessness among minors (under age 18).

DEFINITIONS

In designing preventive interventions and policies, it is first important to distinguish three key subgroups among the overall homeless population: *homeless adults* without children (mostly men in this Encyclopedia), *homeless families* (mostly young women with children under age 10), and *homeless adolescents* (ages 12–17). It is important to recognize that these three subgroups are largely distinct. In most cities in the United States and other developed nations, homeless families only rarely include children of age 10 or over (Masten, Miliotis, Graham-Bermann, Ramirez, & Neemann, 1993) and children (under age 12) are very rarely found homeless "on their own." Largely distinct sets of services and distinct research literatures have developed involving each of these three subgroups, and some recent research has documented that aside from the obvious age differences, the three subgroups are different on many characteristics (Robertson & Toro, 1999; Shinn & Weitzman, 1996; Toro, 1998).

Homeless adolescents are distinguished from homeless adults based on their age (under 18) and from homeless families because they are homeless on their own. Although studies on "*homeless youth*" sometimes include youth who are

18 or older (Cauce et al., 1994; Kipke, O'Conner, Palmer, & MacKenzie, 1995), the legal, policy, and intervention issues are quite different for minors (under age 18) who are homeless on their own, as compared to those 18 or older (Robertson & Toro, 1999). A variety of terms describing homeless adolescents are common in the research literature, among service providers, in the media, and among the general public. These terms include *runaways*, who have left home without parental permission, *throwaways*, who have been forced to leave home by their parents, and *street youth*, who have spent at least some time living on the streets. These are not mutually exclusive groups. In this review, we include all such youth, as long as they are under age 18. It is not always easy to determine if an adolescent "ran away from home" or was "thrown out" by parents. There are cases in which some of each process appears to apply, and there are cases in which neither process applies well (e.g., those initially separated from their families by authorities or those staying at a shelter to "cool off" by mutual agreement with their parents). Furthermore, on most important characteristics, there appear to be more similarities between such cases than differences (MacLean, Embry, & Cauce, 1999).

The definition of homelessness for adolescents is also different from that typically employed for homeless adults and families in that minors away from home without parental permission have a special legal status and must be returned to their parents except under special circumstances (e.g., when there is evidence that they are being abused at home). Once they turn 18, their legal status is very different. Our definition of homelessness among adolescents includes such cases and is, therefore, somewhat broader than the definition for homeless children and single adults. Most homeless adolescents have spent little or no time on the streets. However, some number of "street youth" can be found in some areas (especially large cities on the east and west coasts).

Homeless children are embedded within a family, one that typically includes a single young mother. Unlike homeless adults (and, to some extent, homeless adolescents), the children in such families are not typically homeless due to their own personal, social, or economic problems. Rather, such children are homeless as a result of their *parent's* situation. The parent could end up homeless for a variety of reasons, including extreme poverty, loss of benefits, eviction, domestic violence, or their own personal problems (e.g., substance abuse). Furthermore, homeless families often include multiple siblings. Unlike single homeless adults and, to some extent, homeless adolescents, homeless families are rarely found on the streets. Rather they tend to be found in homeless shelters. Many can also be found temporarily "doubled up" with friends or family. However, most researchers have not considered such cases as "literally homeless." To prevent or otherwise intervene in homelessness among children, we must understand and intervene in a family context. Addressing the child's own educational, mental health, or other needs, as is done in most existing prevention and treatment programs for general populations in our society, may have little if any impact on preventing homelessness, although such programs may have other positive impacts.

Methodological Issues. Although the findings are still rather sparse, researchers in the past 10–15 years have at least learned a great deal about *how* to study homelessness in children and adolescents. An improved understanding of methodological issues has been occurring in at least three basic areas.

Sampling and Measurement. Early studies on both homeless adolescents and families often involved small, nonrepresentative samples and used measures without established reliability or validity. Researchers have begun to use sophisticated approaches to select more representative samples (McCaskill, Toro, & Wolfe, 1998; Shinn et al., 1998; Yapchai, Toro, & McCaskill, 2001). One such general approach, *probability sampling*, involves identifying the proportion of the total homeless population found at many different sites (e.g., shelters, soup kitchens, streets) and sampling from each site relative to its overall estimated contribution to the population (see Burnam & Koegel, 1988; Toro et al., 1999b; Zlotnick, Robertson, & Lahiff, 1999b). Researchers have also developed and adapted measures appropriate for use with homeless children and adolescents and have established their psychometric properties (McCaskill et al., 1998; Yapchai et al., 2001).

Appropriate Comparison Groups. Many studies on both homeless children and adolescents done in the 1980s painted a rather dismal picture of both homeless subpopulations (Rafferty & Shinn, 1991; Robertson, 1991). However, it is known that the broader population of poor children and adolescents generally also shows some of the same problems. A number of recent studies have selected *appropriate comparison groups* in order to distinguish the unique characteristics of the homeless from those of the poor. As in similar studies on homeless adults, homeless adolescents do show many problems, even when compared to carefully matched housed adolescents. For example, they show more conduct and depressive symptoms and come from more disturbed family environments (McCaskill et al., 1998; Toro & Goldstein, 2000; Wolfe, Toro, & McCaskill, 1999). A different picture is emerging from some of the most recent comparison group studies among homeless families: When compared to carefully matched poor housed families, both the children and the mothers in homeless families have *not* shown clear differences although, when compared to large normative groups, both the poor *and* the homeless have differed on a variety of behavioral, cognitive, and other measures (Yapchai et al., 2001; Ziesmer, Marcoux, & Marwell, 1994).

Understanding the Causes and Consequences of Homelessness. As with any harmful outcome we wish to prevent, it is critical to understand the causal mechanisms that produce the outcome. Although we cannot use experimental methods to directly assess the causes of homelessness, there are other methodologies that can provide some useful data. *Comparison group studies* represent one such methodology. For example, based on the studies just described above, it appears that family homelessness may be largely indistinguishable from extreme poverty among families, while homelessness among adolescents may have some antecedents aside from general economic disadvantage. *Longitudinal studies* can track the "natural course" of homelessness and may also help suggest the causes of homelessness. Although there have been several longitudinal studies done recently on homeless adults (Toro et al., 1999a; Zlotnick et al., 1999b), there have been only a few such studies on homeless families (Shinn et al., 1998) and homeless adolescents (Cauce et al., 1994; Toro & Goldstein, 2000). Studies following large numbers of poor or other children or adolescents "at risk" for homelessness over long periods of time would provide even better causal evidence. However, we are aware of no such studies in the existing literature. Finally, *international comparisons* could help us in the search for causes of homelessness. For example, if comparable rates of homelessness could be produced across various nations, then economic, cultural, and other factors possibly associated with the varying rates could be identified. Although there have been some studies on homelessness in other nations, particularly on homeless adults and youth (especially in the United Kingdom; Burrows, Pleace, & Quiliagars, 1998; Fitzpatrick, 2000), we are aware of only a few attempts to compare homelessness across nations (Adams, 1986; Daly, 1990) and only one study that has used firm empirical data for such comparison. Toro, Lombardo, Blume, Yabar, Fournier, and MacKay (2001) found that the 5-year prevalence of literal homelessness (combining all subgroups) was much higher in the United States (3–4 percent) as compared to five European nations (1 percent).

Characteristics of Homeless Children and Adolescents: Race, Social Class, and Other Background Characteristics. Homeless people of all subgroups appear to come disproportionately from poor, urban, and minority populations (Blasi, 1994; Toro, 1998). This is generally true for homeless adolescents (Cauce et al., 1994; McCaskill et al., 1998; Toro & Goldstein, 2000) and may especially be true for homeless children and their mothers (Masten, 1992; Shinn et al., 1998; Yapchai et al., 2001).

Psychological and Developmental Characteristics. As noted above, recent comparison group studies have identified a number of personal problems among homeless adolescents as compared to matched housed adolescents. Such findings have implications for the development of prevention programs. For example, prevention efforts might target youth at risk for or showing early signs of delinquency and/or other problems. Relatively few differences have been found between homeless and carefully matched housed children. However, both groups show a range of deficits as compared to norms, suggesting that poverty may be over-riding any specific impact of homelessness. These findings suggest that preventive and other intervention efforts should be targeted to a wide range of poverty-stricken children and their families.

Family, Social, and Other Contextual Characteristics. Homeless adolescents have shown a wide array of family and social problems, even when compared to carefully matched housed samples. They have shown significantly higher scores on measures of family conflict, parent–child aggression (both verbal and physical), punitive parenting, disorganized home environments, substance use among network members, association with deviant peers, and family housing moves (Toro & Goldstein, 2000; Wolfe et al., 1999). These same studies have also found that homeless youth have lower scores on various positive indicators of family and social functioning (e.g., parental monitoring and warmth, family cohesiveness, perceived social support). A recent study also found that, among homeless and other at-risk urban youth, negative family environments predicted the development of deviant peer relationships and depressive symptomatology, which each then predicted longitudinal outcomes (substance abuse symptoms and risky sexual behaviors; Lombardo & Toro, 2001). Such findings suggest the need to intervene in family systems if we are to prevent harmful outcomes in this subgroup. The fact that many of these same characteristics have also been found to be common in both poor and homeless families suggests that family-oriented preventive interventions could also be effectively targeted to families (Yapchai et al., 2001).

SCOPE

Prevalence of Homelessness among Children and Youth

It has been estimated that the percentage of the homeless population in the United States that involves mothers and their children ranges from 35 percent to 43 percent, and it is widely believed that homeless families represent the fastest growing segment of the overall homeless population (Burt, Aron, Douglas, Valente, Lee, & Iwen, 1999; Shinn & Weitzman, 1996). With current annual prevalence estimates of about 1 percent for the overall homeless population

(Burt et al., 1999), there could be as many as 1 million persons (children and parents) homeless within families at some point during a year's time.

A recent survey of over 6,000 US adolescents, ages 12–17, estimated the annual prevalence of homelessness among this age group to be 7.6 percent (Ringwalt, Greene, Robertson, & McPheeters, 1998). Based on this estimate, it has been suggested that adolescents probably represent the age group in the homeless population with the greatest risk for homelessness (Robertson & Toro, 1999).

The Costs of Homelessness to Society

Two recent studies, both based on large samples, have produced estimates of the costs to society for services rendered to groups of homeless adults. In a two-city study (Buffalo and Detroit) involving a general group of homeless adults (including those homeless with their children), Hong, Toro, and Daeschler (1996) found total annual costs to society of just under $15,000 per person in each city. Culhane, Metraux, and Hadley (2001) found a much higher annual cost to society ($40,449) for homeless mentally ill adults in New York city. Although we are aware of no similar study attempting to estimate the costs of child or adolescent homelessness to society, we believe that such costs might be more similar to those observed in the prior study because the high costs of psychiatric and criminal justice services for the mentally ill adults in the latter study would likely be lower for homeless adolescents and children. While the general sample of homeless adults would likely have higher costs in some areas (e.g., shelter use, free meals, and substance abuse, mental health, and physical health care), homeless children and youth would likely incur higher costs in other areas (e.g., child care, special education, juvenile justice, foster care, public assistance). Even if the annual cost is somewhat lower than the $15,000 reported in the earlier study, the cost of youth/child homelessness to society would be very high.

THEORIES AND RESEARCH

Social Learning Theories

There is a long tradition of applying social learning principles in understanding delinquency, substance abuse, and other poor outcomes among children and youth (Hawkins, Catalano, & Miller 1992; Petraitis, Flay, & Miller, 1995). One of the most influential social learning theories is the one developed by Patterson and his colleagues to explain the development of aggressive and delinquent behavior (Dishion, Patterson, Stoolmiller, & Skinner, 1991; Patterson, 1982; Patterson, DeBaryshe, & Ramsey,

1989). In Patterson's basic model, inept parenting leads to escalating conflict between parent and child. The child learns that highly negative, aggressive behavior can be effective for getting desires met in the short-term within the family, however, this style of interacting leads to negative consequences outside the family. It is not effective in school settings and leads to disengagement, poor performance, and rejection by normal peers. The child thus begins to associate with other aggressive peers who are likely to be involved in deviant behavior. This model indicates that the impact of coercive family processes on delinquency and problem behavior is indirect. The family process operates primarily through its impact on school achievement and peer relationships. This model and modifications of it have been shown to have explanatory power for understanding a number of problematic behaviors in adolescence (Conger, Conger, Elder, Lovenz, Simons, & Whitbeck, 1992; Patterson, Dishion, & Banks, 1984).

Only recently have such theories been applied to homelessness. Whitbeck and Hoyt (1999) describe a "risk amplification" perspective that suggests that early conditions (such as poor parenting) put the adolescent at risk for homelessness. While these early conditions will likely result in negative long-term outcomes, the perspective posits that the experience of homelessness will add to the prediction of outcomes. In support of this perspective, a recent study involving a probability sample of 251 homeless adolescents (initial ages 12–17) and a matched sample of 145 housed adolescents found different longitudinal trajectories for the two samples (Toro & Goldstein, 2000). There are many ways that adolescent homelessness, as well as the conditions that often exist immediately prior to homelessness (e.g., family violence, delinquent acts), could enhance risk. For example, family members, officials and service providers, and the youth themselves may come to see the youth as "troubled." The resulting "stigma" could increase the likelihood of homelessness and other negative outcomes. In addition, the experiences the youth obtain while homeless (e.g., interaction with deviant peers, engaging in risky behaviors such as prostitution) could introduce the youth to lifestyles that make future homelessness and other poor outcomes more likely. Based on the same sample of 251 homeless and 145 housed youth, Lombardo and Toro (2001) used structural equation modeling and found support for a theoretical model similar to that proposed by Patterson.

Homelessness as Trauma

The deleterious effects of stress and trauma have been demonstrated in a long line of research (Cohen & Wills, 1985). Like poverty, homelessness can be thought of as involving a complex and very burdensome set of life stressors.

Although mental and other disorders could well put one at risk for homelessness, Goodman, Saxe, and Harvey (1991) argue that homelessness can also be seen as involving a set of traumatic events that puts one at risk for disorders. Supporting this view are the high levels of stressful events and victimization reported among all subgroups of homeless people (Toro, 1998; Toro & Goldstein, 2000). Milburn and D'Ercole (1991) made a similar set of arguments in considering homeless women (including those with their children). We believe that this theoretical perspective makes particular sense when considering homelessness among children, since they generally are homeless for reasons "not of their own making." The "crisis intervention" approach to preventing homelessness (described below) follows from this perspective.

An Ecological Perspective

Given the complexity of homelessness as a social issue, an ecological perspective has been proposed as a guide for policy and intervention (Toro, Trickett, Wall, & Salem, 1991). This perspective highlights the need to consider both social and other contextual factors, in addition to individual vulnerabilities, when developing interventions. It also points out that interventions need to be considered at multiple levels of analysis, from individually focused interventions to large-scale social policies. The perspective is not a theory in the traditional sense. Rather, it is a general framework that can guide work in the area. A few recent studies on homeless adolescents and families have implicitly or explicitly adopted an ecological perspective (Rabideau & Toro, 1997; Toro & Goldstein, 2000; Wolfe et al., 1999; Yapchai et al., 2001). We believe the ecological perspective may be especially useful in designing preventive interventions. If we can identify the environmental conditions that conspire to create homelessness, we can create approaches that may prevent them.

STRATEGIES THAT WORK

Clear evidence of effectiveness is not yet available on programs to prevent homelessness among children or adolescents.

STRATEGIES THAT MIGHT WORK

In recent years, there has been considerable progress in developing effective preventive interventions. Such interventions have effectively addressed mental disorders, substance abuse, delinquency, and school dropout (see other entries in this volume). In our exhaustive review, we have identified only one intervention explicitly oriented toward the primary prevention of homelessness (Nelson & Sharp, 1995) and a few review papers explicitly addressing the prevention of homelessness (Robertson & Toro, 1999; Shinn & Baumohl, 1999; Toro & Bukowski, 1995). Based on this limited literature, our general knowledge about homeless children and adolescents (reviewed above), and our review of preventive efforts targeted to other problems (e.g., poverty), we have identified a number of potentially effective approaches to preventing homelessness. Since homeless children and youth are typically homeless for very short periods and very few can be considered as "chronically homeless," many of the existing services targeted to both groups could be considered as secondary prevention efforts. We believe that knowledge of such existing services can assist in designing effective primary preventive interventions.

Crisis Intervention

Nelson and Sharp (1995) used trained volunteer mediators to assist clients in their interactions with landlords, utility companies, and service providers. This primary prevention effort was explicitly designed to prevent poor families from becoming homelessness. Their program has been applied to over 1,400 cases, and Nelson and Sharp believe the program empowers clients by teaching them to effectively negotiate various systems. Many shelters for homeless youth and homeless families operate based on crisis intervention approaches. Some provide a range of family services during the shelter stay, and such services sometimes continue afterwards. To the extent that shelters provide intensive and comprehensive services, such as those offered by Nelson and Sharp (1995), they may be working to prevent future homeless episodes (i.e., secondary prevention). It has been suggested that crisis intervention and other types of prevention-oriented programs could be effectively developed in "natural helping" settings, such as churches, neighborhood organizations, after-school programs, drop-in centers, and parenting groups (Cain, 1993; Rothman, 1991). In any event, such approaches have preventive potential and can be relatively low-cost. They deserve careful attention in rigorous program evaluation research.

Family-Oriented and Other Intensive Interventions

One general category of such interventions involves intensive case management. These interventions work closely with homeless or at-risk clients, attempting to meet all of their long- and short-term needs, including permanent housing, education and job training, and linkages to services in mental health, substance abuse, health care, and other relevant areas. Given that homeless families and homeless youth (and their families) often have multiple problems as well as different assets, it is important that such interventions be tailored to individual needs and strengths and be comprehensive in nature. Interventions that can provide only one or two narrow services (e.g., mental health, substance abuse, housing, or employment) may have limited effectiveness with such multi-problem cases. Recent welfare reforms have been criticized for not meeting the complex and long-term needs of poor families (Edelman, 1997). Instead, these reforms have often focused simply on reducing welfare rolls by increasing employment, sometimes in very low-wage jobs. Several authors have suggested that short-term interventions with many types of multi-problem families are unlikely to succeed (Catalano, Gainey, Fleming, Haggerty, & Johnson, 1999; Halfon, Berkowitz, & Klee, 1993; Serketich & Dumas, 1996). In discussing interventions for homeless families, Cain (1993) suggested that programs need to provide employment, income, benefits, prevent eviction, and generally assist those who are losing their homes. Based on the complex array of risk factors identified in the research literature, Toro and Bukowski (1995) have argued for intensive and long-term programs to prevent adolescent homelessness.

A number of family-oriented or otherwise intensive interventions have recently been adapted and carefully evaluated for homeless street youth (Cauce et al., 1994), homeless families (Homan, Flick, Heaton, & Mayer, 1993; James, Smith, & Mann, 1991), the homeless mentally ill (Morse, Calsyn, Allen, Tempelhoff, & Smith, 1992), and general populations of homeless adults and families (Toro et al., 1997). These interventions have often adopted ecological, trauma reduction, and/or social learning perspectives and have targeted multiple types of problems over long periods (often 6 months or more). These interventions have been obtaining some positive outcomes. For example, based on a randomized design, Cauce et al. (1994) found that, relative to youth in a "regular" case management program, youth assigned to an "intensive" case management program showed reduced externalizing behaviors and improved quality of life ratings over the initial 3-months. Note that, although generally secondary preventive or even treatment-oriented, if targeted to persons "at risk" for homelessness (e.g., the poor), such interventions could be primary preventive as well. The Need for More Low-Income Housing: In most large urban areas, there is a critical shortage of quality low-income housing (Shinn, 1992). Policies and interventions that promote the development of such housing and help families to remain in it make great sense as preventive strategies. In recent longitudinal studies on homeless families and adults, housing subsidies and other public benefits have been some of the best predictors of remaining permanently housed over time (Shinn et al., 1998; Zlotnick et al., 1999b). Federally funded Section 8 housing vouchers and other policies that help maintain families in quality housing should be expanded (in many cities there is a long wait-list to obtain such vouchers). The *Habitat for Humanity* program is another example of how low-income housing can be expanded. This program taps interested volunteers in the community to develop low-income housing. It also involves "sweat equity" by requiring the poor families who obtain the free housing to assist in the construction/rehabilitation of their housing. Other examples involve the "supported housing" approaches (Tilsen, 1998; Tsemberis, 1999) that provide homeless and other at-risk people with low-cost permanent housing along with various support services (e.g., job training and placement, medication monitoring) to help them maintain themselves in that housing.

Targeting Those at Risk for Homelessness

A number of studies have suggested that children and youth with histories of residential instability, foster care, and other out-of-home placements are at heightened risk for homelessness during both adolescence and adulthood. Such groups could be special targets for preventive intervention. Adolescents who are "aging out" of the foster-care system appear to be particularly vulnerable to homelessness. One recent follow-up of such youth found that, in the 12 months after "aging out," a full 12 percent of the youth had spent at least some time homeless (Courtney, Piliavin, Grogan-Kaylor, & Nesmith, 1998). Perhaps the age of eligibility for foster care, other placements, and/or support services could be extended to age 21 or later. Foster parents could also be targeted to better assist the foster children (which might, in turn, ultimately prevent homelessness). Zlotnick, Kronstadt and Klee (1999a) showed that intensive case management services provided to foster parents increased their ability to deal with the variety of problems presented by foster care children.

Another salient problem among at-risk families is the high rate of substance abuse, which in turn predicts child maltreatment and places children who grow up in these families at high risk of becoming substance abusers themselves (Wolock & Magura, 1996). Many homeless youth exhibit substance abuse problems and a history of maltreatment (Wolfe et al., 1999). It seems plausible that preventing substance abuse and/or maltreatment in high-risk families could help prevent homelessness. Catalano et al. (1999) randomly assigned methadone-treated parents to either an experimental group that included 33 sessions of family, parent and child training skills combined with 9-months of home-based case management or to a control group that included the standard methadone treatment received at the clinic. The goal was to prevent substance abuse among children and relapse among parents. At 12-month follow-up, the experimental group showed several significant gains compared to the control group, including better problem-solving skills in drug-related situations, a decrease in drug use, and an increase in pro-social involvement of children with parents. Intensive interventions targeted to families at risk for child abuse or neglect (e.g., due to poverty, transience, and/or low education achievement) might also prevent homelessness (Onyskiw, Harrison, Spady, & McConnan, 1999).

Teenage mothers with children have a higher risk of becoming homeless than their peers who do not have children (Greene & Ringwalt, 1998). They tend to drop out of school, thus increasing their chance of unemployment and becoming dependent on social welfare services for economic survival (Ahn, 1994). Fischer (1997) targeted pregnant teens and provided pre- and post-natal care, educational assistance, job training, parent training, intervention aimed at preventing subsequent pregnancies, and services to strengthen support from the family of origin. Compared to teenage mothers receiving only pre- and post-natal care, the girls who received the intensive services showed more educational attainment, better health outcomes, less subsequent pregnancies, and more employment at 18-months. Similarly, using a randomized design, O'Sullivan and Jacobsen (1992) found that teenage mothers receiving intensive services showed a rate of repeated pregnancy less than half that of the control group.

In designing all such interventions, we believe it is important to assess and enhance participants' competencies in addition to trying to prevent various negative outcomes. For example, many women homeless with their children have developed effective coping skills and surprisingly good parenting abilities (Banyard, 1995). These skills can be honed and put to use in primary or secondary prevention programs. For example, women with effective parenting skills could serve as paraprofessional parent trainers or teacher aides in preschool programs, providing the mothers with a meaningful source of employment while also meeting societal needs for more and better childcare services.

School-Based Programs

Early childhood intervention programs, such as Head Start, have demonstrated effectiveness at reducing the harmful developmental outcomes often associated with poverty (Committee on Child Psychiatry, 1999). Such programs have been applied to homeless children and could promote the secondary prevention of homelessness (NAEHCY/NCH, 1999). However, we believe that to accomplish prevention, whether secondary prevention for currently homeless children or primary prevention for non-homeless children at-risk for homelessness, such programs probably need to do more than simply provide day care, educational stimulation, and nutritious meals. While the day-care provided could serve a preventive function (by helping the parent(s) maintain employment, financial viability, and housing), providing

services targeted more directly to the parents (e.g., case management, educational and employment assistance, parent training) could be even more important in preventing future homeless episodes. Again, we emphasize that comprehensive and tailored interventions may be most effective if one wishes to effectively prevent homelessness. Zigler (1994) has, in fact, suggested that Head Start for all children might usefully develop into a more comprehensive program such as what we are advocating here. Given the close apparent connection between homelessness and poverty, especially for homeless children, it is reasonable to consider any program that can reduce poverty and its possible harmful consequences as, in the long-run, also having the potential to prevent homelessness. Homelessness and housing stability could serve as useful outcomes in the evaluations of such programs.

School-based programs also have potential for preventing homelessness among older children and adolescents. Rothman (1991) has suggested that, because teachers and other school personnel often have intimate contact with children and their families, they have opportunities to identify problems before a crisis that produces homelessness emerges. Enhancing school mental health services to play preventive and crisis intervention roles could have great impact on homelessness over time, if done on a large scale. Hendrickson and Omer (1995) discussed the "comprehensive service school" that takes an ecological perspective in examining relationships among students, families, institutions, and communities. Services in such schools include adult education and career development, child care, economic and social services (e.g., helping families find housing, jobs, food assistance), family support services (e.g., parenting classes, support groups), transportation, legal services, health services, and mental health counseling.

STRATEGIES THAT DO NOT WORK

In the rush to deal with the problem in the past two decades, many services for homeless children and youth have been implemented. This growth has been occurring at a fast pace in the United States and United Kingdom and has been somewhat more recent in other developed nations. Few of these services have been carefully evaluated. Most of the services being developed have been oriented towards meeting the immediate needs of homeless children and youth (e.g., food, shelter, health care) and are provided only on a temporary basis. However, based on existing research, we know that homeless children and youth have long-term needs. Emergency services also do little to "stem the tide" of others entering the ranks of the homeless. As such, these services are not effective as prevention strategies.

Dishion, McCord, and Poulin (1999) have recently reviewed a number of studies whose findings converge to suggest that interventions offered to adolescents in a peer-group format may have harmful effects on the development of problem behaviors. These findings are especially relevant because therapy in peer group settings is very common in the juvenile justice system. Given these data and that homeless adolescents share many characteristics of delinquent youth (Robertson & Toro, 1999), we would suggest that peer group approaches to preventing homelessness may have pitfalls.

SYNTHESIS

As with many social problems, emergency and treatment-oriented approaches are unlikely to make a major impact in reducing the prevalence of homelessness. Instead, we must consider preventive interventions and policies that take a comprehensive approach and address the multiple needs that persons at risk for homelessness are likely to have, while also recognizing the competencies of such persons. Crisis intervention, family-oriented, and other intensive interventions have already shown some promise in preventing homelessness in the first place (primary prevention) and/or in preventing various harmful outcomes among children and youth who have already experienced some amount of homelessness (secondary or tertiary prevention). Especially to reduce the prevalence of homeless children (who are generally homeless with their mothers), it will also be important to change policies in order to enhance the stock of low-income housing available in most cities in the United States and other developed nations. By promoting such interventions and policies, then carefully evaluating the prevention efforts, perhaps we will be able to assist in ending homelessness someday.

Also see: Homelessness: Adulthood; Community Capacity.

References

Adams, C.T. (1986). Homelessness in the post-industrial city: Views from London and Philadelphia. *Urban Affairs Quarterly, 21,* 527–549.

Ahn, N. (1994). Teenage childbearing and high school completion: Accounting for individual heterogeneity. *Family Planning Perspectives, 26,* 17–21.

Banyard, V.L. (1995). "Taking another route": Daily survival narratives from mothers who are homeless. *American Journal of Community Psychology, 23,* 871–891.

Baumohl, J. (Ed.). (1996). *Homelessness in America.* Phoenix: Oryx Press.

Blasi, G. (1994). And we are not seen: Ideological and political barriers to understanding homelessness. *American Behavioral Scientist, 37,* 563–586.

Burnam, A., & Koegel, P. (1988). Methodology for obtaining a representative sample of homeless persons: The Los Angeles Skid Row Study. *Evaluation Review, 12,* 117–152.

Burrows, R., Pleace, N., & Quiliagars, D. (1998). *Homelessness and social policy.* London: Routledge.

Burt, M.R., Aron, L.Y., Douglas, T., Valente, J., Lee, E., & Iwen, B. (1999). *Homelessness: Programs and the people they serve (summary report).* Washington, DC: Urban Institute.

Cain, A. (1993). Homeless families. In C. Fawcett (Ed.), *Family psychiatric nursing* (pp. 195–212). St. Louis, MO: C.V. Mosby Co.

Cauce, A.M., Morgan, C.J., Wagner, V., Moore, E., Sy, J., Wurzbacher, K., Weeden, K., Tomlin, S., & Blanchard, T. (1994). Effectiveness of intensive case management for homeless adolescents: Results of a 3-month follow-up. *Journal of Emotional and Behavioral Disorders, 2,* 219–227.

Catalano, R.F., Gainey, R.R., Fleming, C.B., Haggerty, K.P., & Johnson, N.O. (1999). An experimental intervention with families of substance abusers: One year follow up of the focus on families project. *Addiction, 94,* 241–254.

Cohen, S., & Wills, T.A. (1985). Stress, social support, and the buffering hypothesis. *Psychological Bulletin, 98,* 310–357.

Committee on Child Psychiatry. (1999). *In the long run: Longitudinal studies of psychopathology in children.* Washington, DC: American Psychiatric Association.

Conger, R.D., Conger, K., Elder, G.H., Lorenz, F.O., Simons, R.L., & Whitbeck, L.B. (1992). A family process model of economic hardship and influences on adjustment of early adolescent boys. *Child Development, 63,* 526–541.

Courtney, M.E., Piliavin, I., Grogan-Kaylor, A., & Nesmith, A. (1998). *Foster youth transitions to adulthood: Outcomes 12 to 18 months after leaving out-of-home care.* Unpublished manuscript. Institute for Research on Poverty, University of Wisconsin-Madison.

Culhane, D.P., Metraux, S., & Hadley, T. (2001). The impact of supportive housing for homeless people with severe mental illness on the utilization of the public health, corrections, and emergency shelter systems: The New York-New York initiative. *Housing Policy Debate.*

Daly, G. (1990). Programs dealing with homelessness in the United States, Canada, and Britain. In J. Momeni (Ed.), *Homelessness in the United States: Data and issues* (pp. 133–152). New York: Praeger.

Dishion, T.J., McCord, J., & Poulin, F. (1999). When interventions harm: Peer groups and problem behavior. *American Psychologist, 54,* 755–764.

Dishion, T.J., Patterson, G.R., Stoolmiller, M., & Skinner, M.L. (1991). Family, school, and behavioral antecedents to early adolescent involvement with antisocial peers. *Developmental Psychology, 27,* 172–180.

Edelman, P. (1997, March). The worst thing Bill Clinton has done. *Atlantic Monthly,* 43–58.

Fischer, R.L. (1997). Evaluating the delivery of a teen pregnancy and parenting program across two settings. *Research on Social Work Practice, 7,* 350–369.

Fitzpatrick, S. (2000). *Young homeless people.* Basingstoke, UK: MacMillan Press.

Goodman, L., Saxe, L., & Harvey, M. (1991). Homelessness as psychological trauma: Broadening perspectives. *American Psychologist, 46,* 1219–1225.

Greene, J.M., & Ringwalt, C.L. (1998). Pregnancy among three national samples of runaway and homeless youth. *Journal of Adolescent Health, 23,* 370–377.

Halfon, N., Berkowitz, G., & Klee, L. (1993). Development of an integrated case management program for vulnerable children. *Child Welfare, 72,* 379–396.

Hawkins, J.D., Catalano, R.F., & Miller, J.Y. (1992). Risk and protective factors for alcohol and other drug problems in adolescence and early adulthood: Implications for substance abuse prevention. *Psychological Bulletin, 112,* 64–105.

Hendrickson, J., & Omer, D. (1995). School-based comprehensive services: An example of interagency collaboration. In P. Adams & K. Nelson (Eds.), *Reinventing human services: Community and family centered practice. Modern applications of social work* (pp. 145–162). Hawthorne, NY: Aldine de Gruyter.

Homan, S.M., Flick, L.H., Heaton, T.M., & Mayer, M. (1993). Reaching beyond crisis management: Design and implementation of extended shelter based services for chemically dependent homeless women and their children: St. Louis. *Alcoholism Treatment Quarterly, 10*, 101–112.

Hong, T.B., Toro, P.A., & Daeschler, C. (1996, June). *The costs of homelessness: An economic analysis in two cities.* 60th Anniversary Convention, Society for the Psychological Study of Social Issues, Ann Arbor, MI.

James, W., Smith, A., & Mann, R. (1991). Educating homeless children: Interprofessional case management. *Childhood Education, 67*(5), 305–308.

Kipke, M.D., O'Conner, S., Palmer, R., & MacKenzie, R.G. (1995). Street youth in Los Angeles: Profile of a group at high risk for human immunodeficiency virus infection. *Archives of Pediatric Adolescent Medicine, 149*, 513–519.

Lombardo, S., & Toro, P.A. (2001). *Risky sexual behavior and substance abuse among at-risk adolescents.* Unpublished manuscript. Department of Psychology, Wayne State University.

MacLean, M.G., Embry, L.E., & Cauce, A.M. (1999). Homeless adolescents' paths to separation from family: Comparison of family characteristics, psychological adjustment, and victimization. *Journal of Community Psychology, 27*, 179–188.

Masten, A. (1992). Homeless children in the United States: A mark of a nation at risk. *Current Directions in Psychological Science, 1*, 41–44.

Masten, A.S., Miliotis, D., Graham-Bermann, S.A., Ramirez, M., & Neemann, J. (1993). Children in homeless families: Risks to mental health and development. *Journal of Consulting and Clinical Psychology, 61*, 335–343.

McCaskill, P.A., Toro, P.A., & Wolfe, S.M. (1998). Homeless and matched housed adolescents: A comparative study of psychopathology. *Journal of Clinical Child Psychology, 27*, 306–319.

Milburn, N., & D'Ercole, A. (1991). Homeless women: Moving toward a comprehensive model. *American Psychologist, 46*, 1161–1169.

Morse, G., Calsyn, R.J., Allen, G., Tempelhoff, B., & Smith, R. (1992). Experimental comparison of the effects of three treatment programs for homeless mentally ill people. *Hospital and Community Psychiatry, 43*, 1005–1010.

National Association for the Education of Homeless Children and Youth and the National Coalition for the Homeless (NAEHCY/NCH) (1999). *Making the grade: Successes and challenges in providing educational opportunities to homeless children and youth.* Washington, DC: Author.

Nelson, M., & Sharp, W. (1995). Mediating conflicts of persons at risk of homelessness: The Helping Hand Project. *Mediation Quarterly, 12*, 317–325.

Onyskiw, J.E., Harrison, M.J., Spady, D., & McConnan, L. (1999). Formative evaluation of a collaborative community based child abuse prevention project. *Child Abuse and Neglect, 23*, 1069–1081.

O'Sullivan, A.L., & Jacobsen, B.S. (1992). A randomized trial of a health care program for first time adolescent mothers and their infants. *Nursing Research, 41*, 210–215.

Patterson, G.R. (1982). *Coercive family process.* Eugene, OR: Castalia.

Patterson, G.R., DeBaryshe, B.D., & Ramsey, E. (1989). A developmental perspective on antisocial behavior. *American Psychologist, 44*, 329–335.

Patterson, G.R., Dishion, T.J., & Banks, L. (1984). Family interaction: A process model of deviancy training. *Aggressive Behavior, 10*, 253–267.

Petraitis, J., Flay, B.R., & Miller, T.Q. (1995). Reviewing theories of adolescent substance use: Organizing pieces in the puzzle. *Psychological Bulletin, 117*, 67–86.

Rabideau, J.M.P., & Toro, P.A. (1997). Social and environmental predictors of adjustment in homeless children. *Journal of Prevention and Intervention in the Community, 15*(2), 1–17.

Rafferty, Y., & Shinn, M. (1991). The impact of homelessness on children. *American Psychologist, 46*, 1170–1179.

Ringwalt, C.L., Greene, J.M., Robertson, M., & McPheeters, M. (1998). The prevalence of homelessness among adolescents in the United States. *American Journal of Public Health, 88*, 1325–1329.

Robertson, M.J. (1991). Homeless youth: An overview of recent literature. In J.H. Kryder-Coe, L.M. Salamon, & J.M. Molnar (Eds.), *Homeless children and youth: A new American dilemma* (pp. 33–68). London: Transaction.

Robertson, M.J., & Toro, P.A. (1999). Homeless youth: Research, intervention, and policy. In L.B. Fosburg & D.L. Dennis (Eds.), *Practical lessons: The 1998 National Symposium on Homelessness Research* (pp. 3-1–3-32). Washington DC: US Department of Housing and Urban Development and US Department of Health and Human Services.

Rothman, J. (1991). *Runaway and homeless youth: Strengthening services to families and children.* New York: Longman/Addison Wesley Longman.

Serketich, W.J., & Dumas, J.E. (1996). The effectiveness of behavioral parent training to modify antisocial behavior in children: A meta-analysis. *Behavior Therapy, 27*, 171–186.

Shinn, M. (1992). Homelessness: What is a psychologist to do? *American Journal of Community Psychology, 20*, 1–24.

Shinn, M., & Baumohl, J. (1999). Rethinking the prevention of homelessness. Chapter 13 in L.B. Fosburg & D.L. Dennis (Eds.), *Practical lessons: The 1998 National Symposium on Homelessness Research* (pp. 13-1–13-36). Washington DC: US Department of Housing and Urban Development and US Department of Health and Human Services.

Shinn, M., & Weitzman, B.C. (1996). Homeless families are different. In J. Baumohl (Ed.), *Homelessness in America* (pp. 109–122). Phoenix: Oryx Press.

Shinn, M., Weitzman, B., Stojanovic, D., Knickman, J.R., Jimenez, L., Duchon, L., James, S., & Krantz, D.H. (1998). Predictors of entry into and exit from homelessness among families in New York City. *American Journal of Public Health, 88*, 1651–1657.

Tilsen, T. (1998). *Minnesota supportive housing demonstration program: One-year evaluation report.* Minneapolis, MN: Wilder Research Center.

Toro, P.A. (1998). Homelessness. In A.S. Bellack & M. Hersen (Eds.), *Comprehensive clinical psychology: Vol. 9. Applications in diverse populations* (pp. 119–135). New York: Pergamon.

Toro, P.A., & Bukowski, P.A. (1995). Homeless adolescents: What we know and what can be done. *NMHA Prevention Update, 6*(1), 6–7.

Toro, P.A., & Goldstein, M.S. (2000, August). *Outcomes among homeless and matched housed adolescents: A longitudinal comparison.* 108th Annual Convention, American Psychological Association, Washington, DC.

Toro, P.A., Goldstein, M.S., Rowland, L.L., Bellavia, C.W., Wolfe, S.M., Thomas, D.M., & Acosta, O. (1999a). Severe mental illness among homeless adults and its association with longitudinal outcomes. *Behavior Therapy, 30*, 431–452.

Toro, P.A., Lombardo, S., Blume, M., Yabar, Y., Fournier, L., & MacKay, L. (2001, June). *Homelessness in Europe and the US: A comparison of prevalence and public opinion.* Biennial Conference of the Society for Community Research and Action, Atlanta, GA.

Toro, P.A., Rabideau, J.M.P., Bellavia, C.W., Daeschler, C.V., Wall, D.D., Thomas, D.M., & Smith, S.J. (1997). Evaluating an intervention for homeless persons: Results of a field experiment. *Journal of Consulting and Clinical Psychology, 65*, 476–484.

Toro, P.A., Trickett, E.J., Wall, D.D., & Salem, D.A. (1991). Homelessness in the United States: An ecological perspective. *American Psychologist, 46*, 1208–1218.

Toro, P.A., Wolfe, S.M., Bellavia, C.W., Thomas, D.M., Rowland, L.L., Daeschler, C.V., & McCaskill, P.A. (1999b). Obtaining representative samples of homeless persons: A two-city study. *Journal of Community Psychology, 27,* 157–178.

Tsemberis, S. (1999). From streets to homes: An innovative approach to supported housing for homeless adults with psychiatric disabilities. *Journal of Community Psychology, 27,* 225–242.

Whitbeck, L.B., & Hoyt, D.R. (1999). *Nowhere to grow: Homeless and runaway adolescents and their families.* New York: Aldine de Gruyter.

Wolfe, S.M., Toro, P.A., & McCaskill, P.A. (1999). A comparison of homeless and matched housed adolescents on family environment variables. *Journal of Research on Adolescence, 9,* 53–66.

Wolock, I., & Magura, S. (1996). Parental substance abuse as a predictor of child maltreatment reports. *Child Abuse and Neglect, 20,* 1183–1193.

Yapchai, C.J., Toro, P.A., & McCaskill, P.A. (2001). *Behavioral and cognitive functioning among homeless and housed poor children: A comparative study.* Unpublished manuscript under editorial review. Department of Psychology, Wayne State University.

Ziesmer, C., Marcoux, L., & Marwell, B. (1994). Homeless children: Are they different from other low-income children? *Social Work, 39,* 658–668.

Zigler, E. (1994). Reshaping early childhood intervention to be a more effective weapon against poverty. *American Journal of Community Psychology, 22,* 37–47.

Zlotnick, C., Kronstadt, D., & Klee, L. (1999a). Essential case management services for young children in foster care. *Community Mental Health Journal, 35,* 421–430.

Zlotnick, C., Robertson, M.J., & Lahiff, M. (1999b). Getting off the streets: Economic resources and residential exits among homeless adults. *Journal of Community Psychology, 27,* 209–224.

Homelessness, Adulthood

Giri Raj Gupta

INTRODUCTION

During the last three decades, homelessness in the United States has received public attention due to the high visibility of the homeless people across the nation. Diverse groups of homeless in the major cities in the United States attracted the attention of concerned people that the United States is failing to care for some of its most vulnerable citizens. Voluntary organizations such as the National Mental Health Association and the National Coalition of the Homeless have given further visibility to the plight of the homelessness. This entry addresses several relevant issues involved in adult homelessness and reviews current policies and programs directed at reducing the incidence of homelessness in the United States.

DEFINITIONS

Homelessness is a social condition that refers to the absence of a stable place of residence in which a person can live and call home. This conceptualization is generally accepted in the United States and most countries of the Western world. There is considerable disagreement among scholars about the definition of the homeless as political, economic, ethnic, and cultural issues play a vital role in determining who is and who is not a homeless person. The living standards, availability of resources, climatic conditions, and social policies vary in so many ways that classifying a segment of a population homeless in a certain country may be viewed as ethnocentric. Controversies are also associated with explanations of homelessness as some call it as a lifestyle of choice while others view it as a callous disregard by society toward those who are not part of the mainstream.

Researchers generally agree that key issues for the homeless are the absence of stable housing, adequate personal resources, and community ties. Other problems not included in the definition are unemployment, issues regarding a sense of personal responsibility and motivation, marketable job skills, good health, education, and family support.

In 1984, the US Department of Housing & Urban Development defined *homelessness* as a condition of living: (a) in public or private emergency shelters which take a variety of forms—armories, schools, church basements, government buildings, former fire-houses, and where temporary vouchers are provided by public and private agencies, even hotels, apartments, or boarding houses; or (b) in the streets, parks, subways, bus terminals, railroad stations, airports, under bridges or aqueducts, abandoned buildings without utilities, cars, trucks, or any other public or private space that is not designed for shelter. This definition seems to ignore those who are homeless in rural areas where few shelters exist. In many rural areas, the homeless are hidden and are likely to survive by living with relatives, friends, or good-hearted people who help others in distress (US Department of Agriculture, 1996).

Scholars have also attempted to define homelessness on the basis of time, place, and personal situation. For example, some persons with serious mental illnesses have been homeless for long periods. Others have not been able to afford regular housing; they live under difficult housing circumstances constantly threatened by eviction.

SCOPE

Homelessness has existed across history. Its nature and tenure has been determined by the socioeconomic, political, and geographical conditions of a particular country. Although widespread, homelessness has been the result of social, economic, and environmental upheavals including depression, war, political turmoil, and disease. Major natural disasters such as earthquakes, floods, and famine and at times industrial accidents have caused havoc leaving people without places to live or work. Often new problem-solving approaches and social policies have directly contributed to homelessness. For example, deinstitutionalization—the release of people with severe mental disorders, beginning with the 1960s—has contributed to the increasing number of the homeless in the United States. Estimates suggest that there are between 300,000 and 3,000,000 homeless people in the United States (Johnson, 1990, p. 46). The sheer range of estimated homeless indicates how poorly this social problem is understood (National Law Center on Homelessness and Poverty in America, 2000).

The problem of homelessness is not restricted to any one country, nor does it have the same causes. In some countries, such as India, in their large metropolitan centers, between 2 and 10 percent of the population lives on the streets or in temporary shelters built on unauthorized land. In Sudan and Ethiopia, the ongoing political turmoil has disrupted the lives of hundred of thousands of families leaving behind homeless children and a broken people. Many of these people have been forced out of their homes and are on the path to annihilation due to mass starvation and disease. In Bangladesh, over a million people become homeless every year during the monsoon season (*The Economist*, 1998). Due to the ever-increasing number of homeless people around the world, there is a growing concern that more has to be done by voluntary organizations because governments are either not willing or unable to address this problem. For example, in 1996, the Habitat II conference held in Istanbul, Turkey estimated the number of homeless worldwide at 100 million, with over one billion people suffering from inadequate shelter (Wright, 2000, p. 27).

Incidence of Homeless in the United States

Link, Susser, Stueve, Phelan, Moore, and Streuning (1994) conducted a cluster sample survey, using telephone interviews, with 1,507 people living in households in the continental United States. They found a 14 percent lifetime prevalence rate of any type of homelessness—about 26 million people. That is, at some point in their lives, these people either (a) had slept in a park, an abandoned building, etc.; (b) had slept in a shelter for homeless people; or (c) had doubled up at the residence of a relative or friend because they themselves had no home. By restricting the definition to the first two criteria, Link et al. report 7.4 percent were literally homeless, approximately 13.5 million people.

For the 1990 US census, the Census Bureau used several procedures in an attempt to accurately count the homeless population. Census employees worked with a variety of local agencies to identify street locations and shelters, abandoned or boarded up buildings, hotels, motels, and shelters charging less than $12 a night where homeless were known to stay. At the end, 24,000 street sites and 11,000 shelters were included in the count. The data showed that there were a total of 292,178 homeless that included 178,638 persons in emergency shelters; 49,734 were living at street locations, 11,768 were in shelters for abused women; 52,038 were in drug and alcohol abuse group homes (Census of Population and Housing, 1990). It was the most concerted effort to include the homeless in the census. Yet, due to the predetermined nature of the sites and sample, not all the homeless were counted.

Further, the figures on trends in the homeless population are varied and inconsistent. This is because the data were collected at different points of time with certain areas in mind. Compared to 1960s and 1970s, there are more homeless now and the make up of that population has changed.

Age

The new homeless person is younger. The stereotype of older men, who were chronic alcoholics, is being replaced by younger men in their mid-thirties (US Department of Housing & Urban Development, 1984). Families are the fastest growing homeless group with children representing about 40 percent of the people who become homeless. The US Conference of Mayors Report (1998) reports that families constituted 38 percent of the homeless population. This figure is likely to be higher in rural areas where single mothers and children make up the largest homeless group. The US Conference of Mayors' survey of homelessness in 30 cities found that children under the age of 18 accounted for 25 percent of the urban homeless population. This study also reported that unaccompanied minors represented 3 percent of the urban homeless population (US Conference of Mayors Report, 1998).

Gender and Marital Status

The 1990 census reported that women comprised 31.2 percent of the homeless population. High divorce rates, domestic abuse, substance abuse, and emotional problems have contributed to this situation. Between 1980 and 1984, the number of families in shelters more than quadrupled (Kosof, 1988). Homeless women, especially those with children, make up roughly 38 percent of the estimated 3 million homeless people in the United States (Bassuk, 1991). In large cities, such as New York and Los Angeles, families represent 40–45 percent of the homeless population in shelters.

Race and Ethnicity

In contrast to the 1920s when young Caucasian men were most likely to be homeless, the 1998 survey of 30 cities by the US Conference of Mayors' found that the homeless population was 49 percent African American, 32 percent Caucasian, 12 percent Latino, 4 percent Native American, and 3 percent Asian. It appears that the homeless in rural areas are more likely to be White, Native Americans, or migrant Latino workers. In urban areas, African Americans are disproportionately represented among the homeless.

A Short History of Homelessness in the United States

Many of the homeless in the US in the 19th century were White single men with a sense of wanderlust who explored new territories and seized opportunities for wealth (the Comstock silver discovery, the Alaska gold rush, the opening of western farmland). This adventurous homeless soul was replaced during the Great Depression (1929–1939) with displaced families who lost their homes to unemployment, bankruptcies, and foreclosures. Many jobless men, unable to support their families, could not live with loss of their pride and self-worth, and joined the flow of people seeking a livelihood without their families.

One of the earliest sociological reports on the lives of the homeless men was *The hobo* (Anderson, 1923) followed later by *Twenty thousand homeless men* (Sutherland & Locke, 1936). Thomas (1923) described the experiences of young women in Chicago in *The unadjusted girl*, who were either forced out of homes or ran away from familial abuse and often worked as prostitutes on the streets of Chicago. These studies focused on street crime and gangs, impoverished communities, vagrancy, and substance abuse problems. Since then, there have been scores of studies examining various social and economic forces pushing the homeless toward the fringes of society.

In the 1970s, studies of the homeless changed their focus of analysis from sociological factors to individual pathology and underplayed the role of stressful environments that pushed people from their homes onto the street. In the 1980s and 1990s, social research rediscovered the core causes and consequences of homelessness. Surveys by Snow and Anderson (1987, 1993), Rossi (1989), and Wright (1989) went beyond the lives of the homeless on the street to the social, political, and personal factors contributing to people becoming homeless and maintaining a homeless lifestyle. The social processes that drive people into homelessness include persistent family problems, job instability, problems with available housing, and interpersonal difficulties. Homelessness is a complex social problem exacerbated by the following factors.

Housing

The destruction of traditional low income housing, increasing rents, cuts in federal housing programs, and the gentrification of city neighborhoods threaten affordable housing for low-income people. During the 1970s, about half of the nation's single-room occupancy units (SROs) were destroyed, causing severe shortages of housing and leaving former occupants on the streets or in shelters. In 1993, problematic housing for the poor reached an all-time high, affecting 5.3 million households. Each of these households paid more than half of their income for housing or lived in houses with serious maintenance problems.

Income

About 1 in 10 of the extremely poor in the United States become homeless. In 1995, about 36.4 million people in the United States lived at or below the poverty line, facing the risk of becoming homeless. Minimum wage earnings no longer allowed these families to pay rent and meet daily expenses. Although 20 percent of homeless adults are employed (usually in day labor jobs), their income does not allow them to meet basic necessities. Technological acceleration excludes those with lower skill levels from the competitive job market. Reduced public assistance left many homeless or at risk, following the replacement of the Aid to Families with Dependent Children (AFDC) entitlement programs with the non-entitlement block grant programs.

In 1996, in response to the perceived failure of the welfare system, Congress passed the Personal Responsibility and Work Opportunity Reconciliation Act, popularly know as "the Welfare Reform Act." Among its main provisions were the work requirement mandating 2 years of assistance and a significant reduction in the Food Stamp Program. Under this act, states are allowed to drop unwed mothers and their children from the welfare roles unless they attend school and live with an adult. The National Coalition for the Homeless (1997) conducted a national survey and found that only a fraction of the new jobs pay above poverty wages. In Wisconsin's much publicized welfare experiment, nearly two out of three former recipients had lower incomes than during the 3 months before they left welfare. Many factors contribute to these pessimistic data, including transportation problems between suburban job sites and inner city housing, lack of adequate child care facilities, and lack of a culture of experiences on holding a job. In the absence of adequate investment in education and job training, a cohort of people who are unable to meet the new work environment challenges face an increased risk of homelessness.

Health Services

The cost of health care has placed a large number of low-income families at a serious risk of homelessness. Studies of New York City homeless shelter populations found that many homeless people have health problems (Padgett & Struening, 1991). Not surprisingly, the homeless are less likely to have access to adequate health care. About 30 percent of homeless people suffer from chronic mental disorders, but less than 3 percent of the men and 14 percent of the women receive disability benefits.

Domestic Violence

One of the major causes of homelessness is domestic violence. While spousal abuse cuts across all income levels, it disproportionately affects women with annual incomes of less than $10,000. A survey of cities in 1996 reported that 46 percent identified domestic violence as a primary cause of homelessness (Craven, 1996; National Coalition for the Homeless, 1997).

THEORIES AND RESEARCH

There is disagreement among scholars about the origins of homelessness. Some, within the medical community, explain most homelessness using a biological model. That is, many seriously emotionally ill individuals become homeless because of their "brain disorder." Other scholars reject biological and genetic explanations and offer instead an ecological explanation. For these social scientists, homelessness is multicausal and related to personal, family, neighborhood, and larger societal factors. These factors include but are not limited to the break up of families, the unplanned release of the mentally ill from care, unemployment, the lack of affordable housing, and substance abuse. Some sociologists explain homelessness by analyzing the social processes inherent in society. Durkheim (1951/1897) expressed this idea as a lack of cohesiveness among social institutions to regulate behavior, leaving some people on the fringes of society in a state of anomie. Although he did not address homelessness, his views on the creation of new social groups and institutions to provide a sense of belonging as members of a huge, complex, and often impersonal society are as relevant to the homeless as they are to potential suicides.

From a Marxian perspective, the key factor in homelessness would be the alienation of the homeless from the economic engine of society. Hence, they command no influence in society (in the terms of the social exchange theory by Homans (1961) and Blau (1964), they have nothing tangible to exchange) and are perceived as a nuisance, not as a social problem to be solved through socioeconomic changes.

STRATEGIES: OVERVIEW

Ending homelessness involves: (1) providing affordable housing, (2) training the homeless to hold jobs that generate living incomes, (3) taking care of their physical and mental health needs, and (4) creating a social support network for them. Therefore, preventive programs with regard to potential homeless adults and families have to include broad social policies and a national moral consensus; intermediate community-level opportunities and supports; and direct services and encouragements to involved persons to avoid their becoming homeless.

STRATEGIES THAT WORK

At this time, there are no descriptions of programs or research studies that prevent homelessness in adults, which meet the criteria for inclusion in this encyclopedia.

STRATEGIES THAT MIGHT WORK

The following two examples of strategies need evaluation, but are promising in the way they are structured. The New York City's Fountain House is a program operated by and for the homeless. This kind of organization might be more sensitive to the many kinds of needs of the homeless, as well as their strategies that might interfere with the resolutions of their difficulties. According to legend, it was started in the 1950s by three ex-state hospital patients who had nothing to do and took to hanging out at a soda fountain, hence the name. To date, the program has sponsored 50 apartments, a thrift shop, a snack bar, and an employment service. The Fountain is using three of prevention's tools to enable its members to succeed. Those tools are education by teaching job readiness skills, providing social support, and promoting social competency. Learning how to function successfully in the world of work gives rise to feelings of belonging, being valued, and making a meaningful contribution to society.

The second promising program is operated by the Broward County Homeless Assistance Center in Florida. It is a facility that offers job training and placement programs. Unlike many public homeless shelters, the Broward County Homeless Assistance Center was created by the combined efforts of public servants, philanthropists, and taxpayers, who raised the necessary funding and developed a continuum-of-care model for the Florida Miami Dade County. Interestingly,

Miami is one of the very few places where the number of homeless is actually dropping. This program offers participants housing in the residence, free health care, child care, classes in life skills and anger management, and job training. More than 60 percent of the program participants hold jobs outside the shelter, while others work on-site. All are encouraged to gain self-sufficiency. Demanding standards are maintained at the residence, including no drugs or alcohol (Swope, 1999).

There are many other types of shelters and services for the homeless, but few are evaluated and thus we are not making use of these natural experiments to learn what methods are promising with the homeless. In the coming decade, programs should encourage the formation of natural caregiving networks among the homeless.

STRATEGIES THAT DO NOT WORK

There is no information about ineffective strategies identified in the published literature, although we can speculate that merely providing food and shelter does not influence either resolution of existing problems in the homeless, nor does the existence of these limited services prevent future homelessness.

SYNTHESIS

Providing shelter is not enough to solve the homeless problem. What we have learned from the limited literature on this topic is that any preventive effort would benefit from having homeless people actively involved as participants, managers, and supervisors in the program. We have also learned that we need somehow to stir the national conscience about homelessness, and the potential for its prevention. Let's look at what we can learn from the theoretical perspectives.

First, the homeless are ordinary human beings who have experienced more stress than they are able to handle. This still means that they have strengths and resources that should be optimized as part of any overall strategy for the homeless and natural caregiving provide such an opportunity. To the extent that they are involved in the control of their own destiny, they will be less likely crushed and demoralized by the possible progressive deterioration of their situations, especially when it involves dead end food-and-shelter institutional solutions. Primary prevention involves competency promoting activities like connecting with people at high risk of becoming homeless, and taking such actions that are calculated to shore up their own strengths and the resources of others in their primary group circle—before they are labeled as homeless. Labeling a person as homeless is self-defeating and socially defeating.

In general, the best strategies for the future prevention of homelessness involves drawing on the individual's own strengths to the degree possible and augmenting these strengths with naturally existing support systems based on reciprocity, not welfare. It will also be necessary to call upon the larger society to provide the socioeconomic basis for maintaining housing rather than having to pay the fiscal and moral bill of producing yet another generation of homeless.

Also see: Homelessness: Childhood; Community Capacity; Loneliness/Isolation: Older Adulthood.

References

Anderson, N. (1923). *The hobo: The sociology of homeless men.* Chicago: University of Chicago Press.

Blau, P. (1964). *Exchange and power in social life.* New York: Wiley.

Bussuk, E. (1991). Homeless families. *Scientific American, 265,* 66–74.

Census of Population and Housing. (1990). *Population and housing guide.* Washington, DC: US Department of Commerce, Economics and Statistics Administration, Bureau of Census.

Craven, D. (1996). *Female victims of violent crime, selected findings.* Washington, DC: Bureau of Justice Statistics, US Department of Justice.

Durkheim, E. (1951). *Suicide.* (J.A. Spaulding and George Simpson, Trans.). New York: Free Press. (Originally published 1897.)

The Economist. (1998). Drowning. *348,* 8085.43.

Homans, G. (1961). *Social behavior in elementary forms.* New York: Harcourt, Brace and World.

Johnson, A.B. (1990). *Out of bedlam: The truth about deinstitutionalization.* New York: Basic Books.

Kosof, A. (1988). *Homeless in America.* New York: Franklin Watts.

Link, B., Susser, E., Stueve, A., Phelan, J., Moore, R., & Streuning, E.L. (1994). Lifetime and five year prevalence of homelessness in the United States. *American Journal of Public Health, 88,* 1907–1912.

National Coalition for the Homeless. (1997). How many people experience homelessness. NCH Fact Sheet #1 & 2. http://www2.ari.net/home/nch/numbers.html

National Law Center on Homelessness and Poverty in America. (2000) Myths and facts about homeless. <http://www.nlchp.org/h&pusa/htm>http://www.nlchp.org/h&pusa/htm

Padgett, D.K., & Struening, E.L. (1991). Influence of substance abuse and mental disorders on emergency room use by homeless adults. *Hospital and Community Psychiatry, 42,* 834–837.

Rossi, P.H. (1989). *Down and out in America: The origins of homelessness.* Chicago: University of Chicago Press.

Snow, D., & Anderson, L. (1987). Identity work among the homeless: The verbal construction and avowal of personal identities. *American Journal of Sociology, 92,* 1336–1371.

Snow, D., & Anderson, L. (1993). *Down on their luck: A study of homeless street people.* Berkeley: University of California Press.

Sutherland, E., & Locke, H. (1936). *Twenty thousand homeless men: A study of unemployed men in the Chicago shelters.* Philadelphia: J.B. Lippincott.

Swope, C. (1999, December). Beyond shelter. *Governing, 13,* 26.

Thomas, W.I. (1923). *The unadjusted girl.* Boston: Little Brown.

US Conference of Mayors. (1998). A status report on hunger and homelessness in America's cities. Washington, DC: Author.

US Department of Agriculture. (1996). *Rural homelessness: Focusing on the needs of the rural homeless.* Washington, DC: Author.

US Department of Housing & Urban Development. (1984). *Helping the homeless: A resource guide*. Washington, DC: Government Printing Office.

Wright, J. (1989). *Address unknown: The homeless in America*. New York: Aldine DeGruyter.

Wright, T. (2000). Resisting homelessness: Global, national, and local solutions. *Contemporary Sociology, 29*, 27–43.

Homicide, Adolescence

Michael J. Furlong, Tisa C. Jimenez, and Jill D. Sharkey

INTRODUCTION AND SCOPE

The specter of adolescents committing homicide does not bode well for any society because of the social, economic, and cultural damage it causes. Whenever these acts occur, all societies pause to consider why a youth at a stage of life that should involve self-discovery and exploration felt the need to murder another. As an isolated event, adolescent homicides affect relatively few, and are limited to the individuals involved, but when it occurs frequently, broader societal implications are indicated. This entry examines historical trends in adolescent homicide, what is known about adolescents who commit homicide, and prevention programs designed to reduce homicide and behavior leading to its outcome.

In the absence of significant social unrest, conflict, or war, adolescent homicides should be rare events as they are in most industrialized countries. However, as with homicides in general, the adolescent homicide rate in the United States far exceeds those of any other nation. For example, in 1993, the overall homicide rate per 100,000 for ages 15–24 in the United States was 15.3 compared to 3.1 in Canada and 0.4 in Japan (McGonigal, 2001). This pattern holds for adolescents ages 10–17—in 1993, for example, 7 percent of homicides in Canada were attributed to adolescents, which compares to 14 percent in the United States (Heide, 2000). During the late 1980s and early 1990s, the adolescent homicide rate increased dramatically in the United States across all youth ages 14–17 (see Figure 1). These increases were associated with the use of firearms (the availability of which distinguished the United States from other nations) and homicides of known acquaintances and strangers (Snyder & Sickmund,

1999). Family-related homicides, such a parricide, actually decreased. Males (93.4 percent, in 1997) and African Americans (53.9 percent in 1997) were disproportionately involved in adolescent homicides (Snyder & Sickmund, 1999).

Much of the decline in adolescent homicides in the United States in the late 1990s was due to substantial decreases among African American males.

Between the peak years of 1993 and 1999, adolescent homicide arrests in the United States decreased by 68 percent (Snyder, 2000). Putting these figures into perspective, in 1999, there were about 1,400 juveniles (ages 10–17) arrested for homicide in the United States, which compares to 3,800 in 1993. Arrests of juveniles for homicide was about five per 100,000, or at its lowest level since 1980 (Snyder, 2000).[1] In addition, the homicide rate among youths ages 0–14 actually declined steadily from 1980 through 1999, with all increases of youth homicide coming from the 15–17 year-old age group (Dunworth, 2000).

It is encouraging that the US adolescent homicide rate has decreased substantially. Homicides committed by adolescents are rare in non-US countries and studies are often based on case examples. Nevertheless, it is important to examine factors associated with juveniles who commit homicide in other countries in order to have a broad understanding of this phenomenon. One study examined the characteristics of samples of adolescent murderers. Busch, Zagar, Hughes, Arbit, and Bussell (1990) compared a sample of 71 English adolescents convicted of homicide to 71 non-violent adjudicated adolescents. They found that the homicide-convicted group were more likely to: (a) have a criminally violent family member (58 vs. 20 percent), (b) be involved in a youth gang (41 vs. 14 percent), (c) abuse alcohol (38 vs. 24 percent), and (d) have general cognitive ability test scores two standard deviations below the mean (21 vs. 10 percent). In a study of 72 adolescents from the United States, Cornell, Benedek, and Benedek (1987) compared homicide perpetrators to a separate group of non-violent delinquents. The juveniles arrested for homicide were a diverse group with no clear, single behavior pattern. Interestingly, the non-violent juvenile offenders had the most at-risk profile with the poorest mental health status.

---

[1] This entry focuses on juveniles who commit homicide. For perspective sake, in 1997, 2,100 juveniles were the victims of homicide. Fifty percent of these youth were of ages 15–17 and 83 percent of juvenile victims ages 12–17 were killed with a gun. Most of these juvenile homicides, as many as 75 percent, involve an adult perpetrator (Wilson, 2000). In addition, in the United States, female violent crime rates have increased, but female homicide often represents different acts than those of males. Of the slightly more than 100 girls who commit homicide annually, their offenses are more likely than boys to involve interpersonal conflicts as opposed to criminally motivated acts (Loper & Cornell, 1996). Comprehensive adolescent homicide prevention programs should integrate efforts to reduce juvenile perpetration and victimization.

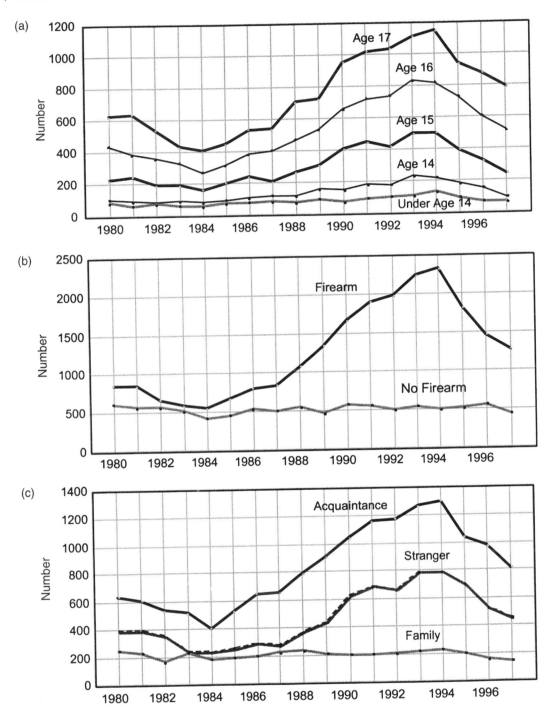

Figure 1. Adolescent homicide trends, United States, 1980–1997.

(Data source: *US Federal Bureau of Investigation. (1999, September). Supplementary homicide reports for the years 1980–1997* [machine-readable data files]. [On-line]. Available: http://www.ojjdp.ncjrs.org)

(a) Age of known juvenile homicide offenders, United States 1980–1997; (b) Firearm related homicides of known juvenile offenders, United States 1980–1997; (c) Relationship of victims to known juvenile homicide offenders, United States 1980–1997

THEORIES

Developmental Pathways toward Violence

Through longitudinal studies, researchers have described the development pathways of boys' delinquent behavior. Youth manifest antisocial behavior by engaging in less serious behaviors at early ages, persisting in these behaviors as they grow up, and later accelerate into more serious antisocial behaviors. In addition, only a small number of youth that begin further along an antisocial pathway end up reaching its advanced stages (Kelley, Loeber, Keenan, & DeLamatre, 1997). Though not focused specifically on youth who commit homicide, these theories provide information about how a child develops antisocial or violent behavior (youth may commit serious aggravated assaults that do not result in the death of the victim). One example of a developmental pathway model is provided by Kelley and colleagues (1997) who described how boys move along toward increasingly deviant behaviors in three distinct but related ways. The Overt pathway includes those youth most likely to commit homicide. Youth enter the Overt pathway at a young age through bullying peers and picking on others. These lower level physical behaviors move into physical fighting, which in turn can lead to other violence such as rape, attack, and homicide. Under this model, boys most likely to reoffend are those with multiple offenses, who begin at an early age, and whose severity of offenses increases over time. Patterson, Reid, and Dishion (1992) also formulated a theory of delinquency centered on stages of development. In this model, poor parenting practices such as lack of management skills, ineffective discipline, and lack of monitoring promotes coercive and manipulative ways of responding to the world. When such a child reaches school age, his or her abrasive manner of interpersonal interaction leads to peer rejection. In addition, the child learns to use coercive techniques to avoid challenging tasks. As the child grows more alienated from peers and school, the natural tendency is to seek out similar peers with whom they continue antisocial behaviors including truancy, substance abuse, and increasingly more delinquent behaviors. In this model, family factors, emotional functioning, academic performance, and substance abuse are all factors correlated with antisocial behaviors, including violence toward others.

RESEARCH

Lipsey and Derzon (1998) provide a review through meta-analysis of predictors of serious and violent offenses from longitudinal research studies. They found that variables differed depending on age at assessment. For offenders between the ages of 6 and 11, committing a general offense ($r = 0.38$) and substance use ($r = 0.30$) were the strongest predictors of future serious and violent offending. For offenders between the ages of 12 and 14, lack of social ties ($r = 0.39$), antisocial peers ($r = 0.37$), and committing a general offense ($r = 0.26$) were the strongest predictors of later serious and violent offending. Additional factors are positively correlated with subsequent offending. Within the realm of antisocial behavior, physical violence, aggression, person crimes, problem behavior, and substance use were identified as predictors. Personal characteristics included having a low IQ, poor school attitude and performance, and psychological conditions such as high activity level, impulsiveness, and psychopathology. Family characteristics included antisocial and abusive parents, poverty, and parent–child relationships characterized by low supervision, low warmth, and punitive discipline. Few social activities and association with antisocial peers were also found to predict antisocial behavior.

Gender

Though violent offenses are most often committed by males, recent studies show that female violence is increasing (Bilchik, 1999a). Research on female perpetrators indicates differences in the types of and motivations for homicide between boys and girls. Loper and Cornell (1996) analyzed data from homicide reports collected between 1984 and 1993 by the FBI in order to investigate this difference. Offense patterns indicate that girls mostly victimized family members, with 54 percent being infant offspring, and 24 percent being a parent. In contrast, only 8 percent of boys' victims were family members. When compared to boys, girls used a firearm significantly less frequently (32.2 vs. 82.3 percent). Girls were also involved more often in conflict-related homicides (79.3 percent) than crime-related homicides (20.7 percent). In contrast, boys were more often involved in crime-related homicides (57.3 percent) than conflict-related homicides (42.7 percent). Boys were also more likely to kill someone of the same gender (86 percent) than were girls (42 percent). These results point to extreme levels of emotional angst being experienced by girls who commit homicide and highlight the need for gender-specific programming. Programs teaching coping skills and the management of stressful life circumstances such as teen pregnancy may be warranted (Loper & Cornell, 1996).

Gangs

Gang-related activities markedly contribute to the incidence of adolescent homicide. For example, in Los Angeles County in 1998, gangs played a role in almost 80 percent of adolescent homicides (Bilchik, 1999a). In addition, only five communities in the United States (Los Angeles, Chicago, Houston, Detroit, and New York), all with a significant gang presence, accounted for 25 percent of all known juvenile homicide offenders in 1997 (Loeber, Farrington, & Waschbusch, 1998). Programs aimed at decreasing rates of homicide must consider gang influences and develop unique treatments to intervene with this population.

Firearms

A majority of US juvenile homicide victims are killed with a firearm, with percentages ranging from 79 to 83 percent in various communities (Bilchik, 1999a). In a Los Angeles survey of adolescent males living in high-risk neighborhoods, 25 percent of youth surveyed indicated that they knew several places to get a gun in their neighborhood, and 7 percent indicated that they could secure one in less than an hour (Bilchik, 1999a). The combination of easy access to firearms and their pivotal role in homicides makes gun accessibility an important issue in considering how to reduce homicide rates.

Gun control is a hotly debated topic in the United States, the only industrialized nation to allow the private possession of handguns (Sherman, 2000). In reviewing the issue of reducing gun violence, Sherman (2000) notes that research into the effects of various gun policies is limited. Epidemiological studies show that using conviction history to control gun sales is not useful because a majority of gun-related crimes are committed by individuals with no criminal history. In addition, it is important to note that most gun violence occurs in areas where gun possession is dense (Sherman, 2000). Such information about the nature of gun crimes allows for the informed analysis of what types of innovative policies may help reduce gun violence. Sherman (2000) argues that what works to reduce gun violence is having police patrol high density gun crime areas and mandating background checks in order to restrict gun sales in stores. What "does not work" includes gun buy-back programs? What is promising includes virtual bans on private handgun ownership and bans on the sale of new assault weapons. Additional ideas for effective programs include: bans on high-caliber guns, ammunition controls, waiting periods for ammunition, and national one-gun-a-month laws.

STRATEGIES: OVERVIEW

All substantial increases of the US adolescent homicide arrests rate between 1984 and 1994 were reversed by the end of 1999. A mixture of public policy, enforcement, and prevention programs played a role in this dramatic reversal (Bilchik, 1999b). No single, narrow-focused intervention has been proven to reduce adolescent homicide, most likely because of its complex etiology and multiple determinants involving the perpetrators and the contexts in which homicide occurs. Consequently, in this section, we describe multi-component programs that have shown promise to reduce adolescent antisocial behaviors and aggression and focus on at-risk youth and their personal social context—precursor conditions of homicide. In addition to discussing these promising efforts, we briefly discuss ineffective strategies. It is important to note that adolescent homicide prevention has focused primarily on males and consequently, the prevention programs discussed generally involved populations of male, at-risk youth.

STRATEGIES THAT WORK

Research in this area has attempted to pinpoint common elements within successful programs that can reduce serious and chronic youth violence (Catalano, Loeber, & McKinney, 1999; Centers for Disease Control and Prevention, 2000; Tolan & Guerra, 1998). Although research has identified various characteristics found in effective intervention programs, only four of the most common are discussed in addition to examples of programs that address these common characteristics. It is important to note that these programs focus on reducing identified risk factors that contribute to aggressive and violent behavior and serious delinquency in their efforts to prevent homicide.

Successful prevention programs target multiple risk factors that affect violent youths and become obstacles toward decreasing their maladaptive behavior (e.g., poverty, serious illness, poor parenting, poor academic achievement, and gang affiliation). Effective delinquency prevention programs typically range from 2 to 5 years in length. Longer intervention programs affect multiple predictors of delinquency, whereas brief interventions might only have time to affect single risk factors (Yoshikawa, 1994). Another aspect of successful programs is that they maintain a level of cultural sensitivity in the support services they provide to delinquent youth and their families. By maintaining this cultural competence, the needs of all youth and families considered "at risk" are addressed. A third aspect of exemplary programs is that they include program evaluation. Studies to evaluate program effectiveness must examine how the interventions were implemented and adequately examine their effectiveness in addressing the needs of high-risk populations (Foote, 1997; Tate, Reppucci, & Mulvey, 1995; Tolan & Guerra, 1998). Finally, successful interventions target risk factors that individual youth encounter in a variety of settings (e.g., within the individual youth, within the youth's close interpersonal relationships, within proximal social contexts, or within greater societal macrosystems; Fraser, 1996; Tolan & Guerra, 1998).

Multisystemic Therapy

One well-researched example of a cross-context intervention is *Multisystemic Therapy* (MST) developed by Henggeler and colleagues (1999). MST focuses on familial problems including difficulties experienced with parenting techniques and family cohesion and organization. It can be considered a prevention program when it is used to intervene with youths who show signs of chronic, violence antisocial behavior in order to prevent future homicide. MST draws upon validated treatment strategies such as strategic family therapy and cognitive behavioral therapy. The program targets interpersonal, familial and extra familial factors, which can contribute to serious violent and delinquent behavior. MST's success in decreasing serious antisocial behavior stems from its highly individualized and flexible interventions. The program uses an individualized treatment-planning strategy to address the unique needs and circumstances of each adolescent and his or her family. When compared to individual therapy, MST has been found to be more effective in decreasing antisocial behaviors and adjustment problems and has established both short- and long-term success with chronic, serious, and violent youth (Borduin, 1999). It has also been used in school settings as part of a broader, multi-component strategy to reduce youth violence (Cunningham & Henggeler, 2001).

Cognitive Behavioral Programs

Programs that focus on particular risk factors that affect youth (e.g., difficulty with self-control and problem-solving skills) are often based on a cognitive-behavioral approach. This approach seeks to decrease antisocial and violent behavior by changing the social cognitive mechanisms linked with such behavior. An example of such an approach is the *Viewpoints Training Program*, which focuses on improving social problem-solving skills, increasing self-control, changing beliefs and attitudes about violence and enhancing perspective taking (Tate et al., 1995; Tolan & Guerra, 1998). This 12-session, small-group training program attempts to teach youth appropriate responses to conflict. Guerra and Slaby (1990) examined the effectiveness of this program with 120 juvenile offenders randomly assigned to the Viewpoints program, an attention-control group, or a no-treatment group. Their results showed decreases in aggressive as well as impulsive behavior, with increases in problem-solving skills for the participants of the Viewpoints program.

Behavior Contingency Programs

Promising programs in this area implement strategies that include behavior modification techniques. These approaches focus on changing behavior through such techniques as direct reinforcement, contingency contracting, and modeling. The volunteer *Buddy System* program is an example of an individualized behavior modification program that partners youths with volunteers to address a range of academic and behavioral problems (Catalano et al., 1999). With the assistance of a volunteer, the youth participates in a variety of weekly behavioral support activities. In addition to 12 hr of initial training, the mentors later attend biweekly training sessions on behavior management throughout the duration of the program. These volunteers work with their assigned youths, submit reports on their youth's behavior, complete weekly logs, and collaboratively complete weekly assignments (Catalano et al., 1999). An evaluation of the program demonstrated a decrease in truancy when mentors implemented various methods of reinforcement for appropriate behaviors (Fo & O'Donnell, 1975).

Social Network-Focused Prevention Programs

Influencing a youth's close interpersonal relations (e.g., family and peers) is a strategy to reduce adolescent violence. Family interventions have repeatedly reduced antisocial behavior by focusing on behavior management and family relations. *Multisystemic Therapy*, previously described in this entry, is a very successful example of a family focused and comprehensive prevention program (Henggeler et al., 1999). Another successful program attentive to the needs of families is the *Prenatal and Infancy Nurse Home-Visitation* program. Each family is assigned an individual nurse who stays with the family during pregnancy. The nurse visits the home once a week after registration into the program for the first month and then every other week through delivery. Once the baby is born, home visits are made once a week for the first 6-weeks, then every other week for the first 2-years of the infant's life. The nurses monitor the health and well being of the mother while providing parenting instruction and other activities in order to promote the physical, cognitive and emotional development of the children in the home (Muller & Mihalic, 1999). This intervention is designed to help mothers manage their children and their own lives more effectively, reducing the stress typically experienced after the birth of their children. This program has been shown to reduce verified reports of child abuse and neglect by 79 percent, reduce maternal behavior problems due to alcohol and drug abuse by 44 percent, and reduce future arrests of the children involved in the program by 56 percent (Olds, Hill, Mihalic, & O'Brien, 1998). Evidence of child abuse, neglect, and parental alcohol and drug abuse are risk factors that have been known to contribute to juvenile violence and chronic delinquency. A third family program is *Functional Family Therapy* (FFT). This is a complete family program that assists families in changing their communication, interaction, and problem solving patterns (Muller & Mihalic, 1999). FFT is a short-term intervention that targets at-risk adolescents, from 11- to 18-years-old, and their families. The program has worked successfully with youth who have a variety of problems from conduct disorders to serious criminal offenses. Depending on the severity of the case, 8–30 hr of direct service are provided by a wide range of interventionists (e.g., degreed mental health professionals, mental health technicians, trained probation officers). FFT has been reported to be a cost effective program, with significant treatment effects including a reduction in recidivism rates from 75 to 40 percent (Alexander et al., 1998).

Social Context Interventions

Other general strategies to prevent adolescent violence and homicides include those interventions that focus on the adolescent's immediate social setting. These programs seek to transform aspects of the youth's social context that encourage or reinforce serious violent or antisocial behavior. An equally important emphasis is on identifying those social influences that interfere with the development of more positive behaviors (Tolan & Guerra, 1998). These programs are community-based and involve schools, neighborhoods, and communities. One such program, that has been recognized as exemplary by the US Office of Education, Safe and Drug-Free Schools Expert Panel, is *Positive Action Through Holistic Education* (PATHE; Gottfredson, 1986). The program's main objective is to improve the school environment so as to enhance students' attitudes toward school, improve academic achievement and consequently reduce juvenile delinquency and violence. Teams of teachers, school staff, students as well as community members implement school improvement programs. These teams participate in ongoing training in and collaborative review of school curriculum and discipline policies. The program promotes various academic, school climate, and career-oriented innovations, and provides counseling and academic services for students demonstrating particular academic or behavioral needs. High school students involved in the PATHE program have demonstrated decreases in delinquency, drug use, school suspensions and punishment (Catalano et al., 1999). Another exemplary program is *Project Care*. This program uses classroom management and cooperative learning techniques to reduce the incidence of delinquent behavior within a middle school setting (Catalano et al., 1999). Teams of teachers, administrators, school staff and parent volunteers are involved in the

program. After 2 years of implementation, students reported a significant decrease in delinquency while teachers found improvements in classroom discipline (Gottfredson, 1987).

Other community and neighborhood programs with promising results have sought to increase the motivation of high-risk students to attend school and participate in prosocial community activities (Tolan & Guerra, 1998). The *Big Brothers, Big Sisters of America* (BBBSA) mentoring program serves at-risk youth from 6- to 18-years-old who are from single-parent homes. The goal of the program is to provide the youth with a consistent and stable relationship (Muller & Mihalic, 1999). An adult volunteer and child meet weekly for 3–5 hr over the course of a year or more. A professional case manager outlines goals identified in an initial interview with the child or adolescent that will guide the activities of the relationship. Goals can include developing stable relationships with adults, siblings, parents, and peers as well as improving school attendance, academic performance and personal hygiene. These goals are developed into an individualized case plan. An 18-month study comparing 500 youth participants of BBBSA with 500 youth randomly assigned to a control group (youth not matched with a BBBSA mentor) found that youth participants were less likely to use drugs or assault another child or adult. BBBSA youth improved their school attendance, grades and their relationships with family members and peers (McGill, Mihalic, & Grotpeter, 1998). A similar mentoring program in Hawaii, *The Buddy System*, previously addressed in this entry, also uses mentoring relationships with at-risk youth to promote appropriate behavior and reduce truancy (Catalano et al., 1999). Mentoring programs, which expose at-risk youth to positive adult role models, serve as a key protection against future violence and antisocial behavior (Centers for Disease Control and Prevention, 2000).

Several community-based programs focus on adolescent drug, smoking, and alcohol use, which are risk factors for delinquency and antisocial behavior in at-risk youth. An example of such a program is the *Midwestern Prevention Project* (MPP) in Kansas City, which is designed to prevent substance abuse in at-risk middle and junior high school students. Over a 5-year period, the program included a media campaign, school curriculum, parent education, community organization, and changes in local health policy supporting the goals of the intervention (Muller & Mihalic, 1999). The program was first introduced in the schools and provided students with direct skills training on resistance to drug use. Teachers and other adults provided indirect skills training on prevention practices while community efforts supported non-drug use. The implementation of MPP had resulted in decreases of daily smoking, marijuana, and alcohol use with students through the 12th grade (Pentz, Mihalic, & Grotpeter, 1998), all behaviors positively associated with aggression. *Project Northland* in Minnesota similarly combines an educational curriculum and community-based interventions, in addition to parent education, in order to prevent alcohol use among at-risk adolescents (Catalano et al., 1999). This 3-year program integrates individual, parent, peer and community training and targets sixth- through eighth-grade students. In the sixth grade, students collaborate with their parents on assignments regarding adolescent alcohol use. In seventh grade, the curriculum emphasizes resistance skills and normative expectations concerning adolescent alcohol use. During eighth grade, students become community activists by making recommendations to the community regarding strategies for the prevention of teen alcohol use. A evaluation found that youth who participated in the program versus those students who had not participated demonstrated lower scores on their tendency to use alcohol, and on peer influence to use alcohol. An increase was noted in scores relating to students' communication with their parents about the consequences of drinking (Catalano et al., 1999).

STRATEGIES THAT DO NOT WORK

As discussed in the previous section, programs with proven effectiveness to reduce adolescent aggressive behavior universally have taken a "contextual" approach. By this, we mean that they have multiple components and they consider most instances of violence, including homicide, to be the result of a long-term developmental process that is influenced by multiple social contexts and circumstances. As such, effective interventions have focused not only on the social competence of the youth, but on family, school, and community contexts as well. Given this status of violence prevention, it is perhaps not surprising that ineffective programs do not take such a holistic and contextual approach. For example, traditional psychotherapy, psychiatric hospitalization, institutional placement, and psychopharmacological management have not shown to consistently prevent adolescent violence or homicide. In addition, group therapy, although considered to be a more cost-effective approach in comparison to individual therapy, has no evidence regarding its effectiveness in reducing antisocial or violent behavior in at-risk youth (Tate et al., 1995; Tolan & Guerra, 1998). Social casework, which combines individual counseling with close supervision and coordination of social services, has not proven to be effective in preventing serious antisocial and violent behavior (Tolan & Guerra, 1998).

SYNTHESIS

Adolescent aggression and homicide is disturbing because when it occurs in any culture, it suggests that some aspects of the youth development and socialization processes have gone awry. Juvenile homicide is a particular problem in the United States, although rates of violence have decreased by more than two thirds between 1994 and 1999 as a result of multi-level prevention programs aimed at high-risk youth. Despite these recent successes, there continues to be recurring incidents of adolescent homicide, most of which are unknown to the public. Given continued public concern about youth violence, there has been a growing interest in profiling the "typical" homicide offender. Such a practice is dubious due to the comparatively low incidence of homicide and the many variations in the types of adolescent homicide (Furlong, Bates, & Smith, 2001). What continues to be needed is an in-depth analysis of homicide in order to learn more about the different types of adolescent homicide (e.g., relationship-based, gang-associated, drug-involved, and revenge-driven killings). Intensive case studies (Gabarino, 2000) are necessary in order to determine what contexts and conditions are associated with homicide. It is crucial to examine contextual and environmental elements in order to understand how to provide preventive support to those at risk for such violent acts.

Several neglected areas in understanding youth antisocial behavior need to be addressed through research. First, the ecology that supports violent behaviors must be examined. Homicide is promoted, in part, by basic beliefs and societal values surrounding violence and used as a means to solve problems. Owning guns is seen as a right, revenge is seen as being appropriate for "evening the score." Perpetrators of extreme acts of violence are highly visible in the media and justified homicide is often glorified (e.g., movie action heroes). These values are prevalent not only in the media, but in our communities, schools, and homes, fostering conditions where violence can occur. Even school shooters receive an abundance of attention for their crimes. Second, it is necessary to better understand the relationship between delinquency, antisocial behaviors, aggression, and homicide for diverse youth. Homicide may be viewed as one possible outcome of a developmental trajectory that begins in early childhood (Moffitt, Caspi, Dickson, Silva, & Stanton, 1996). Factors that maintain this trajectory should be examined for diverse populations of youths, such as females and various cultural groups. Finally, a balanced research focus necessitates the consideration of youth assets as they affect outcomes. The influence of protective factors in decreasing the likelihood of a homicidal act should be investigated in order to increase the sensitivity of screening procedures to determine which components would enhance prevention and treatment programs.

From what is currently known about homicidal behavior, it is clear that multiagency, multi-systematic, and school-community options must be available for those youth showing multiple risk signs. Efforts to prevent homicide should be invested in providing a comprehensive, coordinated continuum of services necessary to respond to youth needs at every level. Successful programming will involve a four-tiered system. At the first level, the targets are community-wide beliefs and values. Expectations of appropriate behavior must be made explicit and demonstrated by adult role models. Second, comprehensive community services must be made available for all youths in need of support where early intervention is key. Third, those youths most at risk for homicide must be provided with more intensive services. These youth are likely to experience extraordinary life challenges from which few children should be expected to thrive without support. Finally, it must be recognized that there are some adolescents who will not respond to prevention efforts throughout childhood and may require more intensive services later in adolescence. These youths may need to be removed from their current environments (community contexts) and provided opportunities to learn new social and life skills in a different social setting. Public resources should be made available to support local community programs that provide a full continuum of services to youth who are beginning to manifest or already are showing warning signs of chronic and violent behaviors.

Programs that have proven the most effective in reducing adolescent violence and homicide are those that include social competence and problem-solving skills training combined with efforts to improve social support across family, community, and school contexts. The successes of these programs support efforts to continue their refinement and their expansion in order to kindle hope for the elimination of adolescent homicide.

Also see: Violence Prevention: Childhood; Intimate Partner Violence: Adulthood.

References

Alexander, J., Barton, C., Gordon, D., Grotpeter, J., Hansson, K., Harrison, R., Mears, S., Mihalic, S., Parsons, B., Pugh, C., Schulman, S., Waldron, H., & Sexton, T. (1998). *Blueprints for violence prevention, book three: Functional family therapy.* Boulder, CO: Center for the Study and Prevention of Violence.

Bilchik, S. (1999a). *Juvenile violence research. Report to congress.* Washington DC: Office of Juvenile Justice and Delinquency Prevention. NCJ176976.

Bilchik, S. (1999b). *Promising strategies to reduce gun violence.* Washington, DC: Office of Juvenile Justice and Delinquency Prevention. NCJ173950.

Borduin, C.M. (1999). Multisystemic treatment of criminality and violence in adolescents. *Journal of the American Academy of Child and Adolescent Psychiatry, 38,* 242–249.

Busch, K.G., Zagar, R., Hughes, J.R., Arbit, J., & Bussell, R.E. (1990). Adolescents who kill. *Journal of Clinical Psychology, 46,* 472–485.

Catalano, R.F., Loeber, R., & McKinney, K.C. (1999). *School and community interventions to prevent serious and violent offending.* Washington, DC: Office of Juvenile Justice and Delinquency Prevention, US Department of Justice.

Centers for Disease Control and Prevention. (2000). *Best practices of youth violence prevention: A sourcebook for community action.* Atlanta, GA: US Department of Health and Human Services.

Cornell, D.G., Benedek, E.P., & Benedek. D.M. (1987). Characteristics of adolescents charged with homicide: Review of 72 cases. *Behavioral Sciences & the Law, 5,* 11–23.

Cunningham, P.B., & Henggeler, S.W. (2001). Implementation of an empirically based drug and violence prevention and intervention program in a public school setting. *Journal of Clinical Child Psychology, 30,* 221–232.

Dunworth, T. (2000). *National evaluation of the youth firearms violence initiative.* Washington, DC: US Department of Justice, National Institute of Justice: Research in the Brief. NCJ184482.

Fo, W.S., & O'Donnell, C.R. (1975). The buddy system: Effect of community intervention on delinquent offenses. *Behavior Therapy, 6,* 522–524.

Foote, J. (1997). *Expert panel issues report on serious and violent juvenile offenders.* Washington, DC: Office of Juvenile Justice and Delinquency Prevention, US Department of Justice.

Fraser, M.W. (1996). Aggressive behavior in childhood and early adolescence: An ecological-developmental perspective on youth violence. *Social Work, 41,* 347–357.

Furlong, M.J., Bates, M.P., & Smith, D.C. (2001). Predicting school weapon possession: A secondary analysis of the Youth Risk Behavior Surveillance Survey. *Psychology in the Schools, 38,* 127–140.

Gabarino, J. (2000). *Lost boys: Why our sons turn to violence and how we can save them.* New York: Vantage.

Gottfredson, D.C. (1986). An empirical test of school based environmental and individual interventions to reduce the risk of delinquent behavior. *Criminology, 24,* 705–731.

Gottfredson, D.C. (1987). An evaluation of an organization development approach to reducing school disorder. *Evaluation Review, 11,* 739–763.

Guerra, N.G., & Slaby, R.G. (1990). Cognitive mediators of aggression in adolescent offenders: 2. Intervention. *Developmental Psychology, 26,* 269–277.

Heide, K.M. (2000). *Young killers: The challenge of juvenile homicide.* Thousand Oaks, CA: Sage.

Henggeler, S.W. et al. (1999). Home-based Multisystemic therapy as an alternative to the hospitalization of youths in psychiatric crisis: Clinical outcomes. *Journal of the American Academy of Child and Adolescent Psychiatry, 38,* 1331–1339.

Kelley, B.T., Loeber, R., Keenan, K., & DeLamatre, M. (1997). *Developmental pathways in boys' disruptive and delinquent behavior.* Washington, DC: OJJDP Juvenile Justice Bulletin, Office of Juvenile Justice and Delinquency Prevention. NCJ165692.

Lipsey, M.W., & Derzon, J.H. (1998). Predictors of violent or serious delinquency in adolescence and early adulthood: A synthesis of longitudinal research. In R. Loeber & D.P. Farrington (Eds.), *Serious and violent juvenile offenders: Risk factors and successful interventions* (pp. 86–105). Thousand Oaks, CA: Sage.

Loeber, R., Farrington, D.P., & Waschbusch, D.A. (1998). Serious and violent offenders. In R. Loeber & D.P. Farrington (Eds.), *Serious and violent juvenile offenders: Risk factors and successful interventions* (pp. 13–29). Thousand Oaks, CA: Sage.

Loper, A.B., & Cornell, D.G. (1996). Homicide by juvenile girls. *Journal of Child and Family Studies, 5,* 323–336.

McGill, D.E., Mihalic, S.F., & Grotpeter, J.K. (1998). *Blueprints for violence prevention, book two: Big brothers and Big sisters of America.* Boulder, CO: Center for the Study and Prevention of Violence.

McGonigal, M.D. (2001). *Violence prevention programs [on-line].* Available: http://www.courses.ahc.umn.edu/medical-school/InMd/Gun%20Violence%20and%20You/sld001.htm

Moffitt, T.E., Caspi, A., Dickson, N., Silva, P., & Stanton, W. (1996). Childhood-onset versus adolescent-onset antisocial conduct in males: Natural history from ages 3–18 years. *Development and Psychopathology, 9,* 399–424.

Muller, J., & Mihalic, S. (1999). *Blueprints: A violence prevention initiative.* Washington, DC: Office of Juvenile Justice and Delinquency Prevention, US Department of Justice.

Olds, D., Hill, P., Mihalic, S., & O'Brien, R. (1998). *Blueprints for violence prevention, book seven: Prenatal and Infancy Home Visitation by Nurses.* Boulder, CO: Center for the Study and Prevention of Violence.

Patterson, G.R., Reid, J.B., & Dishion, T.J. (1992). *Antisocial boys.* Eugene, OR: Castalia.

Pentz, M.A., Mihalic, S.G., & Grotpeter, J.K. (1998). *Blueprints for violence prevention, book one: The Midwestern Prevention Project.* Boulder, CO: Center for the Study and Prevention of Violence.

Sherman, L.W. (2000). *Reducing gun violence: What works, what doesn't, what's promising. Presentation at perspectives on crime and justice: 1999–2000 lecture series, National Institute of Justice, IV.* Washington, DC: US Department of Justice.

Snyder, H.N. (2000, December). *Juvenile arrests 1999.* Washington, DC: OJJDP Juvenile Justice Bulletin, Office of Juvenile Justice and Delinquency Prevention. NCJ 185236.

Snyder, H.N., & Sickmund, M. (1999). *Juvenile offenders and victims: 1999 national report.* Washington, DC: Office of Juvenile Justice and Delinquency Prevention.

Tate, D.C., Reppucci, N.D., & Mulvey, E.P. (1995). Violent juvenile delinquents: Treatment effectiveness and implications for future action. *American Psychologist, 50,* 777–781.

Tolan, P., & Guerra, N. (1998). *What works in reducing adolescent violence: An empirical review of the field.* Boulder, CO: University of Colorado, Center for the Study and Prevention of Violence.

Wilson, J.J. (2000). *Children as victims. 1999 national report series: Juvenile justice bulletin.* Washington, DC: Office of Juvenile Justice and Delinquency Prevention. NCJ 180753.

Yoshikawa, H. (1994). Prevention as cumulative protection: Effects of early family support and education on chronic delinquency and its risks. *Psychological Bulletin, 115,* 28–54.

Homophobia, Adolescence

Chris Downs and Brian M. Judd

INTRODUCTION AND DEFINITIONS

Fear, hatred, and discrimination directed at gay, lesbian, bisexual, transgender, transsexual, transvestite, hermaphrodite, and questioning peoples[1] have been documented across numerous, especially Western, societies and across many centuries (Boswell, 1980; Downs & Hillje, 1993). While a variety of terms and definitions for such reactions have been offered during the last 120 years, the word *homophobia*, coined by Weinberg (1972), has the most widespread usage. He crafted the term based on Greek words for "same" and "fear." *Homophobia*, then, refers to "fear of the same." Many authors have expanded the definition into social constructs, which refer to irrational anxieties about people who have same-sex attractions (MacDonald, 1976) and an irrational worry concerning love of someone of the same sex (Evans, 2000).

Blumenfeld (1992) points out how *cultural homophobia* is evidenced when a society: (a) informally attempts to prevent gay and lesbian people from associating with each other; (b) denies the probable numbers of gays or lesbians in that society so as to deny their significance; (c) tries to hide or minimize the visibility and historical contributions of sexual minority persons; (d) tolerates ghettos, or special places for sexual minority persons; and (e) uses labels and stereotypes to derogate the group. Herek (1984) cites a variety of other terms that seem closely related to homophobia including homoerotophobia, homosexphobia, homosexism, heterosexism, and homonegativism. The common denominator of these terms, and *homophobia* as used in this paper, is a multidimensional construct of attitudes, prejudices, emotional reactions, negative behaviors and fears directed at sexual minority persons. Herek (2000) recently offered the term *sexual prejudice* as a better term than homophobia since it seems to be free of some of the underlying assumptions and motivations for homophobia. In this entry, we retain the term homophobia because of more common usage and understanding about the discriminatory and prejudicial attitudes, behaviors, and feelings displayed against gay and lesbian people.

SCOPE

Homophobia has many manifestations. It can be seen in negative attitudes, stereotypes and labels about gay men and lesbians (Simon, 1998) and in discriminatory behavior, ranging from derogatory joke telling to not granting equivalent legal rights to domestic partnerships and protection

---

[1] Like the term *homophobia*, use of the terms homosexual, lesbian, transsexual, transvestite, queer, bisexual, GLB, GLBTQ, questioning, and so forth have had lengthy and often very divisive and political histories. In this entry, the terms *gay* and *lesbian* will be used to represent all sexual minority peoples. The authors recognize that these terms may not fairly represent some sexual minority peoples. Our intent is to focus on homophobia rather than on the varieties of sexual minority persons. We apologize to those who might feel marginalized by our selection of terms.

from violence and hate crimes (Elze, 1992; Ryan & Futterman, 1998). The prevalence of negative attitudes toward gay men and lesbians has been documented in numerous investigations. These attitudes have been generally analogous in samples from the United States (Herek, 1984, 2000), Canada (Minton, 1997), Brazil (Proulx, 1997), Israel (Ben-Ari, 1998), and Argentina (Vujosevich, Pecheny, & Kornblit, 1997). Homophobic attitudes are especially common in high schools (Smith & Smith, 1998; Walters & Hayes, 1998).

The prevalence of homophobic behavior has been widely reported. Negative reactions directed toward sexual minority adults are among the most frequent motivations behind bias-related violence in society (Comstock, 1991; Hershberger & D'Augelli, 1995). Reactions toward gay and lesbian adolescents are less well-documented but have been reported to be very high, with 50 percent of gay youths in some samples reporting verbal assault (Remafedi, 1987a) and over 40 percent reporting physical attacks during the high school years (Hunter, 1990; Remafedi, Farrow & Deisher, 1991). Some authors have argued that violence and hate crimes are probably more often directed at adolescents, compared with adult sexual minority persons, and more toward sexual minority youths who are also youths of color (Ryan & Futterman, 1998). Recently, Franklin (2000) reported that 10 percent of a large anonymous sample of *noncriminal heterosexuals* reported that they had exhibited physical violence or threats against gay and lesbian people solely because of their sexual orientation.

Hate crimes are the most violent example of homophobic reactions. In the United States, the Federal Bureau of Investigation (FBI) reported that in 1999, there were 1,303 reported hate crimes against sexual minorities, or about 16 percent of all hate crimes reported for that year. Since the FBI believes that two third of all hate crimes go unreported, there are an estimated 4,000 hate crimes against sexual minority persons in the United States each year (Federal Bureau of Investigation, 2000). The Canadian Department of Justice, while reporting difficulty in defining "hate crimes," has indicated that about 11 percent of all Canadian bias crimes are committed against sexual minorities (Duncanson, 1998). Australian hate crime reports are not separated out from other crimes, but in New South Wales, homicides involving gay men have been tracked since 1989. Within a 10-year span, four men per year were murdered because they were gay (Mouzous & Thompson, 2000).

However, not all societies and cultures are homophobic. Williams (1992) describes the Navajo and Polynesian cultures where sexual minority persons are honored and homophobic reactions are comparatively absent. In these societies, numerous benefits of non-homophobic reactions are described, including better quality friendships, more harmonious societies, and stronger supports for child rearing.

Not all victims of homophobic reactions are sexual minority persons. Many heterosexuals are also victimized by these reactions simply because they are perceived as gay, lesbian or as being "gay-friendly" (Thompson, 1992).

THEORIES

There are theories on two basic types of homophobia: externalized and internalized. *Externalized homophobia* is what most think of as homophobia—the negative views, reactions, and behaviors directed by members of society at gay men and lesbians. Some have argued that this type of homophobia is parallel to negative reactions toward other minorities, such as racial groups and women and can be explained in similar ways. Sociocultural views stress the nature, content and operation of stereotypes and how they become reflected in behavior. Motivational theories argue that homophobic reactions provide sources of strength for the actor's personal identity, including intolerant reactions and prejudice. Cognitive views argue that stereotypes provide templates that help people evaluate stimuli in a complex environment. Many religious theories view sexual minority persons as sinners in need of conversion and use negative reactions and propaganda (i.e., homophobic reactions and claims of successful reparative therapies) as methods of helping the unrepentant move toward this goal of conversion. Finally, the biological model argues that homophobia has an evolutionary purpose for heterosexuals when they negatively react to and have some impact on "defective" sexual minorities (Kantor, 1998; Kite, 1994).

Internalized homophobia includes negative reactions and behaviors directed at the self. Theories of internalized homophobia are basically of two sorts: psychodynamic and sociodevelopmental. Psychodynamic theories argue that internalized homophobia is caused by defensive reactions to reduce anxiety associated with same-sex feelings and desires. These reactions can include projection, denial, and identification with an aggressor and rationalization (Kantor, 1998; Shidlo, 1994).

The sociodevelopmental theory of internalized homophobia notes that sexual minority people "lack access to an affirmative reference group (the gay community) and to mentors and role models to help in the development of healthy sociosexual identity" (Meyer & Dean, 1998, p. 162). Youths begin to experience heightened same-sex attractions at the same time that traditional pressures are applied to adolescents to conform to heterosexual norms for dating (D'Augelli, 1998). Potential discovery by peers intensifies internalized barriers against same-sex expression and intensification of homophobic reactions, especially when lacking gay support groups. Some authors have argued that internalized homophobia is a part of the developmental history of all gay men and lesbians reared in heterosexist cultures (Shidlo, 1994).

RESEARCH

Findings from research on the impact of homophobic reactions on gay and lesbian adolescents are very disturbing. Anti-gay attacks begin early in school, often starting with verbal attacks in elementary schools (D'Augelli, 1998). By junior high and high school, attacks and verbal assaults are very frequent with 48–80 percent of adolescents reporting at least one verbal or physical assault (Gross, Aurand, & Adessa, 1988; Pilkington & D'Augelli, 1995).

Numerous investigations have linked gay adolescents' high stress levels brought on by peers' homophobic reactions to higher-risk sexual behaviors, prostitution, substance abuse, running away, and school problems (Savin-Williams, 1994). Some evidence has also linked homophobic reactions toward gay adolescents with larger numbers of suicide attempts (Rotheram-Borus, Hunter, & Rosario, 1994; Savin-Williams, 1994).

Internalized homophobia has numerous negative consequences as well, including lower self-esteem, lower social supports, weaker social networks, greater loneliness, and greater likelihood of seeking therapy (Meyer & Dean, 1998; Shidlo, 1994). Elze (1992) reports that many gay and lesbian adolescents also engage in heterosexual sex in order to "prove" that they are not gay. This further damages self-esteem and increases self-doubt about identity.

STRATEGIES THAT WORK

There are several strategies that might work in preventing homophobia. However, homophobia prevention is a relatively new area of inquiry and prevention strategies have not yet been adequately tested. Promising strategies are covered in the next section. Inquiry on the prevention of homophobia is comparable to the state of inquiry on the prevention of racism in the 1960s and 1970s. Namely, at that time, only a few strategies (including education efforts) had been put forward and none had been thoroughly tested until the late 1970s (Gorman, 1977). After 30 years of research, it is clear that at least two strategies work in the prevention and reduction of racism: reduction of social-environmental stress (Albee, 1995) and anti-racist education (Ruemper, 1996). The promising strategies for preventing homophobia described below may similarly be cited as strategies that might work sometime in the future.

STRATEGIES THAT MIGHT WORK

It is highly likely that anti-homophobia education, including gay-affirmative modules in curricula, might reduce homophobic attitudes. Targeted education for teachers and school counselors may also reduce the perception of support for students' homophobic reactions in high schools (Ryan & Futterman, 1998).

School-based programs educating students about the realities of homosexuality decrease anti-gay sentiments and actions. These programs demystify homosexuality by presenting adolescents with academic curricula and guest speakers providing views into the diverse lifestyles, personalities, backgrounds, and experiences of sexual minorities (Henning-Stout, James, & Macintosh, 2000). Such representations make it difficult to stereotype and de-humanize what is "typical" for gay and lesbian people, thus reducing irrational hatred and violence directed toward them. This education could also help gay and lesbian youth with their coming out process by providing role models from whom they can form a positive, gay identity.

School-based homophobia prevention programs can potentially reach the highest number of adolescents, since they spend much of their daily life in schools. Research on the effectiveness of these programs is sparse but consistent. For example, a study conducted by Serdahely and Ziemba (1985) compared one group of college students whose human sexuality course had a unit on homosexuality against a control group taking the same course, but with no lessons on homosexuality. Although the groups did not differ significantly before the course, the mean scores for each group differed dramatically following the class, with marked reduction in homophobia among students with the unit on homosexuality.

Blumenfeld (1993–1994) was one of the first to report on an emerging movement in high schools called Gay–Lesbian–Straight Education Networks, or GLSENs. These groups are composed of gay, lesbian, bisexual, other sexual minority, and heterosexual adolescents for the purpose of providing a welcoming school environment for students of all sexual orientations and identities. Aspects of homophobia in the school and society are identified and discussed; solutions are proposed and tried. Student victims of homophobic attacks can turn to other network peers for support. All in all, these support groups provide an environment that appears to be the antithesis of the typical, homophobic American high school.

Other educational strategies are currently being tested, including a large, national study being conducted by GLSEN, in which adolescent attitudes toward homosexuality will be measured before and after an intensive educational workshop is presented (J. Kosky, personal communication, 2001).

The impact of anti-homophobia workshops for older learners (e.g., teachers) is still uncertain, but a promising mode of prevention. Such workshops are devoted to helping learners understand the roots of sexual orientation, how to help adolescents come out, and how to resolve differences between religion and sexual orientation (Blumenfeld, 1992). While such workshops may be effective, they may also attract only those who are already inclined to be gay-affirmative.

Gay and lesbian adolescents often suffer the most from homophobia because the normal development of their same-sex expressions and identity is blunted by anti-gay victimization in high schools. D'Augelli (1998) argues that if gay and lesbian adolescents experience a gay-positive environment, their normal developmental trajectory would be supported and the consequent damage inflicted by homophobia would be reduced substantially.

This underscores the need for adolescents to have access to the larger gay community (Meyer & Dean, 1998) since this helps them redefine the (heterosexual) values they have acquired previously for intimacy, identity, and sometimes family. This is supported by evidence that young gay men have much higher levels of overall mental health when they have accepted their sexual orientation, self-identified as gay to significant others, read the local gay newspapers regularly, belonged to a gay social club, or were coupled with a life partner (Meyer & Dean, 1998).

Clearly, one of the best solutions to homophobia is replacing hatred, prejudice, and negative reactions with love, acceptance, and normalcy. Sexual minority persons have been honored in some other cultures and societies. For instance, among the Navajo people, the *Nadle* is an honored sexual minority person who receives much dignity and respect (Williams 1992). Decriminalization of homosexuality and support for equal rights for gay people in many Western countries may lead to lowered levels of homophobic attitudes and behaviors. On September 12, 2000, The Netherlands, known for being among one of the more progressive countries for equal rights for sexual minorities, passed a bill granting full marriage, divorce, and adoption rights to its gay and lesbian citizens (Dutch Legislators, 2000). Earlier that same year, the state of Vermont passed a "civil unions" bill, allowing same-sex couples to receive most of the benefits previously afforded only to heterosexual couples in that state (Vermont's House, 2000). These two landmark laws have created a foundation for further legislation to eliminate prejudice and discrimination toward sexual minorities.

A recent approach to preventing homophobia includes new guidelines from the American Psychological Association (APA) (Division 44, 2000). The APA's original guidelines in 1975 removed homosexuality from its list of mental disorders. The latest guidelines provide very clear guidance on therapy with sexual minority clients, with an emphasis on the special needs of sexual minority youths. These guidelines may make the therapeutic environment more supportive for youths, especially those struggling with internalized homophobia, as they *require* the therapist to regard sexual orientation as a normal part of the person, rather than as a dysfunction. These guidelines also lead therapists to examine how homophobia, whether their own or otherwise, affects their practice with clients.

Many parents of sexual minority adolescents react very negatively when their offspring reveal their sexual orientation (Remafedi, 1987b). Support groups, such as Parents and Friends of Lesbians and Gays (P-FLAG) show great promise of supporting parents during the coming out process; this might also reduce the frequencies with which they inflict homophobic reactions on their children (Henderson, 1998).

The impact of normalizing gay parenting is still relatively unknown with respect to homophobia. Lesbians and gay men choosing to parent may help to bring sexual minorities into the mainstream of child rearing (Raymond, 1992). In addition, one promising area of support for adolescents facing homophobia in their homes of origin is foster parents and foster homes. Specifically, Downs (1998) has reported that gay and lesbian foster parents may be very effective in providing safe homes for sexual minority youths in need of short- or long-term placements. This might prove very helpful when gay and lesbian youth face rejection from their parents when coming out.

STRATEGIES THAT DO NOT WORK

Much like the pre-civil rights movement in the United States, inaction sustains prejudice. While hate crimes statistics are now gathered, many members of western countries ask that sexual minority persons, and especially adolescents, not be given "special rights." The reality is that equal rights are not "special" rights. Such arguments foster complacency, which in turn will not reduce homophobia.

While explicitly condemned by professional associations, conversion therapies continue to be administered to sexual minority persons by "therapists" and "counselors." (Divison 44, 2000). These approaches, often offered by religious groups and the "ex-gay" movement, are designed to convert gay men and lesbians into heterosexuals, or at least non-practicing homosexuals (Khan, 2000). These approaches not only increase homophobia within the culture, but also inflict serious psychological damage, including shame and guilt often leading to suicidal ideation, on the people going through these "therapies" (Shidlo, 1994).

SYNTHESIS

One primary goal provides a common thread connecting all of these prevention strategies: to educate people about homosexuality in order to replace stereotypical, homophobic views of gay and lesbian people with more accurate, complex models of what it means to be a sexual minority in a heterosexist society. Through early child education, homophobic beliefs and actions must be characterized as unacceptable, much like the current intolerance shown for racism and sexism. Without these social lessons, children will be brought up to believe that intolerance toward sexual minorities is acceptable. If we are to continue progressing toward a more just society, we cannot afford the fostering of ignorance toward any group on any level.

The field of homophobia prevention is comparatively new, especially with respect to the impact on adolescents. Much can be learned from racism prevention (Albee, 1995; Ruemper, 1996) and the impact of racism on adolescents of color.

An especially important area of inquiry is the impact of educational efforts that span sexual orientations, such as GLSEN. This effort includes gay, straight, lesbian, bisexual and transgender adolescents in a united effort to combat homophobia in all environments frequented by adolescents, especially high schools. Other educational efforts, sponsored and woven into the educational mainstream require examination as well. For instance, antiracist education, when built into the school curricula, has a large role in combating adolescent racism (Ng, Staton, & Scane, 1995).

Other educational arenas need research attention as well. For instance, the study of anti-homophobia education on older adults, including counselors, teachers, coaches, and mentors is urgently needed.

The impact of APA's recent guidelines on psychotherapy with gay and lesbian clients is a promising area of research inquiry. There are few indicators of the percentages of counselors and therapists who continue to foster homophobic reactions in their adolescent clients and within themselves as part of their work. APA believes these reactions are harmful, especially to adolescents who are forming identities. Research in this area is essential.

As in the arena of the impact of racism on youths of color, homophobia clearly takes a toll on gay and lesbian youth. Researchers should focus on the impact of moderating homophobic environments on subsequent adolescent self-esteem and developmental functioning.

Formal research on the role of support groups, such as P-FLAG, is also greatly needed. These groups seem to play a vital role for parents of gay and lesbian youths. It would be very interesting to assess the influence of these support groups on parental behaviors and attitudes toward their offspring.

Finally, the area of out-of-home care, including foster homes, for gay and lesbian adolescents who have been displaced because of the homophobic reactions of their parents is a promising area of inquiry.

Also see: Homophobia: Adulthood; Sexual Assault: Adolescence; Sexuality: Adolescence.

References

Albee, G.W. (1995). Counseling and primary prevention. *Counseling Psychology Quarterly, 8*(3), 205–211.

Ben-Ari, A.T. (1998). An experiential attitude change: Social work students and homosexuality. *Journal of Homosexuality, 36*(2), 59–72.

Blumenfeld, W.J. (1992). Conducting antiheterosexism workshops: A sample. In W.J. Blumenfeld (Ed.), *Homophobia: How we all pay the price*, (pp. 275–302). Boston: Beacon Press.

Blumenfeld, W.J. (1993–1994). "Gay/straight" alliances: Transforming pain to pride. *High School Journal, 77*(1–2), 113–121.

Boswell, J. (1980). *Christianity, social tolerance, and homosexuality: Gay people in Western Europe from the beginning of the Christian era to the Fourteenth century*. Chicago: University of Chicago Press.

Comstock, G.D. (1991). *Violence against lesbians and gay men*. New York: Columbia University Press.

D'Augelli, A.R. (1998). Developmental implications of victimization of lesbian, gay, and bisexual youths. In G.M. Herek (Ed.), *Stigma and sexual orientation: Understanding prejudice against lesbians, gay men, and bisexuals* (pp. 187–210). Thousand Oaks, CA: Sage.

Division 44. (2000). Guidelines for psychotherapy with lesbian, gay, and bisexual clients. *American Psychologist, 55*(12), 1440–1451.

Downs, A.C. (1998, August). *Gay and lesbian foster parents*. Paper presented at the American Psychological Association, San Francisco. Available E-mail: cdowns@casey.org

Downs, A.C., & Hillje, L.S. (1993). Historical and theoretical perspectives on adolescent sexuality: An overview. In T.P. Gullotta, G.R. Adams, & R. Montemayor (Eds.), *Adolescent Sexuality* (pp. 1–33). Newbury Park: Sage.

Duncanson, J. (1998, September 22). Hate crimes reported up. *Toronto Star*, p. A1.

Dutch legislators approve full marriage rights for gays. (2000, September 13). *New York Times*, p. A4.

Elze, D. (1992). "It has nothing to do with me." In W.J. Blumenfeld (Ed.), *Homophobia: How we all pay the price* (pp. 95–113). Boston: Beacon Press.

Evans, A. (2000). The logic of homophobia. *Gay & Lesbian Review, 7*(3), 19–23.

Federal Bureau of Investigation. (2000). *Crime in the United States* (FBI Publication No. 0-16-048756-0). Washington, DC: US Department of Justice Printing Office.

Franklin, K. (2000). Antigay behaviors among young adults. *Journal of Interpersonal Violence, 15*(4), 339–353.

Gorman, L. (1977). A White nursing faculty member's experiences in training anti-racism content to masters students in nursing. *Journal of Contemporary Psychotherapy, 9*(1), 21–23.

Gross, L., Aurand, S.K., & Adessa, R. (1988). *Violence and discrimination against lesbian and gay people in Philadelphia and the Commonwealth of Pennsylvania*. Philadelphia: Philadelphia Lesbian and Gay Task Force.

Henderson, M.G. (1998). Disclosure of sexual orientation: Comments from a parental perspective. *American Journal of Orthopsychiatry, 68*(3), 372–375.

Henning-Stout, M., James, S., & Macintosh, S. (2000). Reducing harassment of lesbian, gay, bisexual, transgender, and questioning youth in school. *School Psychology Review, 29*(2), 180–192.

Herek, G.M. (1984). Beyond "homophobia": A social psychological perspective on attitudes toward lesbians and gay men. In J.P. DeCecco (Ed.), *Bashers, baiters & bigots: Homophobia in American society* (pp. 1–21). New York: Harrington Park Press.

Herek, G.M. (2000). The psychology of sexual prejudice. *Current Directions in Psychological Science, 9*(1), 19–22.

Hershberger, S.L., & D'Augelli, A.R. (1995). The impact of victimization on the mental health and suicidality of lesbian, gay, and bisexual youths. *Developmental Psychology, 31*(1), 65–74.

Hunter, J. (1990). Violence against lesbian and gay male youths. *Journal of Interpersonal Violence, 5*, 295–300.

Kantor, M. (1998). *Homophobia: Description, development, and dynamics of gay bashing.* Westport, CT: Praeger.

Khan, S. (2000). The "ex-gays": Anatomy of a fraud. *Gay & Lesbian Review, 7*(3), 29–33.

Kite, M.E. (1994). When perceptions meet reality: Individual differences in reactions to lesbians and gay men. In B. Greene & G.M. Herek (Eds.), *Lesbian and gay psychology: Theory, research and clinical applications* (pp. 25–53). Thousand Oaks, CA: Sage.

MacDonald, A.P. (1976). Homophobia: Its roots and meanings. *Homosexual Counseling Journal, 3*(1), 23–33.

Meyer, I.H., & Dean, L. (1998). Internalized homophobia, intimacy, and sexual behavior among gay and bisexual men. In G.M. Herek (Ed.), *Stigma and sexual orientation: Understanding prejudice against lesbians, gay men, and bisexuals* (pp. 160–186). Thousand Oaks, CA: Sage.

Minton, H.L. (1997). Queer theory: Historical roots and implications for psychology. *Theory & Psychology, 7*(3), 337–353.

Mouzous, J., & Thompson, S. (2000). *Gay-hate related homicides: An overview of major findings in New South Wales.* Canberra: Australian Institute of Criminology.

Ng, R., Staton, P., & Scane, J. (1995). *Anti-Racism, feminism, and critical approaches to education.* Chicago: Greenwood Publishing Group.

Pilkington, N.W., & D'Augelli, A.R. (1995). Victimization of lesbian, gay, and bisexual youth in community settings. *Journal of Community Psychology, 23*, 33–56.

Proulx, R. (1997). Homophobia in northeastern Brazilian university students. *Journal of Homosexuality, 34*(1), 47–56.

Raymond, D. (1992). "In the best interests of the child": Thoughts on homophobia and parenting. In W.J. Blumenfeld (Ed.), *Homophobia: How we all pay the price* (pp. 114–130). Boston: Beacon Press.

Remafedi, G. (1987a). Male homosexuality: The adolescent's perspective. *Pediatrics, 79*, 326–330.

Remafedi, G. (1987b). Homosexual youth: A challenge to contemporary society. *Journal of the American Medical Association, 258*, 222–225.

Remafedi, G., Farrow, J.A., & Deisher, R.W. (1991). Risk factors for attempted suicide in gay and bisexual youth. *Pediatrics, 87*, 869–875.

Rotheram-Borus, M.J., Hunter, J., & Rosario, M. (1994). Suicidal behavior and gay-related stress among gay and bisexual male adolescents. *Journal of Adolescent Research, 9*, 498–508.

Ruemper, W. (1996). Models for change: Antiracist education for universities and colleges. *Canadian Review of Sociology & Anthropology, 33*(3), 317–335.

Ryan, C., & Futterman, D. (1998). *Lesbian & gay youth: Care & counseling.* New York: Columbia University Press.

Savin-Williams, R.C. (1994). Verbal and physical abuse as stressors in the lives of lesbian, gay male, and bisexual youths: Associations with school problems, running away, substance abuse, prostitution, and suicide. *Journal of Consulting and Clinical Psychology, 62*, 261–269.

Serdahely, W.J., & Ziemba, G.J. (1985). Changing homophobic attitudes through college sexuality education. In J.P. DeCecco (Ed.), *Bashers, baiters & bigots: Homophobia in American society* (pp. 109–116). New York: Harrington Park Press.

Shidlo, A. (1994). Internalized homophobia: Conceptual and empirical issues in measurement. In B. Greene & G.M. Herek (Eds.), *Lesbian and gay psychology: Theory, research and clinical applications* (pp. 176–205). Thousand Oaks, CA: Sage.

Simon, A. (1998). The relationship between stereotypes of and attitudes toward lesbians and gays. In G.M. Herek (Ed.), *Stigma and sexual orientation* (pp. 62–81). Thousand Oaks, CA: Sage.

Smith, G.W., & Smith, D.E. (1998). The ideology of "fag": The school experience of gay students. *Sociological Quarterly, 39*(2), 309–336.

Thompson, C. (1992). On being heterosexual in a homophobic world. In W.J. Blumenfeld (Ed.), *Homophobia: How we all pay the price*, (pp. 235–248). Boston: Beacon Press.

Vermont's house backs wide rights for gay couples. (2000, March 17). *New York Times*, p. A1.

Vujosevich, J., Pecheny, M., & Kornblit, A.L. (1997). La homofobia en Buenos Aires/Homophobia in Buenos Aires. *Acta Psiquiatrica y Psicologica de America Latina, 43*(3), 212–221.

Walters, A.S., & Hayes, D.M. (1998). Homophobia within schools: Challenging the culturally sanctioned dismissal of gay students and colleagues. *Journal of Homosexuality, 35*(2), 1–23.

Weinberg, G.H. (1972). *Society and the healthy homosexual.* New York: St. Martin's.

Williams, W.L. (1992). Benefits for nonhomophobic societies: An anthropological perspective. In W.J. Blumenfeld (Ed.), *Homophobia: How we all pay the price* (pp. 258–274). Boston: Beacon Press.

Homophobia, Adulthood

Carlton W. Parks

INTRODUCTION

This entry focuses on the prevention of homophobia and sexual prejudice in adulthood. This task is accomplished through an examination of the empirical literature focusing on homophobia/sexual prejudice to ascertain which strategies work and do not work in the reduction of sexual prejudice toward gay men, lesbians, bisexuals, and transgenders. The following three contexts are utilized to facilitate this exploration: (1) sexual prejudice in the workplace, (2) AIDS stigma and discrimination, and (3) sexual prejudice and hate crime victimization.

DEFINITIONS

The term *homophobia*, coined by Weinberg (1972), has been used extensively in the social science literature, since the 1960s, to refer to individual anti-gay attitudes and behaviors (Herek, 2000, p. 19). In contrast, the term *heterosexism* refers to a societal ideological system that denies, denigrates, and stigmatizes any attitudes, behaviors, identity, and community that is non-heterosexual (Herek, 1992a, p. 150). This ideological system fosters prejudicial and discriminatory societal customs and institutions (i.e., cultural heterosexism) as well as individual attitudes and behaviors (i.e., psychological heterosexism) (Herek, 1992a). *Biphobia* is the fear or dislike of people who do not identify or behave as either gay, lesbian, or heterosexual (Hutchins & Kaahumanu, 1991). *Discrimination* is any behavior directed against persons because of their membership in a particular group (Brehm & Kassin, 1996, p. 121).

In response to researchers (e.g., Fyfe, 1983) who challenged the notion that homophobia is an irrational fear of homosexuals and an indicator of individual psychopathology, Herek (2000) coined the term *sexual prejudice* which refers to negative attitudes toward an individual when the target is gay, bisexual, or straight (p. 19). Herek (2000) makes no assumptions about the motivations underlying these negative attitudes and utilizes the social psychological literature on prejudice as the theoretical framework.

Internalized homophobia refers to negative social attitudes concerning gays, lesbians, and bisexuals that are turned inward leading to a devaluation of the self, resulting in internal conflicts, low self-esteem, and is a major component of minority stress for gay men, lesbians, bisexuals, and transgenders. From a global perspective, it is imperative for the reader to comprehend the ethnocentric nature of these terms which are used routinely in the United States. These terms may or may not have any relevance in their ability to accurately reflect the phenomenological experiences of homosexuals, bisexuals, and transgenders (Lumsden, 1996) living in other cultures. For instance, sexual orientation identity in other cultures may be viewed as distinct points along a continuum ("two-spirited people" among Native Americans [Tafoya, 1997]) instead of as a dichotomous variable (i.e., straight vs. gay) (Lumsden, 1996).

SCOPE

The first nationwide survey documenting on anti-gay violence was performed by the National Gay and Lesbian Task Force and sampled 1,420 gay men and 654 lesbians ($n = 2,074$) in eight US cities: Boston, New York, Atlanta, St. Louis, Denver, Dallas, Los Angeles, and Seattle. Nineteen percent reported having been punched, hit, kicked or beaten once in their lives because of their sexual orientation, and 44 percent had been threatened with physical violence. Ninety-four percent reported experiencing some type of victimization (e.g., verbal abuse, physical assault, police harassment), and 84 percent knew other gay or lesbian individuals who had been victimized because of their sexual orientation (National Gay & Lesbian Task Force [NGLTF], 1984).

Most adults in the United States perceived homosexual behavior, in a national telephone survey, as being "wrong" (69.8 percent) and "unnatural" (86.4 percent) (Herek & Capitanio, 1996). Fifty-six percent of the General Social Survey respondents in 1996 regarded homosexuality as "always wrong" (Yang, 1997). Participants responding to the ongoing American National Election Studies rated lesbians and gay men among the lowest of all groups along a 101-point feeling thermometer (Yang, 1997).

Most Americans believe that a gay person should not be denied employment or basic civil liberties (Yang, 1997). However, it is still widely believed that same-sex domestic partners should not be allowed to legally marry or adopt children (Yang, 1997). Interestingly, most Americans in national samples of voters, believe that gays should be allowed to enroll in the military forces (61 percent vs. 31 percent opposed) (Strand, 1998).

Twenty percent of Euro-American lesbians and 33 percent of African American same-gender loving women reported "some guilt" over their sexual activities which are considered to be indicators of the prevalence of internalized homophobia (Shildo, 1994). Chan (1995) has documented the reality that ethnic minority communities (e.g., Asian American/Pacific Islander communities) perceive homosexuality as being a Euro-American Western phenomenon which results in increased reluctance on the part of same-gender loving Asian Americans/Pacific Islanders from "coming out" for fear of possible expulsion from their extended family and their community. The social climate around the world with respect to homophobia ranges from the Netherlands, Denmark, and Sweden, where there is tolerance or indifference to China, Scotland, Russia, and Egypt, where there is repression and open hostility (Buston & Hart, 2001; Chan, 1995).

THEORIES AND RESEARCH

Negative stereotypes about minority groups can be created as the expression of social norms embedded within the social environment and fostered through socialization and peer conformity influences (Duckitt, 1992). Some stereotypes are specific to a particular out-group (e.g., gender-role non-conformity) or reflect cultural ideologies about outsiders (e.g., outsiders perceived as being either threatening and/or inferior to members of the dominant group) (Morales, 1996). These stereotypes develop in an attempt of individuals to integrate varied incoming stimuli in such a manner as to perceive the world as being reasonably stable, predictable, and manageable. One strategy to accomplish this objective in *cognitive theory* is *categorization* wherein one attempts to mentally group different objects (including people according to some common characteristic). A *stereotype* typically represents the inappropriate application of the categorization process to a social group. Hayes and Gelso's (1993) examination of male counselors' reactions to gay male and HIV-infected clients revealed that the counselors' homophobia predicted their discomfort with gay male clients. Counselors experienced greater discomfort with HIV-infected clients than with HIV-negative clients. Similarly, in a sample of Ghanians and Canadians, religious fundamentalism, and right-wing authoritarianism were associated with negative attitudes toward homosexuals with religious fundamentalism being the best predictor of homophobia. Attendance in male-only schools was associated with elevated levels of homophobia. This effect remained significant even when the effects of religious fundamentalism were controlled (Hunsberger, Owusu, & Duck, 1999). These findings support this perspective.

The functional approach to homophobia/sexual prejudice is also grounded within *social psychological theory* (Katz, 1960), and suggests that different individuals can express similar attitudes for entirely different reasons. It is believed that a person's attitudes toward distinct objects can serve different functions. Thus, these attitudes assist individuals in meeting their psychological needs (Katz, 1960). Three major needs appear to be operative when individuals express attitudes toward lesbians and gay men.

First, experiential attitudes categorize social reality on the basis of one's past interactions with homosexual persons. For instance, Herek and Capitanio (1996) revealed that interpersonal contact with lesbians and gay men was reported in a national AIDS telephone survey when the respondents were highly educated, politically liberal, young, and female. Interpersonal contact was associated with positive attitudes toward gay men. Heterosexuals' attitudes were more favorable to the extent that they reported more relationships, closer relationships, and receiving direct disclosure about another's homosexuality.

Second, defensive attitudes help an individual cope with some internal conflict or anxiety by projecting it onto gay men and lesbians. For instance, Adams, Wright, and Lohr (1996) investigated the role of homosexual arousal in exclusively heterosexual men who admitted negative affect toward homosexuals. Homophobic ($n = 35$) and non-homophobic men ($n = 29$) were exposed to sexually explicit erotic stimuli consisting of heterosexual, male homosexual, and lesbian videotapes, and only the homophobic men showed an increase in penile erection when viewing gay male stimuli, as assessed by penile plethysmography, while both homophobic and non-homophobic men exhibited increases in penile circumference to heterosexual and lesbian videos.

Third, symbolic attitudes express abstract ideological concepts that are closely linked to one's own notion of self and to one's social networks and reference groups. Survey findings revealed that individuals with elevated levels of sexual prejudice tend to be older, less educated, live in the South, Midwestern or rural regions of the United States, be traditionally masculine heterosexual males, members of a fundamental religious denomination, and have elevated scores on measures of authoritarianism and conservatism (Herek, 1984).

Gagnon and Simon (1973) have developed *social script theory* that proposes a sociological perspective to explain psychosexual development. The role of society and culture in the expression of the psychosexual development is highlighted in this theory. It presumes that most behavior is heavily influenced by social scripts or previous learning concerning the expectations of what is appropriate behavior and what is not. Sexual scripts dictate the "who, what, when, where, and why" of individual sexual behavior as well as the meaning attached to it. These scripts are heavily influenced by interpersonal interactions that tap psychological, social, and cultural influences that vary from culture to culture. The survey research of Liu, Ng, Zhou, and Haeberle (1997) focusing on sexuality within China supports this perspective.

STRATEGIES: OVERVIEW

This discussion will be restricted to the following three topics: (1) sexual prejudice within the workplace, (2) sexual prejudice and AIDS stigma, and (3) sexual prejudice and hate crime victimization.

STRATEGIES THAT WORK

Presently, there is not sufficient evidence to identify strategies that work.

STRATEGIES THAT MIGHT WORK

The creation of an environment tolerant and respectful of racial, ethnic, and cultural differences on multiple levels by individuals in leadership positions results in a more creative and productive setting (Winfeld & Spielman, 1995). Culturally informed prevention programs designed specifically for ethnic and culturally diverse populations are more effective than generic prevention programs. Winfeld and Spielman (1995) have proposed four strategies for a more culturally tolerant environment, based on their experiences as workplace diversity consultants: (1) nondiscrimination policies that are developed by the Human Resources Department, adhered to and taken seriously by all levels of the organizational structure, (2) educational programs that increase the knowledge base of the population, in question, about sexual orientation identity, both in small and large groups, in community groups as well as in one-to-one interactions. The importance of modifying the use of heterosexist language cannot be overemphasized when developing psychoeducational interventions for the workplace, (3) equitable benefits (e.g., domestic partner benefits) for all employees or independent of their sexual orientation identity, and (4) HIV/AIDS and other sexually transmitted diseases' psychoeducational interventions designed to dispel preexisting myths and stereotypes.

Friskopp and Silverstein (1995) have revealed that interpersonal contact between heterosexuals and sexual minorities is a critical feature for the creation of a culturally inclusive environment. Herek (1992b) has documented the same strategy to reduce the levels of anti-gay violence within the community. Formal and informal social interactions over a sustained period of time between heterosexuals and gay-identified men, lesbians, bisexuals, and transgenders provide opportunities for everyone involved to dispel preexisting negative stereotypes for both participants within a dyadic interaction. This strategy often results in the formation of friendship bonds, particularly in instances where they can collaborate on some cooperative venture (Friskopp & Silverstein, 1995). It will be easier to have an impact upon negative stereotypes related to lesbians as compared to gay male and bisexual men, and/or transgenders (Friskopp & Silverstein, 1995; Herek, 1992b).

Generic psychoeducational interventions over time with no interpersonal contact between heterosexuals, bisexual, and transgenders may work especially when moral and/or religious values are used as the foundation for attitude change (e.g., Wetherford & Wetherford, 1999). Concerted attempts should be made not to duplicate existing prevention education programs in the community, and they should highlight statistics, dispel myths and stereotypes, and address the real fears individuals may have while honestly addressing taboo issues (e.g., drugs, homophobia, racism, sexism, heterosexual AIDS transmission, hate crime incidents, sexual and police harassment). Personal testimonies are frequently quite effective, and connect well with the audience while affirming the ability of individuals to make wise choices (Herek, 1992b; Wetherford & Wetherford, 1999).

The reality of closeted versus "out" gay and lesbian professionals in the workplace is becoming a phenomena that is confronting the workplace environment in the 21st century (Friskopp & Silverstein, 1995). Interestingly, Friskopp and Silverstein (1995) revealed that the ethnic minority same-gender loving men who were "out" at work (in corporate settings) perceived little or no discrimination based on their race or sexual orientation identity. "Out" gay and lesbian professionals can have a significant impact on the workplace environment (e.g., "out" gay and lesbian law clerks working with the Supreme Court Justices) (Murdoch & Price, 2001).

There is a pressing need for prevention researchers to broaden their conceptualization of "at risk" groups. For instance, there exists a need to develop culturally informed prevention programs for HIV positive men within our urban communities to reduce the spread of HIV (Gomez & Shriver, 2001). Upon first glance, this "at risk" group may not appear to be in need of prevention services but that would be far from accurate. Ratti, Bakeman, and Peterson (2000) have revealed that Canadian men, South Asian men, and European men who have sex with other men who reported elevated levels of internalized homophobia were more likely to engage in both high-risk anal and oral sex placing them at risk for becoming HIV positive. Ratti et al. (2000) revealed that South Asian men, as a group, were likely to exhibit elevated levels of internalized homophobia. When these men were less acculturated to the US culture, they were more likely to engage in anal and oral sex once again placing them at risk for becoming HIV positive. Thus, subgroups of same-gender loving ethnically and culturally diverse HIV positive men are in dire need of HIV prevention services that are tailored specifically to their respective subgroups.

STRATEGIES THAT DO NOT WORK

Primary prevention programs that do not address how issues related to self-labeling and sexual orientation identity status dramatically affect our ability to educate diverse populations are doomed to failure. Potential clients may simply ignore the message because they do not perceive themselves as being a "member" of that "at risk" group (Diaz, 1997; Morales, 1996).

Work environments that condone and reinforce instances of harassment, jokes, ridicule, and assaultive behaviors while paying lipservice to a written nondiscrimination policy are not likely to benefit from the creation of a primary prevention program to eradicate discriminatory behavior. The workplace employees will take their lead from how they interpret and process the verbal, non-verbal, and behavioral responses of their administrative leadership with respect to this topic.

SYNTHESIS

For prevention programs to be effective, one needs to conceptualize the implementation of such programs from a macro perspective. The interventions need to eventually incorporate the: (1) individuals, families, peers, (2) racial, ethnic, and cultural groups, (3) institutional structures, (4) neighborhoods, (5) city and state, (6) geographic region, as well as (7) national and international arenas. Care needs to be taken to incorporate the relevant constituency groups into the implementation design of any primary prevention program. Total reliance on a micro perspective (e.g., individual) when developing a primary prevention program will result in a reduced likelihood of producing desired attitudinal and/or behavioral changes.

Sexual prejudice can be prevented through the use of culturally informed programs that exist over a sustained period of time. A critical feature of these programs should be some form of sustained interpersonal contact with the minority population that has been stigmatized, marginalized, and oppressed. The integration of both cognitive and affective dimensions is key to inducing both attitudinal and behavioral change. Having individuals engage in some task that requires cooperative behavior over time is the best way to produce the desired effect. The existence of support groups (e.g., Parents and Friends of Lesbians and Gays [P-FLAG]) can assist in providing sustained interpersonal contact between homophobic individuals and parents and family members of lesbians, gay men, bisexuals, and transgenders that may lead to reductions in elevated levels of homophobia/sexual prejudice.

It is highly unlikely that sporadic educational programs will serve as a catalyst for the sustained reduction in the levels of homophobia. There exists considerable research data that questions the viability of isolated educational programs of short duration and intensity in reducing elevated levels of homophobia/sexual prejudice. Concerted efforts at modifying existing discrimination laws provide those committed citizens and lawmakers opportunities for exposure to gay men, lesbians, bisexuals, and transgenders that may lead to reduced sexual prejudice. The global AIDS epidemic is an arena for the exploration of one's cognitive distortions, dysfunctional attitudes, and beliefs where HIV and homosexuality are intertwined. Individuals grappling with such distortions can utilize interpersonal contact with HIV positive gay or bisexual or transgender individuals as a strategy to successfully eradicate their preexisting homophobic belief systems.

More systematic attention by social scientists to document the phenomenological experiences of "at risk" groups with their multiple identities resulting in multiple oppressions has the potential of yielding more culturally sensitive primary prevention programs in the 21st century within our global community.

Also see: Homophobia: Adolescence; Sexual Harassment: Adulthood; Sexuality: Adolescence; Sexuality: Older Adulthood; Intimate Partner Violence: Adulthood.

ACKNOWLEDGMENTS

The author would like to gratefully acknowledge the assistance of Gregory M. Herek, PhD, Research Professor in the Department of Psychology at the University of California at Davis, in the development of this entry.

References

Adams, H.E., Wright Jr., L.W., & Lohr, B.A. (1996). Is homophobia associated with homosexual arousal? *Journal of Abnormal Psychology, 105*(3), 440–445.

Brehm, S.S., & Kassin, S.M. (1996). *Social psychology* (3rd edn). Boston, MA: Houghton Mifflin Company.

Buston, K., & Hart, G. (2001). Heterosexism and homophobia in Scottish school sex education: Exploring the nature of the problem. *Journal of Adolescence, 24*(1), 95–109.

Chan, C.S. (1995). Issues of sexual identity in an ethnic minority: The case of Chinese American lesbians, gay men, and bisexual people. In A.R.D'Augelli & C.J. Patterson (Eds.), *Lesbian, gay, and bisexual identities over the lifespan: Psychological perspectives* (pp. 87–101). New York, NY: Oxford University Press.

Diaz, R.M. (1997). *Latino gay men and HIV: Culture, sexuality, and risk behavior.* New York, NY: Routledge.

Duckitt, J. (1992). Psychology and prejudice: A historical analysis and integrative framework. *American Psychologist, 47*(10), 1182–1193.

Friskopp, A., & Silverstein, S. (1995). *Straight jobs, gay lives: Gay and lesbian professionals, the Harvard Business School and the American workplace.* New York, NY: Simon and Schuster.

Fyfe, B. (1983). "Homophobia" or homosexual bias reconsidered. *Archives of Sexual Behavior, 12*, 549–554.

Gagnon, J.H., & Simon, W. (1973). *Sexual conduct: The social origins of human sexuality.* Chicago, ILl: Aldine.

Gomez, C.A., & Shriver, M. (2001, April). *The prevention for positive movement and initiatives.* Presented at the First Annual University of California at San Francisco's Center for AIDS Prevention Studies (CAPS) AIDS Research Institute's Conference: Renewing HIV Prevention, San Francisco, California.

Hayes, J.A., & Gelso, C.J. (1993). Male counselors' discomfort with gay and HIV-infected clients. *Journal of Counseling Psychology, 40*(1), 86–93.

Herek, G.M. (1984). Beyond "Homophobia": A social psychological perspective on attitudes toward lesbians and gay men. In J.P. DeCecco (Ed.), *Homophobia: An overview* (pp. 1–21). New York, NY: Haworth Press.

Herek, G.M. (1992a). Psychological heterosexism and anti-gay violence: The social psychology of bigotry and bashing. In G.M. Herek & K.T. Berrill (Eds.), *Hate crimes: Confronting violence against lesbians and gay men* (pp. 149–169). Newbury Park, CA: Sage.

Herek, G.M. (1992b). The community response to violence in San Francisco: An interview with Wendy Kusuma, Lester Olmstead-Rose, and Jill Tregor. In G.M. Herek & K.T. Berrill (Eds.), *Hate crimes: Confronting violence against lesbians and gay men* (pp. 241–258). Newbury Park, CA: Sage.

Herek, G.M. (2000). The psychology of sexual prejudice. *Current Directions in Psychological Science, 9*(1), 19–22.

Herek, G.M., & Capitanio, J. (1996). "Some of my best friends": Intergroup contact, concealable stigma, and heterosexuals' attitudes toward gay men and lesbians. *Personality and Social Psychology Bulletin, 22*(4), 412–424.

Hunsberger, B., Owusu, V., & Duck, R. (1999). Religion and prejudice in Ghana and Canada: Religious fundamentalism, right-wing authoritarianism, and attitudes toward homosexuals and women. *International Journal for the Psychology of Religion, 9*(3), 181–194.

Hutchins, L., & Kaahumanu, L. (Ed.). (1991). *Bi any other name: Bisexual people speak out.* Boston, MA: Alyson.

Katz, D. (1960). The functional approach to the study of attitudes. *Public Opinion Quarterly, 24,* 163–204.

Liu, D., Ng, M.L., Zhou, L.P., & Haeberle, E.J. (1997). *Sexual behavior in modern China: Report on the nationwide survey of 20,000 men and women.* Herndon, VA: Cassell & Continuum.

Lumsden, I. (1996). Institutionalized homophobia. In I. Lumsden (Ed.), *Machos, maricones, and gays: Cuba and homosexuality* (pp. 55–80). Philadelphia, PA: Temple University Press.

Morales, E. (1996). Gender roles among Latino gay and bisexual men: Implications for family and couple relationships. In J. Laird & R. Jay-Green (Eds.), *Lesbians and gays in couples and families* (pp. 272–297). San Francisco, CA: Jossey-Bass.

Murdoch, J., & Price, D. (2001). *Courting justice: Gay men and lesbians v. The Supreme Court.* New York, NY: Basic Books.

National Gay & Lesbian Task Force (NGLTF). (1984). *Anti-gay/lesbian victimization: A study by the National Gay Task Force in cooperation with gay and lesbian organizations in eight US cities.* Washington, DC: Author.

Ratti, R., Bakeman, R., & Peterson, J.L. (2000). Correlates of high-risk sexual behavior among Canadian men of South Asian and European origin who have sex with men. *AIDS Care, 12*(2), 193–202.

Shidlo, A. (1994). Internalized homophobia: Conceptual and empirical issues in measurement. In B. Greene & G.M. Herek (Eds.), *Lesbian and gay psychology: Theory, research and clinical applications* (pp. 176–205). Thousand Oaks, CA: Sage.

Strand, D.A. (1998). Civil liberties, civil rights, and stigma: Voter attitudes and behavior in the politics of homosexuality. In G.M. Herek (Ed.), *Stigma and sexual orientation: Understanding prejudice against lesbians, gay men, and bisexuals* (pp. 108–137). Thousand Oaks, CA: Sage.

Tafoya, T. (1997). Native gay and lesbian issues: The two-spirited. In B. Greene (Ed.), *Ethnic and cultural diversity among lesbians and gay men* (pp. 1–10). Thousand Oaks, CA: Sage.

Weinberg, G. (1972). *Society and the healthy homosexual.* New York, NY: St. Martin's.

Wetherford, R.J., & Wetherford, C.B. (1999). *Somebody's knocking at your door: AIDS and the African-American church.* New York, NY: Haworth Press.

Winfeld, L., & Spielman, S. (1995). *Straight talk about gays in the workplace: Creating an inclusive, productive environment for everyone in your organization.* New York, NY: American Management Association.

Yang, A. (1997). Trends: Attitudes toward homosexuality. *Public Opinion Quarterly, 61,* 477–507.

Housing, Older Adulthood

Nancy W. Sheehan

INTRODUCTION

While the link between housing and health promotion is often ignored, seniors housing offers the potential for creating environments that promote "healthy aging" (MacDonald, Remus, & Laing, 1994; Minkler, Schauffler, & Clements-Nolle, 2000). This entry begins with an overview of the seniors housing industry and the health needs of elderly residents. Next, the value of ecological aging theories for implementing health promotion and disease prevention (HPDP) programs is discussed. Following this introduction, current HPDP strategies are analyzed with recommendations for an overall effective strategy for use in seniors housing.

DEFINITIONS

Seniors housing is a term that refers to any planned residential setting primarily serving older adults. It includes low-income subsidized housing, affluent retirement communities, congregate housing, continuing care retirement communities (CCRCs), and residential care facilities (RCFs). Most often, these housing options are viewed as representing a "continuum" from independent to dependent care facilities. Understanding the differences among these options and the residents they serve is vital for planning successful HPDP initiatives. The following definitions capture the unique features of each housing type.

Subsidized senior housing provides affordable housing for low- or moderate-income elders. Subsidized by either the federal or state government, it provides independent living units to eligible elders. Originally designed to ensure access to affordable housing, there were no provisions for addressing supportive service needs.

Congregate housing combines housing and limited support services for elders who have some difficulty carrying out daily activities. Residents live in individual apartments and receive a core set of services, including at least one meal a day, housekeeping, transportation, and 24-hr emergency response.

Continuing Care Retirement Communities (CCRCs) are residential communities offering a continuum of shelter and care accommodations within the same facility. Levels range from independent apartment units to skilled nursing home beds. While contractual arrangements vary among different types of CCRCs (comprehensive, modified, and fee for service), this multilevel residential approach offers long-term security to relatively affluent elders.

Residential Care Facilities (RCFs) serve as a bridge between independent living and nursing home care. RCFs provide services such as meals, medication supervision or reminders, organized activities, and transportation or help with bathing, dressing, and other activities of daily living. RCFs include board and care homes, assisted living facilities, personal care homes, domiciliary care, and rest homes.

SCOPE

While there is limited evidence that many elders who live in age segregated residential settings encounter a wide range of health-related problems that place them at risk, there are no comprehensive estimates to indicate the extent or scope of residents' problems. In part, the lack of comprehensive data regarding prevalence rates for specific problems among elderly residents may be linked to the widespread variability among residents within and across different residential settings. Further, the complex interdependence between the person and environment in seniors housing complicates efforts to determine the prevalence of physical, psychological, and social problems among elderly residents.

In the absence of comprehensive data regarding the scope of problems that elderly residents encounter, available data suggest that elderly residents in seniors housing represent a vulnerable group. More specifically, as a group, they demonstrate more characteristics associated with risk of nursing home placement. They are older, more likely to be unmarried, female, living alone, have limited informal support, and experience more physical and mental health problems than their community-living age peers. Residents in low-income elderly housing are particularly vulnerable because they are poor, less educated, suffer more functional impairments, report more unmet needs, encounter higher levels of stress, and experience a greater probability of mental health problems. Therefore, given the nature of problems that many residents encounter, HPDP programs in seniors housing frequently target a particularly disadvantaged group of elders. As a result, HPDP programs geared to elders living in seniors housing must be responsive to residents' most basic needs (e.g., poverty, frailty, etc.), if these programs are to succeed (Buchner, Nicola, Martin, & Patrick, 1997; King et al., 1998). Interventions geared toward residents' higher level goals will fail, if they ignore the most basic needs.

Despite the problems posed by the lack of comprehensive data regarding elderly residents' needs for health promotion initiatives (Borgatta, Bulcroft, Montgomery, & Bulcroft, 1990; Buchner et al., 1997), there is growing recognition of the costs of such problems if untreated. From a housing perspective, failure to promote health among elderly residents is linked to increased turnover and relocation in the housing. From a long-term care perspective, the increased probability of relocation is associated with increased long-term care costs. Through efforts to promote health and independence among elderly residents, the probability that residents will need expensive and lengthy nursing home care decreases. Given the escalating costs associated with providing nursing home care, the failure to deploy HPDP strategies in seniors housing will dramatically increase the societal costs of providing institutional care to the growing numbers of elders.

THEORIES

Ecological theories of aging are particularly helpful models for conceptualizing how the environment influences elders' health and the success of HPDP programs. From an ecological perspective, positive health outcomes occur when there is a reasonable balance between individual needs and preferences and environmental demands and supports (Buchner et al., 1997; Minkler et al., 2000). The *competence model of aging* (Lawton & Nahemow, 1973) highlights the dynamic interactions between the person (competence) and environment (environmental press). From this perspective, a residential environment must be reasonably matched to an elderly resident's competence to ensure positive health and well-being. Unlike traditional health promotion models, the point of intervention may be either the person or the environment. Prolonged exposure to mismatched environments progressively results in deteriorating health, progressive loss of functional ability, or onset or exacerbation of mental health challenges. The construct *goodness of fit* between environmental demand and competence is particularly useful for planning HPDP programs (Minkler et al., 2000).

Alternately, the *social ecology approach* as proposed by Moos and his colleagues emphasizes how residential settings influence individual and social change (Moos & Lemke, 1994). According to Moos and Lemke (1994), if residential environments are well planned and managed, they can enhance successful aging. Since the person and environment are interdependent, one cannot be defined without reference to the other. Consequently, the same feature of the environment, such as organized social activities, may be experienced by some as an environmental demand and by others as a resource. Individual characteristics, such as functional level, social resources, etc. influence how residents experience their environment. Opportunities for personal control are more important for more competent tenants.

According to Moos and Lemke (1994, p. 10), "High expectations for independent behavior may promote better functioning among more competent residents but have little influence or even result in lower morale among impaired residents." The model also emphasizes how residential policies, service networks, and variations in the social climate influence residents' health and coping. Overall, propositions derived from ecological theories provide frameworks for developing initiatives to promote residents' health, particularly for elders living in resource-poor environments (Seigley, 1998).

STRATEGIES: OVERVIEW

HPDP initiatives in seniors housing include preventive services (e.g., flu shots, mammography) and health promotion activities (e.g., physical exercise program, health education, empowerment programs). The goals of HPDP programs in seniors housing include to: (1) reduce or delay the onset of chronic diseases, (2) improve the ability to manage chronic diseases, (3) reduce stress, (4) increase physical fitness and activity, (5) prolong residency as appropriate to the person's condition, and (6) enhance social support, self-determination, and quality of life. From a housing industry perspective, HPDP programs may improve marketability, increase worker satisfaction and retention, and reduce resident turnover.

However, there is only limited empirical evidence concerning the impact of HPDP initiatives in seniors housing. In fact, from the long list of recommended initiatives, empirical evidence exists only for physical activity programs, preventive occupational therapy, mental health outreach programs, supportive services, and socialization and empowerment programs. Information derived from these empirically based interventions serves as the foundation for improving knowledge regarding effective strategies for enhancing elderly residents' health and well-being.

STRATEGIES THAT WORK

Given the limited attention paid to health promotion initiatives in seniors housing, few definitive conclusions can be drawn about HPDP strategies that work and those that do not work. Consequently, much more empirical work needs to be completed before substantive conclusions emerge from the literature. However, one example of research strategies that work comes from Clark et al. (1997) where a preventive emphasis is given to a traditional therapeutic method.

Preventive Occupational Therapy in seniors housing is employed to prevent excess disability, improve health and self-esteem, promote meaningful leisure, and enhance overall quality of life. The Well Elderly Study (Clark et al., 1997) evaluated the impact of an intervention using preventive occupational therapy in the lives of elderly residents in federally assisted senior housing. Comparing three groups (preventive occupational therapy, social activity, and non-treatment control), elders receiving preventive occupational therapy demonstrated positive benefits in health, life satisfaction, social functioning, and general mental health. This preventive use of occupational therapy, which extended over 9 months, was associated with either improvements or reduced declines in comparison to the other groups. According to Clark and her colleagues, preventive occupational therapy assisted residents to construct health promoting and meaningful daily routines. In addition, individual monthly contact with preventively oriented occupational therapy provided residents with a personalized approach to intervention.

The lack of empirical research has not limited the number of recommendations for specific HPDP initiatives in seniors housing. These include wellness clinics, physical activity programs, health education programs (e.g., smoking cessation, drug and alcohol education programs, etc.), mental health outreach, and socialization and empowerment programs. In addition, modifications to the residential setting, such as adding support services, deploying a resident service coordinator, and changing residential policy are being recommended by personnel in the field. These types of services await testing in the housing context.

STRATEGIES THAT MIGHT WORK

The present discussion of HPDP strategies that have some demonstrated evidence of effectiveness in seniors housing is organized around the different types of approaches employed. Within each of the following sections, this review presents evidence for the effectiveness of the strategies discussed.

Mental Health Outreach Programs

Addressing the mental health needs of elderly residents is a major challenge due to their high prevalence rates of mental health problems and level of unmet need, particularly among subsidized housing residents (Black, Rabins, German, McGuire, & Roca, 1997; Staebler, 1991). Outreach programs seek to increase the utilization of mental health services, reduce the likelihood of eviction, and create a healthy, normalized life for elders. Most programs have targeted elders living in government-subsidized housing because their mental health needs are exacerbated by poverty, isolation, limited social support, and other factors. Features of successful outreach programs include (1) flexible service provisions,

(2) individualized care plans, (3) cooperation from the housing staff, and (4) repeated outreach visits. Flexible programs recognize that interventions must address residents' medical, social, and psychological problems. The *Community Connections* program, a three-year federally-funded project, targeted the mental health of residents in Seattle's elderly high rise buildings (Staebler, 1991). Using a "friendly visitor" model, outreach staff provided repeat visits to isolated elders. Designed to promote autonomy, staff provided only those services that elders requested. Residents' resistance to receiving mental health services decreased as they established trust. Initial requests for services involved instrumental assistance (e.g., chore service), however, over time, the number of mental health referrals increased. Since the most vulnerable elders are the least likely to reach out for services, "Outreach and engagement services are essential to systems that seek to avoid institutional care as the primary public response" (Staebler, 1991, p. 56).

The *Psychogeriatric Assessment and Treatment in City Housing* (PATCH) program in Baltimore City public housing developments was designed and implemented to meet inner city elderly residents' mental health needs (Black et al., 1997; Robbins et al., 2000). Alarmed that the prevalence rate for mental health problems was four times greater for these residents than community-living elders, the PATCH program was developed to prevent mental health problems and to minimize problems by linking residents with available mental health services. As part of the program, housing personnel were trained to identify residents who were at risk for mental health problems. Through early identification, staff sought to deliver essential services to enable residents to remain living independently. A psychiatric nurse provided home visits, assessments, and referrals. Results revealed a reduction in psychiatric symptoms. Both cooperation with staff and trust with residents were keys to facilitating residents' mental health and delivering services to mentally ill elders. From a public health perspective, however, the program was ineffective in reducing "undesirable" moves to institutional settings (Katz & Coyne, 2000).

Overall, health promotion initiatives to enhance elderly residents' mental health can be effective only when the interventions take into account how the residential environment influences both residents and staff. Therefore, unless HPDP strategies are designed to address the ecological context of the housing, interventions in different types of seniors housing will be ineffective.

Supportive Services and/or Resident Services Coordinators

Non-traditional health promotion interventions in seniors housing seek to create environments that detect problems early, prolong residents' ability to age in place, and promote healthy aging by altering the resources available to residents ("service rich" environments) (Sheehan, 1992). These interventions include adding support services and hiring a resident service coordinator (RSC). Altering the service nature of the housing provides more alternatives to meet residents' needs which may delay relocation to a nursing home. A pilot program bringing supportive services to 12 publicly subsidized elderly housing complexes in Rhode Island reported that after 6 months, the supportive services program positively influenced the health of mentally ill and frail elderly residents. More specifically, services improved the residents' quality of life and health (e.g., better nutrition, closer monitoring of medications, etc.) (Park & Robertson, 1999). After 6 months, residents suffering from mental illness had improved their level of cognitive function to a level comparable to the total resident population. Similarly, an unpublished study examining the impact of bringing assisted living services into congregate housing demonstrated the health enhancing features of the program (Sheehan, 1999). Residents who received services reported improved quality of life and increased social interactions. Help with both instrumental and personal care tasks enabled frail residents to engage in activities that provided them with personal satisfaction and increased their overall sense of social integration.

Socialization and Empowerment Programs

Despite the link between the social environment and promotion of residents' health and well-being, only a handful of interventions have attempted to improve the social climate in seniors housing. Critical features of the social environment include social support and social interaction with residents, family, friends, health professionals, and housing staff, opportunities to exercise control, social integration, and staff expectations. In addition, the social environment reflects the aggregate characteristics of residents, attitudes of staff, and the meaning that residents and staff attribute to the housing. Interventions have sought to either strengthen existing networks or create new meaningful sources of social support and social interaction. Empirical evidence has examined the impact of reminiscence groups (Fielden, 1990), empowerment groups (Cox & Parsons, 1996), and tenant empowerment groups to improve the quality of care (van Geen, 1997). Comparing residents participating in either a reminiscence or "here and now" group, Fielden (1990) found that while the "here and now" had no impact on psychological well-being or life satisfaction, the reminiscence group demonstrated positive changes. Reminiscence group participants also increased their level of social participation. Shared reminiscences provided residents opportunities for personal sharing that

removed barriers preventing engagement in meaningful social interactions.

Cox and Parsons (1996) used an empowerment group intervention with a small group of semi-isolated elderly residents in a low-income senior housing complex. Designed to increase residents' coping mechanisms and understanding of aging, the empowerment group positively influenced residents' sense of safety, feelings of commonality, opportunities for social interaction, and interdependence. Affirmation, mutual aid, and mutual decision-making which took place in the group setting provided residents with feelings of trust, safety, and commonality. These feelings created a basis for building meaningful personal relationships (Fielden, 1990).

Alternately, empowerment interventions address residents' ability to influence their environment and the quality of care they receive. An empowerment program entitled *Measure and Discuss*, developed in the Netherlands established a process for addressing residents' concerns related to the quality of care that they receive (van Geen, 1997). Through group process, residents' concerns were identified and translated into a report with practical recommendations and an action plan for improving the quality of care. The report and its recommendations for action provide a basis for discussion between management and the residents' committee to improve policy (van Geen, 1997). The process of involving residents and management in addressing quality of care issues, not only provides a mechanism for empowering residents, but also develops policies to improve the quality of the residential setting.

Physical Activity Programs

A major goal of health promotion programs in seniors housing is promoting physical activity for older residents. Efforts to increase elderly residents' level of physical activity have yielded mixed results. On the one hand, while most residents who participate in physical activity programs demonstrate positive short-term benefits, the longer term effects are generally disappointing because most discontinue their participation. Further, while elderly residents have a greater need for physical activity programs than other community-living elders, they are more difficult to recruit and retain in such programs (Buchner et al., 1997; Haber, Looney, Babola, Hinman, & Utsey, 2000; Stewart et al., 1997).

The *Community Healthy Activities Model Program for Seniors* (CHAMPS) program designed to increase congregate residents' involvement in community-based physical activity programs illustrates issues involved in successful interventions (Stewart et al., 1997). However, over 40 percent of residents did not increase their level of activity. Further, in comparison to elders recruited from a senior center, residents were less likely to become involved in physical activity

programs, particularly over the long term. They were also in poorer health and reported more functional limitations. Similar disappointing long-term results were reported from a recent study of the impact of health promotion education with overweight, inactive elders recruited from both a congregate housing facility and a senior center (Haber et al., 2000). The 7-week (14-hr) education program provided biweekly sessions on stretching, strength training, and walking, stress management, and nutrition. Short-term benefits included increased involvement in regularly scheduled exercise (walking, flexibility, and strength building), however, the longer term effects were disappointing. Only 10 of the 35 elders continued involvement in regular exercise. Recognizing the difficulties involved in recruiting elderly residents to participate in physical activity programs, concerted outreach efforts are needed to reduce the barriers to participation. Difficulties in recruitment are underscored by Buchner et al. (1997) who employed an outreach worker 8 hr per week for 16 months in a single housing site ($n = 44$ residents) to recruit participants to a physical exercise program. With concerted outreach activities to all 44 residents, only 18 (41 percent) participated at some time and 8–12 became regular users.

In sum, issues surrounding physical activity programs in senior housing are recruitment, retention, and long-term compliance. Successful interventions must involve efforts to (1) understand how residents perceive their health concerns, (2) eliminate barriers that prevent participation (e.g., lack of transportation, etc.), and (3) recruit and motivate residents to maintain involvement (Buchner et al., 1997; Haber et al., 2000; Mills et al., 1996).

STRATEGIES THAT DO NOT WORK

On an encouraging note, housing, and by extension, seniors housing-based HPDP initiatives appear to be so central to the lives of seniors that they offer tremendous opportunities for positive preventive potential. However, health promotion initiatives to enhance elderly residents' health can be effective only when the interventions take into account how the residential environment influences both residents and staff. Therefore, unless HPDP strategies are designed to address the ecological context of the housing, interventions in different types of seniors housing will be ineffective.

SYNTHESIS

At the present time, knowledge about what works, what might work, and what does not work to promote health among senior housing residents is beginning to emerge.

(e.g., identity status, identity exploration, commitment, etc.). Rather, the collection of measures used in these studies stem from a diverse array of theoretical perspectives and orientations, many of which have evolved around the specific constructs measured (e.g., self-esteem, self-efficacy, attachment, autonomy, empowerment, etc.). Nevertheless, a qualitative coding of the labeled indices reported in the Catalano et al. (1999) review using Strauss and Corbin's (1998) method of constant comparative analyses (Montgomery, Ferrer-Wreder, Kurtines, & Cass Lorente, 2001) identified three basic constructs underlying the measures that appear to tap concepts that have traditionally been seen as at the core of identity development or the adjacent psychosocial stages of industry or intimacy, thus supporting the utility of the identity construct in organizing and integrating the diverse array of measures/indices used in the literature.[3]

STRATEGIES THAT DO NOT WORK

Clear evidence of ineffectiveness is not yet available.

SYNTHESIS

For those interested in the implications of identity for preventive intervention, it appears that there is good news and bad news. The *bad news* is that there is still a considerable distance between the prevention and the developmental literature when it comes to the promotion of adolescent identity development. Practical and methodological constraints have to date limited efforts to develop and evaluate interventions that specifically target identity development at a global level. This conclusion, however, is not unexpected in that the types of interventions that have tended to be "well-evaluated" (i.e., that include an experimental or quasi-experimental design, multiple measures, and multiple assessment points, etc.) have been theoretically "diffused" as a group. As a whole, these interventions have typically consisted of relatively brief interventions[4] that do not expressly target global identity and do not follow participants long enough or with enough depth to capture the

impact that the interventions may have had on participants' life course development.

The *good news* is that the idea of fostering positive identity development is alive and well in the intervention literature, as a core organizing concept. Indeed, an umbrella construct such as the concept of identity appears not only useful, but necessary for organizing and making sense of the proliferation of evaluative concepts and constructs (and the burgeoning number of measures and indices) that have been used in evaluation studies. Moreover, the convergence of concern with respect to this issue has the potential to make a contribution to both the prevention and identity literatures—to the prevention literature by providing a workable conceptual framework for developing evaluations of outcomes at a more global level, and to the identity literature by offering the opportunity to explore the empirical significance of the contribution of a large and diverse array of self-related concepts and constructs to the notion to identity development. When coupled with the development of more long-term and intense youth interventions and advances in methods for assessing qualitative and quantitative change (Denzin & Lincoln, 2000; Taylor, Graham, Cumsille, & Hansen, 2001), the news indeed appears encouraging.

The even better news is that the emergence in both the prevention and identity literatures of identity as a concept providing a framework for articulating a diverse array of general indices of positive adjustment and optimal functioning, when combined with the emergence of life course concepts such as life transitions and turning points, provides a very useful vocabulary for complementing and extending concepts such as reducing risk and increasing protective factors. More specifically, the integration of these concepts has the potential to broaden the range of outcomes to include concepts useful in documenting the impact of such interventions in helping young people to turn their lives around and change their life course or life trajectory in positive ways, that is, ways that move them along proactive and prosocial pathways rather than trajectories or pathways that are disruptive and antisocial. Moreover, it provides a vocabulary of concepts that is especially relevant to adolescence. In sum, Eriksonian views of the preventive role of positive identity development appear to have the potential to make a significant contribution to the field of primary prevention intervention in ways consistent with the movement toward a greater emphasis on positive adjustment, optimal functioning, and individuals as contributors to their own development and supporting young people's efforts to develop a consistent and competent view of themselves (Cowan, 2000).

Interventions that illustrate ways in which this potential may be realized have already begun to emerge. The *Changing Lives Program* (CLP; Ferrer-Wreder et al., 2002), provides one such example. This program seeks to

---

[3] The three basic constructs identified in the qualitative coding included variables related to the optimal functioning of the individual as a self-directed agent (core identity variables), optimal interpersonal functioning (core intimacy variable), and personal competence. The individual characterized by a mature identity, as least with respect to the range of variables tapped by these studies, could thus be characterized as self-directed, interpersonally effective, and competent.

[4] The majority of the interventions described in this review intervene for one school year or less. The only exceptions to this general finding are the Growing Healthy—Smith, Redican, and Olson (1992); Know Your Body—Walter, Vaughan, and Wynder (1989), programs that had program activities for up to 2 and 6 years, respectively.

explore the utility of global identity as an organizing concept or construct and to document intervention-related change in the context of life course transitions, namely the transition that many at-risk youth make when they begin to move into more adaptive developmental trajectories or hold course on their current paths. Conducted as part of an ongoing program of co-constructivist theory and research program (Berman, Schwartz, Kurtines, & Berman, 2001; Ferrer-Wreder et al., 2002), this intervention uses the concept of identity as a coherent and integrated self-construction and a concept of human agency consistent with life course theory within a developmental framework. We have found this framework to be useful for articulating and working with a broad band of developmental domains and processes related to identity formation as well as a number of general indices of positive adjustment and optimal functioning.

Specifically, the CLP is a school-based intervention that works with a multiethnic population of troubled high school youth with a history of attendance, behavior, or motivational problems in school (Berman, Kurtines, Silverman, & Serafini, 1996). The program uses participatory and transformative intervention strategies drawn from Freire's (1970/1983) approach to empower marginalized people by creating a context where they could enhance their critical consciousness about their exclusion from the mainstream. Developmental domains targeted for intervention include increasing participants' acceptance of control and responsibility for their lives, the exploration of and commitment to a positive identity, and their active participation in their social contexts. This "bottom-up" approach not only complements those "top-down" prevention models that are designed to intervene at a contextual/ecosystemic level (e.g., with family, peers, school, etc.); it is also consistent with many contemporary views of identity and life course theory, in that adaptive identity development involves making decisions to take control of one's life as well as the exploration of and commitment to one's potential (Berzonsky, 1989; Côté, 1997; Waterman, 1995). In addition, efforts are being taken to draw on advances in qualitative methods (Denzin & Lincoln, 2000; Taylor et al., 2001) to document the power of such interventions to alter the life course of intervention participants.

To date, the program has undergone two short-term efficacy trials using a quasi-experimental design that have indicated the intervention's utility for working with multiethnic and socially marginalized youth in increasing their critical thinking and problem-solving skills and sense of control and responsibility for their lives (Ferrer-Wreder et al., 2002; Ferrer-Wreder, Milnitsky, Kurtines, Cass Lorente, Briones, & Cestari, 2001; Milnitsky, Kurtines, Ferrer-Wreder, Cass Lorente, Briones, & Cestari, 2001). The CLP is undergoing further evaluation as a multi-year school based intervention in the United States and has been integrated as a core component of a 2-year community-based Swedish universal prevention program designed to promote participation in competence-enhancing leisure activities (Koutakis, Ferrer-Wreder, & Stattin, 2000, 2001). It should be noted that there are many different ways in which future interventions may choose to use global identity as an organizational framework and this is just one program option that may prove promising.

Looking to the future, it is our belief that the concept of identity has the potential to open up new ways to enhance the overall developmental prospects of young people. The view of identity as a "steering mechanism" guiding the individual's life course provides a conceptual link between the skills and competencies that intervention efforts often target and the developmental outcomes that these skills and competencies serve. Individuals do not acquire skills and competencies in a vacuum. Positive development involves the acquisition and use of skills and competencies in the service of life goals and values that the individual deems worthy of commitment. Consequently, the next generation of interventions should continue to develop and test broadband programs for promoting youth development. These interventions should be designed to integrate multiple knowledge-based components, including those that target identity issues.

Also see: Self-Esteem: Early Childhood; Self-Esteem: Childhood; Self-Esteem: Adolescence; Family Strengthening: Childhood; Family Strengthening: Adolescence; Life Skills: Adolescence; Risk-Taking: Adolescence; Social Competency: Adolescence; Social and Emotional Learning: Early Childhood; Social and Emotional Learning: Childhood; Social and Emotional Learning: Adolescence.

References

Allen, J.P., Philliber, S., Herrling, S., & Kuperminc, G.P. (1997). Preventing teen pregnancy and academic failure: Experimental evaluation of a developmentally based approach. *Child Development, 64*(4), 729–742.

Archer, S. (1994). *Interventions for adolescent identity development.* Thousand Oaks, CA: Sage.

Battistich, V., Schaps, E., Watson, M., & Solomon, D. (1996). Prevention effects of the Child Development Project: Early findings from an ongoing multisite demonstration trial. *Journal of Adolescent Research, 11*(1), 12–35.

Berman, S., Kurtines, W., Silverman, W., & Serafini, L. (1996). The impact of exposure to crime and violence on urban youth. *American Journal of Orthopsychiatry, 66*(3), 329–336.

Berman, A.M., Schwartz, S.J., Kurtines, W.M., & Berman, S.L. (2001). The process of exploration in identity formation: The role of style and competence. *Journal of Adolescence, 24*(4), 513–528.

Berzonsky, M.D. (1989). The self as a theorist: Individual differences in identity formation. *International Journal of Personal Construct Psychology, 2*(4), 363–376.

Brandtstaedter, J., & Lerner, R.M. (Eds.) (1999). *Action & self-development: Theory and research through the life span.* Thousand Oaks, CA: Sage.

Cardenas, J.A., Montecel, M.R., Supik, J.D., & Harris, R.J. (1992). The Coca-Cola Valued Youth Program. Dropout prevention strategies for at-risk students. *Texas Researcher, 3,* 111–130.

Catalano, R.F., Berglund, M.L., Ryan, J.A.M., Lonczak, H., & Hawkins, J.D. (1999). *Positive youth development in the United States: Research findings on evaluations of positive youth development programs.* Washington, DC: US Department of Health and Human Services.

Clausen, J.A. (1998). Life reviews and life stories. In J.Z. Giele & G.H. Elder (Eds.), *Methods of life course research: Qualitative and quantitative approaches* (pp. 189–212). Thousand Oaks, CA: Sage.

Compas, B.E., Hinden, B.R., & Gerhardt, C.A. (1995). Adolescent development: Pathways and processes of risk and resilience. *Annual Review of Psychology, 46,* 265–293.

Côté, J.E. (1997). An empirical test of the identity capital model. *Journal of Adolescence, 20*(5), 577–597.

Côté, J.E. (2001). The hope and promise of identity theory and research. *Identity, 1*(1), 1–5.

Cowan, E.L. (2000). Psychological wellness: Some hopes for the future. In D. Cicchetti, J. Rappaport, I. Sandler, & R.P. Weissberg (Eds.), *The promotion of wellness in children and adolescents* (pp. 477–503). Washington, DC: CWLA.

Dahlberg, L.L. (1998). Youth violence in the United States: Major trends, risk factors, and prevention approaches. *American Journal of Preventive Medicine, 14*(4), 259–272.

Denzin, N.K., & Lincoln, Y.S. (Eds.) (2000). *The handbook of qualitative research* (2nd ed.). Thousand Oaks, CA: Sage.

Dishion, T.J., French, D.C., & Patterson, G.R. (1995). The development and ecology of antisocial behavior. In D. Cicchetti, D. Cohen et al. (Eds.), *Developmental psychopathology, Vol. 2: Risk, disorder, and adaptation* (pp. 421–471). New York, NY: Wiley.

Elder, G.H. (1998a). The life course and human development. In R.M. Lerner (Ed.), *Handbook of child psychology, Vol 1: Theoretical models of human development.* New York: Wiley.

Elder, G.H. (1998b). The life course as developmental theory. *Child Development, 69*(1), 1–12.

Enright, R.D., Ganiere, D.M., Buss, R.R., Lapsley, D.K., & Olson, L.M. (1983). Promoting identity development in adolescents. *Journal of Early Adolescence, 3,* 247–255.

Enright, R.D., Olson, L.M., Ganiere, D., Lapsley, D.K., & Buss, R.R. (1984). A clinical model for enhancing adolescent ego identity. *Journal of Adolescence, 7,* 119–130.

Erikson, E.H. (1963). *Childhood and society.* New York: Norton.

Erikson, E.H. (1968). *Identity: Youth and crisis.* New York: Norton.

Erikson, E.H., & Erikson, K.T. (1957/1995). The confirmation of the delinquent. In S. Schlein (Ed.), *A way of looking at things: Selected papers from 1930 to 1980.* New York: Norton.

European Monitoring Centre for Drugs and Drug Addiction. (2000). *Annual report on the state of the drugs problem in the European Union.* Luxembourg: Office for Official Publications of the European Communities.

Ferrer-Wreder, L., Cass Lorente, C., Kurtines, W., Briones, E., Bussell, J., Berman, S., & Arrufat, O. (2002). Promoting identity development in marginalized youth. *Journal of Adolescent Research. 17*(2), 168–187.

Ferrer-Wreder, L., Milnitsky, C., Kurtines, W., Cass Lorente, C., Briones, E., & Cestari, L. (2001). *Oficinas Escolhas de Vida: O Raciocínio Crítico e Identidade na Adolescência, Psicologia* [The life choice workshop: Critical thinking and identity issues in adolescence]. Submitted for publication.

Freire, P. (1970/1983). *Pedagogy of the oppressed.* New York: Herder & Herder.

Giele, J.Z., & Elder, G.H. (Eds.). (1998). *Methods of life course research: Qualitative and quantitative approaches.* Thousand Oaks, CA: Sage.

Hahn, A., Leavitt, T., & Aaron, P. (1994). *Evaluation of the Quantum Opportunities Program (QOP). Did the program work? A report on the post secondary outcomes and cost-effectiveness of the QOP Program (1989–1993).* Waltham, MA: Brandeis University Heller Graduate School Center for Human Resources.

Hawkins, J.D., Catalano, R.F., & Miller, J.Y. (1992). Risk and protective factors for alcohol and other drug problems in adolescence and early adulthood: Implications for substance abuse prevention. *Psychological Bulletin, 112*(1), 64–105.

Johnson, L.D., O'Malley, P.M., & Bachman, J.G. (1998). *National survey results on drug use from the Monitoring the Future Study, 1975–1997* (Vol. 1: Secondary school students). Rockville, MD: National Institute on Drug Abuse.

Johnson, K., Strader, T., Berbaum, M., Bryant, D., Bucholtz, G., Collins, D., & Noe, T. (1996). Reducing alcohol and other drug use by strengthening community, family, and youth resiliency: An evaluation of the Creating Lasting Connections Program. *Journal of Adolescent Research, 11*(1), 36–67.

Jones, R.M. (1992). Identity and problem behaviors. In G.R. Adams, T.P. Gullotta, & R. Montemayor (Eds.), *Adolescent identity formation: Advances in adolescent development* (pp. 216–233). Newbury Park, CA: Sage.

Jones, R.M. (1994). Curricula focused on behavioral deviance. In S.L. Archer (Ed.), *Interventions for adolescent identity development* (pp. 174–190). Thousand Oaks, CA: Sage.

Koutakis, N., Ferrer-Wreder, L., & Stattin, H. (2000). *Örebro prevention project.* Presented at the Society for Prevention Research, Montreal, Canada.

Koutakis, N., Ferrer-Wreder, L., & Stattin, H. (2001). *The Örebro Prevention Project: Youth leisure, adjustment, and intervention.* In L. Ferrer-Wreder (Chair), *Nordic intervention work: Recent findings from efficacy/effectiveness trials.* Presented at the Society for Prevention Research, Washington, DC.

Kröger, C., Winter, H., & Shaw, R. (1998). *Guidelines for the evaluation of drug prevention intervention.* Lisbon, Portugal: European Monitoring Centre for Drugs and Drug Addiction.

Kroger, J. (1996). Identity, regression, and development. *Journal of Adolescence, 19,* 203–222.

Kurtines, W.M., & Szapocznik, J. (1996). Family interaction patterns: Structural family therapy in contexts of cultural diversity. In E.D. Hibbs, P.S. Jensen et al. (Eds.), *Psychosocial treatments for child and adolescent disorders: Empirically based strategies for clinical practice* (pp. 671–697). Washington, DC: American Psychological Association.

Lerner, R.M. (1995). *America's youth in crisis: Challenges and options for programs and polices.* Thousand Oaks, CA: Sage.

LoSciuto, L., Freeman, M.A., Harrington, E., Altman, F., & Lanphear, A. (1997). An outcome evaluation of the Woodrock Youth Development Project. *Journal of Early Adolescence, 17*(1), 51–66.

LoSciuto, L., Rajala, A.K., Townsend, T.N., & Taylor, A.S. (1996). An outcome evaluation of Across Ages: An intergenerational mentoring approach to drug prevention. *Journal of Adolescent Research, 11*(1), 116–129.

Marcia, J.E. (1988). Common processes underlying ego identity, cognitive/moral development, and individuation. In D.K. Lapsley & F.C. Power (Eds.), *Self, ego, and identity: Integrative approaches* (pp. 211–266). New York: Springer-Verlag.

Markstrom-Adams, C. (1992). A consideration of intervening factors in adolescent identity formation. In G.R. Adams, T.P. Gullotta et al. (Eds.), *Adolescent identity formation. Advances in adolescent development* (Vol. 4, pp. 173–192). Newbury Park, CA: Sage.

Markstrom-Adams, C., Ascione, F.R., Braegger, D., & Adams, G. (1993). The effects of two forms of perspective-taking on ego-identity formation in late adolescence. *Journal of Adolescence, 16,* 217–224.

Masten, A.S., & Coatsworth, D.J. (1998). The development of competence in favorable and unfavorable environments: Lessons from research on successful children. *American Psychologist, 53*(2), 205–220.

Milnitsky, C., Kurtines, W., Ferrer-Wreder, L., Cass Lorente, C., Briones, E., & Cestari, L. (2001). *Educação Transformadora em Contexto: Os Temas Transversais no Brasil e nos Estados Unidos* [Transformative education in context: The cross discipline themes]. Submitted for publication.

Montemayor, R., Adams, G.R., & Gullotta, T.P. (Eds.). (1994). *Personal relationships during adolescence.* Thousand Oaks, CA: Sage.

Montgomery, M.J., Ferrer-Wreder, L., Kurtines, W.M., & Cass Lorente, C. (2001). Identity interventions: Where are we now? Where are we going? In M.J. Montgomery (Chair), *Intervening to promote identity development: How do we foster and evaluate positive change?* Presented at the Society for Research on Identity Formation. London, Ontario, CA.

Montgomery, M.J., & Sorell, G.T. (1998). Love and dating experience in early and middle adolescence: Grade and gender comparisons. *Journal of Adolescence, 21,* 677–689.

Mrazek, P.J., & Haggerty, R.J. (Eds.). (1994). *Reducing risks for mental disorders: Frontiers for preventive intervention research.* Washington, DC: National Academy Press.

Schinke, S.P., Botvin, G.J., Trimble, J.E., Orlandi, M.A., Gilchrist, L.D., & Locklear, V.S. (1988). Preventing substance abuse among American-Indian adolescents: A bicultural competence skills approach. *Journal of Counseling Psychology, 35*(1), 87–90.

Sherrod, L.R., & Brim, O.G., Jr. (1986). Epilogue: Retrospective and prospective views of life-course research on human development. In A. Sorensen, F.E. Weinert, & L.R. Sherrod (Eds.), *Human development and the life course: Multidisciplinary perspectives* (pp. 557–575). Hillsdale, NJ: Lawrence Erlbaum.

Sloboda, Z., & David, S.L. (1997). *Preventing drug use among children and adolescents: A research-based guide.* Washington, DC: National Institute on Drug Abuse.

Smith, D.W., Redican, K.J., & Olson, L.K. (1992). The longevity of growing healthy: An analysis of the eight original sites implementing the School Health Curriculum Project. *Journal of School Health, 62*(3), 83–87.

Strauss, A., & Corbin, J. (1998). *Basics of qualitative research.* Thousand Oaks, CA: Sage.

Taylor, B.J., Graham, J.W., Cumsille, P., & Hansen, W.B. (2001). Modeling prevention program effects on growth in substance use: Analysis of five years of data from the Adolescent Alcohol Prevention Trial. *Prevention Science, 1,* 183–197.

Tierney, J.P., Grossman, J.B., & Resch, N.L. (1995). *Making a difference: An impact study of Big Brothers/Big Sisters.* Philadelphia, PA: Public/Private Ventures.

Van Dijk, J.J.M., & Mayhew, P. (1992). *Criminal victimization in the industrialized world: Key findings of the 1989 and 1992 international crime surveys.* The Hague: Ministry of Justice, Department of Crime Prevention.

Walter, H.J., Vaughan, R.D., & Wynder, E.L. (1989). Primary prevention of cancer among children: Changes in cigarette smoking and diet after six years of intervention. *Journal of the National Cancer Institute, 81*(3), 995–999.

Waterman, A.S. (1995). Eudaimonic theory: Self-realization and the collective good. In W.M. Kurtines & J.L. Gewirtz (Eds.), *Moral development: An introduction* (pp. 255–278). Boston: Allyn & Bacon.

Injuries, Unintentional, Early Childhood

David Chalmers, Jonathan Kotch, and Viet Nguyen

INTRODUCTION

Unintentional injuries are the leading cause of death among children in the United States over the age of six months. They also cause more childhood disability than any other condition after birth defects and congenital anomalies. For all age groups combined in the United States, unintentional injury is the leading cause of potential years of life lost, outdistancing even cancer, heart disease, and HIV. This is a consequence of unintentional injury's disproportionate toll on young people.

This entry discusses the incidence of unintentional injury among infants and preschool-age children in developed and developing countries; it examines a theory-based approach to prevention, and describes various injury control strategies.

DEFINITIONS

Injury is defined as the physical damage done to a living organism by the rapid exchange of energy, or by sudden interference with a necessary metabolic process. Examples of the former are kinetic, thermal, radiant, ionizing, chemical, and electrical energy. The latter may include poisoning as well as the acute absence of a necessary chemical such as oxygen. An *unintentional injury* is one that is not deliberate or premeditated, although it is not infrequent that intention cannot be determined.

SCOPE

Developed Countries. In the United States, as in most developed countries, unintentional injury is the leading cause of death among children of all ages after the first year of life. In infants, unintentional injuries and adverse events (such as medical errors) are the eighth leading cause. After infancy, however, unintentional injuries and adverse events lead the list (Office of Statistics and Programming, 2000a).

The death rate among children 1–4 years of age in the United States attributable to unintentional injury in 1998 was 11.6 per 100,000 (National Safety Council, 2000). The single most frequent cause of unintentional injury death in the United States among children 0–4 years old is motor vehicle injury, followed by drowning, fires and burns, suffocation by ingestion, and falls. In 1998, firearms and poisoning by liquid or solid substances claimed an equal number of US children in this age group (National Safety Council, 2000).

There are important ethnic and gender differences in the risk of injury death. Crudely speaking, males experience a higher rate of death due to unintentional injury than do females, and non-Whites a higher rate than Whites. In the United States, American Indians and Alaska Natives have the highest rates of all, whereas Asian Americans and Pacific Islanders have the lowest rates (Office of Statistics and Programming, 2000b). Most observers attribute the increased risk of injury death among children of color to socioeconomic, rather than racial or ethnic, differences.

Rates for non-fatal injuries are more difficult to obtain, because in the United States there is no nation-wide surveillance mechanism for them. Estimates are based on local, state, or regional surveillance systems, surveys, or medical care utilization data. Child injury rates, ranked by levels of severity, have been likened to an iceberg: mortality rates are the least frequent, representing the tip of the iceberg, followed by hospital discharge rates, emergency department visit rates, office-based physician visits and finally by injuries which do not enter the medical care system at all (see Figure 1).

The pioneering and most often quoted statewide childhood injury surveillance project in the United States is the Massachusetts' State Childhood Injury Prevention Project (SCIPP). That study collected data from hospitals, emergency departments, and doctors' offices. The investigators concluded that the ratio among deaths, hospital discharges, and emergency department visits was 1:45:1300 (Gallagher, Finison, Guyer, & Goodenough, 1984). The rank order of the most to the least frequent causes of non-fatal child injury is not the same as the rank order for injury death, since injuries differ in their likelihood of causing death. *Drowning* by

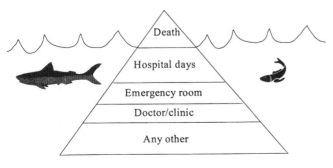

Figure 1. Injury Iceberg.

definition is a fatal event, and non-fatal immersions are relatively uncommon. On the other hand, falls and poisonings in preschoolers are much less likely to be fatal. Therefore, depending upon the data source and the population studied, poisoning and/or falls are more often reported to be the most common causes of non-fatal injury among preschool children than are motor vehicle injuries and drowning.

In New Zealand, injury is the leading cause of death for children from the age of 1 year (Kypri, Chalmers, Langley, & Wright, 2000). For children aged less than 1 year (infants), injury is the fourth leading cause of death. The mortality rates for children aged <1 year, 0–4 years, and 5–9 years are 35.4, 22.5, and 11.4 per 100,000 person years, respectively. The leading causes of injury death for infants are suffocation (unintentional), motor vehicle traffic (MVT) incidents, homicide, fire/flame, and drowning (predominantly in domestic baths). For children aged 1–4 years the leading causes are MVT incidents, drowning (at least half in domestic swimming pools or spa baths), fire/flame and suffocation. For children aged 5–9 years the leading causes are MVT incidents and drowning.

Injury is the fourth leading cause of hospitalization for children aged 0–4 years in New Zealand, where national data are available on hospital discharges, and the leading cause for children aged 5–9 years (Kypri, Chalmers, Langley, & Wright, 2001). The hospitalization rates for children aged <1 year, 0–4 years, and 5–9 years are 926, 1,534, and 1,307 per 100,000 person years, respectively. The leading injury causes of hospitalization for infants are falls, burns from hot objects/substances, suffocation (predominantly from inhalation/ingestion of food or other objects), assault, poisoning, and MVT incidents. For children aged 1–4 years the leading causes are falls, poisoning, burns from hot objects/substances, MVT incidents (54 percent as vehicle occupants, 40 percent as pedestrians), cutting/piercing incidents, striking incidents, and pedal cycle incidents. For children aged 5–9 years the leading causes are falls, MVT incidents (37 percent as vehicle occupants, 43 percent as pedestrians), and pedal cycle incidents.

Developing Countries. In most developing countries, while childhood infectious diseases, the leading cause of death in childhood, decrease, childhood injury has emerged as increasingly more important. According to the World Health Organization (WHO), drowning is the 11th leading cause of death in middle and lower income countries for children under 5, war injuries are 13th and road-traffic injuries 14th. Falls, drowning, war and road-traffic events are the 12th through 15th leading contributors to the burden of disease for 0–4 year olds in these same countries (World Health Organization, 1999).

In China, Mexico, and Thailand, injuries are the leading cause of death in people from age 1–44 (Mock, Abantanga,

Cummings, & Koepsell, 1999). However, very few published studies on injury morbidity and mortality in these countries exist. In Africa, all of the official sources of data are of limited value because of incomplete vital and death registration (Mock, Forjuoh, & Rivara, 1999). A survey in Ghana, however, has shown the annual incidence of transport-related injury to be 997/100,000 in urban areas and 941/100,000 in rural areas. Transport-related mechanisms were a leading cause of child injury (40 percent), follow by falls (27 percent) (UNICEF Vietnam, 2000).

Vietnam has one of the highest physicians per capita ratios in the developing world (1 physician per 2,694 population), and has the most favorable hospital bed-to-population ratio. Vietnamese often hear about the effects of infection disease and malnutrition on child health, but not many people realize that

> ... more Vietnamese children die from poisonings at home than from Japanese Encephalitis B, and more die from falls in their homes than from Dengue Fever. More adolescents die in traffic accidents than from Malaria, and more die by drowning than from all major infectious diseases combined. (UNICEF, n.d.)

There are very few studies on injury in Vietnam and no national data on unintentional injuries among Vietnamese children. Tuong and Quanys (1995) completed one study on child injuries in Hanoi, children under age 15 from three different sources (hospitals, a community, and the Bao Viet Insurance Company). In the hospital setting, they collected data from all 10 hospitals located in Hanoi. In the community, the investigators collected information by interviewing the eldest adult or caregiver in households in the O Cho Dua District of Hanoi, which has a population of 15,000, including 4,157 children under age 15.

This study showed that the unintentional injury incidence rate was 0.078 per child per year (Tuong & Quang, 1995). Falls, traffic injuries, unintentional poisoning, dog bites, burns, and drowning are the leading causes of unintentional injuries in Vietnamese children. Table 1 compares the proportion of injury causes from each of the three settings.

The data from the Bao Viet Insurance Company, the biggest insurance company in Vietnam, showed that in 1990, 3,570 among the 490,000 children covered by the company submitted claims for injuries (Tuong & Quang, 1995). Each child spent about $1.70/year for the insurance premium, compared with the $0.80 per capita that the Vietnamese government spends on health care, which is much lower than all other countries in Asia. The Bao Viet Insurance Company paid approximately $28,000 for 3,570 injuries in 1990, about $8.00 per claim. Although private health care expenditure accounts for 59–69 percent of all health care in Vietnam (Gellert, 1995), the private health practices are not

Table 1. Proportion of Injury Causes from Each of the Three Settings in Hanoi

Injuries	Hospitals total percentage	Community total percentage	Bao Viet insurance total percentage
Traffic injuries	12.91	16.35	21.73
Unintentional poisoning	2.74	*Intentionally blank*	*Intentionally blank*
Falls	48.42	19.14	38.73
Fire and flames	16.88	12.65	4.99
Drowning	0.05	4.01	2.26
Animal bite	0.80	33.33	15.49
Violence	2.08	*Intentionally blank*	9.83
Foreign body	2.69	*Intentionally blank*	*Intentionally blank*
Negligence	1.15	*Intentionally blank*	*Intentionally blank*
Others	12.28	14.51	6.94
Total cases (%)	12,758 (100)	324 (100)*	3,570 (100)*

*Rounded.
Source: Tuong and Quang (1995). Injuries in children under 15 years in Hanoi. *Vietnam Pediatric Association, 4*(2), 38–40.

a reliable source of medical records, making data collected from insurance companies less reliable.

In a city such as Hanoi, there are many injury problems that need to be solved. For drivers, use of seatbelts, observing speed limits, avoiding drinking and driving, and stopping at stop signs are yet to be learned. For the motorcyclist, although helmet use had been introduced in some big cities, it is not yet a common practice. The bicycle is a major mode of transportation, especially in rural areas, but most bicycles are not equipped with lights, and wearing helmets is rare. Government subsidies for the purchase of bicycle helmets are called for.

Basic home injury prevention strategies are needed in developing countries such as Vietnam. In the case of falls, window guards are already widely used, but grab bars in the bathroom and toilet, stair-rails, adequate lighting, and anti-slip devices are lacking. The concept of the "Safe Kitchen" including first aid for burns, is not well understood. Since medicines are still dispensed in paper and/or plastic bags or in bottles without fitted, childproof tops, poisoning is common. Electric shock injury is also quite common due to unsafe cooking habits or poor quality electrical devices.

At present, Vietnam does not have a national program of public safety. The government is beginning to pay attention to the problem by collaborating with the US Embassy, UNICEF and others, to promote safety and reduce injury risk (UNICEF Vietnam, 2000).

THEORY

The theoretical approach to injury prevention parallels the public health model of infectious disease epidemiology,

	Host	Agent	Environment	
			Physical	Social
Pre-event				
Event				
Post-event				

Figure 2. Haddon Matrix.

but the agent of injury is energy rather than a microorganism. Inanimate objects that transfer energy between the host and the environment are called *vehicles*, and animate objects *vectors*. William Haddon combined the epidemiologic triangle (agent, host, environment) with the three levels of prevention (primary, secondary, tertiary) to create what has come to be called the "Haddon Matrix" (Haddon, 1980). When the environment was subdivided into social and physical, a 12-cell matrix for brainstorming injury control strategies resulted (see Figure 2).

Another of Haddon's legacies is his list of 10 countermeasures or strategies for reducing damage from environmental hazards (Haddon, 1980):

1. Prevent the creation of the hazard in the first place (e.g., stop making fireworks).
2. Reduce the amount of hazard brought into being (e.g., reduce the height of playground equipment).
3. Prevent the release of the hazard that already exists (e.g., prevent the discharge of firearms).
4. Modify the rate or spatial distribution of release of the hazard from its source (e.g., brakes on motor vehicles).
5. Separate, in time or space, the hazard and that which is to be protected (e.g., using sidewalks to separate pedestrians from motor vehicles).
6. Separate the hazard and that which is to be protected by interposition of a material barrier (e.g., child resistant containers for poisons).
7. Modify relevant basic qualities of the hazard (e.g., making crib slat spacing too narrow to strangle a child).
8. Make what is to be protected more resistant to damage from the hazard (e.g., increasing physical fitness through exercise).
9. Begin to counter the damage already done by the environmental hazard (e.g., emergency medical care).
10. Stabilize, repair, and rehabilitate the object of the damage (e.g., rehabilitation).

The 10 countermeasures were intended by Haddon to provide an aid for "identifying, considering, and choosing" policies or programs for injury control (Haddon, 1980). Haddon also introduced the notion of "*passive*" versus "*active*" injury control measures. Passive measures are those that require no individual action, while active measures are those that require "much action on the part of individuals" (Haddon, 1980). Examples of passive measures include air bags in motor vehicles and self-closing gates in swimming pool fences. Examples of active strategies include child restraints in motor vehicles and wearing bicycle helmets. Haddon recognized that passive strategies were more effective than active ones (National Committee for Injury Prevention and Control, 1989).

STRATEGIES: OVERVIEW

Although still the leading cause of death among children in developed countries, injury deaths fell by about half between 1970 and 1995 in the 26 countries of the Organization for Economic Cooperation and Development (UNICEF, 2001). How has this been accomplished? Injury prevention strategies take a variety of forms including legislation/enforcement, education/behavior change, and engineering/technology (National Committee for Injury Prevention and Control, 1989). Often a combination of all three approaches is required. For example, occupant protection in motor vehicles began with the development of seat belts and child auto safety restraints, followed by the promotion of the voluntary use of these devices through public education programs and eventually compulsory use through legislation and enforcement.

STRATEGIES THAT WORK

Child Auto Safety Restraints. While many road safety strategies affect motor vehicle occupants of all ages, child safety restraint devices have been shown to work well in reducing the risk of injury to the youngest occupants of motor vehicles. Child restraint devices, or car seats as they are better known, are designed to protect child occupants by securing them to the vehicle so that deceleration in a crash is less abrupt, the impact forces are spread more widely over the stronger parts of the body, and the children are not thrown against the vehicle interior or ejected from the vehicle (Wilson, Baker, Teret, Shock, & Garbarino, 1991). The available evidence indicates that up to 71 percent (depending on age) of occupant deaths for children under the age of 5 years can be prevented through the correct use of an appropriate restraining device (Rivara & Grossman, 1996).

Once correctly seated in a restraint, the device provides passive protection for the child occupant. The correct installation of restraints in motor vehicles and the correct seating of children in restraints require active intervention by parents and other caregivers. Incorrect use reduces the effectiveness of restraints by as much as 59 percent (National Highway Transport Safety Administration [NHTSA], 1999). High levels of incorrect use have been reported in a number of countries. In one US study, for example, Margolis, Wagenaar, and Molnar (1988) found that 65 percent of children in restraints were incorrectly restrained.

Poison-Prevention Packaging. Poisoning is no longer one of the leading causes of death in the 0–5 year age group in developed countries, but it remains a major concern (Baker, O'Neill, Ginsburg, & Li, 1992). For every poisoning death of a child under 6 years of age in the United States, there are an estimated 20,000 ingestions (Litovitz, Schmitz, & Holm, 1989; cited in Baker et al., 1992). Happily, the advent of childproof packaging has sharply reduced the occurrence of poisoning, especially in the toddler age group. In the United States, the Poison Prevention Packaging Act (PPPA) was enacted in 1970 to protect young children from opening containers and ingesting medicines and other hazardous substances stored about the home (Walton, 1982). Clarke and Walton (1979) documented a 48–56 percent reduction in poisoning among under 5-year-olds by ingestion of baby aspirin, and a 43 percent reduction in poisoning by ingestion of adult aspirin, following the introduction child-proof packaging. In a more recent time series study, covering the period 1974–1992, Rodgers (1996) demonstrated an annual reduction in oral prescription drug-related mortality of 1.4 deaths per million children younger than 5 years. Similar reductions have followed the implementation of childproof packaging of petroleum products, caustics and cleaning agents, and other solid and liquid hazards. Walton (1982) conducted a time series analysis of data from the National Electronic Injury Surveillance System (NEISS) for the period 1973–1978. Over this period, ingestion rates declined for products covered by the PPPA (e.g., drain cleaners, oven cleaners, turpentine), from 0.45 to 0.15 incidents per 1,000 children less than 5 years of age. Similar evidence of the effectiveness of child-resistant packaging has been demonstrated in Sweden and the United Kingdom (Assargaard & Sjoberg, 1995; Sibert, Craft, & Jackson, 1977).

Pool Fencing. Drowning is by definition a fatal event, and drowning is one of the leading causes of early childhood injury deaths in both developed and developing countries. In the United States, for example, drowning is the leading cause of injury death among children aged 1–4 years (Wilson et al., 1991). In developed countries with temperate climates, such as Australia, New Zealand, and the United States, a common location for drowning is the domestic or residential swimming pool (Cass, Ross, & Lam, 1996; Kypri et al., 2000; Wintemute, 1990). In fact, 58 percent of drowning among 1–2 year olds, and 51 percent of drowning among 2–3 year olds, took place in "artificial pools" (including swimming pools, jacuzzis, whirlpools, and hot tubs) at homes, parks, apartment complexes, etc. (Brenner, Trumble, Smith, Kessler, & Overpeck, 2001). One "effective primary prevention strategy" (Brenner, Smith, & Overpeck, 1994, p. 1607) for which there is a body of supporting evidence is the erection of barriers around domestic pools, in the form of a fence, "5 and preferably 6 feet high, surrounding all four sides of the pool, with a self-closing and locking gate with a latch near the top" (Wilson et al., 1991, p. 226). Early evidence of the success of this strategy was provided by ecological studies which showed that drowning rates were lower in communities with laws requiring pool fencing than in those without (Milliner, Pearn, & Guard, 1980; Pearn, Wong, Brown, Ching, Bart, & Hammar, 1979). Further evidence of the effectiveness of mandatory pool fencing was provided by case–control studies (Fergusson, Horwood, & Shannon, 1983; Pitt & Balanda, 1991). Pitt and Balanda (1991), for example, reported that the risk of drowning or near-drowning incidents in unfenced pools was four times greater than in fenced pools (RR = 3.76, CI = 2.14–6.62). The Centers for Disease Control and Prevention (CDC) has estimated that 51 percent of the reported drowning and near-drowning among those four-and-under in Maricopa County, Arizona, could have been prevented by fencing (Flood, Aickin, Englender, & Tucker, 1990).

Contrary evidence has recently been reported, however, by Morgenstern, Bingham, and Reza (2000). These researchers found that in Los Angeles County there was no difference in the rate of childhood drowning in pools subject to fencing regulations when compared to those not regulated. They concluded that this may have been because the regulations did not require isolation fencing (i.e., fencing on all four sides of the pool as opposed to fencing which permits direct access from the house to the pool), inadequate operation or maintenance of fences by pool owners, or inadequate enforcement by relevant authorities. A survey of local government agencies responsible for administration of the New Zealand domestic pool fencing law, introduced in 1987, found that there was inadequate monitoring and enforcement of compliance with the law (Morrison, Chalmers, Langley, Alsop, & McBean, 1999). Of the estimated 60,000 domestic swimming pools in New Zealand in 1997, 10 years after introduction of the law, only 47 percent were known to comply with the law, 20 percent were known to be non-compliant, and the status of the remaining 33 percent was unknown. In a time series analysis of drowning in domestic pools in Queensland, Australia, Pitt, and Balanda (1998) found that drowning decreased from 12 per year in

1982–1991 to 2 per year in 1992–1994, following the introduction of mandatory fencing, and then increased to 11 per year in 1995–1997. These and other authors have recommended increased enforcement of pool fencing laws, as well public education in the need for compliance (Cass et al., 1996; Morrison et al., 1999; Pitt & Balanda, 1998).

Smoke Alarms. The risk of death due to housefire is greatest among young children and the elderly (Baker et al., 1992). By providing occupants with an early warning, smoke detectors can substantially reduce the risk of death in residential fires (ISCAIP, 1999). The strongest evidence of this protective effect was provided by a case–control study of risk factors for fatal residential fires reported by Runyan, Bangdiwala, Linzer, Sacks, and Butts (1992). These authors found that 77 percent of fatal and 50 percent of non-fatal fires occurred in homes without smoke detectors and estimated that the risk of dying in a house fire was 3.4 times greater when there was no detector. In a subsequent study involving the same investigators, the presence of a functioning smoke detector was found to significantly reduce the risk of death (OR = 0.39, CI = 0.18–0.83) (Marshall, Runyan, Bangdiwala, Linzer, Sacks, & Butts, 1998). Many countries and states within countries have laws requiring the installation of smoke detectors (ISCAIP, 1999). In a study of two affluent US communities, McLoughlin, Marchone, Hanger, German, and Baker (1985) found that legislation requiring the retrofitting of smoke detectors was successful in increasing the number of homes with detectors and in reducing the risk of residential fire deaths. From a systematic review of controlled trials of interventions, DiGuiseppi and Higgins (2000) concluded that providing safety advice as part of routine child health surveillance increased the likelihood of families owning a smoke detector, having a functioning detector, or of acquiring a detector. Programs in which smoke detectors are given away to residents in high risk neighborhoods have been shown to be successful in increasing the installation of detectors and reducing the risk of fire-related injury (Mallonee et al., 1996; Schwartz, Grisso, Miles, Holmes, & Sutton, 1993). DiGuiseppi and Higgins (2000) argue, however, that because these trials were non-randomized their effects may have been exaggerated. In a recent editorial, Roberts and DiGuiseppi (1999) have cautioned that neither legislation nor giveaway programs "will necessarily increase the prevalence of *functioning* alarms" and have called for more reliable evidence on both the effectiveness and cost-effectiveness of interventions.

STRATEGIES THAT MIGHT WORK

Factors that contribute to the risk of child pedestrian injuries are traffic volume, speed, and socioeconomic status, with children in economically disadvantaged areas being exposed to higher volumes of traffic, traffic traveling at higher speeds, and a greater number of road crossings (Kypri et al., 2000). The most promising solution to this problem appears to be modification of the traffic environment to separate children from motor vehicles or to reduce the volume and/or speed of traffic. A collection of measures commonly known as traffic calming, including closing off residential streets, speed bumps, narrowing of roadways, and substantial reductions in speed limits have been shown to reduce traffic volume and speed in residential neighborhoods (Dowswell, Towner, Simpson, & Jarvis, 1996; Rivara & Grossman, 1996; Van Houten & Malenfant, 1992; Vis, Dijkstra, & Slop 1992). A reduction in pedestrian injuries following the introduction of traffic calming in Denmark has been reported (Engel & Thomsen, 1992).

Many childhood injuries are associated with consumer products such as nursery furniture (cots and cribs), prams and strollers, baby walkers, playground equipment and trampolines (Watson, Ozanne-Smith, & Lough, 2000). A common strategy adopted with regard to consumer products is to develop and promote a safety standard. Compliance with such standards is often voluntary. While this strategy may work, there is little evidence of its effectiveness. For example, New Zealand's mortality rate for infant suffocation is almost twice that of the United States (Kypri et al., 2000; Langley & Smeijers, 1997). The majority of infant deaths from suffocation occur in the sleeping environment and involve wedging/entrapment in components of cribs, suspension between cots and walls or other furniture (e.g., chests of drawers), and strangulation by clothing, toys, or blind and curtain cords. While there are design standards for cribs, there is no evidence of their effectiveness, and maintenance and correct placement (away from walls, other furniture and cords) are dependent on parental action (Nixon, Kemp, Levene, & Sibert, 1995). Warning labels and the implementation of a voluntary standard to remove loops from blind cords appear to have had no impact on infant deaths in the United States (Rauchschwalbe & Mann, 1997).

Another strategy that has been widely adopted but for which little reliable evidence is yet available, is community based injury prevention programs (Dowswell et al., 1996). The model for these is the much-publicized Falkoping (Sweden) *Accident Prevention Programme* (Schelp, 1987). Such programs generally target a range of injuries, involve multiple strategies and promote interagency collaboration. The *Lidkoping Accident Prevention Programme*, a sister to the Falkoping Programme, is claimed to have produced an average reduction in injury hospitalizations of 2 percent per annum over the period 1983–1991 (Svanstrom, Ekman, Schelp, & Lindstrom, 1995). Langley and Alsop (1996), however, have criticized the statistical approach taken by

Svanstrom et al. and have argued that any reduction in injury that might have occurred would have been very modest in relation to the substantial resources put into the program.

STRATEGIES THAT DO NOT WORK

In the overview of strategies provided earlier, we noted that a combination of strategies is often required to achieve success in addressing an injury problem. The examples provided above reinforce this view. From their comprehensive review of "what works" in preventing childhood unintentional injury, Dowswell et al. (1996) concluded that "the most successful interventions seemed to be those where the three approaches (legislation, environmental changes, and education) are combined." What does not appear to work are public relations campaigns alone and education-only interventions. When they can get published, negative examples, such as Rauchschwalbe and Mann (1997), are unequivocal. In an early demonstration of this, Robertson, Kelley, Wixom, Eiswirth, and Haddon (1974) conducted a controlled study of the effect of a television campaign on car safety belt use. They developed a series of television messages promoting safety belt use, which were shown for nine consecutive months on one cable of a dual cable television system designed for marketing research. From observations made of safety belt use in the neighborhoods served by the television system, the investigators concluded that the campaign had no effect on safety belt use. Similarly, an elaborate evaluation of *Boston's Project Burn Prevention* failed to prove that the educational program had any impact on injury incidence or severity (MacKay & Rothman, 1982). From their systematic review of controlled trials of interventions to promote smoke alarms, DiGuiseppi and Higgins (2000) concluded that counseling or education alone was "likely to have only a modest effect, if any, on smoke alarm ownership, function, or acquisition."

Conventional, office-based health education by physicians, by itself, has yet to be shown to have any effect on childhood injury. In a comprehensive review of childhood injury prevention counseling in primary care settings, Bass et al. (1993) identified 65 articles addressing childhood unintentional injury prevention counseling, reduced these to 20 that were original reports from primary care settings, and grouped the 20 according to the quality of the evidence as defined by the US Preventive Services Task Force. Among the 20, seven were randomized controlled studies, and five of these reported some positive effect. Of the five, only two included physician counseling. The positive outcomes for these two, however, did not include injury occurrence. In other words, among those studies of physician counseling whose evidence was obtained from a "properly designed randomized

controlled trial" (Bass et al., 1993, p. 546), there were no effects on child injuries, only on knowledge and behaviors.

SYNTHESIS

Many more studies on injury prevention and control are needed to allow definitive recommendations to be made for effective injury prevention programs. Furthermore, what we know comes mainly from studies in developed countries. The injury picture may look different between developed and developing countries, among developing countries themselves, and between different parts of any given country such as Vietnam. Nevertheless, two strong messages emerge from this review. First is that legislation and regulation are almost always necessary to achieve meaningful injury control policy. A recent report by Deal, Gomby, Zippiroli, and Behrman (2000) contends that implementing policy changes by law to reduce speed limits in residential areas, require children to wear bicycle helmets and force homeowners to erect fences around home swimming pools could eliminate 19,000 deaths and injuries among children ages 1–19 years. Experience with the use of seat belts and child auto safety restraints would suggest that enforcement is necessary for the new laws to have the most effect (Insurance Institute for Highway Safety, 2000).

Second, one may conclude that a combination of legislation, enforcement, education and counseling would be more effective than any one of these alone. Without legislation, education's effects are weak to nil, but with legislation, education and counseling can help inform parents and advise them how to meet the letter and spirit of the law. For example, more than 20 years after Tennessee passed the first child auto safety seat legislation in the United States, the majority of parents still use these safety devices incorrectly (Taft, Mikelide, & Taft, 1999).

Finally, no review of injury prevention can be complete without a comment about alcohol. In the case of adolescents and adults, alcohol use directly increases the risk of virtually every possible serious injury. But alcohol use by adults also increases the risk of injury among the children they care for. This is the case when alcohol impairs the judgment and the reaction time of adults responsible for supervising children playing in water; increases the risk of housefire death (Marshall et al., 1998); and increases the risk of motor vehicle injury because the driver (usually the one in the car with the child, according to Quinlan, Brewer, Sleet, & Dellinger, 2000) is drunk. As with other injury interventions, policy changes rather than education alone are necessary. In addition to increasing the legal drinking age to 21 as has occurred in the United States, increasing the cost of alcohol through taxation and restricting the sale of alcohol around recreational water areas and convenience stores which also sell gasoline and/or service automobiles will be necessary.

Also see: Injuries, Unintentional: Childhood; Injuries, Unintentional: Adolescence; Injuries, Unintentional, Occupational: Adulthood; Environmental Health: Early Childhood.

References

Assargaard, U., & Sjoberg, G. (1995). The successful introduction of child resistant closures for liquid paracetamol preparations. *Safety Science, 21*, 87–91.

Baker, S.P., O'Neill, B.O., Ginsburg, M.J., & Li, G. (1992). *The Injury Fact Book* (2nd ed.). New York: Oxford.

Bass, J.L., Christoffel, K.K., Widome, M., Boyle, Scheidt, P., Stanwick, R., & Roberts, K. (1993). Childhood injury prevention counseling in primary care settings: A critical review of the literature. *Pediatrics, 92*, 544–550.

Brenner, R.A., Smith, G.S., & Overpeck, M.D. (1994). Divergent trends in drowning rates—US 1971–1988. *Journal of the American Medical Association, 271*, 1606–1608.

Brenner, R.A., Trumble, A.C., Smith, G.S., Kessler, E.P., & Overpeck, M.D. (2001). Where children drown, US, 1995. *Pediatrics, 101*(1), 85–90.

Cass, D.T., Ross, F., & Lam, L.T. (1996). Childhood drowning in New South Wales 1990–1995: A population-based study. *Medical Journal of Australia, 165*, 610–612.

Clarke, A., & Walton, W.W. (1979). Effect of safety packaging on aspirin ingestions by children. *Pediatrics, 63*, 687–693.

Deal, L.W., Gomby, D.S., Zippiroli, L., & Behrman, R.E. (2000). Unintentional injuries in children: analysis and recommendations. *The Future of Children, 10*(1), 4–22.

DiGuiseppi, C., & Higgins, J.P. (2000). Systematic review of controlled trials of interventions to promote smoke alarms. *Archives of Disease in Childhood, 82*, 341–348.

Dowswell, T., Towner, E.M.L., Simpson, G., & Jarvis, S.N. (1996). Preventing childhood unintentional injuries—what works? A literature review. *Injury Prevention, 2*, 140–149.

Engel, U., & Thomsen, L.K. (1992). Safety effects of speed reducing measures in Danish residential areas. *Accident Analysis and Prevention, 24*, 17–28.

Fergusson, D.M., Horwood, L.J., & Shannon, F.T. (1983). The safety standards of domestic swimming pools 1980–1982. *New Zealand Medical Journal, 96*, 93–95.

Flood, T.J., Aickin, M., Englender, S.J., & Tucker, D. (1990). Child drownings and near-drownings associated with swimming pools—Maricopa County, Arizona, 1988 and 1989. *Morbidity and Mortality Weekly Report, 39*, 441–442.

Gallagher, S.S., Finison, K., Guyer, B., & Goodenough, S. (1984). The incidence of injuries among 87,000 Massachusetts children and adolescents: results of the 1980–81 Statewide Childhood Injury Prevention Program Surveillance System. *American Journal of Public Health, 74*(12), 1340–1346.

Gellert, G.A. (1995). The influence of market economics on primary health care in Vietnam. *Journal of the American Medical Association, 273*(19), 1498–1502.

Haddon, W. (1980). Advances in the epidemiology of injuries as a basis for public policy. *Public Health Reports, 95*, 411–421.

Insurance Institute for Highway Safety. (2000, December). *Best & worst state traffic safety laws: Some states do a better job than others*

[on-line]. Available: http://www.highwaysafety.org/news_releases/2000/pr122000.htm [cited] July 20, 2001.

ISCAIP Smoke Detector Legislation Collaborators. (1999). International smoke detector Legislation. *Injury Prevention 5*, 254–255.

Kypri, K., Chalmers, D.J., Langley, J.D., & Wright, C.S. (2000). Child injury mortality in New Zealand 1986–95. *Journal of Paediatrics and Child Health, 36*, 431–439.

Kypri, K., Chalmers, D.J., Langley, J.D., & Wright, C.S. (2001). Child injury morbidity in New Zealand, 1987–1996. *Journal of Paediatrics and Child Health. 37*(3), 227–234.

Langley, J.D., & Alsop, J.C. (1996). Lidkoping accident prevention programme: What was the impact? *Injury Prevention, 2*, 131–134.

Langley, J.D., & Smeijers, J. (1997). Injury mortality among children and teenagers in New Zealand compared with the United States of America. *Injury Prevention, 3*(3), 195–199.

Litovitz, T.L., Schmitz, B.F., & Holm, K.C. (1989). 1988 annual report of the American Association of Poison Control Centers National Data Collection System. *American Journal of Emergency Medicine, 7*, 495–545.

MacKay, A.M., & Rothman, K.J. (1982). The incidence and severity of burn injuries following Project Burn Prevention. *American Journal of Public Health, 72*(3), 248–252.

Mallonee, S., Istre, G.R., Rosenberg, M., Reddish-Douglas, M., Jordan, F., Silverstein, P., & Tunell, W. (1996). Surveillance and prevention of residential-fire injuries. *New England Journal of Medicine, 335*(1), 27–31.

Margolis, L.H., Wagenaar, A.C., & Molnar, L.J. (1988). Recognizing the common problem of child automobile restraint misuse. *Pediatrics, 81*, 717–720.

Marshall, S.W., Runyan, C.W., Bangdiwala, S., Linzer, M.A., Sacks, J.J., & Butts, J.D. (1998). Fatal residential fires. Who dies and who survives? *Journal of the American Medical Association, 279*(20), 1633–1637.

McLoughlin, E.M., Marchone, L., Hanger, P.S., German, P.S., & Baker, S.P. (1985). Smoke detector legislation: Its effect on owner-occupied homes. *American Journal of Public Health, 75*, 858–862.

Milliner, N., Pearn, J., & Guard, R. (1980). Will fenced pools save lives? A 10-year study from Mulgrave Shire, Queensland. *Medical Journal of Australia, 2*, 510–511.

Mock, C.N., Forjuoh, S.N., & Rivara, F.P. (1999). Epidemiology of transportation-related injuries in Ghana. *Accident Analysis and Prevention, 31*(4), 359–370.

Mock, C.N., Abantanga, F., Cummings, P., & Koepsell, T.D. (1999). Incidence and outcome of injury in Ghana: A community-based survey. *Bulletin of the World Health Organization, 77*(12), 955–964.

Morgenstern, H., Bingham, T., & Reza, A. (2000). Effects of pool-fencing ordinances and other factors on childhood drowning in Los Angeles County, 1990–1995. *American Journal of Public Health, 90*, 595–601.

Morrison, L., Chalmers, D.J., Langley, J.D., Alsop, J.C., & McBean, C. (1999). Achieving compliance with pool fencing legislation in New Zealand: A survey of regulatory authorities. *Injury Prevention, 5*, 114–118.

National Committee for Injury Prevention and Control. (1989). Injury prevention: Meeting the challenge. *American Journal of Preventive Medicine, 5*(Suppl.), 1–303.

National Highway Transport Safety Administration (NHTSA). (1999). Final economic assessment: Child restraint systems, child restraint anchorage systems. Washington, DC: US Department of Transportation.

National Safety Council. (2000). Injury facts. *Deaths due to unintentional injuries, 1998* [on-line]. Available: www.nsc.org/lrs/statinfo/99008.htm [cited] July 1, 2001.

Nixon, J.W., Kemp, A.M., Levene, S., & Sibert, J.R. (1995). Suffocation, choking, and strangulation in childhood in England and Wales: Epidemiology and prevention. *Archives of Disease in Childhood, 72*(1), 6–10.

Office of Statistics and Programming, NCIPC, CDC. (2000a). *10 leading causes of death, US, 1998, all races, both sexes* [on-line]. Available: http://webapp.cdc.gov/sasweb/ncpic/leadcaus.html [cited] July 1, 2001.

Office of Statistics and Programming, NCIPC, CDC. (2000b). *All injury death rates per 100,000, all races, both sexes* [on-line]. Available: http://webapp.cdc.gov/sasweb/ncpic/mortrate.html [cited] July 1, 2001.

Pearn, J.H., Wong, R.Y., Brown, J., III, Ching, Y.C., Bart, R., Jr., & Hammar, S. (1979). Drowning and near-drowning involving children: A five-year total population study from the City and County of Honolulu. *American Journal of Public Health, 69,* 450–454.

Pitt, R.W., & Balanda, K.P. (1991). Childhood drowning and near-drowning in Brisbane: The contribution of domestic pools. *Medical Journal of Australia 154,* 661–665.

Pitt, W.R., & Balanda, K.P. (1998). Toddler drownings in domestic swimming pools in Queensland since uniform fencing requirements. *Medical Journal of Australia, 169,* 557–558.

Quinlan, K.P., Brewer, R.D., Sleet, D.A., & Dellinger, A.M. (2000). Characteristics of child passenger deaths and injuries involving drinking drivers. *Journal of the American Medical Association, 283*(17), 2249–2252.

Rauchschwalbe, R., & Mann, N.C. (1997). Pediatric window-cord strangulations in the United States, 1981–1995 [see comments]. *Journal of the American Medical Association, 277*(21), 1696–1698.

Rivara, F.P., & Grossman, D.C. (1996). Prevention of traumatic deaths to children in the United States: How far have we come and where do we need to go? *Pediatrics, 97,* 791–797.

Roberts, I., & DiGuiseppi, C. (1999). Smoke alarms, fire deaths, and randomised controlled trials. *Injury Prevention, 5,* 244–245.

Robertson, L.S., Kelley, A.B., Wixom, C.W., Eiswirth, R.S., & Haddon, W. (1974). A controlled study of the effect of television messages on safety belt use. *American Journal of Public Health, 64,* 1071–1080.

Rodgers, G.B. (1996). The safety effects of child-resistant packaging for oral prescription drugs. Two decades of experience. *Journal of the American Medical Association, 275,* 1661–1665.

Runyan, C.W., Bangdiwala, S.I., Linzer, M.A., Sacks, J.J., & Butts, J. (1992). Risk factors for fatal residential fire deaths. *New England Journal of Medicine, 327,* 859–863.

Schelp, L. (1987). Community intervention and changes in accident pattern in a rural Swedish municipality. *Health Promotion, 2,* 109–125.

Schwartz, D.F., Grisso, J.A., Miles, C., Holmes, J.H., & Sutton, R.L. (1993). An injury prevention programme in an urban African-American community. *American Journal of Public Health, 83,* 675–680.

Sibert, J.R., Craft, A.W., & Jackson, R.H. (1977). Child-resistant packaging and accidental child poisoning. *Lancet, 2,* 289–290.

Svanstrom, L., Ekman, R., Schelp, L., & Lindstrom, A. (1995). The Lidkoping Accident Prevention Programme—a community approach to preventing childhood injuries in Sweden. *Injury Prevention, 1,* 169–172.

Taft, C.H., Mikelide, A.D., & Taft, A.R. (1999, February). *Child passengers at risk in America: A national study of car seat misuse.* Washington, DC: National Safe Kids Campaign.

Tuong Chu Van, & Quang Van Tran (1995). Injuries in children under 15 years in Hanoi. *Vietnam Pediatric Association, 4*(2), 38–40.

UNICEF. (n.d.). *The safe Vietnam initiative. Protecting children from preventable injuries* [on-line]. Available: www.unicef.org/vietnam/safevn1.htm [cited] July 1, 2001.

UNICEF. (2001). *A league table of child deaths by injury in rich nations. Innocenti report card 2.* Florence: Unicef Innocenti Research Centre.

Unicef Vietnam. (2000). *The situation of women and children in Vietnam 2000* [on-line]. Available: http://www.unicef.org/vietnam/sitan1.htm [cited] July 19, 2001.

Van Houten R., & Malenfant, L. (1992). The influence of signs prompting motorists to yield before marked crosswalks on motor vehicle-pedestrian conflicts at crosswalks with flashing amber. *Accident Analysis and Prevention, 24*(3), 217–225.

Vis, A.A., Dijkstra, A., & Slop, M. (1992). Safety effects of 30 Km/H zones in the Netherlands. *Accident Analysis and Prevention, 24*(1), 75–86.

Walton, W.W. (1982). An evaluation of the Poison Prevention Packaging Act. *Pediatrics, 69,* 363–370.

Watson, W., Ozanne-Smith, J., & Lough, J. (2000). *Consumer product-related injury to children.* Clayton: Monash University Accident Research Centre.

Wilson, M.H., Baker, S.P., Teret, S.P., Shock, S., & Garbarino, J. (1991). *Saving children: A guide to injury prevention.* New York: Oxford University Press.

Wintemute, G.J. (1990). Childhood drowning and near-drowning in the United States. *American Journal of Diseases of Children, 144,* 663–669.

World Health Organization. (1999). *Injury: a leading cause of the global burden of disease* [on-line]. Available: www.who.int/violence_injury_prevention/injury/InjuryBoDtables.htm [cited] July 1, 2001.

Injuries, Unintentional, Childhood

Kristi Alexander and
Michael C. Roberts

INTRODUCTION

Unintentional injuries (also referred to as non-intentional or inadvertent injuries) are the leading cause of death for children in both the United States (Rodriguez, 1990) and Canada (Canadian Institute of Child Health, 1994). The terms "accident" and "accidental injuries" have been largely abandoned because of the implication inherent in those terms that injuries are unavoidable, random events that cannot be decreased or eliminated (Roberts, 1993; Rosen & Peterson, 1990). Indeed, injuries are perceived by most as resulting from behavioral and environmental factors that interact in such a way as to result in harm to an individual. Consequently, interest in developing effective ways to prevent unintentional injuries has grown significantly. To date, prevention efforts have been focused on three different targets: children, their parents and caregivers, and the environment. Legislative, educational, and other types of interventions have been used to affect these targets. Several programs have been very successful in reducing injury to children, although more work is needed to help children live safe and healthy lives.

DEFINITIONS

In contrast to intentional injuries, *unintentional injuries* are those that result from events that are *not* willfully precipitated by the actions of another person. A child who breaks an arm falling from a scooter is said to have sustained an unintentional injury, while the same injury, resulting from the actions of an abusive parent, is considered to be an intentional injury. This distinction, however, has been recently challenged by Peterson (1994) and others as imprecise, and possibly erroneous, in many instances.

Two general categories of prevention are employed to describe injury control programs: passive and active. *Passive prevention* occurs when the person being protected does not have to do much to gain prevention benefit, whereas in *active prevention* the person must do something on a regular basis in order to prevent injuries. For example, airbags and automatic seatbelts in cars are passive prevention mechanisms because the protection is present whether or not the car passenger does anything. In contrast, having to buckle up every time a person rides in a car is active prevention.

SCOPE

Each year, countless young children experience trauma, disability, and death as the result of an unintended injury. In the United States, approximately 22,000 children die and 30,000 become permanently disabled as the result of unintentional injuries (Rodriguez, 1990). These rates are higher than in other industrialized countries (Tremblay & Peterson, 1999).

Unintentional injuries are not only potentially lethal, they are costly. Care for injuries is the leading cause of medical spending for children from 5 to 21 years of age (Moody-Williams et al., 2000). In 1994, the estimated cost of treatment for pediatric injuries was over 3 billion dollars (Ray & Yuniler, 1994) and when considering both indirect and direct costs, the annual estimated cost of injury to children surpasses 7.5 billion (Rodriguez, 1990).

The costs associated with unintentional injuries are not limited to medical care. Parents and other family members may experience pecuniary penalties as a result of injury to their child. In one study, a month after discharge almost 60 percent of parents whose children had sustained minor injuries and were in the hospital for one day (or less) reported financial and/or work difficulties as a result of the injury (Osberg, Kahn, Rowe, & Brooke, 1996). Middle-income families, according to Osberg et al. (1996), appear to be most financially affected by injury because of limited financial resources and being ineligible for means-based services that may be available to low SES families. Furthermore,

over 40 percent of parents in this study at one month post-injury reported missing time from work because of medical appointments for their injured child and 30 percent reported cutting back time at work to care for their child (Osberg et al., 1996). Changes such as these may result in decreased productivity (Moody-Williams et al., 2000).

Similarly, injuries are expensive for schools. School nurses spend a considerable portion of their workday caring for injured children. In a 2-year period, over 80 percent of elementary school students will visit the nurse for an injury-related problem (SAFE KIDS, n.d.).

Lastly, the emotional toll to children and families from unintentional pediatric injuries cannot be overlooked. Aaron, Zaglul, and Emery (1999) found that one month post-hospitalization for an acute injury, over 22 of children met the diagnostic criteria for Post-Traumatic Stress Disorder (PTSD) and half of all subjects were experiencing "considerable distress" (p. 340). Another study examining the impact of pedestrian injuries found that 25 percent of injured children and 15 percent of parents met the diagnostic criteria for PTSD at 7–12 months post injury (de Vries, Kassam-Adams, Cnaan, Sherman-Slate, Gallagher, & Winston, 1999). The results of a similar study of traffic injuries found that 4–7 months post-injury, 33 percent of children were described by their parents as having a moderate stress reaction, while 11 percent of children were described as severely affected (Ellis, Stores, & Mayou, 1998).

THEORIES AND RESEARCH

One model used to understand injuries and their prevention is the *public health* model of host, agent, and environment. This public health model was first applied to the problem of injuries by Haddon (1980), and then specifically to pediatric injuries by Robertson (1981). In this model, unintentional injuries result when there is a transfer of energy by an agent to a vulnerable host. Inherent in this model is a realization that energy (e.g., electricity, heat, chemicals, etc.) exists, and that a particular agent may or may not serve as a dangerous conduit. For example, while a bottle (the environment) contains potential dangerous toxins (the agent), injuries result when the bottle is not child-safe. Further, inherent in this model is that characteristics of the host influence safety and injury risk. Toddlers with their smaller bodies and developing systems are more susceptible to potential toxins. Children's delicate skin is more vulnerable to burns from hot water than is the skin of an adult.

The use of this model allows a partial understanding of the sex differences in childhood unintentional injuries. Boys, who are at greater risk for unintentional injuries (Rivara, Bergman, LoGerfo, & Weiss, 1982), are more likely to come in contact with agents that increase their risk for injury. For example, boys sustain more bicycle-related injuries because they ride bicycles more than do girls (Rivara et al., 1982).

Another model applied to preventive health behaviors has been *Protection Motivation Theory* (PMT; Rogers, 1975). In this model, protection motivation is directly influenced by one's beliefs in three areas: self-efficacy (beliefs about one's ability to engage in a preventive behavior), response efficacy (beliefs about the effectiveness of a prevention behavior), and response costs (beliefs about the psychological and monetary costs to engage in the preventive behavior). Factors effecting these beliefs include the perception of one's personal vulnerability to a particular threat and the perception of the threat as severe. PMT has been used to predict compliance with a variety of health behaviors such as preventive asthma medication (Bennett, Rowe, & Katz, 1998) and exercise for cardiac patients (Plotnikoff & Higginbotham, 1998), but has been rarely applied to the prevention of unintentional injuries in childhood

One application of PMT to injury prevention examined children's adaptive and maladaptive coping beliefs regarding bicycle helmet use (McElreath, 1995). PMT would predict that children would engage in the preventive behavior if they perceived themselves as able to consistently wear a helmet (self-efficacy) and that wearing a helmet would protect them from injury (response efficacy), but the expected relationships were not found. Another PMT study, also examining bicycle helmet use, targeted caregivers' intentions to purchase helmets for their children (Miller, 1993). Miller found that, although parents' perceptions of their child's risk for head injury and intentions to prevent injury by purchasing a helmet were consistent with PMT, few parents in her study actually engaged in the required behavior. Further applications of PMT to the behavior of parents and other caregivers would appear warranted to understand the factors that inhibit injury control behaviors.

Other psychological theories are mentioned as relevant to injury prevention, such as *social learning theory* and applications of modeling by adults wearing bicycle helmets and demonstrating safe swimming practices, for example. Although safety campaigns have often used high status models to encourage safety actions, apparently very little research has been conducted to demonstrate effectiveness. Undoubtedly, however, safety behavior is imitated everyday (as are unsafe behaviors) and the processes of enhancing modeling effects for positive effects have not been clearly explicated.

Two related theoretical models, the Health Belief Model and the Theory of Planned Behavior, might be applicable to understanding how preventive actions are influenced. Partial evidence has been demonstrated with bicycle helmets and helmets used by college age in-line skaters, but these have not been adequately investigated in terms of childhood injuries (Quine, Rutter, & Arnold, 2000; Williams-Avery & MacKinnon, 1996).

STRATEGIES: OVERVIEW

Parents and other caregivers often try to create safe environments for children where hazards are controlled to reduce injuries such as "safety-proofing" a home or day care center by putting in child-resistant locks on cabinets and inserts or coverings on electrical sockets. There is considerable research evidence for the efficacy of passive and environment prevention. However, not all injuries are amenable to passive prevention. Consequently, active behavioral change may be necessary for the more difficult injury-causing situations. Active prevention in the form of direct supervision is one of the most important applications. Thus, a combination of both active and passive interventions is necessary. Typically considered passive prevention interventions are the overlapping approaches of environmental changes and legislative mandates.

STRATEGIES THAT WORK

Environmental Manipulations.   Infants and children are unable to control their own environments to be safer. Thus, adults need to take preventive action. The introduction of child-proof containers for medications and poisons is a prime example of a most effective intervention of this type. As a result, children are unable to access substances that could harm them, and poisonings have decreased substantially (Walton, 1982). Similarly, installing bars or guards on above ground windows has been shown to prevent falls by toddlers (Spiegel & Lindaman, 1977). Requiring the installation of smoke detectors and fire alarms may be considered an environmental approach to burn prevention that significantly reduces deaths and non-fatal injuries (Hall, 1994).

Legislative Approaches.   As noted, legislation may be passed, rules and standards may be imposed from local, state, and federal governmental bodies in order to protect children. These may regulate consumer products such as making refrigerators easier to open if a child is trapped inside, lowering temperatures for water heaters to prevent burns, mandating flame-retardant sleepwear, regulating crib construction, and installing air bags in cars. Legislation can also regulate behavior, such as speed limit laws, drunk driving laws, or age limits on when children can be left at home unsupervised. State laws requiring children to be buckled into car safety seats at young ages or seat belts at older ages are effective injury control measures (Wagenaar, Maybee, & Sullivan, 1988). Bicycle helmet laws increase their use (Dannenberg, Gielen, Beilenson, Wilson, & Joffe, 1993). Almost any proposed legislation for safety purposes places limitations or financial costs on some person or group (e.g., business) and often raises controversy. Not all unsafe behavior or products can be regulated, but there exists substantial evidence for effectiveness in the relatively few areas where legislation or rule-making has taken place. Given the controversy over regulating behavior or business, and the fact that many unsafe situations are not amenable to effective intervention this way, other forms of injury prevention are implemented.

Caregiver Interventions. Caregivers can take action to improve the safety of children's environments and behaviors. For example, child care centers can put energy-absorbing materials around properly maintained playground equipment and remove hazards. Parents can make similar changes to their homes to improve safety and can be taught to take actions such as lowering water heater temperatures and removing frayed electrical cords (Tertinger, Greene, & Lutzker, 1984). Supervision of children at home and at play is a primary parental responsibility, although research suggests that there is no consensus regarding what is safe and what is not (Peterson, Ewigman, & Kivlahan, 1993).

Community Interventions. Some injury prevention occurs through community-wide programs, often through voluntary alliances or civic groups. For example, a series of projects to reward children with stickers, notebooks, and pizza coupons increased their riding in cars buckled into seatbelts (Roberts, Layfield, & Fanurik, 1991). A school-based intervention for spinal cord injury prevention found improvements in children's knowledge and some behaviors (Richards, Hendricks, & Roberts, 1991). Home visiting programs by nurses where at-risk parents were provided child health and safety information and social support resulted in fewer injuries and poisonings (Olds & Kitzman, 1990). A community-based program on childhood injury prevention in a rural area of Sweden educated parents about safety equipment and behaviors. The results indicated a significant decrease in injuries through use of safety locks, electrical outlet covers, and helmets for cycling and sledding (Schelp, 1987). Zins, Garcia, Tuchfarber, Clark, and Laurence (1994) reported on a successful community intervention promulgated by Cincinnati Children's Hospital. A comprehensive approach through medical settings, loaner programs, law enforcement, and multimedia campaigns resulted in improved safety seat and seat belt use. Similarly, the *Seattle Children's Bicycle Helmet Campaign* used the media, schools, and medical professionals to increase the purchase and use of bicycle helmets. Observed use of the helmets went up, and correspondingly, head trauma requiring medical

attention went down moderately (Bergman, Rivara, Richards, & Rogers, 1990; Rivara et al., 1994). The *Harlem Safe Kids/Health Neighborhoods Injury Prevention Program* is another excellent example of a community public health campaign to reduce falls, assaults, guns, and motor vehicle related injuries (Davidson, Durkin, Kuhn, O'Connor, Barlow, & Heagarty, 1994). A coalition of agencies and civic groups focused on improving and supervising playgrounds along with traffic safety training for children. The involvement by the community in direct action resulted in injury reduction.

STRATEGIES THAT MIGHT WORK

Most effective community programs target specific safety behaviors, other community programs may be more generally applicable to a number of injury causing situations. The national and local SAFE KIDS coalition has not been fully evaluated, but is an example of community interventions to create a general atmosphere of support and knowledge about safety (National Committee for Injury Prevention and Control, 1989). Whether specific or general, community wide programs promote generalizability of safety behaviors.

STRATEGIES THAT DO NOT WORK

Caregiver Focused Interventions. Throughout the history of injury prevention programs, much hope, energy, and financial resources have been devoted to providing information to parents and caregivers about injury and preventive actions in order to educate them to create safe environments. These information activities have been done in physicians' offices and community settings such as malls and schools. Unfortunately, despite their ubiquity, these health education programs have not been shown to be very effective in changing behavior (Cushman, James, & Waclawik, 1991; Dershewitz & Williamson, 1977; Pless & Arsenault, 1985; Thomas, Hasseinen, & Christophersen, 1984). Some of these programs have distributed safety equipment for parents to use such as cabinet locks, smoke detectors, or car safety seats and still have failed to demonstrate consistent effects. Thus, educational campaigns may provide basic information to parents, but are rarely sufficient to motivate safety behavior without significant contingencies.

Child-Focused Interventions. Other safety interventions have targeted the children and adolescents themselves. Adolescents may have increasing ability to control the safety of their environments, however, children rarely do. Much of the focus is to get them to take safety precautions.

Similar to adult education campaigns, mere provision of information to children does not itself change unsafe behaviors. For example, the "Mr. Yuk" campaign, through education and counseling, was designed to reduce poisonings, but did not produce significant effects (Fergusson, Horwood, Beautrais, & Shannon, 1982). The large scale DARE program for drug abuse prevention has yielded few positive results (Ennett, Tobler, Ringwalt, & Flewelling, 1994). Child-oriented safety change can be fostered through behaviorally based skills enhancement interventions such as safe behavior at home alone after school (Peterson, 1989), evacuation of a home in a fire (Hillman, Jones, & Farmer, 1986), and pedestrian street crossing by young children (Yeaton & Bailey, 1978). Some of these appear to work, at least in the short-term, by instilling safer behaviors. However, over time, the performance of these behaviors tends to decline. Monitoring of behavior and booster session may be necessary to maintain behavior change. Some professionals express concern that giving responsibility to children for their own safety is misplaced and inappropriate. Furthermore, there is concern that parents and other caregivers will decrease the vigilance and supervision in the erroneous belief that a child has been "safety-proofed" by swimming lessons, instructions in gun safety, or admonitions to be careful.

SYNTHESIS

Injury prevention remains a difficult, yet essential task for parents, teachers, community leaders, and legislators. Although passive prevention techniques such as childproof containers and automatic seatbelts, are very effective in preventing injuries, their scope is limited. Furthermore, educating caregivers to provide appropriate supervision are necessary for passive prevention techniques to work. Automatic seatbelts will not protect any child, if a caregiver allows a child to bypass the system.

Active prevention techniques that rely solely on both caregiver implementation and application are fraught with difficulties. The most effective interventions appear to involve all levels of the child's world—from parents, to teachers, to community leaders. Raising children safely does "take a village" and without the coordination of efforts, many parents and caregivers are unable to keep children safe and healthy. As stated in the *Injury Prevention: Meeting the Challenge* report, "it is rare that a single intervention will significantly reduce a complex injury problem" such that preventionists "should carefully consider a mix of legislation/ enforcement/education/behavior change, and engineering/ technology interventions that complement each other and increase the likelihood of success" (National Committee, 1989, p. 72). The evidence for the effectiveness

of coordination may be seen in the increased use of appropriate child restraint devices (i.e., carseats, seatbelts, booster seats) by parents. Although the consistent use of carseats was initially viewed as improbable, the combined effects of legislation and education have resulted in high levels of compliance (US Department of Transportation, 1991). Thus, prevention of injuries may be most successful when behavior is mandated through legislative changes as well as encouraged and supported through community efforts.

Continued research of the behaviors that place children at risk and inhibit the implementation of effective injury control programs is needed. Furthermore, evaluating existing prevention programs is necessary to determine if such programs are having the desired effect on children's injury rates. However, research is only one part of the complex prevention picture; dissemination of the knowledge gained, garnering funding for research and program implementation, lobbying for legislation necessary to change the contingencies for unsafe behaviors, and countless other tasks are necessary for effective injury control. Clearly, an interdisciplinary effort is required to decrease injuries to children and will necessarily involve the contributions of numerous scientific disciplines, governmental agencies, non-governmental organizations, and the public in making all aspects of children's environments safer and conducive to health and development.

Also see: Injuries, Unintentional: Early Childhood; Injuries, Unintentional: Adolescence; Injuries, Unintentional, Occupational: Adulthood; Environmental Health: Childhood.

References

Aaron, J., Zaglul, H., & Emery, R.E. (1999). Posttraumatic stress in children following acute physical injury. *Journal of Pediatric Psychology, 24*, 335–344.

Bennett, P., Rowe, A., & Katz, D. (1998). Reported adherence with preventive asthma medication: A test of protection motivation theory. *Psychology, Health & Medicine, 3*, 347–354.

Bergman, A.B., Rivara, F.P., Richards, D.D., & Rogers, L.W. (1990). The Seattle Children's Bicycle Helmet Campaign. *American Journal of Diseases of Children, 144*, 727–731.

Canadian Institute of Child Health. (1994). *The health of Canada's children* (2nd ed.). Ottawa: Author.

Cushman, R., James, W., & Waclawik, H. (1991). Physicians promoting bicycle helmets for children: A randomized trial. *American Journal of Public Health, 81*, 1044–1046.

Dannenberg, A.L., Gielen, A.C., Beilenson, P.L., Wilson, M.H., & Joffe, A. (1993). Bicycle helmet laws and education campaigns: An evaluation of strategies to increase children's helmet use. *American Journal of Public Health, 83*, 667–674.

Davidson, L.L., Durkin, M.S., Kuhn, L., O'Connor, P., Barlow, B., & Heagarty, M.C. (1994). The impact of the safe kids/healthy neighborhoods injury prevention program in Harlem, 1988–1991. *American Journal of Public Health, 84*, 580–586.

Dershewitz, R.A., & Williamson, J.W. (1977). Prevention of childhood household injuries: A controlled clinical trial. *American Journal of Public Health, 67,* 1148–1153.

de Vries, A.P., Kassam-Adams, N., Cnaan, A., Sherman-Slate, E., Gallagher, P.R., & Winston, F.K. (1999). Looking beyond the physical injury: Posttraumatic stress disorder in children and parents after pediatric traffic injury. *Pediatrics, 104,* 1293–1299.

Ellis, A., Stores, G., & Mayou, R. (1998). Psychological consequences of road traffic accidents in children. *European Child & Adolescent Psychiatry, 7,* 61–68.

Ennett, S.T., Tobler, N.S., Ringwalt, C.L., & Flewelling, R.L. (1994). How effective is drug abuse resistance education? A meta-analysis of Project DARE outcome evaluations. *American Journal of Public Health, 84,* 1394–1401.

Fergusson, D., Horwood, L., Beautrais, A., & Shannon, F. (1982). A controlled field trial of a poisoning prevention program. *Pediatrics, 69,* 515–520.

Haddon, W. (1980). Advances in the epidemiology of injuries as a basis for public policy. *Public Health Reports, 95,* 411–421.

Hall, J.R. (1994). The U.S. experience with smoke detectors. *National Fire Protection Association Journal, 88,* 4.

Hillman, H.S., Jones, R.T., & Farmer, L. (1986). The acquisition and maintenance of fire emergency skills: Effects of rationale and behavioral practice. *Journal of Pediatric Psychology, 11,* 247–258.

McElreath, L.H. (1995). Protection motivation theory and children's modes of coping: Relevance to bicycle helmet usage. (Doctoral dissertation, University of Alabama, 1995). *Dissertation Abstracts International, 55,* 5051.

Miller, K.M. (1993). *A test of protection-motivation theory for promoting injury control.* Unpublished masters thesis, Virginia Polytechnic Institute and State University, Blacksburg.

Moody-Williams, J.D., Athey, J., Barlow, B., Blanton, D., Garrison, H., Mickalide, A., Miller, T., Olson, L., & Skripak, D. (2000). Injury prevention and emergency medical services for children in a managed care environment. *Annals of Emergency Medicine, 35,* 245–51.

National Committee for Injury Prevention and Control. (1989). *Injury prevention: Meeting the challenge.* New York: Oxford University Press.

Olds, L.D., & Kitzman, H. (1990). Can home visitation improve the health of women and children at environmental risk? *Pediatrics, 86,* 108–116.

Osberg, J.S., Kahn, P., Rowe, K., & Brooke, M.M. (1996). Pediatric trauma: Impact on work and family finances. *Pediatrics, 98,* 890–897.

Peterson, L. (1989). Latchkey children's preparation for self-care: Overestimated, underrehearsed, and unsafe. *Journal of Clinical Child Psychology, 18,* 36–43.

Peterson, L. (1994). Child injury and abuse-neglect: Common etiologies, challenges, and courses toward prevention. *Current Directions in Psychological Research, 8,* 116–120.

Peterson, L., Ewigman, B., & Kivlahan, C. (1993). Judgments regarding appropriate child supervision to prevent child injury: The role of environmental risk and child age. *Child Development, 64,* 934–950.

Pless, I.B., & Arsenault, L. (1985). The role of health education in the prevention of injuries to children. *Journal of Social Issues, 43,* 87–104.

Plotnikoff, R.C., & Higginbotham, N. (1998). Protection motivation theory and the prediction of exercise and low-fat diet behaviors among Australian cardiac patients. *Psychology & Health, 13,* 411–429.

Quine, L., Rutter, D., & Arnold, L. (2000). Comparing the theory of planned behaviour and the health belief model: The example of schoolboy cyclists. In P. Norman & C. Abraham (Eds.), *Understanding and changing health behaviors: From health beliefs to self-regulation* (pp. 73–98). Amsterdam: Harwood Academic.

Ray, L.U., & Yuniler, J. (1994). *Child and adolescent fatal injury data book.* Washington, DC: Department of Maternal and Child Health Bureau.

Richards, J.S., Hendricks, C., & Roberts, M.C. (1991). Prevention of spinal cord injury: An elementary education approach. *Journal of Pediatric Psychology, 16,* 595–609.

Rivara, F., Bergman, A., LoGerfo, J., & Weiss, N. (1982). Epidemiology of childhood injuries. *American Journal of Disease in Children, 136,* 502–506.

Rivara, F.P., Thomson, D.C., Thompson, R.S., Rogers, L.W., Alexander, B., Felix, D., & Bergman, A.B. (1994). The Seattle Children's Bicycle Helmet Campaign: Changes in helmet use and head injury admissions. *Pediatrics, 93,* 567–569.

Roberts, M.C. (1993). Special section editorial: Explicating the circumstances of nonintentional injuries in childhood. *Journal of Pediatric Psychology, 18,* 99–103.

Roberts, M.C., Layfield, D.A., & Fanurik, D. (1991). Motivating children's use of car safety devices. In M. Wolraich & D. Routh (Eds.), *Advances in developmental and behavioral pediatrics* (Vol. 10, pp. 61–88). London: Jessica Kingsley.

Robertson, L. (1981). Environmental hazards to children: Assessment and options for amelioration. In *Select panel for the promotion of child health—Better health for our children: A national strategy* (Vol. 1) (DHHS, Public Health Service Publication No. 79-55071). Washington, DC: US Government Printing Office.

Rodriguez, J.G. (1990). Childhood injuries in the United States: A priority issue. *American Journal of Diseases of Children, 144,* 625–626.

Rogers, R.W. (1975). A protection motivation theory of fear appeals and attitude change. *Journal of Psychology, 91,* 93–114.

Rosen, B.N., & Peterson, L. (1990). Gender differences in children's outdoor play injuries: A review and integration. *Clinical Psychology Review, 10,* 187–205.

SAFE KIDS. (n.d.). School/playground safety tips and resources. *National SAFE KIDS campaign: Promoting child safety to prevent unintentional injury* [on-line]. Retrieved December 27, 2000. Available World Wide Web: http://www.safekids.org/tier2_rl.cfm?folder_id=177

Schelp, L. (1987). Community intervention and changes in accident patterns in a rural Swedish municipality. *Health Promotion, 2,* 109–125.

Spiegel, C.N., & Lindaman, F.C. (1977). Children can't fly: A program to prevent childhood morbidity and mortality from window falls. *American Journal of Public Health, 67,* 1143–1147.

Tertinger, D.A., Greene, B.F., & Lutzker, J.R. (1984). Home safety: Development and validation of one component of an ecobehavioral treatment program for abused and neglected children. *Journal of Applied Behavior Analysis, 17,* 159–174.

Thomas, K.A., Hasseinen, R.S., & Christophersen, E.R. (1984). Evaluation of group well-child care for improving burn prevention practices in the home. *Pediatrics, 74,* 879–882.

Tremblay, G.C., & Peterson, L. (1999). Prevention of childhood injury: Clinical and public policy changes. *Clinical Psychology Review, 19,* 415–434.

US Department of Transportation, National Highway Traffic Safety Administration. (1991). *Occupant protection trends in 19 cities.* Washington, DC: Author.

Wagenaar, A.C., Maybee, R.G., & Sullivan, K.P. (1988). Mandatory seat belt laws in eight states: A time-series evaluation. *Journal of Safety Research, 19,* 51–70.

Walton, W.W. (1982). An evaluation of the Poison Prevention Packaging Act. *Pediatrics, 69,* 363–370.

Williams-Avery, R.M., & MacKinnon, D.P. (1996). Injuries and use of protective equipment among college in-line skaters. *Accident Analysis and Prevention, 28,* 779–784.

Yeaton, W.H., & Bailey, J.S. (1978). Teaching pedestrian safety skills to young children: An analysis and one year follow-up. *Journal of Applied Behavior Analysis, 11,* 315–329.

Zins, J.E., Garcia, V.F., Tuchfarber, B.S., Clark, K.M., & Laurence, S.C. (1994). Preventing injury in children and adolescents. In R. Simeonsson (Ed.), *Risk, resilience, and prevention: Promoting the well-being of all children* (pp. 183–201). Baltimore: Paul H. Brookes.

Injuries, Unintentional, Adolescence

Barbara Tuchfarber, Victor F. Garcia, and Joseph Zins

INTRODUCTION

This entry describes the epidemiology of unintentional injury among adolescents, the contribution of adolescent risk-taking behaviors to the high incidence and mortality rates, principles of injury prevention, and specific injury prevention approaches that focus on adolescents.

DEFINITIONS

"An injury is no accident" (Doege, 1978). The phrase *unintentional injury* has replaced the word "accident" as the preferred term for injury resulting from an unintended event. Accident implies a random, uncontrollable, unpreventable incident. *Unintentional injuries* show clear patterns and are often associated with specific behaviors. For example, teens exhibit low rates of seat belt use and high rates of exceeding the speed limit. The first factor increases the likelihood of serious injury in the event of a crash and the second increases the likelihood of a crash event occurring. These factors interact to increase the number of unintentional motor vehicle-related injuries during adolescence. Because the individuals and demographic groups at highest risk for unintentional injury can be identified, injuries can be prevented and injury rates decreased, demonstrating that the precipitating events are not occurring at random or by "accident."

SCOPE

US Incidence—Injury Deaths

In 1999, about 14 percent of the US population was between the ages of 10 and 19 years. Although unintentional injury is the leading cause of death among all persons younger than 44 years of age, rates are particularly high during adolescence. Emergency departments annually treat about 5.8 million teens for injury. Each year about 19,000 adolescents die from those injuries. Motor vehicles and firearms are the two most lethal mechanisms of injury for teens. Most firearm deaths result from assault (intentional injury) and are dealt with elsewhere in this volume. Because the number of motor vehicle-related deaths is more than 10 times greater than the second most lethal mechanism, our discussion and examples will focus on motor vehicle crashes. Unintentional injury is a major public health issue in the United States. Overall, unintentional injuries rank as the fifth leading cause of death. Unintentional injury rates are higher among adolescents than any other age group.

Unintentional injury *is the leading cause of death* among adolescents, followed by homicide, suicide, and cancers (Centers for Disease Control and Prevention [CDC], 2001). In 1997, unintentional injury deaths among 13–19-year-olds accounted for 46 percent of all deaths in this age group (Guyer, MacDorman, Martin, Peters, & Strobino, 1998) (Table 1). Injury mortality rates among 15–19-year-olds are four times higher than those in children 5–14-years-old and more than twice as high as rates for children younger than 5 years. In 1997, the unintentional injury mortality rate for teens rose from 10.4/100,000 among 13-year-olds to 41.9/100,000 among 19-year-olds. Mortality peaked at 43.5/100,000 among 21-year-olds (National Safety Council [NSC], 2000).

Injury rates for males are higher than those for females in all age groups with the greatest differences occurring during adolescence (Scheidt, Harel, Trumble, Jones, Overpeck, & Bijur, 1995). Males are almost twice as likely as females to be injured or to die from injuries during the teen years (Rivara & Aitken, 1998). Although unintentional injury

Table 1. Major Mechanisms of Unintentional Injury Deaths During Adolescence (13–19-year-olds)

Mechanism	Number of deaths
Motor vehicle crash occupant[a]	5,033
Drowning[b]	459
Pedestrians[a]	333
Firearms[b]	222
Poison[b]	219
Other vehicles[a]	133
Bicycle/motor vehicle collision[a]	131
Motorcyclists[a]	119
Falls	118
Fires[b]	116
Mechanical suffocation[b]	76
All other	524

Notes
[a] Insurance Institute for Highway Safety (IIHS), 2000 (1999 data).
[b] NSC, 2000 (1997 data).

mortality rates have decreased in all pediatric age groups from 1979 through 1996, adolescent rates have demonstrated the smallest decreases (Rivara & Aitken, 1998).

Canadian Incidence—Injury Deaths

Unintentional injuries are also the leading cause of Canadian teen deaths. In 1997, 146 young Canadian teens (10–14 years; 7.2/100,000) and 529 Canadian teens between 15 and 19 years of age died from unintentional injuries (26.1/100,000) (Health Canada Child Injury Facts, 2001). Injury deaths accounted for 45.8 percent of all mortality among the older adolescents. As in the United States, unintentional mortality rates are about twice as high for males as females. Fifteen percent of all hospitalizations among 15–19-year-olds are for unintentional injury. About 12,240 Canadian teens were hospitalized in 1996–1997. The most frequent mechanisms of fatal injury among 15–19-year-olds are motor vehicle occupants, pedestrian, drowning, firearm, falls, and motorcycles.

As noted previously, *motor vehicles* are the most frequent mechanism of fatal unintentional injuries. Adolescent drivers have the highest crash rates among the driving population and pose a major hazard in all motorized countries. Teens present a serious challenge to public health in the United States. In 1999 there were 5,033 teen deaths due to motor vehicle crashes (IIHS, 2000). During the 1980s, the adolescent population between the ages of 16 and 19 decreased, which dampened the impact of teenage drivers. This trend ended in 1992 and as the population of 16–19-year-olds has increased, so has the incidence of motor vehicle crash-related fatalities (IIHS, 2000).

Most US states grant full-privilege drivers' licenses to teens at younger ages and with less driving experience than other industrialized countries. Crash rate per mile driven is the highest between American 16- and 17-year-olds, three times higher than the rate for 18- and 19-year-olds. High crash rates are directly related to adolescent characteristics. Immaturity and lack of experience behind the wheel contribute to risk-taking behaviors (such as speeding and tailgating) as well as failure to recognize and appropriately respond to hazardous situations. Driver error and speeding are often involved in teenage driver-related crashes. Young drivers are mostly involved in a single-vehicle crash with departure of the vehicle off of the roadway. Because teenage drivers tend to carry adolescent passengers (often in large numbers), teens are disproportionately injured in crashes as passengers as well as drivers (NHTSA & NSC, 2000). About two thirds of all teenagers killed in motor vehicle crashes are males. More than half of teenage motor vehicle-related deaths occur on the weekend (Friday–Sunday). In 1999, 41 percent of these deaths occurred at night (9:00 PM–6:00 AM).

Other risk-taking behaviors also contribute to teenage death toll exacted by motor vehicle crashes. The National Highway Traffic Safety Administration estimates that safety belts save more than 11,000 lives per year. Safety belts reduce the risk of death to front seat passengers by 45 percent and the risk of moderate-to-severe injury by 50 percent. Yet use of safety belts is particularly low among teenagers. Nineteen percent of high school students report rarely or never wearing a safety belt (CDC, 1998). Among students in alternative high schools, 29 percent report rarely or never wearing a safety belt (CDC, 1999).

Alcohol also plays a role in teenage motor vehicle-related deaths. Among drivers too young to legally purchase alcohol (16–20-years-old), about 22 percent of drivers involved in a fatal crash had a blood alcohol concentration at or above 0.10 percent. When a male teenage driver has a blood alcohol concentration between 0.05 percent and 0.08 percent, he is 17 times more likely to be killed in a single-vehicle crash. At blood alcohol concentrations of 0.08–0.10 percent he is 52 times more likely to die in a single-vehicle crash.

The second most common mechanism of fatal injuries during adolescence is *drowning*. More than 2,000 children under the age of 20 die each year by drowning. Drowning rates are highest in the southern and western United States and in Alaska (Baker, O'Neill, & Ginsburg, 1992; Waller, Baker, & Szocka, 1989). The highest mortality rate for drowning occurs among young children under the age of five, who most typically die in a pool or tub (O'Flaherty & Pirie, 1997). The second highest mortality occurs among adolescents and young adults from 15 to 24 years of age. In this age group, drowning is more likely to occur in a natural body of water and often alcohol is a factor in the incident. Most drowning victims during adolescence are males. Drowning among males from 16 to 18 years of age is primarily attributed to the three "Ds"—drinking, drugs, and dares (CDC, 1990). It is estimated that alcohol and/or illicit drug use are involved in 40–50 percent of all adolescent drowning (CDC, 1990).

US Incidence—Morbidity

Adolescents also experience the highest non-fatal injury rates. It is estimated that for every injury death, there are 41 hospitalizations and another 1,100 injuries severe enough to require treatment in a hospital emergency department. Injury is the leading reason for emergency department visits among all adolescent age and gender subgroups.

Motor vehicles are a major reason for injury morbidity. For every one death resulting from a motor vehicle crash, it is estimated that there are 100 non-fatal injuries (NHTSA & NSC, 1994). It is estimated that non-fatal near-drowning incidents occur at a rate of 10–14/100,000 per year. For every one drowning death, there are approximately four hospitalizations for near-drowning and about four emergency department visits for every hospitalization (Fields, 2000).

Sports injuries also account for a large percentage of emergency department visits. Football for males and soccer for females account for the highest number of injuries resulting from participation in high school sports. Basketball, baseball, softball, and track events also account for large numbers of adolescent injuries (Patel & Nelson, 2000).

Injuries occurring in the workplace are an emerging concern. More than 5 million adolescents are legally employed in the United States and several million more work in violation of wage, hour, and safety regulations (Pollack, 1997). About one third of all high school students have a job during the school year and the majority of high school students work at least part-time over the summer months. Most are employed in the retail sector, primarily in restaurants and grocery stores. Students in vocational programs are more likely to be employed in other environments such as auto repair and construction sites. Employment has many benefits to teens beyond providing a paycheck. Jobs teach time management and personal responsibility, development of job-specific skills, and promote self-confidence and self-esteem (Rubenstein, Sternbeck, & Pollack, 1999). However, students who work long hours are less likely to remain in school, more likely to use tobacco and illegal substances, more likely to be involved in other deviant behaviors, often get insufficient sleep and exercise, and tend to spend less time with their families (Wegman & Davis, 1999). Occupational injury rates are almost twice as high among adolescents as adults (4.9/100 workers vs. 2.8/100 workers). It is estimated that about 200,000 adolescents are injured and 70 die each year from job-related injuries (Landrigan & McCammon, 1997).

Prevalence

Injury is generally considered an acute condition, associated with a high incidence but low prevalence. However, injuries can produce chronic sequelae. The NSC estimates that 20.8 million Americans were temporarily or permanently disabled by unintentional injuries in 1999. Injury is also the leading cause of acquired mental retardation (NIH, 1998). Teens are more likely to be injured severely and therefore exhibit more functional impairment. Teens are more likely to spend two or more days in bed, miss school, and have restrictions on role activities than younger children (Rivara, Thompson, Thompson, & Calonge, 1991). At 6 months after discharge, 48 percent of a group of children between the ages of 5 and 17 who had been hospitalized for treatment of injuries were still experiencing limitations in physical function (Wesson, Williams, Spence, Filler, Armstrong, & Pearl, 1989).

Costs

The economic impact of unintentional injury on the 1999 US population was $469.0 billion, about $1700 per person. These expenses included lost wages and productivity (50 percent), medical expenses (16.5 percent), administrative expenses (16.5 percent), motor vehicle damage (8.6 percent), employer cost (4.3 percent), and fire loss (1.8 percent) (NSC, 2000).

Motor vehicle-related injuries accounted for 38.7 percent of unintentional injury-related cost. Injuries occurring in the workplace amounted to 26.1 percent of the total cost, injuries occurring in the home accounted for 21.7 percent, and non-motor vehicle-related injuries occurring in public places accounted for 16.7 percent.

A price tag is also affixed to diminished quality of life. In 1999, lost quality of life was estimated at $1,091.4 billion, raising the comprehensive societal cost for one year of unintentional injury to $1,560.4 billion (NSC, 2000).

THEORIES

Social learning theory (SLT) has been widely applied to understanding human behavior within a social context and may provide some insight into adolescent behaviors contributing to the high rates of unintentional injury. SLT is founded on the concept that an individual's behavior can be understood only by examining interactions among attributes of the individual, other persons in the environment, and key aspects of the environment context (Bandura, 1977a). This model predicts that new behaviors are learned through a combination of: (a) observations of competent models; (b) direct mastery experiences in the performance of the desired behaviors (e.g., through role playing and behavioral rehearsal) with corrective feedback; (c) positive reinforcement for accurate performance. *Modeling* in particular is seen as a powerful means of influencing learning or behavior change principally through its informative function; the modeled activities serve as guides for appropriate performance. Bandura suggests that to learn from behavioral modeling, the learner must attend to what the model is doing, process and remember what the model did, practice what the model did and receive corrective feedback, and begin to use what they have learned at appropriate times. Another key concept in SLT is *reciprocal determinism*, which suggests that individuals are influenced by their environment, and in turn, have an influence on the environment (Bandura, 1977b). For example, teenage children of parents who wear a safety belt are more likely to wear a safety belt themselves. SLT also recognizes the importance of intrapersonal variables such as thoughts, perceptions, and attributions (Bandura, 1982).

Social action theory (SAT) is an extension of the SLT which explicitly relates SLT to desired public health outcomes. The SAT is designed to foster social and contextual analysis of personal behavior change (Evert, 1991). The SAT is particularly relevant because many injuries can be prevented by modifying personal behaviors. The social action perspective integrates social interdependence with personal control of behavior. This theory suggests that a program designed to increase safety belt use among all students attending a given high school might be more successful because it changes the social milieu in the school and makes it more socially acceptable for an individual to begin wearing a safety belt. The more positive social context might also provide positive reinforcement for behavior change from those in the school environment.

RESEARCH

Although the literature contains a myriad of studies describing the high unintentional injury rates among adolescents, few scientifically rigorous studies of interventions to reduce injury rates in adolescents have been conducted (Munro, Coleman, Nicholl, Harper, Kent, & Wild, 1995).

Most injury prevention measures can be classified as educational, legislative, environmental, or engineering. Over the past three decades, the public health approach to injury prevention and control has developed a focus on combinations of these four strategies (National Committee for Injury Prevention and Control, 1989).

The Harborview Injury Prevention Research Center has described four principles of injury control that apply to most injury mechanisms and age groups (Rivara, & Mueller, 1987). The first principle states that narrowly targeted programs are far more likely to be successful than diffuse, broad interventions. Multiple messages are often confusing and the desired action in not clear. The second principle is that strategies requiring repeated behavioral change are less likely to be effective than those which require human action only once or not at all. For example, safety belts require a specific action every time an adolescent enters a car whereas the air bag will deploy automatically in the case of a crash.

The third principle states that resources and efforts should be directed at injury problems that are "important." Criteria for "importance" include:

1. the injury problem should occur frequently,
2. the injury should be severe,
3. there should be a reasonable chance for success in avoiding the accident.

Some well-intentioned persons insist that if an intervention prevents even one child from being injured, the intervention is warranted. However, the same resources required to protect that one child from a rare injury may be able to prevent hundreds of children from being injured equally severely through a more common mechanism.

The fourth principle recognizes that most injury problems have existed for long periods of time and will not be solved quickly. High crash rates among teens have been recognized for decades and have been addressed over the years through a variety of programs. Involvement of young drivers in fatal crashes has decreased from 46.2/100,000 in 1988 to 36.9/100,000 in 1995—yet crash rates remain unacceptably high (CDC, 1996).

These principles are directly relevant to prevention of unintentional injuries among teens. Adolescence is marked by the development of abstract thinking and a strong urge for independence. These traits synergize with self-absorption and a sense of personal immortality to establish adolescents as perhaps the most challenging target population for injury prevention strategies. As noted previously, the leading mechanism of morbidity and mortality during adolescence is motor vehicle-related. Much of the adolescent-specific injury research that has been published focus on this topic.

STRATEGIES THAT WORK

Environmental injury prevention approaches have been effective in reducing adolescent unintentional injury mortality due to crashes but the magnitude of the effect on adolescents as a specific group is difficult to measure. Removal of unforgiving structures (such as trees or boulders) from roadsides, energy-absorbing highway barriers and guardrails, and improved lighting on dark roadways contribute to fewer serious crashes among all drivers (Robertson, 1998).

Airbags and other products of automotive and *safety engineering* have also been helpful in decreasing teen deaths. Air bags reduce driver mortality by about 14 percent and reduce passenger deaths by about 11 percent but are less effective among teens because of the low rate of safety belt use (Committee on Injury and Poison Prevention, American Academy of Pediatrics, 1996). The safety belt is required to hold the occupant in place so that the air bag provides protection as designed and the occupant is not in a position to be injured by the deployment of the bag itself.

Many *legislative interventions* are underway to decrease the number of adolescents injured in motor vehicle crashes. Graduated licensure is perceived as a means of restricting teen driving to lower risk situations, providing the driver time to gain experience and maturity. The expectation is that by the time full driving privileges are granted, the likelihood of driver error and risk-taking behaviors will be decreased (IIHS, 2000). Although it is too early to evaluate the full impact of graduated licensure, crash rates in California and Maryland decreased by about 5 percent among 15–17-year-old drivers and by 16 percent in Oregon following implementation of the program (Jones, 1994).

The Canadian experience with graduated licensure has paralleled that of the United States, demonstrating a 27 percent decrease in the crash rate for 16–19-year-old new drivers. Mortality decreased from 6.6/10,000 among 16-year-old drivers to 1.8/10,000 following implementation of graduated licensure (NHTSA & NSC, 2000).

STRATEGIES THAT MIGHT WORK

The most frequently employed injury prevention approaches are *educational programs*. Such programs are appealing because they are generally inexpensive and can reach large groups of teens at one time. The goal of these programs is behavior change—adoption of a safety behavior (such as buckling a safety belt) or eliminating an unsafe behavior (such as running red lights). Educational programs are often considered the weakest of all strategies, but sometimes they are the only approach available (Robertson, 1998).

Three Canadian injury prevention programs that target adolescent injuries through educational programs are the PARTY Program, the Heroes Program, and Think First. The "PARTY Program" (Prevent Alcohol & Risk-related Trauma in Youth) is designed to help adolescents make informed decisions in potentially hazardous situations (Warnell, 1997). This 6-hr program combines a didactic presentation by a health professional with a tour of a rehabilitation facility and discussion with a traumatic brain injury survivor.

The 1-hr "Heroes Program" provides information through a 1-hr high-tech slide show followed by a presentation from an injury survivor. Two teens from the school end the program by delivering five injury prevention messages: look first, buckle up, drive sober, wear the gear, and get trained. Following the program, 85 percent of students responded that the information they received would affect their future decision-making (Smartrisk Foundation, 1996).

"Think First" is a program designed to reduce brain and spinal cord injury. The 50-min program is presented in classrooms throughout the United States and Canada. This presentation includes videotapes presenting stories of young traumatic brain and spinal cord injury survivors and a didactic presentation by a nurse or other health professional describing central nervous system anatomy and physiology. An uncontrolled pretest–posttest evaluation demonstrated a significant increase in knowledge of nervous system structure and function following the program (Damba, Sam, Depres, Edmonds, & Tator, 1996).

Incorporation of a 5-hr passenger safety program into a high school physics class demonstrated significant increases in self-reported safety belt use as a passenger but not as a driver (Martinez, Levine, Martin, & Altman, 1996).

Such short-term educational programs are considered the weakest forms of injury prevention. Observation of actual behavioral change in lacking and self-reported safety behavior is notoriously inaccurate. There is no reason to believe that a single educational encounter will result in a change in established behaviors. The primary benefit of such programs may be to reinforce previously learned information and to raise awareness of injury as a major threat to well-being.

The incorporation of feedback, rewards, and rehearsal are extremely important if an education program is to be successful (Peterson, 1988). Educational programs which provide a short one-time exposure to a message are less likely to produce an effect than are sustained, interactive, multifaced programs. As discussed in the theory section, SLT suggests that repetition of a clear message and role modeling of the desired behaviors may promote movement in the appropriate direction. Therefore, didactic presentations to large groups would not be expected to produce the same result as interactive, multisensory programs providing modeling behavior, individual rehearsal of the desired behaviors, and responsive feedback. An interesting area for research might be to examine whether such safety programs might be more effective in promoting safety behaviors not currently in use (e.g., wearing a safety belt) than deterring teens from risky behaviors that they might like to engage in (e.g., carrying several passengers or "hill hopping").

STRATEGIES THAT DO NOT WORK

Many injury prevention programs and campaigns target teens but few are evaluated. In the light of continued high injury mortality, it is unlikely that "quick fixes" such as TV campaigns and informational brochures have been effective in encouraging seat belt use or reduced driving speed among adolescents.

A more structured program designed to decrease motor vehicle crash-related injuries is high school driver education. Teens were required to participate in such a program before being licensed by the state on the premise that mandating exposure to information about safe driving would result in better drivers with fewer crashes. In fact, the opposite effect has been observed. Driver education classes did not decrease teen crashes or driving convictions but actually contributed to the problem by encouraging earlier and easier licensure, thereby increasing risk exposure (NHTSA & NSC, 2000).

Legislative interventions may prescribe certain safety behaviors or proscribe risky behaviors (Robertson, 1998). However, laws are only as effective as their enforcement. Although all 50 states have a uniform minimum drinking age of 21 years, 25 percent of the male teens killed in a crash were underage and had been drinking. Eighty percent of these teens were unrestrained at the time of crash, despite laws in 49 states requiring drivers to wear safety belts.

SYNTHESIS

The high rate of unintentional injury, especially motor vehicle crashes, among adolescents emphasizes the need for targeted injury prevention programs. Studies have demonstrated that drivers' education programs have *contributed* to high injury rates by providing inadequate preparation for the road but making a driver's license more readily obtainable for the 16-year-olds at highest risk for poor performance. Media campaigns to increase safety belt use have also been unsuccessful (Robertson, 1998). Legislative efforts to protect teen drivers and passengers have been inadequate but the graduated licensing approach appears to hold considerable promise for reductions in injuries and deaths. Engineering has been very successful in reducing injuries through advances such as making cars heavier and safer, improving occupant protection systems, providing energy-dissipating roadway dividers and guardrails, re-banking dangerous stretches of roadway, analyzing the degree of road curvature, line painting placement and materials, and improved braking systems. Engineering is less likely to solve the problem of risk-taking adolescents who choose to run red lights, drive over the speed limit, carry large numbers of passengers, play "chicken" on the expressway, or drink and drive.

The most effective methodology for reducing the injury toll among adolescents requires integration of education (of both adolescents and parents), legislation, enforcement of existing laws, environmental modification, engineering, and psychosocial injury prevention approaches. Graduated licensure could provide the legislative structure for such an approach if supplemented by educational programs for parents demonstrating their responsibilities in the program, education for teens about the importance of safety belts, vigorous enforcement of safety belt laws, continued environmental and engineering advances in automotive safety, and suggestions for making such behavioral changes palatable to individual teens and to their peer groups.

Also see: Injuries, Unintentional: Early Childhood; Injuries, Unintentional: Childhood; Injuries, Unintentional, Occupational: Adulthood; Accident, Motor Vehicle: Adulthood; Risk-Taking: Adolescence.

References

Baker, S.P., O'Neill, B., Ginsburg, M.J., & Li, G. (1992). *The injury fact book* (2nd edn). NY: Oxford University Press.

Bandura, A. (1977a). *Social learning theory*. Englewood Cliffs, NJ: Prentice-Hall.

Bandura, A. (1977b). Self-efficacy: Toward a unifying theory of behavioral change. *Psychological Review, 84*: 191–215.

Bandura, A. (1982). Self-efficacy mechanism is human agency. *American Psychologist, 37*: 122–147.

Centers for Disease Control and Prevention (CDC). (1990). Fatal injuries to children—United States, 1986. *Morbidity and Mortality Weekly Report, 39*, 443–451.

Centers for Disease Control and Prevention (CDC). (1996). Involvement by young drivers in fatal motor-vehicle crashes—United States, 1988–1995. *Morbidity and Mortality Weekly Report, 45*(48): 1049–1053.

Centers for Disease Control and Prevention (CDC). (1998). Youth risk behavior surveillance—United States, 1997. *Morbidity and Mortality Weekly Report, 47*(SS-3).

Centers for Disease Control and Prevention (CDC). (1999). Youth risk behavior surveillance—National alternative high school youth risk behavior survey, United States, 1988. *Morbidity and Mortality Weekly Report, 48*(SS-7).

Centers for Disease Control and Prevention (CDC). (2001). *Leading causes of death*. http://webapp.cdc.gov/sasweb/ncipc. Accessed 9/3/01

Committee on Injury and Poison Prevention, American Academy of Pediatrics. (1996). The teenage driver. *Pediatrics, 98*(5).

Damba, C., Sam, E.P., Depres, A., Edmonds, V.E., & Tator, C.H. (1996). *An impact evaluation of the Think First Brain and Spinal Cord Injury Prevention School Program*. Toronto, Canada: SportSmart Canada.

Doege, T.C. (1978). An injury is no accident. *New England Journal of Medicine, 298*, 509–510.

Evert, C.K. (1991). Social action theory for a public health psychology. *American Psychologist, 46*, 931–946.

Fields, A.L. (2000). Near-drowning in the pediatric population. *Critical Care Clinic, 8,* 113–129.

Guyer, B., MacDorman, M.F., Martin, J.A., Peters, K.D., & Strobino, D.M. (1998). Annual summary of vital statistics—1997. *Pediatrics, 102*(6), 1333–1349.

Health Canada Child Injury Facts. (2001). www.hc-sc.gc.ca/pphb-dgspsp/injury. Accessed 10/2001

Insurance Institute for Highway Safety (IIHS). (2000). *Fatality facts*. Insurance Institute for Highway Safety.

Jones, B. (1994). The effectiveness of provisional licensing in Oregon: An analysis of traffic safety benefits. *Journal of Safety Research, 25*, 33–46.

Landrigan, P.J., & McCammon, J.B. (1997). *Public Health Report, 112*(6), 466–473.

Martinez, R., Levine, D.W., Martin, R., & Altman, D.G. (1996). Effect of integration of injury control information into a high school physics course. *Annals of Emergency Medicine, 27*(2), 216–224.

Munro, J., Coleman, P., Nicholl, J., Harper, R., Kent, G., & Wild, D. (1995). Can we prevent accidental injury to adolescents: A systematic review of the evidence. *Injury Prevention, 1*, 249–255.

National Committee for Injury Prevention and Control. (1989). Injury prevention: Meeting the challenge. *American Journal of Preventive Medicine, 5*, 1S–303S.

National Highway Traffic Safety Administration (NHTSA), & National Safety Council (NSC). (1994). *Traffic safety facts 1992: A compilation of motor vehicle crash data from the fatal accident reporting system and the general estimating system (revised 1992 data)* (USDOT pub HS-808-022). Washington, DC.

National Highway Traffic Safety Administration (NHTSA), & National Safety Council (NSC). (2000). *Saving teenage lives: The case for graduated driver licensing*. Washington DC: authors.

National Institutes of Health (NIH). (1998, October 26–28). *Rehabilitation of persons with traumatic brain injury: NIH consensus statement, 16*(1), 1–41.

National Safety Council (NSC). (2000). *Injury facts, 2000 edition*. Itasca, IL: Author.

O'Flaherty, J.E., & Pirie, P.L. (1997). Prevention of pediatric drowning and near-drowning: A survey of members of the American Academy of Pediatrics. *Pediatrics, 99*(2), 169–174.

Patel, D.R., & Nelson, T.L. (2000). Sports injuries in adolescents. *Medical Clinics of North America, 84*(4), 983–1007.

Peterson, L. (1988). Preventing the leading killer of children: The role of the social psychologist in injury prevention. *School Psychology Review, 17*, 593–600.

Pollack, S. (1997). Adolescent occupational injuries and exposures: An important role for physicians. In E.A. Emmett and A.L. Frank (Eds.), *The year-book of occupational and environmental medicine*. St. Louis: Mosby.

Rivara, F.P., & Aitken, M. (1998). Prevention of injuries to children and adolescents. *Advances in Pediatrics, 45*, 37–73.

Rivara, F.P., Thompson, R.S., Thompson, D.C., & Calonge, N. (1991). Injuries to children and adolescents: Impact on physical health. *Pediatrics, 88*(4), 783–788.

Rivara, F.P., & Mueller, B. (1987). The epidemiology and causes of childhood injuries. *Journal of Social Issues, 43*(2), 13–31.

Robertson, L. (1998). *Injury epidemiology: research and control strategies* (2nd ed.). New York, NY: Oxford University Press.

Rubenstein, H., Sternbeck, M.R., & Pollack, S.H. (1999). Protecting the health and safety of working teenagers. *American Family Physician, 60*(2), 575–580.

Smartrisk Foundation. (1996). *An evaluation of the heroes program*. Toronto, Canada. Prepared by the Leeds, Grenville, and Lanark District Health Unit.

Scheidt, P.C., Harel, Y., Trumble, A.C., Jones, D.H., Overpeck, M.D., & Bijur, P.E. (1995). The epidemiology of nonfatal injuries among US children and youth. *American Journal of Public Health, 85*(7), 932–938.

Waller, A.E., Baker, S.P., & Szocka, A. (1989). Childhood injury deaths: National analysis and geographic variations. *American Journal of Public Health, 79*, 310–315.

Warnell, P. (1997, September). Injury prevention programs: Do they really make a difference? *AXON*, 6–9.

Wegman, D.H., & Davis, L.K. (1999). Protecting youth at work. *American Journal of Industrial Medicine, 36*(5), 579–583.

Wesson, D.E., Williams, J.I., Spence, L.J., Filler, R.M., Armstrong, P.F., & Pearl, H. (1989). Functional outcomes in pediatric trauma. *Journal of Trauma, 29*, 589–592.

Injuries, Unintentional, Occupational: Adulthood

E. Scott Geller

INTRODUCTION

Unintentional injury is the leading cause of death to people aged 44 and under (US Bureau of Labor Statistics, 1998), and a large portion of these fatalities occur to people on the job. Whether leading to a disabling injury or death, most accidents are caused to some extent by human behavior. Human behavior is influenced by the environmental context in which it occurs and a variety of psychological dimensions, including attitude, perception, personality, and cognition. This entry addresses the human element of occupational injuries by reviewing leading theories and practical applications that need to be considered when designing programs to prevent unintentional injury in the workplace.

DEFINITIONS

An *activator* is an environmental event that precedes behavior and gives it direction.

Ergonomics applies engineering and behavioral science to maximize productivity and minimize employee discomfort at a work station.

Goal setting is technique to direct and motivate behavior by specifying measurable, attainable, and traceable objectives relevant for reaching a desired outcome.

Outcome expectancy is a belief that the ultimate outcome from a prevention strategy is worth the effort required to implement the strategy.

Prevention strategy involves the manipulation of one or more factors or independent variables to increase safe behavior or decrease at-risk behavior in order to reduce the probability of an injury.

Response-efficacy is a belief that a certain prevention strategy will produce a desired outcome.

Risk compensation refers to adjusting behaviors to compensate for a change in risk perception.

Risk perception is selectively viewing environmental or behavioral factors that could contribute to an injury.

Self-efficacy is a personal confidence that one can accomplish a certain task.

Self-management refers to using principles of behavioral science to improve one's own behavior(s).

SCOPE

Every year, an estimated 7,000–11,000 US employees are killed on the job and 2.5–11.3 million are seriously injured (Miller, 1997). This results in 250,000 potential productive years of life lost annually—more than from cancer and cardiovascular disease combined (Leigh, 1995). The overall financial liability of work-related injuries in the United States was estimated at $116 billion in 1992, an increase from the 1989 estimate of $89 billion and dramatically larger than the 1985 estimate of $34.6 billion

(Leigh, 1995). The direct costs include lost wages, medical expenses, insurance claims, production delays, lost time of coworkers, equipment damage, and fire losses (Miller, 1997).

The Workers' Compensation Board of Canada paid over $4.5 billion in benefits for the almost 1 million occupational injuries reported in 1997. The annual total cost of occupational injuries to the Canadian economy is estimated at over $9.1 billion (Human Resources Development Canada, 1997). One Canadian worker out of sixteen was injured on the job in 1997, and that year an average of three occupational fatalities occurred per every workday (Human Resources Development Canada, 1997). That amounted to 1 worker out of 15,750 dying from an occupational incident. In New Zealand, the occupational death rate is slightly lower, averaging 1 death per 25,000 workers in 1994 (New Zealand Environmental and Occupational Health Research Centre, 1999).

Even though all of these losses and cost statistics are enormous, they are likely gross underestimates. Many occupational injuries go unreported, especially at the large number of industrial sites that link prizes or financial bonuses to the absence (or non-report) of an injury. Moreover, the pain and suffering to victims of unintentional injury and their families cannot be quantified, and thus the liabilities from occupational injuries are substantially greater than the estimated financial costs.

THEORIES

Risk Perception

How much risk we perceive determines how much precaution we take to avoid injury. People are generally underwhelmed by risks or safety hazards at work, because our daily experiences on the job lead us to perceive a relatively low level of risk in the workplace. Researchers of risk communication have studied various characteristics of a hazard that influence people's perceptions (Covello, Sandman, & Slovic, 1991), leading to important theory regarding aspects of situations that influence risk perception. Three of these factors are reviewed below, suggesting strategies for increasing employees' perception of risk and their awareness of environmental hazards and unsafe behaviors.

The Power of Choice

Hazards we choose to experience (like driving, skiing, and working) are seen as less risky than ones we feel forced to endure (like food preservatives, environmental pollution, and earthquakes). Of course, the perception of choice is quite subjective, varying dramatically among individuals.

For example, employees who feel they have their pick of places to work generally perceive less risk in a particular work environment than do those who feel compelled to work at the site.

Familiarity Breeds Complacency

Familiarity is probably a more powerful determinant of perceived risk than choice. The more we know about a risk, the less it threatens us. Remember how attentive you were when first learning to drive, or when you were first introduced to the equipment in your workplace? However, it was not long before you lowered your perceptions of risk, and changed your behavior accordingly.

Understood and Controllable Hazards

Hazards we can explain and control cause much less alarm than hazards that are not understood and perceived as uncontrollable. This reveals a problem with explaining hazards as if they can be completely controlled. Safety professionals often state a goal of "zero injuries," implying absolute control over the factors that cause injuries. This actually lowers perceived risk by convincing people all of the causes of occupational injuries are understood and controllable.

Risk Compensation

The basic idea behind this important but controversial theory is quite simple and straightforward. People are presumed to adjust their behavior to compensate for changes in perceived risk. If a job is made safer with machine guards or the use of personal protective equipment (PPE), workers can be expected to reduce their perception of risk and thus perform more recklessly.

Obviously, the notion that an individual's behavior could off-set the safety benefits of PPE is extremely repugnant to a safety professional. Could this mean that efforts to make environments safer with engineering innovations are worthless in the long run? Are safety belts and air bags responsible for increases in vehicle speeds?

Some researchers and scholars are convinced risk compensation is real and detrimental to injury prevention (Peltzman, 1975; Wilde, 1994), while others contend that the phenomenon does not exist (Lehman & Gage, 1995). There is, in fact, scientific evidence that risk compensation or risk homeostasis does occur (Janssen, 1994; Streff & Geller, 1988), but the off-setting or compensating behavior does not negate the benefits of PPE. Although football players increase at-risk behaviors when suited up, for example, they sustain far fewer injuries than they would without the protective gear.

Efficacy Theory

Self-efficacy (Bandura, 1997) is among the most popular theoretical perspectives in clinical psychology, and it can be applied to occupational safety. Self-efficacy reflects a "can do" attitude. It refers to a person's perception that he or she can organize the relevant resources and execute the procedures necessary to reach a certain goal. However, when people have self-efficacy and adequate skills to implement a prevention strategy, they will not do it unless they also have *response-efficacy.*

Response-efficacy refers to one's belief that a certain technique or strategy will actually produce a desired outcome. This concept has critical implications for safety training. Specifically, it is not enough to teach participants the procedural steps for conducting a certain safety process. Trainers need to convince their audience that the technique has the potential to prevent personal injury.

A third type of belief entertained in Bandura's text on self-efficacy is *outcome-expectancy.* This is about the consequence one expects to receive when participating in a particular prevention program. We might believe we can do something and believe what we do will have a certain effect, but we will not perform unless we also believe the effect is worth the effort. In safety, for example, a group might believe their safety record is good enough, given that they see very few coworkers getting seriously injured. The potential gain from an inconvenient safety process might seem too small to justify the amount of extra effort required for implementation.

RESEARCH

Guastello (1993) summarized the evaluation data from 53 different research reports of safety programs conducted in workplace settings since 1977. From this review, he ranked 10 different injury-prevention approaches according to the mean percentage decrease in injury rates. Each approach is defined briefly below, ranked from best to least effective at decreasing occupational injuries.

1. Behavior-Based

Programs in this category consisted of employee training regarding particular safe and at-risk behaviors, systematic observation and recording of the targeted behaviors, and feedback to workers regarding the frequency or percentage of safe versus at-risk behavior. Some of these programs included *goal setting* and/or incentives to encourage an observation and feedback process (average reduction in injuries from seven studies = 59.6 percent).

2. Comprehensive Ergonomics

The *ergonomics* (or human factors) approach to safety refers essentially to any personal or environmental adjustment of working conditions in order to reduce the frequency or probability of an environmental hazard or unsafe behavior (Kroemer, 1991). An essential ingredient in these programs was a diagnostic survey or environmental audit by employees which led to specific recommendations for eliminating hazards that put employees at risk or promoted at-risk behaviors (average injury reduction from three studies = 51.6 percent).

3. Engineering Changes

This category included the introduction of robots and the comprehensive redesign of facilities to eliminate certain at-risk behaviors. It was noted, however, that the robotic approach introduced the potential for new types of workplace injuries, like a robot catching an operator in its work envelope and impaling him or her against a structure. Thus, these changes usually require special protective engineering such as equipment guards, emergency kill switches, radar-type sensors, and workplace re-design to prevent injury from robots (average injury reduction from four studies = 29.0 percent).

4. Group Problem-Solving

For this approach, operations personnel met voluntarily to discuss safety issues and problems, and to develop action plans for safety improvement (Saarela, 1990). This approach is analogous to quality circles where employees who perform similar types of work meet regularly to solve problems of product quality, productivity, and cost (injury reduction from one study = 20.0 percent).

5. Government Action (in Finland)

Two Finnish government agencies responsible for labor production targeted the most problematic occupational groups and implemented certain action strategies, including: (a) disseminating information to work supervisors regarding the cause of workplace injuries and methods to reduce them; (b) setting standards for safe machine repair and use; and (c) conducting periodic work-site inspections (average injury reduction across two studies = 18.3 percent).

6. Management Audits

For programs in this category, designated managers were trained to administer a standard International Safety Rating System (ISRS). This system evaluates work settings according to 20 components of industrial safety, including leadership and administration, management training, planned inspections, task analysis, task observations, emergency preparedness, organizational rules, accident analysis, employee training, PPE, health control, program evaluation, engineering controls, and off-the-job safety (average reduction in injuries across four studies = 17.0 percent).

7. Stress Management

These programs taught employees how to cope with stressors or sources of work stress (Ivancevich, Matteson, Freedman, & Phillips, 1990; Murphy, 1984). Exercise was often a key action strategy promoted as a way to prevent stress-related injuries in physically demanding jobs (cf. Cady, Thomas, & Karwasky, 1985) (average injury reduction across two studies = 15.0 percent).

8. Poster Campaigns

The two published studies in this category evaluated the injury-reduction impact of posting signs that urged workers at a shipyard to avoid certain at-risk behaviors and to follow certain safe behaviors. Most signs were posted at relevant locations and gave specific behavioral instructions like "take material for only one workday," "gather hoses immediately after use," "wear your safety helmet," and "check railing and platform couplings (on scaffolds)" (average reduction in injury across two studies = 14.0 percent).

9. Personnel Selection

This popular but essentially ineffective approach to injury prevention is based on the intuitive notion of *accident proneness*. The strategy is to identify aspects of accident proneness among job applicants and then screen out people with critical levels of certain characteristics. Accident proneness characteristics targeted for measurement and screening have included: anxiety, distractibility, tension, insecurity, beliefs about injury control, general expectancies about personal control of life events, social adjustment, reliability, impulsivity, sensation seeking, boredom susceptibility, and self-reported alcohol use.

Although measuring and screening for accident proneness sounds like a "quick fix" approach to injury prevention, this technique has not worked consistently to prevent workplace injuries because: (a) the instruments or procedures available to measure the proneness characteristics are unreliable or invalid; (b) the proneness characteristics do not necessarily carry across settings, so a person might show them at home but not at work or vice versa; and (c) a person

with a higher desire to take risks (such as a sensation seeker) might be more inclined to take appropriate precautions (like using PPE) to avoid potential injury (average injury reduction across 26 studies = 3.7 percent).

10. Near-Miss Reporting

This approach involved increased reporting and investigation of incidents that did not result in an injury but certainly could have under slightly different circumstances. One program in this category increased the number of corrective suggestions generated, but did not reduce injury rate. The other scientific publication in this category reported a 56 percent reduction in injury *severity* as a result of increased reporting of "near misses," but the overall *number* of injuries did not change (average injury reduction across two studies = 0.0 percent).

STRATEGIES THAT WORK

For almost a decade, behavior-based or behavioral safety has been flourishing in industrial settings nationwide, and more recently throughout the world. Several books have been published which detail the principles and procedures of behavioral safety. They provide solid evidence for the success of this approach to injury prevention (e.g., Geller, 2001b,c; Geller & Williams, 2001; Krause, Hidley, & Hodson, 1996; McSween, 1995; Petersen, 1989). Each of these books is consistent with regard to certain basic principles and methods, as described next.

Principle 1: Focus Intervention on Observable Behavior

The behavior-based approach focuses on what people do, analyzes why they do it, and then applies a research-supported prevention strategy to improve what people do. Improvement results from *acting people into thinking differently* rather than targeting internal awareness or attitudes in order to *think people into acting differently*.

Principle 2: Look for External Factors to Improve Behavior

Certainly we do what we do because of factors in both our external and internal worlds. But given the difficulty in objectively defining internal factors, it is far more cost-effective to identify environmental conditions that influence behavior and to change these factors (even system-wide) when behavior change is called for.

Principle 3: Direct with Activators and Motivate with Consequences

Activators (or events antecedent to behavior) are only as powerful as the *consequences* supporting them. In other words, activators tell us what to do in order to receive a consequence, from the ringing of a telephone or doorbell to the instructions from a training seminar or one-on-one coaching session. But, we follow through with the particular behavior activated (from answering a telephone or door to following a trainer's instructions) to the extent we expect doing so will result in a pleasant consequence or enable us to avoid an unpleasant consequence.

Principle 4: Focus on Positive Consequences to Motivate Behavior

In his classic 1971 book, *Beyond freedom and dignity*, B.F. Skinner writes, "The problem is to free men, not from control, but from certain kinds of control" (p. 41). He goes on to explain why the type of control to reduce in order to increase perceptions of personal freedom is control by aversive consequences. When people work to achieve positive consequences, as opposed to performing to avoid negative events, their attitude is more positive and their desire to look out for the safety of others is stronger.

Unfortunately, the common metric used to rank companies on their safety performance is "total recordable injury rate" (or an analogous count of losses) which puts people in a reactive mindset of "avoiding failure" rather than "achieving success." Behavioral safety provides proactive measures that employees set goals to achieve in order to prevent occupational injury.

Principle 5: Apply the Scientific Method to Improve a Prevention Strategy

The occurrence of a specific behavior can be objectively observed and measured before and after a proactive process is implemented. This application of the scientific method provides critical feedback upon which improvement can build. The acronym "DO IT" can be used to teach and remember this principle of behavioral safety: D = Define the target behavior to increase or decrease; O = Observe the target behavior during a preprogram baseline period to understand natural environmental or interpersonal factors influencing the target behavior (see Principle 1), and to set behavior-improvement goals; I = Intervene to change the target behavior in desired directions; and T = Test the impact of the prevention procedure by continuing to observe and record the target behavior during the injury-prevention program.

After a DO IT process, an intervention can be objectively evaluated for unbiased decision-making. Comparisons between observations taken during baseline and during the test phase might indicate: (a) the intervention should be continued; (b) another prevention strategy should be used; or (c) another behavior should be defined for the DO IT process. The systematic evaluation of a number of DO IT processes can lead to a body of knowledge worthy of integrating into a theory. This is reflected in the next principle.

Principle 6: Use Theory to Integrate Information

After applying the DO IT process, a number of times, you will see distinct consistencies. Certain injury-prevention techniques will work better in some situations than others, by some individuals than others, or with some behaviors than others. You should summarize relationships between intervention impact and specific interpersonal or contextual characteristics. The outcome will be a research-based theory of what is most cost-effective under given circumstances. You are using theory to integrate information gained from systematic behavioral observation.

Principle 7: Design Prevention Strategies with Consideration of Feelings and Attitudes

Feelings and attitudes are influenced indirectly by the type of behavior-based prevention technique implemented, and such relationships require careful consideration by the developers and managers of a behavioral safety process. The rationale for using more positive than negative consequences to motivate behavior (Principle 4) is based on the different feeling states resulting from positive reinforcement versus punishment procedures. Likewise, the way an injury-prevention process is introduced and administered can increase or decrease perceptions of empowerment, build or destroy interpersonal trust, and facilitate or inhibit a sense of interdependency or teamwork.

STRATEGIES THAT MIGHT WORK

Behavior-based safety changes how people talk about occupational safety, and that may be the most important aspect of this approach to injury prevention. In other words, when workers communicate constructively with each other about objective factors or hazards that could lead to an injury, they are activating a prevention process. Factors upstream from property damage or a near miss are then removed. Thus, any strategy that improves the quality of conversations about safety or increases the quantity of such conversations is likely to reap injury-prevention benefits.

Certain approaches ranked relatively low by Guastello (1993) have the potential to improve or increase interpersonal conversations about injury prevention, and thus should not be discounted. For example, group problem-solving, management audits, and near-miss reporting could stimulate constructive communication about environmental hazards and risky behaviors that need to be eliminated or changed. By following the seven behavior-based principles reviewed above, these conversations will not be negative nor confrontational but will be positive, productive, and proactive. Then when observable improvement occurs in the factors identified, these prevention-focused conversations are reinforced and thus likely to continue.

So, how can constructive conversations about injury prevention be activated? Behavioral safety uses the results of an observation and feedback process to stimulate beneficial injury-prevention conversations. A near-miss report or the results of a management audit could also lead to productive communication *if* the focus is proactive fact finding rather than reactive fault finding. For many work cultures, this is a severe paradigm shift from the standard communication about a near miss or management audit. Therefore, proactive and positive conversations about near misses and management audits may not come easy.

A powerful and objective way to stimulate constructive safety conversation is suggested by Bird and Germain (1997). These authors stress the need to investigate incidents resulting in property damage—but no injury. In effect, these are near misses. Then, the property damage needs to be fixed in order to prevent workplace injury. Yet the value of investigating property damage incidents is sorely overlooked. My point here is that property damage—a physical trace of a near miss—could be used to activate the kind of individual and group communication that could prevent injury. And when the property damage is repaired, the proactive conversation is visibly supported.

STRATEGIES THAT DO NOT WORK

It's Not Attitude First

The last basic principle of behavior-based safety emphasizes the importance of individual feeling states, beliefs, and perceptions. As reviewed earlier, people need to believe they can implement certain prevention techniques (self-efficacy) and that the techniques will work (response-efficacy). Also, they need to believe the consequences justify their efforts (outcome-expectancy). Then when people perceive the need to eliminate or reduce environmental or behavioral risks, they will feel empowered to use the prevention techniques they have learned.

As discussed in Principle 1, however, it is not cost-effective to address person states first in an attempt to change workers' behaviors. Thus, prevention strategies are misdirected with the common slogan that "Safety is an Attitude," and the notion that attitude must be changed first before safety-related behaviors can be improved. As reviewed above, behavior-based observation and feedback targets safe and at-risk behavior directly, but delivers and supports the prevention process in such a way that such person states as attitude, belief, and sense of empowerment are benefited indirectly.

Don't Select for Accident Proneness

Related to the ineffective "attitude first" strategy is the personnel selection approach. As reviewed above, the aim here is to define the "accident prone" personality, and then select these individuals out of the workforce. Of the 53 research articles reviewed systematically by Guastello (1993), 26 studies targeted a total of 19,177 employees in an attempt to identify individuals most likely to be injured and use this information to hire "safe" employees or determine job assignments. Some reasons for the failure of this approach were reviewed earlier. In addition, finding correlations between personality characteristics and injury rates does not mean the proneness factors caused changes in an injury rate. Other factors, including cultural factors or environmental events, are more likely to have caused both the injury and the accident-proneness person state. So, again, it is most cost-effective to target the environmental and behavioral factors directly.

Tracking the Wrong Numbers

Many companies address injury prevention in ways that actually cause more harm than good. Specifically, it is common for management at an industrial site to offer employees a financial bonus if their plant shows a reduction in injury rate. Under these circumstances, large signs at industrial sites display the number of days (or hours) worked without an injury. What behavior does this kind of incentive/reward program and tracking process motivate?

Empirical evidence as well as basic common sense indicates that incentive programs based on injuries motivate workers to hide their injuries (referred to as "the bloody pocket syndrome" in many work cultures). Such a focus on remote outcomes (as in "loss control") can also cultivate a sense of "helplessness" about actually preventing injuries. If the only score for safety is a reactive outcome measure (as is, in fact, the case in most industries), employees can feel demotivated and apathetic about safety. Without targeting what people need to do proactively to stay healthy and safe, there is no clear direction or motivation for a work force. Injuries keep happening to "the other guy," and the individual employee feels helpless with regard to preventing future "accidents." In this scenario, the incidents are truly "accidents," meaning "an event occurring by chance" (*The New Merriam-Webster Dictionary*, 1989) and beyond one's immediate control.

Behavior-based safety, as defined above, puts employees in control of safety and builds a sense of empowerment that they can make a difference. The final section offers an integrative model to understand critical relationships among four awareness states, three kinds of behavior, and four prevention strategies.

SYNTHESIS

Three Types of Behavior

Most safety-related behaviors on the job start out as *other-directed*, in the sense that employees follow someone else's instructions. Such direction can come from a training program, an operations manual, or a policy statement. After people learn to do, essentially by memorizing or internalizing the appropriate instructions, their behavior can become *self-directed*. Before performing a behavior, we might talk to ourselves or formulate an image in order to activate the right response.

After performing some behaviors frequently and consistently over a period of time, they become automatic. A *habit* is formed. Some habits are good and some are bad, depending on their short-term and long-term consequences. If implemented correctly, rewards, recognition, and other positive consequences can facilitate the transfer of behavior from the self-directed phase to the habit phase.

Three Kinds of Prevention Strategies

Instructional Strategy

This is typically an activator or antecedent event used to get new behavior started or to move behavior from the automatic (habit) stage to the self-directed stage. Or it is used to improve behavior already in the self-directed stage. The aim is to get the performer's attention and instruct him or her to transition from being *unknowingly risky to knowingly safe*. You assume the person wants to improve, so external motivation is not needed—only external and extrinsic direction.

Supportive Strategy

Once a person learns the right way to do something, practice is important so the behavior becomes part of a regular routine. Continued practice leads to *fluency* and in many cases to automatic or habitual behavior. Practice does not come easily, and benefits greatly from supportive intervention. We need support to reassure us we are doing the right thing and to encourage us to keep going. Thus, when we give people *rewarding feedback* or recognition for performing safe behavior, we are showing our appreciation for their efforts and increasing the likelihood they will perform the behavior again.

Motivational Strategy

When people know what to do and do not do it, they require some external encouragement or pressure to change. Instruction alone is obviously insufficient because they are knowingly doing the wrong thing. This is when a behavior-based *incentive/reward* program is useful. Such a program attempts to motivate a certain target behavior by promising people a positive consequence if they perform it. The promise is the incentive and the consequence is the reward. In safety, this kind of motivational contingency is much less common than a *disincentive/penalty* program. This is when a rule, policy, or law threatens to give people a negative consequence (a penalty) if they fail to comply or take a calculated risk.

A motivational strategy is clearly the most challenging to design and implement, requiring enough external influence to get the target behavior started without triggering a desire to assert personal freedom (cf. Geller, 2001a). Powerful external consequences might improve behavior only temporarily, as long as the behavioral intervention is in place. Hence the individual is knowingly safe, but the excessive outside control makes the behavior entirely other-directed. Excessive control on the outside of people can limit the amount of internal control or self-direction they develop.

The Flow of Behavior Change

Figure 1 depicts relationships among four competency states (unknowingly risky, knowingly risky, knowingly safe, and fluently safe) and four behavior-based prevention strategies (instructional, motivational, supportive, and self-management). When people are unaware of the safe work practice (i.e., they are unknowingly risky), they need repeated instruction until they understand what to do. Then, as depicted at the far left of the figure, the critical question is whether they perform the desired behavior. If they do, the question of behavioral fluency is relevant. A fluent response becomes a habit or part of a regular routine, and thus the individual is fluently safe.

When workers know how to perform a task safely but do not, they are considered knowingly risky or irresponsible. This is when an external motivational strategy is needed, as discussed above. Then when the desired behavior occurs at least once, interpersonal support is needed to get the behavior to a fluent state.

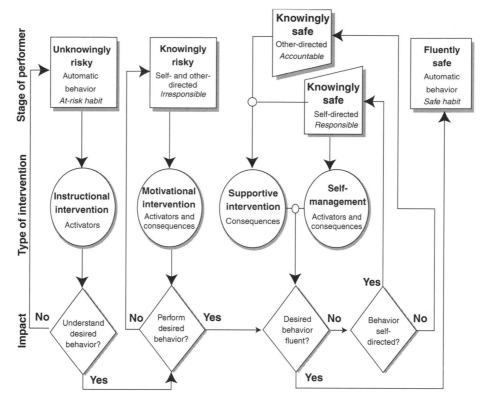

Figure 1. Competency States and Behavior-Based Prevention Strategies.

Self-management (Watson & Tharpe, 2002) essentially involves the application of the DO IT process (Principle 5 above) to one's own behavior. This means: (a) defining one or more target behavior(s) to improve; (b) monitoring these behaviors systematically and objectively; (c) manipulating relevant activators and consequences to increase desired behavior and decrease undesired behavior; and (d) tracking continual change in the target behavior(s) in order to determine the impact of the self-management process.

Accountability versus Responsibility

From the perspective of large-scale safety and health promotion, the distinction in Figure 1 between accountable and responsible is critical, reflecting one of the greatest challenges in the safety profession. When you are held accountable, you are asked to reach a certain objective or goal, often within a designated time period. But you might not feel responsible to meet the deadline. Or you might feel responsible enough to complete the assignment, but that is all. You do only what is required and no more.

There are times, however, when you extend your personal responsibility beyond accountability. You do more than what is required. You go beyond the call of duty as defined by a particular accountability system. This is often essential when it comes to industrial safety and health. To improve safety beyond the current performance plateaus experienced by many companies, workers need to extend their responsibility for safety beyond that for which they are held accountable. They need to transition from an other-directed state to a self-directed state.

Many jobs are accomplished by a lone worker. There is no supervisor or coworker around to hold the employee accountable for performing the job safely. So the challenge for safety professionals and corporate leaders is to build the kind of work culture that enables or facilitates responsibility or self-accountability for safety. I have covered some ways to do this in this entry, but we still have a lot to learn regarding how to help people transition from being held accountable for their safety-related behavior to feeling personally responsible to take extra precautions for injury prevention. Discovering more ways to do this is among the most important research needs in the domain of injury prevention.

Also see: Injuries, Unintentional: Early Childhood; Injuries, Unintentional: Childhood; Injuries, Unintentional: Adolescence; Environment: Foundation.

References

Bandura, A. (1997). *Self-efficacy: The exercise of control.* New York: W.H. Freeman.

Bird, F.E., Jr., & Germain, G.L. (1997). *The property damage accident: The neglected part of safety.* Loganville, GA: FEBCO.

Cady, L.D., Thomas, P.C., & Karwasky, R.J. (1985). Program for increasing health and physical fitness of fire fighters. *Journal of Occupational Medicine, 27,* 110–114.

Covello, V.T., Sandman, P.M., & Slovic, P. (1991). Guidelines for communicating information about chemical risks effectively and responsibly. In D.G. Mayo & R.D. Hollander (Eds.), *Acceptable evidence: Science and values in risk management.* New York: Oxford University Press.

Geller, E.S. (2001a). Sustaining participation in a safety improvement process: Ten relevant principles from behavioral science. *Professional Safety, 46*(9), 24–29.

Geller, E.S. (2001b). *The psychology of safety handbook.* Boca Raton, FL: CRC Press.

Geller, E.S. (2001c). *Working safe: How to help people actively care for health and safety* (2nd ed.). New York: Lewis.

Geller, E.S., & Williams, J. (Eds.). (2001). *Keys to behavior-based safety.* Rockville, MD: Government Institutes.

Guastello, S.J. (1993). Do we really know how well our occupational accident prevention programs work? *Safety Science, 16,* 445–463.

Human Resources Development Canada. (1997). *Occupational injuries and their cost in Canada, 1993–1997.* Ottawa, Ontario: Human Resources Development Canada.

Ivancevich, J.M., Matteson, M.T., Freedman, S.M., & Phillips, J.S. (1990). Worksite stress management interventions. *American Psychologist, 45,* 252–261.

Janssen, W. (1994). Seat belt wearing and driving behavior: An instrumented-vehicle study. *Accident Analysis and Prevention, 26,* 249–261.

Krause, T.R., Hidley, J.H., & Hodson, S.J. (1996). *The behavior-based safety process: Managing improvement for an injury-free culture* (2nd ed.). New York: Van Nostrand Reinhold.

Kroemer, K.H. (1991). Ergonomics. *Encyclopedia of human biology, 3,* 473–480.

Lehman, B.J., & Gage, H. (1995). How much is safety really worth? Countering a false hypothesis. *Professional Safety, 40*(6), 37–40.

Leigh, J. (1995). *Causes of death in the workplace.* Westport, CN: Quorum Books.

McSween, T.E. (1995). *The value-based safety process: Improving your safety culture with a behavioral approach.* New York: Van Nostrand Reinhold.

Miller, T.R. (1997). Estimating the costs of injury to U.S. employees. *Journal of Safety Research, 28*(1), 1–13.

Murphy, L.R. (1984). Occupational stress management: A review and appraisal. *Journal of Occupational Psychology, 57,* 1–16.

New Zealand Environmental and Occupational Health Research Centre. (1999). *Work-related fatal injuries in New Zealand, 1985–1994: Descriptive epidemiology.* Dundein, New Zealand: University of Otago.

Peltzman, S. (1975). The effects of automobile safety regulation. *Journal of Political Economics, 83,* 677–725.

Petersen, D. (1989). *Safe behavior reinforcement.* New York: Aloray.

Saarela, K.L. (1990). An intervention program utilizing small groups: A comparative study. *Journal of Safety Research, 21,* 149–156.

Skinner, B.F. (1971). *Beyond freedom and dignity.* New York: Alfred A. Knopf.

Streff, F.M., & Geller, E.S. (1988). An experimental test of risk compensation: Between-subject versus within-subject analysis. *Accident Analysis and Prevention, 20,* 277–287.

The *New Merriam-Webster Dictionary.* (1989). Springfield, MA: Merriam-Webster.

United States Bureau of Labor Statistics. (1998). *Safety and health statistics.* Occupational Safety and Health Home Page, http://www.bls.gov/stat

Watson, D.L., & Tharpe, R.G. (2002). *Self-directed behavior: Self-modification for personal adjustment* (8th ed.). Belmont, CA: Wadsworth.

Wilde, G.J.S. (1994). *Target risk.* Toronto, Ontario, Canada: PDE.

Intellectual Growth, Childhood

Sandra M. Chafouleas, Melissa A. Bray, and Thomas J. Kehle

INTRODUCTION

This entry focuses on promoting intellectual growth in early childhood, primarily from the perspective of cognitive development. However, we recognize that other factors such as affective, behavioral, and social variables are involved in promoting development, and discuss these as relevant to our major perspective.

DEFINITIONS

Intellectual or cognitive development is influenced by a combination of genetically based and environmental factors. Further, intelligence is a complex construct and has been historically difficult to define. In fact, Sattler (2001) summarized information presented at two major symposia by stating that the struggle continues in trying to find a common definition of intelligence. Despite the difficulty in achieving consensus, Sattler (2001) identified common themes across most definitions that emphasize the ability to adapt to the environment, to learn, and to think abstractly.

Since the creation of the Binet scale at the beginning of the 20th century, psychologists have struggled with the assessment of intelligence. Some theorists support a *g* or general factor (Jensen, 1998) of intelligence as commonly measured by a traditional standardized intelligence test. Others theorists such as Gardner (1983) suggest that there are multiple intelligences that cannot be adequately assessed by such a test. Similarly, Sternberg (1996) proposed a triarchic theory of intelligence that describes intelligence as a combination of analytic, creative, and practical abilities. Carroll's (1993) contemporary theory of intelligence, the three-strata factor analytic theory of cognitive abilities, proposes that although *g* is the all-encompassing level of intelligence, many distinct individual abilities exist to define it.

SCOPE

By definition, in a normal distribution of attributes like intelligence quotient (IQ) scores, 68 percent of the scores fall within 1 standard deviation above and below the mean. Individuals in this range are the focus of this entry on promoting intellectual development.

Costs

Public education is a basic utility for almost all societies in the world. The question of costs and financing of public education, as the fundamental basis for the continuity of society, varies depending on the wealth of a given nation, and the values that it attaches to public education. Investment in public education, as with many other preventive/promotive programs, changes with current events.

THEORIES AND RESEARCH

The study of intellectual growth is primarily undertaken through one of three major theories or approaches: psychometric, cognitive, and information-processing.

The *psychometric approach* to the study of intelligence was an early effort to understand the concept of cognitive differences among people. This approach has a long history and represents a central interest in contemporary psychology (Neisser et al., 1996). The psychometric approach to the study of intelligence focuses on an examination of the structure of an IQ test (Kaplan & Saccuzzo, 2001), such as its reliability, underlying factor structure, and predictive validity. The psychometric tradition is embedded in individually administered, standardized IQ tests such as the Wechsler (1991) scales. Full-scale IQ scores on these indices are predictive of many social and personal variables. For example, a relationship exists between IQ and standardized tests of academic achievement (correlations between 0.5 and 0.7) (Brody, 1992). With respect to predicting job performance in different occupations, the relationship ranges from approximately 0.27 to 0.61, with an average corrected correlation of 0.53. The range of these correlations is a function of job complexity with respect to cognitive demands (Hunter & Hunter [1984] as cited in Brody, 1992). At first impression, this means that the IQ score theoretically explains about a quarter of the variance (calculated with the coefficient of determination) of what influences these variables.

Moreover, younger children show considerably more variability in their scores on IQ tests than older children. That is, with the exception of those children receiving very low scores (Batshaw, 1993), IQ scores obtained during early childhood are not necessarily stable over time. However, as children age, this variability attenuates. For example, studies with monozygotic twins raised apart indicate that the correlations between their full-scale IQ scores increase as they age. That is to say, heritability estimates increase with age, and maximizes at approximately age 14 (Brody, 1992).

There is considerable dispute on the place of psychometric approaches in American society. Some writers argue that general intelligence (or *g* scores) is a relatively stable trait that has good predictive ability, particularly with respect to academic achievement (Herrnstein & Murray, 1994), but this view has received many critiques (Fraser, 1995). For example, Devlin, Daniels, and Roeder (1997) conducted a meta-analysis of the heritability of IQ, and found that genes account for less than 50 percent, which means that environmental interventions offer opportunities for influencing intellectual development. Despite the controversies, it is generally accepted that public concern regarding the social consequences of the use of IQ tests is legitimate. However, the issue is to correctly distinguish between negative consequences for individual children or groups that are due to flaws inherent in the IQ test and its theoretical basis versus flaws that are inherent in the misrepresentation and misuse of IQ tests (Linn & Gronlund, 2000).

The *cognitive approach* to studying intellectual development grew from Piaget's observations of children that led him to create a stage-based theory of cognitive development. Piaget believed that cognitive development progresses sequentially through four stages based on a combination of biological maturation, personal experiences, and the environment. The basic process of cognitive development occurs through adaptation to new information, either through assimilation (incorporate new into existing mental structures or schemata) or accommodation (modify existing schemata to incorporate new).

According to Piaget, the first stage (birth–2 years) involves sensorimotor experiences, which are characterized by learning through sensory information and motor actions with regard to the things learned. Key accomplishments include object permanence (objects continue to exist when they are out of sight), recognition that events cause other events, and symbolic thought (using language to think before acting). The preoperational stage occurs from the ages 2–7 years, and is marked by the ability to use symbols to learn about things that are not present (symbolic function). At this stage, children exhibit animism (attributing human characteristics to inanimate objects), magical thinking (thinking about something will cause it), and egocentrism (inability to take another's perspective). During the third stage, concrete operations (7–11 years), children will be able to use mental operations rather than solely physical to carry out activities. Children grasp the concept of conservation, or the recognition that two equal quantities remain equal as long as nothing is added or taken away. Formal operations (11+ years) comprises the final stage. A person in this stage is able to think abstractly and theoretically. That is, they are able to think about their own thinking. Later research has indicated that cognitive development does not necessarily follow this hypothesized sequence, especially in the later stages. Some of the concepts may be understood by children younger than Piaget had conceptualized, and the ages at which stages are reached may vary for different cultures. However, this approach has been used to guide early education programs (Schweinhart & Weikart, 1988).

The *information processing approach* to studying intellectual growth focuses on describing the process of acquiring information or solving problems. In other words, it examines what people do with information that is perceived. It is a relatively new approach that was prompted in part by research comparing human and computer functioning. Specific processes or tasks such as memory (e.g., recognition, recall) and the use of rules are the focus of interest rather than global intellectual ability. For example, research with young infants and children might focus on tasks related to visual-recognition memory. How quickly infants habituate to familiar stimuli has been found to correlate moderately with later language ability and intelligence tests.

STRATEGIES: OVERVIEW

Many writers have argued that there is evidence that society can influence intellectual growth (Devlin et al., 1997; Zigler, Kagan, & Hall, 1996; Zigler & Styfco, 1993). On the other hand, Brody (1992) suggests that it may be more accurate to state that a particular instructional program may benefit low IQ students, while there are also instructional programs that can impede their educational achievement without influencing the academic achievement of high IQ students. In other words, the interactions between an individual and the environment is complex and yet to be fully understood.

However, there is encouraging evidence from the field of developmental neuroscience, which suggests that the "brain retains its capacity to grow throughout life ... the brain is a complex organ, it does not develop in a homogenous fashion over time." (Thompson & Nelson, 2001, p. 12). Research has clearly identified several biological factors that can impede intellectual growth from conception, such as exposure to teratogens and inadequate nutrition. In addition,

other environmental strategies derived from social science research have also been shown to work as well, like supportive parents and quality preschool. Flynn (1998) suggests that environmental factors have influenced intelligence with his research indicating generational IQ gains in the United States since the 19th century. The problem has been with identifying specific factors. Explanations such as nutrition, TV, early school enrichment, and increased educational opportunities have been suggested, but not validated (Flynn, 1998). For example, some research has indicated that Chinese children's IQ scores early in the 20th century (very much below the national average) became higher than the national average by the end of that century (Flynn, 1991; Lynn, 1991).

The questions facing educators, parents, policy makers, and researchers are how to prevent detrimental biological hazards from occurring, as well as how to maximize the advantages that a quality environment can provide to children.

STRATEGIES THAT WORK

Prenatal and Perinatal Factors

A number of factors during development prior to birth (prenatal) have been associated with negative impacts on intellectual development (Allen, 1993). The most familiar primary prevention efforts have been through public health, education, and social action programs related to limiting exposure to various toxins. These toxins, or teratogens, cross the placental barrier, causing damage to the embryo or fetus. The first trimester is typically the period most susceptible to damage by teratogens. Alcohol and certain drugs are probably the most widely known, given federal legislation requiring cautionary labeling of these items for consumption by pregnant women. In addition, pre- and postnatal exposure to lead has been associated with a number of negative side effects, including delayed cognitive development (Smith, 1998). A common source of lead poisoning is lead-based paint, which may be most often found in houses built prior to 1978. Awareness of possible risks of exposure and preventive actions in the affected environment to remove lead can reduce the incidence of lead poisoning. If exposure is probable or unavoidable, monitoring of lead levels in blood throughout pregnancy and after birth will identify if treatment is necessary. The process of chelating lead from the blood is expensive and unpleasant for the victim.

Another group of risk factors relates to maternal health. Exposure to certain diseases (e.g., Rubella, HIV/AIDS) has been associated with impact on a number of areas of development, including cognitive. In addition, good maternal nutrition is important, particularly during the third trimester (months 6–9). In summary, many prenatal risks associated with delayed cognitive development can be reduced or avoided through careful prenatal monitoring. Unfortunately, the individuals who are most at risk are least likely to obtain high quality prenatal care or adequate nutrition.

In addition, fetal and/or newborn screening can identify genetic factors that can cause delayed intellectual growth. For example, phenylketonuria (PKU) is a condition in which the person lacks an enzyme needed to metabolize phenylalanine, an amino acid. Without early identification of the condition and subsequent dietary restriction, severe mental retardation is possible. Other genetic factors associated with delayed intellectual growth can be identified through screening and genetic counseling. For example, one factor for higher risk of Down's syndrome (trisomy-21), a genetic condition involving an extra chromosome, is increased maternal age. People planning families at older ages should be advised of the risks involved.

Although infrequently occurring, perinatal or birth complications also can have negative consequences for cognitive development. For example, anoxia (oxygen shortage) can occur from an umbilical cord wrapped around a baby's neck. Anoxia can affect cognitive as well as motor development.

Accident Prevention

Accidents such as falls, sports and recreational injuries, and motor vehicle accidents have the potential to create traumatic brain injury (TBI). TBI has been cited as the most common cause of acquired disability in childhood (Michaud, Duhaime, & Batshaw, 1993). Limiting the incidence of accidents and thus TBI is a major strategy of primary prevention with regard to intellectual growth. A primary method of accident prevention is through parent and caregiver education. Education on the proper and necessary use of child safety seats and bicycle helmets are some examples. Laws requiring child safety seats may also be credited with saving large numbers of children from injury and death. In addition, tougher legislation to prevent avoidable accidents such as drunk driving provides another method of primary prevention.

Nutrition

Quality nutrition is important to intellectual growth across the lifespan. For example, poor nutrition has been implicated in adult cognitive deficits, although these deficits are generally restored after nutrition is improved (Botwinick, 1984). For children in particular, the developing brain is especially vulnerable to nutritional inadequacy. The young brain relies heavily upon nutrients such as folic acid, iron, and vitamins to stimulate growth and development (Thompson & Nelson, 2001).

Overall Quality of Care at School and Home

School

Evidence has suggested that an enriched school environment can increase the cognitive functioning of children with low IQ scores (Baumrind, 1993). Further, it has been found that schooling creates schemata that are necessary for continued growth in cognitive and problem-solving skills (Hunt, 1999). The amount of time spent in, or quantity of, school has been related to moderate gains in intelligence (Brody, 1992). In addition to simply being present in school, the amount of time the student is actively engaged in the learning process is related to school success (Gettinger & Stoiber, 1999). Finally, a successful primary prevention strategy for increasing academic achievement is peer tutoring (Greenwood, Delquadri, & Hall, 1989), or individual tutoring by adults.

In addition to these school promotion strategies, a picture of the impact of quality schooling may come from performance-based methods such as curriculum-based assessment (CBA) (Shapiro & Elliott, 1999). CBA allows for the direct evaluation of the student's specific curriculum and subsequent design of instruction to promote academic functioning. CBA probes the areas of spelling, mathematics, written language, and reading. Following the assessment, academic instruction is tailored to the needs of the individual. For example, the area of reading fluency (how accurately and quickly a student reads) may be addressed through implementation of strategies such as cuing, modeling, phrasing, previewing, and repeated readings.

Home

Classic adoption studies (e.g., Scarr & Weinberg, 1976; Skodak & Skeels, 1949), although cited as having methodological flaws, have found that adopted children's performance on intelligence and academic achievement tests were above children who were not adopted yet had similar genetic backgrounds. The variables proposed to contribute to this were high parental involvement, emphasis on independence, teaching of language, engagement in verbal expression, and positive modeling of intellectual interests (Hanson, 1976). For example, literature supporting the importance of reading to your child encompasses virtually all of these variables. In addition, modeling of appropriate verbal and social interactions has been related to promotion of cognitive growth (Levenstein, 1988). Responsiveness or involvement of the caretaker to the child during both distressed and non-distressed states may also be a relevant factor. In summary, one portion of promoting cognitive skills is related to quality of care in the child's environment. The significance of this point is that there are many environmental ways that we know work with regard to promoting intellectual growth and development. The issue is how to organize and deliver these many opportunities.

STRATEGIES THAT MIGHT WORK

Early Intervention Programs

Studies examining the effects of early intervention programs on intelligence test scores have shown mixed results. Some investigations have indicated significant increases in IQ test scores over controls while others have found the advantages are not evident over the long term (Kamphaus, 2001). Part of the difficulties in making conclusions about the potential of intervention programs may lie in faulty evaluation practices (Gilliam, Ripple, Zigler, & Leiter, 2000), inconsistent implementation of high-quality programming (Ramey, 1999), and the relatively short-term nature of some programs (Zigler & Styfco, 2000). In addition, long-term advantages may not be found when the quality of teaching and home support does not continue what early intervention programs had begun. Zigler and Styfco (2001) assert that appropriate environmental support services need to target not only the preschool environment, but also the entire ecology in which the child is raised.

It is also important to note that increases in IQ test scores do not represent a complete picture of growth. For example, although enrollment in high quality pre-school experiences such as the *Perry Preschool Project* may not have resulted in long-term increases in IQ test scores, it certainly resulted in socially valued outcomes (Schweinhart & Weikart, 1988). In a 25-year follow-up, Barnett (1993) reported lower rates of delinquency and higher levels of work (and tax paying) for young people having this pre-school experience compared to randomly selected controls.

In summary, a complete picture of promoting intellectual growth occurs not simply from enrollment in an early intervention program. Enrollment in a carefully planned and sequenced school program coupled with coordinated family and community support (e.g., housing, health) over the long term may be the best course of action, although research is needed on how best to coordinate and organize all of these supports.

STRATEGIES THAT DO NOT WORK

Tracking

Tracking refers to the placement of students in homogenous groups based on ability. That is, lower ability students are grouped with similar students and vice versa. In general, the effects of tracking have suggested a type of self-fulfilling prophecy. That is, negative effects on achievement as well as motivation can be evident for those students in lower tracks. Overall, it is suggested that heterogeneous grouping (no tracking) tends to be beneficial for lower ability groups with, at worst, no impact on higher ability groups (Oakes, 1985).

SYNTHESIS

> Development is not a disease to be treated. It is a process that needs constant nurturance. There is no reason to expect that an intensive program of early stimulation is an inoculation against all further developmental problems. No one would predict that a child given an adequate amount of vitamin C at two years of age will not have vitamin C deficiency at 10 years of age. Currently, according to the most viable model of development that applies to both at-risk and normal children, developmentally functional stimulation is desirable at every period of development and not only in early years (Horowitz & O'Brien, 1989, p. 444).

The Horowitz and O'Brien (1989) quote drives our synthesis, or understanding, of best practices regarding the primary prevention of the promotion of intellectual growth. Although there are certainly many strategies (e.g., prenatal and postnatal factors, quantity of schooling) that help assure a child's intellectual growth would not be thwarted, particular strategies to increase this potential have been difficult to isolate from within a comprehensive approach to quality care in a mass society.

Other factors in addition to intelligence contribute to the prediction of life's desired outcomes, and may be more amenable to modification. The promotion of intellectual growth through early childhood may be facilitated through the modification of environmental factors that support intelligent behavior, building on the strongest biological foundation (e.g., freedom from tetragons) possible. The task of the future is how to coordinate and organize all of these factors in promoting intellectual development in young children, and then, continuing, over the course of the entire lifespan. For example, Begley (2001) summarized research on promoting adult intelligence, and found that an individual should strive to reduce stress, be socially and intellectually active, and adhere to the tenets of good physical health. These results have their parallels in the suggestions made for promoting intellectual development in children. Promoting intellectual growth is a lifelong process. A good beginning in early childhood is a vital first step.

Also see: Culture, Society, and Social Class: Foundation; Politics and Systems Change: Foundation; Academic Success: Adolescence; Child Care: Early Childhood; Environmental Health: Early Childhood; Environmental Health: Childhood; Family Strengthening: Childhood; Family Strengthening: Adolescence; Media Habits: Childhood; Nutrition: Early Childhood; Nutrition: Childhood.

References

Allen, M.C. (1993). The high-risk infant. *The Pediatric Clinics of North America, 40,* 479–490.

Barnett, W.S. (1993). Benefit–cost analysis of preschool education: Findings from a 25-year follow-up. *American Journal of Orthopsychiatry, 63,* 500–508.

Batshaw, M.L. (1993). Mental retardation. *The Pediatric Clinics of North America, 40,* 507–521.

Baumrind, D. (1993). The average expectable environment is not good enough: A response to Scarr. *Child Development, 64,* 1299–1337.

Begley, S. (2001, Fall/Winter). The brain in winter. *Newsweek* (Special edition, Health for life), 24–29.

Botwinick, J. (1984). *Aging and behavior.* New York: Springer.

Brody, N. (1992). *Intelligence* (2nd ed.). San Diego, CA: Academic Press.

Carroll, J.B. (1993). *Human cognitive abilities: A survey of factor-analytic studies.* New York: Cambridge University Press.

Devlin, B., Daniels, M., & Roeder, K. (1997). The heritability of IQ. *Nature, 388,* 468–471.

Fraser, S. (Ed.). (1995). *The bell curve wars: Race, intelligence, and the future of America.* New York: Basic Books.

Flynn, J.R. (1991). *Asian Americans: Achievement beyond IQ.* Hillsdale, NJ: Lawrence Erlbaum Associates.

Flynn, J.R. (1998). IQ gains over time: Toward finding the causes. In U. Neisser (Ed.), *The rising curve: Long-term gains in IQ and related measures* (pp. 25–66). Washington, DC: American Psychological Association.

Gardner, H. (1983). *Frames of mind: The theory of multiple intelligence*s. New York: Basic Books.

Gettinger, M., & Stoiber, K.C. (1999). Excellence in teaching: Review of instructional and environmental variables. In C.R. Reynolds & T.B. Gutkin (Eds.), *The Handbook of School Psychology* (3rd ed., pp. 933–958). New York, NY: Wiley.

Gilliam, W.S., Ripple, C.H., Zigler, E.F., & Leiter, V. (2000). Evaluating child and family demonstration initiatives: Lessons from the comprehensive child development program. *Early Childhood Research Quarterly, 15,* 41–59.

Greenwood, C.R., Delquadri, J.C., & Hall, R.V. (1989). Longitudinal effects of classwide peer tutoring. *Journal of Educational Psychology, 81,* 371–383.

Hanson, R.A. (1975). Consistency and stability of home environmental issues related to IQ. *Child Development, 46,* 470–480.

Herrnstein, R.J., & Murray, C. (1994). *The bell curve.* New York, NY: The Free Press.

Horowitz, F.D., & O'Brien, M. (1989). A reflective essay on the state of our knowledge and the challenges before us. *American Psychologist, 44,* 441–445.

Hunt, E. (1999). Intelligence and human resources: Past, present, and future. In P.L. Ackerman, P.C. Kyllonen, & R.D. Roberts (Eds.), *Learning and individual differences: Process, trait, and content determinants* (pp. 3–30). Washington, DC: Author.

Jensen, A.R. (1998). The g factor and the design of education. In R. Sternberg & W. Williams (Eds.), *Intelligence, instruction and assessment: Theory into practice* (pp. 111–131). Mahwah, NJ: Lawrence Erlbaum Associates.

Kamphaus, R.W. (2001). *Clinical assessment of child and adolescent intelligence* (2nd ed.). Needham Heights, MA: Allyn & Bacon.

Kaplan, R.M., & Saccuzzo, D.P. (2001). *Psychological testing* (5th ed.). Belmont, CA: Wadsworth.

Levenstein, P. (1988). *Messages from home: The mother–child home program and the prevention of school disadvantage.* Columbus, OH: Ohio State University Press.

Linn, R.L., & Gronlund, N.E. (2000). *Measurement and assessment in teaching* (8th ed.). Upper Saddle River, NJ: Prentice-Hall.

Lynn, R. (1991). Race differences in intelligence: A global perspective. *Mankind Quarterly, 31,* 254–296.

Michaud, L.J., Duhaime, A., & Batshaw, M.L. (1993). Traumatic brain injury in children. *The Pediatric Clinics of North America, 40,* 553–565.

Neisser, U., Boodoo, G., Bouchard, T.J., Boykin, A.W., Brody, N., Ceci, S.J. et al. (1996). Intelligence: Knowns and unknowns. *American Psychologist, 51,* 77–101.

Oakes, J. (1985). *Keeping track: How schools structure inequality.* New Haven, CT: Yale University Press.

Ramey, S.L. (1999). Head Start and preschool education: Toward continued improvement. *American Psychologist, 54,* 344–346.

Sattler, J.M. (2001). *Assessment of children: Cognitive applications* (4th ed.). San Diego, CA: Jerome M. Sattler.

Scarr, S., & Weinberg, R.A. (1976). The influence of "family background" on intellectual attainment. *American Sociological Review, 43,* 674–692.

Schweinhart, L.J., & Weikart, D.P. (1988). The High/Scope Perry Preschool Program. In R. Price et al. (Eds.), *14 ounces of prevention.* Washington, DC: American Psychological Association.

Skodak, M., & Skeels, H.M. (1949). A final follow-up study of one hundred adopted children. *The Journal of Genetic Psychology, 75,* 85–125.

Shapiro, E.S., & Elliott, S.N. (1999). Curriculum-based assessment and other performance-based assessment strategies. In C.R. Reynolds & T.B. Gutkin (Eds.), *The handbook of school psychology* (3rd ed., pp. 383–408). New York, NY: Wiley.

Smith, C.R. (1998). *Learning disabilities: The interaction of learner, task, and setting* (4th ed.). Needham Heights, MA: Allyn & Bacon.

Sternberg, R.J. (1996). *Successful intelligence.* New York: Simon & Schuster.

Thompson, R.A., & Nelson, C.A. (2001). Developmental science and the media: Early brain development. *American Psychologist, 56,* 5–15.

Wechsler, D. (1991). *WISC-III manual.* San Antonio, TX: The Psychological Corporation.

Zigler, E., Kagan, S.L., & Hall, N.W. (Eds.). (1996). *Children, families, and government: Preparing for the twenty-first century.* Cambridge: Cambridge University Press.

Zigler, E., & Styfco, S.J. (1993). *Head Start and beyond: A natural plan for extending childhood intervention.* New Haven, CT: Yale University Press.

Zigler, E., & Styfco, S.J. (2000). Pioneering steps (and fumbles) in developing a federal preschool intervention. *Topics in Early Childhood Special Education, 20,* 67–70.

Zigler, E., & Styfco, S.J. (2001). Extended childhood intervention prepares children for school and beyond. *Journal of the American Medical Association, 285,* 2378–2380.

Intimate Partner Violence, Adulthood

Audrey Begun

INTRODUCTION

Intimate partner violence (IPV) is a complex social problem of great significance to individuals, families, neighborhoods, communities, service delivery systems, and society. There are no adequate simple, linear explanatory models of IPV. Hence, the prevention endeavor is complex to plan, implement, and evaluate. The literature is rife with controversy concerning the nature of vulnerability, risk, resilience, and protective factors related to IPV. There is also debate over the effectiveness of various intervention efforts. This entry provides an overview of the primary prevention issues related to IPV, although this necessarily involves some explorations into interventions with the perpetrators of IPV.

DEFINITIONS

IPV is the use of violence, and/or its threatened use within the context of intimate partner relationships. It refers to physical acts of aggression, as well as sexual, psychological, and emotional abuse. Less inclusive, but related terms are spouse abuse, domestic violence, dating violence/date rape, battering, and marital violence/marital rape. IPV relates to intimate partnerships between heterosexual, as well as same-sex partners, and involves boyfriend/girlfriend, cohabiting, married, and ex-partners.

SCOPE

It is difficult to determine the scope of IPV because of variability in definitions and measurement approaches (e.g., use of victim reports, perpetrator self-reports, hospital emergency visit data, public surveys, arrests and/or police contacts). Unreported incidents may be as much as three to five times the total of those reported (Tjaden & Thoennes, 2000). In addition, IPV incidence figures can be reported differentially as the numbers of abusive acts perpetrated, new individuals victimized, new perpetrating individuals, or new relationships in which IPV has occurred. Prevalence figures may reflect the number of individuals who have ever been the victim or perpetrator of IPV or only those who continue to perpetrate or be victimized. Disparities in these reporting approaches make comparisons between studies and across populations exceedingly difficult.

Incidence and Prevalence Reports

During each year between 1992–1996, an average of 8 in 1,000 US women aged 12 or more experienced IPV (Greenfield et al., 1998). Annually in the United States, between 1.8 and 4.4 million women are battered by an intimate partner (Campbell & Soeken, 1999). While in 85 percent of incidents the victims were women, and women are approximately six times more likely than men to experience

IPV, approximately 1 in 1,000 men experienced violence perpetrated by a current or former intimate partner (Bureau of Justice Statistics, 2000). There were approximately 2,000 lethal incidents of IPV during 1996; 30 percent of all female and 3 percent of male murder victims were killed by an intimate partner (Federal Bureau of Investigation [FBI], 1996). Approximately 15 percent of men and 11 percent of women in cohabiting same-sex partnerships experience IPV (Tjaden & Thoennes, 2000), where the apparent reversal in victim rates by gender actually continues to reflect higher perpetration rates by males than by females.

IPV occurs in all strata of American society, although its occurrence may not be proportionally equal across groups. The average annual rate (1994–1996) of victimization through IPV is about 8.2 per 1,000 among White women, 11.7 per 1,000 among Black women, 7.2 per 1,000 among Latino women. And, while IPV occurs in households across all economic strata, its frequency may increase as household income declines (Flowers, 2000).

IPV is international in scope. Each country that reported to The Fourth United Nations International Conference on Women identified IPV within their borders, but there was tremendous variability in the reporting approaches adopted (United Nations, 1996). In Nicaragua, 52 percent of women aged 15–49 had been victims of IPV at some point in their lives (Ellsberg, Caldera, Herrera, Winkvist, & Kullgren, 1999). In Chile, 25 percent of metropolitan women aged 22–55 were currently beaten by an intimate partner (McWhirter, 1999). The statistics reported for post-Soviet Russia demonstrate an alarming trend: the number of women killed by a domestic partner has been rising from approximately 14,500 during 1993 to 16,000 during 1995 (Horne, 1999).

Costs to Individuals and to Society

The direct costs related to IPV are immense, beginning with the health and welfare of the individuals who are abused. Assault by an intimate is the leading cause of injury among women and frequently results in significant physical injury, chronic physical health problems, permanent disability, sexually transmitted diseases, unplanned pregnancies, pregnancy complications, serious psychological disturbances, and death (Campbell & Soeken, 1999; Parker, McFarlane, Soeken, Silva, & Reel, 1999; Wiehe, 1998). Furthermore, significant negative effects are experienced by children and others who witness incidents of IPV, and IPV has been associated with increased probabilities for other forms of family and community violence as well (Walker, 1999; Wiehe, 1998; Wolak & Finkelhor, 1998).

The costs to individuals, families, communities, and society include direct and indirect economic costs of physical injuries and emotional or psychological sequelae (e.g., "Battered Woman Syndrome," post-traumatic stress, depression, anxiety, headaches, sleep disruption, difficulties in concentration, suicidal thoughts and attempts, substance abuse, temporary or permanent disability, sexually transmitted diseases). In addition, legal expenses (court expenses and fines, victim service/protection expenses, relationship dissolution costs) and employment interference (loss of employment, lost work time for medical or legal reasons, interruption of work due to partner's harassment) must be considered. Annual medical costs related to IPV are estimated at $1.3 billion, costs of lost work combined with medical costs is estimated at $5–10 billion, and costs to the criminal justice system approach $67 billion (Giles-Sims, 1998).

THEORIES

In order to understand the host of theories pertaining to the etiology of IPV, one must first distinguish between those pertaining to *becoming a victim* and to *becoming a perpetrator*. Models also differ in their emphasis on *proximal* (e.g., unemployment, social support, personal stress, and substance abuse) or *distal* (e.g., witnessing violence in the family of origin, parental substance and child abuse patterns, and social attachment) factors. Because most studies are correlational rather than longitudinal, we have a poor understanding of the actual developmental processes involved in the emergence of IPV and the factors that might protect against it.

The risk of perpetrating IPV has been associated with a host of personality/character traits, biological/hereditary/genetic predispositions, social learning/modeling, social skills, self-esteem, and cultural norms. A wide range of risk factors have been explored, including gender-role attitudes, substance abuse, serotonin or androgen/testosterone levels, past history of witnessing abuse, delinquency, stress responses, depression, and general hostility (Begun, 1999; Kantor & Jasinski, 1998). A relatively recent area of attention is the development of batterer typologies, distinguishing among "family only," "generally violent," and "borderline personality" batterers (Healey, Smith, & O'Sullivan, 1998) or between individuals demonstrating different aspects or stages in a behavioral change cycle, which is the process of intentionally changing one's behaviors (Begun, Shelley, Strodthoff, & Short, 2001). Accurate typologies and staging may eventually increase the likelihood of matching interventions to target groups, thereby enhancing intervention effectiveness.

Several *etiological models* for the perpetration of IPV have each garnered at least partial support. *Social learning theory* suggests that individuals may learn to perpetrate IPV in two general ways. First, individuals may witness IPV behavior in their parents' or other significant individuals' relationships. In addition, as a child, an individual may be a direct or indirect target of parental maltreatment. Thus, a cycle of violence is perpetuated across generations through *imitation of social models*, and through an *absence of models for positive intimate partner relationships*. Second, individuals may learn IPV through the classic *learning paradigms*. For example, if an act of aggression is "rewarded" by the partner's submission, it is instrumental in achieving a goal, and an individual is increasingly likely to aggress in future situations with intimate partners. Furthermore, a person's inhibitions against aggressing in general may become weakened through *desensitization from overexposure to violence* (e.g., family, peer group, neighborhood, media, etc.). This *disinhibition* can result in a generalized tendency toward violence that will be directed at intimate partners, as well as others in the social environment.

Biological models of aggression suggest that some individuals are predisposed to aggression in their social interactions. Biological models tested in primate development suggest that an individual's early developmental environmental context has a significant impact on later arousal responses and hyperaggressiveness. The effects of genetic, hormonal and central nervous system pathways in humans are only beginning to be understood in relation to the expression of IPV, but leave few options for its primary prevention.

Closely related to the biological models are the effects of *substance abuse*. Certain substances that individuals may abuse—particularly alcohol, cocaine, amphetamines, phencylidine, and opiate withdrawal—can cause hyperaggressive behavior, which may be directed toward an intimate partner or anyone else in proximity. Some substances can result in disinhibition so that a person ignores the likely consequences for IPV. Still other IPV situations may occur as a result of a partner being perceived as interfering with access to substances to which an individual is addicted.

Personality theory also suggests ways in which certain individuals may become equipped with a predisposition to IPV behavior. *Social skills deficits* and certain *social cognitions* (thoughts and beliefs about the social world) have also been explored as contributors to IPV. For example, individuals who believe that they have a right and/or responsibility to control others are more likely to impose their control over a partner through IPV. And, individuals who have poor mastery of positive social skills are likely to rely on brute force to achieve their social interaction goals when communication, negotiation, self-expression, or empathy fail.

Cultural models related to IPV indicate that values and belief systems that permeate many societies are forces that condone IPV and fail to deter its expression. Patriarchal and highly "traditional," dominance-related sex-role beliefs may be associated with approval, or at least a lack of disapproval, for IPV. When IPV is conceptualized as an international human rights issue, nations are called upon to deal with and eliminate the social conditions that breed violence against women, rather than focusing strictly on intervention services for victims (Walker, 1999). This includes targeting cultural and state sanctions for men's (and military) use of violence to control women, patriarchal cultural systems and strict gender role socialization, community tolerance of violence to resolve conflicts, women's acceptance of violence as a normative part of life, acceptance of violence as a manifestation of love, women's lack of independent access to resources, and male control of legal systems, social services, and the media (Ellsberg et al., 1999; Horne, 1999; McWhirter, 1999).

Theories pertaining to the risk of becoming the victim of IPV address factors such as guilt and self-blame, low self-esteem and learned helplessness, ambiguous paternity of children, use of defensive violence, substance abuse, family of origin experiences with violence (either witnessing or being the target of maltreatment). Critical, too, is the nature of the potential victim's economic, legal, emotional, spiritual and/or physical dependence on another individual. Such dependency might arise from emotional and psychological roots, or may be due to youthfulness, disability, aging, immigrant status, cultural/religious beliefs, fear/terror of the abusive person, relying on the abusive person for protection from others, lack of resources or reasonable alternatives (Begun, 1999; Wiehe, 1998). The risk of victimization does not necessarily diminish with termination of the relationship, since IPV is often directed at ex-partners and victims may find new partners who are abusive.

RESEARCH

Evidence that "Prevention Works" might be implied by the decline in reports of IPV toward women between 1993–1996, from 1.1 million to 840,000 (Greenfield et al., 1998). Unfortunately, there is no conclusive evidence that the trend is strictly a function of national and regional preventive intervention efforts (e.g., the 1994 Violence Against Women Act, NIJ and CDC collaborative initiatives to prevent IPV, etc.). The reductions may be attributed to the health of the economy and low unemployment or to shifts in the reporting practices that are being employed.

STRATEGIES: OVERVIEW

IPV is a field of study where there exist some gray areas in distinguishing prevention from treatment. Information and activities directed toward young adults and other community members not yet affected by the problem would be the conventional meaning of primary prevention efforts. However, services to victims of IPV may be *both* treatment (dealing with immediate or delayed physical and/or mental health problems that result) *and* prevention (addressing future incidents of IPV unrelated to the present or past events). Furthermore, adolescent interventions may not be primary prevention because some of these individuals have been engaged in IPV behaviors. Thus, this entry discusses prevention in both the conventional sense of primary prevention, and in the expanded sense of *both* treatment *and* prevention, as explained above. While punishing a perpetrator for a specific act of IPV may represent a form of treatment (or retribution), some individuals view batterer treatment efforts as prevention because they may deter individuals from new incidents of IPV with other people.

STRATEGIES THAT WORK

Strong and convincing evidence does not currently exist to suggest that any particular strategies work as primary prevention of IPV.

STRATEGIES THAT MIGHT WORK

There are three major IPV prevention approaches: (1) primary prevention efforts directed at adolescents so as to prevent the emergence of violent relationships in adulthood; (2) community-wide prevention efforts; and (3) indicated prevention directed to individuals who have been victims of IPV and/or to those identified as being "at risk."

Primary Prevention with Adolescents

School-based preventive education programs have been developed for implementation with middle and high school populations. The rationale behind this approach is that adolescents might (1) avoid becoming victims of IPV if, prior to their intensive involvement in intimate partner relationships, they are made aware of the warning signs and signals of potentially abusive relationships—such as these general points: isolating a person from contacts with friends and family; controlling what a person does, wears, whom he/she talks to; denying the person access to money; threatening to harm self if they break up; and publicly humiliating the person and (2) avoid becoming IPV perpetrators if they are made aware that it is unacceptable and that there are constructive, successful alternative behaviors. Hence, some of these interventions are geared toward preventing IPV in the future, as the adolescents become adults, and others are geared toward preventing IPV in the "here and now" adolescent dating relationships. Many of these relationship violence prevention programs are components of general violence prevention programs based in the schools.

Adolescent-focused interventions generally address issues of awareness and recognition of IPV/dating violence, and counter adolescents' beliefs that IPV represents love, is the victim's fault, or is normative relationship behavior (Wekerle & Wolfe, 1999). Some indicated prevention programs extend batterer's treatment to adolescents who are "at risk" of perpetrating IPV because dating violence in adolescence and young adulthood appears to be an important juncture in the emergence of adult IPV (Wekerle & Wolfe, 1999). In addition, some battered women's support programs have developed indicated prevention interventions for the children and adolescents who witness IPV among their parents, both as a means of preventing the inter-generational transmission of IPV to the children and as a means of preventing the psychological sequelae associated with the experiences (Chalk & King, 1998).

Several studies have demonstrated desirable changes in adolescents' knowledge and attitudes about IPV as the result of brief school-based educational preventive interventions (Hamby, 1998; Macgowan, 1997; Wekerle & Wolfe, 1999). However, what has yet to be addressed is the weak persistence of effects over time, differential impacts on boys and girls, and possible developmental differences between middle- and high-school audiences. Furthermore, there is not yet convincing evidence that actual adolescent dating behavior or later intimate partner relationships as adults are affected by the interventions, but only that known risk factors have been modified.

Long-term, intensive IPV preventive intervention programs are rare. Wekerle and Wolfe (1999) recommended that preventive intervention with "at risk" adolescents be multilevel in nature, that they include a relationship-basis and bi-directional dialogues, and that they be associated with identified cultural, familial, and social influence risk factors. Successful programs in youth violence prevention are those using broad-based approaches targeting multiple issues in multiple domains, addressing the behavior within the social context, and coordinating strategies across social domains (Reppucci, Woolard, & Fried, 1999).

Community-Wide Prevention Strategies

Community-wide prevention efforts are generally designed to influence values, beliefs, and norms concerning IPV-related issues. The objectives include consciousness-raising, problem awareness, and initiating social action, along with replacing IPV-promoting norms with non-acceptance of IPV and informing the public about available options. Before launching into the development and implementation of community-wide preventive interventions, it is essential to first assess the community's readiness for the change effort. Fawcett, Heise, Isita-Espejel, and Pick (1999) have delineated a "stages of change" model for community assessment, with accompanying behavioral descriptors associated with the various levels of readiness to engage in efforts to change IPV. Once an adequate assessment has been made, the change agents have a basis for action-planning that is tailored to the specific make-up of the community. Campaigns that have demonstrated effectiveness should be considered for transfer to other, similar types of communities and considered for modification, tailoring them to other types. Furthermore, because communities are heterogeneous in nature, campaigns might be tailored for sub-populations using directed marketing strategies (e.g., distinct campaigns for ethnic groups, different age groups, by gender).

Several public media campaigns have been launched in recent years. Hotline calls from victims and perpetrators, as well as calls for general information and volunteer opportunities increased dramatically each time the campaign was disseminated over a 3-year period. However, call rates returned to baseline at the end of each campaign.

There currently exists a strong push for the development of coordinated community responses to IPV (also called coordinated community action models; Hamby, 1998). The philosophy behind this push is that the effectiveness of many prevention and intervention approaches can be intensified if each approach occurs within the context of a coordinated system of strategies. In part, this requires a collaborative effort between the various health care, social service, and criminal justice systems in each community (e.g., coordinated reporting, imposing penalties for treatment non-compliance, ensuring victim safety, long-term follow-up with perpetrators and victims, etc.). In concert, these agents can better ensure the delivery of consistent non-violence messages and sanctions against IPV, as well as efficient utilization of resources.

Hamby (1998) suggests that there is a cumulative effect for each successive intervention experienced by the perpetrator—successful prosecution, probation, and completion of counseling services together accounted for 25 percent lower recidivism than any one isolated approach. At the core of a successful coordinated community response is the coordination of criminal justice responses to IPV-responses from law enforcement officers, selected prosecutors, pretrial services personnel, victim advocates, judges, probation officers, and batterer treatment programs to which individuals are referred (Healey et al., 1998). In addition, a coordinated community response would permit the addressing of IPV issues through any of the various contexts in which the problem may appear (e.g., child welfare and substance abuse programs). Coordinating the community's response to IPV may minimize the potential for re-victimization of and discrimination against those who have been the targets of IPV, as well as ensuring a seamless continuity-of-care approach to victims. One such model system is the Domestic Abuse Counseling Center of Pittsburgh (Healey et al., 1998). The coordinated community action model (CCAM) is another type of coordinated response (Hamby, 1998). Because of their relative novelty, there is little systematic evaluation data to support their use, but one element in particular appears critical in launching a successful coordinated community response: the community has to have an ability to provide a sufficient array of options to victims, perpetrators, at-risk adolescents/young adults, and the community as a whole.

Indicated Interventions for Victims of IPV

Victim-oriented interventions are designed to prevent or minimize negative consequences to victims (ensuring victims' present needs for safety and victim support services) and to support them in their efforts to prevent future violence in their relationships. Most victim services are crisis-oriented with a short-term focus; IPV prevention may require long-term support of victims toward self-sufficiency, advocacy and legal services, safety planning, as well as long-term follow-up, mental health care, and economic assistance (Burt, Newmark, Olson, Aron, & Harrell, 1997). In addition, it is imperative that preventive services be accessible and acceptable to economically, regionally, ethnically, and age diverse populations. Currently, identification and treatment interventions predominate over preventive, proactive strategies (Chalk & King, 1998).

STRATEGIES THAT DO NOT WORK

Preventive interventions with adolescents do not have a long-term effect when they are single-dose, non-interactive training exposures. Preventive interventions at the community level do not work when the level of sophistication in the messages is too basic to teach people new ways of viewing and responding to IPV. Preventive interventions with victims do not work unless they are economically, legally, physically, psychologically, socially, and emotionally empowered to change their risky living situations. Encouraging them to end their relationships also does not work, and may make certain victims more vulnerable to escalated violence. Preventive interventions with perpetrators do not work when they occur in a vacuum, without the reinforcement of a consistent set of contextual sanctions, and when immediate results are demanded (Begun et al., 2001). In sum, there is little or no preventive benefit to providing single dose interventions randomly, in an uncoordinated, unsystematic fashion. There

is also little benefit to providing preventive interventions that cannot be sustained over time or cannot be targeted to specific subgroups in diverse communities.

Batterer interventions, designed to prevent future incidents of IPV, generally involve either individualized and/or group psycho-educational and/or cognitive behavioral programs. Although some programs incorporate couples counseling, the safety and effectiveness of this practice is hotly debated. Such intervention programs have been criticized for having little recognizable, long-lasting positive preventive impact (Chalk & King, 1998; Healey et al., 1998; Scott & Wolfe, 2000). Others, however, have suggested that as many as 67–87 percent of men who complete such programs remain violence-free 3–12 months later and that 60 percent may not have recidivated 4 years after completing the intervention (Healey et al., 1998; Wiehe, 1998). Unfortunately, these success statistics only apply to those who complete the program; participant "drop out" rates range between 40 and 75 percent (Wiehe, 1998).

Arrest as a preventive strategy with perpetrators of IPV also has had mixed reviews. In the widely cited Minneapolis Domestic Violence Experiment (Sherman & Berk, 1984), arrest was associated with an almost-50 percent reduction in subsequent assault, attempted assault, and property damage in comparison with ordering a party out of the house or police advising the couple. Since then, however, research has suggested that arrest is often associated with an increase in violence or has no meaningful impact, and that different types of individuals might react differently to arrest (Hamby, 1998). Unfortunately, arrested offenders have been inconsistently prosecuted, thereby undermining any potential long-term deterrence effects of arrest. Mandatory arrest policies, along with other mandatory strategies, have been criticized because they eliminate a victim's power for self-determination in managing the situation.

One mandate of the Violence Against Women Act (VAWA) is that states spend at least 25 percent of their federal Services, Training, Officers, Prosecutors (STOP) grant funds for victim support services. Services that combine advocacy with social support for victims of IPV have demonstrated a need for a variety of resources in this population (Reppucci et al., 1999) and a number of socioemotional gains associated with the receipt of such services. Unfortunately, there was little impact on further abuse rates, even among those who were no longer with the assailant. The greatest preventive impact lies in the minimization of IPV sequelae.

SYNTHESIS

Progress has been and continues to be made in understanding the basic science aspects of IPV. Research has expanded our understanding of the etiologic factors related to risk and vulnerability to perpetrating and becoming a victim of IPV. However, we are still at the beginning stages in developing empirically based preventive solutions that have practical import. There is a need for longitudinal study of the processes by which individuals become perpetrators and victims of IPV, in order to identify earlier key, *nodal points* in the process so as to prevent predictable problems from taking place.

Increasing the regional, national, and international coordination of community-wide campaigns would serve to reinforce the messages delivered and conserve campaign development resources. Coordination efforts might also be directed toward supporting policy changes that minimize the public's exposure to IPV incidents in entertainment media and maximize exposure to positive behavior models. Reinforcement of multi-disciplinary efforts and interventions that span social service systems (e.g., mental health, criminal justice, child welfare, welfare, and domestic violence) should be strongly encouraged and evaluated.

School-based IPV prevention programs might be advised to adopt approaches consonant with the recommendations for school-based violence prevention programs (Henrich, Brown, & Aber, 1999). These recommendations include: (1) assuring implementation fidelity and a sound theoretical basis of the intervention, (2) assuring sufficient dosage (frequency and intensity of sessions) and duration of exposure (extending across at least two school years seems to have the most significant lasting impact), and (3) appropriate qualitative and quantitative evaluation of short-, medium-, and long-term effects. Furthermore, it is likely that there exists a developmental process to the perpetration of IPV such that interventions targeted at the early emergence of violent and controlling behavior (bullying, peer harassment, sexual harassment, and community violence) may be significant in preventing dating violence (Bennett & Fineran, 1997).

An important caution to reliance on school-based efforts is offered: many of the students "at risk" for becoming perpetrators of IPV have poor school attendance and may not respond well to interventions delivered by educational authorities. It is essential to develop ways of engaging these students with the content, involving them in discourse rather than didactics. Furthermore, it may prove important that violence-free principles be incorporated across the school curricula (Krajewski, Rybarik, Dosch, & Gilmore, 1996) rather than relying on single-dose exposures, and that schools develop an unambiguous climate of non-tolerance for IPV behaviors (e.g., through coordinated responses by faculty, staff, administrators, and peer groups, and adolescent public media messages). In addition, the incorporation of a social action component to the interventions, where adolescents act to design and implement social action projects related to IPV (e.g., fund-raising, information and resources alerts, and linkages with community agencies) may be associated with more dramatic retention of the intervention impact (Wekerle & Wolfe, 1999).

Finally, ensuring that entire school (and workplace) cultures are shaped to reflect principles that support nonviolent alternatives to IPV behavior will provide adolescents (and adults) with an immersion experience rather than a spotty, "chance-encounter" IPV preventive experience. Efforts might include teacher and staff training about unambiguous IPV prevention messages and recognition of early warning signs, development of adolescent-directed media campaigns to reinforce positive beliefs and attitudes counter to IPV behavior, and implementation of non-stigmatizing, adolescent-centered, targeted interventions for individuals who are identified as being "at risk."

Additional Efforts

A number of federal, state, and local projects related to the prevention of IPV have been initiated, too recently to be able to report on their impact. For up-to-date information regarding their efforts, several websites merit review. These include the National Institute of Justice (www.ojp.usdoj.gov/nij), the Centers for Disease Control and Prevention—National Center for Injury Prevention (www.cdc.gov), the National Violence Against Women Prevention Research Center (www.vawprevention.org), and national as well as state Coalitions Against Domestic Violence.

Also see: Aggressive Behavior: Adolescence; Anger Regulation: Adolescence; Criminal Behavior: Adulthood; Marital Satisfaction: Adulthood; Sexual Assault: Adolescence.

References

Begun, A.L. (1999). Intimate partner violence: An HBSE perspective. *Journal of Social Work Education, 35*(2), 239–252.

Begun, A.L., Shelley, G., Strodthoff, T., & Short, L. (2001) Adopting a stage of change approach in intervention with individuals who are violent with their intimate partners. *Journal of Aggression, Maltreatment & Trauma, 5*(2), 105–127. (Published concurrently in R.A. Geffner & A Rosenbaum (Eds.), *Domestic violence offenders: Current interventions, research, and implications for policies and standards* (pp. 105–127). New York: Haworth Press.)

Bennett, L., & Fineran, S. (1997, July). *Sexual and severe physical violence of high school students: Power beliefs, gender, and relationship.* Paper Presented at the Fifth International Conference on Family Violence Research, Durham, NH.

Bureau of Justice Statistics. (2000). NCJ 178247, www.ojp.usdoj.gov/bjs and www.ojp.usdoj.Gov/bjs/cvict_c.htm.

Burt, M.R., Newmark, L.C., Olson, K.K., Aron, L.Y., & Harrell, A.V. (1997). The Violence Against Women Act of 1994: Evaluation of the

STOP formula grants to combat violence against women. Washington, DC: The Urban Institute Report to the National Institute of Justice.

Campbell, J.C., & Soeken, K.L. (1999). Women's responses to battering: A test of the model. *Research in Nursing and Health, 22,* 49–58.

Chalk, R. & King, P.A. (Ed.). (1998). Violence in families: Assessing prevention and treatment programs. Washington, DC: National Academy Press.

Ellsberg, M., Caldera, T., Herrera, A., Winkvist, A., & Kullgren, G. (1999). Domestic violence and emotional distress among Nicaraguan women: Results from a population-based study. *American Psychologist, 54,* 30–36.

Fawcett, G.M., Heise, L.L., Isita-Espejel, L., & Pick, S. (1999). Changing community responses to wife abuse. *American Psychologist, 54*(1), 41–49.

Federal Bureau of Investigation (FBI). (1996). *Crime in the United States—1996. Uniform Crime Reports: 1996* (p. 17).

Flowers, R.B. (2000). *Domestic crimes, family violence and child abuse: A study of contemporary American society.* Jefferson, NC: McFarland & Co.

Giles-Sims, J. (1998). The aftermath of partner violence. In J.L. Jasinski & L.M. Williams (Eds.), *Partner violence: A comprehensive review of 20 years of research* (pp. 44–72). Thousand Oaks, CA: Sage.

Greenfield, L.A., Rand, M.R., Craven, D., Flaus, P.A., Perkins, C.A., Ringel, C., Warchol, G., Maston, C., & Fox, J.A. (1998). Violence by intimates: Analysis of data on crimes by current or former spouses, boyfriends, and girlfriends. *Bureau of Justice Statistics Factbook* (NCJ-167237). Washington, DC: US Department of Justice, Bureau of Justice Statistics.

Hamby, S.L. (1998). Partner violence: Prevention and intervention. In J.L. Jasinski & L.M. Williams (Eds.), *Partner violence: A comprehensive review of 20 years of research* (pp. 210–258). Thousand Oaks, CA: Sage.

Healey, K., Smith, C., & O'Sullivan. (1998). Batterer intervention: Program approaches and criminal justice strategies. Washington, DC: National Institute of Justice.

Henrich, C.C., Brown, J.L., & Aber, J.L. (1999). Evaluating the effectiveness of school-based violence prevention: Developmental approaches. *Social Policy Report, XIII*(3). Society for Research in Child Development.

Horne, S. (1999). Domestic violence in Russia. *American Psychologist, 54*(1), 55–61.

Kantor, G.K., & Jasinski, J.L. (1998). Dynamics and risk factors in partner violence. In J.L. Jasinski & L.M. Williams (Eds.), *Partner violence: A comprehensive review of 20 years of research* (pp. 1–43). Thousand Oaks, CA: Sage.

Krajewski, S.S., Rybarik, M.F., Dosch, M.F., & Gilmore, G.D. (1996). Results of a curriculum intervention with seventh graders regarding violence in relationships. *Journal of Family Violence, 11*(2), 93–112.

Macgowan, M.J. (1997). An evaluation of a dating violence prevention program for middle school students. *Violence and Victims, 12*(3), 223–235.

McWhirter, P.T. (1999). La Violencia Privada: Domestic violence in Chile. *American Psychologist, 54,* 37–40.

Parker, B., McFarlane, J., Soeken, K., Silva, C., & Reel, S. (1999). Testing an intervention to prevent further abuse to pregnant women. *Research in Nursing & Health, 22,* 59–66.

Reppucci, N.D., Woolard, J.L., & Fried, C.S. (1999). Social, community, and preventive interventions. *Annual Reviews of Psychology, 50*(1), 387–418.

Scott, K.L., & Wolfe, D.A. (2000). Change among batterers: Examining men's success stories. *Journal of Interpersonal Violence, 15*(8), 827–842.

Sherman, L.W., & Berk, R.A. (1984). The specific deterrent effects of arrest for domestic assault. *American Sociological Review, 49,* 261–272.

Tjaden, P., & Thoennes, N. (2000). Extent, nature, and consequences of intimate partner violence: Findings from the National Violence Against Women Survey (NCJ-181867). Washington, DC: US Department of Justice, Office of Justice Programs.

United Nations. (1996). The Beijing Declaration and the platform for action. NY: United Nations (United Nations Department of Public Information, DPI/1766/Wom).

Walker, L.E. (1999). Psychology and domestic violence around the world. *American Psychologist, 54*(1), 21–29.

Wekerle, C., & Wolfe, D.A. (1999). Dating violence in mid-adolescence: Theory, significance, and emerging prevention initiatives. *Clinical Psychology Review, 19*(4), 435–456.

Wolak, J., & Finkelhor, D. (1998). Children exposed to partner violence. In J.L. Jasinski & L.M. Williams (Eds.), *Partner violence: A comprehensive review of 20 years of research* (pp. 73–111). Thousand Oaks, CA: Sage.

Wiehe, V.R. (1998). *Understanding family violence: Treating and preventing partner, child, sibling, and elder abuse.* Thousand Oaks, CA: Sage.

L

Life Challenges, Older Adulthood

Avis M. Bernstein

INTRODUCTION

Facing our own and our family's aging present a multitude of challenges. This entry focuses on these challenges, and how they have been, and continue to be, addressed. All will be presented with an eye on promoting health and preventing disease, examining ways to modulate the potential negative impact of aging on the family, and exploring approaches that optimize the positive aspects of this final process of development.

DEFINITIONS

Older Adults or the *Elderly* refer to persons aged 65 or older, although both lower (55) and higher ages (70) have been used in the literature. Several other distinctions are made: the "young-old" (65 to 75 or 80); the "middle old" or the "old-old" (75 or 80 to 90); and the "very old" or "oldest old" (85 or 90 and older) (Schaie & Willis, 1986).

According to the US census, a *family* is a group of two or more people who reside together and who are related by birth, marriage, or adoption. In gerontology literature, a common residence is not required.

Care Recipient is the person receiving physical, psychological, and/or social assistance. *Caregiver* is the person primarily responsible for organizing and/or providing for the physical, psychological, and social needs of the care recipient.

ADL (activities of daily living) includes walking, dressing, eating, using the toilet, bathing, and getting into and out of bed. *IADL* (instrumental activities of daily living) includes meal preparation, grocery shopping, making phone calls, taking medications, and money management. *ALE* (active life expectancy) refers to the probable period of life free of disability including independence in ADLs (Katz et al., 1983).

Caregiver Burden refers to the adverse consequences of caregiving viewed as an accumulation of stress consisting of "objective burden" involving tangible assistance (e.g., providing for personal hygiene needs and/or meal preparation), and "subjective burden," referring to the caregiver's perceived stress in providing such assistance.

Long-Term Care is the provision of services to those who can no longer function independently in terms of ADLs and/or IADLs due to the presence of chronic conditions and/or diseases, associated disabilities and functional limitations. *Respite Care* is the temporary relief for caregivers through provision of in- or out-of-home services to the elderly care recipient.

SCOPE

The "graying of America" continues to be heralded, as the "baby boomers" become the "elderly boomers." An estimated 34.7 million Americans, or 13 percent of the population, aged 65+ in 1997, are projected to increase to 53.2 million by 2020 (Takamura, 1998), and to 70 million by 2030, when 20 percent of the US population will be 65 years or older (APA Working Group on the Older Adult, 1998; National Center for Health Statistics [NCHS], 1999).

Of this number, an estimated 79 percent of non-institutionalized persons aged 70 and over report at least one of seven chronic conditions (arthritis, hypertension, diabetes, respiratory illness, heart disease, stroke, and cancer (NCHS, 1999). Approximately one third of these chronically ill elderly receive help from a caregiver, with the percentage receiving assistance increasing with age (NCHS, 1999). To this must be added those 2 to 4 million suffering from Alzheimer's disease (AD) (US General Accounting Office, 1998), the prevalence of AD is estimated to be 5–10 percent of elderly, increasing to 25–50 percent in the very old (American Psychiatric Association, 1997). As the population of elderly care recipients rise, the proportions of caregivers dwindles (Frudenheim, 1996). The majority, 55 percent, of the elderly lives with their spouses (US Census Bureau, 2000), who provide the primary support. However, with increasing age these percentages change significantly, 64 percent of persons under 75 live with a spouse as compared to only 44 percent of those 75 and older (US Census Bureau, 2000). Surprisingly, over the past decade, the responsibility of caring for the elderly has been shifting from institutions to family members (Covinsky, Goldman, & Cook, 1994; Gutner, 1997; Vladeck, 1997). Based upon the National Caregiver Survey in 1997, 22.4 million US households or nearly a quarter of the population contain someone caring for an older relative or friend (National Alliance of Caregiving, 1997). Takamura (1998) estimates the cost to the nation for services being rendered by caregivers range from $45 to $95 billion per year. The impact that caregiving has on total cost to business ranges from a "conservative estimate" of $11.4 billion to $29 billion per year (National Alliance of Caregiving, 1997). Add to this the undetermined costs for the health care of the caregivers themselves, described as "hidden patients" (Schultz, Visintainer, & Williamson, 1990), and the problem expands exponentially.

It should be noted that although much of the literature addresses the issues of the elderly (the care recipient) and those who provide care (the caregiver) as separate entities facing their own unique challenges, this is often done for heuristic purposes. The actual persons involved may well take umbrage at being called caregiver or recipient, preferring to maintain their own designation as wife or husband, mother or father.

The *elderly* are often viewed as a single entity, a misconception leading to stereotyping for which activists against "ageism" such as Maggie Kuhn of the Gray Panthers have been trying to eliminate since the 1960s (Schaie & Willis, 1986). Aside from individual variations, such as race, culture, ethnicity, religious beliefs, and socio-economic status (SES),

the "elderly" span 35+ years. The problems faced by the very old—including the 100,000 centenarians (Takamura, 1998)—such as failing health and loss of support, are quite different than those faced by the young old entering retirement and themselves facing the challenges of being caregivers to grandchildren and elderly parents. Yet, by and large, the elderly still continue to be studied as a monolith.

The APA Working Group on Older Adults (1998) reports these common age-associated changes: physical changes include hearing impairment, visual changes, decreased reaction time, increased risk of multiple chronic conditions including arthritis, hypertension, cataracts, heart disease, diabetes, and osteoporosis, and facing death from heart disease, cancer, cerebrovascular disease, pneumonia and influenza, and chronic obstructive pulmonary disease. Cognitive changes including: speed of information processing resulting in a slower learning rate and greater need for repetition of new information; cognitive flexibility in terms of dividing attention between two simultaneous tasks, switching attention and filtering out irrelevant information, recall of remote memory, word-finding, visual-spatial tasks, abstraction and mental flexibility with preservation of language abilities. Although physical symptoms predominate in the concerns of the elderly and, excluding cognitive impairments, as a group they evidence fewer diagnosable psychiatric disorders than do younger persons, they remain vulnerable to the same psychological issues and disorders effecting younger adults.

Despite common physical difficulties, the ALE in 1991 for a 65 year old man is 11–13 years; for a 65 year old women, 15–17 years (Branch et al., 1991); and three fourths of community-dwelling people aged 65 to 74 and two thirds of those aged 75 and over reported their health to be good to excellent compared with others their age (APA Working Group on the Older Adult, 1998). Although the elderly will be discussed here as "care recipients," oftentimes these people are caregivers either to their elderly spouses, or to their children and/or grandchildren. Many people in industrialized countries are living longer healthier lives than ever before so that aging does not automatically imply deterioration and increased dependency. It is no longer sufficient to focus on quantity of life without simultaneously focusing on improving the quality of life.

Finally, the average age of the care recipient is 77, and most likely has a chronic condition that will require an average of 4.5 years of care (Family Caregiving in the US, 1997) presenting a number of challenges to the family members who care for them.

The Caregiver

Caregivers are even more heterogeneous than the elderly population for whom they care. To the individual, gender, racial, cultural, ethnic, religious, and SES differences is added the divergent age span encompassing a range of developmental stages. The middle-aged caregiver is sandwiched between the burdens and benefits of intergenerational care (Bergtson, Rosenthal, & Burton, 1995). Bearing the responsibilities of caring for their own children and their parents, this person has very different issues to address than does the elderly caregiver who, like the care recipient, faces her/his own health concerns and functional limitations. To these groups can be added the emerging trend of young adults serving as primary caregivers of the elderly (Dellman-Jenkins, Blankemeyer, & Pinkard, 2001). A healthy respect for all groups' psychological and developmental needs is required in order to provide beneficial assistance to the family as a whole. These differences have a tremendous impact upon the quality of caregiving and the stress felt by members of the dyad. Additional factors effecting care include: type of illness and differing prognoses (e.g., relatively stable condition as with stroke versus gradual or acute progression as with Alzheimer's disease or cancer, respectively); extent of functional impairment and level of required care (e.g., caring for IADL's, such as checking accounts, vs. ADL's, such as feeding and bathing); numbers of other stressors (e.g., providing care to young children, financial limitations, work-load and associated job duties); type and quality of relationship (e.g., emotionally close spouse vs. emotionally detached adult child; extent of role reversals where the traditional caregiver now becomes the care recipient).

Caring for an elderly parent or spouse places significant stress upon the caregiver who must take time and energy from other responsibilities. Caregiving affects the physical, mental, and emotional health of the caregiver. Takamura (1998) reports that one third of all caregivers of the elderly described their own health as poor. Elevated rates of depression are one of the most consistent findings in research on the caregiver (Schulz, Newsom, Fleissner, DeCamp, & Nieboer, 1997; Schulz, O'Brien, Bookwala, & Fleissner, 1995; Schulz & Williamson, 1991). And although differing widely in reactions to the caregiving experience (Williamson & Schulz, 1993), caregivers are at risk for poorer mental health outcomes than their non-caregiving peers (Schulz et al., 1995; Wright, Clipp, & George, 1993). The effect of the stress of caregiving has been shown to suppress immune function (Robinson-Whelen, Kiecolt-Glaser, & Glaser, 2000) placing caregivers at increased risk for disease.

The caregiver is most likely a woman who is the elderly wife of the care recipient or the middle-aged daughter or daughter-in-law (NCHS, 1999; Stone, Carrerata, & Sangl, 1987). Schulz and Beach (1999) note that the mental and emotional strain experienced by the elderly spousal caregiver was reported to be an independent risk factor for mortality. Stress plays out not only in increased health risks for the caregiver, but is considered a contributing factor to the approximate 450,000 elderly living in domestic settings who are yearly abused or neglected (National Center on Elder Abuse, 1998).

THEORIES

There appears to be no over-riding theory that addresses the multitude of factors involved in health promotion (HP) and disease prevention (DP) in the elderly. Geriatricians have viewed Engel's (1977) *Biopsychosocial Model* as sufficiently comprehensive to recognize all components of health, and, therefore, capable of addressing issues such as quality of life, functional status, autonomy, dignity, among others (Yoshikawa, Cobbs, & Brummel-Smith, 1998). Only by viewing individuals in the context of their environment can we hope to address the health needs of older persons (Calkins, Boult, Wagner, & Pacala, 1999; Taylor, 1999). This is true for the caregiver, too.

A second theory to consider when addressing concerns of the elderly is Erikson's (1968) *psychosocial model*, which provides increased appreciation for the developmental tasks faced by the elderly who are seeking to balance a sense of integrity (associated with perceived meaningfulness) with feelings of despair. At the same time, Erikson's model allows for increased understanding of the caregiver's developmental tasks ranging from the young caregiver confronting the challenges of career development, differentiating from the family, and establishing intimate relationships; the middle-aged addressing issues of generativity involving career and child-rearing; and the elderly caregiver facing the same developmental tasks as the care recipient. Based on Erikson's work, Havighurst's (1972) "developmental tasks of late life" provide an overview of primary issues to be addressed by the elderly:

1. Adjusting to decreasing physical strength and health;
2. Adjusting to retirement and reduced income;
3. Adjusting to death of spouse;
4. Establishing an explicit association with one's age group;
5. Adopting and adapting social roles in a flexible way; and
6. Establishing satisfactory physical living arrangements.

The above reveal direct challenges for the elderly that need to be considered by the caregiver (Eyetsemitan, 2000).

Brooks (1998) presents a comprehensive model for the elderly, which uses Antonovsky's (1979) salutogenic (i.e., health promoting) concept as a framework that is of sufficient scope to guide research directed towards successful aging, focused on prolonging independent functioning in the elderly and alleviating caregiver burden. The emphasis is on facilitating health by studying those who are successfully coping either with the process of aging or with the role of caregiver. Two concepts "generalized resistance resources," which are defined as personal, group, and environmental characteristics facilitating the effective management of stress, and "sense of coherence" (SOC), which refers to a general orientation towards, and self-perception of, life as manageable, meaningful, and comprehensible (pp. 230–231), are discussed as factors that affect one's ability to adapt and effectively cope with life events.

Hypotheses based upon this model were supported with regard to the elderly in that the SOC was correlated with the three dimensions of successful aging (life satisfaction, social health, and overall physical health). Research on caregivers, however, is needed (Chiriboga, Weiler, & Nielsen, 1990).

A Model of Care for the Caregiver

Haley and his associates (Haley, Levine, Brown, & Bartolucci, 1987; Haley et al., 1996) propose a stress process model for examining the relationships among caregivers' stressors, psychosocial resources, and well-being. Based on the work of Lazarus and Folkman (1984), this model identifies multiple psychosocial factors that mediate caregiving stress including caregiver appraisals of primary stressors, coping responses, and social support such that the more benign the appraisals of primary stressors, the higher the self-efficacy ratings, increased problem- (vs. emotion-) focused coping, and greater social support, the better one's state of well-being. This model provides insight into a number of venues to assist the caregiver. Pearlin, Mullan, Semple, and Skaff (1990) suggested that "caregiver stress" be dichotomized into *primary stressors* (the *objective burden*) arising directly from the specific responsibilities of caregiving, distinguished from *secondary stressors* (the *subjective burden*) arising from the effects of caregiving on other activities and obligations (e.g., as an employee, mother, grandmother). This is most evident in the "sandwich generation" (Davis, 1981) providing care to both elderly parents and children. The primary stressors are further broken down into stress experienced from direct care while assisting with IADLs and ADLs, and stress from handling behavioral problems caused by disinhibition and leading to anger outbursts, dangerous or inappropriate and embarrassing behaviors and/or cognitive deficits leading to disorientation and repetitive questions (Goode, Haley, Roth, & Greg, 1998; Haley et al., 1987; Schulz et al., 1995).

STRATEGIES THAT WORK

Given the inter-relationship between care recipient and caregiver, it can be inferred that what is helpful to the elderly recipient will be helpful to the caregiver and visa versa. Both the elderly and the family member have crucial roles to play, individually and in collaboration, in efforts to maximize their own and each other's functioning.

Interventions to reduce and/or eliminate health-risk behaviors while establishing health-promoting behaviors in the elderly have met with varying success. Murphy and Cicilline (1999) offer an overview of studies on prevention in the elderly. Primary prevention strategies that work include education for alcohol and smoking cessation (noting that even minimal counseling by a health care provider has proven beneficial); increasing exercise; improving diet; preventing injury from accidents (use of seat belts and helmets; home safety issues; refraining from drinking and driving); interventions to avoid unnecessary medications; immunoprophylaxis for influenza, pneumonia and tetanus; and chemoprophylaxis such as using aspirin to reduce thrombotic stroke, myocardial infarction, and possibly reducing risk of colorectal cancer and estrogen replacement therapy to decrease risk of coronary heart disease, osteoporosis, possibly prevent colorectal cancer and AD, and improve sexual function and cosmesis (refers in medicine to the affects of surgery on one's facial appearance).

STRATEGIES THAT MIGHT WORK

In another review on preventing frailty in the elderly and prolonging the period of independent functioning, Buchner (1999) indicates the advantages of a multiple risk factor approach again including the promotion of physical activity, proper nutrition, home safety, screening of body weight, vision, hearing, affect, and cognition. In these efforts, the primary care physician has a crucial role to play, as the elderly tend to follow medical recommendations. The problem is in the follow-through and this is where the family, support network, and community can have an impact (Taylor, 1999). We do not yet have research on how to deliver this follow-through most effectively.

STRATEGIES THAT DO NOT WORK

Sometimes efforts undertaken with the best of intentions may not be helpful. For example, Krause (1997) revealed that social ties for the elderly entail psychosocial costs in reduced self-reliance, individual achievement, and autonomy resulting in detrimental effects on health and well-being.

SYNTHESIS

The stress process model (Goode et al., 1998) is used as a framework to discuss the multiple approaches presented in the health promotion and disease prevention literature on the elderly and caregiver.

First, practical suggestions for problem-focused coping specifically directed toward the caregiver include promoting one's own health by taking time for regular exercise, proper nutrition; decreasing health risk behaviors; actively seeking support by joining a support group; taking advantage of respite care; and increasing one's willingness and ability to delegate responsibilities to others (National Alliance of Caregiving, 1977). In order to do this, caregivers must be willing to reprioritize needs to simplify their life as much as possible and, thereby, reduce the number of stressors. Brooks (1998) also suggested paying closer attention to healthy aging, those who have aged gracefully by employing effective coping mechanisms to maintain mental health, general life satisfaction, and a positive outlook, what Brooks calls a sense of coherence. These elderly epitomize problem-focused coping, challenging themselves with social and/or solitary activities (e.g., playing bridge, working crossword puzzles), engaging in mental activities and employing compensatory skills (e.g., list making and using mnemonic devices to assist with memory); participating in available mood and memory workshops; modifying tasks and their environment to accommodate physical changes; drawing strength from personal spirituality; cultivating creativity, optimism, hope; seeking support from family, friends, neighbors, and other peer groups.

Centenarians demonstrate another useful problem-focused coping strategy in their ability to handle whatever life experiences come their way, what Lehr (1982) calls "resiliency" and, as such, once again provide excellent examples for long-term survival (Pascucci & Loving, 1997).

Second, providing time for "life review" (Butler, 1975; Haight, Michael, & Hendrix, 2000) may serve not only the elderly but can be useful to younger family members in learning about their history and possibly prevent regrets of not obtaining information prior to this person's death. Life review or reminiscence has been shown to contribute to life satisfaction (Cook, 1998; Ghusn, Hyde, Stevens, & Hyde, 1996). However, the benefits obtained may have more to do with the social activity involved than with the specific content (Brennan & Steinberg, 1983–1984).

These interventions fit into what Rosenberg and McCullough (1981) have called "mattering," pertaining to an individual's perceptions of their value by making a difference to the lives of others, perhaps most beneficial in being able to assist their own family (Pearlin, Aneshensel, Mullan, & Whitlatch, 1996). Caregivers themselves can learn how better to approach their own aging; they are exposed to models of healthy aging by which to encourage the care recipient to enhance independence and thereby offset demands placed upon them; the relationship between caregiver and care recipient is enhanced; and, by perceiving the elderly as "teachers," they can begin to change their own appraisal of their caregiving role (i.e., seeing the benefit of interactions and observations of aging family members).

Third, caregiver stress may be appraised in light of actual demands and perceived resources with which to cope. Either of these two factors is modifiable. The actual demands can be reframed to enhance the benefits not only through learning from the elderly by witnessing how well they cope with daily challenges but by seeing how they do not—learning behaviors to cull as well as to avoid. The role of "altruism" and the benefits of being able to provide help to the family should not be ignored (Louderback, 2000) and could well be useful in reducing stress. The benefits of caregiving have been evidenced in even what could be considered by most extreme cases of caring for terminal patients, providing what Enyert and Burman (1999) termed a sense of "self-transcendence."

Fourth, social support offered to the families in their own environment (Caplan, Caplan, & Erchul, 1994) takes a variety of forms including: *instrumental support* consisting of tangible assistance, information, resources, and services; *expressive support* providing emotional reassurance; and *appraisal support* helping an individual understand the nature of the stressful event, the resources and coping strategies better address it (Pearlin et al., 1996; Taylor, 1999). Each of these social supports may help improve or maintain the quality of life, emphasizing the prolongation of independent functioning. Emphasis must be placed upon the importance of mutual respect and collaborative efforts to resolve challenges, increasing a sense of independence for the care recipient and, thereby, helping to alleviate the burden of caregiving. By identifying and targeting caregivers and care recipients at risk, efforts can be made to increase the quality of life for both of the parties involved and thereby the family as a whole.

Also see: Caregiver Stress: Older Adulthood; Chronic Disease: Older Adulthood; Crises Intervention: Older Adulthood; Health Promotion: Older Adulthood; Retirement Satisfaction: Older Adulthood; Sexuality: Older Adulthood.

References

American Psychiatric Association. (1997). Guidelines for the treatment of patients with Alzheimer's disease and the other dementias of late life. *American Journal of Psychiatry, 154*(Suppl.), 1–39.

Antonovsky, A. (1979). *Health, stress, and coping: New perspectives on mental and physical well-being.* San Francisco: Jossey-Bass.

APA Working Group on the Older Adult. (1998). What practitioners should know about working with older adults. *Professional Psychology: Research and Practice, 29*(5), 413–427.

Bergtson, V., Rosenthal, C., & Burton, L. (1995). Paradoxes of families and aging. In R.H. Binstock & L.K. George (Eds.), *Handbook of aging and the social sciences* (4th ed., pp. 254–275). San Diego, CA: Academic Press.

Brennan, P.L., & Steinberg, L.D. (1983–1984). Is reminiscence adaptive? Relations among social activity level, reminiscence, and morale. *International Journal of Aging & Human Development, 18*(2), 99–110.

Branch, L.G., Guralnik, J.M., Foley, D.J. et al. (1991). Active life expectancy for 10,000 Caucasian men and women in three communities. *Journal of Gerontology, 46*, M145–M15.

Brooks, J.D. (1998). Salutogenesis, successful aging, and the advancement of theory on family caregiving. In H.I. McCubbin, E.A. Thompson et al. (Eds.), *Stress, coping, and health in families: Sense of coherence and resiliency* (pp. 227–248). Thousand Oaks, CA: Sage.

Buchner, D.M. (1999). Prevention of Frailty. In E. Calkins, C. Boult, E.H. Wagner, & J.T. Pacala (Eds.), *New ways to care for older people: Building systems based on evidence* (pp. 3–19). New York: Springer.

Butler, R.N. (1975). *Why Survive?* New York: Harper & Row.

Calkins, E., Boult, C., Wagner, E.H., & Pacala, J.T. (Eds.). (1996). *Introduction to new ways to care for older people: Building systems based on evidence.* New York: Springer.

Caplan, G., Caplan, R.B., & Erchul, W.P. (1994). Caplanian mental health consultation historical background and current status. *Journal of Consulting Psychology, 46*(4), 2–12.

Chiroboga, D.A., Weiler, P.G., & Nielsen, K. (1990). The stress of caregivers. In D.E. Biegel & A. Blum (Eds.), *Aging and caregiving: Theory, research, and policy* (pp. 121–138). Newbury Park, CA: Sage.

Cook, E.A. (1998). Effects of reminiscence on life satisfaction of elderly female nursing home residents. *Health Care for Women International, 19*, 109–118.

Covinsky, K.E., Goldman, L., & Cook, F. (1994). The impact of serious illness on patients' families. *Journal of the American Medical Association, 272*, 1839–1844.

Davis, R.H. (1981). The middle years. In R.H. Davis (Ed.), *Aging: Prospects and issues* (3rd ed.). Los Angeles: Andrus Gerontology Center.

Dellmann-Jenkins, M., Blankemeyer, M., & Pinkard, O. (2001). Incorporating the elder caregiving role into the developmental tasks of young adulthood. *International Journal of Aging and Human Development, 52*(1), 1–18.

Engel, G.L. (1977). The need for a new medical model: A challenge for biomedicine. *Science, 196*, 129–136.

Enyert, G., & Burman, M.E. (1999). A qualitative study of self-transcendence in caregivers of terminally ill patients. *American Journal of Hospital Palliative Care, 16*(2), 455–462.

Erikson, E.H. (1968). *Identity: Youth and crisis.* New York: W.W. Norton & Company.

Eyetsemitan, F. (2000). Care of the elderly persons in the family: An approach based on a developmental model. *Psychological Reports, 86*(1), 281–286.

Family Caregiving in the US. (1997). *Findings from a national survey. Final report.* Washington, DC: National Alliance for Caregiving and the American Association of Retired Persons.

Freudenheim, E. (Ed.). (1996). *Chronic care in America: A 21st century challenge.* Princeton, NJ: Robert Wood Johnson Foundation.

Ghusn, H.F., Hyde, D., Stevens, E.S., & Hyde, M. (1996). Enhancing life satisfaction in later life: What makes a difference for nursing home residents? *Journal of Gerontological Social Work, 26*, 27–47.

Goode, K.T., Haley, W.E., Roth, D.L., & Greg, R.F. (1998). Predicting longitudinal changes in caregiver physical and mental health: A stress process model. *Health Psychology, 17*(2), 190–198.

Gutner, T. (Ed.). (1997). Farewell to the nursing home: a host of alternatives help the aging live independently. *Business Week*, 100–101.

Haight, B.K., Michel, Y., & Hendrix, S. (2000). The extended effects of the life review in nursing home residents. *International Journal of Aging and Human Development, 50*(2), 151–168.

Haley, W.E., Levine, E.G., Brown, S.L., & Bartolucci, A. (1987). Stress, appraisal, coping, and social support as predictors of adaptational outcome amount dementia caregivers. *Psychology and Aging, 2*, 323–330.

Haley, W.E., Roth, D.L., Coleton, M.I., Ford, G.R., West, C.A.C., Collins, R.P., & Isobe, T.L. (1996). Appraisal, coping, and social support as mediators of well-being in Black and White family caregivers of patients with Alzheimer's disease. *Journal of Consulting and Clinical Psychology, 64*, 121–129.

Havighurst, R.J. (1972). *Developmental tasks and education* (3rd ed.). New York: McKay.

Katz, S., Branch, L.G., Branson, M.L. et al. (1983). Active life expectancy. *New England Journal of Medicine, 309*, 1218–1224.

Krause, N. (1997). Received support, anticipated support, social class, and mortality. *Research on Aging, 19*, 387–422.

Lazarus, R.S., & Folkman, S. (1984). *Stress, appraisal, and coping.* New York: Springer.

Lehr, U.M. (1982). Social-psychological correlates of longevity. *Annual Review of Gerontology and Geriatrics, 3*, 102–147.

Louderback, P. (2000). Elder care: a positive approach to caregiving. *Journal of the American Academy of Nurse Practice, 12*(3), 97–99.

Murphy, J.B., & Cicilline, M. (1999). Prevention for older persons. In J.J. Gallo, J. Busby-Whitehead, P.V. Rabins, R.A. Silliman, & J.B. Murphy (Eds.), *Reichel's care of the elderly: Clinical aspects of aging* (5th ed.). Philadelphia: Lippincott Williams & Wilkins.

National Alliance for Caregiving and the American Association of Retired Persons. (1997). *Family caregiving in the US findings from a national survey. Final report.* Bethesda, MD: National Alliance for Caregiving.

National Center for Health Statistics (NCHS). (1999). *Health, United States 1999 with health and aging chartbook.* (DHHS Publication (PHS) 99-1232). Hyattsville, MD.

National Center on Elder Abuse at The American Public Human Services Association in collaboration with Westat I. (1998). *The National Elder Abuse Incidence Study—Final Report.* Washington, DC: The Administration on Aging.

Pascucci, M.A., & Loving, G.L. (1997). Ingredients of an old and healthy life. A centenarian perspective. *Journal of Holistic Nursing, 15*(2), 199–213.

Pearlin, L.I., Aneshensel, C.S., Mullan, J.T., & Whitlatch, C.J. (1996). Caregiving and its social support. In R.H. Binstock and L.K. George (Eds.), *Handbook of aging and the social sciences* (4th ed.). San Diego, CA: Academic Press.

Pearlin, L.I., Mullan, J.T., Semple, S.J., & Skaff, M.M. (1990). Caregiving and the stress process: An overview of concepts and their measures. *Gerontologist, 30*, 583–591.

Robinson-Whelen, S., Kiecolt-Glaser, J.K., & Glaser, R. (2000). Effects of chronic stress on immune function in the elderly. In S.B. Manuck & R. Jennings (Eds.), *Behavior, health, and aging* (pp. 69–82). Mahwah, New Jersey: Lawrence Erlbaum.

Rosenberg, M., & McCullough, B.C. (1981). Mattering: Inferred significance and mental health among adolescents. *Research in Community and Mental Health, 2*, 163–182.

Schaie, K.W., & Willis, S.L. (1986). *Adult Development and Aging.* Boston: Little, Brown, & Co.

Schulz, R., & Beach, S.R. (1999). Caregiving as a risk factor for mortality: The caregiver health effects study. *Journal of the American Medical Association, 282*(23), 2215–2219.

Schulz, R., Newsom, J.T., Fleissner, K., DeCamp, A.R., & Nieboer, A.P. (1997). The effects of caregiving: The cardiovascular health study. *Annals of Behavioral Medicine, 19,* 110–116.

Schulz, R., O'Brien, A.T., Bookwala, J., & Fleissner, K. (1995). Psychiatric and physical morbidity effects of Alzheimer's disease caregiving: Prevalence, correlates, and causes. *Gerontologist, 35,* 771–791.

Schulz, R., Visintainer, P., & Williamson, G.M. (1990). Psychiatric and physical morbidity effects of caregiving. *Journal of Gerontology, 45,* 181–191.

Schulz, R., & Williamson, G.M. (1991). A 2-year longitudinal study of depression among Alzheimer's caregivers. *Psychology and Aging, 6,* 569–578.

Stone, R., Carrerata, G.L., & Sangl, J. (1987). Caregivers of the frail elderly: A national profile. *Gerontologist, 27,* 616–626.

Takamura, J.C. (1998). An aging agenda for the 21st century: The opportunities and challenges of population longevity. *Professional Psychology: Research and Practice, 29*(5), 411–412.

Taylor, S.E. (1999). *Health psychology* (Vol. 4). Boston: McGraw Hill.

United States Census Bureau. (2000). *Statistical Abstract of the United States: 2000* (120th ed.). Washington, DC.

United States General Accounting Office. (1998). *Alzheimer's disease. Estimates of prevalence in the United States.* GAO/HEHS. 98-16.

Vladeck, B.C. (1997). *On reforming Medicare home health benefit.* Statement before the House Commerce Committee, Subcommittee on Health and Environment. Washington, DC: HCFA.

Williamson, G.M., & Schulz, R. (1993). Coping with specific stressors in Alzheimer's disease caregiving. *The Gerontologist, 33,* 747–755.

Wright, L.K., Clipp, E.C., & George, L.K. (1993). Health consequences of caregiver stress. *Medicine, Exercise, Nutrition, and Health, 2,* 181–195.

Yoshikawa, T.T., Cobbs, E.L., & Brummel-Smith, K.B. (1998). *Practical ambulatory geriatrics* (2nd ed., pp. 4–5). St. Louis: Mosby.

Life Skills, Adolescence

Gilbert J. Botvin and
Kenneth W. Griffin

INTRODUCTION AND DEFINITIONS

Drug abuse is a serious threat to public health in the United States and throughout the world. Alcohol, tobacco, and other drug use frequently begin during early adolescence and increase in frequency and quantity during the adolescent years. When drug abuse appears among adolescents in a community, it is often of great concern to parents, educators, and other adults. In this entry, we review the epidemiology and etiology of adolescent drug abuse and focus on the role of social and personal competence skills in the initiation and escalation of substance use. In this context, *competence* refers to generic self-management and social skills that enable an individual to confront and master life problems and succeed in developmental tasks. Deficits in these life skills play a central role in the etiology of adolescent drug abuse because poorly competent youth are often highly vulnerable to the social, environmental, and intrapsychic forces that support drug abuse.

Fortunately, evidence has shown that competence enhancement approaches that teach life skills along with drug-specific social resistance skills can effectively prevent adolescent drug abuse. Below we review theory and evidence regarding two contemporary approaches to adolescent drug abuse prevention that are effective in changing behavior: competence enhancement approaches and social resistance training approaches. Also, we describe traditional prevention approaches such as information dissemination techniques that are still commonly used despite evidence showing they are ineffective in changing behavior. Finally, we review literature which suggests that, in addition to preventing drug abuse, competence enhancement approaches may hold promise for preventing interpersonal violence and other adolescent risk behaviors and promoting positive youth development.

SCOPE

Survey data has shown that adolescents often begin to use alcohol, tobacco, and other drugs during the middle school years, with a smaller number experimenting with substance use during elementary school. In the United States, national survey data from the Monitoring the Future study (Johnston, O'Malley, & Bachman, 2001) reveal that rates of substance use frequently increase over the course of adolescence and that most young people report engaging in the use of one or more substances by the time they are in secondary school. Alcohol and tobacco are the most commonly used substances by teenagers, with about one in three twelfth graders reporting drunkenness, binge drinking (i.e., five or more drinks in a row), or smoking cigarettes in the past month. Findings also indicate that almost half of high school students report using marijuana in their lifetime and more than one fourth report using marijuana in the past month. Indeed, marijuana is the most commonly used illegal drug among American secondary school students. Other drugs used by substantial numbers of adolescents in the United States include amphetamines, barbiturates, and Ecstasy (MDMA). Ecstasy has seen a dramatic increase in use— from 6 percent of adolescents reporting lifetime use in 1996 up to 11 percent in 2000. In fact, Ecstasy is currently used by more American teenagers than cocaine and there are few signs that the growing popularity of Ecstasy will subside in the near future.

THEORIES AND RESEARCH

Several theoretical models outline how risk and protective factors contribute to the development of adolescent drug abuse (Petraitis, Flay, & Miller, 1995). *Social learning theories* (e.g., Bandura, 1977) emphasize how young people often imitate the behavior of role models that use drugs, while *social attachment theories* focus on how youth withdraw from parents or school and turn to deviant peer groups that support drug abuse (e.g., social development model; Hawkins & Weis, 1985). Cognitive theories such as the *health belief model* (Becker, 1974) describe the role of poor decision-making processes in weighing perceived risks and benefits, while others such as the *self-medication hypothesis* (Khanzian, 1997) emphasize the role of affective or personality characteristics that can lead to drug abuse. Broader social psychological theories have been developed that attempt to integrate the many determinants of adolescent drug use. One of the most prominent is *problem behavior theory* (Jessor & Jessor, 1977), which proposes that adolescents engage in drug use and similar behaviors in order to achieve developmental goals that they believe they cannot achieve in more adaptive ways. For example, from the point of view of an adolescent with poor interpersonal or self-management skills, the use of alcohol, tobacco, and other drugs may serve an important function by helping them to gain acceptance by peers or attract attention from adults. As described below, this component of problem behavior theory has clear implications regarding the importance of developing competence skills as a way to prevent adolescent drug abuse and promote positive youth development.

Protective Role of Competence Skills: Implications for Prevention

Adolescence is an important transitional period in the lives of young people. Virtually all youth must contend with a variety of new academic, social, and vocational challenges during this time of life. Adolescents negotiate these developmental challenges with varying degrees of success. Those with poor competence skills are less likely to succeed in these tasks, and when failures are repeated over time, these experiences can reduce self-efficacy, confidence, and self-esteem. Poorly competent youth may become overwhelmed when faced with important decisions, new opportunities, or the need to cope with major and minor life events. They may make short-term or maladaptive decisions without thinking through the consequences. One of these decisions may be to initiate alcohol, tobacco, or other drug use.

Conversely, youth with good social and personal competence skills are likely to be more successful in meeting the developmental challenges they face. Because these youth have greater social, cognitive, and behavioral self-management skills, they may be more effective decision-makers, more persistent in setting and reaching goals, more capable of responding appropriately to challenges, and better at garnering social support from peers and adults compared to youth with poor competence skills. Successes in these domains may serve a protective function by contributing to a well-developed sense of personal mastery, psychological well-being, and self-esteem. These factors may in turn reduce susceptibility to environmental, social, and intrapsychic forces that promote substance use.

Several etiologic studies have shown that social and personal competence skills play an important protective role in adolescent substance use. In addition to a direct protective effect of competence, recent research has begun to provide some important insights into the mediating mechanisms by which competence skills are protective. For example, research has found that competent youth engage in less substance use because they have fewer positive expectancies regarding the social benefits of use (Griffin, Epstein, Botvin, & Spoth, 2001), are more likely to experience a sense of well-being that is protective (Griffin, Scheier, Botvin, & Diaz, 2001), and are better equipped to utilize drug-specific refusal skills (Epstein, Griffin, & Botvin, 2000).

STRATEGIES THAT WORK

Over the past two to three decades, the focus of adolescent drug abuse prevention programming has shifted as knowledge concerning the etiology of drug abuse has accumulated. The most promising contemporary approaches focus on interactive skills training techniques and are conceptualized within a theoretical framework that incorporates the known risk and protective factors for adolescent drug use (Hawkins, Catalano, & Miller, 1992). Several different approaches to drug abuse prevention have been implemented, mostly in school settings. Schools have become the major focus of prevention activities because they offer access to youth during the time when they typically initiate substance use. Contemporary prevention approaches can be grouped into two general categories: (1) competence enhancement or life skills approaches and (2) social influence approaches.

Effective Strategy: Promoting Life Skills

According to the competence enhancement approach, drug use is conceptualized as a socially learned and functional behavior that is the result of an interplay between social and personal factors. Drug use is learned through a process of modeling, imitation, and reinforcement, and is influenced by an adolescent's prodrug cognitions, attitudes, and beliefs. These factors, in combination with poor personal and social skills, are believed to increase an adolescent's susceptibility to influences that promote drug use (Botvin, 2000).

The most effective competence enhancement approaches to adolescent drug abuse prevention emphasize the teaching of generic personal self-management skills and social coping skills in combination with social resistance skills training (Botvin, 2000). Examples of the kind of competence skills included in this prevention approach are decision-making and problem-solving skills, cognitive skills for resisting interpersonal and media influences, skills for enhancing self-esteem (goal-setting and self-directed behavior change techniques), adaptive coping strategies for dealing with stress and anxiety, general social skills (complimenting, conversational skills, and skills for forming new friendships), and general assertiveness skills. The most effective way to teach these skills are by using cognitive-behavioral skills training methods: instruction and demonstration, role-playing, group feedback and reinforcement, behavioral rehearsal (in-class practice) and extended (out-of-class) practice through behavioral homework assignments.

Over the years, a number of evaluation studies have tested the efficacy of the competence enhancement or life skills approach to drug abuse prevention. These studies have demonstrated behavioral effects on smoking, alcohol, marijuana use as well as the use of multiple substances and illicit drugs. The magnitude of these effects has typically been relatively large, with reductions in drug use behavior in the range of 40–80 percent. Long-term follow-up data indicate that the prevention effects of these approaches can last for up to 6 years (Botvin, Baker, Dusenbury, Botvin, & Diaz, 1995; Botvin, Griffin, Diaz, & Ifill-Williams, 2001). Recent studies have shown that this approach is effective with inner-city minority youth (Botvin et al., 2001) with minimal modifications (e.g., graphics, language, and role-play scenarios appropriate to the target population). Overall, the strongest behavioral effects across studies have been found when programs are delivered with high integrity by trained providers and when booster sessions are provided to reinforce the material after the initial intervention.

Effective Strategy: Social Resistance Skills Training

According to the social resistance skills approach, adolescent drug use results from various social influences including the direct modeling of drug use behavior, particularly that of peers. Other important social influences include persuasive advertising appeals and media portrayals encouraging alcohol, tobacco, and other drug use. Therefore, social influence programs focus extensively on teaching youth

how to recognize and resist pressures to use drugs using a variety of resistance skills training exercises. The goal of these exercises is to have students learn ways to avoid high-risk situations where they are likely to experience pressure to smoke, drink, or use drugs, as well as acquire the knowledge, confidence, and skills needed to handle social pressure in these and other situations. Also, because adolescents tend to overestimate the prevalence of drug use, social resistance programs often attempt to correct normative expectations that nearly everybody smokes, drinks alcohol, or uses drugs. In fact, resistance skills training may be ineffective in the absence of clear social norms against drug use because adolescents are less likely to resist if the norm is to engage in drug use (Donaldson et al., 1996).

Evaluation research has shown that social resistance skills programs are generally effective. A comprehensive review of resistance skills studies published from 1980 to 1990 reported that the majority of prevention studies (63 percent) had positive effects on drug use behavior, with fewer studies having neutral (26 percent) or negative effects on behavior (11 percent); and several studies finding no effects had inadequate statistical power to detect program effects (Hansen, 1992). Furthermore, several follow-up studies of social resistance skills interventions have reported positive behavioral effects lasting for up to 3 years. Longer-term follow-up studies have shown that these effects gradually decay over time, suggesting the need for ongoing intervention or booster sessions.

STRATEGIES THAT MIGHT WORK

Despite the literature of studies supporting the effectiveness of the social resistance skills prevention approach, recent research has called into question the efficacy of interventions that focus solely on social influences. Because the etiology of alcohol, tobacco, and other drug use among adolescents is multifactorial, preventive interventions that incorporate a variety of the most salient risk and protective factors are likely to be more effective than programs that focus on one or two of these factors. The *Hutchinson Smoking Prevention Project* (HSPP) is an example of a focused social influence-based smoking prevention curriculum that was ineffective in changing smoking behavior. The HSPP was implemented from the third grade through high school among a sample of youth in Washington state (Peterson, Kealey, Mann, Marek, & Sarason, 2000). Despite its length, findings indicated that students in the prevention group had essentially the same smoking rates as the students in the control group at the end of the 12th grade. The article received a great deal of attention from researchers, policy makers, and the press, some of whom suggested that the findings illustrate that social influence programs in general do not work. However, the only conclusion that can appropriately be drawn is that this particular intervention (the HSPP program) was ineffective.

Prevention strategies are more likely to work when they are based on a set of underlying assumptions that accurately reflect the many pathways that lead young people to drug use. Competence enhancement and social resistance approaches differ somewhat in the scope of their assumptions about adolescent substance use. Social influence approaches have a more focused set of assumptions, primarily that young people do not want to use drugs but lack the skills or confidence to refuse drug offers. However, as shown by a large and growing scientific literature, the etiology of adolescent drug use is complex, and using drugs may not be simply a matter of yielding to peer pressure. Competence enhancement approaches have a broader set of assumptions that also recognize that drug use may have a functional purpose for some youth, for example, by helping them deal with anxiety, low self-esteem, or a lack of comfort in social situations.

STRATEGIES THAT DO NOT WORK

Where contemporary prevention approaches such as social resistance and competence enhancement programs focus more interactive skills training techniques, traditional approaches focus on didactic instruction and the dissemination of information about drug abuse and the negative health, social, and legal consequences of abuse. Indeed, simply providing students with factual information about drugs and alcohol remains the most commonly used approach to drug abuse education. Some information dissemination approaches attempt to dramatize the dangers of using drugs with the use of fear-arousal techniques designed to attract attention and frighten individuals into not using drugs with vivid portrayals of the severe adverse consequences of drug abuse. Evaluation research and meta-analytic studies of informational approaches to drug abuse prevention have consistently failed to show any impact on drug use behavior or intentions to use drugs in the future (Tobler & Stratton, 1997). It has become increasingly clear that the etiology of drug and alcohol abuse is complex and prevention strategies that rely primarily on information dissemination are not effective in changing behavior.

Project *Drug Abuse Resistance Education* (DARE), is the most popular school-based prevention program in the United States, where it is provided in over two thirds of school districts. DARE uses trained uniformed police officers in the classroom to teach the drug prevention curriculum. Despite its popularity, research has shown that DARE has little impact on drug use behavior (Rosenbaum & Hanson, 1998). DARE may be ineffective for a number of reasons, including the fact that it is less interactive than more successful programs as well as the simple fact that teenagers may "tune out" what is seen as an expected message from an ultimate authority figure.

SYNTHESIS

Research suggests that several adolescent problem behaviors including substance use, early sexual activity, and antisocial behavior tend to co-occur in the same individuals and share common etiological factors (Donovan & Jessor, 1985). This suggests that enhancing social and personal competence skills may be a useful prevention approach for a variety of negative behaviors during adolescence. Indeed, several previous studies have shown that youth with good competence skills have lower rates of substance use, depression, delinquency, aggression, and other problem behaviors, and that skills training programs that promote social and personal competence can effectively prevent many of these behaviors drug use, antisocial and aggressive as well as promote overall school success (Dalley, Bolocofsky, & Karlin, 1994; Frey, Hirschstein, & Guzzo, 2000; Weissberg, Barton, & Shriver, 1997; Zins, Elias, Greenberg, & Weissberg, 2000).

In particular, competence enhancement may be a useful approach to preventing youth violence. Like drug abuse, interpersonal violence is a major public health problem that contributes substantially to morbidity and mortality rates, particularly among youth (Koop & Lundberg, 1992). A recent study of over 4,500 youth attending high school found that 43 percent of respondents reported hitting or threatening to hit someone in the past year, 14 percent reported attacking someone, and 13 percent reported carrying a hidden weapon (Ellickson, Saner, & McGuigan, 1997). Programs designed to prevent violence and aggression have traditionally been developed and implemented independently of adolescent drug abuse prevention programs. However, because substance use and interpersonal violence share similar etiological factors, a common prevention approach may be able to address the underlying determinants of these behaviors and possibly other risk behaviors. It does appear to be critical that training in generic life skills be combined with behavior-specific material in order to teach youth to apply new skills to specific behavioral outcomes. One study showed that a prevention program that taught generic competence skills without domain-specific material concerning the primary behavioral outcome was only minimally effective in reducing alcohol use (e.g., Caplan, Weissberg, Grober, Sivo, Grady, & Jacoby, 1992).

In summary, alcohol, tobacco, and other drug use are important problems among young people. Fortunately, substantial progress has been made in drug abuse prevention programs. Traditional prevention approaches that simply provide information about the negative consequences of drug abuse are not effective. Prevention approaches have been shown to be effective when they teach social and personal life skills along with skills to identify and resist pro-drug influences, contain information to correct inaccurate or exaggerated normative beliefs regarding the prevalence of drug use, and address other important risk and protective factors associated with drug use. Research has shown that prevention programs that include all of these components can reduce drug use for up to several years, including until the end of high school. However, further research is needed to examine how to maximize these effects and make them last, increase our understanding of the mediating mechanisms of effective prevention approaches, and to determine how to extend competence enhancement of life skills approaches to new problem behaviors.

Also see: Risk-Taking: Adolescence; Identity Promotion: Adolescence; Peer Relationships: Adolescence; Self-Esteem: Early Childhood; Self-Esteem: Childhood; Self-Esteem: Adolescence.

References

Bandura, A. (1977). *Social learning theory*. Englewood Cliffs, NJ: Prentice Hall.

Becker, M.H. (1974). *The health belief model and personal health behavior*. Thorofare, NJ: Slack.

Botvin, G.J. (2000). Preventing drug abuse in schools: Social and competence enhancement approaches targeting individual-level etiological factors. *Addictive Behaviors, 25*, 887–897.

Botvin, G.J., Baker, E., Dusenbury, L., Botvin, E.M., & Diaz, T. (1995). Long-term follow-up results of a randomized drug abuse prevention trial in a White middle-class population. *Journal of the American Medical Association, 273*, 1106–1112.

Botvin, G.J., Griffin, K.W., Diaz, T., & Ifill-Williams, M. (2001). Drug abuse prevention among minority adolescents: One-year follow-up of a school-based preventive intervention. *Prevention Science, 2*, 1–13.

Caplan, M., Weissberg, R.P., Grober, J.S., Sivo, P., Grady, K., & Jacoby, C. (1992). Social competence promotion with inner-city and suburban young adolescents: Effects of social adjustment and alcohol use. *Journal of Consulting & Clinical Psychology, 60*, 56–63.

Dalley, M.B., Bolocofsky, D.N., & Karlin, N.J. (1994). Teacher-ratings and self-ratings of social competency in adolescents with low- and high-depressive symptoms. *Journal of Abnormal Child Psychology, 22*, 477–485.

Donaldson, S.I., Sussman, S., MacKinnon, D.P., Severson, H.H., Glynn, T., Murray, D.M., & Stone, E.J. (1996). Drug abuse prevention programming: Do we know what content works? *American Behavioral Scientist, 39*, 868–883.

Donovan, J.E., & Jessor, R. (1985). Structure of problem behavior in adolescence and young adulthood. *Journal of Consulting & Clinical Psychology, 53*, 890–904.

Ellickson, P., Saner, J., & McGuigan, K.A. (1997). Profiles of violent youth: Substance use and other concurrent problems. *American Journal of Public Health, 87*, 985–991.

Epstein, J.A., Griffin, K.W., & Botvin, G.J. (2000). Role of general and specific competence skills in alcohol use among inner-city adolescents. *Journal of Studies on Alcohol, 61*, 379–386.

Frey, K.A., Hirschstein, M.K., & Guzzo, B.A. (2000). Second step: Preventing aggression by promoting social competence. *Journal of Emotional & Behavioral Disorders, 8*, 102–112.

Griffin, K.W., Epstein, J.A., Botvin, G.J., & Spoth, R.L. (2001). Social competence and substance use among rural youth: Mediating role of social benefit expectancies of use. *Journal of Youth & Adolescence, 30*, 485–498.

Griffin, K.W., Scheier, L.M., Botvin, G.J., & Diaz, T. (2001). The protective role of personal competence skills in adolescent substance use: Psychological well-being as a mediating factor. *Psychology of Addictive Behaviors, 15*, 194–203.

Hansen, W.B. (1992). School-based substance abuse prevention: A review of the state of the art in curriculum, 1980–1990. *Health Education Research: Theory & Practice, 7*, 403–430.

Hawkins, J.D., Catalano, R.F., & Miller, J.Y. (1992). Risk and protective factors for alcohol and other drug problems in adolescence and early adulthood: Implications for substance abuse prevention. *Psychological Bulletin, 112*, 64–105.

Hawkins, J.D., & Weis, J.G. (1985). The social development model: An integrated approach to delinquency prevention. *Journal of Primary Prevention, 6*, 73–97.

Jessor, R., & Jessor, S.L. (1977). *Problem behavior and psychosocial development: A longitudinal study of youth*. San Diego, CA: Academic Press.

Johnston, L.D., O'Malley, P.M., & Bachman, J.G. (2001). *Monitoring the future national results on adolescent drug use: Overview of key findings, 2000*. (NIH Publication No. 01-4923). Bethesda, MD: National Institute on Drug Abuse.

Khanzian, E.J. (1997). The self-medication hypothesis of substance use disorders: A reconsideration and recent applications. *Harvard Review of Psychiatry, 4*, 231–244.

Koop, C.E., & Lundberg, G.D. (1992). Violence in America: A public health emergency. *Journal of the American Medical Association, 267*, 3076–3077.

Peterson, A.V., Kealey, K.A., Mann, S.L., Marek, P.M., & Sarason, I.G. (2000). Hutchinson smoking prevention project: Long-term randomized trial in school-based tobacco use prevention—Results on smoking. *Journal of the National Cancer Institute, 92*, 1979–1991.

Petraitis, J., Flay, B.R., & Miller, T.Q. (1995). Reviewing theories of adolescent substance use: Organizing pieces in the puzzle. *Psychological Bulletin, 117*, 67–86.

Rosenbaum, D.P., & Hanson, G.S. (1998). Assessing the effects of school-based drug education: A six-year multilevel analysis of Project D.A.R.E. *Journal of Research in Crime & Delinquency, 35*, 381–412.

Tobler, N.S., & Stratton, H.H. (1997). Effectiveness of school-based drug prevention programs: A meta-analysis of the research. *Journal of Primary Prevention, 18*, 71–128.

Weissberg, R.P., Barton, H.A., & Shriver, T.P. (1997). The social-competence promotion program for young adolescents. In G.W. Albee, T.P. Gullotta et al. (Eds.), *Primary prevention works. Issues in children's and families' lives* (pp. 268–290). Thousand Oaks, CA: Sage.

Zins, J.E., Elias, M.J., Greenberg, M.T., & Weissberg, R.P. (2000). Promoting social and emotional competence in children. In K. Minke & G. Bear (Eds.), *Preventing school problems—promoting school success: Strategies and programs that work* (pp. 71–99). Bethesda, MD: National Association of School Psychologists.

Literacy, Childhood

Pia Rebello Britto, Allison Sidle Fuligni, and Jeanne Brooks-Gunn

INTRODUCTION

Children begin the process of learning long before they enter school. The home has been cited as a significant place for learning, as illustrated by links between the provision of learning experiences by families and children's academic success. This entry examines the home environment as a context for promoting young children's literacy development and academic achievement.

DEFINITIONS

Literacy refers to activities that involve print, such as reading and writing. However, according to the recently published definition of literacy by the National Academy of Science Report on Preventing Reading Difficulties in Young Children, literate behaviors, in addition to reading, include "... writing and other creative or analytic acts that at the same time invoke particular bits of knowledge and skill in specific subject matter..." (Snow, Burns, & Griffin, 1998, p. 42). The concept of *emergent literacy* is based on the notion that children acquire literacy skills not only as a result of direct instruction, but as a product of a stimulating and responsive environment that exposes children to the functionality and uses of print, and motivates and encourages them to engage with printed materials. Emergent literacy consists of skills, knowledge, and attitudes that are developmental precursors to conventional forms of reading and writing (Whitehurst & Lonigan, 1998). Therefore the emergence of literacy skills is often seen before children begin formal schooling.

SCOPE

The problem of low levels of literacy and lowered academic achievement is not new. According to the 1991 Carnegie Foundation report, *Ready to Learn: A Mandate for the Nation*, over a third of children in the United States enter public schools with skill levels lower than required for success in school and therefore are at risk for early academic difficulties. Based on a national longitudinal study of beginning kindergartners' knowledge and skills it was ascertained that 66 percent of the children were proficient in recognizing letters, and 29 percent proficient in associating the beginning letter of a word with the corresponding sound (National Center for Education Statistics, 2000). However, our knowledge of the scale of the early academic achievement problems is limited by the lack of national data on kindergartners. In terms of reading achievement, only a third of fourth graders were rated as proficient readers based on a national assessment of reading progress (National Assessment of Educational Progress, 1998).

In the United States, children reared in poverty tend to be over-represented in low literacy populations. They often perform below normative standards on school, state, and national assessments of reading achievement. On average, 13 percent of 9-year-olds eligible for the national school lunch program (an indicator of income poverty) were rated as proficient readers compared to 40 percent of those who were ineligible (National Assessment of Educational Progress, 1998). The influence of poverty on children's verbal ability as measured by standardized test scores during early childhood years is approximately a standard deviation below the normative mean. Other indices of poor academic achievement, such as grade retention, also suggest that children from poor families tend to fare worse in elementary school. Data from a national survey indicate that in 1995, 10 percent of second-graders from poor families repeated a grade compared to 7 percent of second-graders from non-poor families (poor families were defined in terms of the ratio between the total number of household members and estimates of household income; National Center for Education Statistics, 1995).

Internationally, problems of literacy and academic achievement are vast and complex. However, they are of a different scale and cannot be addressed completely within the scope of this entry. In developing countries rates of literacy among young children are very low, especially in the regions of sub-Saharan African and South East Asia. Some regions, for example, South Asia, estimate that approximately 65 percent of their female population is illiterate. Worldwide there are 113 million school-aged children out of school, 97 percent of them in less developed regions and 70 percent of them girls (World Education Forum, 2000). Equally dismal are the enrollment rates for primary school (47 percent) and for secondary school (12 percent). Globally, grade retention is a widely accepted indictor of academic achievement. Based on a UNESCO study, a wide range was noted in grade repetition rates for children enrolled in primary school (2 percent in the Republic of Korea to 35 percent in Togo), with the average retention rate at about 15 percent.

THEORIES AND RESEARCH

Several theories have been put forth regarding preventing low literacy and promoting academic achievement in young children. They range from focusing on genetic problems, to cognitive deficiencies, to school and home environments. In this entry we focus on environmental influences, such as the home environment, from an *ecological perspective*. In particular, the discussion centers around the multilayered context within which a child develops literacy and academic skills.

The family context is clearly central to children's development from infancy through the adolescent years (Bronfenbrenner, 1979). In addition to socioeconomic factors such as household income and parental education, other characteristics of parents, such as parenting behaviors, play an important role in children's early literacy development and academic achievement. For instance, shared book reading between parents and children, an iconic aspect of parenting behavior, promotes young children's early academic skills. Children who are read to regularly at home in early childhood enter school with a leg up and in the elementary school years, they tend to score higher on standardized tests of reading ability than those who are not read to so frequently (Bus, van IJzendoorn, & Pellegrini, 1995; Saracho, 1997; Snow et al., 1998).

The home environment is comprised of several aspects—language, learning, social and emotional, and physical (Bradley, 1994). In this entry we focus on the former two aspects given their significant associations with children's literacy and academic outcomes.

Three decades of extensive research has demonstrated that children who are exposed to a richer linguistic environment earlier on in life demonstrate a richer vocabulary, have a steeper language and literacy developmental trajectory, and perform better on standardized tests of reading achievement during the school years (Snow, 1993).[1] For instance, in the United States, an extensive longitudinal investigation by Hart and Risley (1995) has demonstrated the association between words used at home and young children's developing literacy skills. In their sample of 42 families from a range of socioeconomic backgrounds, they noted great variability in the amount and types of words children were exposed to at home. Through hierarchical regression analyses, Hart and Risley found that the language diversity in the home prior to 3 years of age was predictive of children's vocabulary use at age 3, which, in turn, was predictive of children's receptive vocabulary scores as measured by the PPVT-R (Peabody Picture Vocabulary Test-Revised) at ages 9–10.

The limitation of the Hart and Risley study was its small sample size, which has been overcome in larger scale, nationally representative studies demonstrating similar results, albeit without the benefit of being able to document language use per se. These studies suggest that language and cognitive stimulation in the home are generally more predictive of young children's cognitive, verbal, and early school achievement. For instance, reading to children predicts child outcomes during elementary school. These findings remain significant controlling for a host of demographic characteristics, such as maternal verbal ability, parental education, marital status of the mother, family income, number of children, ethnicity and mother's age (Smith et al., 1997).

Measuring shared book reading has been considered one of the primary ways to assess language and cognitive stimulation in the home. In terms of frequency of parent and child shared book reading, in the Commonwealth Fund Survey of Parents with Young Children 45 percent of the parents of 1- to 3-year-olds reported reading to their children daily and 37 percent reported reading more than once a day (Britto, Fuligni, & Brooks-Gunn, 2002). Although, reading to children at home during the preschool years is considered an important precursor for the development of literacy skills, the manner in which parents interact with their children during book reading seems to have a greater impact on the child's emerging literacy than actual time spent reading. Mothers employ a variety of individual reading styles and strategies during shared book reading to facilitate their child's literacy and language development and maintain their child's interest in the activity. For instance, some mothers simply read the text to their child while others engage their children in discussions during the reading activity (Heath & Branscombe, 1985). Differences in maternal reading styles have been associated with variability in child outcomes, namely language usage, word recall, and story comprehension (Sénéchal & LeFevre, 2001).

A related area of study is children's exposure to learning opportunities. This line of research is slightly different from studies that have used observational instruments such as the Home Observation for Measurement of the Environment inventory (HOME[2]) or survey measures to

---

[1] One concern raised in the literature is that parental language behavior may be in part due to parental genetics (i.e., good readers are likely to speak and read more to children as well as to have more printed material in the home), which itself is associated with children verbal and reading achievement. However it is especially noteworthy that some studies have been able to control for maternal verbal ability in their models as a partial way to separate out nature versus nurture effects (Smith, Brooks-Gunn, & Klebanov, 1997). These studies still show strong associations, suggesting that parental genetics may not be the sole contributors to children's verbal and reading skills.

[2] The HOME combines parent interview and observation to evaluate such features as parent–child literacy activities and the number of stimulating books and materials in the home (Bradley, 1994).

assess reading interaction. Exposure to learning opportunities in the home typically has been measured in terms of availability and exposure to printed matter in the home, such as the presence of books, newspapers, magazines, crayons, and coloring books. Based on a national assessment of reading proficiency and presence of various types of reading materials in the home (such as newspaper subscription, magazine subscription, more than 25 books, and an encyclopedia in the home), a significant difference was noted in the reading proficiency of children who had more materials in the home compared to children who had fewer (National Center for Education Statistics, 1992). Some 9-year-olds with none to two of these types of materials in the home were able to carry out simple reading tasks and follow brief descriptions, whereas 9-year-olds with four or more different types of reading materials in the home demonstrated more complex intellectual abilities, such as understanding and combining ideas from different subjects, and making inferences about short uncomplicated passages and specific or sequentially related information.

Other common measures of learning experiences in the first few years of life center around frequent use of printed matter in the home, parental modeling of literacy behaviors, and frequency of engagement in learning-focused activities. Parents use printed matter in a variety of ways while interacting with their children—as a source of entertainment; a skill to be learned; and/or as an integral ingredient of daily life. Children whose parents tend to view and use reading as a source of entertainment appear to have a more positive attitude and better reading skills compared to children of parents who tend to use more direct skill instruction while engaging their children with print (Baker, Scher, & Mackler, 1997). The home learning environment has also been assessed in terms of parental modeling of reading and writing behaviors. It is hypothesized that children who see their parents reading and writing purposefully and enjoying the activity are more likely to engage in such behaviors themselves.

Few studies have integrated the three approaches discussed, that is, actually analyzing maternal speech, measuring language and cognitively stimulating experiences (with a focus on shared book reading), and assessing the availability of exposure to printed material in the home more generally. In one such study, the Newark Young Family Study, the differential and relative importance of these approaches were studied in conjunction with each other in a sample of low-income, African American, female-headed, families with preschool aged children (Britto & Brooks-Gunn, 2001). The results suggest that all three dimensions are important for children's emerging literacy (expressive and receptive vocabulary) and school readiness skills. However, their relative importance varies depending on the skill being acquired. For instance, preschoolers' expressive vocabulary was associated with the language and verbal interactions and academic stimulation and support in the home.

Despite connections between low-income and low literacy, variability in language, literacy, and school achievement outcomes have been noted in low income preschool and elementary school aged populations. Among the potential explanations for the heterogeneity in child outcomes, the home environment has been cited as a portentous influence on the development of literacy and school readiness skills (Snow, Barnes, Chandler, Hemphill, & Goodman, 1991). Differences in provision of learning experiences in the home have been associated with variability in outcomes for children reared in poverty. An observation of the home environment of over 300 Head Start low-income families indicated tremendous variation in the literacy environments based on frequency of parent and child shared book reading, number of books in the home, frequency of parent–child library visits, and enjoyment of parent self-reading (Payne, Whitehurst, & Angell, 1994).

Data from the National Longitudinal Study of Youth–Child Supplement (NLSY–CS) indicate that a greater provision of stimulating and developmentally appropriate learning environments was associated with higher school achievement and verbal ability in the children of low-income families (Sugland et al., 1995). Data from other longitudinal samples, such as a sample of low-income, low education families headed by teenage mothers, show associations between the learning aspect of the home environment and preschool-aged children's emergent literacy skills. In particular, maternal assistance and informal teaching around a puzzle solving activity was strongly linked with the children's school readiness and expressive vocabulary (Britto & Brooks-Gunn, 2001).

STRATEGIES: OVERVIEW

Concern over the lower literacy and school-readiness skills of children from low-income families when they enter school, and recognition of the links discussed above between home learning environments and children's emerging literacy skills, have led to the creation of several models of early intervention programs designed to enhance family literacy practices. These programs seek to improve school readiness and later school success of children who, by virtue of poverty, are at-risk of lower academic outcomes. Although approaches vary, these programs tend to target family literacy either as their primary outcome or as one of several outcomes they strive to improve.

In the United States, family literacy programs vary in terms of their service delivery method, as well as their approaches to improving family literacy. Programs may be primarily home-visiting, center-based, or may combine both home-visiting and center-based services into a comprehensive package of services for young children and families. In the *home-visiting model*, a professional or para-professional visits the family on a regular basis with the frequency of visits ranging from weekly to monthly, to provide parenting and child development information on a one-on-one basis to parents. Home visitors may model specific activities that engage the child, provide books, materials, or toys for the family; and/or serve as a resource for addressing specific family needs and concerns. Two large-scale home visiting programs in the United States that are specifically geared towards improving family and child literacy are the *Parents as Teachers* (PAT) program for parents of diverse socioeconomic backgrounds with children aged three and younger (Wagner & Clayton, 1999), and the *Home Instruction Program for Preschool Youngsters* (HIPPY) that is designed to teach low-income parents of preschoolers how to engage in academically-oriented activities with their children (Baker, Piotrkowski, & Brooks-Gunn, 1998).

Center-based models tend to address child development more directly through offering high-quality early childhood education services. Additionally, they may seek to improve family literacy through regular group sessions with parents that focus on literacy and cognitively stimulating activities with children. When the primary goal of the program is improving parent–child learning interactions and the home learning environment, services are likely to be delivered directly to parents through home visits; therefore, a combination of center-based and home-visiting services is often seen. *Even Start* is a federal family literacy program that provides a combination of primarily center-based early childhood education, adult education, and parenting education services to improve intergenerational family literacy (St. Pierre, Swartz, Gamse, Murray, Deck, & Nickel, 1995). Another example of an educationally oriented early intervention programs that has combined center-based and home-visiting approaches in the first few years of life is the *Infant Health and Development Program* (IHDP, 1990).

Efforts at improving parenting practices during the early years are also in place outside of the United States. In its report on "The State of the World's Children 2001," UNICEF calls for governments worldwide to invest in parent training programs to help parents provide their young children with the appropriate stimulation and nurturance to optimize children's brain development and ability to learn throughout childhood (UNICEF, 2001). One example is the Early Childhood Development (ECD) component of the *Strong Beginnings* program currently operating in several countries in Asia, Africa, and South America. Strong Beginnings, a global educational initiative, was launched by Save the Children in 1990 in response to the World Conference on Education for all, in order to provide children and adults with equal access to quality education. The ECD component focuses on children from birth to 7 years of age and aims to teach parents and caregivers ways to stimulate children's early learning, including cognitive and language development, within the social and cultural context of the country, through local community involvement. For instance in their program in Bangladesh (where three fourths of the women are illiterate and thirty million children are living in absolute poverty), they reinforce traditional positive child rearing practices and build on parents' self-esteem to create a stimulating and productive environment for children. In El Salvador community involvement in ECD sparked the concept of "schools for parents" with the intention of strengthening enriched home learning environments for children (Wood, 1998).

STRATEGIES THAT WORK

Research on these programs for children's home learning environments and their ultimate school success suggests that these approaches can be beneficial to children and families. Early childhood programs serving children directly tend to have the strongest effects on children's language and cognitive development (see Fuligni & Brooks-Gunn, 2000). Home-visiting programs that incorporate a specific focus on child development, such as PAT and HIPPY, has documented positive child outcomes in these areas as well, but the more traditional home-visiting model without such a focus have not (Gomby, Culross, & Behrman, 1999). Numerous early childhood intervention programs for children at risk of poor academic outcomes have documented program effects on children's language and cognitive test scores, including the IHDP (Brooks-Gunn, 1995; Brooks-Gunn et al., 1994; IHDP, 1990), as well as the specifically literacy-focused Even Start program (St. Pierre et al., 1995).

In addition, programs providing parent education services have shown effects on parents' provision of a stimulating home literacy environment. This outcome has been measured by a standard assessment of the home environment, the HOME, as well as through single item indicators of the number of literacy materials present, or the number and types of literacy activities in which parents and children engage. For instance, Even Start has shown positive effects on the number of reading materials for children in the home in comparison to randomly-assigned control group families, and significant improvements over time for participating families in terms of learning activities in the home (St. Pierre et al., 1995), although there were no program-control group differences on home learning activities.

The intensity of services that families receive may be linked to programs' effects on family literacy practices.

In IHDP, families who showed greater program participation, on their own volition, had improved home environment scores when children were 12 months old and higher child IQ scores when the children were 3 years old, as assessed by the intervention program (Liaw, Miesels, & Brooks-Gunn, 1995). This relationship between participation and outcomes may alternatively be explained by greater motivation and/or commitment of the participants, however, because degree of program participation in this instance was voluntary.

Early childhood intervention programs that include a parent-focused component often aim to improve child outcomes both directly and indirectly through their effects on parenting practices. However, very few program evaluations actually test the pathway of effects through the parent or home environment. A handful of studies to date have done so, with mixed findings (Brooks-Gunn, Berlin, & Fuligni, 2000). IHDP has documented both significant direct effects on children's outcomes, as well as a pathway between the program and child outcomes mediated by its effects on the home environment (Linver & Brooks-Gunn, in preparation). The *Abecedarian* and *Project CARE* programs found that improved home environments were associated with children's test scores, but could not show a mediated link between program effects on the home environment and children's outcomes (Burchinal, Campbell, Bryant, Wasik, & Ramey, 1997).

STRATEGIES THAT MIGHT WORK

School-Transition Services

The large body of research showing links between early childhood education interventions and children's school-readiness-related outcomes has often been qualified by findings that program effects tend to diminish over time as control group members enter school and begin to "catch up" with children who participated in intervention programs before school entry (e.g., Royce, Darlington, & Murray, 1983). This pattern is not altogether surprising given that many children from low-income families who receive early intervention services go on to attend schools of substantially lower quality than do children from higher income families. One response to this problem is to provide children and families with ongoing support services as the children enter formal schooling. School-age supports may include home visits, a home-school coordinator to help improve communication between family and school, and after-school care. The *Head Start Transition* program has conducted a demonstration of such a program, offering comprehensive services to children and families to enhance their experiences as the children enter kindergarten and continuing support through the third grade (Head Start Bureau, 1996). *Equal Access*

to Success in Education (Project EASE) is another such project that has demonstrated the potential for schools to support parents to enrich their children's literacy development through providing parents information about strategies for doing so (Head Start Bureau, 1996). Although research has not yet linked such programs to family learning environments, this is a direction for future research. It is likely that parents can benefit from ongoing guidance on the provision of a stimulating and enriching home environment as children progress through formal schooling.

Neighborhood-Based Programs

Researchers have hypothesized that neighborhood-level SES may have both direct and indirect effects on children's outcomes (Fuligni & Brooks-Gunn, 2000). For very young children, most effects are likely to be indirect, as parents control the child's access to neighborhood resources, relationships, and collective norms (Leventhal & Brooks-Gunn, 2000).

Indeed, living in a poor neighborhood has been linked to less cognitively-stimulating home environments for 3–4-year-olds in the IHDP and NLSY, and less maternal warmth in the IHDP (Klebanov, Brooks-Gunn, Chase-Lansdale, & Gordon, 1997), setting the stage for indirect effects on children through these parenting variables. These studies have also linked parenting characteristics (cognitively stimulating environment and maternal warmth) to preschoolers' cognitive outcomes. Although the complete model, showing neighborhood effects on cognitive outcomes being mediated by home learning environments, was not statistically significant for preschoolers, it was for young school-aged children. In both the IHDP and NLSY, living in a neighborhood with affluent neighbors was associated with higher verbal and ability scores as well as lower behavior problem scores, and these effects were mediated by the cognitive stimulation parents provided in the home (Klebanov et al., 1997).

There is a question, then, of how neighborhood residence might influence parental provision of stimulating experiences, sensitivity, and warmth. Neighborhoods vary with respect to institutional resources, such as availability of learning, social and recreational activities, child care, and schools. Institutional resources may be of most interest regarding children's achievement outcomes, as the availability of libraries, museums, and learning programs in the community may affect the ease or difficulty of parents' provision of such experiences outside the home, and, in turn, children's school readiness and achievement. Additionally, unequal access to print resources (such as signs, logos, labels in public places) in low-income and middle-income neighborhoods has important implications for young children's early literacy development.

Second, there are several ways parental relationships might mediate the links between neighborhood characteristics and child outcomes. For instance, neighborhood poverty affects parental mental health, which influences parenting behaviors, and ultimately, child outcomes. Parental warmth, sensitivity, harshness, supervision, and monitoring are all dimensions of parenting that could both be affected by neighborhood characteristics and affect child outcomes.

Thus, faced with growing evidence that neighborhood environments may operate independently of family characteristics to influence child outcomes, an argument could be made for focusing intervention for low SES children on improving the characteristics of poor neighborhoods. Interventions focusing on the neighborhood (as opposed to focusing on individuals or families) are emerging, and are termed "comprehensive community initiatives" (CCIs). These initiatives target the physical, economic, and social conditions of neighborhoods in order to improve the lives of the low-income individuals and families living there (Roundtable on Comprehensive Community Initiatives for Children and Families, 1997). Thus, comprehensive community initiatives expect to directly influence individuals, families and communities, and they also expect to have an indirect effect on individuals and families through their effect on communities. CCIs might directly and indirectly support young children's development by creating more supportive home and out-of-home experiences.

It is important to reiterate, however, that much of the research on neighborhood influences, as well as the focus of many CCIs, has been on adolescent development. At this point, there is no existing research to support the effectiveness of the CCI approach in improving the developmental outcomes of low SES children or parenting of young children. However, such initiatives might be beneficial for poor children if: (a) they do, in fact, improve the community characteristics that have been found to influence children's healthy development, such as neighborhood income and employment levels, and (b) they include high-quality child care as a form of direct service to young children. Additional research is required to determine whether such an approach is intensive enough to have effects on young children.

STRATEGIES THAT DO NOT WORK

The clearest message that may be gleaned from the multitude of studies on early interventions is that programs that provide only low-intensity services have not been successful in improving parenting and the home environment or children's developmental outcomes (e.g., Gomby et al., 1999). Low levels of service intensity can be a problem among programs that are only designed to provide low levels of service,

as well as among those that intend to provide high levels of service but find that participation rates are lower than intended. For instance, across three well-known home-visiting programs (Hawaii Healthy Start, Parents as Teachers, and the Nurse Home Visiting Program), families received only 38–56 percent of the intended number of home visits (Gomby et al., 1999). Rates of service receipt have implications both for delivery of the intended curriculum and for the extent to which families become engaged in the program and develop trusting relationships with service providers.

As noted above, home-visiting programs that do not incorporate a specific focus on child development also appear to be relatively ineffective in supporting children's language and cognitive development (Gomby et al., 1999).

SYNTHESIS

The family environment has been identified as an important context for early learning, with children from disadvantaged families tending to experience less cognitive and linguistic stimulation in the home. A burgeoning body of research suggests that different aspects of the home environment may have differential influences on young children's emerging skills. Interventions, particularly those focused directly on parents, parenting styles, and home environments, seeking to ultimately improve the academic prospects of disadvantaged children have shown evidence of their promise in raising the academic and literacy-related skills of such children. Program services that focus directly on children have also shown positive results in terms of enhancing children's language and cognitive development. These services, by taking into account the associations between specific aspects of the environment and specific skill development, could further improve child literacy and school achievement outcomes.

Second, in terms of service delivery, the location of services (i.e., home-based or center-based) does not appear to matter as much as the intensity of services themselves. Greater program participation on the part of parents and families has been linked to positive effects on home environments and child cognitive development. On the other hand, programs providing only low levels of services to parents and children have not had as much success in influencing parenting or child outcomes. Finally, we have discussed two additional avenues worthy of additional research for improving children's home literacy environment and school-related outcomes—comprehensive services to families supporting their child's transition into schooling, and comprehensive community initiatives aiming to improve child and family well-being through improvement of the larger neighborhood community.

Also see: Academic Success: Adolescence; Family Strengthening: Childhood; Family Strengthening: Adolescence; School Absenteeism: Childhood; School Drop-outs: Adolescence

ACKNOWLEDGMENTS

We would like to thank the Spencer foundation for their support in the writing of this chapter.

References

Baker, A., Piotrkowski, C.S., & Brooks-Gunn, J. (1998). The effects of the home instruction program for preschool youngsters (HIPPY) on children's school performance at the end of the program and one year later. *Early Childhood Research Quarterly, 13,* 571–588.

Baker, L., Scher, D., & Mackler, K. (1997). Home and family influences on motivations for reading. *Educational Psychologist, 32,* 69–82.

Bradley, R.H. (1994). The HOME inventory: Review and reflections. In H.W. Reese (Ed.), *Advances in child development and behavior* (pp. 242–288). New York: Academic Press.

Britto, P.R., & Brooks-Gunn, J. (2001). Beyond shared book reading: Dimensions of home literacy and low-income African-American preschoolers' skills. In P.R. Britto & J. Brooks-Gunn (Eds.), *New directions for child and adolescent development, Vol. 92, The role of family literacy environments in promoting young children's emerging literacy skills* (pp. 73–90). San Francisco, CA: Jossey Bass.

Britto, P.R., Fuligni, A., & Brooks-Gunn, J. (2002). Reading, rhymes, and routines: American parents and their children. In N. Halfon, K. McLearn, and M. Schuster (Eds.), *The health and social conditions of young children in American families* (pp. 117–145). New York: Cambridge University Press.

Bronfenbrenner, U. (1979). *The ecology of human development: Experiments by nature and design.* Cambridge, MA: Harvard University Press.

Brooks-Gunn, J. (1995). Strategies for altering the outcomes for poor children and their families. In P.L. Chase-Lansdale & J. Brooks-Gunn (Eds.), *Escape from poverty: What makes a difference for children?* (pp. 87–117). Cambridge: Cambridge University Press.

Brooks-Gunn, J., Berlin, L.J., & Fuligni, A.S. (2000). Early childhood intervention programs: What about the family? In J.P. Shonkoff & S.J. Meisels (Eds.), *Handbook of early childhood intervention* (2nd ed., pp. 549–588). New York: Cambridge University Press.

Brooks-Gunn, J., McCarton, C., Casey, P., McCormick, M., Bauer, C., Bernbaum, J., Tyson, J., Swanson, M., Bennett, F., Scott, D., Tonascia, J., & Meinert, C. (1994). Early intervention in low birth weight, premature infants: Results through age 5 years from the Infant Health and Development Program. *Journal of the American Medical Association, 272,* 1257–1262.

Burchinal, M.R., Campbell, F.A., Bryant, D.M., Wasik, B.H., & Ramey, C.T. (1997). Early intervention and mediating processes in cognitive performance of children of low-income African-American families. *Child Development, 68,* 935–954.

Bus, A.G., van IJzendoorn, M.H., & Pellegrini, A.D. (1995). Joint book reading makes success in learning to read: A meta-analysis on intergenerational transmission of literacy. *Review of Educational Research, 65,* 1–21.

Fuligni, A.S., & Brooks-Gunn, J. (2000). The healthy development of young children: SES disparities, prevention strategies, and policy opportunities. In B.D. Smedley & S.L. Syme (Eds.), *Promoting health: Intervention strategies from social and behavioral research* (pp. 170–216). Washington, DC: National Academy Press.

Gomby, D.S., Culross, P.L., & Behrman, R.E. (1999). Home visiting: Recent program evaluations—analysis and recommendations. *The Future of Children, 9*(1), 4–26.

Hart, B., & Risley, T.R. (1995). *Meaningful differences in the everyday experience of young American children.* Baltimore, MD: Brookes.

Heath, S.B., & Branscombe, A. (1985). The book as a narrative prop in language acquisition. In B. Schieffelin & P. Gilmore (Eds.), *The acquisition of literacy: Ethnographic perspectives* (pp. 16–34). Norwood, NJ: Ablex.

Head Start Bureau. (1996). *Head Start children's entry into public school: An interim report on the National Head Start-Public School Early Childhood Demonstration Study.* Washington, DC: Department of Health and Human Services.

Infant Health and Development Program (IHDP). (1990). Enhancing the outcomes of low-birth-weight, premature infants. *Journal of the American Medical Association, 263,* 3035–3042.

Klebanov, P.K., Brooks-Gunn, J., Chase-Lansdale, P.L., & Gordon, R.A. (1997). Are neighborhood effects on young children mediated by features of the home environment? In J. Brooks-Gunn, G.J., Duncan, & J.L. Aber (Eds.), *Neighborhood poverty: Vol. 1. Context and consequences for children* (pp. 79–118). New York: Russell Sage Foundation Press.

Leventhal, T., & Brooks-Gunn, J. (2000). The neighborhoods they live in: The effects of neighborhood residence on child and adolescent outcomes. *Psychological Bulletin, 126,* 309–337.

Liaw, F., Meisels, S., & Brooks-Gunn, J. (1995). The effects of experience of early intervention on low birth weight, premature children: The Infant Health and Development Program. *Early Childhood Research Quarterly, 10,* 405–431.

Linver, M., & Brooks-Gunn, J. (in preparation). Parenting as mediating early intervention effects upon young children.

National Assessment of Education Progress. (1998). *1998 reading report card for the Nation and the States.* Washington, DC: US Department of Education.

National Center for Education Statistics. (1992). *National assessment of education progress, 1992 trends in academic progress.* Washington, DC: Department of Education.

National Center for Education Statistics. (1995). *National education longitudinal study of 1988, second follow-up.* Washington, DC: US Department of Education.

National Center for Education Statistics. (2000). Family characteristics of 6- to 12-year olds. *Education Statistics Quarterly, 2*(1), 48–50.

Payne, A.C., Whitehurst, G.J., Angell, A.L. (1994). The role of home literacy environment in the development of language ability in preschool children from low-income families. *Early Childhood Research Quarterly, 9,* 427–444.

Roundtable on Comprehensive Community Initiatives for Children and Families. (1997). *Voices from the field: Learning from the early work of comprehensive community initiatives.* Washington, DC: The Aspen Institute.

Royce, J.M., Darlington, R.B., & Murray, H.W. (1983). Pooled analyses: Findings across studies. In *As the twig is bent...Lasting effects of preschool programs.* Hillsdale, NJ: Erlbaum.

Saracho, O.N. (1997). Prespectives on family literacy. *Early Child Development and Care, 127–128,* 3–11.

Sénéchal, M., & LeFevre, J. (2001). Storybook reading and parent teaching: Links to language and literacy development. In P.R. Britto & J. Brooks-Gunn (Eds.), *New directions for child and adolescent development, Vol. 92, The role of family literacy environments in promoting young children's emerging literacy skills* (pp. 39–52). San Francisco, CA: Jossey-Bass.

Smith, J.R., Brooks-Gunn, J., & Klebanov, P.K. (1997). The consequences of living in poverty for young children's cognitive and verbal ability and early school achievement. In G.J. Duncan & J. Brooks-Gunn (Eds.), *Consequences of growing up poor* (pp. 132–189). New York: Russell Sage Foundation Press.

Snow, C.E. (1993). Families as social contexts for literacy development. In C. Daiute (Ed.), *The development of literacy through social interaction* (pp. 11–24). San Francisco: Jossey-Bass.

Snow, C.E., Barnes, W.S., Chandler, J., Hemphill, L., & Goodman, I.F. (1991). *Unfulfilled expectations: Home and school influences on literacy.* Cambridge, MA: Harvard University Press.

Snow, C.E., Burns, M.S., & Griffin, P. (Eds.). (1998). *Preventing reading difficulties in young children.* Washington, DC: National Academy Press.

St. Pierre, R., Swartz, J., Gamse, B., Murray, S., Deck, D., & Nickel, P. (1995). *National evaluation of the Even Start Family Literacy Program: Final report.* Washington, DC: US Department of Education.

Sugland, B.W., Zaslow, M., Smith, J.R., Brooks-Gunn, J., Coates, D., Blumenthal, C., Moore, K.A., Griffin, T., & Bradley, R. (1995). The Early Childhood HOME inventory and HOME-Short Form in differing racial/ethnic groups: Are there differences in underlying structure, internal consistency of subscales, and patterns of prediction? *Journal of Family Issues, 16,* 632–663.

UNICEF (2001). The state of the world's children 2001. New York: UNICEF.

Wagner, M.M., & Clayton, S.L. (1999). The parents as teachers program: Results from two demonstrations. *The future of children, Vol. 9. Home visiting: Recent program evaluations* (pp. 91–115).

Whitehurst, G.J., & Lonigan, C.J. (1998). Child development and emergent literacy. *Child Development, 69*(3), 848–872.

Wood, F. (1998). Alternative perspectives on ECD. *Early Childhood Matters, 88,* 12–17.

World Education Forum. (2000). *Education for all 2000 assessment.* New York: UNESCO.

Loneliness/Isolation, Older Adulthood

Melanie Gironda and James Lubben

INTRODUCTION

Loneliness and social isolation have been shown to be of increasing significance to the quality of life among older populations. Research on loneliness has greatly expanded in the last 25 years since the seminal work on loneliness by Weiss (1973). The groundbreaking study by Berkman and Syme (1979) demonstrating that social isolation was associated with increased mortality spawned a surge in research on social support networks. This entry provides a conceptual framework for distinguishing between loneliness and social isolation as well as to provide the reader with current theories to explain loneliness and social isolation among aging populations. Finally, this entry delineates the state of the art in terms of prevention strategies for combating loneliness and social isolation among older adults.

DEFINITIONS

Differentiating loneliness from isolation is often challenging. *Isolation* is defined as an insufficient social network from which a person may draw from or exchange social supports. Structural dimensions of *social networks* include size, density, source of ties, member homogeneity, frequency of contacts, geographic proximity, durability, intensity, and opportunity for reciprocal exchange of supports (Ell, 1984; Vaux, 1988). *Social support* is the fulfillment of the basic ongoing requirements for well-being as well as the fulfillment of more time limited needs that arise from adverse life events or circumstances (Cutrona & Russell, 1986). *Loneliness* is defined as the expression of dissatisfaction with a low number of social contacts. More specifically, Perlman (1987) maintains that loneliness is a discrepancy between one's desired and achieved levels of social contacts. Loneliness is identified as a subjective experience, whereas isolation is defined as an objective condition that involves a lack of integration into social networks (Rook, 1984).

SCOPE

Loneliness Literature

Although the extent of loneliness is difficult to establish, it is a serious problem for perhaps a quarter of retired people (Jerrome, 1991; Weiss, 1973). One of the largest studies done on loneliness was the survey conducted by Louis Harris and Associates for the National Council on Aging. They found that although loneliness was perceived as a "very serious" problem for older adults among 45 percent of those surveyed, in fact only 13 percent reported it to be a "very serious problem" in their own personal experience (Harris and Associates, 1981).

Loneliness has been associated with ill health (de Jong-Gierveld, 1987; Jones, Victor, & Vetter, 1985; Long & Martin, 2000; Mullins, Smith, Colquitt, & Mushel, 1996); increased nursing home admissions (Russell, Cutrona, & Wallace, 1997); and depression (Koropeckyj-Cox, 1998; Mullins et al., 1996). In a review of literature, Wenger (1996) looked at a range of studies on loneliness and found the prevalence of loneliness in adults aged 65+ to range from 2 to 16 percent among various populations.

Social Isolation Literature

Much of the literature on social isolation among older adult populations pertains to the link between social isolation and physical health and well-being (Auslander & Litwin, 1991; Berkman & Syme, 1979; Chappell & Badger, 1989; Jackson & Antonucci, 1992; Lubben & Gironda, 1996; Lubben, Weiler, & Chi, 1989; Mullins et al., 1996). Some stronger social networks are also related to better psychological health (Mor-Barak & Miller, 1991).

Research on social support and social isolation has grown over the years. One of the seminal studies was that of Berkman and Syme (1979) who found that the age adjusted mortality rates for socially isolated older adults were two to three times higher than the age adjusted rates for socially integrated adults. Public health experts now posit that the association between support networks and health is now as strong as the epidemiological evidence linking smoking and health (House, Landis, & Umberson, 1988; Kaplan, Seeman, Cohen, Knudsen, & Guralnik, 1987; Lubben et al., 1989; Rook, 1994). One recent study even suggested that people with more social ties are less susceptible to the common cold (Cohen, Doyle, Skoner, Rabin, & Gwaltney, 1997).

Inadequate social support is associated with an increase in mortality (Berkman & Syme, 1979; House et al., 1988), morbidity (Berkman, 1985; Ell, 1984; Torres, McIntosh, & Kubena, 1992), psychological distress (Hurwicz & Berkanovic, 1993), and a decrease in overall general health and well-being (Chappell, 1991; Chappell & Badger, 1989; Cutrona & Russell, 1986).

Although few large-scale empirical studies have been conducted among elderly populations, a significant relationship also appears to exist between an elder's level of social networks and health risk (Kaplan et al., 1987; Lubben et al., 1989). In a clinical trial of social health risks among a large community dwelling elderly population, 66 percent of the study sample were at low risk for social isolation, another 16 percent were rated at moderate risk, 10 percent were rated at high risk, and 8 percent were rated as isolated. Details of the study are found elsewhere (Dorfman et al., 1995; Rubinstein, Lubben, & Mintzer, 1994). In a study among older American veterans, those at high or moderate risk for social isolation were 4–5 times more likely to be re-hospitalized within a year than low isolation risk veterans (Mistry, Rosansky, McGuire, McDermott, & Jarvik, 2001).

THEORIES AND RESEARCH

Loneliness Theories

Weiss (1973) introduced the concept of loneliness with an emphasis on *attachment theory* that has as one of its basic assumptions that disruptions in childhood relationships lead to emotional and interpersonal difficulties (including loneliness) in adulthood. Another body of research doing similar theoretical lines, expanded on child attachment to suggest that there is a continuity of sociability patterns over long periods of time or over the life cycle (Antonucci & Akiyama, 1987; Skolnick, 1986). Expanding on this avenue of research, other theorists suggested a stronger emotional behavioral/personality component to loneliness (de Jong-Gierveld, 1987; Dykstra, 1995; Perlman & Peplau, 1982). They argued that some form of deficit in one's social relationships influences loneliness. For example, some people may have never learned how to meaningfully connect to anyone throughout their lives and find themselves lonely in old age. Therefore, loneliness is more of an affective state in which an individual is subjectively responding to the experience of being emotionally apart from others.

One distinguishing aspect of loneliness is that it is often times uninterrupted by social activity (Weiss, 1973). The idea that one may feel lonely while in the midst of a crowd is often used to capture the quality of loneliness. Rokach (2000) in an investigation of how terminally ill persons cope with the loneliness that accompanies life-threatening and socially feared diseases, describes loneliness as including feelings of self-alienation, emptiness, and a sense of meaninglessness.

Weiss (1973) identified two types of loneliness: emotional and social. *Emotional loneliness* is a lack of truly intimate ties stemming from emotional detachment described in Bowlby's attachment theory. The remedy for this type of loneliness is the integration of another emotional attachment or the reintegration of the one lost. *Social loneliness*, on the other hand, is a lack of a network of involvement with family, peers, friends, and neighbors for which the remedy is access to an engaging social network.

It is in this social loneliness domain that social isolation presents as a critical issue for older adults who have lost access to significant parts of their social network. In elderly cohorts, we often see social loneliness as a result of isolation. In particular, certain subpopulations of elders are at risk for social isolation including people who are among the oldest old, in poorer health, not married, and with lower levels of income and education (Kaufman & Adams, 1987). Gironda, Lubben, and Atchison (1999) also report that childless older adults and those without proximal children are at increased risk for both isolation and loneliness. Therefore the social, physical, and economic contexts in which loneliness occurs is an important consideration in determining at risk groups. For example, Long and Martin (2000) found that for the oldest-old, affectionate relationships with children were of prime importance as a buffer to loneliness. Mullins, Sheppard, and Anderson (1991) in their research highlight two divergent directions of the relationship between subjective and objective loneliness. They report that older adults desire the perceived availability of family and peer contacts but not necessarily the actual contact. Further, Mullins and associates noted that although older persons may desire ongoing contact with family members, they prefer social contacts with peers.

As people grow older, their social network may become limited due to such factors as outliving relatives and friends, increasing chronic health problems that limit mobility, and limited social opportunities, resulting in social isolation. However, not all socially isolated older adults experience social loneliness. Perception of isolation has a stronger influence on loneliness than absolute isolation (Hoeffer, 1987).

Isolation Theories

A number of theories have been proposed to account for the apparent relationship between social isolation and health. For example, social ties may serve to stimulate the *immune system* to ward off illnesses more effectively. Similarly, a *buffering effect theory* suggests that strong social ties may reduce the susceptibility of an individual to stress-related illnesses (Cassel, 1976; Cobb, 1976; Krause, Herzog, & Baker, 1992; Krause & Jay, 1991; Mor-Barak & Miller, 1991; Thoits, 1982). A third theory suggests that since social networks provide essential *support* needed during times of illness, thereby contributing to better adaptation and quicker recovery time, socially isolated elders are at increased risk for illness-related complications and are more likely to have a slower recovery time (Cohen & Syme, 1985). Yet a fourth theory posits that *social networks* are instrumental in adherence to good health practices and the cessation of bad ones (Kelsey, Earp, & Kirkley, 1997; Potts, Hurwicz, & Goldstein, 1992).

Link between Loneliness and Social Isolation

Research suggests that lonely persons report smaller and less satisfying social networks (e.g., fewer friends and companions) and they are less likely to engage in social activities (Perlman & Peplau, 1982). Townsend (1968) introduced the idea that isolation and loneliness are not necessarily coincidental, rather they influence and affect each other. For the purpose of this presentation, the focus is on the connection between social loneliness and social isolation. Wenger (1996) found the following correlates of both social isolation and loneliness: age, gender, widowhood, singleness, living alone, childlessness, retirement migration, poor health, restricted mortality, and low morale. In a study by Lubben and Gironda (1996) comparing three measures

of social integration, an inter-scale comparison showed a shared variance of 34 percent between the isolation measure (Lubben Social Network Scale) and the loneliness measure (UCLA-Loneliness Scale). This suggests that both loneliness and isolation can be used to explain a common element of social integration. Another study found social network variables, as well as individual differences variables contribute to self-reported loneliness (Stokes, 1985).

Measures of social isolation and loneliness exist in the gerontological literature; however, they are frequently operationalized using different standards. For example, Chappell and Badger (1989) identify the following common indicators in the literature of isolation; live alone, no confidant, no companions, no children, unmarried, and various combinations of these. Wenger (1996) reported that isolation was associated with marital status, network type, and social class, whereas loneliness was associated with network type, household composition, and health.

A widely used instrument to measure loneliness is the Revised UCLA Loneliness Scale (Russell, Peplau, & Cutrona, 1980). It is a 20-item, self-report measure. A shortened 4-item version has also been developed (Hays & DiMatteo, 1987). Another commonly used loneliness measure is the 9-item Loneliness–Deprivation Scale (de Jong-Gierveld, 1987). This scale is used to assess the intensity of deprivation feelings concerning relationships with others. An alternative to formal scales is to use a single item such as "How often one feels lonely?" with a Likert-type response pattern (Wenger, 1996).

Due in part to the high complexity of social relationship phenomena, there lacks agreement on definitions and preferred measures for social support networks (Ell, 1984; House et al., 1988; Lin, Te, & Ensel, 1999; Lubben & Gironda, 1996; Vaux, 1988; Wenger, 1996). Few of these measures actually establish cut-point for social isolation. One that does is the Lubben Social Network Scale (LSNS) (Lubben, 1988). It has been used in applied and research settings to evaluate social isolation (Dorfman et al., 1995; Mor-Barak, 1997; Okwumabua, Baker, Wong, & Pilgrim, 1997; Rubinstein et al., 1994). The LSNS is a 10-item scale. A 6-item scale version (LSNS-6) has recently been developed by Lubben and Gironda (2000) for use in health risk appraisal instruments.

STRATEGIES THAT WORK

A common strategy that works with lonely and/or isolated older adults is to first identify those at risk. One area where this should take place is in health promotion and wellness programs for older adults where screening for social isolation and loneliness can be conducted. Some of the assessment instruments described earlier can be readily incorporated into health screening instruments and used by a variety of health professionals in various health care settings.

Besides inclusion in health screening instruments, general assessment regimes should also be adapted to include at least a few items that might alert the health care provider of potential social isolation and/or loneliness. Increased sensitivity of providers to the importance of social support networks for well-being in old age might help flag those elders in need of a more comprehensive assessment by a social worker or other practitioner.

One review of the literature suggests that loneliness is least common among those who are married or cohabitating and those elderly who tend to be most lonely are widowed, divorced, or separated. However, it is noted that marriage is not a safeguard against loneliness and being single should not be equated with being lonely (Dykstra, 1995). Three practical interventions for individuals include: (1) making regular phone and in-person contact with older family members and neighbors, (2) ensure that older people feel needed and valued, and (3) include older friends and neighbors in family gatherings (Hall & Havens, 1999).

The availability of appropriate resources is another strategy for minimizing loneliness and isolation in older adult populations. Studies show that clubs, groups, and associations formed and run by older adults seem to be an effective intervention for loneliness and isolation in part due to the sense of control attained by the elders who must decide for themselves the nature of terms of the group experience (Hall & Havens, 1999; Jerrome, 1991). Outreach programs provided by Area Agencies on Aging (AAAs), such as meals-on-wheels, phone-a-friend, or lifeline services are other ways in which loneliness and social isolations are successfully minimized.

STRATEGIES THAT MIGHT WORK

One strategy that has withstood the test of time, yet is in need of some more empirical testing is in the area of caregiving contributes to loneliness and isolation. Caregivers are often referred to as the "hidden victims" of not only loneliness and isolation, but diminished health and well-being as well. Caregiving tasks are often 24 hr a day and 7 days a week, which severely limits the level of social involvement needed to maintain social connectedness. One researcher suggests that since large numbers of older adults are subject to frequent contact with health care providers, it is also of value to examine care-giving practices that may precipitate or mitigate the loneliness experience in this age group (Ryan & Patterson, 1987). The earlier the detection of loneliness and

isolation happens and an intervention strategy is identified, the hope is that the duration and intensity of the loneliness and/or isolation experience is reduced.

Respite care is another intervention strategy for loneliness and isolation suffered by the caregiver and care recipient. It gives the caregiver an opportunity to reconnect with important members of his/her social support system as a secondary benefit. It can give the care recipient an opportunity to interact with people other than the caregiver. Some spouses become so burdened with caretaking responsibilities that they no longer see their own friends. Cognizant of the importance of friendship to mental health, it is clear that spousal and other overburdened elder caretakers need a break.

The use of computer technology such as the Internet is a possible remedy for isolation among older people. However, the jury is still out on its actual effectiveness. Rokach (2000) points to a small, but growing body of research that suggests that although access to people thousands of miles away is accomplished in seconds, real intimacy which combats loneliness and social isolation remains illusive. Some studies have shown that increased use of the Internet leads to shrinking social support and increased loneliness. These criticisms may be remedied in the future as technology improves.

STRATEGIES THAT DO NOT WORK

One strategy that clearly does not work is to apply a "one approach fits all" model to the problem of loneliness and/or isolation. The amount of social contact needed by older people will vary depending on personality patterns. Johnson and Mullins (1989, p. 113) define different levels and types of social contact needed to prevent the development of loneliness using a concept they call the "*loneliness threshold.*" More than one type of intervention will be needed to address the diversity of social isolates and strengthen social support networks. First, not all isolates are alike and different interventions need to be developed to address distinctive types and profiles of isolates. For example, respite programs might be an appropriate strategy for older adults whose social contacts have become impaired due to caregiving responsibilities, whereas self-help groups might work best for those whose isolation is attributed to bereavement. Second, a wide array of services is available for older adults, but changing populations, cohorts, and circumstances determine the types of services utilized. Third, many older individuals do not participate in programs and activities for a variety of reasons including gender, ethnicity, health status, class and income, social skills, environment, technology, and transportation.

Another strategy that does not work is what might be referred to as benign neglect of those at risk. The Northridge, California earthquakes of 1994 and the Chicago, Illinois heat wave of 1995 are but two examples, where some older persons suffered great injury and were even at increased risk of death as a direct result of their isolation. These isolated older adults may have appeared to be self-sufficient but their isolation contributed to their increased risk of morbidity and mortality in these extreme crisis situations.

Along this same line of thinking, a third strategy that does not work is to glamorize the idea of isolation into a notion of healthful solitude. Whether isolation is sought or endured, those that endure solitude should not be characterized as having achieved a desired state but should instead be identified as a population at potential risk. The glamorization of solitude when it is actually loneliness is analogous to the argument of the "model minority," often heard when referring to Asian American groups that do not need help because they are expected to "take care of their own." In his book entitled *The solitude of loneliness*, Woodward suggests that when solitude is not something chosen, loneliness is the product. For example, the social outcasts, including abandoned elderly living alone are just some of the casualties of forced solitude (Woodward, 1988).

SYNTHESIS

Loneliness and social isolation are detrimental to the health and well-being of older populations. However, loneliness and social isolation are relatively distinct constructs suggesting the need for separate measures of each. From an applied gerontological research perspective, there is growing pressure to develop short and efficient scales. As discussed by Kohut, Berkman, Evans, and Cornoni-Huntley (1993), elderly populations with specific physical or cognitive limitations may not do well with long questionnaires. Therefore, parsimonious and effective screening tools need to be developed for detecting loneliness and isolation.

Geriatric practice should include regular screening for loneliness and isolation that facilitate more timely intervention to modify these health risk factors. Future research needs to more specifically ascertain the causes of loneliness and isolation as well as evaluate interventions tailored for the various types of loneliness and isolation. Finally, clinical trials should be implemented to evaluate these various approaches so that practice can be informed as to what works best and for whom.

Also see: Community Capacity; Depression: Childhood; Depression: Adolescence; Depression: Adulthood; Depression: Older Adulthood.

References

Antonucci, T.C., & Akiyama, H. (1987). Social networks in adult life and a preliminary examination of the convoy model. *Journal of Gerontology, 42*, 519–527.

Auslander, G.K., & Litwin, H. (1991). Social networks, social support, and self-ratings of health among the elderly. *Journal of Aging and Health, 3*(4), 493–510.

Berkman, L.F. (1985). The relationship of social networks and social supports to morbidity and mortality. In S. Cohen & S.L. Syme (Eds.), *Social support and health* (pp. 241–262). Orlando, FL: Academic Press.

Berkman, L.F., & Syme, S.L. (1979). Social networks, host resistance, and mortality: A nine year follow-up study of alameda county residents. *American Journal of Epidemiology, 109*, 186–204.

Cassel, J. (1976). The contribution of the social environment to host resistance. *American Journal of Epidemiology, 104*, 107–123.

Chappell, N.L. (1991). The role of family and friends in quality of life. In J.E. Birren, J.E. Lubben, J.C. Rowe, & D.E. Deutchman (Eds.), *The concept and measurement of quality of life in the frail elderly* (pp. 171–190). New York: Academic Press.

Chappell, N.L., & Badger, M. (1989). Social isolation and well-being. *Journal of Gerontology: Social Sciences, 44*, S169–S176.

Cobb, S. (1976). Social support as a moderator of life stress. *Psychosomatic Medicine, 38*, 300–314.

Cohen, S., Doyle, W.J., Skoner, D.P., Rabin, B.S., & Gwaltney, J.M. (1997). Social ties and susceptibility to the common cold. *Journal of the American Medical Association, 277*, 1940–1944.

Cohen, S., & Syme, S.L. (1985). *Social support and health*. New York: Academic Press.

Cutrona, C., & Russell, D. (1986). Social support and adaptation to stress by the elderly. *Psychology of Aging, 1*, 47–54.

de Jong-Gierveld, J. (1987). Developing and testing a model of loneliness. *Journal of Personality and Social Psychology, 53*(1), 119–128.

Dorfman, R.A., Lubben, J.E., Mayer-Oakes, A., Atchison, K.A., Schweitzer, S.O., Dejong, J., & Matthais, R. (1995). Screening for depression among a well elderly population. *Social Work, 40*, 295–304.

Dykstra, P.A. (1995). Loneliness among the never and formerly married: The importance of supportive friendships and a desire for independence. *Journal of Gerontology: Social Sciences, 50B*(5), S321–S329.

Ell, K. (1984). Social networks, social support, and health status: A review. *Social Service Review, 58*, 133–149.

Gironda, M.W., Lubben, J.E., & Atchison, K.A. (1999). Social support networks of elders without children. *Journal of Gerontological Social Work, 27*, 63–84.

Hall, M., & Havens, B. (1999, November). *The effect of social isolation and loneliness on the health of older women*. Presented at GSA.

Harris, L. and Associates. (1981). *Aging in the eighties: America in transition*. Washington, DC: National Council on Aging.

Hays, R.D., & DiMatteo, M.R. (1987). A short form measure of loneliness. *Journal of Personality Assessment, 51*(1), 69–81.

Hoeffer, B. (1987). A causal model of loneliness among older single women. *Archives of Psychiatric Nursing, 1*(5), 366–373.

House, J.S., Landis, K.R., & Umberson, D. (1988). Social relationships and health. *Science, 241*, 540–545.

Hurwicz, M.L., & Berkanovic, E. (1993). The stress process of rheumatoid arthritis *Journal of Rheumatology, 20*, 1836–1844.

Jackson, J.S., & Antonucci, T.C. (1992). Social support processes in health and effective functioning of the elderly. In M.L. Wykle, E. Kahana, & J. Kowal (Eds.), *Stress and health among the elderly* (pp. 72–95). New York: Springer.

Jerrome, D. (1991). Loneliness: Possibilities for intervention. *Journal of Aging Studies, 5*(2), 195–208.

Jones, D., Victor, C., & Vetter, N. (1985). The problem of loneliness in the elderly in the community. *Journal of Royal College of General Practitioners, 35*(272), 136–139.

Johnson, D.P., & Mullins, L.C. (1989). Religiosity and loneliness among the elderly. *The Journal of Applied Gerontology, 8*(1), 110–131.

Kaplan, G.A., Seeman, T.E., Cohen, R.D., Knudsen, L.P., & Guralnik, J. (1987). Mortality among the elderly in the Alameda county study: Behavioral and demographic risk factors. *American Journal of Public Health, 77,* 307–312.

Kaufman, A.V., & Adams, J.P. (1987). Interaction and loneliness: A dimensional analysis of the social isolation of a sample of older southern adults. *Journal of Applied Gerontology, 6*(4), 389–404.

Kelsey, K., Earp, J.L., & Kirkley, B.G. (1997). Is social support beneficial for dietary change? A review of the literature. *Family & Community Health, 20,* 70–82.

Kohut, F.J., Berkman, L.F., Evans, D.A., & Cornoni-Huntley, J. (1993). Two shorter forms of the CES-D depression symptoms index. *Journal of Aging and Health, 5*(2), 179–193.

Koropeckyj-Cox, T. (1998). Loneliness and depression in middle and old age: Are the childless more vulnerable? *Journal of Gerontology: Social Sciences, 53B*(6), S303–S312.

Krause, N., Herzog, A.R., & Baker, E. (1992). Providing support to others and well-being in late life. *Journal of Gerontology: Psychological Sciences, 47,* P300–P311.

Krause, N., & Jay, G. (1991). Stress, social support, and negative interaction in later life. *Research on Aging, 13,* 333–363.

Lin, N., Te, X., & Ensel, W.M. (1999) Social support and depressed mood: A structural analysis. *Journal of Health and Social Behavior, 40,* 344–359.

Long, M.V., & Martin, P. (2000). Personality, relationship closeness, and loneliness of oldest old adults and their children. *Journal of Gerontology: Psychological Sciences, 55B,* P311–P319.

Lubben, J.E. (1988). Assessing social networks among elderly populations. *Family Community Health, 11,* 42–52.

Lubben, J.E., & Gironda, M.W. (1996). Assessing social support networks among older people in the United States. In H. Litwin (Ed.), *The social networks of older people* (pp. 143–161). Westport, CT: Greenwood.

Lubben, J.E., & Gironda, M.W. (2000). Social support networks. In D. Osterweil, K. Brummel-Smith, & J.C. Beck (Eds.), *Comprehensive geriatric assessment* (pp. 121–137). New York, NY: McGraw Hill.

Lubben, J.E., Weiler, P.G., & Chi, I. (1989). Health practices of the elderly poor. *American Journal of Public Health, 79,* 371–374.

Mistry, R., Rosansky, J., McGuire, J., McDermott, C., & Jarvik, L. (2001). Social isolation predicts re-hospitalization in a group of older American veterans enrolled in the UPBEAT program. *International Journal of Geriatric Psychiatry, 16,* 950–959.

Mor-Barak, M.E. (1997). Major determinants of social networks in frail elderly community residents. *Home Health Care Service Quarterly, 16,* 121–137.

Mor-Barak, M.E., & Miller, L.S. (1991). A longitudinal study of the causal relationship between social networks and health of the poor frail elderly. *The Journal of Applied Gerontology, 10*(3), 293–310.

Mullins, L.C., Smith, R., Colquitt, M., & Mushel, M. (1996). An examination of the effects of self-rated objective indicators of health condition and economic condition on the loneliness of older persons. *The Journal of Applied Gerontology, 15*(1), 23–37.

Mullins, L.C., Sheppard, H.L., & Anderson, L. (1991). Loneliness and social isolation in Sweden: Differences in age, sex, labor force status, self-rated health, and income adequacy. *The Journal of Applied Gerontology, 10*(4), 455–468.

Okwumabua, J.O., Baker, F.M., Wong, S.P., & Pilgrim, B.O. (1997). Characteristics of depressive symptoms in elderly urban and rural African Americans. *Journals of Gerontology: Biological Sciences and Medical Sciences, 52A,* M241–M246.

Perlman, D. (1987). Further reflections on the present state of loneliness research. *Journal of Social Behavior and Personality, 2*(2), 17–26.

Perlman, D., & Peplau, L.A. (1982). Theoretical approaches to loneliness. In L.A. Peplau & D. Perlman (Eds.), *Loneliness: A sourcebook of current theory, research, and therapy* (pp. 123–134). New York: Wiley Interscience.

Potts, M.K., Hurwicz, M.L., & Goldstein, M.S. (1992). Social support, health-promotive beliefs, and preventive health behaviors among the elderly. *The Journal of Applied Gerontology, 11*(4), 425–440.

Rokach, A. (2000). Terminal illness and coping with loneliness. *The Journal of Psychology, 134*(3), 283–296.

Rook, K.S. (1984). *Loneliness, social support and social isolation.* Prepared for the Office of Prevention, National Institute of Mental Health.

Rook, K.S. (1994). Assessing the health-related dimensions of older adults' social relationships. In M.P. Lawton & J.A. Teresi (Eds.), *Annual review of gerontology and geriatrics* (pp. 142–181). New York: Springer.

Rubinstein, R.L., Lubben, J.E., & Mintzer, J.E. (1994). Social isolation and social support: An applied perspective. *The Journal of Applied Gerontology, 13*(1), 58–72.

Russell, D., Peplau, L.A., & Cutrona, C.E. (1980). The revised UCLA loneliness scale: Concurrent and discriminant validity evidence. *Journal of Personality and Social Psychology, 39,* 472–480.

Russell, D.W., Cutrona, C.E., & Wallace, R.B. (1997). Loneliness and nursing home admission among rural older adults. *Psychology and Aging, 12*(4), 574–589.

Ryan, M.C., & Patterson, J. (1987). Loneliness in the elderly. *Journal of Gerontological Nursing, 13*(5), 6–12.

Skolnick, A. (1986). Early attachment and personal relationships across the life course. In P. Batles, D. Featherman, & R. Lerner (Eds.), *Life-span development and behavior* (Vol. 7, pp. 173–206). Hillsdale, NJ: Lawrence Erlbaum.

Stokes, J.P. (1985). The relation of social network and individual difference variables to loneliness. *Journal of Personality and Social Psychology, 48*(4), 981–990.

Thoits, P.A. (1982). Conceptual, methodological and theoretical problems in studying social support as a buffer against life stress. *Journal of Health and Social Behavior, 23,* 145–159.

Torres, C.C., McIntosh, W.A., & Kubena, K.S. (1992). Social network and social background characteristics of elderly who live and eat alone. *Journal of Aging and Health, 4,* 564–578.

Townsend, P. (1968). Isolation, desolation and loneliness. In E. Shanas, P. Townsend, D. Wedderburn, H. Friis, P. Milhoy, & J. Stenhouwer (Eds.), *Old people in three industrial societies.* London: Routledge.

Vaux, A. (1988). *Social support: Theory, research and intervention.* New York: Praeger.

Weiss, R.S. (1973). *Loneliness: The experience of emotional and social isolation.* Cambridge: MIT Press.

Wenger, G.C. (1996). Social isolation and loneliness in old age: Review and model refinement. *Aging and Society, 16,* 333–358.

Woodward, J.C. (1988). *The solitude of loneliness.* Massachusetts: Lexington Books.

M

Marital Enhancement, Adulthood

Chien Liu

INTRODUCTION

Marital sexual life is a very important part of marriage, and it is central to the institution of the family since it can either promote or destabilize a marriage. A married person can have two types of partnered sex, marital sex and extramarital sex; both have a tremendous impact on marriage. Good marital sex can enhance marital happiness and thus promote marriage, while extramarital sex poses a threat to marital stability. In the past half century, though marital sex has been studied extensively by social scientists, the study of extramarital sex remains limited (Christopher & Sprecher, 2000). This entry summarizes the findings of recent research on marital sex and extramarital sex and suggests some strategies to enhance marital sex and to prevent extramarital sex, thus achieving the goal of protecting and promoting marriage. Although this entry focuses on marital sexual life, the analysis and strategies presented are applicable to other types of adult sexual relationships such as cohabitation.

DEFINITIONS AND SCOPE

Marriage is a contract; each party explicitly or implicitly agrees to recognize certain rights of the other (England &

Farkas, 1986). One such right is an individual's right to restrict his/her spouse's sexual action. Specifically, in a marriage, each party agrees to give up his/her own right to have a sexual relationship with a third party, in return for the right to restrict his/her spouse's sexual action. Within this structure of rights, neither party should have sex with another person but his/her spouse. This right to control a spouse's sexual action must be either implicitly or explicitly recognized by each party. The fact that more than 90 percent of the Americans think that extramarital sex is always or almost always wrong (Smith, 1994) (i.e., people do not have the right to engage in extramarital sex, a cultural norm) indicates that the right to control a spouse's sexual action does exist in reality. Without this right, a husband or wife will suffer from serious, negative consequence or externalities of their spouse's involvement in extramarital sex, including but not limited to sexually transmitted disease, hardship in determining paternity, the possibility of supporting another man's child, jealousy, decline in companionship, and possible dissolution of the marriage. (A negative externality arises when the action of one party imposes costs on another party.)

Individuals invest in *human capital* whenever they sacrifice something desirable in the present (e.g., money, time) to develop a personal attribute which will pay off in the future, whether in a job or household relationship (England & Farkas, 1986). General human capital includes accumulated investments in such activities as education, job training, and migration. They are general in that knowledge and skills acquired can be used for various positions. For example, a well-trained economist can work as a professor, economic analyst, advisor, policy maker, and so on. Similarly, those qualities helpful in person-to-person interaction can be viewed as a form of human capital, for example, the ability to provide empathy, companionship, sexual and intellectual pleasure, and so on. They are relationship-specific in that they have value only within the current relationship, and would be of no benefit in a different one (England & Farkas, 1986). For example, a married man has acquired a skill to please his current wife, but this skill may not please another woman.

Marital sex refers to sexual actions between a husband and wife for physical pleasure and/or for emotional satisfaction.

Extramarital sex is any sexual behavior between a married individual and a third person other than his/her spouse.

THEORIES AND RESEARCH

Understanding the Declining Frequency of Marital Sex

Since Kinsey and his colleagues reported the decline in the frequency of marital sex in the 1940s and 1950s (Kinsey, Pomeroy, & Martin, 1948; Kinsey, Pomeroy, Martin, & Gebhard, 1953), the frequency of marital sex has been extensively studied by scholars from various disciplines. Their studies consistently report that the frequency of marital sex declines with marital duration (Blumstein & Schwartz, 1983; Call, Sprecher, & Schwartz, 1995; Greenblat, 1983; James, 1981; Jasso, 1985; Masters, Johnson, & Kolodny, 1992; Trussell & Westoff, 1980; Udry, Deven, & Coleman, 1982). The National Survey of Sexual Attitudes and Lifestyle (NSSAL) conducted in Britain in 1994 also reports that frequency of marital sex declines with marital duration (Wellings, Field, Johnson, Wadsworth, & Bradshaw, 1994). Although advancing age is correlated with this decline, Blumstein and Schwartz (1983) find that the impact of age and duration are approximately equal. Moreover, it has been discovered that the declining frequency of marital sex cannot be accounted for by "background" variables such as premarital sex, education, income, and religion (Greenblat, 1983; Masters et al., 1992).

The phenomenon of declining frequency of marital sex, which is often called the "honeymoon effect," can be explained by applying the law of diminishing marginal utility that social scientists widely use to explain human behavior. According to this law, other things being equal, the marginal utility (or satisfaction) derived from consuming a good or service (i.e., each extra unit of the satisfaction derived from consuming each additional unit of a good or service) diminishes as the consumption of that good or service increases. Applying this law to marital sex, we have the following explanation: marital sexual actions between a husband and a wife initially bring about a relatively high level of satisfaction; therefore, one can expect sexual activity to be more frequent. As marital sex increases,

the level of satisfaction lowers; thus fewer resources (including time, physical, or emotional inputs) will be allocated to it; consequently, the frequency of marital sex declines (Liu, 2000).

Understanding the Motivation to Engage in Extramarital Sex

In the United States, about 25 percent of married men and 13 percent of married women engage in extramarital sex (Laumann, Gagnon, Michael, & Michaels, 1994). The NSSAL also reports that married men are much more likely to engage in extramarital sex than are women in Britain (Wellings et al., 1994). Extramarital sex has enormous disruptive potential for a marriage; it is frequently cited by divorced persons as a reason for marital dissolution (South & Lloyd, 1995). Therefore, preventing extramarital sex is of great importance to the goal of protecting marriage. However, to prevent extramarital sex, we need to understand what motivates people to engage in it. In this section, theories and research that attempt to explain the motivation of extramarital sex are presented. Since men are twice more likely to engage in extramarital sex than are women, the analysis below takes into account this gender difference.

As a married individual's satisfaction with his/her marital sex declines, this person will have stronger incentive to engage in extramarital sex and to seek a higher level of satisfaction from sexual variety because, other things being equal, the marginal satisfaction of a sexual action with a new partner is higher than that of a sexual action with an old partner (Liu, 2000). However, the declining satisfaction and frequency of marital sex alone are not sufficient for extramarital sex to occur. This is because extramarital sex can be very costly in terms of search for a partner, concealment, and dissolution of marriage. Research shows that individuals actually make a calculated decision on whether or not to engage in extramarital sex. For example, Lawson (1988) reports that a wife makes a quick negative and positive checklist, and a husband asks himself: "Why am I doing this? What will I get out of it? How does this affect the status quo?" This example shows that husbands and wives do consider costs and benefits and engage in a strategic interaction when facing extramarital options.

Previous research shows that a person's credibility to sanction his/her spouse for engaging in extramarital sex is an important factor that affects extramarital sexual behavior: if a person's threat to sanction his/her spouse for engaging in extramarital sex is not credible, his/her spouse is more likely to engage in extramarital sex (Brown, 1991; Liu, 1996). This argument partly explains why men are more likely to engage in extramarital sex. In the United States, about 40 percent of married women do not work in the market; in addition, men typically contribute more to family income. These facts suggest that a large number of married women depend on their husbands for financial support. It follows that it costs wives more to sanction their husbands than it does for husbands to sanction their wives. If a married man is sanctioned for engaging in extramarital sex by a divorce, he can still "live on his earnings, purchase some of the domestic services his wife was providing, and his earnings are a resource that improves his 'rating' in the market for new partners" (England & Farkas, 1986, p. 56). In contrast, non-working housewives typically invest more heavily in the relationship-specific human capital and depend on their husbands for financial support (England & Farkas, 1986, pp. 55–56). Therefore, their act of sanctioning their husbands for having extramarital sex (e.g., divorce) also imposes high costs on themselves. These costs may include losing the financial support from their husbands and losing the future return from their investments in the marriage-specific human capital because such investments are not easily transferable to a single life or a new relationship (England & Farkas, 1986, pp. 57–58). Thus, their threat to carry out the sanctions is hardly credible because the cost of the sanction is so high that carrying out the sanction is not in their interest. This is one reason why married men are less constrained and are more likely to engage in extramarital sex. For the same reason, men are more likely to impose sanctions on their wives for engaging in extramarital sex because such sanctions would cost them less; as a result, married women are less likely to engage in extramarital sex (Liu, 1996). Previous research also shows that middle-aged men are more likely to engage in extramarital sex because their wives' threat of sanctioning their husbands becomes less credible since they have made heavy investments in their marriage and their remarriage prospects have declined (Brown, 1991).

The likelihood of a person's involvement in extramarital sex not only depends on his/her sexual interests and the credibility of his/her spouse's threat of sanction, but also depends on the opportunities, shared network, nonpermissive values, and religiosity. Treas and Giesen (2000) report that befriending a partner's family is associated with a 26 percent decrease in the odds of sexual infidelity because in a shared social network, one must go to greater lengths to keep sexual infidelity secret. Church attendance negatively affect an individual's involvement in extramarital sex (Liu, 2000; Treas & Giesen, 2000). This is because, first, a person who belongs to and attends church is regularly exposed to sexual norms that proscribe extramarital sex; therefore, he or she is more likely to internalize such norms and adhere to them. Thus, extramarital sex may incur a heavy cost of internal sanctions. Second, those who regularly attend church services form a closure of social networks. This closure is

featured by frequent communication among its members and is indispensable for sanctioning a target actor who violates norms (Coleman, 1990). Thus, those who go to church regularly are more likely to be sanctioned for engaging in extramarital sex.

STRATEGIES THAT WORK: PROMOTING MARITAL SEX

The declining frequency of marital sex is troublesome to many couples (Rubin, 1992); it can also affect marital stability by increasing the probability of extramarital sex. Recent research on marital sex suggests some ways to remedy the declining frequency.

Marriage is a long-term relationship in which both partners have incentives to invest in the marriage-specific human capital—abilities to provide empathy, companionship, intellectual pleasure, and sexual pleasure; the accumulation of such human capital raises expected gains from the marriage and makes both parties better off (Becker, 1991; England & Farkas, 1986). Specifically, the human capital stock associated with marital sex includes the "spouse-specific" skills that enhance the enjoyment of marital sex and the knowledge about the spouse's sexual preferences, desires and habits, that is, what pleases the spouse, what excites, what frustrates, and what angers (Laumann et al., 1994). With such knowledge and skills, couples can better their coordination in sexual actions and thus achieve higher satisfaction. As marital sex increases, so does the human capital stock, which in turn increases the marginal satisfaction with marital sex.

Satisfaction with marital sex has two dimensions—physical pleasure and emotional satisfaction. Couples can invest in their marriage-specific human capital so that their marital sex is vested with affective elements—"to create socioemotional closeness and exchange rather than just psychophysiological pleasure and relief" (Posner, 1992, p. 112). As a result, the loss in physical pleasure can be compensated by an increase in emotional satisfaction, namely, comfort, companionship, safety, and intimacy that couples value highly (Rubin, 1992). Data from the National Health and Social Life Survey (NHSLS) conducted by the National Opinion Research Center (NORC) support this hypothesis. The NHSLS data show that married people report mean levels of sexual actions about twice as high as a single person; in addition, they report significantly higher levels of physical as well as emotional satisfaction with their sexual life. These differences are due to the fact that married individuals typically invest more in their marital sex than do single people in their sexual lives (Laumann et al., 1994). This finding suggests that investment in relationship-specific human capital has a positive effect on both the frequency of and satisfaction with marital sex.

However, like other investments, the marginal return of the investment in marriage-specific human capital decreases as the investment increases, ceteris paribus. There are two reasons for this decline. First, as the number of ways explored by a couple to enhance their marital sexual satisfaction increases, the number of the methods that can be potentially explored in the future decreases. Second, any new method will eventually lose its novelty. For example, Rubin (1992) reports that couples try different ways (i.e., investing in the human capital) to enhance their marital sexual satisfaction; however, satisfaction progressively diminishes; Jasso (1985) finds that the frequency of marital sex declines less and less steeply. These findings indicate that though the investment in human capital can lower the rate of the decline in the frequency of marital sex, it appears to be unable to stop it.

STRATEGIES THAT WORK: PREVENTING EXTRAMARITAL SEX

In any social relationships, there are individuals who attempt to violate others' rights for their own benefits. For example, a person's rights specified by law are regularly violated by criminals even though such rights are protected by law enforcement agencies. One must protect his/her property right by using a lock, installing an alarm system, etc. Similarly, a married individual must protect his/her right to control his/her spouse's sexual action. Typically, rights are enforced by sanctions. That is, an individual must be able to sanction (e.g., to divorce) his/her spouse for engaging in extramarital sex. If he/she is unable to impose a sanction on his/her spouse who violates the right or if the threat of sanction is not credible, this individual may lose the right if the spouse benefits from violating it (e.g., engaging in extramarital sex).

As far as the strategies to prevent extramarital sex are concerned, there is little empirical evidence that shows what works and what does not. Therefore, the best we can do is derive some strategies to prevent extramarital sex from the theory and research findings on extramarital sex. The analysis specifies two conditions under which extramarital sex is likely to occur: a married person is likely to engage in extramarital sex (1) if for him/her, the marginal satisfaction of marital sex is significantly lower than that of sexual action with a third party, and (2) if his/her spouse's threat of sanctioning him/her for engaging in extramarital sex is not credible. These two conditions point to two corresponding strategies to prevent extramarital sex: (1) to increase the quality of one's marital sex and (2) to make one's threat of

sanctioning the spouse's cheating behavior credible. The first strategy has been discussed earlier; this section focuses on the second strategy—how to increase the credibility of one's threat of sanctioning. Treas and Giesen (2000) find that being male increases the odds of having engaged in extramarital sex by 79 percent, suggesting that an effective strategy to prevent extramarital sex is more important to women than to men. Therefore, the following discussion on the strategy targets women primarily, though the strategies developed are equally applicable to men.

1. To make one's threat of sanctioning his/her spouse for engaging in extramarital sex credible, one needs to decrease his/her financial and emotional dependence on the spouse. One way to increases one's independence is to invest in human capital—education. Education not only helps one raise his/her value on the labor market but also provides one with the abilities and skills to improve his/her personal life. Specifically, in contrast to non-working married women, working women are financially independent, contribute more to their family income, and can live on their own earnings if their marriage dissolves. In addition, compared with non-working married women, well-educated and financially independent women are more independent mentally or emotionally because they are more capable of managing damage in that they know where to get information and professional help if necessary. As a result, their threat of sanctioning their husbands for cheating behavior is credible, and the credible threats of sanctioning will deter their husbands from engaging in extramarital sex. Empirical research shows that other things being equal, for both men and women who work in the labor market, their spouses are less likely to engage in extramarital sex (Liu, 1996).

2. The analysis also implies that if an individual detects his/her spouse's cheating behavior but fails to impose effective sanction on the spouse, the spouse will continue to cheat. Thus, one strategy to prevent extramarital sex from occurring repeatedly is to apply effective sanctions once extramarital sex is detected.

3. Since social network decreases the likelihood of extramarital sex, one can lower the likelihood of his/her spouse's involvement in extramarital sex by involving the spouse in close family ties (e.g., encourage the spouse to enjoy one's kinship and friendship networks) and community ties (e.g., church attendance).

Finally, research reports that some intervention programs that emphasize communication and problem-solving skills, clarifying and sharing expectations and sensual and sexual enhancement help prevent the development of marital distress and thus promote marriage (Markman, Floyd, Stanley, & Storaasli, 1988; Markman, Renick, Floyd, Stanley, & Clements, 1993).

SYNTHESIS

The following general statements can be made based on the above analysis.

1. To promote one's marriage and enhance marital sex, one needs to make marriage-specific human capital; namely, to learn his/her spouse's sexual preferences and habits so that one is able to do what pleases the other party and avoid doing what displeases him/her.

2. Although the investment made by a couple in their marital-specific human capital does have a positive effect on the quality of their marital sex, one should be realistic about the extent of such an effect. The decline in the frequency of marital sex seems to be inevitable, which is a built-in defect of monogamy. Therefore, one needs to form a realistic view or expectation of his/her marital sex because higher expectation lowers one's rating of a sexual event (Laumann et al., 1994). Rubin (1992) reports that for those couples who have a realistic view of marital sex, the declining frequency of marital sex does not negatively affect their marriage. Finally, since marriage involves many other aspects of life, for example, empathy, companionship, intellectual pleasure, earnings, and children, a couple can explore mutual interests in these aspects so that the gain in these areas can offset the loss in marital sex, thereby achieving the goal of protecting and promoting marriage.

3. In one's life, an individual generally invests in two types of human capital: general human capital (i.e., education and career) and marriage-specific human capital. Both are indispensable for one's welfare. On the one hand, if an individual just invests in education and career, his/her marital life may not be happy because a good marriage depends on both parties' investment in the marriage. On the other hand, if one just invests in marriage-specific human capital, he/she will become vulnerable to his/her spouse's cheating behavior and other abuses. Thus, a balanced investment in the two types of human capital helps one protect or promote his/her marriage.

Also see: Marital Satisfaction: Adulthood; Intimate Partner Violence: Adulthood.

ACKNOWLEDGMENT

I thank Edmund Worthy for his comments and for kindly editing the entry.

References

Becker, G. (1991). *A treatise on the family.* Cambridge: Harvard University Press.

Blumstein, P., & Schwartz, P. (1983). *American couples.* New York: William Morrow.

Brown, E. (1991). *Patterns of infidelity and their treatment.* New York: Brunner-Mazel.

Call, V., Sprecher, S., & Schwartz, P. (1995). The incidence and frequency of marital sex in a national sample. *Journal of Marriage and the Family, 57,* 639–652.

Christopher, S., & Sprecher, S. (2000). Sexuality in marriage, dating, and other relationships: A decade review. *Journal of Marriage and the Family, 62,* 999–1017.

Coleman, J. (1990). *Foundations of social theory.* Cambridge: Belknap Press of Harvard University Press.

England, P., & Farkas, G. (1986). *Households, employment, and gender: A social, economic and demographic view.* New York: Aldine.

Greenblat, C. (1983). The salience of sexuality in the early years of marriage. *Journal of Marriage and the Family, 45,* 289–298.

James, W.H. (1981). The honeymoon effect on marital coitus. *The Journal of Sex Research, 17,* 114–123.

Jasso, G. (1985). Marital coital frequency and the passage of time: Estimating the separate effects of spouses' ages and marital duration, birth and marriage cohorts, and period influences. *American Sociological Review, 50,* 224–241.

Kinsey, A.C., Pomeroy, W., & Martin, C.E. (1948). *Sexual behavior in the human male.* Philadelphia: W.B. Saunders.

Kinsey, A.C., Pomeroy, W., Martin, C.E, and Gebhard, P.H. (1953). *Sexual behavior in the human female.* Philadelphia: W.B. Saunders.

Laumann, E., Gagnon, J.H., Michael, R., & Michaels, S. (1994). *The social organization of sexuality: Sexual practices in the United States.* Chicago: The University of Chicago Press.

Lawson, A. (1988). *Adultery: An analysis of love and betrayal.* New York: Basic Books.

Liu, C. (1996). *A theory of the gender difference in extramarital sexual behavior.* Paper Presented at the Annual Meeting of American Sociological Association in New York City.

Liu, C. (2000). A theory of marital sexual life. *Journal of Marriage and the Family, 62,* 363–374.

Markman, J.H., Floyd, J.F., Stanley, M.S., & Storaasli, D.R. (1988). Prevention of marital distress: A longitudinal investigation. *Journal of Consulting and Clinical Psychology, 56,* 210–217.

Markman, J.H., Renick, J., M., Floyd, J.F., Stanley, M.S., & Clements, M. (1993). Preventing marital distress through communication and conflict management training: A 4- and 5-year follow-up. *Journal of Consulting and Clinical Psychology, 61,* 70–77.

Masters, W., Johnson, V., & Kolodny, R. (1992). *Human sexuality.* New York: HarperCollins.

Posner, R. (1992). *Sex and reason.* Cambridge: Harvard University Press.

Rubin, L. (1992). Sex and the coupled life. In A.S. Skolnick & J.H. Skolnick (Eds.), *Family in transition* (pp. 137–150). New York: HarperCollins.

Smith, T. (1994). Attitudes toward sexual permissiveness: Trends, correlates, and behavioral connections. In A.S. Rossi (Ed.), *Sexuality across the life course.* Chicago: University of Chicago Press.

South, S., & Lloyd, K.M. (1995). Spousal alternatives and marital dissolution. *American Sociological Review, 60,* 21–35.

Treas, J., & Giesen, D. (2000). Sexual infidelity among married and cohabiting Americans. *Journal of Marriage and the Family, 62,* 48–60.

Trussell, J., & Westoff, C. (1980). Contraceptive practice and trends in coital frequency. *Family Planning Perspectives, 12,* 246–249.

Udry, R., Deven, F., & Coleman, S. (1982). A cross-national comparison of the relative influence of male and female age on the frequency of marital intercourse. *Journal of Biosocial Science, 14,* 1–6.

Wellings, K., Field, J., Johnson, A., Wadsworth, J., & Bradshaw, S. (1994). *Sexual behaviour in Britain: The national survey of sexual attitudes and lifestyles.* London: Penguin Books.

Marital Satisfaction, Adulthood

Benjamin Silliman, Walter Schumm, Robyn Parker, and Michele Simons

INTRODUCTION AND DEFINITIONS

Promotion of marital satisfaction requires a clear understanding of relationship processes and outcomes as well as prevention and intervention strategies. Relationships are assessed by instruments focused on subjective *satisfaction* or perceived *quality*. Observational measures typically focus on processes including *interactive behaviors* such as verbal and nonverbal communication, conflict resolution, or problem-solving exchanges. *Adjustment* indicates satisfaction, successful task completion, coping or adaptation, or togetherness. *Stability*, marked by absence of thoughts or steps toward separation or divorce and *marital duration* often serve as proxy for success, although they may inadequately describe relationship adjustment (Bradbury, Fincham, & Beach, 2000; Gottman & Notarius, 2000; Huston, 2000). *Prevention/competence-building resources* include self-help books, tapes, or web sites, couple- or professional-directed workshops or support groups, or needs assessments designed to prevent conflict or divorce and promote marital adjustment. These *marriage education or psychoeducational* strategies are usually distinguished from but can be incorporated in marital therapy.

Marital distress and divorce remain at high levels in the United States and are rising worldwide. Despite these trends, marriage remains the most popular voluntary institution in the free world. The incidence of marriage in new cases per year is reflected in number and rate of marriages, which are highest in the United States (4.5 million weddings; 8.8/1000 rate), substantial in Australia (114,316 weddings; 6.0 rate), Canada (160,256; 5.5 rate), Britain (5.5 rate), Germany (5.1 rate), Sweden (3.8 rate), and France (4.8 rate) (Australian Bureau of Statistics, 2000). The prevalence of divorce, reflected in divorce rate, is highest in the United States (4.3/1000), but substantial in Britain (2.9), Australia (2.8), Canada (2.6), Sweden (2.4), Germany (2.1), and France (1.9). Marriage education addresses both trends as it promotes postponement of marriage, reduces divorce, and increases positive marital interaction (Markman, Floyd, Stanley, & Storaasli, 1988). Since relationship growth entails ongoing challenges (Mace, 1983) educational resources may benefit the majority of the adult population in developed nations that is currently married (53 percent in the United States) or cohabiting (5 percent of all homes in the United States), in addition to those approaching first marriage or remarriage (US Census Bureau, 2000).

Costs of marital distress and divorce for partners include poorer physical, mental, and economic health. Children of divorce and distress experience these difficulties as well as lower school performance and higher rates of delinquency, violence, and relationship breakup for children (Halford, 2000, p. 5; Waite & Gallagher, 2000). An Australian study found direct costs to governments for social security payments, family court costs, legal aid, and child support at least $3 billion per annum (House of Representatives Standing Committee on Legal and Constitutional Affairs, 1998, p. 51). Workplace productivity and social capital in the community decline among distressed and divorcing couples. Since most distressed couples who stay together seem to resolve differences satisfactorily, marriage promotion before crises, and investment in crisis intervention would seem a cost-effective alternative to high divorce rates. Domestic violence occurs in less than 10 percent of marriages and overall, married women are less frequently victimized than unmarried. Rates of couple violence are much higher among unmarried and cohabitating and among separated partners and those raised in violent families (Waite & Gallagher, 2000, pp. 152–156). Medical treatment for adult victims alone accounted for $740 million in the United States in 1993 (Miller, Cohen, & Wiersema, 1996). Intangibles, including fear of additional attacks, depression, and cynicism about relationships, represent more profound and long-term costs to partners and society.

THEORIES

A wide variety of theories underlie efforts to understand and improve marriages. The traditional macrosociological perspective, *structural functionalism* (SF), is still employed by conservative scholars to interpret trends and policy implications for promoting marriage. *Symbolic interaction* (SI) theory, focusing on partner self-concept, role and value systems, and interpersonal communication has been more often employed to explain dyadic adjustment and satisfaction. During the late 1940s, *family development*, notably the A–B–C–X mid-range theory, integrated the element of generational time with the best aspects of SF and SI to explain how partner attributions, coping, and support resources impact adjustment within or between stages of the family career. Adaptation of *attachment theory* from human development further expanded the explanatory and educational potential of *SI* and *developmental* theories (Karney & Bradbury, 1995).

Social exchange theory has been widely employed by scholars to explain patterns of cost and reward that sustain or erode marriages. Over the past two decades, scholars and clinicians using exchange and *cognitive behavioral theory* in psychology have identified key components of interpersonal reward patterns that predict sustained adjustment or a "cascade toward divorce." Overall, these findings suggest that high negative reciprocity (e.g., a cycle of hostility) together with low levels of affection or dedication, triggers a downward spiral of declining satisfaction and investment, often ending in divorce. Positive interaction, equitable rewards, and successful adjustment, particularly in the context of moral or social barriers to divorce, reduces search for alternatives and increases investments and couple growth (Bagarozzi & Wodarski, 1978). Following these insights, *psychoeducational programs* seek to establish realistic and shared expectations (e.g., cognitive reframing) and improve skills in communication, problem solving, and conflict resolution (e.g., reduce negative, enhance positive interaction).

Family systems theory is increasingly employed to study and influence the dynamics of change and balance (Broderick, 1990). A dissatisfied spouse may seek change through enforcing current rules (level 1: "if you come home late, you will be yelled at"), to modify or elaborate current rules (level 2: "call first if you are going to be late"), change the priority of rules used (level 2: "adjusting dinner time to match return time"), or develop new rules (level 3: "dinner will be served without you"). At a higher systemic level, families may change priorities, goals, or values (level 4: "let's work out a new schedule together, not just react"). Lower level changes are easier but less effective over the long term. Recently, attention to social, community, and family system influences beyond couple interaction (Huston, 2000) is expanding the understanding of feedback mechanisms and contexts which affect couple change processes.

Feminist theory focuses on dynamics of power and support within relationships and society as a whole that influence equity or oppression in families (Walker, 1999). Increasing awareness of oppressive and alternative structures and taking action to establish equitable, supportive communities, and relationships is central to implementation of feminist family life education. Amid the emergence of such postmodern theories, many researchers and practitioners continue to be guided by traditional frameworks such as *psychodynamic* and *humanistic* theories.

RESEARCH

Scholars and practitioners from several fields, working at the community, institutional, family, couple, and individual level contribute to understanding and promotion of marital satisfaction. Sociological research indicates that marital satisfaction tends to be higher for couples in favorable economic, social, and developmental conditions (Larson & Holman, 1994). Thus social policy or economic progress which enhances income adequacy and stability, social support networks and pro-marriage attitudes, or quality child care, schools, and health might indirectly strengthen marriage. However, marital interaction *and* social trends are so complex that indirect approaches (e.g., economic, social policy, or legal changes in individual actions) often produce slow, disproportionate, or even counterproductive changes in marital quality and stability across the population in the short run.

Psychological and clinical research suggests that *individual* education or therapy that enhances competence (e.g., knowledge, mental health, differentiation, interpersonal skills) will indirectly contribute to marital stability and quality (Karney & Bradbury, 1995). Couples education via intensive, high-quality programs provides a direct approach to improve marital quality and stability. The most thoroughly tested model is *Premarital Relationship Enhancement and Prevention* (PREP), a 12–24-hr sequence of cognitive–behavioral skill training (Stanley, Blumberg, & Markman, 1999). PREP yielded improvements in both support/validation and withdrawal-negative communication at posttest, sustained to 3 years. PREP participants show lower divorce and separation rates than controls at 5 years (8 vs. 19 percent) and 12 years (19 vs. 28 percent), with relationship skills and satisfaction sustained as long as 12 years. Similar programs in Germany and Australia produced significant gains in communication, conflict management, and satisfaction at posttest and at 1 and 3 years follow-up.

Relationship Enhancement (RE), a humanistic model teaching disclosure and empathy skills in a structured 16–24 hr format (Guerney & Maxson, 1990), produced immediate gains for college couples in empathy and problem solving and sustained gains in disclosure and empathy and communication. Relationship skills workshops improved conflict resolution skills of treatment couples through 15-hr teaching–training–discussion small groups (Bader & Sinclair, 1983). The *Couple Communication Program* (CCP), a 12-hr systems-based awareness and skill-training showed improved self- and other-awareness and support (Miller, Wackman, & Nunnally, 1983), although less effectively than RE (Brock & Joanning, 1983).

All three models showed couple skill gains under community professionals, lay leaders, or student instructors (Silliman & Schumm, 1999) nearly equal to those in clinical or lab settings. College (Laner & Russell, 1994; Long, Angera, Carter, Nakamoto, & Kalso, 1999; Sharp & Ganong, 2000) and church-based (Center for Marriage and Family, 1995; Russell & Lyster, 1992) courses also show promise for building realistic attitudes, interpersonal skills, and knowledge of marriage issues. Marriage enrichment programs help well-adjusted couples build skills and satisfaction (Dyer & Dyer, 1999). More extensive reviews of marriage education programs are available elsewhere (Berger & Hannah, 1999; Guerney & Maxson, 1990; Silliman & Schumm, 2000).

Markman et al. (1988) suggest useful four criteria for evaluating program success: (a) absence of withdrawal-reactivity cycles; (b) partner emotional investment in growth; (c) optimism regarding marital transition; and (d) relationship efficacy. Worldwide, the vast majority of programs lack scientific evidence for medium and long-term impacts (Halford, 2000).

STRATEGIES THAT WORK

Strategies for promotion of marital satisfaction include *(Pre)marriage education* (Hunt, Hof, & DeMaria, 1998) which are often (para)professional-led information and skill training workshops or couple consultations; couple-led *enrichment* skill-building and support groups; or *(pre)marital counseling or therapy*, professionally guided clinical and educational efforts to foster growth or address crisis (Berger & Hannah, 1999; Stahmann & Hiebert, 1998). *Informational approaches* such as books, fact sheets, tapes, web sites, newspaper articles, and *(pre)marriage assessment* (Larson, Holman, Klein, Busby, Stahmann, & Petersen, 1995) of realistic expectations, personality compatibility, knowledge or skills, can be used separately and in combination with programming. No consistent terminology has emerged and practice in the United States and Australia often reflects discipline-specific and eclectic approaches (House of Representatives Standing Committee on Legal and Constitutional Affairs, 1998; Silliman & Schumm, 1999). At best, community-based programs apply adult education, learner-centered and facilitative delivery (Harris, Simons, Willis, & Barrie, 1992) and adapt curricula to cultural and couple needs.

Skills-based training is the most effective strategy to date (Halford, 2000). At least 12 hr of intensive practice (e.g., role play, interactive rehearsal and coaching) with highly trained leaders, focused on empathy, problem-solving, or conflict resolution seems key to breaking cycles of escalation, invalidation, withdrawal, and negative interpretation and to establishing cycles of active listening and collaborative problem solving. Effects of specific techniques such as active listening are debated (Gottman, Carrere, Swanson, & Coan, 2000; Stanley, Bradbury, & Markman, 2000). Premarital couples seem to gain more than married couples, males more than females. Skill training is most effective with non-distressed couples in early marriage (vs. pre-marriage), and where partners share deep and mutual commitment (Silliman & Schumm, 1999) and where booster sessions reteach and reinforce skills. In addition, participation may encourage later help-seeking (Bader & Sinclair, 1983; Harris et al., 1992) and self-directed growth. Most studies involve White, middle-class, volunteer couples, raising questions of generalizability (Parker, 1999). Nevertheless, application of skills, especially in high-stress settings, is critical to training impact. Couples engaging in marital violence require additional skill training, but can benefit from educational programs (Holtzworth-Munroe et al., 1995).

Marriage enrichment incorporates many of the skill-practice and mutual support components of skills training (Dyer & Dyer, 1999). Well-trained leaders and motivated volunteer couples in organizations such as Association of Couples in Marriage Enrichment (ACME) and Marriage Encounter (ME) help explain the success of the movement. While most such programs are not evaluated, several models provide evidence for increasing interpersonal skills, marital closeness and satisfaction (Worthington, Buston, & Hammonds, 1989). Such programs were designed for non-distressed couples, yet there is evidence that at-risk couples may experience growth and support as well (Guerney & Maxson, 1990) in marriage enrichment workshops.

Targeting developmental transitions such as engagement and early marriage, first child, empty nest (Stanley, Blumberg, & Markman, 1999), and crises captures the "teachable moment" and provides more opportunities for application of skills and insights. In Australia, a series of eight newsletters between pre- and post-wedding trainings increased contact, satisfaction, and post-wedding participation of couples (Andrews, Crawford, & Reiter, 2000).

While educational and therapeutic approaches for promoting marital satisfaction are still in their infancy, research in the past decade points to several effective strategies. Skills-based trainings in religious organizations, colleges, workplaces, military, and community settings show promise although they have not been extensively evaluated. Client preferences (Morris, Cooper, & Gross, 1999; Silliman & Schumm, 1999), as well as availability, provider skill (or effectiveness, with training), and continuing support (Stanley et al., 2001) recommend these local providers as naturally occurring training networks. Government-funded, independently evaluated couples programs in Australia have strengthened existing efforts in religious organizations and expanded offerings by civil marriage celebrants, in defense forces, non-English-speaking communities, and through distance education and self-directed programs to rural areas. Program satisfaction is high, although relationship impacts are not yet known (Halford, 2000). While never tested, resources and programs which enhance parents' capacities to model and teach marriage skills would fit teens' and young adults' learning preferences (Silliman & Schumm, 1999).

Skills-based courses are currently being introduced voluntarily and by mandate in high school classes (Hunt et al., 1998). Preliminary findings suggest that *Connections: Relationships and marriage, RQ: Relationship intelligence, and the art of loving well* (Mack, 2000) represent the best curricula for teens but note that most curricula "…fail to educate students about important social, legal, economic, child-rearing, and religious dimensions in marriage." While several violence prevention programs for teens are effective for increasing skills and decreasing interpersonal conflict and harm (Foshee, Bauman, Arriaga, Helms, Koch, & Fletcher-Linder, 1998), long-term outcomes have not been examined.

Retrovaille, a crisis-recovery and couple support model, has been acclaimed in popular (McManus, 1993) circles, but not professionally evaluated. Programs for at-risk couples, including those from violent or divorced parents, health or social traumas, teen marriages, low-income, ethnic minority, and recent immigrants are desperately needed.

Community marriage policies show client report and anecdotal success in lowering divorce rates and increasing participation in premarital training in Roman Catholic churches (Center for Marriage and Family, 1995) and in several communities with strong support from ministerial alliances (McManus, 1993). Such policies have the potential to build public awareness and support, promote improvements in training and curricula, and encourage couple participation and family support for high-quality learning experiences. More extensive evaluation research is needed to verify anecdotal claims of marriage policy proponents. Given the demands and turnover among religious and human service providers, numbers of client couples, and costs in time and effort for training, impact, and sustainability require collaborative partnerships under stable leadership.

Mentoring of newlyweds by mature and supportive couples has been well received (McManus, 1993; Parrott & Parrott, 1999) but not formally evaluated. Like all mentoring programs, effective screening, training, and matching, combined with consistent positive contact and referral when needed will be key to benefits for both mentors and mentees.

STRATEGIES THAT MIGHT WORK

Covenant marriage laws like those in Louisiana and Arizona are well-founded in principle but supported by an inadequate infrastructure of qualified trainers, supportive mentors, or communities deeply committed to pro-marriage policies and practices. Because they operate on a smaller scale within consensual communities, marriage policies at the organization or community level are more likely to reduce divorce and violence and promote marital satisfaction.

STRATEGIES THAT DO NOT WORK

Unfortunately, the most popular approaches to marriage preparation and maintenance are largely ineffective or counterproductive. Self-directed strategies including imitating parent role models and cohabitation typically lack the guidance needed to build stable, growing bonds. The "natural learning" assumption that parents' successes, a happy childhood, or romantic love will produce a happy marriage correctly identify correlates of marital satisfaction. However, these beliefs underestimate the ongoing work and dedication needed for adjustment from stage-to-stage. Cohabitation, which produces few of the benefits of marriage, more often ends in breakup, and is related to higher personal and social costs than divorce. Cohabitants who marry generally experience lower satisfaction and stability, likely due to lower commitment, tensions and role stereotypes, and lower social support carried over from their cohabitation period (Waite & Gallagher, 2000).

Traditional efforts of organizations such as churches, schools, and agencies to enrich marriage tend to lack intensity or relevance. Fact sheets, books, magazines, and web sites are often too general and too casually used to enhance marital outcomes. If their information is reliable, understanding and application are likely inconsistent across consumers. While popular material is more often based on research today than a decade ago, popular attitudes (e.g., "I'll do it if it sounds good"), lack of skill practice (e.g., "Oh, that was interesting but I never did it"), and media entertainment focus (e.g., "This was fun, but now on to real life") limit the educational potential of many materials. Lecture classes focusing mostly on knowledge (e.g., explaining communication, sexuality, finances) without skill practice and discussion lead to learner disengagement. Combinations of lecture, discussion, and skill rehearsal can be effective, however. Some research suggests that couples become more frustrated when courses increase awareness without enhancing skills. Traditional church-based consultation, with little or no attention to couple skills and emphasis on wedding arrangements, church membership, or marital roles does not equip couples with realistic expectations and competencies (Silliman & Schumm, 1999).

SYNTHESIS

While the past decade produced several empirically supported and promising practices, both marital satisfaction

(Bradbury et al., 2000) and marriage education (Silliman & Schumm, 2000) research are in their infancy. Promotion of marital satisfaction would be greatly advanced by an integrated, multidimensional strategy guiding research and practice. Since marital satisfaction is often construed in subjective terms, scholars and practitioners ought to be more concerned with promoting interactive processes resulting in positive marital adjustment. In short, the growth orientation and capacity of the marital system, or the family and community network which supports it, are much more important than partners' current satisfaction with marriage. An ecosystem framework (Huston, 2000) emphasizes this focus on processes of interaction, adjustment, and development between partners and within the family and community context. Macrosystem interventions could include public and organizational policies, cultural messages about relationships and values, and social awareness of the traits and benefits of effective marriage and education programs. While governmental and societal initiatives can shape attitudes and behavior in broad ways over the long term, they may inadequately address complex circumstances or individual needs. Governments can strengthen legal support for marriage via repealing the marriage penalty, welfare reform support for two parent families, enforcement of child support, and incentives for marriage education. Government can also intensify efforts to prosecute and prevent domestic violence and sexual assault. Marriage movement organizations can provide public service messages and provider-training campaigns to build awareness of the benefits of marriage and education programs. Government and foundation funding for basic research and program evaluations would improve the knowledge base for further policy, education, and public awareness efforts (Stanley & Markman, 1997).

Institutional or mesosystem interventions might include organizational or professional policies, initiatives, and attitudes regarding marriage and family life. Religious, professional, and community organizations can do much to expand high-quality training and resources (e.g., face-to-face, print, and electronic) for providers and couples, strengthen support networks, especially for couples at high risk, and promote prevention and lifelong education attitudes among members. Microsystem interventions can include efforts of families, friends, and informal groups to improve knowledge, skill, or family interaction (e.g., house or group rules). Parents must become more intentional about role-modeling positive interaction and commitment through crisis. In addition, involved parents can do much to shape prosocial behavior and teach empathy and problem-solving skills in the context of their children's friendship and dating experiences. Strengthening social support and mentoring networks should expand the practical and emotional resources available to both parents and youth.

Additional Issues

Both demographic trends such as marriage and divorce rates and program outcomes commend prevention education for promotion of marital satisfaction. Several issues are critical for effective prevention, including funding, provider qualifications, recruitment, dissemination of model programs, and cross-training of providers.

Funding remains a central concern in the testing and dissemination of effective strategies. Religious organizations traditionally sponsored most marriage education, although governments in Australia, Britain, Norway, and several states in the United States fund courses for marriage and cohabitation and urge participation for teens, couples preparing for marriage, seeking growth, or experiencing crisis. Issues of values and privacy are still being worked out (Harris et al., 1992; Stanley & Markman, 1997). Qualifications of providers remain a central issue for effective programming. A wide variety persons conduct relationship education but a growing specialization in roles and training needs is underway (Simons & Harris, 1997). Interdisciplinary teams or community family centers are supporting healthy family development across the lifespan in Australia, Britain, and the United States. Recruitment and retention are critical to quality and quantity of impact where marriage education is voluntary. Funding and improving program quality are increasing participation rates, although couples most at risk are least likely to complete courses. Multimedia awareness campaigns show promise and would likely be more successful with greater television and radio coverage (Andrews et al., 2000). While laboratory-based programs show positive outcomes, replication at the community level is rare (Stanley et al., 2001). Fidelity to program models, with room for individualizing standards to fit local needs is critical to replication of any model program. Audience needs, including practical adjustments, developmental and cultural appropriateness, and provider creativity often result in variations from proven approaches and reductions in effectiveness. Finally, cross-training of practitioners can enhance collaboration and individual effectiveness. In many places, teams of practitioners including clergy, educators, attorneys, and financial planners maximize expertise while minimizing individual effort. In other instances, couples skills are being integrated into parenting, family strengths, and other educational programs (Sanders, 2000) as well as therapy (Berger & Hannah, 1999).

The past decade brought a fresh awareness of the significance of marriage in personal and social life, together with the recognition that satisfaction within a companionate model of marriage will require a more committed, skill-focused effort by couples and educators. As marriage education moves beyond social–political–religious rhetoric and laboratory-based model programs, communities around the world can more effectively strengthen couple and family bonds, thus promoting individual mental health and community social and economic success.

Also see: Marital Enhancement: Adulthood; Family Strengthening: Childhood; Family Strengthening: Adolescence; Parenting: Early Childhood; Parenting: Adolescence; Parenting, Single Parent: Adolescence; Parenting: Adulthood.

References

Andrews, K., Crawford, C., & Reiter, M. (2000). From wedding to marriage: Developing an integrated pre and post-wedding program. *Threshold, 63*, 24–27.

Australian Bureau of Statistics. (2000). *Marriages and divorces* (Cat. No. 3310.0). Canberra: Author.

Bader, E., & Sinclair, C. (1983). The critical first year of marriage, In D.R. Mace (Ed.), *Prevention in family services: Approaches to family wellness* (pp. 77–86). Beverly Hills, CA: Sage.

Bagarozzi, D.A., & Wodarski, J.S. (1978). Behavioral treatment of marital discord. *Clinical Social Work Journal, 6*, 135–154.

Berger, R., & Hannah, M.T. (Eds.). (1999). *Preventive approaches in couples' therapy*. Philadelphia: Brunner-Mazel.

Bradbury, T.N., Fincham, F.D., & Beach, S.R.H. (2000). Research on the nature and determinants of marital satisfaction: A decade in review. *Journal of Marriage and the Family, 62*(4), 964–980.

Brock, G.W., & Joanning, H. (1983). A comparison of the relationship enhancement and the Minnesota couples communication program. *Journal of Marital and Family Therapy, 4*(9), 13–27.

Broderick, C.B. (1990). Family process theory. In J. Sprey (Ed.), *Fashioning family theory* (Ch. 6, pp. 171–206). Newbury Park, CA: Sage.

Center for Marriage and Family. (1995). *Marriage preparation in the Catholic Church: Getting it right*. Omaha, NE: Author, Creighton University.

Dyer, P.M., & Dyer, G.H. (1999). Marriage enrichment: A.C.M.E-Style. In R. Berger & M.T. Hannah (Eds.), *Preventive approaches in couples' therapy* (pp. 29–54). Philadelphia: Brunner-Mazel.

Foshee, V.A., Bauman, K.E., Arriaga, X.B., Helms, R.W., Koch, G.G., & Fletcher-Linder, G. (1998). An evaluation of safe dates, an adolescent dating violence prevention program. *American Journal of Public Health, 88*(1), 45–50.

Gottman, J., Carrere, S., Swanson, C., & Coan, J.A. (2000). Reply to "From basic research to interventions." *Journal of Marriage and the Family, 62*(1), 265–273.

Gottman, J.M., & Notarius, C.I. (2000). Decade review: Observing marital interaction. *Journal of Marriage and the Family, 62*(4), 927–947.

Guerney, B.G., Jr., & Maxson, P. (1990). Marital and family enrichment research: A decade review and a look ahead. *Journal of Marriage and the Family, 52*(4), 1127–1135.

Halford, W. (2000). *Australian couples in Millennium Three*. Department of Family and Community Services, Canberra.

Harris, R., Simons, M., Willis, P., & Barrie, A. (1992). *Love, sex, and waterskiing: The experience of pre-marriage education in Australia*. Centre for Human Resource Studies, University of South Australia, Adelaide.

Holtzworth-Munroe, A., Markman, H.J., O'Leary, K.D., Neidig, P., Leber, D., Heyman, R.E., Hulbert, D., & Smultzer, N. (1995). The need for marital violence prevention efforts: A behavioral-cognitive secondary prevention program for engaged and newly married couples. *Applied and Preventive Psychology, 4*, 77–88.

House of Representatives Standing Committee on Legal and Constitutional Affairs. (1998). *To have and to hold: Strategies to strengthen marriage and relationships*. Canberra: The Parliament of the Commonwealth of Australia.

Hunt, R.A., Hof, L., & DeMaria, R. (1998). *Marriage enrichment: Preparation, mentoring, and outreach*. Thousand Oaks, CA: Sage.

Huston, T.L. (2000). The social ecology of marriage and other intimate unions. *Journal of Marriage and the Family, 62*(2), 298–321.

Karney, B.R., & Bradbury, T.N. (1995). The longitudinal course of marital quality and stability: A review of theory, method, and research. *Psychological Bulletin, 118*, 3–34.

Laner, M.R., & Russell, J.N. (1994). Course content and change in students: Are marital expectations altered by marriage education? *Teaching Sociology, 22*, 10–28.

Larson, J., Holman, T.B., Klein, D.M., Busby, D.M., Stahmann, R.F., & Petersen, D. (1995). A review of comprehensive questionnaires used in premarital education and counseling. *Family Relations, 44*, 245–252.

Larson, J.H., & Holman, T.B. (1994). Premarital predictors of marital quality and stability. *Family Relations, 43*, 228–237.

Long, E.C.J., Angera, J.J., Carter, S.J., Nakamoto, M., & Kalso, M. (1999). Understanding the one you love: A longitudinal assessment of an empathy training program for couples in romantic relationships. *Family Relations, 48*(3), 235–242.

Mace, D.R. (1983). Training families to deal creatively with conflict. In D.R. Mace (Ed.), *Prevention in family services: Approaches to family wellness* (pp. 190–200). Beverly Hills: Sage.

Mack, D. (2000). *Hungry hearts: Evaluating the new curricula for teens on marriage and relationships*. New York: Institute for American Values.

Markman, H.J., Floyd, F.J., Stanley, S.M., & Storaasli, R.D. (1988). Prevention of marital distress: A longitudinal investigation. *Journal of Consulting and Clinical Psychology, 56*, 210–217.

McManus, M.J. (1993). *Marriage savers*. Grand Rapids, MI: Zondervan.

Miller, T.R., Cohen, M.A., & Wiersema, B. (1996). *Victim costs and consequences: A new look* (Publication No. NJC 155282). Washington: DCL National Institute of Justice.

Miller, S., Wackman, D.B., & Nunnally, E. (1983). Couple communication: Equipping couples to be their own best problem solvers. *The Counseling Psychologist, 11*(3), 73–77.

Morris, M.L., Cooper, C., & Gross, K.H. (1999). Marketing factors influencing the overall satisfaction of marriage education participants. *Family Relations, 48*(3), 251–261.

Parker, R. (1999). *A framework for future research in pre-marriage education*. Melbourne: Australian Institute for Family Studies.

Parrott, L., & Parrott, L. (1999). Preparing couples for marriage: The SYMBIS model. In R. Berger & M.T. Hannah (Eds.), *Preventive approaches in couples' therapy* (pp. 237–254). Philadelphia: Brunner-Mazel.

Russell, M., & Lyster, R. (1992). Marriage preparation: Factors associated with consumer satisfaction. *Family Relations, 41*, 446–451.

Sanders, M. (2000). *Effects of parenting interventions on marital relationships*. Paper Presented at the International Conference on Personal Relationships, Brisbane, Australia.

Sharp, E.A., & Ganong, L.H. (2000). Raising awareness about marital expectations: Are unrealistic beliefs changed by integrative teaching? *Family Relations, 49*(1), 71–76.

Silliman, B., & Schumm, W.R. (1999). Improving practice in marriage preparation. *Journal of Sex and Marital Therapy, 25*, 23–43.

Silliman, B., & Schumm, W.R. (2000). Marriage preparation programs: Literature review. *The Family Journal, 8*(2), 128–137.

Simons, M., & Harris, R. (1997). *Analysis of the roles of marriage and relationship educators. Development and validation of competency standards*. Centre for Research in Education, Equity and Work, University of South Australia, Adelaide.

Stahmann, R.F., & Hiebert, W.J. (1998). *Premarital and remarital counseling*. San Francisco: Jossey-Bass.

Stanley, S.M., Blumberg, S.L., & Markman, H.J. (1999). Helping couples fight for their marriages: The PREP approach. In R. Berger & M.T. Hannah (Eds.), *Preventive approaches in couples' therapy* (pp. 270–303). Philadelphia: Brunner-Mazel.

Stanley, S.M., Bradbury, T.N., & Markman, H.J. (2000). Structural flaws in the bridge from basic research on marriage to interventions for couples. *Journal of Marriage and the Family, 62*(1), 256–264.

Stanley, S.M., & Markman, H.J. (1997). *Can governments save marriage?* Unpublished manuscript, University of Denver/PREP.

Stanley, S.M., Markman, H.J., Prado, L.M., Olmos-Gallo, P.A., Tonelli, L., St. Peters, M., Leber, B.D., Bobulinski, M., Cordova, A., & Whitton, S.W. (2001). Community-based premarital preparation: Clergy and lay leaders on the front lines. *Family Relations, 50*(1), 67–76.

US Census Bureau. (2000). Current population reports. *Statistical Abstract of the United States*. Washington, DC: US Department of Commerce.

Waite, L., & Gallagher, M. (2000). *The case for marriage*. New York: Doubleday.

Walker, A.J. (1999). Gender and family relationships. In M. Sussman, S.K. Steinmetz, & G.W. Peterson (Eds.), *Handbook of Marriage and the Family* (Ch. 16, pp. 439–474). New York: Plenum.

Worthington, E.L., Buston, B.G., & Hammonds, T.M. (1989). A component analysis of marriage enrichment: Information and treatment modality. *Journal of Counseling and Development, 67*, 555–560.

Media

Joshua Fogel

INTRODUCTION

Nearly everyone loves gadgets—especially electronic ones. Increasingly, primary-prevention practitioners are capitalizing on this popularity and are incorporating technology into their work (Table 1). This entry discusses the use of different technologies to conduct educational campaigns on an individual and group basis. It examines the existing evidence-based knowledge to determine the usefulness and the potential of these tools and their impact on health.

First, a cautionary statement is in order. Media technology almost exclusively makes use of the preventive tool of education to inform and entertain. We know from an extensive literature cited across many entries in this encyclopedia that education alone is not enough to promote health and prevent illness. It is true that education will increase knowledge. It will occasionally change attitudes, however, it rarely changes behavior. Rather, the combination of education with natural caregiving, environmental change, and social-competency promotion will work towards achieving lasting health changes.

DEFINITIONS

Mass media as used in health promotion and illness prevention includes anything that delivers a planned message to an identified audience. Usually it involves relatively simple content, delivered by an expert, with the intent to persuade the audience—to change their attitudes, beliefs, and actions in the direction of desired goals. Mass media includes commercial advertising (e.g., cereal boxes with sports heroes consuming the presumably healthy product) or the non-commercial placement of messages (e.g., the cautionary notices on packages of cigarettes). The experts may be opinion groups (e.g., anti-abortion or pro-life car bumper stickers) or governmental groups (e.g., signs to "buckle up—it's the law").

SCOPE

Technology is an integral part of society. Older forms of technology such as radio and television are present and used in almost every home in North America and other developed nations (Jason, 1998). In 1985, television was already the dominant communication medium in the United States (Meyers, Graves, Whelan, & Barclay, 1996).

Computers and the Internet have developed into the newest technology to become part of many homes in the United States. These new media have many of the same properties of radio and television with two important differences. The first is the potential for increased interaction. The second is the ability of anyone using the Internet to gain access to a national and even an international audience. For all age groups, this offers an opportunity for primary prevention and health promoting activities (Wartella & Jennings, 2000).

In the United States, in homes with children ages 2–17, home computer ownership increased from 48 percent in 1996 to 70 percent in 2000. Internet connections jumped from 15 percent to 52 percent during that same time. On average, children in the United States use the computer for 34 min each day (Shields & Behrman, 2000). About 65 percent of US households have a computer. Of those, 19 percent of households are multi-computer households. About 43 percent of US households have an Internet connection (Nie & Erbring, 2000).

Computer and video games have become a central part of life with 60 percent of the population in the United States

Table 1. Technology Primary-Prevention Interventions

Authors	Sample, location	Intervention	Theory	Results
Community-level approaches				
Svenkerud et al. (1999)	5,587 adults, Tanzania	Radio	SCT, two-step flow model	Used an HIV/AIDS prevention method such as condoms.
Stephenson et al. (1999)	1,601 adolescents, Lexington, KY	Television	SCT, activation model of information exposure	Less lifetime marijuana use, less increases in pro-marijuana occasional use beliefs and occasional use attitudes, but not less increases in pro-marijuana regular use beliefs and regular use attitudes.
Flynn et al. (1992, 1994); Worden et al. (1996)	5,458 children and adolescents, VT, MT, NY	Radio, television	SCT	Reductions in cigarette smoking, less increases in attitudes and beliefs related to smoking. Two-year follow-up showed they smoked less and had a lower risk of smoking cigarettes.
Ramirez et al. (1999)	212 adult Latina women, Brownsville, TX	Radio, television, newspapers, pamphlets	SCT, diffusion theory	Increased PAP screening adherence.
Individual-level approaches				
Harvey-Berino (1998)	166 adults, Burlington, VT	Television (distance learning)	Behavioral theory	Changed eating behaviors, exercise behaviors, and weight loss similar to other behavioral interventions but no differences between the intervention and control groups.
Kalichman et al. (1999)	117 African American adult men, Atlanta, GA	Video	SCT, information–motivation–behavioral skills model	Greater risk-reduction skills, sexual risk reduction, and condom use—but most changes not maintained at 6-month follow-up. Only the risk-reduction skills of planning ahead of time to have sex and talking with a sex partner about condoms remained significant. No differences on measures of AIDS knowledge, condom attitudes, or behavioral intentions.
Winzelberg et al. (1998)	57 university student women, CA	Computer	Cognitive–behavioral theory	Improved body image and these results maintained at a 3-month follow-up. Other measures of the Eating Disorders Inventory, Eating Disorders Examination, and body mass index did not differ between the groups.
Patrick et al. (2001)	117 adolescents, San Diego, CA and Pittsburgh, PA	Computer	SCT, transtheoretical model	Increased physical activity, fruit and vegetable consumption, and decreased fat consumption, while vigorous physical activity only approached significance.
Hornung et al. (2000)	209 children, NC	Computer	SCT	Increased knowledge regarding dangers of ultraviolet radiation overexposure, and changed attitudes toward tanning, but no changed behavioral practices.
Winett et al. (1999)	180 adolescent girls, VA	Internet	SCT	Overall increases in eating a variety of healthy foods, decrease in regular sodas, increase in exercise, but no change in high-fat dairy foods or unhealthy snacks.
Celio et al. (2000)	76 university student women, CA	Internet	Cognitive–behavioral theory	Reduced weight/shape concerns, drive for thinness differing from wait-list control but not active control group. Results maintained at 3-month follow-up with differing from wait-list control but not active control group.

Note: All locations are in the United States unless specified in a different country. SCT = Social Cognitive Theory.

playing these games. Game playing is not limited to children; 70 percent of the most frequent users of computer games are those ages 18 and above, with 40 percent of users over age 35 (IDSA, 2001).

Besides using a computer for games, computers are used to connect with the Internet. The Internet can be a source not only for general information, but also for health information topics. A 1997 survey in the United States found that nearly half of Internet users spent some time looking for health information on the web (Eng, Maxfield, Patrick, Deering, Ratzan, & Gustafson, 1998). In the United States in 2000, 41 million individuals (*On Monthly*, 2001) and in 2001, 100 million individuals sought health information online (Taylor & Leitman, 2001).

In the former communist Eastern European countries, the Internet has not made the impact on society that it has in the United States and Western Europe. Romania, with only 7 percent of the population using the Internet, has one of the higher percentages of Internet use. Although Russia has 4 million Internet users, that comprises only 3 percent of its population (Kennedy, Hegerl, Bussfeld, & Seemann, 2001). With the emergence and penetration of technology in these developing areas, Internet use will likely become prevalent and popular worldwide.

THEORY

There are several relevant theories: some focus on how messages are delivered/received (communication theory) and what receivers do with them (input overload). Other theories focus on the receiver, such as social cognitive theory, social marketing theory, and the stages of change model (transtheoretical model); these inform prevention-program designers of the "how and when" to deliver a specific message.

Prevention campaigns using *innovation-diffusion theory* (Rogers, 1983) or the *two-step flow model* (Rogers, 1995) are among the more successful communication theory-based programs. *Innovations* refer to individuals perceiving ideas, objects, and/or behaviors as new, while *diffusion* is the process by which the innovation is transmitted over time to community members. Interpersonal channels such as *change agents* are individuals who offer specialized information that otherwise may not be readily available to the public through mass media. For example, a community can perceive condom use for casual sex as an innovation. Over a few months this idea can diffuse and become more accepted through promotion in the mass media. The change agents can be those local health workers who make contact with individuals or groups, distribute pamphlets, and discuss the importance of condom use for the prevention of STDs.

According to *social cognitive theory* (Bandura, 1986), two factors influence the likelihood that preventive steps will be taken. First, individuals must appraise that the benefits of performing the behavior outweigh the costs. For example, they listen to messages heard on the television about stopping smoking. They decide that it is worth the stress involved to stop smoking because the benefits include immediate changes (like reducing bad breath and increasing lung capacity) and minimizing the long-term risks of contracting lung cancer.

Second, individuals must have a sense of *self-efficacy*, which involves the belief that one has the ability to deal with a specific challenging event in life. An important part of this theory is *modeling*, which relies on observational learning.

The *stages of change model* (*transtheoretical model*) (Prochaska, Norcross, & DiClemente, 1994) describes five stages of change. These stages are precontemplation, contemplation, preparation, action, and maintenance. These stages tell us what kind of message is needed for a person at a given stage.

There are few substantive theories of how technology works in primary prevention. There may be a parallel in the religious model of sin-and-absolution (M. Bloom, personal communication, 2001). For example, in constructing a health-oriented poster, designers would present: (1) "a hook"—a catchy picture or phrase that makes the viewer feel guilt or desirous of something, (2) a symbol—something the viewer can hold onto after the message has passed, and (3) the resolution—information that the viewer can act on to resolve the hook. One example of this approach is the poster with three parts: the top suggests that "Vanessa was in a fatal accident last night. But she does not know that yet" (the hook). This statement sounds strange and stimulates your curiosity. You then look further at the large picture with Vanessa and her boyfriend kissing passionately in a car (the symbol). At the very bottom of the page are some other words that direct the viewer to get more information on HIV transmission and its prevention (the resolution). Technology combines these attributes and can be applied for primary prevention.

RESEARCH

One classic primary prevention project using the media was a community-based cardiovascular disease prevention study. The Stanford Three Community Study (Farquhar, 1991; Farquhar et al., 1994) delivered media health messages to two small communities, and not to a third (the control). Media communication includes television, radio, newspapers, newsletters, booklets, and self-help kits. The Stanford Five City Project extended the research findings from the Stanford Three Community Study (Shea & Basch, 1990a,b). It focused on smoking, diet, high blood pressure, exercise, and obesity. Interventions were delivered through the media as well as in other forms. Over 6 years, adults in the participating communities received approximately 26 hr of message exposure. Principles of modeling and involving community organizations also helped to modify behavior. The results of these studies showed reduction in blood pressure, cigarette use, cholesterol, and improved physical activity for the experimental communities as compared to the control community.

As part of these studies, mass media interventions were combined with natural caregiving and competency promotion. Rimal, Flora, and Schooler (1999) analyzed what were the key aspects to the successful interventions in the Stanford Five City Project. They found that the booklets, health columns, and television programming were significant predictors of information seeking and interpersonal communication about cardiovascular disease. These results were true even when controlling for demographics and other interventions.

Another area involves the programmatic studies conducted by Jason (1998) with media and primary prevention. He and his colleagues have developed a multi-system, multilevel approach that moves closer to solving the multidimensional puzzle of community interventions for primary prevention. For example, some of his programs successfully involved information about smoking cessation delivered by television, and print information that was available in neighborhood hardware stores.

Representative Strategies.   Primary prevention programs for health use technology as either part of the intervention or as the sole basis of the intervention. Below are representative studies showing a variety of primary prevention efforts using these technologies. Readers will notice the relative lack of effective outcomes.

Radio.   In Tanzania (Svenkerud, Rao, & Rogers, 1999), a radio-soap opera named, "Twende na Wakati" was broadcasted for 30 mins twice weekly on prime time. As part of this show, there was a discussion of HIV/AIDS prevention, family planning, spousal communication, and gender equality. After 2 years, 52 percent of adults in the experimental region listened to this show. Half of those who listened discussed the topics of the radio show with others— a form of social support. As compared to the control group of individuals in an area where the show was not broadcast, individuals in the experimental condition were more likely to adopt an HIV/AIDS prevention method such as condom use. Also, those who discussed these topics with others were more likely to adopt an HIV/AIDS prevention method than those who listened but did not discuss the topics mentioned on the show. This study is an example of information and discussion helping to modify risky behaviors. It also cautions us to limit our expectations about information alone as being effective in producing behavioral change.

Television.   In the United States, public service announcements were televised for 4 months (Stephenson, Palmgreen, Hoyle, Donohew, Pugzles Lorch, & Colon, 1999). Each public service announcement used models to show one or more negative consequences of marijuana use (e.g., lower grades, or poor relationships with friends and family). At the 8-month follow-up, adolescent participants in the experimental city had less lifetime marijuana use, less increases in pro-marijuana occasional use beliefs and pro-marijuana

occasional use attitudes, but no less increase in pro-marijuana regular use beliefs and pro-marijuana regular use attitudes than did adolescents in the control city. Again, caution in depending only on mass media is indicated.

Distance Learning via Television.   Participants in a health promotion class were taught behavioral strategies using an interactive television system for 12 sessions (Harvey-Berino, 1998). An audio hookup activated a video system that allowed participants to see others who participated. The control group received the same intervention through a traditional live-contact group-training format. The results showed that both groups had changed eating behaviors, exercise behaviors, and weight loss, but there were no significant differences between groups. The interactive television group did not offer any additional benefits over standard treatment and was more expensive.

Video.   African American men saw educational and motivational enhancement videos that used African American models and had group discussions on HIV prevention for two 3-hr sessions (Kalichman, Cherry, & Browne-Sperling, 1999). Compared to a control group using a community standard educational format of the same time duration, experimental participants showed greater risk-reduction skills (e.g., almost always using condoms, talking with a partner about AIDS), and lower rates of unprotected vaginal intercourse, but these were not maintained at the 6-month follow-up. Only the risk-reduction skills of planning ahead of time to have sex and talking with a sex partner about condoms remained significant. No differences existed between the groups for measures of AIDS knowledge, condom attitudes, or behavioral intentions after the intervention, and at the 3-month and 6-month follow-ups.

Computer.   An interactive CD-ROM program with audio and video content titled, "Student Bodies" was developed for women and offered psycho-educational material on body image dissatisfaction, excessive weight concerns, and dieting or restricted eating patterns (Winzelberg, Taylor, Sharpe, Eldredge, Dev, & Constantinou, 1998). Study participants also had the choice of participating in an e-mail support group moderated by a clinical psychologist. After completing the computer program, participants had greater improvements in body image than a wait-list control group. These results continued at a 3-month follow-up. The other measures of the Eating Disorders Inventory, Eating Disorders Examination, and body mass index did not differ between groups. The overall results of this study are mixed. Further work is warranted with attention given to the potential value that the e-mail support group added to the intervention.

In a second study using CD-Rom technology, adolescents participated in a primary care computer assessment program named "PACE+" that helped them identify their health motivation level and develop a specific self-change plan incorporating goal-setting, social support, and problem solving (Patrick et al., 2001). Their health-care providers gave verbal and written endorsement of this computer-developed plan. About 4 months later, participants had increased physical activity, fruit and vegetable consumption, and decreased fat consumption, while vigorous physical activity was not significant. This individualized computer-based intervention needs follow-up data and the use of a control group to demonstrate its effectiveness.

Finally in an attempt to reduce children's harmful exposure to the sun, a group of children saw for 18 min a CD-ROM titled, *Playing it Safe in the Sun* (Hornung, Lennon, Garrett, DeVellis, Weinberg, & Strecher, 2000). Three different cartoon characters modeled three different sun-safety behaviors. After completing this program, children had greater knowledge about the dangers of ultraviolet radiation overexposure and changed attitudes regarding tanning as compared to a group of those taught this information with standard educational didactic methods and a standard control group. However, no differences existed among the three groups for behavioral practices of ultraviolet radiation protection. At the 7-month follow-up, the computer group differed from the control group but not the standard group only on knowledge about the dangers of ultraviolet radiation overexposure. This study illustrates the cautions expressed at the beginning of this entry that increased knowledge may have little relationship to behavioral change.

Internet.   To improve healthy eating behaviors, adolescent girls completed a 5-module weekly web-based program named, *Eat4Life* (Winett, Roodman, Winett, Bajzek, Rovniak, & Whitely, 1999). Each module provided a brief assessment of nutritional practices and offered strategies to change specific practices. After the 5-week program, there was an increase in eating healthy foods, and exercise and a decrease in soda consumption as compared to a control group of those educated by a teacher using a didactic format. No changes existed after the intervention for eating high-fat dairy foods or unhealthy snacks.

In another health promotion study, women used an interactive program with text, audio, and video content titled *Student Bodies* that was revised for the Internet (Celio et al., 2000). Unlike the CD-ROM version (Winzelberg et al., 1998), this program had structured 8-week sessions, on-line self-monitoring journals, behavior change exercises, defined homework assignments, and a required discussion group. Three of the sessions were face-to-face and photos of the participants were linked to the online discussion group

sessions. An incentive of receiving a passing or failing grade on a college course was used to encourage adherence. Results found participants had reduced weight/shape concerns and a reduced drive for thinness as compared with a wait-list control group. However, these reductions were no different than an active control group involving a classroom program. At a 3-month follow-up, these results still existed between the wait-list and the experimental groups. Also, participants had reduced eating concerns as compared to the wait-list control group. As before, there were no differences between the experimental group and the active control group involving a classroom program.

Mixed Interventions Using and/or Including Technology.   Smoking cessation campaigns often combine different media interventions. One 4 year study targeted children and adolescents with radio and television messages discussing the harmful effects of cigarette smoking. The results demonstrated significant reductions in smoking for those who saw these messages and attended the classes on the harmful effects of cigarette smoking as compared to a control group who just attended classes (Flynn, Worden, Secker-Walker, Badger, Geller, & Costanza, 1992). Further, there were fewer increases in positive attitudes and beliefs related to smoking in the combined mass media and class group (Worden, Flynn, Solomon, Secker-Walker, Badger, & Carpenter, 1996). These results were maintained in a 2-year follow-up (Flynn et al., 1994).

Another study concerned with PAP smear testing had Latina women see television, radio, and newspaper messages discussing how and why women get PAP smears and other cancer screening services (Ramirez, Villarreal, McAlister, Gallion, Suarez, & Gomez, 1999). Also, peer educators distributed monthly pamphlets on these topics. After 2 years, the results showed that women in the geographic area receiving these messages had an increase in PAP screening compared to women who did not receive these messages.

TECHNOLOGY AND THE FUTURE

What does this collection of studies suggest? One lesson is that media messages alone rarely result in desired behavioral change. Next, information retention drops sharply as soon as the media campaign ends. Third, presently radio delivers information inexpensively and in areas where other technologies are not available.

In the near future, television technology will improve so as to offer new opportunities for prevention programming. DeJong and Winsten (1990) in their review of mass media campaigns, state that an obstacle with television health promotion is access to specialized groups. With the advent of digital television, it becomes possible to target specific messages for specific individuals. Digital television will allow individuals to choose from hundreds of channels and health promotion messages could be tailored for each channel based on the profile of its viewers. However, the current consumer profiling capabilities being used by advertising researchers as with the Internet can be used for both good and evil.

Are there potential good uses for this technology—yes. For example, with cell phones and Internet access, individuals might willing choose to have their health monitored daily, and be coached via voice messaging on health promoting behaviors. As Internet technology and costs decline, voice and picture transmission should spur the wider use of this technology for natural caregiving, the improvement of information dissemination, and even efforts at competency promotion. On the other hand, the imagination does not need to wander far to see how these same examples could be used for evil purposes like tracking given individuals and monitoring their behavior without their knowledge. Time will tell what will happen, but the key to staying ahead and appealing to the many individuals fascinated with technology is to utilize these technological advances for primary prevention, while protecting civil liberties.

Also see: Media Habits: Childhood.

References

Bandura, A. (1986). *Social foundations of thought and action: A social cognitive theory*. Englewood Cliffs, NJ: Prentice-Hall.

Celio, A.A., Winzelberg, A.J., Wifley, D.E., Eppstein-Herald, D., Springer, E.A., Dev, P., & Taylor, C.B. (2000). Reducing risk factors for eating disorders: Comparison of an Internet- and a classroom-delivered psychoeducational program. *Journal of Consulting and Clinical Psychology, 68*(4), 650–657.

DeJong, W., & Winsten, J.A. (1990). The use of mass media in substance abuse prevention. *Health Affairs, 9*(2), 30–46.

Eng, T.R., Maxfield, A., Patrick, K., Deering, M.J., Ratzan, S.C., & Gustafson, D.H. (1998). Access to health information and support: A public highway or a private road? *Journal of the American Medical Association, 280*(15), 1371–1375.

Farquhar, J.W. (1991). The Stanford cardiovascular disease prevention programs. *Annals of the New York Academy of Sciences, 623*, 327–331.

Farquhar, J.W., Maccoby, N., Wood, P.W., Alexander, J.K., Breitrose, H., Brown, B.W., Jr., Haskell, W.L., McAlister, A.L., Meyer, A.J., Nash, J.D., & Stern, M.P. (1994). Community education for cardiovascular disease. In A. Steptoe & J. Wardle (Eds.), *Psychosocial processes and health: A reader* (pp. 316–324). New York: Cambridge University Press.

Flynn, B.S., Worden, J.K., Secker-Walker, R.H., Badger, G.J., Geller, B.M., & Costanza, M.C. (1992). Prevention of cigarette smoking through mass media intervention and school programs. *American Journal of Public Health, 82*(6), 827–834.

Flynn, B.S., Worden, J.K., Secker-Walker, R.H., Pirie, P.L., Badger, G.J., Carpenter, J.H., & Geller, B. (1994). Mass media and school interventions for cigarette smoking prevention: Effects 2 years after completion. *American Journal of Public Health, 84*(7), 1148–1150.

Harvey-Berino, J. (1998). Changing health behavior via telecommunication technology: Using interactive television to treat obesity. *Behavior Therapy, 29*, 505–519.

Hornung, R.L., Lennon, P.A., Garrett, J.M., DeVellis, R.F., Weinberg, P.D., & Strecher, V.J. (2000). Interactive computer technology for skin cancer prevention targeting children. *American Journal of Preventive Medicine, 18*(1), 69–76.

IDSA. (2001). Sixth annual consumer survey on games. Retrieved August 1, 2001 from the World Wide Web: http://www.idsa.com/consumersurvey2001.html

Jason, L.A. (1998). Tobacco, drug, and HIV prevention media interventions. *American Journal of Community Psychology, 26*(2), 151–187.

Kalichman, S.C., Cherry, C., & Browne-Sperling, F. (1999). Effectiveness of a video-based motivational skills-building HIV risk-reduction intervention for inner-city African American men. *Journal of Consulting and Clinical Psychology, 67*(6), 959–966.

Kennedy, R.S., Hegerl, U., Bussfeld, P., & Seemann, O. (2001). Psychiatry via the Internet: Benefits, risks, and perspectives. *Techmed, 1*(1). Retrieved August 5, 2001 from the World Wide Web: http://www.medscape.com

Meyers, A.W., Graves, T.J., Whelan, J.P., & Barclay, D.R. (1996). An evaluation of a television-delivered behavioral weight loss program: Are the ratings acceptable? *Journal of Consulting and Clinical Psychology, 64*(1), 172–178.

Nie, N.H., & Erbring, L. (2000). Internet and society: A preliminary report. *Stanford Institute for the Quantitative Study of Society*. Retrieved February 27, 2000 from the World Wide Web: http://www.stanford.edu/group/siqss

On Monthly (2001, March 5). pp. 37, 43.

Patrick, K., Sallis, J.F., Prochaska, J.J., Lydston, D.D., Calfas, K.J., Zabinski, M.F., Saelens, B.E., & Brown, D.R. (2001). A multi-component program for nutrition and physical activity change in primary care: PACE+ for adolescents. *Archives of Pediatric and Adolescent Medicine, 155*(8), 940–946.

Prochaska, J.O., Norcross, J.C., & DiClemente, C.C. (1994). *Changing for good*. New York: Avon.

Ramirez, A.G., Villarreal, R., McAlister, A., Gallion, K.J., Suarez, L., & Gomez, P. (1999). Advancing the role of participatory communication in the diffusion of cancer screening among Hispanics. *Journal of Health Communication, 4*, 31–36.

Rimal, R.N., Flora, J.A., & Schooler, C. (1999). Achieving implements in overall health orientation. *Communication Research, 26*(3), 322–348.

Rogers, E.M. (1983). *Diffusion of innovations*. New York: Free Press.

Rogers, E.M. (1995). *Diffusion of innovations* (4th ed.). New York: Free Press.

Shea, S., & Basch, C.E. (1990a). A review of five major community-based cardiovascular disease prevention programs. Part I: Rationale, design, and theoretical framework. *American Journal of Health Promotion, 4*(3), 203–213.

Shea, S., & Basch, C.E. (1990b). A review of five major community-based cardiovascular disease prevention programs. Part II: Intervention strategies, evaluation methods, and results. *American Journal of Health Promotion, 4*(4), 279–287.

Shields, M.K., & Behrman, R.E. (2000). Children and computer technology: Analysis and recommendations. *Children and Computer Technology, 10*(2), 4–30.

Stephenson, M.T., Palmgreen, P., Hoyle, R.H., Donohew, L., Pugzles Lorch, E., & Colon, S.E. (1999). Short-term effects of an anti-marijuana media campaign targeting high sensation seeking adolescents. *Journal of Applied Communication Research, 27*, 175–195.

Svenkerud, P.J., Rao, N., & Rogers, E.M. (1999). Mass media effects through interpersonal communication: The role of "Twende na

Wakati" on the adoption of HIV/AIDS prevention in Tanzania. In W.N. Elwood (Ed.), *Power in the blood: A handbook on AIDS, politics, and communication* (pp. 243–253). Mahwah, NJ: Erlbaum.

Taylor, H., & Leitman, R. (2001). eHealth traffic critically dependent on search engines and portals. *Health Care News, 1*(13), 1–3.

Wartella, E.A., & Jennings, N. (2000). Children and computers: New technology—old concerns. *Children and Computer Technology, 10*(2), 31–43.

Winett, R.A., Roodman, A.A., Winett, S.G., Bajzek, W., Rovniak, L.S., & Whitely, J.A. (1999). The effects of the Eat4Life Internet-based health behavior program on the nutrition and activity practices of high school girls. *Journal of Gender, Culture, and Health, 4*(3), 239–254.

Winzelberg, A.J., Taylor, C.B. Sharpe, T., Eldredge, K.L., Dev, P., & Constantinou, P.S. (1998). Evaluation of a computer-mediated eating disorder intervention program. *International Journal of Eating Disorders, 24*, 339–349.

Worden, J.K., Flynn, B.S., Solomon, L.J., Secker-Walker, R.H., Badger, G.J., & Carpenter, J.H. (1996). Using mass media to prevent cigarette smoking among adolescent girls. *Health Education Quarterly, 23*(4), 453–468.

Media Habits, Childhood

Robert Hampton and Lucia Magarian

INTRODUCTION

When the American Bill of Rights was adopted in 1791, the importance of the media to the American lifestyle and culture was irrevocably established. From the simple text, "Congress shall make no law abridging the freedom of speech, or of the press" today, has spawned a multi-billion dollar industry with the capacity to affect the fortunes of every citizen in this country. In an open and democratic society, this feature of public life is critical for our sustained common good. The media serve to unite people; to teach about customs, values, and beliefs; to present news and events; to advocate and investigate; and to entertain in times of peace, and to enable us to rally and mourn in times of tragedy and war.

However, with such power comes responsibility—not only by the industry itself to act as a good citizen, but on each recipient, to hold this industry accountable for its actions—especially with regard to vulnerable children. This entry focuses on the relationship between the media and children (media habits), its effects (on health), and what families, institutions, government and the industry can do to address some of the issues that have been raised.

DEFINITIONS

The term *media* includes the following forums: television, videos, films, music, magazines, comic books, newspapers, electronic games, computer games, and the Internet by which information is communicated to a large audience in a planned manner. The phrase *media habits* is meant to encompass the entire complex of acts involving any use of, or access to, media.

The phrase *healthy habits* as related to media consumption means those habits that promote a balanced diet, plenty of activity, good personal hygiene, and proper rest are critical for the growing child's healthy physical development. Healthy habits also include those that stimulate intellectual curiosity, reinforce affection, teach self-discipline, and promote interaction with peers. These help a child to gain a sense of herself and to develop self-esteem and self-control in relationships with others, which are the building blocks to mature relationships, and ultimately, to good citizenship.

SCOPE

Many children in the United States are not only failing to thrive physically, but they are developing *unhealthy* habits that have negative effects in the present time and over their life span. On the cognitive and social level, many of these habits translate into sleep deficits, under-functioning in school, poor grades, and/or increased aggression. This is due, in part, to the amount of time children engage in most media behavior (e.g., watching television, surfing the Internet, or playing with electronic games). Conservative estimates report that 60 percent of today's children spend 3 or more hours a day watching television (American Academy of Child and Adolescent Psychiatry, Fact Sheet, no. 54). Add into this mix children's addiction to electronic games that, according to one report published by the Senate Committee on the Judiciary (1999, p. 9) can be upwards of 90 min a day, with the increased amount of time our youth spend surfing the web, and it becomes clear why public health officials and institutions have identified a sedentary lifestyle as a major health concern for youth. In fact, some researchers estimate that obesity affects 25–30 percent of pre-adolescent children in the United States (Field Camargo, Taylor, Berkey, Roberts, & Colditz, 2001; Crespo et al., 2001), and that it is directly linked to the amount of time children spend watching television, playing video games, surfing the web, or reading fashion magazines (Faith et al., 2001; Field, Cheung, Wolf, Herzog, Gortmaker, & Colditz, 1999; Harrison & Cantor, 1997; Jeffrey & French, 1998). Additionally, secondary health problems, such as high blood pressure, poor circulation, carpal tunnel syndrome, high cholesterol, fatigue, sleep disorders, and seizures, have been linked to excessive media exposure (Anderson, 2000; Austin, 1999; Austin, Pinkleton, & Fujioka, 2000; Graf, Chatrian, Glass, & Knauss, 1994; Thomas, 1999).

Moreover, indiscriminate and unsupervised exposure to a variety of media stimuli has societal implications on family well-being and community stability. In a recent survey on parent and teen perceptions of family life, one factor consistently stood out (Global Strategy Group, 2000). Parents overwhelmingly seemed to believe they were more involved in their children's lives than they actually were. For instance, the survey reported that,

> Parents often say that they frequently monitor their teen's time in front of the TV and on the Internet, but their children don't agree. 85% of parents say they frequently monitor what their kids watch on TV. 61% of children say they are watching TV without any parental supervision. 71% [of parents] assert that they frequently monitor their child's use of the Web. However, 45% of teens say they surf the Web "all the time/often" without a watchful parental eye.

The cumulative effect of such long-term exposure to the media and its unexamined values can result in unhealthy and/or fatal social behaviors—especially for many adolescents, who may come from vulnerable households (e.g., poverty, child abuse or neglect). Three areas of particular concern are teen substance abuse, especially the consumption of alcohol; increased early, sexualized behavior; and incidents of violence and aggression. According to the National Institute on Drug Abuse (NIDA), in 2000 the annual rates for illicit drug use for 10th and 12th graders were 26 and 41 percent, respectively; and the annual use of alcohol was 65 and 73 percent, respectively. Given these data, it is not surprising that the National Highway Safety Administration reported that in 1999 "Motor vehicle crashes were the leading cause of death for 15–20 year olds (p. 1) [and] 21 percent of the young drivers who were killed in crashes were intoxicated" (p. 4). More disturbingly is that even *eighth* graders, were annually using alcohol at a rate of 41 percent (NIDA). To understand the allure of alcohol, Robinson, Chen, and Killen (1998) conducted a study of over 1500 ninth graders to examine the "associations between media exposure and alcohol use in adolescents." The students were assessed initially as to their media and alcohol use, and then followed up 18 months later for comparative analysis. The researchers concluded that the "onset of drinking was significantly associated with baseline hours of television viewing" (1998, p. 354).

Similarly, there appears to be a small but growing number of studies examining the correlation of sexual beliefs and behavior to the number of hours spent watching television, particularly soap operas and talk shows (Strasburger & Donnerstein, 1999; Ward & Rivadeneyra, 1999) where there

is little connection between sexual activity, intimacy, and personal responsibility. The American Academy of Pediatrics (2001, p. 191) reported that , "American adolescents will view nearly 14,000 sexual references per year, yet only 165 of these references deal with birth control, self-control, abstinence, or the risk of pregnancy or STDs." The consequence of this overexposure is that children—especially teenage girls—are often sexually anesthetized. Zillman (2000, p. 42) calls this the development of "sexual callousness" and analyzes its effect:

> that prolonged exposure to erotica leads to perceptions of exaggerated sexual activity in the populace. Dispositional changes include diminished trust in intimate partners, the abandonment of hopes for sexual exclusivity with partners, evaluation of promiscuity as the natural state, and the apprehension that sexual inactivity constitutes a health risk. Cynical attitudes about love emerge, and superior sexual pleasures are thought attainable without affection towards partners.

The result is that women and children are more at risk for rape and other acts of sexual exploitation and abuse at increasingly younger and younger ages. The National Institute of Justice, Centers for Disease Control and Prevention reported the following: "More than half (54 percent) of female rape victims identified by the survey were under 18 years of age when they first experienced rape; 32% were between the ages of 12 and 17, and 22% were children under the age of 12" (Tjaden & Thoennes, 1998, p. 2).

Lastly, the repetitive viewing of "real life" traumatic and/or violent events is another area where children, youth, and young adults are vulnerable. The "24/7" news coverage of singular, catastrophic events, such as the Twin Towers and Pentagon disasters in the United States, is a prime example of media over-exposure which can have long-term consequences on the health of children. According to FEMA's web resources for parents, "Children who experience an initial traumatic event before they are 11 years old are three times more likely to develop psychological symptoms than those who experience their first trauma as a teenager or later." **[website:]** FEMA suggests that limiting the amount of exposure to the event, including watching the news, can be one useful method in preventing children from developing many of the symptoms associated with post-traumatic stress syndrome.

Globalization and the Media

Each of the above health and social concerns is not limited to the United States. From Europe to the Asia, the effects of overexposure to the media are the same. For instance, in Canada, the problem of childhood obesity mirrors the same trend in the United States, with a 57 percent increase in the prevalence of overweight affecting young girls during a fifteen year time span (Anderson, 2000; Tremblay & Williams, 2000). In Spain, Caviedes, Quesada, and Herranz (2000) conducted an extensive survey of children's television viewing habits. Like their American counterparts, Spanish parents underestimated the amount of time their children spent watching television as well as the nature of the programs consumed. This overexposure often has a domino affect: the children are over stimulated which results in less restful sleep and tiredness during the next day in school. Researchers at Tel Aviv University conducted a study of 72 boys and 68 girls from grades 2 through 6, and they discovered that "the sleep of infants, children, and adolescents is sensitive to environmental stress" (Sadeh et al., p. 298). The issue for parents and educators is what constitutes environmental stress. Daily media consumption appears to be such a contributing factor, as Owens, Maxim, McGuinn, Nobile, Msall, and Alario (1999, p. 327) discovered in their study of 495 children between kindergarten and fourth grade. They report, "television viewing habits associated most significantly with sleep disturbance were increased daily television view, viewing amounts and increased television viewing at bedtime. The sleep domains that appeared to be affected most consistently by television were bedtime resistance, sleep onset delay, and anxiety around sleep, followed by shortened sleep duration."

THEORIES AND RESEARCH

The three predominate theories most cited as being influential to the way children relate to the media are cognitive–behavioral approach, social learning theory, and, more recently, cultivation theory.

As children mature and become more aware of their world, they begin to form social relationships, and, thus, learns to model their behavior on important others and the responses they receive for their actions (Bandura, 1999, p. 31). However, as Bandura (1999, p. 29) writes, the "influences from peers, family members, the mass media, and the broader society are often in conflict," which makes the development of self-identity more difficult. The question for parents, teachers, and others to grapple with is when, what type, and how much intervention is necessary between the child and these media stimuli. To illustrate power of the media on our children's developmental growth, we examine the issue of violence in this context.

Groves (1997, p. 81) writes that our children have neither the cognitive nor emotional structures to understand the context of the violence. They do not understand the motives

for the violence, nor do they grasp the consequences of the behavior. Finally, children who see violence on television begin to see the world as a dangerous place. This worldview is a troubling message to send to young children and may discourage the kind of curiosity and exploration that leads to knowledge, self-confidence, and mastery.

Media violence may increase a child's susceptibility to the somatic effects of trauma, for example, increased anxiety, sleeplessness, and aggression. Singer, Slovak, Frierson, and York (1998) studied the responses of children between the grades of three and eight to ascertain if there was any association between television viewing and trauma symptomology. They found that children who watched more than 6 hr of television a day had higher total trauma scores and reported higher levels of violent behavior than their peers who watched less television. Not surprisingly, those "children who preferred 'actions and fighting' shows, also, reported higher levels of violent behaviors" (Singer et al., 1998, p. 1043).

Grossman (1999, p. 68) compares children's early exposure to violence to the way the military desensitizes its new recruits as they are trained to become soldiers.

> Something very similar to this desensitization toward violence is happening to our children through violence in the media—but instead of 18 years old, it begins at the age of 18 months when a child is first able to discern what is happening on television. At that age, a child can watch something… and mimic the action. But it isn't until children are six or seven years old that the part of the brain kicks in that lets them understand where the information comes from. Even though young children have some understanding of what it means to pretend, they are developmentally unable to distinguish clearly between fantasy and reality.

The *cultivation perspective* developed by Gerbner, Gross, Morgan, and Signorielli (1994), posits that the longer an individual is exposed to a medium and a message, the more the individual will begin to adopt that particular worldview as representing the predominate perspective of social reality. The implication of such an act is that this perspective is encoded by the child as having society's approval, even if that is not true, in fact.

RESEARCH

A brief survey of the research on media violence reveals the extent to which exposure to media violence affects the behavior and perceptions of children. Nathanson and Cantor (2000) devised a simple but effective methodology to determine the effects of watching fantasy violence on aggressive behavior with and without an actual mediator present. They divided their sample of students from grades two through six into three groups. Two of the groups watched a brief clip from a Woody Woodpecker cartoon. However, one group was given a specific intervention before watching the cartoon. They were asked to think about the other character (i.e., the "victim" of the violence) throughout the viewing. The third group served as the "control" and did not view any clip. All the groups were then asked to complete a questionnaire designed to assess their reactions and their aggressive tendencies. Interestingly, boys were the most affected by the mediator. The group that just watched the clip showed a marked increase in aggressiveness without mediation, whereas those boys who were given the message to consider the victim increased their awareness of the victim's suffering, which "seemed to help them resist accepting aggressive attitudes or feelings after viewing" (Nathanson & Cantor, 2000, p. 137).

Moliter and Hirsch (1994) document their attempt to duplicate the Drabman and Thomas studies from the 1970s that demonstrated a correlation between viewing aggressive behavior in films and a subsequent desensitization to real life aggression. They worked with fourth and fifth grade students in a controlled experiment to ascertain how quickly they would respond to real life violence depending upon the kind of stimulus (a moderately violent film clip versus a scene from a Summer Olympic match) to which each had been exposed. The researchers offered this sobering conclusion: "Children tend to tolerate the violence of others—in this case, younger children—more if they have seen TV/film violence" (p. 202).

Film, television, and music are not the only sources for negative stimulus. Video games are another vehicle for exposure to violence or misogynist behavior. Because a child is a participant in the process by virtue of playing the game, many (Grossman, 1999; Funk, 1999; Song & Anderson, 2001) fear the cumulative effects from such interactive behavior. Often these games involve the user "acting out" a position within the violent fantasy sequences vis à vis, by blowing up figures, killing and shooting at targets and then being rewarded for such acts by advancing to the next level. Funk, Flores, Buchman, and Germann (1999) conducted research with fourth graders to ascertain their awareness of and preferences for the different types and categories of electronic games. They discovered that most children would rather play violent games (males preferred human or sports violence; girls preferred fantasy violence) over educational selections, an indication of how widespread the acceptability of violence is.

Thus, a teenager who is exposed to frequent television viewing of violent shows, plays violent video games, and listens to lyrics that promote violence is more apt to display aggression and to believe that he/she is conforming to society's framework than one who has more limited access

to such content. DuRant and his colleagues (1997, pp. 443–448) conducted a random content analysis of music videos airing on Music Television (MTV) and Black Entertainment Television (BET) airing over a 4-week period in 1997 to determine how widespread violence was represented. They discovered that in 46.5 percent of the videos, the main actor carried a weapon and engaged in violence and in 41.1 percent of the videos the background characters were also violent and carried a weapon. But, even more disturbingly, in those videos where the background characters were engaged in violence, 72 percent of these characters were *portrayed as children* carrying a weapon and 63 percent of them were portrayed as children engaged in some form of violence (pp. 443–448).

Similar studies have been conducted regarding other social behaviors, such as early adolescent sexuality (Steele, 1999), alcohol consumption (Robinson et al., 1998), and cigarette use (Schooler & Feighery, 1996). For instance, Austin et al. (2000) conducted a cross-sectional study of more than 500 ninth and twelfth grade students in two public high schools in California to determine the influence of media messages about alcohol on adolescent beliefs and behavior. They found, "expectancies—beliefs about the benefits of drinking alcohol—develop over time and are influenced by perceptions of media messages even more than by media exposure itself" (p. 348).

The same result applies to long-term exposure to violence, body image messages, and sexual exploration. Brown (2000) has developed a *media practice model* that helps identify some of the key factors in the process of adolescent's use of the media: First, they are active in consciously selecting their choices and medium, for example, television or music; second, they are not passive recipients of the message, but rather actively engage the content and process it within each individual's unique personal framework; and third, that this framework comprises the individual's current values *plus* his or her desired identity to reflect a certain image or identity. In other words, Brown believes "adolescents (and probably others as well) choose media and interact with media based on who they are or who they want to be" (p.35).

Huesmann and Moise (1996, p. 6), writing about violence, have identified five ways exposure to media affects our youth. These are: *imitative*, that is, they mimic the actions of "media heroes, especially when the action is rewarded"; *desensitized*, that is, a child is more apt to "become aggressive ... and to become suspicious and expect others to act violently" in return or preemptively; *justified*, meaning that a child then looks to television to mitigate feelings of guilt and to seek approval for his or her aggressiveness; *cognitive priming or cueing*, repeated exposure can result in subconscious associations between an act or object that, in turn, triggers aggression; and *arousal*, which suggests that "viewing violence is unpleasant at first, but children who constantly watch violent television become habituated, and their emotional and physiological responses decline."

What is the result of such an omnipresent influence by the media on our children and society? Pawlowski (2000) identifies seven roles that television has usurped from parents and other leaders. These include: family manager, cultural narrator, gender mentor, sexual advisor, hero, arbitrator, and friend. Moreover, Kane, Taub, and Hayes (2000) argue the media have become the de facto arbiters of societal values by the sheer volume of their interactions with children, youths, and adults. While the authors acknowledge that the media rejects this role, they counter with the observation that, "the media teach even when they do not intend to do so" (p. 59). Thus, they assert that the media are assumed to play a role in transmitting, maintaining, and reinforcing the societal and cultural consensus" (p. 57) and consequently, "Even if the media do not intend to contribute to the formation of values, they most assuredly do" (p. 62).

STRATEGIES THAT WORK

The need to promote healthy media habits is beyond debate. The question is, how to do it best? Strasburger and Donnerstein (1999) suggest there are four arenas in which to seek solutions: control the access and the way children view the media (parent's role); intervene at the public health level (physician's or mental health worker's role); regulate the standards and industry (government's role) and improve the content (media industry's role). The first approach is the most direct method for intervention with children as it requires parents to take a more proactive stance towards media consumption in general. This would involve limiting the amount of time children are allowed to engage in all media activities during the week and promoting alternative activities that would increase a child's overall quality of life. Jason and Brackshaw (1999) provide an example of this, where an obese child was required to use an exercise bike to earn time to watch TV, minute for minute. Results showed both weight loss and reduction in TV viewing.

The second approach is to implement strategies that would counter the effects of media violence and encourage children to become more critically aware of the messages being sent. Nathanson and Cantor's (2000) study provides empirical evidence that the latter approach would be very effective. They demonstrated that mediation works both to de-escalate aggression and to increase empathy for victims—especially in young boys. The benefit of teaching parents how to act as mediator with their children is obvious. "This kind of mediation required only two sentences. As a result, it is a simple strategy that parents could easily use

when they watch violent programs with their children … [and] this may help children develop critical viewing skills that they can use each time they view, regardless of whether a parent is present or not."

The third and fourth arenas are best epitomized in the public policy debate and responses as have been evidenced in the aforementioned hearings held in the US Congress. While Strasburg and Donnerstein advocate a proactive response to the media, the practical implications of this strategy is best demonstrated at the grassroots level by individual involvement in parent and community groups as media activists and advocates. Examples of such activism can be realized by simply monitoring the books and videos being promoted in the public library, the use of computer technology in the classroom, the enforcement of admission policies at the local movie house, or the songs that are airing constantly on the radio. Such activism raises serious civil liberties issues.

STRATEGIES THAT MIGHT WORK

Public service announcements (PSAs) are predicated on the advertising concept that consistent exposure to a product or particular message (dose), over time (duration), will affect the behavior of the consumer. Recent research suggests that PSAs might be as effective at changing the behavior of children and teens as traditional advertising, but only if they are carefully developed and targeted to the developmental life stage of these viewers and if they follow certain criteria. For instance, traditional PSAs were designed as informational resources, and the assumption was that simply by exposure to content, viewers would adjust their behavior. However, because adolescence is the time when peer approval is a necessary component of developing an identity, PSAs which are constructed around social approval messages are more likely to be attended to by young viewers (Schoenbachler & Whittler, 1996).

A sub-category of adolescents, identified as "thrill seeking," are more likely to be attracted to risk taking behaviors, such as alcohol consumption, cigarette smoking, and drug use. Schoenbachler and Whittler (1996) conducted a study with 371 seventh and eighth grade students. They write, "Our findings also confirm the importance of sensation seeking as a targeting variable for antidrug PSAs. A high sensation seeker is not only more likely to use drugs, but responds differently to antidrug PSAs than a low sensation seeker. The high sensation seeker reacts negatively to antidrug messages, feels he/she is immortal, and tends to view drugs favorably. PSA producers must recognize that reaching these at-risk individuals is a necessary but difficult task. Our results provide some guidance by showing social threat messages to be more persuasive than physical threat messages with such an audience" (p. 52). Yet, persuasive is still no guarantee of performance. As Carr and Sarvela (1991) write, "the primary role of mass media is reinforcement. It is important to supplement health promotion campaigns with face to face contact strategies as well as grass roots participation."

STRATEGIES THAT DO NOT WORK

Two ineffective methods of dealing with media consumption and children's health are self-regulation, as in allowing an industry to define its own ratings' system, and self-monitoring, as in allowing children to voluntarily monitor their own behavior. In both instances, these methods often appeal to overworked and stressed parents who have little time to engage in close supervision of their children's media habits.

A voluntary ratings system for movies, television, music, and games has become a popular and politically expedient way to appease parents, who want more help with managing the media consumption of their children, as well as the various industries, who want to restrict the government's involvement in their right to produce and market their products freely and without censorship. Yet, often these ratings have the opposite effect. Instead of discouraging children from accessing inappropriate material, it helps to highlight which products are more forbidden.

Moreover, parents are often unaware of just how inaccurate the ratings' system is at defining a product as being violent or sexually explicit. For example, Funk et al. (1999) conducted a study with 1,000 fourth grade to eighth grade students who were asked to play video games in order to "to determine whether commercial ratings reflect consumer perceptions of game content" (p. 284). Not surprising, they discovered that all of the children were able to correctly identify the videos that were rated violent..." and they were "more likely than adults to place these games into one of the violence categories" (p. 301). This is not surprising when, as the authors note, "It is unrealistic to expect that parents will personally view the full spectrum of content throughout a game. Many games take more than 100 hours to play to the end, where the content may be dramatically different than at the beginning" (p. 296).

SYNTHESIS

The best recommendation for developing healthy media habits for children is for parents to be proactive and assertive in monitoring and assessing their children's media consumption (American Academy of Pediatrics, Media Education, 1999; Media Violence, 1995). Minimally, this would involve:

- limiting the amount of time children can engage in media consumption of all kinds such as television, electronic games, surfing the web;
- engaging the children in discussions about the content of the products and discussing the truth of what is presented and/or the values that are promoted therein;
- planning alternative activities to balance the time that would have been spent engaging the media;
- screening, in advance, content of music lyrics, videos, web sites, and other outlets for appropriateness;
- participating together in watching programs, listening to music, or playing video games;
- eliminating easy access to television and computers, for example, removing televisions from children's bedrooms or moving the computer into a family area where it can be viewed easily by everyone.
- networking with others, such as teachers, pediatricians, religious community, and other parents, to share information, regulate access, and monitor the types of media to which children are being exposed; and
- becoming more civilly active by lobbying Congress and demanding accountability from the media industry.

Children are remarkably resilient and responsive. They need to be nurtured, molded, and guided in order to fulfill their greatest potential. Therefore, healthy media consumption is best understood within the context of a parental environment that is involved, committed, and vigilant about the messages that are given to their children. When this occurs parents have the potential power to help children develop critical thinking skills and empathic responses by vicariously experiencing situations beyond their immediate environment. In the absence of such control, the long-term effects on a child's health, well-being, and future social functioning is insidiously at risk.

Also see: Media; Academic Success: Adolescence; Family Strengthening: Childhood; Family Strengthening: Adolescence.

References

American Academy of Child and Adolescent Psychiatry. (1996) "Children and watching TV." Fact sheet No. 54. Available online: http://www.aacap.org/web/aacap/publications/factsfam/tv.htm

American Academy of Pediatrics. (2001). Sexuality, contraception, and the media. *Pediatrics, 107*, 191–194. Available Online Database: Medline.

American Academy of Pediatrics. (1999). Media education. *Pediatrics, 104*, 341–343. Available online database: Medline.

American Academy of Pediatrics. (1995). Media violence. *Pediatrics, 95*, 949–950. Available Online Database: Medline.

Anderson, R.E. (2000). The spread of the childhood obesity epidemic. *Canadian Medical Association Journal, 163*, 1461–1462. Available online database: Academic Search Elite.

Austin, E. (1999). Is t.v. keeping your kid up? *Child, 14*, 92–94.

Austin, E.W., Pinkleton, B.E., & Fujioka, Y. (2000). The role of interpretation processes and parental discussion in the media's effects on adolescents' use of alcohol. *Pediatrics, 105*, 343–349. Available online database: Ovid.

Bandura, A. (1999). Exercise of personal and collective efficacy in changing societies. *Self-efficacy in changing societies.* Cambridge: Cambridge University Press.

Brown, J.D. (2000). Adolescents' sexual media diets. *Journal of Adolescent Health, 27S,* 35–40. Available online database: Ovid.

Carr. K. and Sarvela, P. (1991). Marketing and promotions. *Wellness Perspectives, 7,* 126–139. Available online database: Academic Search Elite.

Caviedes, A., Quesada, F., & Herranz, J.L. (2000). La television y los ninos: es responsible la television de todos los males que se le atribuyen? [Television and children: is television responsible for all the evils attributed to it?] *Aten Primaria (Atencion primaria/Sociedad Espanola de Medicina de Familia y Comunitaria), 25,* 142–147. Abstract in English: Available online database: Medline Full article available: NIH.

Crespo, C.J., Smit, E., Troiano, R., Bartlett, S., Macera, C., & Anderson, R. (2001). Television Watching, energy intake, and obesity in US children. *Archives of Pediatrics & Adolescent Medicine, 155,* 360–365.

DuRant, R.H., Rich, M., Emans, S.J., Rome, E.S., Woods, E.R., Rome, E.A., & Woods, E.R. (1997). Violence and weapon carrying in music videos, a content analysis. *Archives of Pediatric and Adolescent Medicine, 151,* 443–448. Available online database: Ovid and Health Reference Center.

Faith, M.S., Berman, N., Heo, M., Pietrobelli, A., Gallagher, D., Epsetin, L., Eiden, M.T., & Allison, D.A. (2001). Effects of contingent television on physical activity and television viewing in obese children. *Pediatrics, 107,* 1043–1049. Available online database: EBSCOHost.

Field, A.E., Camargo, C.A., Jr., Taylor, C.B., Berkey, C.S., Roberts, S.B., & Colditz, G.A. (2001). Peer, parent, and media influences on the development of weight concerns and frequent dieting among preadolescent and adolescent girls and boys. *Pediatrics, 107,* 54–60. Available online database: Lexis-Nexis Academic Universe.

Field, A.E., Cheung, L., Wolf, A.M., Herzog D.B., Gortmaker, S.L., & Colditz, G.A. (1999). Exposure to the mass media and weight concerns among girls. *Pediatrics, 103,* 660. Available online database: Academic Search Elite.

Funk, J., Flores, G., Buchman, D., & Germann, J. (1999). Rating electronic games. *Youth & Society, 30,* 283–313. Available online database: Academic Search Elite. 1–21.

Gerbner. G., Gross, L., Morgan, M., & Signorielli, N. (1994). Growing up with television: The cultivation persepective. In J. Bryant & D. Zillmann (Eds.), *Media Effects: Advances in Theory and Research* (pp. 17–42). Hillsdale: Lawrence Erlbaum.

Global Strategy Group, Inc. (2000). *Talking with teens: The YMCA parent and teen survey final report* (pp. 1–4) [on-line]. Available http://www.ymca.net/presrm/research/teensurvey.htm

Graf, W.D., Chatrian, G., Glass, S.T., & Knauss, T.A. (1994). Video game-related seizures: a report on 10 patients and a review of the literature. *Pediatrics, 93,* 551–556. Available online database: Lexis-Nexis.

Groves, B.M. (1997). Growing up in a violent world: the impact of family and community violence on young children and their families. *Topics in Early Childhood Special Education, 17,* 74–102. Available online database: Health Source Plus and Academic Search Elite.

Grossman, D. (1998). We are training our kids to kill. *Saturday Evening Post, 27*(4), 64. Available online database: Academic Search Elite. 1–7.

Harrison, K., & Cantor, J. (1997). The relationship between media consumption and eating disorders. *Journal of Communications, 47,* 40–67. Available online database: EBSCOHost.

Huesman, L.R., & Moise, J. (1996). Media violence: A demonstrated public health threat to children. *Harvard Mental Health Letter, 12*(12), 5–8. Available online database: Health Source Plus. 1–4.

Jason, L.A., & Brackshaw, E. (1999). Access to T.V. contingent on physical activity: Effects on reducing T.V.-viewing and body-weight. *Journal of Behavior Therapy and Experimental Psychiatry, 30,* 145–151.

Jeffrey, R., & French, S. (1998). Epidemic obesity in the United States: are fast foods and television viewing contributing? *American Journal of Public Health, 88,* 277–281. Available online database: Academic Search Elite.

Kane, H.D., Taub, G., & Hayes, B.G. (2000). Interactive media and its contribution to the construction and destruction of values and character. *Journal of Humanistic Counseling Education & Development, 39,* 58–66. Available online database: Academic Search Elite. 1–7.

Moliter, F., & Hirsch, K.W. (1994). Children's toleration of real-life aggression after exposure to media violence: A replication of the Drabman and Thomas studies. *Child Study Journal, 24,* 191–208. Available online database: Health Source Plus. 1–10.

Nathanson, A., & Cantor, J. (2000). Reducing the aggression-promoting effect of violent cartoons by increasing children's fictional involvement with the victim: A study of active mediation. *Journal of Broadcasting & Electronic Media, 44,* 125–143. Available online database: Academic Search Elite. 1–15.

National Highway Traffic Safety Administration. (1999). *Traffic saftety facts, 1999—Young drivers* [on-line]. Available: http://www.nhtsa.dot.gov/people/ncsa/pdf/young99.pdf.

National Institute on Drug Abuse (NIDA) of the US Department of Health and Human Services. (2000). *High school and youth trends* [on-line]. National Institute on Drug Abuse (NIDA) Infofax. Available: http://www.nida.nih.gov/inforfax/HSYouthtrends.html.

Owens, J., Maxim, R., McGuinn, M., Nobile, C., Msall, M., & Alario, A. (1999) "Television-viewing habits and sleep disturbance in school children." *Pediatrics, 104,* e27. Available online database: Medline.

Pawlowski, C. (2000). *Glued to the Tube.* Naperville, IL: Sourcebooks.

Robinson, T.N., Chen, H.L., & Killen, J.D. (1998). Television and music video exposure and risk of adolescent alcohol use. *Pediatrics, 102e,* 54. Available online database: Ovid.

Sadeh, A., Raviv, A., & Gruber, R. (2000). Sleep patterns and sleep disruptions in school-age children. *Developmental Psychology. 36,* 291–301.

Schoenbachler, D., & Whittler, T. (1996). "Adolescent processing of social and physical threat communications." *Journal of Advertising, 25,* 37–55. Available online database: EBSCOhost.

Schooler, C., & Feighery, E. (1996). Seventh graders' self-reported exposure to cigarette marketing and its relationship to their smoking behavior. *American Journal of Public Health, 86,* 1216–1222.

Senate Committee on the Judiciary. (1999). *Children, violence, and the media* (pp. 1–21) [on-line]. Available: http://www.senate.gov.

Singer, M., Slovak, K., Frierson, T., & York, P. (1998). Viewing preferences, symptoms of psychological trauma, and violent behaviors among children who watch television. *Journal of American Academy of Child and Adolescent Psychiatry, 37*(10), 1041–1048.

Song, E., & Anderson, J. (2001) How violent video games may violate children's health. *Contemporary Pediatrics, 18,* 102–113.

Steele, J.R. (1999). Teenage sexuality and media practice: factoring in the influences of family, friends, and school. *Journal of Sex Research, 36,* 331–341. Available online database: Academic Search Elite.

Strasburger, V.C., & Donnerstein, E. (1999). Children, adolescents and the media: Issues and solutions. *Pediatrics, 103,* 129–140. Available online database: Academic Search Elite.

Sustein, C. (2000). Marketing of violent media to children. Statement before the Senate Judiciary Committee. *FDCH Congressional Testimony, 9/20/2000* (pp. 1–8). Available online database: Academic Search Elite.

Thomas, S.G. (1999). Kids wrists at risk. *US News and World Report, 127,* 62–63.

Tjaden, P., & Thoennes, N. (1998). *Prevention, incidence, and consequences of violence against women: Findings from the National*

Violence Against Women Survey. Washington, DC: National Institute of Justice, Centers for Disease Control and Prevention.

Tremblay, M.S., & Williams, J.D. (2000). Secular trends in the body mass index of Canadian children. *Canadian Medical Association Journal, 163,* 1429–1433. Available online database: PubMed.

Ward., L.M., & Rivadeneyra, R. (1999). Contributions of entertainment television to adolescents' sexual attitudes and expectations: the role of viewing amount versus viewer involvement. *The Journal of Sex Research, 36,* 237–249.

Zillmann, D. (2000). Influence of unrestrained access to erotica on adolescents' and young adults' dispositions toward sexuality. *Journal of Adolescent Health, 27S,* 41–44. Available online database: Ovid.

Mental Health, Adulthood

James E. Maddux, C.R. Snyder, and David B. Feldman

INTRODUCTION

This entry reviews theory and research on promoting mental health in adulthood through a focus on promoting happiness rather than preventing mental disorder. Most of the entry discusses of the various roles that goals and goal-related beliefs play in the construction of satisfying, fulfilling, and "mentally health" lives.

DEFINITIONS

Any discussion of how to promote "mental health" needs to begin with a definition of that term. The many definitions offered over the years have ranged from freedom from mental disorder to the attainment of optimal psychological functioning (self-actualization) (Korchin, 1976). Traditional approaches to promoting mental health have focused primarily on the prevention of mental illness or disorder. The *Diagnostic and statistical manual of mental disorders-IV-TR* (American Psychiatric Association [APA], 2000) defines "mental disorder" as "a clinically significant behavioral or psychological syndrome or pattern that occurs in an individual and that is associated with present distress ... or disability ... or with a significantly increased risk of suffering, death, pain, disability, or an important loss of freedom" (p. xxxi). Given this definition of "mental disorder," the traditional approach to promoting mental health would consist of preventing distress, suffering, pain, disability,

death, or loss of freedom and the prevention of one or more of the hundreds of syndromes described in the *DSM*.

This traditional definition of mental health and the traditional preventive approach are too narrow and limited. They emphasize preventing disability and deficient functioning rather than promoting strengths and optimal functioning. Thus, the research discussed in this entry is not concerned with preventing "suffering, death, pain, disability, or an important loss of freedom" (APA, 2000, p. xxxi) or specific mental disorders, but with enhancing people's feelings of well-being and their satisfaction with their lives and themselves—typically referred to as *happiness.*

Quite a bit is known about the predictors of happiness, but less is known about its causes. This article focuses on those predictors that appear to be causes. People have considerable control over *what* they try to accomplish in life and *how* they try to accomplish it. Therefore, most of this entry discusses the relationship between happiness and people's *goals* (what people are trying to accomplish in life) and their *expectations* for attaining goals (their beliefs about their ability to achieve their goals). Related terms to be discussed include *hope* (the belief that there are means to attain goals and the belief that one can implement those means), *regret* (goals people wish they had pursued but did not), *flow* (loss of self-awareness during goal-related activity), *linking* (the perceived relationship between attainment of a goal and happiness), and *rumination* (obsessive thinking and worrying about unfulfilled goals). The entry also discusses how various *types of goals* are related to happiness.

SCOPE

Statistics on the prevalence of mental disorder and unhappiness depend largely on how those terms are defined. Most studies of the prevalence of mental disorder use the diagnostic criteria described in one of the various editions of the *DSM*. These studies suggest that up to 50 percent of people in the United States will experience a diagnosable mental disorder sometime during their lives and that up to 30 percent will experience such a disorder in a given 12-month period (Kessler et al., 1994). Studies of happiness usually ask people how satisfied they are with their lives or simply ask them how happy they are. A recent survey of adults in the United States found that the average life satisfaction rating was 7.73 on a 10-point scale (Diener, 2000). In another survey, 60 percent of adults in the United States reported that they were "pretty happy," yet 10 percent said that they were "not too happy" (Lykken, 1999).

Several questions remain concerning the relationship between unhappiness and mental disorder. For example, what percentage of people who consider themselves unhappy meet the diagnostic criteria for a *DSM* mental disorder? Likewise, what percentage of people who meet the diagnostic criteria for a mental disorder nonetheless consider themselves happy?

THEORIES

The use of the word "happiness" immediately raises philosophical and scientific issues that can be only touched on here. One of the major controversies in the study of happiness concerns the distinction between the *hedonic* approach, which focuses on the attainment of pleasure and the avoidance of pain, and the *eudaimonic* approach (from "daimon," meaning "true self"), which focuses on meaning and self-realization (Ryan & Deci, 2001). Choosing between these two approaches is not a matter that can be settled by science because the choice is between two different conceptual definitions that reflect different sets of values. The approach we take in this entry is more eudaimonic than hedonic because we are concerned with people's satisfaction with themselves and their lives—that is, the degree to which they feel good about themselves and their lives, not just the degree to which they "feel good." The term *subjective well-being* (Diener, Suh, Lucas, & Smith, 1999), which is has both cognitive (evaluative or eudaimonic) and affective (emotional or hedonic) components (Diener et al., 1999), probably captures this idea best. For convenience, however, we will use the term "happiness."

The other major controversy involves the distinction between "bottom–up" and "top–down" theories of happiness. According to the bottom-up theory, happiness is primarily the result of the accumulation of objectively positive life experiences (Feist, Bodner, Jacobs, Miles, & Tan, 1995). According to the top–down view, happiness results from one's tendency to interpret life experiences in positive or negative ways (Feist et al., 1995). Science can shed some light on the utility of these different approaches, and research thus far primarily supports the top–down theory (Lyubomirsky, 2001).

RESEARCH

A *genetic predisposition* may account for as much as half of the variance in current happiness and as much as 80 percent of the variance in long-term (i.e., 10 years) happiness (Lykken & Tellegen, 1996). Genetics may strongly influence the establishment of a happiness set point to which a person returns following a rise or fall in happiness resulting from a positive or negative life event (Diener et al., 1999).

One way that genes influence happiness is through their influence on *extraversion* and *agreeableness*. Extraverted people are generally happier than introverted people (Diener et al., 1999), and highly agreeable people are usually happier than less agreeable people (DeNeve, 1999; DeNeve &

Cooper, 1998). Perhaps the genetic factors that predispose one to happiness also predispose one to extraversion and agreeableness; perhaps happiness makes individuals more sociable and agreeable; or perhaps being with people and being agreeable while with people makes most people happier.

Optimism is associated with happiness. People who expect favorable outcomes and believe that they can produce those outcomes are happier than people who tend to expect and believe otherwise (Diener et al., 1999; Schneider, 2001). Optimism is not an immutable trait but a set of beliefs and expectations that can be learned and self-taught (Seligman, 1991). One reason optimistic people may be happier is that their optimism leads them to remain engaged in life tasks and in efforts to achieve valued goals (Schneider, 2001). This assertion is supported by research on related constructs such as hope, self-efficacy, expectancy for control, and "positive illusions" (Diener et al., 1999).

Health is not strongly related to happiness. The relationship between physical health and happiness is strong when people rate their own health (subjective ratings) but weak or nonexistent when their health is rated more objectively, such as by their physicians (Diener et al., 1999; Okun & George, 1984). Perhaps because happy people also are optimistic, they view their health more positively than do less happy people.

Religious people are happier than non-religious people, especially when religiosity is measured by behavior rather than by attitude scales (Diener et al., 1999; Ellison, 1991). This research has been conducted mostly with Christians in the United States, however, and the extent to which the same associations hold true for other religions is uncertain. Religiosity may increase happiness because it helps people find meaning and purpose, increases optimism, and usually provides opportunities to be with other people, all of which are associated with greater happiness.

Intelligence (measured by traditional IQ tests) does not appear to be related to happiness, especially if the relationship between intelligence and demographic factors is statistically controlled (Diener et al., 1999).

Married people are generally happier than never married, divorced, separated, or widowed people (Diener et al., 1999). Although happier people may be more likely to get married than are less happy people, marriage does indeed seem to lead to greater happiness (Headey, Veenhoven, & Wearing, 1991), but only if one is happily married (Diener et al., 1999). Living together while not married also seems to increase happiness as long as such arrangements are not inconsistent with cultural norms (Diener et al., 1999).

Age is related to happiness in complex ways, but it is certainly not true that happiness diminishes with age. Although people become less joyful as they age (Charles, Reynolds, & Gatz, 2001), they report decreases in negative affect (Charles et al., 2001) and greater satisfaction with their lives (Diener & Suh, in press). The frequency of positive emotions appears to diminish slightly beginning in the 1960s, but so do loneliness, depression, and boredom (Charles et al., 2001). Aging extroverts fare better than aging introverts (Charles et al., 2001).

Gender does not seem to be related to happiness (Diener et al., 1999). Although the incidence of depression is higher among women than men, this tendency to experience greater and more frequent negative affect than do men may be offset by the tendency of women to experience more frequent and strong positive emotions (Lee, Seecombe, & Shehan, 1991).

Employed people are generally are happier than unemployed people, and this difference does not seem to be related to income differences (Diener et al., 1999). Those who are satisfied with their jobs are happier than those who are dissatisfied with their jobs, although happier people may simply be happier wherever they are (Stones & Kozma, 1986).

Education is weakly associated with happiness, although this association is stronger among lower-income people and people in poor countries (Campbell, 1981). This association may be due to the positive impact of education on occupational status, as well as on people's abilities to pursue their personal goals (Diener et al., 1999).

Wealth is associated only weakly with happiness. In the United States, very rich people are only slightly happier than the non-rich (Diener, Horowitz, & Emmons, 1985). Increases in income are sometimes associated with increases in happiness, but not always (Brickman, Coates, & Janoff-Bulman, 1978). Between 1946 and 1990, the average purchasing power of the citizens of France, Japan, and the United States doubled, but average happiness did not increase (Diener & Suh, 1997). Within nations, the correlation between income and happiness averages about 0.17 (Haring, Okun, & Stock, 1984). Although the association between income and happiness is strongly positive across nations, this may be due to the fact that wealthier countries are usually more democratic, free, and egalitarian than poorer ones (Diener et al., 1999).

Social comparisons may influence happiness (Diener & Fujita, 1997). Happier people are more likely to compare themselves only to worse off others (downward comparison), whereas less happy people compare themselves both to those who are worse off and to those who are better off than they are (upward comparison) (Lyubomirsky & Ross, 1997).

Finally, people who believe that they have a *purpose in life* and who report clearly defined *goals* on which they are making progress are generally happier than people who do not (Brunstein, 1993; Snyder, in press). In keeping with our focus on the contributors to happiness that people can control, the remainder of this entry deals with the relationship between goals and happiness.

Goals and the Construction of Happy Lives

As noted previously, research supports the top–down theory of happiness—that happiness does not just happen and does not seem to be caused directly by specific life events but, instead, is constructed. Happy people seem to be those people who actively construct their lives so as to get what will bring them happiness and who actively construe life events in ways that promote happiness (Lyubomirsky, 2001). One important way in which people construct their lives is by setting goals and working toward them. Goals influence happiness in a number of ways. Goals influence happiness through their relationships with positive and negative emotions, hope, regret, flow, linking, and goal-related rumination. Happiness is influenced also by the types of goals people choose to pursue.

Goals and Emotions

To a large extent, happiness involves experiencing positive emotions more often than negative emotions. When people perceive that they are successfully pursuing desired goals, they experience positive emotions (Snyder, Sympson, Ybasco, Borders, Babyak, & Higgins, 1996), and when they perceive barriers that impede goal pursuits, they experience negative emotions (Emmons, 1986). Furthermore, people's perceived lack of progress toward major goals seems to be the cause of reductions in well-being, rather than vice versa (Brunstein, 1993).

Hope: Goals and the Future

Goals will enhance happiness only if people believe that they can attain them—that is, if they have *hope*. Snyder et al. (1991) have defined hope as involving three interrelated cognitive components: goals, pathways, and agency. A *goal* is an imagined end-point or state that the person wants to attain (e.g., a college degree) or avoid (e.g., illness). *Pathways* beliefs are appraisals of one's proficiency in generating plausible plans to attain desired goals. Thoughts of multiple pathways often become available when encountering impediments to goals. When facing impediments, high-hope people: (1) see themselves as being able to come up with alternate routes; and (2) actually do produce more alternative routes than do low-hope individuals (Irving, Snyder, & Crowson, 1998).

Agency is the perceived capacity to use the routes to desired goals. Agency is manifest in affirmative thoughts regarding one's ability to initiate *and* sustain movement along pathways to desired goals (Snyder, LaPointe, Crowson, & Early, 1998). Agency and pathway thoughts influence each other such that an increase in pathways thinking is likely to increase agency which, in turn, fuels further pathway thinking, and so on. Agentic thinking is particularly important when initial routes are blocked and motivation must be redirected to alternate pathways (Snyder, 1994).

Hope is related to a number of dimensions of psychological adjustment (Snyder et al., 1991). Hopeful people are more likely than persons with lower hope to view impediments in goal-pursuit as challenges rather than as threats, to focus their attention on the consequences of success rather than of failure, and to estimate a greater probability of attaining success (Snyder, in press). Accordingly, higher hope has been associated with superior academic performance, better athletic performance, and more favorable psychotherapy outcomes (Snyder, in press). Hope is also associated with health-related benefits, such as adjustment to cancer and other chronic diseases (Snyder, Feldman, Taylor, Schroeder, & Adams, 2000). In addition, optimism and self-efficacy, constructs theoretically related to hope, are associated with a number of aspects of psychological and physical well-being (Bandura, 1997; Maddux, 1995; Maddux & Meier, 1995; Scheier & Carver, 1992). Finally, hope is closely associated with people's perceptions that their lives are filled with meaning (Feldman & Snyder, 2001).

Goals, however, do not achieve themselves. Goal-pursuit is a process that demands intense cognitive activity; it entails the construction and implementation of pathways, and the generation of self-mobilizing agentic thoughts. When people hold strong beliefs that they can attain a goal, they are more likely to initiate goal-related action, persist in the face of difficulties, and actually achieve what they set out to achieve (Bandura, 1997; Maddux, 1995). Thus, hope is a future-focused construct, but one through which people construct meaningful, satisfying, and happy existences in the here and now.

Regret: Goals and the Past

Happiness is influenced not only by our beliefs about what could be (hope) but also by our beliefs about what might have been. Goals that people wish they had actively pursued, but did not, are called *regrets* (Lecci, Okun, & Karoly, 1994). Regrets influence happiness when the person worries about what could have been to the detriment of hopeful and constructive thinking and planning about what realistically still could be (i.e., current goals; Klinger, 1977).

Regrets have not been studied extensively, but the findings so far are illuminating. In one study, college students were asked to rate both their most important life regret and their most important current goal along such dimensions as importance, attainability, distress, and disappointment (Lecci et al., 1994). They also completed measures of subjective well-being, life satisfaction, and negative affect.

Among older subjects (age 33+), the number of regrets correlated negatively with subjective well-being. Among younger subjects (18–32), however, subjective well-being was positively associated with the belief that they could have attained the discarded goals if they had decided to pursue them. Thus, younger people may feel less regretful about an abandoned goal if they believe they could have attained it but chose not to, rather than if they believe they gave up because they lacked the ability and means to attain it. This suggests that people are distressed less by an abandoned goal if they maintain a strong sense of self-efficacy and some hope that they might one day be able to attain it.

The finding that happiness is more strongly associated with construal of regrets than with number of regrets suggests that regrets are not all equal. A random telephone survey in a medium-sized city (Gilovich & Medvec, 1994) asked 60 adults whether their biggest regrets were regrets of *action* (i.e., things they did, but now wish they had not done) or regrets of *inaction* (i.e., things they did not do, but now wish they had done). Three fourths said they regretted most those actions not taken. In addition, 77 others adults were asked to describe the biggest regrets of their lives, but with no mention of the action-inaction distinction. They reported almost twice as many regrets of inaction as regrets of action (63 vs. 37 percent). In another study, adults were asked to describe their biggest regret of the past week and the biggest regret of their lives. Slightly more than half of these adults reported that their biggest regrets of the past week were actions taken that turned out badly, but 84 percent said that the biggest regrets of their lives were actions they *failed* to take or goals they failed to pursue. Among the most common regrets of inaction were missed opportunities for education, romance, time with family, and intellectual or artistic pursuits, as well as a general failure to take risks or "seize the moment."

Flow: Goals and the Present Moment

Hope is a future-centered construct, consistent with Western civilization's notion that happiness is something to be attained in one's journey toward the future. Eastern philosophies such as Taoism and Zen Buddhism, however, teach us that happiness is not something to be earned but something to be discovered by immersing ourselves in the present moment. According to Czikszentmihalyi's (1990) research, "the best moments of our lives are not the passive, receptive, and relaxing times [but times] when a person's body or mind is stretched to the limits in a voluntary effort to accomplish something difficult and worthwhile" (p. 3). These are the times "in which people are so involved in an activity that nothing else seems to matter; the experience itself is so enjoyable that people will do it even at great cost, for the sheer sake of doing it" (p. 4). He refers to this experience as flow, and suggests that happiness depends on the degree to which people experience flow in daily life.

Flow is dependent on two basic conditions—that the activity is *goal-directed* and has clear *rules*. Without goals and rules, we cannot get feedback on how well we are doing. Without the experience of continuous and immediate feedback, the kind of engrossment in an activity that leads to loss of self-consciousness, temporary freedom from worries and frustrations, and alteration in the sense of time is impossible.

In Czikszentmihalyi and LeFevre (1989), over 100 men and women working full-time at a variety of occupations wore electronic pagers for one week. The pagers were triggered at random, eight times daily. Each time the pagers sounded, subjects recorded in a booklet what they were doing and how they were feeling at that time, including indicating (on a 10-point scale) how many challenges they faced at the moment and how many skills they believed they were using. An individual was considered to be "in flow" whenever he or she indicated that both challenge level and skill level were above the mean for the week (a liberal definition of flow, the authors concede). As predicted, the amount of time spent in flow during the week was correlated positively with the overall quality of subjects' reported experience. During flow, subjects typically reported feeling strong, activated, creative, and motivated. When challenges and skills were both high, subjects reported feeling happier, more cheerful, stronger, and more active; they concentrated more; and, they felt more creative and satisfied.

An unexpected finding was the frequency with which people reported flow situations at work relative to leisure. People reported being in flow 54 percent of the time when signaled while working (actually working, not simply at their place of work), but only 18 percent of the time when engaged in leisure activities such as reading, watching TV, socializing, or dining at a restaurant. The leisure responses were typically in the range the authors called *apathy*, which was characterized by below-average levels of both challenges and skills and by reports of feeling passive, weak, dull, and dissatisfied. Most of the time while at leisure (52 percent), subjects were in this state of apathy; when working, however, only 16 percent of subjects' responses were in the apathy region. Thus, we have a paradoxical situation: On the job, people often feel both challenged and skillful and, therefore, relatively happy, strong, creative, and satisfied. In their free time, however, people usually feel that there is generally not much to do and that their skills are not being used; therefore, they tend to feel more sad, weak, dull, and dissatisfied. Ironically, work is actually easier to enjoy than free time, because it often boasts built-in goals, rules, feedback, and challenges, all of which encourage involvement in one's activities, concentration, and losing oneself in the present moment. Nonetheless, most people say that they would like to work less and spend more time in leisure!

Certainly people value work and devote time and energy to work for reasons other than its capacity for leading to a flow experience. Our society, for example, places a high premium on productivity and rewards devotion to work. This notion, however, can explain only why people spend so much time at work, not why they report enjoying it more than their leisure time. People also may spend more time working to avoid the relative emptiness and ennui of leisure time, which they may find unrewarding and even distressing because of its lack of structure and engrossment and the uncomfortable self-awareness that emerges.

Happiness may be the result not of goal attainment but of being absorbed in goal-directed activity—that is, in flow. The paradox of goals and happiness, therefore, is that without the goal, attainment of flow and happiness is impossible; yet when we find ourselves consciously aware of the goal and our goal-directed activity, flow is disrupted, and we are no longer happy. Thus, having goals is essential to achieving happiness, but thinking about our goals while working toward them interferes with happiness. This notion also suggests that hope will produce happiness if it leads to active engagement in goal-directed activities rather than passive daydreaming.

Linking and Ruminating: Obsessing over Goals Unfulfilled

Support for the paradox described previously is provided by recent research on the role of goal-related *linking* and *rumination* in unhappiness. Linking refers to the degree to which a person believes that attainment of a particular goal is essential for happiness (Martin & Tesser, 1989). Rumination refers not to productive planning and strategizing but to what most people call "worrying" and "obsessing" (Martin & Tesser, 1989). Rumination occurs when progress toward a highly valued goal has been blocked and we become unpleasantly aware of the discrepancy between what we want and what we have. Rumination is most likely to occur in response to perceptions of failure to attain a higher-order abstract goal such as happiness (Martin & Tesser, 1989). Thus, the non-attainment of a lower-order goal will lead to rumination to the extent that the person believes that attainment of this goal is essential to happiness (Brothers & Maddux, in press). This linking of a goal with happiness will lead to rumination even when people believe that they are on the right track toward goal attainment. Rumination is unpleasant. In addition, rumination makes flow impossible because flow requires intense attention, concentration, and absorption in the task at hand. Thus, the belief that a certain goal is essential to happiness is likely to diminish happiness because this linkage leads to rumination, which interferes with flow.

Types of Goals and Happiness

The concept of flow suggests that any strongly desired goal can be conducive to the attainment of the flow experience and thus to happiness. Yet common sense, experience, and psychological theory (e.g., Deci & Ryan, 1985; Maslow, 1962) suggest that some goals are more conducive to happiness than others. For example, extrinsic goals that depend on external reward or the reactions of others may be related less strongly to happiness than intrinsic goals based on deeply held values (e.g., Emmons, 1991). This view is consistent with the eudaimonic approach to happiness noted previously.

People whose goals are congruent with their general motives and values report greater life satisfaction than people whose goals are less consistent with their motives and values (Brunstein, Schultheiss, & Maier, 1999). Also, people whose goals are congruent with each other (i.e., non-conflicting) and coherently organized are generally happier than people with goals that are less organized and less congruent (Emmons & King, 1988; Sheldon & Kasser, 1995).

Kasser and Ryan (1993) investigated four types of goals derived from theory and research: *self-acceptance* goals (psychological growth, self-esteem, and autonomy); *affiliation* goals (securing satisfying personal relationships); *community feeling* goals (altruistic commitments and making the world a better place); and *financial success* goals (attaining wealth and material success). They found that people who placed greater emphasis on self-acceptance, affiliation, and community feeling than on financial goals were happier than people who placed greater emphasis on financial goals. These results are consistent with the general finding that income and standard of living are not associated with happiness once a person has sufficient income to meet basic needs (Diener et al., 1999). These findings also are consistent with the finding that the vast majority of people's biggest regrets concern personal development and relationships (Gilovich & Medvec, 1994).

Thus, simply having goals may not guarantee happiness. What those goals are and on what values they are based may be equally or more important. Striving for self-improvement, healthy relationships, and a place for oneself in one's community (however defined) seem more likely to bring peace of mind than striving for financial and material success.

STRATEGIES THAT WORK

Research has not yet provided us with sure-fire recipes for happiness and mental health, so we can offer none here.

STRATEGIES THAT MIGHT WORK

Fortunately, the causes of happiness suggested by research are ones over which people have considerable control. This research suggests that happiness is likely to be attained by:

- Keeping in mind that happiness does not just happen. Happy lives are actively constructed. If people simply wait for happiness, it probably will not come; but if they get busy trying to construct happy lives, they are likely to have some success.
- Developing and nurturing close relationships. Most people will accomplish this by getting married or finding a domestic partner. If this is not a viable or desirable option, developing and nurturing a small network of very close friends and family members is an alternative pathway.
- Striving to be more hopeful, optimistic, and self-efficacious. Like happiness, these attitudes and beliefs can be learned and practiced.
- Developing a sense of religiosity or spirituality, and perhaps even joining a group of people with similar beliefs.
- Reducing or eliminating upward comparisons—that is, comparisons to people who are "better off" in some way or another. Instead, people should compare their lots to those less fortunate and "count their blessings."
- Accepting growing older with grace and even gratitude. Because people's sense of control, self-satisfaction, peace, and contentment usually increase they get older, aging is now something to which more and more people can truly look forward.
- Working. Working need not refer only to full-time employment for pay. Work comes in many varieties, including community service and other volunteer activities. Continuing education and many hobbies can be viewed as forms of work. What is important is to become engaged in endeavors that are consistent with one's values, give meaning and purpose to life, and provide the challenge, rules, and feedback necessary for experiencing flow.
- Finding meaning and purpose. This is best done by developing goals that serve one's personal values and motives, generating plans for attaining them, and getting down to work.
- Developing hope. Once you have chosen your goals, actively look for a variety of strategies (pathways) for accomplishing them, and actively develop strong self-efficacy beliefs (agency) by paying attention to what you have done well and to small bits of progress and improvement.

- Remembering that not all goals are equally conducive to happiness. Most important, research suggests that money does not buy happiness and that the best moments in life are those that leave people feeling competent, worthwhile, self-sufficient, and connected with others.
- Remembering that, in the long run, the biggest regrets are often over actions not taken and goals not pursued rather than over actions taken that turned out badly and goals that were pursued but not attained.

STRATEGIES THAT DO NOT WORK

The happiness-construction approach and the research reviewed here suggests that happiness (and thus mental health) will not be attained by:

- Wishing and hoping. Passivity and inactivity are likely to be ineffective and counterproductive because they are incompatible with being in flow and because they are likely to lead to rumination about unfulfilled goals.
- Passing the buck (euro). The pursuit of financial goals seems to be inversely related to satisfaction with life and self.
- Having it all. It is not the attainment of goals themselves that determine happiness but the experience of flow while actively engaged in attaining them.
- Playing it safe. The vast majority of unhappiness-inducing regrets are not over goals that were pursued but not attained but over goals that were envisioned but never pursued.
- Going it alone. Introverted people are not as happy as extraverted people, and people without close relationships are not as happy as those with close relationships.
- Killing time. People are more like to experience flow and thus feel happy and satisfied when they are working than when they are at leisure because, for most people, leisure time is idle time—that is, goal-less and unstructured.

SYNTHESIS

Future research on promoting mental health in adulthood needs to make a radical shift from the assumptions that have guided psychology and psychiatry for the past century. The first important shift is from the assumption that the best way to promote mental health is to prevent psychological disorders to the assumption that the best way to promote mental health is to enhance happiness. The new "positive psychology" movement (Snyder & Lopez, 2001) provides a philosophical and scientific foundation for changing our focus from the prevention of human psychological disabilities and weaknesses to the enhancement of human abilities and strengths, including the capacity for happiness. This is essentially a change away from the "illness ideology" that has shaped clinical psychology and psychiatry for the past hundred years (Maddux, 2001).

The second basic shift is from the assumption is that happiness is the result of what happens to people to the assumption that happiness is constructed through the choices people make about what they do with their lives and how they construe what happens to them. This shift will be as much (if not more so) a shift that non-professionals need to make in their understanding of mental health as a shift in what professionals assume or believe. Research on how people actively construct happiness in the various ways noted previously should add much to our knowledge of how to promote mental health among adults, beginning with promoting it among children.

People cannot always control what happens to them, but they can exert considerable control over the goals toward which they aspire, the activities in which in they engage to move them toward their goals, and the meanings they ascribe to life events that may be beyond their control. Thus, this combined happiness-promotion/happiness-construction approach requires that researchers focus less identifying the life events that produce happiness and unhappiness and focus more on identifying the happiness-promoting aspects of life over which people can exert some control, including their construal of so-called positive and negative life events.

Also see: Culture, Society, and Social Class: Foundation; Politics and System Change: Foundation; Children, Parents with Mental Illness: Childhood; Depression: Childhood; Depression: Adolescence; Depression: Adulthood; Depression: Older Adulthood; Families with Parental Mental Illness: Adolescence; Family Strengthening: Childhood; Family Strengthening: Adolescence.

ACKNOWLEDGMENT

The first author would like to thank Ernest Mundell, Patricia Rippetoe, and Gregory Pence for their helpful comments on an earlier version of this entry.

References

American Psychiatric Association (APA). (2000). *Diagnostic and statistical manual of mental disorders* (4th ed., text revision).

Bandura, A. (1997). *Self-efficacy: The exercise of control.* New York: W.H. Freeman and Co.

Brickman, P., Coates, D., & Janoff-Bulman, R. (1978). Lottery winners and accident victims: Is happiness relative? *Journal of Personality and Social Psychology, 36,* 917–927.

Brothers, S.C., & Maddux, J.E. (in press). The goal of biological parenthood and emotional distress from infertility: Linking parenthood to happiness. *Journal of Applied Social Psychology.*

Brunstein, J.C. (1993). Personal goals and subjective well-being: A longitudinal study. *Journal of Personality and Social Psychology, 63*(5), 1061–1070.

Brunstein, J.C., Schultheiss, O.C., & Maier, G.W. (1999). The pursuit of personal goals: A motivational approach to well-being and life adjustment. In J.C. Brandtstaedter & R.M. Lerner (Eds.), *Action & self-development: Theory and research through the life span* (pp. 169–196). Thousand Oaks, CA: Sage.

Campbell, A. (1981). *The sense of well-being in America: Recent patterns and trends.* New York: McGraw-Hill.

Charles, S.T., Reynolds, C.A., & Gatz, M. (2001). Age-related differences and change in positive affect over 23 years. *Journal of Personality and Social Psychology, 80,* 136–151.

Czikszentmihalyi, M. (1990). *Flow.* New York: Harper Perennial.

Czikszentmihalyi, M., & LeFevre, J. (1989). Optimal experience in work and leisure. *Journal of Personality and Social Psychology, 56*(5), 815–822.

Deci, E.L., & Ryan, R.M. (1985). *Intrinsic motivation and self-determination in human behavior.* New York: Plenum Press.

DeNeve, K.M. (1999). Happy as an extraverted clam? The role of personality for subjective well-being. *Current Directions in Psychological Science, 8,* 141–144.

DeNeve, K.M., & Cooper, H. (1998). The happy personality: A meta-analysis of 137 personality traits and subjective well-being. *Psychological Bulletin, 124,* 197–229.

Diener, E. (2000). Subjective well-being: The science of happiness and a proposal for a national index. *American Psychologist, 55,* 34–43.

Diener, E., & Fujita, F. (1997). Social comparisons and subjective well-being. In B. Buunk & R. Gibbons (Eds.), *Health, coping, and social comparison* (pp. 329–357). Mahwah, NJ: Erlbaum.

Diener, E., Horowitz, J., & Emmons, R.A. (1985). Happiness of the very healthy. *Social Indicators Research, 16,* 263–274.

Diener, E., & Suh, E.M. (1997). Measuring quality of life: Economic, social, and subjective indicators. *Social Indicators Research, 40,* 189–216.

Diener, E., & Suh, E.M. (Eds.). (in press). *Subjective well-being across cultures.* Cambridge, MA: MIT Press.

Diener, E., Suh, E.M., Lucas, R.E., & Smith, H.L. (1999). Subjective well-being: Three decades of progress. *Psychological Bulletin, 125,* 276–302.

Ellison, C.G. (1991). Religious involvement and subjective well-being. *Journal of Health and Social Behavior, 32,* 80–99.

Emmons, R.A. (1986). Personal strivings: An approach to personality and subjective well-being. *Journal of Personality and Social Psychology, 51,* 1058–1068.

Emmons, R.A. (1991). Personal strivings, daily life events, and psychological and physical well-being. *Journal of Personality, 59,* 453–472.

Emmons, R.A., & King, L.A. (1988). Conflict among personal strivings: Immediate and long-term implications for psychological and physical well-being. *Journal of Personality and Social Psychology, 54,* 1040–1048.

Feldman, D.B., & Snyder, C.R. (2001). *Hope and meaning in life: A new approach to an old problem.* Unpublished manuscript.

Feist, G.J., Bodner, T.E., Jacobs, J.F., Miles, M., & Tan, V. (1995). Integrating top–down and bottom–up structural models of subjective well-being: A longitudinal investigation. *Journal of Personality of Social Psychology, 68,* 138–150.

Gilovich, T., & Medvec, V.H. (1994). The temporal pattern to the experience of regret. *Journal of Personality and Social Psychology, 67,* 357–365.

Haring, M.J., Okun, M.A., & Stock, W.A. (1984). A quantitative synthesis of literature on work status and subjective well-being. *Journal of Vocational Behavior, 25,* 316–324.

Headey, B., Veenhoven, R., & Wearing, A. (1991). Top–down versus bottom–up theories of subjective well-being. *Social Indicators Research, 24,* 81–100.

Irving, L.M., Snyder, C.R., & Crowson, J.J., Jr. (1998). Hope and the negotiation of cancer facts by college women. *Journal of Personality, 66,* 195–214.

Kasser, T., & Ryan, R.M. (1993). A dark side of the American dream: Correlates of financial success as a central life aspiration. *Journal of Personality and Social Psychology, 65*(2), 410–422.

Kessler, R.C., McGonagle, K.A., Zhao, S., Nelson, C.B., Hughes, M., Eshleman, S., Wittchen, H., & Kendler, K.S. (1994). Lifetime and 12-month prevalence of *DSM-III-R* psychiatric disorders in the United States. *Archives of General Psychiatry, 51,* 8–19.

Klinger, E. (1977). *Meaning and void: Inner experience and incentives in people's lives.* Minneapolis: University of Minnesota Press.

Korchin, S.J. (1976). *Modern clinical psychology.* New York: Basic Books.

Lee, G.R., Seecombe, K., & Shehan, C.L. (1991). Marital status and personal happiness: An analysis of trend data. *Journal of Marriage and the Family, 53,* 839–844.

Lecci, L., Okun, M.A., & Karoly, P. (1994). Life regrets and current goals as predictors of psychological adjustment. *Journal of Personality and Social Psychology, 66*(4), 731–741.

Lykken, D. (1999). *Happiness.* New York: Golden Books.

Lykken, D., & Tellegen, A. (1996). Happiness is a stochastic phenomenon. *Psychological Science, 7,* 186–189.

Lyubomirsky, S. (2001). Why are some people happier than others? The role of cognitive and motivational processes in well-being. *American Psychologist, 56,* 239–249.

Lyubomirsky, S., & Ross, L. (1997). Hedonic consequences of social comparison: A contrast of happy and unhappy people. *Journal of Personality and Social Psychology, 73,* 1141–1157.

Maddux, J.E. (1995). Self-efficacy theory: An introduction. In J.E. Maddux (Ed.), *Self-efficacy, adaptation, and adjustment: Theory, research and application* (pp. 3–33). New York: Plenum.

Maddux, J.E. (2001). Stopping the "madness": Positive psychology and the deconstruction of the illness ideology and the *DSM.* In C.R. Snyder & S.J. Lopez (Eds.), *Handbook of positive psychology.* New York: Oxford University Press.

Maddux, J.E., & Meier, L.J. (1995). Self-efficacy and depression. In J.E. Maddux (Ed.), *Self-efficacy, adaptation, and adjustment: Theory, research and application* (pp. 143–169). New York: Plenum.

Martin, L.L., & Tesser, A. (1989). Toward a motivational and structural theory of ruminative thought. In J.S. Uleman & J.A. Bargh (Eds.), *Unintended thought: The limits of awareness, intention, and control* (pp. 306–326). New York: Guilford.

Maslow, A.H. (1962). *Toward a psychology of being.* Princeton, NJ: Van Nostrand.

Okun, M.A., & George, L.K. (1984). Physician- and self-ratings of health, neuroticism, and subjective well-being among men and women. *Personality and Individual Differences, 5,* 533–539.

Ryan, R.M., & Deci, E.L. (2001). On happiness and human potential: A review of research on hedonic and eudaimonic well-being. *Annual Review of Psychology, 52,* 141–166.

Scheier, M.F., & Carver, C.S. (1992). Effects of optimism on psychological and physical well-being: Theoretical overview and empirical update. *Cognitive Therapy and Research, 16*(2), 201–228.

Schneider, S.L. (2001). In search of realistic optimism. *American Psychologist, 56,* 250–263.

Seligman, M.E.P. (1991). *Learned optimism.* New York: Knopf.

Sheldon, K.M., & Kasser, T. (1995). Coherence and congruence: Two aspects of personality integration. *Journal of Personality and Social Psychology, 68,* 531–543.

Snyder, C.R. (1994). *The psychology of hope: You can get there from here.* New York: Free Press.

Snyder, C.R. (in press). Hope theory: Rainbows in the mind. *Psychological Inquiry.*

Snyder, C.R., Feldman, D.B., Taylor, J.D., Schroeder, L.L., & Adams, V., III. (2000). The roles of hopeful thinking in preventing problems and enhancing strengths. *Applied and Preventive Psychology, 15,* 262–295.

Snyder, C.R., Harris, C., Anderson, J.R., Holleran, S.A., Irving, L.M., Sigmon, S.T., Yoshinobo, L., Gibb, J., Langelle, C., & Harney, P. (1991). The will and the ways: Development and validation of an individual-differences measure of hope. *Journal of Personality and Social Psychology, 60,* 570–585.

Snyder, C.R., LaPointe, A.B., Crowson, J.J., Jr., & Early, S. (1998). Preferences of high- and low-hope people for self-referential input. *Cognition & Emotion, 12,* 807–823.

Snyder, C.R., & Lopez, S.J. (2001). *Handbook of positive psychology.* New York: Oxford University Press.

Snyder, C.R., Sympson, S.C., Ybasco, F.C., Borders, T.F., Babyak, M.A., & Higgins, R.L. (1996). Development and validation of the State Hope Scale. *Journal of Personality and Social Psychology, 70,* 321–335.

Stones, M.J., & Kozma, A. (1986). "Happy are they who are happy...": A test between two causal models of happiness and its correlates. *Experimental Aging Research, 12,* 23–29.

N

Nuclear Families, Childhood

Gary W. Peterson and Hilary A. Rose

INTRODUCTION

Families with a mother and father who reside together with biologically related children remain a common setting for socializing school-age youngsters in our society. A much debated, but common presumption in the existing scholarship is that these nuclear families are the optimal environments for children against which the efficacy of all other types of families are measured (Popenoe, 1993, 1996). Observers frequently identify the potential advantages of nuclear families as: (a) parents mutually supporting each other in child-rearing, (b) parents sharing the responsibilities of child-rearing by structuring a division of labor (e.g., traditional or egalitarian role divisions), (c) parents and children profiting from long-term, biologically-based ties that provide continuous support and guidance, and (d) parents and children benefiting from the socioeconomic advantages provided by two adult wage earners. Although the actual realization of these advantages varies widely among nuclear families, this type of family structure has often been studied in reference to how it protects children from developing problem behaviors and how it fosters children's healthy development.

DEFINITIONS

The concept *nuclear family* refers to a specific family structure in which a mother and father reside in the same household (often due to marriage) with children who are either biologically related or adopted. Besides the purely structural benefits frequently ascribed to nuclear families (Popenoe, 1993), much of the literature on socialization within nuclear families has been focused on internal dynamics within the parent–child relationship that convey nurturance, provide companionship, and exercise moderate control, all of which foster social competence in children (Baumrind, 1980, 1991; Burgess, 1926; Parsons, 1944; Peterson & Hann, 1999).

Social competence is viewed as a set of attributes or psychological resources that assist children in adapting to their social circumstances and in coping sufficiently with everyday life to ward off problematic behavior (i.e., externalizing and internalizing behavior) (Baumrind, 1991; Peterson & Hann, 1999). A general definition of *social competence* is the ability of children to function adaptively in relationships with peers, parents, and others. Recent conceptions of social competence identify some of its subdimensions as: (a) a balance between autonomy and connectedness (i.e., emotionally close bonds and being receptive to parental influence) in reference to parents, (b) psychological or cognitive resources (e.g., self-esteem and problem-solving skills), and (c) social skills with peers and other interpersonal relationships (Peterson & Hann, 1999; Peterson & Leigh, 1990). Cultural and ethnic differences in children's social competence exist to the extent that different socialization priorities are assigned to becoming autonomous from others, conforming to authority figures, and the extent to which children's self-concepts are defined according to themes of individuality versus connections with others (Peterson, 1995).

Internalizing and externalizing behavior, two general categories of problematic outcomes, can be viewed as collections of attributes that contradict social competence. Externalizing behaviors refer to psychological difficulties that take the form of behavior problems (e.g., conduct disorder) reflecting the tendencies of children to "act out" against society. Internalizing behaviors, on the other hand, are those in which the difficulties of children become evident as psychological disturbances that focus on the self (e.g., depression or social withdrawal).

Most of the existing research also identifies a multidimensional pattern of socialization, *authoritative parenting*, as the primary approach that fosters social competence in children (Baumrind, 1991; Peterson & Hann, 1999). Authoritative parenting also appears to prevent the development of at-risk behavior (i.e., internalizing and externalizing behavior) by children during the elementary school years. An important means of preventing externalizing and internalizing behavior in the young child is through the tendency of authoritative parenting to foster social competence, the components of which function as protective factors that prevent the onset of problem behavior. When conceptualized in terms of component behaviors, authoritative parenting can include parental support, reasoning, limit setting, monitoring, and firm control, but contrasts with punitive or permissive approaches to parental control (Baumrind, 1991; Patterson & Capaldi, 1991; Peterson & Hann, 1999). Although significant questions remain about the generalizability of authoritative parenting to a broad range of ethnic-minority and socioeconomic populations (Demo & Cox, 2000), empirically supported prevention strategies for nuclear families often use concepts that are either based on or compatible with this conception of child-rearing.

SCOPE

Specific kinds of domestic arrangements, commonly referred to as nuclear families, have declined proportionately in our society at the same time that families of varied structural and relationship arrangements (e.g., mother-only families, the matriarchal structure of African American families, cohabitational families, stepfamilies, and families with gay parents) have increased as social venues for the socialization of children (Teachman, 2000). Some observers argue that children have become increasingly at-risk as nuclear families have declined proportionately in the population (Popenoe, 1993). Frequently cited are high divorce rates since the 1960s, increases in single-parent families, diminishing numbers of fathers who reside with their children,

and rising numbers of children who live in poverty within the context of mother-headed families (Amato & Booth, 1996; McLanahan & Sandefur, 1994; Popenoe, 1996). The primary problem, according to Popenoe (1993), is that our base-line form of the family (i.e., the nuclear family) is declining, with the result being that alternative family structures cannot provide such things as affection, companionship, and child socialization to the same degree of effectiveness.

Others provide a contrasting view by pointing to flaws in the view that declines in nuclear families inherently mean that "the family" is declining and that structural changes are the root of today's problems for many children. These critics point, in particular, to the excessive preoccupation with equating co-resident or nuclear families with the "normative" manifestation of "the family" (Allen, Fine, & Demo, 2000; Coontz, 1991, 1997). Instead, traditional nuclear families are viewed as being anachronistic for postmodern society by reinforcing the prominence of male "breadwinners," traditional gender role divisions of labor, and by restricting the economic and social emancipation of women. Other aspects of this argument involve acceptance of constant social change, the emergence of diverse family structures, and proposals that such alternative circumstances such as divorce and stepparenting have become normalized (Coontz, 1991; Osmond & Thorne, 1993; Stacey, 1993, 1996).

Dealing more specifically with the parent–child relationship is substantial evidence that parental competence varies widely within nuclear families (Peterson & Hann, 1999). Furthermore, only modest if any differences in children's social and personality outcomes have been traced specifically to variations in family structure (Demo & Cox, 2000; Teachman, 2000). Moreover, rather than having roots in specific family structural variations, children's psychosocial differences are often linked more precisely to socioeconomic disadvantages and the minimal support systems available to alternative families in our society (Coontz, 1997; Demo & Cox, 2000; Teachman, 2000).

The most frequent alternative to "structural explanations" for children's socialization, however, is the substantial body of evidence supporting the view that social psychological aspects of parent–child relationships are more relevant to children's prosocial or problematic outcomes than are family structural variables. These social psychological dimensions of parent–child relationships within nuclear families are conceptualized as being more directly predictive of children's psychosocial characteristics than are the more remote influences of family structure (Peterson & Hann, 1999). Rather than differing fundamentally, therefore, both nuclear and alternative families tend to have much in common in reference to the social psychological means of socializing children. Consequently, effective prevention strategies are not designed frequently to address the relative merits of family structural variations per se, but seek instead to improve the quality of parent–child relationships within nuclear families in a direct manner. A closely related strategy is to provide some form of support to parents so they, in turn, can cope more effectively and maintain effective child-rearing approaches with their children. A central conclusion in the current parent–child research within nuclear families is that a primary means of preventing children's problematic outcomes is to encourage parents in nuclear families to use child-rearing strategies that foster social competence (Baumrind, 1991; Peterson & Hann, 1999).

THEORIES AND RESEARCH

Attachment Theory

Attachment theory underscores the importance of early social bonding and the centrality of warm, supportive relationships between children and parents. The formation of secure attachment relationships is thought to promote social competence and prevent the eventual development of internalizing and externalizing behavior in children. An area of particular focus in this perspective is the importance of emotionally close relationships early in the lives of children as prototypes for later interpersonal associations. Drawing from ethological, evolutionary, neopsychoanalytic, and cognitive theories, the view is provided that human nature includes the inclination of the young to form strong emotional bonds with adults (Bowlby, 1988; Price & Rose, 2000). Attachment processes are thought to be rooted partially in genetic propensities of the young to seek attachment objects so that protection from harm and problematic circumstances can result.

Attachment theory proposes that infants and young children often develop proximity-seeking, emotionally-based ties with primary attachment objects, most frequently mothers, but also fathers and other adults. These early attachment relationships become models for later interpersonal associations and give rise to expectations for self and others in relationships. Consequently, a child's attachment increasingly consists of internalized representations of relationships that protect children from problematic involvements by "connecting" the young to supportive adults.

Central to this perspective is the proposal that secure emotional bonds with parents provide an essential basis for the development of adaptive autonomy—a complementary balance of two attributes that form an essential aspect of social competence (Peterson & Hann, 1999). Problems in development are more likely to occur for children when attachment bonds within the parent–child relationship are either disrupted or insecure. These problematic relationship

circumstances place the young at greater risk for developing personal and social adjustment problems (Bowlby, 1988).

Socialization Theory

Another prevention framework, the socialization perspective, also focuses specifically on the importance of high quality parent–child relationships within nuclear families as a means of discouraging problem behaviors in children. Socialization perspectives are eclectic in origin, with roots in such general frameworks as social learning theory in psychology and symbolic interaction theory in sociology. These perspectives provide the conceptual basis for the idea that child-rearing behaviors by parents help to either encourage or inhibit the development of social competence in children. The basic concept is that the child-rearing strategies of parents operate as part of children's social environments to change their behavior, attitudes, and attributes through principles of learning and processes of internalization (Patterson & Capaldi, 1991; Peterson & Hann, 1999).

Two major dimensions of parental behavior, support and control, have been the focus of these perspectives. The most common conceptualization of this theory proposes that parental behaviors associated with the "authoritative" style make effective contributions to social competence and inhibit the development of internalizing and externalizing behavior in young children. Specifically, problematic behavior in children tends to be prevented when parents use firm, rationally based forms of control (i.e., limit setting, monitoring, reasoning) in combination with encouragement and support (Patterson & Capaldi, 1991; Peterson & Hann, 1999). This contrasts with styles of parenting that emphasize either more "authoritarian" (i.e., arbitrary punitive control and diminished support) or more "permissive" approaches (diminished control combined with high support) that are commonly associated with reduced social competence and higher frequencies of psychosocial problems (Baumrind, 1991).

Clearly, however, substantial debate exists about the generalizability of authoritative parenting beyond European American populations to parents and children of diverse ethnic-minority backgrounds (Demo & Cox, 2000). Some observers report, for example, that authoritative parenting is less characteristic of and less effective in fostering youthful social competence within African American families (Avenevoli, Sessa, & Steinberg, 1999), whereas other research demonstrates that African American parents also use reasoning and other child-centered strategies commonly associated with an authoritative approach (Bluestone & Tamis-Lemonda, 1999; Kelley, Power, & Wimbush, 1992). Another illustrative critique is that of Chao (1994) who argues that the application of authoritative parenting to Chinese and other Asian populations is an example of ethnocentrism. Thus, although the generalizability of authoritative parenting is considerable, especially when socioeconomic variations are accounted for, substantial attention should be devoted to tailoring prevention programs for parents and children who have cultural values that vary from those of the mainstream.

Ecological Perspectives

The most comprehensive way of conceptualizing family-based prevention strategies is to view parent–child relationships within nuclear families as subcomponents of much larger social environments. These "ecological" perspectives can provide insight for a broad range of prevention strategies aimed at levels of society ranging from dyadic relationships within nuclear families (e.g., parenting programs) to macro-level institutions (e.g., social policy) (Bronfenbrenner, 1979; Lerner, 1995). Thus, children are viewed as being nested within a complex array of interconnected systems that encompass individual, family, and extrafamilial (e.g., peer, school, and neighborhood) settings. Both problematic and socially competent outcomes are viewed as products of reciprocal exchanges between children and their diverse settings in addition to the interconnections among the social systems in which children develop (Bronfenbrenner, 1979).

The ideal circumstance, from an ecological perspective, occurs when children are exposed to constructive developmental experiences within each of these settings and none of these environments contradict the other. Problems occur, however, when children are exposed to socialization experiences (e.g., high parental punitiveness) that inhibit social competence and encourage externalizing or internalizing behavior. Difficulties in socialization are further amplified when children's developmental settings (e.g., the nuclear family and the neighborhood) contradict each other. This circumstance may occur, for example, when the values and behaviors of deviant peers in school contradict the prosocial values and behaviors of parents.

Ecological theories embody a general view of development that serves as the basis for comprehensive, community-based approaches, key aspects of which are within the parent–child relationship. Such multi-component programs are illustrated by the *Child Development Project* (CDP), a prevention effort aimed at reducing risk behavior by changing the social ecology of elementary schools to create "caring communities of learners" (Battistich, Schaps, Watson, & Solomon, 1996). This program combines school-wide community building activities with parent involvement activities such as interactive homework assignments that reinforce the family–school partnership. Another example is the *Linking the Interests of Families and Teachers* (LIFT) program aimed at aspects of the social ecology that reduce future violence and delinquency. The specific ecological arenas addressed by this program are the parent–child relationship, the individual classroom, and the peer group. Specific components include parent education to foster consistent limit setting and parental involvement, combined with training for children in social and problem-solving skills to resist negative peer group influences, and approaches to reduce inappropriate physical aggression on the playground (Reid, Eddy, Fetrow, & Stoolmiller, 1999).

Risk and Resiliency Theory

Closely related to ecological perspectives is another systemic orientation commonly referred to as "risk and resiliency" (or risk and protective factors) theory (Garmezy, 1983; Hawkins, Catalano, & Miller, 1992; Petraitis, Flay, & Miller, 1995). This perspective was developed specifically to identify the many potential hazards that children face and the resources they have to ward off the more perilous aspects of their social development. An important use of risk and resiliency models is to emphasize the need for prevention efforts within multiple aspects of social development to discourage the emergence of internalizing and externalizing behavior. This perspective identifies risk and protective factors within the parent–child relationship and conceptualizes family-based prevention as an essential component of comprehensive community-based models.

This model seeks to identify how risk and protective factors may operate and accumulate in the lives of children within individual, family, peer, school, neighborhood, and community circumstances. The first of the two general categories of social developmental phenomena, risk factors, is based on epidemiological models of disease development, such as efforts to identify the multiple hazards that lead to chronic diseases. The second general category of social phenomena, protective factors (or sources of wellness), are individual capabilities or social-environmental resources that enhance the abilities of youngsters to function in adaptive ways in the face of stressful or risky circumstances (Garmezy, 1985; Hawkins et al., 1992; Petraitis et al., 1995). At the parent–child level of analysis, risk factors would include such social behaviors as parental punitive and neglectful behavior, whereas protective factors include consistent parental monitoring, limit setting, reasoning, supportiveness, or dimensions of children's social competence that contribute to wellness (e.g., social skills and self-esteem).

The main goal of this perspective is to understand how risk and protective factors operate in children's lives so that prevention approaches can be designed to diminish the hazards and build upon sources of resiliency. Prevention efforts that implement the ideas of this theory and address an array of risk and protective factors to prevent problem behaviors are the *Preparing for the Drug Free Years Program and the Iowa Strengthening Family Programs* (Redmond, Spoth, Shin, & Lepper, 1999; Spoth, Redmond, Shin, 1998).

STRATEGIES THAT WORK

A small number of effective prevention programs for children in nuclear families have been aimed at improving the quality of parent–child relations, enhancing social competence and reducing the risk of negative child outcomes such as conduct disorder, school failure, and substance abuse and violence. For the most part, these programs derive from theoretical models that are based in socialization models, with elements that are developmental, ecological in nature, and that emphasize risk and resiliency. For example, several theories (e.g., Catalano, Kosterman, Hawkins, Newcomb, & Abbott, 1996) posit that children learn both prosocial and antisocial behaviors from socialization agents such as the family, school, and peers. Furthermore, precursors of later behavior problems are evident as early as the preschool years, with developmental trajectories leading either to social competence and school success, or to social deficits and school failure (Conduct Problems Prevention Research Group, 1992). The most successful programs designed to foster children's social competence, therefore, must be comprehensive in nature and begin early enough to make a difference (Tremblay, Pagani-Kurtz, Masse, Vitaro, & Pihl, 1995).

Effective prevention programs for children in this age group are comprehensive in that they target not just the individual child, but the family and school contexts as well. In addition to providing information, the programs offer participants specific training and practice in parenting and prosocial skills. Although few prevention approaches involving school-age children have been thoroughly evaluated to date (e.g., Hogue & Liddle, 1999), we briefly review several programs that have thus far demonstrated considerable achievements.

School-Based Intervention Program Against Bullying

Following the suicides of three teen boys (as a consequence of severe bullying by peers) in the 1980s, the Norwegian Ministry of Education launched a nationwide campaign against bullying in schools. Olweus developed and evaluated, a comprehensive school-based program against bullying (Olweus, 1993, 1994) that is also notable for having a family component consisting of parental involvement. The *School-Based Intervention Program Against Bullying* is aimed at reducing the levels of children's bullying/victim problems during grades 4–7 in

Bergen, Norway. The program is multi-component, focusing on the individual level (including meetings with the parents of victims and bullies), the classroom level (e.g., classroom rules against bullying), and the school level (e.g., Parent–Teacher Association meetings). The ultimate goal is to create a school (and ideally home) environment that is authoritative—that is, warm but firm—with respect to the bully/victim problem. Meetings with parents about the program and their children's participation are one of the core components of the program. The program evaluations have been positive (e.g., Olweus, 1994) through demonstrated reductions in bullying and other antisocial behavior (e.g., fighting, vandalism). Moreover, improvements emerged in the "social climate" of the classroom (e.g., cooperation, discipline) and students' attitudes toward school. Findings were obtained for both girls and boys, with the effects of the program being stronger after 2 years than after 1 year. This program illustrates how involving school and family contexts in prevention strategies can enhance the quality and experiences of children within learning environments.

Preparing for the Drug-Free Years (PDFY) Program

Based on a social developmental model, the goals of the *Preparing for the Drug Free Years Program* are to enhance protective parent–child interactions (e.g., anger management) and reduce children's risk for early initiation of substance use (Spoth et al., 1998). The 5-week-long program involved families of sixth graders from rural midwestern schools. Parents were instructed in risk factors for substance abuse and in parenting techniques consistent with an authoritative approach such as developing guidelines for substance use, monitoring compliance with guidelines, enhancing parent–child bonding (supportiveness), enhancing child involvement in family activities, as well as managing anger and family conflict. Social competence is also fostered directly by teaching children social skills that are useful for resisting peer pressure. Evaluation results have demonstrated that hypothesized intervention effects for the targeted parenting behaviors were statistically significant both on posttest (Spoth et al., 1998) and 1-year follow-up measures (Redmond et al., 1999).

Iowa Strengthening Families Program (ISFP)

The *Iowa Strengthening Families Program* is aimed at enhancing family protective factors and reducing risk factors associated with negative child outcomes (Spoth et al., 1998). Like the PDFY program, the 7-week-long ISFP is family-based, involving families of sixth graders who attended 33 participating schools located in the rural Midwest. Parents were instructed about parenting techniques and communication skills consistent with an authoritative approach, clarifying developmentally appropriate expectations, and using non-physical discipline. Children were instructed about interpersonal skills and how to resist peer pressure, while family members practiced conflict resolution and communication skills. Evaluation results have demonstrated that hypothesized intervention effects on the targeted parenting behaviors were statistically significant both for posttest results (Spoth et al., 1998) and for 1-year follow-up measures (Redmond et al., 1999).

FAST (Families and Schools Together) Track Program

Based on a developmental model, the goals of the *FAST Track Program* are to promote family competence, prevent the development of conduct disorders, and reduce school failure (Conduct Problems Prevention Research Group, 1992). This program illustrates how a large population of young children with very early signs of problematic behavior can be dealt with from prevention rather than a treatment approach, in part, within nuclear families.

FAST Track is a multi-component prevention effort: one component is classroom-based and universal in scope, whereas other components are individual- and family-based and selective in scope. This program was implemented with a population of kindergartners from selected schools in four regions of the United States who had high rates of conduct problems (Durham, NC, Nashville, TN, Seattle, WA, and rural Pennsylvania). The children were screened for disruptive behavior and poor peer relations based on parent and teacher ratings. As a result, 10 percent of the children and their families were invited to participate in this multi-site, multi-component program, with the goal being to identify children with potential for conduct disorder at an early stage and prevent its further development. Classmates of the selected children also participated in the universal classroom intervention component.

The program involves a 22-session parent training curriculum (e.g., using strategies consistent with authoritative parenting to promote developmentally-appropriate expectations for their child's behavior), biweekly home visits, children's social -skills training (e.g., interpersonal skills), academic tutoring in reading, and a universal classroom intervention (e.g., problem-solving skills). Results from an evaluation study for the program's initial year demonstrated that children who received the intervention, relative to those in the control group, improved both in interpersonal skills and school grades in the language arts (Conduct Problems Prevention Research Group, 1999a). Parents reported less physical discipline, greater warmth, and more school

involvement, while teachers in intervention classrooms (compared to teachers in control classrooms) rated their students as having fewer conduct problems (Conduct Problems Prevention Research Group, 1999b). A final important result was that "intervention" classrooms were rated as having more positive atmospheres than control classrooms. Consequently, these initial findings are supportive of the strategies used in the FAST Track program.

STRATEGIES THAT MIGHT WORK

Montreal Longitudinal-Experimental Study

Based on a developmental model, the Montreal Longitudinal-Experimental Study is a 2-year prevention program aimed at reducing disruptive behavior, delinquency, and enhancing school retention, and delinquency in French Canadian boys (Tremblay et al., 1995). A key aspect of this program was that kindergarten teachers identify disruptive boys from schools in lower socioeconomic areas of Montreal, Canada. Subsequently, 30 percent of these boys (and their families) were designated as being at risk for later antisocial behaviors and invited to participate. Parents were trained in techniques consistent with authoritative parenting (e.g., monitoring children's behavior, non-physical discipline) during as many as 46 sessions as required, whereas the boys were given social skills training for 2 years (from ages 7 to 9). Although teachers rated treatment group boys as less disruptive than control group boys until age 13, this difference was found not to be statistically significant. Moreover, until age 13, treatment group boys were more likely than control group boys to be members of age-appropriate classrooms. By age 15, however, this difference had disappeared, with only 40 percent of the boys remaining in age-appropriate classrooms. An important confirming result, in turn, was that, at 1–6 years after the end of the intervention, boys in the treatment group reported fewer delinquent behaviors than boys in the control group. Consequently, mixed results and qualified support has been provided for the efficacy of strategies composing the Montreal Longitudinal-Experimental Study.

Child Development Project (CDP)

Based on a risk/resiliency model, the *Child Development Project* is a multi-component effort to reduce risk and promote resiliency in children by helping schools become "caring communities of learners" (Battistich, Schaps, Watson, & Solomon, 1996; Solomon, Watson, Battistich, Schaps, & Delucchi, 1996). Two of the five key components of the program involve parents and families of students in elementary schools in six school districts throughout the United States. Not only are parents and other family members included in school activities designed to reduce competition and hierarchical divisions between older and younger students, and between teachers and parents, families are also encouraged to participate in students' "homeside" activities. These activities are designed to build bridges between home and school, and foster communication between students and parents. For example, students interview parents about their family histories and culture and then share the information with other students in the class. Early evaluations found modest reductions in drug use and delinquent behavior such as skipping school and carrying a weapon (Battistich et al., 1996), and gains in students' social and ethnic attitudes and values (Solomon et al., 1996). Program effects, however, were limited to those schools that were most successful in implementing the program and thus establishing a caring community in the school.

STRATEGIES THAT DO NOT WORK

Prevention programs for school-age children that fail to achieve their goals often share one or more of the following characteristics: (a) a non-developmental focus, (b) a lack of focus on the larger social ecology of children's development, (c) a primary focus on instilling fear, (d) an exclusively information-based approach without skill training, (e) implementation at a later phase of development, and (f) one-shot programs of brief duration. Programs that ignore children's developmental levels (or the developmental trajectory of problem behaviors) run the risk of being irrelevant at best. Likewise, programs that ignore the multiple contexts (or the social ecology) of development (e.g., family, peers, school, community, society) also ignore potential protective and risk factors that influence and are influenced by developing behavior problems (Conduct Problems Prevention Research Group, 1992). Programs that are fear-based (i.e., employ scare tactics) or solely information-based (i.e., present factual information without application) may, in fact, backfire and encourage the very behaviors (e.g., smoking, drinking, sexual initiation) that these approaches were designed to discourage (Hogue & Liddle, 1999; Rollin, Anderson, & Buncher, 1999). Finally, programs of short-term duration, or that target older children to address behaviors having their roots in early childhood may simply be "too little, too late."

SYNTHESIS

Family-based prevention approaches within nuclear families can be important components of broader ecological strategies for fostering the welfare of school-age children. The primary focus of prevention efforts within nuclear families should be to improve the quality of parenting within families so that children's social competence is fostered. Prevention models should focus on internal social psychological processes of families rather than trying to reverse patterns of inevitable structural change in families and the emergence of diverse family living arrangements. A focus on the problems of school-age children through "structural deficit" models (i.e., using the nuclear family as the ideal type) has questionable theoretical and empirical linkages to children's developmental outcomes. Instead, the most effective prevention strategies should focus on the common issues that generalize across family structural variations, rather than focusing on supposed "deficits" of alternative forms of the family.

Prevention programs aimed at fostering authoritative (or closely related) parenting so that social competence in children is encouraged have considerable empirical support, both in terms of basic research on parent–child relationships and the applied scholarship on prevention. The components of authoritative parenting (i.e., nurturance, firm control, monitoring, use of reason, clear communication, conflict management skills, and low use of arbitrary punitiveness) are protective factors that provide important targets for the design of prevention programs. The most effective prevention programs are those that teach specific skills to parents and provide ample practice sessions to increase the possibility that behavioral change is stable.

The success of family-based approaches is best accomplished, however, within the context of a larger ecological design that begins early in children's development and addresses more than one developmental setting simultaneously. Family, school, community, and societal contexts can be used to reinforce socially competent outcomes through complementary approaches that diminish risk factors and capitalize on the potential for resiliency provided by protective factors. Prevention strategies based within nuclear families can be vital components of larger ecological strategies that encourage the effective progress of adolescents into adulthood by fostering the development of social competence through improvements in the quality of parenting.

Prevention strategies within nuclear families should be part of a larger strategy involving the implementation of compatible programs, at least within families and schools, if not also youth peer groups, neighborhoods, and the larger community. Externalizing and internalizing behavior have complex etiologies and no single program component is likely to prevent these problematic outcomes. Greater progress is likely to be made through an array of coordinated strategies that are long-term in nature and designed specifically for the circumstances of each community.

Also see: Parenting: Early Childhood; Parenting: Adolescence; Parenting, Single Parent: Adolescence; Parenting: Adulthood; Prosocial Behavior: Early Childhood.

References

Allen, K.R., Fine, M.A., & Demo, D. (2000). An overview of family diversity: Controversies, questions, and values. In D.H. Demo, K.R. Allen & M.A. Fine (Eds.), *Handbook of family diversity* (pp. 1–14). New York: Oxford University Press.

Amato, P.R., & Booth, A. (1996). A prospective study of divorce and parent–child relationships. *Journal of Marriage and the Family, 52*, 347–360.

Avenevoli, S., Sessa, F.M., & Steinberg, L. (1999). Family structure, parenting practices, and adolescent adjustment: An ecological examination. In E.M. Hetherington (Ed.), *Coping with divorce, single parenting, and remarriage* (pp. 65–90). Mahwah, NJ: Erlbaum.

Battistich, V., Schaps, E., Watson, M., & Solomon, D. (1996). Prevention effects of the Child Development Project: Early findings from an ongoing multi-site demonstration trial. *Journal of Adolescent Research, 11*, 16–35.

Baumrind, D. (1980). New directions in socialization research. *American Psychologist, 35*, 639–652.

Baumrind, D. (1991). Effective parenting during the early adolescent transition. In P.A. Cowan & M. Hetherington (Eds.), *Family transitions* (pp. 111–163). Hillsdale, NJ: Lawrence Erlbaum.

Bluestone, C., & Tamis-Lemonda, C.S. (1999). Correlates of parenting styles in predominantly working- and middle-class African American mothers. *Journal of Marriage and the Family, 61*, 881–893.

Bowlby, J.A. (1988). *A secure base: Parent–child attachment and healthy human development.* New York: Basic Books.

Bronfenbrenner, U. (1979). *The ecology of human development.* Cambridge: Harvard University Press.

Burgess, E.W. (1926). The family as a unity of interacting personalities. *The Family, 7*, 3–9.

Catalano, R.F., Kosterman, R., Hawkins, J.D., Newcomb, M.D., & Abbott, R.D. (1996). Modeling the etiology of adolescent substance use: A test of the social development model. *Journal of Drug Issues, 26*, 429–455.

Chao, R. (1994). Beyond parental control and authoritarian parenting style: Understanding Chinese parenting through the cultural notion of training. *Child Development, 65*, 1111–1119.

Conduct Problems Prevention Research Group. (1992). A developmental and clinical model for the prevention of conduct disorder: The FAST track program. *Development and Psychopathology, 4*, 509–527.

Conduct Problems Prevention Research Group. (1999a). Initial impact of the Fast Track prevention trial for conduct problems: I. The high-risk sample. *Journal of Consulting and Clinical Psychology, 67*, 631–647.

Conduct Problems Prevention Research Group. (1999b). Initial impact of the Fast Track prevention trial for conduct problems: II. Classroom effects. *Journal of Consulting and Clinical Psychology, 67*, 648–657.

Coontz, S. (1991). *The way we never were.* New York: Basic Books.

Coontz, S. (1997). *The way we really are: Coming to terms with America's changing families.* New York: Basic Books.

Demo, D.H., & Cox, M.J. (2000). Families with young children: A review of research in the 1990s. *Journal of Marriage and the Family, 62*, 876–895.

Garmezy, N. (1983). Stressors of childhood. In N. Garmezy & R. Rutter (Eds.), *Stress, coping, and development in children* (pp. 43–84). New York: McGraw-Hill.

Garmezy, N. (1985). Stress-resistant children: The search for protective factors. In J.E. Stevenson (Ed.), *Recent research in developmental psychopathology* (pp. 213–233). Oxford, England: Pergamon Press.

Hawkins, J.D., Catalano, R.F., & Miller, J.Y. (1992). Risk and protective factors for alcohol and other drug problems in adolescence and early adulthood: Implications for substance abuse prevention. *Psychological Bulletin, 112*, 64–105.

Hogue, A., & Liddle, H.A. (1999). Family-based preventive intervention: An approach to preventive substance use and antisocial behavior. *American Journal of Orthopsychiatry, 69*, 278–293.

Kelley, M.L., Power, T.G., & Wimbush, D.D. (1992). Determinants of disciplinary practices in low-income black mothers. *Child Development, 63*, 573–582.

Lerner, R. (1995). *America's youth in crisis: Challenges and options for programs and policies.* Thousand Oaks, CA: Sage.

McLanahan, S., & Sandefur, M. (1994). *Growing up with a single parent.* Cambridge, MA: Harvard University Press.

Olweus, D. (1993). *Bullying at school: What we know and what we can do.* Oxford, England: Basil Blackwell.

Olweus, D. (1994). Annotation: Bullying at school: Basic facts and effects of a school based intervention program. *Journal of Child Psychology and Psychiatry, 35*, 1171–1190.

Osmond, M.W., & Thorne, B. (1993). Feminist theories: The social construction of gender in families and society. In P.G. Boss, W.J. Doherty, R.W. LaRossa, W.R. Schumm, & S.K.Steinmetz (Eds.), *Sourcebook of family theories and methods: A contextual approach* (pp. 591–623). New York: Plenum.

Parsons, T. (1944). The social structure of the family. In R.N. Anshen (Ed.), The family: Its function and destiny (pp. 173–201). New York: Harper.

Patterson, G.R., & Capaldi, D.M. (1991). Antisocial parents: Unskilled & vulnerable. In P.A. Cowan & E.M. Hetherington (Eds.), *Family transitions* (pp. 195–218). Hillsdale, NJ: Lawrence Erlbaum Associates.

Peterson, G.W. (1995). Autonomy and connectedness in family. In R.D. Day, K.R. Gilbert, B.H. Settles, & W.R.Burr (Eds.), *Research and theory in family science* (pp. 20–41). Pacific Grove, CA: Brooks Cole.

Peterson, G.W., & Hann, D. (1999). Socializing parents and children in families. In M. Sussman & S.K. Steinmetz (Eds.), *Handbook of marriage and the family* (pp. 471–507). New York: Plenum Press.

Peterson, G.W., & G.K. Leigh (1990). The family and social competence in adolescence. In G. Adams & R. Montemayor (Eds.), *Developing social competency in adolescence: Advances in adolescent development* (pp. 97–138). Newbury Park, CA: Sage.

Petraitis, J., Flay B., & Miller, T.Q. (1995). Reviewing theories of adolescent substance use: Organizing pieces in the puzzle. *Psychological Bulletin, 177*, 67–86.

Popenoe, D. (1993). American family decline, 1960–1990: A review and appraisal. *Journal of Marriage and the Family, 55*(3) 527–555.

Popenoe, D. (1996). *Life without father: Compelling new evidence that fatherhood and marriage are indispensable for the good of children and society.* New York: Free Press.

Price, C.A., & Rose, H.A. (2000). Caregiving over the life course of families. In S.J. Price, P.C. McKenry, & M.J. Murphy (Eds.), *Families across time: A life course perspective* (pp. 145–159). Los Angeles: Roxbury.

Redmond, C., Spoth, R., Shin, C., & Lepper, H.S. (1999). Modeling long-term parent outcomes of two universal family-focused prevention interventions: One-year follow-up results. *Journal of Consulting and Clinical Psychology, 67*, 975–984.

Reid, J.B., Eddy, J.M., Fetrow, R.A., & Stoolmiller, M. (1999). Description and immediate impacts of a preventive intervention for conduct problems. *American Journal of Community Psychology, 27*, 483–517.

Rollin, S.A., Anderson, C.W., & Buncher, R.M. (1999). Coping in children and adolescents: A prevention model for helping kids avoid or reduce at-risk behavior. In E. Frydenberg (Ed.), *Learning to cope: Developing as a person in complex societies* (pp. 299–321). Melbourne: Oxford University Press.

Solomon, D., Watson, M., Battistich, V., Schaps, E., & Delucchi, K. (1996). Creating classrooms that students experience as communities. *American Journal of Community Psychology, 24*, 719–748.

Spoth, R., Redmond, C., & Shin, C. (1998). Direct and indirect latent-variable parenting outcomes of two universal family-focused preventative interventions: Extending a public health-oriented research base. *Journal of Consulting and Clinical Psychology, 66*, 385–399.

Stacey, J. (1993). Is the sky falling? *Journal of Marriage and the Family, 55*, 555–559.

Stacey, J. (1996). *In the name of the family: Rethinking family values in the postmodern age.* Boston: Beacon Press.

Teachman, J.D. (2000). Diversity of family structure: Economic and social influences. In D.H. Demo, K.R. Allen, & M.A. Fine (Eds.), *Handbook of family diversity* (pp. 32–58). New York: Oxford University Press.

Tremblay, R.E., Pagani-Kurtz, L., Masse, L.C., Vitaro, F., & Pihl, R.O. (1995). A bimodal preventive intervention for disruptive kindergarten boys: Its impact through mid-adolescence. *Journal of Consulting and Clinical Psychology, 63*, 560–568.

Nutrition, Early Childhood

David L. Katz, Ming-Chin Yeh, and Kinari Webb

INTRODUCTION

Nutritional status between conception and the age of 5 is strongly associated with growth and development. Children in this age group are uniquely vulnerable to the adverse effects of dietary deficiencies, both physiologically, because of high metabolic demand, and socially, because of lack of autonomy. This age group may be particularly vulnerable to the long-term sequelae of overnutrition as well, with increasing evidence that overweight early in life predicts later obesity. The primary prevention of short and long term sequelae of both over- and under-nutrition in this age group is achievable through the application of health and nutrition knowledge, the provision of social services, and the exercise of political will.

DEFINITIONS

In-utero growth and development is divided into the *embryological period* (approximately first 12 weeks following conception) during which organ systems are forming, and the *fetal period* (the latter two trimesters of pregnancy) during which organ systems have all formed and are maturing. The *neonatal period* refers to the first 1 month of life following birth. *Infancy* begins at the end of the neonatal period and lasts until 12 months of age.

Malnutrition generally refers to deficient intake of macronutrients (i.e., protein, carbohydrate, fat) and/or micronutrients (i.e., vitamins, minerals). However, adverse nutriture (nutrition) may be either deficient or excessive; *overnutrition* is also a form of malnutrition. *Marasmus* refers to severe wasting that is due to a lack of adequate calorie intake, and *kwashiorkor* refers to severe malnutrition that is associated predominantly with edema. *Kwashiorkor* was at one time thought to be due to a lack of protein, but further research strongly indicates that this is not the case. Supplementation with high protein diets may increase mortality in patients with *kwashiorkor*. *Kwashiorkor* is likely to occur due to increased oxidant stress in an already malnourished child. This increased stress could occur from systemic illness, bacterial diarrhea, aflatoxins, or gut flora overgrowth. Children with *kwashiorkor* have very low levels of antioxidants such as glutathione, vitamin E, carotene, and selenium and also have high levels of nitrous oxide (Fechner, Bohme, Gromer, Funk, Schirmer, & Becker, 2001; Golden, 1998).

SCOPE

There are approximately 129,434,000 pregnancies brought to term each year worldwide (World Health Organization, 1999). Variation in the perinatal and neonatal survival rate among countries relates in part to the adequacy of nutrition for mother and baby during and following pregnancy (Ceesay et al., 1997), although many other factors pertain as well. The infant mortality rate is highest in Sierra Leone, at 170 deaths per 1,000 live births, and lowest in Japan, at 4 deaths per 1,000 live births. The rate in Canada is 6 deaths per 1,000 live births, and in the United States it is 7 deaths per 1,000 live births (World Health Organization, 1999).

Within the United States there is marked variation among different populations, likely related to socioeconomics predominantly, although often characterized in terms of ethnicity (Chima, 2001). The infant mortality rate among African Americans in the United States is 13.8 deaths per 1,000 live births, among Latinos it is 5.8 deaths per 1,000 live births, and among non-Latino Whites, it is 6.0 deaths per 1,000 live births (US Department of Health and Human Services, 2000). The degree to which nutrition influences survival beyond infancy is variable, but it may be an important mediator in developing countries (Ceesay et al., 1997).

Optimal nutrition has the potential to promote cognitive and physical development and to prevent infectious disease or mitigate its consequences (Tomkins, 2000). In contrast, varying degrees of sub-optimal nutrition threaten physical and cognitive development, impair sensory organ function and impair immune function, and increase susceptibility to infectious disease and its consequences. Prevalent hazards of malnutrition during the period from conception through early childhood include malnutrition (kwashiorkor, marasmus); specific nutrient deficiency syndromes (deficiencies of vitamin A resulting in xerophthalmia; of iron resulting in anemia; of zinc leading to increased respiratory infections and diarrhea, etc.); low birth weight; macrosomia; dietary excess associated with obesity development; and sub-optimal nutriture, such as relative deficiency of Omega-3 fatty acid intake without overt deficiency signs.

Excess energy intake, a particular threat in countries of the West, has the potential to promote childhood obesity, diabetes, and susceptibility to other chronic degenerative diseases in adulthood. There is some evidence to suggest that maternal malnutrition intra-partum and low birth weight may predispose to obesity and/or insulin resistance later, particularly with subsequent exposure to a nutrient-dilute, energy-rich food supply (Osmond & Barker, 2000). This risk is greatest in indigent and ethnic minority groups.

It is estimated that 2 billion people worldwide subsist on diets lacking essential nutrients needed for growth, development, and physiological maintenance, and 780 million people are undernourished, lacking sufficient food to meet their basic nutritional needs for protein and energy. On the contrary, people from western, affluent countries suffer mainly from overnutrition. In the United States alone, it is estimated that national health care expenditures for 1990 totaled $666 billion, of which 30 percent were related to inappropriate diet (Bidlack, 1996). However, these estimates are crude, as the actual costs over time of, for example, subtle impairments in cognitive function attributable to sub-optimal nutriture at a population level are largely incalculable (Pollitt, Saco-Pollitt, Jahari, Husaini, & Huang, 2000).

THEORIES AND RESEARCH

The US Department of Health and Human Services has provided guidelines in its *Healthy People 2010* objectives for promoting overall health for women and children (US Department of Health and Human Services, 2000). Objective 16 pertains to maternal, infant, and child health, and objective 19 to nutrition issues. Infant mortality is an important indicator of a nation's health and an indicator of health status and social well-being worldwide. Although a downward trend has been observed in the 1980s and 1990s in the United States, the rate of infant mortality in the United States remains among the highest in industrialized countries

(National Center for Health Statistics, 1999). Objective 16-1c calls for reduction in infant deaths from 7.2 per 1,000 live births in 1998 to 4.5 per 1,000 live births in 2010. Race disparity is evident in infant mortality (US Department of Health and Human Services, 2000).

Healthy People 2010 objective 19-4 focuses on reducing growth retardation (i.e., stunting or low height for age) among low-income children under age 5 years to 5 percent or less by 2010. Although growth retardation is not a problem for most of the young children in the United States, eight percent of low-income children under age 5 were found to have growth retardation in 1997 (Centers for Disease Control and Prevention [CDC], 1998a). The growth retardation rate for African American children of low-income families was as high as 15 percent.

Low birth weight (LBW, less than 2500 gm) is the risk factor most closely related to neonatal death. In addition, studies have shown that LBW infants are more likely to experience long-term developmental and neurological disabilities than are normal birth weight infants (Hack, Klein, & Taylor, 1995). Objective 16-10a calls for reduction in low birth weight to 5 percent in 2010, compared to 7.6 percent in 1998. Again, race is an important factor related to low birth weight. In 1998, the rate of low birth weight was 6.5 percent for children born to a non-Latino White mother, whereas for those born to an African American mother the rate was 13.0 percent.

The *Special Supplemental Food Program for Women, Infants, Children* (WIC) program is designed to meet the nutritional needs of women and infants in the United States and assists nearly 1 million women annually in meeting nutritional needs during pregnancy. WIC supplements tend to be shared with family members, so that the nutrient intake of pregnant women in this population often is sub-optimal and requires close scrutiny to assure optimal pregnancy outcomes. Overall, the increased micronutrient requirements of pregnancy exceed the increased energy requirements. Therefore, vitamin supplementation during pregnancy is universally indicated, and the nutrient density of foods assumes increased importance.

Approximately 7 percent of all infants born in the United States are under 2500 gm. The energy reserves of a term infant of normal size are enough to withstand nearly a month of starvation, while those of a 1000 gm infant would last only 4–5 days. Adequate nutrition is likely to be critical to normal cognitive development in premature and LBW infants in particular. The caloric and protein density of formula generally allows for more rapid catch-up growth, but evidence to date suggests that breast milk may reduce the risk of infections and confer a range of other benefits as well, including superior visual acuity and cognition. Energy needs of LBW infants are estimated at 120 kcal/kg/day. Protein intake and weight gain are directly related in LBW infants; a protein intake in the range of 3 gm/kg/day is recommended. For a variety of reasons, insensible water loss of LBW infants tends to be approximately twice that of normal weight term infants; fluid intake of approximately 140 cc/kg/day is recommended.

Anemia is the most common nutrient-related abnormality of pregnancy and is attributable to iron deficiency nearly 90 percent of the time, with the remainder due primarily to folate deficiency. Maternal hemoglobin at sea level during pregnancy should consistently be higher than 11 gm/dl to assure adequate oxygen delivery to the fetus. Nutritional causes of anemia should be considered if the hemoglobin falls below this level and another explanation is not evident. A microcytic anemia suggests iron deficiency, while a macrocytic anemia suggests folate or B12 deficiency; the former is more common.

Iron deficiency anemia has been found to be associated with LBW, pre-term births, and developmental delays in infants and children (Idjradinata & Pollitt, 1993). In 1996, 29 percent of low-income pregnant women in their third trimester were anemic, and the target for Healthy People 2010 is to reduce the number to 20 percent or less. There are three objectives in Healthy People 2010 that are related to iron deficiency and anemia in young children and women. Objective 19-12 is to reduce iron deficiency among young children and females of childbearing age; objective 19-13 is to reduce anemia among low-income pregnant females in their third trimester; and objective 19-14 calls for a reduction in iron deficiency among pregnant females. Young children, especially toddlers and minority children (African Americans, Latinos), had the highest rate of iron deficiency (Looker, Dallman, Carroll, Gunter, & Johnson, 1997). During the period of 1988–1994, the rates of iron deficiency were 9 percent for children aged 1–2 years and 4 percent for children aged 3–4 years. The goals are to reduce the rates to 5 percent and 1 percent for these respective age groups by 2010.

There is definitive evidence that periconceptional folate supplementation decreases the incidence of neural tube defects (Thompson, Torres, Stevenson, Dean, & Best, 2000). The maternal diet is often deficient in calcium, iron, and other micronutrients, and supplementation with a prenatal vitamin throughout pregnancy is indicated. Vitamin A at doses in the range of 10,000 IU per day is teratogenic, and to be avoided during pregnancy. Carotenoids with vitamin A activity are safe. Caloric needs rise in pregnancy, but excessive weight gain is potentially disadvantageous to both mother and fetus. Underweight in the mother is associated with low-birth weight, while maternal overweight is associated with increased risks of gestational hypertension, diabetes, and toxemia.

A recent study of more than 170,000 women demonstrated that weight gain during pregnancy in ranges recommended by the Institute of Medicine decreased the incidence of LBW babies for lean White and Latino women. The data were less consistent with regard to Black women. Low birth weight was uncommon among obese or high BMI White and Latino women, and the benefit of recommended weight gain in these groups was unclear (Schieve, Cogswell, & Scanlon, 1998). Nutritional support of malnourished women during pregnancy is, in general, approached as is malnutrition under other circumstances. The topic has been recently reviewed (Hamaoui & Hamaoui, 1998).

In general, pregnancy requires a calorie increase over baseline of approximately 300 kcal/day, and lactation requires 500 kcal/day. Nutrients for which the recommended daily allowance (RDA) is specifically raised in pregnancy include: total protein, total energy, magnesium, iodine, zinc, selenium, vitamin E, vitamin C, thiamin, niacin, iron, calcium, and folate. Lactation requires further increases in protein, zinc, vitamin A, vitamin E, vitamin C, and niacin. Requirements for iron and folate actually decline. These adaptations in the maternal diet are necessary to assure optimal nutrition for the fetus/newborn.

Immediately post-partum for a period of approximately 3–5 days, human mammary glands produce colostrum, a fluid rich in sodium, chloride, and immune globulins that confer passive immunity to the newborn. Colostrum is replaced by milk, which is rich in lactose and protein, and comparatively low in sodium and chloride. Milk volume consumed by the neonate is 50 cc per day at birth, 500 cc by day 5, and 750 cc at 3 months. Milk production is maintained by infant suckling. The first 4 months of lactation consume, and convey to the infant, a comparable amount of energy as the entire gestational period. Human milk is appropriate as the sole source of infant nutrition for up to 6 months provided it is free of dangerous contaminants or pathogens (e.g., the HIV virus). There is uncertainty whether milk meets all of the infant's nutritional needs beyond this point. Breastfeeding, under most circumstances, is the preferred nutritional source for neonates. A generous intake of dietary calcium, and continued use of prenatal vitamins, is indicated throughout the period of lactation.

Breast milk and infant formulas differ substantially in a variety of nutrients (Huisman, van Beusekom, Lanting, Nijeboer, Muskiet, & Boersma, 1996). The significance of all of the differences has yet to be established. The prevailing view is that breast milk favors optimal brain development, and breast-feeding is associated with greater intelligence, at least during childhood, although such observations are subject to confounding (Uauy & Andraca, 1995). There is interest in the role breast-feeding may play in preventing the development of atopy (allergy). The data are to date preliminary (Vandenplas, 1997). Evidence is convincing that breast-feeding confers protection against infections, although the mechanisms by which breast milk influences infant immunity remain under study (Garofalo & Goldman, 1998; Hamosh, 1998). Provided that a sanitary water supply is available, the safety of formula is generally not of concern. Soy-based formulas are available for infants intolerant of bovine milk protein. Properly nourished, the healthy infant should double in weight by 4–5 months, and triple in weight by 12 months. Demand feeding is the preferred method of assuring adequate energy intake.

The epidemiology of nutrition-related health problems in children in developed countries has changed dramatically in the latter half of the 20th century. Childhood obesity is considerably more common in the United States than is growth retardation (Kennedy & Powell, 1997). Most children still consume fat in excess of recommendations and fail to consume the recommended quantities of fruits and vegetables. National surveys have revealed excessive intake of both total and saturated fat in children over the age of 1 year (Kimm, Gergen, Malloy, Dresser, & Carroll, 1990). Dietary fat intake was excessive in children as young as 6 months in the Bogalusa Heart Study, which also demonstrated important racial differences in dietary patterns in young children, with African American children consuming more total energy and fat than their white counterparts (Nicklas et al., 1987).

Niinikoski and colleagues conducted a randomized, prospective study in which over 500 7-month olds were assigned to a dietary counseling intervention aimed at reducing fat intake and promoting compliance with adult dietary guidelines or to a control group. At 3 years, cholesterol was lower in the intervention subjects (significantly in males, not significantly in females) than the controls, with no discernible differences in height, weight, or rate of growth (Niinikoski et al., 1997). The intervention produced significant reductions in total and saturated fat intake by 13 months, and this effect was sustained thereafter (Niinikoski et al., 1997), while growth was preserved despite a decline in energy intake.

In Canada, a working group derived from the membership of the Canadian Paediatric Society and Health Canada was convened to address the appropriateness of adult nutritional guidelines for children. The group concluded that the provision of adequate energy and nutrients to assure growth and development should be the highest priority, and that foods should not be eliminated on the basis of fat content during childhood (Joint Working Group of the Canadian Paediatric Society and Health Canada, 1995). The group advocates a transition during childhood to a diet with 30 percent or less of calories from fat, and 10 percent or less of calories from saturated fat (Joint Working Group of the Canadian Paediatric Society and Health Canada, 1995.) Dietary guidelines need not be specifically advocated as a priority until linear growth has stopped. The Canadian guidelines encourage a common eating pattern for families, with the implication that the fat content in the diets of children might decline, and encourage the promotion of regular physical activity and fruit and vegetable consumption during childhood (Zlotkin, 1996).

STRATEGIES THAT WORK

Optimal development in-utero is associated with several nutrients in particular. Supplementation with approximately 400 µg of folic acid per day beginning prior to conception markedly reduces the risk of neural tube defects, including anencephaly and spina bifida. Evidence for this association has been extensively reviewed and is considered definitive (Bendich, Deckelbaum, Locksmith, & Duff, 1998; Czeizel, 1997). Ingestion of more than 1 mg per day of folate is generally not recommended. However, in women with prior pregnancies leading to neural tube defects, the ingestion of up to 4 mg per day of folate may confer additional benefit.

Pregnancy consumes approximately 1040 mg of iron in total, of which 200 mg are recaptured after pregnancy from the expanded red cell mass, and 840 mg are permanently lost. The iron is lost to the fetus (300 mg), the placenta (50–75 mg), expanded red cell mass (450 mg), and blood loss at parturition (200 mg). Only about 10 percent of ingested iron is absorbed in the non-pregnant state, but pregnancy may enhance absorption up to 30 percent. There was initial concern that supplementing iron in areas with malaria might increase the risk of malaria during pregnancy, although recent studies have not shown this to be the case. Therefore, an intake of between 13 and 40 mg per day is recommended during the third trimester for all women. Vitamin/mineral supplements generally contain 30 mg of iron, and diet (in the United States) provides an additional 15 mg, easily meeting the needs of most women without anemia. Women with iron deficiency anemia during pregnancy require increased intake to replete bone marrow stores and still provide for the metabolic needs of the fetus. In this situation, daily intake of between 120 and 150 mg of iron is typically required. Iron supplementation prior to conception will facilitate meeting the iron needs of pregnancy and lactation, which together result in a net loss of between 420 and 1030 mg of elemental iron. Iron supplementation should continue post-partum, both to provide iron for breast milk and to replenish losses due to bleeding at delivery. Strategies useful in the prevention of iron deficiency among children include promoting breastfeeding, using iron-fortified formulas if formulas are used, and introducing age appropriate, iron rich solid foods (CDC, 1998b).

The fatty acid composition of human milk varies with maternal dietary intake. With the exception of iodine and selenium, there is little evidence that the levels of minerals and trace elements in milk vary with maternal diet. In contrast, vitamin levels in milk are responsive to dietary intake, with the strength of the relationship varying by nutrient. Both fat and water soluble vitamin levels in milk vary in proportion to maternal intake. Calcium and folate, and possibly other nutrients, are preserved in milk at the expense of maternal stores when maternal intake is less than daily requirements. Energy requirements to sustain lactation are based on the caloric density of human milk (approximately 70 kcal/100 cc), the metabolic cost of milk production, and total milk volume. The consensus view that lactation requires 500 kcal per day above the energy required to maintain maternal weight assumes that approximately 200 kcal per day of milk production energy will derive from pregnancy-related fat stores. Weight loss of 0.5 to 1 kg per month is common during lactation, while loss in excess of 2 kg per month generally implies inadequate nutrition unless such weight loss is intentional. Maintenance of weight and weight gain during lactation are not uncommon.

Maternal diet strongly influences the fatty acid and vitamin composition of breast milk but generally exerts a modest influence on minerals (Bates & Prentice, 1994; Emmett & Rogers, 1997). Iodine and selenium are exceptions, varying substantially in response to maternal intake (Picciano, 1998). Vitamins D and K are generally at low levels in breast milk, and supplementation is recommended (Jensen, Ferris, & Lammi-Keefe, 1992). However, a recent study suggests that low vitamin D intake in breast-fed neonates may not adversely affect bone metabolism (Park, Namgung, Kim, & Tsang, 1998). A recent study of 52 lactating women suggests that intake of calcium, zinc, folate, vitamin E, vitamin D, and pyridoxine may tend to be deficient in this group in the United States (Mackey, Picciano, Mitchell, & Smiciklas-Wright, 1998.) Continued use of prenatal vitamins during lactation is indicated.

Recommended daily allowances (RDAs) have been established for essential nutrients for both the first and second 6-month intervals of life. For ongoing revisions of dietary reference intakes by the National Research Council, see: http://www.nas.edu/nrc/. Iron deficiency is the most common nutrient deficiency in early childhood. Iron absorption from breast milk is apparently particularly efficient, as iron deficiency rarely occurs in breast-fed infants despite the lower levels of iron in breast milk than in formula (Heird, 1996). Increased use of iron-fortified infant formula among non-breast fed babies has substantially reduced the incidence of iron deficiency in this age group. Iron requirements may relate to vitamin E and polyunsaturated fat content of the diet. Supplementation is recommended in non-breast fed infants until age 2. Vitamin deficiencies are rare in adequately nourished infants. Vitamin K is provided by injection at or near the time of birth to prevent neonatal hemorrhage; subsequently, deficiency is uncommon.

By 6 months of age, gastrointestinal physiology is substantially mature, and infants metabolize most nutrients comparably to adults. Nutrient needs can be met with breast milk or formula, but most authorities advocate the gradual introduction of solid foods beginning at or around 6 months. As infant foods begin to replace breast milk or formula, the nutrient density of the diet is apt to decline, and the introduction of a multivitamin supplement is indicated (Heird, 1996). Completion of weaning to solid food by 1 year of age is common practice and appropriate.

The nutrient recommendations for infants 6–12 months of age are based largely on extrapolation from the first 6-month period; less is known about the nutrient needs of infants 6–12 months old. There is currently debate regarding the optimal level of energy intake, with some recommending a reduction from 95 to 85 kcal/kg per day (Heird, 1996). Adequate growth is apparently maintained at the lower energy intake level.

Means of assuring optimal nutritional exposure for all children up to age 5 are elusive. Practices of clear value in the prevention of nutritional deficiencies include: food-supply fortification (e.g., folate); widespread use of prenatal vitamin supplementation; nutrient supplements for lactating women; nutrient supplements for children at weaning; use of commercial infant formulas rather than bovine milk as breast-milk alternatives; and the continued efforts of food assistance programs in the United States (e.g., WIC) and abroad to protect access to an adequate supply of food energy and nutrients.

STRATEGIES THAT MIGHT WORK

Preliminary evidence suggests that high consumption of marine oils is associated with longer gestation, and that dietary supplementation with n-3 polyunsaturated oils may increase the proportion of term births in diverse populations (Scholl & Hediger, 1997). There is evidence that n-3 fatty acids are important in the normal development of eye and brain function (Lteif & Schwenk, 1998; Uauy-Dagach, Mena, & Peirano, 1997). A recent case-control study in Greece supports the hypothesis that n-3 fatty acids may be especially important in fetal brain development, and that low maternal fish consumption may elevate risk of cerebral palsy (Petridou et al., 1998). Increased consumption of n-3 fatty acids may therefore confer health benefits to both mother and baby. Relative to the prehistoric dietary pattern, the modern diet is deficient in n-3s (Eaton, Eaton, & Konner, 1997) lending the support of an evolutionary context to the hypothesis that increased intake may be beneficial.

Essential fatty acids are of particular interest with regard to early childhood development. The n-3 content of breast milk is mediated by maternal intake. Long-chain polyunsaturated fatty acids (PUFAs) are particularly concentrated in the brain and retina. Eicosapentneoic acid (EPA) and docosahexanoic acid (DHA) are relatively abundant in human breast milk and prominently incorporated into the developing brain (Koletzko & Rodriguez-Palmero, 1999). DHA in particular is considered essential to healthy brain development (Horrocks & Yeo, 1999). Impaired cognitive development in premature babies may relate in part to insufficient availability of DHA during a critical period of brain development (Gordon, 1997). Breast-feeding is associated with enhancement of both IQ and visual acuity in infants (Golding, Rogers, & Emmett, 1997). The apparent health benefits of breast-feeding relative to formula feeding may relate in part to the DHA content of breast milk. Increasingly, long-chain PUFAs including DHA are being added to commercial formulas (Smith, 1998). Although the essential fatty acid, α-linolenic acid, is a precursor to DHA as well as EPA, conversion to DHA in particular appears to be limited and variable. The putative benefits of DHA apparently require that it be administered directly in the diet (Gerster, 1998). While health benefits of DHA supplementation are likely on the basis of confluent lines of evidence, they are as yet not conclusively proved (Morley, 1998).

The amino acid pattern of breast milk is species-specific. For this and other reasons, human milk might make unique contributions to early development (Sarwar, Botting, Davis, Darling, & Pancharz, 1998). Breast milk contains more than 100 different oligosaccharides. There is current interest in the influence these carbohydrates have on intestinal flora of the infant, and their capacity to play a role in the prevention of infection (McVeagh & Miller, 1997).

Maternal diet influences the flavor of breast milk and thereby serves as a means of introducing the neonate to a variety of taste experiences (Mennella, 1995; Mennella & Beauchamp, 1998). Strong flavors, and the familiarity or novelty of such flavors, may influence the feeding behaviors of infants. Thus, variation in the maternal diet during lactation may play some role in determining childhood food preferences. There is some evidence to suggest that breast-feeding, especially if protracted, may confer protection against the later development of obesity (Butte, 2001), although this remains controversial.

While the principal goal of nutrition management in early childhood is the preservation of optimal growth and development, children in the United States and other developed countries are increasingly susceptible to the adverse effects of dietary excess, particularly obesity. As a result, there is intense interest regarding the age at which dietary restrictions might first be safely imposed. In general, restriction of macronutrients (dietary fat being of particular concern) is discouraged prior to age 2, with increasing evidence that restrictions comparable to those recommended for adults may be safe and appropriate after age 2. The establishment of health-promoting diet and activity patterns in childhood may be of particular importance, as preferences established early in life tend to persist. Proponents of dietary fat restriction beginning at age 2 cite evidence that atherosclerosis begins in childhood, and that a diet with not more than 30 percent of calories from fat beginning at age 2 is compatible with optimal growth (Kleinman, Finberg, Klish, & Lauer, 1996). Others in the United States argue for the Canadian approach, with a gradual transition to lower fat intake and attention to the type and distribution of dietary fat (Lifshitz & Tarim, 1996). Controversy on the optimal dietary recommendations for young children has persisted for more than a decade (Taras, Nader, Sallis, Patterson, & Rupp, 1988).

There is increasing evidence that efforts to modify the diets of children to reduce long-term cardiovascular risk are likely to be safe. Whether or not such diets do reduce long-term risk is less clear. Obviously, evidence of long-term outcome effects is difficult to obtain. To be considered in the debate is the importance of providing a single, consistent dietary pattern for a family, as well as the issue of dietary patterns tracking over time. Data from the Bogalusa Heart Study demonstrate that there is tracking, between the ages of 6 months and 4 years, of both dietary pattern and cardiovascular risk factors (Nicklas et al., 1988). In light of these considerations, it appears that the recommendation in the United States to advocate a similar diet for everyone over the age of 2 years is reasonable and safe (Kennedy & Powell, 1997) and may offer long-term benefits. While there is some evidence that a comparable diet may be safe even prior to age 2, consensus opinion in the United States, and prudence, argue against the imposition of macronutrient restrictions in this age group. Conclusive evidence of benefit from early dietary modification efforts will accrue very slowly.

STRATEGIES THAT DO NOT WORK

Children over the age of 1 year will tend to eat an appropriate variety of foods/nutrients when provided access to such. However, balance may not be achieved on any given day. Provided the child continues to be provided reasonable food choices, balance will be achieved over several days. Parents should be reassured that a balanced diet need not be measured on a per meal or even per day basis. A reasonable approach is to avoid any major distinction between snacks and meals, so that healthy food can be eaten when the child is hungry, and meal size can be adjusted to account for snacking.

The prudence of advocating the same diet for adults and children has been challenged, largely based on the lack of evidence that dietary restrictions in childhood prevent chronic disease in adults (Lifshitz, 1992). However, obtaining evidence that dietary interventions in early childhood prevent chronic disease in late adulthood is a daunting challenge. Indirect, epidemiologic, and inferential evidence may be the best guidance available. The safety of the American Heart Association Step 1 diet for children over the age of 2 has received fairly widespread support (Dobrin-Seckler & Deckelbaum, 1991).

The provision of adequate, let alone optimal, nutrition to all of the world's children requires that lines of supply be secure and reliable. In myriad settings around the world, child nutrition is compromised by social upheavals that prevent access to an appropriate food supply. Assistance programs do not adequately correct this problem, as food delivered to a site of great need may not reach those individuals for whom it is intended. Thus, strategies that fail to contend with social and political barriers to food access are ill-fated.

In the industrialized world, children are early exposed to a vast array of nutrient-dilute, energy-dense foods. Vast sums of money are spent by the food industry on advertisements aimed at children. It is against this backdrop that an epidemic of childhood obesity is developing, and progressing. Providing "guidelines" on healthy eating in a "toxic" nutritional environment is clearly ineffective. A recent Cochrane review failed to find quality evidence supporting any particular strategy for the prevention of childhood obesity (Campbell, Waters, O'Meara, & Summerbell, 2001).

SYNTHESIS

The provision of optimal nutrition during infancy and early childhood is of vital importance to growth and development and is likely related to a wide array of health outcomes in later life. The establishment of good nutriture for an infant begins in-utero, during which maternal dietary practices may influence fetal metabolism. The most reliable way to assure optimal nutrition for a newborn is breast-feeding. Therefore, based on the confluence of multiple lines of evidence, breast-feeding for a period of 6 months is advisable unless the practice is contraindicated by communicable disease. The maintenance of salutary maternal nutrition during lactation is of importance to the health of both mother and baby. While commercial infant formulas provide generally balanced nutrition, there is concern that they are deficient in long-chain PUFAs, DHA in particular. As evidence of the importance of DHA and other essential fatty acids continues to accrue, the composition of commercial formulas will likely be revised. In the interim, there is preliminary evidence that both cognition and vision are enhanced by breast as compared to formula feeding.

Weaning to solid food should generally begin at approximately 6 months; earlier weaning may increase the risk of food allergies. Weaning from breast milk or formula is generally complete by around 12 months, although such practices are culturally determined; medically, weaning at 12 months is appropriate. Children will generally self-select foods that meet micronutrient requirements when provided with an array of healthy food choices. This practice is to be encouraged. In the developing world, the transition from breast milk to solid food may represent a period of particular vulnerability to malnutrition. This can be due to the poor nutrient quality of the food the children will be switched to, the lack of adequate amounts of food for a growing child (children are sometimes only fed twice a day in the developing world), and to the increased risk of infection. Diarrheal illnesses are particularly common during the switch to solid food due largely to the lack of adequate hygiene. Once a child becomes ill, he or she often has less appetite and because of cultural taboos is sometimes given less food. This can lead to a spiraling effect where illness leads to inadequate nutrition, which then leads to increased susceptibility to disease. Policies and programs aimed at providing balanced nutrition to children in this age group and improved hygiene are thus of vital importance.

Children with access to an adequate diet reliably meet their energy needs, although energy intake may vary considerably by meal and even day. Parents should be reassured in this regard and discouraged from placing too great an emphasis on "plate-cleaning". Whether or not such a practice contributes to later obesity is unknown, but an association is plausible.

There is persistent controversy regarding the optimal timing for approximating adult dietary guidelines in children. There is evidence that adult dietary recommendations are safe for children as young as 7 months of age, although few in the United States would endorse such a practice. Evidence is more definitive that the imposition of such guidelines beginning at age 2 years is safe and reasonable. This provides the added benefit of unifying family dietary practices earlier. There is evidence that dietary preferences established in childhood tend to persist, highlighting the importance of establishing a prudent dietary pattern early. Therefore, the diet that should be advocated to adults and older children to promote health may be provided promptly, or approximated gradually, in children beginning at age 2. Micronutrient supplementation with a multivitamin/mineral tailored for children is a reasonable practice. Vitamin A supplementation in subsistence populations is among the more cost-effective health practices known, and evidence is accumulating that zinc supplementation decreases respiratory infections and diarrheal illnesses. When plausible, regular consumption of fish should be encouraged. The consistent intake of DHA may offer considerable health benefits, supported by preliminary, but accumulating, evidence.

With regard to the prevention of overnutrition and its consequences among children in the industrialized world, there is support for the promotion of breast-feeding for 6–12 months as appropriate, and for efforts to promote physical activity. However, there is little evidence of true effectiveness for any strategy to date. Increasingly, and appropriately, attention is turning to modification of a "toxic" nutritional environment, in which young children are exposed and acclimated to a dietary pattern linked to a host of chronic diseases in adulthood. The combination of improved nutrition education and modification of the environment to support improved dietary and activity patterns offers promise for the future.

Also see: Nutrition: Childhood; Nutrition: Adulthood; Nutrition: Older Adulthood.

ACKNOWLEDGMENT

The authors acknowledge with gratitude the technical assistance of Mrs. Michelle Larovera.

References

Bates, C., & Prentice, A. (1994). Breast milk as a source of vitamins, essential minerals and trace elements. *Pharmacology & Therapeutics, 62*, 193–220.

Bendich, A., Deckelbaum, R.J., Locksmith, G., & Duff, P. (1998). Preventing neural tube defects: The importance of periconceptional folic acid supplements. *Obstetrics and Gynecology, 91*, 1027–1034.

Bidlack, W. (1996). Interrelationships of food, nutrition, diet and health: The National Association of State Universities and Land Grant Colleges White Paper. *Journal of the American College of Nutrition, 15*, 422–433.

Butte, N. (2001). The role of breastfeeding in obesity. *Pediatric Clinics of North America, 48*, 189–198.

Campbell, K., Waters, E., O'Meara, S., & Summerbell, C. (2001). Interventions for preventing obesity in children. *Cochrane Database of Systematic Reviews, 2*, CD001871.

Centers for Disease Contol and Prevention (CDC). (1998a). *Pediatric nutrition surveillance, 1997. Full report.* Atlanta, GA: HHS, CDC.

Centers for Disease Contol and Prevention (CDC). (1998b). Recommendations to prevent and control iron deficiency in the United States. *Morbidity and Mortality Weekly Report, 47*, 1–29.

Ceesay, S., Prentice, A., Cole, T., Foord, F., Weaver, L., Poskitt, E., & Whitehead, R. (1997). Effects on birth weight and perinatal mortality of maternal dietary supplements in rural Gambia: 5 year randomized controlled trial. *British Medical Journal, 315*, 786–790.

Chima, F. (2001). Infant mortality, class, race and gender: Implications for the health profession. *Journal of Health and Social Policy, 12*, 1–18.

Czeizel, A. (1997). Folic acid-containing multivitamins and primary prevention of birth defects. In Bendich & Deckelbaum (Eds.), *Preventive nutrition: The comprehensive guide for health professionals.* Totowa, NJ: Humana Press.

Dobrin-Seckler, B., & Deckelbaum, R. (1991). Safety of the American heart association Step 1 diet in childhood. *Annals of the New York Academy of Sciences, 623*, 263–268.

Eaton, S., Eaton S., III, & Konner, M. (1997). Paleolithic nutrition revisited: A twelve-year retrospective on its nature and implications. *European Journal of Clinical Nutrition, 51*, 207–216.

Emmett, P., & Rogers, I. (1997). Properties of human milk and their relationship with maternal nutrition. *Early Human Development, 49*, s7–s28.

Fechner, A., Bohme, C., Gromer, S., Funk, M., Schirmer, H., & Becker, K. (2001). Antioxidant status and nitric oxide in the malnutrition syndrome kwashiorkor. *Pediatric Research, 49*, 237–243.

Garofalo, R., & Goldman, A. (1998). Cytokines, chemokines, and colony-stimulating factors in human milk: The 1997 update. *Biology of the Neonate, 74*, 134–142.

Gerster, H. (1998). Can adults adequately convert alpha-linolenic acid (18:3n-3) to eicosapentaenoic acid (20:5n-3) and docosahexaenoic acid (22:6n-3)? *International Journal for Vitamin and Nutrition Research, 68*, 159–173.

Golden, M. (1998). Oedematous malnutrition. *British Medical Bulletin, 54*, 433–444.

Golding, J., Rogers, I., & Emmett, P. (1997). Association between breast feeding, child development and behaviour. *Early Human Development, 49*, S175–S184.

Gordon, N. (1997). Nutrition and cognitive function. *Brain Development, 19*, 165–170.

Hack, M., Klein, N., & Taylor, H. (1995). Long-term developmental outcomes of low birth weight infants. *Future Child, 5*, 176–196.

Hamaoui, E., & Hamaoui, M. (1998). Nutritional, assessment and support during pregnancy. *Gastroenterology Clinics of North America, 27*, 89–121.

Hamosh, M. (1998). Protective function of proteins and lipids in human milk. *Biology of the Neonate, 74*, 163–176.

Heird, W. (1996). Nutritional requirements during infancy. In E. Ziegler & L. Filer, Jr. (Eds.), *Present knowledge in nutrition* (7th ed.). Washington, DC: ILSI Press.

Horrocks, L., & Yeo, Y. (1999). Health benefits of docosahexaenoic acid. *Pharmacological Research, 40*, 211–225.

Huisman, M., van Beusekom, C. M., Lanting, C., Nijeboer, H., Muskiet, F., & Boersma, E. (1996). Triglycerides, fatty acids, sterols, mono- and disaccharides and sugar alcohols in human milk and current types of infant formula milk. *European Journal of Clinical Nutrition, 50*, 255–226.

Idjradinata, P., & Pollitt, E. (1993). Reversal of developmental delays in iron deficiency anemic infants treated with iron. *Lancet, 341*, 1–4.

Jensen, R., Ferris, A., & Lammi-Keefe, C. (1992). Lipids in human milk and infant formulas. *Annual Review of Nutrition, 12*, 417–441.

Joint Working Group of the Canadian Paediatric Society and Health Canada. (1995). Nutrition recommendations update: Dietary fats and children. *Nutrition Reviews, 53*, 367–375.

Kennedy, E., & Powell, R. (1997). Changing eating patterns of American children: A view from 1996. *Journal of the American College of Nutrition, 16*, 524–529.

Kimm, S., Gergen, P., Malloy, M., Dresser, C., & Carroll, M. (1990). Dietary patterns of US children: Implications for disease prevention. *Preventive Medicine, 19*, 432–442.

Kleinman, R., Finberg, L., Klish, W., & Lauer, R. (1996). Dietary guidelines for children: US recommendations. *The Journal of Nutrition, 126*, 1028s–1030s.

Koletzko, B., & Rodriguez-Palmero, M. (1999). Polyunsaturated fatty acids in human milk and their role in early infant development. *Journal of Mammary Gland Biology and Neoplasia, 4*, 269–284.

Lifshitz, F. (1992). Children on adult diets: is it harmful? Is it healthful? *Journal of the American College of Nutrition, 11*, 84s–90s.

Lifshitz, F., & Tarim, O. (1996). Considerations about dietary fat restrictions for children. *The Journal of Nutrition, 126*, 1031S–1041S.

Looker, A., Dallman, P., Carroll, M., Gunter, E., & Johnson, C. (1997). Prevalence of iron deficiency in the United States. *Journal of the American Medical Association, 277*, 973–976.

Lteif, A., & Schwenk, W.F., 2nd. (1998). Breast milk: Revisited. *Mayo Clinic Proceedings, 73*, 760–763.

Mackey, A., Picciano, M., Mitchell, D., & Smiciklas-Wright, H. (1998). Self-selected diets of lactating women often fail to meet dietary recommendations. *Journal of the American Dietetic Association, 98*, 297–302.

McVeagh, P., & Miller, J. (1997). Human milk oligosaccharides: Only the breast. *Journal of Paediatrics and Child Health, 33*, 281–286.

Mennella, J. (1995). Mother's milk: A medium for early flavor experiences. *Journal of Human Lactation, 11*, 39–45.

Mennella, J., & Beauchamp, G. (1998). Early flavor experiences: Research update. *Nutrition Reviews, 56*, 205–211.

Morley, R. (1998). Nutrition and cognitive development. *Nutrition, 14*, 752–754.

National Center for Health Statistics. (1999). *Health, United States, 1999*. Hyattsville, MD: US Department of Health and Human Services.

Nicklas, T., Farris, R., Major, C., Frank, G., Webber, L., Cresanta, J., & Berenson, G. (1987). Dietary intakes. *Pediatrics, 80*, 797–806.

Nicklas, T., Farris, R., Smoak, C., Frank, G., Srinivasan, S., Webber, L., & Berenson, G. (1988). Dietary factors relate to cardiovascular risk factors in early life. Bogalusa heart study. *Arteriosclerosis, 8*, 193–199.

Niinikoski, H., Lapinleimu, H., Viikari, J., Ronnemaa, T., Jokinen, E., Seppanen, R., Terho, P., Tuominen, J., Valimaki, I., & Simell, O. (1997). Growth until 3 years of age in a prospective, randomized trial of a diet with reduced saturated fat and cholesterol. *Pediatrics, 99*, 687–694.

Osmond, C., & Barker, D.J. (2000). Fetal, infant, and childhood growth are predictors of coronary heart disease, diabetes, and hypertension in adult men and women. *Environmental Health Perspectives, 108*, 545–553.

Park, M., Namgung, R., Kim, D., & Tsang, R. (1998). Bone mineral content is not reduced despite low vitamin D status in breast milk-fed infants versus cow's milk based formula-fed infants. *Journal of Pediatrics, 132*, 641–645.

Petridou, E., Koussouri, M., Toupadaki, N., Youroukos, S., Papav assiliou, A., Pantelakis, S., Olsen, J., & Trichopoulos, D. (1998). Diet during pregnancy and the risk of cerebral palsy. *British Journal of Nutrition, 79*, 407–412.

Picciano, M. (1998). Human milk: Nutritional aspects of a dynamic food. *Biology of the Neonate, 74*, 84–93.

Pollitt, E., Saco-Pollitt, C., Jahari, A., Husaini, M., & Huang, J. (2000). Effects of an energy and micronutrient supplement on mental development and behavior under natural conditions in undernourished children in Indonesia. *European Journal of Clinical Nutrition, 54*, S80–S90.

Sarwar, G., Botting, H., Davis, T., Darling, P., & Pancharz, P. (1998). Free amino acids in milks of human subjects, other primates and non-primates. *The British Journal of Nutrition, 79*, 129–131.

Schieve, L., Cogswell, M., & Scanlon, K. (1998). An empiric evaluation of the Institute of Medicine's pregnancy weight gain guidelines by race. *Obstetrics and Gynecology, 91*, 878–884.

Scholl, T., & Hediger, M. (1997). Maternal nutrition and preterm delivery. In A. Bendich & R.J. Deckelbaum (Eds.), *Preventive nutrition: The comprehensive guide for health professionals*. Totowa, NJ: Humana Press.

Smith, K. (1998). Recent developments in infant formulae: 1—The addition of LCPs. *Prof Care of Mother and Child, 8*(151), 154–156.

Taras, H., Nader, P., Sallis, J., Patterson, T., & Rupp, J. (1988). Early childhood diet: Recommendations of pediatric health care. *Journal of the American Dietetic Association, 88*, 1417–1421.

Thompson, S., Torres, M., Stevenson, R., Dean, J., & Best, R. (2000). Periconceptional vitamin use, dietary folate and occurrent neural tube defected pregnancies in a high risk population. *Annals of Epidemiology, 10*, 476.

Tomkins, A. (2000). *Malnutrition, morbidity and mortality in children and their mothers*. Paper presented at the Proceedings of the Nutrition Society.

Uauy, R., & Andraca, I.D. (1995). Human milk and breast feeding for optimal mental development. *Journal of Nutrition, 125*, 2278s–2280s.

Uauy-Dagach, R., Mena, P., & Peirano, P. (1997). Dietary polyunsaturated fatty acids for optimal neurodevelopment. In A. Bendich & R. Deckelbaum (Eds.), *Preventive nutrition: The comprehensive guide for health professionals*. Totowa, NJ: Humana Press.

US Department of Health and Human Services. (2000). *Healthy people 2010*. Washington DC: US Government Printing Office.

Vandenplas, Y. (1997). Myths and facts about breastfeeding: Does it prevent later atopic disease? *Acta Paediatrica, 86*, 1283–1287.

World Health Organization. (1999). *The world health report 1999: Making a Difference* [on-line]. Available: http://www.who.int/whr/1999/index.htm

Zlotkin, S. (1996). A review of the Canadian "Nutrition recommendations update: Dietary fat and children." *Journal of Nutrition, 126*, 1022s–1027s.

Nutrition, Childhood

David L. Katz, Kinari Webb, and Ming-Chin Yeh

INTRODUCTION

The nutritional status of children between the ages of 5 and 12 is strongly associated with physical and cognitive development. The primary prevention of both short-term developmental delays, and long-term sequelae of over- and undernutrition is possible with optimal nutritional patterns during this period.

DEFINITIONS

Malnutrition, the inadequacy of micronutrients, macronutrients, or both, takes many forms. *Macronutrients* are the three major classes from which nutrient energy is derived: carbohydrate, fat, and protein. *Micronutrients* are the myriad organic and inorganic constituents of food that play a role, essential or otherwise, in metabolism. *Marasmus* is severe malnutrition without edema (excessive tissue water retention) that is secondary to inadequate total energy intake. *Kwashiorkor* refers to malnutrition with edema that is thought to occur because of increased oxidant stress. *Rickets* is an impaired skeletal growth and associated stunting and deformity resulting from vitamin D deficiency. *Xerophthalmia* is the scarring of the eyes induced by inadequate intake of vitamin A; this condition can lead to blindness. While also a form of adverse dietary exposure, *overnutrition* tends to be defined independently of malnutrition. In general, the term refers to intake of macronutrients, although excessive intake of micronutrients, such as sodium, also occurs. Overnutrition is associated with the development of *overweight* (more than 10 percent above ideal weight for height) and *obesity* (more than 20 percent above ideal weight for height).

SCOPE

There are approximately 129,434,000 additions to the global human population yearly. World Health Organization (WHO) statistics from 1999 indicate that more than one of three children become malnourished and 43 percent become stunted in their growth as a result. In industrialized countries, children are more often subject to overnutrition than deficiency. The prevalence of overweight among children in the United States varies with the definition applied (Flegal, Ogden, Wei, Kuczmarski, & Johnson, 2001), but is clearly rising and in the range of 15–25 percent.

The costs of suboptimal nutriture among 5–12-year-olds are uncertain. The direct consequences of severe malnutrition, such as xerophthalmia, marasmus, and kwashiorkor, are more readily measured than are potential long-term subtle cognitive deficits resulting from mild-moderate malnutrition, or micronutrient deficiencies. Similarly, the costs associated with chronic disease, including cancer, referable in part to childhood dietary patterns, are impossible to measure due to the multitude of interposing variables. The best estimates of the impact of nutrition during this period of life on society are cast in terms of simple assumptions rather than dollars. The evidence suggests that diets established in childhood have long-term health effects either directly, or because of their tendency to track into adulthood. One may assume, as is often done in trans-cultural analyses, that all cultures/societies (barring specific genetic predispositions to disease) could achieve or approach the lowest rate for any particular disease seen among the populations of the world by adopting the pertinent salutary behaviors and/or environmental conditions. Under the constraints of such supposition,

improvements in childhood nutrition could be projected to reduce dramatically the incidence of many infectious diseases, blindness, skeletal deformity, obesity, diabetes, cardiovascular disease, and cancer, to name only a few of the more evident physiologic benefits. Improved nutrition in developing countries could also have potentially far-reaching positive ramifications by increasing the physical and mental capacities of the individuals living there. The financial implications of such projections are incalculable.

THEORIES AND RESEARCH

The link between nutrition and healthy childhood development is sufficiently self-evident as to be largely atheoretical. Theoretical aspects of childhood nutrition relate less to the nature of existing problems, and more to the interventions best suited to their resolution. With regard to undernutrition, there is little debate that cognitive development is threatened when nutrient intake is grossly inadequate. Cognitive development encompasses a broad range of outcomes. Various studies have documented a small but significant decrease in overall IQ, school performance, fine motor skills, and exploration of the environment as well as increased apathy and attention deficit disorder (Galler, Ramsey, Morely, Archer, & Salt, 1990; Gardner, Grantham-McGregor, Himes, & Chang, 1999; Grantham-McGregor, 1990). Less certain, however, is the impact of mild to moderate malnutrition and how important the age of the child is and the duration of malnutrition. It appears that malnutrition earlier in life (less than 2 years of age) is more deleterious, but there is unlikely to be a sharp age cut-off and longer periods of malnutrition later in childhood may have equally deleterious effects (Galler & Ross, 1993; Sigman, McDonald, Neumann, & Bwibo, 1991). The human brain is, however, remarkably resilient and given enough nutrition and psychosocial stimulation, children appear to be able to recover essentially completely both in growth and cognitive development (Grantham-McGregor, 1995). Thus, the degree of malnutrition, the duration, the timing, and the quality of the subsequent environment all interact in complex ways that are not yet fully elucidated, to determine the long-term mental and physical outcomes of children who have been malnourished.

There is also debate regarding the role of early malnutrition, in particular in utero, on the development of cognitive and physical parameters. There is some evidence that decreased availability of intrauterine nutrients leading to growth restriction may increase insulin resistance (Forsen, Eriksson, Tuomilehto, Reunanen, Osmond, & Barker, 2000). Generally associated with overnutrition and obesity, insulin resistance may be induced by physiologic stresses that contribute to or manifest as low birth weight (Osmond & Barker, 2000).

A wide array of theoretical considerations also relates to the control of overnutrition in childhood and is the issue that is more likely to be encountered in much of the developed world. There was little concern with the restriction of energy intake in children until the latter half of the 20th century, with most prior effort directed toward securing dietary adequacy. With the advent of increasing childhood obesity (Flegal, 1999), establishment of a link between dietary fat intake and cardiovascular disease risk in adults (Keys et al., 1966), and evidence that incipient atherosclerosis is evident in late childhood or early adolescence (McGill, 1998), the control of overnutrition in childhood emerged as a public health concern.

Over recent decades, recommendations in the United States and Canada have emphasized unrestricted diets in children under age 2. The American Academy of Pediatrics endorsed a diet consistent with adult guidelines for children over age 2 in 1998 (American Academy of Pediatrics Committee on Nutrition, 1998). However, some authorities still favor gradual approximation of adult dietary guidelines by the age of 6 (Lifshitz, 1992; Lifshitz & Tarim, 1996). In contrast, there is evidence, largely from Scandinavia, that a fat-restricted diet may be suitable for children as young as 7 months, and thus there is some support for the approximation of adult guidelines at weaning.

The determination and alteration of dietary preferences and patterns are informed by several related theories. Social scientists contend that dietary preferences derive in part from familiarity, and are reinforced by it. Factors underlying the selection of a particular diet, and thus its becoming familiar, include palatability, accessibility, convenience, and cost. These factors influence adult selection that, in turn, influences childhood exposure. Taste preferences in childhood are apparently the product of both nature and nurture. A preference for sugar in the diet is innate (Birch, 1998), while other taste preferences are more likely to be acquired. Diets high in fat or salt, for example, may tend to reinforce themselves. Children apparently tend to prefer diets similar to their earliest exposures, including the maternal diet during pregnancy and lactation.

Theories directed at the control of overnutrition in childhood are comparable to those applied to adults. The maintenance of near ideal weight for height is considered desirable. There is general consensus that the total number of fat cells (adipocytes) one has influences susceptibility to obesity, and thus may influence the capacity for obesity control. Variation in weight in adults is more related to changes in the size of a fixed number of fat cells; when obesity results from enlargement of fat cells, it is referred to as *hypertrophic obesity*. Children are much more vulnerable to increases in the number of fat cells when nutrient energy intake exceeds need; this condition is referred to as *hyperplastic obesity*. Fat cells seem to have a normal, or desirable, size range. Thus, losing weight by "shrinking" relatively few, large fat cells back to their normal size is far easier than losing weight by decreasing an excessive number of fat cells to below their normal size. Thus, the control of body fatness (adiposity) in childhood is thought to portend future weight control. The formula for weight control in childhood is, as in adulthood, predicated on the balance between energy consumption and energy expenditure, with allowance for vertical growth. Because of the needs to sustain growth, energy requirements per kilogram are greater in children than adults.

Regular physical activity in childhood is thought to be protective against obesity. Television viewing and other sedentary activities such as computer use are thought to contribute to obesity risk. Dietary fat restriction is thought to help control weight in children as in adults, as is compliance with guidelines for intake of fruits and vegetables. Practical strategies for achieving adherence to guidelines at the population level are lacking to date. In addition, there is increasing interest in the role of specific fatty acid classes in human health. N-3 fatty acid (Omega-3) intake in childhood may be of particular importance to cognitive development, susceptibility to allergies, and immune function.

Finally, to the extent that a theory- or model-based understanding of childhood dietary behavior is required to inform efforts at dietary modification, there is increasing support for the consideration of evolutionary biology. While there are substantial uncertainties regarding human ancestry (Hippel, 1998), and even greater uncertainties regarding particular behaviors, including dietary behaviors, of paleolithic humans, there is sufficient anthropologic consensus to support a model (Milton, 1999). This model may be of use in explaining the basis for dietary tendencies and preferences in children, and thus in suggesting means of promoting more judicious diets when such are indicated.

Children over the age of 1 year will tend to eat an appropriate variety of foods/nutrients when provided access to such; however, balance may not be achieved on any given day. Provided the child continues to be provided reasonable food choices, balance will be achieved over several days. Parents should be reassured that a balanced diet need not be measured on a per meal or even per day basis. A reasonable approach is to avoid any major distinction between snacks and meals, so that healthy food can be eaten when the child is hungry, and meal size can be adjusted to account for snacking.

The prudence of advocating the same diet for adults and children has been challenged, based largely on the lack of evidence that dietary restrictions in childhood prevent chronic disease in adults (Lifshitz, 1992). However, obtaining evidence that dietary interventions in early childhood prevent chronic disease in late adulthood is a daunting challenge. Indirect, epidemiologic, and inferential evidence may be the best guidance available. The safety of the American Heart Association (AHA) Step 1 diet for children over the age of 2 has received fairly widespread support (Dobrin-Seckler & Deckelbaum, 1991).

National surveys in the United States have revealed excessive intake of both total and saturated fat in children over the age of 1 year (Kimm, Gergen, Malloy, Dresser, & Carroll, 1990). In Canada, a working group derived from the membership of the Canadian Paediatric Society and Health Canada was convened to address the appropriateness of adult nutritional guidelines for children. The group concluded that the provision of adequate energy and nutrients to assure growth and development should be the highest priority, and that foods should not be eliminated on the basis of fat content during childhood (Joint Working Group of the Canadian Paediatric Society and Health Canada, 1995). The group advocates a transition during childhood to a diet with 30 percent or less of calories from fat, and 10 percent or less of calories from saturated fat (Joint Working Group of the Canadian Paediatric Society and Health Canada, 1995); dietary guidelines need not be specifically advocated as a priority until linear growth has stopped. The Canadian guidelines encourage a common eating pattern for families, with the implication that the fat content in the diets of children might decline, and encourage the promotion of regular physical activity and fruit and vegetable consumption during childhood (Zlotkin, 1996).

Proponents of dietary fat restriction beginning at age 2 cite evidence that atherosclerosis begins in childhood, and that a diet with not more than 30 percent of calories from fat beginning at age 2 is compatible with optimal growth (Kleinman, Finberg, Klish, & Lauer, 1996). Others in the United States argue for the Canadian approach, with a gradual transition to lower fat intake, and attention to the type and distribution of dietary fat (Lifshitz & Tarim, 1996).

A recent rise in the saturated fat consumption of children has been noted in an Italian population with a traditionally health-promoting "Mediterranean" diet (Greco, Musmarra, Franzese, & Auriccio, 1998). A study of 100 Finnish school children demonstrated that the intake of several important nutrients tended to be lower among the children with the highest fat intake (Rasanen & Ylonen, 1992). Niinikoski and colleagues studied over 500 7-month-olds assigned to a dietary counseling intervention aimed at reducing fat intake and promoting compliance with adult dietary guidelines, or to a control group. At 3 years, cholesterol was lower in the intervention subjects (significantly in males, not significantly in females) than the controls, with

no discernible differences in height, weight, or rate of growth (Niinikoski et al., 1997). Of note is that growth was preserved despite a decline in energy intake associated with the intervention. While the debate in the United States and Canada has focused on the safety of restricting dietary fat after age 2, this study would suggest that such an intervention may be safe at even a much earlier age (Niinikoski et al., 1996).

Thus, there is increasing evidence that efforts to modify the diets of children to reduce long-term cardiovascular risk are likely to be safe. Whether or not such diets do reduce long-term risk is less clear. Obviously, evidence of long-term outcome effects is difficult to obtain. To be considered in the debate is the importance of providing a single, consistent, dietary pattern for a family, as well as the issue of dietary patterns tracking over time. Data from the Bogalusa Heart Study demonstrate that there is tracking, between the ages of 6 months and 4 years, of both dietary pattern and cardiovascular risk factors (Nicklas et al., 1988). In light of these considerations, it appears that the recommendation in the United States to advocate a similar diet for everyone over the age of 2 years is reasonable and safe, and may offer long-term benefits. Conclusive evidence of benefit from early dietary modification efforts will accrue very slowly.

Even in the midst of overall nutritional excess, there is some threat of nutrient deficiencies, incipient or overt, in children living in industrialized nations. Long-chain n-3 polyunsaturated fatty acids are particularly concentrated in the brain and retina. Docosahexaenoic acid (DHA) in particular is considered essential to healthy brain development (Horrocks & Yeo, 1999). Although the essential fatty acid, α-linolenic acid, is a precursor to DHA as well as eicosapentaenoic acid (EPA), conversion to DHA, in particular, appears to be limited and variable; the putative benefits of DHA apparently require that it be administered directly in the diet (Gerster, 1998). While health benefits of DHA supplementation are likely on the basis of confluent lines of evidence, they are as yet not conclusively proven (Morley, 1998). There is evidence of widespread nominality, if not deficiency, of zinc in both adults and children, and that supplementation may enhance immune function (Tomkins, 2000). Girls are particularly subject to inadequate calcium intake and its long-term sequelae, a susceptibility greatly compounded if low levels of body fat induce amenorrhea; calcium supplementation may be indicated. Other nutrients likely to be consumed at less than optimal levels in this age group include B vitamins (particularly folate), vitamin A, and possibly vitamin D; multivitamin/mineral supplementation is not an unreasonable practice, although lacking substantiating evidence.

Indigent populations in industrialized nations and general populations in developing nations are susceptible to malnutrition and nutritional deficiency states. Children who are susceptible to malnutrition benefit from the provision of a diet providing variety and, in particular, animal fat and protein (Sigman et al., 1991). Micronutrient supplements are generally appropriate, especially of vitamin A to protect against xerophthalmia, vitamin D where sun exposure is limited, and certain minerals. For example, nominal zinc deficiency may be fairly widespread, even in developed countries as noted above, and zinc supplementation may enhance immune function in children (Tomkins, 2000). Selenium supplementation is likely beneficial in certain populations, such as Chinese in rural areas, subject to selenium deficiency; evidence of benefit in others is lacking. Iron deficiency contributes to both cognitive impairment and anemia, and is very common in developing nations; supplementation in children is appropriate (Pollitt, 1995). The threshold relationship between malnutrition and cognitive development (e.g., IQ, communication skills, social skills, fine and gross motor skills among others) remains to be fully elucidated.

STRATEGIES THAT WORK

The primary prevention of adverse effects of suboptimal nutrition (either deficient, excessive, or a combination of both) in childhood requires knowledge of the optimal dietary pattern for children, the age-appropriateness of dietary recommendations, the population-specific barriers to achieving the desired pattern, and the means to overcome such impediments. Gaps in this knowledge, and/or the means to execute what is known, continue to preclude the achievement of optimal nutrition for all the worlds' children and the attendant prevention of nutrition-related disease.

The recommended diet for adults and children over the age of 2 is schematically represented by the USDA food pyramid (Figure 1). The foundation of the recommended diet is cereal grains. Fruits and vegetables should be consumed in variety and abundance, with the National Cancer Institute's "5 a day" representing a minimal recommendation. The consumption of fat-restricted and preferably fat-free dairy products is advisable to increase calcium intake; full-fat dairy product intake should be restricted. Meats should generally be eaten as peripherals to vegetable-based meals. With regard to macronutrient distribution, guidelines call for 30 percent of total calories from fat, 55–60 percent from carbohydrate, and 10–15 percent from protein. More specific recommendations with regard to fat generally suggest an intake of monounsaturates at approximately 10–15 percent of total calories, polyunsaturates at approximately 10 percent of total calories, and saturated fat below 10 percent of total calories, and preferably lower still. Specific recommendations for the intake of trans fat are lacking, but the

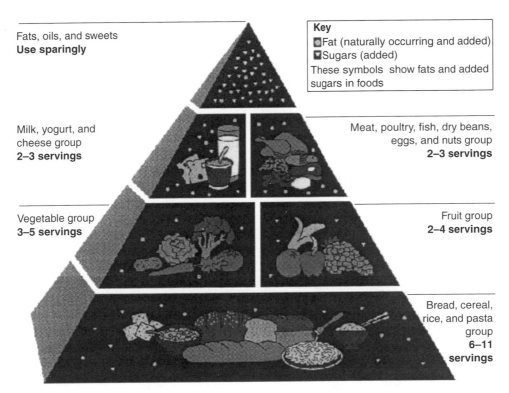

Figure 1. Recommended Diet for Adults and Children as Represented by the USDA Food Pyramid.

evidence suggests that trans and saturated fat should be combined and collectively restricted to below 10 percent of total caloric intake. Total calorie consumption should be that required to maintain a healthful body weight. Sodium intake should be restricted to not more than 3 grams per day, a figure supported by recommendations to eat processed foods sparingly.

There is persistent controversy regarding the optimal timing for approximating adult dietary guidelines in children. There is evidence that adult dietary recommendations are safe for children as young as 7 months of age, although few in the United States would endorse such a practice. Evidence is more definitive that the imposition of such guidelines beginning at age 2 is safe and reasonable. This provides the added benefit of unifying family dietary practices early.

In the United States, and increasingly in all industrialized nations, the average child is at greater risk of nutritional excess and obesity than of macronutrient deficiencies. Restrictions of dietary fat and alterations in the type of fat consumed in the West are strongly supported by an extensive literature (Lichtenstein et al., 1998). An association between dietary fat intake and obesity is similarly supported by an extensive literature, including observational and interventional studies (Lichtenstein et al., 1998; Lissner & Heitman, 1995). King and Blundell (1995) have shown that ad libitum consumption of high-fat food following vigorous exercise exceeds the energy expended, while low-fat food preserves an energy deficit. There is evidence from blinded experiments that the energy density of food is an important determinant of energy intake, indicating that abundant dietary fat is likely to play a role in positive energy balance (Rolls & Bell, 1999). While there is general agreement that restricting fat intake in isolation is insufficient to control or prevent obesity, fat restriction is considered by most experts to be an essential aspect of the dietary management of obesity in both children and adults (Bray & Popkin, 1998). Long-term weight losses are achieved more successfully in children than in adults (Epstein, McKenzie, Valoski, Klein, & Wing, 1994; Jeffery, 1998; Schonfeld-Warden & Warden, 1997). Evidence supports the inclusion of dietary change, behavior modification, parental involvement, and follow-up in a pediatric obesity program (Epstein, Valoski, Koeske, & Wing, 1986; Johnson et al., 1997). Programs have emphasized both reduction in sedentary behaviors (Israel, Guile, Baker, & Silverman, 1994), and dietary modification (Schonfeld-Warden & Warden, 1997). Childhood food preferences are greatly influenced by parents' food choices and eating habits, therefore family-based approaches are encouraged (Phillips & Snowdon, 1985). A recent randomized controlled trial designed to reduce television, videotape, and video game use among third and fourth graders showed statistically significant decreases in BMI in the intervention group as compared with controls after the 6-month intervention (Stamler et al., 1987). While clear evidence of effective strategies to prevent or reverse childhood overweight and obesity is scant, there is support for the promotion of breastfeeding until age 1, restriction of television viewing, encouraging or requiring (in school) regular physical activity, and providing a diet at home and in school that corresponds with guidelines (Centers for Disease Control and Prevention, 1996).

Even in the context of overnutrition, deficiencies of select micronutrients appear to be quite common. Deficiencies of iron, calcium, zinc, folate, vitamin D, vitamin A, and vitamin C are particularly common, although other nutrients probably are not consumed at truly optimal levels. While a balanced diet provides the needed micronutrients, social pressures at adolescence tend to favor a particular pattern of dietary imbalance, with excessive intake of processed and fast foods, and consequently sugar, salt, and fat. A multivitamin/mineral supplement is an appropriate recommendation, although clearly not compensatory for an imprudent dietary pattern. Evidence of health benefits of multivitamin/mineral supplements is lacking at the population level; support for the practice is largely inferential.

In developing nations and among the indigent in industrialized nations, strategies for the prevention or amelioration of malnutrition vary with culture and environment. It has been asserted that famines are unknown in countries with a free press and competitive elections. Distribution of food is all too often used as a political tool to harm the economically and politically disenfranchised (Scrimshaw, 1987). In urban areas, access to food may be limited by purchasing power but not distance; subsidy and aid programs for families such as food stamps or food drives have been shown to be helpful in the United States (Rose, 1999). In rural areas both in developed and developing nations, adequate distribution of existing food stores may be more limiting than cost. Access to food with high nutrient content, such as fresh produce or in some areas meat protein, is precluded by poor distribution, the expense of travel or inconvenience (Dillinger, Jett, Macri, & Grivetti, 1999; Vaughan, Benyshek, & Martin, 1997). In the developing world, female literacy has also been associated with a lower prevalence of stunting, suggesting that more educated mothers may be finding creative ways to increase the food that their children get (Frongillo, de Onis, & Hanson, 1997). Some supplementation programs such as the provision of vitamin A by the WHO, are well established and have been shown to be beneficial. Ideally the dietary pattern recommended for children in the West is an appropriate goal for children worldwide. However, political accountability may be a necessary prerequisite before any substantive changes in access to adequate nutrition occurs for the majority of the world.

STRATEGIES THAT MIGHT WORK

Children will generally self-select foods that meet micronutrient requirements when provided with an array of healthful food choices; this practice is to be encouraged. Children also reliably meet their energy needs when sufficient nutrient energy is available, although energy intake may vary considerably by meal and even day. Parents should be reassured in this regard, and discouraged from placing too great an emphasis on "plate-cleaning"; whether or not such a practice contributes to later obesity is unknown, but an association is plausible.

There is evidence that dietary preferences established in childhood tend to persist, highlighting the importance of establishing a prudent dietary pattern early. Therefore, the diet that should be advocated to adults and older children to promote health may be provided promptly, or approximated gradually, in children beginning at age 2. Micronutrient supplementation with a multivitamin/mineral tailored for children is a reasonable practice, although definitive evidence of long-term benefit is lacking. Regular consumption of fish should be encouraged in non-vegetarians; the consistent intake of DHA may offer considerable health benefits, supported by preliminary, but accumulating, evidence.

The single most important principle in dietary health promotion is that a single diet is appropriate for the prevention of most diseases. Children at eventual risk of cardiovascular disease may be at risk of diabetes, cerebrovascular disease, hypertension, renal insufficiency, and cancer, and are constantly vulnerable to infectious disease. If each disease required a different diet, consistent recommendations could not be made to an individual, let alone to a population. The emergence of a "one diet" approach to nutritional health is a logical outgrowth of confluent lines of evidence, and the clinical and public health imperative for consistent and practicable advice. That families tend to eat at least some meals together argues for dietary recommendations for adults and children that are comparable, if not identical. The benefits of a health-promoting diet should be combined with regular physical activity for maximal benefit; a sedentary lifestyle may undermine many of the potential health benefits of an otherwise salutary dietary pattern in childhood.

Methods to achieve widespread compliance with recommendations for dietary and physical activity patterns in children remain speculative for the most part; limited success has been achieved. Among the practices that warrant both further study and, on the basis of such evidence as has been gathered, current application are: distribution of food, and in particular, food sources of protein of high biologic value, to displaced children and families; vitamin A supplementation throughout the developing world; widespread use of multivitamin/mineral supplements in both industrialized and developing nations; encouragement of breastfeeding (other than when it represents an infectious disease risk) for the first year of life; the provision of school food choices that reflect nutrition guidelines; and the promotion, both in school and at home, of regular physical activity in children.

STRATEGIES THAT DO NOT WORK

The obstacles to combating under- and overnutrition effectively are generally quite distinct. Among undernourished children, especially among members of a displaced population, barriers to optimal nutrition are more likely to be environmental and political than either cultural or behavioral. In such populations, food distribution programs may or may not achieve their goals depending on how distribution channels are controlled. Problems of sanitation or facilities for storage may also compromise the effectiveness of a well-intended program. Nonetheless, so long as children and adults are subject to social upheavals and poverty, such programs are clearly indicated, with every effort made to ensure that food is both culturally appropriate (e.g., no meat is provided to a vegetarian culture) and delivered to its intended recipients.

Barriers to the prevention of overnutrition represent a constellation of environmental, sociocultural, and behavioral factors. The environment in developed countries provides convenient access to energy-dense, nutrient-dilute food, and technology that largely obviates the need for physical activity, and even lures children from physically active pursuits (e.g., video games). This is compounded by a food industry that spends large sums on advertising directed at children. Schools often enter into financial relationships with food or beverage distributors, and as a result, do not practice the nutrition that is preached to the children. Physical activity is increasingly de-emphasized in schools, and as there has been little improvement in the rate of physical activity among adults in the United States over the past decade, few adults set an example in this regard worthy of emulation. Efforts to promote salubrious diet and activity patterns in children in such an environment are largely ineffective. Given the worsening epidemic of obesity and diabetes among children as well as adults in the United States, one may conclude without undue pessimism, that virtually nothing being done to combat overnutrition and underactivity to date is effective at the population level. However, the failure of efforts to promote individual behavior change against the resistance of environmental factors is generating increasing attention to social and environmental determinants of dietary patterns, which offer promise for the future.

SYNTHESIS

There are two principal considerations in determining best strategies to promote optimal nutrition among the world's children. The first is what the dietary pattern should be, and second is to ensure that it is adopted.

Estimates of our ancestral dietary intake pattern suggest that we are adapted to a fat intake of approximately 25 percent of total calories (Eaton & Konner, 1997). Further, our ancestral intake of trans fat was negligible, and saturated fatty acid intake is thought to have made up less than 5 percent of total calories. Nearly half of the fat in our "natural" diets is derived from polyunsaturated fat, with an Omega-3 to Omega-6 ratio of between 1:1 and 1:4. The other half is derived from monounsaturated fat. Approximating this pattern of fat intake may confer health benefits, and is consistent with the weight of modern scientific evidence. The inclusion of adequate Omega-3 fatty acids in the diet may be particularly important during childhood.

On the basis, therefore, of both evidence and theory, a recommendation may be made to children and adults to consume approximately 25 percent of total calories as fat, in a nearly even distribution between poly- and monounsaturated fatty acids. The combination of trans and saturated fat should be kept below 5 percent of total calories. This can be achieved in part by following the consensus recommendations captured in the food guide pyramid emphasizing intake of grains, vegetables, and fruit. However, unless fish consumption is very consistent, n-3 fatty acid intake is apt to be lower than optimal given the near complete elimination of n-3s from the flesh of domestic food animals. Consumption of soybeans and seeds, in particular flaxseeds, as a means of raising n-3 fatty acid intake is recommended. The use of flaxseed oil, totaling about $1/2$ to 1 tablespoon a day, is recommended. A multivitamin/mineral supplement for most children is a reasonable practice, and regular physical activity among children should be encouraged.

The second consideration, the means to achieving these goals, is considerably more intractable. For children subject to malnutrition, food subsidy programs are a transient, discontinuous, and incomplete solution. Social interventions directed at the sources of poverty and displacement, while beyond the scope of this chapter, are clearly the definitive interventions for malnutrition. For children subject to overnutrition, education about eating well in the midst of a toxic nutritional environment is a tepid and ineffective response. Dietary guidelines, not convenience or financial expediency, should be the basis for school nutrition programs. Physical activity should be promoted by schools both during and after hours. Nutrient-dense, energy-dilute foods should be made as available and appealing to children as fast food now is, although the political and financial opposition to such reforms may be insurmountable in the short term. Until or unless the political will is gathered to modify the toxic nutritional environment in which children are being raised, we may realistically expect that relatively few will know the benefits of truly optimal nutrition. If such diets can be widely achieved among the world's children, the benefits to long-term health are likely to be profound.

Also see: Nutrition: Early Childhood; Nutrition: Adulthood; Nutrition: Older Adulthood.

ACKNOWLEDGMENT

The authors acknowledge with gratitude the technical assistance of Mrs. Michelle LaRovera.

References

American Academy of Pediatrics Committee on Nutrition. (1998). Cholesterol in childhood. *Pediatrics, 101*, 141–147.

Birch, L.L. (1998). Psychological influences on the childhood diet. *Journal of Nutrition, 128*, 407S–410S.

Bray, G., & Popkin, B. (1998). Dietary fat intake does affect obesity! *American Journal of Clinical Nutrition, 68*, 1157–1173.

Centers for Disease Control and Prevention. (1996). Guidelines for school health program to promote lifelong healthy eating. Centers for Disease Control and Prevention. *MMWR, 45*, 1–41.

Dillinger, T., Jett, S., Macri, M., & Grivetti, L. (1999). Feast or famine? Supplemental food programs and their impacts on two American Indian communities in California. *International Journal of Food Sciences and Nutrition, 50*, 173–187.

Dobrin-Seckler, B., & Deckelbaum, R. (1991). Safety of the American Heart Association Step 1 Diet in Childhood. *Annals New York Academy of Science, 623*, 263–268.

Eaton, S., & Konner, M. (1997). Paleolithic nutrition revisited: A twelve-year retrospective on its nature and implications. *European Journal of Clinical Nutrition, 51*, 207–216.

Epstein, L.H., McKenzie, S.J., Valoski, A., Klein, K.R., & Wing, R.R. (1994). Effects of mastery criteria and contingent reinforcement for family-based child weight control. *Addictive Behavior, 19*, 135–145.

Epstein, L.H., Valoski, A., Koeske, R., & Wing, R.R. (1986). Family-based behavioral weight control in obese young children. *Journal of the American Dietetic Association, 86*, 481–484.

Flegal, K. (1999). The obesity epidemic in children and adults: current evidence and research issues. *Medical Science Sports Exercise, 31*, s509–s514.

Flegal, K., Ogden, C., Wei, R., Kuczmarski, R., & Johnson, C. (2001). Prevalence of overweight in US children: Comparison of US growth charts from the Centers for Disease Control and Prevention with other reference values for body mass index. *American Journal of Clinical Nutrition, 73*, 1086–1093.

Forsen, T., Eriksson, J., Tuomilehto, J., Reunanen, A., Osmond, C., & Barker, D. (2000). The fetal and childhood growth of persons who develop type 2 diabetes. *Annual Internal Medicine, 133*, 176–182.

Frongillo, E., de Onis, M., & Hanson, K. (1997). Socioeconomic and demographic factors are associated with worldwide patterns of stunting and wasting of children. *Journal of Nutrition, 127*, 2302–2309.

Galler, J., Ramsey, F., Morely, D., Archer, E., & Salt, P. (1990). The long-term effects of early kwashiorkor compared with marasmus. IV. Performance on the national high school entrance examination. *Pediatrics Research, 28*, 235–239.

Galler, J., & Ross, N. (1993). Malnutrition and mental development. In R.M. Suskind & L. Lewinter-Suskind (Eds.), *Textbook of pediatric nutrition* (2nd ed.). New York: Raven Press.

Gardner, J., Grantham-McGregor, S., Himes, J., & Chang, S. (1999). Behavior and development of stunted and nonstunted Jamaican children. *Journal of Child Psychology and Psychiatry, 40*, 819–827.

Gerster, H. (1998). Can adults adequately convert alpha-linolenic acid (18:3n-3) to eicosapentaenoic acid (20:5n-3) and docosahexaenoic acid (22:6n-3)? *International Journal of Vitamin Nutrition Research, 68*, 159–173.

Grantham-McGregor, S. (1990). Malnutrition, mental function and development. In R. Suskind & L. Lewinter-Suskind (Eds.), *The malnourished child*. New York: Raven Press.

Grantham-McGregor, S. (1995). Review of studies of the effect of severe malnutrition and mental development. *Journal of Nutrition, 125*, 2233s–2238s.

Greco, L., Musmarra, R., Franzese, C., & Auriccio, S. (1998). Early childhood feeding practices in southern Italy: Is the Mediterranean diet becoming obsolete? Study of 450 children aged 6–32 months in Campania, Italy. *Acta Paediatric, 87*, 250–256.

Hippel, A. (1998). *Human evolutionary biology: Human anatomy and physiology from an evolutionary perspective*. Anchorage, AL: Stone Age Press.

Horrocks, L., & Yeo, Y. (1999). Health benefits of docosahexaenoic acid. *Pharmacology Research, 40*, 211–225.

Israel, A.C., Guile, C.A., Baker, J.E., & Silverman, W.K. (1994). An evaluation of enhanced self-regulation training in the treatment of childhood obesity. *Journal of Pediatric Psychology, 19*, 737–749.

Jeffery, R. (1998). Prevention of obesity. In G. Bray, C. Bouchard, & W. James (Eds.), *Handbook of obesity* (pp. 819–829). NY: Marcel Dekker.

Joint Working Group of the Canadian Paediatric Society and Health Canada. (1995). Nutrition recommendations update: Dietary fats and children. *Nutrition Review, 53*, 367–375.

Johnson, W.G., Hinkle, L.K., Carr, R.E., Anderson, D.A., Lemmon, C.R., Engler, L.B., & Bergeron, K.C. (1997). Dietary and exercise interventions for juvenile obesity: Long-term effect of behavioral and public health models. *Obesity Research, 5*, 257–261.

Keys, A., Aravanis, C., Blackburn, H., Buchem, F.V., Buzina, R., Djordjevic, B., Dontas, A., Fidanza, F., Karvonen, M.J., Kimura, N., Lekos, D., Monti, M., Puddu, V., & Taylor, H.L. (1966). Epidemiological studies related to coronary heart disease: Characteristics of men aged 40–59 in seven countries. *Acta Medica Scandanavia Supplement, 460*, 461–392.

Kimm, S., Gergen, P., Malloy, M., Dresser, C., & Carroll, M. (1990). Dietary patterns of US children: Implications for disease prevention. *Preventive Medicine, 19*, 432–442.

King, N., & Blundell, J. (1995). High-fat foods overcome the energy expenditure induced by high-intensity cycling or running. *European Journal of Clinical Nutrition, 49*, 114–123.

Kleinman, R., Finberg, L., Klish, W., & Lauer, R. (1996). Dietary guidelines for children: US recommendations. *Journal of Nutrition, 126*, 1028s–1030s.

Lichtenstein A.H., Kennedy, E., Barrier, P., Danford, D., Ernst, N., Grundy, S., Leveille, G., van Horn, L., Williams, C., & Booth, S. (1998). Dietary fat consumption and health. *Nutrition Review, 56*, s3–s28.

Lifshitz, F. (1992). Children on adult diets: Is it harmful? Is it healthful? *Journal of the American College of Nutrition, 11*, 84s–90s.

Lifshitz, F., & Tarim, O. (1996). Considerations about dietary fat restrictions for children. *Journal of Nutrition, 126*, 1031S–1041S.

Lissner, L., & Heitman, B. (1995). Dietary fat and obesity: Evidence from epidemiology. *European Journal of Clinical Nutrition, 49*, 79–90.

McGill, H. (1998). Nutrition in early life and cardiovascular disease. *Current Opinion Lipidol, 9*, 23–27.

Milton, K. (1999). Nutritional characteristics of wild primate foods: Do the diets of our closest living relatives have lessons for us? *Nutrition, 15*, 488–498.

Morley, R. (1998). Nutrition and cognitive development. *Nutrition, 14*, 752–754.

Nicklas, T., Farris, R., Smoak, C., Frank, G., Srinivasan, S., Webber, L., & Berenson, G. (1988). Dietary factors relate to cardiovascular risk factors in early life. Bogalusa Heart Study. *Arteriosclerosis, 8*, 193–199.

Niinikoski, H., Lapinleimu, H., Viikari, J., Ronnemaa, T., Jokinen, E., Seppanen, R., Terho, P., Tuominen, J., Valimaki, I., & Simell, O. (1997). Growth until 3 years of age in a prospective, randomized trial of a diet with reduced saturated fat and cholesterol. *Pediatrics, 99*, 687–694.

Niinikoski, H., Viikari, J., Ronnemaa, T., Lapinleimu, H., Jokinen, E., Salo, P., Seppanen R., Leino A., Tuominen J., Valimaki I., & Simell, O. (1996). Prospective randomized trial of low-saturated-fat, low-cholesterol diet during the first 3 years of life. The STRIP Baby Project. *Circulation, 94*, 1386–1393.

Osmond, & Barker. (2000). Fetal, infant, and childhood growth are predictors of coronary heart disease, diabetes, and hypertension in adult men and women. *Environmental Health Perspect, 108*, 545–553.

Phillips, R.L., & Snowdon, D.A. (1985). Dietary relationships with fatal colorectal cancer among Seventh-Day Adventists. *Journal National Cancer Institute, 74*, 307–317.

Pollitt, E. (1995). Functional significance of the covariance between protein energy malnutrition and iron deficiency anemia. *Journal of Nutrition, 125*, 2272S–2277S.

Rasanen, L., & Ylonen, K. (1992). Food consumption and nutrient intake of one- to two-year-old Finnish children. *Acta Paediatric, 81*, 7–11.

Rolls, B., & Bell, E. (1999). Intake of fat and carbohydrate: Role of energy density. *European Journal of Clinical Nutrition, 53*, s166–s173.

Rose, D. (1999). Economic determinants and dietary consequences of food insecurity in the United States. *Journal of Nutrition, 129*, 517S–520S.

Schonfeld-Warden, N., & Warden, C.H. (1997). Pediatric obesity. An overview of etiology and treatment. *Pediatric Clinics of North America, 44*, 339–361.

Scrimshaw, N. (1987). The phenomenon of famine. *Annual Review of Nutrition, 7*, 1–21.

Sigman, M., McDonald, M., Neumann, C., & Bwibo, N. (1991). Prediction of cognitive competence in Kenyan children from toddler nutrition, family characteristics and abilities. *Journal of Child Psychology and Psychiatry, 32*, 307–320.

Stamler, R., Stamler, J., Grimm, R., Gosch, F.C., Elmer, P., Dyer, A., Berman, R., Fishman, J., Van Heel, N., Civinelli, J. et al. (1987). Nutritional therapy for high blood pressure. Final report of a four-year randomized controlled trial—the Hypertension Control Program. *Journal of the American Medical Association, 257*, 1484–1491.

Tomkins, A. (2000). *Malnutrition, morbidity and mortality in children and their mothers*. Paper Presented at the Proceedings of the Nutrition Society.

Vaughan, L., Benyshek, D., & Martin, J. (1997). Food acquisition habits, nutrient intakes, and anthropometric data of Havasupai adults. *Journal of the American Dietetic Association, 97*, 1275–1282.

World Health Organization (1999). http://www.who.int/nutgrowthdb/ [web site]

Zlotkin, S. (1996). A review of the Canadian "Nutrition Recommendations Update: Dietary Fat and Children." *Journal of Nutrition, 126*, 1022s–1027s.

Nutrition, Adulthood

Sarah C. Couch, Grace A. Falciglia, and Richard J. Deckelbaum

INTRODUCTION

In the past decade, interest in nutrition has increased dramatically as diet is now recognized as a major contributor to 4 of the 10 leading causes of death in the United States—coronary heart disease, cancer, stroke, and diabetes (National Center for Health Statistics, 1996). A number of different behaviorally focused nutritional interventions have been employed to promote optimal nutrition and disease prevention in adults. These include national or community-based media campaigns, comprehensive community interventions, community programs in supermarkets, restaurants, and worksites, and programs that target the individual at high risk for disease. The following review of selected nutrition studies (published primarily over the last decade) provide data to address the following questions—Which elements in the program worked, which have the potential to be effective, and which strategies did not work in promoting healthy diet-related behavior changes in adults?

DEFINITIONS

The popular concept that different diets are recommended to prevent cancer, heart disease, diabetes, and stroke has been reinforced by the publication of separate dietary guidelines by several official and voluntary health organizations. This has purportedly led to much public confusion over what is considered an optimal diet for the primary prevention of chronic diseases. For example, in 1987, NHIS Cancer Epidemiology Supplement survey found that 48 percent of individuals who had not made any diet change for reasons of health in the past 5 years reported that they felt confused over which set of dietary recommendations to follow (Cotugna, Subar, Heimendinger, & Kahle, 1992).

Recently, however, efforts have been made toward consolidation of dietary recommendations from several health agencies to form a more unified set of common strategies. The Nutrition Committee of the American Heart Association, together with the Council on Cardiovascular Disease in the Young, and the Council on Epidemiology and Prevention (Deckelbaum et al., 1999) reviewed the dietary recommendations from various health organizations and agencies and the scientific evidence in support of the recommendations, and published a consensus statement summarizing common dietary recommendations for the prevention of atherosclerosis, cancer, diabetes, and obesity. These included consuming ≤ 30 percent of calories from total fat, <10 percent of calories from saturated fat, ≤ 10 percent of calories from polyunsaturated fat, ≤ 15 percent of calories from monounsaturated fat, and ≤ 300 mg of cholesterol each day. In addition, carbohydrate intake was recommended to be consumed at a level ≥ 55 percent of calories, salt intake limited to <6 g per day and total calories at a level to achieve and maintain desirable weight. When translated into food practices, these nutrient guidelines were compatible with and encompassed in the most recent version of the Dietary Guidelines for Americans (US Department of Agriculture [USDA], 2000). Thus, to promote healthy eating patterns across the US population, the primary goal of nutritional efforts should be to achieve the recommendations set forth in the Dietary Guidelines for Americans. Use of one common set of dietary recommendations may help to alleviate public confusion over diverse dietary messages and assist Americans in adopting more healthy eating habits.

SCOPE

The American diet is not consistent with most of the dietary recommendations in spite of clear dietary recommendations targeted at the general public to promote health and prevent diet-related chronic diseases (USDA, 2000). For example, while it is suggested that total fat intake be limited to 30 percent or less of calories, and saturated fat to less than 10 percent, mean daily intake of calories from total and saturated fat were estimated to be 34 and 12 percent, respectively, for males 20–65 years old, and 33 percent and 11 percent, respectively, for females in the same age group (USDA, 1997). The National Cancer Institute recommends consuming up to 30 g of fiber in the diet daily (Butrum, Clifford, & Lanza, 1988). However, Americans were estimated to consume on average 14 g of fiber for women and 18 g for men (USDA, 1997). Diets of both men and women were reported to be very low in fruits and dark green and yellow vegetables, with white potatoes serving as the primary vegetable (USDA, 1997). Additionally, while food consumption data from the National Health and Nutrition Examination Survey (NHANES) II (1976–1980) and NHANES III (1988–1994) showed a decrease in energy intake leveling off in 1990 (Lichtenstein, Kennedy, & Barrier, 1998), the prevalence of overweight and obesity among adults has increased (overweight prevalence: 47 percent in 1976–1980 increased to 56 percent in 1988–1994; obesity prevalence: 32 percent in

1976–1980 increased to 33 percent in 1988–1994) (National Center for Health Statistics, 2000).

The problem with achieving national dietary recommendations for adults is not unique to the United States. National dietary recommendations for dietary fat, fiber, and servings from the different food groups are similar for Canadians and Americans. While Canadians are faring better with respect to meeting goals for total and saturated fat for adults, age 18–65 years, mean intake of fiber, and servings of fruits, vegetables, and grain products for males and females in this age group were much below Canadian dietary recommendations (Gray-Donald, Jacobs-Starkey, & Johnson-Down, 2000). Given the very important role of diet in the prevention of chronic diseases, further improvements in the diet of adults are needed.

THEORIES AND RESEARCH

There is general agreement among nutrition educators that to achieve a desired dietary and/or diet-related behavior change, an intervention must be theory-driven with specific end-points. A theory-based approach can both guide program development and provide a foundation for the evaluation of impact and the identification of areas in need of further work. Several theoretical models have been used for adult behavioral interventions to predict changes in dietary behavior. These include the *health belief model, the social learning theory, the stages of change model, the social marketing theory, and community organization models.*

The *health belief model* (Maiman & Becker, 1974) indicates that readiness to change behavior is more likely if actions to be taken are feasible, the benefits are recognized, and the barriers to adopting the new behaviors are low. The basic tenet of the *social learning theory* is that a person both affects and is affected by his/her environment (Bandura, 1986). According to this theory, behavior change can be achieved if an intervention increases an individual's awareness of important factors in their environment affecting healthful food choices, enhances the value an individual places on the desired health-related behavior ("*expectancy*"), provides the knowledge and skills necessary for an individual to perform the desired behavior ("*behavioral capability*"), instills an individual with the confidence to perform a particular behavior ("*self-efficacy*"), and provides rewards or incentives for achieving and/or maintaining the desired health-related behavior ("*reinforcement*"). Many of the interventions reviewed below contain these elements.

The *stages of change model* complements the aforementioned theories, proposing that people who change behaviors do so through a series of stages along a continuum of change-readiness: *pre-contemplation, contemplation,*

determination/preparation, action, and maintenance (Prochaska & DiClemente, 1982). A person's position on the continuum determines which types of educational approaches should be used in an intervention to change their behavior. Mass media campaigns in particular use the *social marketing theory,* which is based on theories of consumer behavior (Kotler & Zaltman, 1974). The theory suggests that individuals will change behavior in exchange for perceived benefits, such as reducing disease risk. According to the theory, the behavior change occurs only when the perceived benefits meet or exceed the perceived costs. Social marketing also centers on the idea that consumer research is critical to identifying the target audience for a program, their needs and wants, and the factors that go into their decision-making processes.

Recent community-based approaches to behavior change recognize the importance of empowering the community or organization to direct the nature, design the scope, and identify the process for an intervention, a concept central to *community organization models* for community change (Minkler, 1990). In worksite interventions, for example, organizational empowerment often takes the form of mobilizing and training employees to plan, promote, and implement interventions to enhance the likelihood that employees will participate in the programs. Additional key elements of community organization models include fostering a community's ability to collaborate effectively on problem identification and resolution, promoting community involvement and participation in program activities, and changing perceived norms for healthy behaviors within the infrastructure of an organization (Minkler, 1990). Most of the community-based interventions reviewed below include one or a combination of these models to better understand and facilitate the behavioral change process.

STRATEGIES THAT WORK

Mass Media Campaigns

Social marketing theory was the major developmental force behind three national health campaigns that have successfully increased public awareness of health-promoting behaviors that may reduce risk of cancer, hypertension and cardiovascular disease. *The National High Blood Pressure Education Program* (NHBPEP) and the *National Cholesterol Education Program* (NCEP) have permeated the media for over a decade focusing on the link between high blood pressure and high cholesterol and cardiovascular disease. Based on formative research involving national survey data, focus groups, and concept tests with the public, these campaigns have effectively conveyed the message that high blood pressure and high cholesterol are seriously linked to illness, but have no symptoms and can occur in anyone (Bellicha & McGrath, 1990; Ward, 1984). Additionally, these programs have encouraged the general public to "know your numbers" by participating in cholesterol and blood pressure screening programs. A recent progress report by the National Institutes of Health showed a 60 percent decline in mortality and morbidity rates for stroke and coronary heart disease since the inception of the NHBPEP in 1972 (Frohlich, 1997). Both programs have reported an increased awareness of the link between high blood pressure and cholesterol and heart disease, and the number of individuals that have been screened. The success of these media efforts has been attributed, in part, to the simplicity and specificity of the message, and the reliance on consumer guidance to tailor the communication elements of the intervention (Contento et al., 1995).

The national *5 A Day for Better Health Program*, a joint project of the National Cancer Institute and the Produce for Better Health Foundation, has used the media, community, and retail efforts to increase the number of daily servings of fruits and vegetables that Americans eat to five or more. Based on extensive consumer research, the program chose as its target those adults who were already eating some fruits and vegetables each day (Eisner, Loughrey, Hadley, & Doner, 1992). These individuals were identified as likely "changers" according to the stages of change model. The program highlighted the benefits of eating fruits and vegetables, and offered easy, practical strategies to include these foods in the diet. The concept of *benefit*, defined as a reward that the consumer expects to gain from participating in the program, is central to social marketing theory (Andreasen, 1995). Using focus groups, benefits determined as likely to encourage increased consumption of fruits and vegetables were immediate benefits (e.g., feeling more energetic vs. more long-term benefits such as reducing health risks) (Balch, Loughrey, Weinberg, Lurie, & Eisner, 1997). Additionally, removing perceived barriers to achieving dietary benefits, such as lack of time and money, were identified by consumers as being essential to promoting increased fruit and vegetable intake (Balch et al., 1997). The 5 A day media campaign has effectively raised public awareness that fruits and vegetables help reduce disease risk, has increased fruit and vegetable consumption in major population segments, and has created ongoing partnerships between public health and agribusiness (National Cancer Institute, 1995). The success of the program has underscored the importance of direct consumer research to ensure that program messages and strategies are appropriate and relevant to the target audience.

Mass media campaigns have also been used to target one of the primary sources of saturated fat in the American diet— whole milk. Reger, Wootan, and Booth-Butterfield, (1999) used paid advertising and a public relations campaign (several press conferences and taste test events) to encourage individuals in Wheeling, West Virginia to switch from high-fat to low-fat milk. In developing the campaign, focus groups and consumer surveys were used to create a message that was focused on a single behavior and could be communicated easily to the public. The effectiveness of the "1% Or Less" campaign was evaluated by collecting milk sales data from supermarkets and conducting pre- and post-intervention telephone surveys in the intervention city. These results were compared to the same data collected from a city of equal demographics that received the media campaign plus community-based educational activities, and a city of comparable demographics that received no intervention. Similar significant increases in milk sales and number of people switching to low-fat milk were documented after 6 months in the cities receiving the media-only intervention and the media plus community activities compared with the city receiving no intervention. Importantly, the results obtained with the media-only approach were not sustained after the ads stopped airing. Thus, while mass media campaigns that are simple, focused on a single behavior and based on consumer research may be an effective means of reaching a large number of people quickly to promote a desired health-related behavior change, the effect may be short-lived if the program is not combined with additional programming to continuously reinforce and support the advocated behavior change.

Community Interventions

Three large, multi-risk factor community trials spanned more than a decade (1980–1992). Each had as a primary purpose cardiovascular disease prevention: the *Stanford Five City Project* (Farquhar, Fortmann, & Maccoby, 1990; Fortmann, Tahor, Flora, & Winkleby, 1993); the *Minnesota Heart Health Program* (Luepker, Murray, Jacobs, Mittlemark, Bracht, & Carlaw, 1994); and the *Pawtucket Heart Health Program* (Elder, McGraw, & Abrams, 1986). These multimillion-dollar trials addressed the prevention and treatment of smoking, hypertension, poor diet quality, obesity, and physical inactivity. Using components of social marketing theory, social learning theory, and community organization theories, these programs were designed to improve participant's nutrition knowledge, attitudes, and behaviors by providing them with the skills necessary to lower the total fat and cholesterol in their diets. Participants were exposed to a variety of educational messages in the form of television, radio, and print media (media here was used to support other programming rather than as the focus of the intervention), seminars, and classes. Additionally, collaborations with existing community agencies were sought to develop a lasting health promotion structure within the community.

Although penetration of nutrition-related risk reduction information was high in all three community trials, nutrition-related behavior change as measured by reduced dietary intake of total fat and cholesterol was no greater than in control communities in the Stanford Program (Fortmann et al., 1993). Both control and intervention communities showed significant reductions in consumption of these "unhealthy" nutrients. Dietary intake was not reported in the Minnesota and Pawtucket programs. All three programs reported increased screening behavior, decreased serum cholesterol levels (although marginal in two of the studies) and smoking prevalence in intervention communities compared to control sites (Elder et al., 1986; Fortmann et al., 1993; Luepker et al., 1994). While changes in serum cholesterol were less than anticipated in all three studies, from a public health perspective even a small change in diet-related risk factors at the community level can lead to large effects on disease risk. Importantly, a high contact rate, coupled with even a small intervention effect, has the potential to produce substantial changes in diet-related risk factors at the community level (Sorensen & Pechacek, 1990).

The lack of a direct dietary change in the Stanford community intervention was disappointing given the comprehensive nature of the nutrition component of the program. Fortmann et al. (1993) provided several possible explanations for the results: (1) dietary assessment methodology was not sensitive enough to detect small changes in diet over time; (2) dietary baseline data were not comparable among study sites; and (3) the nutrition-related risk reduction information was not pervasive or powerful enough to make a noticeable difference in eating behavior above the wide range of other health promotion activities initiated in that particular community over the same decade.

High-Risk Interventions

Dietary interventions directed at free-living, high-risk adults are too numerous to review in detail. However, several exemplary studies will be described in brief to illustrate the point that individually directed interventions can produce significant changes in dietary habits and diet-related behaviors when the program is targeted at highly motivated individuals. The Trials of Hypertension Prevention study was a multi center, randomized trial designed to examine the efficacy of sodium and weight reduction in reducing blood pressure over a 3-year period (Trials of Hypertension Prevention Collaborative Research Group, 1997). The intervention component of the program was delivered in the form of weekly group or individual counseling sessions over a 3-month period. Follow-up was implemented through telephone and biweekly or monthly in-person group or individual meetings. A series of short refresher and enrichment courses of 3–6 sessions supplemented by participant-initiated contacts were provided in years 2 and 3 of the program. Participants were guided through a behavioral change process that focused on

action goals, and knowledge and behavioral skills necessary to make and maintain reductions in body weight and sodium. In normal weight and overweight adults with high–normal blood pressure, weight loss and reduction in sodium intake were successfully achieved by the intervention and the dietary changes resulted in significant lowering of both systolic and diastolic blood pressure. Significant reductions in diastolic blood pressure were maintained in the weight loss group, while systolic changes were maintained for both the weight loss and sodium groups.

The Women's Health Trial, initiated by the National Cancer Institute in three centers in the United States (Henderson, Kushi, & Thompson, 1990) and a similar dietary intervention trial conducted in Toronto, Canada (Boyd, Martin, Beaton, Cousins, & Kriukov, 1996) were designed to study the effects of a low-fat, high-carbohydrate diet on the incidence of breast cancer in women at elevated risk for the disease. The interventions consisted of an 8–10-week intensive phase of group meetings that focused on skill building, motivation, and decision-making, followed by less intensive monthly meetings to reinforce the same information over a 1-year period. In both studies, participants were able to reduce their fat intake by approximately 13 percent, and maintain this change for 1 year. Factors contributing to adherence in the Women's Health Trial included attendance at the educational classes and consequent knowledge of skills necessary to make changes, education level, and frequency of face-to-face contact with a dietitian. Results from these studies suggest that even short periods of intensive dietary counseling may have prolonged effects on diet if the intervention is targeted at a highly motivated, at-risk population.

STRATEGIES THAT MIGHT WORK

The marginal diet-related behavior changes made by expensive community-based health promotion interventions may also be attributed to insufficient or non-sustained environmental support for the programs. Community interventions that seek to form networks of collaborations with a variety of existing state and county-level agencies and businesses are suggested to hold the most promise for achieving more substantial and lasting dietary change within a community. One program that has been particularly successful in this endeavor is the *Kansas LEAN Project* (Johnston, Marmet, Coen, Fawcett, & Harris, 1996). One hundred organizations and businesses across Kansas, including food distributors, media, private industry, and volunteer health agencies, have joined forces to form a unique coalition for the primary purpose of changing unhealthy dietary habits to prevent chronic disease. The members have succeeded in developing and distributing nutrition education resources, implementing community-level nutrition interventions, and designing an evaluation element for the program. Additionally, the coalition has cost communities almost no money, because of numerous grants and donations received to carry out its mission. Although data are still forthcoming on the effectiveness of the program, it is anticipated that this type of intervention will have substantial environmental impact and make a significant contribution to promoting healthy eating habits across the state and elsewhere.

Point-of-Choice Interventions have been used to promote healthful food purchasing behavior with some degree of success at supermarkets and restaurants. In general, supermarket programs that involved active participation of the individual in changing unhealthy food buying behavior (Carson & Hedl, 1998; Shannon, Mullis, Pirie, & Pheley, 1990), gave feedback on food purchases with specific goals for change (Winnett, Wagner, & Moore, 1991), educated consumers about healthy food preparation methods, and provided nutrition information along with the potential health benefits of specific foods (Davis-Cherven, Rogers, & Clark, 1985), had a significantly positive impact on individual food purchases. Supermarket programs that were strictly educational campaigns, such as those using poster displays, shelf signs, and brochures to promote healthy foods and brand names, often changed consumer awareness and knowledge about unhealthy foods but did not change buying behavior (Russo, Staelin, Nolan, Russell, & Metcalf, 1986). In restaurants, interventions have primarily focused on nutrient labeling to promote healthful food items. These efforts have reportedly increased sales of the targeted food item during the intervention, but the effects generally disappear almost immediately after the intervention has ceased (Anderson & Haas, 1990). Point-of-choice interventions may be especially useful as adjuncts to other comprehensive community efforts.

Worksites have been used extensively for health promotion efforts among adults and offer several distinct advantages over other community-based settings. Worksites are an ideal channel for promoting change in large segments of the adult population and there are social support systems to reinforce health behavior changes. Additionally, worksite interventions can be offered repeatedly, increasing the likelihood of motivating behavior change in persons who are at various stages of readiness (Sorensen et al., 1999). Of particular importance is the effect that worksite risk reduction programs can have on less educated workers and those in low-status jobs, among whom diet-related behavioral risk factors are particularly high (USDA, 2000).

Over the past decade, five multiple-risk factor intervention trials have been conducted at the worksite that combine individually oriented programs directed at promoting healthy nutrition and lifestyle practices with organizational-level strategies designed to support healthy behavior. These studies were similar in research design (randomized, match-pair), duration (15–24 months), and theoretical basis (included elements of social learning theory, health belief model, and community organization models). The *Working Well Trial* (Patterson et al., 1997), the Treatwell *5 A Day Study* (Sorensen et al., 1999), the *Take Heart Program II* (Glasgow, Terborg, Strycker, Boles, & Hollis, 1997), the *Next Step Trial* (Tilley, Glanz, Kristal, Hirst, Vernon, & Myers, 1999), and the *WellWorks Study* (Sorensen et al., 1998) included worker participation in the planning and implementation of the intervention, utilized an array of health education programs and materials targeting individual behavior change strategies (some more extensive than others), and incorporated worksite environmental changes as specified by an employee advisory panel. The nutrition focus in all but the Take Heart Program II was similar—increasing fruits, vegetables, and fiber and decreasing total fat intake. The Take Heart Program II focused only on decreasing total dietary fat. The results of the interventions were variable. Of those studies with a multicomponent nutrition focus, fruit and vegetable consumption increased in all studies, fiber intake increased in three, and total dietary fat decreased marginally in only two. The Take Heart Program II showed a more significant decrease in mean total fat intake among worksite employees, possibly because nutrition education programs focused on that particular nutrient. Nutrition educators have suggested that adopting a low-fat diet is a complex set of behaviors requiring that an individual be able to change basic food selection and preparation patterns and often limit intake of many favorite foods (Patterson et al., 1997). Conversely, the message to eat more fruits and vegetables is positive, simple and may be more successfully translated in worksites and other community-based interventions.

STRATEGIES THAT DO NOT WORK

We have learned a variety of important lessons from worksite interventions, including what does not work. The duration and intensity of the individual program components and the degree to which the intervention considers an individual's social context in relation to eating behavior correlated with the success of the effort. Of the worksite programs that evaluated nutrition behavior change in relation to program duration and intensity, there was general agreement that long-term, interactive intervention efforts (such as contests and classes) resulted in more positive nutrition-related behavior changes than one-time activities (kick-offs) or passive efforts (use of print materials) (Glasgow et al., 1997; Patterson et al., 1997; Sorensen et al., 1998). Further, interventions that attempted to bring about health-promoting changes in the worksite environment (e.g., food availability, point-of-choice nutrition information) were able to sustain changes in eating behavior longer than those that focused on individually based approaches only. The Treatwell 5 A Day study incorporated a family education component into the worksite based health promotion program, along with changes in the worksite environment. The significant dietary behavior changes achieved by this study over other programs demonstrates that the effectiveness of nutrition interventions can be enhanced when programs take into account an individual's social context, including the home and worksite (Sorensen et al., 1999). To the extent that these factors are not considered, then success is made less likely.

SYNTHESIS

There is general agreement that Americans need to eat better to improve their chances for a healthier life. However, research demonstrates that many individuals are confused about current recommendations from different health organizations on healthy ways to eat to prevent chronic disease. Further, it appears that, for some, this confusion has resulted in dietary inaction. A first step in accelerating efforts to improve America's diet and health may be for nutritionists and other health professionals to assist the public in recognizing that dietary recommendations from diverse US health organizations are in agreement in their major principles:

> to choose a diet that is low in saturated fat and cholesterol, moderate in total fat, moderate in salt, includes a variety of grains, fruits and vegetables, and contains an appropriate energy-level to achieve a healthy weight.

National implementation of the Dietary Guidelines for Americans (USDA, 2000) may help to alleviate public confusion and promote action toward achieving a more healthful diet across the United States.

Contemporary theories related to individual, social, and environmental change have proven to be critical in formulating effective dietary interventions and corresponding program evaluations. In brief, campaigns using social marketing were most effective if they considered the perceived needs, aspirations, and personal motivators of the target audience. Further, attempts to modify dietary behaviors using this approach worked most often if the campaign message was simple, specific, and combined with additional community programming to support the advocated dietary behavior change. More recent community interventions were based on the health belief model, the social learning theory, the stages of change theory, as well as models of community organization and participation. Community programs most likely to be effective were those that were sustained over a long duration, included educational strategies that were motivating,

taught skills necessary to change behavior, and considered the individual's social context (home, work, and community) in relation to eating behavior. Successful interventions directed at high-risk individuals utilized many of these same theories and strategies as well as individualized interpersonal counseling and education.

In summary, to promote a healthful diet in adults, strategies based on theory that empower the individual through a simple and unified message, motivating and skill building activities, and continuous social and environmental support, should be the basis for the development of future dietary intervention approaches for the primary prevention of chronic disease.

Also see: Nutrition: Early Childhood; Nutrition: Childhood; Nutrition: Older Adulthood.

References

Anderson, J., & Haas, M.H. (1990). Impact of a nutrition education program on food sales in restaurants. *Journal of Nutrition Education, 22,* 232–238.

Andreasen, A.R. (1995). *Marketing social change: Changing behavior to promote health, social development, and the environment.* San Francisco: Jossey-Bass.

Balch, G.I., Loughrey, K.L., Weinberg, L., Lurie, D., & Eisner, E. (1997). Probing consumer benefits and barriers for the National 5 A Day Campaign: Focus group findings. *Journal of Nutrition Education, 29,* 178–183.

Bandura, A. (1986). *Social foundations of thought and action: A social cognitive theory.* Englewood Cliffs, NJ: Prentice-Hall.

Bellicha, T., & McGrath, J. (1990). Mass media approaches to reducing cardiovascular disease risk. *Public Health Reports, 105,* 247–252.

Boyd, N.F., Martin, L.J., Beaton, M., Cousins, M., & Kriukov, V. (1996). Long-term effects of participation in a randomized trial of a low-fat, high-carbohydrate diet. *Cancer Epidemiology, Biomarkers and Prevention, 5,* 217–222.

Butrum, R., Clifford, C., & Lanza, E. (1988). NCI dietary guidelines: Rationale. *American Journal of Clinical Nutrition, 48,* 888–895.

Carson, J.S., & Hedl, J.J. (1998). Smart shopper tours: Outcome evaluation. *Journal of Nutrition Education, 30,* 323–331.

Contento, I., Balch, G.I., Bronner, Y., Lytle, L., Maloney, S., Olson, C., Sharaga, & Swadener, S. (1995). Nutrition education for adults. *Journal of Nutrition Education, 27,* 312–328.

Cotugna, N., Subar, A., Heimendinger, J., & Kahle, L. (1992). Nutrition and cancer prevention knowledge, beliefs, attitudes and practices: The 1987 National Health Interview Survey. *Journal of the American Dietetic Association, 92,* 963–968.

Davis-Cherven, D., Rogers, T., & Clark, M. (1985). Influencing food selection with point-of-choice nutrition information. *Journal of Nutrition Education, 17,* 18–22.

Deckelbaum, R.J., Fisher, E.A., Winston, M., Kumanyika, S., Lauer, R.M., Pi-Sunyer, F.X., St. Jeor, S., Schaefer, E.J., Weinstein, I.B. (1999). Summary of a scientific conference on preventive nutrition: Pediatrics to geriatrics. *Circulation, 100,* 450–456.

Eisner, E., Loughrey, K., Hadley, L., & Doner, L. (1992). *Understanding benefits and barriers to fruit and vegetable consumption.* Bethesda, MD: National Cancer Institute.

Elder, J.P., McGraw, S.A., & Abrams, D.B. (1986). Organization and community approaches to community-wide prevention of heart disease: The first two years of the Pawtucket Heart Health Program. *Preventive Medicine, 14*, 107–117.

Farquhar, J.S., Fortmann, S.P., & Maccoby, N. (1990). Effects of community-wide education on cardiovascular disease risk factors: The Stanford Five-City Project. *Journal of the American Medical Association, 264*, 359–365.

Fortmann, S.P., Tahor, C.B., Flora, J.A., & Winkleby, M.A. (1993). Effects of community-wide education on plasma cholesterol levels and diet: The Stanford Five-City Project. *American Journal of Epidemiology, 137*, 1039–1055.

Frohlich, E.D. (1997). The sixth report of the Joint National Committee: An appropriate celebration of the 25th anniversary of the National High Blood Pressure Education Program. *Hypertension, 30*, 1305–1306.

Glasgow, R.E., Terborg, J.R., Strycker, L.A., Boles, S.M., & Hollis, J.F. (1997). Take Heart II: Replication of a worksite health promotion trial. *Journal of Behavioral Medicine, 20*, 143–160.

Gray-Donald, K., Jacobs-Starkey, L., & Johnson-Down, L. (2000). Food habits of Canadians: Reduction in fat intake over a generation. *Canadian Journal of Public Health, 91*, 381–385.

Henderson, M.M., Kushi, L.H., & Thompson, D.J. (1990). Feasibility of a randomized trial of a low-fat diet for the prevention of breast cancer: Dietary compliance in the Women's Health Trial Vanguard Study. *Preventive Medicine, 19*, 115–133.

Johnston, J.A., Marmet, P.F., Coen, S., Fawcett, S.B., & Harris, K.J. (1996). Kansas LEAN: An effective coalition for nutrition education and dietary change. *Journal of Nutrition Education, 28*, 115–118.

Kotler, P., & Zaltman, G. (1974, July). Social marketing: An approach to planned social change. *Journal of Marketing*, 3–12.

Lichtenstein, A.H., Kennedy, E., & Barrier, P. (1998). Dietary fat consumption and health. *Nutrition Reviews, 56*, S3–S19.

Luepker, R.V., Murray, D.M., Jacobs, D.R., Mittlemark, M.B., Bracht, N., & Carlaw, R. (1994). Community education for cardiovascular disease prevention: Risk factor changes in the Minnesota Heart Health Program. *American Journal of Public Health, 84*, 1383–1393.

Maiman, L.A., & Becker, M.H. (1974). The Health Belief Model: Origin and correlates in psychological theory. In B.H. Becker (ed.), *The health belief model and personal health behavior* (pp. 9–26). Thorofare, NJ: Charles Slack.

Minkler, M. (1990). Improving health through community organization. In K. Glanz, F.M. Lewis, B.K. Rimer (eds.), *Health behavior and health education: Theory, research and practice* (pp. 257–287). San Francisco: Jossey-Bass.

National Cancer Institute, Office of Cancer Communications. (1995). *Five A Day for better health: NCI media campaign*. Bethesda: Author.

National Center for Health Statistics. (1996, October). *Monthly vital statistics report*, p. 31.

National Center for Health Statistics. (2000). Prevalence of overweight and obesity among adults: United States, 1999. http://www.cdc.gov/nchs/products/pubs/pubd/hestats/obese/obse99.htm

Patterson, R.E., Kristal, A.R., Glanz, K., McLerran, D.F., Herbert, J.R., Heimemdinger, J., Linnan, L., Probart, C., & Chamberlain, R.M. (1997). Components of the Working Well Trial intervention associated with adoption of healthful diets. *American Journal of Preventive Medicine, 13*, 271–276.

Prochaska, J.O., & DiClemente, C.C. (1982). Transtheoretical therapy: Toward a more integrative model of change. *Psychotherapy: Theory, Research and Practice, 19*, 276–288.

Reger, B., Wootan, M.G., & Booth-Butterfield, S. (1999). Using mass media to promote healthy eating: A community-based demonstration project. *Preventive Medicine, 29*, 414–421.

Russo, J.E., Staelin, R., Nolan, C.A., Russell, G.J., & Metcalf, B.L. (1986). Nutrition information in the supermarket. *Journal of Consumer Research, 12*, 48–70.

Shannon, B., Mullis, R.M., Pirie, P.L., & Pheley, A.M. (1990). Promoting better nutrition in the grocery store using a game format: The Shop Smart Game Project. *Journal of Nutrition Education, 22*, 183–188.

Sorensen, G., & Pechacek, T. (1990). Occupational and worksite comparisons of smoking and smoking cessations. *Journal of Occupational Medicine, 28*, 360–364.

Sorensen, G., Stoddard, A., Hunt, M.K., Herbert, J.R., Ockene, J.K., Avrunin, J.S., Himmelstein, J., & Hammond, S.K. (1998). The effects of a health promotion–health protection intervention on behavior change: The WellWorks Study. *American Journal of Public Health, 88*, 1685–1690.

Sorensen, G., Stoddard, A., Peterson, K., Cohen, N., Hunt, M.K., Stein, E., Palombo, R., & Lederman, R. (1999). Increasing fruit and vegetable consumption through worksites and families in the Treatwell 5-a-Day Study. *American Journal of Public Health, 89*, 54–60.

Tilley, B.C., Glanz, K., Kristal, A.R., Hirst, K., Li, S., Vernon, S.W., & Myers, R. (1999). Nutrition intervention for high-risk auto workers: Results of the Next Step Trial. *Preventive Medicine, 28*, 284–292.

Trials of Hypertension Prevention Collaborative Research Group. (1997). Effects of weight loss and sodium reduction intervention on blood pressure and hypertension incidence in overweight people with high–normal blood pressure. *Archives of Internal Medicine, 157*, 657–667.

US Department of Agriculture (USDA), Agricultural Research Service. (1997). *1994–1996 Continuing Survey of Food Intake by Individuals* [CD-ROM]. NTIS Accession Number PB98-500457

US Department of Agriculture (USDA), Agricultural Research Service, Dietary Guidelines Committee. (2000). *Dietary Guidelines for Americans* (5th ed.) (USDA, Home and Garden Bulletin No. 232).

Ward, G.W. (1984). The national high blood pressure education program: An example of social marketing in action. In L.W. Fredericken, L.J. Solomon, & K.A. Brehony (eds.), *Marketing health behavior: Principles, techniques and applications*. New York: Plenum Press.

Winnett, R.A., Wagner, J.L., & Moore, J.F. (1991) An experimental evaluation of prototype public access nutrition information system for supermarkets. *Health Psychology, 10*, 75–78.

Nutrition, Older Adulthood

Monica J. Belyea, Michelle B. Pierce, and Carol J. Lammi-Keefe[1,2]

INTRODUCTION

Optimal nutrition permits older adults to maintain health, treat and rehabilitate chronic conditions, and secure

[1] Supported in part by funds made available through the Hatch Act and the University of Connecticut Family Nutrition Program.
[2] Represents scientific contribution number 2021, Storrs Agricultural Experiment Station, University of Connecticut, Storrs, Connecticut.

functional independence by helping to maintain lean body mass, immune function, and prevent chronic disease without excessive weight gain or loss (American Dietetic Association, 2000). While life span may not be significantly extended through improved dietary patterns instituted during later years, preventing morbidity—"adding life to years" (Minkler, Schauffler, & Clements-Nolle, 2000)—is an important goal of nutrition promotion activities.

DEFINITIONS

An *optimal diet* for older adults is typified by nutrient dense foods including fruits, vegetables, whole grains, low-fat dairy products, and low-fat protein foods (Russell, Rasmussen, & Lichtenstein, 1999). Additionally, reduced sodium intake can benefit older adults by helping to prevent the blood pressure elevation commonly experienced by older adults (Chobanian & Hill, 2000). *Nutrient dense* foods are those which have a relatively high nutrient content for the energy they provide. *Malnutrition* includes both *undernutrition*, a lack of nutrients, and *overnutrition*, an excess of nutrients. Undernutrition of micronutrients and overnutrition of macronutrients is most commonly seen in the United States. *Micronutrients* include vitamins, minerals, and phytochemicals. *Macronutrients* include protein, carbohydrate, fat, and water. The *US Dietary Guidelines* are science-based recommendations put forth by the US Department of Agriculture (USDA) and US Department of Health and Human Services (2000) in an attempt to synthesize current research into optimal dietary recommendations based on common nutrition-related problems associated with underconsumption of micronutrients and overconsumption of macronutrients for a healthy US public. These guidelines, much like those of other western countries, set forth a pattern of food intake rather than nutrient recommendations.

SCOPE

The prevalence of malnutrition is widespread among older adults in the United States. Typically, protein intakes are marginal; vitamin E, B_6, calcium, magnesium, and zinc are inadequate; total fat, saturated fat, and sodium are high; and fiber is insufficient. Nationally representative data from the *Continuing Survey of Food Intakes of Individuals 1989–1991* showed that 34–89 percent of US older adults consumed below recommended intakes for energy and 10 nutrients including protein, vitamins E, C, niacin, and B and the minerals calcium, phosphorous, magnesium, iron, and zinc (Weimer, 1998). Similarly, studies in Canada, Japan, and Europe confirm a decreased energy intake and general

micronutrient underconsumption in older adults (Bogan, 1997; de Groot van den Broek, & van Staveren, 1999; Nakatsuka et al., 1999)

Older adults have a much higher rate of nutrition-related chronic disease than younger populations. The costs associated with malnutrition among older adults include both decreased quality of life and increased care dollars. The US Department of Health and Human Services (1999) quantified the cost to older adults in personal health care expenditures in 1995 for heart disease and diabetes alone at $84 billion.

THEORIES

Nutrition promotion, like all aspects of health promotion for older adults, should be developed based on a thorough assessment and understanding of the target audience and sound health behavior theory. In program planning, practitioners often substitute methods of education for behavior theories to the detriment of the learning experience and participant outcomes.

Adult learning theory can been used successfully as the basis for developing materials and physical environments for older adults (Taylor-Davis et al., 2000). Behavior change theories have been proposed for the promotion of nutrition (Doner, 1997). These include Social learning theory, the Transtheoretical model or Stages of change, and the Health belief model. Although knowledge of optimal nutrition and positive attitudes toward nutrition do not always lead to optimal behaviors, the two constructs should not be summarily dismissed. They can explain in part nutrition behavior among older adults (Fischer, Crockett, Heller, & Skauge, 1991).

Social learning theory characterizes individual health behavior based on three determinants: (1) personal factors, such as attitudes and values; (2) environment influences, such as social relationships and physical environment; and (3) factors associated with the behavior itself, such as perceived capability to perform the behavior and outcomes expected for performing the behavior. This theory can be used to design interventions that help older adults work through the barriers and benefits of eating nutrient dense foods.

The *Transtheoretical model* or *Stages of change* considers behavior change in a series of cognitive steps: precontemplation, contemplation, preparation, action, maintenance, and termination. According to the theory, effective nutrition interventions should be tailored to the step or stage of the participants. Interestingly, in a recent investigation of the application of this model, Nigg et al. (1999) found that when asked about eating high fiber, a cohort of older adults fell into precontemplation or maintenance stages only; no one indicated contemplation, preparation, action, or termination.

Similar results were found when older adults were asked about avoiding fat.

Based on our experience, elderly cohorts, like other consumers, can often state ideal nutrition constructs; however, they are unable to translate the message into practice. For example, while older adults may recognize that a low-fat diet is healthful and may believe they are following a low-fat diet, they do not know how to select lower fat cuts of meat. More accurate self-assessments can be achieved after complex nutrition behaviors such as "eating low fat" have been adequately described.

The *Health belief model* may be effective with older adults because of their proximity to disease morbidity. According to this model, an individual will take action to avoid disease because of perceived susceptibility to the disease and perceived severity of the disease. Variables within a person's environment modify these perceptions and affect the likelihood of preventive measures.

RESEARCH

The new Dietary Reference Intakes are being developed to replace the Recommended Dietary Allowances by the Standing Committee on the Scientific Evaluation of Dietary Reference Intakes of the Food and Nutrition Board, Institute of Medicine (1997). The new standards reflect a growing body of literature specific to older adults and include two life stage groups, 51–70 years and 71+ years. Nutrient recommendations consider physiological changes specific to older adults. Research provides evidence that elderly are not consuming adequate nutrients and that their requirements for some nutrients are higher than previously believed. The factors that affect nutrient intake are complex involving physical activity, food security, socioeconomic status, and life course. Other factors that can affect nutritional states are drug–nutrient interactions, changes in smell, taste, and thirst, and diet-related chronic conditions (Haller, 1999).

Nutrient Intake

The interrelationship of nutrient adequacy and health in older adults has been reviewed by Blumberg (1997) and Haller (1999). Low caloric intakes, commonly seen in older adults, make it difficult for this population to consume adequate nutrients. Micronutrient intakes may not be low enough to cause a clinical abnormality or deficiency, but low intakes combined with an illness or other morbidity can lead to subclinical deficiency and affect daily function and morbidity.

Nutrients of concern, both because they are typically underconsumed and because some are needed in high quantity, include protein, water, fiber, the minerals calcium and zinc, and vitamins D, B_{12}, B_6, folate, and carotenoids. Older adults need slightly more dietary protein to maintain lean body mass. The recommendation is 1–1.25 g/kg/day compared to the 1989 RDA of 0.8 g/kg/day for all adults (Evans & Cyr-Campbell, 1997). Adequate fluid intake is necessary to compensate for decreased thirst perception and increased likelihood of constipation and decreased intestinal absorption of water.

Recommended calcium intake for older adults has been increased to 1,200 mg per day. This increase reflects research that demonstrates that adequate calcium intake can prevent bone mineral loss, delay osteoporosis, and ultimately reduce bone fractures. Vitamin D recommendations have been increased to 400 International Units per day to ensure adequate calcium absorption and help regulate bone minerals. Decreased skin production of this vitamin with age and the need to protect skin from sun exposure put older adults at risk for deficiency (Food and Nutrition Board, Institute of Medicine, 1997).

Vitamin B_{12} is a targeted nutrient for older adults because a chronic deficiency can lead to dementia and permanent neurological damage. Changes in gut acidity and decreased Intrinsic Factor production, required for digestion of B_{12}, has led to the recommendation that this age group consume synthetic B_{12} sources such as fortified foods or supplements (Food and Nutrition Board, Institute of Medicine, 1997).

Reducing sodium intake below 2,400 mg per day, the national recommendation, has been shown to help safely lower blood pressure in older adults. This recommendation has not been widely accepted for any other population group (Chobanian & Hill, 2000).

Physical Activity

Decreased physical activity is often cited as the cause for decreased energy needs in older adults. Evidence shows that a decrease in caloric needs and loss of lean mass is not inherent to the aging process. Increased physical activity, including strength training and aerobic exercise, can help maintain caloric requirements, lean mass, usual glucose uptake and insulin sensitivity, and normal blood pressure (Evans & Cyr-Campbell, 1997).

Socioeconomic Status

Weimer (1998) analyzed data from the Continuing Survey of Food Intakes of Individuals 1989–1991, a nationally representative survey conducted by the USDA. Older adults with lower incomes and less education, as well as Blacks, and women, had lower quality diets. Similarly, Keller, Ostbye, and Bright-See (1997) reported an association between dietary intake and education, income, social support, and level of happiness in a cohort of older Canadians.

Food Stamp Participation

A discouraging note from Weimer's (1998) report is that participation in the USDA Food Stamp program had no effect on diet quality. It may be that only the most financially insecure, hungry or poorly functioning older adults participate in the Food Stamp program. Those older adults with relatively better situations, but who also qualify, may choose not to participate in the Food Stamp program and thereby miss an opportunity to purchase high quality foods. Wolfe, Olson, Kendall, and Frongillo (1996) examined the perceptions of rural versus urban older adults. They determined that many of the rural older adults who might benefit from food stamps could not bring themselves to apply because of the stigma associated with using government assistance. Many of the urban seniors were more willing to participate but only qualified for the minimum benefit of $10 per month. For this group, the effort of applying was not worth the small benefit.

Eating Alone

Eating alone is considered a risk factor for poor intake, but it is not strong enough by itself to produce an effect. As reviewed in Pierce (2000), living alone may have a slight, negative impact on food intake patterns, especially for males. It is suggested that gender and living arrangements are indicators of larger social forces. In this elderly cohort, females had been the traditional providers of food and nutrition. Simultaneously, females had shouldered the responsibilities of maintaining social networks. The poor diet quality of elderly men who live alone may result from limited knowledge of food procurement and preparation methods. An inadequate support network may further exacerbate the situation.

Life Course

The research of Falk, Bisogni, and Sobal (1996) supports the influence of life course, or life experience, on variation in nutrient intake among older adults. In rural older adults, the effect of life course on food choice was most prominent through its influence on the development of ideals. Ideals included participants' beliefs about the content of "proper" meals, which included meat and potatoes. Also important was eating the foods they were served whether it be at a meal program, church supper, or at someone's home. This ideal was more important than health restrictions, personal preferences, or other ideals. The complex model takes into consideration value negotiations of ideals and is discussed by Falk et al. (1996).

STRATEGIES THAT WORK

There is a paucity of studies documenting positive nutrition behavior changes by older adults. Successful programs have taken a client-centered approach and employed print media, intensive and interactive programs, some with personal assessment and feedback. Some placed the nutrition promotion activities within a larger health promotion program. Many of the successful and unsuccessful nutrition education programs are reviewed by Contendo et al. (1995). More recent or non-traditional nutrition promotion approaches are reviewed here.

Print Materials

As reviewed by Contendo et al. (1995), print materials have been successfully employed to influence nutrition outcomes. Researchers have used focus groups to obtain a client perspective on appropriate topics and the manner of delivery that would be well received for nutrition messages and related recipes in senior newspapers. In a random survey of older adults within the readership market, 68 percent reported reading the articles and 26 percent of those reported changing an eating or food-buying habit as a result of the articles.

A second approach employed print materials delivered exclusively through the mail as part of a comprehensive health promotion intervention for retirees. The intervention included health risk appraisals completed by participants every 6 months, feedback letters based on the appraisals and self-management materials. Nutrition assessment and feedback were given in the context of general health promotion. The intervention group was rated as significantly better on several health indicators, including fat intake, than the control group who received only the risk appraisals. Possible effective elements of this intervention included personal assessment, targeted suggestions for improvement, and a total health context. Taylor-Davis et al. (2000) found that a nutrition newsletter designed using focus group testing and known elements to make it senior-friendly could affect knowledge, attitude, and behavior. Interventions included: (1) newsletters only, (2) newsletters plus a process evaluation administered by telephone, and (3) control group. Both interventions produced significantly greater positive changes in knowledge, perceived knowledge, interest in nutrition, stages of change for fiber and the "avoid fat" behavior over the control group. In addition, the newsletter plus telephone interview produced greater effects over the newsletter alone. These findings show that with the addition of personal contact, an impersonal newsletter can have additional benefits for older adults.

Interactive and Intensive Interventions

Another program, reviewed in Contendo et al. (1995), the Senior Gardening Project, used an intensive theory-based intervention which combined nutrition and gardening education with support elements. The intervention included bimonthly group nutrition and gardening education sessions, personal assessment, development of personal action plans with support from peers, acknowledgment of personal experience and successes, and home visits. In addition, raised bed gardens were built for each participant. Behavior changes included increase in the consumption of water, whole grains and starchy vegetables, vegetables and fruits, iron-rich foods, and vitamin C-rich vegetables/fruits and dairy.

Herman, Brown, and Heintz (2000) evaluated an eight-session "Healthy Living" program. The program emphasized the US Dietary Guidelines with their messages of balance, variety, and moderation, as well as a positive approach to foods and food choices. Sessions included knowledge and skill elements including recipe demonstrations, handouts, visuals, activities, and resources. There were significant increases in the number of servings consumed in the bread, vegetable, and milk food groups, a decrease in fat consumption and a decrease in blood cholesterol.

STRATEGIES THAT MIGHT WORK

Potentially helpful services and programs have been under-utilized by older adults or inadequately researched vis-à-vis behavior change and primary prevention. Registered dietitians, physicians, and food programs have the potential to help older adults achieve optimal nutrition, but their full potential has not been tested.

Registered dietitians are qualified to provide preventive nutrition guidance; however, their services are rarely covered by health insurance. Medicare has only recently been expanded to include nutrition services for older persons with diabetes or renal disease. Cost of service is likely prohibitive to many older adults. Lack of knowledge, on the part of physicians and older clients, about the quality of low-cost/free community nutrition programs may prevent referral and utilization of these potentially beneficial resources. Furthermore, physicians tend to view nutrition services as part of the treatment of chronic disease rather than prevention (Shawver & Cox, 2000).

Medical nutrition therapy, as delivered by registered dietitians, has been shown to help older adults achieve better health outcomes (Food and Nutrition Board, Institute of Medicine, 1999). When compared to similar efforts by physicians, patient outcomes were better when a registered dietitian offered nutrition guidance. These types of services are well documented for treating diseases and presumably reduce prescription drug costs for patients. The effect of these services for primary prevention of disease has not yet been examined.

Primary care providers are an important source of nutrition guidance and can positively influence health behaviors (Hiddink, Hautvast, van Woerkym, Fieren, 1997). The role of physicians in preventive nutrition behavior is strongest as gatekeeper. The primary care provider holds the power of referral and can offer legitimacy to preventive nutrition behaviors in the minds of older adults as well as their supportive network (Pierce, 2000).

In addition to offering nutrition education to older adults, efforts should be directed toward educating the nutrition-related support network. Daughters are the most frequent source of information for older women. Other network members, both formal and informal, who assist with food acquisition may benefit from nutrition education to assist with dietary adequacy as well (Pierce, Sheehan, & Ferris, 2001). An important improvement in diet quality is achieved when the social support networks of elderly living in subsidized housing includes managers, near-by store clerks, and other residents (Minkler et al., 2000).

Food coupons and alternative food provision programs have great potential. As discussed in Contendo et al. (1995), the Farmers' Market Coupon Program for low-income elderly can help older adults access fresh, seasonal produce. Similar to the WIC Farmers' Market Coupon Program, the senior coupons are distributed by each state to limited-income, older adults. Usually each older adult receives between $5 and $15 in low-denomination coupons to spend during one season at the WIC certified farmers' markets. Further study is needed to see if this type of program can improve a senior's diet quality and access to foods that promote health. Wolfe et al. (1996) found that older adults did not perceive using food pantries as a form of social welfare support and were far more willing to accept food donations than participate in formal types of programs like Food Stamps.

Older adults desire to reciprocate for help received. Thus, programs that request an *exchange of services*, such as SHARE or SERVE New England, are more likely to be used (Pierce, 2000). These programs are cooperative food purchasing programs that offer participants a half price bag of groceries in exchange for a small commitment of community service. When these programs are combined with service opportunities designed to meet the physical limitations of elders, they can be very successful. The provision of meals through the Elderly Nutrition Program improves the dietary quality of those who participate. However, it does not affect their food choice or consumption outside of the meal site. More importantly, the majority of seniors do not participate in these programs including high-risk seniors who reported difficulty buying food (Klesges, Pahor, Shorr, Wan, Williamson, & Guralnik, 2001). Additional investigation with non-participants is needed to provide insight into program redesign or alternatives.

Having food sources close to home, adequate transportation services for food shopping, manufacturing food items in convenient sizes and with optimal nutritional quality, and adaptive packaging, kitchens and appliances to make food preparation easier may improve diet quality (Minkler et al., 2000).

Social marketing uses traditional marketing principals to affect a health behavior. Less of a theory than a method of action, it involves a thorough understanding of the target audience and the issues they face when making decisions about health behaviors. Messages are developed based on this understanding and placed where they will be accessed by the target audience. As used in health or nutrition education, the beneficiary of the campaign is the individual or society rather than a profit-making organization (Doner, 1997). Some of the barriers to participation in the programs and services described above may be overcome by using social marketing.

STRATEGIES THAT DO NOT WORK

Changing the way people eat is not a simple matter. Strategies that work and might work require a strong commitment and active involvement. Strategies that have not worked share commonalties with those that succeeded but have lacked this commitment. For example, in their study of nutrition screening combined with one targeted nutrition counseling session, Benedict et al. (1999) were not able to affect nutrition outcomes. Participants in the counseling session often did not have any nutrition questions or understand that they were at nutritional risk. In addition, though many reported the session to be valuable in improving their nutritional health, only a small percentage had sought the services to which they were referred during the session.

Active participation in the nutrition intervention by participants choosing to attend a group education program is also important as demonstrated by Bedell and Shackleton (1989). Their intervention, which included four lectures with question and answer periods, had no effect on the 24 participants they surveyed.

As described above, government benefit programs, including the Food Stamps program and the Elderly Nutrition Program, are not widely utilized. There is a need to improve participation and ensure that older adults have adequate access to the foods they need.

SYNTHESIS

Optimal nutrition adopted later in life can reduce morbidity, adding quality and life to years. An optimal intake of nutrients and optimal dietary patterns can reduce chronic disease. Unfortunately, malnutrition exists among older adults. Bringing reduced energy needs in line with nutrient requirements can be difficult for many older adults to achieve.

Nutrition promotion should be, first and foremost, client-centered beginning with a thorough understanding of issues and solutions as perceived by the target population. Nutrition promotion for older adults should include strong, theory-based educational activities as well as environmental and system changes that help older adults overcome barriers to good nutrition. Additional documentation of approaches that work well with this population and increased vocalization of their perspective are needed.

All people do not learn or motivate in the same way. It is reasonable to expect to use multiple approaches with subgroups of older adults. Approaches may include group and individual education programs, printed materials, and mass media. Additional outcomes research should be conducted in all areas to help improve methods and better understand the food choice processes and limitations of older adults.

Successful educational programs and materials will include positive messages about food choices that are desirable to the target group; they will define the desired behaviors clearly and simply; they will offer participants an opportunity to assess their current behaviors and select priority behaviors to improve. Skill teaching and opportunities to reflect on and validate personal experience are also important aspects of successful education programs. This level of involvement by the participants and commitment by the educators can be a barrier to success. New research should determine levels of intensity required to achieve cost-effective programs.

Environmental and system changes should start with a better understanding of the barriers that older adults face when trying to access services and programs. Determining and changing factors that prevent older adults from participating in congregate meals and the Food Stamp program, increased reimbursement by Medicare and insurance companies for early preventive nutrition services, increased physician education related to preventive nutrition and the role of registered dietitians, as well as increased funding of nutrition-related support services, for example, grocery shopping for younger, higher functioning older adults, can all impact diet quality of older adults. Nutrition promoters need to look beyond typical nutrition education and begin to study these supportive mechanisms to determine the level of benefit that is achievable.

Also see: Nutrition: Early Childhood; Nutrition: Childhood; Nutrition: Adulthood.

References

American Dietetic Association. (2000). Position of the American Dietetic Association: Nutrition, aging, and the continuum of care. *Journal of the American Dietetic Association, 100*, 580–595.

Bedell, B.A., & Shackleton, P.A. (1989). The relationship between a nutrition education program and nutrition knowledge and eating behaviors of the elderly. *Journal of Nutrition for the Elderly, 8*, 35–45.

Benedict, J.A., Wilson, D., Snow, G., Nipp, P., Remig, V., Spoon, M., Leontos, C., & Read, M. (1999). Use of nutrition screening to develop and target nutrition education interventions for Nevada's elderly. *Journal of Nutrition for the Elderly, 19*, 31–47.

Blumberg, J. (1997). Nutritional needs of seniors. *Journal of the American College of Nutrition, 16*, 517–523.

Bogan, A.D. (1997). Nutrient intakes of senior women: Balancing the low-fat message. *Canadian Journal of Public Health, 88*, 310–313.

Chobanian, A.V., & Hill, M. (2000). National Heart, Lung, and Blood Institute workshop on sodium and blood pressure: A critical review of current scientific evidence. *Hypertension, 35*, 858–863.

Contendo, I., Balch, G.I., Bronner, Y.L., Paige, D.M., Gross, S.M., Bisignani, L., Lytle, L.A., Maloney, S.K., White, S.L., Olson, C.M., & Swadener, S.S. (1995). Special issue: The effectiveness of nutrition education and implications for nutrition education policy, programs, and research. *Journal of Nutrition Education, 27*, 339–346.

de Groot, C.P., van den Broek, T., & van Staveren, W. (1999). Energy intake and micronutrient intake in elderly Europeans: Seeking the minimum requirement in the SENECA study. *Age and Aging, 28*, 469–474.

Doner, L. (Ed.). (1997, February 28). *Charting the course for evaluation: How do we measure the success of nutrition education and promotion in food assistance programs?* (Summary of proceedings). Washington, DC: US Department of Agriculture, Food and Consumer Service, Office of Analysis and Evaluation.

Evans, W.J., & Cyr-Campbell, D. (1997). Nutrition, exercise, and healthy aging. *Journal of the American Dietetic Association, 97*, 632–638.

Falk, L.W., Bisogni, C.A., & Sobal, J. (1996). Food choice processes of older adults: A qualitative investigation. *Journal of Nutrition Education, 28*, 257–265.

Fischer, C.A., Crockett, S.J., Heller, K.E., & Skauge, L.H. (1991). Nutrition knowledge, attitudes, and practices of older and younger elderly in rural areas. *Journal of the American Dietetic Association, 91*, 1398–1401.

Food and Nutrition Board, Institute of Medicine. (1997). *Dietary reference intakes for calcium, phosphorus, magnesium, vitamin D, and fluoride.* Washington, DC: National Academy Press.

Food and Nutrition Board, Institute of Medicine. (1999). *The role of nutrition in maintaining health in the nation's elderly: Evaluating coverage of nutrition services for the Medicare population.* Washington, DC: National Academy Press.

Haller, J. (1999). The vitamin status and its adequacy in the elderly: An international overview. *International Journal of Vitamin Nutrition Research, 69*, 160–168.

Herman, J., Brown, B., & Heintz, S. (2000). Impact of a nutrition promotion program on dietary behaviors, dietary intake, and health measures in adults over fifty-five years of age. *Journal of Nutrition for the Elderly, 19*, 1–14.

Hiddink, G.J., Hautvast, J.G.A.J., van Woerkym, S.M.J., & Fieren, C.J. (1997). Consumers' expectations about nutrition guidance: The importance of primary care physicians. *American Journal of Clinical Nutrition, 65*(Suppl.), 1947S–1949S.

Keller, H.H., Ostbye, T., & Bright-See, E. (1997). Predictors of dietary intake in Ontario seniors. *Canadian Journal of Public Health, 88*, 305–309.

Klesges, L.M., Pahor, M., Shorr, R.I., Wan, J.Y., Williamson, J.D., & Guralnik, J.M. (2001). Financial difficulty in acquiring food among elderly disabled women: Results from the women's health and aging study. *American Journal of Public Health, 91*, 68–75.

Minkler, M., Schauffler, J., & Clements-Nolle, K. (2000). Health promotion for older Americans in the 21st century. *American Journal of Health Promotion, 14*, 371–379.

Nakatsuka, H., Satoh, H., Watanabe, T., Yamamoto, R., Satoh, R., Imai, Y., Abe, K., & Ikeda, M. (1999). Poorer nutritional status of the older-generation in a Japanese farming village, as related to fewer types of food consumed. *Public Health, 113*, 251–253.

Nigg, C., Burbank, P.M., Dufresne, R., Rossi, J.S., Velicer, W.F., Laforge, R.G., & Prochaska, J.O. (1999). Stages of change across ten health risk behaviors for older adults. *Gerontologist, 39*, 437–482.

Pierce, M.B. (2000). *Nutrition support to elderly women: Influence on diet quality.* New York: Garland.

Pierce, M.B., Sheehan, N.W., & Ferris, A.M. (2001). Older women living in subsidized housing report low levels of nutrition support. *Journal of the American Dietetic Association, 101*, 251–254.

Russell, R.M., Rasmussen, H., & Lichtenstein, A.H. (1999). Modified food guide pyramid for people over seventy years of age. *Journal of Nutrition, 129*, 751–753.

Shawver, G.W., & Cox, R.H. (2000). Need for physician referral of low-income, chronic disease patients to community nutrition education programs. *Journal of Nutrition for the Elderly, 21*, 17–33.

Taylor-Davis, S., Smiciklas-Wright, H., Warland, R., Achterberg, C., Jensen, G.L., Sayer, A., & Shannon, B. (2000). Responses of older adults to theory-based nutrition newsletters. *Journal of the American Dietetic Association, 100*, 656–664.

US Department of Agriculture, & US Department of Health and Human Services. (2000). *Nutrition and your health: Dietary guidelines for Americans* (5th ed., Home and Garden Bulletin No. 232). Washington, DC: US Government Printing Office.

US Department of Health and Human Services. (1999). *Health, United States, 1999* (PHS Publication No. 99-1232). Washington, DC.

Weimer, J. (1998). *Factors affecting nutrient intake of the elderly* (Agricultural Economic Report No. 769). Washington, DC: US Department of Agriculture.

Wolfe, W.S., Olson, C.M., Kendall, A., & Frongillo, E.A., Jr. (1996). Understanding food insecurity in the elderly: A conceptual framework. *Journal of Nutrition Education, 28*, 92–100.

Nutrition and Physical Activity, Adolescence

Andrea Bastiani Archibald,
Erin O'Connor, Julia A. Graber,
and Jeanne Brooks-Gunn

INTRODUCTION

The adolescent years are a time when attitudes and behaviors associated with a healthy lifestyle can be introduced and established. As an adolescent is still undergoing rapid physiological growth, this may be an ideal period to intervene and correct damage due to prior unhealthy practices, as well as to promote healthy behaviors with the goal of improving health immediately (in adolescence) and into adulthood. In particular, adequate nutrition and regular physical activity have been linked to decreasing an adolescent's risk of developing chronic illnesses such as cardiovascular disease (CVD), obesity, cancers, as well as osteoporosis in later life (Sallis, 1993). Similarly, late childhood and the entry into adolescence are important periods in the development of health patterns that may result in either healthy food intake or precursors for eating problems and disorders and obesity.

DEFINITIONS

The term *prevention*, as we are using it, is in reference to deterring the onset of subclinical eating problems (contributing to over and underweight) and risks for chronic illness. *Subclinical eating problems* include strict dieting, occasional bingeing and purging, overeating, excessive exercising, and/or having a negative/distorted body image. *Primary prevention initiatives* are generally universal, and therefore implemented with all adolescents, or all adolescents in particular communities or settings. *Health promotion programs*, which are the focus of this entry, require an emphasis on the enhancement of adaptive skills or an emphasis on competency rather than on problems and pathology (Compas, 1993) so these programs usually target all youth in a classroom, grade, or of a particular age. In other words, adolescents can learn and practice skills that they can utilize when confronting the numerous challenges of adolescence. Health promotion encompasses the development of health in multiple domains, including physical health, psychological health, and social health (Graber, Archibald, & Brooks-Gunn, 1999). Health promotion efforts with adolescents have primarily been used in programs targeting smoking, alcohol and other drug use, and sex education. More recently, promoting physical health has been an emphasis of nutrition education programs that had formerly focused only on teaching adolescents and children about nutritional requirements and healthy foods (Graber et al., 1999).

Additional factors which are crucial in health promotion are: self-efficacy, social support, and health knowledge (Johnson, Niklas, Webber, & Berenson, 1997). Appropriate incentives to change unhealthy behaviors should also be provided (Killen et al., 1996). Furthermore, sociocultural factors should be explored in relation to their impact on nutrition and food availability, norms for physical activity,

and the related areas of weight and body shape. For example, the media glorifies a thin body ideal while at the same time advertising foods high in fat and calories. Therefore, recognition of persuasion tactics in the media is essential in health promotion programs so adolescents may be aware of social influence processes and thus may use resistance skills learned through such programs.

SCOPE

Nutrition and Dietary Intake Patterns

Like American adults, children and adolescents in the United States consume excess amounts of dietary fat (over 40 percent of daily caloric intake) and cholesterol (in excess of 300 mg per day) (King, Telch, Robinson, Maccoby, Taylor, & Farquhar, 1988). Furthermore, only 23 percent of the American population consumes the recommended level of fruit and vegetable consumption. This is of concern as studies have indicated an association between higher levels of fruit and vegetable intake and lowered risk for a multitude of cancers (Havas et al., 1995). Fruit and vegetable tastes and intake patterns develop in childhood and adolescence and continue into the adult years.

The transition to adolescence is particularly important in the development of eating patterns as precursors of adult CVD, and related problems (e.g., high blood pressure) develop in childhood (Johnson et al., 1997). Along these lines, by young adulthood, risk factors may develop to the extent they set the stage for clinical manifestations in the fifth and sixth decades of life (Johnson et al., 1997). Thus, the presumption is that keeping in check the risk factors in childhood and young adulthood may reduce the likelihood of developing CVD (Johnson et al., 1997), though few studies to date have actually tested this hypothesis. Despite the severity of this problem, national studies indicate that the diets of adolescents are high in saturated fat (Kimm, Gergen, Malloy, Dresser, & Carroll, 1990). Adolescents frequently do acknowledge that they are not eating a healthy diet (Archibald, Graber, Harris, & Brooks-Gunn, in process) and identify lack of time and poor self-discipline as barriers to healthy eating (Sallis, 1993). High consumption of fast food, which is cheap and convenient for adolescents, also contributes to high fat and sodium content of diets among adolescents.

Physical Activity Patterns

Physical activity patterns are also less than optimal for adolescents. Approximately, only 66 percent of individuals 10 through 17 engage in regular physical activity. Thus, at the same time that they are consuming foods higher in fat and calories, American adolescents appear to be gaining weight due to increased physical inactivity (Johnson et al., 1997). Research indicates that physical activity decreases over the adolescent decade. Contributing to this problem is the fact that there are significant barriers to children and adolescents acquiring appropriate amounts of physical activity. This is especially the case for the less affluent who may not have access to gyms and youth sports (McKenzie et al., 1995). Females also may have limited access to organized physical activity leading to girls decreasing their time spent in vigorous physical activity in preadolescence. While school physical education (PE) classes could provide enjoyable and beneficial physical activity for students, research indicates that the middle- and high-school PE classes being offered have declined, and those that exist are infrequent and students are rather inactive in them (McKenzie et al., 1996). Low levels of physical exercise are associated with coronary heart disease, hypertension, non-insulin dependent diabetes mellitus, osteoporosis, obesity, stroke, and colon cancer (Johnson et al., 1997). Furthermore, physical activity may increase HDL (good) cholesterol in adolescents (McKenzie et al., 1996).

Eating Problems and Disorders

Girls in particular, are more likely to use dietary restraint to control body shape leading to extremely deficient nutrient intake, and are more prone to obesity and eating disorders than males. Eating disorders (which include anorexia nervosa and bulimia) are relatively uncommon for later childhood and adolescent females (approximately 1 percent of girls 12–18 years old). However, subclinical eating problems amongst adolescent girls, are more prevalent. Perhaps 20 percent of all adolescent girls will engage in less extreme, but still unhealthy dieting behaviors (Story, Rosenwinkel, Himes, Resnick, Harris, & Blum, 1991). These subclinical problems include strict dieting, occasional bingeing and purging, and excessive exercising. Negative perceptions of weight and appearance also increase during the early adolescent years and may pose adjustment problems or be predictive of eating problems for some girls. Additionally, 2–3 percent of adolescent girls demonstrate elevated symptoms of Binge Eating Disorders (BED) and significant proportion may be considered clinically obese (Gortmaker, Dietz, Sobol, & Wehler, 1987). Thus, it is important and appropriate to address the related area of eating problems in health programs promoting nutrition and physical activity. However, it should be noted that inclusion of information related to this area need not be limited to prevention of eating disorders per se. Instead, programs might more subtly address issues associated both with the development of eating disorders and nutrition/physical activity by discussing not taking nutrition or physical activity to

"extreme levels," but maintaining a healthy, balanced level of each, as well as, body image, media literacy, etc. While it is especially important to include such information in programming targeting adolescent girls, both boys and girls would be well-served by such information.

Knowledge of the health risks present in later childhood and adolescence indicate the necessity of effective prevention and health promotion programs, and schools have repeatedly been cited as appropriate venues for health education and promotion programs (Johnson et al., 1997). School-based health promotion and education programs may be conducted within existing group settings leading to cost efficiency and normative support for changed behavior. In school, physical education classes can provide activity during class time and may reduce gender differences in access to physical activity by providing equitable opportunities and practical skills for participation in health-related physical activity for males and females (McKenzie et al., 1996). School-aged adolescents are appropriate targets for preventive and health promotion efforts since the major risks for eating problems, CVD and osteoporosis often begin in later childhood and adolescence. Thus the school community is an excellent environment for health instruction and behavior modification (Johnson et al., 1997).

THEORIES

Adolescents in different stages of development face unique pressures, needs and concerns that should be attended to in health promotion programs. Theory and research indicate that during early adolescence pubertal development, issues of independence and family relationships, peer interactions, achievement pressures related to the transition from elementary school to middle school or junior high school, and development of a self-image are prevalent concerns (Feldman & Elliot, 1990). Cognitively, *early adolescents* are most likely to still think about health in very concrete ways; thus, it is appropriate that prevention strategies developed for this age group provide specific information appropriate for the developmental tasks at hand. Particular areas which should be addressed include information about the following: changes in body fat which occur during adolescence (Story et al., 1991), realistic body weights, healthy and unhealthy uses of food, drugs and alcohol, problem-solving and time management skills, and increased pressures regarding peer interactions. In addition, because peer acceptance is extremely important in this developmental stage and because adolescents engage in eating and physical activities within peer groups, negotiating with peers around these areas of health should be incorporated into prevention efforts. Behavioral training in assertiveness and relaxation may also be helpful in assisting young adolescents in learning healthy means to control their emotions.

Primary developmental concerns in *middle adolescence* appear to be focused on friendships, achievement pressures relating to school and future career goals, developing a positive self-esteem and achieving a balance between a need for independence and relationships. Middle adolescence is categorized by an increased ability for abstract thinking. Concerns over puberty lessen at this time, however, prevention strategies should continue to address nutrition, self-regulation, and peer relationships addressed during early adolescence. Several additional elements, however, must be added to prevention programs for this age group. Shisslak and Crago (1994) recommend teaching female adolescents in particular, to critique gender-role expectations in order to evaluate negative effects of attempting to live up to superwoman expectations. Images of women in the media may be an effective point of discussion about pressures facing women. In addition, building on factual information related to nutrition and weight, females may now start to investigate issues surrounding body image as they relate to health and self-esteem.

Concerns regarding eating behavior and attitudes continue through *late adolescence*. During this stage, women face additional transitions relating to separation as they prepare to graduate from high school, enter college or the job market and enter into new friendships and romantic relationships. Thus, issues surrounding connection and separation arise again. Furthermore, females are acutely faced with society's image of the superwoman and society's ideal body image for women. At this stage it is crucial to maintain presenting young women with factual information regarding healthy body weight, exercise, and nutrition.

Health promotion with minority adolescents should additionally take into account cultural issues. Successful participation in health promotion is likely based on gaining an insight of multiple culture's eating patterns, standards of beauty, as well as individual health concerns (Earls, 1993) through program lessons and activities. Thus, it is crucial that students be able to use and feel comfortable using health strategies learned in promotion programs in their own families and communities. For example, a nutrition lesson will be less effective if a Latino adolescent is learning about healthy foods listed in the USDA food pyramid, but does not have those foods frequently available to her at home because her family eats a traditional Mexican diet. Healthy foods from all cultures should be introduced and discussed, as such.

RESEARCH

While the combination of nutrition and physical activity seems obvious, remarkably few programs targeting both promotion of nutrition *and* physical activity have been developed for adolescents and tested. To follow, five programs are reviewed, with three addressing nutrition only, and two addressing both nutrition and physical activity as targets of the programs. Strategies that "work," "might work," as well as those that "do not work" will then be considered.

A Review of Nutrition and Physical Health Promotion Programs: King and colleagues (1988) developed and evaluated a school-based, behaviorally focused dietary change program for 10th graders. Behavioral change objectives encompassed raising the intake of complex carbohydrates and lowering the intake of saturated fats, sugar, and salt. Snack food choices were a main focus because much of teenagers' daily caloric intake is from high-fat, high-salt snacks. The dietary curriculum was taught by a masters level health professional trained in the program with regular classroom teachers present. The program was composed of a 3 week, 5-session curriculum created to give students dietary knowledge as well as cognitive-behavioral strategies to change dietary practices. Overall, slide presentations, contests and food preparation and tastings gained students' attention and maintained their interest in course content. Homework assignments encouraged dietary change behaviors outside of the classroom (King et al., 1988). All students demonstrated increases in knowledge especially in the areas of starches and proteins, where students had first demonstrated the greatest deficits. Also, a significantly greater number of students in the program made a positive, healthy change in their snack choices and indicated greater availability of healthful foods at home, following the intervention. However, at 1-year follow-up, only knowledge changes were found to be durable. This demonstrates the necessity for continued reinforcement and practice of health related behaviors and skills in order to maintain healthy behaviors when faced with conflicting messages and demands (King et al., 1988).

The *Great Sensations Program* (Coates et al., 1985) is another nutrition-education program for high-school students intended to decrease students' intake of salty snacks and to increase students' intake of fresh fruit snacks. The program had demonstrated positive outcomes with predominately White populations; however, a recent evaluation of the program tested its applicability to predominantly Black, inner-city high school students. The program in total consisted of six sessions conducted over a 4-week period by a research staff member in the presence of a regular teacher. Each class session was created to include five strategies to support behavior change: models of desired behavior, behavioral rehearsal, goal specification, and feedback of results of reinforcement for behavioral change. A parental involvement component was also included to instruct parents on the program and to gain their support, to prompt parents to make heart-healthy, as opposed to salty, snacks available and to instruct parents on label reading and cost analysis of salty versus healthy snacks. Two 5-min telephone calls and three brochures were the extent of the parent component. As well, a school-wide media program was incorporated to give out of class support for changes in food intake. Posters were displayed throughout the school, cafeteria cashiers were instructed to encourage students who bought low-salt snacks, and announcements over the public address system motivated students to consume low-salt snacks (Coates et al., 1985).

The results of this study demonstrate the necessity of classroom instruction for the maintenance of changes in target food consumption. While all students in the intervention school demonstrated immediate reduction in salty food content only those who received classroom instruction maintained these reductions until the end of the school year. Furthermore, only students not receiving classroom instruction demonstrated a gain in the consumption of other snack foods. Interestingly, parental involvement indicated mixed results. Initially, parents in the intervention did make desired changes in food availability; however, by the beginning of the subsequent school year, students in the parental involvement cohort consumed fewer target snacks than those whose parents were not in the program (Coates et al., 1985).

Gimme 5: A fresh nutrition concept for students was a school-based health-education program designed to increase adolescent's consumption of fruits and vegetables (Johnson et al., 1997). It was created to develop an environment in which predisposing, enabling and reinforcing factors act to increase student's intake of fruits and vegetables. The contents of the program addressed the following steps to behavior change: awareness development, interest stimulation, skills training, reinforcement, application, and maintenance. The intervention consisted of four parts: workshops and associated activities, school meal and snack modification, a school media and marketing campaign, and parental involvement. Experts in education and health delivered five workshops over 4 years. The workshops included an introduction to healthy consumption of fruits and vegetables, eating healthy for appearance and athletic performance, snacking healthy, how to eat healthy in fast food restaurants and healthy microwave cooking. Lessons in other classes complemented information communicated in the workshops. For example, in French class students learned French words for fruits and vegetables. In addition, fruit and vegetable options were increased in the school cafeteria. The media campaign through brochures, videotapes, posters, pubic service announcements, games, rap-songs, drama skits, and marketing stations reinforced the consumption of fruits and vegetables. Parents, through activities and printed materials, were instructed on how to increase their children's consumption of fruits and vegetables. In baseline assessment approximately one third of the fruit and vegetable knowledge questions

were answered correctly. Correct responses were higher for girls than boys and for Whites compared to other racial groups. Only 12 percent of students reported eating five or more daily servings of fruits and vegetables. Students were also assessed in terms of their stage of behavior change. More females than males were at a stage of preparing for dietary change, and more males than females were unaware of the necessity for change. Interestingly, none of the students reported actively changing their diets or behavior. In terms of self-efficacy about 40 percent of students were very or extremely confident that they could consume five daily servings of fruits/vegetables (Johnson et al., 1997).

Killen and colleagues (1988) developed a school-based health-promotion program targeting both dietary and physical activity changes. Their goal was to increase adolescents' motivation to accept and use healthy weight-regulation practices by providing them with skills to combat social influences that promote dieting and an overemphasis on weight and body shape, and to help students gain weight-regulation strategies. In addition, the program targeted CVD risk factors. The objectives of the program were to have students reduce caloric consumption and foods high in saturated fats, cholesterol and salt, to increase levels of aerobic and physical activities and the intake of complex carbohydrates, to decrease heart rate, blood pressure, body mass index, and skin fold thickness, and to decrease other CVD risk factors, such as cigarette smoking. The program emphasized immediate consequences of health behavior based on research which has indicated that adolescent students' interests in health are based primarily on personal appearance and physical conditioning. The intervention was composed of 20 sessions organized around five program modules: physical activity, nutrition, cigarette smoking, stress, and personal problem-solving (Killen et al., 1988). Each module gave students information on the impact of health practices in order to make healthful lifestyles attractive to students, cognitive and behavioral skills to help students alter their personal behavior, specific skills to help resist social influences and practice in utilizing skills in order to better performance (Killen et al., 1988). Results of the evaluation with 10th grade boys and girls demonstrated that the intervention produced positive results regarding physical fitness, nutrition practices, and weight regulation. Females, in the study, reduced their heart rates and body mass index, in comparison to females in a control group. Cardiovascular risk factor knowledge was significantly greater among students receiving the intervention than control subjects. A greater proportion of individuals in the intervention than the control group, who were not exercising regularly at baseline, indicated regular exercise at follow-up. Students in the intervention were also more likely than control subjects to choose "heart-healthy" snacks. In addition, more students, from the intervention group, who at baseline were experimental smokers reported quitting at follow-up than students in the control group. Also, a significantly smaller percentage of baseline experimental smokers in the treatment became regular smokers, compared to the control group.

Finally, our group is currently conducting a pilot evaluation of *the Building Bodies and Better Eating* (BBBE) school-based curriculum for 7th–10th grade girls (Archibald et al., in process). The BBBE program has two parts; the first part is a seminar, which includes interesting, interactive lessons and activities about adolescent girls' health, development, fitness and wellness. These seminars meet once a week throughout the school year, last for approximately 30 min, and are lead by trained fitness educators and instructors. The second part is a 1-hr physical education class, following the seminar that reinforces concepts presented earlier. In order to address the different developmental needs, abilities, and interests of younger and older adolescents, two-seminar curriculum were developed: one for 7th and 8th grade girls, and the other for 9th and 10th grade girls. Each curriculum was designed to improve girls' health- and fitness-related knowledge, attitudes, and behaviors. The 7th and 8th grade curriculum includes topic-specific material concerning nutrition and healthy food choices for young women, fitness and exercise, dieting, pubertal development, and body image. The 8th and 9th grade curriculum includes topic-specific material concerning body image and media literacy, fitness-related self-care and hygiene, fitness-related nutrition, effects of tobacco, alcohol, and drug use on fitness and health, stress reduction and anger management for a healthy lifestyle, sportswomanship, and careers in health and fitness. Both curriculums included more general information on decision-making and goal setting. Curriculums also included limited parental involvement through homework activities for the adolescent and parents to complete together. Effectiveness is currently being evaluated in a sample of Black, White, and Latino girls from New York City.

STRATEGIES THAT WORK

Comprehensive health promotion programs targeting either or both, nutrition and physical activity, have only recently been attempted with adolescents, resulting in limited information on which to base any debate over the merits of different elements of programs. However, it does appear that classroom-based strategies (as opposed to individual workshops or solely school-wide media based programs) are most effective in promoting health in these areas (Coates et al., 1985; Killen et al., 1988; King et al., 1988), and particularly in knowledge gained. This suggests that students need to be actively and regularly engaged in learning about the health benefits of nutrition and physical activity in their typical learning environment. Clear evidence of the effectiveness of other program elements is not yet available.

STRATEGIES THAT MIGHT WORK

A particular strategy that might work is the addition of parental-involvement components to classroom-based programs. Findings specific to parental involvement are mixed (Coates et al., 1985), or not yet tested (Archibald et al., in process; Johnson et al., 1997) in the programs reviewed previously. However, prior work (Perry et al., 1989) on education programs in nutrition with children has reported significantly more behavioral changes in programs that have involved parents in addition to the target child. Even though this effect did not persist in longer follow-ups, the work of Perry and her colleagues demonstrates the feasibility of parent involvement and the possibility for enhanced treatment effects. As maternal attitudes toward eating, weight, and dieting have demonstrated some associations with adolescent girls' behaviors and attitudes (Byely, Archibald, Graber, & Brooks-Gunn, 2000; Pike & Rodin, 1991), mother involvement in particular, may prove to be critical for altering an adolescents' behavior.

Research on health promotion with children conducted by Perry and her colleagues (1989) has demonstrated that parents are willing to participate in these types of programs with a majority of families beginning and completing the program. Perry and others (e.g., Nader, Sallis, Patterson, Abramson, & Rupp, 1989) have used a "Home Team" program in which students are given assignments to be conducted with parents at home. Hence, rather than expecting parents to spend time away from home and, in fact, spend less time with their children, the parents and children complete tasks together at home. In the later weeks of the program, "Fun Nights" at school are conducted at which time more experiential programs can be conducted. Experiential components often include role-play activities that aid in the development of conflict resolution and communication skills, which may be particularly useful for parents and adolescents. These approaches have demonstrated effectiveness in attracting and maintaining parent participation as well as in influencing nutrition in children and smoking behaviors in young adolescents (Perry et al., 1989).

STRATEGIES THAT DO NOT WORK

As stated previously, health promotion programming in the area of nutrition and physical activity is relatively new. As such, evidence of the specific lack of effectiveness of individual program strategies is not yet available.

SYNTHESIS

Research and practice suggests that health promotion programming targeting nutrition and physical activity can have a significant positive impact on an adolescent's health knowledge, likelihood of making nutritious food choices, having a healthy attitude about nutrition, physical activity, self-efficacy, and body image, as well as reducing risk factors for CVD, obesity, osteoporosis, eating problems, and related illnesses. While potentially simpler in scope, targeting only nutrition or physical activity with the goal of improving overall health and reducing risk of eating problems and illness seems an incomplete and thus, ineffective message for adolescents, as the improvement of both areas is necessary for optimal physical health and well-being.

Effective programs should furnish social and physical environments that encourage physical activity, adequate information on a variety of healthy food options, repeated messages that foster healthful dietary and physical activity practices, as well as information on decision-making. Those most effective programs are classroom-based, and also target related, developmentally timely concerns of adolescents, such as the influence of families and peers on engaging in healthy behaviors. Furthermore, sociocultural factors should be explored in relation to their impact on nutrition and food availability, norms for physical activity, and the related areas of weight and body shape. While it has less frequently been examined, the incorporation of program elements including parents, even if only through homework and individual group sessions, appears an important and potentially fruitful area for future program development and investigation. Finally, successful programs also have demonstrated the necessity for continued reinforcement and practice of health-related behaviors and skills in order to maintain healthy behaviors when faced with conflicting messages and demands in the adolescent culture and beyond.

Also see: Nutrition: Early Childhood; Nutrition: Childhood; Nutrition: Adulthood; Nutrition: Older Adulthood.

References

Archibald, A.B., Graber, J.A., Harris, J., & Brooks-Gunn, J. (in process). Pilot evaluation of the *Building Better Eating* program.

Byely, L., Archibald, A.B., Graber, J.A., & Brooks-Gunn, J. (2000). A prospective study of familial and social influences on girls' body image and dieting. *International Journal of Eating Disorders, 28,* 155–164.

Coates, T.J., Barofsky, I., Saylor, K.E., Simons-Morton, B., Huster, W., Sereghy, E., Straugh, S., Jacobs, H., & Kidd, L. (1985). Modifying the snack food consumption patterns of inner city high school students: The great sensations study. *Preventive Medicine, 14,* 234–247.

Compas, B.E. (1993). Promoting positive mental health during adolescence. In S.G. Millstein, A.C. Petersen, & E.O. Nightingale (Eds.), *Promoting the health of adolescents* (pp. 159–179). New York: Oxford University Press.

Earls, F. (1993). Health promotion for minority adolescents: Cultural considerations. In S.G. Millstein, A.C. Petersen, & E.O. Nightingale (Eds.), *Promoting the health of adolescents* (pp. 159–179). New York: Oxford University Press.

Feldman, S.S., & Elliot, G.R. (Eds.). (1990). *At the threshold: The developing adolescent.* Cambridge, MA: Harvard University.

Gortmaker, S.L., Dietz, W.H., Sobol, A.M., & Wehler, C.A. (1987). Increasing pediatric obesity in the United States. *American Journal of Diseases in Children, 141*(5), 535–540.

Graber, J.A., Archibald, A.B., & Brooks-Gunn, J. (1999). The role of parents in the emergence, maintenance, and prevention of eating problems and disorders. In N. Piran, M.P. Levine, & C. Steiner-Adair (Eds.), *Preventing eating disorders: A handbook of interventions and special challenges* (pp. 44–62). New York: Bruner/Mazel.

Havas, S., Heimendinger, J., Damron, D., Nicklas, T.A., Arnette, C., Beresford, S.A.A., Sorensen, G., Buller, D., Bishop, D., Baranowski, T., & Reynolds, K. (1995). 5 a day for better health-nine community research projects to increase fruit and vegetable consumption. *Public Health Reports, 110*(1), 68–79.

Johnson, C.C., Nicklas, T.A., Webber, L.S., & Berenson, G.S. (1997). Health Promotion. In R.T. Ammerman & M. Hersen (Eds.), *Handbook of prevention and treatment with children and adolescents: Intervention in the real world context.* New York: John Wiley & Sons.

Killen, J.D., Taylor, C.B., Hayward, C., Haydel, K.F., Wilson, D.M., Hammer, L. et al. (1996). Weight concerns influence the development of eating disorders: A 4-year prospective study. *Journal of Consulting and Clinical Psychology, 64*(5), 936–940.

Killen, J.D., Telch, M.J., Robinson, T.N., Maccoby, N., Taylor, B., & Farquhar, J.W. (1988). Cardiovascular disease risk reduction for tenth graders: A multiple-factor school-based approach. *Journal of the American Medical Association, 260*(12), 1728–1733.

Kimm, S.Y., Gergen, P.J., Malloy, M., Dresser, C., & Carroll, M. (1990). Dietary patterns of US children: Implications for disease prevention. *Preventive Medicine, 19,* 432–442.

King, A.C., Saylor, K.E., Foster, S., Killen, J.D., Telch, M.J., Farquhar, J.W., & Flora, J.A. (1988). Promoting dietary change in adolescents: A school-based approach for modifying and maintaining healthful behavior. *American Journal of Preventive Medicine, 4*(2), 68–74.

McKenzie, T.L., Feldman, H., Woods, S., Romero, K., Dahlstrom, V., Stone, E. et al. (1995). Children's activity levels and lesson context during third grade physical education. *Research Quarterly Exercise and Sport, 66,* 184–193.

MacKenzie, T.L., Nader, P.R., Strikmiller, P.K., Yang, M., Stone, E.J., Perry, C.L. et al. (1996). School physical education: Effect of the child and adolescent trial for cardiovascular health. *Preventive Medicine, 25,* 423–431.

Nader, P.R., Sallis, J.F., Patterson, T.L., Abramson, I.S., & Rupp, J.W. (1989). A family approach to cardiovascular risk reduction: Results from the San Diego Family Heart Project. *Health Education Quarterly, 16,* 229–244.

Perry, C.L., Luepker, R.V., Murray, D.M., Hearn, M.D., Halper, A., Dudovitz, B., Maile, M.C., & Smyth, M. (1989). Parent involvement with children's health promotion: A one-year follow-up of the Minnesota Home Team. *Health Education Quarterly, 16,* 171–180.

Pike, K.M., & Rodin, J. (1991). Mothers, daughters and disordered eating. *Journal of Abnormal Psychology, 100,* 198–204.

Sallis, J.F. (1993). Promoting healthful diet and physical activity. In S.G. Millstein, A.C. Petersen, & E.O. Nightingale (Eds.), *Promoting the health of adolescents*. New York: Oxford University Press.

Shisslak, C.M., & Crago, M. (1994). Toward a new model for the prevention of eating disorders. In P. Fallon, M.A. Katzman, & S.C. Wooley (Eds.), *Feminist perspectives on eating disorders* (pp. 419–437). New York: Guilford.

Story, M., Rosenwinkel, K., Himes, J.H., Resnick, M., Harris, L.J., & Blum, R.W. (1991). Demographic and risk factors associated with chronic dieting in adolescents. *American Journal of Diseases of Children, 145*, 994–998.

O

Obesity, Adolescence

Cynthia H. Ledford

INTRODUCTION

Obesity is a rapidly growing health concern that is reaching epidemic proportions. The prevalence of this disease has escalated over the last 20–30 years, largely due to sedentary lifestyles and high-fat energy dense foods.

DEFINITIONS

Experts participating in the World Health Organization Consultation on Obesity in June 1997 agreed on Body Mass Index (BMI) as the international standard for measurement of overweight and obesity. BMI is defined as weight (in kilograms) divided by the square of the height (in meters): kg/m^2. For adult populations, the definitions of overweight and obesity are as follows:

Overweight: $BMI = 25–29.9 \ kg/m^2$
Obese: $BMI = 30 \ kg/m^2$ or more

Obesity can be further categorized as:

Category I: $BMI = 30–34.9 \ kg/m^2$
Category II: $BMI = 35–39.9 \ kg/m^2$
Category III: $BMI = 40 \ kg/m^2$ or more

In children, *overweight*, or more specifically *adiposity*, is not as clearly defined. Children in the top 5 percent in adiposity or 95th percentile are considered overweight. For children and adolescents the distribution of BMI by age is a useful tool for identifying overweight that correlates with other markers of fatness. A child with a BMI greater than the 95th percentile is overweight. Children with BMI in the 85th to 95th percentile are considered at risk of becoming overweight. The Center for Disease Control has growth curves available for the distribution of BMI for different ages in the United States (CDC, 2000). BMI does not correlate with adiposity as well for children (Pietrobelli, Faith, Allison, Gallagher, Shiumello, & Heymsfield, 1998; Troiano & Flegal, 1998) or older adults (Bedogni et al., 2001) as it does for the general adult population.

SCOPE

Worldwide obesity is a growing concern. The Global Database on Obesity and BMI in Adults survey data estimates the global prevalence of obesity in the year 2000 as 8.2 percent or 302.1 million people. The prevalence is highest in more developed countries (WHO Global Database, 2001).

In the United States, 55 percent of all adults over 19 years of age are overweight. An estimated 97 million adults in the United States are overweight or obese. Minority groups, people of lower income levels, and less educated adults are more likely to be obese. Results from the 1999 National Health and Nutrition Examination Survey estimate that 13 percent of children 6–11 years of age and 14 percent of children 12–19 years of age are overweight. This is a significant increase from the results in 1963–1970 when only 4–5 percent of children were overweight. In 1998–1999, close to one third of the Canadian population aged 15 or older was overweight and 14 percent were obese. In this population, the prevalence of overweight increased with age, then declined slightly for seniors (Canadian Health Reports, 2000).

Obesity is costly in terms of medical complications, premature loss of life, loss of productivity, and social stigmatization and discrimination. The medical complications of obesity include hypertension, diabetes mellitus, dyslipidemias, coronary atherosclerosis, stroke, gallbladder disease, osteoarthritis, sleep apnea, and cancers of the endometrium, breast, prostate gland, and colon (Clinical Guidelines on the Identification, Evaluation, and Treatment of Overweight and Obesity, 1998). Obesity is estimated to be the second leading external factor leading to death in the United States (McGinnis & Foege, 1993). Total annual costs (medical and lost productivity) attributable to obesity alone in the United States is estimated as more than $99 billion dollars. These costs increase with increasing degrees of obesity.

THEORIES

A key to identifying potential prevention strategies is to identify a causal or sequential risk model for the problem. The simplest concept of causality for this problem is that obesity is the result of excessive caloric intake relative to the physical activity sustained. Within an individual or population however the behaviors and environmental factors that determine dietary intake and physical activity are complex and not fully understood. The approaches to prevention and treatment of obesity are grounded in various theoretical frameworks including a medical model, social cognitive, and social ecological theory. Interventions involve nutrition, physical activity, or both. Prevention activities target an entire community, the general population within a segment of the community such as workplace, school, or healthcare center, or groups of individuals identified as at risk. The endpoints for these programs are both the prevention of obesity and the prevention of progression of obesity. More immediate surrogate endpoints are promotion of healthy dietary habits and increased physical activity and fitness.

Theorizing from a medical model, genetics has been studied as a determinant of obesity. An inherited gene causes obesity in only a very small number of obese children and adults. The concept of inheriting a susceptibility to obesity that is neither necessary nor sufficient alone to the development of obesity better explains the observations within a population. This genetic concept proposed by Greenberg (1993) suggests that genetics might lower the threshold for development of obesity but that non-genetic determinants of caloric intake and energy expenditure are crucial for the development of this disease. The role of genetics in prevention of

obesity is limited to identification of at-risk individuals. The recent rapid increase in the prevalence of obesity globally and in certain populations, such as the United States, supports the importance of non-genetic causes of obesity. Preventive measures that are based on a medical model advise individuals about healthy physical activity and nutrition as a means of counteracting these non-genetic causes of obesity.

Environmental factors contributing to obesity may be political, socioeconomic, cultural, and physical. The social cognitive theory of obesity recognizes that the environment influences the behaviors of individuals. These behaviors, in turn also affect the environment. Prevention strategies based on the social cognitive theory include efforts to modify the environment. The social ecological model of prevention asserts that the environment sets limits on the behaviors of individuals. With social ecology, the environmental factors are the primary target.

Common elements of prevention strategies emerge, regardless of whether the strategy approaches the problem from a medical, social cognitive, or social ecological model or whether the study targets at risk individuals, selected groups, or the general population. The basic elements of obesity prevention strategies are the promotion of healthy food intake, prevention of unhealthy food intake, the promotion of physical activity, and the prevention of sedentary activity (Figure 1).

Methods to change behaviors related to nutrition or physical activity can focus on the individual through education and behavior modification or focus on the environmental factors that influence these behaviors (Figure 2). For example, fruit and vegetable consumption can be promoted through behavior modification techniques working with individuals at risk of obesity or by changing the environment and offering more choices of fruits and vegetables at a reduced price. In the area of nutrition, prevention programs targeting environmental factors promote appeal, availability, convenience, and cost of healthy food choices and prevent exposure to high fat and energy dense foods. Interventions might increase physical activity through targeting barriers such as lack of neighborhood safety preventing outdoor activities or adding to physical education programs in the schools.

RESEARCH

Examples of research in the prevention of obesity are diverse in their strategies, target populations, outcomes measured, and quality. No single prevention strategy has emerged as most effective. Often the strategies have multiple components. This makes it difficult to identify the elements that are exerting the effect. Strategies that are effective in one context may not transfer to another context

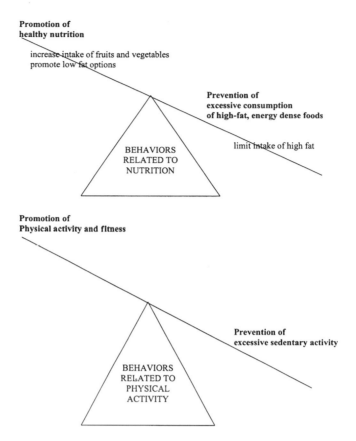

Figure 1. Common Elements of Obesity Prevention Strategies.

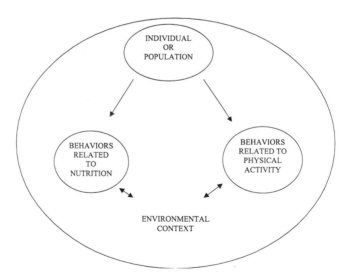

Figure 2. Factors Determining Behaviors Related to Nutrition and Physical Activity.

due to differences in the political, socioeconomic, cultural, and physical factors involved.

Several strategies successfully promote healthy nutrition. The fruit and vegetable consumption of families with children at risk for obesity is increased through behavior modification techniques (Epstein, Gordy, Raynor, Beddome, Kilanowski, & Paluch, 2001). Modification of school lunch in rural schools improves the diet of children and attenuates obesity (Donnelly et al., 1996). In a cafeteria setting, the consumption of fruit and salad triples with increased availability and reduced pricing of these options (Jeffery, French, Raether, & Baxter, 1994). In workplace and high school vending machines, the purchase of low-fat options increases through promotional signs, labeling, and price reduction (French, Jeffery, Story, Breitlow, & Baxter, 2001).

Other strategies prevent excessive high fat and energy dense intake. An intervention with African American mothers and daughters in Chicago results in reduced saturated fat intake and less calories from fat (Stolley & Fitzgibbon, 1997). Behavior modification to reduce high fat and sugar intake in families with children at risk of obesity successfully changes dietary patterns (Epstein et al., 2001). A tailored, computer-generated message to improve dietary behavior through healthcare providers reduces the total fat intake by 23 percent (Campbell, DeVellis, Ammerman, DeVellis, & Sandler, 1994). The *Minnesota Heart Health* program used a community-wide educational effort to target a number of cardiovascular risk factors including reducing dietary fat and reducing body weight, unfortunately after 7 years no effect on BMI was found (Jeffery, 2001).

Several strategies promote physical activity. The Minnesota Heart Health Program included an educational component addressing increased physical activity. The *First Body Owner's* program built on a successful fitness-based physical education program for children in South Australia schools (Dwyer, Coonan, Leitch, Hetzel, & Baghurst, 1983). The *Singapore Fit and Trim* program also documents success in increasing fitness and physical activity in school children. In one study, 52 percent of patients report adopting regular physical activity 6 weeks after structured physician counseling (Calfas, Sallis, Oldenburg, & French, 1997).

Other preventive measures attempt to reduce sedentary activity. Epstein describes a reduction in sedentary activity through lifestyle exercise programming (Epstein, Valoski, Wing, & McCurly, 1994). Through an intervention titled *Planet Health*, reduced television viewing mediated the reduction in obesity prevalence seen in the treatment group (Gortmaker et al., 1999).

From these examples of research, the evidence emerges for what works well, what strategies show great promise and what strategies do not work. The greatest limitation of the evidence available is that often success is documented in short-term surrogate outcomes, but not in terms of weight or BMI.

STRATEGIES THAT WORK

No single preventive strategy has emerged as most effective. Several approaches prove to be effective in several studies.

1. The school is an effective setting from which to launch strategies for prevention of childhood obesity. Several very

different studies have shown promising results in the school setting. Many researchers have successfully used this setting to address either nutrition or physical activity levels or both in an attempt to prevent obesity. The successful programs have ranged from the preschool through high school settings.

Several strategies successfully modify the nutritional intake of students in the schools. Donnelly and colleagues show that modification of the school lunch program can attenuate obesity (Donnelly et al., 1996). Promotional signs and price reduction in high school vending machines can increase the purchase of low-fat options (French et al., 2001). A program of counseling and support by peers linked with lunchbox examination for nutritional and caloric content of foods and positive reinforcement resulted in statistically less weight gain for the targeted obese children over a 12-week period (Foster, Wadden, & Bownell, 1985). Other successful strategies include nutrition as a component, combined with physical activity interventions.

Several strategies document success of school-based interventions targeting physical activity. A school-based exercise program in Thailand decreases the obesity indexes of kindergarten children (Mo-suwan, Pougprapai, Junjana, & Puetpaeboon, 1998). The Singapore Fit and Trim program aimed at ensuring that all school children have regular physical activity at school has documented population-wide increased fitness and decrease in obesity rates (World Health Organization [WHO], 1999). South Australia's First Body Owners program includes daily physical activity in comparison to the usual three half-hour physical education periods per week to successfully lower skin fold measurements and BMI (Dwyer et al., 1983). A Dance for Health intervention uses a three times a week aerobic dance pilot to change attitudes toward physical activity and lower BMI in at-risk minority students (Flores, 1995).

Several school-based interventions document success with multiple strategies. The *Stanford Adolescent Heart Health* program uses the tenth grade classroom to target behavior modification with specific motivating messages, vignettes, and incentives to learn that results in improved knowledge of nutrition and physical activity benefits, self-reported healthy behaviors, and BMI (Killen et al., 1989). The *Child and Adolescent Trial for Cardiovascular Health* (CATCH) intervenes with primary school students through food service modifications, enhanced physical education and health curricula resulting in improved dietary content and increased physical activity measures (Luepker et al., 1996). Planet Health uses behavioral choice and social cognitive theory to change four behaviors: television viewing, physical activity, high-fat food consumption, and fruit and vegetable consumption. The prevalence of obesity of female students significantly declined in the intervention versus the control schools (Gortmaker et al., 1999).

All of these interventions document the effectiveness of the school setting for prevention of obesity. This success may be attributed to the captive audience, ability to control environmental factors, daily exposure and potential for interventions over time.

2. *Fitness-based physical education can improve the fitness of the general school-based population.* The Singapore Fit and Trim program, Australia's First Body Owner's programs, Dance for Health, and other interventions provide evidence for successful promotion of physical activity in school children. The Singapore Fit and Trim program ensures regular physical activity for every school child in Singapore. Since this program began in 1992, the school population as a whole has shown significant improvements in fitness and a reduction in obesity rates (WHO, 1999). Australia's First Body Owner's program replaced the usual three half hours a week of physical education with an intervention of daily physical activity for one and a quarter hours vigorous enough to increase the heart rate. With this daily physical activity, the fitness group experienced a decline in skin fold thicknesses and lower BMI (Dwyer et al., 1983). In Dance for Health, the physical activity intervention consists of three 50-min sessions per week of a dance-oriented aerobic activity. Students in the intervention had a significantly lower BMI compared to those in the usual physical education class (Flores, 1995).

These interventions document that incorporating regular or daily physical activity into the routine of an environmental setting, such as the school, can reduce the obesity in the entire population. The outcomes that these studies measure are short-term improvements in adiposity and fitness. Further research is needed to evaluate whether changes can be sustained outside the school environment. These programs need to be studied to discover whether they can be transferred to other countries or communities with diverse political and cultural contexts.

3. *Modification of school, cafeteria, and vending machines options through selection, pricing, and promotion can effectively change the diet of children and adults.* Several strategies have shown short-term success in modifying the dietary consumption by modifying the options available at schools or workplaces. Modification of school lunch improves the diet of children (Donnelly et al., 1996). Reducing prices and expanding options increases the consumption of fruit and salads (Jeffery et al., 1994). Promotional signs, labeling, and price reduction increases the purchase of low-fat options in vending machines (French et al., 2001). In settings where access to food options is limited, offering and promoting healthier dietary choices can improve the consumption of these items in both children and adults.

STRATEGIES THAT MIGHT WORK

A variety of strategies show great promise. The following are promising strategies for changing behaviors related to nutrition:

1. Use of behavior modification to increase fruit and vegetable consumption of families and adults (Epstein et al., 2001). This is accomplished by targeting the entire family of at-risk children with a strategy to reinforce the selection and consumption of a larger number of fruits and vegetables.
2. Modification of school lunch to promote healthy nutrition (Donnelly et al., 1996). The menu of the school cafeteria can be altered to exclude non-nutritious options, reduce fat-intake to desirable levels, and increase the fruit and vegetable choices, resulting in increased consumption of healthy options.
3. Use of pricing, selection, and promotion to positively affect diet changes (Donnelly et al., 1996; French et al., 2001). Offering a wider selection of fruits, vegetables and low fat foods at a lower price than the high fat and unhealthy options will increase the consumption of the healthier foods.
4. Increasing the consumption of fruit and salad through increased availability and reduced pricing of these options, in a cafeteria setting (Jeffery et al., 1994). Offering a larger selection of fruits and salad selections at a reduced price in the cafeteria setting will increase the consumption of these healthier options.
5. Use of labeling and promotion to encourage selection of low fat options (French et al., 2001). Consumption of low fat foods increases with promotion through signage and labeling of these options.
6. Use of behavior modification to reduce consumption of high fat, energy dense foods (Stolley & Fitzgibbon, 1997). A culturally sensitive intervention to discourage high fat food consumption that includes an exploration of options at local food sources and modifies individual cooking habits reduces the consumption of fat and calories.
7. Use of behavior modification to reduce high fat and sugar intake in families with children at risk of obesity (Epstein et al., 2001). Targeting the entire family of at risk children to reinforce the selection of lower fat and sugar intake through behavior

modification techniques lowers the consumption of these energy dense, low nutrient foods.

8. A tailored intervention through the healthcare setting can reduce fat intake (Campbell et al., 1994). Use of a computer-generated message to tailor recommendations for behavior change related to diet reduces fat intake by 23 percent.

Other strategies show promise in changing behaviors related to physical activity.

1. Healthcare provider counseling to promote physical activity (Calfas et al., 1997). Advice about increasing physical activity from a healthcare provider, coupled with telephone calls to reinforce recommendations increases patients' self-reported physical activity.
2. Programmed physical activity to reduce sedentary activities (Epstein et al., 1994). Promotion of non-aerobic, less vigorous forms of physical activity reduce the time spent in sedentary activities.
3. Reduction of television viewing reduces obesity (Gortmaker et al., 1999). Behavior modification techniques directed at reducing television viewing decreases the prevalence of obesity seen in the target population.

STRATEGIES THAT DO NOT WORK

Education alone has not been shown to be effective. While health education interventions have shown success in reducing other risk behaviors, health education directed toward preventing obesity has not shown much success. While the educational programs add to the population or an individual's knowledge about healthy nutrition and physical activity, the individuals behaviors related to obesity do not change. Only directed, specific behavioral modification techniques have shown some success.

Several large community based studies have used educational measures to prevent obesity. The Minnesota Heart Healthy program used mass media, adult educational programs, school and workplace interventions, and risk screening to promote exercise and healthy diet, among other desired outcomes. Unfortunately the BMI of the population continued to increase unchecked by the intervention. The Pound of Prevention program sought to slow the progression of obesity through an educational program supported by newsletters and incentives. While participation was excellent, obesity was not prevented (Jeffery, 2001). The lack of effect for these educational programs suggests that knowledge of the benefits of nutrition and physical fitness by itself is not sufficient to protect against obesity.

SYNTHESIS

We are only beginning to understand the causal relationships between complex environmental factors and the population's behaviors related to nutrition and physical activity. Clearly these environmental factors have a significant impact upon the development of obesity within a population. The epidemic of obesity in more developed countries is evidence of these environmental factors. While we can speculate that easy access to low-nutrient, energy-dense foods and increasingly sedentary activities are key factors, the relative importance and effect of these environmental factors on our eating behaviors and activity is poorly understood. A greater understanding of these factors can only improve our efforts to counteract these influences and prevent the development of obesity.

While some studies show success in modifying an individual's behaviors related to nutrition and physical activity. Efforts based on a medical model alone are unlikely to succeed in the long term. Particularly if these individuals live in environments with significant obstacles to continued healthy behaviors.

A successful long-term prevention strategy will need to create an environment conducive to healthful nutrition and sustainable physical fitness. Unfortunately, we do not yet know how to do this. We have been most successful in accomplishing this in the school setting. Here both nutrition and physical activity can be changed through control of environmental factors and targeting the population through education and behavior modification. We need to further explore the effectiveness of these strategies for prevention of obesity and promotion of healthy behaviors. As we gain greater understanding of effective strategies, these strategies can be applied to other settings such as the workplace, the healthcare center, community centers, residential communities, or the community-at-large.

The greatest limitation faced in interpreting our current studies is that many successful interventions use only short-term outcomes that measure change in behaviors related to nutrition or physical activity. Many do not include the BMI as an endpoint, choosing surrogate short-term markers instead. Some that have used population-based BMI as a marker have been disappointing in their effect. Perhaps in part because the prevention strategy had insufficient power to overcome the other as yet poorly defined environmental factors that promote unhealthy eating behaviors and sedentary lifestyle. The overwhelming effects of fast food and snack food appeal and the draw to sedentary activities such as television watching and computers may be difficult to overcome.

Future directions for research include acquiring a better understanding of the factors driving the current epidemic of obesity, expanding upon the successes in the school setting, and further attempts to modify the environmental factors influencing both behaviors related to nutrition and behaviors related to physical activity. The preventive strategies need to use both short-term markers of behavior change and the direct marker of obesity, BMI. The prevention strategies need to be evaluated for a sustained protective effect over time.

Also see: Nutrition: Early Childhood; Nutrition: Childhood; Nutrition: Adulthood; Nutrition: Older Adulthood; Nutrition and Physical Activity: Adolescence.

References

Bedogni, G., Pietrobelli, A., Heymsfield, S.B., Borghi, A., Manzieri, A.M., Morini, P., Battistini, N., & Salvioli, G. (2001). Is the body mass index a measure of adiposity in elderly women? *Obesity Research, 9*(1), 17–20.

Calfas, K.J., Sallis, J.F., Oldenburg, B., & French, M. (1997). Mediators of change in physical activity following an intervention in primary care: PACE. *Preventive Medicine, 26*, 297–304.

Campbell, M.K., DeVellis, B.M., Ammerman, A.S., DeVellis, R.F., & Sandler, R.S. (1994). Improving dietary behavior: The effectiveness of tailored messages in primary care setting. *American Journal of Public Health, 84*(5), 783–797.

Canadian Health Reports. (2000). *Statistics Canada, Catalogue 82-003, 12*(3), 1–20.

Center for Disease Control (CDC). (2000). *Growth charts: United States.* Developed by the National center for Health Statistics in collaboration with the National Center for Chronic Disease Prevention and Health Promotion Available: http://www.cdc.gov

Clinical Guidelines on the Identification, Evaluation, and Treatment of Overweight and Obesity in Adults—The Evidence Report (1998). *The National Heart, Lung and Blood Institute* (NHLBI).

Donnelly, J.R., Jacobsen, D.J., Whitley, J.E., Swift L.L., Cherrington, A., Polk, B., Tran, A.V., & Reed, G. (1996). Nutrition and physical activity program to attenuate obesity and promote physical and metabolic fitness in elementary school children *Obesity Research, 4*, 229–243.

Dwyer, T., Coonan, W.E., Leitch, D.R., Hetzel, B.S., & Baghurst, R.A. (1983). An investigation of the effects of daily physical activity on the health of primary school students in South Australia. *International Journal of Epidemiology, 12*(3), 308–313.

Epstein, L.H., Gordy, C.C., Raynor, H.A., Beddome, M., Kilanowski, C.D., & Paluch, R. (2001). Increasing fruit and vegetable intake in families at risk for childhood obesity. *Obesity Research, 9*(3), 171–177.

Epstein, L.H., Valoski, A., Wing, R.R., & McCurly, J. (1994). Ten-year outcomes of behavioral family-based treatment for childhood obesity. *Health Psychology, 13*(5), 373–383.

Flores, R. (1995). Dance for health: Improving fitness in African-American and Hispanic adolescents. *Public Health Reports, 110*(2), 189–193.

Foster, G.D., Wadden, T.A., & Bownell, K.D. (1985). Peer-led program for the treatment and prevention of obesity in the schools. *Journal of Consulting and Clinical Psychology, 53*(4), 538–540.

French, S.A., Jeffery, R.W., Story, M., Breitlow, K.K., & Baxter, J.S. (2001). Pricing and promotion effects on low-fat vending snack purchases: The CHIPS study. *American Journal of Public Health, 9*(1), 112–117.

Gortmaker, S.L., Peterson, K., Wiecha, J., Sobol, A.M., Dixit, S., Fox, M.K., & Laird, N. (1999). Reducing obesity via a school-based interdisiplinary intervention among youth: Planet Health. *Archives of Pediatric and Adolescent Medicine, 153*, 409–418.

Greenberg, D.A. (1993). Linkage analysis of "necessary" disease loci versus "susceptibility loci." *American Journal of Human Genetics, 52*, 135–145.

Jeffery, R.W. (2001). Public health strategies for obesity treatment and prevention. *American Journal for Health Behavior, 25*(3), 252–259.

Jeffery, R.W., French, S.A., Raether, C., & Baxter, J.E. (1994). An environmental intervention to increase fruit and salad purchases in a cafeteria. *Preventive Medicine, 23*, 788–792.

Killen, J.D., Robinson, T.N., Telch, M.J., Saylor, K.E., Maron, D.J., Rich, T., & Sryson, S. (1989). The Stanford Adolescent Heart Health program. *Health Education Quarterly, 16*(2), 263–283.

Luepker, R.V., Perry, C.L., McKinlay, S.M., Nader, P.R., Parcel, G.S., Stone, E.J., Webber, L.S., Elder, J.P., Felman, H.A., Johnson, D.D., Kelder, S.H., & Wu, M. (1996). Outcomes of a field trial to improve children's dietary patterns and physical activity: The child and adolescent trial for cardiovascular health (CATCH). *Journal of the American Medical Association, 275*(10), 768–776.

McGinnis, J.M., & Foege, W.H. (1993). Actual causes of death in the United States. *Journal of the American Medical Association, 270*(18), 2207–2211.

Mo-suwan, L., Pongprapai, S., Junjana, C., & Puetpaeboon, A. (1998). Effects of a controlled trial of a school-based exercise program on the obesity indexes of preschool children. *American Journal of Clinical Nutrition, 68*, 1006–1011

Pietrobelli, A., Faith, M.S., Allison, D.B., Gallagher, D., Shiumello, G., & Heymsfield, S.B. (1998) Body mass index as a measure of adiposity among children and adolescents: A validation study. *Journal of Pediatrics, 132* (2), 204–210.

Stolley, M.R., & Fitzgibbon, M.L. (1997). Effects of an obesity prevention program on the eating behavior of African American mothers and daughters. *Health Education & Behavior, 24*(2), 152–164.

Troiano, R.P., & Flegal, K.M. (1998). Overweight children and adolescents: description, epidemiology, and demographics. *Pediatrics, 101*, 497–504.

World Health Organization (WHO). (1997). *"Obesity epidemic puts millions at risk form related diseases"* World Health Organization Press Release, June 12, 1997. Information from the World Health Organization Consultation on Obesity (Geneva, June 3–5, 1997).

World Health Organization (WHO). (1999). *Obesity: Preventing and managing the global epidemic. Report of a WHO consultation on obesity.*

WHO Global Database on Obesity and Body Mass Index (BMI) in Adults. (2001). Available: http://www. who.int/nut/db_bmi.htm

Oral Health, Early Childhood

Tegwyn L. Hughes, Georgia G. dela Cruz, and R. Gary Rozier

INTRODUCTION

In his report "Oral Health in America", the US Surgeon General identified a "silent epidemic" of dental disease

Table 1. Glossary of Selected Terms

Determinants of health.   The forces predisposing, enabling, and reinforcing lifestyles, or shaping environmental conditions of living, in ways that affect the health (Green & Kreuter, 1999).

Enabling factor.   Any characteristic of the environment that facilitates action and any skill or resource required to attain a specific behavior populations (Green & Kreuter, 1999).

Fluoride.   An element that is found naturally throughout the environment and has been identified by the Institute of Medicine as a nutrient which is essential for maintaining health (IOM, 1997). It is most commonly available in toothpaste or drinking water, where it can occur naturally or be added to bring its concentration to an optimal level to prevent dental caries. It also can be used in dietary supplements, or applied professionally, or individually to the teeth in pastes, gels, and varnishes.

Framework.   Sometimes referred to as a model, it provides a set of concepts believed to be related to a particular public health problem. It helps explain health and the factors that influence it. Usually it is formed by more than one theory and is conceptualized at multi-levels, from micro to macro (Sogaard, 1993).

Off-label use.   The use of approved drugs for a condition or patient category for which they are, as of yet, unapproved. "Unapproved" does not imply improper or illegal use, or contraindication based on positive evidence of lack of safety or efficacy (AAP, 1996).

Predisposing factor.   Any characteristic of a person or population that motivates behavior prior to the occurrence of the behavior (Green & Kreuter, 1999).

Prevalence.   The number of persons with disease or an attribute at a specified point in time (Last & Abramson, 1995).

Primary teeth.   Also know as deciduous teeth or milk teeth, these are the first teeth that erupt into the mouth, generally between 6 months and 3 years of age. These teeth enable young children to eat solid foods, aid in speech development and serve as space holders for the permanent dentition.

Reinforcing factor.   Any reward or punishment following or anticipated as a consequence of a behavior serving to strengthen the motivation for or against the behavior (Green & Kreuter, 1999).

Risk assessment.   A method used to identify individuals and/or communities at high risk of disease using a combination of causal and predictive factors related to a specific disease. These factors could be environmental, behavioral, or biological, which if present, increase the probability of a disease occurring, and if absent or removed, reduce the probability. Terms often used to describe these factors are: risk factors, risk indicators, demographic risk factors, and risk markers/predictors (Beck, 1998).

within the United States (US Department of Health and Human Services [USDHHS], 2000). Children in poor families bear a particularly heavy burden, with many unable to achieve their full potential because tooth decay and other dental diseases interfere with their well-being and functioning. Poor oral health is all the more tragic because safe, effective and low-cost preventive methods are available for use by the public, health professionals and related groups. This entry reviews the scope of dental problems faced by children 0–5 years of age, the preventive methods available to address these problems, the evidence for their effectiveness, and recommendations for their use.

DEFINITIONS

A number of diseases and conditions affect the teeth, mouth, face, and surrounding structures. This entry focuses largely on tooth decay because it is so widespread. Tooth decay, also known as *dental caries*, is a carbohydrate-modified bacterial disease that can affect individuals throughout life. It is considered to be an infectious disease because decay-causing bacteria in the infant are obtained from the primary caregiver. In children younger than 6 years of age, dental caries is referred to as *Early Childhood Caries* (ECC), a name that is beginning to replace terms such as nursing

caries and baby bottle tooth decay (Drury, Horowitz, Ismail, Maertens, Rozier, & Selwitz, 1999). Other terms used in this entry are defined in Table 1.

SCOPE

The dental and craniofacial health of children during the first 6 years of life results from a series of complex interactions among many biological, behavioral, and environmental factors beginning at conception. As many as 360 inherited genetic diseases or disorders involve the mouth and craniofacial structures. Fortunately, these inherited diseases are rare, with only about 2 infants in every 1,000 live births having some type of birth defect, about half of which are clefts of the lip or palate. Treatment costs for these children, however, can approach $1 billion a year (Slavkin, 1998). Other children suffer from trauma, cancer, or infectious diseases involving the oral and facial areas.

ECC is the most common oral health problem of childhood. It also is the most common of all chronic diseases of childhood, with a prevalence five times greater than that of asthma (USDHHS, 2000). Overall, 18 percent of 2–4-year-old US children have had one or more cavities. But dental disease is not evenly distributed among the population, being concentrated among those living in poverty. All 1-year-old infants found to be affected in the most recent national survey belonged to families classified as poor or near poor (Kaste, Drury, Horowitz, & Beltran, 1999). These disparities by socioeconomic status observed in infants continue as children get older (Vargas, Crall, & Schneider, 1998). In the last few years, the overall severity of ECC has gotten worse in the average child (Brown, Wall, & Lazar, 2000). Adding to the problem, as much as 80 percent of dental disease goes untreated in young children who live in poverty.

The annual dental bill to restore all children's decayed teeth exceeds $2 billion in the United States, making it one of the most expensive uncontrolled diseases of childhood (Lewit & Monheit, 1992). Severe ECC, a major reason for hospitalization of infants and toddlers, is estimated to cost at least $100 million a year for hospital charges alone (Health Resources and Services Administration [HRSA], 1998). Children with severe, untreated ECC can be underweight, fail to thrive, and have impaired speech development. Later in life their performance in school may be reduced (Office of Health Promotion and Disease Prevention, 2000).

THEORIES

No comprehensive model exists for the promotion of oral health in early childhood. We chose to adapt a framework for use in this entry proposed by Green and Kreuter (1999).

It is often used to plan and evaluate interventions designed to influence behaviors that result in poor health outcomes, as well as the living conditions and other environmental factors that influence these behaviors or their outcomes.

We chose the Green–Kreuter framework as a guide for this entry for several reasons. First, it recognizes that health and health risks have multiple determinants, which applies to oral problems, particularly ECC. Second, because it assumes that health risks and outcomes are caused by multiple factors, it recognizes that efforts to affect behavioral, environmental, and social change must be multidimensional. The prevention and control of diseases and conditions of the mouth and the promotion of oral health require a complex set of strategies involving individual practices, personal medical and dental health services, public health activities and health policy initiatives. Most efforts to understand the etiology of ECC and address its causes have focused on biological processes or clinical care, not the constellation of factors that predispose the child to problems or enable or reinforce these causal or predictive factors. The model leads us to expand our consideration of prevention strategies beyond those that are proven to prevent and control oral diseases, and to critically examine those risk factors for which we have little evidence for effective interventions. Finally, the model includes the entire population of children and their caregivers, not just those who use dental or medical services or have significance disease.

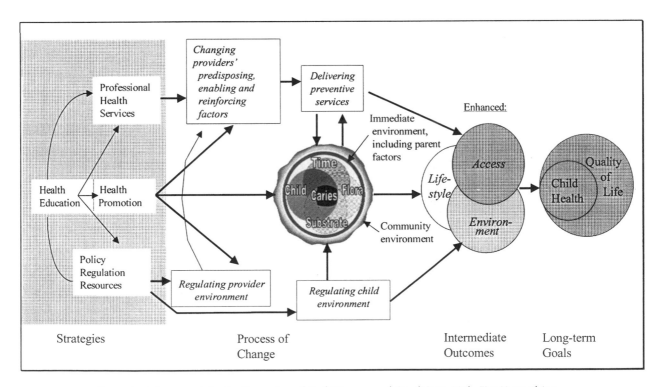

Figure 1. A Framework for the Prevention of Oral Diseases and Conditions, Birth–Five Years of Age.

Our adaptation of the framework (Figure 1) emphasizes three primary categories of preventive strategies: (1) community, professional, and individual health education and health promotion; (2) professional health services; and (3) policy making. These strategies establish a process of change to influence factors that a professional or caregiver might provide for the child. A number of factors can predispose (e.g., knowledge), enable (e.g., skill), and reinforce (e.g., patient feedback) preventive services provided by the health care professional. Likewise, a number of factors can predispose (e.g., motivation), enable (e.g., transportation), and reinforce (e.g., family attitudes) preventive services provided by the caregiver. Immediate outcomes of any intervention that sets this process of change in motion are enhanced children's access to health services, lifestyle, or environment. The long-term outcome is improved oral health and quality of life.

At the center of this framework is the young child and dental caries, the primary focus of this entry. The dental caries process is well understood (Featherstone, 2000). The necessary components of the process are the tooth itself, decay-causing bacteria, carbohydrates, and time. Acid is produced in the mouth as a by-product when decay-causing bacteria in a film (plaque) on the teeth metabolize fermentable carbohydrates. When the tooth is exposed to this acid environment it loses minerals (calcium and phosphorous). This process takes place at a microscopic level and can be reversed within minutes when saliva buffers the acid environment or transports replacement minerals to the tooth structure. This cycle of initiation and reversal can begin each time carbohydrates are introduced into the mouth, usually several times each day. If pathologic factors predominate for a sufficient length of time without the removal of bacteria or sufficient buffering by saliva, the tooth defenses are overwhelmed and the process can progress to the point that it is not reversible. With further advancement, the tooth structure collapses and a hole (cavity) develops.

Multiple prevention strategies seek to interfere with the convergence of the three necessary components of the dental caries process—carbohydrates (e.g., frequency of sucrose), bacteria (e.g., levels of infection with mutans streptococci and lactobacilli), and host factors (e.g., fluoride, calcium, and phosphorous in saliva and plaque). Caregivers play a crucial role in filtering the interaction between children and their environment through the type of food they feed the child and the oral hygiene care and other preventive services that they make available to the child. Predisposing, enabling, and reinforcing factors affect the caregiver's effectiveness in filtering out caries causing factors and supplying caries promoting factors. Factors that support caregivers in poor families are particularly important in helping them raise healthy children.

An understanding of the process of change in our framework and how to influence that process requires theories from many disciplines, including economics, sociology, behavioral sciences, and political science as well as knowledge of biology, and preventive sciences. However, few general theories have been empirically validated in etiological studies of ECC or its prevention.

RESEARCH

The safety and effectiveness of methods available to prevent dental caries and other diseases in children have been reviewed extensively in the literature. A number of recent reviews followed protocols for systematic reviews, and some meta-analyses of study results have been performed. Recent reviews and recommendations by organizations in the United States have addressed the various types of fluoride use (Centers for Disease Control and Prevention [CDC], 2001), methods used by dental health professionals for the prevention of dental caries in high risk individuals (Bader et al., 2000) or the general population (Rozier, 2001), and community-based methods for prevention of a number of dental diseases (USDHHS, 2000). Both the US Preventive Services Task Force (US Preventive Services Task Force [USPSTF], 1996) and the Canadian Task Force on the Periodic Health Examination (Lewis & Ismail, 1995) have reviewed the evidence for the primary prevention of dental diseases, primarily aimed at the medical profession. Systematic reviews of preventive methods for a number of dental diseases are soon to be released by the US Task Force on Community Preventive Services (http://www. thecommunityguide.org) and the Cochrane Collaboration (http://cochrane.hcn.net.au/).

While the literature on the prevention of dental disease is extensive, few randomized controlled trials have been conducted with preschool-aged children and their parents. The only extensive review of methods specifically for the prevention of ECC did not follow a rigorous protocol for systematic reviews, but did grade the evidence and recommendations according to methods used by the USPSTF (Ismail, 1998). Thus, many of the recommendations for use presented in this entry, if followed, must be considered "off-label" use because randomized controlled trials have not established effectiveness in young children (American Academy of Pediatrics [AAP], 1996). Use of a particular therapy off-label does not necessarily mean that it is not effective, just that it has not been tested sufficiently to support an evidence-based recommendation. Often these recommendations are supported by expert opinion alone.

Table 2. Recommendations for Preventing Oral Diseases in Children 0–5 years of Age, and Strength of Evidence Supporting Recommendations

Intervention strategy and setting	Strength of evidence supporting recommendation[a]	Recommendation and target population[b]	References supporting recommendation[c]
Medical office			
Screening and referral as needed	Insufficient	All persons	1
Counseling	Insufficient	All persons	1
Dental office			
Regular visit	Fair	All persons	1
Prophylaxis (cleaning)	Insufficient	High-risk persons	2
Counseling	Insufficient	All persons	1,2
Fluoride gel and varnish	Good	High-risk persons	3,4
Dental sealant	Good	High-risk persons	2,4
Community			
Water fluoridation	Fair	All communities	1,3,4
Education	Insufficient	High-risk communities	d
Organization and development	Insufficient	High-risk communities	d
Individual Environment			
Oral hygiene	Insufficient	All persons	1,4
Fluoridated toothpaste	Good	All persons	3,4
Diet	Good	All persons	1,4
Fluoride supplements			
Pregnant women	Good	None	3,4
Children aged < 6 years	Insufficient	High-risk persons	3,4

[a] Criteria for strength of recommendation designations are adapted from the US PSTF (1996). Most ratings are inferred from studies of older children because of the lack of randomized controlled trials in children birth to 5 years of age.
[b] Evidence for targeting some strategies to children or communities at high risk is derived from opinions of experts, the weakest evidence in support of a recommendation, and is based mostly on considerations of costs rather than evidence for effectiveness. The systematic review by Bader et al. (2000) found fair evidence to support use of fluoride varnish in caries-active individuals.
[c] *References* (Full references provided in the reference list at end of chapter.)
(1) US PSTF (1996). Guide to clinical preventive services.
(2) Lewis & Ismail (1995). Canadian task force on the periodic health examination.
(3) Centers for Disease Control and Prevention. (2001). Recommendations for using fluoride to prevent and control dental caries in the United States.
(4) US Department of Health and Human Services (2000). Oral health in America: A report of the Surgeon General.
[d] Recommendation not supported by published systematic review.

STRATEGIES: OVERVIEW

The characteristics of ECC and the availability of preventive methods support primary prevention as an important strategy to address this important pediatric health problem and its serious consequences. The following pages focus on exposures that children have to prevention services through their interactions with health professionals, their families, and their communities, all of which are supported by health policies. Recommendations for most of these strategies and the strength of the evidence supporting them are summarized in Table 2.

STRATEGIES: EVIDENCE FOR EFFECTIVENESS

Oral Health Policies, Regulations, and Resources

The United States has prevention policies in a number of areas that can affect the oral health of young children. Policies relate to the provision of clinical and community prevention services, financing of professional dental services and establishment of delivery systems, guidelines and performance standards for the delivery of dental services and other quality improvement methods, professional education and public health core functions. The following paragraphs describe public policies that relate to the oral health and welfare of young children. The effects of the various policies are rarely studied for their causal relationship to young children's oral health and quality of life. However, we know from those that have been studied that the effects are mixed.

National Prevention Policies

The Healthy People initiative has provided a national strategic plan for improving health over the last two decades. An evaluation of the extent to which national oral health objectives for 2000 were met provides an assessment of the overall success in our national prevention efforts. Only one of 17 objectives was completely met during the last decade, and that one did not involve young children (USDHHS, 2000). Healthy People 2010 provides direction for the present decade. Among its 28 chapters is one devoted to oral health. It contains 17 objectives, three of which are specifically targeted to preschool aged children. These objectives set benchmarks for reducing the prevalence of dental caries in young children, increasing treatment for caries, and the identification and referral of infants and children with cleft lips, cleft palates, or other craniofacial anomalies. Objectives for broader age groups include young children, and relate to expanding community water fluoridation and public health treatment programs, increasing the use of personal health services, specifically preventive services in low-income children, and providing for oral health surveillance.

Water fluoridation is a cornerstone of US prevention policy for young children. This policy has been supported for more than half a century by statements from the US Surgeon General, scientific reviews, grants to states and communities to expand coverage, surveillance and training to ensure quality, and a National Fluoride Plan. Fluoridation is not legislated at the federal level and is perceived in most states as a local issue, but ten states and Puerto Rico have enacted legislation mandating water fluoridation. While full coverage for the nation has not been achieved, it is considered a major factor responsible for improvements in dental caries prevalence during the second half of the last century (CDC, 1999).

Financing of Clinical Preventive Dental Services

Public policy provides for the payment for dental services delivered by dentists in private practice or in public clinics. The largest of these programs is Medicaid, established by amendments to the Social Security Act in 1965. More than 1 out of every 5 children younger than 6 years of age or about 9 million children, most of whom are poor, are enrolled in the program. After some initial success, utilization of dental care for children enrolled in Medicaid has faltered, and it now fails to provide dental services to most of those who are eligible. Only 16 percent of 1–5-year-old Medicaid children receive any preventive care (USDHHS, 1996). Young children and their families face particularly difficult circumstances, and a large percentage of young children with ECC receive only emergency dental services, at best. One study found that only 2 percent of 3-year-old children enrolled in Medicaid in one state received comprehensive care in a 12-month period (Cashion, Vann, Jr., Rozier, Venezie, & McIver, 1999).

Direct Provision of Clinical Preventive Services

Several federal, state, and local agencies provide direct educational and clinical services to children and their families. Most notable among the federal agencies is the Indian Health Service (IHS), which operates a mostly rural primary care system for 1.5 million American Indians and Alaskan natives, and the Health Resources and Services Administration, which funds a relatively small network of community health centers in medically underserved areas that provides services to slightly more than 1.2 million low-income patients. A report to the US Congress by the General Accounting Office (2000) concluded that these two programs, plus the IHS loan repayment program and the National Health Service Corps, which places dentists in underserved areas, have a limited effect on providing access to dental services.

Professional Interventions

Health care professionals provide a number of preventive services important to maintaining the oral health of young children. About 3,600 dentists in the United States have specialty training in the care of children, supplying only about 1 pediatric dentist for every 5,300 children younger than 5 years of age. This ratio of pediatric dentists to children underscores the important role that not only general dentists, but primary care physicians and other child health care providers can play in providing access to preventive dental services, particularly for very young children and those who do not have access to dental care. The following paragraphs describe professional preventive dental services that can be provided in primary care medical offices and thus take full advantage of partnerships between the dental and medical communities, and then those that a dental professional provides.

Primary Care Medical Visit

The medical office provides an important setting where provision of oral health preventive services can take place. Caregivers should be advised on a number of practices that can affect their children's oral health. Guidelines for education conducted by medical personnel are available in which broad dental messages are keyed to milestones in the child's development, such as the eruption of the first tooth (Casamassimo, 1996), or in which educational messages are more limited and specific to particular risk factors or disease (USPSTF, 1996). Avoidance of sugary foods, use of fluorides, good oral hygiene practices, and dental visits are considered important in preventing dental disease and anticipatory guidance is recommended, even though the effectiveness of primary care health professionals in providing advice on these behaviors has not been evaluated.

The medical visit also provides a key access point for dental screenings to determine elevated risk, actual disease or injuries, the need for referrals to dentists and assistance in finding a dentist. Children who have reached the age where they should be seen by a dentist, or a child of any age who is believed to have elevated risk of ECC, already has signs of ECC such as discolored or broken teeth, or has dental pain should be referred to a dentist. Children can be at increased risk for dental disease if they are from low-income families, have experienced caries in the past, have early signs of carious lesions such as white spots or discolored tooth surfaces, or have visible plaque (Tinanoff, 1995). Some prevention services should be limited to those children who are at high risk. For example, professionally prescribed daily doses of fluoride tablets or drops are recommended for children who are at least 6 months old, who have inadequate water fluoridation (<0.6 mg/L), and who are otherwise determined to be at high risk for ECC. The accuracy of medical clinicians' screening results or their success in assisting caregivers obtain dental care for their children is unknown. Nevertheless, it is prudent for clinicians to screen children for oral disease and act on their findings.

Recommendations for the age at which the child's first visit to a dentist should occur vary from around age 1 (American Academy of Pediatric Dentistry [AAPD], 2000) to 3 years of age (AAP, 1995). Dental caries can start soon after the first tooth comes into the mouth at around 6 months of age, so an early dental visit is important to provide caregivers with anticipatory guidance at critical times in the oral health development of a child. The early dental visit should be seen as the foundation on which a lifetime of preventive education and dental care can be built.

Table 3. Anticipatory Guidance for Children's Oral Health
(Modified from: Nowak & Casamassimo, 1995)

Content area for counseling	Dental professional's role
Oral development	
Eruption of first tooth	Review teething facts and myths
Development of permanent dentition	Review patterns and timing of eruption
Concepts of occlusion, arch length and, spacing	Describe oral anatomic landmarks and tooth position
	Discuss oral stimulation
Fluoride	
Fluoride toxicity and safety	Assess fluoride status-determine if supplements needed
Topical and systemic fluoride action	Discuss appropriate fluoride vehicles and delivery
Fluoride sources (water, food, outside the home)	Discuss fluoride toxicity and management of ingestion
Oral hygiene/health	
Oral bacteria innoculation	Review oral hygiene for infants:
Mouth-cleaning techniques	Soft toothbrush and no dentifrice or pea-sized amount
Periodicity of dental visits	Parental supervision and compliance with oral hygiene
Role of child and parent in brushing	Plan for next dental visit by risk assessment
Frequency and timing of oral hygiene	Explain dental radiographs
Habits	
Non-nutritive sucking/pacifier use/thumbsucking	Review pacifier use, safety, and hygiene
Breastfeeding and oral health	Discuss role of the mouth in infant exploration
	Discuss thumbsucking effects on oralfacial growth
	Discuss breastfeeding effects on oral health
	Discuss discontinuation strategies of non-nutritive sucking
Nutrition and diet	
Nursing bottle tooth decay/inappropriate feeding	Encourage weaning at appropriate time
Role of sugar and carbohydrates in dental caries	Discuss role of sugar/carbohydrates/milk in dental caries
Frequency of feeding/snacking	Discuss plaque development and dental caries
	Discuss a healthy diet
	Discuss frequency of intake in dental caries
Injury prevention	
Oral trauma/tooth trauma	Review normal oral and dental anatomy with parents
Electric cord injury	Reinforce electrical cord safety, home child-proofing, bike helmet, and use of car seats
Home child-proofing/falls	Develop plan for oral trauma management at home or day care: post emergency numbers
Bicycle safety	
Car safety	

Primary Care Dental Visit

Like the medical clinician, dentists and their staff provide oral health education and preventive services, but in addition provide comprehensive diagnostic and treatment services, thus preventing more serious outcomes in those who are already affected (Kanellis, 2000). Guidelines for use by dental professionals in providing anticipatory guidance for young children and their caregivers are available (Nowak & Casamassimo, 1995). They recommend education on specific items related to growth and development, fluoride, oral hygiene, oral habits, diet, and injury prevention (Table 3). In general, studies suggest that education in the primary care dental setting can improve knowledge and behaviors, but few studies have been done on the effectiveness of educating caregivers in the dental care setting on these targeted behaviors or health outcomes.

The dental visit also provides the opportunity for a professional cleaning, and in appropriate cases other preventive services such as fluoride treatments (Klimek, Prinz, Hellwig, & Ahrens, 1985). The cleaning removes debris and stain from the teeth, but its clinical support comes from the opportunity to provide individually based risk assessment, preventive advice, and feedback to both the parent and child. It is not supported by evidence of caries prevention unless a fluoride treatment is provided during the visit. A professional cleaning also provides an opportunity for the child to become accustomed to oral health services.

Professional applications of fluoride to the teeth using gels or varnishes are safe and effective (Kanellis, 2000). Fluoride varnish is particularly appropriate for use in young children because it can be painted on the teeth at any age. It reduces the occurrence of new carious lesions in primary teeth by 37–44 percent and is effective in halting the progression of already existing small lesions (Autio-Gold & Courts, 2001; Holm, 1979). The use of topical fluorides in the office and the prescription of fluoride supplements for use at home should be based on the caries risk of the child. Primary teeth in high-risk children also may need dental sealants, a plastic material placed on the chewing surfaces of teeth to keep decay-causing bacteria out of the pits and fissures of teeth. Sealant is most commonly used for prevention of caries in permanent teeth of children older than 5 years of age, where reductions average 71 percent, but it is effective when applied to the primary teeth of high-risk children (Hardison, Collier, Sprouse, Van Cleave, & Hogan, 1987).

Community Interventions

Proven community interventions to promote oral health in infancy and early childhood are limited in number. However, they can influence the child's environment and address predisposing and enabling factors, particularly those of the parent and others who provide child care services.

Community Water Fluoridation

Fluoridation is considered by the Centers for Disease Control and Prevention as one of the 10 greatest public health achievements of the 20th century (CDC, 1999). It has proven again and again to be an effective and safe method for the prevention of dental caries. The costs for fluoridation are less than the money it would take to treat the disease it prevents. Fluoridation benefits people of all ages, particularly young children, and it helps reduce disparities in dental caries. Reductions in the severity of ECC from fluoridation now range from 13 to 68 percent, with the most common value being between 50 and 60 percent (Locker, Lawrence, & Jokovic, 1999). It provides an important environmental factor in the control of ECC. Currently 62 percent of the population has access to community water systems containing fluoride.

Community Oral Health Education

Most community-based dental health education interventions do not result in behavior changes or oral health outcomes proportionate to the resources that are expended. Therefore, widespread, single component interventions such as mass media campaigns cannot be recommended for the general population. For high risk communities whose members may have low educational levels, ethical considerations require the provision of community health education so that caregivers will have the necessary knowledge and support to make decisions regarding appropriate preventive actions on behalf of their children (USDHHS, 2000). Effective strategies might involve education on preventing ECC in programs such as WIC (Special Supplemental Food Program for Women, Infants, and Children) or other settings. A recent randomized controlled community trial found that regular home visits by dental health educators to mothers with high caries risk infants, commencing during the first year of life, reduced disease in children by 83 percent (Kowash, Pinfield, Smith, & Curzon, 2001).

Community Development

Community development "recognises the social, economic, and environmental causes of ill health and links user involvement and commissioning to improve health and reduce inequalities" (Fisher, Neve, & Heritage, 1999). It involves developing appropriate and accessible services through: identifying health needs; increasing the number or types of needed services that are provided by health care workers; and identifying and coordinating services with existing community networks, programs and agencies. Community development potentially can improve children's oral health by altering the physical environment of the parent and child. It can assist caregivers in obtaining a dental home for their children, with case management and with transportation (Watson, 2000).

Evidence of effectiveness for community organization and development in improving oral health of young children is insufficient because few interventions have implemented simultaneously all of the necessary aspects of a comprehensive program. Those programs that have come closest to the ideal have not been fully evaluated using control populations and for their effects on disease outcomes. However, improvements in the use of preventive dental services in one project indicate that an emphasis on community development may help improve oral health of children living in high-risk communities (Milgrom, Hujoel, Grembowski, & Fong, 1999).

Individual Interventions

The knowledge, skills, and appropriate decision-making of an adult are required to ensure that children receive proper diet, hygiene, and other services to promote their oral health and prevent disease. For this reason, we focus on individual preventive practices performed by the parent or caregiver on behalf of their child.

Oral Hygiene

Most studies of the effect of oral hygiene education on dental caries have failed to produce a lasting effect. However, numerous studies have shown an association between poor oral hygiene and dental caries, and the earlier tooth brushing begins, the less likely children are to develop tooth decay (Creedon & O'Mullane, 2001). Parents should begin cleaning an infant's gums with a moistened cloth or cotton gauze before teeth erupt. Brushing should begin once teeth start to erupt. Because of the nature of plaque, the teeth should be cleaned at least twice a day, preferably in the morning and the evening. Children should participate in the brushing routine at an early age, but parents should supervise brushing at all times and brush the child's teeth themselves at least once a day until the child is 8 years of age.

Fluoride

Use of fluoridated toothpaste by children is an extremely important practice to prevent ECC. It should be used by most children during brushing beginning at 2 years of age, when parents should use a pea-sized amount of toothpaste (0.25 g) no more than twice a day. Children should be

encouraged to spit out excess toothpaste. Those children who are at risk for ECC may need to start using fluoridated toothpaste before 2 years of age, but it should be started only on the advice of a dentist or physician. Parents should not allow their children to place toothpaste on the brush unsupervised because excessive use by children younger than 8 years of age can lead to discoloration of the permanent teeth (CDC, 2001).

Diet and Nutrition

The importance of nutrition in the child's oral health begins before birth. Adequate maternal nutrition is important for proper formation of the craniofacial structures and teeth (USDHHS, 2000). Once born, a child's consumption of sweet snacks or beverages between meals increases the risk of tooth decay (Tinanoff & Palmer, 2000). Because bacterial digestion of sugar produces the acid that causes cavities, parents should limit the frequency and amount of sugary foods or beverages that their children consume. Otherwise healthy liquids such as formula and unsweetened fruit juices sometimes contain sugar that can produce tooth decay if they are sipped frequently. For this reason, parents should discontinue bottle use by 12 months and should not allow their child to have constant access to a cup containing these liquids, especially during sleep times.

Parents can take two important steps to ensure that their children receive the recommended dietary allowances of fluoride (Institute of Medicine [IOM], 1997). First, they should be aware of the fluoridation status of their drinking water. Local or state health departments can provide information on whether community water supplies are fluoridated. They also usually offer low or no cost water-testing services for those who are not using a public drinking water source and thus the fluoride content of water is unknown. Second, parents who use drinking water that is not optimally fluoridated should inform their dentist or health care provider and discuss the need for intensified ECC prevention options such as dietary fluoride supplements.

Oral Habit

Oral habits such as digit sucking, lip sucking, or pacifier use can disrupt normal dental and facial development if they are conducted forcefully or for extended periods of time (Nowak & Warren, 2000). These habits can interfere with the normal eruption of anterior teeth and may set the stage for constricted growth of the upper jaws. Both of these problems may require expensive orthodontic intervention in adolescence. It is generally recommended that parents offer pacifiers to infants who attempt to engage in digit or lip sucking behavior. Pacifier use can be gradually decreased after 2 years of age more easily than a digit habit because pacifier availability can be controlled by the caregiver.

SYNTHESIS

This entry has used a broad framework to examine strategies that can prevent dental diseases and promote oral health in young children. Fluorides provided in community programs, by primary health care professionals or by caregivers are particularly effective in the prevention of ECC. Less evidence exists for the effectiveness of other interventions and diseases, largely because prevention research in dentistry has not concentrated on this age group. Many interventions are recommended because they address well-understood components of the biological process by which ECC is established and because experts believe that they are effective in reducing ECC, not because good evidence from controlled clinical trials is available.

Historically, the oral health of young children has not been the focus of major disease prevention and health promotion initiatives in the United States. Less than 1 percent of a total budget of $409 billion for eight federal agencies in the Department of Health and Human Services is devoted to oral health (USDHHS, 2000). The public health infrastructure in states likewise is severely limited, with dental public health expenditures for all ages and all services amounting to only 38 cents per person (Lockwood & Malvitz, 1995). Recently, national attention has been focused on the oral health of children and the deficit in our knowledge base for oral health promotion. The Office of the US Inspector General, the General Accounting Office, the American Dental Association, the American Public Human Services Administration, the Urban Institute, and the National Governor's Association are among the dozens of organizations that have issued detailed reports on what might be done to improve oral health. Many promising activities that should contribute to young children's oral health are already underway.

Arguably the most significant public policy seeking to improve access to medical and dental care since the enactment of Medicaid is the State Children's Health Insurance Program (S-CHIP). This 1997 legislation is designed to provide public insurance for the approximately 10 million children birth to 19 years of age who exceed Medicaid income eligibility guidelines but cannot afford private health insurance. All states elected to accept Federal funds, which amounts to $48 billion over 10 years, and now have started programs. Programs in all but two of these states include dental benefits. States have implemented S-CHIP in one of three ways—by raising the income eligibility criteria for Medicaid and thus in effect expanding enrollment in that program, creating an insurance program separate from Medicaid, or some combination of these two options. Fourteen states chose to model S-CHIP after private insurance programs or other delivery systems not currently in use by Medicaid. Most of these programs have comprehensive dental benefits similar to Medicaid but with reimbursements for dentists that are closer to market rates. Preliminary evidence shows that these programs result in improvements in access to dental services for low-income children, and that those closely tied to Medicaid continue their poor performance (Almeida, Hill, & Kenney, 2001).

Advances are also being made in the biological area. The transmission of decay-causing bacteria from the parent to the child is the first step toward ECC. However, to date we do not have effective antimicrobial therapies to combat this important aspect of the etiology of ECC. Promising methods such as the use of varnishes and rinses containing chlorohexidine or povidone-iodine with children or parents to prevent colonization currently are being tested. Other research is testing vaccines designed to develop specific immune defenses against decay-causing bacteria and the oral application of genetically engineered or plant-derived antibodies to these bacteria (Slavkin, 1999).

Of great potential significance to the oral health of children is the release of the US Surgeon General's report on oral health and the two conferences he held following its release. His workshop and conference resulted in 24 recommendations that provide a strong foundation for oral health promotion and disease prevention activities. Prevention is emphasized, along with recommendations to start these activities early in each child's life, involve parents in these activities, and integrate them into primary care. The Surgeon General has called for the establishment of a national oral health plan to eliminate disparities in oral health and access to care for all Americans, but especially children. The plan is under development (Evans, 2001), and it should build on these recommendations to provide a blueprint for the promotion of oral health in young children.

Also see: Child Care: Early Childhood; Community Capacity.

References

Almeida, R., Hill, I., & Kenney, G. (2001). *Does SCHIP spell better dental care access for children? An early look at new initiatives.* Retrieved August 6, 2001, from http://newfederalism.urban.org

American Academy of Pediatrics (AAP). (1995). Committee on Practice and Ambulatory Medicine. Recommendations for pediatric health care. *Pediatrics, 96,* 833.

American Academy of Pediatrics (AAP), Committee on Drugs. (1996). Unapproved uses of approved drugs: the physician, the package insert, and the Food and Drug Administration: subject review. *Pediatrics, 98,* 118–123.

American Academy of Pediatric Dentistry (AAPD). (2000). 2000–2001 American academy of pediatric dentistry reference manual. *Pediatric Dentistry, 22*(Suppl.), 1–119.

Autio-Gold, J.T., & Courts, F. (2001). Assessing the effect of fluoride varnish on early enamel carious lesions in the primary dentition. *Journal of the American Dental Association, 132*, 1247–1253.

Bader, J.D., Shugars, D.A., Rozier, R.G. et al. (2000). *Diagnosis and management of dental caries: Evidence report* (Vols. 1 & 2). Research Triangle Park, NC: Research Triangle Institute.

Beck, J.D. (1998). Risk revisited. *Community Dentistry and Oral Epidemiology, 26*, 220–225.

Brown, J.L., Wall, T.P., & Lazar, V. (2000). Trends in untreated caries in primary teeth of children 2 to 10 years old. *Journal of the American Dental Association, 131*, 93–100.

Casamassimo, P.S. (1996). *Bright futures in practice: Oral health*. Arlington, VA: National Center for Education in Maternal and Child Health.

Cashion, S.W., Vann, W.F., Jr., Rozier, R.G., Venezie, R.D., & McIver, F.T. (1999). Children's utilization of dental care in the NC Medicaid program. *Pediatric Dentistry, 21*, 97–103.

Centers for Disease Control and Prevention (CDC). (1999). Achievements in public health, 1900–1999: fluoridation of drinking water to prevent dental caries. *Morbidity and Mortality Weekly Reports, 48*(41), 933–940.

Centers for Disease Control and Prevention (CDC). (2001). Recommendations for using fluoride to prevent and control dental caries in the United States. *MMWR Recommendations and Reports, 50*(RR14), 1–42.

Creedon, M.I., & O'Mullane, D.M. (2001). Factors affecting caries levels amongst 5-year-old children in County Kerry, Ireland. *Community Dental Health, 18*, 72–78.

Drury, T.F., Horowitz, A.M., Ismail, A.I., Maertens, M.P., Rozier, R.G., & Selwitz, R.H. (1999). Diagnosing and reporting early childhood caries for research purposes: Report of a workshop sponsored by the National Institute of Dental and Craniofacial Research, Health Resources and Services Administration, and Health Care Financing Administration. *Journal of Public Health Dentistry, 59*, 191–197.

Evans, C.A. (2001). Opportunity: Creating a national oral health plan. *Journal of Dental Research, 80*, 1784.

Featherstone, J.D.B. (2000). The science and practice of caries prevention. *Journal of the American Dental Association, 131*, 887–899.

Fisher, B., Neve, H., & Heritage, Z. (1999). Community development, user involvement, and primary health care. *British Medical Journal, 318*, 749–750.

General Accounting Office. (2000). *Oral health: Factors contributing to low use of dental services by low-income populations*. GAO/HEHS-00-72.

Green, L.W., & Kreuter, M.W. (1999). *Health promotion planning: An education and ecological approach* (3rd ed.). Mountain View, CA: Mayfield.

Hardison, J.R., Collier, D.R., Sprouse, L.W., Van Cleave, M.L., & Hogan, A.D. (1987). Retention of pit and fissure sealant on the primary molars of 3- and 4-year-old children after 1 year. *Journal of the American Dental Association, 114*, 613–615.

Health Resources and Services Administration (HRSA). (1998). *Oral disease, a crisis among children in poverty*. Retrieved September 15, 2001, from http://www.hrsa.gov/oralhealth

Holm, A.K. (1979). Effect of fluoride varnish (Duraphat) in preschool children. *Community Dentistry and Oral Epidemiology, 7*, 241–245.

Institute of Medicine (IOM), Food and Nutrition Board. (1997). *Dietary reference intakes: Calcium, phosphorus, magnesium, vitamin D, and fluoride*. Washington, DC: National Academy Press.

Ismail, A.I. (1998). Prevention of early childhood caries. *Community Dentistry and Oral Epidemiology, 26*(Suppl. 1), 49–61.

Kanellis, M.J. (2000). Caries risk assessment and prevention: Strategies for Head Start, Early Head Start, and WIC. *Journal of Public Health Dentistry, 60*, 210–217.

Kaste, L.M., Drury, T.F., Horowitz, A.M., & Beltran, E. (1999). An evaluation of NHANES III estimates of early childhood caries. *Journal of Public Health Dentistry, 59*, 198–200.

Klimek, J., Prinz, H., Hellwig, E., & Ahrens, G. (1985). Effect of a preventive program based on professional toothcleaning and fluoride application on caries and gingivitis. *Community Dentistry and Oral Epidemiology, 13*, 295–298.

Kowash, M.B., Pinfield, A., Smith, J., & Curzon, M.E.J. (2001). Effectiveness on oral health of a long-term health education programme for mothers with young children. *British Dental Journal, 188*, 2001–2005.

Last, J.M., & Abramson, J.H. (1995). *A dictionary of epidemiology* (3rd ed.). New York, NY: Oxford University Press.

Lewis, D.W., & Ismail A.I. (1995). Periodic health examination, 1995. Update: 2. Prevention of dental caries. Canadian Task Force on the Periodic Health Examination. *Canadian Medical Association Journal, 152*, 836–846.

Lewit, E.M., & Monheit, A.C. (1992). Expenditures on health for children and pregnant women. In: Center for the Future of Children. *US health care for children*. Los Altos, CA: Center for the Future of Children, David and Lucile Packard Foundation.

Locker, D., Lawrence, H., & Jokovic, A. (1999). *Benefits and risks for water fluoridation*. Report prepared for Ontario's public consultation on water fluoridation levels. Toronto, CN: University of Toronto.

Lockwood, S.A., & Malvitz, D.M. (1995). Trends in state agency oral health and public health expenditures, 1984 through 1989. *American Journal of Public Health, 85*, 1266–1268.

Milgrom, P., Hujoel, P., Grembowski, D., & Fong, R. (1999). A community strategy for Medicaid child dental services. *Public Health Report, 114*, 528–532.

Nowak, A.J., & Casamassimo, P.S. (1995). Using anticipatory guidance to provide early dental intervention. *Journal of American Dental Association, 126*, 1156–1163.

Nowak, A.J., & Warren, J.J. (2000). Infant oral health and oral habits. *Pediatric Clinics of North America, 47*, 1043–1066.

Office of Disease Prevention and Health Promotion. (2000). Healthy People 2010. Retrieved September 12, 2001, from http://www.health.gov/healthypeople/Document/HTML/Volume2/21Oral.htm#_Toc489700403

Rozier, R.G. (2001). Effectiveness of methods used by dental professionals for the primary prevention of dental caries. *Journal of Dental Education, 65*, 1067–1077.

Slavkin, H.C. (1998). Meeting the challenges of craniofacial-oral-dental birth defects. Retrieved September 15, 2001, from www.nidcr.nih.gov/slavkin/birth%5Fdf.htm

Slavkin, H.C. (1999). Streptococcus mutans, early childhood caries and new opportunities. *Journal of the American Dental Association, 130*, 1787–1792.

Sogaard, A.J. (1993). Theories and models of health behavior. In L. Schou & A.S. Blinkhorn (Ed.), *Oral health promotion* (pp. 25–64). New York: Oxford Medical.

Tinanoff, N. (1995). Critique of evolving methods for caries risk assessment. *Journal of Dental Education, 59*, 980–995.

Tinanoff, N., & Palmer, C.A. (2000). Dietary determinants of dental caries and dietary recommendations for preschool children. *Journal of Public Health Dentistry, 60*, 197–206.

US Department of Health and Human Services (USDHHS). (2000). Oral health in America. A report of the Surgeon General. Rockville, MD: US Department of Health and Human Services, National Institute of Dental and Craniofacial Research, National Institutes of Health.

US Department of Health and Human Services (USDHHS), Office of the Inspector General. (1996). *Children's dental services under Medicaid. Access and utilization.* San Francisco: Office of Evaluation and Inspection; Publication No. OE1-09-93-00240.

US Preventive Services Task Force (USPSTF). (1996). *Guide to clinical preventive services* (2nd ed.). Baltimore: Williams and Wilkins.

Vargas, C.M., Crall, J.J., & Schneider, D.A. (1998). Sociodemographic distribution of pediatric dental caries: NHANES III, 1988–1994. *Journal of the American Dental Association, 129*, 1229–1238.

Watson, M.R. (2000). Response to Kanellis: Caries risk assessment and prevention, strategies for Head Start, Early Head Start, and WIC. *Journal of Public Health Dentistry, 60*, 218–220.

Oral Health, Older Adulthood

H. Asuman Kiyak, Angus W.G. Walls, and Michael I. MacEntee

INTRODUCTION

This entry addresses improvements in oral health status and the reasons for these changes over the past 40 years among older cohorts in the United States, Canada, and the United Kingdom. Differences across population groups, and theoretical models that might explain these differences will be discussed. It should be noted that not all elders have benefited from the improvements in public health efforts and increased attention to diseases of the orofacial region. Risk factors for poor oral health are examined. Finally, some recent clinical studies aimed at improving the oral health of older adults at greatest risk are discussed.

The oral health of older persons has been improving with each successive cohort in most Western countries. This phenomenon is attributable to increased awareness and interest in dental care among adult populations, local and national public health efforts aimed at improving the oral health of communities, as well as greater access to dental services. In this entry, we focus on older adults in the United States, Canada, and the United Kingdom; but the improvements described for these countries reflect the status of many other countries in Europe, Australia, and Japan. The countries selected for examination have available large, nationally or regionally representative epidemiological data recently collected on the oral health status of their populations, and in some cases, offer comparable data on previous cohorts of older adults.

DEFINITIONS

Most people assume that *oral* means dental, and focus only on the number of natural teeth, the extent to which these teeth have active decay or filled surfaces, and if they have been replaced with partial or complete dentures. However, dental professionals have a broader concept of oral health that includes teeth, periodontal and other soft tissues, salivary glands, the tongue, and the impact of these components of the mouth on functional health and psychosocial well-being. The ability to speak and eat without pain, to avoid dry mouth associated with some medical conditions and/or the medications used to treat these conditions, all result from the status of one's oral health. Furthermore, the appearance of teeth and smile influences perceptions of facial attractiveness and social acceptance. Researchers have demonstrated an association between social acceptance and malocclusion, missing or discolored front teeth, and bad breath due to caries and periodontal disease (Brunette, 1996). Regardless of age, people with straight white teeth, well-maintained gums and teeth, and without chronic bad breath caused by oral disease are evaluated as more attractive by others.

The components of oral health addressed in this entry are defined below:

1. *Edentulism* refers to tooth loss in either the upper (maxilla) or lower (mandible) jaw or both. Most researchers agree that tooth loss in adulthood and old age is attributable to *caries* or *periodontitis* (Baelum, Laun, Chen, & Fejerskov, 1997; Hawkins, Main, & Locker, 1997; Johnson, 1993; MacEntee, 1994; Ong, 1996; Steele, Treasure, Pitts, Morris, & Bradnock, 2000). Older people who retain most of their teeth have generally practiced a lifetime of conscientious brushing, flossing, seeking professional dental care, and avoiding refined carbohydrates in their diets.

2. *Caries* or dental decay is the primary disease affecting teeth, in which the enamel, root surfaces, or pulp are damaged by bacterial infection. It is prevalent at all ages. Decay is initiated and sustained by a combination of bacteria in the mouth; acidity of the diet; and resistance of the teeth to demineralization (Thylstrup & Fejerskov, 1986). Bacteria produce acids when they metabolize carbohydrates and sugars on the surface of teeth. Eventually, a cavity opens when the enamel matrix of the tooth collapses, and an abscess develops in the jawbone around a tooth when bacteria invade the root canal. It occurs on the roots of the teeth when these same bacteria attack the roots of teeth if any root surfaces have been exposed because of gingival tissue (gum) protecting them receding. Older adults who have a high intake of sugar and refined carbohydrates in snacks or

drinks, especially those suffering from *dry mouth*, are at greatest risk for caries. If the decayed surfaces are not filled, the upper portion or crown of the tooth can break off and leave a *root fragment*. Fortunately, the carious process is slowed substantially, or prevented altogether, in those who have had access to fluoridated water. In addition, annual or semi-annual visits to a dentist can help pinpoint the problem and initiate preventive care such as dietary interventions, new techniques in brushing and flossing, sometimes including electric toothbrushes, and fluoride rinses or varnishes. For those who develop a cavity, it can be filled before it proceeds to the pulp.

3. Dry mouth (or *xerostomia*) was once thought to result from the normal process of aging, but today there is extensive evidence that saliva production does not decline with aging under normal circumstances. The primary culprit appears to be medications that many older adults use, including some antihypertensives, diuretics, antidepressants, and antihistamines. Indeed, a review of the most commonly prescribed medications concluded that over 400 list this as a side effect (Sreebny & Swartz, 1997). In such cases, xerostomia may be alleviated by substituting the offending medication with another one that does not have such effects, in consultation with the patient's physician.

Another cause of xerostomia that cannot be so easily resolved is radiation used to treat head and neck cancers. Unfortunately, the radiation does not simply inhibit salivary secretion, but actually destroys the salivary glands.

4. *Periodontal diseases* include *gingivitis*, which affects the gums, versus *periodontitis*, which involves all of the soft tissue and bone that support the teeth. Gingivitis is far more common in adulthood than is the more severe disease, periodontitis. There are many factors involved in the etiology of gingivitis, including bacteria. These bacteria result in an inflammation of the gums, characterized by redness, swelling, and bleeding. But the condition rarely increases sensitivity and tenderness of these tissues, so most who have the condition experience no pain. In the more severe form of periodontal disease, bacterial activity gradually destroys the ligament and bone supporting the tooth. This can leave a deeper than normal periodontal pocket between the tooth and adjacent soft tissue. As the pocket grows deeper, the teeth loosen and are exfoliated.

The severity of periodontal destruction can be measured with a periodontal probe to assess the depth of the periodontal pocket to the point of resistance (*probing depth [PD]*). Clinical attachment loss (AL) is also an indicator of the amount of gingiva that is detached from the teeth. Epidemiological studies use these indices to assess the extent and severity of periodontal disease; higher levels indicate more destruction.

SCOPE

The primary sources of epidemiological studies on oral health in the United States are the National Health and Nutrition Examination Surveys (NHANES), conducted by the National Center for Health Statistics (NCHS). The surveys were completed in 1971–1974 (NHANES I), 1984–1985 (NHANES II), and 1988–1994 (NHANES III); they included extensive clinical assessments and interviews on oral health. In addition, the 1982–1985 Adult Dental Health Survey, conducted by the National Institute of Dental and Craniofacial Research (NIDCR), one of the National Institutes of Health, provides a useful epidemiological "snapshot" of the oral health status of working younger and middle-aged adults, as well as retired elders. Together, these data offer insights into trends in oral diseases among American adults, and projections for future cohorts.

In England and Wales, national data have been collected every 10 years since 1968. Known as the Adult Dental Health Surveys (ADHS), these studies obtain information from residents throughout the United Kingdom on the number of natural teeth remaining, functional dentition, and use of dental services, as well as their socioeconomic and other demographic characteristics. Data are available for 1968, 1978, 1988, and 1998. In addition, a specific study of older adults was undertaken in 1995 as part of the UK National Diet and Nutrition Survey (NDNS) series, focusing on people aged 65 and over (Steele, Sheiham, Marcenes, & Walls, 1998).

None of these national surveys followed individuals longitudinally, so incidence data are not available. Only the prevalence of diseases in a given cohort of adults is available from these studies; incidence data have been collected by smaller scale studies. In Canada, epidemiological data on oral health status are not available at the national level. However, regional studies among community-dwelling and institutionalized populations in Canada provide useful information. The following sections will describe recent trends in tooth loss, decayed and filled teeth, and periodontal disease among older cohorts in these three countries.

Tooth Loss Among Older Cohorts

While the goal of medicine and medical care is to prevent death for as long as possible, the goal of dentistry is to prevent tooth loss due to disease. As described above, most tooth loss in adults is attributable to caries and periodontitis. American dental public policy makers have emphasized preventing edentulism to the extent that the primary objective related to older adults in the document, *Healthy People 2000*, was to "reduce the number of adults who have lost all their natural teeth" (objective #13.4). Between 1989 and 1999, policy makers could claim some success; they reported a decline in total edentulism from 36 to 30 percent over 10 years. While this was not as dramatic as the stated goal of 20 percent, the trend was certainly in the direction of more adults maintaining their natural teeth into advanced old age (US Department of Health and Human Services [USDHHS], 2000).

Edentulism rates have declined over a 20-year period in both the United States and the United Kingdom. In comparing American adults aged 65–74 in 1974 with their counterparts in 1994, researchers found a decline from 45.6 to 28.6 percent with no natural teeth (USDHHS, 2000). A similar reduction was observed in the 55–64 age group, from 33.3 percent edentulous in 1974 to 20 percent in 1994. The UK comparison of adults aged 65–74 or 55–64 in 1978 versus 1998 revealed similar declines over 20 years, from approximately 72 to 36 percent, and from 42 to 18 percent, respectively (Steele et al., 2000). A survey of 521 adults aged 70 and older in Vancouver, British Columbia demonstrates similar rates; only 30 percent in this older group were edentulous (MacEntee, Stolar, & Glick, 1993).

The lower rate of edentulism among younger cohorts in the United States and the United Kingdom bodes well for the future, when this cohort will retain most of their natural teeth into their 60s, 70s, and beyond. Indeed, not only are more people keeping their teeth, but more teeth than ever before are surviving. In the Adult Dental Health Survey, British elders (ages 65–74) had retained an average of 17 teeth, compared with almost 20 for those aged 55–64. Older Americans who retained their teeth in the 1988–1994 NHANES III had, on average, 6.5 teeth, compared with 7.9 among 55–64-year-olds (NCHS, 1996). It is noteworthy that a greater proportion of US elders have some remaining teeth; but older adults in the United Kingdom who retain *any* teeth have almost three times as many as their counterparts in the United States.

These dramatic improvements in tooth survival can be explained at several levels of health promotion. At the population level, there is increased awareness among successive cohorts that tooth loss is not inevitable with aging, and that one can control one's own changes of retaining natural teeth. At the individual level, this awareness has resulted in greater attention to preventive dentistry. Cohorts born before 1930 were more likely to view dental visits as unnecessary or triggered by dental pain. Cohorts born between 1930 and 1950 benefited from increased attention to preventive dental care by dental professionals and reimbursement for these services by health insurers. Cohorts born since 1950 have also benefited from widespread efforts to fluoridate community water supplies, school-based preventive dental programs, and application of dental sealants to primary teeth. These changes, combined with increased dietary choices (e.g., sugarfree beverages) have increased the likelihood that adults will be more aware and capable of preventing tooth decay, periodontal disease, and ultimately tooth loss, so that people can enhance their oral health into advanced old age.

Decayed and Filled Teeth

To the extent that natural teeth can survive intact into later adulthood, with no active decay or filled surfaces, the older person has been successful in maintaining good oral health. This also reduces the chances of tooth loss due to caries. Among older adults examined in 1971–1974 in NHANES I, an average of 12 permanent teeth had no decay or fillings, compared with 9.6 teeth free of caries or fillings in the later NHANES III. It is somewhat surprising to find *lower* numbers of intact teeth in the later survey, but this may reflect the greater use of dental services among newer cohorts of elders. It may also indicate that a greater proportion of older adults are struggling to retain teeth that would previously have been extracted, and these are being restored. In this latest survey, almost 25 percent of women and 33 percent of men aged 65–74 had untreated dental tooth decay, with higher rates among 75–84-year-olds (NCHS, 1996). This suggests that the teeth retained into old age are at risk for caries, and that more than a quarter of older Americans do not obtain treatment for this condition. These US findings are mirrored by data from the National Diet and Nutritional Survey (NDNS) in the United Kingdom, where increasing age was associated with an increased proportion of decayed teeth. In a subsequent section of this entry, we discuss some risk factors for tooth loss and the development of caries among older persons, and why utilization of dental services varies in this population.

Periodontal Health

The primary indicator of periodontal health or disease in epidemiological studies is periodontal AL. Although older adults in NHANES III had more periodontal surfaces with AL greater than 4 and 6 mm than their younger counterparts, the rates were relatively low in both groups. For example, among those aged 65–74, 55 percent had at least one site with AL of 4 mm or more, and only 23.4 percent had at least one site with 6 mm or more. In contrast, among the sample aged 55–64, 50.2 percent had one or more sites with AL 4 mm or more, and only 19 percent had a 6 mm or greater pocket. Men in both age groups generally were more likely to have worse periodontal health, or 30 percent compared to 17.7 percent of women among 65–74-year-olds, and 25 versus 13.6 percent, respectively among 55–64-year-olds (Burt & Eklund, 1999; NCHS, 1996). Even so, it is remarkable that only 30 percent of young-old men and 18 percent of young-old women can be described as having periodontal disease.

These data do not provide longitudinal evidence for improved periodontal health with age, but suggest that the teeth most at risk from AL are extracted. They may also mean that the same factors that have resulted in greater tooth survival are also helping older people avoid periodontal disease. These include greater use of home care aids such as floss, and electric devices designed to clean into the gum line, such as Sonicare®. Age-associated changes in immune function also appear to alter the pattern of periodontal disease progression. These changes reduce the impact of this disease process in older populations (Grbic & Lamster, 1992; Grbic, Lamster, Celenti & Fine, 1991).

Data from the ADHS in the United Kingdom, where older subjects who had any teeth had, on average, more teeth than their US counterparts, show a progressive *increase* in the proportion of adults with both 4 and 6 mm AL. Kelly, Steele, Nuttal, Bradnock, Morris, and Nunn (2000) found at least one site with AL >6 mm among 10 percent of people they examined who were aged 45–54, 17 percent of 55–64-year-olds, and 31 percent of those 65 and over. These statistics are slightly higher than rates of periodontal disease in the United States. Despite some increase with age, less than 1/4 show evidence of advanced disease in US surveys.

THEORIES AND RESEARCH

Protective versus Risk Factors

The declines in edentulism, caries, and periodontal disease described above have not been observed in all segments of the US, UK, or Canadian populations. The comparisons by gender suggest that older women are more likely to have retained teeth, to have fewer tooth surfaces with active caries, and fewer periodontal pockets with significant loss of attachment in the United States, whereas in the United Kingdom, edentulism is higher and numbers of teeth lower in older women compared with men. What are some other risk factors for poor oral health in old age? In this section, we will discuss demographic and socioeconomic characteristics that have emerged from epidemiological studies, as well as psychological variables that predict oral health versus disease.

Demographic Differences

The World Health Organization has conducted two major epidemiological studies of oral health in several countries, known as the International Collaborative Studies (ICS). The most recent survey, conducted in 1988–1992 (comparable to the NHANES III data collection period), is known as ICS II (Chen, Andersen, Barmes, Leclerq, & Lyttle, 1997). It collected data from children aged 12–13,

adults aged 35–44, and elders aged 65–74. Both clinical and interview data were obtained from communities in Germany, Poland, New Zealand, Japan, as well as Whites and African Americans in Baltimore, Whites and Latinos in San Antonio, and American Indians on the Navajo and Lakota reservations. In this large, international survey, the proportion of edentulous elders ranged from 16 percent in San Antonio to 59 percent in New Zealand. There were significant variations even within the United States communities, with edentulism rates of only 16 percent among African Americans and 25 percent among Whites in Baltimore, but as high as 54 percent among Lakota Indians (Marcus, Reifel, & Nakazono, 1997). This is consistent with findings of NHANES III. Regional differences emerged, such that 48 percent of participants aged 65 and older in West Virginia were edentate, compared with 14 percent of those examined in Hawaii (Tomar, 1997). Such regional differences also occur in the United Kingdom, with more elders retaining their natural teeth in Southern England and fewer in Wales or Scotland (Steele et al., 2000). These differences have been attributed to both socioeconomic variations and treatment philosophies in different regions of each country. Access to dentists is greater in regions with more clinicians per 100,000 population, with Medicaid funding for dental care of low income populations, and with greater awareness in the community about ways to prevent caries, periodontal disease, and tooth loss.

Ethnic differences have emerged in rates of tooth loss between Whites, Blacks, and Mexican Americans (NCHS, 1996). Tooth decay and periodontal disease rates also differ across ethnic groups in epidemiological studies. In the NHANES III sample, after controlling for income levels, African Americans had the greatest number of tooth surfaces with untreated decay, followed by Mexican Americans, then whites in the non-poor group (30.2 percent, 21.9 percent, 8.6 percent, respectively had one or more decayed tooth surfaces). Among adults who were categorized as poor, higher rates of active decay were found in all three groups. Differences emerged again in the same order of ethnicity: 46.7 percent of Blacks, 46.9 percent of Mexican Americans, and 27 percent of Whites had untreated caries. Blacks also were twice as likely as the other two groups to have evidence of periodontal disease (at least one periodontal surface with AL measures of 6 mm or worse). In a more recent study of low income adults aged 60–90 in Seattle, Washington, with a large Asian population, Asians and African Americans were found to have more signs of periodontal disease than Latinos or non-Latino Whites who were in the same socioeconomic group (Persson, Persson, Kiyak, & Powell, 1998).

In the ICS II described above, proportionately more Navajo and Lakota Indians aged 65–74 had at least one periodontal site with AL scores greater than 6 mm (23 and 25 percent, respectively) than did elders in Poland or Germany (6 and 5 percent, respectively). In this case, ethnicity may be confounded with poverty, because many of the elders examined on the Navajo and Lakota reservations were categorized as poor, compared to a more middle-class population in Poland and Germany. However, even when ethnicity and socioeconomic status can be separated, as in the NHANES III described above, both untreated decay and periodontal disease rates were worse in poorer adults in all ethnic groups beyond age 25 (Burt & Eklund, 1999). Among those aged 75 and older, 36.2 percent of those in the low socioeconomic group had signs of periodontal disease, compared with 23.3 percent of elders in the higher socioeconomic group.

It appears from these epidemiological studies that ethnicity and socioeconomic background have an additive effect on oral health status. The problem is compounded in older persons, who have a lifetime accumulation of oral diseases and tooth loss due to neglect and lack of treatment. These findings are consistent with the results of the 1998 Adult Dental Health Survey in the United Kingdom. In the United Kingdom, however, social class differences were greater among older men than women, especially when comparing elders who had worked at manual labor with those who had done other types of work (Kelly et al., 2000). These differences suggest that dental values and practices are more important than financial adequacy in adults' use of dental services.

Predictors of Preventive Dental Service Utilization

It is generally agreed in dentistry that regular dental service utilization is essential for maintaining good health and preventing disease before it becomes severe enough for tooth loss. In the ICS II Survey, adults aged 65–74 who reported making one or more visits to a dentist in the past year for preventive check-ups and cleaning were three to seven times more likely to have some natural teeth remaining (with some variation by community) than were those who had made no dental visits in the past year. This was a far better correlate of dentition status than sociodemographic characteristics (although ethnicity was a close second), smoking or dietary behaviors (Atchison & Andersen, 2000). Although the nature of these visits was not specified, most semi-annual and annual visits include professional cleaning of teeth, diagnostic x-rays, some oral health education in the form of chairside reminders of home care, and treatment of small carious lesions and periodontal pockets before they become severe.

Nevertheless, individual differences persist in the public's beliefs about the benefits of preventive procedures such as cleaning, exams, and radiographs. In the NHANES III sample, the highest preventive utilization rates were found among college-educated women, at about twice the rate of adults with less than a high school education, and somewhat higher than for college-educated men. Clearly, income alone does not explain these differences. This pattern emerged in all ethnic groups, although the ethnic differences persisted, with Whites more likely than Blacks, who were more likely than Latinos to use dental services. Dental insurance also was associated with regular use of dental services among working adults, but this was less important in the older sample because most are not covered by dental insurance in the United States.

Even when free or reduced fee dental services are available, many older persons do not use these services. Dental care is heavily subsidized for all and free to some in the United Kingdom. Nevertheless, attendance rates decline; perceived need for care and measured disease both increase with increasing age. Attendance rates among edentulous elders has been found to be particularly low in the UK National Dental Service Program, according to Steele et al. (1998). Only 7 percent of this group had sought dental care in the past year. The institutionalized elderly population is most likely to be edentulous, and least likely to seek dental care. As shown in a study of long-term care facilities in Vancouver, approximately one fourth of residents have no teeth or dentures in at least one jaw (Wyatt & MacEntee, 2001). Among those with any natural teeth, at least half had some untreated caries. This situation of poor oral conditions among institutionalized elders is not unusual in all three countries. Despite the large number of US nursing homes with regular visits by a dentist to the facility, only a small proportion of residents avail themselves of these services.

Evidence from studies of community-dwelling elders who qualify for reduced fee dental services but do not use them suggests that psychosocial variables are better predictors of utilization than the individual's demographic characteristics. For example, among those aged 65 and older in NHANES III, the primary reasons given for non-utilization were "no teeth" (49.7 percent) or "no dental problems" (31.2 percent). These responses were consistent among Whites, Blacks, and Mexican Americans. Cost was mentioned by less than 5 percent in all three ethnic groups. In the next section, we will discuss attitudes and values that distinguish older adults who practice healthy dental behaviors from those who do not.

STRATEGIES

Given the significant role that professional dental services plays in the maintenance of good oral health and prevention of caries, periodontal disease, and tooth loss, researchers have devoted considerable energy to understanding what variables are most important in predicting utilization. The epidemiological studies described above highlight the impact of ethnicity, socioeconomic status, and costs of dental care on the oral health status of older adults and their decisions to seek care. Perhaps the most widely tested conceptual model to assess the relative impact of these and other variables on dental service use was first developed by Andersen and Newman (1973) to predict medical service utilization. This model includes three components: (1) *predisposing* characteristics such as socioeconomic status, ethnicity, gender, and perceived general health; (2) *enabling* characteristics, which include access, income, and dental insurance; and (3) *need variables*, which are both objective and perceived indicators of need for dental care.

Over the past 20 years, this health behavior model has been modified in various ways and applied to dental service utilization. For example, a series of studies by Kiyak and colleagues (Diehnelt, Kiyak, & Beach, 1990; Kiyak, 1987) expanded the list of predisposing variables to include *attitudes toward oral health*, using the Fishbein and Ajzen (1972) model of attitudes (i.e., a summative score based on beliefs regarding a concept and the relative value or importance attached to each belief). These studies demonstrated that the best predictor of utilization among various groups of low-income elders who had access to free or low cost dental care was the *importance* component of attitudes. This variable could significantly discriminate between users and non-users, and could predict subsequent utilization by previous non-users in a 6-month follow-up. The only other components of the Andersen and Newman model that explained a significant proportion of variance in utilization patterns were *perceived need* and *number of natural teeth* remaining. This was consistent with the findings of NHANES III, described above.

In the ICS II, the Andersen and Newman model was again utilized in dental research, serving as a framework to assess the relationship between individual characteristics and oral health outcomes. The research team reports a slightly different set of explanatory variables for each ethnic group (Andersen & Davidson, 1997). For example, White elders in Baltimore who were *more educated*, had *more teeth*, had a *usual source of dental care*, and had some *oral pain* were most likely to have used dental services in the past 12 months, whereas for their African American counterparts, all the same predictors emerged except educational level. The *perceived importance* of oral health was a significant predictor only for the Navajo elders in that study.

In the United Kingdom, dental utilization rates were higher in *women*, those from more *affluent* social backgrounds and people who were either *retired or employed part-time*. People from manual socioeconomic backgrounds

had particularly poor attendance patterns, 15–20 percentage points lower than those from non-manual backgrounds.

Self-efficacy is another psychological variable that has been shown to distinguish users of dental services from non-users. It can also predict the development of new caries and periodontal disease in older adults (Kiyak, 1996; Persson et al., 1998). This is a valuable concept that provides the clinician with an indication of the individual's perceived ability to control and modify his/her own health. It has been found to be a useful predictor of other health behaviors, and may be a useful focal point for intervention studies.

To date, there has been little effort to enhance older adults' self-efficacy in oral health promotion efforts. Indeed, there have been few systematic studies of oral health promotion in general. Research by the first author demonstrates that oral health self-efficacy can be improved through hands-on educational programs. A 6-week, twice weekly program compared the effectiveness of an oral health-focused versus an integrated health promotion intervention, both using active learning methods in small groups. Outcomes included oral health knowledge, attitudes, recognition of oral disease symptoms, and self-efficacy. The focused program was effective, resulting in significant increases from pre- to post-intervention in oral health knowledge, recognition of symptoms, and oral health self-efficacy. Of the three dimensions of self-efficacy measured in that study, oral health was the lowest at baseline, and highest at the immediate and six-month post-intervention. These beneficial effects faded after 6 months, suggesting a need for a "booster series" that might consist of 2–4 sessions several months later, repeating key concepts learned initially, thereby maintaining any gains achieved.

Another method to help elders retain this information and self-efficacy in the long-term is to provide an opportunity for them to teach others. Pilot research by the first author supports the efficacy of such an approach, especially when elders teach children (Kiyak & Mjelde-Mossey, 1997). This may also reduce attrition if participants know they will be asked to teach children. A new community-based health promotion study by the first author will use these principles to train Latino and Caucasian elders as oral health educators of fourth and fifth graders.

SYNTHESIS

The field of geriatric preventive dentistry is slowly entering a stage of testing behavioral interventions, where attempts are being made to change some of the barriers to positive oral health outcomes. Research by the authors in the United States, United Kingdom, and Canada demonstrates that the oral health of newer cohorts of elders is improving on a population basis because of community-wide, school-based efforts for children, and educational campaigns by product manufacturers. Nevertheless, significant differences remain across ethnic and socioeconomic groups and communities. Small-scale efforts aimed at older persons provide strong evidence that oral health promotion for elders works. These improvements can lead to better oral health behaviors and tooth survival. However, a successful oral health promotion effort must include the following elements:

1. small groups with hands-on learning opportunities;
2. multiple sessions focused on specific aspects of oral health;
3. booster sessions several months later to reinforce learning;
4. possibly the opportunity to teach other elders or children this information.

Unfortunately, such an oral health promotion program requires more concentrated efforts than a public service campaign or occasional lectures by dental professionals to senior groups. Nevertheless, community-based programs can be effective if advocates and representatives of elders are trained in these topics, then teach others in small groups, who in turn can educate other elders or children. This approach could result in significant improvements in the oral health of underserved populations of elders and children alike.

Also see: Crises Intervention: Older Adulthood; Health Promotion: Older Adulthood.

References

Andersen, R.M., & Davidson, P.L. (1997). Ethnicity, aging, and oral health outcomes: A conceptual framework. *Advances in Dental Research, 11*(2), 203–209.

Andersen, R.M., & Newman, F.J. (1973). Societal and individual determinants of medical care utilization in the U.S. *Milbank Memorial Fund Quarterly, 51*, 96–120.

Atchison, K.A., & Andersen, R.M. (2000). Demonstrating successful aging using the International Collaborative Study for oral health outcomes. *Journal of Public Health Dentistry, 60*(4), 282–288.

Baelum, V., Laun, W.M., Chen, X., & Fejerskov, O. (1997). Predictors of tooth loss over 10 years in adult and elderly Chinese. *Community Dentistry and Oral Epidemiology, 25*, 204–210.

Brunette, D.M. (1996). Effects of baking soda-containing dentifrices on oral malodours. *Compendium of Continuing Education in Dentistry, 17*(Suppl. 19), S22–S32.

Burt, B.A., & Eklund, S.A. (1999). *Dentistry, dental practice, and the community*. Philadelphia: W.B. Saunders.

Chen, M., Andersen, R.M., Barmes, D.E., Leclerq, M.H., & Lyttle, C.S. (1997). *Comparing oral health systems*. Geneva: World Health Organization. WHO/ORH/ICS II/97.1

Diehnelt, D., Kiyak, H.A., & Beach, B. (1990). Predictors of oral health behaviors among elderly Japanese-Americans. *Special Care in Dentistry, 10*, 114–120.

Fishbein, M., & Ajzen, I. (1972). Attitudes and opinions. *Annual Review of Psychology, 23*, 487–544.

Grbic, J.T., & Lamster, I.B. (1992). Risk indicators for future clinical attachment loss in adult periodontitis: Tooth and site variables. *Journal of Periodontology, 63*, 262–269.

Grbic, J.T, Lamster, I.B., Celenti, R.S., & Fine, J.B. (1991). Risk indicators for future clinical attachment loss in adult periodontitis: Patient variables. *Journal of Periodontology, 62*, 322–329.

Hawkins, R.J., Main, P.A., & Locker, D. (1997). The normative need for tooth extractions in older adults in Ontario, Canada. *Gerodontology, 14*, 75–82.

Johnson, T.E. (1993). Factors contributing to dentists' extraction decisions in older adults. *Special Care in Dentistry, 13*, 195–199.

Kelly, M., Steele, J.G., Nuttal, N., Bradnock, G., Morris, J., & Nunn, J. (2000). *Adult dental health survey: Oral health in the United Kingdom 1998*. London: The Stationery Office.

Kiyak, H.A. (1987). An explanatory model for older persons' use of dental services: Implications for health policy. *Medical Care, 25*(10), 936–952.

Kiyak, H.A. (1997). Measuring psychosocial variables that predict older persons' oral health behavior. *Gerodontology, 13*, 69–75.

Kiyak, H.A., & Mjelde-Mossey, L. (1997). Exploring elders' potential as health educators of children (abstract). *The Gerontologist, 37*, 234.

Kiyak, H.A., & Weidenfeld, S. (1991). Increased self-efficacy: A new approach to health promotion (published abstract). *The Gerontologist, 31*, 83.

MacEntee, M.I. (1994). How severe is the threat of caries to old teeth? *Journal of Prosthetic Dentistry, 71*, 473–477.

MacEntee, M.I., Stolar, E., & Glick, N. (1993). Influence of age and gender on oral health and related behaviour in an independent elderly population. *Community Dentistry and Oral Epidemiology, 21*, 234–239.

Marcus, M., Reifel, N.M., & Nakazono, T.T. (1997). Clinical measures and treatment needs. *Advances in Dental Research, 11*(2), 263–271.

National Center for Health Statistics (NCHS). (1996). *National Health and Nutrition Examination Survey (NHANES III) reference manuals and reports*. Hyattsville, MD: NCHS/USDHHS/Centers for Disease Control.

Ong, G. (1996). Periodontal reasons for tooth loss in an Asian population. *Journal of Clinical Periodontology, 23*, 307–309.

Persson, R.E., Persson, G.R., Kiyak, H.A., & Powell, L.V. (1998). Periodontal effects of a biobehavioral prevention program. *Journal of Clinical Periodontology, 25*, 322–329.

Sreebny, L.M., & Swartz, S.S. (1997). A reference guide to drugs and dry mouth—2nd edition. *Gerodontology, 14*, 33–48.

Steele, J.G., Sheiham, A., Marcenes, W., & Walls, A.W.G. (1998). *National Diet and Nutrition Survey: People aged 65 years and over. Vol 2: Report of the oral health survey*. London: Stationery Office.

Steele, J.G., Treasure, E., Pitts, N.B., Morris, J., & Bradnock, G. (2000). Total tooth loss in the United Kingdom in 1998 and implications for the future. *British Dental Journal, 189*(11), 598–603.

Thylstrup, A., & Fejerskov O. (1986). Pathology of dental caries. In A. Thylstrup & O. Fejerskov (Eds.), *Textbook of cariology* (pp. 204–234). Copenhagen: Munksgaard.

Tomar, S. (1997). Total tooth loss among persons aged greater than or equal to 65 years. Selected states: 1995–1997. *Morbidity Mortality Weekly Reports, 48*, 206–210.

US Department of Health and Human Services. (2000). *Oral health in America: A report of the Surgeon General*. Rockville, MD: USDHHS/NIDCR/NIH.

Wyatt, C.C.L., & MacEntee, M.I. (2001). Oral health among residents of Canadian long-term care facilities. *Journal of Dental Research, 80*(Special Issue), Abstract #1784.

P

Parenting, Early Childhood

Donald G. Unger, Margaret Brown, and Elizabeth Park

In countries such as the United States and Canada, great value, pride, and approval is placed on parents' being self-sufficient and able to provide the resources their children need. In these countries, society's role has been as a backup for those requiring temporary help to achieve or regain independent lifestyles (Bullen, 1991; Peters, 1980). The assumption is that parents are "in charge" of this childrearing responsibility. Most parents, however, are middle managers or "weakened executives" (Keniston, 1977). Even under ideal situations, becoming a parent enters the adult(s) and child into dynamic, evolving transactions among: (a) themselves, (b) their family and social networks, (c) programs that serve children, (d) work settings that regulate parent schedules, (e) communities that have resources and risks, (f) social, moral, and political climates of neighborhoods, regions, and countries of origin, and (g) traditions and values of previous generations that together send parents mixed messages about childrearing (Collins, Maccoby, Steinberg, Hetherington, & Bornstein, 2000).

THE NEED FOR COMMUNITY-BASED PREVENTION AND SUPPORT INTERVENTIONS

While many parents effectively navigate this complex environment for childrearing, others experience difficulties, placing their children at risk for health and developmental problems. In the United States, for example, there has been an increasing incidence of parental substance abuse, HIV/AIDS, and divorce. One million children experience abuse and/or neglect annually, with children under the age of 3 being the largest single age group of maltreatment victims (US Department of Health and Human Services, 2000). Such conditions have resulted in substantially higher rates of young children being raised by grandparents. More children live away from their parents in foster care; a third of these children are preschoolers, with African American and Latino children being disproportionately represented. About a third of births in the United States are to unmarried mothers, many of whom are teenagers. The teen birth rate in the United States remains higher than in most other developed countries, including Canada, Israel, Australia, Japan, and the United Kingdom. Infant mortality rates are also high compared with other industrialized nations. African American babies are more than twice as likely to die than white infants.

Increasing numbers of American parents are in need of quality child care since a majority of mothers and fathers who have preschool aged children are in the workplace (Child Health USA, 2000). The number of parents who are working yet still raising their children in poverty has increased by a third over the past decade in the United States. In fact, the child poverty rate in the United States is among the highest in the developed world (one in four children under 6 years of age live in poverty) (KIDS Count, 2000).

To respond to these contemporary needs of parents and young children, voluntary prevention and support programs have developed over the past three decades. The major objectives of these support and prevention programs are: (a) to enable and assist parents in the care of their children and (b) to promote the development and well-being of children and their families. While the goals and activities of parent support and prevention programs are very diverse, they generally focus on strengthening one or more of six parental roles discussed below. In this entry, the term "parent" refers to a person or persons who assumes primary responsibility for carrying out these roles (including biological parents and grandparents, adoptive parents, and non-relative caregivers).

ROLES OF PARENTS: THE FOCUS OF COMMUNITY-BASED PARENT SUPPORT AND PREVENTION PROGRAMS

A primary parental role is providing for a child's basic needs including adequate nutrition, health care, shelter, and clothing. Acquiring early prenatal care increases the likelihood of a healthy, full-term birth. Using folic acid and abstaining from tobacco, alcohol and illicit drug use can promote healthy births. Ensuring up-to-date immunizations can prevent potentially severe or fatal illnesses such as measles, mumps, rubella, polio, meningitis, diphtheria, whooping cough, hepatitis, and tetanus. Positioning babies on their backs or sides while sleeping can prevent Sudden Infant Death Syndrome (SIDS). Providing children with well baby checkups and screening for metabolic disorders, vision and hearing, iron deficiency and sickle cell anemia, motor and language development, and lead exposure can identify those who need early intervention services.

A second parental role is protecting children from psychological and physical harm. Parents are responsible for their children's safety and can prevent injuries by reducing exposure to potential injury risks. For example, proper use of child auto safety seats and seat belts protects children from motor vehicle injuries, the single leading cause of children's deaths. Safety applies to monitoring play spaces, peer relationships, and neighborhood areas, as well as providing a lead free and smoke free environment. Equally critical is finding ways to discipline children without harming them.

A third role is to guide the child's cognitive, emotional, physical, sexual, social, moral, religious, and spiritual development. Parents of young children accomplish this in various ways, but usually by: (a) encouraging exploration, (b) mentoring in basic skills, (c) celebrating developmental advances, (d) rehearsing and extending new skills, (e) comforting

and communicating, and (f) providing limits (Ramey & Ramey, 1999). Parents also model prosocial behaviors and are socialization agents for a child's ethnic identity, religious beliefs and values, and understanding of gender roles and racism.

Fourth, parents play an important role in a child's school/child care life. Choosing good quality child care (as indicated by group size, staff–child ratios, caregiver training, caregiver behavior toward children) can have a positive influence on school readiness and school success in the early elementary years, particularly for children with psychosocial risk factors. Parents also help children prepare for school entry through activities such as family excursions and family rituals that provide learning opportunities for children. Among Asian Americans, the teaching role of parents is one of the most highly valued responsibilities.

Fifth, parents advocate within the wider community on behalf of their children to promote safe neighborhoods and communities, good schools, adequate recreational facilities, and to receive quality services from preschools and service delivery systems. Advocacy is necessary because policies of delivery systems, organizations, and communities that parents navigate to help their children often do not meet the needs of parents and/or children. For instance, parents act as child and family advocates when they live in communities where environmental toxins threaten the health of their children, where there is limited availability of services for children, where homophobia threatens the adjustment of children of lesbian or gay parents, or when laws prevent foster parents and grandparents caring for children to act in ways they believe are in the best interests of these children.

Sixth, parents need to develop effective self-care skills for themselves. Inadequate support systems, emotional distress, ineffective coping skills, and a limited sense of mastery and efficacy adversely affect parenting (Cochran & Niego, 1995). Establishing and maintaining a system of supportive relationships with a partner, extended family, and/or friends helps to buffer parenting stress, reduce isolation, and provide respite opportunities. Married fathers particularly value marital relationships where each parent's childrearing judgments, values, and roles are respected. Divorced, separated, and never-married fathers can benefit from developing non-marital social supports that promote involvement with their children. Grandparents who become the primary caregivers of children need to find ways to cope with the new demands on their time and energy. Lastly, developing a sense of parenting efficacy or self-agency (i.e., the belief that they have an influence on their children's development and/or confidence in their ability to be successful in their role as parent) enables parents to carry out supportive childrearing practices and model appropriate behaviors.

COMMUNITY-BASED MODELS TO SUPPORT PARENTING ROLES

There are essentially four models or frameworks that are used to support these parental roles. They include: (a) parent education, (b) parent support, (c) family resources and support, and (d) family preservation. In *parent education*, parents receive information to promote their understanding of child development, and they may also learn techniques for managing stress and relationship difficulties. Parents typically engage in activities to enhance parent–child relationships and parenting skills, and opportunities are provided to try alternate approaches to childrearing. A *parent support* approach focuses on establishing relationships between parents and others to strengthen parents' abilities to draw upon available resources for the well-being of themselves and their families. Helping parents develop long-term support systems, manage stress, access community resources, and strengthen the home–preschool link are important aspects of parent support. *Family resource and support interventions* use a combination of these parent education and parent support models. They also systematically and intentionally reach out to the child's family, extended family, and community to promote development within the individual, family, and community. They involve parents, volunteers, professionals, and paraprofessionals, and offer numerous family services that build upon family and community strengths. Lastly, *family preservation* programs provide intensive clinical and concrete short-term support services to families whose children are at risk for out-of-home placements.

METHODS TO SUPPORT PARENTS WITH YOUNG CHILDREN

Community-based parent education and supportive models are quite diverse in the methods that are used. All four types of models use one or more of the following methods of programming.

Home visiting

Home visiting has received increased attention in the past decade. However, the impact of home visiting with universal and indicated populations, including families with children at risk of imminent foster care placement, has not been as profound as had been hoped. Findings are inconsistent across programs and populations served (Gomby, Culross, & Behrman, 1999; Human Services Policy, 2001). The most promising results have been from the Nurse Home Visitation Program that has demonstrated reductions in preterm births, in the percentage of low birth weight infants, in subsequent pregnancies and births, and in problems resulting from substance abuse (Olds, Henderson, Kitzman, Eckenrode, Cole, & Tatelbaum, 1999). Preliminary results from Early Head Start programs delivering home visiting services are also encouraging and suggest both child and family gains. Lastly, home visiting programs grounded in attachment theory and utilizing professional visitors have demonstrated positive effects on infant attachment behavior and attachment security (Heinicke, Fineman, Ruth, Recchia, Guthrie, & Rodning, 1999).

Early Intervention and Preschool Programming

For high risk and teen parent families, combining intensive child-focused early intervention with high quality parent and family-focused services has significant potential for improved child and family outcomes (Ramey, Campbell, Burchinal, Skinner, Gardner, & Ramey, 2000). Early intervention programs for children with disabilities and children at risk for developmental delays have increasingly adopted a family centered philosophy that addresses family needs and goals for the child and family, provides choices in services for parents, and promotes collaborative, trusting relationships between parents and professionals (Dunst, Trivette, & Deal, 1994). Also, some preschool programs offer literacy training and general education for parents, becoming a "two generation" program, based on the premise that children's educational experience is closely tied to parent literacy (Smith & Zaslow, 1995).

Parent Education and Support Groups

These groups are conducted by parents and/or professionals and often are organized around parent and/or child concerns (e.g., parents with children with cancer, teen parenting, adults transitioning to parenthood, parents in lesbian relationships). Parent education and support groups can reinforce and enhance parents' existing competencies, provide information about development and available resources, and increase coping skills to reduce the stresses of childrearing (Rosenberg & Reppucci, 1990).

Outreach to Fathers

Some support programs reach out specifically to fathers, most often to African American fathers who are 18–25 years of age with limited formal education. These programs assume that parenting programs do not typically address the unique needs of fathers, particularly young, low-income African American men. No common set of objectives or best practices for fatherhood programs have yet been identified. However, programs that promote collaborative co-parenting provide opportunities for fathers to learn from each other, and focus on critical transitions such as the birth of a child or divorce appear more successful.

Premarital and Marital/Relationship Enrichment

These educational programs help partners learn conflict resolution and other relationship skills. The *Prevention and Relationship Enhancement* Program (PREP), for example, enhances partner relationships and family communication (Markman, 1995). Focuses on skills in addition to knowledge are critical components of effective programs.

Advocacy

Programs frequently focus on helping parents mobilize resources to change organizations and policies affecting their families, and/or to receive services to which parents and their children are entitled, but have difficulty accessing due to system barriers. Parent resource centers for parents with children with disabilities and the Citizen's Clearinghouse for Hazardous Waste are two examples of interventions offering parents technical assistance and advocacy skills.

Preconception and Birth Spacing Counseling

Longer birth intervals and preconception counseling have been associated with better infant and maternal health outcomes. Preconception counseling is included in many parent education and support programs, particularly those with teen parents who are less likely to delay subsequent births and are at risk for adverse health consequences.

IMPLEMENTATION: THE KEY TO SUCCESSFUL OUTCOMES

Based upon current research, it is not possible to identify what framework or method, or combination of parent support and prevention methods, will be most likely to achieve specific child, family, and/or community outcomes. However, whichever models, methods, and measures are used, intended outcomes appear most apt to be achieved when programs have a good fit and ongoing "refitting" between the program, service providers, children, families, and their communities (Powell, 1988). Identifying strategies for successfully achieving this good fit has been a major challenge for conducting (and evaluating) parent education and support programs. Several strategies that appear necessary, but perhaps not sufficient, for successful implementation are discussed below.

Services Need to Be Relevant by Initiating Them at Developmental Transitions and Targeting Appropriate Life Span Issues

The prenatal and early postpartum periods are optimal times to provide services. Times of divorce and stepfamily formation are other important transition periods for services. Goals must be age-appropriate for parents and their children and also relevant to the life stages of family members (e.g., adolescence, young adulthood, older adulthood). Child-focused curricula will more likely be perceived as relevant when programs move beyond a focus on "normal" development to recognizing that, while children may be of the same age, they can be quite different and present unique challenges to caregivers. A child with a difficult temperament, or with a poor "fit" with a parent's temperament, may not respond to parents in the same way as do children whose temperaments are more moderate. A child who is born premature has greater need for care than full-term infants, is typically less responsive, and presents more complex opportunities for initial bonding, particularly if the child remains hospitalized for an extended period of time. A child that has a developmental disability or is medically fragile creates additional demands for parents whose world now includes a wide range of services involving specialists and additional financial and time demands.

Programs Are More Likely to Engage Parents and Develop Trusting Relationships When They Take into Account a Range of Parental Emotional and Developmental Needs

First, parents who are depressed employ fewer preventive health and safety measures for their children and find it difficult to develop new relationships. Teen parents, for example, often struggle with depression during the first year of parenthood. Second, alcoholism and drug abuse compromise parents' abilities to fulfill their parenting and familial responsibilities. Alcoholic parents may alternate between neglecting their children during intemperate periods and overindulging them when sober. Third, regardless of income, stressful life events and family distress can affect parenting behaviors. With an increase in the number and intensity of stressors and family discord, empathy, family cohesion, and positive attitudes about discipline are likely to decline. Fourth, parents may not know how to be emotionally responsive as parents or how to build social support networks for themselves. Emotional deprivation resulting from neglect, family violence, or aggression learned as a victim or witness of abuse may contribute to neglectful or violent behavior as a parent.

Fifth, confronting the compatibility of one's parenting beliefs and values on the one hand with those of previous generations and the intervention program on the other can be confusing and difficult. Second-generation immigrant parents, for example, are often faced with the emotional challenge of finding acceptable ways of responding to their parents' beliefs and values from their countries of origin, the expectations of the dominant culture, and their personal and familial desires and preferences. Lastly, how parents fit with their cohort of men and women of similar ages may influence the nature and quality of their support systems and their coping. Men in their twenties and early thirties who choose to delay occupational achievement in order to spend time as a child's primary caregiver may be out-of-step with their peers, who are devoting their energies to establishing their careers. Grandparents becoming the primary caregivers of their children's children, often feel socially isolated. In contrast to their peers, they find themselves returning to work for more family income; others leave their jobs and depend on government assistance, savings, and/or pensions.

Interventions Need to Build Parent-Program Relationships That Are Based on Positive, Culturally Competent Approaches and Trust

Especially with high-risk parents, the relationship between the parent and the service provider(s) is crucial to the success of the intervention. Needed are approaches that involve and collaborate with parents in choosing program design and content and incorporate cultural beliefs and practices of parents. Intentional, systematic efforts are needed that build on parents' existing strengths, rather than deficits or failures. Developing a relationship with some parents, however, may be especially difficult, compounded by parents' prior experiences of prejudice, racism, and unavailability of culturally competent community services. Services delivered by those of a different race and ethnicity are often suspect due to the continued presence of prejudice and racism in communities. Cultural values of family privacy, language barriers, and gender bias may also influence parent/program relationships. Service providers need to be

culturally sensitive and competent in helping parents acquire the information and support they need to work toward their expectations for their children and themselves.

Differences within, as well as between, groups need to be understood and respected. Program planning for Latino families, for example, requires attention to the diversity and similarities among people of Puerto Rican, Mexican American and Cuban origins, and from other Central American, South American and Caribbean countries. Parents may also be cautious to develop relationships with the program because of negative experiences and beliefs about services. Parents with mental retardation, for example, are apt to be mistrustful and reluctant to receive parent education services because of fears that their children will be removed from them. Finally, the sex and gender roles and values of the program leader(s)/home visitor and other participants may make a difference to some parents in the process of building relationships. Parents with more traditional gender roles may relate differently with providers who tend to be more androgenous. Parenting programs that include mothers with fathers may provide opportunities to communicate more openly about parenting issues and changes in personal goals that come about by becoming a parent.

Retention of Participants Must Be a Priority and Addressed with Proactive Planning

Special attention to retention issues is warranted because of the high rate of dropouts often reported by prevention and support programs. Practical barriers to participation need to be addressed, such as time constraints and competing responsibilities. In populations with limited resources, providing transportation, child care, convenient times and locations, and meals or refreshments may improve retention. Fathers, in particular, might be recruited where they work or participate in recreational activities. Programs can also be provided in conjunction with job training and vocational counseling. Interested but very busy parents may gain as much from learn-at-home formats such as newsletters, which can be adapted to individual schedule needs and challenges. Lastly, incentives for continued participation—and rewards to celebrate milestones—may be effective, especially in populations with limited economic resources.

A Continuum of Multidisciplinary Services Needs to Be Available in Order to Meet the Diverse Needs of Parents and Their Families

Parents with multiple risk factors may need more intensive and comprehensive services. Combining home visiting services, for instance, with a broader set of services for families with young children is most apt to be successful (Gomby et al., 1999). Programs that target only one domain such as the health of the child do not recognize the complexity of human development or parenting and are unlikely to be effective. Needed are a set of strategies or a "menu" of services that is available to parents in order to address the numerous demands of parenting. Expertise is required from service providers with different areas of training including medicine, public health, family life education, and mental health. Ongoing availability of these services and follow-up is necessary, given the difficulty of changing parent and child behaviors, and the dynamic (and often unpredictable) nature of family life. Parents will benefit from a service delivery system where programs collaborate and link parents with needed services.

Programs Need to Be Flexible Yet Have a Curriculum

Flexibility is needed to respond to family crises and stresses while at the same time having a curriculum; social support is not enough. Determining how to balance support services and program protocol is a constant challenge. Programs must support positive parenting and family functioning in the context of stress and economic hardship. For parents who are stressed by personal and environmental conditions, programs must address these concerns and obstacles in their environment.

Curricula Need to Be Presented with Methods That Fit with Parents' Learning Styles

Classes, reading, and group discussions, which are typical formats for middle-class parents, may be unfamiliar and/or uncomfortable for other parents. Similarly, role-playing, modeling, and coaching demonstration methods may be better suited for some parents' learning styles than others. When printed material is used, the reading level must be geared to the audience. For audiences with limited literacy skills, videos can provide information and modeling with the added advantage of being available for repeat viewing.

Program Personnel Need to Demonstrate Both Personal and Employment-Relevant Competencies, Receive Ongoing Training and Supervision, and Be Supported by Their Host Organization

Staff need excellent interpersonal and facilitative skills. They must also be extremely well trained in order to serve families that face multiple, complex issues. Whether the optimal service providers are paraprofessionals or professionals is unclear from the available research. Paraprofessionals may be better able to engage high-risk participants because of shared cultural and social experiences. However, higher turnover rates among paraprofessionals than among professionals may threaten the success of interventions, partly due to the disruption of trust in the parent/provider relationship. Programs that do employ paraprofessional home visitors must provide significant training and supervision to help them sort out the complex issues they confront when working with families who are difficult to engage, as well as to deal with their own reactions to emotionally charged situations. (Similar support is needed for professionals). The ratio of supervisor-to-staff must be small enough to permit frequent interaction to discuss the complexity of situations, identify the strengths upon which to build, and determine how to reduce the specific risks in each family. Lastly, programs require strong leadership from the organization that is the host of the intervention so that systemic demands to serve more families for less cost do not detract from the necessary time and resources for training and supervision.

Parent Education and Support Services should Be Offered in the Context of Family and Community Diversity

Multiple caregivers that include not only fathers and mothers but grandmothers, aunts, and other kin need to be recognized as important caregivers. In some Native American and African American families, caregiving is shared with non-relative community members. Including grandmothers is especially important in helping teen parents and their families' deal with the discrepancies that may exist between the parenting practices promoted in the program and practices used to rear earlier generations. Parenting education and support similarly must respond to diversity in the needs of caregivers. Parents who choose to have children late or early in life, who are gay or lesbian, conceive through in-vitro fertilization with donor egg or sperm, adopt their children, provide temporary foster care, or add grandchildren to their parenting responsibilities will have differing needs from parent education and support programs. Lastly, programs offered in the community must be "of" the community so that effective linkages with resources in the community can be made and community values and norms can be understood and respected by making variations in service delivery strategies.

ONGOING PROGRAM EVALUATION IS CRUCIAL

Program evaluation can be used to guide program implementation, assess program fidelity, monitor the integrity of program implementation, identify and address barriers to implementation, identify areas in which additional training is needed, and determine what program modifications are needed (Reppucci, Britner, & Woolard, 1997). Evaluation can also help to target services by identifying which parents benefit the most from which specific programs and from which components of a program. Approaches such as empowerment and participatory evaluation are needed that can accommodate the complexity of service provision and the need for flexible and responsive programming.

In closing, parent support and prevention programs have developed in response to the changing nature of parenting and society. In order to identify those strategies that are most likely to assist parents in successfully raising their children, greater attention needs to be given to: (a) program implementation, (b) diversity among children, parents, and communities, and (c) the specific parenting roles and behaviors that are the focus of the intervention. Evaluation research that takes into account the interface of child and adult development, gender, family diversity, and program and community context will be the most helpful for developing effective parent support and prevention programs.

Also see: Parenting: Adolescence; Parenting, Single Parent: Adolescence; Parenting: Adulthood; Child Care; Early Childhood; Environmental Health: Early Childhood; Family Strengthening: Childhood; Prosocial Behavior: Early Childhood.

References

Bullen, J. (1991). J.J. Kelson and the "New" Child-savers: The genesis of the children's aid movement in Ontario. In R. Smandych, G. Dodds, & A. Esau (Eds.), *Dimensions of childhood: Essays on the history of children and youth in Canada* (pp. 135–158). University of Manitoba: Legal Research Institute.

Child Health, USA 2000. (2000). Washington, DC: US Government Printing Office.

Cochran, M., & Niego, S. (1995). Parenting and social networks. In M.H. Bornstein (Ed.), *Handbook of parenting* (Vol. 3, pp. 393–418). Mahwah, NJ: Lawrence Erlbaum Associates.

Collins, W.A., Maccoby, E.E., Steinberg, L., Hetherington, E.M., & Bornstein, M.H. (2000). Contemporary research on parenting: The case for nature and nurture. *American Psychologist, 55*, 218–232.

Dunst, C.J., Trivette, C.M., & Deal, A.G. (1994). *Supporting and strengthening families.* Cambridge, MA: Brookline.

Gomby, D.S., Culross, P.L., & Behrman, R.E. (1999). Home visiting: Recent program evaluations—analysis and recommendations. *The Future of Children, 9,* 4–26.

Heinicke, C.M., Fineman, N., Ruth, G., Recchia, S., Guthrie, D., & Rodning, C. (1999). Relationship based intervention with at-risk mothers: outcome in the first year of life. *Infant Mental Health, 20,* 349–374.

Human Services Policy. (2001). *Evaluation of family preservation and reunification programs: Interim report.* Washington, DC: Office of Assistant Secretary for Planning and Evaluation, US Department of Health and Human Services.

Keniston, K. (1977). *All our children.* NY: Harcourt Brace Jovanovich.

KIDS Count Data Book. (2000). Baltimore, MD: Annie E. Casey Foundation.

Markman, H. (1995). Strengthening marriages and preventing divorce: New directions in prevention research. *Family Relations, 44,* 392–401.

Olds, D., Henderson, C.R., Kitzman, H.J., Eckenrode, J.J., Cole, R.E., & Tatelbaum, R.C. (1999). Prenatal and infancy home visitation by nurses: Recent findings. *The Future of Children, 9,* 44–65.

Peters, D.L. (1980). Social science and social policy and the care of young children. Head Start and after. *Journal of Applied Developmental Psychology, 1,* 7–20.

Powell, D. (1988). Challenges in the design and evaluation of parent–child intervention programs. In D. Powell (Ed.), *Parent education as early childhood intervention: Emerging directions in theory, research and practice* (pp. 229–237). Norwood, NJ: Ablex.

Ramey, C.T., & Ramey, S.L. (1999). *Right from birth: Building your child's foundation for life.* New York: Goddard Press.

Ramey, C.T., Campbell, F.A., Burchinal, M., Skinner, M.L., Gardner, D.M., & Ramey, S.L. (2000). Persistent effects of early childhood education on high-risk children and their mothers. *Applied Developmental Science, 4,* 2–14.

Reppucci, N.D., Britner, P.A., & Woolard, J.L. (1977). *Preventing child abuse and neglect through parent education.* Baltimore, MD: Brookes.

Rosenberg, M.S., & Reppucci, N.D. (1990). Primary prevention of child abuse. *Journal of Counseling and Clinical Psychology, 53,* 576–583.

Smith, S., & Zaslow, M. (1995). Rationale and policy context for two-generation interventions. In S. Smith (Ed.), *Two generation programs for families in poverty* (pp. 1–36). Norwood, NJ: Ablex.

US Department of Health and Human Services, Administration on Children, Youth and Families. (2000). *Child maltreatment 1998.* Washington, DC: US Government Printing.

Parenting, Adolescence

Gary W. Peterson and Kevin R. Bush

INTRODUCTION

Adolescents currently grow up in a great diversity of family circumstances, one of which is the domestic structure referred to as the nuclear family. Regardless of specific structural characteristics, however, families must prepare adolescents psychologically and socially for greater autonomy from parents and the transition to adulthood (Grotevant, 1998; Steinberg, 1990). The developmental period of adolescence and its associated family relationships are typically portrayed as fraught with dangers and difficult transitions for nuclear families. Such problematic issues for youth and their families include complicated identity issues, the onset of sexual activity, diminished adult influence, the greater influence of "deviant" peers, as well as risks for substance abuse, violence, delinquency, depression, and suicide (Dryfoos, 1998; Furstenberg, 2000). Rather than focusing on how adolescents construct positive identities, become interpersonally competent, and master skills for adulthood, the frequent image portrayed is that of competent adolescents being only the fortunate few who somehow dodge the many "social bullets" of this "perilous" time (Furstenberg, 2000).

A more balanced view of this "time of trouble" perspective is based on substantial research indicating that most youngsters cope effectively with being an adolescent, have positive relationships with parents, and make transitions to adulthood fairly unscathed (Furstenberg, 2000; Peterson & Leigh, 1990). Although many adolescents do experiment with risky activities like alcohol use and minor forms of delinquent behavior (e.g., curfew violations, minor property damage), most of these activities are only temporary and fairly harmless for long-term developmental outcomes (Jessor, 1993). A key influence on the extent to which adolescence is either a constructive or problematic period of development, therefore, is the quality of parent–adolescent relationships provided within nuclear families (Peterson, Madden-Derdich, & Leonard, 2000).

DEFINITIONS

A general definition of *social competence* is the ability of adolescents to function adaptively in relationships with peers, parents, and other interpersonal relationships. Prevention programs that focus on increasing prosocial behavior and social skills, while reducing problem behaviors in adolescents often deal directly or indirectly with aspects of social competence (Dishion, Patterson, & Kavanaugh, 1992; Kumpfer, Molgard, & Spoth, 1996; Tremblay, Masse, Pagani-Kurtz, & Vitaro, 1991). A key point is that focusing on the use of certain kinds of parenting strategies is an indirect means of fostering social competence by manipulating aspects of adolescents' immediate social context within nuclear families.

Social competence consists of a set of attributes or psychological resources that help adolescents adapt to their social circumstances and cope with everyday life sufficiently to ward off problematic behavior while engaging in constructive possibilities (i.e., externalizing and internalizing behavior) (Baumrind, 1991; Peterson & Hann, 1999). Recent conceptions of social competence identify some of its subdimensions as: (1) a balance between autonomy and connectedness in reference to parents (and others), (2) psychological or cognitive resources (e.g., self-esteem, identity, achievement, and problem-solving skills), and (3) social skills with peers and other interpersonal relationships (Peterson & Hann, 1999). Cultural and ethnic differences in adolescents' social competence exist when different priorities are assigned to such valued socialization outcomes as autonomy versus conformity in reference to authority figures. Moreover, cultural diversity in social competence becomes manifest when the social self of adolescents is fostered in terms of different cultural themes. The most commonly discussed difference in cultural themes for the self is that of the European–American emphasis on such values as individuality, the private self, and personal autonomy versus a focus on alterative cultural orientations consisting of collectivism, the connected self, and group-focused values (Arnett, 1995; Peterson, 1995; Peterson, Bush, & Supple, 1999).

Two general categories of problematic outcomes, *internalizing and externalizing behavior*, can be viewed as the other side of the coin in reference to social competence. Internalizing behaviors are those in which the difficulties of adolescents become evident due to psychological disturbances that focus on the self (e.g., depression, suicidal thoughts, and eating disorders). Externalizing (or problem) behaviors, in turn, refer to psychological difficulties that take the form of behavior problems (e.g., vandalism and violent acts) reflecting the tendencies of adolescents to "act out" against society. Extensive involvement in externalizing and internalizing behavior can be a major obstacle to successful progress through adolescence and the transition to adulthood.

Most of the existing research also identifies a multidimensional pattern for socializing adolescents, *authoritative parenting*, as the primary approach that fosters social competence and prevents the development of at-risk behavior (i.e., internalizing and externalizing) by adolescents (Baumrind, 1991; Peterson & Hann, 1999). When conceptualized broadly in terms of component strategies, authoritative parenting can encompass such behaviors as parental support, reasoning, monitoring (or supervision), limit setting, and firm control (Baumrind, 1991; Patterson, Reid, & Dishion, 1991; Peterson & Hann, 1999). Implied components of authoritative parenting include interpersonal capacities to encourage, offer rational parental guidance (i.e., reasoning), engage in effective communication with adolescents, manage parent–adolescent conflict, and prevent coercive cycles (Dishion et al., 1992; Patterson et al., 1991;

Peterson & Hann, 1999). Compared to younger children, the greater cognitive sophistication of adolescents makes verbal exchanges with parents involving abstract thought (e.g., reasoning and communication) more appropriate as part of an effective socialization strategy. Although questions remain about the generalizability of authoritative parenting to a broad range of ethnic-minority and socioeconomic populations (Demo & Cox, 2000), empirically supported prevention strategies for families often use concepts that are either based on or compatible with this conception of parental socialization strategies.

SCOPE

Despite remaining quite prevalent in our society, substantial declines have occurred in nuclear families in which both parents are married for the first time, continuing to reside with each other, and are related to their children biologically or through adoption (Teachman, 2000). Declining numbers of nuclear families are a great worry to some observers who argue that adolescents are increasingly placed at risk because of this trend (Popenoe, 1993, 1996). A controversial but frequent assumption is that nuclear families are the normative benchmark against which all other family structures are compared. Nuclear families are often viewed as being more capable of socializing, protecting, nurturing, and providing companionship to children because co-resident parents can share the responsibilities of child-rearing, mutually support each other, provide long-term ties, and have socioeconomic advantages (Baumrind, 1989, 1991; Burgess, 1926; Parsons, 1944; Peterson & Hann, 1999; Popenoe, 1993, 1996).

Other observers offer the contrasting view that fewer nuclear families, combined with increased alternative family forms, signify that family life, like most social phenomena, will inevitably change over time. Families are viewed as changing, or more precisely, adapting to meet the demands of a constantly changing society (Allen, Fine, & Demo, 2000; Coontz, 1997). Some of these critics argue even further that nuclear families have lost some of their relevance for postmodern society by reinforcing the prominence of male "breadwinners," traditional family divisions of labor, and by restricting the economic and social emancipation of women (Coontz, 1991, 1997; Osmond & Thorne, 1993; Stacey, 1993, 1996).

A related idea is that only modest if any differences in adolescents' social and personality outcomes can be traced specifically to structural variations in families (Demo & Cox, 2000; Teachman, 2000). Instead of structural explanations, much of the research has focused on the dynamic or social psychological dimensions of family and parent–adolescent

relationships. These interpersonal aspects are viewed as being more directly predictive of adolescents' psychosocial characteristics than are the more remote influences of family structure (Grotevant, 1998; Peterson & Hann, 1999). Moreover, from a social–psychological standpoint, both nuclear and alternative families do not differ fundamentally, but have much in common in reference to interpersonal issues involved in socializing adolescents.

Family-based prevention strategies that address these issues do not usually seek to address the relative merits of family structural variations, but are more likely to target the quality of parent–adolescent relationships. A good working hypothesis, therefore, is that prevention strategies are most effective when the goals are to help parents cope more effectively with their circumstances, become more involved with their young, and use effective socialization strategies with adolescents. Specifically, the desired outcome of these family-based programs is high quality parental involvement, which takes the form of authoritative socialization strategies, the management of parent–adolescent conflict, and effective parent–youth communication (Baumrind, 1991; Grotevant, 1998; Peterson & Hann, 1999; Furstenberg, 2000). An associated consequence of improving the socialization performance of parents, in turn, is greater social competence by the young in the form of social problem-solving, higher self-esteem, adaptive autonomy, and effective achievement (Dishion, Andrews, Kavanaugh, & Soberman, 1996). The development of social competence provides adolescents with healthy psychosocial attributes that help to ward off problematic outcomes in the form of internalizing and externalizing behavior (Peterson & Hann, 1999; Peterson & Leigh, 1990). Consequently, family-based prevention programs are needed to encourage forms of parent–adolescent relationships that both occur naturally within some (but certainly not all) nuclear families and that foster social competence in the young.

THEORIES

Family Systems Theory

The fundamental importance of systems perspectives is to focus attention on the importance of family relationships and, more specifically the parent–adolescent subsystem, as sources of either well-being or problematic behavior by adolescents. According to a systems viewpoint, all aspects of families and their members are interrelated through dynamic, mutual, and circular processes (Broderick, 1993). The family systems perspective is especially useful for conceptualizing reciprocal processes that are unique to families, such as patterns of communication and conflict that occur between parents and adolescents. Communication and conflictual processes help to define the structure and meaning of the relationships that develop between parents and adolescents within families. These processes tend to be associated either with the development of social competence or with the advent of internalizing/externalizing behavior in youth (Broderick, 1993). Consequently, family systems theory is important for highlighting the special role of family processes and the need for family-based strategies as key elements of comprehensive prevention programs.

Socialization Theory

A second theoretical framework, the socialization perspective, focuses specifically on the importance of high quality parent–adolescent relationships as a means of discouraging problem behaviors in adolescents. This is complicated by the fact that adolescents confront their elders with increased expectations to grant them autonomy and spend an increasing amount of time without direct parental supervision (Furstenberg, 2000). Socialization perspectives are eclectic in nature, with roots in such general frameworks as social learning and symbolic interaction theories. These perspectives provide the conceptual basis for the idea that parents' socialization behaviors help to either encourage or inhibit the development of social competence in adolescents. The primary idea here is that the child-rearing strategies of parents operate as part of the social environment to change the behavior, attitudes, and attributes of adolescents through principles of learning and processes of internalization (Maccoby & Martin, 1983; Patterson et al., 1991; Peterson & Hann, 1999).

Two major dimensions of parental behavior, control and support, have been the focus of these perspectives. The most common conceptualization proposes that parental behaviors consistent with the "authoritative" style both foster social competence most effectively and inhibit the development of problematic behavior in adolescents. Specifically, problematic behavior by adolescents tends to be prevented when parents use firm, rationally based forms of control in combination with encouragement and support (Baumrind, 1989, 1991; Maccoby & Martin, 1983; Patterson et al., 1991; Peterson & Hann, 1999). This contrast with styles of parenting that emphasize either more "authoritarian" (i.e., arbitrary, punitive control, and diminished support) or more "permissive" approaches (i.e., diminished control and high support) that are commonly associated with reduced social competence and higher frequencies of psychosocial problems (Baumrind, 1991).

Ecological Perspectives

The most comprehensive way of conceptualizing family-based prevention strategies is by viewing the parent–adolescent relationship within nuclear families as a subcomponent of much larger social environments. These "ecological" perspectives can provide insight for a broad range of prevention strategies aimed at social levels ranging from dyadic relationships within nuclear families (e.g., parenting programs) to macro-level societal institutions (e.g., social policy) (Bronfenbrenner, 1979; Lerner, 1995). That is, adolescents are viewed as being nested within a complex array of interconnected systems that encompass individual, family, and extrafamilial (e.g., peer, school, neighborhood, community, and societal) settings. Both socially competent and problematic outcomes are viewed as products of reciprocal exchanges between adolescents and their diverse settings. Moreover, adolescent social competence and the quality of parent–adolescent relations are either supported or hindered by the degree of interconnection among the social systems in which adolescent development occurs (Bronfenbrenner, 1979).

From an ecological perspective, the ideal circumstance occurs when adolescents are exposed to constructive developmental experiences within each of these settings and when none of these environments contradict the other. Problems occur, therefore, when adolescents are exposed to socialization experiences (e.g., high punitiveness) that inhibit social competence and encourage internalizing or externalizing behavior. Difficulties in socialization are further amplified when adolescents' developmental settings (e.g., the nuclear family and the neighborhood) contradict each other—as when the deviant values of neighborhood gangs contradict constructive socialization practices of parents. Ecological theories embody a multifaceted view of development that supports comprehensive, community-based approaches, the key aspects of which are those that focus on the parent–adolescent relationship within families (Garbarino & Kostelny, 1993). Ecological models can be used to understand layers of influence on human behavior and target aspects of development for appropriate prevention strategies.

Risk and Resiliency Theory

Closely related to ecological perspectives is another systemic orientation commonly referred to as "risk and resiliency" (or risk and protective factors) theory (Hawkins, Catalano, & Miller, 1992; Petraitis, Flay, & Miller, 1995; Garmezy, 1983, 1985). This perspective was developed specifically to identify the many potential hazards that adolescents face and the resources they have to ward off the more difficult obstacles to development. An important use of risk and resiliency models is to emphasize the need for prevention efforts within multiple domains of development as a means of discouraging the emergence of internalizing and externalizing behavior. This perspective identifies several risk and protective factors that are based within the parent–adolescent relationship and conceptualizes family-based prevention as being an essential component of comprehensive community-based models (Hawkins, Catalano, Kosterman, Abbott, & Hill, 1999).

Recent findings in risk and resiliency research suggest that mental health problems, social behavioral problems, and health-risk involvements often co-occur as an organized pattern of risk behaviors (Dryfoos, 1990, 1998; Elliot, Huizinga, & Menard, 1989; Jessor, Donovan, & Costa, 1991). Conceptualizing risk factors as being interrelated has led to an overall strategy of targeting multiple factors simultaneously, with the intent of having a more large-scale impact than simply moderating the influence of a single risk factor. Consequently, because risk factors overlap and may predict a variety of outcomes, prevention strategies may have the potential to ameliorate a diverse array of problematic developments (Coie et al., 1993).

This model seeks to identify the various risk and protective factors for adolescents within individual, family, peer, school, neighborhood, and community circumstances. The first of two general social categories from this perspective, risk factors, is based on epidemiological models of disease development, such as efforts to identify the multiple hazards that influence heart disease (e.g., sedentary life style, smoking, and a high fat diet). The second general category of social phenomena, protective factors (or sources of wellness), are individual capabilities or social-environmental resources that enhance the abilities of adolescents to function in adaptive ways in the face of stressful or risky circumstances (Garmezy, 1983, 1985; Hawkins et al., 1992; Petraitis et al., 1995). At the parent–adolescent level of analysis, risk factors would include such social behaviors as exposure to parental punitive and permissive behavior, whereas protective factors (or sources of resiliency) include consistent parental monitoring, reasoning, supportiveness, secure parental attachment, or dimensions of adolescents' social competence that contribute to resiliency (e.g., self-esteem and social skills) (Peterson et al., 2000).

The primary objective of this perspective, therefore, is to understand how risk and protective factors operate so that prevention approaches can be designed to diminish the hazards and build upon adolescents' sources of resiliency. From this perspective, prevention designs are most effectively directed at patterns of risk and protective factors rather than at problematic psychosocial characteristics of adolescents. Consequently, the most efficacious approach is to target multiple negative outcomes within the context of a coordinated set of programs (Greenberg, Domitrovich, & Bumbarger, 2001).

STRATEGIES THAT WORK

Substantial research evidence establishes that aspects of parent–adolescent relationships closely associated with authoritative parenting are: (1) significant contributors to dimensions of adolescent social competence and (2) should be targeted for family-based prevention/intervention approaches. Parental support, for example, provides affection and encouragement to adolescents that help to foster connections with parents, self-confidence for greater personal responsibility (autonomy), and a sense of security used to sustain achievement efforts and feelings of personal self-efficacy (i.e., dimensions of social competence) (Peterson & Hann, 1999). Parents who use aspects of firm control such as limit setting, monitoring (supervision), reasoning, along with two-way communication, often provide the needed guidance for youthful behavior, the internalization of prosocial norms, appropriate levels of autonomy, and sufficient structure for healthy self-concept development (i.e., dimensions of social competence) (Baumrind, 1991; Grotevant, 1998). The use of firm, rational, and supportive behavior by parents, in conjunction with clear communication, helps to manage conflict and avoid escalating cycles of punitive or coercive exchanges between parents and adolescents (Patterson et al., 1991). Moreover, dimensions of adolescent social competence function as psychological and social resources that prevent the development of problematic behavior by the young (Peterson & Leigh, 1990). Consequently, aspects of parent–adolescent relationships and dimensions of adolescent social competence should be targeted as areas of great potential for family-based prevention/intervention strategies.

Adolescent Transitions Program

An initial example of a multifaceted prevention program that focuses both on improving parents' socialization practices and aspects of adolescent social competence is the *Adolescent Transitions Program* (ATP) developed by researchers at the Oregon Social Learning Center (OSLC). Based on substantial evidence supporting the "coercive family process model" (Dishion, Patterson, & Kavanaugh, 1992), researchers at the OSLC have developed, implemented, and evaluated the ATP to prevent or reduce youthful antisocial behavior by fostering prosocial behavior, improve parental practices (supportiveness, limit setting, monitoring), and avoid the escalation of coercive processes (i.e., unmanaged conflict) between the young and their parents (Dishion et al., 1992, 1996). This program teaches adolescents and their parents relationship skills aimed at reducing problem behavior and preventing its reoccurrence in families of early adolescents.

The adolescent and parent components of the ATP are designed to parallel one another, with practice sessions for relationship skills development being an integral feature of the program. The parent component focuses on assisting parents to develop and/or enhance such parenting practices as monitoring, limit setting, dyadic skills, and social reinforcement (supportiveness) that foster prosocial behavior (Dishion et al., 1996). The adolescent component of the ATP teaches at-risk youth to set appropriate goals consistent with developing social competence through gaining peer support, acknowledging limits, learning dyadic skills, providing positive reinforcement, and acquiring problem-solving skills. Over the years, the OSLC group have demonstrated the empirical success of the ATP through improved parenting strategies and decreased frequencies of antisocial behavior among early adolescents and preadolescents (Dishion et al., 1992, 1996).

More recent prevention efforts at the OSLC have incorporated a school component into the ATP (Dishion et al., 1996). A major advantage of including a school component along with adolescent and parent/family components is to address more of the risk and protective factors in a concerted fashion. Moreover, the goal of linking school and family emphasizes the importance of interconnected systems that support each other by facilitating communication between parents and schools to establish common rules, consequences, discipline, and positive reinforcements (Conduct Problems Prevention Research Group, 1999; Dishion et al., 1996). Continuity across social contexts offsets the possibility that prevention efforts implemented in one social context (e.g., school context) will be contradicted in the other setting (e.g., family). For example, without a component addressing parental involvement to encourage school achievement and adjustment issues, the positive impacts of parent and adolescent (family-based) components are more likely to be undermined (Conduct Problems Prevention Research Group, 1999; Dishion et al., 1996).

An important aspect of the school component consists of training teachers to become school–family liaisons through attendance at both the parent and teacher components of the ATP (Dishion et al., 1996). These liaisons record the student's behaviors and performances in school (positive and negative) and then share this information with parents, providing an ongoing linkage between the two social settings. School liaisons also attend adolescent component meetings and provide school-based contingencies for self-regulation skills taught in ATP. Teachers' ratings of adolescents' externalizing behaviors indicate that school-based implementations of the ATP produced lower levels of problem behavior. Moreover, parents' involvement with the schools was shown to be an effective strategy for decreasing adolescent drug use and improving student behavior overall.

School-based programs that foster social competence in childhood and adolescence can be important complements to family-based strategies by affirming ecological models and reinforcing similar outcomes in more than one setting. A school-based program can teach cognitive, behavioral, and affective skills for dealing with everyday challenges, problems, and decisions encountered during adolescence and early adulthood (Weissberg, Barton, & Shriver, 1997). The specific focus may be social problem-solving and peer interaction skills that prevent risk-taking involvements. Socially competent behaviors reinforced in more than one setting are: (1) more likely to function as protective factors and (2) elicit constructive socialization practices from parents (i.e., as a child effect) that are encouraged in family-based prevention strategies (Peterson & Hann, 1999).

Strengthening Families Program

A second project similar to the ATP is the *Strengthening Families Program* (SFP). Originally designed for families of methadone maintenance patients with school-aged children and early-adolescents (6–12 year olds), the SFP is aimed at reducing the youngsters' vulnerability to drug use (Kumper et al., 1996). The SFP has three main components: (1) parent training based on Patterson's (Patterson et al., 1991) coercive family process model and other prevention models, (2) children's social skills training, and (3) family skills training.

The parent component of the SFP includes: (1) teaching parents effective communication and problem-solving skills, (2) alcohol and drug education, (3) effective discipline strategies, and (4) development and implementation of behavior programs for children and adolescents. The children's skill training that addresses social competence includes teaching youth social skills such as: (1) attending to circumstances, problem-solving and effective communication, (2) how to resist peer pressure, (3) how to comply with parental rules, (4) how to understand and cope with emotions, (5) how to use available coping resources, and (6) the application of conflict management strategies.

The family skills component allows parents and youth to apply the skills they have been taught in practice sessions through structured play therapy (i.e., the Child's Game), communication skill practice sessions, and parenting strategy practice sessions (Kumpfer et al., 1996). Experimental studies evaluating the effectiveness of the SFP suggest that, when all three components are implemented together, significant reductions in the targeted risk factors occurred. More specifically, children's problem behaviors decreased, prosocial skills were enhanced, effective parenting strategies increased, family rules became clearer, and family conflict was diminished (Kumpfer et al., 1996).

Recently, the SFP has been renamed the Iowa Strengthening Families Program (ISFP) and modified to serve low income families having youngsters in sixth and seventh grades. Experimental and longitudinal studies indicate that the ISFP produces significant changes in the targeted parenting behaviors and the outcomes of youth, both at posttest and 1-year follow-up assessments (Redmond, Spoth, Shin, & Lepper, 1999).

STRATEGIES THAT MIGHT WORK

Montreal Longitudinal-Experimental Study

Another extremely promising program is the "Montreal Longitudinal-Experimental Study," a preventive approach that targets kindergarten boys at risk for developing delinquency during adolescence. The program consists of both a parent-training component and an adolescent social skills training component (Tremblay, Pagani-Kurtz, Masse, Vitaro, & Pihl, 1995). Based on Patterson's model (Patterson et al., 1991), the parent-training component involves individualized home-based training sessions to encourage parental involvement, monitoring, positive reinforcement of prosocial behavior, effective discipline, and conflict management. The adolescent component was provided in participating schools and focused on teaching social skills to enhance problem solving, encourage conflict management, reduce negative interactions with others, and increase prosocial behavior. Teachers were involved by reporting children's behaviors and the degree of parental involvement. Analyses of yearly follow-up assessments (i.e., boys aged 10–15) indicated that treatment group participants reported significantly less delinquency compared to control group boys (Tremblay et al., 1995).

STRATEGIES THAT DO NOT WORK

Evidence is mounting that "individual strategies" which fail to focus on the broader social ecology or provide family-based approaches are not effective prevention strategies. For example, The *Drug Abuse Resistance Education* program (DARE), an individually focused approach, is the most frequently used drug education program in the United States, with approximately 70 percent of school districts employing this program (Rosenbaum & Hanson, 1998). Numerous evaluations of DARE programs, however, conclude that the program does not produce long-term changes (Ennett, Tobler, Ringwalt, & Flewelling, 1994; Rosenbaum & Hanson, 1998). The DARE program is operated by trained uniformed officers who visit classrooms and teach: (1) knowledge about the negative effects of drugs; (2) responsible decision-making skills; (3) assertiveness; (4) a sense of values; and (5) self-esteem. The assumption here is that increased knowledge, cognitive resources, and interpersonal skills will lower the likelihood of drug use. A recent experimental study with longitudinal components revealed an absence of positive treatment effects, and particularly an absence of long-term outcomes (Rosenbaum & Hanson, 1998).

SYNTHESIS

Family-based prevention models for nuclear families should be focused on the social pychological dynamics of nuclear families, rather than being preoccupied with the relative merits of diverse family forms (i.e., structural deficit models) as targets for programs. A considerable amount of research establishes that authoritative (or closely related) socialization behaviors by parents tend to inhibit the development of problem behaviors by encouraging adolescents to become socially competent. The specific dimensions of social competence (e.g., self-esteem, social problem-solving skills, autonomy, and attachment to parents and others) as well as components of authoritative parenting (nurturance, firm control, monitoring, use of reason, clear communication, conflict management skills, and rejection of arbitrary punitiveness) are protective factors that provide important targets for the design of prevention programs.

This is best accomplished, however, within the context of a larger ecological design that addresses more than one developmental setting of adolescents simultaneously. Family, school, and other community contexts should be used to reinforce prosocial outcomes through complementary approaches for diminishing risk factors and capitalizing on the potential resiliency provided by protective factors. Family-based approaches can be an important element of a broader ecological strategy that seeks to foster the effective transition of adolescents into adulthood by improving the quality of parenting within families so that adolescent social competence is fostered. Prevention programs should capitalize on the strengths of nuclear families and encourage the involvement of both parents, with particular focus on the participation of fathers. Another consideration for prevention strategies is that many family-based risk factors have their origins in periods of development earlier than adolescence. Consequently, those who design prevention strategies may wish to focus on earlier periods of development to most effectively ameliorate problematic outcomes that become evident in adolescence

Family-based prevention approaches should occur as part of a larger strategy that involves components that are implemented across at least the family and school environments, if not also involving the peer group and the larger community. Such a broad-based strategy recognizes that no single program component can prevent multiple risk behaviors. Instead, greater success will be attained through a package of coordinated approaches designed for each community circumstance.

Also see: Parenting: Early Childhood; Parenting, Single Parent: Adolescence; Parenting: Adulthood; Social Competency: Adolescence; Family Strengthening: Adolescence; Identity Promotion: Adolescence; Life Skills: Adolescence.

References

Allen, K.R., Fine, M.A., & Demo, D. (2000). An overview of family diversity: Controversies, questions, and values. In D.H. Demo, K.R. Allen & M.A. Fine (Eds.), *Handbook of family diversity* (pp. 1–14). New York: Oxford University Press.

Arnett, J. (1995). Broad and narrow socialization: The family in the context of cultural theory. *Journal of Marriage and the Family, 54*, 339–373.

Baumrind, (1989). Rearing competent children. In W. Damon (Ed.), *Child development today and tomorrow* (pp. 349–378). San Francisco: Jossey-Bass.

Baumrind, D. (1991). Effective parenting during the early adolescent transition. In P.A. Cowan & M. Hetherington (Eds.), *Family transitions* (pp. 111–163). Hillsdale, NJ: Lawrence Erlbaum.

Broderick, C.B. (1993). *Understanding family process: Basics of family systems theory*. Newbury Park, CA: Sage.

Bronfenbrenner, U. (1979). *The ecology of human development*. Cambridge: Harvard University Press.

Burgess, E.W. (1926). The family as a unity of interacting personalities. *The Family, 7*, 3–9.

Coie, J.D., Watt, N.F., West, S.G., Hawkins, J.D., Asarnow, J.R., Markman, H.J., Ramey, S.L., Shure, M.B., & Long, B. (1993). The science of prevention: A conceptual framework and some directions for a national research program. *American Psychologist, 48*, 1013–1022.

Conduct Problems Prevention Research Group. (1999). Initial impact of the Fast Track prevention trial for conduct problems: II, Classroom effects. *Journal of Consulting and Clinical Psychology, 67*(5), 648–657.

Coontz, S. (1991). *The way we never were*. New York: Basic Books.

Coontz, S. (1997). *The way we really are: Coming to terms with America's changing families*. New York: Basic Books.

Demo, D.H., & Cox, M.J. (2000). Families with young children: A review of research in the 1990s. *Journal of Marriage and the Family, 62*(4), 876–895.

Dishion, T.J., Andrews, D.W., Kavanaugh, K., & Soberman, L.H. (1996). Preventive interventions for high-risk youth: The adolescent transitions program. In R.D. Peters & R.J. McMahon (Eds.), *Preventing childhood disorders, substance abuse, and delinquency* (pp. 184–214). Thousand Oaks, CA: Sage.

Dishion, T.J., Patterson, G.R., & Kavanaugh, K.A. (1992). An experimental test of the coercion model: Linking theory, measurement, and intervention. In J. McCord & R.E. Tremblay (Eds.), *Preventing antisocial behavior: Interventions from birth through adolescence* (pp. 253–282). New York: Guilford Press.

Dryfoos, J.G. (1990). *Adolescents at risk: Prevalence and prevention*. New York: Oxford University Press.

Dryfoos, J.G. (1998). *Making it through adolescence in a risky society: What parents, schools, and communities can do*. New York: Oxford University Press.

Elliot, D.S., Huizinga, D., & Menard, S. (1989). *Multiple problem youth: Delinquency, substance use, and mental health problems*. New York: Springer-Verlag.

Ennett, S.T., Tobler, N.S., Ringwalt, C.L., & Flewelling, R.L. (1994). How effective is drug abuse resistance education? A meta-analysis of project D.A.R.E. outcome evaluations. *American Journal of Public Health, 84*, 1394–1401.

Furstenberg, F.F. (2000). The sociology of adolescence and youth in the 1990s: A critical commentary. *Journal of Marriage and the Family, 62*(4), 896–910.

Garbarino, J., & Kostelny, K. (1993). Neighborhood and community influences on parenting. In T. Luster & L. Okagaki (Eds.), *Parenting: An ecological perspective* (pp. 203–226). Hillsdale, NJ: Lawrence Erlbaum.

Garmezy, N. (1983). Stressors of childhood. In N. Garmezy & R. Rutter (Eds.), *Stress, coping, and development in children* (pp. 43–84). New York: McGraw-Hill.

Garmezy, N. (1985). Stress-resistant children: The search for protective factors. In J.E. Stevenson (Ed.), *Recent research in developmental psychopathology* (pp. 213–233). Oxford, England: Pergamon Press.

Greenberg, M.T., Domitrovich, C., & Bumbarger, B. (2001). The prevention of mental disorders in school-aged children: Current state of the field. *Prevention and Treatment, 4*, 1–84.

Grotevant, H.D. (1998). Adolescent development in family contexts. In W. Damon & N. Eisenberg (Eds.), *Handbook of child psychology* (5th ed., pp. 1097–1149). New York: John Wiley & Sons.

Hawkins, J.D., Catalano, R.F., & Miller, J.Y. (1992). Risk and protective factors for alcohol and other drug problems in adolescence and early adulthood: Implications for substance abuse prevention. *Psychological Bulletin, 112*(1), 64–105.

Hawkins, J.D., Catalano, R.F., Kosterman, R., Abbott, R., & Hill, K. (1999). Preventing adolescent health-risk behaviors by strengthening protection during childhood. *Archives of Pediatrics and Adolescent Medicine, 153*, 226–234.

Jessor, R. (1993). Successful adolescent development among youth in high risk settings. *American Psychologist, 48*(2), 117–126.

Jessor, R., Donovan, J.E., & Costa, F.M. (1991). *Beyond adolescence: Problem behavior and young adult development*. New York: Cambridge University Press.

Kumpfer, K.L., Molgard, V., & Spoth, R. (1996). The strengthening families program for the prevention of delinquency and drug use. In R.D. Peters & R.J. McMahon (Eds.), *Preventing childhood disorders, substance abuse, and delinquency* (pp. 241–267). Thousand Oaks, CA: Sage.

Lerner, R. (1995). *America's youth in crisis: Challenges and options for programs and policies*. Thousand Oaks, CA: Sage.

Maccoby, E.E., & Martin, J.A. (1983). Socialization in the context of the family: Parent–child interaction. In E.M. Hetherington (Ed.), *Handbook of child psychology: Socialization, personality, and social development* (Vol. 4, pp. 1–101). New York: Wiley.

Osmond, M.W., & Thorne, B. (1993). Feminist theories: The social construction of gender in families and society. In P.G. Boss, W.J. Doherty, R.W. LaRossa, W.R. Schumm, & S.K. Steinmetz (Eds.), *Sourcebook of family theories and methods: A contextual approach* (pp. 591–623). New York: Plenum.

Parsons, T. (1944). The social structure of the family. In R.N. Anshen (Ed.), *The family: Its function and destiny* (pp. 173–201). New York: Harper.

Patterson, G.R., Reid, J.B., & Dishion, T.J. (1991). *A social learning approach: Vol. 4. Antisocial boys*. Eugene, OR: Castalia.

Peterson, G.W. (1995). Autonomy and connectedness in family. In R.D. Day, K.R. Gilbert, B.H. Settles, & W.R. Burr (Eds.), *Research and theory in family science* (pp. 20–41). Pacific Grove, CA: Brooks Cole.

Peterson, G.W., & Hann, D. (1999). Socializing parents and children in families. In M. Sussman & S.K. Steinmetz (Eds.), *Handbook of marriage and the family* (pp. 471–507). New York: Plenum Press.

Peterson, G.W., & Leigh, G.K. (1990). The family and social competence in adolescence. In T.P. Gullotta, G.R. Adams, & R. Montemayor (Eds.), *Developing social competency in adolescence: Advances in adolescent development* (pp. 97–138). Newbury Park, CA: Sage.

Peterson, G.W., Bush, K.R., & Supple, A. (1999). Predicting adolescent autonomy from parents: Relationship connectednes and retrictiveness. *Sociological Inquiry, 69*, 431–457.

Peterson, G.W., Madden-Derdich, D., & Leonard, S. (2000). Parent–child relations across the life course: Autonomy within the context of connectedness. In S.J. Price, P.C. McKenry, & M.J. Murphy (Eds.), *Families across time: A life course perspective.* Los Angeles, CA: Roxbury.

Petraitis, J., Flay B., & Miller, T.Q. (1995). Reviewing theories of adolescent substance use: Organizing pieces in the puzzle. *Psychological Bulletin, 177*(1), 67–86.

Popenoe, D. (1993). American family decline, 1960–1990: A review and appraisal. *Journal of Marriage and the Family, 55*(3), 527–555.

Popenoe, D. (1996). *Life without father: Compelling new evidence that fatherhood and marriage are indispensable for the good of children and society.* New York: Free Press.

Redmond, C., Spoth, R., Shin, C., & Lepper, H.S. (1999). Modeling long-term parent outcomes of two universal family-focused preventive interventions: One-year follow-up results. *Journal of Consulting and Clinical Psychology, 67*(6), 975–984.

Rosenbaum, D.P., & Hanson, G.S. (1998). Assessing the effects of school based drug education: A six-year multilevel analysis of project D.A.R.E. *The Journal of Research in Crime and Delinquency, 35*(4), 381–412.

Stacey, J. (1993). Is the sky falling? *Journal of Marriage and the Family, 55,* 555–559.

Stacey, J. (1996). *In the name of the family: Rethinking family values in the postmodern age.* Boston: Beacon Press.

Steinberg, L. (1990). Interdependence in the family: Autonomy, conflict, and harmony in the parent–child relationship. In S.S. Feldman & G.L. Elliot (Eds.), *At the threshold: The developing adolescent* (pp. 255–276). Cambridge: Harvard University Press.

Teachman, J.D. (2000). Diversity of family structure: Economic and social influences. In D.H. Demo, K.R. Allen, & M.A. Fine (Eds.), *Handbook of family diversity* (pp. 32–58). New York: Oxford University Press.

Tremblay, R.E., Pagani-Kurtz, L., Masse, L.C., Vitaro, F., & Pihl, R.O. (1995). A bimodal preventive intervention for disruptive kindergarten boys: Its impact through mid-adolescence. *Journal of Consulting and Clinical Psychology, 63,* 560–568.

Tremblay, R.E., Masse, L.C., Pagani-Kurtz, L., & Vitaro, F. (1996). From childhood aggression to adolescent maladjustment: The Montreal prevention experiment. In R. DeV. Peters & R.J. McMahon (Eds.), *Preventing childhood disorders, substance abuse, and delinquency* (pp. 268–298). Thousand Oaks, CA: Sage.

Weissberg, R.P., Barton, H.A., & Shriver, T.P. (1997). The social-competence promotion program for young adolescents. In G.W. Albee & T.P. Gullotta (Eds.), *Primary prevention works* (pp. 268–290). Thousand Oaks, CA: Sage.

Parenting, Single Parent, Adolescence

Bonnie L. Barber

INTRODUCTION

For a substantial minority of children in single-parent families, adolescence is a period of less than optimal growth characterized by increases in conduct problems, depression, and a decline in academic performance. However, for many others, it is a time of enhanced responsibility, mature self-reliance, and identification with positive goals and values. Why do some adolescents develop successfully in single-parent families while others experience serious difficulties? What interventions with single-parent families are associated with positive developmental outcomes during adolescence? In the past decade, a number of family processes have been identified as mediators of family structure effects on adolescent adjustment (Amato, 1993; Buchanan, Maccoby, & Dornbusch, 1996; Emery, 1999; Hetherington et al., 1992). However, intervention programs have not consistently been guided by these findings and basic research on mediating processes is limited (Grych & Fincham, 1992). This entry highlights possible mechanisms one could target to promote healthy development of adolescents in single-parent families, and the efficacy of existing programs that use related approaches.

DEFINITIONS

In the existing literature, the effects of parental divorce and those of living with a single parent can be difficult to disentangle. These two family contexts are frequently confounded, and it is often difficult to tell which effect is operating in any given study. Much of the research on adolescents in single-parent families has been done with divorced families, so this entry focuses heavily on divorce, with references to never-married parents and to separated parents when possible.

SCOPE

Although the majority of adolescents in the United States, Canada, Australia, United Kingdom, and New Zealand live with two parents, a growing number live with single-parents. For the last three decades, there have been increasing numbers of single-parent households, and at current rates, 50–60 percent of all US children born in the early 1980s will live with only one parent for at least a year before reaching the age of 18 years (Martin & Bumpass, 1989). Between 1970 and 1999, the proportion of US children in two-parent families decreased from 85 to 68 percent, and by 1999, 23 percent of children lived with their mother only and 4 percent lived with their father only (US Department of Health and Human Services, 2000). Single parents were more likely to be never married (40 percent of single mothers and 33 percent of single fathers) or divorced (34 and 44 percent) than widowed (4 and 4 percent) or separated (21 and 18 percent) (US Census Bureau, 2001).

Single parenting has also increased in Canada, with almost one in five children in Canada living with a single parent in 1996. Divorce and separation are accounting for an increasing proportion of single parenthood in Canada (roughly a third of single parents were divorced in 1996, and roughly a fifth were separated) (Statistics Canada, 1997). Australian trends moved in the same direction, with the proportion of children in single-parent families increasing steadily from 12 percent in 1989 to 18 percent in 1997 (Kilmartin, 1997). Similarly, the prevalence of single-parent families among parenting households increased—from 7 percent in 1971 to 18 percent in 1991 in the United Kingdom and from 9 percent in 1976 to 19 percent in 1991 in New Zealand (Ringen, 1997; Shirley, Koopman-Boyden, Pool, & St. John, 1997).

THEORIES AND RESEARCH

In all family types, early adolescence is a challenging developmental period for family members, as parent–child relationships are renegotiated to reflect the increasing maturity of the adolescent. Because single parents are the sole adult authority figure in the home, they are likely to face special difficulties in parenting during their children's transition to adolescence. Decision-making, responsibility, discipline, and communication are central family issues at this time, and there are distinct challenges, but also unique opportunities, in parenting an adolescent alone (Barber & Eccles, 1992). Thus, single parents and their early adolescent children are an especially important target population for education and training. Considering divorced families, Grych and Fincham (1992) suggested that developing parallel intervention groups for parents and children might be the most effective way to influence post-divorce family processes. However, despite the importance of involving parents, divorce intervention programs are usually school based, and target the individual child.

Divorce and Adolescent Adjustment

The lack of health promotion efforts for adolescents and divorced parents is troubling, in view of the fact that parental divorce has been implicated in several areas of adolescent maladjustment. Adolescents from divorced single-mother families are more likely to engage in externalizing, aggressive, non-compliant, and deviant behavior than those in married families (Amato & Keith, 1991; Dornbusch et al., 1985; Hetherington et al., 1992). Increased depression is also found in adolescents in divorced families, but the magnitude of average differences between family types is not large (Amato & Keith, 1991). Divorce has been linked to lower adolescent cognitive and scholastic performance, less

attachment to school, and higher drop-out rates (Hetherington et al., 1992). These negative effects of divorce are most common around the period of the divorce and many children and families recover from the initial distress and resume normal functioning within a few years (Hetherington, Cox, & Cox, 1982). However, a substantial number of adolescents in divorced-mother families remain at a disadvantage even 4–6 years after the divorce when compared to their peers in two-parent families, particularly in the areas of achievement, self-esteem, depression, and risky behavior (Allison & Furstenberg, 1989; Hetherington et al., 1992). Some research has also focused on self-evaluation (competency beliefs) and personal adjustment (self-esteem). The differences in self-esteem between children in divorced and always-married families are not large, and within-group variability is far greater than between-group differences. Self-evaluation, with such individual variability, may provide a domain where mental health promotion efforts might capitalize on the unique opportunities afforded for responsibility and self-direction to youth in divorced families. Thus, a framework for health promotion efforts should include adolescent adjustment in the areas of conduct problems, internalizing, intellectual functioning, and self-evaluation, and self-esteem. All of these domains have been indicated as areas in which adolescents in divorced families may be less well adjusted, and they are domains that are likely to be influenced by parenting practices (Barber, 1995; Emery, 1999).

Maternal Depression and Parenting Efficacy

Efforts to promote adolescent well-being in single-parent families should be informed by the wealth of research on family processes that are likely to enhance adjustment. However, Barber (1995) suggested that working to influence parenting is unlikely to be sufficient for promoting change. Effective functioning requires both skills and self-efficacy beliefs to use them well (Bandura, 1994). Because parental mental health problems and low sense of parenting efficacy have been found to undermine effective parenting behaviors (Furstenberg, Cook, Eccles, Elder, & Sameroff, 1999), intervention efforts should consider single parents' lower sense of parenting efficacy and higher levels of depressed mood as potential mechanisms linking divorce and less promotive parenting strategies. Equipping single parents with skills and experiences to exercise personal control over their parenting could strengthen their sense of efficacy and increase psychological well-being.

Adolescent Intrapersonal Resources

Differences in self-efficacy between divorced and married families are not limited to mothers. Nastasi and

Guidubaldi (1987) have reported that children in divorced families had lower self-efficacy than those with married parents. This difference is important, in view of the fact that efficacy is predictive of adjustment in the domains of academic achievement and successful interpersonal relationships (Nastasi & Guidubaldi, 1987). Kurdek (1988) also found that generalized feelings of mastery and control were related to positive divorce adjustment, and recommended that future intervention efforts should have a cognitive focus. Other intrapersonal characteristics have been found to relate to adolescent adjustment in divorced families, including specific competencies such as divorce-related problem-solving skills, as well as emotional well-being such as a sense of isolation and stigma (Pedro-Carroll & Cowen, 1985). Thus, intervention programs involving adolescents in divorced families should target not only the family environment, but also intrapersonal strengths, such as their sense of self-efficacy, problem-solving capabilities, and understanding of divorce.

Decision-Making, Discipline, and Control

In two parent families, both adults can collaborate on, and reinforce each other's decisions about rules and discipline. Alternatively, they may work against each other, undermining the discipline process. Single-parent families have a different authority structure. Responsibilities are redistributed, and this change may provide an opportunity for the adolescent to have more control in negotiations over rules.

Adolescents, especially boys, in divorced mother families have reported experiencing greater opportunity for involvement in several areas of decision-making and less parental control (Dornbusch et al., 1985). This greater responsibility and input into decision-making may have either positive or negative consequences, depending on its timing and its embeddedness in a detached or authoritative family climate. If it is too early for the adolescent's level of maturity, increased independence in single-parent families may lead to negative outcomes. Independence may put too much pressure on a relatively immature adolescent or it can be associated with inadequate monitoring and increased susceptibility to peer pressure (Dornbusch et al., 1985). If the increase in adult-like responsibility and decrease in parental control are timed appropriately and embedded in a warm, authoritative family environment, they can have positive consequences associated with increased self-esteem, confidence, and a sense of contribution to the family (Barber, 1995).

Processes such as parental control, discipline, and decision-making are related to family structure, and these processes can influence outcomes posited to be more negative in divorced families, such as poor school performance, problem behavior, and maladjustment (Forgatch, Patterson, &

Skinner, 1988; Patterson, 1986), or those considered to be more positive such as independence and self-esteem (Weiss, 1979). Research on these family processes suggests that providing normative developmental information about adolescence and the changing nature of family relationships during this period, in addition to exploring decision-making, monitoring techniques, and negotiation strategies, would be potentially worthwhile components of health promotion efforts for single parents and adolescents.

Expectancies

Divorced mothers have been found to have lower expectations for their children's school performance as well as satisfaction with lower school grades. Reduced expectancies such as these can play a mediating role between divorce and adolescents' lower achievement outcomes (Barber, 1995). In order to reduce these negative self-fulfilling prophesies, prevention efforts could provide information to parents and teachers about the negative effects of lowered expectations, along with the knowledge that lower achievement is not inevitable for children after divorce. Program components could address maternal expectations and standards as well as discipline issues and could focus on distinguishing between short-term (or current) and long-term (or future-oriented) expectations and standards. For example, a short-term standard may be related to what is expected relative to homework. A long-term standard has more to do with how the parents would like their adolescents lives to be in the future (e.g., hopes for their children in the future relative to family and employment). Parents' future-oriented expectations for their children are especially relevant for an adolescent-focused program, because adolescence is a developmental period characterized by the search for identity, and parents are frequently involved in that process (Barber & Eccles, 1992).

Parent–Child Relationships

During adolescence, there is a transformation in parent–adolescent relationships, including increased autonomy and conflict, but there is also substantial continuity in connection to parents (Grotevant, 1998). Across family types, adolescent development is enhanced by a warm, supportive relationship with a parent, accompanied by standards for mature behavior and consistent discipline. In single-parent families the relationship with the residential parent is crucial, because there is only one parent in the home, and that parent's connection to the adolescent may have more impact than when there is also daily input from a second parent. Because parent–adolescent support, communication, and closeness are linked to adolescent well-being, the quality of the relationship should be an important consideration in program efforts for single-parent families (Barber, 1995).

STRATEGIES: OVERVIEW

There has been very little research evaluating the efficacy of programs for children in single-parent families (Emery, 1999), and evaluations that have been published are about programs specifically for divorced families. Even less is known about promoting adolescent well-being in these families, because programs typically target younger children. One program, by Wolchik and her colleagues (1993, 2000), has demonstrated program efficacy in the early adolescent age group using a strong research design, so this work is summarized in the first section, as a strategy that works. There are other promising approaches, but they cannot be conclusively accepted as effective for adolescents given the data available so far, and are reviewed in the section on "Strategies that might work". The first group of these is the programs that are effective in enhancing adjustment of younger children in divorced families. These programs provide empirically supported strategies that may be modified in application with adolescents. Second, promising programs that target divorced parents and the family environment are discussed, including dual-component programs for mothers and their children.

STRATEGIES THAT WORK

Wolchik and colleagues (1993, 2000) have proposed a "small theory" for how a parenting program can prevent post-divorce child adjustment problems. The theory was developed from a strong base in the empirical divorce literature, and guided program development and evaluation. The *Children of Divorce Parenting Intervention* targets five components of parenting hypothesized to be mediating factors in the relationship between divorce and child adjustment: parent–child relationships, interparental conflict, discipline, contact with and support from non-parental adults, and contact with the non-custodial parent (Wolchik et al., 1993). Their first evaluation included a randomized field trial with children ages 8–15, and positive changes were found in participants' parenting practices, which in turn mediated program effects on children's adjustment and behavior (Wolchik et al., 1993). In a second trial, Wolchik and colleagues (2000) evaluated a dual component model for divorced mothers and their children ages 9–12. The mother program and the dual component program for mothers and children were both effective in improving mother–child relationships, particularly for those who entered the program with worse

relationships. The parenting program for mothers was also linked to more effective discipline strategies, and to reductions in maternal reports of internalizing and externalizing problems in their children. The program effects on externalizing were maintained at the 6-month follow-up, particularly for those with greater problems before they entered the program. The dual component program led to few additive effects over and above the mother-only program. The evaluation approach of Wolchik and her colleagues (2000) provides important information for future efforts with single parents and adolescents, in that it identifies family characteristics empirically connected to child and adolescent maladjustment, targets those for change, and includes a theory-driven evaluation.

STRATEGIES THAT MIGHT WORK

Child-Focused Divorce Programs

Programs for children of divorce are generally school based to maximize availability for children, and they typically have educational as well as therapeutic goals for the children (Pedro-Carroll, 1997; Pedro-Carroll & Cowen, 1985; Stolberg & Cullen, 1983). However, the extent to which programs are evaluated is quite limited (Grych & Fincham, 1992). Two well-evaluated programs have been reported: Stolberg and colleagues' *Divorce Adjustment Project* (DAP) for children and single parents (Stolberg & Garrison, 1985; Stolberg & Walsh, 1988), and Pedro-Carroll and Cowen's (1985) Children of Divorce Intervention Project (CODIP). The two programs target intrapersonal processes and resources. Both programs are based on the assumptions that divorce is a stressful event in children's lives, and that post-divorce adjustment can be facilitated by teaching cognitive–behavioral skills and providing emotional support. In particular, they emphasize acquiring specific competencies for dealing with divorce-related challenges.

The DAP consists of two components: the Child Support Group (CSG) and the Single-Parent Support Group (SPSG, described in next section on parent-focused programs). The CSG is a 12-session psychoeducational support group for 7–13 year olds to help them deal with the behavioral and emotional demands of the divorce. Part 1 of the 1-hr session involved discussion of specific topics; part 2 focused on teaching, modeling, and rehearsing specific skills. The DAP has been evaluated using four groups: child as participant, parent as participant, child and parent together, and a no-treatment control group (Stolberg & Garrison, 1985). The immediate post-group evaluation indicated higher self-esteem in the child-only group, and at the 5-month follow-up, this same group showed more positive social skills. Non-random assignment and pre-existing group differences (combined group children were better adjusted prior to the program) may have accounted for less improvement in the combined group.

The CODIP was based on the CSG, but places more emphasis on emotional support and problem-solving skills, divorce-related feelings, less on anger control, and relies more on experiential exercises such as discussions and role plays. The evaluation of this program has been extensive, beginning with an initial field trial with fourth- to sixth-grade children that found benefits in conduct, adjustment, and anxiety (Pedro-Carroll & Cowen, 1985). Replications (Pedro-Carroll, Alpert-Gillis, & Cowan, 1992; Pedro-Carroll, Cowen, Dirk Hightower, & Guare, 1986) have supported CODIP's role in enhancing post-divorce adjustment. CODIP has also been modified for use with younger, urban children, to reflect the developmental and sociocultural characteristics of the sample. This extension supported the program's contribution to improved child outcomes for the more heterogeneous young sample (Alpert-Gillis, Pedro-Carroll, & Cowen, 1989).

These two stress and coping interventions have proven to be quite promising for children of divorce. However, despite the strengths of the CSG and CODIP, they were initially limited to children. There is, unfortunately, very limited research on programs for adolescents.

Adolescent-Focused Divorce Programs

The CODIP has most recently been modified for use with early adolescents (Pedro-Carroll, 1997). The 12-session school-based program aims to reduce the stress of parental divorce for adolescents and to foster coping through skill building (Pedro-Carroll & Black, 1993). The early adolescent version is comprised of objectives common to all CODIP programs, such as supportive group climate, expression of feelings, and problem solving. In addition, the objectives for early adolescents incorporated age appropriate targets of promoting realistic hopes for future relationships and the capacity to trust, as well as teaching strategies for disengaging from parent conflict and being "caught in the middle." Program techniques included role-playing and creative dramatics (Pedro-Carroll, 1997). Pre-post evaluation of a pilot program suggested improved home environment and increases in adolescents' emotional adjustment, interpersonal skills, anger management, and hopefulness about future relationships and responsibilities (Pedro-Carroll & Black, 1993). The CODIP model seems to be a promising approach for early adolescents in divorced families, although further evaluation with a control group is needed to provide more compelling evidence of effectiveness.

Short (1998) reported an outcome evaluation of the *Stress Management and Alcohol Awareness Program (SMAAP)* revised somewhat for children in divorced families. The 12-session program for fifth and sixth grade students was originally designed to improve coping and assertiveness skills, modify alcohol expectancies, and increase self-esteem in children of alcoholics. Program participants reported increased problem-focused coping and self-esteem, and decreased anxiety, anti-social behavior and substance use compared to a control group. Replication of these findings with adolescents in junior high school or middle school (seventh and eighth grades) would be useful.

Parent-Focused Divorce Programs

In addition to these programs for children and adolescents in divorced families, there have been some efforts to support the single parents themselves (usually for mothers). The two types of intervention for these single women target either the efficacy of the mothers' parenting practices (family-environment focus), as in the Wolchik program described in the previous section, or the women's own adjustment to the divorce and/or single parenting (individual-level focus). Those programs aimed at adjustment of the single mother, and not directly at modifying parenting behaviors, are based on the assumption that better adjustment in the mother will lead to better parenting. One such program is the *Single-Parent Support Group* (SPSG) (Stolberg & Garrison, 1985; Stolberg & Walsh, 1988) which is a 12-week support program for divorced custodial mothers. Evaluation results show that participants displayed better divorce adjustment than did those who did not receive the program. However, no changes in child adjustment were found.

Dual Component Programs Targeting Single Mothers and Adolescents

Barber and her colleagues have developed an empirically based family intervention program designed to increase effective functioning of divorced-parent female-headed families and enhance development of early adolescents in those families (Barber, Meschke, & Zweig, 1996). *FAST* consists of two components: the Teen Awareness Group (TAG) and Effective Single Parenting (ESP). Both the mother and adolescent components have four broad goals that drove the development of program sessions. Goals 1 and 2 focus on the participants' sense of efficacy, and their attitudes and perceptions about what it means to live in a divorced family. Goal 3 focuses on expectations—present standards and future goals for the adolescent. Goal 4 targets parent–adolescent interaction directly, focusing on communication and group problem solving and negotiation. In addition, participants in the TAG and ESP groups discuss the changing nature of their relationship as the adolescent has matured, in terms of both self-disclosure and more democratic decision-making.

The program drew from strategies used in successful programs, such as interactive methods and opportunities to try out or practice new skills (Pedro-Carroll & Cowen, 1985). Activities for the adolescents in TAG were very structured, and included ice-breakers, games, role-plays, and group discussions. The ESP group for mothers was less formal, and included mostly discussion, some role plays, and brief (5–10 min) didactic presentations on adolescent developmental issues and parenting strategies considered effective during the transition to adolescence. Pre- and posttests were administered to mothers and adolescents. Mothers reported substantial decreases in depression from pretest to posttest. They also reported decreased conflict with their adolescent, and increased efficacy for helping their adolescent with schoolwork. Adolescents reported a decrease in their mothers' negative disclosure and more positive and accepting attitudes about divorced families.

FAST has now been implemented with single mothers in Australia (Pike, Nicholls, Campbell, & Sheehan, 2000). A descriptive evaluation of two FAST groups in Australia revealed substantial decreases in maternal depression and anxiety over the course of the program. Adolescent outcomes were encouraging as well, with mothers reporting decreases in adolescent internalizing and externalizing, and increased adolescent competence (Pike et al., 2000). These results are very promising, but need to be replicated with a larger sample and a comparison group.

Some studies report success for prevention programs for a broad range of child ages, without indicating whether they were differentially successful for younger children or adolescents. Soehner and his colleagues reported positive results of the Single-Parent Family Project, including decreased behavior problems and stress, and increased self-esteem and competency, for children ages 6–17 (Soehner, Zastowny, Hammond, & Taylor, 1988). It is not clear from their report, however, if the program worked for all ages, or whether the adolescent program sessions differed from the child sessions.

Divorcing-Parent Education

A number of US states have begun to mandate parent education classes for divorcing parents. However, despite widespread implementation, few evaluation studies have been conducted, and it is not known if children or adolescents benefit from their parents' attendance at these classes (Emery, 1999). Pedro-Carroll and Frazee (2001) reported on a follow-up study of ACT—For the Children (Assisting Children through Transition). This skills-based parent education program was not targeted specifically to parents of

any one age group, but the results suggest reductions in parent conflict, increases in cooperative parenting behaviors, and improved child outcomes.

STRATEGIES THAT DO NOT WORK

Intervention programs for divorcing families are, at best, moderately effective (Emery, 1999). Those with the most compelling evidence for positive outcomes have been described in the two preceding sections. The efficacy of many other programs has yet to be evaluated. Published accounts of programs that do not work are rare. In one such account, Hughes and colleagues (Hughes, Clark, Schaefer-Hernan, & Good, 1994) describe an intervention that provided divorced mothers with a series of 14 research-based newsletters on divorce-related issues and parenting. Despite the mothers' overall satisfaction with the newsletters, there were no differences found in coping, psychological well-being, or parenting between control and treatment groups.

SYNTHESIS

Adolescence is a developmental period characterized by changes in all social contexts as well as dramatic individual changes in physiology and cognitive capabilities. Early adolescence is an optimal time to intervene, given the nature, quantity, and potential synchrony of developmental transitions. Despite being a time of heightened autonomy needs, as well as of increasing susceptibility to influence from peers, early adolescence is still a period in which family influences are important, making it ideal for programs that target both the youth and the parent. For adolescents with single parents, the family is a logical and essential context to include in prevention efforts. In particular, the residential parent (most often the mother) should be a primary consideration in program implementation.

The research summarized in this entry has provided evidence regarding important influences on adolescent development in divorced families, and on the gaps in the intervention efforts for divorced families. For example, at the family level, several factors have been identified as important predictors of maladjustment. Key among these factors seems to be indicators of developmentally appropriate family environments. But, the extent to which intervention efforts for divorced families use a developmental theoretical approach is quite limited. Future health promotion programs for divorced parents could make a contribution by focusing specifically on the developmental transitions associated with early adolescence. Specifically, it will be important to consider the normative age-graded transition into junior high school, and accompanying age-related increases in family conflict, particularly over autonomy and control issues (Eccles et al., 1993). Such an approach should emphasize divorced mothers' ability to provide a developmentally responsive family context, with adequate control and monitoring, but also with opportunities for adolescent participation in family decision-making processes.

In addition to lacking an adolescent developmental focus, the few programs designed for mothers seem to come from a remedial perspective, assuming deficits in the parenting skills of divorced women. They do not focus on or work to build on the strengths of divorced-mother families, provide supports to otherwise competent but stressed mothers, and they usually do not include an emphasis on dispelling the stereotypes predominant in our culture about the pervasive negative effects of divorce. These gaps in programming provide the opportunity for a health promotion program to make an innovative contribution to both applied and basic research involving adolescents in divorced families.

In conclusion, we know that some adolescents do not fare well following parental divorce. Although growing up in a single-parent family appears to be difficult for some adolescents, there are effective existing programs designed for children that may be usefully adapted for use with adolescents. In addition, there are a few programs designed to be developmentally facilitative for adolescents, though they need to be more thoroughly evaluated before their efficacy is known. Such evaluations will provide insights into whether empirically derived prevention efforts targeting developmentally appropriate parenting practices can facilitate healthy adolescent development.

Also see: Parenting: Early Childhood; Parenting: Adolescence; Parenting: Adulthood.

References

Allison, P.D., & Furstenberg, F.F. (1989). How marital dissolution affects children: Variations by age and sex. *Developmental Psychology, 25*, 540–549.

Alpert-Gillis, L.J., Pedro-Carroll, J.L., & Cowen, E.L. (1989). The children of divorce intervention program: Development, implementation, and evaluation of a program for young urban children. *Journal of Consulting and Clinical Psychology, 57*, 583–589.

Amato, P.R. (1993). Children's adjustment to divorce: Theories, hypotheses, and empirical support. *Journal of Marriage and the Family, 55*, 23–38.

Amato, P.R., & Keith, B. (1991). Consequences of parental divorce for the well-being of children: A meta-analysis. *Psychological Bulletin, 110*, 26–46.

Bandura, A. (1994). *Self-efficacy: The exercise of control.* New York: Freeman.

Barber, B.L. (1995). Preventive intervention with adolescents and divorced mothers: A conceptual framework for program design and evaluation. *Journal of Applied Developmental Psychology, 16*, 481–503.

Barber, B.L., & Eccles, J.S. (1992). Long-term influence of divorce and single parenting on adolescent family- and work-related values, behaviors, and aspirations. *Psychological Bulletin, 111*, 108–126.

Barber, B.L., Meschke, L.L., & Zweig, J.M. (1996, November). *"Are we having fun yet?": Challenges of delivering and evaluating a theory-driven program for early adolescents and their mothers.* Paper presented at the annual conference of the National Council on Family Relations, Kansas City.

Buchanan, C.M., Maccoby, E.E., & Dornbusch, S.M. (1996). *Adolescents after divorce.* Cambridge, MA: Harvard University Press.

Dornbusch, S.M., Carlsmith, J.M., Bushwall, S.J., Ritter, P.L., Leiderman, H., Hastorf, A.H., & Gross, R.T. (1985). Single parents, extended households, and the control of adolescents. *Child Development, 56*, 326–341.

Eccles, J.S., Midgley, C., Wigfield, A., Miller Buchanan, C., Reuman, D., Flanagan, C., & Mac Iver, D. (1993). Development during adolescence: The impact of stage-environment fit on young adolescents' experiences in schools and in families. *American Psychologist, 48*, 90–101.

Emery, R.E. (1999). *Marriage, divorce, and children's adjustment.* Thousand Oaks, CA: Sage.

Forgatch, M.S., Patterson, G.R., & Skinner, M.L. (1988). A mediational model for the effect of divorce on antisocial behavior in boys. In E.M. Hetherington & J.D. Arasteh (Eds.), *Impact of divorce, single parenting, and stepparenting on children* (pp. 135–154). Hillsdale, NJ: Erlbaum.

Furstenberg, F.F., Cook, T.D., Eccles, J., Elder, G.H., & Sameroff, A. (1999). *Managing to make it: Urban families and adolescent success.* Chicago: University of Chicago Press.

Grotevant, H.D. (1998). Adolescent development in family contexts. In W. Damon (Editor-in-chief) & N. Eisenberg (Vol. Ed.), *Handbook of child psychology: Vol. 3. Social, Emotional and personality development* (5th ed., pp. 1097–1149). New York: Wiley.

Grych, J.H., & Fincham, F.D. (1992). Interventions for children of divorce: Toward greater integration of research and action. *Psychological Bulletin, 111*, 434–454.

Hetherington, E.M., Cox, M., & Cox, R. (1982). Effects of divorce on parents and children. In M. Lamb (Ed.), *Nontraditional families* (pp. 233–288). Hillsdale, NJ: Erlbaum.

Hetherington, E.M., Clingempeel, W.G., Anderson, E.R., Deal, J.E., Hagan, M.S., Hollier, E.A., & Lindner, M.S. (1992). Coping with marital transitions: A family systems perspective. *Monographs of the Society for Research in Child Development, 57*, 1–24.

Hughes, R., Jr., Clark, C.D., Schaefer-Hernan, P., & Good, E.S. (1994). An evaluation of a newsletter intervention for divorced mothers. *Family Relations, 43*, 298–304.

Kilmartin, C. (1997). Children, divorce, and one-parent families. *Family Matters, 48*, 34–35.

Kurdek, L.A. (1988). Cognitive mediators of children's adjustment to divorce. In S.A. Wolchik & P. Karoly (Eds.), *Children of divorce: Empirical perspectives on adjustment.* New York: Gardner Press.

Martin, T.C., & Bumpass, L.L. (1989). Recent trends in marital disruption. *Demography, 26*(1), 37–51.

Nastasi, B.K., & Guidubaldi, J. (1987, April). *Coping skills as mediators of children's adjustment in divorced and intact families.* Paper presented at the biennial meeting for the Society for Research in Child Development, Baltimore, MD.

Patterson, G.R. (1986). Performance models for antisocial boys. *American Psychologist, 41*, 432–444.

Pedro-Carroll, J. (1997). The Children of Divorce Intervention Program: Fostering resilient outcomes for school-aged children. In G. W. Albee & T.P. Gullotta (Eds.), *Primary prevention works* (pp. 213–238). Thousand Oaks: Sage.

Pedro-Carroll, J., & Black, A.E. (1993). *The children of divorce intervention program: Preventative outreach to early adolescents* (Final report to the Gottschalk Mental Health Research Grant). Rochester, New York: University of Rochester, Center for Community Study.

Pedro-Carroll, J.L., & Cowen, E.L. (1985). The Children of Divorce Intervention Program: An investigation of the efficacy of a school based prevention program. *Journal of Consulting and Clinical Psychology, 53*, 603–611.

Pedro-Carroll, J.L., Alpert-Gillis, L.J., & Cowen, E.L. (1992). An evaluation of the efficacy of a preventative intervention for 4th–6th grade urban children of divorce. *Journal of Primary Prevention, 13*, 115–130.

Pedro-Carroll, J.L., Cowen, E.L., Dirk Hightower, A., & Guare, J.C. (1986). Preventive intervention with latency-aged children of divorce: A replication study. *American Journal of Community Psychology, 41*, 277–290.

Pedro-Carroll, J.P., & Frazee, E. (2001). Program can help protect children in break-ups. *New York Law Journal.*

Pike, L., Nicholls, W., Campbell, R., & Sheehan, M. (2000, February). *Families and successful teens: A preventative intervention approach to single parent families. Report on a pilot programme.* Paper Presented at the Helping Families Change Conference, Queensland University, Brisbane, Australia.

Ringen, S. (1997). Great Britain. In S.B. Kamerman & A.J. Kahn (Eds.), *Family change and family policies in Great Britain, Canada, New Zealand, and the United States* (pp. 29–102). Oxford: Clarendon Press.

Shirley, I., Koopman-Boyden, P., Pool, I., & St. John, S. (1997). New Zealand. In S.B. Kamerman & A.J. Kahn (Eds.), *Family change and family policies in Great Britain, Canada, New Zealand, and the United States* (pp. 207–304). Clarendon Press: Oxford.

Short, J.L. (1998). Evaluation of a substance abuse prevention and mental health promotion program for children of divorce. *Journal of Divorce & Remarriage, 28*(3/4), 139–155.

Soehner, G., Zastowny, T., Hammond, A., & Taylor, L. (1988). The Single Parent Family Project: A community-based, preventive program for single-parent families. *Journal of Child & Adolescent Psychotherapy, 5*(1), 35–43.

Statistics Canada. (1997). *The Daily—1996 census: marital status, common-law unions and families* [on-line database]. (October 14, 1997). Available: http://www.statcan.ca/Daily/English/971014/d971014.htm

Stolberg, A.L., & Cullen, P.M. (1983). Preventive interventions for families of divorce: The Divorce Adjustment Project. In L.A. Kurdek (Ed.), *Children and divorce: New directions for child development* (No. 19, pp. 71–81). San Francisco: Jossey Bass.

Stolberg, A.L., & Garrison, K.M. (1985). Evaluating a primary prevention program for children of divorce. *American Journal of Community Psychology, 13*, 111–124.

Stolberg, A.L., & Walsh, P. (1988). A review of treatment methods for children of divorce. In S.A. Wolchik & P. Karoly (Eds.), *Children of divorce: Empirical perspectives on adjustment.* New York: Gardner Press.

US Census Bureau. (2001). *Population profile of the United States: 1999* (Current Population Reports, Series P23-205). Washington, DC: US Government Printing Office.

US Department of Health and Human Services. (2000). *Trends in the well-being of America's children and youth.* Washington, DC: US Government Printing Office.

Weiss, R.S. (1979). Growing up a little faster: The experience of growing up in a single-parent household. *Journal of Social Issues, 35*, 97–111.

Wolchik, S.A., West, S.G., Westover, S., Sandler, I.N., Martin, A., Lustig, J., Tein, J., & Fisher, J. (1993). The children of divorce parenting intervention: Outcome evaluation of an empirically based program. *American Journal of Community Psychology, 21*, 293–331.

Wolchik, S.A., West, S.G., Sandler, I.N., Tein, J., Coatsworth, D., Lengua, L., Weiss, L., Anderson, E.R., Greene, S.M., & Griffin, W.A. (2000). An experimental evaluation of theory-based mother and mother–child programs for children of divorce. *Journal of Consulting and Clinical Psychology, 68*, 843–856.

Parenting, Adulthood

Mark E. Feinberg and Gregory S. Pettit

INTRODUCTION

Although recent research and debate has challenged the view that parenting is a key influence on children's development and adjustment, the importance of positive parenting is accepted by most developmental researchers. This entry summarizes some of the important views on how parenting can be conceptualized, factors that influence parenting, and programs that have achieved some success in helping parents learn and use more positive parenting behaviors.

DEFINITIONS

Authoritarian refers to parenting that is high in limit setting but low in open communication. *Authoritative* parenting is high in limit setting but also high in communication. *Lax* or *negligent* parenting is low in both limit setting and communication.

Differential parenting refers to parents who frequently treat siblings with differing levels of warmth or negativity. Although this may be an indication of favoritism, there is also evidence that parents may be responding to different characteristics in the children.

Monitoring involves knowledge of the child's whereabouts, activities, and companions; efforts directed to obtaining such knowledge through solicitation of information and creating a climate conducive to child disclosure; and actual, successful regulation and management of child behavior.

Social Skills Coaching/Teaching involves parents who provide information and guidance about peer relationships and feedback on children's efforts to initiate and sustain peer interaction.

Proactive Involvement refers to parents who anticipate possible problem behaviors and employ pre-emptive strategies such as distraction, positive engagement, humor, and conversation to minimize its occurrence.

Coercive Cycle occurs when a parent and child attempt to achieve victory in a confrontation through coercive means. Typically, escalation of negative, punitive, or aversive behavior takes place until one individual gives in. If a child is able to achieve certain goals often enough through such means, reinforcement of coercive behavior is believed to take place and it becomes more frequent.

THEORIES

"Parenting" is a set of complex behaviors parents enact toward children that have multiple aspects, including physical, verbal, and emotional displays of affection and negativity; monitoring, discipline, and punitiveness; sensitivity and responsivity; teaching and guiding; direct childcare (feeding, clothing, bathing) and other tasks (securing medical care, arranging for childcare and schooling). There are three types of theory relevant to this broad category of parenting: theories of what aspects of parenting are important for child development, theories of what factors influence parenting, and theories of change in parental attitudes and behaviors.

Theorists from different orientations agree that emotionally warm, sensitive parenting that additionally includes clearly articulated and enacted limits is most beneficial for children. For example, *attachment theory* suggests that consistent, responsive, care-taking influences the quality—the security—of the attachment relationship that develops between parent and child. From this relationship, children are thought to develop a set of expectations and beliefs that serve as a guide for relations with others over the life course. Responsive care-taking requires a sensitivity to emerging issues and challenges in early development, including helping children to manage anxiety-provoking experiences, such as being frightened or being left alone for brief periods. Although the parenting attributes underlying attachment quality evolve and become more complex over the course of the childhood years, at root is a core sense of security that the child–parent relationship will provide for consistent management of needs and protection from environmental threats. These core elements of the attachment relationship are hypothesized to form the framework within which relationships develop with others throughout the life cycle.

Another perspective on parenting and its role in children's adjustment emphasizes the interlocking nature of child behavior and parental response, and points out how reinforcement contingencies can foster the development of distinct behavioral patterns in both children and parents. Adopting a *social learning perspective*, Patterson, Capaldi, and Bank (1991) have convincingly demonstrated that if

certain kinds of behaviors (such as child noncompliance to parental requests) lead to sufficient reinforcement (such as parents' capitulating or "giving in" in the face of child resistance), then such behaviors will tend to persist, even if the reinforcement is accompanied by negative experiences. Even though reinforcement is only probabilistic, over time children learn to repeat and refine these behaviors. In this vein, the work of Patterson and colleagues on antisocial behavior in children has highlighted the importance of effective limit setting in reducing the likelihood of coercive exchanges between parent and child.

The role of *behavioral contingencies* in maladaptive development also has been emphasized by Wahler and colleagues (e.g., Wahler & Bellamy, 1997; Wahler & Megennis, 1997). As pointed out by Wahler (1997), interpersonal encounters in families with behavior-problem children are more likely to be volatile and unpredictable, creating a climate in which coherent social "rules" are difficult to discern. Some children may attempt to create greater predictability and interactional coherence by engaging in negative behaviors designed to elicit some reaction—even a punitive reaction—from parents. Making parents more aware of the connections between their actions and their children's responses appears to be one potentially useful way of reducing children's disruptive behavior.

Many theorists have attempted to devise a typology of parenting based on essential aspects of parenting. One of the most widely cited is Baumrind's *responsive/demanding typology*, which involves consideration of both the level of openness of communication, warmth, or responsiveness with a child, as well as the level of direction, demandingness, or limit setting (Baumrind, 1991). The level of responsiveness refers to the degree to which parents are open to, or accommodate to the child's particular needs and concerns. The level of demandingness refers to the degree to which parents demand that the child conform to, or is assimilated into, standards and norms set by the parents, family, and society. Crossing responsiveness and demandingness yields a fourfold typology: authoritative (high on both aspects), authoritarian (low responsiveness, high limit setting), neglectful (low on both), and permissive (high responsiveness, low limit setting).

It has been noted that parenting "types" reflect a mixture of different parenting behaviors and styles, and that examining the role of these individual constituents may be an important direction for understanding the ways in which parenting may influence children (Darling & Steinberg, 1993). The stylistic qualities of parenting, such as warmth and firmness, may be associated with certain kinds of child outcomes by virtue of their shared association with specific parenting practices. For example, authoritative parents may have children who excel academically because authoritative parents encourage and monitor academically relevant activities. Likewise, warm and responsive parents may have socially skilled children because such parents provide good models of interpersonal effectiveness and provide explicit guidance in, and support of, social skills and competencies (Mize & Pettit, 1997).

In examining the influences on parenting, Belsky has offered a comprehensive *contextual-familial model* of the determinants of parenting that involves three domains: parent characteristics, child characteristics, and the social context (Belsky, 1984). Individual parent characteristics include personality traits and emotional health/psychopathology (e.g., depression). To some extent, parental characteristics that influence both parental styles and parental behavior may themselves be partly influenced by heritable factors. For example, behavioral genetic research suggests that parent's genetic factors may influence aspects of parenting such as overprotection and care, and may influence mothers' parenting more than fathers' parenting (Perusse, Neale, Heath, & Eaves, 1994). It should be noted that behavioral genetic research is often pointed to as a guide for determining where intervention targets may lie; that is, if certain behaviors are strongly influenced by genetic factors and not environmental ones, those behaviors may not be amenable to intervention. Conversely, behaviors under predominantly environmental control are thought to be appropriate targets of change. This use of behavioral genetic research is not completely appropriate as a means of identifying intervention targets, as estimates of genetic and environmental contributions are made within the existing genetic and environmental parameters in which a population develops. Interventions change the environmental parameters, and as such may alter the relative contributions of genetic and environmental factors (Maccoby, 2000).

In any case, parents' own *experiences* growing up in their family of origin also influence parenting behaviors. Additionally, individual's experiences are important contributors to parental cognitions—for example, knowledge, beliefs, and attitudes about children and childrearing—which are thought to influence parenting. For example, in an attributional schema, parents' attributions of their children's behavior has been theorized to link child behavior with parental response (McGillicuddy-De Lisi & Sigel, 1995). Parental knowledge of child development and expectations for their own children also are theorized as important. For example, parents who have expectations of children that are not in line with developmental limitations and progress are more frequently abusive toward children (Bavolek, 1989).

Some researchers have suggested that characteristics of children also influence parenting. For example, parenting behaviors that are more directive and punitive may be evoked by children who are defiant or aggressive. Such influences are known as "child effects," and empirical research has shown that some aspects of parenting are partly influenced by child behaviors (Feinberg, Neiderhiser, Howe, & Hetherington, 2000a; Lytton, 1990). It also appears that parental cognitions—including beliefs about the importance of social skills and behaviors, and the modifiability of those behaviors—stem partly from parents' experiences with their children. Parents of socially competent children tend to believe that social skills are important attributes for children to develop, that such skills can be taught, and that parents' efforts to teach such skills are instrumental in their development (Eron *et al.*, 2002).

Relationships within the family, especially martial conflict, also influence parenting (Emery, 1982; Feinberg, submitted). When conflict is intense and frequent, parents may become too emotionally involved in their own conflict to provide consistent warmth and discipline for their children. The negativity of marital interactions may also spill over and parents may become negative to children as well. Recently, theorists and researchers have focused on the coparenting alliance as an influence on parenting. The coparental alliance refers to the relationship of parents to each other in their roles as parents (e.g., supportive vs. undermining), and is conceptually and empirically distinct from the marital relationship. A positive coparenting alliance may alleviate the negative effects of marital conflict on parenting and child adjustment.

Important influences on parenting are also found within the wider social context or social environment (Bronfenbrenner, 1986). Social networks and social support (Crnic & Greenberg, 1987; Cutrona, 1996; Dunn, 1988) are very important influences on parents' ability to manage stress and provide warm and responsive parenting. Socioeconomic factors also influence parenting. Although this brief review is oversimplified, lower socioeconomic status (SES) parents may be generally more concerned about child conformity with accepted standards and are more directive, controlling, restrictive, and disapproving with children (Dodge, Pettit, & Bates, 1994); higher SES parents tend to place greater value on initiative and independence, and are generally more verbal with their children. Such differences may be related to values and strategies for success at work and in the world that parents learn in the context of their social and work relationships. Regardless of SES, relationships and stress at work may also influence parenting at home. Finally, cultural attitudes and beliefs among ethnic, religious, or other groups are also important influences on parenting and on the ways that children interpret parenting behavior. Such group differences are important for interventionists to recognize in program design.

The third area of theory relates to how parents change. From a cognitive perspective, Goodnow proposes that parents may anticipate parenting decisions and seek information before they need it. This information-gathering period may be the best time to influence parental cognitions (Goodnow, 1995). Goodnow also proposes that change in parenting is most likely when the prevailing mood is positive, and when seeking information or change does not incur judgments from others. Change is also most likely when the new parenting model or skill is in line with a parent's conception of his or her role and social identity.

Some researchers have broached the subject of what typical pattern of change during an intervention demonstrates the best prognosis for maintenance of improved parenting skills. Some researchers have suggested and found that parents who are initially resistant to new ideas and behaviors, but then work through the issues associated with adopting new methods of parenting, do better at follow-up than parents who simply adopt the new skills from the beginning of a program and show linear improvement (Hanish & Tolan, 2001). The process of initial resistance and struggle to accept a new set of behaviors may indicate a deeper level of processing and assimilation of the new behaviors into the parent's complex behavior pattern.

Owing to space considerations, we are unable to detail the many and varied facets of parenting that may bear on many important outcomes such as children's cognitive competence, independent initiative, empathy, conscience, positive peer relations, and other developmental outcomes. But it should be recognized that effective parenting in these domains is frequently associated with the dual accomplishment of balancing warmth/sensitivity with the ability to set firm limits when necessary.

RESEARCH

Research suggests that mothers and fathers are similarly suited to provide warm and sensitive parenting (Lamb, 1995). In many cases, however, social attitudes and the greater amount of time mothers spend with infants lead mothers to become more sensitive to infant cues, with the effect that mothers come to be seen as more expert in the area of caring for children. Consistent with this premise is evidence suggesting role specialization in childrearing, with mothers more typically assuming nurturing and caregiving roles and fathers more typically assuming the role of playmate and disciplinarian (Russell & Saebel, 1997). Moreover, when parents enact the same role or set of behaviors, their actions may have differing consequences for their children. For example, Pettit, Brown, Mize, and Lindsey (1998) showed that mothers' (but not fathers') social teaching was associated with children's social skillfulness, whereas fathers' (but not mothers') playful involvement was associated with

children's peer competence. To the extent that either parent adopts one style to the exclusion of the other, child adjustment will likely suffer. Research utilizing Baumrind's responsive/demanding typology demonstrates that employing both sensitivity, warmth, and open communication with firm limit setting and discipline is optimal for child development.

However, more recent efforts aimed at understanding the role of parenting in children's development have shifted away from the typological approach popularized by Baumrind so as to illuminate the critical constituents of broad parenting types and to trace their links with differing kinds of child adjustment outcomes. Barber (1996), for example, drew attention to the distinction between psychological (i.e., autonomy stunting) and behavioral forms of parental control, and showed that child and adolescent delinquent behavior was associated more strongly with lack of behavioral control, whereas anxiety, depression, and related internalizing problems was associated more strongly with psychological control (e.g., guilt induction, intrusiveness). The roots of these differing forms of parenting were examined by Pettit, Laird, Bates, Dodge, and Criss (2001). Proactive parenting in early childhood forecasted effective behavioral regulation and monitoring in early adolescence, whereas early harsh discipline predicted later use of psychological control.

That effective parenting is multidimensional has now received considerable support in the literature. Patterson, Reid, and Dishion (1992) demonstrated that positive reinforcement, problem solving, and involvement were separate and distinguishable forms of positive parenting. Pettit and colleagues (Pettit, Bates, & Dodge, 1993, 1997) have reported that positive parenting is both multidimensional and empirically nonredundant with negative parenting in its relations with child adjustment. Building on the style versus practice distinction (Darling & Steinberg, 1993), Mize and Pettit (1997; Pettit & Mize, 1993) found that socially competent preschoolers had mothers who displayed a synchronous, responsive interaction style and who also engaged in constructive coaching of social skills. In other words, both the interactional climate or milieu that parents engineer, as well as the specific content of teaching and coaching, appear to be important contributors to child adjustment and well-being.

The critical dimensions of parenting are still much debated, but accumulating evidence suggests that consistency, responsiveness, and affective positivity figure prominently in effective parenting. Specific parenting practices also may be important, although the specification of those practices that might be central for the development of particular skills, competencies, and orientations is as yet incomplete.

STRATEGIES THAT WORK

The use of nurses or paraprofessionals to visit mothers during pregnancy and the early childhood years has a long history, and such programs are widespread and relatively well-supported by state and federal agencies and private foundations. However, few home visiting programs have demonstrated substantial effects in rigorous research studies. David Old's program of *prenatal home visitation* by nurses is an often-cited exception (Olds, 1999). The program targets high-risk mothers (e.g., low income, single) for biweekly visits during pregnancy and the first 2 years of the child's life (with more frequent visits immediately postpartum, and less frequent during the last 3 months). The home visitors employ a range of strategies and techniques to enhance prenatal health, child health, maternal responsiveness and parenting, and maternal life-course (repeat pregnancy, education, work).

Evidence from trials of this program in New York, Tennessee, and Colorado, indicate that the program has positive effects on pregnancy outcomes, child development, and maternal life course. In the present context, the program's effects on maternal caregiving are highlighted. Results indicate that among women with low incomes or identified as having relatively few psychological resources, nurse home visiting results in fewer emergency health care visits for injuries and ingestions, and fewer verified child abuse and neglect reports. In the Tennessee trial, nurse-visited women held fewer beliefs associated with child abuse, and had homes rated as more conducive to healthy child development. The children of nurse-visited women were observed as more communicative and responsive to their mothers. It is important to note that the Olds' program had positive long-term effects on the children of poor unmarried women (but not for the children of other women) at age 15 in the New York trial, including outcomes such as arrest, sexual activity, alcohol, and drug use.

Although more study of long-term effects are needed, several behavioral and cognitive–behavioral parent training programs have demonstrated success in promoting positive parenting. A meta-analysis reported that studies have shown behavioral parent training to be fairly effective in reducing antisocial behavior in children and improving parental personal adjustment (Serketich & Dumas, 1996). For example, Webster-Stratton's *Incredible, Years* program has demonstrated a high level of effectiveness in reducing family management problems, and thus reducing antisocial behavior in children. The series of group sessions focuses on teaching parents, through videotaped vignettes and discussion, how to set clear expectations for children's behavior, monitor and reward behavior, play in a positive way with children, avoid or ignore misbehavior, and use time out and other consequences effectively. One-year follow-up of treatment groups in parent training, child training, and both parent and child training formats have demonstrated fewer negative and more positive behaviors, and less spanking than at baseline. Improved positive parenting strategies and interactions were observed in home visits (Webster-Stratton & Hammond, 1997).

Two other group format parent training programs— The *Iowa Strengthening Families Program* (ISFP) and *Parenting for the Drug Free Years* (PDFY; Kosterman, Hawkins, Spoth, Haggerty, & Zhu, 1997; Spoth, Redmond, & Shin, 1998)—have also been demonstrated as effective in fostering positive parenting behaviors. Like The Incredible Years, PDFY utilizes videotapes to standardize presentation and demonstrate concepts through vignettes. Both ISFP and PDFY are relatively short (5–7 sessions) and intended to be delivered universally. Both also include a component that helps parents (and their children) develop skills to keep children away from drugs and alcohol. An evaluation of these programs found that their influence on targeted parenting behaviors (involvement of children in family decisions; anger management; supportive communication) mediated the program's influence on more general behaviors and parenting styles, such as affective quality, monitoring, and consistent discipline.

A comprehensive behavioral approach to fostering positive parenting has been created by Sanders and colleagues in Australia. *Triple P (Positive Parenting Program)* involves a series of graded levels of interventions (Sanders, 1999). A video series, program guide, and other materials describing positive behavioral parenting techniques represent the first, universal level of intervention. The subsequent levels of indicated and selected interventions may be delivered by health care professionals trained to deliver Triple P in pediatricians' offices. At a second level of intervention, the provider may provide brief advice or consultation to parents in the context of a routine health check-up in reference to a discrete, mild child behavior problem. More extensive behavioral skill training for parents may take place at a third level of intervention involving 1–4 training sessions. The fourth level is designed for parents with children who have more severe behavioral problems; a more intensive parent skills training program is conducted. In the "standard" format, 10 clinic sessions are combined with home visits. An 8-week group format has also been created, along with a self-directed workbook study format. The group and self-directed formats may be supplemented by brief consultation phone calls. The self-directed format may be especially useful for rural families where transportation issues are problematic. Finally, for families in which child behavior problems coexist with family dysfunction, a combination of clinic sessions and home visits focuses on parenting, mood management, stress coping, and partner support skills.

Triple P has demonstrated effectiveness in repeated evaluations. Parents watching the 12 episodes of the television series on videotape, but not a control group, reported a significant and substantial reduction of disruptive child behaviors, increased parenting confidence, and a decrease in negative parenting practices. The more intensive delivery formats have also shown significant effects on child and parent outcomes (Sanders, 1999). Sanders and colleagues have also designed extensions of the basic Triple-P model for parents with depression, stepfamilies, and other specific situations. In addition, a school-based program has been designed to help parents provide positive encouragement to children during the transition to school.

STRATEGIES THAT MIGHT WORK

The quality of the mother–infant relationship in the first months of life is an important relational foundation that has implications for future development. One simple technique that may be effective in promoting this early relationship is the mother's use of front-pack carriers to hold and carry infants. Infants whose mothers were given a front-pack carrier, compared to those given an infant seat, demonstrated substantially higher rates of secure attachment at 13 months in one study (Anisfeld, Casper, Nozyce, & Cunningham, 1990). Further examination of this simple intervention is warranted.

More active promotion of parent–child attachment security through individual intervention seems to hold promise. For example, in one study, mothers of irritable infants were provided with only three, 2-hr home-visit intervention sessions when the babies were between 6 and 9 months old (van den Boom, D., 1997; van den Boom, D.C., 1995). The mothers were helped to attend and sensitively respond to their infants. After the intervention, and at follow-up when the infant was 12, 18, 24, and 42 months, the intervention group mothers were more sensitive, stimulating, and attentive than in the control group; the intervention group babies were more securely attached, more cooperative, and more positive in peer relations than control infants.

The strategy of helping parents to attend to the temperamentally influenced individual characteristics of their infants is also utilized in the *STEEP* program (Erickson, Korfmacher, & Egeland, 1993). The program involves the use of videotape recordings of mother–infant interaction. The interventionist uses the videotapes as a reference point in asking parents about how the baby is communicating as

well as their own strengths in responding. Initial data indicate that the program is effective.

One of the recurrent problems in parent programs is obtaining adequate parent interest and motivation to prevent high rates of attrition. Techniques to engage parents and motivating them to be part of the behavior change process are a neglected aspect of prevention. In general, program designers have used incentives such as money, food, or coupons, and facilitated participation through child care and transportation assistance. A relatively new and promising approach is the Family Check Up, developed as part of the *Adolescent Transitions Programs* (Dishion et al., 2002; Dishion & Andrews, 1995), and based on a program focusing on adult problem drinking. The basic notion is that motivational interviewing techniques are embedded in a three session, home-visit format (although sessions can also be held in a clinic or school office as well). The first session is an introductory intake interview in which rapport is built with the family. The second session involves standardized assessment procedures. The third session, building on the rapport established in the first sessions, focuses on feedback in a framework in which the family becomes an interactive partner and opens into consideration of whether several intervention options might be useful.

Another area of recent interest is the relationship of the parents to each other and how that affects their parenting and the child. For at least 20 years, it has been known that the marital relationship, especially conflict, influences parenting and child outcomes (Emery, 1982). More recently, researchers have begun to examine the relationship of husbands and wives to each other specifically in their roles as parents. This element of the overall marital relationship, the coparenting alliance, appears to play an important role in affecting the quality of parenting. The Cowans' *Becoming a Family* project helped focus attention on the transition to parenthood period as a time when intervention can focus on the marital or coparental relationship. Because of the intensive nature of the intervention used in their study (25 pre- and post-natal sessions, two psychologists as facilitators in each group of four couples), their program is not a realistic model for widespread prevention. However, the program did demonstrate strong effects in improving parents' experience during the transition period—for example, depression and separation/divorce were lower among the intervention group compared to a control group (although the effects appear to dissipate over the course of several years; Cowan & Cowan, 2000).

The Cowans' work has encouraged others to develop other programs that may be more easily disseminable. For example, Feinberg (2001) is developing a preventive intervention designed to enhance coparenting relations during the transition to parenthood. In addition, several established marital intervention researchers are currently adapting their programs to the prenatal and infancy periods.

STRATEGIES THAT DO NOT WORK

Given the file drawer problem in academic social science research (i.e., researchers and journal editors have little inclination to publish non-significant findings), it is difficult to detail interventions that do not work to promote parenting. Further, the absence of significant effects may not be due to an unsound intervention design, but rather problems in implementation, contextual issues, or a mismatch of the program and the target population. Interventions that do not seem to work are typically not replicated in a variety of contexts and with a number of cultural, ethnic, and social class strata. Thus, it is easier to determine what interventions do work than which ones do not.

One recent exception to this scientific bias is a report about a parenting program that *increased* child aggression only in those schools that were located in inner-city neighborhoods (Tolan, 2001). This report follows on recent research suggesting that aggregating high-risk youth into groups for interventions may have negative effects, probably as a result of increased "deviancy training" within the resulting group (Dishion, McCord, & Poulin, 1999). In the parenting program case, a school-based program for youth had positive effects, as did a full package of youth and parent programs in non-inner city schools. However, the addition of the parenting program in the inner city schools led to negative effects, perhaps as a result of overloading already stressed parents with one more service/program obligation, or perhaps as a result of aggregating parents with attitudes toward violence rooted in social conditions that promoted a view of aggression as a self-defensive strategy in a hostile or dangerous environment.

A recent report indicated that two welfare-to-work comprehensive "support" programs for young, single, poor mothers that included parenting classes had little positive benefit, but instead negative effects on families (Reichman & McLanahan, 2001). For example, the New Chance program, which included weekly parenting and life-skills classes, increased mothers' stress and aggravation with their children. Mothers who had high depression symptom scores at the beginning showed the highest increases in stress. These studies are important as they indicate that parenting interventions may have negative effects; that highly stressed parents may feel overwhelmed rather than helped by additional programs; and that comprehensive social programs may lead to positive changes in some areas, such as mothers' pursuit of education or employment, but lead to higher levels of family- and child-related stress.

SYNTHESIS

Many strategies have been used in an attempt to foster positive parenting, and several have been demonstrated to be effective. The most successful models combine a focus on specific parenting behaviors, a comprehensive approach addressing the needs of families with differing levels of risk, and program delivery through established institutional structures that do not involve stigmatization, and attention to the cultural and ecological contexts of the target population.

Behavioral interventions have generally demonstrated the greatest positive effects in studies of treatment for child and family dysfunction (Lochman, 1990). Thus it is not surprising that behavioral interventions have also generally been shown to be most effective in prevention programs. The relative success of behavioral interventions targeting specific parenting behaviors and practices may be due to two factors: First, it is easier to change such behaviors, rather than general parent characteristics and styles. Second, more general characteristics may change as a result of specific behavioral improvements. Researchers interested in altering parents' own working models of attachment in order to change their caregiving capacity, for example, have sometimes used a broader psychodynamic strategy in which the relationship between parent and intervention staff is seen as the change agent. Such strategies may be useful when delivered in an intensive design, utilizing skilled staff, and integrated with cognitive–behavioral techniques (Heinicke, 1993).

As examples of programs that have had negative effects on families have emerged, it is important to consider such a possibility. Typically, program developers consider no benefit to be the worst-case scenario. However, actually causing harm to already stressed parents and families is a distinct possibility. To guard against the development of programs that lead to negative effects, program developers and implementers should be careful to consider the perceptions and feedback from participants: Do they feel the program is beneficial or burdensome? Do they agree with the goals and techniques promoted? Focus groups may be a useful way of gauging participant responsivity to the planned intervention before implementation. And, of course, researchers should consider and assess whether aspects of interventions have had negative effects—and report such results for the benefit of the prevention field.

As mentioned above, one of the common difficulties faced by family-focused prevention programs is the typically low rate of participation and high rate of dropout. One obstacle is that parents, in their role as parents, are generally busy. The importance of the issue of participation cannot be underestimated: if programs only succeed in reaching families most disposed to participating in the first place, higher risk families will not be included. Programs that have succeeded in achieving high rates of participation often seek out parents in their own homes, or provide a combination of incentives and amenities. Further, programs often succeed when they involve parents at key transition points—such as the transition to parenthood itself, or the child's transition to school. Parents may be more open and interested in learning at these times. Finally, similarity of parent and staff person characteristics, as well as relevant life experiences of the staff person, were shown to be related to parent engagement with home visiting family coordinators in the FAST TRACK program, which was then related to parent participation in group sessions (Orrell-Valente, Pinderhughes, Valente, & Laird, 1999).

Another common feature of successful programs is the maintenance of program fidelity. One of the reasons the Olds' home visiting program has been more successful than other similar programs may be partly due to attention to this issue. The use of videotapes to convey concepts and information to parents in programs is another way that fidelity has been fostered; however, the use of videotapes is not the only means by which fidelity can be achieved in group settings. Facilitators should undergo training, receive supervision, and meet minimal skill requirements.

Given the difficulties of engaging families in prevention programs, and given the obstacles to disseminating prevention programs generally, the delivery of family focused prevention through pre-existing institutional structures may be most effective. Thus, the Triple P's implementation through the health care system, which is universally utilized and entails no stigma, is a leading example of how this can be achieved. To facilitate the widespread use of Triple P or other such programs, however, systemic changes in insurance coverage are needed that would reimburse providers for the delivery of empirically supported prevention models. Another delivery mechanism, perhaps the most common one, is the promotion of parent training and intervention through the school system. Frequently, school-based programs have utilized a family component in the context of comprehensive, multicomponent programs (e.g., FAST TRACK, Chicago Metropolitan Area Study, ATP). However, limitations of design and cost have prevented the accumulation of much data on the *value-added* potential of a family component in a larger, school-based intervention program.

The economic value of prevention is now a key question. As in other fields of prevention, programs have now been designed and shown to be effective. The future of widespread dissemination of effective prevention programs for parents and families may hinge on the ability of preventionists to attract ongoing funding for institutionalized programs. To attract or argue for such funding, however, preventionists need better data on long-term effects and on the cost/benefit ratio of the programs. The ability of promoters to demonstrate cost/benefit data has helped the dissemination of Olds' nurse home visiting program, for example. Moving research in these directions requires collaboration and political organization among preventionists and child/family advocates to prompt funding agencies to earmark resources to such long-term, high-quality studies. Thus, the prevention field is in a state in which researchers need community and political support, as much as community and political advocates need researchers' to focus on practical issues.

Also see: Parenting: Early Childhood; Parenting: Adolescence; Parenting, Single Parent: Adolescence; Single-Parent Families: Childhood; Marital Satisfaction: Adulthood.

References

Anisfeld, E., Casper, V., Nozyce, M., & Cunningham, N. (1990). Does infant carrying promote attachment? An experimental study of the effects of increased physical contact on the development of attachment. *Child Development, 61*, 1617–1627.

Barber, B.K. (1996). Parental psychological control: Revisiting a neglected construct. *Child Development, 67*, 3296–3319.

Baumrind, D. (1991). The influence of parenting style on adolescent competence and substance use. *Journal of Early Adolescence, 11*, 56–95.

Bavolek, S.J. (1989). Assessing and treating high-risk parenting attitudes. *Early Child Development and Care, 42*, 99–112.

Belsky, J. (1984). The determinants of parenting: A process model. *Child Development, 55*, 83–96.

Bronfenbrenner, U. (1986). Ecology of the family as a context for human development: Research perspectives. *Developmental Psychology, 22*, 723–742.

Cowan, C.P., & Cowan, P.A. (2000). *When partners become parents: The big life change for couples.* Mahwah, NJ: Lawrence Erlbaum Associates.

Crnic, K., & Greenberg, M.T. (1987). Maternal stress, social support, and coping: Influences on the early mother–infant relationship. In C.F.Z. Boukydis (Ed.), *Research on support for parents and infants in the postnatal period* (pp. 25–40). Norwood, NJ: Ablex.

Cutrona, C.E. (1996). *Social support in couples: Marriage as a resource in times of stress.* Thousand Oaks, CA: Sage.

Darling, N., & Steinberg, L. (1993). Parenting style as context: An integrative model. *Psychological Bulletin, 113*, 487–496.

Dishion, T.J., & Andrews, D.W. (1995). Preventing escalation in problem behaviors with high-risk young adolescents: Immediate and 1-year outcomes. *Journal of Consulting and Clinical Psychology, 63*, 538–548.

Dishion, T.J., Kavanagh, K., Schneiger, A., Nelson, S., & Kaufman, N.K. (2002). Preventing early adolescent substance use: A family-centered strategy for the public middle school. *Prevention Science, 3*, 1981–202.

Dishion, T.J., McCord, J., & Poulin, F. (1999). When interventions harm: Peer groups and problem behavior. *American Psychologist, 54*, 755–764.

Dodge, K.A., Pettit, G.S., & Bates, J.E. (1994). Socialization mediators of the relation between socioeconomic status and child conduct problems. *Child Development, 65*, 649–665.

Dunn, J. (1988). Relations among relationships. In S.W. Duck (Ed.), *Handbook of personal relationships* (pp. 193–209). England: John Wiley & Sons.

Emery, R.E. (1982). Interparental conflict and the children of discord and divorce. *Psychological Bulletin, 92*, 310–330.

Erickson, M.F., Korfmacher, J., & Egeland, B.R. (1992). Attachments past and present: Implications for therapeutic intervention with mother–infant dyads. *Development and Psychopathology, 4*, 495–507.

Eron, L., Huesmann, R., Spindler, A., Guerra, N., Henry, D., & Tolan, P. (2002). A cognitive-ecological approach to preventing aggression in urban ettings: Initial outcomes for high-risk children. *Journal of Consulting and Clinical Psychology, 70*, 179–194.

Feinberg, M.E. (2002). Coparenting and prevention at the transition to parenthood. *Clinical Child and Family Psychology Review, 5*, 173–195.

Feinberg, M., Neiderhiser, J.M., Howe, G.W., & Hetherington, E.M. (2002a). Adolescent, parent, and observer perceptions of parenting: Genetic and environmental influences on shared and distinct perceptions. *Child Development, 72*, 1266–1284.

Goodnow, J. (1995). Parents' knowledge and expectations. In M.H. Bornstein (Ed.), *Handbook of Parenting* (Vol. 3, pp. 305–332). Mahwah, NJ: Erlbaum.

Hanish, L.D., & Tolan, P.H. (2001). *Patterns of change in family-based aggression prevention.*

Heinicke, C.M. (1993). Factors affecting the efficacy of early family intervention. In N.J. Anastasiow, S. Harel et al. (Eds.), *At-risk infants: Interventions, families, and research* (pp. 91–100). Baltimore, MD: Paul H. Brookes.

Kosterman, R., Hawkins, J.D., Spoth, R., Haggerty, K.P., & Zhu, K. (1997). Effects of a preventive parent-training intervention on observed family interactions: Proximal outcomes from preparing for the drug free years. *Journal of Community Psychology, 25*, 337–352.

Ladd, G.W., & Pettit, G.S. (in press). Parents and children's peer relationships. In M.H. Bornstein (Ed.), *Handbook of parenting: Practical issues of parenting*. Mahwah, NJ: Erlbaum.

Lamb, M.E. (1995). The changing roles of fathers. In J.L. Shapiro & M.J. Diamond (Eds.), *Becoming a father: Contemporary, social, developmental, and clinical perspectives. Springer series, focus on men* (Vol. 8, pp. 18–35). New York, NY: Springer.

Lochman, J.E. (1990). Modification of childhood aggression. In M. Hersen, R.M. Eisler et al. (Eds.), *Progress in behavior modification* (Vol. 25, pp. 47–85). Newbury Park, CA: Sage.

Lytton, H. (1990). Child and parent effects in boys' conduct disorder: A reinterpretation. *Developmental Psychology, 26*, 683–697.

Maccoby, E.E. (2000). Parenting and its effects on children: On reading and misreading behavior genetics. *Annual Review of Psychology, 51*, 1–27.

McGillicuddy-De Lisi, A.V., & Sigel, I.E. (1995). Parental beliefs. In M.H. Bornstein (Ed.), *Handbook of Parenting* (Vol. 3, pp. 333–358). Mahwah, NJ: Lawrence Erlbaum Associates.

Mize, J., & Pettit, G.S. (1997). Mothers' social coaching, mother–child relationship style, and children's peer competence: Is the medium the message? *Child Development, 68*, 311–322.

Olds, D. (1999). "Long-term effects of nurse home visitation on children's criminal and antisocial behavior: 15-year follow-up of a randomized controlled trial": Reply. *Journal of the American Medical Association, 281*, 1377.

Orrell-Valente, J.K., Pinderhughes, E.E., Valente, E., Jr., & Laird, R.D. (1999). If it's offered, will they come? Influences on parents' participation in a community-based conduct problems prevention program. *American Journal of Community Psychology, 27*, 753–783.

Patterson, G.R., Capaldi, D., & Bank, L. (1991). An early starter model for predicting delinquency. In D.J. Pepler & K.H. Rubin (Eds.), *The development and treatment of childhood aggression* (pp. 139–168). Hillsdale, NJ: Lawrence Erlbaum Associates.

Patterson, G.R., Reid, J., & Dishion, T.J. (1992). *Antisocial boys.* Eugene, OR: Castilia.

Perusse, D., Neale, M.C., Heath, A.C., & Eaves, L.J. (1994). Human parental behavior: Evidence for genetic influence and potential implication for gene-culture transmission. *Behavior Genetics, 24*, 327–335.

Pettit, G.S., Bates, J.E., & Dodge, K.A. (1993). Family interaction patterns and children's conduct problems at home and school: A longitudinal perspective. *School Psychology Review, 22*, 401–418.

Pettit, G.S., Bates, J.E., & Dodge, K.A. (1997). Supportive parenting, ecological context, and children's adjustment: A seven-year longitudinal study. *Child Development, 68*, 908–923.

Pettit, G.S., Brown, E.G., Mize, J., & Lindsey, E. (1998). Mothers' and fathers' socializing behaviors in three contexts: Links with children's peer competence. *Merrill-Palmer Quarterly, 44*, 173–193.

Pettit, G.S., Laird, R.D., Bates, J.E., Dodge, K.A., & Criss, M.M. (2001). Antecedents and behavior-problem outcomes of parental monitoring and psychological control in early adolescence. *Child Development, 72*, 583–598.

Pettit, G.S., & Mize, J. (1993). Substance and style: Understanding the ways in which parents teach children about social relationships. In S. Duck (Ed.), *Understanding relationship processes: Vol. II. Learning about relationships* (pp. 118–151). Newbury Park, CA: Sage.

Reichman, N.E., & McLanahan, S.S. (2001). *Self-sufficiency programs and parenting interventions: Lessons from new chance and the teenage parent demonstration* (pp. 3–13). Society for Research in Child Development.

Russell, A., & Saebel, J. (1997). Mother–son, mother–daughter, father–son, father–daughter: Are they distinct relationships? *Developmental Review, 17*, 1–37.

Sanders, M.R. (1999). Triple P—Positive Parenting Program: Towards an empirically validated multilevel parenting and family support strategy for the prevention of behavior and emotional problems in children. *Clinical Child and Family Psychology Review, 2*, 71–90.

Serketich, W.J., & Dumas, J.E. (1996). The effectiveness of behavioral parent training to modify antisocial behavior in children: A meta-analysis. *Behavior Therapy, 27*, 171–186.

Spoth, R., Redmond, C., & Shin, C. (1998). Direct and indirect latent-variable parenting outcomes of two universal family-focused preventive interventions: Extending a public health-oriented research base. *Journal of Consulting and Clinical Psychology, 66*, 385–399.

Tolan, P.H. (2001). *A cognitive-ecological approach to preventing aggression in urban settings.*

van den Boom, D.C. (1995). Do first-year intervention effects endure? Follow-up during toddlerhood of a sample of Dutch irritable infants. *Child Development, 66*, 1798–1816.

van den Boom, D. (1997). Sensitivity and attachment: Next steps for developmentalists. *Child Development, 68*, 592–594.

Wahler, R.G. (1997). On the origins of children's compliance and opposition: Family context, reinforcement, and rules. *Journal of Child and Family Studies, 6*, 191–208.

Wahler, R.G., & Bellamy, A. (1997). Generating reciprocity with conduct problem children and their mothers: The effectiveness of compliance teaching and responsive parenting. *Journal of Social and Personal Relationships, 14*, 549–564.

Wahler, R.G., & Megennis, K.L. (1997). Strengthening child compliance through positive parenting practices: What works? *Journal of Clinical Child Psychology, 26*, 433–440.

Webster-Stratton, C., & Hammond, M. (1997). Treating children with early-onset conduct problems: A comparison of child and parent training interventions. *Journal of Consulting and Clinical Psychology, 65*, 93–109.

Peer Relationships, Childhood

Cynthia A. Rohrbeck

INTRODUCTION

Peers play a different role in a child's development than family members. Although peer relationships may not be as long lasting or intense as familial relationships, they tend to be more egalitarian. Indeed, developmental theorists (e.g., Piaget, 1951; Sullivan, 1953) have suggested that the development of peer relationships is important for developing social competence and a sense of justice. Peers provide opportunities for socialization, relationships, and a sense of belonging separate from the family—a kind of independence as a distinct person, especially as children develop and spend more time with peers than family.

As children in Western cultures move through the elementary school-age years, peer interactions dramatically increase to around 30 percent of all social interactions. The size of the peer group enlarges and peer interactions become less supervised by adults. As they develop, children gradually interact with a more diverse set of peers and encounter peers in settings other than home or school. Aggressive behaviors toward peers become less physical and more verbal. In addition, positive behaviors increase.

Several decades of research have suggested that children's peer relationships predict future psychological adjustment or maladjustment. Friendship and peer acceptance predict socioemotional success, while peer rejection and aggression increases children's risk for maladjustment (Parker & Asher, 1993). Poor peer relationships have been related to aggression, poor social skills, and lack of empathy. Indeed, a child's ability to form peer relationships may be the best single predictor of adult adaptation. Retrospective studies indicate that early peer adjustment variables predict psychologically disordered from non-disordered adults while many other variables do not (e.g., Cowen, Pedersen, Babigian, Izzo, & Trost, 1973).

The subgroup of children most at risk for future problems might be those who are rejected by their peers. Rejected children tend to be unhappy, alienated, poor achievers, and low on self-esteem. Peer rejection is correlated with poor school performance, dropping out, antisocial behavior, and delinquency in adolescence, and criminality in adulthood (Bagwell, Newcomb, & Bukowski, 1998; Parker, Rubin, Price, & DeRosier, 1995). Other children at risk include those who are victimized. Peer victimization leads to adjustment difficulties, including depression, loneliness, and school avoidance (Ladd, Kochenderfer, & Coleman, 1997).

Peer friendships are also strongly linked to academic success or failure. Studies since the 1950s have suggested that peer acceptance or rejection predicts academic difficulties and dropout rates. More recent longitudinal studies suggest a causal link between friendship and academic outcome (Ladd, 1999). In addition, a child's peer group, if "deviant," may encourage poor school-related outcomes.

DEFINITIONS

Peer refers to those with equal standing; when using the word with children, it typically refers to those relatively equal in age. In Western cultures, peer relationships are more often age-graded than in other cultures such as India or Africa, where older peers may assume care taking as well as playmate responsibilities (Edwards, 1992).

By *peer acceptance*, researchers usually mean "like ability," or the extent to which age mates want a child as a social playmate or partner. Researchers have identified four categories of peer acceptance—*popular children*, those that many children like, *rejected children*, those actively disliked, *controversial children*, who are liked by some and disliked by others, and *neglected children*, those neither liked nor disliked by their peers. Children who are severely rejected may experience peer victimization, and become targets of verbal or physical abuse by their peers. Although such sociometric classifications are often used when studying peer relations, some researchers have warned that looking only at sociometric indicators as evidence of social competence, neglects other abilities such as a child's ability to participate in group activities. In addition to dyadic peer relations, children also relate in social groups such as cliques.

Cliques are typically defined as groups based on shared friendships, instead of groups assigned by adults such as classroom work groups or extracurricular activities. As children make the transition from childhood to adolescence, almost half of their peer interactions take place within cliques (Crockett, Losoff, & Peterson, 1984).

Although peer relationships are influenced by child characteristics, parenting, culture, stress, and social support, most research has focused on the impact of children's social skills and social competence. *Social skills* can be defined as behaviors that help children solve social tasks or achieve social success. Such behaviors include simple observable behaviors such as making eye contact and introductions, to more complex skills such as the ability to understand others' emotions and intentions, and understanding how to express positive and negative feelings in appropriate ways. *Social competence*, a broader term, refers to the ability to form effective and socially acceptable relationships with others, or "the ability to achieve personal goals in social interaction while simultaneously maintaining positive relationships with others over time and across situations" (Rubin & Rose-Krasnor, 1992; cited in Rubin, Bukowski, & Parker, 1998, p. 645).

SCOPE

It would be difficult to estimate incidence or prevalence when discussing healthy peer relationships. It is easier to speak of the incidence or prevalence of certain disorders that may be the outcome of poor peer relationships. For example, antisocial peer relationships or groups contribute to the development and maintenance of aggressive behaviors, while the act of leaving antisocial peer groups and joining more prosocial groups may decrease antisocial behaviors. Aggression, combined with peer rejection, predicts later delinquency—not just aggression. At an extreme, aggressive behaviors may stabilize into conduct disorder that is estimated to occur in more than 5 percent of boys aged 6–11. Conduct disorder tends to be a stable disorder, continuing over time, and in some cases, leading to a substance abuse disorder. This may be because peer groups provide an important contextual role in predicting alcohol abuse (Mrazek & Haggerty, 1994).

THEORIES AND RESEARCH

Social learning theory is often used to explain the development of peer relationships. This approach accounts for behavior learned as a function of modeling or imitation. Peers influence each other in several ways throughout childhood. First, peers provide social models for each other. In particular, children learn social skills by modeling after more dominant, popular, and socially skilled members of their group. They internalize rules of a social setting and help to maintain the social setting by imitation. Second, peers can serve as a source of reinforcement and punishment to each other. Studies have shown that when peers attend to only certain types of behaviors (e.g., helping behaviors) and ignore other behaviors (e.g., aggressive ones), that there can be significant behavioral changes in social skills (Furman & Gavin, 1989). For aggressive and withdrawn children, rejection by their peers may result in fewer opportunities to learn social skills, and contribute toward a cycle whereby such children become less and less socially competent. Although older children, adolescents and adults can also serve as models for the development of social relationships, peers may provide the strongest model for social skills.

Social-cognitive theory includes the role of individual thoughts when interacting with peers. Many children who are unpopular have both cognitive and behavioral deficits. Peer interactions involve the ability to understand others'

behaviors, or to interpret cues that other children send, steps that would occur before a behavioral response (Crick & Dodge, 1994). Research suggests that children who are disliked attribute negative intent to others. Such attributions can lead to negative or aggressive responses, and ultimately to fewer healthy peer relationships. Peers also provide a basis for social comparison by serving as standards against which children evaluate themselves. Such comparisons can influence a child's self-esteem.

Finally, at a broader level, *social interactional theory* suggests that peer relationship patterns vary depending upon their context. For example, specific contexts, such as interparental conflict or hostile family interactions, combined with poor parental monitoring, can lead to relationships with deviant peers and subsequent substance use.

STRATEGIES THAT WORK

Several strategies to increase healthy peer interactions or relationships have empirical support. Such interventions have often been implemented in the schools—a logical site for programs that promote peer relationships because school is where students spend the most time with peers. The first group of interventions described below, have, as their primary goal, the promotion of healthy peer relationships. In the second set of studies, healthy peer relationships are also a targeted outcome, but in the context of preventing a potentially diagnosable disorder.

Early interventions to promote healthy peer relationships tended to use a social learning approach. Socially isolated or rejected children were directly coached and helped to acquire social skills such as reinforcing others, initiating interactions, and communicating. Other helpful characteristics that were modeled and taught included persistence when faced with rejection, and the ability to be flexible, or use alternative strategies when initiating interactions. For example, research by Oden and Asher (1977) directly targeted peer relationships for improvement. They selected socially isolated third and fourth graders and coached them in verbal and nonverbal friendship skills relevant to cooperation, communication, and providing support. Children who were coached made significant improvements in their sociometric ratings and those improvements were maintained in a 1-year follow-up. Likewise, Ladd (1981) intervened with third graders, coaching them to ask positive questions, offer suggestions, and make supportive statements. After eight sessions across 3 weeks with both adult coaching and practice with classmates, children's popularity increased. In summary, researchers have trained children who are low in sociometric acceptance to interact with peers using prosocial skills, and have found significant differences postintervention on friendships and peer acceptance compared to children in control groups (Mize & Ladd, 1990).

Recent programs that build on these original interventions, tend to include a more comprehensive training of social competence skills. One program that has substantial empirical support is the Improving Social Awareness–Social Problem Solving (ISA–SPS) Project in New Jersey (Elias & Clabby, 1992). In this program, elementary school children are trained in social competence skills, including how to share feelings with a group, ask for and provide help, receive and give praise, productively criticize, choose friends and engage in perspective taking (Elias & Clabby, 1992). ISA–SPS has been widely disseminated. In addition to helping students make the transition to middle school and decrease the likelihood of negative behaviors in the future (e.g., violence, cigarette smoking, vandalism), students trained in this approach also made gains on sociometric ratings (Elias & Tobias, 1996).

Another program that has received substantial empirical support for fostering healthy peer relationships is the Child Development Project. This program has a goal of improving peer relationships, and uses strategies designed to meet that goal (e.g., use of cooperative learning to encourage teamwork). In addition to improving peer relationships, the program attempts to change the overall school climate and produce a more caring community by fostering supportive relationships between school staff and students. One of several large-scale longitudinal evaluations (Battistich, Solomon, Watson, Solomon, & Schaps, 1989) showed positive changes on several social relationship outcomes, including cooperative activities, social understanding, helping activities, and social problem-solving skills such as interpersonal sensitivity.

A second set of state-of-the-art programs encourages healthy peer relationships, but in the context of preventing undesirable outcomes, such as diagnosable disorders. For example, Olweus' (1994) program of research in Norway is designed to prevent the incidence and prevalence of peer victimization, while at the same time attempting to prevent future cases of conduct disorder. His interventions prevent bullying behaviors by changing school rules for acceptable interactions across all domains of the school environment, including the playground. Olweus (1994) notes that developing a school code against bullying, engaging and asking parents for help in changing both bullies' and victims' behavior, and moving aggressive children to other classes or schools, can significantly decrease bullying, which accounts for a large portion of peer aggression in middle childhood. In addition to decreases in bullying and other antisocial behaviors, students in his programs have reported improvements in their social relationships.

Similarly, Bierman and Greenberg's (1996) Fast Track program is a multicomponent social-competency-based intervention designed to prevent conduct disorder and future adolescent problem behaviors in young children at risk. Fast Track (Families and Schools Together) used a randomized clinical trial involving 50 elementary schools in four different locations. Components that would presumably promote peer relationships include social skills training for high-risk children and a peer-pairing program designed to improve social skills and positive peer relationships. Major goals of the program included preventing school failure and conduct problems. With regard to the formation of healthy peer relationships, results suggested greater peer liking on sociometric measures.

The Seattle Social Development Program (SDP) aims to reduce later aggression, delinquency, and drug use by strengthening prosocial attachments in young children (Hawkins & Catalano, 1992). This multicomponent program incorporates parent training, teachers' use of classroom management techniques, mastery-oriented teaching, cooperative learning, and social skills training to achieve its objectives. The program began as children enter first grade. After following children from first to sixth grade, there were significant gains for both boys and girls on a variety of school interest, drug and alcohol use, and delinquent behavior measures. In addition, students in the intervention group, particularly boys, showed improvement in social skills (O'Donnell, Hawkins, Catalano, Abbott, & Day, 1995).

STRATEGIES THAT MIGHT WORK

Promising strategies for improving peer relationships include comprehensive programs that, given real-world research constraints, might not be as strongly empirically supported as those previously described. An example is the New Haven Social Development Project, a comprehensive social development curriculum designed to prevent future high-risk behaviors for children in kindergarten through twelfth grade in the New Haven public school system. One of the five broad goals of this program was to help students become more socially skilled and have more positive relationships with peers. Relevant skills taught during the classroom lessons included social problem solving, conflict resolution, and communication skills. As one of many outcome measures, teacher ratings indicated that social skills improved for the majority of students (K through third grade). Although this program has lacked a comparison group, it is a good example of a school–district-wide intervention (Weissberg & Greenberg, 1998).

Several academic interventions have also improved peer relationships, or have the potential to improve peer relationships. In some cases, interventions have been designed to improve particular relationships (e.g., race relations), while in other cases, peer relationships have been used as the medium for academic gains, and only examined tangentially. Given that researchers have found positive relationships between academic performance and peer relations, interventions that focus on improving academic skills may also indirectly foster peer relationship skills (Durlak, 1997).

There are hundreds of examples of cooperative or collaborative learning interventions in the literature; although most are designed to foster academic gains, there are also some empirically supported programs that target peer relationships. Representative programs include Aronson's Jigsaw classroom (Aronson & Gonzalez, 1988) and Slavin's Teams-Games-Tournaments (Slavin, Karweit, & Wasik, 1994). In these cooperative learning programs, students work together in small groups (usually 3–6 students) in order to master academic subjects such as social studies and spelling. Both programs have shown gains on academic outcomes and on peer relationship variables (e.g., liking for group members, improved race relations). Cooperative learning interventions as a group include a large variety of interventions, and other studies with slightly different programs have shown more mixed results on peer relationship outcomes. Therefore, it is difficult to determine the overall efficacy of cooperative learning interventions in promoting healthy peer relationships at this time.

Another academic approach that uses peer relationships as a vehicle to increase academic outcomes is peer tutoring. Reviews of programs in which peer dyads engage in one-way or reciprocal peer-tutoring have suggested that such approaches are effective for fostering academic gains, both for the tutors and those tutored (e.g., Fantuzzo, Polite, & Grayson, 1990). A subgroup of peer tutoring interventions have also targeted aspects of peer-relationships as outcome variables. For example, Trapani and Gettinger (1989) provided fourth through sixth-grade learning-disabled boys with social skills training and cross-age (older tutors) peer tutoring and found increases in achievement and ability to work with others. Most peer-tutoring interventions use same-age tutoring, in which one peer teaches another or both engage in reciprocal instruction. An example of a same-age tutoring program that found positive changes in peer relations in addition to academic gains was completed by Fantuzzo, King, and Heller (1992). A recent meta-analysis of same-age cooperative learning and peer tutoring studies supports occasional individual study findings that students improve on both academic achievement and indicators of healthy peer relationships, such as social skills and sociometric ratings (Ginsburg-Block, Rohrbeck, & Fantuzzo, 2001).

Use of parents to promote healthy peer relationships appears to be another promising approach for improving peer relationships. Research has shown that parents can serve as models for appropriate social interactions, both directly with their children, and indirectly in relationships with others. Parents can also directly coach or educate their children in social skills. Finally, parents can also provide opportunities for their children to interact with peers, both by choosing neighborhood and school settings that increase or decrease opportunities for peer contact, and also by directly arranging peer contacts. Despite this promise, research using parents to promote healthy peer relationships is lacking in the literature.

STRATEGIES THAT DO NOT WORK

At this time it is difficult to state specific examples of interventions that fail to improve peer relationships. Such examples may suffer from publication bias. In other cases, there are examples of an intervention approach that works, and others that do not, without the ability to disentangle the necessary and effective components from those that have been successful. It does appear that mere exposure to peers, without instruction in social skills (e.g., coaching) or specific required peer interactions (e.g., peer-tutoring), is not enough to lead to improvements in peer relationships.

SYNTHESIS

Programs that seek to foster children's competencies seem to be more effective when they attempt to change the overall relationship patterns and support systems in the intervention setting, as opposed to limiting the intervention to individual child cognitions and behaviors. They are also more effective when incorporated into school curricula, beginning in preschool (or kindergarten) and continuing through twelfth grade (Weissberg & Greenberg, 1998). This is also likely true for interventions that promote healthy peer relationships. If the primary goal is to enhance healthy peer relationships, there are several exemplary interventions that appear to reach that goal (e.g., ISA–SPS and the Child Development Project). In such cases, it is important that outcomes include sufficient indicators of healthy peer relationships (i.e., not just sociometric measures). In other cases, interventions may seek to promote broad social competence skills and also prevent later symptoms or diagnosable disorders. When there are such multiple, diverse goals, programs such as Fast Track or the Social Development Program may be more likely to show change on multiple outcome variables.

Also see: Peer Relationships: Adolescence; Self-Esteem: Childhood; Social and Emotional Learning: Childhood; Sport: Childhood.

References

Aronson, E., & Gonzalez, A. (1988). Desegregation, jigsaw, and the Mexican-American experience. In P.A. Katz & D.A. Taylor (Eds.), *Eliminating racism: Profiles in controversy. Perspectives in social psychology* (pp. 301–314). New York: Plenum.

Bagwell, C.L., Newcomb, A.F., & Bukowski, W.M. (1998). Preadolescent friendship and peer rejection as predictors of adult adjustment. *Child Development, 69*, 140–153.

Battistich, V., Solomon, D., Watson, M., Solomon, J., & Schaps, E. (1989). Effects of an elementary school program to enhance prosocial behavior on children's cognitive-social problem-solving skills and strategies. *Journal of Applied Developmental Psychology, 10*, 147–169.

Bierman, K.L., & Greenberg, M.T. (1996). Conduct Problems Prevention Research Group. Social skills training in the Fast Track Program. In R.D. Peters & R.J. McMahon (Eds.), *Preventing childhood disorders, substance abuse, and delinquency. Banff international behavioral science series* (Vol. 3, pp. 65–89). Thousand Oaks, CA: Sage.

Cowen, E.L., Pedersen, A., Babigian, H., Izzo, L.D., & Trost, M.A. (1973). Long-term follow-up of early detected vulnerable children. *Journal of Consulting and Clinical Psychology, 41*, 438–446.

Crick, N.R., & Dodge, K.A. (1994). A review and reformulation of social information processing systems in children's social adjustment. *Psychological Bulletin, 115*, 774–801.

Crockett, L., Losoff, M., & Peterson, A.C. (1984). Perceptions of the peer group and friendship in early adolescence. *Journal of Early Adolescence, 4*, 155–181.

Durlak, J.A. (1997). *Successful prevention programs for children and adolescents.* New York: Plenum.

Edwards, C.P. (1992). Cross-cultural perspectives on family–peer relations. In R.D. Parke & G.W. Ladd (Eds.), *Family–peer relationships: Modes of linkage* (pp. 285–316). Hillsdale, NJ: Erlbaum.

Elias, M.J., & Tobias, S.E. (1996). *Social problem-solving interventions in the schools.* New York: Guilford.

Elias, M.J., & Clabby, J.F. (1992). *Building social problem-solving skills: Guidelines from a school-based program.* San Francisco: Jossey-Bass.

Fantuzzo, J.W., King, J.A., & Heller, L.R. (1992). Effects of reciprocal peer tutoring on mathematics and school adjustment: A component analysis. *Journal of Educational Psychology, 84*, 331–339.

Fantuzzo, J.W., Polite, K., & Grayson, N. (1990). An evaluation of reciprocal peer tutoring across elementary school settings. *Journal of School Psychology, 28*(4), 309–323.

Furman, W., & Gavin, L.A. (1989). Peers influence on adjustment and development. In T.J. Berndt & G.W. Ladd (Eds.), *Peer relationships in child development.* New York: Wiley.

Ginsburg-Block, M., Rohrbeck, C.A., & Fantuzzo, J.W. (2001). *Social and emotional outcomes of peer assisted learning strategies with elementary school students: A meta-analysis.* Manuscript in preparation. Minneapolis, MN: University of Minnesota.

Hawkins, J.D., & Catalano, R.F., Jr. (1992). *Communities that care: Action for drug abuse prevention.* San Francisco: Jossey-Bass.

Ladd, G.W. (1981). Effectiveness of a social learning method for enhancing children's social interaction and peer acceptance. *Child Development, 52*, 171–178.

Ladd, G.W. (1999). Peer relationships and social competence during early and middle childhood. *Annual Review of Psychology, 50*, 333–359.

Ladd, G.W., Kochenderfer, B.J., & Coleman, C.C. (1997). Classroom peer acceptance, friendship, and victimization: Distinct relationship systems that contribute uniquely to children's school adjustment? *Child Development, 68*, 1181–1197.

Mrazek, P., & Haggerty, R.J. (Eds.). (1994). Institute of Medicine (Institutional author). *Reducing risks for mental disorders: Frontiers for preventive intervention research.* Washington, DC: National Academy Press.

Mize, J., & Ladd, G.W. (1990). Toward the development of successful social skills for preschool children. In S.R. Asher & J.D. Coie (Eds.), *Peer rejection in childhood* (pp. 338–361). New York: Cambridge University Press.

Oden, S., & Asher, S.R. (1977). Coaching children in social skills for friendship making. *Child Development, 48*, 495–506.

O'Donnell, J., Hawkins, J.D., Catalano, R.F., Abbott, R.D., & Day, L.E. (1995). Preventing school failure, drug use, and delinquency among low-income children: Effects of a long-term prevention project in elementary schools. *American Journal of Orthopsychiatry, 65*, 87–100.

Olweus, D. (1994). Bullying at school: Basic facts and effects of a school-based prevention program. *Journal of Child Psychology and Psychiatry, 35*, 1171–1190.

Parker, J.G., & Asher, S.R. (1993). Friendship and friendship quality in middle childhood: Links with peer group acceptance and feelings of loneliness and social dissatisfaction. *Developmental Psychology, 29*, 611–621.

Parker, J.G., Rubin, K.H., Price, J., & DeRosier, M.E. (1995). Peer relationships, child development, and adjustment: A developmental psychopathology perspective. In D. Cicchetti & D. Cohen (Eds.), *Developmental psychopathology: Vol. 2. Risk, disorder, and adaptation* (pp. 96–161). New York: Wiley.

Piaget, J. (1951). *Play, dreams and imitation in childhood.* New York: Norton.

Rubin, K.H., & Rose-Krasnor, L. (1992). Interpersonal problem-solving. In V.B. Van Hassett & M. Hersen (Eds.), *Handbook of social development* (pp. 283–323). New York: Plenum Press.

Rubin, K.H., Bukowski, W., & Parker, J.G. (1998). Peer interactions, relationships, and groups. In W. Damon (Editor-in-Chief) & N. Eisenberg (Vol. Ed.), *Handbook of child psychology, Vol. 3. Social, emotional, and personality development* (5th ed., pp. 619–700). New York: Wiley.

Slavin, R.E., Karweit, N.L., & Wasik, B.A. (Eds.). (1994). *Preventing early school failure: Research, policy, and practice.* Needham Heights, MA: Allyn & Bacon.

Sullivan, H.S. (1953). *The interpersonal theory of psychiatry.* New York: Norton.

Trapani, C., & Gettinger, M. (1989). Effects of social skills training and cross-age tutoring on academic achievement and social behaviors of boys with learning disabilities. *Journal of Research and Development in Education, 23*, 1–9.

Weissberg, R.P., & Greenberg, M.T. (1998). School and community competence-enhancement and prevention programs. In W. Damon (Editor-in-Chief), I.E. Sigel & K.A. Renninger (Vol. Eds.), *Handbook of child psychology, Vol 4. Child psychology in practice* (5th ed., pp. 877–954). New York: Wiley.

Peer Relationships, Adolescence

Cynthia A. Rohrbeck

INTRODUCTION

As children enter into adolescence, the amount of time they spend with peers increases. Peer groups become the most important socializing influence on adolescent behavior and values and peer relationships serve as a bridge as adolescents move away from their parents and toward independent adult functioning. In industrialized nations, adolescents spend most of each weekday with age equivalent peers in school, and in the United States, they also spend much out-of-school time together. Indeed, diaries and self-reports suggest that adolescents spend twice as much time with peers as they do with parents and other adults, even ruling out time in the classroom (Larson, Csikszentmihalyi, & Freeman, 1984).

Peers influence adolescents in positive and negative ways. Peers can promote academic achievement and prosocial behaviors as well as problem behaviors like alcohol use and delinquency. Such influence is rarely coercive; rather, adolescents are influenced by peers because they use them as models for their behavior.

While the number of reported friendships decreases in adolescence, relationships become more intimate. Peer group crowds emerge during early adolescence and are often defined by stereotypes (e.g., jocks, nerds). Smaller cliques, or friendship groups, form around shared interests. Crowds and cliques are formed by adolescents and thus differ from groups formed in the past by adults. Adolescents who are rejected or ostracized from such groups may become victims or begin to affiliate with more deviant peers. Peer victimization can lead to poor self-concepts as well as internalizing and externalizing problems (Steinberg & Morris, 2001). Although deviant peer group gangs may promote identity and friendship for some adolescents, teens involved in such groups, or gangs, are more likely to be involved in violent offenses (Thornberry, Krohn, Lizotte, & Chard-Wierschem, 1993). Friendships with deviant peers can lead to delinquency, high-risk behaviors and school problems, including dropping out of school.

DEFINITIONS

Most of the definitions regarding healthy peer relationships in adolescence are similar to those previously discussed in the child section. In addition to dyadic relationships, groups become important as children move into adolescence. Unlike adult initiated groups, *cliques* are friendship or activity-based groups that develop in early adolescence. They seem to be important for identity purposes in early adolescence, and their importance decreases in later adolescence.

SCOPE

It is difficult to estimate the incidence or prevalence of healthy peer relationships. It is easier to note possible outcomes, including diagnosable disorders, of unhealthy peer relationships. For example, affiliation with deviant or aggressive peers can lead to increases in conduct disorder. More than 10 percent of adolescent boys and 4 percent of adolescent girls have been diagnosed with conduct disorder in community samples (Mrazek & Haggerty, 1994). This is cause for concern, as 50 percent of adolescents diagnosed with conduct disorder show antisocial disorders in adulthood. In addition to such diagnosable disorders, research indicates that peers can exert a negative social influence on adolescents, leading them to engage in high-risk behaviors, such as unsafe sex, illegal substance use, and delinquency (Dryfoos, 1990).

THEORIES AND RESEARCH

Social interactional theory suggests that the interaction patterns between adolescents and their peers vary depending upon the context. For example, a context that includes coercive parent–child interactions, combined with inadequate parental monitoring, might lead to affiliation with deviant peers and subsequent substance use or other high-risk activities (Dasheen & Patterson, 1997).

Social learning theory and *social-information-processing theory* (Dodge, Pettit, McClaskey, & Brown, 1986) suggests that behavior is learned through modeling and imitation. Behavior is influenced by observation of role models, especially when the role models are rewarded for their behavior. Typical important role models for adolescents include friends, older peers, and popular media figures. Curricula based on this theory include "social resistance skills training programs" that help adolescents understand peer pressures and teach them how to resist those pressures (Dusenbury & Falco, 1997). Knowledge that adolescents can serve as role models, combined with research suggesting peer teachers learn as much about the subject they are teaching as the students they are teaching, suggests the value of using adolescent peers in educational and health-promotion interventions.

STRATEGIES THAT WORK

There are few empirically supported programs that primarily intend to foster healthy peer relationships. One of the strongest examples is the Social-Competence Promotion Program for Young Adolescents (SCPP-YA; Weissberg, Barton, & Shriver, 1997). Over half of the 45 "lessons" in SCPP-YA are focused on social problem-solving (SPS) skills such as self-control, stress-management, responsible decision-making, social problem solving, and communication skills.

Lessons focusing on those skills are followed by lessons that teach middle school students to apply those skills to prevent aggressive behaviors, substance abuse, and high-risk sexual behaviors. In the substance abuse component, adolescents become aware of social influences that contribute to drug use, and are taught assertiveness skills to resist peer pressures to experiment with alcohol and drugs. Multiple studies have shown the effectiveness of the SCPP-YA program. With regard to peer relationship outcome variables, the SCPP-YA program has found changes in social problem solving, teacher ratings of popularity, and teacher ratings of peer relations (Caplan, Weissberg, Gorber, Sivo, Grady, & Jacoby, 1992; Weissberg & Greenberg, 1998).

STRATEGIES THAT MIGHT WORK

Other promising programs designed to foster social competence, such as The New Haven Social Development Project, have been less rigorously evaluated. That project was designed to prevent high-risk behaviors among students by implementing a comprehensive social development curriculum for youth K–12. One of the five broad goals of this program was to help students become more socially skilled and develop positive relationships with peers. Relevant skills taught during the classroom lessons included social problem solving, conflict resolution, and communication skills. As one of many outcome measures, teacher ratings indicated that social skills improved for the majority of students (K through third graders) in the intervention. This program is a good example of a school–district-wide intervention, but its evaluation is hampered by the lack of a comparison group (Weissberg & Greenberg, 1998).

Competence enhancement programs that promote peer relationships have sometimes been criticized for not necessarily having an impact on preventing dysfunctional behavior. Likewise, programs designed to focus on the prevention of specific problems, may, or may not, promote healthy peer relationships, even if they incorporate peer relationship components. One peer relationship component frequently used is social resistance skills training. It has been hypothesized that teaching "resistance skills" (skills to resist social and interpersonal pressures to use drugs) and "life skills" (more general coping and interpersonal skills) will prevent problems such as tobacco and drug use (Dusenbury & Falco, 1997).

The Life Skills Training Program is an example of a preventive intervention that teaches resistance skills. The program's goal is to provide junior high school students with refusal and assertion skills so that those students can refuse peer pressures to smoke. In one version, eleventh and twelfth graders are used as peer leaders. Findings from multiple evaluations indicate that program students show reductions in

alcohol, tobacco, and other drug use, compared to students in control groups (Botvin, Schinke, & Orlandi, 1995). As with other such interventions, it is difficult to determine the degree to which a focus on peer relations (compared to other components) is responsible for the outcomes. In addition, although one component of the program includes teaching social skills, evaluations do not include dependent measures of peer relations.

Other programs have incorporated resistance skills into their curricula. Project Northland used a social resistance skills approach to alcohol prevention for students in grades 6–8. A 3-year evaluation study with approximately 2,000 students suggested that alcohol and tobacco use were significantly reduced (Perry et al., 2000). Similarly, The Midwestern Prevention Project, or MPP (Pentz et al., 1989), used a social resistance skills training approach for students in grades 5–8. (It also included other socializing influences such as parents, community leaders, school administrators, and mass media.) Close to 5,000 students comprised an evaluation study sample that showed significant reductions in alcohol, tobacco, and marijuana use throughout the 3 years of the study. Change in perceptions of friends' tolerance of drug use was the most substantial mediator of program effects on drug use (MacKinnon et al., 1991).

Other programs have taught social resistance skills to prevent high-risk sexual behaviors like the Postponing Sexual Involvement Program (PSIP; Howard & McCabe, 1992). In this program, older teen leaders in eleventh and twelfth grades teach eighth grade students to understand social pressures, learn where to go for information about sexuality, their personal rights in relationships, how to behave assertively in pressure situations, and how to postpone sexual involvement. Although social skills resistance training is included in the aforementioned programs, they do not include evaluations of their impact on peer relationships.

"Life skills," typically different than social resistance skills, are the focus of the Going for the Goal (GOAL) program. In this program, young adolescents are taught life skills (how to seek social support in order to achieve their individual goals) by high school peer teachers. Initial results include positive self-reports of change in social behaviors (for boys) and a decrease (compared to controls) in health-compromising behaviors such as smoking and drinking alcohol (for boys) (Danish, 1997). Again, this program's impact on peer relationships was not evaluated.

In contrast to these interventions, which focused mostly on teaching adolescents intrapersonal and interpersonal skills, the School Transitions Environment Project (STEP) takes an ecological approach and alters students' environments. STEP was developed to reduce stress and increase relationship and support for high-risk students transferring to junior high or high schools (Felner et al., 1993).

Incoming students are assigned to groups of students to create a feeling of smaller schools within the school and homerooms of students remain together for the majority of core academic classes during the school day. Furthermore, classrooms for those high-risk students are located in close proximity to each other. Outcome measures have suggested that this intervention has promise (students in the high-risk group do not show as much of an increase in problem behaviors as comparison students). As with many of the programs discussed above, outcomes are not focused on peer relationships, per se. Therefore, although this intervention would appear to promote healthy peer relationships and a sense of social support, it is not clear how well it succeeds in that domain.

Another set of interventions that might promote healthy peer relationships includes peer mediation and peer tutoring. Peer mediation refers to programs that train students to resolve peer conflicts. Peer mediation programs have shown initial signs of success. Further, students in these programs appear to generalize mediation skills to home and community settings (Johnson & Johnson, 1996).

Peers can also serve as teachers while learning academic subject material. In some cases, they might be "experts," as when older peers tutor or teach younger peers. In other cases, they might engage in same-age peer tutoring, or even reciprocate, or alternate, tutoring with each other. Adolescents have served as teachers when engaged in cooperative learning programs, in which different parts of the assignment are distributed to several students who then must teach each other about their portion of the assignment (Aronson, 1994). Most of the studies evaluating peer tutoring or cooperative learning focus on elementary school students; however, similar tutoring and cooperative learning programs exist for middle/junior high and high school students. One would expect that these programs would lead not only to academic increases, but also to improvements in peer relationships. Unfortunately, many interventions do not include peer relationship variables as outcome measures. In addition, adolescent peer-assisted learning interventions vary tremendously and have not been recently reviewed.

STRATEGIES THAT DO NOT WORK

At this time it is difficult to identify interventions that do not promote healthy peer relationships for several reasons. First, studies that failed to promote healthy peer relationships may not have been published. Second, programs that would logically be expected to improve peer relationships, given components that make use of peer relationships (i.e., many of those summarized under "Strategies that might work"), have not been adequately evaluated. Next, programs

that use peers may actually result in potential negative impact or harm to participants. That is, peer support or values might undermine the goals of prevention programs. For example, research has indicated that while suicidal adolescents confide more in peers than adults, those peers are not always supportive or helpful. Similarly, peers in interventions designed to promote healthy eating behaviors (for eating-disordered adolescents), have modeled poor eating behaviors and valued excessive weight loss.

SYNTHESIS

Based on the characteristics of programs that have successfully improved peer relationships, several suggestions can be made for future interventions. First, programs should focus on relationships and support systems in the intervention setting (usually the school), rather than just focusing on changing individual students' social skills. Second, they should be incorporated into the schools' curricula, and span as many grades as possible, so that students can build on prior learning and consolidate skills during different developmental phases (Weissberg & Greenberg, 1998).

When attempting to prevent high-risk behaviors in adolescents, the use of peer modeling and support by peers with prosocial norms, continue to merit consideration (Durlak, 1997; IOM, 1994). It also appears helpful to include information about social influences that could lead toward high-risk behaviors and encourage resistance skills to enable youth to avoid those influences.

Weissberg and Greenberg (1998) suggest that comprehensive programs that address multiple outcomes have a better chance to succeed in schools than short-term programs with only one target. If so, such programs should measure the impact of hypothesized peer-mediating variables, and include peer relations as an outcome variable to know whether or not such programs truly promote healthy peer relationships.

Also see: Peer Relationships: Childhood; Resilience: Childhood; Risk-Taking: Adolescence; Self-Esteem: Adolescence; Social Competency: Adolescence; Social and Emotional Learning: Adolescence.

References

Aronson, E., (1994). *The social animal* (7th ed.). San Francisco: W.H. Freeman.

Botvin, G.J., Schinke, S., & Orlandi, M.A. (1995). School-based health promotion: Substance abuse and sexual behavior. *Applied and Preventive Psychology, 4,* 167–184.

Caplan, M., Weissberg, R.P., Gorber, J.S., Sivo, P.J., Grady, D., & Jacoby, C. (1992). Social competence promotion with inner-city and suburban young adolescents: Effects on social adjustment and alcohol use. *Journal of Consulting and Clinical Psychology, 60,* 56–63.

Danish, S.J. (1997). Going for the goal: A life skills program for young adolescents. In G.W. Albee & T.P. Gullotta (Eds.), *Primary prevention works* (pp. 291–312). New-bury Park, CA: Sage.

Dasheen, T.J., & Patterson, G.R. (1997). The timing and severity of antisocial behavior: Three hypotheses within an ecological framework. In D.M. Stoff, J. Breiling, & J. Maser (Eds.), *Handbook of antisocial behavior* (pp. 205–217). New York: Wiley.

Dodge, K.A., Pettit, G.S., McClaskey, C.L., & Brown, M.M. (1986). Social competence in children. *Monographs of the Society for Research in Child Development, 51*(2, Serial No. 213).

Dryfoos, J.G. (1990). *Adolescents at risk: Prevalence and prevention.* New York: Oxford University Press.

Durlak, J.A. (1997). *Successful prevention programs for children and adolescents.* New York: Plenum.

Dusenbury, L., & Falco, M. (1997). School-based drug abuse prevention strategies: From research to policy and practice. In R.P. Weissberg, T.P. Gullotta, R.L. Hampton, B.A. Ryan, & G.R. Adams (Eds.), *Enhancing children's wellness* (pp. 47–75). Thousand Oaks, CA: Sage.

Felner, R.D., Brand, S., Adan, A.M., Mulhall, P.F., Flowers, N., Sartain, B., & DuBois, D.L. (1993). Restructuring the ecology of the school as an approach to prevention during school transitions: Longitudinal follow-ups of the School Transitional Environmental Project (STEP). *Prevention in Human Services, 10,* 103–136.

Howard, M., & McCabe, J.A. (1992). An information and skills approach for younger teens: Postponing Sexual Involvement program. In B.C. Miller, J. J. Card, R.L. Paikoff, & J.L. Peterson (Eds.), *Preventing adolescent pregnancy: Model programs and evaluations* (Sage focus ed., Vol. 140, pp. 83–109). Thousand Oaks, CA: Sage.

Johnson, D.W., & Johnson, R.T. (1996). Conflict resolution and peer mediation programs in elementary and secondary schools: A review of the research. *Review of Educational Research, 66,* 459–506.

Larson, R., Csikszentmihalyi, M., & Freeman, M. (1984). Alcohol and marijuana use in adolescents' daily lives: A random sample of experiences. *International Journal of the Addictions, 19,* 367–381.

MacKinnon, D.P., Johnson, C.A., Pentz, M.A., Dwyer, J.H., Hansen, W.B., Johnson, C.A., Pentz, M.A., & Dwyer, J.H. (1991). Mediating mechanisms in a school-based drug prevention program: First-year effects of the Midwestern Prevention Project. *Health Psychology, 10,* 164–172.

Mrazek, P.J., & Haggerty, R.J. (Eds.). (1994). *Reducing risks for mental disorders: Frontiers for preventive intervention research.* Washington, DC: National Academy Press.

Pentz, M.A., Dwyer, J.H., MacKinnon, D.P., Flay, B., Hansen, W.B., Wang, E.Y., & Johnson, C.A. (1989). A multicommunity trial for primary prevention of adolescent drug abuse. *Journal of the American Medical Association, 261,* 3259–3266.

Perry, C.L., Williams, C.L., Komro, K.A., Veblen-Mortenson, S., Forster, J.L., Bernstein-Lachter, R., Pratt, L.K., Dudovitz, B., Munson, K.A., Farbakhsh, K., Finnegan, J., & McGovern, P. (2000). Project Northland high school interventions: Community action to reduce adolescent alcohol use. *Health Education and Behavior, 27,* 29–49.

Steinberg, L., & Morris, A.S. (2001). Adolescent development. *Annual Review of Psychology, 52,* 83–110.

Thornberry, T.P., Krohn, M.D., Lizotte, A.J., & Chard-Wierschem, D. (1993). The role of juvenile gangs in facilitating delinquent behavior. *Journal of Research in Crime and Delinquency, 30,* 55–87.

Weissberg, R.P., Barton, H.A., & Shriver, T.P. (1997). The social competence promotion program for young adolescents. In G.W. Albee & T.P. Gullotta (Eds.), *Primary prevention works* (pp. 268–290). Thousand Oaks, CA: Sage.

Weissberg, R.P., & Greenberg, M.T. (1998). School and community competence-enhancement and prevention programs. In W. Damon (Editor-in-Chief), I. E. Sigel & K.A. Renninger (Vol. Eds.), *Handbook of child psychology: Vol 4. Child psychology in practice* (5th ed., pp. 877–954). New York: Wiley.

Perceived Personal Control

Ciporah S. Tadmor

INTRODUCTION

For the last 20 years, a novel crisis intervention model has been successfully implemented by physicians and nurses in a general hospital setting for populations at risk to develop emotional impairment. This preventive intervention model is directed at the prevention of emotional dysfunction for a population free of psychiatric symptomatology. This model, known as the Perceived Personal Control (PPC) Crisis Intervention Model, has been empirically verified (Tadmor, 1983; Tadmor & Brandes, 1984; Tadmor, Brandes, & Hofman, 1987), and is designed to serve as a generic, preventive intervention model to be implemented by professional caregivers to populations at high risk of encountering emotional dysfunction in the fields of medicine, education, and the military.

The PPC preventive intervention model evolved from the pioneering work of Lindemann (1944) and Caplan (1961, 1964). As early as 1960, psychiatrists in different parts of the world were exploring an alternative approach to the medical/psychiatric model that located the problems inside the individual. These new ideas coincided with the emergence of a social learning theory that placed the source of mental disorder in the interaction between the individual, key community institutions, and people in his or her social surround (Albee, 1969). This was exemplified by a shift in orientation from case finding, diagnosis, and treatment to identifying and dealing with pathogenic factors within the community to reduce and prevent the incidence of mental disorder (e.g., Caplan, 1964, 1974). The underlying assumption of this preventive approach is that building psychological strength is more beneficial than trying to counteract entrenched symptomatology or to reduce existing dysfunction.

Findings about human help-seeking behavior highlight the important role that other care giving professionals can play in the prevention of emotional dysfunction.

To illustrate, a recent study by Wang, Berglund, and Kessler (2000) suggests that primary care physicians treat nearly twice as many patients with depression, panic disorder, and general anxiety compared to other mental health specialists. These data are especially true for individuals with lower educational levels. These findings highlight the significant role of "gatekeeper" that physicians play in providing mental health services to individuals in need (Swindle, Heller, Pescosolido, & Kikuzawa, 2000).

Concern has been expressed by some mental health specialists that caregivers, such as physicians and teachers, are not sufficiently trained to be entrusted with handling an individual in distress. This argument misses the point by ignoring reality that there are insufficient professional resources to meet the need at hand and many people would rather bring their personal problems to caregivers than to mental health specialists.

The PPC model was developed to deal with this reality, namely, to develop new approaches such as consultation, training programs, support systems, and to strengthen the ability of caregivers in the community so they can help the individual when he or she needs it most and can benefit from it most when he or she is in a state of crisis and open to

influence. This network of helping agents consists of doctors, nurses, clergymen, teachers, lawyers, social workers, and counselors who are the major source of community aid to people in crisis.

THE PPC THEORETICAL CRISIS MODEL

The PPC model is a theoretical model of crisis. It explains the locus and intensity of crisis as a function of the PPC of the individual (Figure 1). PPC is defined as the availability of a response to modify the stressor and/or to modify its threatening characteristics (Averill, 1973). PPC comprises the availability of perceived control on the emotional, cognitive, and behavioral levels. These are assumed to be the mediating or buffering factors between the individual's perception of a stressful life event and the quality of the crisis outcome. Hence, the PPC construct provides a generalized measure of resistance, irrespective of the specific threat or the pre-crisis personality of the individual.

The PPC model is a synthesis derived from Lazarus' (1968) idea of idiosyncratic perception of the stressor and Caplan's (1964) notion of availability of a coping response

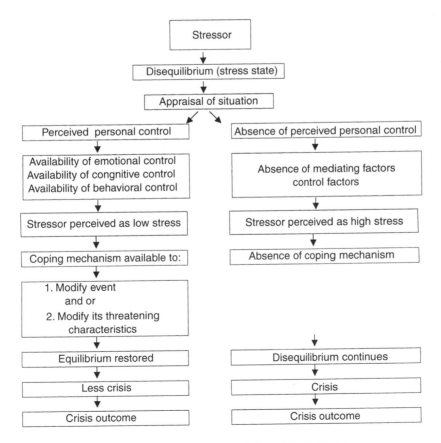

Figure 1. The Perceived Personal Control Crisis Model.

that mediate between the individual's appraisal of the event and his or her response to it. Implied in the concept of PPC are both the availability of a coping response and the perception of the event as low stress, since its threatening characteristics lend themselves to modification. It is assumed that the beneficial potential of the PPC is derived from the combination of perceived control on the cognitive, emotional, and behavioral levels, with the understanding that individual differences may determine the weight of the various sources of control. The notion of PPC is linked on the one hand with success or failure in dealing with similar events in the past and, on the other hand, with the inherent characteristics of the event (Tadmor, 1983).

THE PPC PREVENTIVE INTERVENTION MODEL

The PPC model has significant implications for crisis intervention. It calls for manipulation of situational variables, such as natural and organized support systems, information, anticipatory guidance, and the person's share in the decision-making process, as well as task-oriented activity, geared to enhance emotional, cognitive, and behavioral control, respectively. The PPC model is designed to tackle risk factors in the environment for populations free of psychiatric symptomatology in key community institutions in order to minimize the emotional sequelae encountered. Furthermore, it is geared to assist individuals in accomplishing specific psychological tasks through the mediating services of natural and organized support systems.

The PPC model adheres to the goals of primary prevention and implies short-term and long-term intervention on two distinct and yet complementary levels: (a) crisis intervention administered by a network of natural and organized support systems denoted as Personal Interaction, and (b) introduction of changes in policies, structures, and services conducive to positive mental health, denoted as Social Action (Caplan, 1974).

Personal Interaction refers to attempts to change the emotional forces in the person's environment, or the way the individual solves his or her life problems by direct intervention with him/her, or people around him/her. This program stresses the identification of "key members" in the community who, by virtue of their ascribed roles in society, have a potent effect on the mental health of many people. These key members, or "caregivers," are comprised of physicians, nurses, teachers, and clergymen who have ready access to individuals early in the unfolding of crisis and who are in the unique position to time appropriate intervention to coincide with the peak of the client's openness for maximal results. The reality is such that professional caregivers, despite their lack of mental health training, are called on to provide

interpersonal assistance to individuals grappling with life challenges. Thus, the quality of care that they are able to deliver has significant consequences on the subsequent mental health of their clients, since they provide services for individuals during the crisis interval and can tip the balance between psychological growth and emotional impairment. The PPC model suggests dealing with this reality in the most promising way: (a) by taking part in their pre-professional training; (b) by providing on-the-job training for professional caregivers in principles of crisis theory and intervention techniques, with special emphasis on the specific psychological tasks involved in each specific crisis and the range of healthy and unhealthy patterns of accomplishing them (Caplan, 1974); and (c) by recruiting professional caregivers in the implementation of preventive intervention geared to answer the specific psychological needs of their respective target populations.

On the Social Action level, the PPC model calls for analysis of key institutions in the community, identification of policies, services, regulations, and structures that are detrimental to the mental health of various target populations, and introduction of desirable changes that will facilitate personal growth. Social action is aimed at benefiting target populations in two ways: (a) on the institutional level, by manipulation of environmental conditions and promotion of policies and services geared to answer the specific psychological needs of the target population; and (b) on the political level, by bringing about modification of political, social, and legislative policies to enforce regulations, structures, and laws compatible with positive mental health. This implies that the study of growth producing rehabilitating systems, such as the family, hospitals, schools, prisons, and communities, are of prime interest in the theoretical conceptualization of PPC preventive action.

The PPC model is designed to be implemented in a community setting, such as a general hospital, by community caregivers in general and physicians in particular. The PPC model identifies medical caregivers as the key community caregivers because of their esteemed position in society. Implementation of crisis intervention by medical caregivers is facilitated by the fact that generic crisis intervention does not require psychological sophistication and the unveiling of underlying conflicts, and also by the enhanced affiliation and dependency needs of the individual-in-crisis that speeds up the establishment of the trusting intimate relationship which characterizes the doctor–patient relationship.

PPC preventive intervention, like other empowerment models, seeks to augment the individual's emotional strength, familiarizing the person with the nature of the impending hazard, involving the person in the decision-making process, and equipping the person with task-oriented activities to master the predicament and to minimize its emotional sequelae (Gullotta, 1987; Swift & Levin, 1987).

The short-term objective of the PPC model is resolution of the immediate crisis and restoration of the pre-crisis state. The broader hope is to promote personality growth beyond the crisis level by enhancing the individual's adaptive potential to deal successfully with similar situations in the future.

PPC CRISIS INTERVENTION FOR PEDIATRIC LEUKEMIA PATIENTS

The PPC preventive intervention model has been implemented at Rambam Medical Center in Haifa, Israel, since 1980 and has been successfully applied to the following populations at risk from a mental health point of view: (a) caesarean birth mothers (Tadmor, 1983, 1988); (b) mothers of premature infants (Tadmor & Brandes, 1986); (c) mothers who encounter neonatal death (Tadmor, 1986); (d) pediatric surgery patients and their parents (Tadmor, Bar-Maor, Birkhan, Shoshany, & Hofman, 1987); (e) medical staff dealing with terminally ill patients; (f) pediatric leukemia patients (Tadmor, 1997, 2001; Tadmor & Weyl Ben Arush, 2000); (g) intervention in the school for children with cancer (Tadmor & Weyl Ben Arush, in press); (h) children with cancer at the end-of-life (Tadmor, in preparation).

In this entry, I will explore how the PPC model can be used with respect to a very difficult situation trying to find preventive solutions for a population of pediatric leukemia patients.

The Physiological and Psychological Difficulties Encountered by Children with Leukemia

Recent advances in the treatment of pediatric cancer have dramatically improved the prognosis of children diagnosed with cancer. Childhood cancer has gradually evolved from a rapidly progressing fatal disease to a life-threatening chronic illness (Varni, Katz, Colgrove, & Dolgin, 1995). Today, most children survive for 5 years or longer (Bleyer, 1990) and achieve long-term disease-free survival. With the increase in long-term survival of pediatric cancer patients, quality of life issues have come to assume a more prominent role in their comprehensive treatment. This trend has led to a shift from psychological emphasis on crisis intervention confronting imminent death to facilitating coping with a serious life-threatening disease (Varni & Katz, 1987) to primary prevention of emotional dysfunction (Tadmor & Weyl Ben Arush, 2000).

Focus on a primary prevention approach to children with cancer in general and pediatric leukemia patients in particular is justified as their mental health and quality of life is at risk because of intensive and aggressive chemotherapy regimens with difficult side effects. The treatment protocol for acute lymphoblastic leukemia (ALL) requires intensive chemotherapy in the Day Care Clinic for 6 or 7 months, during which the child may encounter neutropenia (suppressed immune system), which requires isolation from school and peers for long periods of time. The treatment protocol for acute myeloid leukemia (AML) or for high-risk pediatric ALL patients is even more aggressive, requiring prolonged hospitalization followed by bone marrow transplantation.

Children with cancer encounter physiological pain and psychological distress. Pain is derived from four basic categories: (a) treatment-related pain, such as with intramuscular (IM) injections; (b) pain related to side effects of chemotherapy and radiation, such as nausea, mucositis (mouth sores), neuropathia (leg pain), and abdominal pain; (c) procedure-related pain derived from painful, invasive medical procedures, such as bone marrow aspiration (BMA), lumbar puncture (LP), bone biopsy (BB), and postoperative pain; (d) cancer-related pain due to infiltration of the tumor into various organs or tissues (Ljungman, Gordh, Sorensen, & Kreuger, 2000). Treatment- and procedure-related pain have been shown to be a greater problem than cancer pain (McGrath, Hsu, Cappelli, Luke, Goodman, & Dunn-Geier, 1990), thus, most pain experienced by children with cancer is iatrogenic (Ljungman, Gordh, Sorensen, & Kreuger, 1999), namely of medical origin and, therefore, preventable.

Psychological distress is derived from: (a) the pain encountered; (b) the anxiety of having cancer and the threat of losing one's life; (c) the threat of losing quality of life; (d) the fear of losing a function or an organ; (e) the fear of death; (f) the grief of losing one's friends; (g) the threat of losing one's autonomy; (h) the impaired self-image due to the side effects of chemotherapy, such as hair loss; and (i) the fear of social isolation from peers.

The psychological problems encountered reflect the developmental stages of children. Preschoolers mostly exhibit regression, characterized by bedwetting, increased use of pacifiers, thumb sucking, and temper tantrums. School-age children exhibit fear and acting out, while adolescents, threatened by the loss of autonomy and impaired self-image, exhibit aggressive and negativistic behavior, reactive depression and, in many cases, withdrawal from their social surround and friends. The promotion of mental health and enhancing the quality of life of children with malignant disease are complementary and inseparable facets of preventive intervention to help children with ALL and AML to cope with their illness.

The Rationale for the Formulation of Preventive Intervention for Pediatric Leukemia Patients

In 1982, when I started working in the Hematology Day Care Clinic, children with leukemia were not aware of their diagnosis, the chemotherapy protocol, or its side effects. This was due to the objection of parents as well as the resistance of the medical and nursing staff which had difficulty imparting the bad news of having cancer to the adult patient population, let alone to children. Frightened children of all ages waited in a long, narrow corridor with adult patients, and were treated in the same room separated by curtains. This encounter was detrimental to both children and adults.

At every clinic appointment, a different nurse treated the child and a painful intravenous (IV) line was inserted for chemotherapy treatment. Invasive medical procedures, such as LP, were performed without premedication. BMA and BB were carried out with injection of a local anesthetic, yet remained extremely painful. The only consolation was the strong hug of the nurse holding down the screaming child. The parents waited outside the door, listening to their child screaming, feeling helpless, guilty, and desperate. Some parents reported that their children woke up in the middle of the night screaming, as waking from a nightmare.

When requiring surgery, unsuspecting children were snatched from the arms of their parents at the entrance to the Operating Room (OR) by unfamiliar staff members, triggering mistrust and separation anxiety in the children, and helplessness in the parents. In the OR, the bewildered child, wide-awake in spite of the premedication, refused to comply, making induction of anesthesia quite violent at times. The psychological problems, such as nightmares and sleeping and eating difficulties, may very well have originated in the OR. After surgery, the child was received by anxious parents only when coming out of the Recovery Room, wide-awake and usually tearful. After surgery, due to prevailing myths and fallacies, the child's pain was not attended to as required.

When in need of hospitalization due to side effects of chemotherapy, such as fever, children were hospitalized randomly according to vacancy in any one of the two pediatric wards in the hospital. Prior to each hospitalization, the child had to undergo the long and tedious bureaucratic procedure of the Emergency Room. Adolescents were hospitalized in the adult internal wards, their developmental tasks blocked by the fearful encounter with suffering in adult patients. This disturbing description was not typical only to Rambam, but also to other medical centers at that time. The preventive intervention implemented was geared to answer these concerns and assist children with leukemia to accomplish their specific psychological tasks, to secure a positive crisis outcome, and to promote their mental health.

PPC Preventive Intervention for Pediatric Leukemia Patients

Intervention on the Personal Interaction Level

On the personal interaction level, the focus is on the child and family. Preventive intervention is implemented by a multidisciplinary team of physicians, nurses, psychologists, social workers, and child life workers, and is designed to enhance the PPC of the child and the parents on emotional, cognitive, and behavioral levels and secure a positive crisis outcome.

PPC on the Emotional Level. On the emotional level, PPC is attained by gathering a network of natural and organized support systems. The natural support system, namely, the parents accompany the child throughout treatment. Parents are present during all medical procedures, even invasive ones such as BMA, LP, and BB, in order to provide the child with support, security, and control. In addition, two kinds of organized support systems are supplied: (a) a primary care physician and a primary care nurse are assigned to each child, securing continuity of care for each child; and (b) arranging an encounter with a veteran, namely a child who has experienced a similar disease and can serve as a role model, enhancing medical compliance and a positive expectancy for the parents and child alike.

PPC on the Cognitive Level. On the cognitive level, PPC is attained by three strategies. The first is the provision of factual information regarding diagnosis and treatment protocols to parents, siblings, and the sick child him/herself, according to his/her developmental level. Provision of accurate diagnosis to children allows them (a) to be more in control and, consequently, to enhance medical compliance; (b) to release energy otherwise used to keep the diagnosis secret; and (c) to open channels of communication among the child, caregivers, and family members.

The second strategy calls for provision of anticipatory guidance, namely providing, in advance, detailed information concerning the physiological and psychological side effects of chemotherapy, such as loss of hair, loss of appetite, neutropenia (suppressed immune system), fever, hospitalization, and fears. Anticipatory guidance allows the child and family (a) to do the "worry work" in advance and to recruit their resources to deal with the expected side effects when they occur (Caplan, 1976); (b) to reduce anxiety derived from uncertainty (Averill, 1973); (c) to enhance the credibility of factual information (Staub & Kellet, 1972); and (d) to increase medical compliance.

The third strategy used to enhance cognitive control is the child's share in the decision-making process. For example, the child is encouraged to decide how he/she wants to be anesthetized for insertion of the Broviac catheter and at times, unexpected medical procedures are postponed, if possible, to allow the child to prepare him/herself psychologically.

PPC on the Behavioral Level. On the behavioral level, PPC is attained by both task-oriented activity (Gal & Lazarus, 1975) and non-task-oriented activity (Chodoff, Friedman, & Hamburg, 1964). The former involves activities such as physiotherapy, relaxation, and guided imagery, opening and closing the clasp of the Broviac catheter through which chemotherapy is administered, removal of the dressing, and monitoring of the pain medication (patient-controlled analgesia), while the latter suggests activities such as free play, computer games, television, videos, creative work, art, and music. Task-oriented activities are designed to allow the child to become an active participant in the process, while non-task-oriented activities are designed to distract the child's attention and divert him or her from painful procedures or discomfort.

Psychological Intervention

Psychological intervention for children with cancer and their parents is qualitatively and quantitatively different along the illness continuum. While psychological support is constant throughout the course of the disease, the objective of psychological intervention in the induction phase is promotion of mental health by enhancing PPC and building strengths and resources (Tadmor, 2001), and the objectives of psychological intervention at the end of the child's life is to relieve fear, anxiety, depression, and loneliness, allowing the child to die peacefully, without pain and fear, surrounded by his/her loved ones, preferably at home (Tadmor, in press).

Intervention on the Social Action Level

Intervention in the social action realm focuses on the system and is based on three principles: (a) education and training of the medical and nursing staff; (b) education and training of the child and his or her family; and (c) introduction of changes in policies and structures, and allocation of resources and services geared to promote the mental health and quality of life of children with ALL and AML.

Seminars for Medical and Nursing Staff. As early as 1982, a series of 6–10 seminars with the medical and nursing staff of the Hematology and Pediatric Departments was initiated, followed by anesthetists, operating room, and pediatric surgery nurses. These were conducted by the hospital-based psychologist, emphasizing crisis theory and practice, the psychological tasks of cancer patients, burnout, and other relevant topics.

Seminars for Children and Parents. A series of six seminars for children and parents was initiated and conducted by a multidisciplinary team of physicians, nurses, psychologists, social workers, and a dietitian, each in his or her field of expertise. The workshops are ongoing, serving new children and families, and centering on the following topics: (a) leukemia, its course and treatment; (b) side effects of chemotherapy; (c) coping with cancer; (d) coping in the community and at school; (e) nutrition; (f) innovative treatments such as bone marrow transplantation; and (g) an encounter between new patients and their parents with parents and children who have completed treatment and are years in remission.

Introduction of Changes in Policies, Structures, and Allocation of Resources and Services on the Departmental Level. The following changes were introduced in the years 1982–2001 in the Hematology Day Care Clinic, the Departments of Pediatrics, Pediatric Surgery, Pediatric Hemato-Oncology, the OR, and the Recovery Room, which care for pediatric leukemia patients in order to enhance their mental health and quality of life.

Convening All Children with Leukemia on the Same Day. As early as 1982, all sick children and all pediatric hematologists were convened in the Hematology Day Care Clinic on the same day. The underlying rationale for this change in policy was twofold: (a) to separate pediatric from adult patients, to the benefit of both populations; and (b) to utilize child life workers to cater to the needs of the children. This change in policy was facilitated by the chemotherapy regimen employed at the time that required ALL patients to attend the Day Care Clinic only once a week. In January of 1989, the Berlin–Frankfurt–Münster (BFM) protocol for pediatric ALL patients (Reiter et al., 1994) was adopted by the Department of Hematology at Rambam Medical Center, demanding a more intensive chemotherapy regimen that required children to attend the Day Care Clinic more frequently, thus highlighting the need for a separate day care clinic for leukemia patients, which is currently being completed.

Allocation of a Playroom

Convening children on the same day in the Hematology Day Care Clinic highlighted the need for a playroom, esthetically designed and well-equipped with games, computers, doctor's corner, television, etc. The playroom is operated by child life workers and its purposes are (a) to distract the children while waiting for medical tests and treatment; (b) to prepare the children for medical procedures; and (c) to equip the children with coping responses and allow them to express their feelings through play therapy, art therapy, and bibliotherapy.

Weekly Multidisciplinary Meeting. As early as 1982, a multidisciplinary staff comprising of physicians and a psychologist began meeting weekly to discuss hospitalized adult and pediatric hematology patients. Gradually, social workers, nurses, and pediatric hemato-oncologists joined the weekly meetings, allowing for a more holistic approach to hospitalized patients.

Admission of Children to the Same Pediatric Department. Adoption of the BFM protocol (Reiter et al., 1994) for pediatric ALL patients, considered to be more intensive and aggressive, implied that (a) chemotherapy was to be administered not only on an out-patient basis; and (b) more hospitalizations could be expected between chemotherapy treatments, as a result of fever and infections due to neutropenia. These new developments required hospitalizing children in the same Pediatric Department to safeguard continuity of care and familiarization with the medical and nursing staff in charge of their care. Furthermore, in order to shorten the admission procedure, children were admitted directly to their respective departments, eliminating the need to be admitted via the Emergency Room.

Hospitalizing Adolescents in the Pediatric Departments. A significant change in policy was introduced that allowed for the hospitalization of adolescents up to 19 years of age in the pediatric departments rather than in the adult wards of internal medicine. The underlying rationale was that the quality of individual care and the facilities of the pediatric departments exceeded those in the adult departments. Nevertheless, hospitalizing adolescents in the pediatric departments and subsequently in the newly established Department of Pediatric Hemato-Oncology also has its drawbacks. The psychological needs of adolescents are, on one hand, threatened by exposure to younger children and, on the other hand, blocked by exposure to adults. Consequently, in the future establishment of a separate adolescent hemato-oncology unit is a high priority.

Insertion of Broviac Catheter before Initiation of Chemotherapy. A significant change in the policy of the Hematology Department was the insertion under general anesthesia of the Broviac catheter, through which chemotherapy is administered. Before the use of the Broviac catheter, chemotherapy was administered intravenously (IV), causing pain and discomfort to children. About 8 years ago, Broviac catheters were inserted into preschoolers and occasionally to some children after initiation of chemotherapy. Only in 1995 was the policy of the Hematology Department changed to require the insertion of a catheter before initiation of chemotherapy not only for children but also for adult patients.

Preparing Children for Surgery According to their Developmental Needs. As early as 1983, a program for preparing children for surgery, based on the PPC model, was initiated in the Department of Pediatric Surgery by the hospital-based psychologist. As a result of the research findings, premedication was cancelled, and preparation is done according to the psychological and developmental needs of the pediatric surgery patients: (a) the source of trauma for preschoolers is derived from separation from parents; therefore, induction of anesthesia is carried out in the presence of parents, and the children are awakened in the presence of their parents in the Recovery Room; and (b) the source of trauma for school-age children is derived from loss of control and fear of the unknown; therefore, these children receive psychological preparation (Tadmor et al., 1987). These policies have been adopted by at least a dozen pediatric surgery departments throughout Israel.

Eliminate Children's Pain. As early as 1984, an educational process was initiated in the Department of Pediatric Surgery to enhance the sensitivity of the medical and nursing staff to children's pain. As a result, a campaign was launched to differentiate between necessary pain, when pain is used as a symptom and a prerequisite to reach an accurate diagnosis, and unnecessary painful procedures. In 1984, the use of Emla cream that anesthetizes the skin was introduced. Consequently, Emla cream has been used since then before every insertion of an IV line, before BMA, LP, and other invasive medical procedures, in order to reduce pain in children. Furthermore, a more liberal approach to pain medication for children after surgery has been adopted by the medical and nursing staff of the Pediatric Surgery Department, along with the introduction of patient-controlled analgesia. Since 1984, esophageal dilation is performed under general anesthesia rather than under conscious sedation and, for the last 8 years, the dressings of children with burns are changed under deep sedation to ameliorate pain and fear.

Performing Invasive Procedures under Conscious or Deep Sedation. Until recently, invasive medical procedures in the Hematology Day Care Clinic were not carried out under sedation for children with leukemia. Throughout the years, the psychologist prepared children for the medical invasive procedures and equipped them with various techniques to divert their attention from the painful procedures.

In this context, guided imagery, music, story-telling, and relaxation techniques were employed, coupled with the support derived from the presence of the parent, the primary care physician, the nurse, and the psychologist. However, it became evident that these techniques were only partially effective and that children exhibited fears and repeated loud objections to the invasive medical procedures. Furthermore, parents reported nightmares by some of the preschoolers. Consequently, the policy of invasive medical procedures as performed had to be evaluated. As a result, the need for a combination of a psychological and a pharmacological approach became evident in order to reduce pain and ameliorate the emotional sequelae. In 1993, conscious sedation, in which communication is maintained with the child (Murphy, 1997), was employed for preschoolers and occasionally for uncooperative children; only in 1995 was it introduced to all children and occasionally also to the adult population. Currently, all invasive medical procedures are conducted in the Pediatric Hemato-Oncology Department under deep sedation, where the child does not respond to verbal command (Murphy, 1997), in the presence of a pediatric anesthetist for all children except those who prefer otherwise. This practice allows for the amelioration of pain and fear as well as the memory of pain and fear in all children and contributes to their well-being.

The Establishment of a Pediatric Hemato-Oncology Department. In 1995, a Department of Pediatric Hemato-Oncology was established as a separate entity in the children's building to maximize the efficacy of treatment for children with malignant disease who live in northern Israel. The availability of a separate unit to cater to pediatric cancer patients was facilitated by the decision of the Israel Ministry of Health to set up specific expertise in the field of Pediatric Hemato-Oncology.

Liberal Visitation Practices. During the last few years, there has been a gradual change in the attitude of the pediatric hemato-oncologists that allows far more liberal visitation practices of friends and siblings, except during bone marrow transplantation, to prevent alienation of the child from his or her social surround.

Shortening of Hospitalization. Shortening of hospitalization is another positive development recently entertained by pediatric hemato-oncologists. Consequently, hospitalized children are allowed to leave the hospital between chemotherapy regimens and to continue antibiotics as well as total parenteral nutrition at home. Short leaves of absence even between antibiotic regimens during the day are encouraged. This policy, highly appreciated by the children, has been facilitated by the establishment of a continuity-of-care unit in the community.

Assignment of a Teacher-Counselor. As early as 1982, we invited the teacher of every newly diagnosed child with leukemia to come to the hospital to discuss the child's treatment regimen and prognosis and allowed us to learn about the child and initiate tutorial services at home. In 1995, a teacher-counselor was assigned from the Israel Ministry of Education. After the initial visit of the teacher, principal, and nurse to the hospital, an interdisciplinary staff consisting of a physician, nurse, psychologist, or social worker, and the teacher-counselor visit the child's school, with his or her permission, and make a presentation to his or her classmates. Each staff member presents information from his or her area of expertise. The mental health specialist discusses the children's misconceptions about cancer and opens up channels of communication between the child with cancer and his or her peers. In many instances, the sick child attends the presentation and provides personal information. At the end of the session, the sick child joins his or her classmates in drawing pictures that he/she will take home as a reminder of the encounter. This meeting alleviates the fears of the classmates, eases tension, prevents social isolation, and facilitates the sick child's return to school. Intervention in the school has proven to be very significant in the context of primary prevention of mental dysfunction. Recent studies have indicated that the two significant predictors of adaptive coping for children with cancer are peer support (Varni, Katz, Colgrove, & Dolgin, 1994) and school attendance (Hockenberry-Eaton, Manteuffel, & Bottomly, 1997). To date, we have had 95 class presentations and they have always been considered a "peak experience" for all who attend. We have reached Arab villages where, until recently, even the sick child's mother was unaware of her child's diagnosis. The same holds true for orthodox religious communities that have gradually opened up to deal with the diagnosis of cancer (Tadmor & Weyl Ben Arush, 2000).

Monthly Interdisciplinary Meeting. Once monthly, an interdisciplinary meeting is held in the Hematology Day Care Clinic, attended by the psychologist, social workers, and child life workers, to discuss the children in treatment and coordinate a holistic intervention plan. If special concerns arise, meetings can be scheduled more frequently on short notice.

CONCLUSIONS

The PPC model is a flexible model applicable to target populations that deal with life and death events. Indeed, most of the PPC preventive intervention at Rambam Medical Center is implemented for populations dealing with life and death situations and although one has no control over either event, the PPC model tackles risk factors in the environment that interfere with the accomplishment of the specific psychological tasks and hinder reaching a positive crisis outcome. Preventive intervention initiates attachment and bonding for caesarean birth mothers or mothers of premature babies, setting them on a course of positive childrearing practices, or allows mothers who encounter neonatal death to complete the "grief work," preparing for a new baby in her own right. Similarly, PPC preventive intervention safeguards the quality of life of the terminally ill child with cancer as s/he approaches the end-of-life, assisting the child to die without fear and pain, surrounded by loved ones, preferably at home. As the child's death nears, fears are confronted openly and frankly. Parents and siblings are started on anticipatory grief, watching for premature closure, bringing parents to the realization of identifying the point of no return and letting go of the child, preventing additional pain derived from futile aggressive treatments. At the same time, preventive intervention prevents guilt from unfolding, along with marital discord.

In this entry, an illustrative account of PPC preventive intervention for children with leukemia is discussed. It is implemented by medical and nursing caregivers trained in the principles of preventive intervention in a general hospital setting. However, it is applicable to other target populations in other key community institutions, provided the following necessary conditions are secured: (a) it is imperative that one can identify a target population, caregivers in charge, and a system that caters to the target population; (b) it is essential that PPC preventive intervention is implemented in its entirety, namely, on the Personal Interaction and Social Action levels; and (c) it is important that the cooperation of the caregivers is attained.

The PPC model calls for a redefinition of the role of the mental health professional and presents a challenge for the field in setting up innovative action. In the Personal Interaction realm, the mental health specialist is responsible for studying the specific psychological tasks of high-risk populations and for identifying, recruiting, and training non-psychiatric caregivers, family members, and self-help groups. In the Social Action domain, the mental health worker engages in analysis of systems in key community institutions and identifies policies and structures detrimental to mental health of the target population. He or she then introduces desired changes geared to answer the specific psychological needs of a normal population, who is grappling with an ordinary stressful life event, but is at high risk of encountering emotional dysfunction, in order to promote mental health.

Also see: Social Competency: Adolescence; Social and Emotional Learning: Early Childhood; Social and Emotional Learning: Childhood; Social and Emotional Learning: Adolsecence.

ACKNOWLEDGMENTS

I would like to express my appreciation to the medical and nursing staff at Rambam Medical Center for their active participation in the implementation of primary prevention programs, without whom this work would not have been accomplished. Special thanks go to the former and current directors of the hospital, Professors J.M. Brandes and M. Revah, to the former and current directors of the Hematology Department, Professors I. Tatarsky and J. Rowe, and to the late Dr. R. Sharon, the former director of the Pediatric Hematology Out-Patient Clinic, and to Professor M. Weyl Ben Arush, the director of Hemato-Oncology Department, and Dr. R. Elhasid, in charge of pediatric hematology patients. In addition, I would like to thank Professor J.A. Bar-Maor and Dr. G. Shoshany, the former and current directors of the Pediatric Surgery Department and to Professors J. Birkhan and B. Rozenberg, the former and current directors of the Anesthesiology Department, and Dr. E. Usim, pediatric anesthetist. Last, but not least, I would like to thank Professor G. Caplan for his support and guidance throughout this work.

References

Albee, G.W. (1969). The relation of conceptual models of disturbed behavior to institutional and manpower requirements. In F.N. Arnhoff, E.A. Rubenstein, & J.C. Speisman (Eds.), *Manpower and mental health*. Chicago: Aldine.

Averill, J.R. (1973). Personal control over aversive stimuli and its relation to stress. *Psychological Bulletin, 80*, 286–303.

Bleyer, W.A. (1990). The impact of childhood cancer on the United States and the world. *Ca: A Cancer Journal for Clinicians, 40*, 355–367.

Caplan, G. (1961). *Prevention of mental disorders in children*. New York: Grune & Stratton.

Caplan, G. (1964). *Principles of preventive psychiatry*. New York: Basic Books.

Caplan, G. (1974). *Support systems and community mental health: Lectures on concept development*. New York: Behavioral publications.

Caplan, G. (1976, May). *Crisis theory and crisis intervention*. Paper Presented at a Seminar at Harvard University, Boston.

Chodoff, P., Friedman, S.B., & Hamburg, D.A. (1964). Stress defenses and coping behavior: Observations in parents of children with malignant disease. *American Journal of Psychiatry, 120*, 743–749.

Gal, R., & Lazarus, R.S. (1975). The role of activity in anticipating and confronting stressful situations. *Journal of Human Stress, 1*, 4–20.

Gullotta, T.P. (1987). Prevention's technology. *The Journal of Primary Prevention, 8*(1&2), 4–24.

Hockenberry-Eaton, M., Manteuffel, B., & Bottomly, S. (1997). Development of two instruments examining stress and adjustment in children with cancer. *Journal of Pediatric Oncology Nursing, 14*(3), 178–185.

Lazarus, R.S. (1968). Emotions and adaptations conceptual and empirical relations. In W.J. Arnold (Ed.), *Nebraska Symposium on Motivation*. Lincoln, NE: University of Nebraska Press.

Lindemann, E. (1944). Symptomatology and management of acute grief. *American Journal of Psychiatry, 101,* 141–148.

Ljungman, G., Gordh, T., Sorensen, S., & Kreuger, A. (1999) Pain in pediatric oncology: Interviews with children, adolescents, and their parents. *Acta Paediatrica, 88,* 623–630.

Ljungman, G., Gordh, T., Sorensen, S., & Kreuger, A. (2000). Pain variations during cancer treatment in children: A descriptive survey. *Pediatric Hematology and Oncology, 17,* 211–221.

McGrath, P., Hsu, E., Cappelli, M., Luke, B., Goodman, J., & Dunn-Geier, J. (1990). Pain from pediatric cancer: A survey of an outpatient oncology clinic. *Journal Psychosocial Oncology, 8,* 109–124.

Murphy, M.S. (1997). Sedation for invasive procedures in paediatrics. *Archives of Disease in Childhood, 77,* 281–286.

Reiter, A., Schrappe, M., Ludwig, W.D. et al., (1994). Chemotherapy in 998 unselected childhood acute lymphoblastic leukemia patients: Results and conclusions of the multicenter trial. ALL-BFM.86. *Blood, 84,* 3122–3133.

Staub, E., & Kellet, D.S. (1972). Increasing pain tolerance by information about aversive stimuli. *Journal of Personality and Social Psychology, 21,* 198–203.

Swift, C., & Levin, G. (1987). Empowerment: An emerging mental health technology. *The Journal of Primary Prevention, 8*(1&2), 71–94.

Swindle, R., Heller, K., Pescosolido, B., & Kikuzawa, S. (2000). Responses to nervous breakdown in America over a 40-year period. Mental health implications. *American Psychologist, 55,* 740–749.

Tadmor, C.S. (1983). *The perceived personal control crisis intervention model: Training of and application by physicians and nurses to a high risk population of caesarean birth in a hospital setting.* Doctoral dissertation. Hebrew University, Jerusalem.

Tadmor, C.S. (1986). A crisis intervention model for a population of mothers who encounter neonatal death. *The Journal of Primary Prevention, 7*(1), 17–26.

Tadmor, C.S. (1988). The perceived personal control preventive intervention for a caesarean birth population. In R.H. Price, E.L. Cowen, R.P. Lorian, & J. Ramos-McKay (Eds.), *14 ounces of prevention: A casebook for practitioners* (pp. 141–152). Washington, DC: American Psychological Association.

Tadmor, C.S. (1997, November 4). *Changes in the policies of the department of Hematology (1982–1997) designed to promote the mental health of children with leukemia and enhance their quality of life.* Paper Presented at the 2nd Northern Israel Annual Meeting in Pediatric Hematology Oncology, Technion, Faculty of Medicine, Haifa, Israel.

Tadmor, C.S. (2001, April). *Changes in the policies of the Department of Hematology at Rambam Medical Center, 1982–2001, designed to promote the mental health of children with leukemia and enhance their quality of life.* Paper Presented at the Promised Childhood Congress, Tel-Aviv, Israel.

Tadmor, C.S. (in press). Preventive intervention for children with cancer and their families at the end-of-life. *Journal of Primary Prevention.*

Tadmor, C.S., & Brandes, J.M. (1984). The perceived personal control crisis intervention model in the prevention of emotional dysfunction for a high risk population of caesarean birth. *The Journal of Primary Prevention, 4,* 240–251.

Tadmor, C.S., & Brandes, J.M. (1986). Premature birth: A crisis intervention approach. *The Journal of Primary Prevention, 6,* 244–255.

Tadmor, C.S., Bar-Maor, J.A., Birkhan, J., Shoshany, G., & Hofman, J.E. (1987). Pediatric surgery: A preventive intervention approach to enhance mastery of stress. *Journal of Preventive Psychiatry, 3*(4), 365–392.

Tadmor, C.S., Brandes, J.M., & Hofman, J.E. (1987). Preventive intervention for a caesarean birth population. *Journal of Preventive Psychiatry, 3*(4), 343–364.

Tadmor, C.S., & Weyl Ben Arush, M. (2000). Changes in the policies of the department of hematology, 1982–1998, designed to promote the mental health of children with leukemia and enhance their quality of life. *Pediatric Hematology and Oncology, 17,* 67–76.

Tadmor, C.S., & Weyl Ben Arush, M. (in press). School and education of the sick child: Learning and reintegration into the school. In S. Kreitler & M. Weyl Ben Arush (Eds.), *Psychosocial aspects of pediatric oncology.* New York: Wiley.

Varni, J.W., Katz, E.R., Colgrove, R.J., & Dolgin, M. (1994). Perceived social support and adjustment of children with newly diagnosed cancer. *Journal of Developmental and Behavioral Pediatrics, 15*(1), 6–20.

Varni, J.W., Katz, E.R., Colgrove, R.J., & Dolgin, M. (1995). Perceived physical appearance and adjustment of children with newly diagnosed cancer: A path analytic model. *Journal of Behavioral Medicine, 18,* 261–278.

Wang, P.S., Berglund, P., & Kessler, R.C. (2000). Recent care of common mental disorders in the United States. Prevalence and conformance with evidence-based recommendations. *Journal of General Internal Medicine, 15,* 284–292.

Physical Fitness, Adulthood

James E. Maddux and Kimberley A. Dawson

INTRODUCTION AND DEFINITIONS

Physical fitness (consisting of cardiopulmonary capacity, muscle strength and endurance, and flexibility) is one of the keys to a longer, healthier, happier life; and regular *exercise* is one of the most important keys to physical fitness and the prevention of a host of physical and psychological problems. This entry provides a summary of research on the *prediction* of exercise behavior and on *interventions* designed to facilitate the initiation and maintenance of regular exercise. It is not concerned with research on the relationship between specific types of exercise and specific aspects of physical fitness but with research on how to motivate people to do whatever they have already decided they should do to improve their physical fitness. The research on the prediction of exercise is considerable, but the research on the effectiveness of interventions to encourage exercise is scant. Therefore, much of what this entry suggests for facilitating the initiation and maintenance of regular exercise is based as much on prediction research as on intervention research.

Regular exercise has significant physical and psychological benefits. It reduces the risk of heart disease, colon cancer, Type 2 diabetes, osteoporosis, and hypertension

(US Department of Health and Human Services [USDHHS], 1996). It enhances weight control; maintenance of healthy bones, muscles, and joints; physical strength and endurance (USDHHS, 1996). It can also enhance self-esteem and feelings of subjective well-being and reduce depression, anxiety, and stress (Dishman & Duckworth, 1998; Tkachuk & Martin, 1999). To accrue these benefits, the USDHHS' Centers for Disease Control and Prevention recommends a regimen of a half-hour of moderate exercise (e.g., walking) five times a week or 20 min of vigorous exercise (e.g., running) three times a week. (These recommendations have been called into question, however, as we will discuss briefly at the end of this entry.) Yet, despite these proven benefits, in 1998 only 25.4 percent of adults in the United States exercised at the frequency and intensity recommended by the CDC, a figure that was unchanged from 1990 (Centers for Disease Control and Prevention, 2000). In Canada, 35 percent of adults are sedentary or only somewhat active (Tremblay, 1996). *Attrition* (dropping out) from formal and informal exercise regimens averages about 50 percent (Dishman, 1994).

SCOPE

Demographic data are not particularly good predictors of exercise behavior for children or adults (Lee, 1993; Sallis, Prochaska, Taylor, Hill, & Geraci, 1999). Some relationships, however, have been found. For example, beginning at around age 6, physical activity generally declines with age (Lee, 1993; Malina, 1996; Stephens, Jacobs, & White, 1985). At all ages, males are more active, on the average, than females (Stephens et al., 1985; USDHHS, 1996). Men are more likely than women to maintain changes in exercise following formal or structured interventions (Marcus et al., 2000). Men and women sometimes have different notions of what "exercise" means. For example, women are more likely than men to consider walking a form of exercise and to believe that it will enhance health (Lombard, Lombard, & Winett, 1995). Single people of both genders are more active than are married people (Wankel, 1987). Poorer people (incomes < $10,000) are less active than are wealthier people (income > $50,000) (41.5 percent inactive and 17.8 percent inactive, respectively) (USDHHS, 1996).

Exercise also is associated with race and ethnicity. Among African American youth, 15.3 percent are inactive, compared to 9.3 percent of Caucasian youth, and the differences between young African American and Caucasian girls is even more striking (21.4 percent inactive vs. 11.6 percent, respectively) (USDHHS, 1996). Sedentary behavior is more common among African American adults (38.5 percent) than among Latino adults (34.8 percent) and Caucasian adults (26.8 percent).

THEORIES AND RESEARCH

Biological Factors

Biological characteristics may limit a person's ability to exercise and to reap its benefits. Brownell (1991) warns us about our tendency to "overstate the impact of personal behavior on health" (p. 303) and reminds us that "some bodies are not made to run, and some individuals live with genetic barriers that keep them from having the prevailing ideal for weight and shape" (p. 308).

Consistent with this notion, *weight* influences adherence to exercise programs. Overweight people are more likely than normal weight people to drop out of group-based exercise programs, perhaps because of embarrassment about their appearance (King, Kiernan, Oman, Kraemer, Hull, & Ahn, 1997).

Personality Factors

The search for personality traits that predict health behavior in general and exercise in particular has not uncovered much useful information (e.g., Willis & Campbell, 1992). The personality trait that has been investigated the most is *locus-of-control*—the general belief that one's behavior has an impact on one's environment. The more specific notion of *health locus-of-control* (that one's behavior can have an impact on one's health) also has received considerable attention. Research suggests, however, that measures of general locus-of-control and health locus-of-control are not good predictors of who will exercise and who will not (Biddle, 1999; Sallis & Owen, 1999).

People who score higher on measures of *optimism* exercise more than those scoring lower (Kavussanu & McAuley, 1995), but what is not clear is whether being more optimistic leads one to exercise more or whether exercise makes one more optimistic. Optimism probably is associated with the belief that exercise will produce desirable benefits, that one can perform exercise behavior, and that one can overcome the barriers to exercising that are common in daily life. These exercising optimists then reap the additional psychological and emotional benefits of their exercise.

Cognitive Factors

Cognitions are what people think and believe. The vast majority of research on the cognitive predictors of exercise has been based on one or more of the various *social cognitive theories* such as protection motivation theory, the health belief model, self-efficacy theory, the theories of reasoned action and planned behavior, and stages of change theories. (See Maddux, 1993, for review.) The most important assumption of these models is that situational events, environmental events, cognition, emotion, and behavior are mutually interacting influences and that a complete understanding of human behavior in any situation requires an understanding of all of these sources of influences and how they interact. A second crucial assumption is that people engage in *self-regulation* (intentional control over one's own behavior) by envisioning *goals* and by using these goals to create *incentives* and *plans* that motivate and guide their behavior. These models share several basic conceptual building blocks: (1) behavior-outcome expectancy, (2) outcome value, (3) self-efficacy expectancy, and (4) intention.

A *behavior-outcome expectancy* is a belief about the contingency between a specific behavior and a specific outcome (result, consequence) or set of outcomes (Maddux, 1999). People who exercise to reduce risk of heart disease want to prevent these illnesses because they are painful, debilitating, and possibly deadly. In addition, the major desired outcomes that lead people to exercise regularly are feelings of physical and psychological well-being, and the major costs associated with exercise are non-volitional responses such as discomfort and pain.

Behavior-outcome expectancies are good predictors of exercise behavior (Courneya, 1995; Lee, 1993). People are likely to drop out of exercise programs if they have unrealistic expectations about the immediacy of its benefits (Desharnais, Bouillon, & Godin, 1986). People's expectations that they will encounter practical barriers to regular exercise also predicts their level of physical activity (Lee, 1993).

Outcome value is the importance attached to specific outcomes in specific situations (Maddux, 1999). An outcome can be valued because a person wishes to attain it (e.g., a trimmer physique, better health) or because the person wishes to avoid it (e.g., cancer, obesity). The importance of outcome value in health-related behavior has been demonstrated by a considerable body of research (e.g., Rogers & Prentice-Dunn, 1997; Strecher, Champion, & Rosenstock, 1997).

The values of outcomes are not static but can change over time. For example, people often begin exercise programs for the expected physical health and appearance benefits, but over time mood enhancement and social benefits become increasingly important incentives (Hsiao & Thayer, 1997).

A *self-efficacy expectancy* or belief is a judgment concerning one's ability to execute a behavior or course of action. Self-efficacy for performing specific exercise behaviors, scheduling exercise sessions, and overcoming barriers to exercising are all good predictors of exercise (Courneya, 1995; Dawson & Brawley, 2000; Dawson, Brawley, & Maddux, 2000; McAuley & Courneya, 1993). Self-efficacy beliefs are important because they influence the goals people set and people's persistence in pursuing their goals, as well as their emotional reactions to perceived success and failure (Bandura, 1997). In addition, people who believe that physical ability can be enhanced through practice are less likely to experience negative affect and are more likely to persist in the face of difficulty than those who believe that physical ability is immutable (Kasimatis, Miller, & Marcussen, 1996).

An *intention* is what one says one will do. An intention is not a goal, although one can intend to attain a goal. Instead, intentions are concerned with the behaviors one might engage in to attain a goal (Maddux, 1999). Intentions are robust predictors of exercise (e.g., Dawson, Brawley, & Maddux, 2000; DuCharme & Brawley, 1995; Rosen, 2000). Of particular importance are *implementation intentions* or intentions to perform specific behaviors in specific situations because they increase the probability that the person will perform a goal-related behavior when provided the opportunity to do so (Gollwitzer, 1996).

Situational Cues

Situational cues influence behavior in two ways. First, a situation may contain *action cues* such that a behavior performed frequently in that situation may eventually come to be automatically triggered in that situation without the individual's intention or awareness. We call such behaviors *habits* (Bouton, 2000; Ouellette & Wood, 1998). For example, someone might automatically lock the doors and fasten the seatbelt when getting into the driver's side of his or her own automobile. Second, for other behaviors, including most health behaviors, certain situations may contain *decision cues* that elicit the cognitive factors involved in the formation of intentions and action plans (Bouton, 2000; Ouellette & Wood, 1998; Maddux, 1993). For example, clear weather or the sight of one's running shoes or bicycle may initiate a process of deciding whether or not to go for a run or a ride. Seeing a television commercial for athletic gear or a health club may be a cue for deciding whether or not to exercise.

Social Influences

Almost two thirds of adults who exercise regularly do so with other people (Stephens & Craig, 1990), and the exercise behavior of men, women, and children is strongly influenced by the reactions of people (Oka, King, & Young, 1995; Sallis et al., 1999; Tucker & Mueller, 2000). Spouses can encourage exercise by modeling the behavior, discussing health-related issues, and providing emotional support (Tucker & Mueller, 2000). Providing reassurances of worth, attachment, and guidance can enhance attendance at exercise classes (Duncan et al., 1993). For some people, the support provided by fitness clubs members and staff are more important than support from family and friends

(DuCharme, Widmeyer, Dorsch, & Hoar, 1996). In exercise groups, the cohesion of the group is an important predictor of adherence (King, Taylor, Haskell, & DeBusk, 1990), especially in the early phases of adoption.

Social support is effective because other people influence our beliefs about cognitive factors such as self-efficacy beliefs (Carron, Hausenblas, & Mack, 1996; Duncan & McAuley, 1993). In addition, the desire for the approval of important others can influence the motivation to adhere to exercise regimens. Many people exercise because it offers an opportunity to be with other people. As noted previously, the social incentives for exercising increase in importance with time and experience.

Program Factors

Exercise behavior can be influenced by *type* of program and by the *match* between person and type of exercise program. Adherence is likely to be better across all formats if people's preferences for one format over another are taken into account, particularly in the initial stages of a program (King et al., 1997, p. 388). Adherence is often greater for *group programs* than for *individual programs* (Massie & Shephard, 1971), and long-term adherence (2 years) among both men and women is better for *supervised home-based programs* than for group programs (King, Haskell, Young, Oka, & Stefanick, 1995; King et al., 1997). Home-based programs have been shown to be more effective in producing long-term adherence than supervised programs that take place outside the home (Garcia & King, 1991).

The relationship between intensity and adherence seems influenced by frequency. A recent study (King et al., 1995) found greater maintenance at 2 years for a high-intensity home-based program than for a low-intensity home-based program, perhaps because the high-intensity regimen required a lower frequency than the low-intensity program.

The *accessibility* of the location where exercise occurs (e.g., a gym or health club) and its distance from home or work can influence exercise; more accessible and closer locations produce greater adherence rates (Cox, 1984; Wankel, 1985). Likewise, *physical characteristics* of an exercise facility such as layout, size, and age influence attendance (Willis & Campbell, 1992). Finally, simple reminders or *prompts* (e.g., weekly phone calls, mailings) are effective in increasing and maintaining physical activity (e.g., King et al., 1990; Lombard et al., 1995).

Life Events

The maintenance of an exercise regimen can be derailed by *life events* both minor and major. Minor daily *hassles* (e.g., hurrying to meet a deadline, too many responsibilities)

can disrupt the performance of planned exercise, reduce the time spent exercising, and diminish self-efficacy for and satisfaction with exercise (Stetson, Rahn, Dubbert, Wilner, & Mercury, 1997). *Major life events* can significantly disrupt long-term (2-year period) maintenance of exercise regimens (Oman & King, 2000). These major life events seem to be a greater threat to long-term maintenance (e.g., after the first 6 months and up to 2 years) than to the adoption phase (roughly the first 6 months). Two major life events are usually insufficient to cause major disruption of an exercise regimen, but three or more events usually will do the trick (Oman & King, 2000).

Stage or Phase of Change

The factors that influence exercise behavior in the *adoption phase* are not always the same as those factors that affect exercise in the *maintenance phase* (Bandura, 1997; Dishman & Sallis, 1994; Rothman, 2000). As Bandura (1997) has stated, "Adoption relies on factors that facilitate acquisition of knowledge, requisite sub-skills, and generative capabilities, whereas maintenance rests heavily on the ability to motivate oneself to use habitually what one has learned" (p. 410). For example, self-efficacy beliefs may be more important predictors of behavior for beginning exercisers than for experienced or habitual exercisers (Dawson & Brawley, 2000). Similar patterns have been found for social support, intentions, and goals.

STRATEGIES THAT WORK

Research has not yet suggested foolproof strategies for motivating people to not only begin but also to maintain a regular exercise program that will enhance physical fitness.

STRATEGIES THAT MIGHT WORK

Knowing what predicts exercise behavior is useful only if this knowledge can be used to design strategies to increase exercise behavior. To put a spin on an old adage, what is needed is the knowledge to change what can be changed, acceptance of what cannot be changed, and the wisdom to know the difference. Genetically endowed biological capacities, personality traits, gender, age, ethnicity, income, and marital status are resistant to change, to say the least. For this reason, most of the research on interventions to has focused on what can be changed—*cognitive factors* and *program factors*. Unfortunately, this research has not been as plentiful or fruitful as the research on prediction. Many of these interventions have produced robust changes in cognitions (e.g., expected benefits, self-efficacy) but few have produced significant changes in behavior (Baranowski, Anderson, & Carmack, 1998). Research on program factors has fared a little better, as noted previously.

Thus, we are left to engage in considerable speculation about how to convince people to begin to exercise regularly and to maintain this behavior over time. The suggestions below are based on: (1) research on the predictors of exercise behavior; (2) research on exercise interventions; (3) research on other health-related behaviors (e.g., smoking, wearing seatbelts, using condoms); and (4) psychological theory on health behavior in general.

Simply providing information about the benefits of exercise is not sufficient to produce behavior change. Providing additional information on how to change behavior more systematically (e.g., instructions on self-monitoring, scheduling of activities) may be sufficient to motivate some people to initiate behavior change. Such people, however, are likely to be those who already are good self-regulators in other areas of their lives. In addition, encouraging people to exercise with a partner or in a group will probably get some people off the sofa and into the gym or onto the jogging trail. The more recalcitrant among the sedentary (probably the majority), however, are not likely to be motivated into action by either of these strategies. In addition, those who begin are still likely to flounder and quit within a few months, as suggested by the research on attrition.

What is most likely to work is a structured, multiple-component intervention that employs a variety of strategies derived from, as noted above, research on exercise, research on other health behaviors, and the social cognitive theories briefly noted earlier in this entry.

1. *Information.* People must be informed about the numerous physical and psychological benefits of exercise and the perils of a sedentary lifestyle. This information usually takes the form of the behavior-outcomes expectancies and outcome values found in all the major health behavior theories. Information about the dangers of inactivity should be designed to raise concern but not to instill terror because doing so may lead to avoidance rather than constructive action.

2. *Setting Goals.* Effective behavior change requires clear and specific goals. Therefore, people must decide which of the many benefits of exercise are most important to them: making new friends; enhancing health and athletic prowess; increasing physical attractiveness; recovering from an illness or injury; preventing disease and disability; or managing stress, anxiety, or depression. Setting clear and specific goals and subgoals makes it easier for people to gather information about their progress (feedback) and to modify their behavior in a way that facilitates progress toward the goal.

3. *Choosing an Exercise Program.* A careful match of the exercise regimen with the person's needs, preferences, and lifestyle will enhance adherence. Various options include structured programs (e.g., classes), unstructured solo programs (e.g., walking or running alone), team sports (e.g., basketball and soccer leagues), and informal group activities (e.g., running clubs). In addition, the demands of work and family may require a more flexible program for some people than for others. People who are easily bored with repetitive activity may be better suited for team sports than for solo exercising or a regularly scheduled aerobics class. Some people enjoy exercising alone, while others prefer the social benefits of a small group. Gender differences should be considered. As noted previously, men are less likely than women to view walking as "exercise" and may fare better in an activity that is sport-related.

4. *Developing a Plan of Action.* People must develop a plan that includes at least the following components.

(a) A breakdown of long-term goals into manageable *short-term goals. Graded mastery experiences* that increase in frequency, duration, and/or intensity will help people experience initial success, which leads to greater self-efficacy, which in turn encourages people to set slightly higher goals and to persevere toward them.

(b) The identification of what behaviors must be performed and in what situations (where and when) they should be performed. As noted previously, this specificity leads to the development of *implementation intentions* (intentions to perform specific behaviors in specific situations), which increase the probability that the person will engage in goal-directed behavior when given the opportunity to do so.

(c) A time-management strategy. Deliberately scheduling exercise periods into one's weeks and days is more effective than simply hoping to "get around to it" when one has taken care of other responsibilities. The benefits of scheduling derive partly from the influence of implementation intentions. Time management is particularly important at the beginning of an exercise program when many people have difficulty envisioning the possibility of making time in their busy schedules for exercise.

(d) A strategy for harnessing the assistance and *support* of friends, family, fellow exerciser, or a trainer. The support of important others should not be assumed; it should be arranged. The novice exerciser should tell other people what he/she is trying to accomplish and then should tell them how they can be supportive.

(e) A strategy for getting regular *feedback* on progress from a friend or family member (if an informal program) or trainer or group leader (if a formal program). Goals are ineffective without feedback. Positive feedback about performance can enhance self-efficacy, which can, in turn, increase positive effect and decrease negative effect during exercise, especially in the early stages of exercise adoption. This may, in turn, result in lower attrition and fewer missed exercise sessions.

(f) Arranging situational *decision cues*. As noted previously, exercise is not likely to become a habit that is automatically triggered by situational cues. Cognitions about exercise, however, can be triggered by situational cues, and one is more likely to exercise if one is thinking about it than if one is not. For this reason, people can arrange for situational cues that trigger thoughts about exercising, such as leaving one's exercise equipment and exercise clothing where they can be seen and not avoided, posting reminder notes, and sending oneself email or voice mail *prompts* (reminders).

(g) A list of potential exercise *barriers*—that is, situations and events likely to result in *relapse* (e.g., fatigue, emotional distress, daily hassles, major life events, working late, inclement weather, travelling) and a *strategy* for overcoming each of these barriers. Novice exercisers should remind themselves continually that success is not linear, that setbacks and relapses are a normal part of process, and that relapses should be viewed not as failures but as opportunities to exercise their self-regulatory abilities. Acknowledging the inevitability of relapses will increase the probability that the person will recover from the relapse and get back to his or her routine rather than view the relapse as an indication of personal failure or physical incapability.

STRATEGIES THAT DO NOT WORK

Perhaps the most frequently employed strategy to encourage regular exercise that does *not* work is simply to provide people with information about the perils of a sedentary lifestyle, the benefits of a more active lifestyle, and the behaviors they need to perform, and then assume or hope that they will make the necessary behavior changes. Such educational or exhortative strategies, when used alone, rarely have been shown to be effective in changing health behavior of any kind. Most adults are already well aware that regular exercise is good for them, yet relatively few engage in it. Simply repeating such information is unlikely to have much of an impact on most sedentary people. Nor is nagging by friends and family, another version of the exhortative strategy. Likewise, it is unwise to encourage people to start too strenuously because injuries or pain will likely be counterproductive.

SYNTHESIS

The goal of much research on exercise has been to encourage everyone to exercise at the USDHHS recommended levels of intensity and frequency, as noted at the beginning of this entry. Research on attrition, however, suggests that this goal is unrealistic. Most people simply will not maintain exercise regimens at those recommended levels, and if people believe that those levels are necessary to reap meaningful health benefits, they are likely to return to unhealthy sedentary lifestyles. Fortunately, compliance with USDHHS recommendations may be viewed in graduated steps, rather than in all or nothing terms. For example, recent evidence suggests that some of the traditional and accepted notions about the sheer volume of exercise that is necessary for maximum health benefits may be inaccurate (Winett, 1998). This evidence suggests that traditional exercise prescriptions are too time-consuming, provide minimal benefits, and may even be counterproductive or harmful. It also suggests that a focus on less frequent (once or twice a week), briefer (20–25 min sessions), and higher intensity (higher percentage of maximum heart rate and oxygen uptake) training may produce not only better results but also better adherence (Winett, 1998). Recent research also suggests that even the smallest increases in exercise (e.g., brief walks scattered throughout the day) will result in some improvements in health. Even if further research does indeed indicate that we have been asking people to do not just more than they are willing to do, but also more than they need to do, then what we have learned so far about promoting adherence to exercise regimens will nonetheless prove valuable.

Therefore, research on exercise motivation and adherence should focus less on how to get people to adhere to USDHHS standards as such and more on how to encourage people to make small changes in exercise behavior toward those standards based on more realistic expectations derived from each individual's goals, abilities, and limitations. The probability of enhancing physical fitness in the general population will be increased with well-planned and carefully executed interventions to encourage the initiation and maintenance of regular exercise regimens that take into consideration individual differences in ability, personal preferences, and lifestyle. Program planners (including researchers and healthcare professionals) need to make sure that they are trying to get people do to what really works and that they are not asking people to do more than they really need to do to attain their own desired level of fitness. Doing so will increase the likelihood that sedentary people will make at least some modest changes and maintain them over time. We might not end up with a nation of athletes, but we might at least increase the length and quality of the lives of the vast majority of average citizens, most of whom have no desire to become athletes.

Also see: Chronic Disease: Adulthood; Health Promotion: Older Adulthood; Nutrition and Physical Activity: Adolescence; Sport: Childhood.

References

Bandura, A. (1997). *Self-efficacy: The exercise of control.* New York: W.H. Freeman.

Baranowski, T., Anderson, C., & Carmack, C. (1998). Mediating variable framework in physical activity interventions. How are we doing? How might we do better? *American Journal of Preventive Medicine, 15*(4), 260–297.

Biddle, S.J.H. (1999). Motivation and perceptions of control: Tracing its development and plotting its future in exercise and sport psychology. *Journal of Sport and Exercise Psychology, 21*, 1–23.

Bouton, M.E. (2000). A learning theory perspective on lapse, relapse, and maintenance of behavior change. *Health Psychology, 19*, 57–63.

Brownell, K.D. (1991). Personal responsibility and control over our bodies: When expectations exceed reality. *Health Psychology, 10*, 303–310.

Carron, A.V., Hausenblas, H.A., & Mack, D. (1996). Social influence and exercise: A meta-analysis. *Journal of Sport and Exercise Psychology, 18*, 1–16.

Centers for Disease Control and Prevention. (2000). *National health and nutrition examination survey.* Atlanta, GA: US Department of Health and Human Services, Centers for Disease Control and Prevention, National Center for Health Statistics.

Courneya, K.S. (1995). Understanding readiness for regular physical activity in older individuals: An application of the theory of planned behavior. *Health Psychology, 14*, 80–87.

Cox, M.H. (1984). Fitness and lifestyle-programs for business and industry: Problems in recruitment and retention. *Journal of Cardiac Rehabilitation, 4*, 136–142.

Dawson, K.A., & Brawley, L.R. (2000). Examining the relationship between exercise goals, self-efficacy, and overt behaviors with beginning exercisers. *Journal of Applied Social Psychology, 30*, 315–329.

Dawson, K.A., Brawley, L.R., & Maddux, J.E. (2000). Examining the relationships among concepts of control and exercise attendance. *Journal of Sport and Exercise Psychology, 22*, 131–144.

Desharnais, R., Bouillon, J., & Godin, G. (1986). Self-efficacy and outcome expectations as determinants of exercise adherence. *Psychological Reports, 59*, 1155–1159.

Dishman, R.K. (Ed.). (1994). *Advances in exercise adherence.* Champaign, IL: Human Kinetics.

Dishman, R.K., & Sallis, J.F. (1994). Determinants and interventions for physical activity and exercise. In C. Bouchard, R.J. Shephard, & T. Stephens (Eds.), *Physical activity, fitness, and health: International proceedings and consensus statement* (pp. 214–238). Champaign, IL: Human Kinetics Press.

Dishman, R.K., & Duckworth, J. (1998). Exercise psychology. In J.P. Williams (Ed.), *Applied sport psychology: Personal growth to peak performance* (pp. 445–464). London: Mayfield.

DuCharme, K.A., & Brawley, L.R. (1995). Predicting the intentions and behavior of exercise initiates using two forms of self-efficacy. *Journal of Behavioral Medicine, 18*, 479–497.

DuCharme, K.A., Widmeyer, W.N., Dorsch, K., & Hoar, S. (1996). The relationship of social support and self-efficacy to exercise intentions and attendance at a private fitness club. *Journal of Sport and Exercise Psychology, 18*, 27.

Duncan, T.E., & McAuley, E. (1993). Social support and efficacy cognitions in exercise adherence: A latent growth analysis. *Journal of Behavioral Medicine, 16*, 199–217.

Duncan, T.E., McAuley, E., Stoolmiller, M., & Duncan, S.C. (1993). Serial fluctuations in exercise behavior as a function of social support and efficacy cognitions. *Journal of Applied Social Psychology, 23*(18), 1498–1522.

Garcia, A.W., & King, A.C. (1991). Predicting long-term adherence to aerobic exercise: A comparison of two models. *Journal of Sport and Exercise Psychology, 13*, 394–410.

Gollwitzer, P.M. (1996). The volitional benefits of planning. In P.M. Gollwitzer & J.A. Bargh (Eds.), *The psychology of action: Linking cognition and motivation to behavior* (pp. 287–312). New York: Guilford Press.

Hsiao, E.T., & Thayer, R.E. (1997). Exercising for mood regulation: The importance of experience. *Personality and Individual Differences, 24*, 829–836.

Kasimatis, M., Miller, M., & Marcussen, L. (1996). The effects of implicit theories on exercise motivation. *Journal of Research in Personality, 30*, 510–516.

Kavussanu, M., & McAuley, E. (1995). Exercise and optimism: Are highly active individuals more optimistic? *Journal of Sport and Exercise Psychology, 17*, 246–258.

King, A.C., Haskell, W.L., Young, D.R., Oka, R.K., & Stefanick, M.L. (1995). Long-term effects of varying intensities and formats of physical activity on participation rates, fitness, and lipoproteins in men and women aged 50 to 65 years. *Circulation, 9*, 2596–2604.

King, A.C., Kiernan, M., Oman, R.F., Kraemer, H.C., Hull, M., & Ahn, D. (1997). Can we identify who will adhere to long-term physical activity? Signal detection methodology as a potential aid to clinical decision making. *Health Psychology, 16*, 380–389.

King, A.C., Taylor, C.B., Haskell, W.L., & DeBusk, R.F. (1990). Identifying strategies for increasing employee physical activity levels: Findings from the Stanford/Lockheed exercise survey. *Health Psychology, 17*, 269–285.

Lombard, D.N., Lombard, T.N., & Winett (1995). Walking to meet health guidelines: The effect of prompting frequency and prompt structure. *Health Psychology, 14*, 164–170.

Lee, C. (1993). Attitudes, knowledge, and stages of change: A survey of exercise patterns in older Australian women. *Health Psychology, 12*, 476–480.

Maddux, J.E. (1993). Social cognitive models of health and exercise behavior: An introduction and review of conceptual issues. *Journal of Applied Sport Psychology, 5*, 116–140.

Maddux, J.E. (1999). Expectancies and the social-cognitive perspective: Basic principles, processes, and variables. In I. Kirsch (Ed.), *How expectancies shape experience.* Washington, DC: American Psychological Association.

Marcus, B.H., Dubbert, P.M., Forsyth, L.H., McKenzie, T.L., Stone, E.J., Dunn, A.L., & Blair, S.N. (2000). Physical activity behavior change: Issues in adoption and maintenance. *Health Psychology, 19*, 32–41.

Malina, R.M. (1996). Tracking of physical activity and physical fitness across the lifespan. *Research Quarterly for Exercise and Sport, 57*, 48–57.

Massie, J.F., & Shephard, R.J. (1971). Physiological and psychological effects of training. *Medicine and Science in Sports, 3,* 110–117.

McAuley, E., & Courneya, K.S. (1993). Adherence to exercise and physical activity as health-promoting behaviors: Attitudinal and self-efficacy influences. *Applied and Preventive Psychology, 2,* 65–77.

Oka, R.K., King, A.C., & Young, D.R. (1995). Sources of social support as predictors of exercise adherence in women and men ages 50 to 65 years. *Women's Health: Research on Gender, Behavior, and Policy, 1,* 161–175.

Oman, R.F., & King, A.C. (2000). The effect of life events and exercise program format on the adoption and maintenance of exercise behavior. *Health Psychology, 19,* 605–612.

Ouellette, J.A., & Wood, W. (1998). Habit and intention formation in everyday life: The multiple processes by which past behavior predicts future behavior. *Psychological Bulletin, 124,* 54–74.

Rogers, R.W., & Prentice-Dunn, S. (1997). Protection motivation theory. In D. Gochman (Ed.), *Handbook of health behavior research: Vol. 1: Personal and social determinants* (pp. 113–132). New York: Plenum.

Rosen, C.S. (2000). Integrating stage and continuum models to explain processing of exercise messages and exercise intention among sedentary college students. *Health Psychology, 19,* 172–180.

Rothman, A.J. (2000). Toward a theory-based analysis of behavioral maintenance. *Health Psychology, 19,* 64–69.

Sallis, J.F., & Owen, N. (1999). *Physical activity and behavioral medicine.* Newbury Park, CA: Sage.

Sallis, J.F., Prochaska, J.J., Taylor, W.C., Hill, J.O., & Geraci, J.C. (1999). Correlates of physical activity in a national sample of girls and boys in grades 4 through 12. *Health Psychology, 18,* 410–415.

Stephens, T., & Craig, A.V. (1990). *The well-being of Canadians: Highlights of the 1988 Campbell's Survey.* Ottawa: Canadian Fitness and Lifestyle Research Institute.

Stephens, T., Jacobs, D.R., & White, C.C. (1985). A descriptive epidemiology of leisure-time activity. *Public Health Reports, 100,* 147–158.

Stetson, B.A., Rahn, J.M., Dubbert, P.M., Wilner, B.I., & Mercury, M.G. (1997). Prospective evaluation of the effects of stress on exercise adherence in community-residing women. *Health Psychology, 16,* 515–520.

Strecher, V.J., Champion, V.L., & Rosenstock, I.M. (1997). The health belief model and health behavior. In D. Gochman (Ed.), *Handbook of health behavior research: Vol. 1: Personal and social determinants* (pp. 71–92). New York: Plenum.

Tkachuk, G.A., & Martin, G.L. (1999). Exercise therapy for patients with psychiatric disorders: Research and clinical applications. *Professional Psychology: Research and Practice, 30,* 275–282.

Tremblay, M. (1996). Time to take off the gloves and get tough on physical activity. Ottawa, Ontario: Media release circulated by the Canadian Association for Health, Physical Education, Recreation, and Dance.

Tucker, J.S., & Mueller, J.S. (2000). Spouses' social control of health behaviors: Use and effectiveness of specific strategies. *Personality and Social Psychology Bulletin, 26,* 1120–1130.

United States Department of Health and Human Services. (1996). *Physical activity and health: A report of the Surgeon General.* Atlanta, GA: US Department of Health and Human Services, Centers for Disease Control and Prevention: National Center for Chronic Disease Prevention and Health Promotion.

Wankel, L.M. (1985). Personal and situational factors affecting exercise involvement: The importance of enjoyment. *Research Quarterly for Exercise and Sport, 56*(3), 275–282.

Wankel, L.M. (1987). Enhancing motivation for involvement in voluntary exercise programs. In M.L. Maher (Ed.), *Advances in motivation and achievement: Enhancing motivation* (pp. 239–286). Greenwich, CT: JAI Press.

Willis, J.D., & Campbell, L.F. (1992). *Exercise psychology.* Champaign, IL: Human Kinetics.

Winett. R.A. (1998). Developing more effective health-behavior programs: Analyzing the epidemiological and biological basis for activity and exercise programs. *Applied and Preventive Psychology, 7,* 209–224.

Physical Health, Early Childhood

David Wood, Felicia K. Macik, and Jeff Brown

INTRODUCTION

Interventions in child health care to promote the physical health of children from birth to 5 years of age are multiple and diverse. Recommendations for these interventions have been published by the American Academy of Pediatrics (AAP), the American Academy of Family Physicians (AAFP), the Canadian Task Force on Preventive Health Care (CTFPHC), the US Preventive Healthcare Task Force, and others. The degree to which the different interventions have been studied for effectiveness is varied. Some recommended interventions, such as the periodic, unclothed physical examination, have a paucity of evidence of any kind to determine their efficacy, yet they are still recommended as the standard of care. Other interventions, including childhood vaccinations, have a wealth of evidence to support their efficacy. In this entry, we summarize the evidence from a population perspective for a selection of interventions commonly undertaken by child health providers to promote the physical health of children.

It should be said that a lack of quality evidence to support an intervention's effectiveness does not necessarily mean that the diagnostic or curative intervention is not effective or worthwhile. The lack of evidence in child health more commonly means that the studies have yet to be performed, and we must rely on the collective experience of clinician experts, which is still the dominant force in setting standards of practice, to guide their use.

Table 1 summarizes the strength of the evidence for screening approaches for important physical health conditions detectable and treatable in early childhood.

Some screening approaches (and the resultant interventions) are appropriate only at specific ages, and these are noted in the chart. Others are recommended for multiple ages according to a "periodicity schedule," as published by the AAP and AAFP or the CTFPHC. The evidence for or against screening for the particular condition is graded according to

Table 1. Summary of Evidence for Physical Health Promotion Screening in Children, Birth to 5 Years of Age

Disease or condition	Levels of evidence *For* screening: Good (A), fair (B), poor (C) *Against* screening: Fair (D), good (E)*
Genetic diseases screening in newborns	
• Hypothyroidism	• Good (A)
• Phenylketonuria (PKU)	• Good (A)
• Hemoglobinopathies	• Good (A)
Visual acuity screening	
• Screening all high-risk children	• Good (A)
• Formal screening prior to school	• Good (A)
Hearing screening	
• In newborns	• Good (A)
• After age 3	• From poor (C) *for* screening to fair (D) *against* screening
Dental screening and prophylaxis	
• Water supply fluoridation	• Good (A)
• Fluoride food supplements targeting high-risk children 6–16 years of age	• Good (A)
• Fluoride toothpaste	• Good (A)
• Avoid bedtime baby bottle	• Fair (B)
• Periodic dental examination	• Fair (B)
• Professionally applied fluoride	• Poor (C)
• Tooth brushing without fluoride containing toothpaste	• Poor (C)
Screening for developmental dysplasia of the hip (DDH)	• Good (A) to fair (B)
Anemia screening	
• General child population	• Poor (C)
• High-risk populations	• Good (A)
Lead exposure screening	
• Universal screening in the US or Canada	• Poor (C)
• Screening "high-risk" areas/children in the US	• Good (A)
• Screening high-risk children in Canada	• Fair (B)
TB screening	
• Universal screening in US	• Poor (C)
• Screening "high-risk" children	• Good (A)
Routine growth monitoring	
In developing countries	
• monitoring for growth disorders	• Poor (C)
In developed countries	
• monitoring for growth disorders	• Poor (C)
• Obesity screening and prevention	• Poor (C)

Table 1. Continued

Childhood immunizations	• Good (A) evidence for all childhood immunizations currently recommended by the AAP/AAFP/Centers for Disease Control (CDC) (see schedule in section on immunizations)
Anticipatory guidance	• Fair (B)

Table 2. Grades of Recommendations Used by Both the Canadian Task Force for Preventive Health Care and the US Preventive Services Task Force (USPSTF)

A	Good evidence to support the recommendation that the condition be specifically considered in a PHE
B	Fair evidence to support the recommendation that the condition be specifically considered in a PHE
C	Poor evidence regarding inclusion or exclusion of a condition in a PHE, but recommendations may be made on other grounds
D	Fair evidence to support the recommendation that the condition be specifically excluded from consideration in a PHE
E	Good evidence to support the recommendation that the condition be specifically excluded from consideration in a PHE

Table 3. Quality of Published Evidence, Used by Both the Canadian Task Force for Preventive Health Care and the US Preventive Services Task Force

I	Evidence from at least one properly randomized controlled trial (RCT)
II-1	Evidence from well-designed controlled trials without randomization
II-2	Evidence from well-designed cohort or case-control analytic studies, preferably from more than one center or research group
II-3	Evidence from comparisons between time or place with or without the intervention. Dramatic results in uncontrolled experiments could also be included here
III	Opinions of respected authorities, based on clinical experience, descriptive studies or reports of expert committees

Source: Canadian Task Force on the Periodic Health Examination. (1979). The periodic health examination. *Journal of the Canadian Medical Association, 121*, 1193–1254.

the scale developed by the CTFPHC and adapted by the US Preventive Health Care Task Force (Tables 2 and 3).

PREVENTIVE INTERVENTION

Genetic Screening: Congenital Hypothyroidism

Congenital hypothyroidism, or the congenital absence of thyroid hormone, occurs in about 1 out of every 3,500–4,000 newborns (Beaulieu, 1994). It has been known for many years that failure to identify and treat this disorder within the first few months of life is likely to result in irreversible mental retardation and a variety of neuropsychological deficits comprising the syndrome of cretinism (Postellon & Abdallah, 1986). Eight cohort studies showed that affected infants who were identified and treated had significantly higher mean IQ scores than historical and concurrent controls (Glorieux, Dussault, Van Vliet, 1992).

Screening for congenital hypothyroidism in neonates is performed on whole blood obtained by a heel-prick applied to filter paper using a radioimmunoassay for T4 (thyroxine) and/or thyroid stimulating hormone (TSH) from heel-prick specimens applied to filter paper. In the United States, T4 is measured initially on all specimens and TSH is then measured if the T4 level is low (USPSTF, 1989). In Europe and elsewhere, TSH is measured first. Newborn screening for congenital hypothyroidism is mandatory in all states and is recommended by most authorities including the Canadian Task Force, the AAP, and American Thyroid Association. Currently in the United States, only 1 of 120 neonates with congenital hypothyroidism escapes detection, usually as a result of biological factors or screening errors (Fisher, 1987; Holtzman, Slazyk, & Cordero, 1986).

Genetic Screening: Congenital Phenylketonuria

Hyperphenylalaninemia results from a defect in the L-phenylalanine hydroxylase (PAH) enzyme, the gene for which is located on the long arm of chromosome 12: 12q22–q24 (AAP, 2000a). This defect, equally distributed between males and females, is inherited in an autosomal recessive pattern. Persistently elevated phenylalanine concentrations impair the development of the central nervous system. In the absence of treatment during infancy, most persons with this disorder develop severe, irreversible mental retardation. Many experience neurobehavioral symptoms such as seizures, tremors, gait disorders, athetoid movements, and psychotic episodes and autism. Its incidence is 1 in 10,000–25,000 births in the United States (Baldwin & Wilson, 1989).

Dietary phenylalanine restriction is successful in preventing the above problems in over 95 percent of children with PKU and allows them to develop normal or near-normal intelligence (Kotch, Yusin, & Fishler, 1985). The efficacy of dietary treatment has never been proved in a properly designed, controlled trial, and the performance of such a study in the future is unlikely for ethical reasons. Nevertheless, the compelling contrast in outcome between children receiving treatment and historical controls prompted most Western governments to require routine neonatal screening as early as the late 1960s. Neonatal screening for PKU is mandated by law for all hospitals in the United States and Canada (Baldwin & Wilson, 1989; Somens & Favreau, 1982).

Automated blood phenylalanine determinations have been the principal screening tests for phenylketonuria. However, their sensitivity is influenced by the age of the newborn when the sample is obtained. The blood level of phenylalanine is typically normal in affected neonates immediately after birth (due to maternal metabolism of excess phenylalanine), but it increases rapidly after protein feeds have been instituted. The current trend toward early discharge from the nursery (resulting in PKU screening being performed as early as a few hours of age) has raised concerns that there may be insufficient time for phenylalanine levels to rise into the positive range before the test is performed. Therefore, children discharged before 24 hours of age should return to hospital or to a provider's office to have PKU screening within the first week of life.

Genetic Screening: Hemoglobinopathies

Hemoglobinopathies are a group of genetic disorders characterized by the production of abnormal hemoglobin β chains or structural variants, such as HbS and HbC, due to single-amino acid substitutions (i.e., missense mutations). The beta globin gene is located at chromosome 11p15.5 (AAP, 2000a). Affected individuals have lifelong hemolytic anemia with acute and chronic tissue damage secondary to the blockage of blood flow produced by the abnormally shaped red blood cells. Additional clinical manifestations include sepsis, infections, and bone marrow aplasia. Sickle cell disease affects an estimated 50,000 African Americans with an additional 2 million Americans having sickle cell trait. One in 375 African American live births have HbSS, 1 in 835 have HbSC, and 1 in 1667 have HbS β-thalassemia. Based on universal screening data from California, New York, and Texas, sickle cell disease occurs in 1 in 40,000–60,000 births to non-African Americans (Ashley-Koch, Quanhe, & Olney, 2000). The estimated 700,000 Blacks in Canada are predominantly individuals of Caribbean (carrier rate 10–14 percent) and African (carrier rate 20–25 percent in West Africa) origin, in which HbS carrier rates are higher than in US Blacks. Therefore, screening is recommended for this population, but is not universal, in Canada (Goldbloom, 1994).

The other major class of hemoglobinopathies consists of the thalassemias, all of which are characterized by a reduced rate of synthesis of one or more of the globin chains of hemoglobin and are related to a variety of different mutational events. β-thalassemia occurs primarily among individuals of Mediterranean, Southeast Asian, or African descent. The heterozygous carrier state is present in about 1.5 percent of American Blacks, 3–4 percent of Italian Americans, 5 percent of Greek Americans, and about 3–9 percent of Southeast Asians. The exact prevalence of α-thalassemia minor or trait (one or two genes affected) is uncertain, but it is estimated to be 5–30 percent among Blacks and 15–30 percent among Southeast Asians.

Infants with HbSS or HbS/β thalassemia have splenic impairment early in life making them susceptible to overwhelming sepsis by certain encapsulated bacteria. To prevent this, at the time of diagnosis, they should be put on daily penicillin prophylaxis for life. They should also be immunized against pneumococcal, *Hemophilus influenza*, and meningococcal infections. These interventions greatly reduce the rate of death and morbidity from overwhelming sepsis. Death from acute splenic sequestration and aplastic crisis may be prevented or reduced further by transfusion therapy and aggressive treatment of infections.

Evidence for the effectiveness of screening for hemoglobinopathies at birth is good (A). Although hemoglobinopathies occur almost exclusively among defined ethnic and racial groups, experts advocate universal newborn screening to insure the detection of persons whose ethnicity is uncertain (Holtzman & Watson, 1997). As of July 2000, 41 US states have mandated universal testing for hemoglobinopathies, and 5 states are piloting either universal or focused testing. The sensitivity and specificity of the most commonly used test combination (isoelectric focusing, high-performance liquid chromatography) are 100 percent. Prospective studies are currently in progress to evaluate the impact of screening programs on the impact on prognosis of early diagnosis and vigorous treatment.

Vision Screening

Amblyopia (lazy eye) and strabismus (ocular misalignment) rates in young children are estimated to be between 2 and 5 percent in both the United States and Canada (AAP, 1996a). Several times that number will have simple refractive errors by age 16. Amblyopia and strabismus usually develop between the first and sixth year of life. There is convincing evidence that early detection and treatment of visual problems in infants and young children improves the prognosis for normal eye development. Detection and treatment of strabismus and amblyopia by age 1–2 can increase the likelihood of developing normal or near-normal binocular vision and may improve fine motor skills. Interventions for amblyopia and strabismus are significantly less effective if started after age 5 (AAP, 1996a). Late diagnosis and treatment increase the risk for developing irreversible amblyopia, ocular misalignment, loss of depth perception and binocularity, cosmetic defects, and educational and occupational restrictions.

Tests used in children under three to examine the eye include visual inspection, retinal examination by ophthalmoscopy, and the cover–uncover test for amblyopia and strabismus. For children 4 years of age and older, tests of visual acuity and stereoacuity can be used including the Snellen eye chart, the tumbling E, Allen picture cards, and others. The sensitivity and specificity of most visual acuity tests is low for detecting strabismus and amblyopia. For example, the Snellen letters test has a sensitivity of only 25–37 percent. Thus, simple acuity tests may miss many cases of amblyopia and strabismus. Stereograms such as the Random Dot E (RDE) are more effective than visual acuity tests and are quick, requiring only 1 min to perform. The RDE has an estimated sensitivity of 64 percent and a specificity of 90 percent. Combining all of the above tests (visual inspection, visual acuity, and stereoacuity testing) has a negative predictive value of 98.7 percent for amblyopia, strabismus, and/or high refractive errors and a positive predictive value of 72 percent (USPSTF, 2001).

In summary, examination of the eyes can be performed at any age, beginning in the newborn period, and should be done at all well infant and well child visits. Infants at risk for eye problems (e.g., prematurity, a family history of congenital cataracts, retinoblastoma, metabolic and genetic diseases) should have ophthalmologic examinations in the nursery and frequent follow-up. For low-risk children, the AAP recommends external examination and an evaluation of visual following ability and the pupillary light reflex in the newborn period and once again during the first 6 months. Testing of visual acuity, ocular alignment, and ocular disease is recommended by the Academy at ages 4, 5–6, and at less frequent intervals thereafter. The Canadian Task Force recommends an eye examination and the cover–uncover test at ages 1 week, 2 months, and, along with a vision chart test, at ages 2–3 years and 5–6 years (Feighter, 1994a).

Hearing Screening

Significant (>35 dB) bilateral hearing loss is present in approximately 1–3 per 1,000 newborn infants in the well-baby nursery population, and 2–4 per 100 infants that leave neonatal intensive care units (AAP, 1999; CDC, 1997). Undetected and untreated hearing loss can impede speech, language, and cognitive development (Yoshinaga-Itano, Sedey, Coulter, & Mehl, 1998). It is important to identify children early in the first year of life and augment communication in order to optimally support critical early development. Unfortunately, the average age of detecting significant hearing loss is during the second year of life, when parents are expecting language development to occur. In the past, limited screening, restricted to high-risk children (e.g., premature infants, those with a family history of deafness) identified only half of children with early significant hearing loss (National Institutes of Health, 1993).

Fortunately, effective hearing screening tools have been developed that allow hearing screening to be performed as early as the first day of life. Evoked Otoacoustic Emissions (EOAE) and Auditory Brainstem Response (ABR) are the two proven methodologies for newborn hearing screening. Both are noninvasive, quick (<5 min), and easy to perform. EOAE screening is quicker and easier to perform than ABR. However, EOAE may be affected by debris or fluid in the external and middle ear, resulting in a higher false positive rate. All positive EOAE tests should be confirmed by ABR before the screening is considered truly positive. The ABR alone or the EOAE/ABR combination has a very high sensitivity (>95 percent) and specificity (>98 percent). The tests are also inexpensive when applied on a population basis (AAP, 1999). In summary, the evidence for the effectiveness of universal newborn hearing screening is very good.

On the other hand, there is insufficient evidence of benefit to recommend for or against formal audiologic hearing screening (pure tone audiometry) of asymptomatic children beyond the age of 3. Hearing screening in children over three detects a larger proportion of conductive hearing loss due to self-limited episodes of acute otitis media with effusions that generally resolve spontaneously within 6–8 weeks of onset. Since the critical period of language development has passed at this age, these episodes appear to have little impact on educational performance. A variety of recommendations have been issued for screening preschool and school-aged children. The Canadian Task Force recommends against including formal hearing screening in routine preschool examinations (Feighter, 1994b). The AAP recommends pure tone audiometry at 4 and 5 years of age, while the American Speech–Language Hearing Association recommends annual pure tone audiometry for children 3–10 years of age (AAP, 1999; National Institutes of Health, 1993). It is unclear whether the detection of infrequent cases of persistent hearing loss over age 3 outweighs the costs of false-positive referrals and labeling for many children with self-limited disease. At the same time, there is insufficient evidence of harm to discourage current clinical practice or hearing screening efforts by local school systems and private organizations.

Dental Caries Screening and Prophylaxis Against Dental Caries

A large proportion of the US child population suffers from dental caries (tooth decay). US data show that 20–25 percent of children have significant tooth decay (National Institute of Dental Research, 1981). Longitudinal trials in Ontario, Canada, found similar results in "high-risk" children. Those 6–7 years of age had 11 or 12 decayed, missing, or filled tooth surfaces per child (Lewis & Ismail, 1995).

There is *good* (Grade A) evidence that the following interventions are effective in preventing dental caries

(CDC, 2001a):

1. Regular use of fluoride-containing toothpaste has been shown in randomized controlled trials (RCTs) to be both effective in preventing caries and to be of low cost. In fact, the decline in the incidence of caries in developed countries during the past 15–20 years is invariably ascribed to the use of fluoride toothpastes.
2. The incidence of caries has been reduced significantly by the fluoridation of community water supplies. However, only approximately half of US communities have optimally fluoridated water (Lewis & Banting, 1994; Newbrun, 1989).
3. Fluoride supplements for high-risk children aged 6–16 in areas where there is a low level (0.3 ppm or less) of fluoride in the drinking water. While this intervention is proven to be effective, provider compliance in prescribing supplements may be poor. In addition, parent compliance in administering supplements has not been evaluated.

There is fair evidence (Grade B) that advising parents to put infants and toddlers to bed without a bottle may reduce the risk of baby bottle tooth decay (Ripa, 1988). However, the effect of counseling on this practice has not been evaluated (Weinstein, Milgrom, & Melnick, 1989). There is *poor* evidence (Grade C) that professionally applied topical fluoride or the use of fluoride mouth rinses for low-risk patients prevents caries (CDC, 2001a).

Screening for DDH

The acronym DDH includes hips that are unstable, subluxed, dislocated, and/or have malformed acetabula. A hip is unstable when the tight fit between the femoral head and the acetabulum is lost, and the femoral head is able to move within (subluxed) or outside (dislocated) the confines of the acetabulum. A dislocation is a complete loss of contact of the femoral head with the acetabulum. Dislocations are divided into two types, teratologic and typical. Teratologic dislocations occur early in utero and often are associated with neuromuscular disorders, such as arthrogryposis and myelodysplasia, or with various dysmorphic syndromes. The typical dislocation occurs in an otherwise healthy infant and may occur parentally or postnatal. A stable relationship between the femoral head and the acetabulum is necessary for normal hip growth and development (Goldberg, 2000).

The baseline estimate of DDH based on orthopedic screening is 11.5/1,000 infants, with four times the risk for girls compared to boys (rate of 4.1/1,000 in boys and 19/1,000 in girls). Infants with a positive family history (affected first-degree relative) or who are born breech (feet first) are at significantly increased risk. It is important to detect DDH early because the risk for avascular necrosis of the hip and ultimate hip dysfunction in DDH increases with age—2.5/1,000 in infants treated before 2 months of age versus 109/1,000 in infants treated after 2 months of age (Hema, 2001). However, current screening as practiced by generalists and pediatricians in the perinatal period only detects DDH in 1 out of 20 cases. This is due to both poor technique and failure to consistently perform the screening at birth and during the first 2 months of life. However, for proper application of the screening method, both the AAP and the Canadian Task Force agree that there is fair evidence to suggest that serial clinical examination of the hips by a trained clinician is effective at detecting DDH (Hema, 2001).

Anemia Screening

Screening for anemia in childhood, defined by the CDC as a hemoglobin of <11.0 mg/dL, has become a standard in the routine health care for children in the United States (CDC, 1989). Despite the lack of evidence to support or refute the value of screening low risk, asymptomatic populations (with a 3 percent prevalence rate of anemia), universal screening is recommended by both the AAP and the AAFP based on the theoretical risk of impaired growth and cognitive development which may result from chronic mild iron deficiency anemia. Conflicting evidence exists regarding the validity of this concern or whether or not early nutritional intervention results in measurable differences in outcome. Strong support does exist, however, for screening all high-risk children. Currently the Canadian Task Force endorses screening only children at risk for anemia (Feighter, 1994a).

Increased risk for anemia in infancy and childhood occurs among children that are born prematurely, are of low birth weight, low socioeconomic status, immigrate from developing countries, children who consume cow's milk before one year of age (or have excessive consumption of cow's milk at any age), are not breast fed, and/or have inadequate consumption of iron fortified foods like cereals and formulas (CDC, 1998). In addition, African American or children of Alaskan native or native American descent, in whom the prevalence of anemia may approach 30 percent, are also considered high risk. The USPSTF as well as the CTFPHC strongly endorses screening high-risk children for anemia before the age of one (USPSTF, 1989). Currently no well-defined global anemia screening protocols exist for children in the developing world where anemia is extremely common secondary to malnutrition, lack of access to iron fortified foods, and highly prevalent intestinal parasite infections.

Lead Screening

Both short and long-term exposure to lead can be toxic to human beings. However, it is the long-term, lower level exposure in developing children that poses the greatest public health risk. No lower threshold for the toxic effects of lead has been identified. The impact of even low levels of lead exposure on cognition in young children (blood lead levels [BLLs] ≥10 μg/dL) has been amply demonstrated (AAP, 1998). Over the past several decades, much has been done in the United States, Canada, and the world to reduce human exposure to lead by removing lead from gasoline, paint, and food cans. In the most recent study to evaluate lead exposure in the United States (1991–1994), the National Health and Nutrition Examination Survey (NHANES) found the percentage of US children 1–5 years of age with BLLs ≥ 10 μg/dL was 4.4 percent, down from 8.4 percent in 1977. Children aged 1–5 years were more likely to have elevated BLLs if they were poor, of non-Latino Black race, or lived in older housing. The prevalence of elevated BLLs was higher among non-Latino Black children (21.9 percent) and Mexican American children (13.0 percent) living in housing built before 1946 than among non-Latino White children (5.6 percent) living in such older housing. Risk for an elevated BLL was higher among low-income children living in housing built before 1946 (16.4 percent) than among high-income children living in older housing (0.9 percent) (CDC, 2000).

In 1991, the CDC recommended universal lead screening for children 9–72 months of age. Since that time, however, studies have identified many geographic areas where the prevalence of elevated BLLs is so low that selective screening is more appropriate than universal screening. In consideration of these data, the CDC revised its 1991 guidelines for universal screening to be limited in areas with ≥27 percent of housing built before 1950 and in populations in which the percentage of 1- and 2-year-olds with elevated BLLs is ≥ 12 percent. The revised CDC guidelines allow public health authorities to base their screening programs on local blood lead survey data and/or housing data collected by the US Bureau of the Census (CDC, 2000).

Another targeted population are children on Medicaid who, according to analyses of the NHANES, account for 60 percent of children aged 1–5 years with BLLs ≥10 μg/dL and 83 percent of young children with levels ≥20 μg/dL. Despite longstanding requirements for lead screening in the Medicaid program, surveys show that less than 20 percent are screened in the recommended age range. As a result, most children in the United States with elevated BLLs are not identified and, therefore, do not receive appropriate treatment or environmental intervention. To address this, the CDC and other federal agencies are urging states to implement strategies to improve lead screening for all children on Medicaid. The federal government is also urging states to implement innovative blood lead screening strategies in areas where conventional screening services have been ineffective (CDC, 2000).

Surveys conducted in Canada show that only a small percentage of Canadian children have blood lead levels above 10 μg/dL and that the levels of lead exposure have declined in recent years. Therefore, the CTFPHC concluded that there is insufficient evidence to recommend universal screening for lead exposure (Feldman & Randel, 1994).

Tuberculosis Screening

Most tuberculosis infections in children are asymptomatic or latent when detected with a positive tuberculin skin test (TST). Early clinical manifestations of active disease in children are less often pulmonary and can include fever, weight loss, cough, lymphadenopathy, meningitis, and other extra pulmonary manifestations (AAP, 1996b). Case rates of tuberculosis disease in children are highest in foreign-born children, first generation immigrants from high-risk countries (Asia, Africa, and Latin America), and children exposed to adults with active TB, such as homeless children, Native American children, and children living in other poor and overcrowded conditions. As opposed to adults, the diagnosis of active TB in a child rarely represents reactivation of latent disease and should be considered as evidence of recent transmission of *M. tuberculosis* in the community.

The Mantoux TST is the gold standard in screening for infection or exposure to the human tubercle bacillus. For testing, 0.1 mL of standardized purified protein derivative (PPD-T, Connaught Laboratories) containing 5 tuberculin units (TU) is injected intradermally in the forearm and examined at 48–72 hr. The transverse diameter of the induration (not erythema) in millimeters is determined by inspection and palpation. There is no clear point of separation between a positive and a negative test, although cut-off points have been established by comparing reactions among and between infected and uninfected individuals. The CDC, the AAP, and other groups now recommend the use of cut-off values based on a specific population's risk of infection. For children suspected of having TB (suggestive X-ray and/or history) or contacts of infectious cases, the recommended cut-off value is 5 mm. For children younger than 4 years of age or a child of any age who is a member of a high-risk group, the cut off is >10 mm. For children 4 years of age or older without any risk factors, the cut off is increased to 15 mm (CDC, 2001b).

According to reviews by the AAP and the CTFPHC, the evidence for the effectiveness of screening of the general population is poor (Pickering, 2000). Specific screening

questionnaires, comprised of questions directed at risks described above, have been proposed to identify children at higher risk. These questionnaires have been found to be fairly sensitive (80+ percent) and specific (80+ percent). However, due to the low incidence of positive TB tests even among high-risk children, their positive predictive value is low (<10 percent) (Ozuah, Ozuah, Stein, Burton, & Mulvihill, 2001).

Routine Child Health Visits for Growth Monitoring

Routine growth monitoring is widely accepted and strongly supported by health providers and is a standard component of community pediatric services throughout the world (AAP, 2000b). Growth monitoring consists of measuring the height and weight of children regularly throughout childhood, plotting the information on a growth chart to compare with population norms, and intervening with the family if growth is abnormal. The recommendations for the number and spacing of visits for growth monitoring vary across the world (Dickin et al., 1997). In developing countries, the United Nations Children's Fund recommends monthly growth monitoring for all children up to 18 months (UNICEF, 1990). This appears to be based in part on a large volume of narrative endorsements of growth monitoring found in the literature (Morley, 1973). In developed countries, growth monitoring is conducted less frequently, the purpose is different, and the outcomes anticipated are more modest.

A randomized controlled trial in Canada, involving healthy term neonates in intact families from all social classes, compared 5 or 6 visits versus 10 visits during the first 2 years. No differences were found using extensive measures of physical health and other outcomes (Feldman, 1994). In the United States, the AAP recommends measurement and assessment of height and weight at each of the 13 recommended preventive care visits from birth up to 5 years (AAP, 2000b). However, there is no good evidence to show that growth monitoring of this frequency is effective. In a Cochrane review of growth monitoring conducted in 2000, the authors found insufficient evidence that routine growth monitoring has any impact on child health in either developing or developed countries (cited in Panpanich & Garner, 2001).

Growth Monitoring for Obesity

Obesity has been defined as being 20 percent or more above desirable body weight. However, measures of height and weight (with comparison to standard growth charts) are imprecise, subject to significant measurement error, and only approximate the extent of overweight. Moreover, the criteria for desirable body weight are a matter of controversy among experts and vary considerably as presented in different weight-for-height tables (Hall, 1996). The prevalence of obesity among children is uncertain, but it is estimated to be between 5 and 25 percent in the United States and is increasing. There is also very good evidence that childhood obesity commonly leads to adult obesity.

The US Preventive Healthcare Task Force concluded, "Periodic height and weight measurements, although not proven to be effective, are inexpensive, rapid, and acceptable to patients." They may also be useful for the detection of medical conditions causing unintended weight loss, weight gain, or other growth abnormalities. The CTFPHC Services found insufficient evidence to include or exclude in the periodic health examination of infants and children measurement of height and weight to detect obesity (Feldman, 1994). Also, there is insufficient evidence to recommend including or excluding more involved screening for obesity using skin-fold thickness, body-mass index, or other measures. Well-designed studies are needed that examine a range of monitoring approaches and effective interventions for obesity.

Routine Childhood Immunizations

An abundance of evidence exists to support the administration of routine childhood immunizations. The policy in the United States of vaccinating every child has resulted in a dramatic decrease in the incidence of vaccine preventable infectious childhood illnesses, despite significant variation in up-to-date rates across racial, socioeconomic, and geographic groups. The recommended immunization schedule, developed jointly by the AAP, the Advisory Committee on Immunization Practices (ACIP) of the CDC, and the AAFP defines the standard of care with regard to the administration of childhood vaccines (see Figure 1). The schedule, updated and published each 6 months in January and July, currently recommends routine immunization, barring specific contraindications, against measles, mumps, rubella, paralytic poliomyelitis, diphtheria, tetanus, pertussis, Haemophilus influenza type b, Varicella, pneumococcal disease, and hepatitis B (AAP, 2001b). Additional recommendations exist for selective immunization of at-risk children against hepatitis A (CDC, 1999).

Generally, all immunizations are administered before 24 months of age with select booster immunizations scheduled at 4–12 years of age. It is strongly recommended that children who have not been previously immunized against hepatitis B initiate the series at the earliest possible date (CDC, 1995). Although the risk of contracting hepatitis B is extremely low in infancy and childhood, the vaccine is given

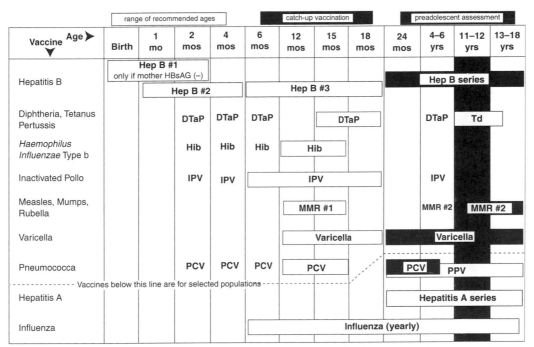

This schedule indicates the recommended ages for routine administration of currently licensed childhood vaccines, as of December 1, 2001, for children through age 18 years. Any doses not given at the recommended age should be given at any subsequent visit when indicated and feasible. The areas in black indicate age groups that warrant special effort to administer those vaccines not previously given. Additional vaccines may be licensed and recommended during the year. Licensed combination vaccines may be used whenever any components of the combination are indicated and the vaccine's other components are not contraindicated. Providers should consult the manufacturers' package inserts for detailed recommendations. (Approved by the Advisory Committee on Immunization Practices, the American Academy of Pediatrics, and the American Academy of Family Physicians)

Figure 1. Recommended Childhood Immunization Schedule: United States, 2002.

for protection in adolescence and adulthood when high-risk behaviors have a significant impact on infection rates. Additionally, children older than one year of age who have not received the Varicella vaccine and who do not have a reliable history of having a prior chickenpox infection should be immunized against Varicella. Despite chickenpox generally being considered a mild illness, vaccination against Varicella has been shown to have a favorable cost–benefit ratio (reducing missed school days, missed days from work) and prevent the occurrence of severe disease and death (there are approximately 50 deaths each year as a complication of Varicella infection in the United States), especially among older children, adolescents, and adults that contract Varicella (Zimmerman, 1996).

Similar routine childhood immunization policies have been adopted by Canada and Mexico as part of their public health programs but with some variances in recommendations and degrees of success. The CTFPHC promotes a schedule almost identical to that of the United States, including recommending Varicella and use of the inactivated polio vaccine rather than oral polio vaccine because of the small but real risk of inducing vaccine-associated paralytic poliomyelitis (Gold & Martell, 1994). Targeted vaccination for hepatitis A and provision of the pneumococcal conjugate vaccine is not included in the Canadian guidelines. Immunization rates in Canada currently approach 90 percent of the targeted population. Mexico utilizes a schedule strongly influenced by the Expanded Program on Immunizations (EPI) advocating the administration of OPV and the Bacillus Camille Guerin (BCG) vaccination for preventing specific types of tuberculosis, as recommended by the World Health Organization (WHO) for endemic areas. The pneumococcal conjugate, Varicella, and hepatitis A vaccines are not included in Mexico's current mass immunization guideline (WHO, 2001). However, the remaining recommendations closely resemble those of the US schedule. Statistics from WHO indicate that just over 40 percent of Mexico's children have been appropriately immunized.

Anticipatory Guidance

Anticipatory guidance has traditionally been a hallmark of the well child visit in the developing and developed world. Parents expect a physician or other health care professional to educate them about expectations for their child's development, safety concerns, and strategies for health promotion in an effort to assist them with providing the best possible care for their child. Surprisingly very few well-designed controlled studies have been undertaken to determine the effectiveness of counseling children and their families during well child health care visits.

Despite this lack of evidence, the USPSTF, AAP, AAFP, and the CTFPHC each encourage some form of anticipatory guidance for parents of children aged' birth through 5 and beyond (Feldman, 1994; USPSTF, 1989). The AAP and AAFP strongly endorse educational efforts directed toward parents, and the two professional associations have expended significant energy and resources to educate physicians about the importance of this aspect of well childcare. Anticipatory guidance may include discussions about sudden infant death syndrome (SIDS) prevention (CDC, 1996), the benefits of breastfeeding (Moreland & Coombs, 2000), proper nutrition, injury prevention (AAP, 1994), the importance of exercise, preventive services (immunizations, periodic physical and dental exams etc.), dosing of over-the-counter medications (specifically those such as Tylenol® that are potentially toxic) (AAP, 2001a), emergency access to care, environmental dangers, first aid, behavioral issues, and family planning among others. A variety of standards for anticipatory guidance based on age are available. Generally, a physician determines what is relevant for individual patients and presents information appropriate for age, health status, social environment, and level of education.

As expected, wide variances exist between recommendations for the developed and developing world (e.g., counseling a family about fluoridated water in the third world would not be productive but discussing safety of drinking water would be critical). The provision of anticipatory guidance is a low-cost and low-risk intervention offering the potential to significantly impact the overall health of a child (especially in populations with limited access to care). It represents an important opportunity to promote the health of children through their own education and education of their families.

Also see: Environmental Health: Early Childhood; Nuclear Families: Childhood.

References

American Academy of Pediatrics. (1994). Committee on injury and prevention: Office-based counseling for injury prevention. *Pediatrics, 94,* 566–567.
American Academy of Pediatrics. (1996a). Eye examination and vision screening in infants, children and young adults (RE9625). *Pediatrics, 98,* 153–157.
American Academy of Pediatrics. (1996b). Update on tuberculosis skin testing of children (RE9605). *Pediatrics, 97,* 282–284.
American Academy of Pediatrics. (1998). Committee on environmental health: Screening for elevated blood lead levels (RE9815). *Pediatrics, 101,* 1072–1078.
American Academy of Pediatrics. (1999). Newborn and infant hearing loss: Detection and intervention (RE9846). *Pediatrics, 103,* 527–530.

American Academy of Pediatrics. (2000a). Newborn screening: A blueprint for the future. A call for a national agenda on state newborn screening programs. *Pediatrics, 106*(Suppl. 2), 389–422.

American Academy of Pediatrics. (2000b). Recommendations for preventive pediatric health care (RE9939). *Pediatrics, 105*, 645.

American Academy of Pediatrics. (2001a). Acetaminophen toxicity in children. *Pediatrics, 108*, 1020–1024.

American Academy of Pediatrics. (2001b). Recommended childhood immunization schedule (RE0057). *Pediatrics, 107*, 202.

Ashley-Koch, A., Quanhe, Y., & Olney, R.S. (2000). Hemoglobin S allele and sickle cell disease. *American Journal of Epidemiology, 151*, 839–845.

Baldwin, R., & Wilson, M.E.H. (1989). Screening for phenylketonuria (ch. 44). In US Preventive Services Task Force *Guide to clinical preventive services: An assessment of the effectiveness of 169 interventions.* Baltimore, MD: Williams and Wilkins.

Beaulieu, M.D. (1994). Screening for congenital hypothyroidism. In *Canadian task force on the periodic health examination* (pp. 190–194). Ottawa: Health Canada.

Centers for Disease Control. (1989). Current trends: CDC criteria for anemia in children and childbearing aged women. *Morbidity Mortality Weekly Reports, 38*(22), 400–404.

Centers for Disease Control. (1995). Recommendations to prevent hepatitis B virus transmission. *Morbidity Mortality Weekly Reports, 44*(30), 574–575.

Centers for Disease Control. (1996). Sudden infant death syndrome—United States 1983–1994. *Morbidity Mortality Weekly Reports, 45*, 859–863.

Centers for Disease Control. (1997). Serious hearing impairment among children aged 3–10 years—Atlanta, Georgia, 1991–1993. *Morbidity Mortality Weekly Reports, 46*, 1073–1076.

Centers for Disease Control. (1998). CDC guidelines for prevention, detection, and treatment of iron deficiency anemia. *Morbidity Mortality Weekly Reports, 47*(RR-3), 1–36.

Centers for Disease Control. (1999). Prevention of hepatitis A through active or passive immunization: Recommendations of the advisory committee on immunization practices. *Morbidity Mortality Weekly Reports, 48*(RR-12), 1–7.

Centers for Disease Control. (2000). Prevention recommendations for blood lead screening of young children enrolled in Medicaid: Targeting a group at high risk. *Morbidity Mortality Weekly Reports, 49*(RR14), 1–13.

Centers for Disease Control. (2001a). Recommendations for using fluoride to prevent and control dental caries in the United States. Fluoride recommendations work group. *Morbidity Mortality Weekly Reports, 50*(RR14), 1–42.

Centers for Disease Control. (2001b). Targeted tuberculin testing and treatment of latent tuberculosis infection: ATS/CDC statement committee on latent tuberculosis infection membership. *Morbidity Mortality Weekly Reports, 49*(RR06), 1–54.

Dickin, K., Black, M., Engle, P., Habicht, J.P., Pelletier, D., Pelto, G.H., & De Onis, M. (1997). *Promoting healthy growth and development: A review of child development and nutrition interventions.* Geneva, Switzerland: World Health Organization, Division of Child Health and Development.

Feighter, J.W. (1994a). Prevention of iron deficiency anemia in infants. *Canadian Task Force on the Periodic Health Examination* (pp. 244–255). Ottawa: Health Canada.

Feighter, J.W. (1994b). Routine preschool screening for visual and hearing problems. *Canadian Task Force on the Periodic Health Examination* (pp. 298–304). Ottawa: Health Canada.

Fisher, D.A. (1987). Effectiveness of newborn screening programs for congenital hypothyroidism: Prevalence of missed cases. *Pediatric Clinical North America, 34*, 881–890.

Feldman, W. (1994). Well-baby care in the first 2 years of life. *Canadian Task Force on the Periodic Health Examination* (pp. 258–266). Ottawa: Health Canada.

Feldman, W., & Randel, P. (1994). Screening children for lead exposure in Canada. *Canadian Task Force on the Periodic Health Examination* (pp. 268–288). Ottawa: Health Canada.

Glorieux, J., Dussault, J., & Van Vliet, G. (1992). Intellectual development at age 12 years of children with congenital hypothyroidism diagnosed by neonatal screening. *Journal of Pediatrics, 121*, 581–584.

Gold, R., & Martell, A. (1994). Childhood immunizations. *Canadian Task Force on the Periodic Health Examination* (pp. 372–384). Ottawa: Health Canada.

Goldberg, M.J. (2000). Clinical practice guideline: Early detection of developmental dysplasia of the hip. *Pediatrics, 105*, 896–905.

Goldbloom, R.B. (1994). Screening for hemoglobinopathies in Canada. *Canadian Task Force on the Periodic Health Examination* (pp. 206–218), Ottawa: Health Canada.

Hall, D.M.B. (1996). *Health for all children. Report of the third joint working party on child health surveillance* (3rd ed.). Oxford, England: Oxford University Press.

Hema, P. (2001). Preventive health care, 2001 update: Screening and management of developmental dysplasia of the hip in newborns. *Canadian Medical Association Journal, 164*, 1669–1677.

Holtzman, C., Slazyk, W.E., & Cordero, J.F. (1986). Descriptive epidemiology of missed cases of phenylketonuria and congenital hypothyroidism. *Pediatrics, 78*, 553–538.

Holtzman, N.A., & Watson, M.S. (Eds.). (1997). *Promoting safe and effective genetic testing in the United States: Final report of the task force on genetic testing.* Bethesda, MD: National Institutes of Health.

Kotch, R., Yusin, M., & Fishler, K. (1985). Successful adjustment to society by adults with phenylketonuria. *Journal of Inherited Metabolic Disorders, 8*, 209–211.

Lewis, D.W., & Banting, D.W. (1994). Water fluoridation: Current effectiveness and dental fluorosis. *Community Dental Oral Epidemiology, 22*, 153–158.

Lewis, D.W., & Ismail, A.I. (1995). Periodic health examination, 1995 update: Prevention of dental caries. *Canadian Medical Association Journal, 152*, 836–846.

Moreland, J., & Coombs, J. (2000). Promoting and supporting breastfeeding. *American Family Physician, 61*, 2093–2100.

Morley, D. (1973). *Paediatric priorities in the developing world.* London: Butterworths.

National Institute of Dental Research. (1981). *The prevalence of dental caries in United States children 1979–80. The National Dental Caries Prevalence Survey.* (Publication No. DHHS (NIH) 82–2245). Bethesda, MD: Author.

National Institutes of Health. (1993). *Early identification of hearing impairment in infants and young children. NIH Consensus Statement.* Bethesda, MD.

Newbrun, E. (1989). Effectiveness of water fluoridation. *Journal of Public Health Dentistry, 49*, 279–289.

Ozuah, P.O., Ozuah, T.P., Stein, R.E., Burton, W., & Mulvihill, M. (2001). Evaluation of a risk assessment questionnaire used to target tuberculin skin testing in children. *Journal of the American Medical Association, 285*, 451–453.

Panpanich, R., & Garner, P. (2001). Growth monitoring in children (Cochrane Review). In *The Cochrane Library, 3.* [Oxford: Update Software]. Web address: http://www.update-software.com/Cochrane/default.HTM

Pickering, L.K. (2000). Tuberculosis. In L.K. Pickering (Ed.), *2000 Red book: Report of the AAP committee on infectious disease.* Elk Grove Village, IL: American Academy of Pediatrics.

Postellon, D.C., & Abdallah, A. (1986). Congenital hypothyroidism: Diagnosis, treatment, and prognosis. *Comprehensive Therapy, 12*, 67–71.

Ripa, LW. (1988). Nursing caries: A comprehensive review. *Pediatric Dentistry, 10*, 268–282.

Somens, D.G., & Favreau, L. (1982). Newborn screening for phenyl-ketonuria: Incidence and screening procedures in North America. *Canadian Journal of Public Health, 73*, 206–207.

UNICEF. (1990). *Strategy for improved nutrition of children and women in developing countries.* New York: United Nations Children's Fund.

US Preventive Services Task Force. (1989). *Guide to clinical preventive services: An assessment of the effectiveness of 169 interventions.* Baltimore, MD: Williams and Wilkins.

US Preventive Services Task Force. (2001 update). *Screening for diminished visual acuity. Guide to clinical preventive services: An assessment of the effectiveness of 169 interventions.* Baltimore, MD: Williams and Wilkins.

Weinstein, P., Milgrom, P., & Mclnick, S. (1989). How effective is oral hygiene instruction? Results after 6 and 24 weeks. *Journal of Public Health Dentistry, 49*, 32–38.

World Health Organization. (2001). Immunization profile—Mexico. Geneva. Web address: http://wwwnt.who.int/vaccines/globalsummary/Immunization/CountryProfileSelect.cfm

Yoshinaga-Itano, C., Sedey, A.L., Coulter, D.K., & Mehl, A.L. (1998). Language of early- and later-identified children with hearing loss. *Pediatrics, 102*, 1161–1171.

Zimmerman, R.K. (1996). Varicella vaccine: Rationale and indications for use. *American Family Physician, 53*, 647–651.

Pregnancy, Adolescence*

Douglas Kirby and Brent C. Miller

INTRODUCTION, DEFINITIONS, AND SCOPE

In the United States, teen pregnancy is an important problem. In 1997, the last year for which accurate estimates are available, about 896,000 young women under the age of 20 became pregnant. Among 15–19-year-old women, 94 per 1,000 became pregnant (Ventura, Mosher, Curtin, Abma, & Henshaw, 2001). This pregnancy rate is higher for African Americans (170 per 1,000) and Latinos (149 per 1,000) than for Whites (65 per 1,000) (Darroch & Singh, 1999). However, much of this ethnic variation reflects differences in poverty. Because annual pregnancy rates are cumulative for each individual, more than 40 percent of young women in the United States become pregnant one or more times before they reach 20 years of age (National Campaign to Prevent Teen Pregnancy, 1997).

* This article is adapted from Kirby (2001).

The US teen pregnancy rate is much higher than rates in other western industrialized countries. For example, the US rate of 94 pregnancies per 1,000 girls is nearly twice as high as rates for Canada (52) and England and Wales (55), four to five times as high as rates in France (23) and Germany (19), and approximately seven times the teen pregnancy rates in Italy, Spain, and the Netherlands, all of which have a rate of 14 per 1,000 (Singh & Darroch, 2000).

On the positive side, the 1997 teen pregnancy rate in the United States is the lowest pregnancy rate since it was first measured in the 1970s (Ventura, Mosher et al., 2001). However, it has fluctuated considerably during the last three decades, reflecting both changing percentages of youth who have sex and improved use of contraception among those having sex (Alan Guttmacher Institute, 1994; Darroch & Singh, 1999; Flanigan, 2001).

While the *teenage pregnancy* rate is, by definition, based upon female teenagers, this does not mean that all the males involved in these pregnancies are teenagers. Indeed, in 1994, while 11 percent of 15–19-year-old females became pregnant, only 5 percent of 15–19-year-old males caused a pregnancy (Darroch, Landry, & Oslak, 1999).

How are teen pregnancies resolved? In 1997, 15 percent ended in miscarriages, 29 percent ended in legal abortions, and 55 percent ended in births (Ventura, Mosher et al., 2001).

Consistent with the pregnancy data, the US teen birth rate is very high by absolute standards (49.6 births per 1,000 15–19-year-old females in 1999) (Curtin & Martin, 2000), is much higher than that in other Western industrialized countries (Henshaw, 1999; Singh & Darroch, 2000), but is at an all-time low for the United States (Curtin & Martin, 2000).

Among *unmarried* teens aged 15–19, the birth rate rose from 22 per 1,000 in 1970 to 40 per 1,000 in 1999 (Ventura, Martin, Curtin, Menacker, & Hamilton, 2001). Similarly, among mothers under the age of 20, the percent of births that occur out of wedlock has risen dramatically from 15 percent in 1960 to 79 percent in 1999 (Ventura, Martin et al., 2001). This large increase in and high rate of non-marital childbearing has alarmed many people and motivated many efforts to reduce teenage pregnancy.

Consequences of Adolescent Childbearing

When teenagers, especially younger teenagers, give birth, their future prospects decline on a number of dimensions (Maynard, 1996). They become less likely to complete school, more likely to have large families, and more likely to be single parents. They work as much as women who delay childbearing for several years, but their earnings must provide for a larger number of children.

However, it is the children of teenaged mothers who may bear the greatest brunt of their mothers' young age. In particular, children born to mothers aged 15–17 in comparison with those born to mothers aged 20 or 21 have less supportive and stimulating home environments, poorer health, lower cognitive development, worse educational outcomes, higher rates of behavior problems, and higher rates of adolescent childbearing themselves (Maynard, 1996).

Although the greatest costs are to the families directly involved, adolescent childbearing leads to considerable cost to taxpayers and society more generally. Estimates of these costs are in the billions (Maynard, 1996).

Adolescent Sexual and Contraceptive Behavior

Obviously, teens become pregnant because they have sex without using contraception effectively. In the United States, the proportion of teens who have ever had sexual intercourse increases steadily with age. In 1995, among girls, the percentage was 25 percent among 15-year-olds and 77 percent among 19-year-olds, while among males, it was 27 percent among 15-year-olds and 85 percent among 19-year-olds (Moore, Driscoll, & Lindberg, 1998). Among students in grades 9–12 across the United States in 1999, 50 percent reported sexual experience (Centers for Disease Control and Prevention [CDC], 2000).

Most sexually experienced teenagers use contraception, at least part of the time (e.g., 69 percent reported using contraception the last time they had sex) (Terry & Manlove, 2000). Condoms and oral contraceptives are the two most common methods, but small and increasing percentages of teens use long-lasting contraceptives such as Depo-Provera or Norplant (Darroch & Singh, 1999).

However, like some adults, many sexually active teenagers do not consistently use contraceptives properly, thereby exposing themselves to risks of pregnancy or STDs. For example, among 15–19-year-old girls relying upon oral contraceptives as their main contraceptive, only 70 percent took a pill every day (Abma, Chandra, Mosher, Peterson, & Piccinino, 1997). Similarly, among sexually experienced teen boys using condoms, only 45 percent used a condom during every act of intercourse in the last year (Sonenstein, Ku, Lindberg, Turner, & Pleck, 1998).

THEORY AND RESEARCH

Important Risk and Protective Factors of Sexual Risk-Taking and Pregnancy

Many researchers have studied the antecedents of adolescent sexual risk-taking and pregnancy, both to identify youth at high risk of pregnancy and to identify the risk and protective factors programs must address in order to reduce

sexual risk-taking and pregnancy (Kirby, 2001; Miller, 1998). These studies reveal that a very large number of antecedents has been linked to one or more sexual or contraceptive behaviors, or pregnancy. They characterize not only individual teens themselves, but also important groups within their environment, for example, their partners, peers, families, schools, communities, and even states as well as the teens' relationships to these important people and groups. Together, the antecedents paint a complex portrait of the factors affecting sexual risk-taking among adolescents.

In part because so many antecedents are related to sexual risk-taking, few antecedents are *very highly* related to behavior. Rather, most of the antecedents are weakly or, in some instances, moderately related to behavior. This means that pregnancy prevention programs that target only one or a small number of antecedents are not likely to have a marked impact upon teen pregnancy. Programs, either singly or in combination, need to address multiple antecedents.

Teens are more likely to engage in sex, less likely to use contraception or more likely to become pregnant when the following occur: (1) they live in communities with lower levels of education, employment, and income and thereby have fewer opportunities; (2) the teens' parents have low levels of education and income; (3) the teens live with only one or neither parent and believe they have little parental support, feel disconnected from their parents, and are inappropriately supervised or monitored by their parents; (4) the parents either express permissive values or model behavior consistent with sexual risk-taking or early childbearing by having sex outside of marriage, giving birth outside of marriage, or giving birth at an early age; (5) the *siblings* of teens model early childbearing by giving birth at an early age; (6) the peers of teens obtain poor grades, are less attached to school, and engage in non-normative behaviors; (7) the teens believe their peers are having sex and fail to use contraceptives consistently; (8) the teens, themselves, are less attached to school, do poorly in school, and lack plans for higher education; (9) the teens, themselves, use alcohol and drugs, engage in other problem or risk-taking behaviors, and have evidence of emotional distress; (10) they begin dating at an early age, date frequently, have a greater number of romantic partners, go steady at an early age, and especially have a romantic partner three or more years older; (11) they were previously sexually abused; and perhaps most important (12) they have permissive attitudes toward premarital sex, lack self-efficacy to avoid sex or to use contraception consistently, do not accept the fact that they are having sex, are less knowledgeable about contraception, have more negative attitudes toward contraception, and are ambivalent about pregnancy and childbearing.

More generally, all of the factors affecting sexual risk-taking and pregnancy can be divided into those that involve some aspect of sexuality (e.g., beliefs and values about teen sex and contraceptive use) and those that do not involve sexuality (e.g., community opportunity and teen success in school). In turn, programs to reduce sexual risk-taking and pregnancy can also be divided into those that focus upon the sexual risk-factors (e.g., sex and HIV education programs) and those that do not (e.g., service learning programs). The effects of these two broad groups of programs are discussed in order.

STRATEGIES THAT WORK, MIGHT WORK, OR DO NOT WORK

Abstinence-Only and Sex and HIV Education Programs

Some curriculum-based sex education programs stress abstinence as the only acceptable choice for preventing pregnancy (often called abstinence-only programs), while others emphasize both abstinence and methods of protection against pregnancy and STD (often called abstinence-plus or sexuality education programs). This latter group can be further divided into those that address both pregnancy and STD/HIV (sometimes called sexuality education programs) and those that focus primarily on STD/HIV prevention (appropriately called HIV education programs).

In a review of all abstinence, sex education and HIV education programs meeting certain criteria (e.g., used an experimental or quasi-experimental design, had a sample size of at least 100, and measured impact upon behavior), Kirby (2001) found that only three abstinence-only studies met these criteria and none of these three programs had a significant impact upon behavior. They did not delay sex, reduce the number of sexual partners, reduce the frequency of sex or affect contraceptive use one way or the other.

Given the great diversity of abstinence-only programs, the small number of studies, and the limitations of these studies, the proper conclusion to draw from these three studies is not that abstinence-only programs cannot reduce sexual risk-taking, but rather that there is too little evidence to determine whether or not they can effectively change sexual behavior. In other words, the jury is still out. Moreover, given the diversity of abstinence-only programs, it seems likely that some do delay the onset of sex, but it is simply not known at this time which programs are most effective.

That same review (Kirby, 2001) found strong evidence that sex and HIV education programs that emphasize abstinence and also discuss condoms and contraceptives in a balanced and medically accurate manner, do not increase any measure of sexual activity and that some programs delay or decrease sexual activity. Twenty-eight studies examined the impact of middle school, high school, or community sexuality or HIV education programs on the *initiation* of intercourse. Nine of them (or about one third) found that the programs delayed the initiation of sex, 18 found no significant impact, and only 1 study out of 28 found that it hastened the initiation of sex. Overall, this is very strong evidence that these programs, as a group, do not hasten the onset of sex, and that some of them actually delay first intercourse.

Nineteen studies examined the impact of sexuality and HIV education programs on the *frequency* of intercourse. Five studies found that they reduced the frequency of sex, 13 found no significant impact, and 1 of 19 studies found a significant increase in frequency. Finally, of the 10 studies that examined impact on *number of sexual partners*, 3 found a significant decrease in partners, 7 found no impact and none found a significant increase. Again, this is strong evidence that these programs do not increase the frequency of sex or number of sexual partners.

These studies also demonstrate that some, but not all, of the programs increased condom use or contraceptive use more generally. Of the 18 programs whose impact on condom use was evaluated, 10 programs (or more than half) significantly increased some measure of condom use. Similarly, 4 of 11 programs significantly increased contraceptive use more generally. None of the programs reduced either condom or contraceptive use.

Not only are there a substantial number of studies indicating that some sex and HIV education programs can reduce sexual risk-taking, the evidence for the effectiveness of some sex and HIV education programs is enhanced by other qualities of these studies. First, there are now three studies with random assignment, large sample sizes, long-term follow-up, measurement of behavior and proper statistical analyses that have shown statistically significant and programmatically important reductions in adolescent sexual risk-taking behavior (Coyle et al., 2001; Jemmott, Jemmott, & Fong, 1998; St. Lawrence, Jefferson, Alleyne, Brasfield, O'Bannon, & Shirley, 1995). Thus, high quality studies also reveal programmatic impact. Second, several studies found lasting effects for 1 year, some found effects for about 18 months, and one study found effects over 31 months (Coyle et al., 2001). Third, there are at least two independent studies in different states indicating that the same curriculum, *Reducing the Risk*, delayed the onset of sexual intercourse and increased condom or contraceptive use among some groups of youth (Hubbard, Giese, & Rainey, 1998; Kirby, Barth, Leland, & Fetro, 1991). Finally, one study has estimated the cost-effectiveness and cost-benefits of a sex education program; it found that for every dollar invested in *Safer Choices*, the program saved $2.65 in total medical and social costs by preventing pregnancy, HIV, and other STDs (Wang, Davis, Robin, Collins, Coyle, & Baumler, 2000).

While some sex and HIV education programs were effective at reducing sexual risk-taking, others were not. When the effective programs were compared with the ineffective ones, they shared 10 common characteristics. Effective programs:

1. focused on reducing one or more sexual behaviors that lead to unintended pregnancy or HIV/STD infection;
2. were based on theoretical approaches that have been demonstrated to be effective in influencing other health-related risky behaviors and that identified specific important sexual antecedents to be targeted (e.g., cognitive behavior theory, theory of reasoned action, and theory of planned behavior);
3. gave a clear message about abstaining from sexual activity and using condoms or other forms of contraception and continually reinforced that message;
4. provided basic, accurate information about the risks of teen sexual activity and about methods of avoiding intercourse or using protection against pregnancy and STD;
5. included activities that address social pressures that influence sexual behavior;
6. provided modeling of and practice with communication, negotiation, and refusal skills;
7. employed a variety of teaching methods designed to involve the participants and help them personalize the information;
8. incorporated behavioral goals, teaching methods, and materials that were appropriate to the age, sexual experience, and culture of the participants;
9. lasted a sufficient length of time to complete important activities adequately;
10. selected teachers or peer leaders who believed in the program they were implementing and then provided them with training.

Family Planning Services

The primary objectives of family planning clinics or family planning services within other health settings are to provide contraception and other reproductive health services and to provide patients with the knowledge and skills to use their selected methods of contraception. Thus, they are based upon the common sense beliefs that providing knowledge about contraceptives, access to contraceptives, and skills to use the chosen methods will increase contraceptive use.

According to a 1992 national survey of family planning clinics, many family planning organizations have special clinics for teenagers, three fourths encourage their counselors to spend extra time with clients under age 18, four fifths have outreach programs for teenagers, many have programs for teenage parents as well as for the parents of these teenagers, and many have sex education training programs (Henshaw & Torres, 1994).

Large numbers of sexually active female teenagers obtain family planning services each year. Many of these young women received oral contraceptives and to a lesser extent other contraceptives that are more effective than condoms or other non-prescription contraceptives. Accordingly, these family planning services undoubtedly prevented many adolescent pregnancies. However, because of important limitations in research, the actual impact of these family planning services on adolescent pregnancy rates has not been accurately estimated.

Clinician–Patient Protocols and Instructional Strategies

Several studies have examined the impact of improving the protocols for patient visits to a health clinic, and quite consistently they found a positive impact upon behavior. In one revised protocol for STD patients, a nurse discussed STDs with the aid of a pamphlet, modeled how to put a condom on a banana (and got the patient to practice), and engaged the patient in a brief role play involving a woman getting her partner to use a condom. As a result, condom use increased (Orr, Langefeld, Katz, & Caine, 1996). A second program included a 15-min audio-taped risk assessment and education program, brochures (e.g., on skills and ways to avoid unprotected sex), a physician–patient review of the patient's risk behaviors, and focused discussions of methods of avoiding unprotected sex. Again, condom use increased (Boekeloo, Schamus, Simmens, Cheng, O'Connor, & D'Angelo, 1999). Finally, Winter and Breckenmaker (1991) showed that a family planning clinic can substantially improve its clinic protocol for adolescents and increased contraceptive use by placing greater focus upon non-medical problems, providing more information and more counseling, delaying the medical examination until the second visit, giving more attention to partner and parent involvement, and designating one staff person as a teen counselor.

Overall, these studies are encouraging, suggesting that even modest clinic interventions or changes in protocols can increase condom or contraceptive use, and that medical providers should review their instructional protocols with youth and spend more time talking with individual adolescent patients about their sexual and contraceptive activity.

School-Based Health Centers and School-Linked Reproductive Health Clinics

School-based health centers are clinics located on school grounds that offer services to students in their schools. The purpose of these clinics is to provide primary health care services that are affordable and accessible to students who otherwise might not have ongoing access to such services. Consequently, all of these clinics provide basic primary health care services. In 1999, there were at least 1,135 school-based health centers in schools and 70 percent of these served students in grades 7–12 (Making the Grade, 2000).

While most (90 percent) clinics in secondary schools provide at least one reproductive health service (such as gynecologic exams, birth control counseling, pregnancy testing, and STD diagnosis and treatment), only 29 percent of these clinics write prescriptions for birth control pills that can be filled elsewhere, and only 18 percent actually dispense birth control pills (Fothergill & Feijoo, 2000). About 28 percent dispense condoms.

When school-based clinics make contraception available to students, many sexually experienced students obtain contraceptives from the clinics. For example, in a study of four clinics that provided prescriptions or actually dispensed contraceptives, the proportion of sexually experienced females who obtained contraceptives through the clinic varied from 23 to 40 percent (Kirby, Waszak, & Ziegler, 1991).

Several studies have examined the impact of these clinics upon sexual risk-taking and birth rates. Although their quasi-experimental designs were not strong, multiple studies have consistently demonstrated that the provision of contraceptives in school-based health centers did not hasten the onset of sexual intercourse nor increase its frequency (Kirby et al., 1991; Kisker, Brown, & Hill, 1994). However, given the relatively wide availability of contraceptives in most communities, school-based clinics, especially those that did not focus on pregnancy or STD prevention, did not appear to markedly increase the school-wide use of contraceptives—that is, there appears to be a substitution effect such that students obtained contraception from school rather than from other sources. Consistent with the lack of school-wide impact on contraceptive rates, the provision of contraceptives through school-based clinics did not appear to decrease the school-wide pregnancy or birth rates in those sites. In contrast, in two sites, a school-based clinic and a school-linked family planning clinic focused much more on contraception and apparently did increase the use of contraception, suggesting that a clear focus may have been needed for these clinics to have a school-wide impact (Kirby, Barth et al., 1991; Zabin, Smith, Streett, & Hardy, 1986).

School Condom-Availability Programs

Given the threat of AIDS, other STDs, and pregnancy, more than 300 schools without school-based clinics have made condoms available through school counselors, nurses, teachers, vending machines, or baskets (Kirby & Brown,

1996). These schools are in addition to about 100 schools that make condoms available to students through school-based clinics. These programs are based upon the beliefs that making condoms accessible and free of charge will decrease barriers to obtaining condoms and may improve school-wide norms regarding condom use among those having sex.

When schools made multiple brands of condoms available in baskets in convenient and private locations and without any restrictions, students obtained many more condoms than when there were restrictions (e.g., when students could only obtain a small number of condoms from school personnel at specified times after brief counseling).

According to multiple studies, the provision of condoms in schools did not hasten the onset of sexual intercourse nor increase its frequency. However, studies of school condom availability programs provide conflicting results regarding their impact upon condom use. Some found that the programs increased condom use, while other studies did not. This variation in results may reflect methodological limitations in the studies, differences in the availability of condoms in the respective communities or differences in the programs themselves.

Community-Wide Pregnancy or HIV Prevention Initiatives with Multiple Components

During the last two decades, there has been a growing belief that to markedly change teen pregnancy rates, it may be necessary to change the communities in which teenagers live. Thus, many communities have developed community-wide collaboratives or initiatives with the goal of reducing teen pregnancy.

Seven different studies examined the impact of these programs. All of them measured impact on community-wide measures of sexual or contraceptive behavior or pregnancy or birth rates; they did not measure the impact on the individual teens directly served. Although this is the proper approach, it is a very challenging and demanding one.

One study evaluated the impact of a mass communications campaign to emphasize abstinence and delay sex among young teens in Monroe County, New York. It included paid television and radio advertising, billboards, posters, guides to process the posters for schools, educational materials for parents, and an educational series in some schools and community settings. The evaluation suggested that it delayed sex and decreased pregnancy rate (Doniger, Riley, Utter, & Adams, 2001).

Another study examined the impact of a large, comprehensive social marketing campaign called Project Action (Polen & Freeborn, 1995). Public service announcements were aired multiple times on television, condom vending machines were installed in locations recommended by youth, and teenagers were trained to facilitate small-group workshops that focused on decision-making and assertiveness skills. Results indicated that the campaign did not increase the proportion of higher risk youth who had ever had intercourse, nor did it increase their acquisition of condoms or their use of condoms with their main partners. However, after the campaign began, there was a significant increase in their use of condoms with casual sexual partners; after the campaign ended, this condom use returned to baseline levels. A similar campaign was implemented in Seattle, but it did not increase either sexual activity or condom use (Alstead, Campsmith, Halley, Hartfield, Goldbaum, & Wood, 1999).

An intensive, multiple component program in rural South Carolina appeared to decrease teen pregnancy (Koo, Dunteman, George, Green, & Vincent, 1994; Vincent, Clearie, & Schluchter, 1987). The program included the following components: teachers, administrators, community leaders, and peer counselors were given training in sexuality education; sex education was integrated into all grades in the schools; the school nurse counseled students, provided male students with condoms, and took female students to a nearby family planning clinic; and local media, churches, and other community organizations highlighted special events and reinforced the messages of avoiding unintended pregnancy. After the program was implemented, the pregnancy rate for 14–17-year-olds declined significantly for several years. After parts of the program ended, the pregnancy rate returned to pre-program levels. It is not clear which of the program components or other unknown factors produced the changes over time in pregnancy rates. However, when different investigators attempted to implement this model in Kansas, there were no consistent *and* significant changes in sexual behavior, condom use, pregnancy rates or birth rates (Paine-Andrews et al., 1999).

These results are modestly encouraging; they suggest that there were some successes and some failures. The most effective programs were clearly the most intensive. However, when others attempted to replicate the South Carolina program, they did not have consistent positive effects. Furthermore, the effects of both Project Action and the South Carolina program also suggest that programs must be maintained if they are to continue to have an effect. Notably, the Monroe County program was maintained over several years.

Programs that Focus Primarily on Non-Sexual Antecedents

Correlational data suggest that improving young women's education and life options reduces their pregnancy and birth rates. In many countries throughout the world, as young women's educational levels and employment opportunities have increased, their fertility rates have declined.

In this country, between the mid-1950s and the mid-1970s, increasingly large percentages of young women pursued both higher education and more challenging professional careers and therefore postponed marriage and childbearing (Alan Guttmacher Institute, 1994). As noted in the antecedents discussion above, among today's adolescents there remains a strong relationship between educational and career plans and adolescent pregnancy. Observing these trends, some professionals working with youth believe that one of the most promising approaches to reducing teen pregnancy is to improve educational and career opportunities for youth.

Service Learning Programs

By definition, service learning programs include: (1) voluntary or unpaid service in the community (e.g., tutoring, working as teachers' aide, working in nursing homes or helping clean up or fix up parks and recreation areas) and (2) structured time for preparation and reflection before, during, and after service (e.g., group discussions, journal writing, or papers). Often the service is voluntary, but sometimes it is prearranged as part of a class. And often, but not always, the service is linked to academic instruction in the classroom.

Service learning programs may have stronger evidence that they reduce teen pregnancy rates while youth are in the programs than any other type of intervention. Four different studies, three of which evaluated programs in multiple locations, have consistently indicated that service learning reduces either sexual activity or teen pregnancy (Allen, Philliber, Herrling, & Kuperminc, 1997; Melchior, 1998; O'Donnell et al., 1999, 2000; Philliber & Allen, 1992).

It is not known why service learning reduces teen pregnancy, but several suggestions have been given for the positive results: some participants developed ongoing relationships with caring program facilitators; some may have developed greater autonomy and felt more competent in their relationships with peers and adults; some may have realized that they could make a difference in the lives of others and thereby felt empowered; and some may have reflected more upon their futures. It may also be that both supervision and alternative activities structured many hours of adolescents' time and simply reduced the opportunity for participants to engage in problem behaviors, including unprotected sex. After all, these programs were time intensive—the average number of hours in an academic year that youth spent in them ranged from 46 hr in one program to about 90 hr in another.

Other Youth Development Programs

Several studies have rigorously studied vocational education programs (e.g., the Conservation and Youth Service

Corps, the Job Corps, and JOBSTART) (Cave, Bos, Doolittle, & Toussaint, 1993; Jastrzab, Masker, Blomquist, & Orr, 1997; Schochet, Burghardt, & Glazerman, 2000). These programs combined remedial, academic, and vocational education and thus addressed some of the important non-sexual antecedents. To varying extents, these programs also provided other support services, for example, life skills education, health education, health care, child care, and job placement assistance. All three programs focused on disadvantaged youth. All three studies incorporated strong experimental designs and consistently failed to find an impact upon long-term childbearing at 15–48 months. It is not clear why these rather intensive vocational education programs that were designed to address some of the important non-sexual antecedents of sexual risk-taking did not have an impact upon childbearing, while intensive service learning programs did have an impact.

Programs that Focus on Both Sexual and Non-Sexual Antecedents

Whereas the programs discussed in the previous sections focused primarily on sexual antecedents or primarily on non-sexual antecedents, some programs attempt to do both. One of the best examples is the *Children's Aid Society Carrera* program (CAS-Carrera) (Philliber, Kaye, Herring, & West, 2000). It was a long-term and intensive program operating 5 days a week and lasting throughout high school; participants spent an average of 16 hr per month in the program. The CAS-Carrera program used a holistic approach and provided multiple services and components: (1) family life and sex education; (2) an education component that included individual academic assessment, tutoring, help with homework, preparation for standardized exams, and assistance with college entrance; (3) a work-related intervention that included a job club, stipends, individual bank accounts, employment, and career awareness; (4) self-expression through the arts; and (5) individual sports. In addition, the program provided mental health care and comprehensive medical care, including reproductive health and contraception. Throughout all these components, staff tried to create close caring relationships with the participants. Although the program focused on youth, it also provided services for the participants' parents and other adults in the community.

After 3 years, the program significantly delayed the onset of sexual intercourse among girls, increased their use of condoms with another highly effective method of contraception, and reduced their pregnancy rate by half. Among males, the program did not have significant positive behavioral effects. This is the first and only study to date with a strong evaluation design that found a positive impact on sexual and contraceptive behavior, and pregnancy and births among girls for as long as 3 years.

SYNTHESIS

Although many studies reviewed in this paper have important methodological limitations, these studies do support several conclusions:

1. Both the studies of antecedents and the evaluations of programs indicate that there are no single, simple approaches that will markedly reduce adolescent pregnancy across the country. That is, there are no "magic bullets."
2. A number of programs appear to reduce sexual risk-taking, pregnancy or childbearing, and they can be classified in three groups. The first group includes those programs that address the sexual antecedents of sexual risk-taking behavior (e.g., school- or community-based sex and HIV/AIDS education programs, and some health clinic programs), the second group primarily addresses non-sexual antecedents (e.g., service learning programs), and the third group addresses both groups of antecedents (e.g., the CAS-Carrera program).
3. Abstinence and use of contraception are compatible goals and approaches with adolescents. There are two ideas behind this simple statement. First, the overwhelming weight of the evidence demonstrates that programs that focus on sexuality and discuss contraception, including sex and AIDS education programs, school-based clinics, and condom availability programs, do not increase sexual activity. Second, programs that emphasized abstinence, that gave it clear prominence, and that presented it as the safest and best approach while also emphasizing condoms or contraceptives for sexually active youth, did not decrease contraceptive use.
4. Relatively little is known about the impact of programs that stress abstinence as the only acceptable behavior for unmarried teens.
5. Studies of some sex and HIV education programs have produced credible evidence for reductions in sexual risk-taking either by delaying the onset of sex, reducing the frequency of sex, reducing the number of sexual partners, or increasing the use of condoms or other forms of contraception. Some studies found these positive effects to endure for periods as long as 31 months. Studies of other sex and AIDS education programs have failed to find positive effects on behavior.

In comparison with the ineffective programs, effective programs have the 10 characteristics described above.

6. Family planning clinics prevent a large, but unknown, number of teen pregnancies.

7. Several studies suggest that when clinics provide improved educational and media materials, discuss the adolescent patient's sexual and condom or contraceptive behavior, give a clear message about that behavior, and incorporate other components into the clinic visit, clinics can increase condom or contraceptive use, although not always for a prolonged period of time.

8. School-based and school-linked clinics and school condom availability programs do not increase sexual activity, but because of a substitution effect do not always increase condom and contraceptive use or reduce unintended pregnancy.

9. Across the different types of effective programs that addressed sexual antecedents, a common theme was that they clearly focused on sexual behavior and condom or contraceptive use, and they gave a clear message about abstaining from sex and/or using protection against STD and pregnancy.

10. The programs with the strongest evidence that they actually reduced teen pregnancy are service learning programs; vocational education programs did not decrease childbearing.

11. The only program which intensively addressed both the sexual and non-sexual antecedents of disadvantaged youth over a prolonged period of time (the CAS-Carrera program) substantially reduced teen pregnancy reported by girls over a long period of time and had other positive effects.

All in all, these findings bring good news, because they mean that quite different approaches to reducing sexual risk-taking are emerging. Some programs that address sexuality directly and some programs that address youth development more broadly can reduce sexual risk-taking or pregnancy. This increases the choices for communities. To reduce teen pregnancy, communities can (1) replicate much more broadly and with fidelity those programs with the greatest evidence for success with populations similar to their own; (2) replicate more broadly programs incorporating the common qualities of programs effective with populations similar to their own; and (3) design and implement programs that effectively address the important antecedents of sexual risk-taking.

Also see: HIV/AIDS: Adolescence; Sexual Assault: Adolescence; Sexuality: Adolescence; Sexually Transmitted Disease: Adolescence.

References

Abma, J., Chandra, A., Mosher, W., Peterson, L., & Piccinino, L. (1997). Fertility, family planning, and women's health: New data from the 1995 National Survey of Family Growth. *Vital and Health Statistics, 23*(19).

Alan Guttmacher Institute. (1994). *Sex and America's teenagers.* New York: Author.

Allen, J.P., Philliber, S., Herrling, S., & Kuperminc, G.P. (1997). Preventing teen pregnancy and academic failure: Experimental evaluation of a developmentally-based approach. *Child Development, 64*(4), 729–742.

Alstead, M., Campsmith, M., Halley, C.S., Hartfield, K., Goldbaum, G., & Wood, R.W. (1999). Developing, implementing, and evaluating a condom promotion program targeting sexually active adolescents. *AIDS Education and Prevention, 11*(6), 497–512.

Boekeloo, B.O., Schamus, L.A., Simmens, S.J., Cheng, T.L., O'Connor, K., & D'Angelo, L.J. (1999). A STD/HIV prevention trial among adolescents in managed care. *Pediatrics, 103*(1), 107–115.

Cave, G., Bos, H., Doolittle, F., & Toussaint, C. (1993). *JOBSTART: Final report on a program for school dropouts.* New York: Manpower Demonstration Research Corporation.

Centers for Disease Control and Prevention. (2000, June 9). CDC Surveillance Summaries, *Morbidity and Mortality Weekly Report, 49*(No. SS-5).

Coyle, K.K., Basen-Enquist, K.M., Kirby, D.B., Parcel, G.S., Banspach, S.W., Collins, J.L., Baumler, E.R., Caravajal, S., & Harrist, R.B. (2001). Safer choices: Reducing teen pregnancy, HIV, and STDs. *Public Health Reports, 116*(Suppl. 1), 82–93.

Curtin, S.C., & Martin, J.A. (2000). Births: Preliminary data for 1999. *National Vital Statistics Report, 48*(14). Hyattsville, MD: National Center for Health Statistics.

Darroch, J.E., Landry, D.J., & Oslak, S. (1999). Age differences between sexual partners in the United States. *Family Planning Perspectives, 31*(4), 160–167.

Darroch, J.E., & Singh, S. (1999). *Why is teenage pregnancy declining? The roles of abstinence, sexual activity and contraceptive use*, Occasional Report. New York: The Alan Guttmacher Institute, No. 1.

Doniger, A.S., Riley, J.S., Utter, C.A., & Adams, E. (2001). Impact evaluation of the "Not Me, Not Now" abstinence-oriented, adolescent pregnancy prevention communications programs, Monroe County, NY, *Journal of Health Communication, 6*(1): 45–60.

Flanigan, C. (2001). *What's behind the good news: The decline in teen pregnancy rates during the 1990s.* Washington, DC: National Campaign to Prevent Teen Pregnancy.

Fothergill, K., & Feijoo, A. (2000). Family planning services at school-based health centers: Findings from a national survey. *Journal of Adolescent Health, 27*(3), 166–169.

Henshaw, S.K. (1999). *US teenage pregnancy statistics with comparative statistics for women aged 20–24.* New York: Alan Guttmacher Institute.

Henshaw, S.K., & Torres, A. (1994). Family planning agencies: Services, policies, and funding. *Family Planning Perspectives, 26*, 52–59, 82.

Hubbard, B.M., Giese M.L., & Rainey, J. (1998). A replication of Reducing the Risk, a theory-based sexuality curriculum for adolescents. *Journal of School Health, 68*(6), 243–247.

Jastrzab, J., Masker, J., Blomquist, J., & Orr, L. (1997). *Youth corps: Promising strategies for young people and their communities.* Cambridge, MA: Abt Associates.

Jemmott, J.B., III, Jemmott, L.S., & Fong, G.T. (1998). Abstinence and safer sex: A randomized trial of HIV sexual risk-reduction interventions for young African-American adolescents. *Journal of the American Medical Association, 279*(19), 1529–1536.

Kirby, D. (2001). *Emerging answers: Research findings on programs to reduce sexual risk-taking and teen pregnancy.* Washington, DC: National Campaign to Prevent Teen Pregnancy.

Kirby, D., Barth, R., Leland, N., & Fetro, J. (1991). Reducing the risk: A new curriculum to prevent sexual risk-taking. *Family Planning Perspectives, 23*(6), 253–263.

Kirby, D., & Brown, N. (1996). School condom availability programs in the United States. *Family Planning Perspectives, 28*(5), 196–202.

Kirby, D., Waszak, C., & Ziegler, J. (1991). Six school-based clinics: Their reproductive health services and impact on sexual behavior. *Family Planning Perspectives, 23*(1), 6–16.

Kisker, E.E., Brown, R.S., & Hill, J. (1994). *Health caring: Outcomes of the Robert Wood Johnson Foundation's school-based adolescent health care program.* Princeton, NJ: Robert Wood Johnson Foundation.

Koo, H.P., Dunteman, G.H., George, C., Green, Y., & Vincent, M. (1994). Reducing adolescent pregnancy through school and community-based education: Denmark, South Carolina, revised 1991. *Family Planning Perspectives, 26*(5), 206–217.

Making the Grade. (2000, Summer). National census survey identifies 1,135 school-based health clinics nationwide. *Access.*

Maynard, R.A. (1996). *Kids having kids: A Robin Hood Foundation Special Report on the costs of adolescent childbearing.* New York: The Robin Hood Foundation.

Melchior, A. (1998). *National evaluation of learn and serve America school and community-based programs.* Waltham, MA: Center for Human Resources, Brandeis University.

Miller, B.C. (1998). *Families matter: A research synthesis of family influences on adolescent pregnancy.* Washington, DC: National Campaign to Prevent Teen Pregnancy.

Moore, K.A., Driscoll, A.K., & Lindberg, L.D. (1998). *A statistical portrait of adolescent sex, contraception, and childbearing.* Washington, DC: National Campaign to Prevent Teen Pregnancy.

National Campaign to Prevent Teen Pregnancy. (1997). *Whatever happened to childhood? The problem of teen pregnancy in the United States.* Washington, DC: Author.

O'Donnell, L., Stueve, A., Doval, A.S., Duran, R., Haber, D., Atnafou, R., Johnson, N., Grant, U., Murray, H., Juhn, G., Tang, J., Piessens, P. (1999). The effectiveness of the Reach for Health community youth service learning program in reducing early and unprotected sex among urban middle school students. *American Journal of Public Health, 89*(2), 176–181.

O'Donnell, L., Stueve, A., O'Donnell, C., Duran, R., Doval, A.S., Wilson, R.F., Haber, D., Perry, E., & Pleck, J.H. (2000). *Long-term reduction in sexual initiation and sexual activity among urban middle school participants in the Reach for Health community youth service learning HIV prevention program.* Unpublished manuscript.

Orr, D.P., Langefeld, C.D., Katz, B.P., & Caine, V.A. (1996). Behavioral intervention to increase condom use among high-risk female adolescents. *Journal of Pediatrics, 128*(2), 288–295.

Paine-Andrews, A., Harris, K.J., Fisher, J.L., Lewis, R., Williams, E.L., Fawcett, S.B., & Vincent, M.L. (1999). Effects of a replication of a multi-component model for preventing adolescent pregnancy in three Kansas communities. *Family Planning Perspectives, 31*(4), 182–189.

Philliber, S., & Allen, J.P. (1992). Life options and community service: Teen outreach program. In B.C. Miller, J.J. Card, R.L. Paikoff, & J.L. Peterson (Eds.), *Preventing adolescent pregnancy* (pp. 139–155). Newbury Park, CA: Sage.

Philliber, S., Kaye, J.W., Herring, S., & West, E. (2000). *Preventing teen pregnancy: An evaluation of the Children's Aid Society Carrera program.* Accord, NY: Philliber Research Associates.

Polen, M.R., & Freeborn, D.K. (1995). *Outcome evaluation of Project ACTION.* Portland, OR: Kaiser Permanente Center for Health Research.

Schochet, P.Z., Burghardt, J., & Glazerman, S. (2000, February 9). *National Job Corps study: The short-term impacts of Job Corps on participants' employment and related outcomes.* Report and Evaluation Report Series 00-A. Washington, DC: US Department of Labor, Employment and Training Administration.

Singh, S., & Darroch, J. (2000). Adolescent pregnancy and childbearing: Levels and trends in developed countries. *Family Planning Perspectives, 32*(1), 14–23.

Sonenstein, F.L., Ku, L., Lindberg, L.D., Turner, C.F., & Pleck, J.H. (1998). Changes in sexual behavior and condom use among teenaged males: 1988 to 1995. *American Journal of Public Health, 88*(6), 956–959.

St. Lawrence, J.S., Jefferson, K.W., Alleyne, E., Brasfield, T.L., O'Bannon, R.E., III, & Shirley, A. (1995). Cognitive-behavioral intervention to reduce African American adolescents' risk for HIV infection. *Journal of Consulting and Clinical Psychology, 63*(2), 221–237.

Terry, E., & Manlove, J. (2000). *Trends in sexual activity and contraceptive use among teens.* Washington, DC: National Campaign to Prevent Teen Pregnancy.

Ventura, S.J., Martin. J.A., Curtin, S.C., Menacker, F., & Hamilton, B.E. (2001). Births: Final data for 1999. *National Vital Statistics Reports, 49*(1).

Ventura, S.J., Mosher, W.D., Curtin, S.C., Abma, J.C., & Henshaw, S. (2001, June). Trends in pregnancy rates for the United States, 1976–97: An update. *National Vital Statistics Reports, 49*(4).

Vincent, M., Clearie, A., & Schluchter, M. (1987). Reducing adolescent pregnancy through school and community-based education. *Journal of the American Medical Association, 257*(24), 3382–3386.

Wang, L.Y., Davis, M., Robin, L., Collins, J., Coyle, K., & Baumler, E. (2000). Economic evaluation of safer choices. *Archives of Pediatric Adolescent Medicine, 154*(10), 1017–1024.

Winter, L., & Breckenmaker, L.C. (1991). Tailoring family planning services to the special needs of adolescents. *Family Planning Perspectives, 23*(1), 24–30.

Zabin, L.S., M.B., Smith, E.A., Streett, R., & Hardy, J.B. (1986). Evaluation of a pregnancy prevention program for urban teenagers. *Family Planning Perspectives, 18*(3), 119–126.

Prosocial Behavior, Early Childhood

Jannette Rey

INTRODUCTION

The development of prosocial behavior in early childhood is a key developmental task for later successful interactions. Children with prosocial reputations tend to be high in socially appropriate behavior, coping, attentional regulation, and low in negative emotionality (Eisenberg et al., 1996). Interferences in the development of prosocial skills greatly diminishes the protective factors that have been found to be integral to successful adaptation and resiliency (Masten & Coatsworth, 1998).

In this entry, we provide an overview of the nature and course of prosocial development in early childhood (i.e., 0–5 years) and the factors that impede or enhance healthy development in this area. Discussion then turns to interventions that have been employed to promote prosocial behavior in young children.

DEFINITIONS

Social skills are commonly defined as a repertoire of specific behavioral skills (e.g., ability to initiate conversations, ability to provide feedback to others in a socially appropriate manner) that facilitate social interactions. Rather than a set of discrete social behaviors, *social competence* is characterized by those behavioral, cognitive, and affective factors that contribute to successful adaptation to and navigation within and across social interactions. *Prosocial behavior*, a critical indicator of social competence, is characterized by behaviors that promote positive interactions and convey positive regard for others such as sharing, reciprocity (verbal and/or nonverbal), sensitivity to others' distress, and socially appropriate behavior.

SCOPE

Prosocial behavior encompasses the integration of affect, behavior, and cognition and takes on different forms depending on the age and development of the child. Until the infant is approximately 18 months old, social interactions with the environment primarily involve the primary caregiver and are characterized by orientedness to immediate stimuli in the environment and behaviors that engage the caregiver. During toddlerhood (e.g., 18–36 months), typical development is characterized by early signs of play (e.g., imitating, showing toy), and an increasing use of language, and emerging prosocial behaviors (e.g., sharing, reacting to distress of others). As children reach preschool-age (ages 3–6), normative prosocial skill development is largely influenced by the increase in language development, role-taking and problem-solving ability, and emotional regulation. Children in this age range begin to participate in more coordinated patterns of play, friendship-building becomes more meaningful, and social competence within the peer group becomes an important task. As the toddler matures, prosocial actions become increasingly marked by same-sex reciprocity. The emergence of empathy during this period has also been associated to prosocial behavior. In terms of cognitive and social development, children can consistently

make social judgments by age three and resolve story dilemmas in a prosocial manner (Guerra, Nucci, & Huesmann, 1994). Socially competent preschool-aged children, then, show high levels of social engagement, agreeabilty, reciprocity, good communicational skills, and emotional regulation (LaFreniere & Sroufe, 1985).

Although few gender differences in prosocial behavioral patterns have been found in very young children (Hay, 1994), it is suggested that socialization with female children may be easier due to several factors. Not only do girls generally develop communication skills at earlier ages than boys, but there are empirical data that suggest that female preschoolers demonstrate higher levels of empathy than same-aged boys and better skills in decoding and encoding nonverbal cues (Hall, 1990).

Cross-cultural studies of prosocial development revealed several differences in the patterns and expression of prosocial behavior. For example, in a comparison of US and Japanese parent–infant populations, researchers found a wider variety of infant temperamental patterns and parent tolerance for these behaviors in the Japanese parent–infant dyads (Fogel, Toda, & Kawai, 1988). While girls from both cultures expressed more prosocial themes than did boys, research from several other countries, including Finland, Israel, Italy, Poland, and the United Kingdom, have that females exceed males in their rates of "indirect aggression" or "relational aggression" (Crick & Grotpeter, 1995; Osterman et al., 1998; Owen, 1996).

While the developmental nature of several problem behaviors may reflect normal developmental changes, it is generally accepted that 12–20 percent of children exhibit significant behavior problems during *early* childhood (Mathieson & Sanson, 2000). Direct costs to society of children who are deficient in their social competencies can include such aspects as disruption of healthy development, development of more serious delinquent and/or risky behaviors (e.g., substance abuse, property damage), adult criminality and resulting costs of incarceration, and perpetuation of risk to their offspring.

THEORIES

There are a number of theories that have contributed to our current understanding of prosocial development and the factors that enhance it at the individual, family, and environmental/contextual level. In developmental theory, a child's prosocial nature is described as an organizational construct that develops over time and shapes the social demands and reactions by caregivers and peers. Relatedly, cognitive-developmental theory highlights the link between the child's ability to control and maintain attention and socioemotional development (Eisenberg et al., 1996). The reformulated theory of social information processing explains a child's social actions and adjustment as a result of number of steps in processing (e.g., attention, encoding) and interpretation of social cues (Crick & Dodge, 1994). Research has found that the action selected reflects the child's degree of competence in the particular social situation and that higher quality of problem-solving strategies is associated with social competence. Young aggressive children have been shown to process social cues differently than their prosocial counterparts, resulting in higher rates of inaccurate and hostile attributions regarding others' behaviors and, in turn, higher rates of aggressive responding.

Recent conceptualizations of infant temperament highlight how a child's emotional reactivity and ability to regulate emotion affect cognitive processing, thereby influencing the quality of social behaviors. More specifically, a child's prosocial behavior can be triggered by cues that evoke particular emotions, attributions, and/or schemas. Early childhood environments, then, that contain moderate degrees of emotional expressivity by others provide opportunities for a child's exploration of the relationships between emotional situations and internal and external cues, allowing for better development of emotion knowledge. In a similar way, theories of personality have identified empathy as a key factor in the development of prosocial thought, perspective and role-taking ability, and emotional responsiveness that can inhibit or mitigate antisocial behavior (Miller & Eisenberg, 1988).

Theories regarding parent–child attachment and mutual reciprocity between caregiver and child lend to the understanding of the development of prosocial behavior during early childhood. In fact, it is during the establishment of this "first" of social relationships with the caregiver that the child begins to solidify social skills (e.g., use of nonverbal cues to engage others) (Belsky, Woodworth, & Crnic, 1996). Poor attachment, however, can impair internal representations of the world and lead to negative attributions of the self and, thus, higher vulnerability to feelings of helplessness and depression. From social learning, ecological, and transactional models of development, both family and peer experiences contribute to the development of a young child's social functioning (Sroufe, Egeland, & Carlson, 1999). While parental insistence, warmth, and sensitivity play key roles in the promotion of social competence, child behavior problems appear to be associated with power-assertive parenting, maternal depression and/or anxiety mothers, and family adversity and stress (Rapee, 1997). Similarly, peer relationships in early childhood are strongly reflective of the nature of the parent–child relationship early in life and predictive of social competence in middle and later childhood.

RESEARCH

Empirical investigations of prosocial development have examined direct, additive, and interactional effects of child, parent, family, and environmental contextual factors. Children with inaccurate social schemas have been found to misinterpret social cues and utilize more rigid processing in problem-solving, leading to patterns of social problems (Saarni, 1999). Several components of the parent–child relationship that influence a child's level of social competence include patterns of attachment, childrearing styles, emotional expressiveness, parent–child play, and the parent's directiveness in the child's peer environment (Patterson, 1982). For example, caregivers may help their toddlers utilize behaviors that help produce positive social interactions (e.g., gestures, appropriate affect, verbal behavior). Similarly, research has found that caregivers' responsivity during early childhood has been found to influence their toddler's attention, language development, play complexity, and cooperation (Smith, Landry, & Swank, 2000). Studies of preschool-aged children have found higher levels of social skills and social competence for those children whose mothers emphasized social skills (Prinstein & LaGreca, 1999). In fact, research with adoptive parent–child dyads has demonstrated that even children with predisposed risk for poor social competence based on difficult temperament have achieved better outcomes when placed with well-adjusted adoptive parents who provide adaptive transactional processes in the parent–child relationship (Cadoret, Yates, Troughton, Woodworth, & Stewart, 1995).

Prosocial behavior has been shown to be a key antecedent of peer acceptance and a precursor of school and social adjustment (Rimm-Kaufman Pianta, 2000). However, children who develop aggressive behavioral patterns early in childhood are at risk for continued reliance on aggressive strategies in the absence of alternative prosocial behaviors. Researchers have examined the impact of supportive parenting (e.g., warmth and positive engagement, proactive teaching, inductive discipline) and family adversity on children's later social and school adjustment. Their findings suggest that high levels of positive and supportive parenting not only predicted healthy child adjustment years later, but mitigated the effects of family adversity on behavioral functioning and increased the children's sense of social responsibility and positive relationships with peers. Conversely, harsh and controlling parental discipline practices have strong associations with the development of child behavioral and emotional difficulties (Patterson, 1982). Moreover, while socially skilled children interact well with their peer group and are adept at initiating and maintaining friendships, the quality of these relationships plays an important role in overall adjustment (Hartup, 1999). It is this status of friends, versus nonfriends, that provides unique opportunities that contribute to better outcomes during periods of developmental transitions.

The influence of more global environmental factors, such as poverty and other environmental adversities, have been found to increase children's risk of poor developmental outcomes. Significant differences in the rates of conduct problems for children aged 5 and 6 years residing in disadvantaged neighborhoods has been found even after controlling for sociodemographic family factors (Brooks-Gunn, Duncan, Klebanov, & Sealand, 1993). Patterson, Reid, and Dishion (1992) found that economically disadvantaged children are rejected by peers more often than middle socioeconomic status (SES) counterparts. The specific developmental outcomes that result from exposure to community violence are, however, influenced by both community and individual factors. Findings by O'Kane (1998), for example, suggest that factors such as the child's social cognitions may function as either protective or risk factors for the development of aggression depending upon the quality and accuracy of social information processing.

STRATEGIES: OVERVIEW

The goal of prevention in prosocial development is to prevent, reduce, or eliminate behavioral problems while targeting skill development and social competence. Comprehensive preventive interventions (i.e., multicomponent, multimodal) that are guided by theory, whereby theory guides how the specific interventions reduce risk factors and promote protective factors, increase the likelihood of maintenance of treatment gains (Hawkins, Catalano, Morrison, O'Donnell, Abbott, & Day, 1992). As such, effective strategies target child, family, and environmentally focused risk factors.

STRATEGIES THAT WORK

Effective interventions designed to prevent and/or reduce aggression include elements to improve social reasoning skills, encourage bonding relationships, teach social skills, and increase social competence and peer interactions to improve social reasoning skills. Family-focused interventions address risk-related areas such as family climate, parental functioning, and parental knowledge and beliefs about parenting and child development. These have been shown to be especially critical for high-risk populations given that these families often do not respond to traditional parent training interventions that fail to address contextual factors. Parent–infant focused interventions commonly intervene with those parents whose emotional responsiveness to

their infants is challenged. *Home-based visitation* (Olds, 1997) is a widely studied and empirically supported preventive program that consists of pre- and postnatal (up to 1 year) health and child care education provided by nurse home visitors or master's level family therapists to families that are identified as being "at-risk" for poor health and social outcomes. Home visits have been found to be effective in improving parent–child interactions and child development.

Interventions geared toward socialization of the child via a parent's responding to affective cues have also demonstrated effectiveness for prosocial development. *The Incredible Years Parenting Training Program* (Webster-Stratton, 1990) is a preventive intervention designed to improve parent–child interactions, reduce preschoolers negative behaviors, and improve children's prosocial behavior via parent and teacher training. Both the parent and teacher intervention is comprised of multiple training series that include didactic discussion and videotaped modeling of essential behavior management strategies, as well as ways to improve child prosocial behavior. Findings with children demonstrating clinic-level behavioral problems indicate significant reductions in problematic behaviors and improved parenting. Additional programming to improve parent–teacher bonding was recently evaluated with results indicating higher bonding between parent–teacher dyads in the treatment group as compared to the controls.

Given the numbers of young children enrolled in childcare and preschool programs, early childhood educators have also become key agents for promoting healthy psychosocial and emotional development in young children. The *Perry Preschool Program* (Berrueta-Clement, Schweinhart, Barnett, Epstein, & Weikart, 1984) provides high-quality home visitation and early childhood education to disadvantaged children (ages 3 and 4) in order to promote children's intellectual, social, and physical development. Program staff receive ongoing instruction and are trained in early childhood development and education. Children who participated in the program demonstrated less antisocial behavior at follow-up in elementary and secondary school levels. One such approach is through *Interpersonal Cognitive Problem-Solving* (ICPS) training programs (Shure & Spivack, 1979) that are specifically targeted to social–cognitive skill development through the improvement of the child's cognitive processing with respect to interpersonal challenges and conflict. Via didactic games led by an adult, ICPS programs foster the child's ability to generate numerous and, ultimately, high quality problem-solving strategies. Post-treatment and follow-up outcome data indicate a decline in rates of acting out behaviors of children with self-control deficits, and positive changes for overly inhibited children who became more socially engaged and rated as likeable by peers (Youngstrom, Wolpaw, Kogos, Schoff, Ackerman, & Izard, 2000). Another effective intervention targeted to social–cognitive skill development is *Skillstreaming*—one of the first psychoeducational curricula available for social skills training (McGinnis & Goldstein, 1990). The curriculum, guided by social learning theory, incorporates modeling, behavioral rehearsal, and social reinforcement for the development and enhancement of specific social skills. Outcome evaluations of Skillstreaming revealed that children's social competence and self-concept demonstrate significant enhancement after participation in the program when significant others in the child's environment also participate. The *I Can Problem Solve* (Shure, 1992) program, an example of an effective school-based intervention, focuses on the development of problem-solving abilities (e.g., generating possible solutions, considering consequences, accurately identifying emotions) for children in childcare and kindergarten settings. The program is designed to be delivered in small groups and targets skill-building in problem-solving language, emotion identification, and problem-solving practice in real and hypothesized situations. Treatment outcome evaluations indicate that participating students demonstrated less impulsivity and better problem-solving skills as compared to a peer control group at 1- and 5-year follow-ups. Similarly, *Stop and Think!* (Rosenthal, 1997), also targets problem-solving ability and was designed to teach young children with developmental delays how to interact cooperatively and utilize effective interactional strategies. Children participating in the program were rated as more socially skilled at post-treatment (Rosenthal, 1997).

STRATEGIES THAT MIGHT WORK

A promising approach in effective prosocial promotion is the *Yale Child Welfare Project*, an early childhood intervention, also designed to improve parent–child bonding and interactional patterns via team-based support to disadvantaged families (Seitz & Apfel, 1994). Through the enhancement of resources otherwise limited in this population, the program seeks to improve child development and overall family functioning from pregnancy until the infants reach 30 months of age. A 10-year follow-up revealed better social adjustment for boys across several dimensions (i.e., school, peer interactions, home life). Another promising intervention for the promotion of childhood prosocial behaviors through parent–child relationship building is the *Parent Child Development Program* (Johnson & Breckenridge, 1982). The intervention is multidimensional and is designed especially for low-income families to help mothers become more effective in childrearing. Program components include psychoeducational parent training regarding critical aspects of child development, in-home parenting sessions, continuing education courses, health and social services, and therapeutic feedback regarding communication and interaction skills.

Outcome studies indicate improvements in the positiveness of parent–child interactions, improved parental disciplinary practices, and fewer behavior problems exhibited by participating children at 1-, 2-, and 3-year follow-ups. The *First and Best Teacher* program (Evans et al., 2000), adapted from models of childcare center programming to prevent antisocial behavior, is a training and mentoring program for early childhood educators of children aged 3–5 years. The program is designed to build skills and competencies in preschool children by teaching child care center staff to effectively identify and address early behavior problems and work with children to cultivate pro-social behavior, improve problem-solving and conflict resolution skills, and improve linkages between school and home. Initial program findings suggest that the curriculum is promising in its effectiveness for increasing caregiver knowledge regarding child development which, in turn, increases their competency in promoting prosocial child behavior (Evans et al., 2000). A similar program, the *Resilient Children Making Healthy Choices Project* (Dubas, Lynch, Galano, Geller, & Hunt, 1998), is also designed to promote health and social competence in young children through the integration of resiliency-based skill-building strategies in the teaching practices of the early childhood educators. Analysis of outcome data from a pre/post-comparison group design revealed increases in teacher interactional skills designed to enhance children's resiliency, and improvements in children's prosocial behaviors (Dubas et al., 1998). *Toddler–Parent Psychotherapy* (TPP; Lieberman, 1992) has demonstrated some promise in effective prevention of maladaptive cognitive development in toddlers. TPP, based on attachment theory, involves participation of the parent and child in therapy sessions in which the focus is on improvement of the parent–child relationship, parental affective communication, and maternal responsivity to the child. Treatment outcome studies of toddlers aged 20 months have shown normative cognitive developmental patterns and functioning at age 3 (Cicchetti, Rogosch, & Toth, 2000). Similarly, the *Syracuse Family Development Research Program* (Lally, Mangione, Honig, & Wittner, 1988) is designed to improve parent–child interactions, particularly for economically disadvantaged families via weekly home visits to assist mothers in developing effective behavior management and socialization strategies that promote prosocial behavior (e.g., cooperation, empathy) in their young children. Outcome data indicate higher ratings regarding prosocial behaviors of program children as well as higher child-reported rates of positive self-concept.

STRATEGIES THAT DO NOT WORK

In the area of prosocial skill development in early childhood, current empirical support points to a need for multimodal, multifaceted intervention approaches. Further, interventions that directly target skill enhancement and provide formal teaching opportunities for the use and refinement of social skills have yielded positive effects for increased social competence. Conversely, strategies that are unifocused (e.g., child-focused, parent-focused) and/or rely on instruction that occurs solely outside of the child's natural environment, fail to produce significant change effects on prosocial behavior.

SYNTHESIS

Effective promotion of prosocial development during early childhood can be achieved through a variety of means. Primary target areas for intervention address: communication, social skills (sharing, cooperation), friendship-building skills (i.e., initiating and maintaining peer interactions), and/or problem-solving and conflict resolution skills that can mediate social interaction. Recent research has indicated that successful programs: (a) utilize a program of longer duration, (b) synthesize a number of successful approaches, (c) incorporate a developmental model, (d) provide greater focus on the role of emotions and emotional development, (e) provide increased emphasis on generalization techniques, (f) provide ongoing training and support for implementation, and (g) utilize multiple measures and follow-ups for assessing program effectiveness.

Although the field of social skills training has advanced over the decades, generalization and social validity remain critical indices of effective programming. Through comprehensive and intensive intervention efforts within a larger context of long-term efforts, many dimensions of child development, including prosocial behavior, can be enhanced. It is key, however, that the selection of an intervention to promote prosocial behavior follow careful assessment of the nature of the deficiencies in social competence. In response to reformulated national educational goals, school-based interventions are required to prepare children in those competencies that maximize healthy adjustment and resiliency (Zigler & Hall, 2000). In addition to preventive interventions applied at the level of the parent–child system, the promotion of prosocial development within school settings, where increasingly more early intervention programs are located "in-house" (e.g., pre-K and preschool programs), remains a critical venue for prevention efforts.

Also see: Child Care: Early Childhood; Family Strengthening: Childhood; Self-Esteem: Early Childhood; Self-Esteem: Childhood; Self-Esteem: Adolescence; Social and Emotional Learning: Early Childhood; Social and Emotional Learning: Childhood; Social and Emotional Learning: Adolescence.

References

Belsky, J., Woodworth, S., & Crnic, K. (1996). Troubled family interaction during toddlerhood. *Development and Psychopathology, 8*, 477–495.

Berrueta-Clement, J.R., Schweinhart, L.J., Barnett, W.S., Epstein, A.S., & Weikart, D.P. (1984). Changed lives: The effects of the Perry Preschool Program on youths through age 19. *Monographs of the High/Scope Educational Research Foundation, 8*, Ypsilanti, MI: High/Scope Press.

Brooks-Gunn, J., Duncan, G.J., Klebanov, P.K., & Sealand, N. (1993). Do neighborhoods influence child and adolescent development? *American Journal of Sociology, 99*, 353–395.

Cadoret, R.J., Yates, W.R., Troughton, E., Woodworth, G., & Stewart, M.A. (1995). Genetic environmental interaction in the genesis of aggressivity and conduct disorders. *Archives of General Psychiatry, 52*, 916–924.

Cicchetti, D., Rogosch, F.A., & Toth, S.L. (2000). The efficacy of toddler–parent psychotherapy for fostering cognitive development in offspring of depressed mothers. *Journal of Abnormal Child Psychology, 28*, 135–148.

Crick, N.R., & Dodge, K.A. (1994). A review and reformulation of social information processing mechanisms in children's social adjustment. *Psychological Bulletin, 115*, 74–101.

Crick, N.R., & Grotpeter, J.K. (1995). Relational aggression, gender, and social–psychological adjustment. *Child Development, 67*, 1003–1014.

Dubas, J.S., Lynch, K.B., Galano, J., Geller, S., & Hunt, D. (1998). Preliminary evaluation of a resiliency-based preschool substance abuse and violence prevention project. *Journal of Drug Education, 28*, 235–255.

Eisenberg, N., Fabes, R.A., Karbon, M., Murphy, B.C., Wosinki, M., Polazzi, L., Carlo, G., & Juhnke, C. (1996). The relations of children's dispositional prosocial behavior to emotionality, regulation, and social functioning. *Child Development, 67*, 974–992.

Evans, G.D., Rey, J., Hemphill, M.H., Beaulieu, L.J., Perkins, D.F., Austin, W., Racine, P., & Hammett, M. (2000). *First and Best Teacher: An early childhood violence prevention trial.* Manuscript in preparation.

Fogel, A., Toda, S., & Kawai, M. (1988). Mother infant face-to-face interaction in Japan and the United States: A laboratory comparison using 3-month-old infants. *Developmental Psychology, 24*, 398–406.

Guerra, N.G., Nucci, L., & Huesmann, L.R. (1994). Moral cognition and childhood aggression. In L.R. Huesmann (Ed.), *Aggressive behavior: Current perspectives* (pp. 13–33). New York: Plenum Press.

Hall, J.A. (1990). *Nonverbal sex differences: Accuracy of communication and expressive style.* Baltimore, MD: Johns Hopkins University Press.

Hartup, W.W. (1999). Constraints on peer socialization: Let me count the ways. *Merrill Palmer Quarterly, 45*, 172–183.

Hawkins, J.D., Catalano, R.F., Morrison, D.M., O'Donnell, J., Abbott, R.D., & Day, L.E. (1992). The Seattle Social Development Project: Effects of the first four years on protective factors and problem behaviors. In J. McCord & R.E. Tremblay (Eds.), *Preventing antisocial behavior: Interventions from birth through adolescence* (pp. 139–161). NY: The Guilford Press.

Hay, D.F. (1994). Psychosocial development. *Journal of Child Psychology and Psychiatry, 35*, 29–71.

Johnson, D.L., & Breckenridge, J.N. (1982). The Houston Parent–Child Development Center and the primary prevention of behavior problems in young children. *American Journal of Community Psychology, 10*, 305–316.

LaFreniere, P.J., & Sroufe, A.L. (1985). Profiles of peer competence in the preschool: Interrelations between measures, influence of social ecology, and relation to attachment history. *Developmental Psychology, 21*, 56–69.

Lally, J.R., Mangione, P.L., Honig, A.S., & Wittner, D.S. (1988). More pride, less delinquency: Findings from the ten-year follow-up study of the Syracuse University Family Development Research Program. *Zero to Three, 8*(4), 13–18.

Lieberman, A.F. (1992). Infant–parent psychotherapy with toddlers. *Development and Psychopathology, 4,* 559–574.

Masten, A.S., & Coatsworth, J.D. (1998). The development of competence in favorable and unfavorable environments: Lessons from research on successful children. *American Psychologist, 53,* 205–220.

Mathieson, K.S., & Sanson, A. (2000). Dimensions of early childhood behavior problems: Stability and predictors of change from 18 to 30 months. *Journal of Abnormal Child Psychology, 28,* 15–31.

McGinnis, E., & Goldstein, A.P. (1990). *Skill-streaming in early childhood: Teaching prosocial skills to the preschool and kindergarten child.* Champaign, IL: Research Press.

Miller, P.A., & Eisenberg, N. (1988). The relation of empathy to aggressive and externalizing/antisocial behavior. *Psychological Bulletin, 103,* 324–344.

O'Kane, J.B. (1998). Exposure to violent events: The impact of social information on children's cognitive appraisal. *Dissertation Abstracts International Section A: Humanities and Social Sciences, 59,* 1343.

Olds, D. (1997). The Prenatal/Early Infancy Project: Fifteen years later. In G.W. Albee & T.P. Gullotta (Eds.), *Primary prevention works. Issues in children's and families' lives* (pp. 41–67). Thousand Oaks, CA: Sage.

Osterman, K., Bjorkqvist, K., Lagerspetz, K.M.J., Kaukiainen, A., Landau, S.F., Fraczek, A., & Caprara, G.V. (1998). Cross-cultural evidence of female indirect aggression. *Aggressive Behavior, 24,* 1–8.

Owen, L.D. (1996). Sticks and stones and sugar and spice: Girls' and boys' aggression in schools. *Australian Journal of Guidance and Counselling, 6,* 45–55.

Patterson, G.R. (1982). *Coercive family process.* Eugene, OR: Castalia.

Patterson, G.R., Reid, J.B., & Dishion, T.J. (1992). *Antisocial boys.* Eugene: Castalia.

Prinstein, M.J., & LaGreca, A.M. (1999). Links between mothers' and children's social competence and associations with maternal adjustment. *Journal of Clinical Child Psychology, 28,* 197–210.

Rapee, R. (1997). Potential role of childrearing practices in the development of anxiety and depression. *Clinical Psychology Review, 17,* 47–67.

Rimm-Kaufman, S.E., & Pianta, R. (2000). An ecological perspective on the transition to kindergarten: A theoretical framework to guide empirical research. *Journal of Applied Developmental Psychology, 21,* 491–511.

Rosenthal, M. (1997). Stop and think!: Using metacognitive strategies to teach students social skills. *Exceptional Children, 29,* 29–31.

Saarni, C. (1999). *The development of emotional competence.* New York: The Guilford Press.

Seitz, V., & Apfel, N.H. (1994). Parent-focused intervention: Diffusion effects on siblings. *Child Development, 65,* 677–683.

Shure, M.B. (1992). *I Can Problem Solve: An interpersonal cognitive problem-solving program: Preschool.* Champaign, IL: Research Press.

Shure, M.B., & Spivack, G. (1979). Interpersonal cognitive problem solving and primary prevention: Programming for preschool and kindergarten children. *Journal of Clinical Child Psychology, 8,* 89–94.

Smith, K.E., Landry, S.H., & Swank, P.R. (2000). The influence of early patterns of positive parenting on children's preschool outcomes. *Early Education and Development, 11,* 147–169.

Sroufe, A.L., Egeland, B., & Carlson, E.A. (1999). One social world: The integrated development of parent–child and peer relationships. In W. A. Collins & B. Laursen (Eds.), *Relationships as developmental contexts* (pp. 241–261). Mahwah, NJ: Lawrence Erlbaum Associates.

Webster-Stratton, C. (1990). Enhancing the effectiveness of self-administered videotape parent training for families with conduct-problem children. *Journal of Abnormal Child Psychology, 18,* 479–492.

Youngstrom, E., Wolpaw, J.M., Kogos, J.L., Schoff, K., Ackerman, B., & Izard, C. (2000). Interpersonal problem solving in preschool and first grade: Developmental change and ecological validity. *Journal of Clinical Child Psychology, 29,* 589–602.

Zigler, E.F., & Hall, N.W. (2000). *Child development and social policy: Theory and applications.* New York: McGraw-Hill.

R

Racial and Ethnic Disparities, Adulthood

Harold W. Neighbors and
Briggett C. Ford

INTRODUCTION AND DEFINITIONS

The existence of racial and ethnic health disparities is a major problem for the United States. Whether identified by the construct of "excess deaths" (HHS, US, 1985) or Years of Potential Life Lost (YPLL) (LaVeist, 2000), the differences in morbidity and mortality between US ethnic minority groups and European Americans has been a source of concern and embarrassment since the early 1900s (Thomas & Quinn, 2001). Statistics on racial and ethnic health disparities are inconsistent with notions of social justice and equality. Racial and ethnic health disparities are also problematic because they may suggest to some that groups of color are deficient or inferior with regard to health and mental health, when in fact, the cause of the disparities could very well be due to social, cultural, economic, and political factors, reflected in the pattern of discrimination minority groups experience (Williams & Neighbors, 2001).

Although the concept of *disparity* is defined neutrally as population group differences in epidemiologic data, it must be recognized that for many, these differences are felt

with such passion that the issue becomes an indicator for the health of a nation and its fundamental philosophical bases. In this entry, we identify the scope of ethnic disparities in health and mental health, provide a conceptual perspective on these matters, and consider strategies by which we might prevent future disparities.

SCOPE

Using the indicator YPLL, LaVeist (2000) reported that in 1992, Black men had the highest number of YPLL-65, 102.3 years per 1,000 compared to White men (50.1 years), followed by Black women (48.6 years) and then White women (24.0 years). Among Black men, homicide was the largest contributor to YPLL-65, adding eight times as many YPLL years as for White men and five times as many years as for Black women. YPLL due to stroke was also higher for Black men and women in comparison to Whites. LaVeist used the YPLL measure to compute Black/White ratios separately for males and females across six leading indicators of death. The most striking finding was the fact that not one of these twelve comparisons fell to a value of 1.0, an indication of no racial health disparity. The largest of the Black–White YPLL ratios occurred for HIV among females where the rate for Black women was 8.4 times that of White women.

LaVeist also provided a 10-year update to the *Secretary's Task Force on Black and minority health* (HHS, US, 1985) by calculating the excess deaths for African Americans per 1,000 population for 1996. This analysis showed that 36 percent of all deaths for African Americans were in "excess." meaning greater than what would be expected based on their proportion in the total population. Cancer accounted for 13.7 percent and HIV for 11 percent;

and for homicide almost 80 percent of the deaths were excess. Heart disease, the leading cause of the excess mortality, accounted for 28 percent of the total excess deaths. Heart disease is the leading cause of death in the United States. Except for African Americans, all other ethnic minority groups have lower rates than Whites (Williams, 2001). In fact, while the rates have declined since 1950 for both Blacks and Whites, the Black/White ratio increased between 1950 and 1995. In 1995 all minority groups except Asians/Pacific Islanders had higher death rates due to diabetes than Whites. Black rates have been rising, going from 17.2 per 100,000 in 1950 to 28.5 per 100,000 in 1995. Recent increases for Blacks, Native American/Alaskan Natives and Latinos were higher than the increases for Whites leading to a current larger minority/white ratio in 1995 (Williams, 2001).

Black–White comparisons in Life Expectancy (LE) at age 45 for men and women by family income show that while White men and women can expect to live longer than Blacks at all levels of family income, the difference is larger at the lowest income levels (Pamuk, Makuc, Heck, Reuben, & Lochner, 1998). In 1998, White males lived 6.4 years longer than Black males; White women lived 4.4 years longer than Black women. The leading causes of death that contributed to the disparity in LE were heart disease (27.4 percent), cancer (19.4 percent), homicide (9.7 percent), and stroke (8.1 percent). While homicide ranked 13th among causes of death and accounted for less than 1 percent of all US deaths in 1998, homicide accounted for 10 percent of the Black–White LE differential (HHS, US, 2001).

Studies of mental health typically focus on well-being, psychological distress, and discrete mental disorders. Blacks typically report lower levels of life satisfaction, happiness, and marital happiness than Whites (Hughes & Thomas, 1998). It is important to note that these racial disparities in the quality of life remain, even after socioeconomic status differences are controlled. Blacks, on the other hand, have comparable or better mental health than Whites in terms of psychological distress (Neighbors & Williams, 2001; Williams & Harris-Reid, 1999). Moreover, Blacks have comparable or lower rates of mental disorder, such as major depression than Whites. Taken together, national epidemiologic estimates show that the prevalence of serious mental illness in African Americans is equivalent or below that of Whites (Neighbors & Williams, 2001).

THEORIES AND RESEARCH

The Individualized Behavior/Lifestyle Model

The Secretary's Task Force Report (HHS, US, 1985) emphasized the important role of health education and personal behavior in its recommendations on how to address racial health disparities. Decisions about whether to exercise, choices about what to eat, or the use of seat belts are, to some extent, under the individual's direct control. However, these "personal" decisions are influenced by discrimination, as well as economic, and political factors. For example, being restricted to certain minimal-paying job opportunities limits one's income, which reduces choice of foods to eat, places to live, etc.

The Afrocentric Model

Airhihenbuwa's (1995) PEN-3 Afrocentric model is based on the assumption of fundamental differences between African Americans and European Americans in values, family, and community. The PEN-3 model consists of three interdependent dimensions: health education, diagnosis of health behavior, and cultural appropriateness of health behavior. Within each of these three components is a focus on the person, the environment, and the neighborhood. PEN-3 offers a useful guiding framework for developing health education and intervention programs designed to help health educators develop programs that fit better with the belief systems and practices of African American communities. Applicability of the model depends, of course, on the degree of acculturation and assimilation of particular African American communities and the extent to which its residents are indeed distinctly different from European Americans. Nevertheless, PEN-3 offers one of the best set of procedures for the development of culturally tailored practice.

The Socioeconomic Status (SES) Model

This model suggests that SES is a more important factor than race or ethnicity in determining a person's health or mental health. Both racial status and SES are positively correlated as are many morbidity outcomes. In fact, the higher overall prevalence of morbidity among African Americans (and other minorities) is often attributed to the fact that ethnic minorities are disproportionately represented in the lower socioeconomic strata of US American society (Dressler, 1993). While it is true that race and SES are correlated, they are not the same thing. Although adjusting for SES when making racial comparisons is clearly an improvement over reporting simple bivariate associations between race and health, the practice is not without its critics (Anderson & Armstead, 1995). Many of the criticisms of controlling for SES argue that traditional SES indicators (income, education, occupation) do not mean the same thing to ethnic minorities as they do to European Americans (Kaplan, Everson, & Lynch, 2000; LaVeist, 2000). Controlling for SES is, however, useful if for no other reason than to underscore the fact that race and ethnicity really do matter for health because taking SES into account eliminates some but not all racial and ethnic differences in health. It is not clear, however, how precisely race or ethnicity per se account for these remaining differences.

Genetic Perspective

Race has been conceptualized traditionally as representing distinct genetic differences between population groups. As a result, race has been used by racists as the basis for negative stereotyping entire groups of people, which in turn has been used to justify acts of discrimination. In fact, recently a new generation of writers has emerged speculating on whether the Human Genome Project will ultimately explain racial disparities (Taylor, 1998). Recognizing that time, events, and rates of intermarriage have so blended population groups as to constitute continually emerging and changing social entities (i.e., people who at any point in time feel that they share a common heritage, language, beliefs, or values), the vast majority of health researchers define race and ethnicity from a social constructionist perspective. To paraphrase Landrine and Klonoff (1996, pp. 11–14), races are simply ethnic groups that have been socially defined as such on the basis of physical criteria as identified by some other, more powerful, ethnic group. It is for these reasons that in this entry, we use the terms race and ethnicity interchangeably even though these are complex terms whose meanings are extensively debated in the literature.

The Early Exposure Hypothesis

Geronimus' (1992) "weathering" (or early exposure and long-term effect) hypothesis focuses on the ways in which social inequalities affect differentially the maternal health of women across race and the ways in which these race-based exposures are compounded with age. Weathering suggests that socioeconomically disadvantaged ethnic minority women are subjected to many health risks that accumulate over time. Similar to weathering is the position taken by Williams (Williams & Collins, 1995), Lynch (Lynch, Kaplan, & Salonen, 1997), and others who argue that racial health disparities, particularly (but not exclusively) at the middle and upper socioeconomic strata, may result from race differences in early life negative exposures. According to this perspective, racial disparities exist at all levels of SES because the damage of these early exposures cannot be easily overcome despite the upward social mobility of some individuals of color (Kaplan et al., 2000; Lynch et al., 1997; Williams, 1990; Williams, 2001; Williams & Collins, 1995).

The Cultural Model

Although the above stress-exposure models help to understand the disparities between African Americans and European Americans, they do less well when multigroup comparisons are employed. Many times, adding a third (or fourth) population group, Latinos or Asians for example, creates what some have called paradoxical findings (Abraido-Lanza & Dohrenwend, 1999; Markides & Coriel, 1986). It is at this point that writers typically turn to the notion of culture. The cultural model focuses more explicitly on the search for behaviors, attitudes, or customs that are unique (i.e., different from an unspecified US mainstream culture) or indigenous to a particular ethnic group. Often, these cultural factors are hypothesized to be protective of health in some way. For example, religion may provide integrative forces that bind individuals together with the larger group and thus protect them from self-destructive influences or the pressures from the larger society. It is difficult to identify particular cultural risk or protective factors in African Americans, in part because they may participate in a wide range of cultures, including mainline white culture, no one of which provides clear protection from the stresses they experience.

STRATEGIES: OVERVIEW

In order to prevent or reduce racial health disparities, we need to identify the best available research and demonstration programs describing strategies that worked or are promising but in need of further study. We also have to identify what does not work to reduce these health disparities. We are using criteria of selection that include clear specification of the risk factors, an adequate description of the theory-guided intervention, a research design that includes a control or comparison group, and adequate measures of morbidity outcomes. We have discovered few studies that reach these criteria, which underlines the need for more and better research in this area.

STRATEGIES THAT WORK

The *Cardiovascular Dietary Education System (CARDES)*, a community-based nutrition education program designed to reduce dietary fat, cholesterol, and sodium among African Americans was introduced during office visits for nonnutritional concerns (Kumanyika et al., 1999). Participants used the program in a self-directed manner along with the assistance of a nutritionist. The program resulted in a decrease in total cholesterol, LDL levels, and blood pressure. Women improved lipid levels throughout the follow-up period. Men experienced significant decreases in cholesterol.

The *North Carolina Black Churches United for Better Health* (BCUBH) Project was a 4-year intervention project focused on increasing the consumption of fruits and vegetables among African Americans (Campbell et al., 1999, 2000). Churches in the five intervention counties received the Five-a-Day intervention, while churches in the delayed intervention counties did not receive any program activities until after the 2-year follow-up survey. The Five-a-Day intervention ran for twenty months and was based on the stages-of-change transtheoretical model, social cognitive theory and social support models. Services offered by lay health advisors, pastor support, and grocer–vendor involvement were examples of reinforcing factors. Researchers found that at 1-year follow-up those churches participating in the intervention had increased their fruit and vegetable consumption. The increase in fruit and vegetable consumption in the intervention group continued at the 2-year follow-up.

The *High/Scope Educational Research Project* studied 123 African American children living in poverty and at risk of school failure (Schweinhart, Barnes, & Weikart, 1993). At ages 3 and 4 the children were randomly assigned to a group that received an active learning preschool program and a group that received no program. The active learning program included daily classes and weekly home visits. Teachers trained in the High/Scope curriculum taught children in the program group by assisting them in completing activities that they planned. Parents were involved in the program through weekly home visits. Children participating in the project were followed until the age of 27. Progress of the intervention group was significantly different from controls in the areas of social responsibility, earnings and economic status, educational performance, marriage, and return on investment. Researches found that only 7 percent of those children assigned to the intervention group had been arrested five or more times and that only 7 percent of the participants in the program group were ever arrested for drug dealing during adulthood. In contrast, 35 percent of the children in the no program group had been arrested five or more times and 25 percent of the no program participants were arrested for drug dealing at some point during adulthood. Almost 30 percent of those in program group earned $2,000 or more per month, including 42 percent of the males. Thirty-six percent of program group participants owned their own homes and 30 percent owned two cars. Over 70 percent of those in the program group graduated from regular or adult high school or received a GED. Males participating in the program group had been married for an average of 6.2 years in comparison to the 3.3 years for the children in the control group. These results show that providing a preschool program such as High/Scope can significantly increase children's ability to contribute positively to society.

STRATEGIES THAT MIGHT WORK

One promising example of a church-based intervention program with implications for prevention research is the *Baltimore Church High Blood Pressure Program* (CHBPP) (Kumanyika & Charleston, 1992). This weight loss program focuses on overweight women with a history of high blood pressure. Group members talked to a dietitian, participated in behavioral modification activities, completed dietary logs, and took part in low impact aerobic exercise. Women participating in this study lost on average 3–9 pounds and gained no weight at the 6-month follow-up assessment. Women also experienced a decrease in blood pressure that was sustained at 6-month follow-up. In contrast, only 32–34 percent of women in the CHBPP who did not participate in the weight control program experienced no change or a decrease in blood pressure. There were no comparisons made for weight loss between the groups.

The *Heart, Body and Soul (HBS)* program was developed as a coalition between the City of Baltimore, the Center for Health Promotion at the Johns Hopkins School of Medicine and the Clergy United for the Renewal of East Baltimore (CURE). CURE is an organization of 200 churches that was formed to address the health needs of the East Baltimore community. The original intervention consisted of exit interviews within the hospital clinics to clarify and reinforce treatment, family or peer education to enhance social support, and small group participation to enhance motivation and commitment. Comparisons were made to a 50-patient control group (Levine et al., 1992). During the 5-year period of the study there was a significant improvement in the control of hypertension within the intervention group. The rate of hypertension control doubled and there were significant decreases in both hospitalization and mortality due to uncontrolled hypertension. This is a promising prevention program because the theory and methods are also applicable to healthy populations of African Americans, identified in some way before they develop hypertension, for example, with younger people in schools or clubs.

STRATEGIES THAT DO NOT WORK

There is very little information at all about preventing health disparities in minority populations, and none that we could identify that proved to be ineffective. Most of the programs surveyed were relatively limited in scope, and did not attempt to deal with the whole ecology in which health disparities exist. So, working on one small part may be less than effective, since other factors not addressed may be pushing in the opposite direction. In short, a more systematic and multisystem approach might be more useful than piece-meal programs.

SYNTHESIS

Given that the early childhood environment is important to the health and mental health of all individuals, what can be done to improve that environment for all, particularly those who now are disproportionately at risk? We recommend that the most realistic way to prevent future health disparities for ethnic minorities is to focus on preventive and promotive efforts with children and adolescents, while taking stopgap or treatment measures in reducing current disparities among adults. First, we recommend preventing predictable problems facing minority children, including concerns about physical, mental, and social health. A sound mind in a sound body flourishes best in a social context that encourages healthy development for all citizens. Second, we encourage the protection of existing strengths in young people and their parents and friends. The literature verifies that ethnic minorities possess many personal and social assets. However, it is also the case that these assets need to be protected in order to be actualized. Third, we urge creative thinking about desired goals for minority children that will enable them to fulfill their potential. Without the promotion of these goals, the social energy and skills that minority children have to offer will be wasted.

There is much potential for prevention of health problems and the promotion of strengths in early childhood health and education experiments like Head Start. Such programs should be able to reach a large section of minority youth and will have many positive repercussions for these individuals as well as for the entire society. These kinds of programs directly address young children with stimulating educational challenges that have positive implications for both physical and mental health. They also offer opportunities for parents to connect with available social resources (Zigler & Styfco, 1993). When minority children reach school age, the skills acquired from participating in Head Start and similar programs must be sustained in high quality schools. Reality has to catch up with the rhetoric that no child should be left behind (e.g., see the entries in the *Encyclopedia* on academic achievement, drop out, and other issues that impinge directly on the education of minority youth). High quality schools are essential for providing minority youth with the skills necessary to participate constructively in the wider society. When adolescents graduate from high school, they face the world of work for which

society owes them a reasonable opportunity for adequate employment with liveable wages. This obligation stems from the society's need for regeneration as well as its sense of social justice. Short changing the educational and work opportunities of any portion of that future work force is self-defeating. Relatively soon, a majority of that American work force will be composed of ethnic minorities. We must understand that it takes a serious, long-term commitment to educate an increasing diverse work force. Affirmative action legislation can help ensure a level playing field for minority youth, free of discrimination that is not only harmful to the targeted individuals, but also to the entire society that does not benefit fully from their labor.

Discrimination will, no doubt, persist in many forms. Minority groups should participate in organizations that can buffer them from some of the extremes of discrimination while promoting unique cultural values and ethnic pride. It will be necessary for Civil Rights organizations to help maintain a constant vigilance against discrimination. Churches can be especially effective in reaching young people and adults with a supportive message, which could also include health messages delivered over long periods of time in friendly surroundings. There is a long and rich tradition in African American communities for using Black churches as an organizational base for health, mental health, and civil rights. Minorities are more likely to be actively involved in prevention programs if the church and community persons are enlisted because both emotional and material support can be provided to individuals attempting to alter their behavior.

Local community centers and churches could also provide a safe comfortable environment for program participants to exercise and learn more about living a healthy lifestyle. Another way in which future prevention programs can more effectively address racial disparities is to provide educational materials that are culturally appropriate for the target group. For example, the CARDES program showed that the use of ethnically specific videotapes helped to increase understanding and adaptation of healthy eating behaviors. All educational materials need to be carefully reviewed for accurate translation and reading level appropriateness. In order to be more effective in reducing racial disparities future prevention programs need to thoroughly address the psychosocial factors that influence disease. Programs such as the Diabetes Prevention Project, Women's Healthy Lifestyle Project, and CARDES showed that including family and friends into the intervention process increases the likelihood that individuals will adopt a healthier lifestyle.

To make progress toward the elimination of racial health disparities, we must also conduct better prevention research. For much of the disparities literature Whites continue to serve as the criterion against which other groups are compared. From this perspective, African Americans continue to do comparatively poorly on most indicators of risk, morbidity, and mortality. This is not, however, universally true. Black youth are less likely than White and Latino youth to smoke or to be heavy users of illicit drugs. Similarly, the prevalence of major depression is lower among African Americans and Blacks are also less likely to commit suicide. Unfortunately we still know very little about why these "positive disparities" exist. Speculation centers on the role of the family, religion, and racial identity but more studies are needed before we can effectively incorporate these factors into programs and policies designed to protect and enhance such existing states of minority healthy behavior. Finally, training more health care professionals from underrepresented groups will also continue to be an important part of the strategy to close health disparities (Smedley, Stith, Colburn, & Evans, 2001).

The issues discussed in this entry cut across many diseases, risk factors, social problems, and population groups. This complexity and diversity also make it difficult to conclude definitively that we know "what works" with respect to programs designed to eliminate racial health disparities. Unfortunately, the patterns observed in the epidemiologic data make it clear that the interventions we have been able to implement over the past two decades have not been very effective. We need a prevention strategy that does a better job of integrating the importance of behavior and lifestyle within ethnic cultural context and addresses the social changes necessary to address the structural processes that also contribute to health disparities. We can only hope that the next decade of minority health research will be more effective in closing the health gaps among all racial and ethnic groups.

Also see: African American Youth: Adolescence; Resilience: Childhood; Child Care: Early Childhood; Environmental Health: Early Childhood; Environmental Health: Childhood; Health Promotion: Older Adulthood; Culture, Society, and Social Class: Foundation; Politics and Systems Change: Foundation; Diversity: Foundation.

References

Abraido-Lanza, A., & Dohrenwend, B. (1999). The Latino mortality paradox: A test of the "Salmon Bias" and healthy migrant hypotheses. *American Journal of Public Health, 89,* 1543–1548.

Airhihenbuwa, C.O. (1995). *Health and culture: Beyond the Western paradigm.* Thousand Oaks, CA: Sage.

Anderson, N.B., & Armstead, C.A. (1995). Toward understanding the association of socioeconomic status and health: A new challenge for the biopsychosocial approach. *Psychosomatic Medicine, 57*(3), 213–225.

Campbell, M.K., Demark-Wahnefried, W., Symons, M., Kalsbeek, W.D., Dodds, J., Cowan, A., Jackson, B., Motsinger, B., Hoben, K., Lashley, J., Demissie, S., & McClelland, J.W. (1999). Fruit and vegetable consumption and prevention of cancer: The Black Churches United for Better Health Project. *American Journal of Public Health, 89*(9), 1390–1396.

Campbell, M.K., Motsinger, B.M., Ingram, A., Jewell, D., Makarushka, C., Beatty, B., Dodds, J., McClelland, J., Demissie, S., & Demark-Wahnefried, W. (2000). The North Carolina Black Churches United for Better Health Project: Intervention and process evaluation. *Health Education & Behavior, 27*(2), 241–253.

Dressler, W.-W. (1993). Health in the African American community: Accounting for health inequalities. *Medical Anthropology Quarterly (New Series), 7*(4), 325–345.

Geronimus, A.T. (1992). The weathering hypothesis and the health of African-American women and infants: Evidence and speculations. *Ethnicity & Disease, 2*(3), 207–221.

HHS, US. (1985). *Report of the Secretary's Task force on Black and minority health.* Washington, DC: US Government Printing Office.

HHS, US. (2001). Influence of homicide on racial disparity in life expectancy—United States, 1998. *Morbidity & Mortality Weekly Report, 50*(36), 780–783.

Hughes, M., & Thomas, M.E. (1998). The continuing significance of race revisited: A study of race, class, and quality of life in America, 1972 to 1996. *American Sociological Review, 63,* 785–795.

Kaplan, G.A., Everson, S.A., & Lynch, J.W. (2000). The contribution of social and behavioral research to an understanding of the distribution of disease: A multilevel approach. In B.D. Smedley & S.L. Syme (Eds.), *Promoting health: Intervention strategies from social and behavioral research* (pp. 37–80). Washington, DC: National Academy Press.

Kumanyika, S.K., Adams-Campbell, L., Van Horn, B., Ten Have, T.R., Treu, J.A., Askov, E., Williams, J., Achterberg, C., Zaghloul, S., Monsegu, D., Bright, M., Stoy, D.B., Malone-Jackson, M., Mooney, D., Deiling, S., & Caulfield, J. (1999). Outcomes of a cardiovascular nutrition counseling program in African-Americans with elevated blood pressure or cholesterol level. *Journal of the American Dietetic Association, 99*(11), 1380–1391.

Kumanyika, S.K., & Charleston, J.B. (1992). Lose weight and win: A church-based weight loss program for blood pressure control among Black women. *Patient Education & Counseling, 19*(1), 19–32.

Landrine, H., & Klonoff, E.A. (1996). *African American acculturation: Deconstructing race and reviving culture.* Thousand Oaks: Sage.

LaVeist, T.A. (2000). African Americans and health policy: Strategies for a multiethnic society. In J.S. Jackson (Ed.), *New directions: African Americans in a diversifying nation* (pp. 144–161). Washington, DC: National Policy Association.

Levine, D., Becker, D., Bone, L., Stillman, F., Tuggle, M., Prentice, M., Carter, J., & Filippeli, J. (1992). A partnership with minority populations: A community model of effectiveness research. *Ethnicity & Disease, 2*(3), 296–305.

Lynch, J.W., Kaplan, G.A., & Salonen, J.T. (1997). Why do poor people behave poorly? Variation in adult health behaviours and psychosocial characteristics by stages of the socioeconomic lifecourse. *Social Science & Medicine, 44*(6), 809–819.

Markides, K., & Coriel, J. (1986). The health of Hispanics in the southwestern United States: An epidemiologic paradox. *Public Health Reports, 101,* 253–265.

Neighbors, H.W., & Williams, D.R. (2001). The epidemiology of mental disorder: 1985–2000. In R.L. Braithwaite & S.E. Taylor (Eds.), *Health issues in the Black community* (2nd ed., pp. 99–128). San Francisco: Jossey-Bass.

Pamuk, E., Makuc, D., Heck, K., Reuben, C., & Lochner, K. (1998). *Socioeconomic status and health chartbook.* Hyattesville, Maryland: National Center for Health Statistics.

Schweinhart, L.J., Barnes, H.V., & Weikart, D.P. (1993). *Significant benefits: The High-Scope Perry preschool study through age 27.* Ypsilanti, MI: High/Scope Press.

Smedley, B., Stith, A., Colburn, L., & Evans, C. (2001). *The right thing to do, the smart thing to do: Enhancing diversity in the health professions*. Washington, DC: National Academy Press.

Taylor, J. (Ed.). (1998). *The real American dilemma: Race, immigration, and the future of America*. Oakton, VA: New Century Foundation.

Thomas, S., & Quinn, S. (2001). Closing the gap: Eliminating health disparities. In R. Braithwaite & S. Taylor (Eds.), *Health issues in the Black community* (2nd ed., pp. 543–560). San Francisco: Jossey-Bass.

Williams, D.R. (1990). Socioeconomic differentials in health: A review and redirection. *Social Psychology Quarterly: Special Issue: Social structure and the individual, 53*(2), 81–99.

Williams, D.R. (2001). Racial variations in adult health status: Patterns, paradoxes, and prospects. In N.J. Smelser, W.J. Wilson, & F. Mitchell (Eds.), *American becoming: Racial trends and their consequences* (pp. 371–410). Washington, DC: National Academy Press.

Williams, D.-R., & Collins, C. (1995). US socioeconomic and racial differences in health: Patterns and explanations. *Annual Review of Sociology, 21*, 349–386.

Williams, D.R., & Harris-Reid, M. (1999). Race and mental health: Emerging patterns and promising approaches. *A handbook for the study of mental health: Social contexts, theories, and systems* (pp. 295–314). New York, NY: Cambridge University Press.

Williams, D., & Neighbors, H. (2001). Racism, discrimination and hypertension: Evidence and needed research. *Ethnicity and Disease, 11*, 800–816.

Zigler, E., & Styfco, S. (1993). *Head Start and beyond: A national plan for extending childhood intervention*. New Haven, CT: Yale University Press.

Religion and Spirituality, Childhood

Wendy Kliewer, Nathaniel G. Wade, and Everett Worthington, Jr.

INTRODUCTION

Children around the world today face a range of stressors—both acute and chronic—that heighten their risk for mental and physical maladjustment. Yet not all children are at equal risk for developing adjustment problems. Some children show resilience, which refers to a dynamic process encompassing positive adaptation within the context of significant adversity (Luthar, Cicchetti, & Becker, 2000). Others, while not technically "resilient," are better able to cope than are most. The religiosity and spirituality of a child (or a child's family) are factors that may help children weather the stressors and crises that come their way. Unfortunately, relatively little is known about how religiosity and spirituality affect a child's ability to cope with stressors, or how religiosity and spirituality influence normative development.

DEFINITIONS

Religion and spirituality are like poetry, it is easier to point to examples than adequately and comprehensively define them. This is reflected in the multiplicity of definitions that have been offered for religion (which can be grouped into functional or structural definitions) (Paloutzian, 1996), and the many ways that religion has been operationally defined. "Religion" consists of religious experiences (public and private), religious coping (positive and negative), religious commitment, religious practice (e.g., prayer, service attendance), and religious beliefs. Spirituality has been studied as spiritual feelings, experiences, beliefs, and well-being. For our entries, we adopt definitions consistent with those offered by Larson, Swyers, and McCullough (1997) after they reviewed empirical studies of religion, spirituality, and health. Spirituality is "the feelings, thoughts, experiences, and behaviors that arise from a search for the sacred" (Larson et al., 1997, p. 21). Sacred refers to that which is considered holy, venerated, or hallowed—a divine being, ultimate reality, or ultimate truth. Religion or religiousness is spirituality—the individual search for the sacred—that occurs within an identifiable group of people and may include the "search … for non-sacred goals (such as identity…)" (Larson et al., 1997, p. 21). Our definitions are as follows. *Religion* is defined as the individual and corporate search for the sacred that has been formalized into an institution. *Spirituality* is defined as the search of the sacred, which might or might not exist within an institution.

Others concur with this attempt to delineate religion and spirituality without dichotomizing. They state that the tendency to dichotomize religion and spirituality, respectively, into opposing concepts, such as corporate versus individual, stagnant versus vital, and external versus internal, incorrectly devalues religion and diminishes the power of authentic spirituality (Hill & Hood, 1999; Hill et al., 2000; Pargament, 1997; Seybold & Hill, 2001). Grimes (1999) agreed that spirituality and religion are distinct, yet overlapping concepts. Thus, spirituality is a "practiced attentiveness aimed at nurturing a sense for the interdependence of all beings sacred and all things ordinary" (p. 157). Religion, he claimed, is "spirituality sustained as a tradition or organized into an institution" (p. 158). In each definition, the primary distinction is the corporate or institutionalized aspects of the "search for the sacred." For the purposes of this and the three subsequent entries, we characterize religion as both an individual and corporate "search for the sacred" that has been formalized into an institution.

Spirituality is the search for the sacred, which might exist within an institution, but the institution is not a necessary part of spirituality.

SCOPE

The percentage of children (preadolescents) in the United States or elsewhere that consider themselves either religious or spiritual has not been quantified. However, the majority of adults in the United States (Zinnbauer et al., 1997) report themselves to be both religious and spiritual. In the largest national survey conducted on religious affiliation in the United States, over 92 percent of the respondents identified themselves as religious (Goldman, 1991). Koenig, McCullough, and Larson (2001) estimated that 151 million US adults were Christian, 3 million were Jewish, one half million were Muslim, 0.4 million were Buddhist, and one quarter million were Hindu. The World Almanac (1997) estimated that, in the world, 1.9 billion adults were Christian, 14 million were Jewish, 1 billion were Muslim, 324 million were Buddhist, and 781 million were Hindu. Further, results from a 15-nation study of religious beliefs indicate that in religious nations, both a nation's religious environment and family religiosity shape children's religious beliefs (Kelley & DeGraaf, 1997).

Estimating spirituality is more speculative given its essentially individual nature. Recall that most religious people—at least in the United States—also consider themselves spiritual; the number of people who consider themselves religious but not spiritual is small (Zinnbauer et al., 1997). Martin Marty suggested five types of spirituality along with estimates of the fraction of people in the United States who might identify with each (cited in Koenig et al., 2001). *Humanistic spirituality* focuses on the human spirit without reference to the divine or a higher power (about 7 percent of the population). *Unmoored* (to traditional religions) *spirituality* focuses on individualistic but transcendent experiences such as "new age" spirituality (about 7 percent). *Moored spirituality—Eastern type* (less than 3 percent) is spirituality within Buddhist, Hindu, or other Eastern traditions. *Moored spirituality—Western type I* (about 25 percent) involves spirituality within theologically conservative religious traditions, such as evangelicals, conservative Roman Catholics, Eastern Orthodox Jews, and Muslim believers. *Moored spirituality—Western type II* includes most Roman Catholics and mainline Protestant denominations (about 60 percent). These are estimates, not survey data and consequently only approximate 100 percent.

It is important to consider the religiosity and spirituality of the parents when considering the spirituality of the child (Clark, Worthington, & Danser, 1988; Danser,

Worthington, Clark, & Berry, 1988). Most children have little choice about whether and to what extent they will participate in religious activities within or outside of the home. Parents determine whether and where the family will attend religious services, to which and how many religious activities the child will be exposed, and how, when, and how often religious activities will be incorporated within the home. Parents decide whether children will attend public or religious schools, or (increasingly) whether children will be home schooled. Parents decide who the majority of playmates of their children are. In addition, parents determine the degree to which religious experiences that the child is exposed to will be more a matter of form (which might promote a low-spirituality religious orientation in the child) or warm personal experiences (which might promote vibrant religious commitment and spirituality).

Of course, how the child will ultimately respond to the early religious or spiritual experiences also depends on the child's personality and disposition, which in turn is dependent on both genes and experiences. Is the child fundamentally agreeable? Perhaps the child will go along with the parents more than a child who is not agreeable. Is the child conscientious? Perhaps the child will filter his or her experiences to be more receptive to conscientiousness-based religions (Worthington, Berry, & Parrott, 2001). Is the child extraverted? People-oriented influences might be received more readily than less people-oriented influences. Is the child fundamentally open to experience? Perhaps the child will be more influenced by peers and other adults and less so by parents. Is the child high on neuroticism (i.e., emotional instability)? Perhaps the child will react strongly and emotionally to salient religious experiences.

THEORIES

A variety of theorists have speculated about how people develop faith. Some apply most directly to childhood (e.g., Elkind, 1970). Others apply more to adolescence (Fowler, 1981), adulthood (Whitehead & Whitehead, 1979; Wilber, 2000), or older adulthood (Jung, 1933). Others apply throughout the life span (e.g., Fowler, 1981). In the present entry and the subsequent three entries, we will review only aspects of theories most pertinent to the time period of focus. For a more thorough summary of each of the theories, even aspects not mentioned in the present review, see Worthington (1989).

In childhood, the primary theories of interest are Elkind's (1970) and Fowler's (1981). Elkind (1970) based his theorizing on his empirical research, which was informed by Piagetian theory. Elkind found that a child's learning of object permanence in early childhood prepared him or her for the notion of a God who is not physically present. School-aged children who became aware of death—even though death might not have actually touched their experience—"solved" their problem of loss by developing the notion of life after death. The need to "conserve" life provided a platform for developing theological conceptions, regardless of whether children were raised in explicitly religious families. Elkind also found the emergence of logical thinking readied children to think of how God might be represented symbolically and perhaps worshipped.

Fowler (1981) posited seven stages in the development of faith. He also has supported his theorizing by extensive research. In undifferentiated faith (Stage 0), children have religious conceptions, if any, that are preverbal. In intuitive–projective faith (Stage 1), children project the characteristics of adult care-givers onto a divine being or onto a nondeistic conception of ultimate concerns. In mythic–literal faith (Stage 2), children begin to impose order on stories, beliefs, rules, and attitudes. They develop a system of religion and spirituality based on narratives, experiences, and stories. Religious concepts are not well elaborated. Fowler theorized that most children do not progress past Stage 2 until adolescence or beyond. We will continue our discussion of Fowler in the next entry, on adolescents.

Mechanisms of Influence by Religion and Spirituality

Parents with spiritual or religious commitments may be hypothesized to encourage more healthy coping. There are a number of mechanisms through which the religiosity or spirituality of a child or of a child's parents could possibly affect a child's physical and emotional well-being. Kliewer, Sandler, and Wolchik (1994) have discussed three theoretical mechanisms by which parents influence children's coping processes, and these can be used to understand how parental spirituality might affect children's well-being.

First, parents might influence children by *coaching* them to engage in particular ways of thinking about and responding to stressors. That is, parents suggest to children how they might interpret events that occur, and suggest options for how they might respond. Parents with spiritual or religious commitments may tend to encourage more healthy coping (e.g., seeking support, thinking about the situation, forgiving others) and discourage coping that is less adaptive (e.g., avoidant and aggressive behavior). They may help their children find meaning in the events that occur to them by suggesting that their children interpret events from a spiritual or religious viewpoint. This conceptual framework that religious parents can provide actually goes far beyond helping children merely cope with life events. The religious narrative adopted within a family can provide a cognitive

scaffold on which the child's worldview might be constructed—having wide-ranging effects on the remainder of the child's life (McAdams, 1996).

Parental coaching may apply to physical, as well as emotional, needs. Most religions are associated with a host of pro-health behaviors and discourages behaviors that are unhealthy. While spirituality might be associated with pro-health lifestyles, the research, at this point, is unclear. Parents who are spiritual might coach their children to engage in healthier habits (e.g., eating right, taking care of one's body, sleeping enough) than parents who are less spiritual. The spiritual and religious values of parents undergird the coaching messages they relay to their children.

Second, parents might influence children through *modeling*. Parents who are spiritually or religiously committed may be more likely than parents who are not to cope adaptively with life stressors (e.g., seek support, pray, forgive others, take action to solve the problem, not turn to drugs or alcohol) and to take good care of their own physical needs (e.g., eat right, exercise, have regular medical care). For adults, strong and replicable intercorrelations have been found between religious measures and positive health behaviors (McCullough, Hoyt, Larson, Koenig, & Thoresen, 2000). In addition, parents with spiritual commitments might be more likely than other parents to model prosocial behavior in the community. (Again, virtually all the research has been on religion, not spirituality.) Children observe their parents' behavior and imitate them, particularly when they are young. As parents participate in activities that lead to enhanced physical and emotional well-being and that foster community connectedness, children will benefit. Further, by coping adaptively and taking care of themselves, parents who are spiritual may enjoy better physical and emotional adjustment, which enables them to be more effective at attending to their children's needs. Parents who are spiritually committed may be more intentional about modeling particular ways of coping and interacting with the community to their children than other parents.

Third, parents might influence children by creating a *context* in which behaviors are learned and enacted. Parents are architects of the home environment. The extent to which the home is a safe haven in which family members communicate and care about one another is largely the responsibility of adults in the home. Parental spirituality and religious commitment might affect the context in which children are raised in a myriad of ways depending on their beliefs. For example, spiritual parents might make greater efforts than parents who are not spiritual at protecting their children from environmental stressors. This might be particularly true of those embracing what Marty called humanistic spirituality or perhaps those whose religious beliefs emphasize keeping themselves isolated from people who believe differently.

If parents have the financial means, spiritual parents may locate in environments that are less toxic (e.g., less crime ridden or less value-discrepant). If parents have little choice about where they live, they may invest in creating what they consider to be spiritually safe and healthy environments within the confines of their home. As another example, parents with spiritual commitments might be more likely to invest in their child's development and have more effective parenting styles than less spiritual parents. For instance, spiritual or religious parents may be more loving and accepting of and less hostile toward their children, more likely to establish boundaries that provide security, and more able to provide support to their children. On the other hand, spiritual or religious parents might also have some prejudices or harmful beliefs that are associated with their religious or secular spiritual beliefs. Those too might be likely to be transmitted to children. At present, there is little empirical evidence that bears on these hypotheses.

In addition to parental influences, children's own spirituality may influence their well-being in several ways. First, children's spirituality may provide them with a sense of support, either from God or from members of a religious community to which they belong (George, Larson, Koenig, & McCullough, 2000). This support may buffer children from stressors by enhancing their sense of control or esteem, or bolstering their connections with others (Sandler, Miller, Short, & Wolchik, 1989). Second, children who are spiritual (who understand and engage in the "search for the sacred" themselves), might be more likely than children who are not spiritual to exhibit traits such as respect for authority and community that will encourage them to follow the prescriptions and example of their parents and communities. The interaction between the child's personal religious or nonreligious spirituality and his or her community's religious or nonreligious spirituality further encourages positive behaviors that lead to healthy outcomes. Thus, a child's religion or spirituality might act as a protective factor by encouraging and fostering healthy behaviors, which in turn serve as additional protective factors, even in the face of difficult cultural, environmental, or personal situations.

Third, a child's religion or spirituality may provide him or her with a sense of coherence or meaning, that can assist with coping with difficult situations. Pargament (1997) has identified two kinds of religious coping. One type is *conservative coping*. Children can employ religious coping strategies to resolve a stressful situation and return to equilibrium. The level of a child's personal religiosity or spirituality will likely provide the motivation to engage in such conservative religion-based coping. The child's religious and spiritual cognitive framework will likely provide the content of many of the coping mechanisms. Second, when conservative coping strategies are insufficient to solve the child's problem,

the child might engage in *transformative coping*. Transformative coping strategies are those that break starkly with the existing conceptual framework of the child. The child might come to see God differently, might have a religious conversion experience, might reject the religion of the parents, or might decide to change the place or style of worship. The context that parents have established during the childhood years, as well as the child's own spirituality, are vital in whether and to what extent the child is likely to engage in different types of coping.

RESEARCH

Discerning the impact of religion or spirituality on physical or mental health has traditionally been difficult. The problem is that religion is intimately intertwined with numerous variables related to health and mental health (Koenig, McCullough, & Larson, 2001). Religion is not necessarily causal, but it seems to be part of a package that is bundled together. Researchers have typically taken a statistically conservative approach to discerning the effects of religion. Usually, the health effects on religion of social support, risky health behaviors (e.g., delinquency), and the like have been removed statistically or controlled experimentally. Then the residual effect of religion has been measured (see McCullough et al., 2000). In a way, because religious commitment and many health-promoting and health-risk-preventing behaviors are packaged together, the effects of religion on health and mental health might have been systematically underestimated for parents and children. Conservative statistical strategies have nonetheless revealed a substantial unique correlation between religion and both physical and mental health.

As noted above, there is limited evidence linking parent or child *spirituality* to children's well-being. However, there is evidence indicating that parental spirituality within their religiosity affects marital adjustment (Bahr & Chadwick, 1985; Wilson & Filsinger, 1986) and parenting behavior (Strayhorn, Weidman, & Larson, 1990); that individual and community spirituality foster a sense of support (Haight, 1998); that children who live in religious environments tend to adopt the religious beliefs and customs of their community (Kelley & DeGraaf, 1997); and that the sense of meaning children gain from spirituality acts as a protective factor (Coles, 1990; Garbarino, 1999b; Werner, 1993).

Evidence that parental religiosity is associated with particular parental behaviors is found in a study of 199 families with children in a Head Start program (Strayhorn et al., 1990). Strayhorn et al. found that religiousness in parents was related to more positive parenting techniques and to less hostility and depression in parents. In a more direct test of linkages between parental religiosity and child adjustment among rural, two-parent, African American families, Brody, Stoneman, and Flor (1996) found that greater formal religiosity was directly related to more cohesive family relationships, lower levels of inter-parental conflict, and fewer externalizing and internalizing behaviors among the 9–12-year olds in the study. Formal religiosity was also indirectly associated youth self-regulation through its positive relationship with family cohesion and negative relationship with inter-parental conflict.

A 4-year ethnographic study of spirituality as a protective factor in an African American community (Haight, 1998) provided evidence that spirituality was fostered or socialized in children, and that individual and community religious spirituality fostered a sense of support. This sense of support is used to deal with chronic stressors such as racism, inadequate education, and limited occupational opportunities.

Evidence that children's spirituality and the sense of meaning that it generates is protective comes from several studies. In Werner's (1993) classic study of children born on the island of Kauai, two of the many factors that were protective for children were religious involvement and the emotional support received from church groups or leaders. Further, a sense of coherence gained from this religious involvement helped children acquire a faith that their lives had meaning and they had control over their fate. In a landmark book on the spirituality of children, Coles (1990) examined the spiritual experiences and beliefs of children around the world. He interviewed individuals and groups, held discussion groups with children on spirituality, and asked children to draw pictures that represented spiritual or religious concepts. Coles asserted that while children do follow their parents' and community's lead with regard to spirituality, they also have their own distinctive spirituality. In many cases, this understanding is much greater than adults usually ascribe to children and can serve as a great source of meaning and direction during difficult times (Coles, 1990). After numerous interviews across many cultures, Coles (1990) believes that "children try to understand not only what is happening to them, but why; and in doing that, they call upon the religious life they have experienced, the spiritual values they have received, as well as other sources of potential explanation" (p. 159).

Finally, Garbarino argues that not only is children's spirituality a protective factor against potentially negative outcomes, negative events themselves spur children toward greater spirituality. In extensive work with children in difficult circumstances, from the horrors of war to the struggle of poverty, Garbarino (1999b) observed that trauma can create in some children a desire for answers that leads to a spiritual quest. This search for meaning in response to a traumatic event will often lead to personal growth and answers that allow for better functioning later in life.

STRATEGIES THAT WORK

The extant literature is silent when it comes to proven ways of enhancing children's health through religiosity or spirituality. Although there is adequate correlational evidence linking parent and child religiosity, and parent religiosity and well-being, there have been no "clinical trials" documenting how change in a child's religiosity or spirituality affects well-being, nor studies documenting the efficacy of attempts to enhance child religiosity or spirituality.

STRATEGIES THAT MIGHT WORK

In contrast to the above, there is much correlational and clinical evidence to suggest that encouraging children to explore the spiritual has beneficial effects. The literature documents robust associations between parental spirituality and religious commitment and better parental well-being, greater family cohesion and marital harmony, and more positive parenting techniques. Further, children's religiosity and spirituality is linked to better adjustment. Given these associations, a viable avenue to promoting health in preadolescents seems to be promoting more religiosity and spirituality in children or parents who desire to become more spiritual or religious (or both). Obviously, it would be a moral and ethical transgression for professionals to conduct a religious or spiritual intervention on people who do not give informed consent or who are coerced to accept a religious intervention. The "how" by which one (such as a parent, church worker, or professional working consistently with a parents' bidding) might intentionally promote increased religion or spirituality among normally developing children has not been explored much empirically, and we offer some places to begin in our synthesis section.

Much of work that has shown children to be spiritual and that has advocated spiritual interventions for children has emanated from studies of children facing trauma, including serious illness and potential death. Parents and caregivers can play an important role in fostering spiritual development in children who are confronting these types of stressors. Professionals can intervene more tentatively and only after informed consent. One stressor can serve as an example. Children with cancer have unique spiritual needs. Hart and Schneider (1997) encourage oncology nurses to enact interventions that assist children with cancer in finding meaning and purpose in life, continuing relationships, and transcending beyond the self. In addition, professionals might also incorporate the search for the sacred into traditional therapies that are used with chronically ill children, such as art therapy (Koepfer, 2000). Finally, Garbarino (1999b) has noted that exposure to trauma is often the impetus for children to begin seeking meaning for the events they have observed or experienced. As adults are sensitized to this tendency, they can aid children in their quest for answers. Further, Garbarino (1999a) notes that spiritual exploration is one of the factors that contributes to the success of lost boys—boys who have turned to violence, substance use, and other behaviors that compromise their well-being. Because spiritual exploration contributes to success, Garbarino argues that spiritual literacy should be a part of educational program for boys at risk. Once this spiritual foundation is in place, then traditional intervention strategies (educational programs, vocational experiences, counseling, or psychotherapy) can help children move to a more positive life path.

STRATEGIES THAT DO NOT WORK

In terms of strategies that *do not* appear to promote children's health via spirituality, there is little evidence that religious school for elementary school children affects their religious development (Greeley & Gockel, 1971). What parents coach and model is much more relevant to preadolescents' spiritual development.

Harsh parenting practices likely impede the development of childhood spirituality (Bromley & Cress, 1998; Larzelere, 1998). In fact, ineffective discipline and low emotional support each contribute to generally poor child outcomes and specifically to children who might respond poorly to God because they might identify God with parents.

SYNTHESIS

In this section, we offer our own views on the best mechanisms to promote children's health through religiosity and spirituality. (Obviously, people who are not religious or spiritual might have many ways of promoting their children's health.) From the outset, we must acknowledge that it is impossible to investigate experimentally (within the bounds of ethics) whether becoming religious when one has not been religious or becoming spiritual when one has no interest in spirituality *causes* better health or mental health outcomes. One cannot randomly assign nonreligious or nonspiritual people to an intervention that is focused on promoting religion or spirituality, respectively. One cannot ethically assign a, for example, Jewish person to an intervention to promote Christianity or a, for example, Christian

to an intervention aimed at increasing nonreligious spirituality. Neither intervention would likely be acceptable to the participant.

However, one might experimentally investigate the effectiveness or efficacy of value- and belief-congruent religious or spiritual interventions with those who are already minimally religious or spiritual and who agree to the possibility of being assigned to a religious or spiritual intervention. For example, a religiously tailored intervention to reduce hypertension could be compared to a nonreligious intervention within a religious community; people could be randomly assigned to either of the treatment conditions and compared to people assigned to a no-treatment or waiting-list control condition. Whereas such designs have been used in studying religious psychotherapy (see Worthington, Kurusu, McCullough, & Sandage, 1996; Worthington & Sandage, 2002, for reviews) in adults, they have not been employed with children to date. Thus, most of the suggestions we make (see below) assume that interventions can be made and studies can be conducted in faith-based communities where people might want to increase their religion or spirituality in hopes of affecting their physical or mental health—not in the general population where people might be assigned to interventions or studies that are not congruent with their values or beliefs.

We acknowledge that discussing strategies to promote health or mental health by promoting religion are problematic. First, religion is not, nor (we would argue) should it be, entirely a matter of individual choice. Religion indeed requires individual choice, but it is choice exercised within a community. Religion is communal and involves community standards, structures, and norms. Families are part of the systems of interlocking communities within which individuals embrace religion. Families and broader communities thus "impose" a value framework on both children and adults, and those communities have a right to expect allegiance and impose sanctions for deviant behaviors. Interventions that strengthen behavioral norms of a religious community could be considered interventions that work. We have elected not to consider such "interventions." Rather, we have considered interventions narrowly to be efforts by professionals (or other helpers) to promote people's existing religious beliefs or values in value-consistent ways. As such, few of these narrowly conceived interventions have been shown definitively to work. Few have even been seriously proposed—so strong is US philosophy that characterizes religion as requiring choice. Those that have been proposed are considered those that "might work."

We believe a primary strategy that would likely promote children's religiosity and spirituality is to assist parents (who wish to do so) in developing spiritual values and commitments themselves. This recommendation is based on cross-national evidence showing that children, particularly children who reside in less religious nations, are strongly influenced by family religiosity (Kelley & DeGraaf, 1997). Further, a study of religiosity inheritance documented the importance of family context in transmitting family values (Myers, 1996). In that study, several factors aided in the transmission of religiosity to children: parental religiosity, parental marital happiness, parent–child support, moderate strictness, and a traditional family structure. Thus, it is important to note that parental religious and spiritual commitments cannot be divorced from other aspects of parenting in order to promote health in children. As part of a strategy to enhance children's health through religiosity and spirituality, parents should be encouraged to *coach* children to (a) look for spiritual meaning in events that happen to them using developmentally appropriate concepts, (b) help children recognize they have coping resources that are outside of their own capabilities, and (c) use religious coping strategies when appropriate (e.g., prayer, forgiveness). Parents should also be encouraged to teach their children directly about God and other religious concepts that are a part of their worldview.

In addition to coaching, parents should be encouraged to *model* their religious commitments and values in their own pursuit of what is sacred; the way they cope with their own stresses; and in how they interact with their children, other members of the household, and people with whom they come in contact outside the home. For example, if parents want their children to be prayerful, they will be most effective if they both encourage their children to pray and model a prayerful life themselves. If parents want their children to be forgiving, they should model forgiveness, including not being reticent to ask their own children for forgiveness. The values that are core to their religious and spiritual commitments should be reflected in daily interactions with others around them.

Spiritual routines and family activities that are consistent with parents' religious values should also be encouraged in parents. Children gain security and a sense of control from routines (Boyce, Jensen, James, & Peacock, 1983). Religious routines provide children with a sense of security but also help them to develop spiritual habits that can be built on as children mature and begin to explore their own spiritual values. Engaging in activities as a family that enact parental spiritual values, such as serving the community, is also a way to actively transmit spiritual values to children.

A second strategy to strengthen children's health and mental health through promoting children's spirituality and religion is to encourage parents to commit to a faith community. There are benefits to children of belonging to a faith community that are different from merely having parents with a strong religious or spiritual commitment. Communities of faith can reinforce what parents are trying to communicate to their children about spiritual issues, provide emotional and instrumental support for children (Haight, 1998; Werner, 1993), and act as a buffer between parents and children when parents are undergoing a lot of stress. Faith communities may also provide a sense of working together for a common goal. Health can be affected through (a) affecting children's health behaviors, (b) providing increased social support, and (c) reducing risky health-compromising behaviors.

A third strategy that would likely promote children's spirituality is to encourage children to develop friendships with other children who have spiritual sensitivities. Research shows that while parents remain important in children's lives as they enter adolescence, peers gain influence (Harris, 1998). If children interact with peers who support, rather than denigrate spirituality, children may be more likely to engage in the search for the sacred. This suggestion is slightly different than strategy two. Children can be members of a faith community without having close friends or peers in that community.

A fourth strategy that would likely promote children's spirituality is to directly encourage children to explore these issues, independent of parental religious or spiritual commitment. Webster (1998) has advocated using stories, poetry, and art in the context of the educational system to foster spirituality. Webster's ideas might be incorporated into the curriculum of youth organizations (e.g., Boy Scouts, Girl Scouts, 4-H) or after-school programs (e.g., Boys and Girls clubs).

In summary, there is a fair amount of evidence that parental spiritual and/or religious commitments are strongly associated with child spirituality, and that child religion (and to a lesser degree) spirituality is protective for children. While the efficacy of interventions to enhance children's religiosity and spirituality are unknown, research from the parenting literature suggests that encouraging parents to develop spiritual and religious commitments themselves, to become involved with a faith community, and to encourage their children to interact with peers who have spiritual interests, will likely help foster religious and spiritual development in children and perhaps physical and mental health. Further, directly encouraging children themselves to explore the sacred, either as a part of regular educational or extracurricular activities, or in response to trauma, illness, or poor life choices may help promote spiritual development. Research is needed that critically evaluates these types of efforts in awakening children to religious and spiritual possibilities.

Also see: Religion and Spirituality: Adolescence; Religion and Spirituality: Adulthood; Religion and Spirituality: Older Adulthood.

References

Bahr, H.M., & Chadwick, B.A. (1985). Religion and family in Middletown, USA. *Journal of Marriage and the Family, 47*, 407–414.

Boyce, W.T., Jensen, E.W., James, S.A., & Peacock, J.L. (1983). The Family Routines Inventory: Theoretical origins. *Social Science and Medicine, 17*, 193–200.

Brody, G.H., Stoneman, Z., & Flor, D. (1996). Parental religiosity, family processes, and youth competence in rural, two-parent African American families. *Developmental Psychology, 32*, 696–706.

Bromley, D.G., & Cress, C.H. (1998). The logic of child discipline in two social worlds. *Marriage and Family: A Christian Journal, 1*, 152–164.

Clark, C.A., Worthington, E.L., Jr., & Danser, D.S. (1988). The transmission of religious beliefs and practices from parents to first-born early adolescent sons. *Journal of Marriage and the Family, 50*, 463–472.

Coles, R. (1990). *The spiritual life of children.* Boston: Houghton-Mifflin.

Danser, D.S., Worthington, E.L., Jr., Clark, C.A., & Berry, J.T. (1988). Effects of theological belief and church attendance and parental beliefs and behaviors in families of preadolescent first sons. *Family Perspective, 22*, 87–104.

Elkind, D. (1970). The origins of religion in the child. *Review of Religious Research, 12*, 35–42.

Fowler, J.W. (1981). *Stages of faith.* New York: Harper & Row.

Garbarino, J. (1999a). *Lost boys.* New York: The Free Press.

Garbarino, J. (1999b). The effects of community violence on children. In L. Balter, C.S. Lawrence, Tamis-LeMonda et al. (Eds.), *Child psychology: A handbook of contemporary issues* (pp. 412–425). Philadelphia, PA: Psychology Press.

George, L.K., Larson, D.B., Koenig, H.G., & McCullough, M.E. (2000). Spirituality and health: What we know, what we need to know. *Journal of Social and Clinical Psychology, 19*, 102–116.

Goldman, A.L. (1991, April 10). Portrait of religion in US holds dozens of surprises. *New York Times*, pp. A1, A11.

Greeley, A.M., & Gockel, G.L. (1971). The religious effects of parochial education. In M.P. Strommen (Ed.), *Research on religious development* (pp. 264–301). New York: Hawthorne Books.

Grimes, R.L. (1999). Forum: American spirituality. *Religion and American Culture, 9*, 145–152.

Haight, W.L. (1998). "Gathering the spirit" at First Baptist Church: Spirituality as a protective factor in the lives of African American children. *Social Work, 43*, 213–221.

Harris, J.R. (1998). *The nurture assumption: Why children turn out the way they do.* New York: The Free Press.

Hart, D., & Schneider, D. (1997). Spiritual care for children with cancer. *Seminars in Oncology Nursing, 13*, 263–270.

Hill, P.C., & Hood, R.W., Jr. (Eds.). (1999). *Measures of religiosity.* Birmingham, AL: Religious Education Press.

Hill, P.C., Pargament, K.I., Hood, R.W., Jr., McCullough, M.E., Swyers, J.P., Larson, D.B., & Zinnbauer, B.J. (2000). Conceptualizing religion and spirituality: Points of commonality, points of departure. *Journal for the Theory of Social Behaviour, 30*, 51–77.

Jung, C. (1933). *Modern man in search of soul.* New York: Harcourt Brace Jovanovich.

Kelley, J., & DeGraaf, N.D. (1997). National context, parental socialization, and religious belief: Results from 15 nations. *American Sociological Review, 62*, 639–659.

Kliewer, W., Sandler, I.N., & Wolchik, S.A. (1994). Family socialization of threat appraisal and coping: Coaching, modeling, and family context. In F. Nestmann & K. Hurrelmann (Eds.), *Social networks and social support in childhood and adolescence.* Berlin: De Gruyter.

Koenig, H.G., McCullough, M.E., & Larson, D.B. (2001). *Handbook of religion and health.* Oxford: Oxford University Press.

Koepfer, S.R. (2000). Drawing on the spirit: Embracing spirituality in pediatrics and pediatric art therapy. *Art Therapy, 17*, 188–194.

Larson, D.B., Swyers, J.P., & McCullough, M.E. (1997). *Scientific research on spirituality and health: A consensus report.* Rockville, MD: National Institute for Healthcare Research.

Larzelere, R.E. (1998). Effective vs. counterproductive parental spanking: Toward more light and less heat. *Marriage and Family: A Christian Journal, 1*, 179–192.

Luthar, S.S., Cicchetti, D., & Becker, B. (2000). The construct of resilience: A critical evaluation and guidelines for future work. *Child Development, 71*, 543–562.

McAdams, D.P. (1996). Personality, modernity, and the storied self: A contemporary framework for studying persons. *Psychological Inquiry, 7*, 295–321.

McCullough, M.E., Hoyt, W.T., Larson, D.B., Koenig, H.G., & Thoresen, C. (2000). Religious involvement and mortality: A meta-analytic review. *Health Psychology, 19*, 211–222.

Myers, S.M. (1996). An interactive model of religiosity inheritance: The importance of family context. *American Sociological Review, 61*, 858–866.

Paloutzian, R.F. (1996). *Invitation to the psychology of religion* (2nd ed.). Needham Heights, MA: Allyn & Bacon.

Pargament, K.I. (1997). *The psychology of religion and coping: Theory, research, practice.* New York: Guilford Press.

Sandler, I.N., Miller, P., Short, J., & Wolchik, S.A. (1989). Social support as a protective factor for children in stress. In D. Belle (Ed.), *Children's social networks and social supports.* New York: John Wiley and Sons.

Seybold, K.S., & Hill, P.C. (2001). The role of religion and spirituality in mental and physical health. *Current Directions in Psychological Science, 10*, 21–24.

Strayhorn, J.M., Weidman, C.S., & Larson, D.B. (1990). A measure of religiousness and its relation to parent and child mental health variables. *Journal of Community Psychology, 18*, 34–43.

Webster, D. (1998). Fostering the spiritual dimension of education in young children. *Early Childhood Development and Care, 146*, 13–20.

Werner, E.E. (1993). Risk, resilience, and recovery: Perspectives from the Kauai longitudinal study. *Development and Psychopathology, 5*, 503–515.

Whitehead, E.E., & Whitehead, J.D. (1979). *Christian life patterns: The psychological challenges and religious invitations of adult life.* New York: Image Books (Doubleday).

Wilber, K. (2000). *Integral psychology: Consciousness, spirit, psychology, therapy.* Boston: Shambhala.

Wilson, M.R., & Filsinger, E.F. (1986). Religiosity and marital adjustment: Multidimensional interrelationships. *Journal of Marriage and the Family, 48*, 147–151.

World Almanac. (1997). *World Almanac and book of facts.* New York: World Almanac Books.

Worthington, E.L., Jr. (1989). Religious faith across the life span: Implications for counseling and research. *The Counseling Psychologist, 17*, 555–612.

Worthington, E.L., Jr., Berry, J.W., & Parrott, L. III. (2001). Unforgiveness, forgiveness, religion, and health. In T.G. Plante & A. Sherman (Eds.), *Faith and health: Psychological perspectives.* (pp. 107–138). New York: Guilford Press.

Worthington, E.L, Jr., Kurusu, T.A., McCullough, M.E., & Sandage, S.J. (1996). Empirical research on religion and psychotherapeutic processes and outcomes: A ten-year review and research prospectus. *Psychological Bulletin, 119*, 448–487.

Worthington, E.L., Jr., & Sandage, S.J. (2002). Religion and spirituality. In John C. Norcross (Ed.), *Psychotherapy relationships that work.* New York: Oxford University Press.

Zinnbauer, B.J., Pargament, K.I., Cole, B., Rye, M.S., Butter, E.M., Belavich, T.G., Hipp, K.M., Scott, A.B., & Kadar, J.L. (1997). Religion and spirituality: Unfuzzying the fuzzy. *Journal for the Scientific Study of Religion*, 36, 549–564.

Religion and Spirituality, Adolescence

Wendy Kliewer, Nathaniel G. Wade, and Everett Worthington, Jr.

INTRODUCTION

Adolescents around the world today face normal developmental challenges such as adjusting to their new cognitive capacities, individuating from the family, developing their own sense of identity, and dealing with the addition of new members to their social network. In addition, some adolescents must cope with poverty, violence, and pressures to engage in health-compromising behaviors. The period of adolescence is one of the most stressful in the lifespan. Many teens (15–20 percent) have clinical levels of adjustment difficulties (Arnett, 1999). However, many adolescents do well or even thrive in the face of significant challenges. These adolescents are *resilient*, which refers to a dynamic process encompassing positive adaptation within the context of significant adversity (Luthar, Cicchetti, & Becker, 2000). Others, while not technically "resilient," still cope well. Numerous individual-, family-, and community-level factors contribute to adolescents' resilience. Religiosity and spirituality—of adolescents, their families, and their communities—are factors associated with positive adjustment in the face of adversity as well as with more adaptive behavior.

DEFINITIONS AND SCOPE

Religion is defined here as the individual and corporate search for the sacred that has been formalized into an institution. *Spirituality* is defined as the search for the sacred, which might or might not exist within an institution.

The percentage of adolescents in the United States or elsewhere who consider themselves either religious or spiritual has not been accurately measured. However, most adults in the United States (Zinnbauer et al., 1997) report themselves to be both religious and spiritual. Further, Kelley and DeGraaf (1997) conducted a 15-nation study of religious beliefs. They found that both a nation's religious environment and family religiosity shape children's and adolescents' religious beliefs (Kelley & DeGraaf, 1997). A relatively recent, large (32,129 participants) study of religion and well-being in adolescents (Donahue & Benson, 1995) found that the average level of religiousness of US adolescents has not declined in the last two decades.

The Role of Religion of the Parents

It is important to consider the religiosity and spirituality of the parents when considering the spirituality of the adolescent (Clark, Worthington, & Danser, 1988), even though adolescents, relative to younger children, are given more autonomy with regard to everyday choices. The religious family traditions and rituals parents have had in place, including whether, where, and how often the family attends religious services, and how often religious activities have been incorporated within the home, shape adolescents' worldviews and expectations about their own spiritual development. Parents also determine the degree to which religious experiences to which children are exposed will be more a matter of form (which might promote a religious orientation in the child but low religious spirituality) or warm personal experiences (which might promote vibrant religious commitment and spirituality). These childhood experiences serve as a backdrop against which adolescents will examine religious identity (McAdams, 1996). Likewise, the schooling to which adolescents have been exposed—public, religious, or home schooling—is largely determined by parents and affects the paradigms with which adolescents evaluate the world.

Parenting is not the entire story, of course. As transactional models of development espouse, adolescent interest in spiritual development stems from an interaction of parenting behavior, extra-familial influences, and their own personality. There is good evidence that genetic and personality influences play a larger role in shaping behavior in adolescence, relative to early or even middle childhood (Plomin & Petrill, 1997). Studies of the relation between the Big Five model of personality (i.e., a factor analytic solution of data from numerous trait measures that identifies five major personality traits that underlie all other second-order personality traits) and religiosity in adolescents have found that *agreeableness* and *conscientiousness* were related to religiosity, particularly an *intrinsic* (i.e., religion-for-its-own-sake) orientation to religion (Kosek, 1999; Taylor & MacDonald, 1999), while *extraversion* was associated with *extrinsic* (i.e., religion as a means to other ends such as dates, acceptance, etc.) religiosity (Kosek, 1999) in middle adolescence, but not late adolescence (Taylor &

MacDonald, 1999). *Openness* and *neuroticism* were not found to be related to religion.

THEORIES

Several theories are relevant to understanding how adolescent spirituality and religious commitment might develop. First, Erikson's (1968) notions of *identity formation* are germane. The major psychosocial task of adolescence, according to Erikson, is to resolve the crisis of identity versus role confusion. As adolescents near adulthood, they struggle to achieve an identity that will allow them to become a part of the adult world. The crisis of identity versus role confusion involves attempts to balance trying out many possible selves with selecting a single self. Adolescents deliberately experiment with different selves to learn more about possible identities. Much of this testing is career oriented, some is romantically oriented, and still other exploration involves religious and political beliefs (King, Elder, & Whitbeck, 1997). The literature is clear. Committing to an identity without having personally explored options is less optimal than exploring alternatives and then committing. Parenting plays a role in adolescents' identity formation. Overall, adolescents are most likely to establish a well-defined identity in a family atmosphere where the parents encourage the children to explore alternatives on their own but do not pressure them (Harter, 1990).

A second theory relevant to understanding adolescent spirituality is Fowler's (1981) theory that describes *stages of the development of faith*. According to Fowler (1981), faith develops in seven invariant stages that represent successively more complex ways of organizing meaning. Preadolescent children typically move through undifferentiated faith (Stage 0) to intuitive-projective faith (Stage 1). Adolescents are typically in Stage 2 (i.e., mythic-literal faith), which is characterized by attempts to impose order on the stories, beliefs, rules, and attitudes in one's environment, or in Stage 3, which Fowler calls synthetic-conventional faith. Faith in Stage 3 is conformist. It emerges as adolescents apply formal operational thinking (abstract reasoning) to literal thoughts and beliefs and as they discover apparent contradictions that cannot be explained. Faith in Stage 3 is sensitive to the beliefs and expectations of others in the adolescent's social world. Some adolescents, particular late adolescents, may move to Stage 4, which Fowler calls individuative-reflective faith. The movement to Stage 4 is often driven by the desire to make sense of contradictions between two or more valued authorities or by encounters with experiences or perspectives that promote critical reflection on one's beliefs and values. There is evidence (Vianello, 1991) that as youth move from early to middle adolescence they begin to consider religion in a personalized, critical, and autonomous way.

Mechanisms of Influence by Religion and Spirituality

In addition to theories that address how and why adolescents develop spirituality, there are theories developed primarily with adults in mind that are useful in thinking about the processes by which the spirituality of an adolescent and his or her family and community might be associated with sustained physical and mental health. Based on their review of the research, George, Larson, Koenig, and McCullough (2000) theorized that religiosity (measured as religious commitment or attendance at religious services) might positively affect health by (a) encouraging positive health behaviors and discouraging negative health behaviors, (b) facilitating social support, and (c) giving individuals a sense of coherence or meaning in their life.

Parental religiosity and spirituality could affect adolescent well-being directly, via providing adolescents with resources that meet their spiritual, emotional, and physical needs, by (a) suggesting that they engage in behaviors that are more, versus less, adaptive, (b) providing instrumental and emotional support, and (c) helping adolescents interpret events from a spiritual or religious viewpoint. Indirectly, parental religiosity and spirituality could affect adolescent well-being via (a) modeling positive behaviors that relate to spiritual, emotional, and physical well-being and abstaining from behaviors that compromise health, (b) creating a home environment that promotes communication, is cohesive, is low in conflict, and deals forthrightly with issues from a religious perspective, and (c) having input into the adolescent's peer group. In much the same way, the religious community of which adolescents are a part may affect well-being by (a) sanctioning behaviors that are health-promoting and discouraging or prohibiting behaviors that compromise well-being, (b) providing a context in which to have relational needs met, (c) providing a paradigm by which to interpret events that occur on the individual, family, or community level, and (d) providing a peer-community of religious adolescents.

Adolescents' own behavioral choices may emanate from their religious and spiritual commitments. Adolescents may find their religious and spiritual commitments a source of support and comfort, particularly if they have peers within the religious community to which they belong. In making sense of the confusion of adolescence, religious and spiritual commitments may give youth a paradigm from which to ascribe meaning. Pargament's (1997) work on types of religious coping is relevant in this regard. Pargament has identified two types of religious coping.

One type is *conservative coping*. Adolescents can employ conservative religious coping strategies to resolve a stressful situation and return to equilibrium. The level of an adolescent's personal spirituality will likely provide the motivation to engage in such conservative religion-based coping, and the adolescent's religious and spiritual framework will likely provide the content of many of the coping mechanisms. Importantly, the conservative coping strategies seek to conserve the fundamental belief and value system. However, through struggling with a difficult life stressor, the adolescent (or adult) can deepen his or her faith and understanding, moving to more sophisticated levels of faith while maintaining fundamental beliefs and values. However, when conservative coping strategies are insufficient to solve the problem, the adolescent might engage in *transformative coping*. Transformative coping strategies are those that break starkly with the existing conceptual framework of the adolescent. The adolescent might come to see the sacred differently, might have a religious conversion experience (perhaps more common in adolescence than in any other life stage), might reject the religion of the parents, or might decide to change their place or style of worship. The context that parents have established during the childhood years is vital in whether and to what extent the adolescent is likely to engage in different types of coping.

Fowler's (1981) theory of stages of faith development implies that coping experiences are what move individuals from less advanced (e.g., Stage 2) to more advanced (e.g., Stages 3 and 4) understandings of faith. These might result in either conservative or transformative coping.

RESEARCH

There is a growing body of work documenting associations of parental religiosity or spirituality to parenting behavior and adolescent well-being. For example, Giesbrecht (1995) explored the relationship between parental religious commitment, parenting styles, and spousal agreement in parenting style to adolescent religious commitment in a sample of 132 adolescents and their parents. Although parental religious commitment was not significantly related to adolescents' religious commitment, authoritative and supportive parenting and spousal agreement in parenting style were associated with intrinsic religious commitment among adolescents. Permissive parenting was significantly related to extrinsic religious commitment, primarily among males.

Using data from 486 families from the Nonshared Environment Study, Lindner Gunnoe, Hetherington, and Reiss (1999) found that religiosity of mother and father was associated with authoritative parenting. Structural equation modeling indicated both direct and indirect effects of parental religiosity on adolescent (ages 10–18) social responsibility.

Litchfield, Thomas, and Li (1997) used data from two longitudinal studies of over 1,500 adolescents (ages 11–18) to examine connections between parent–child interactions, adolescent religiosity, and adolescent deviance. Parental behaviors were correlated with adolescents' public and private religiosity, and their expectations of future religious activity, which in turn were related to reduced deviant behavior. Expectations of future religious activity reduced subsequent deviance more than either public or private religiosity. The authors suggest that adolescents construct a view of their future patterns of religious activity and behave in ways that are consonant with that view. Taken together, these representative articles illustrate how parental religiosity is correlated with adolescent adjustment.

There is an even larger body of research correlating levels of adolescent religiosity, and to a lesser extent, spirituality, with various health and mental health outcomes (e.g., less risk-taking behavior, more negative attitudes towards and less use of drugs, less delinquency, less voluntary sexual activity, less depression, greater psychosocial maturity, and greater pro-social values and behavior). Wallace and Forman (1998) used a large, nationally representative sample of high school seniors to examine the relationship between religious importance, attendance, and affiliation and behaviors that compromise or enhance adolescents' health. Relative to their peers, religious youth described themselves as less likely to engage in behaviors that compromised their health. For example, they were less likely to carry weapons, get into fights, or drink and drive. Religious youth also described themselves as more likely to behave in ways that enhanced their health, such as getting proper nutrition, exercise, and rest. Importantly, these patterns persisted after controlling for demographic factors.

Many studies have linked adolescent religiosity to lower substance use. Using a random sample of 13,250 adolescents, Bahr, Maughan, Marcos, and Li (1998) examined relations among parent–child bonding, parental monitoring, family aggression, drug problems, adolescent religiosity, and adolescent use of alcohol, marijuana, and amphetamines. Mother–adolescent bonding and family drug problems had modest, indirect associations on the likelihood of adolescent drug use. Father–adolescent bonding, parental monitoring, and family aggression were weakly associated with adolescent drug use. Students who were religious tended not to use drugs or to have close friends who did. Patterns were similar across gender and type of drug investigated. Miller, Davies, and Greenwald (2000) examined religiosity and substance use and abuse among a nationally representative sample of 676 adolescents aged 15–19.

Use and dependence on a range of illegal substances were associated with lower levels of personal religious devotion (a personal relationship with the sacred) and affiliation with less fundamentalist denominations. Personal conservativism (a personal commitment to teaching and living according to creed) was associated with less use of alcohol only. In an exceptionally large (> 32,000), representative sample of adolescents (ages 12–18), Donahue and Benson (1995) found that with respect to substance use, religiosity was negatively associated with use of both illicit drugs and alcohol. Interestingly, religious attendance was more strongly negatively associated with binge drinking, marijuana use, and cigarette smoking than was the personal importance of religion to the adolescent. Collectively, the above articles suggest several mechanisms for the relation between adolescent religiosity and substance use. Donahue and Benson (1995) also found a negative association between religious attendance and delinquency and between personal importance of religion (closer to religious spirituality) and delinquency.

Holder, Durant, Harris, Daniel, Obeidallah, and Goodman (2000) investigated the association between religion (and spirituality) and adolescent sexual activity with 141 11–25-year olds. Eight dimensions of religion and spirituality were assessed, including the usual religious variables plus existential aspects of spirituality and spiritual interconnectedness. Adolescents who were less sexually active reported greater importance of religion and higher spiritual interconnectedness with friends. In the Donahue and Benson (1995) study, teens who were more religious were less likely to have ever engaged in sexual intercourse.

In a related vein, adolescent religiosity was associated with fewer depressive symptoms among 451 adolescents (Wright, Frost, & Wisecarver, 1993). However, Donahue and Benson (1995) uncovered weak associations between religious attendance and importance of religion and suicide ideation and attempts.

Several studies have looked at the relation between adolescent religiosity and positive behavior. Markstrom (1999) studied the relation between religious involvement and psychosocial development, including ego strength and esteem, among 125 high school juniors. Markstrom found that the ego strengths of hope, will, purpose, fidelity, love, and care, as well as school esteem (but not general self-esteem) were significantly associated with religious involvement and participation. In the Donahue and Benson (1995) study noted previously, religiosity was significantly and positively correlated with altruistic values and behavior.

Evidence that adolescent's spirituality and the sense of meaning that it generates is protective comes from several studies. In Werner's (1993) classic study of children born on the island of Kauai, spiritual and religious involvement and the emotional support received from church groups or leaders were two among many protective factors. Further, a sense of coherence gained from this religious involvement helped children acquire a faith that their lives had meaning and they had control over their fate. In his studies of the effects of violence on children, Garbarino (1999a) observed that not only is an adolescent's spirituality a protective factor against potentially negative outcomes, negative events themselves spur youth toward greater spirituality. In extensive work with children and adolescents in difficult circumstances, from the horrors of war to the struggle of poverty, Garbarino (1999b) observed that trauma can create in some youth a desire for answers that leads to a spiritual quest, which might lead to personal growth and answers that allow for better functioning later in life.

STRATEGIES THAT WORK

Our review of the psychological literature revealed no empirical studies evaluating efforts to enhance adolescent's spirituality in an effort to promote their physical or emotional well-being. However, there are strong theoretical reasons to believe that certain approaches will result in enhanced religious and spiritual commitments by adolescents and possibly enhanced well-being. These will be considered under the next heading.

Second, the literature on parenting is very clear that an authoritative parenting style in which parents encourage adolescents to examine their religious commitments and values, and a family context where communication is valued will promote adolescent exploration of religious and spiritual identity (Harter, 1990). Thus, parents could be encouraged to use authoritative parenting (moderate amounts of both warmth and reasoned control) with their adolescents, and to create open lines of communication within the home. Investigations of the efficacy of such interventions should be undertaken.

STRATEGIES THAT MIGHT WORK

Fowler's (1981) perspective on faith development suggests that once adolescents have the ability to reason abstractly (i.e., middle adolescence), they should be encouraged to think about their faith, ask hard questions, and engage in dialog with parents and others. Adolescents for whom faith is personal and important also make behavioral choices that promote good adjustment. Garbarino (1999a) notes that spiritual exploration is one of the factors that contributes to turn-around for boys who have turned to violence, substance use, and other behaviors that compromise their well-being. Because spiritual exploration contributes to positive outcomes, Garbarino argues that spiritual literacy should be a part of educational program for boys at risk, providing a foundation for educational programs, vocational experiences, counseling, and psychotherapy.

The extant empirical literature points to several possibilities that may affect adolescents' religiosity or spirituality, and perhaps their well-being. Although religious education is not related to spiritual development in children, it does appear to have positive effects for adolescents (Greeley & Gockel, 1971). Therefore, providing formal religious education for adolescents might enhance their own spiritual quest. Second, parents should encourage adolescents to develop friendships with peers and adults outside the home who have spiritual sensitivities. Research shows that while parents remain important in children's lives as they enter adolescence, peers gain influence (Harris, 1998).

For youth confronted with significant stress (e.g., trauma, chronic illness), parents, caregivers, and professionals can play an important role in fostering spiritual development in these adolescents. For example, children with cancer have unique spiritual needs. Hart and Schneider (1997) encourage oncology nurses to enact interventions that assist children and adolescents with cancer in finding meaning and purpose in life, continuing relationships, and transcending beyond the self. Professionals might also incorporate the search for the spiritual into traditional therapies that are used with chronically ill children, such as art therapy (Koepfer, 2000).

Some faith-based programs seek to help adolescents control substance abuse or avoid other life-controlling problems. *Teen Challenge* reaches out to people in juvenile settings such as jails, and prisons. It also presents drug information via the web and in school programs, and it conducts weekly support group meetings. Some programs assist the local church to establish an effective, on-going, biblically based, small group ministry to help people overcome or remain free of life-controlling problems. DiIulio (1994) has found that community interventions by faith-based organizations has cut adolescent delinquency dramatically. Parochial schools in economically disadvantaged communities has similarly resulted in positive outcomes for students and communities. While these reports are encouraging, they do not have enough evidence supporting their effectiveness to suggest that they work. At present, they are considered promising.

STRATEGIES THAT DO NOT WORK

In terms of strategies that do not appear to promote adolescent health through promoting adolescent spirituality, forcing adolescents to adopt parental religious views and commitments does *not* lead to a sense of personal religious identity or ownership. Further, harsh and restrictive parenting or permissive parenting is negatively associated with intrinsic religious commitments.

SYNTHESIS

It is clear that, for adolescents, religious commitment and spirituality is highly intercorrelated with the restraint of many health-risk behaviors (e.g., not smoking, not drinking to excess, not engaging in risky sexual behavior, not engaging in juvenile delinquency). It is less clear that religious commitment or spirituality is associated with directly health-promoting behaviors (e.g., good diet, exercise, etc.). It is also clear that religion is associated with many indirectly health promoting factors (e.g., positive family interactions, social support, etc.). Nonreligious and nonspiritual people may engage in the same positive behaviors as do religious adolescents and their families and many religious adolescents and their families still take risks and behave unwisely. Many religious youth probably behave well for a variety of reasons and religion happens to be part of the pro-social package. However, there appears also to be a subset of adolescents who behave well and healthily *because* they are religious. Studies are needed to discern the characteristics of adolescents for whom religion is either causal, correlational as part of an integrated package, or correlational but epiphenomenal. At the present, no research has sought to disentangle those groups of adolescents. We have discussed different aspects of this causality-correlation conundrum in other entries on religion and spirituality.

From the correlational evidence we have presented, it would seem wise to make use of religious activities as possible influences that teach adolescents how to make more effective choices, to avoid risks, and to move toward positive mental and physical health. Other interventions that might possibly be helpful and health-promoting might not be specifically religious but might be done in a religious context because the adolescent is comfortable in that context (e.g., basketball leagues of teams from faith-based communities). Interventions should also be targeted separately at parents of the adolescents, community (e.g., peers, school, community organization), and individual adolescents.

Our reading of the literature leads us to suggest that one route to adolescent health through religiosity and spirituality is to encourage parents to belong to a faith community, and to engage in activities within that community that strengthen family ties as well as give adolescents the opportunity to explore their religious identity. Being part of a faith community may provide adolescents with security and support as they develop and "own" religious commitments for themselves.

Further, adolescent religious commitments and activities appear to be protective in a number of domains, although the mechanisms by which they operate are unclear. Interventions to enhance adolescent's spirituality and health have not been investigated. We suspect that effective interventions will eventually help adolescents themselves to explore the sacred, either as a part of regular educational activities, or in response to trauma, illness, or poor life choices. Those interventions will be religiously tailored to the consonant with family and religious doctrine for adolescents. Research is needed that critically evaluates these types of efforts in awakening adolescents to spiritual possibilities.

Also see: Religion and Spirituality: Childhood; Religion and Spirituality: Adulthood; Religion and Spirituality: Older Adulthood.

References

Arnett, J.J. (1999). Adolescent storm and stress, reconsidered. *American Psychologist, 54*, 317–326.

Bahr, S.J., Maughan, S.L., Marcos, A.C., & Li, B. (1998). Family, religiosity, and the risk of adolescent drug use. *Journal of Marriage and the Family, 60*, 979–992.

Clark, C.A., Worthington, E.L., Jr., & Danser, D.S. (1988). The transmission of religious beliefs and practices from parents to first-born early adolescent sons. *Journal of Marriage and the Family, 50*, 463–472.

DiIulio, J.J. (1994). America's ticking crime bomb. *Wisconsin Interest, 3*(1), 16–17.

Donahue, M.J., & Benson, P.L. (1995). Religion and the well-being of adolescents. *Journal of Social Issues, 51*, 145–160.

Erikson, E.H. (1968). *Identity: Youth and crisis.* New York: Norton.

Fowler, J.W. (1981). *Stages of faith.* New York: Harper & Row.

Garbarino, J. (1999a). *Lost boys.* New York: The Free Press.

Garbarino, J. (1999b). The effects of community violence on children. In L. Balter, C.S. Lawrence, Tamis-LeMonda et al. (Eds.), *Child psychology: A handbook of contemporary issues* (pp. 412–425). Philadelphia, PA: Psychology Press.

George, L.K., Larson, D.B., Koenig, H.G., & McCullough, M.E. (2000). Spirituality and health: What we know, what we need to know. *Journal of Social and Clinical Psychology, 19*, 102–116.

Giesbrecht, N. (1995). Parenting style and adolescent religious commitment. *Journal of Psychology & Christianity, 14*, 228–238.

Greeley, A.M., & Gockel, G.L. (1971). The religious effects of parochial education. In M.P. Strommen (Ed.), *Research on religious development* (pp. 264–301). New York: Hawthorne Books.

Harris, J. (1998). *The nurture assumption: Why children turn out the way they do.* New York: The Free Press.

Hart, D., & Schneider, D. (1997). Spiritual care for children with cancer. *Seminars in Oncology Nursing, 13*, 263–270.

Harter, S. (1990). Self and identity development. In S.S. Feldman & G.R. Elliott (Eds.), *At the threshold: The developing adolescent.* Cambridge, MA: Harvard University Press.

Holder, D.W., Durant, R.H., Harris, T.L., Daniel, J.H., Obeidallah, D., & Goodman, E. (2000). The association between adolescent spirituality and voluntary sexual activity. *Journal of Adolescent Health, 26*, 295–302.

Kelley, J., & DeGraaf, N.D. (1997). National context, parental socialization, and religious belief: Results from 15 nations. *American Sociological Review, 62*, 639–659.

King, V., Elder, G.H., & Whitbeck, L.B. (1997). Religious involvement among rural youth: An ecological and life-course perspective. *Journal of Research on Adolescence, 7*, 431–456.

Koepfer, S.R. (2000). Drawing on the spirit: Embracing spirituality in pediatrics and pediatric art therapy. *Art Therapy, 17*, 188–194.

Kosek, R.B. (1999). Adaptation of the Big Five as a hermeneutic instrument for religious constructs. *Personality & Individual Differences, 27*, 229–237.

Lindner Gunnoe, M., Hetherington, M.E., & Reiss, D. (1999). Parental religiosity, parenting style, and adolescent social responsibility. *Journal of Early Adolescence, 19*, 199–225.

Litchfield, A.W., Thomas, D.L., & Li, B.D. (1997). Dimensions of religiosity as mediators of the relations between parenting and adolescent deviant behavior. *Journal of Adolescent Research, 12*, 199–226.

Luthar, S.S., Cicchetti, D., & Becker, B. (2000). The construct of resilience: A critical evaluation and guidelines for future work. *Child Development, 71*, 543–562.

Markstrom, C.A. (1999). Religious involvement and adolescent psychosocial development. *Journal of Adolescence, 22*, 205–221.

McAdams, D.P. (1996). Personality, modernity, and the storied self: A contemporary framework for studying persons. *Psychological Inquiry, 7*, 295–321.

Miller, L., Davies, M., & Greenwald, S. (2000). Religiosity and substance use and abuse among adolescents in the National Comorbidity Survey. *Journal of the American Academy of Child and Adolescent Psychiatry 39*, 1190–1197.

Pargament, K.I. (1997). *The psychology of religion and coping: Theory, research, practice.* New York: Guilford Press.

Plomin, R., & Petrill, S.A. (1997). Genetics and intelligence: What's new? *Intelligence, 24*, 53–77.

Taylor, A., & MacDonald, D.A. (1999). Religion and the five factor model of personality: An exploratory investigation using a Canadian university sample. *Personality and Individual Differences, 27*, 1243–1259.

Vianello, R. (1991). Religious beliefs and personality traits in early adolescence. *International Journal of Adolescence and Youth, 2*, 287–296.

Wallace, J.M., & Forman, T.A. (1998). Religion's role in promoting health and reducing risk among American youth. *Health Education and Behavior, 25*, 721–741.

Werner, E.E. (1993). Risk, resilience, and recovery: Perspectives from the Kauai longitudinal study. *Development and Psychopathology, 5*, 503–515.

Wright, L.S., Frost, C.J., & Wisecarver, S.J. (1993). Church attendance, meaningfulness of religion, and depressive symptomatology among adolescents. *Journal of Youth and Adolescence, 22*, 559–568.

Zinnbauer, B.J., Pargament, K.I., Cole, B., Rye, M.S., Butter, E.M., Belavich, T.G., Hipp, K.M., Scott, A.B., & Kadar, J.L. (1997). Religion and spirituality: Unfuzzying the fuzzy. *Journal for the Scientific Study of Religion, 36*, 549–564.

Religion and Spirituality, Adulthood

Nathaniel G. Wade, Everett L. Worthington, Jr., and Wendy L. Kliewer

INTRODUCTION

Do religion and spirituality prevent dysfunction or lead to it? Can religion and spirituality promote physical and mental health or leave people susceptible to greater health problems? Psychological research into these questions has a sporadic and irregular past (Paloutzian, 1996). However, recently researchers have shown a growing interest in both religion and spirituality as predictors of different physical and mental health outcomes (Koenig, McCullough, & Larson, 2001; Larson, Swyers, & McCullough, 1997). This is also reflected in the growing awareness of and interest in religious and spiritual diversity and its impact on prevention and intervention efforts (Richards & Bergin, 1997, 2000).

DEFINITIONS

While existing definitions span a broad spectrum, we have chosen the following: *Religion* is the individual and corporate search for the sacred that has been formalized into an institution. *Spirituality* is the search for the sacred, which may or may not exist within an institution.

The scope of religious and spiritual variables is complex, making measurement difficult. Empirical studies have isolated particular aspects of religion, exploring religious experiences (public and private), religious coping (positive and negative), religious commitment, religious practice (e.g., prayer, service attendance), and religious beliefs. Spirituality has been even more difficult to define operationally. It has been measured as spiritual feelings, experiences, beliefs, and well-being. Research on religion has accumulated, albeit in fits and starts, for over 100 years. We can now confidently say many things about its relationship to mental and physical health. Not so with spirituality. Little research has been completed on its health promoting effects. While interest in the empirical study of spirituality is increasing, it is too soon for reliable findings to have accumulated. In the following entry, we focus primarily on the research relating religion to the prevention of dysfunction and the promotion of health in adults. We include spirituality where applicable and speculate about the possible implications of spirituality on prevention and health promotion.

SCOPE

Regarding information about the general scope of the potential, religion is a slippery animal. In the United States and the United Kingdom religious questions are not asked as part of the national census (in the United States it is actually forbidden by law). However, other research groups and agencies have examined the extent of religious belief and practice, typically reporting the percentages of people adhering to different religious faiths. For example, according to the *American Jewish yearbook*, approximately 2.3 percent of the US population define themselves as Jewish in religious practice as well as cultural heritage (American Jewish Community, 1998). National surveys conducted by the Gallup Organization also intimate at the scope of the religious beliefs and practices in the United States. In May, 2001, a Gallup survey estimated that in the United States approximately 55 percent of adult Americans are Protestant, 24 percent are Catholic, 3 percent are Jewish, and 9 percent indicated some other religious affiliation. Only 9 percent indicate no religious affiliation. The degree to which these 91 percent who claim religious affiliation actually engaged in meaningful religious practices and beliefs is less certain. According to surveys conducted in the spring of 2001, approximately 57 percent of Americans report that religion is "very important" to their lives. In addition, 65 percent of Americans are a member of a church or synagogue, and about 53 percent attend religious services at least once a month (Gallup Organization, 2001).

The extent of religious belief and practice in countries other than the United States is more difficult to assess. For example, while in the United Kingdom the Church of England claims a membership of 27 million, this does not accurately reflect the actively religious (Gallagher, 1999). This may also be true for other countries throughout the world where religion has a strong cultural as well as religious component. Gallagher (1999) reports "forty percent of Americans attend services weekly—an astounding rate when contrasted with the United Kingdom's 2 percent, say, or Italy's 5 percent" (p. 17). These statistics provide a rough estimate of the scope of the potential influence of religion on health.

THEORIES

Several theories that relate to religious and spiritual development have been proposed from a Western scientific perspective. Erikson's psychosocial stages and Fowler's stages of faith are two prominent theories that have direct implications for religious and spiritual development. Both theories apply throughout the adult years. For parsimony, we discuss these theories in Religion and Spirituality, Older Adulthood. In the present entry, we consider a theory that is probably more prevalent in adults of middle or early adulthood. Wilber integrates theories and scholarly work from both Eastern and Western sources in an integrative theory of spirituality and consciousness. Citing and integrating work from a vast number of authors and sources, Wilber (2000) presents a stage model of spirituality. The lower stages are more heavily influenced by Western religion and psychology. The latter stages are heavily Eastern in philosophy and religion. The latter four of his six stages are particularly relevant to adult religion and spirituality and are reviewed below.

The first stage of relevance to adults is the "mythic-literal" stage of development. This is closely linked to Piaget's concrete operational stage of cognitive development. In this stage individuals see myth and symbol as literal and factual. There is limited ability to understand the deeper aspects of life or spirituality that the myth or symbol represents or is used to convey. For instance, "Our Father in Heaven" is literally understood as an immense paternal figure living in the clouds.

Wilber's next two stages beyond mythic-literal are associated with the post-conventional stage of moral development (Kohlberg, 1980). In these stages, individuals choose morally responsible behavior based on what they think and feel is the right thing to do, regardless of community sentiments. The first of these two stages is "rational-universal." In this stage, the adult has gained the capacity for rational thought that Piaget identified as "formal operational." This includes the cognitive capacity to take another's perspective, to understand the figurative meaning of words, symbols, and myth, and to embrace belief and practice for oneself. These advanced cognitive skills can lead to myth and symbol being treated rationally, the rejection of "thoughtless" belief, and at advanced stages a respect for and acceptance of a plurality of worldviews and perspectives.

Wilber's next stage of development associated with (Kohlberg's) post-conventional morality is the "integral-holistic" stage. Post-formal thought (Sinnott, 1998) also characterizes this stage. The integral-holistic stage is the most advanced stage prior to what Wilber (2000) calls the "transpersonal." The integral-holistic stage is associated with a focus beyond what the mind or rational processes can accomplish. It is an integration of the rational mind with the spirit or soul. Individuals in this stage purportedly have a greater capacity to understand a multiplicity of perspectives and can utilize this complex perspective-taking to approach life and others with a universal or holistic belief system. While Wilber admits that most people do not attain integral-holistic spiritual development (estimating that less than one percent of people attain this level), his connections among various spiritual and religious traditions make these stages an interesting speculation.

The final stage of spirituality, "transpersonal spirituality," is comprised primarily of spiritual experience and is made up of four substages. This stage corresponds to the stages of mystical experience described by Underhill (1961). It includes concepts derived from systems such as Mahamudra'a stages of meditation, St. Teresa's seven stages of interior life, and Funk's contact with the numinous.

RESEARCH

The foci of the present entry are to explore the degree and direction of relationship between religion and spirituality

and (1) the prevention of dysfunction and (2) the promotion of physical and mental health. Research has established that many people claim to use religion and spirituality as resources for the prevention of numerous difficulties and for promoting mental and physical health during life's most difficult moments (George, Larson, Koenig, & McCullough, 2000; Koenig et al., 2001; Pargament, 1997). For example, Fitchett, Rybarczyk, and DeMarco (1999) found that among 96 medical rehabilitation patients in a Midwest city, 78 percent reported that they "received a great deal of strength and support from religion" in dealing with their medical problems (p. 340).

While people might report using both religion and spirituality to deal with difficulty, are either or both effective? Reviews of empirical studies of religion and spirituality over the last decade have largely concluded that religion is associated with positive health and well-being (George et al., 2000) although some findings disagree (see below). Positive relationships have also been found between religious variables and physical health (Larson et al., 1997; Levin, 1994). This relationship is stable whether researchers consider onset of physical illness (e.g., disability) (Idler & Kasl, 1992) or duration of and recovery from illness (e.g., recovery from hip surgery) (Pressman, Lyons, Larson, & Strain, 1990).

For example, McCullough, Hoyt, Larson, Koenig, and Thoresen (2000) recently conducted a meta-analysis of studies examining the relationship between religious involvement and mortality. They found that, across the 42 samples that they reviewed, people who were more religiously involved were more likely to be alive at follow-up than people who were not religiously involved. This relationship was observed even after controlling for a host of other health-related variables (e.g., diet, smoking, drinking, social support, marital status, etc.). McCullough et al. (2000) calculated an odds ratio between religious involvement and mortality of 1.26, indicating that people with more religious involvement were more likely to be alive at follow-up than people with less religious involvement. To put this in perspective, religious attendance had the same chance of extending life and reducing early mortality as (a) avoiding exposure to carcinogens such as benzene, or (b) giving up smoking nearly a pack of cigarettes per day. In addition, religion has been correlated with physical health (and lack of disease) in many studies. Koenig et al. (2001) summarized the data from 30 studies on coronary heart disease, 3 studies on cholesterol, 34 studies on hypertension, 6 studies on cerebrovascular disease, 5 studies on immune system functioning, 11 studies on neuroendocrine functioning, 13 studies on cancer, 12 studies on physical disability, 10 studies on pain and somatic symptoms, and 25 studies on health behaviors. Overwhelmingly, religion has been correlated with healthy outcomes, rarely with ill-health. Typically, incidence of disease is less in highly religious people than less religious or nonreligious people. In addition, coping with the disease has been better for religious than other people. Some denominational differences exist.

Koenig (1999) has put forth a hypothesized model to explain the potential causal mechanisms involved in the correlational findings. Religion was hypothesized to act through direct effects on mental health, production of social support, and stimulating positive health behaviors. Mental health in turn was hypothesized to affect autonomic nervous system and disease detection and treatment compliance strongly and to affect stress hormones and high-risk health behaviors (e.g., smoking and overdrinking) less strongly. Social support was hypothesized to affect disease detection and treatment compliance strongly and immune system functioning less strongly. Health behaviors were thought to affect high-risk health behavior strongly and immune system functioning more weakly. Those mechanisms were each implicated in producing physical diseases and mitigating their progress after detection.

A variety of measures of mental health have been found to be associated with degree of religiosity (Koenig et al., 2001). For example, of 100 studies relating religiosity and psychological well-being, 80 had at least one positive correlation. About 80 percent of the studies found a positive relationship between religion and either hope or optimism. Fifteen of 16 found that more religious people have a greater sense of meaning in life. Religiosity was positively associated with higher self-esteem in 16 of 29 studies, with lower self-esteem in only 2. The remainder showed either no relationship or mixed results. In 8 of 17 studies, higher religiosity was related to better adaptation to bereavement. Of 20 studies relating religion and social support, 19 reported at least one positive relationship.

Higher religiosity has also consistently been related to fewer or less severe mental health problems. For suicide, 57 of 66 studies found low religiosity more predictive of suicide than high religiosity. The remainder of the studies were inconclusive. A similar strong relationship existed with drug and alcohol abuse. Of 86 studies, 76 found lower religiosity related to drug and alcohol abuse. Only two studies found the opposite. Only 8 studies were inconclusive.

In about two thirds of 89 studies ($n = 60$), low religiosity was related to depression. Only 16 of the 89 studies found the opposite. Only 13 were inconclusive. The pattern for anxiety was almost identical to the pattern for depression. For anxiety, just under two thirds (49 of 76) found a relationship between low religiosity and anxiety disorders. Only 10 studies found the opposite. Seventeen studies were inconclusive.

In one other mood problem (loneliness) and with schizophrenia, the results are less definitive. Four of 10 studies found low religiosity to be related to loneliness; one of the studies found high religiosity to be related to loneliness. In half of the 10 studies, the findings were inconclusive. The same pattern held with schizophrenia. Four of the 10 studies found low religiosity to be related to schizophrenia. One of 10 found the opposite; 5 studies were inconclusive.

Spiritual variables are also related to positive outcomes in physical illness. In a longitudinal study of 155 adults admitted to a rehabilitation hospital, Kim, Heinemann, Bode, Sliwa, and King (2000) found that spiritual well-being (at admission) was positively associated with life satisfaction at each measurement point. While changes in patients' motor functioning over time were observed, no analyses were reported on the connection between motor functioning and spiritual well-being. Spiritual variables appear to be important components of recovery from substance-use disorders. Programs that make extensive use of spiritual teachings, attitudes, and beliefs (such as Alcoholics Anonymous) have been among the most successful for helping people overcome addiction (Miller, 1998). In fact, because of the influence of 12-step programs that stress spirituality but do not identify this with religion, the research on treatment of alcohol- and drug-related problems has been the most fecund area for results related to nonreligious spirituality (Miller & Bennett, 1997).

Some studies, however, indicate mixed or negative results between spiritual and religious variables and health outcomes. For example, the relationship between spiritual beliefs and medical outcome was investigated in 250 patients admitted to a London hospital. Participants with more self-reported spiritual beliefs at admission were 2.2 times more likely to have stayed the same or gotten worse medically at a 9-month follow-up than were patients with fewer spiritual beliefs (King, Speck, & Thomas, 1999), even controlling for age, social class, ethnicity, type of condition and social functioning. Another study investigated the impact of religiosity, religious coping, and spirituality on physical and mental health outcomes in 96 people rehabilitating from a medical condition (Fitchett et al., 1999). This longitudinal analysis found no evidence that religiosity (public or private) or spirituality (positive or negative) at admission were related to regaining more activities in living, greater general health, or greater mobility. Public religiosity, religious coping, and spirituality at admission were correlated with life satisfaction at discharge (Fitchett et al., 1999).

As the field continues to grow, more will undoubtedly be learned about spirituality. The current state of the research suggests, however, that religion and perhaps spirituality are related to the prevention of dysfunction and promotion of health. Research has been conducted by scientists seeking to "prove" religion is helpful or is hurtful. It has been studied by those who are disinterested and by those who treat the data fairly despite biases. A remarkably clear and consistent picture has emerged (Koenig et al., 2001). A vast proportion of the time religion (and to a lesser extent, spirituality) has been associated with positive physical- and mental-health indices. Occasionally, no relationship or a negative relationship has been found. As yet, analyses have not been fine-grained. Researchers still need to determine which specific variables reliably lead to positive, negative, or neutral correlations.

STRATEGIES THAT WORK

While this knowledge described above is important and useful, a deeper understanding of the potential causal links among these variables is crucial in conducting research to deliberately prevent dysfunction and promote health. At the present time, there are no empirical studies in primary prevention indicating that interventions that promote or are heavily contextualized using religion or spirituality prevent dysfunction or promote health.

STRATEGIES THAT MIGHT WORK

In the entry on children, we argued that professional interventions to promote health and mental health by promoting stronger religion ought ethically to be done within value-congruent formats or with clearly informed consent. Thus educational, or physical health-promoting interventions that seek to influence a person's religious or spiritual life should be either religiously tailored within a person's faith community or faith perspective or the religious nature of the intervention should be clearly disclosed to a person whose values are not congruent and free choice should be given prior to the onset of an intervention.

Perhaps the area in which faith-congruent interventions have been most used has been religious counseling or psychotherapy. Religious counseling has involved pastoral counseling (i.e., counseling done by a cleric) and professional counseling or psychotherapy that is specifically accommodated to religious clients. Often the accommodation involves adaptation of secular psychotherapeutic procedures. For 30 years, the research on religious clients, counselors, and interventions has been systematically reviewed (Arnold & Schick, 1979; Richards & Bergin, 1997, 2000; Worthington, 1986; Worthington, Kurusu, McCullough, & Sandage, 1996; Worthington & Sandage, 2002). Since 1970, over 350 studies have investigated religious clients, counselors, and interventions. Worthington et al. (1996) concluded that the *understanding* of religious clients and counselors is consonant with other fields in degree of understanding and methodological sophistication. However, the efficacy of religious psychotherapeutic interventions was not as clear. Nonetheless, we would suggest that borrowing from religious counseling or psychotherapy may provide some fruitful strategies for primary prevention.

Worthington and Sandage (2002) investigated religious counseling and concluded that religious counseling or psychotherapy *might* work to promote better mental health. In fact, the task force of the American Psychological Association that evaluates empirically supported psychotherapeutic interventions recently classified religiously accommodated psychotherapy as having "insufficient evidence" to classify it as empirically supported. Worthington and Sandage (2002) concluded that religiously accommodated psychotherapy and specifically religious counseling (such as pastoral counseling or use of ecclesiastically based interventions such as prayer) have virtually identical mental health outcomes with secular empirically supported psychotherapies (such as cognitive therapy for depression). Actually no studies found secular treatments better with religious clients and one study found a religiously accommodated treatment superior in mental health outcomes. The evidence has accumulated supporting a *preference* of many highly committed religious clients for religious psychotherapy. Evidence exists that religious psychotherapy does not challenge religious clients' religious values (although it might challenge their beliefs) whereas secular psychotherapy has resulted in the erosion of religious clients' religious beliefs.

Church-based community health screenings have recently been proposed as ways to prevent health problems or detect problems early in the disease. As of now, a little evidence is available to suggest effectiveness, which qualifies this as a promising method needing more study (Ferdinand, 1997; Kumanyika & Charleston, 1992; Smith, 1992; Smith, Merritt, & Patel, 1997).

Marriage longevity and satisfaction have been found to be related to both physical and mental health (Koenig et al., 2001). Thus interventions to strengthen marriage may be related to increases in physical and mental health over the lifespan. Most religions are theologically pro-marriage. Religiously tailored marriage-enrichment interventions or preparation-for-marriage preventive programs are likely to affect physical and mental health through affecting the marriage. There is initial evidence that effective preparation-for-marriage interventions can be delivered by lay people as effectively as by professional trainers (Stanley et al., 2001). Marital therapy interventions based on effective secular approaches have been tailored for Christians, but they have not been empirically tested and cannot rely on tests of secular approaches to substantiate their efficacy (Ripley & Worthington, 1998).

There are other promising interventions. Johnson, Larson, and Pitts (1997) have found that religious environments within prisons have produced numerous positive outcomes. Prisoners who participate in religious programs not only cause less trouble while in prison, but they also have lower rates of recidivism than other prisoners. While these reports are encouraging, at present insufficient evidence supports their effectiveness to unambiguously designate them as interventions that work.

STRATEGIES THAT DO NOT WORK

The study of the use of religiously trained interventions to promote physical health is in its infancy. Simply because few interventions have been studied, almost none have been shown to be ineffective.

SYNTHESIS

There appears to be a stable positive correlation between religion and both health and mental health. Logically, there are four possibilities. First, the correlation could be spurious. This is unlikely given that over 500 studies have been conducted (Koenig et al., 2001).

Second, good health and good mental health might cause people to adopt religion. For most people, though, it appears that the opposite is occurring. People tend to be drawn to religion more often when they develop health problems or mental health disorders as a mechanism of coping with adversity (Pargament, 1997) than they seek religion in times of plenty. People in low socioeconomic statuses (SES) throughout the world tend to be more religious than those of high SES, and low SES is more often related to health problems. Certainly some people do escape from abject poverty or poor health and find the freedom to pursue religion, but these cases seem to be rarer than the opposite.

Third, there might be other variables that cause both religion and health outcomes. Still, even when the variance from such variables is removed, the relationship between religion and health remains.

Fourth, there are likely some mechanisms by which religion causes better health and mental health. Theoretical work has identified three mechanisms that might be responsible for connections between religion, spirituality, and positive health indices (Idler, 1995). Religion might be *protective*. Religion and spirituality may protect people from the symptoms and experiences that lead to or prolong negative health. Religion might be *consoling*. Religion and spirituality may provide solace, comfort, and support for people dealing with negative life events, ill health, and

adversity. Religion might encourage *perspective-taking*, or positive reframing of experience. Religion and spirituality may help individuals view their lives more positively or from a more meaningful perspective, and so experience a better quality of life even if they have poor mental or physical health.

Religion Might Prevent Problems by Being Protective

Potential Mechanisms of Protection

The protective aspect of religious and spiritual variables has received the most attention from researchers. At times it appears as an unspoken assumption that seems to drive some research. Religious and spiritual variables are expected to protect against sickness, dysfunction, and dissatisfaction and encourage positive health. Thus, the more religious or spiritual an individual is the better physical or mental health outcomes she or he would be expected to have. Based on their review of the research, George et al. (2000) described three potential mechanisms that might account for the protective effect of spirituality and religion.

Prescription of Healthy Behaviors. First, most religions prescribe healthy behaviors. People with spiritual or religious commitments tend to encourage positive health behavior and discourage (if not outright ban) unhealthy behavior. For example, many religious communities encourage adherents to drink alcohol in moderation or abstain. This might reduce alcohol-related risks such as cirrhosis (one of the top five causes of death in the United States for men and women), addiction, motor vehicle accidents, and violence (which can be disinhibited when people drink). Religions often discourage smoking, which has been consistently related to many diseases. Religions also tend to discourage illicit drug usage and out-of-wedlock sexual behavior. Religions are typically pro-marriage, which has been related to better health than are divorce or single status.

Religion and spirituality might also encourage more positive behaviors. For example, religious or spiritual adults might receive more support and encouragement from their religious orientations to be invested in their child's development and to use more effective parenting styles. In a study of 199 families with children in a Head Start program, parental religiousness was related to more positive parenting behavior and less hostility and depression in parents (Strayhorn, Weidman, & Larson, 1990). These positive outcomes not only affect the parent or adult, but also benefit their children.

Social Support. Second, religion and spirituality might affect health by promoting social support. Religion is positively correlated with social support. The more religious an individual, the more social support he or she experiences (George et al., 2000). Religion not only provides local communities of believers but can also help people to feel connected to something global or universal. Nouwen (1999), a monk well known for his spiritual guidance, described the joy of praying not only with those in his faith community, but with the monks and nuns, the clergy and laypeople throughout the country and world. Prayer, as well as other religious practices, might encourage social connection and support.

However social support is activated for the individual, it is hypothesized to help deal with problems and difficulties of life. The relationships between social support, religion, and health were investigated in a national survey of 883 Black and 1,667 White adults (Ferraro & Koch, 1994). Health status was predicted by two measures of social support—self-report of emotional support from significant others and amount of voluntary association in social organizations. This relationship remained after shared variance with other variables such as race, gender, SES, and religious practice and identity was accounted for (Ferraro & Koch, 1994).

In an African American community, Haight (1998) concluded that individual and community spirituality fostered a sense of social support that African Americans used to deal with racism, inadequate education, and limited occupational opportunities. Further, Haight (1998) suggested that the spirituality itself was fostered, or socialized in the children within the faith community that she studied. Not only did the community's spirituality bring them together and create greater social networks, but also the community itself fostered spirituality.

Coherence and Meaning. Third, religion might affect health by providing a sense of coherence and meaning. Spirituality, as defined above, is the search for the sacred. One of the primary results of this search can be a sense of coherence or meaning in one's life. Spirituality and religion can provide answers (although at times incomplete ones) to the most basic questions and issues of life. Spirituality is at least the journey toward (the search for) understanding and meaning for one's (or one's community's) existence.

Batson (1976) has identified an orientation toward religion that emphasizes the search for meaning, the "quest religious orientation." Questing for answers and perhaps finding answers can contribute to physical and mental health if the quest is for a limited time or engaged in with a spirit of *joie de vivre*. However, one can also quest as a manifestation of cynicism, skepticism, nihilism, or general unrest. Such a questing might not be associated with positive health outcomes (Batson, Schoenrade, & Ventis, 1993). In a review of religious orientation and mental health, Ventis (1995) identified and summarized the mixed associations between

mental health and the quest orientation. Ventis first identified seven definitions of mental health used in the studies he reviewed, such as absence of illness or freedom from worry and guilt. The quest religious orientation was related only to open-mindedness and flexibility. While a questing orientation may not be specifically related to outcomes, the coherence and meaning that religion or spirituality can provide has been hypothesized to facilitate positive mental and physical health outcomes (George et al., 2000). For example, for 40 male adults dealing with different degrees of HIV and AIDS, finding a sense of meaning within the disease experience predicted better health and longevity (Taylor, Kemeny, Reed, Bower, & Gruenewald, 2000).

One recent study investigated the role of religious and spiritual coping in 33 elderly women who had been recently diagnosed with breast cancer (Feher & Maly, 1999). Analysis of qualitative interviews suggested that these women coped with their cancer by using their religious and spiritual beliefs to marshal emotional and social support needed to deal with the difficulty of the diagnosis and to help them find meaning in their experience. The authors concluded further that the ability to find meaning reduced the anxiety and stress of the diagnosis and increased subjective well-being.

In a longitudinal study of 698 people followed from infancy to adulthood, risk and protective factors were analyzed for a variety of outcomes, such as academic and occupational accomplishments (Werner, 1993). One of the protective factors that surfaced in this 32-year study was spiritual and religious involvement and the emotional support received from church groups or leaders. Further, Werner contends that the coherence from these activities led to resiliency and recovery. "With their help, the resilient children acquired a faith that their lives had meaning and they had control over their fate" (Werner, 1993, p. 505).

Religion Might Prevent Problems by Being Consoling

The second hypothesized causal mechanism whereby religion affects health is that religion is consoling (Fitchett et al., 1999; Idler, 1995). Religion often provides coping mechanisms for dealing with negative life events, including physical and mental illness. If religion and spirituality are activated during distress, then a negative relationship between health and religion would be expected (Idler, 1995). As people suffer more negative life events, sickness, or adversity, they will use more religious or spiritual resources. Thus, as health or positive experiences decline, religious involvement should increase to the extent that it helps people cope. In a national survey of 3,617 adults, consolation (defined as seeking spiritual support for difficulties in life) was negatively related to health status (Ferraro & Kelley-Moore, 2000). For example, greater consolation was associated with greater depression and more chronic conditions. The authors argued that, as individuals experience more sickness, they are more likely to turn to religion for support.

Religious coping is a well-established area of research that also supports the consolation hypothesis (Pargament, 1997). Pargament and his colleagues have conducted over 50 empirical studies examining the ways that people use religion to cope and the outcomes related to this coping. Based on these and other related studies, Pargament (1997) distinguishes between two motives for coping. In the face of stress (defined as a demand for change) most people employ religious coping mechanisms for *conservative* motives. That is, they handle the difficulty by removing the demand for change (stressor) or dealing with it in a way that settles them back into the original, prestress state. If such efforts fail, people may employ *transformative* coping mechanisms. People may use religious coping mechanisms to move to a different— often dramatically different—state. Religious conversions under stress (toward or away from religion) can result from transformative coping motives (Pargament, 1997).

The effectiveness of religious coping for dealing with adversity is difficult to interpret. Most studies have simply examined the correlation between health and consolation, seeking a negative relationship to support the hypothesis (Ferraro & Kelley-Morre, 2000; Ferraro & Koch, 1994; Idler, 1995). Whether religious coping actually provides relief, solace, or comfort has been more difficult to determine. In fact, some forms of religious coping seem to make matters worse. In a recent study, 49 Roman Catholic adults and 196 university students reported on a negative life event, mental health and well-being, and aspects of religious coping (Pargament, Zinnbauer, Scott, Butter, Zerowin, & Stanik, 1998). In reaction to the negative life event they identified, participants from both samples who reported more doubts about their religious beliefs, more anger at God, and more apathy about themselves and their religion showed less mental health (measured as less self-esteem, less problem-solving skills, and greater anxiety). In addition, these three variables were related to greater negative mood and poorer general health outcomes (Pargament et al., 1998).

Religion Might Prevent Problems by Promoting Perspective-Taking

Idler (1995) has suggested that religion might promote positive health outcomes through stimulating positive perspective-taking. Idler suggests that perhaps religion enables people living in difficult experiences to maintain a more positive outlook than they might without religion. Applied to physical health problems, religious and spiritual aspects of life might enable people to gain meaningful, "nonphysical senses of self" (Idler, 1995, p. 686). By developing a sense of self that is less dependent upon physical health, patients with even serious illnesses or conditions might report good "health" and well-being. If people's lives have meaning apart from their physical health, disease or illness might not make a dramatic impact in their overall quality of life or general well-being. Further, religion and spirituality would be related to well-being above and beyond illness to the extent that they help people to develop a sense of self that is independent from physical health.

In a direct analysis of these hypotheses, Idler (1995) investigated 200 outpatients of an urban rehabilitation clinic. Participants completed self-report measures of health, religiosity, mental health, social support, and a scale to measure one's "nonphysical sense of self." One's nonphysical sense of self was related to both self-rated religiosity and self-rated health. Those participants who had greater nonphysical senses of self reported more religiosity and better health. However, the analyses do not rule out other variables that might account for the relationship. While it does appear that a sense of oneself independent of physical health contributes to a greater sense of well-being, these results must be considered preliminary until more precise investigations can be conducted.

How Much Effect Does Religion Have?

Up to now we have attempted to show that religion might be a kind of master variable that affects physical and mental health by influencing numerous related pro-health variables. We have scrupulously avoided discussing how much health-promoting or problem-preventing effect it actually has. One answer may be found in McCullough et al. (2000) who meta-analyzed 42 longitudinal samples involving over 125,826 participants. Even after removing the effects of the variables we have discussed above as protecting, consoling, and promoting perspective-taking, McCullough et al. (2000) found an odds ratio of 1.26 between religious involvement and mortality (which might be about the equivalent of ceasing smoking a pack of cigarettes per day).

What Is Happening in the "Pure Effect" of Religion on Health?

As a major working hypothesis we suggest that religion is beneficial to a person's health. It is related to many pro-health behaviors and, even with the variance from those removed, it still rivals such acts as ceasing smoking in the amount it can extend life. Why? One possible reason might have to do with the effect of religious spirituality. People who are religiously spiritual might experience peace and calm, which frequently activate the relaxation response (Benson, 1997). Other naturalistic mechanisms might be at work as well, such as psychoneuroimmunological effects.

The assumptions that most scientists usually adhere to is that any effect (such as the link between religion and health) is, in principle, 100 percent explainable naturalistically. They might or might not believe that a divine being is at work supernaturally (in parallel with the natural). An alternative hypothesis, however, is that some of the unexplained variance might be due to supernatural reasons. This is a difficult position for an empirical scientist to take (because it can paralyze future scientific investigation if taken to an extreme), but it is a position to which many religions advocate and most lay people are sympathetic.

Several clinical researchers have attempted to measure health effects of religion that are not accounted for by naturalistic causes (to the extent the causes can be experimentally controlled). For example, Byrd (1988) attempted to study the health effects of prayer. He used a double-blind study in which neither physician nor patient (in cardiac surgery) knew whether the patient was being prayed for. Distance prayer predicted better outcomes on several "hard" variables than did no prayer. Byrd's study was criticized because it did not strictly control for Type I error.

Matthews (2000) has attempted to replicate (and improve) Byrd's (1988) design using patients with rheumatoid arthritis. Patients were randomly assigned to distance or in-person prayer. Physicians and assessors did not know the experimental condition to which the patients were assigned. When distance prayer was used, the patients did not know whether they were prayed for by a designated prayer team. The patients receiving in-person prayer showed more improvement than those not receiving in-person prayer. Distance prayer (beyond any that the patient might normally have received, which was controlled by random assignment) did not affect outcomes. Other efforts are currently underway to investigate the efficacy of distance prayer. This is one illustration of the efforts to take supernatural claims seriously and investigate their veracity with the most rigorous scientific standards extant.

In sum, religion has been shown to be related to positive health. This might be because it prevents problems, aids in recovery when problems do occur, helps people cope, or simply is bundled with other pro-health behaviors and life circumstances. Many, but not all of the mechanisms have been identified, explaining this correlation. For spirituality, however, the jury is still out. Until methodical problems are solved to operationalize spirituality rigorously and a corpus of empirical research on spirituality and health grows, the claims of positive health effects of spirituality are tenuous. Thus, adult spirituality may or may not effectively prevent dysfunction or promote health.

Also see: Religion and Spirituality: Adolescence; Religion and Spirituality: Childhood; Religion and Spirituality: Older Adulthood.

References

American Jewish Community. (1998). *American Jewish yearbook.* Philadelphia: Jowich Publication Society of America.

Arnold, D., & Schick, C. (1979). Counseling by clergy: A review of empirical research. *Journal of Pastoral Counseling, 14*, 76–101.

Batson, C.D. (1976). Religion as prosocial: Agent or double agent? *Journal for the Scientific Study of Religion, 15*, 29–45.

Batson, C.D., Schoenrade, P., & Ventis, W.L. (1993). *Religion and the individual.* New York: Oxford University Press.

Benson, H. (1997). *Timeless healing: The power of biology and belief.* New York: Simon & Schuster.

Byrd, R.C. (1988). Positive therapeutic effects of intercessory prayer in a coronary care unit population. *Southern Medical Journal, 81*, 826–829.

Feher, S., & Maly, R.C. (1999). Coping with breast cancer in later life: The role of religious faith. *Psycho-Oncology, 8*, 408–416.

Ferdinand, K.C. (1997). Lessons learned from the Healthy Heart Community Prevention Project in reaching the African American population. *Journal of Health Care for the Poor and Underserved, 8*, 366–371.

Ferraro, K.F., & Kelley-Moore, J.A. (2000). Religious consolation among men and women: Do health problems spur seeking? *Journal for the Scientific Study of Religion, 39*, 220–234.

Ferraro, K.F., & Koch, J.R. (1994). Religion and health among black and white adults: Examining social support and consolation. *Journal for the Scientific Study of Religion, 33*, 362–375.

Fitchett, G., Rybarczyk, B.D., & DeMarco, G.A. (1999). The role of religion in medical rehabilitation outcomes: A longitudinal study. *Rehabilitation Psychology, 44*, 333–353.

Gallagher, W. (1999). *Working on God.* New York: Random House.

Gallup Organization. (2001). *Religion in American.* Available: http://www.gallup.com/poll/indicators/indreligion.asp

George, L.K., Larson, D.B., Koenig, H.G., & McCullough, M.E. (2000). Spirituality and health: What we know, what we need to know. *Journal of Social and Clinical Psychology, 19*, 102–116.

Haight, W.L. (1998). "Gathering the spirit" at First Baptist Church: Spirituality as a protective factor in the lives of African American children. *Social Work, 43*, 213–221.

Idler, E.L. (1995). Religion, health, and nonphysical senses of self. *Social Forces, 74*, 683–704.

Idler, E.L., & Kasl, S.V. (1992) Religion, disability, depression, and the timing of death. *American Journal of Sociology, 97*, 226–238.

Johnson, B., Larson, D.B., & Pitts, T.C. (1997). Religious programs, institutional adjustment, and recidivism among former inmates in prison fellowship programs. *Justice Quarterly, 14*(1), 145–166.

King, M., Speck, P., & Thomas, A. (1999). The effect of spiritual beliefs on outcome from illness. *Social Science and Medicine, 48*, 1291–1299.

Kim, J., Heinemann, A.W., Bode, R.K., Sliwa, J., & King, R.B. (2000). Spirituality, quality of life, and functional recovery after medical rehabilitation. *Rehabilitation Psychology, 45*, 365–385.

Koenig, H.G. (1999). The healing power of faith: Science explores medicine's last great frontier. New York: Simon and Schuster.

Koenig, H.G., McCullough, M.E., & Larson, D. (2001). *Handbook of religion and health.* London: Oxford University Press.

Kohlberg, L. (1980). Stages of moral development as a basis for moral education. In B. Munsey (Ed.), *Moral development, moral education, and*

Kohlberg: Basic issues in philosophy, psychology, religion, and education (pp. 15–98). Birmingham, AL: Religious Education Press.

Kumanyika, S.K., & Charleston, J.B. (1992). Lose weight and win: A church-based weight loss program for blood pressure control among Black women. *Patient Education and Counseling, 19*, 19–32.

Larson, D.B., Swyers, J.P., & McCullough, M.E. (1997). *Scientific research on spirituality and health: A consensus report*. Rockville, MD: National Institute for Healthcare Research.

Levin, J.S. (1994). Religion and health: Is there a relationship, is it valid, and is it causal? *Social Science and Medicine, 38*, 1475–1482.

Matthews, D. (2000, February). *Interim report on a study of distance and in-person prayer*. Paper Presented at the Advisory Board Meeting of the John Templeton Foundation.

McCullough, M.E., Hoyt, W.T., Larson, D.B., Koenig, H.G., & Thoresen, C. (2000). Religious involvement and mortality: A meta-analytic review. *Health Psychology, 19*, 211–222.

Miller, W.R. (1998). Researching the spiritual dimensions of alcohol and other drug problems. *Addictions, 93*, 979–990.

Miller, W.R., & Bennett, M.E. (1997). Alcohol/drug problems. In D.B. Larson, J.P. Swyers, & M.E. McCullough (Eds.), *Scientific research on spirituality and health: A consensus report* (pp. 55–67). National Institute for Healthcare Research. Rockville, MD: Templeton Foundation Press.

Nouwen, H. (1999). In W. Greer (Ed.), *The only necessary thing: Leading a prayerful life*. New York: Crossroads.

Paloutzian, R.F. (1996). *Invitation to the psychology of religion*. Boston: Allyn & Bacon.

Pargament, K.I. (1997). *The psychology of religion and coping: Theory, research, practice*. New York: Guilford Publications.

Pargament, K.I., Zinnbauer, B.J., Scott, A.B., Butter, E.M., Zerowin, J., & Stanik, P. (1998). Red flags and religious coping: Identifying some religious warning signs among people in crisis. *Journal of Clinical Psychology, 54*, 77–89.

Pressman, P., Lyons, J.S., Larson, D., & Strain, J.J. (1990). Religious belief, depression, and ambulation status in elderly women with broken hips. *American Journal of Psychiatry, 147*, 758–760.

Richards, P.S., & Bergin, A.E. (1997). *A spiritual strategy for counseling and psychotherapy*. Washington, DC: American Psychological Association.

Richards, P.S., & Bergin, A.E. (Eds.). (2000). *Handbook of psychotherapy and religious diversity*. Washington, DC: American Psychological Association.

Ripley, J.S., & Worthington, E.L., Jr. (1998). What the journals reveal about Christian marital counseling: An inadequate (but emerging) scientific base. *Marriage and Family: A Christian Journal, 1*, 375–396.

Sinnott, J.D. (1998). *The development of logic in adulthood: Post-formal thought and its applications*. New York: Plenum.

Smith, E.D. (1992). Hypertension management with church-based education: A pilot study. *Journal of the National Black Nurses Association, 6*, 19–28.

Smith, E.D., Merritt, S.L., & Patel, M.K. (1997). Church-based education: An outreach program for African Americans with hypertension. *Ethnic Health, 2*, 243–253.

Stanley, S.M., Markman, H.J., Prado, L.M., Olmos-Gallo, P.A., Tonelli, L., St. Peters, M., Leber, B.D., Bobulinski, M., Cordova, A., & Whitton, S. (2001). Community based premarital prevention: Clergy and lay leaders on the front lines. *Family Relations, 50*, 67–76.

Strayhorn, J.M., Weidman, C.S., & Larson, D.B. (1990). A measure of religiousness, and its relation to parent and child mental health variables. *Journal of Community Psychology, 18*, 34–43.

Taylor, S.E, Kemeny, M.E., Reed, G.M., Bower, J.E., & Gruenewald, T.L. (2000). Psychological resources, positive illusions, and health. *American Psychologist, 55*, 99–109.

Underhill, E. (1961). *Mysticism: A study in the nature and development of man's spiritual consciousness*. New York: Dutton.

Ventis, W.L. (1995). The relationship between religion and mental health. *Journal of Social Issues, 51*, 33–48.

Werner, E.E. (1993). Risk, resilience, and recovery: Perspectives from the Kauai longitudinal study. *Development and Psychopathology, 5*, 503–515.

Wilber, K. (2000). *Integral psychology: Consciousness, spirit, psychology, therapy*. Boston: Shambhala.

Worthington, E.L., Jr. (1986). Religious counseling: A review of empirical research. *Journal of Counseling and Development, 64*, 421–431.

Worthington, E.L., Jr., Kurusu, T., McCullough, M.E., & Sandage, S. (1996). Empirical research on religion and psychotherapeutic processes and outcomes: A 10-year review and research prospectus. *Psychological Bulletin, 199*, 448–487.

Worthington, E.L., Jr., & Sandage, S.J. (2002). Religion and spirituality: Therapist consultations and responsiveness to patients. In J.C. Norcross (Ed.), *Psychotherapy relationships that work* (pp. 383–399). New York: Oxford University Press.

Religion and Spirituality, Older Adulthood

Nathaniel G. Wade, Everett L. Worthington, Jr., and Wendy L. Kliewer

INTRODUCTION AND DEFINITIONS

Any exploration of religion and spirituality must begin with explicit definitions of concepts. While existing definitions span a broad spectrum, we have chosen the following: *Religion* is the individual and corporate search for the sacred that has been formalized into an institution. *Spirituality* is the search for the sacred, which may or may not exist within an institution.

SCOPE

Prevalence

To our knowledge, no prevalence data specifically on spirituality in older adults exists. Rather, one must extrapolate from the data available on the prevalence of religious experience. This would seem justified based on findings by Zinnbauer et al. (1997). In a survey of 346 adults in the United States, Zinnbauer et al. (1997) found that a majority of people report themselves as both religious and spiritual. Few of their participants reported being spiritual but not religious.

This is consistent with Marty's estimates that 14 percent of US adults consider themselves as spiritual but not traditionally religious (as reported in Koenig, McCullough, & Larson, 2001). Furthermore, the elderly are more likely to have retained connections to traditional Western religion because most elderly were not greatly influenced by Eastern religions, which entered US culture in force in the 1960s. For the elderly, the 1960s was after their adolescence and early adulthood, when people are most open to new religious ideas. This cohort effect does not preclude the elderly from being attracted to Eastern religions, but it makes the likelihood less. On the other side of the equation, immigration of elderly Asians to the United States has increased the prevalence of Buddhists, Hindus, and Asian religions.

With so much overlap between religious and spiritual definitions and experiences, an analysis of the health-related correlates, causes, and consequences of spirituality in older adults would not be complete without including studies investigating religious variables as well. As a note of caution, among the very elderly, physical limitations may reduce their ability to attend religious services. Thus, some nonattenders might still be quite religious (and spiritual). In a large-scale national survey of older adults in the United States, 75 percent of respondents reported that "religion is very important to them" (Koenig, 1995, p. 12). Further, 50 percent of the older adults said they attend religious services at least once a week, and approximately 40 percent said they engage in personal prayer apart from mealtimes several times per week.

A similar survey explored the religious practices and coping strategies of 178 Latino older adults in the southwest United States (Maldonado, 1995). Of the respondents, 75 percent reported weekly attendance at some religious service, although 80 percent had attended some service the week of the survey. Of this group, only 3 percent reported that they were not at all religious. The older adults reported using their religion in times of difficulty. Seventy-six percent of men and 96 percent of women indicated that they "turn to prayer" when they feel stress or sadness (Maldonado, 1995, p. 127).

Koenig (1995) also reported that, when asked specifically whether they use religion to cope with adversity, approximately 90 percent of elderly people responded positively. To avoid response biases that might arise from being asked directly about whether people use religious coping, other interviewers have asked elderly adults simply how they cope with life's difficulties. In a study of 339 elderly men admitted to a VA medical center, 24 percent spontaneously reported using religion to cope (Koenig, 1995). In a sample of 100 White older adults, 45 percent reported some form of religious coping (Koenig, 1995).

Religion appears to be a common and important aspect of the lives of older adults. Not only do a large portion of elderly individuals engage in religious practices (such as attending religious services and praying), but they also turn to their religion as a source of strength and support during times of difficulty. The prevalence and quality of older-adult spirituality can only be inferred from the data on religious experience and practice. However, it seems reasonable to expect that most older adults consider themselves spiritual and value their spirituality as an important part of their lives.

THEORIES

In a review of some of the influential theories related to spiritual development of older adults, Vogel (1995) described and compared the theories of Levinson, Erikson, and Fowler. Levinson and Erikson both explained aspects of human development in terms of stages. When adults enter the stage that Levinson called the middle-adult era, they are faced with what Erikson termed the challenge of *generativity versus stagnation*. In this stage, adults must negotiate such transitions as valuing wisdom versus physical power, socializing versus sexualizing human relationships, and maintaining mental flexibility versus rigidity (Vogel, 1995). The overall task of this stage according to Erikson relates to engaging in the future of younger generations by providing guidance, support, and help (i.e., generativity) rather than disengaging from relationships, focusing on self, and failing to pass on some form of legacy (i.e., stagnation). The psychological tasks associated with this stage are similar to aspects of spirituality, such as finding meaning outside the self, engaging in community with others, and valuing wisdom and spiritual truth over the physical or material aspects of life (Vogel, 1995).

The next, and last, stage described by Levinson, the late-adult era, corresponds with Erikson's final stage of human development—the conflict between *integrity and despair*. Erikson hypothesized that older adults face the struggle to find worth and meaning in their lives, to *integrate* all the aspects and experiences of their lives, and to find some peace. Failure to integrate life experiences results in despair, which often develops from guilt and regret for life choices, a desire to hold onto the past and deny the present, or the inability to find worth and meaning in life. These are not only emotional or psychological in nature but are related to spiritual tasks.

Fowler (1981, 1986) suggests seven stages of faith development (see earlier entries). In particular, four are most pertinent to the elderly. First, in synthetic-conventional faith, Stage 3 adults reflect the faith system of their community as a means for connecting with a higher power. Stage 3 is marked by the ability to take another's perspective and to view oneself from outside the self. This leads to the ability to seek values and beliefs that are acceptable to important significant others as a means of structuring life and gaining approval (Fowler, 1986). In the stage of individuative-reflective faith, Stage 4, adults are aware of their own religious identity within a particular ideology, begin to embrace a faith system (or lack of one) that they choose, and tend to "demythologize" the symbols and myths of religious faith. While people in Stage 4 often have difficulty tolerating ambiguity and complexity, they have achieved a level of religious or spiritual individuation.

In the next stage of faith development, conjunctive faith, Stage 5, adults have developed the capacity to accept their own ideas and beliefs without demanding that others believe as they do. These adults are capable of experiencing deeper meanings of their faith communities while simultaneously understanding the limitations of those meanings. With maturity in faith come the abilities to accept ambiguity without giving up understanding, embrace complexity while living a simple faith, and experience autonomy within the context of a community (Fowler, 1981, 1986). In the final stage, universalizing faith, Stage 6, adults move beyond the self as the source for faith, knowledge, and values. "A radical process of decentration from the self as the epistemological and valuational reference point for construing the world" is completed in this stage (Fowler, 1986, p. 31). Not seeing the self as one's center frees the individual to find her or his source of love and value in a power beyond the self.

Stages of adult development, such as Levinson's and Erikson's theories of psychosocial development, focus primarily on ego integration, which might be described as finding an integrated context for the self. This can also be said of Fowler's theory with the possible exception of his final stage, universalizing faith. This ego-centric focus has been criticized as missing the crucial nature of spiritual development in the elderly (Tornstam, 1994). Tornstam (1994) proposed that *transcendence* rather than integration is the primary and optimal goal of older adult spirituality. Transcendence (or "gero-transcendence") is defined as "a shift in meta-perspective, from a materialistic and rational vision to a more cosmic and transcendent one..." (Tornstam, 1994, p. 203). This theory suggests that the core of spiritual development in older adults is redefining themselves, others, and the world in less materialistic and more cosmic or universal terms than in earlier stages. Transcendence is hypothesized to be a natural part of aging, although the cultural context in which older adults live may influence the expression of the transcendence.

This perspective of transcendence versus ego integration is supported and refined by Wilber's (2000) analysis and review of cross-cultural stage theories of spiritual development (see adult entry). Wilber claims that one's definition of "ego" is paramount to understanding whether the stages are accurately describing older adult development. He claims

that if "ego" means "an exclusive identification with the personal self...," then ego is definitely not strengthened or integrated during the final stages of adult spirituality (p. 91). However, if by ego one means the aspect of self that relates to the external world, is capable of witnessing the self, or integrates aspects of life and experience, then ego is retained and often strengthened in advanced stages of development.

STRATEGIES: OVERVIEW

Self-Initiated Strategies

Research has established that many people (including the elderly) claim to use religion and spirituality as resources for preventing numerous difficulties and for promoting mental and physical health during life's most difficult moments (Idler, 1995; Pargament, Smith, Koenig, & Perez, 1998; for reviews see George, Larson, Koenig, & McCullough, 2000; Pargament, 1997). If we can judge by mere usage, people must at least believe that religious coping works to mitigate adversity or reactions to it. Older adults might utilize religious practice for coping more than any other age group (for reviews see Koenig, 1994; Paloutzian, 1996). For example, in a national survey of 883 Black and 1,667 White adults, age was used to predict the use of personal spirituality during times of difficulty (Ferraro & Koch, 1994). Older age was associated with greater use of spiritual comfort in handling adversity, even after controlling for other factors such as ethnicity, SES, religious affiliation, and geographic location.

Although many older people claim to utilize both religion and spirituality for dealing with difficulty, we might question whether such efforts are effective. Reviews of the empirical studies of religious and spiritual variables over the last decade have generally concluded that these variables are associated with positive physical health and well-being in adults of all ages (George et al., 2000; Koenig et al., 2001) and specifically in older adults (Koenig, 1994, 1995). For example, in his review of the health correlates of religion, Koenig (1995) identified hypertension and heart disease as two conditions that are less frequent among elderly people who are highly religious service attenders. In contrast, the incidence and recovery from cancer does *not* seem to be associated with religious beliefs or behaviors (Koenig, 1995). Finally, studies of longevity and mortality have suggested relationships of each to religion. A recent meta-analysis by McCullough, Hoyt, Larson, Koenig, and Thoresen (2000) found that across the 42 samples that they reviewed, people who were more religiously involved were more likely to be alive at follow-up than people who were not religiously involved. This relationship was observed even after controlling for a host of other related variables. As in other entries on religion and spirituality such evidence is correlational, not causal.

The relationship between religious variables and mental health outcomes has been found to be positive for all-aged adults (Bergin, 1983; Worthington, Kurusu, McCullough, & Sandage, 1996) and specifically older adults (Koenig, 1994, 1995). In particular, religious attendance and involvement predicts fewer anxiety disorders, less depression, less incidence of substance-use disorders, less fear of death, and less suicide (Koenig et al., 2001).

Two recent studies investigated the effect of spirituality on coping with difficulty. Feher and Maly (1999) examined the relationship between spirituality and coping with illness in 33 elderly women who had been recently diagnosed with breast cancer. Analysis of qualitative interviews suggested that these women coped with their cancer by using their religious and spiritual beliefs to marshal emotional and social support needed to deal with the difficulty of the diagnosis and to help them find meaning in their experience. The authors concluded further that the ability to find meaning appeared to reduce the anxiety and stress of the diagnosis and was associated with better subjective well-being.

Gamino, Sewell, and Easterling (2000) investigated the role of spirituality in dealing with the loss of a loved one in 85 adults referred from a psychiatric outpatient clinic, self-help grief support groups, and a hospital chaplain service. Intrinsic spirituality (Kass, Friedman, Leserman, Zuttermeister, & Benson, 1991) was one of the four significant factors that predicted personal growth as an outcome of the bereavement. Adults who exhibited greater intrinsic spirituality were found to experience more personal growth after the death of a loved one than did adults who exhibited less intrinsic spirituality. This may have particular relevance for older adults because they often must cope with the multiple losses through death of loved ones that often occur at advanced ages.

STRATEGIES THAT WORK

Secular Therapies Accommodated to Religious or Spiritual People

Professionally administered interventions that include spiritual and religious components have received some notable attention recently. For example, recent books have described spiritual or religious interventions in medical (King, 2000) and psychological (Richards & Bergin, 2000) contexts. Most "spiritual" or "religious" interventions to date are simply secular therapies that include a few spiritual

exercises or use some limited religious language. These types of interventions use spiritual or religious content to make the recipients more comfortable with treatment or to connect with their religious or spiritual values. For practitioners, sensitivity toward religious diversity is important, and efforts are being made to inform treatment providers in both medicine and psychology of this need (Richards & Bergin, 2000). It is important that practitioners not attempt to design interventions that mix religions or mix religion with secular (or humanistic) spirituality. As a result the bulk of these interventions are framed as a way to be sensitive to *a particular* religious heritage or background the way one would be sensitive to particular ethnicity or gender issues. To use an analogy, an ethnically sensitive practitioner would not design a group that mixed African American and Asian American traditions. Similarly, a religiously sensitive practitioner would not mix Jewish and Buddhist or Christian and "new age" interventions. Spiritual and religious interventions are often not used "across the board" as a general intervention strategy. Both religious and nonreligious people would probably consider this inappropriate.

There are some exceptions to this general trend of religiously "spinning" secular interventions. In a review of religious and spiritual interventions, Thoresen, Worthington, Swyers, Larson, McCullough, and Miller (1997) identified a list of nine types of largely religious or spiritual interventions, including: prayer, meditation, religious bibliotherapy, 12-step fellowships, ritual, forgiveness, willingness and letting go, cognitive–behavioral therapies incorporating spiritual themes, and religious or spiritual dance. Of these, several stand alone as a means of intervention that have received adequate empirical attention and utilize spiritual or religious components in more than a perfunctory manner. These include: meditation and 12-step fellowships, which are considered to have accumulated enough empirical study to say that they "work." Importantly, each religious tradition might employ meditation, yet it would probably be a mistake to teach Buddhist meditation to Christians or to Hindus. Each of these interventions may be specifically helpful to older adults in helping them handle the challenges particular to their age group.

Meditation is a form of concentrated relaxation that includes reducing activity, focusing mental activity, and freeing the mind from distraction. It has been a part of many different religious traditions for thousands of years. Buddhists have used meditation as a method for clearing the mind and focusing on that which is thought to be real. Hindus have used meditation to achieve high levels of religious experience and aim to empty the mind. Christians have utilized meditation to achieve higher levels of communion with God and as a means of focusing on God or Jesus.

Over the last several decades, meditation in some form has been incorporated into treatments for mental illnesses, such as anxiety and depression, and for physical illnesses, such as recovery from cardiac surgery and hypertension. Programs that are intended to promote mental and physical health, such as the transcendental mediation movement, have also used meditation. The application of meditation as an intervention is a form of spiritual practice that has been successfully employed to prevent illness and promote health (Thoresen et al., 1997).

Meditation (consistent with one's religious or spiritual tradition) may be an important intervention for the elderly. Meditation in the treatment of physical difficulties has been identified as a useful adjunct to traditional treatments, particularly with chronic illnesses (Thoresen et al., 1997). Because older people in western cultures are living longer due to improved healthcare, they are also experiencing a rise in chronic health conditions (Koenig, 1994). Thus, meditation might be particularly relevant for them in coping with these difficulties.

Twelve-Step Fellowships

Another intervention that utilizes spirituality is the 12-step fellowships. Starting with Alcoholics Anonymous in the middle of the last century and growing to millions of members and dozens of offshoot organizations (e.g., Narcotics Anonymous, Over-Eaters Anonymous), 12-step fellowships are important sources of support and treatment to people suffering from addictions. At the core of the interventions are the 12 Steps, which guide the progress that members make through the fellowship. The 12 Steps are spiritual. For example, after stating in the first step their "powerlessness" over their addiction and life, members state that they "came to believe that a power greater than [them]selves could restore [them] to sanity" (Alcoholics Anonymous, 1952). Themes of powerlessness, transformation, faith, and community, in short, spiritual themes, pervade the 12-step fellowships.

Twelve-step fellowships have a place in elderly communities. Koenig (1994) reports that 1 in 10 older adults might have some form of substance abuse problem, most who abuse misuse alcohol. Their abuse of alcohol might be the result of a long-standing problem as often as a result of dealing with the challenges of growing old (Koenig, 1994, 1995). Twelve-step fellowships might also play a generative role in the lives of older adults. Older members of these fellowships are often given special status as sponsors of newer members and leaders of local meetings. As people within the fellowships age, they might find a place where they can give back to others. Miller (1998) has found that evidence exists supporting the effectiveness of 12-step approaches for those who come to agree with its philosophy.

STRATEGIES THAT MIGHT WORK

Promotion of Forgiveness

Another type of intervention that incorporates spiritual principles in general is the promotion of forgiveness. There is a growing literature on interventions that are specifically aimed at helping people overcome the bitterness, hurt, and sadness of interpersonal offenses. The majority of these interventions are effective in helping people forgive (see Worthington, Kurusu, Collins, Berry, Ripley, & Baier, 2000, for a meta-analysis).

Paradoxically, forgiveness has been valued by all of the major religious traditions (Dorff, 1998; Marty, 1998; Rye et al., 2000), yet only one of the interventions evaluated scientifically to date has been tailored to a religious clientele (Rye & Pargament, 2002). Despite its conceptual association with religions, especially Christianity, forgiveness has broad acceptability to many nonreligious people.

Forgiveness interventions consistently utilize spiritual concepts and practices in order to assist people in the healing process. For example, one well-studied intervention encourages people who have been hurt by another to (a) gain empathy for their offenders, (b) increase their humility and gratitude by recalling times they have hurt others, and (c) contemplate the possibility of giving an altruistic gift of forgiveness (i.e., Pyramid Model to REACH forgiveness) (Worthington, 2001). Each of these interventions is reconcilable with spirituality. Increasing empathy, humility, and gratitude, and contemplating the benefits of an altruistic act are compatible with the kinds of actions, emotions, and thoughts often accompanying a healthy spirituality. Enright and Fitzgibbons (2000) summarize research on Enright's intervention, which promotes behavioral, cognitive, and affective aspects of forgiveness. Enright's and Worthington's model—indeed, interventions by McCullough, Worthington, and Rachal (1997), DiBlasio (1998), Luskin and Thoresen (1998), and Rye and Pargament (in press)—share many more similarities than differences. Worthington et al. (2000) plotted a dose–effect curve (i.e., graph relating time spent forgiving to a standardized measure of forgiveness) for 19 experimental conditions and found a correlation of 0.75 irrespective of whose intervention was used. McCullough, Worthington, & Rachal (1997) have suggested that a victim's experience of empathy for the transgression is the key element in whether forgiveness takes place.

How might interventions that promote forgiveness apply specifically to older adults? One study investigated this question by examining the effectiveness of a general forgiveness intervention with 24 elderly women who were all over 65 years of age (Hebl & Enright, 1993). Through an 8-week intervention, women in the forgiveness group were more successful at dealing with past hurts and offenses than were their counterparts in the control group. By resolving past hurts, some of these women were able to restore broken relationships or move on from a painful experience in the past. Hebl and Enright's study has important implications for the application of forgiveness interventions for older adults. The gero-transcendence model described above focused on the change of perspective that can occur in the elderly. Forgiveness interventions might be one method through which this change could be fostered. To the degree that forgiveness enables people to overcome the past, move beyond hurtful relationships and events, and embrace a broader and more life-affirming attitude, forgiveness interventions would be appropriate and important for helping some older adults put away the past and grow spiritually.

STRATEGIES THAT DO NOT WORK

Few preventive strategies have been scientifically investigated with regard to promoting health and preventing dysfunction among older adults. Religion and spirituality might indeed affect anyone in ways that produce negative mental health outcomes (e.g., prejudice in some groups, suspicion, anxiety, hyper-scrupulosity) and physical health outcomes (e.g., refusal of medical treatment, unwillingness to take reasonable health precautions).

SYNTHESIS

To understand the role of spirituality in an individual's life, one must distinguish between spirituality as the *cause* and as the *consequence* of an intervention or of other factors naturally occurring in life. Most research on spirituality focuses on it as a cause that prescribes processes by which other outcomes might occur.

In previous entries, we have discussed the correlational versus causal nature of the relationship between religion and spirituality and health. We have taken several lines of argument. In this final entry, we seek to summarize the possibilities in a model.

Much of the intervention research in particular attempts to promote increased religious commitment and/or spirituality in hopes that this will produce one or more beneficial outcome (e.g., better mental or physical health). This is seen in the meditation, 12-step fellowships, and forgiveness interventions. They attempt to facilitate aspects of spirituality (though not necessarily religious spirituality) to encourage abstinence and recovery, healing and forgiveness, or peaceful emotional states. The implied reasoning is that increased spirituality (or at least aspects of it) will produce a beneficial effect upon some biological (e.g., reduced heart rate), psychological (e.g., reduced anxiety or depression), or social factor (e.g., improved family relationships), thus leading to better mental or physical health (or both).

This relationship between spirituality (as cause) and other factors is represented in path A in Figure 1. Religious or spiritually tailored interventions are hypothesized to have

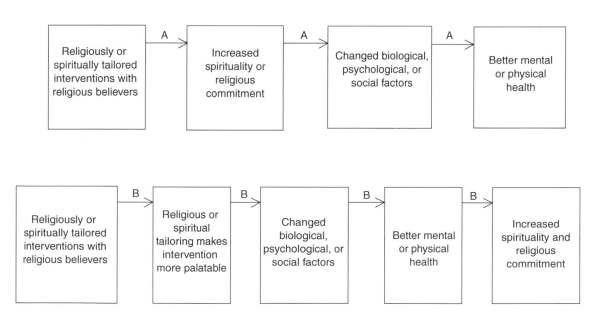

Figure 1. Causal Mechanism Between Spirituality and other Outcomes. A and B are Paths Indicating Hypothesized Causal Direction.

a direct and causal effect on a variety of factors. In a review of the research on spirituality and health, George et al. (2000) describe three potential causal mechanisms. First, they suggest that greater spirituality may cause people to avoid specific negative health behaviors (e.g., smoking) that are associated with disease and other negative outcomes. This might be particularly important to older adults, since the negative effects of bad health behaviors are not typically experienced until later life. In a longitudinal study of 3,968 older adults, attendance at religious service and private religious behaviors (such as prayer) were negatively related to smoking (Koenig, George, Cohen, Hays, Larson, & Blazer, 1998).

The second causal mechanism (see Figure 1, path A) that George et al. (2000) hypothesized was that spirituality might increase social support, which then would positively influence biological, psychological, and social factors. Social support has been consistently identified in the research as a positive force that helps ameliorate and mitigate the effects of mental and physical health problems (for reviews see George et al., 2000; Uchino, Uno, & Holt-Lunstad, 1999).

Finally, spirituality is expected to have a salutatory effect on health outcomes by providing people with a sense of meaning or coherence to their lives. We have defined spirituality as a search for the sacred. Often what drives that search is the desire for meaning in life, to find connection with someone or something that is greater than the self. Some have even argued that the search for meaning is in fact more important and helpful for individuals than the actual outcome of the search (Marrone, 1999). George et al. (2000) indicated that this mechanism appeared to account for the most variance in positive health outcomes. Facilitating meaning and coherence might also positively affect other areas of life such as mental health, well-being, relationships with significant others, work performance, and cognitive functioning. The potential correlates among spirituality, meaning or coherence, and factors other than health have yet to be examined. Spirituality appears to be implicated in several causal mechanisms that have beneficial effects on health, and likely many other psychological and social factors.

Further, interventions may also play a critical role in the causal mechanism between spirituality and other outcomes (see Figure 1, path A). For example, the interventions discussed above—meditation, 12-step, and forgiveness interventions—might all facilitate spirituality, which might have a positive effect upon biological, psychological, or social factors. At various ages throughout the life cycle, religiously or spiritually tailored interventions might affect spirituality directly. For example, comforting children who are undergoing a health trauma, encouraging adolescents to explore their spirituality, providing adolescents with peer-based religious education, using religiously tailored peer

communities for adolescent delinquents or drug or alcohol abusers, and providing adults with religious education or counseling are all examples of interventions that appear primarily to affect religion or spirituality and produce subsequent changes in mental or physical health through biological, psychological, or social mechanisms.

The second pathway is represented by path B in Figure 1. Theories described above indicate that spirituality *develops* or changes over time, becoming more mature and potentially more useful for the individual. Path B (Figure 1) indicates that religiously or spiritually tailored interventions can be made more palatable by framing them in religious terminology. Biological, psychological, and social effects can result from the intervention. Because the intervention was framed as religious, the positive changes in mental and physical health can also lead to changes in religiosity or spirituality. That is, when a person attributes change to his or her religion, the person's religious attributions are strengthened and the person's faith might be strengthened (as well as the person's personal sense of spirituality). Thus, in path B (Figure 1) we are stressing that explicitly framing an intervention as religious or spiritual might have the effect of strengthening a person's spirituality or religious faith (if positive health and mental health outcomes are experienced) or weakening the person's spirituality or religious faith (if negative health or mental health outcomes are experienced).

Some evidence exists for the causal mechanisms of path B (Figure 1)—that is, events can cause people to become more religious or spiritual. One theory—the consolation hypothesis—indicates that as people experience negative life events, they tend to turn more to spiritual (and religious) sources for help and support (Fitchett, Rybarczyk, & DeMarco, 1999; Idler, 1995). Religious interventions and religion itself become more attractive. People thus become more religious. Empirical evidence supports this. For example, in a national survey of 3,617 adults, consolation (defined as seeking spiritual support for difficulties in life) was negatively related to health status (Ferraro & Kelley-Moore, 2000). Greater depression and more chronic conditions were related to greater consolation.

Biological (e.g., health problems), psychological (e.g., emotional difficulty), or social factors (e.g., struggling marriage) might therefore cause one's spirituality to become more intense (Figure 1, path B). In addition, life events (whether positive or negative) might spur some (previously nonspiritual) people to investigate spiritual beliefs and practices (Frankl, 1963).

On the other hand, life experiences might also negatively affect one's spirituality. In response to trauma, difficulty, or unmet needs some might respond with negative thoughts and emotions that derail the search for the sacred. Recent literature has begun to investigate the reactions to negative life events that lead to reduced spirituality. One of the first studies of this type investigated the spiritual reactions to negative life events in two samples, 49 Roman Catholic adults and 196 college students all who had experienced some negative life event within the previous two years (Pargament, Zinnbauer, Scott, Butter, Zerowin, & Stanik, 1998). Both experiencing anger at God and feeling religious doubts as a result of the negative event were associated with less self-esteem, lower problem solving, more anxiety, and poorer general health in both samples.

Finally, interventions might influence and change the events in people's lives or the way that they experience those events (path B in Figure 1). Thus interventions could have a causal impact on spirituality. For example, a medical intervention might treat a physical illness, by providing a hip replacement for an elderly female, allowing her more energy, mobility, and emotional and mental strength to be invested in her religious or spiritual development. A psychological intervention might help alleviate an older man's debilitating depression after the loss of his wife, enabling him to return to social support and activities that bolster his spirituality. A social intervention might provide safe housing to low-income retired people, freeing them from the immediate concern of shelter and allowing time and energy for religious or spiritual activities, growth, and investment.

In the four entries we have written, we suggested numerous interventions that have empirical evidence suggesting that they might (a) be palatable because they are religiously framed, (b) affect mental or spiritual health, and (c) as a result affect a person's spirituality and religiosity. Parenting interventions for children, religious peer groups for adolescents, religiously tailored counseling, community-based health programs, and marriage interventions are some examples.

For many, spirituality is a critical aspect of growing old. Not only does the development of spirituality continue through old age, but spirituality is often used to cope with the difficulties and trials of aging. Interventions to promote spirituality and assist older adults are existent, but are under-utilized and under-investigated. With religious and spiritual experience so prevalent among older adults, these limitations are almost tragic. The spirituality of older adults is a mother lode of resources awaiting research and intervention strategies. However, part of realizing this resource is understanding the recursive nature between interventions, spirituality, and other factors. Spirituality might be utilized to promote good outcomes, but it is likely to be shaped and changed in the process. Attending to the potential causes as well as consequences of spirituality is crucial for both researchers and intervention providers.

Also see: Religion and Spirituality: Adolescence; Religion and Spirituality: Childhood; Religion and Spirituality: Adulthood.

References

Alcoholics Anonymous. (1952). *Twelve steps and twelve traditions.* New York: Alcoholics Anonymous World Series.

Bergin, A.E. (1983). Religiosity and mental health: A re-evaluation and meta-analysis. *Professional Psychology: Research and Practice, 14,* 170–184.

DiBlasio, F.A. (1998). The use of decision-based forgiveness intervention within intergenerational family therapy. *Journal of Family Therapy, 20,* 77–94.

Dorff, E.N. (1998). The elements of forgiveness: A Jewish approach. In E.L. Worthington, Jr. (Ed.), *Dimensions of forgiveness: Psychological research and theological perspectives* (pp. 29–55). Philadelphia: Templeton Foundation Press.

Enright, R.D., & Fitzgibbons, R.P. (2000). *Helping clients forgive: An empirical guide for resolving anger and restoring hope.* Washington, DC: American Psychological Association Press.

Feher, S., & Maly, R.C. (1999). Coping with breast cancer in later life: The role of religious faith. *Psycho-Oncology, 8,* 408–416.

Ferraro, K.F., & Kelley-Moore, J.A. (2000). Religious consolation among men and women: Do health problems spur seeking? *Journal for the Scientific Study of Religion, 39,* 220–234.

Ferraro, K.F., & Koch, J.R. (1994). Religion and health among Black and White adults: Examining social support and consolation. *Journal for the Scientific Study of Religion, 33,* 362–375.

Fitchett, G., Rybarczyk, B.D., & DeMarco, G.A. (1999). The role of religion in medical rehabilitation outcomes: A longitudinal study. *Rehabilitation Psychology, 44,* 333–353.

Fowler, J.W. (1981). *Stages of faith: The psychology of human development and christian faith.* San Francisco: Harper & Row.

Fowler, J.W. (1986). Faith and the structuring of meaning. In C. Dykstra & S. Parks (Eds.), *Faith development and Fowler* (pp. 15–42). Birmingham, AL: Religious Education Press.

Frankl, V.E. (1963). *Man's search for meaning.* New York: Pocket Books.

Gamino, L.A., Sewell, K.W., & Easterling, L.W. (2000). Scott and White Grief Study—Phase 2: Toward an adaptive model of grief. *Death Studies, 24,* 633–660.

George, L.K., Larson, D.B., Koenig, H.G., & McCullough, M.E. (2000). Spirituality and health: What we know, what we need to know. *Journal of Social and Clinical Psychology, 19,* 102–116.

Grimes, R.L. (1999). Forum: American spirituality. *Religion and American Culture, 9,* 145–152.

Hebl, J.H., & Enright, R.D. (1993). Forgiveness as a psychotherapeutic goal with elderly females. *Psychotherapy, 30,* 658–667.

Idler, E.L. (1995). Religion, health, and nonphysical senses of self. *Social Forces, 74,* 683–704.

Kass, J.D., Friedman, R., Leserman, J., Zuttermeister, P.C., & Benson, H. (1991). Health outcomes and new measures of spiritual experience. *Journal for the Scientific Study of Religion, 30,* 203–211.

King, D.E. (2000). *Faith, spirituality, and medicine: Toward the making of the healing practitioner.* London: Haworth Pastoral Press.

Koenig, H.G. (1994). *Aging and God: Spiritual pathways to mental health in midlife and later years.* New York: Haworth Press.

Koenig, H.G. (1995). Religion and health in later life. In M.A. Kimble et al. (Eds.), *Aging, spirituality, and religion* (pp. 9–29). Minneapolis, MN: Fortress Press.

Koenig, H.G., George, L.K., Cohen, H.J., Hays, J.C., Larson, D.B., & Blazer, D.G. (1998). The relationship between religious activity and cigarette smoking in older adults. *Journals of Gerontology. Series A, Biological Sciences and Medical Sciences, 53A,* M426–M434.

Koenig, H.G., McCullough, M.E., & Larson, D. (2001). *Handbook of religion and health.* London: Oxford University Press.

Luskin, F., & Thoresen, C. (1998). *Effectiveness of forgiveness training on psychosocial factors in college-aged adults.* Unpublished manuscript, Stanford University, Stanford, CA.

Maldonado, D. (1995). Religion and persons of color. In M.A. Kimble et al. (Eds.), *Aging, spirituality, and religion* (pp. 119–128). Minneapolis, MN: Fortress Press.

Marrone, R. (1999). Dying, mourning, and spirituality: A psychological perspective. *Death Studies, 23,* 495–519.

Marty, M.E., (1998). The ethos of Christian forgiveness. In E.L. Worthington, Jr. (Ed.), Dimensions of forgiveness: Psychological research and theological speculations (pp. 9–28). Philadelphia: The Templeton Foundation Press.

McCullough, M.E., Worthington, E.L., Jr., & Rachal, K.C. (1997). Interpersonal forgiving in close relationships. *Journal of Personality and Social Psychology, 73,* 321–336.

McCullough, M.E., Hoyt, W.T., Larson, D.B., Koenig, H.G., & Thoresen, C. (2000). Religious involvement and mortality: A meta-analytic review. *Health Psychology, 19,* 211–222.

Miller, W.R. (1998). Researching the spiritual dimension of alcohol and other drug problems. *Addictions, 93,* 979–990.

Paloutzian, R. (1996). *Invitation to the psychology of religion* (2nd ed.). Boston: Allyn & Bacon.

Pargament, K.I. (1997). *The psychology of religion and coping: Theory, reseach, practice.* New York: Guilford Press.

Pargament, K.I., Smith, B.W., Koenig, H.G., & Perez, L. (1998). Patterns of positive and negative religious coping with major life stressors. *Journal of the Scientific Study of Religion, 37,* 710–724.

Pargament, K.I., Zinnbauer, B.J., Scott, A.B., Butter, E.M., Zerowin, J., & Stanik, P. (1998). Red flags and religious coping: Identifying some religious warning signs among people in crisis. *Journal of Clinical Psychology, 54,* 77–89.

Richards, P.S., & Bergin, A.E. (Eds.). (2000). *Handbook of psychotherapy and religious diversity.* Washington, DC: American Psychological Association.

Rye, M.S., Pargament, K.I., Ali, M.A., Beck, G.L., Dorff, E.N., Hallisey, C., Narayanan, V., & Williams, J.G. (2000). Religious perspectives on forgiveness. In M.C. McCullough, K.I. Pargament, & C.E. Thoresen (Eds.), Forgiveness: Theory, research, and practice (pp. 17–40). New York: Guilford.

Thoresen, C., Worthington, E.L., Jr., Swyers, J.P., Larson, D.B., McCullough, M.E., & Miller, W.R. (1997). Religious/spiritual interventions. In D.B. Larson, J.P. Swyers, & M.E. McCullough (Eds.), *Scientific research on spirituality and health: A consensus report* (pp. 105–128). Rockville, MD: National Institute for Healthcare Research.

Tornstam, L. (1994). Gero-transcendence: A theoretical and empirical exploration. In L.E. Thomas & S.A. Eisenhandler (Eds.), *Aging and the religious dimension* (pp. 203–225). Westport, CT: Auburn House.

Uchino, B.N., Uno, D., & Holt-Lunstad, J. (1999). Social support, physiological processes, and health. *Current Directions in Psychological Science, 8,* 145–148.

Vogel, L.J. (1995). Spiritual development in later life. In M.A. Kimble et al. (Eds.), *Aging, spirituality, and religion* (pp. 74–86). Minneapolis, MN: Fortress Press.

Wilber, K. (2000). *Integral psychology: Consciousness, spirit, psychology, therapy.* Boston: Shambhala.

Worthington, E.L., Jr. (2001). *Five steps to forgiving: The art and science of forgiving.* New York: Crown Books.

Worthington, E.L., Jr., Kurusu, T., Collins, W., Berry, J.W., Ripley, J.S., & Baier, S.N. (2000). Forgiveness usually takes time: A lesson learned by studying interventions to promote forgiveness. *Journal of Psychology and Theology, 28,* 3–20.

Worthington, E.L., Jr., Kurusu, T., McCullough, M.E., & Sandage, S. (1996). Empirical research on religion and psychotherapeutic processes and outcomes: A 10-year review and research prospectus. *Psychological Bulletin, 119,* 448–487.

Zinnbauer, B.J., Pargament, K.I., Cole, B., Rye, M.S., Butter, E.M., Belavich, T.G., Hipp, K.M., Scott, A.B., & Kadar, J.L. (1997). Religion and spirituality: Unfuzzying the fuzzy. *Journal for the Scientific Study of Religion, 36,* 549–564.

Resilience, Childhood

Peter A. Wyman, JoAnne Pedro-Carroll, and Emma L. Forbes-Jones

INTRODUCTION

Children vary in how they adapt to life adversity. Some children develop problems that impede their development over time. Other children demonstrate considerable competence despite adversities and, in some cases, appear strengthened by mastering challenges they face. The concept of resilience has been developed to describe positive adaptation among individuals in adverse environments. Most research undertaken to illuminate resilience has been conducted with children in the contexts of psychosocial adversity (e.g., family discord, poverty). Developmental changes throughout childhood provide ideal opportunities to observe differences in children's mastery of challenges. Resilience is an important component within the fields of prevention and psychological wellness (Cowen, 1994) for several reasons. Resilience focuses attention to processes that promote healthy outcomes among groups of children at high risk of problems, directs attention to empirical knowledge about protective factors, emphasizes building on strengths, and implies a focus on both promoting positive outcomes and decreasing problems (Luthar & Cicchetti, 2000). Knowledge from research on children's resilience has relevance for preventive interventions for children who face multiple, chronic adversities (e.g., poverty, ongoing violence) and for those who face specific adaptive challenges such as parental divorce and family restructuring after divorce (Pedro-Carroll, 2001).

Several decades ago terms such as "invulnerable" or "invincible" were used to describe competent children in highly unfavorable environments. Although those evocative terms vivified the fact that some children are competent in adversity, the concept of invulnerability was unsuitable for several reasons. Invulnerability implied a mistaken view that some children were immune to the effects of stressors or trauma and directed attention exclusively to protective attributes within children. Resilience is a more useful term because it better accounts for the wide continuum and changing nature of children's adjustment and the diversity of resources that promote coping and mastery.

DEFINITIONS

Based on present knowledge, *resilience* is best defined as a diverse set of processes that promote adaptive transactions between children and their environments in ways that reduce the potential negative effects of adversities on children (e.g., reduce distress, promote effective behavioral responses) and promote their competence. Distinctions among different types of adaptive processes should be recognized. For example, *protective processes* reduce the potential negative effects of stressors, as for example parenting practices that reduce children's exposure to conflict during divorce. *Protective-enhancing processes* help children to engage with adversities in ways that strengthen competence, such as developing cognitive skills for understanding problems, which also enhance academic success (Luthar, 1991). Another important distinction is revealed between groups of at-risk children who demonstrate ongoing positive development versus children who recover from maladjustment. Ongoing competence and recovery represent different developmental patterns and different resilience processes.

SCOPE

To what extent can children's problems be prevented by enhancing their resilience to life adversities? Children exposed to significant stressors are more likely to develop diagnosable problems (e.g., higher rates of mental health and substance use problems) and are less likely to attain positive developmental outcomes (e.g., competent educational outcomes) (Wolchik & Sandler, 1997). Many children face considerable challenges, including children whose family environments fail to provide average, expectable parenting experiences. For example, between 1.5–5 percent of children in the United States each year experience sexual abuse, physical abuse, or prolonged neglect (Emery & Laumann-Billings, 1998). Other life adversities are less catastrophic but can significantly affect children's well-being. For example, approximately 3.5 percent of children in the United States experience death of a parent during childhood (US Bureau of the Census, 1990). Some common adversities

also can initiate problems for children. Nearly one half of first marriages in the United States now end in divorce, and, as a result, about one million children are affected by marital dissolution each year (Cherlin, 1992).

Across nations, the nature and frequency of adverse conditions for children varies widely (Save the Children, 2001). For example, whereas about 1 in 1,000 children will have a parent die in childbirth or from pregnancy-related complications in developed nations (e.g., Europe, Japan, United States), that risk is about 1 in 48 for children living in developing nations. In many nations girls experience gender-specific adversities at high rates. For example, 17 percent of girls were married before age 10 in 1993 in parts of rural India, a practice that reduces educational opportunities. Moreover, each year an estimated 1–2 million girls and women are trafficked around the world for forced labor or for other exploitation.

Although it is imperative for societies to reduce the occurrence of assaults to children's development, it is also vital to promote practices and conditions that enhance well-being for children who experience adverse conditions. For example, by reducing the negative effects on children associated with divorce or death of a parent, a significant proportion of conduct problems or childhood depressions may be decreased. Although parental divorce only modestly increases a child's risk for developing conduct problems, so many children experience divorce that this stressor is estimated to account for up to 22 percent of classifiable conduct disorders. Death of a parent affects far fewer children but significantly increases the likelihood that a child will become depressed and therefore accounts for up to 19 percent of childhood depressions (Wolchik & Sandler, 1997).

Individual life adversities often have far-reaching, negative rippling effects across a child's social environment. For example, problems that bring a family into poverty (e.g., job loss, parent substance use) often affect children in multiple ways. Children of families below the poverty line are more likely to have a depressed parent, to witness violence, and to be exposed to environmental toxins (McLoyd, 1998). Children who experience multiple life adversities develop problems at much higher rates than children who experience only one or two life stressors (Rutter, 1979).

THEORIES AND RESEARCH

Decades ago, pioneering investigators of children at risk for serious psychiatric problems, children in families exposed to war or natural disasters, and children in poverty observed that many children expected to develop psychopathology did not (e.g., Elder, 1974). This recognition stimulated interest in studying mastery and competence as independent topics of inquiry. A second underpinning to risk and resilience research was found in studies of normal development and coping, such as the Berkeley Development Project, and the Harvard Preschool Project (White, 1978). The Harvard Preschool Project, for example, investigated the foundations of social competence in young children from diverse ethnic and socioeconomic status (SES) backgrounds and highlighted interwoven relationships between children's personal attributes, their experiences with primary caregivers, and their social development over time.

The pioneering study of a group of approximately 700 children on the Hawaiian Island of Kauai (Werner & Smith, 1982, 1992) served as a model for a first generation of researchers of resilience. The Kauai project was unique in several respects. The study group consisted of a large proportion of children born in a single year on this small Pacific island with low mobility rates and high rates of poverty and was ethnically diverse, including children of Hawaiian, Chinese, Anglo, and Filipino extraction. In addition, the study group was followed for over two decades.

One important observation from the Kauai study was that nearly 30 percent of the sample of children (204 of 698) had developed serious problems between birth and age 18. However, a group of 70 children demonstrated a contrary pattern. Although all 70 had experienced four or more life adversities (e.g., poverty, parent problems) before age 2, children in this group demonstrated competence in major adjustment domains at age 18. The study's core analyses compared those 70 children at several age periods with children who developed problems (Werner & Smith, 1982).

Although factors that distinguished children demonstrating resilience from those demonstrating maladjustment differed somewhat for boys and girls, three clusters of resources consistently predicted positive development: (1) Early childhood competencies such as social responsiveness, adaptability to change, and positive mood. Those early characteristics may be in part due to differences in temperament. (2) A family environment that provided a consistent, warm relationship to children. Few well-adapting children had extended separations from parents in early childhood. (3) A child's access to adult sources of interest and support outside the immediate family, including teachers, neighbors, and religious leaders.

The knowledge base about risk and resilience has been increased by studies of children in different environments (e.g., rural, urban settings) and by studies of differences in pathways toward competence (e.g., Luthar, 1991; Masten, Best, & Garmezy, 1990). Two principal domains of resources have been linked to positive outcomes for children in challenging environments.

(1) *Social system resources and resilience.* The extent to which family environments continue to satisfy children's emotional needs (e.g., for responsiveness, connection) and provide structure, despite disrupting and challenging conditions, is an important factor accounting for children's positive development (Masten & Coatsworth, 1998; Wyman, Cowen, Work, Hoyt-Meyers, Magnus, & Fagen, 1999). This conclusion is based on studies of children exposed to a range of problems, including financial hardship and parent dysfunction. Parenting responsiveness and continuity promote in children a foundation of self-regulating behavior (e.g., the ability to manage feelings effectively and control behavior) in ways that better equip them to manage subsequent life stressors and challenges to development (Egeland, Carlson, & Sroufe, 1993). Parenting competence also reduces the escalation of ongoing stressful conditions and can prevent new stressors from occurring in children's lives (Gest, Neeman, Hubbard, Masten, & Tellegen, 1993).

During middle childhood and adolescence, children interact in increasingly broader social contexts (e.g., schools, peer groups) that also provide them with opportunities for enhanced adaptation, including new relationships and roles for experiencing competence (e.g., through a job or structured activity). These new opportunities, or "turning points," can stimulate resilience for many youths. For example, studies by investigators in Great Britain showed that many at-risk youths from inner-city neighborhoods and from institutions for orphan children improved in conduct and in overall functioning if they formed a relationship with a prosocially oriented partner in young adulthood (Quinton, Pickles, Maughan, & Rutter, 1993).

(2) *Child-based resources and resilience.* Children who develop well within unfavorable environments are characterized by competencies that tend to support their mastery of developmental objectives (e.g., educational success, relationship formation) and enhance their ability to manage challenges. In general, these competencies are associated with sound development among children in both favorable and unfavorable environments (Masten, 2001). They include: (a) *positive mastery beliefs*, including perceptions of personal competence; self-efficacy (i.e., children's beliefs that they can achieve desired outcomes when they face challenges); and positive expectations for the future (Werner & Smith, 1982; Wyman, Cowen, Work, & Kerley, 1993); (b) *social–emotional competence*, such as affective attunement to peers; behaviors that promote social acceptance, and realistic understanding of events over which children have limited control (Cowen, Work, Wyman, Parker, Wannon, & Gribble, 1992); and (c) *sound intellectual ability*, including an early positive start in school (Masten & Coatsworth, 1998).

Although there are commonalities in resources that promote adaptation for children across settings, children adapt to specific life challenges in different ways. Therefore caution must be exercised in generalizing about resilience processes across groups of children. For example, research with children who had histories of maltreatment indicated that those children who showed improved adaptation over time were more likely to draw on personal mastery experiences for promoting competence compared to children without histories of maltreatment, who were more likely to draw on support from relationships (Cicchetti & Rogosch, 1997). In addition, attributes associated with competence for many children may not promote competence in all children and, in fact, may be counterproductive in some contexts. For children with histories of conduct problems, perceptions of high personal competence (which exceed ability) have been linked to higher aggression and lower levels of school engagement (Hughes, Cavell, & Grossman, 1997). Whereas positive self-views appear to promote striving in many children, those beliefs may reduce some children's ability to receive and effectively use feedback about their behaviors.

STRATEGIES: OVERVIEW

Research on resilience in childhood suggests that one approach for prevention is fostering competencies that promote effective mastery of life stressors while simultaneously reducing risks for children at key phases of development or during major life transitions. This approach has been termed "cumulative protection" and "cumulative competence promotion and stress protection" (Masten & Coatsworth, 1998; Wyman, Sandler, Wolchik, & Nelson, 2000). The goal of this strategy is to strengthen children's capacity to effectively navigate challenges throughout childhood. This framework is useful for families dealing with marital transitions and for understanding how preventive interventions for those families are effective.

Divorce, for example, typically initiates a series of stressful transitions, ranging from emotional readjustment to changes in residence, which pose ongoing challenges for children and their families. A review of over 92 studies comparing children living in divorced single-parent families with children living in continuously married families indicated that children who experienced parental divorce had lower average functioning on a variety of adjustment indices, including academic achievement and behavioral conduct (Amato & Keith, 1991). It is important to emphasize that the average difference in adjustment between children from divorced and nondivorced families is modest and that many children manage the transitions following divorce effectively. However, not all divorces pose equal challenges for children. Children of parents in highly conflictual marriages or post-divorce situations face substantially greater

challenges and, as a result, have higher rates of emotional and behavioral problems (Davies & Cummings, 1994). Conflict between parents is a key risk factor for all children; thus, the potential benefit to children from reducing risk exposure and promoting competence is substantial.

A number of protective factors are associated with positive adjustment for children who experience parental divorce. Many of these protective factors are similar to those identified in research with children in other adverse circumstances. Some of these factors are potentially modifiable which make them particularly relevant for incorporating into interventions.

Individual factors. How children perceive and cope with the often unwanted, uncontrollable, and unexpected experiences of divorce influences their adjustment. Realistic appraisal of control and accurate understanding about the reasons for the break-up predict better adjustment in school-aged children (Pedro-Carroll & Cowen, 1985). Similarly, children who use active coping approaches and can draw on positive thinking (i.e., not catastrophizing) are less likely to be depressed and their beliefs that their coping will be successful stimulates effective use of active coping strategies (Sandler, Tein, & West, 1994).

Family factors. Better outcomes for children occur when parents reduce children's exposure to conflict, and in particular limit children's exposure to aggressive conflict that involves child-related issues (Davies & Cummings, 1994). Other important protective factors are parents' emotional well-being, continuity of parenting quality and emotional responsiveness, and noncustodial fathers' maintaining close emotional bonds with their children and utilizing authoritative (i.e., emotionally warm but structured) parenting practices (Chase-Lansdale & Hetherington, 1990).

Extended family/community factors. Although predictors of children's post-divorce adjustment are typically considered only in terms of their families of origin, positive relationships with peers, grandparents, and other adults promote positive adjustment (e.g., Cowen, Pedro-Carroll, & Alpert-Gillis, 1990).

STRATEGIES THAT WORK

The knowledge base on children and families in transition underscores the potent protective processes that can occur through strengthening secure connections between parents and children, promoting children's access to support and enhancing children's own coping resources.

Two different interventions demonstrate benefits of enhancing parenting competence following divorce. The *New Beginnings* program (Wolchik et al., 1993) teaches custodial mothers effective discipline strategies, positive family activities, listening skills, and use of positive reinforcement, including one-on-one time in which the parent expresses pleasure with their interactions with the child as they engage in a shared activity. Another effective intervention model for parents developed by Forgatch and DeGarmo (1999) emphasizes parents' use of noncoercive discipline practices and setting limits on children's inappropriate behavior. Results of evaluations of these programs support their efficacy in improving parenting, reducing children's adjustment problems, and enhancing their competence. Evaluation of the New Beginnings Program showed that improved parenting accounted for positive outcomes in children's well-being after six months and later in adolescence (Wolchik et al., 2000).

A child-focused intervention shown to effectively strengthen children's coping and mastery of divorce-related challenges is the *Children of Divorce Intervention* program. This structured group intervention reaches children in school-settings who might otherwise not receive services. The program was initially developed for 4th–6th grade children and aims to reduce children's misperceptions of divorce and their isolation and strengthen their capacities to address and solve specific divorce-related challenges (e.g., loyalty conflicts). Evaluation of the program demonstrated its effectiveness in both enhancing children's skills (e.g., accurate understanding of family changes) and their behavior and emotional adjustment (Pedro-Carroll & Cowen, 1985). The program has been extended to younger children and to early adolescents and has been implemented effectively with children of diverse sociocultural backgrounds (e.g., Alpert-Gillis, Pedro-Carroll, & Cowen, 1989). After 2 years young children who participated in the program had fewer school adjustment problems and more competencies than their demographically matched peers in a nonprogram control group (Pedro-Carroll, Sutton, & Wyman, 1999).

STRATEGIES THAT MIGHT WORK

There are several promising approaches that might work to bolster the protective factors linked to children's healthy adjustment following parental divorce. The recent proliferation of court-based parent education programs for separating couples is an excellent example of an approach with much potential to provide information and skills to help parents protect their children from risk factors such as ongoing conflict. There is some evidence that parent education programs that provide specific skills training to enhance effective parenting practices and protect children from interparental conflict may promote more positive parent–child relationships over time and increase parents' efficacy (Pedro-Carroll, 2001). However, more research is needed to provide an evidence base for such programs and to identify essential content and a model for best practices.

STRATEGIES THAT DO NOT WORK

At this time, there is not a sufficient knowledge base to identify approaches that clearly do not work in promoting positive outcomes and resilience for children and families following divorce.

SYNTHESIS

Research on resilience has moved beyond identifying general protective factors to more specificity in understanding protective processes and cumulative competence enhancement throughout stages of childhood. Integrating research on resilience and the effects of divorce on children can inform new directions for research, practice, and policy. While the integration of these two areas of research holds promise, numerous challenges remain. Like children in chronic adverse circumstances, children dealing with marital conflict, divorce, and life in a single parent family (including, possibly, remarriage) represent a diverse population with different needs for protective resources and competence promotion. A worthy, yet challenging goal is to help children not only survive, but also thrive in the aftermath of divorce and in the context of other life challenges. The protective pathways for children in different family circumstances are varied, requiring multifaceted solutions and resources over time. Some examples of ways that processes of resilience may be promoted in children and families are given below.

1. Interventions that enhance competencies and resources for children across more than one level of their developmental context are more likely to have enduring effects. For example, interventions that simultaneously enhance young children's health and mothers' parenting competence are more likely to build strengths that reverberate throughout family contexts. Evaluations of comprehensive programs need to adopt a broad perspective, with the expectation that successful programs may change individual children, their families, and larger systems, when implemented on a community basis.

2. Protecting children from the corrosive effects of ongoing parent conflict. Educational interventions for parents can be effective in supporting parents' efforts to encapsulate conflict and not allow it to erode relationships with their child. Preventive interventions can serve parents well by incorporating skills for conflict resolution, anger management, adopting a more business-like approach, and disengaging from inflammatory verbal exchanges and interactions (Pedro-Carroll, 2001).

3. Developing effective strategies to enhance parents' and children's functioning and well-being during major transitions. It is clear that marital disruptions pose risks to adults' physical and emotional well-being, and having a well functioning parent is a potent protective pathway to children's healthy development. Parent education programs and preventive interventions should be proactive in emphasizing to parents the importance of attending to their physical and emotional health so they can best care for their children. Information about the pitfalls of using substances to relieve stress and suggestions for healthy stress reduction merit inclusion in such programs, as well as efforts to link parents with additional supportive resources once a program has ended. Schools can provide outreach through supportive interventions for children and proactive policies that encourage the active involvement of both parents in children's school success. The legal/judicial system can have a positive impact on divorcing parents by containing conflict and providing alternatives to adversarial proceedings and costly litigation.

4. Foster solid, supportive parent–child relationships through interventions across the span of childhood. Research on resilience for children in adverse circumstances has recurring themes in common with research on children and divorce: the importance of a supportive relationship between children and at least one parent or caregiver. Equally important is the finding that a healthy relationship with one parent has the potential to buffer children from a negative relationship with the other parent. These high quality relationships can enhance children's felt security, reduce fears, and promote competencies that equip children to master challenges on their own. Interventions targeted to separating parents that teach effective parenting practices and strengthen relationships hold much promise for stress protection and fostering resilience.

Our efforts to reach out to families in transition must be informed by current research, evidence-based interventions, and policies that keep children's developmental needs a top priority. Numerous challenges remain but current research suggests some promising approaches to fostering children's resilience and capacity to cope effectively with challenging life circumstances.

Also see: Academic Success; Identity Promotion; Self-Esteem.

References

Alpert-Gillis, L.J., Pedro-Carroll, J.L., & Cowen, E.L. (1989). Children of Divorce Intervention Program: Development, implementation and evaluation of a program for young urban children. *Journal of Consulting and Clinical Psychology, 57,* 583–587.

Amato, P.R., & Keith, B. (1991). Consequences of parental divorce for children's well being: A meta-analysis. *Psychological Bulletin, 110,* 26–46.

Chase-Lansdale, P.L., & Hetherington, E.M. (1990). The impact of divorce on life-span development: Short and long term effects. In P.B. Baltes, D.L. Featherman, & R.M. Lerner (Eds.), *Life-span development and behavior* (Vol. 10, pp. 105–150). Hillsdale, NJ: Lawrence-Erlbaum.

Cherlin, A.J. (1992). *Marriage, divorce, and remarriage.* Cambridge: Harvard University Press.

Cicchetti, D., & Rogosch, F.A. (1997). The role of self-organization in the promotion of resilience in maltreated children. *Development and Psychopathology, 9,* 797–815.

Cowen, E.L. (1994). The enhancement of psychological wellness: Challenges and opportunities. *American Journal of Community Psychology, 22,* 149–179.

Cowen, E.L., Pedro-Carroll, J.L., & Alpert-Gillis, L.J. (1990). Relationships between support and adjustment among children of divorce. *Journal of Child Psychology and Psychiatry, 31,* 727–735.

Cowen, E.L., Work, W.C., Wyman, P.A., Parker, G.R., Wannon, M., & Gribble, P. (1992). Test comparisons among stress-affected, stress-resilience, and nonclassified fourth-through sixth-grade urban children. *Journal of Community Psychology, 20,* 200–214.

Davies, P.T., & Cummings, E.M. (1994). Marital conflict and child adjustment: An emotional security hypothesis. *Psychological Bulletin, 116,* 387–411.

Egeland, B., Carlson, E A., & Sroufe, L.A. (1993). Resilience as process. *Development and Psychopathology, 5,* 517–528.

Elder, G.H., Jr. (1974). *Children of the Great Depression.* Chicago: University of Chicago Press.

Emery, R.E., & Laumann-Billings, L. (1998). An overview of the nature, causes, and consequences of abusive family relationships: Toward differentiating maltreatment and violence. *American Psychologist, 53,* 121–135.

Forgatch, M.S., & DeGarmo, D.S. (1999). Parenting through change: An effective prevention program for single mothers. *Journal of Consulting and Clinical Psychology, 67,* 711–724.

Gest, S.D., Neeman, J., Hubbard, J.J., Masten, A.S., & Tellegen, A. (1993). Parenting quality, adversity and conduct problems in adolescence: Testing process oriented models of resilience. *Development and Psychopathology, 5,* 663–682.

Hughes, J.N., Cavell, T.A., & Grossman, P.B. (1997). A positive view of self: Risk or protection for aggressive children? *Development and Psychopathology, 9,* 75–94.

Luthar, S.S. (1991). Vulnerability and resilience: A study of high-risk adolescents. *Child Development, 62,* 600–616.

Luthar, S.S., & Cicchetti, D. (2000). The construct of resilience: Implications for interventions and social policies. *Development and Psychopathology, 12,* 857–885.

Masten, A.S., Best, K.M., & Garmezy, N. (1990). Resilience and development: Contributions from the study of children who overcome adversity. *Development and Psychopathology, 2,* 425–444.

Masten, A.S., & Coatsworth, J.D. (1998). The development of competence in favorable and unfavorable environments: Lessons from research on successful children. *American Psychologist, 53,* 205–220.

McLoyd, V. (1998). Socioeconomic disadvantage and child development. *American Psychologist, 53,* 185–204.

Pedro-Carroll, J.L. (2001). The promotion of wellness in children and families in transition: Challenges and opportunities. *American Psychologist, 56,* 993–1004.

Pedro-Carroll, J.L., & Cowen, E.L. (1985). The Children of Divorce Intervention Project: An investigation of the efficacy of a school-based prevention program. *Journal of Consulting and Clinical Psychology,* *53,* 603–611.

Pedro-Carroll, J.L., Sutton, S.E., & Wyman, P.A. (1999). A two-year follow-up evaluation of a preventive intervention program for young children of divorce. *School Psychology Review, 28,* 467–476.

Quinton, D., Pickles, A., Maughan, B., & Rutter, M. (1993). Partners, peers, and pathways: Assortative pairing and continuities in conduct disorder. *Development and Psychopathology, 5,* 763–783.

Rutter, M. (1979). Protective factors in children's responses to stress and disadvantage. In M.W. Kent & J.E. Rolf (Eds.), *Primary prevention of psychopathology: Social competence in children* (Vol. 3, pp. 49–74). Hanover, NH: University Press of New England.

Rye, M. S., & Pargament, K. I. (2002). Forgiveness and romantic relationships in college: Can it heal the wounded heart? *Journal of Clinical Psychology, 54,* 419–441.

Sandler, I.N., Tein, J., & West, S.G. (1994). Coping, stress and psychological symptoms of children of divorce: A cross sectional and longitudinal study. *Child Development, 65,* 1744–1763.

Save the Children. (2001). *State of the world's mothers 2001.* New York: Author.

US Bureau of the Census. (1990). *Statistical abstracts of the US, 1990* (110th ed.). Washington, DC: US G trafficking in women and girls: An international human rights violation. Washington, DC: US Government Printing Office.

Werner, E.E., & Smith, R.S. (1982). *Vulnerable but invincible: A study of resilient children.* New York: McGraw-Hill.

Werner, E.E., & Smith, R.S. (1992). *Overcoming the odds: High-risk children from birth to adulthood.* Ithaca, NY: Cornell University Press.

White, B.L. (1978). *Experience and environment: Major influences on the development of the young child* (Vol. 2). Englewood Cliffs, NJ: Prentice Hall.

Wolchik, S.A., & Sandler, I.N. (1997). *Handbook of children's coping: Linking theory and intervention.* New York: Plenum Press.

Wolchik, S.A., West, S.G., Sandler, I.N., Tein, J.-Y., Coatsworth, D., Lengua, L., Weiss, L., Anderson, E., Greene, S., & Griffin, W. (2000). The New Beginnings program for divorced families: An experimental evaluation of theory-based single-component and dual-component programs. *Journal of Consulting and Clinical Psychology, 68,* 843–856.

Wolchik, S.A., West, S.G., Westover, S., Sandler, I. N., Martin, A., Lustig, J., Tein, J.-Y., & Fisher, J. (1993). The Children of Divorce Parenting Intervention: Outcome evaluation of an empirically based program. *American Journal of Community Psychology, 21*(3), 293–331.

Wyman, P.A., Cowen, E.L., Work, W.C., & Kerley, J.H. (1993). The role of children's future expectations in self-system functioning and adjustment to life-stress. *Development and Psychopathology, 5,* 649–661.

Wyman, P.A., Cowen, E.L., Work, W.C., Hoyt-Meyers, L.A., Magnus, K.B., & Fagen, D.B. (1999). Caregiving and developmental factors differentiating young at-risk urban children showing resilient versus stress-affected outcomes: A replication and extension. *Child Development, 70,* 645–659.

Wyman, P.A., Sandler, I, Wolchik, S., & Nelson, K. (2000). Resilience as cumulative competence promotions and stress protection: Theory and intervention. In D. Cicchetti, J. Rappaport, I. Sandler, & R. Weissberg (Eds.), *The promotion of wellness in children and adolescents.* Washington, DC: CWLA Press.

Risk-Taking, Adolescence*

Aleta L. Meyer

INTRODUCTION

The term "risk-taking" in the field of prevention typically refers to negative behaviors youth engage in that have a high likelihood of resulting in harm to their future development (DiClemente, Hansen, & Ponton, 1996). These risks often involve behaviors that break societal norms for their age group—behaviors such as underage drinking or driving or precocious sexual activity. From the perspective of youth, many of these behaviors are highly reinforcing, often because of the physical thrill they provide or because they are behaviors youth expect to engage in as adults. For these reasons, and others, primary prevention efforts that try to curtail risk-taking behavior all together can fall short of their goals.

DEFINITIONS

Primary prevention programming can benefit from the appeal risk-taking has for adolescents by thinking of risk-taking behavior in two categories: *Negative risk-taking* can refer to challenging activities that have a high likelihood of negative consequences for the youth or others though highly reinforcing; *positive risk-taking* can refer to challenging activities that have a high likelihood of positive consequences for the youth or others (Meyer, Farrell, Northup, Kung, & Plybon, 2000). Because activities that are perceived to be challenging usually involve uncertain yet desirable outcomes, as well as the acceptance of personal responsibility for the outcome, they can arouse high levels of emotion, such as exhilaration, anticipation, and fear in youth who attempt them. Examples of positive risk-taking for youth include challenging activities such as testing their personal limits, demonstrating mastery in an area of life, developing close relationships, engaging in fun and exciting modes of learning, and discovering their place in the larger community. A key assumption of positive risk-taking is that of *challenge*

*This work was supported in part by a cooperative agreement (#U81/CCU309966) and a center grant (#R49/CCR318597-01) from the Centers for Disease Control and Prevention (CDC). The research and interpretations reported are the sole responsibility of the author and are not necessarily endorsed by CDC or represent the views, opinions, or policies of the CDC or their staff.

by choice (Rohnke, 1984) whereby individual youth control a major part of the degree of challenge or risk they will take and are kept aware of that control throughout the experience.

SCOPE

When attempting to explain the undesirably high levels of unhealthy behaviors that youth exhibit today (US Department of Health and Human Services, 2000), some authors point to the lack of meaningful developmental milestones (e.g., rites of passage) that include both physical and cognitive challenges (Blumenkrantz, 1992; Taibbi, 1991; Oldfield, 1987). They have argued that, without constructive challenges, youth who are motivated toward risk are likely to meet their needs for challenge through behaviors such as delinquency and experimentation with drugs and alcohol, whereas students who do not feel comfortable with risk may withdraw and become socially isolated and/or depressed. If such an argument is valid, one could measure the potential of positive risk-taking in adolescence in terms of the negative behaviors that may be displaced by increased participation in behaviors expected of adults. For example, familiar "thrill-seeking" efforts at adult behavior that often lead to car crashes, unprotected sex, and drinking might be replaced by the equally challenging behaviors of trying out for a sport team, writing an essay, resolving a conflict, climbing a mountain, painting a landscape, or preparing a meal for someone special.

THEORIES

At the individual level, one way to conceptualize the contribution of positive risk-taking to primary prevention is to consider the role of emotion in *social-information processing* (Lemerise & Arsenio, 2000). In a comprehensive overview of theory and research on the relationship between cognitions and emotions in personal-social decision-making, Lemerise and Arsenio (2000) describe how emotions can serve to help organize thoughts and motivate behaviors through *emotion–event* links that facilitate adaptive goal-directed behavior. For example, if a child is in a certain situation and responds in a way that results in a positive emotion (e.g., something valuable is attained), that emotion becomes linked to that type of situation and facilitates recollection of the same response in similar situations. Given that any challenge has an infinite number of solutions, a person's having had success or failure with previous strategies, as well as having current priorities, provides concrete markers to those options that allow a person to quickly restrict the number of options in any given situation. Unfortunately, although

crucial in the development of effective prevention programs, previous models of social-information processing have not fully articulated the role of emotions (Crick & Dodge, 1994) and, hence, social cognitive interventions have not fully utilized this component of effective decision-making. Even though practicing a decision-making model with a hypothetical situation may help students to understand the value of certain strategies over others, it may not provide the affect–event link that is needed for students to recall those effective strategies in a real life situation—thus limiting the transferability of social skills across contexts. In contrast, the heightened emotional experience of using a decision-making model within the context of a structured and supervised situation such as a peer mediation session or a high-ropes course may provide the affect–event link that allows students to transfer problem-solving skills to new situations.

An additional individual level conceptualization of the potential of positive risk-taking is to consider the benefits of youth having goals focused on increasing competence (i.e., learning goals) over having goals focused on gaining positive appraisals from others and/or avoiding negative ones (e.g., performance goals) (Dweck, 1986). While people with either type of goal are motivated to seek challenge and persist when they are feeling confident, their level of motivation differs when confidence in their ability is low. For example, in response to an experience of failure and a decreased sense of confidence, a person who focuses on learning goals stays on task and persists. In contrast, a person who focuses on performance goals is likely to disengage. Because adulthood is saturated with new and unexpected demands, in order to thrive and prosper in our rapidly changing world, youth need to learn how to persist in the face of challenge and failure, no matter how confident they feel. Experiences such as responsibly supervised rock-climbing can provide concrete metaphors of the benefits of a learning goal over a performance goal. For example, a person climbing up a rock-face has to stay focused on the individual hand-holds and foot placements to reach the top, rather than focused on the top of the climb itself, or that person will literally slip back to the last place where he or she was firmly planted. In the same way, if someone wants to achieve a higher grade in a math course, he or she has to stay focused on the tasks of completing homework assignments on time and asking for help when needed, rather than on the higher grade, or else one's exam scores will reflect a level of achievement below that of the uncompleted homework assignments. An additional benefit to youth for having learning goals is the correlation between having those types of goals and the belief that intelligence is malleable, not fixed (Dweck, 1986). With such a belief system, previous achievement or being better than someone else is not requisite to developing competencies in multiple domains, a hallmark of responsible adult behavior (Garbarino, 1982).

Another way to conceptualize positive risk-taking is at the community/cultural level as a reframed form of rites of passage that can help facilitate a continuous transition to adulthood. In a cross-cultural comparison of the ways in which adolescents are socialized to their roles of adulthood, Benedict (1934) noted differences in how abruptly or smoothly children were moved into their adult roles across cultures as well as how consistent messages were about expected adult behavior. Cultures such as that of the United States frequently have inconsistent messages about adult behavior and when one becomes an adult these are manifested in discontinuous transitions into adulthood. Perhaps most striking is the way in which an 18-year-old male in the United States is old enough to join the military and to vote, yet is not old enough to legally drink alcohol. Such a dynamic is not only inconsistent about when one becomes an adult, it sets up alcohol consumption as the last marker of adulthood, giving it extremely high value as an adult behavior. Because of the fun and excitement drinking alcohol represents, not to mention the highly reinforcing nature of alcohol consumption (Leigh & Stacy, 1993) and its potential negative impact on a young life, it may take an extremely challenging and equally fun counter activity to diffuse the attraction of a negative risk like underage drinking (Levanthal & Keeshan, 1993). Such an activity would need to have components of the thrill of alcohol consumption as well as the status of expected adult behavior to fully substitute. If well facilitated and followed up over time, a 5-day trek in the mountains may achieve this, wherein youth face dangers, learn to trust and respect each other, have fun, and take responsibility for their own safety and that of their peers. Because these types of structured and supported positive-risk activities are often lacking in the lives of youth, youth may seek out dangerous activities instead. For example, a negative risk behavior related to rites of passage in college fraternities is binge-drinking (Arnold & Kuh, 1992), a behavior that facilitates a good time and bonding with friends. While it may also provide an opportunity to learn to cope with and take responsibility for deadly accidents, STD's from unprotected sex while drunk, and alcoholism itself (Commission on Substance Abuse at Colleges and Universities, 1994).

RESEARCH

In addition to the aforementioned research areas focused on the role of emotion in social-information processing, the impact of goal orientation on motivation, and transitions to adulthood, other bodies of research that support the concept of risk as something valuable for primary prevention come from work on adolescent experimentation and substance abuse (Baumrind, 1991; Shedler & Block,

1990), the function of violence in adolescence (Fagan & Wilkinson, 1998), experiential education (Henton, 1996), and spirituality as a key dimension of positive youth development (Catalano, Berglund, Ryan, Lonczak, & Hawkins, 1998). In a longitudinal study of adolescent development, Shedler and Block (1990) found that the most psychologically healthy adolescents in their study were those who had experimented with marijuana as compared to those who either abstained or abused marijuana. Similarly, Baumrind (1991) found that experimenters and rational abstainers were more psychologically healthy than substance abusers or irrational abstainers. One of the shared conclusions these authors derived from their respective research was that experimentation itself is a valuable behavior and that sometimes a youth's lack of experimentation with substances may have more to do with a generalized fear of the unfamiliar than with sound decision-making.

In a similar turn from conventional wisdom, Fagan and Wilkinson's (1998) examination of research on the meaning and social context of violence in adolescence challenges the perspective that youth who engage in violence are merely deficient in social problem-solving skills. Instead, their review indicated that violence was often the means to the ends of gaining social status, honor, and respect, particularly for youth in under-resourced areas such as the inner city. When violence is the result of this type of dynamic, either in isolation or in combination with social skill deficits, the prevention of violence may require finding replacement activities for those youth that provide means for achieving and maintaining high status (i.e., positive risks).

Viewing adventure within the experiential learning cycle (Henton, 1996) is another angle for considering empirical support for the benefits of positive risk-taking. In the tradition of experiential learning (Dewey, 1938), the full experience is viewed as necessary to learning. Moreover, use of the experiential learning cycle of the physical activity itself, reflection on the activity, generalizing and abstracting from the activity, and transferring the learning to other areas of life provides educational opportunities for youth no matter what their learning style preference (Kolb, 1985). In other words, adults providing youth with fully engaging activities (i.e., positive risks) and then enacting the experiential learning cycle to process those activities may be the optimal educational experience.

The final parallel between positive risk-taking and other bodies of research taps into the unpredictable nature of risk itself and the fact that Catalano et al.'s (1998) comprehensive review of research on positive youth development specifies the fostering of spirituality as a key process. The aspect of spirituality referred to here is that of trusting in a power greater than oneself, particularly in situations where the outcome is unknown (Meyer & Lausell, 1996). By practicing the process of trusting and letting go in a safe and supportive context with activities perceived to be dangerous (i.e., positive risks), youth may develop their personal spirituality.

STRATEGIES THAT WORK

While clear evidence of the impact of promoting positive risk-taking in adolescence per se is not yet available, there is evidence to support the positive impact of many structured activities that can be thought of as manifestations of positive risk-taking. These include experiential education (Dewey, 1938; Kolb, 1985), rite of passage experiences (Blumenkrantz & Gavazzi, 1993), peer mediation (Jones, 1998), sports (Danish, Hale, & Petispas, 1990), and alternative substance use prevention programming (Tobler, 1986). These bodies of research, however, do not hone in on the risk-taking aspect of these activities as key processes for prevention.

STRATEGIES THAT MIGHT WORK

While not focused on prevention in adolescence, research on adventure as a key process of change can be found in literature on the efficacy of organizational development activities combined with outdoor adventure for adults in corporate settings. A review of evaluation studies on the impact of these activities by Priest and Gass (1997) indicates that initial changes in desired behavior (e.g., teamwork, clarity on mission and purpose) which occur after group outdoor adventure interventions are maintained when there is follow-through and repeated modeling of the facilitation process by corporate leaders *within* the corporate organization over an extended period of time. This research is consistent with the theory regarding the transference of lessons learned in the wilderness to every day settings, whereby activities must (1) be designed with specific objectives related to personal change; (2) provide opportunities to practice while on the adventure; (3) provide opportunities to reflect on the experience; (4) include significant others in the experience; (5) utilize naturally occurring consequences for behavior; (6) place responsibility for learning on the participants; (7) use techniques to process each experience; (8) include participants who have successfully completed similar adventures; and (9) provide follow-up experiences (Gass, 1984). From a social cognitive perspective (Bandura, 1986), this follow-through and modeling provides the opportunity for skill practice within a framework of social support. It is reasonable to infer that optimal transference of learning with adolescents from an adventure setting to other settings in life would require similar contingencies. Therefore, the most efficacious use of positive risk-taking with adolescents

might be in the context of a long-term learning agenda provided by supportive and consistent peers and adults.

A simple manifestation of this partnership might involve increased communication and collaboration between field trip and prevention staff that work with the same youth. For example, prior to taking students on a week-end retreat, staff who are leading the retreat could take time to meet with health instructors that implement smoking prevention and other prevention curricula in the school to learn the language being taught for examining self-talk, calming down, and problem-solving. Then, after a situation in which students start to panic (e.g., feeling lost during a supervised hike), the supervising adult might say something such as, "I was talking with Mr. So-and-so about what to do when you start getting really upset. He told me about this stuff you are learning in your health class about ways to calm down and talk to yourself. Do you think that might be helpful now? What do we need to do?" Similarly, when the students are back in the classroom, Mr. So-and-so might ask students for examples from the retreat when they used the skills of stopping and calming down and whether or not that was helpful. A parent could use similar strategies of reflection and application to help his or her child optimize a positive risk experience such as traveling to a foreign country.

A more involved and possibly synergistic combination could involve systematically pairing research-validated primary prevention programming (see US Department of Education, 2001, for a list of promising and exemplary programs) with specific positive risk-taking activities. For example, to internalize the value of social cognitive problem-solving skills for conflict resolution taught in a research-validated violence prevention program, a school might implement a peer mediation program. Similarly, to demonstrate the value of goal-setting for academic achievement within a research-validated social competence program, a school might enroll its students in a series of progressively more difficult rock-climbing activities led by staff who use the language of that social competence program during facilitation.

Another strategy for incorporating positive risk-taking in prevention is to build positive risk activities into the curriculum itself. Such an approach has been taken for extending the long-term positive effects of the sixth grade *Responding In Peaceful and Positive Ways* violence prevention program (RIPP-6) (Farrell, Meyer, & White, 2001; Meyer et al., 2000). In the seventh grade program (RIPP-7) (Meyer et al., 2000), activities from the nonviolent martial art of Aikido (Crum, 1987) are used in explicit fashion for demonstrating the centering, perspective-taking, and goal-setting skills of the curriculum. The eighth grade program (RIPP-8) (Meyer et al., 2000) takes an even more literal approach by focusing on taking positive risks during the transition to high school as a tool for violence prevention.

These risks are designed at both the group and the individual level. At the individual level, youth are encouraged to explore positive risks such as setting academic goals, trying something they have always wanted to do but have never tried, and forgiving someone. At the group level, an adventure activity called the Raccoon Circle (Smith, 1996), made of an 11-foot piece of webbing tied in a loop, serves as a metaphor for taking risks in a safe and supportive environment.

Other strategies for promoting positive risk focus explicitly on rites of passage. Ideally, these programs systematically parallel adolescent development from puberty to graduation. The *Rite of Passage Experience* (ROPE) is a community-based example of such a program (Blumenkrantz & Gavazzi, 1993) while *Journey to Adulthood* (J2A) is a church-based example of such a program (Hughes, 1993). The *Timbertop Extended Stay Outdoor Adventure School* is shorter in duration, but more intensive, with youth spending the entire ninth grade academic year in the Australian Bush (Gray, Patterson, & Linke, 1993).

STRATEGIES THAT DO NOT WORK

Given the contingencies for optimizing the impact of positive risk-taking, one-time adventure experiences with no reflection and/or long-term follow-through are of minimal benefit (Priest & Gass, 1997). What is more important to note, yet perhaps less evident from the previous discussion, is that poorly facilitated positive risk activities can have a significant negative impact (Priest & Gass, 1997). For example, if a youth is forced, coerced, or bribed to do something by an adult and/or peer, a violation of the challenge by choice principal (Rohnke, 1984), not only physical safety is compromised, but most of the intrinsic reward for participating in the activity is diminished (Priest & Gass, 1997). Even though dominating approaches to leadership, which often coexist with a mentality of conquering nature (Humberstone, 1989), have been all but abandoned in the professional outdoor adventure field and replaced with challenge by choice and a focus on being with nature (Mitten, 1992), they are not infrequent in the lay outdoor adventure enthusiast and should be addressed, if necessary. In other words, before signing youth on for positive risk-taking activities, adults need to take a close look at the training, facilitation style, and experience of those leading the activities.

SYNTHESIS

Even though risk is rarely framed in a positive light in prevention and education literature, the psychosocial processes which positive risk-taking may facilitate are considered crucial to optimal adolescent development.

Moreover, in our rapidly changing world, it may be more important than ever to prepare youth to cope with and adapt to the unexpected. If positive risk-taking activities increase the affect–behavior link of problem-solving skills as well as a learning orientation towards goals, they might be expected to improve the long-term impact of research-validated prevention programs. Moreover, thoughtful incorporation of positive risk-taking into prevention may be an extremely effective strategy given the potential of positive risk behavior for diffusing the power and appeal of behaviors such as substance abuse, precocious sex, and violence. In summary, helping young people feel comfortable with success in areas that are personally valuable through a prevention strategy of structured and supervised activities that at first seem scary may be a contemporary solution to the age-old desire to be a hero in our own time (Campbell, 1949).

ACKNOWLEDGMENT

The author would like to acknowledge outdoor adventure educator Kathleen Konrad for thoughtful dialogue regarding possibilities for combining social cognitive prevention programming and positive risk-taking.

Also see: Academic Success; Peer Relationships (adolescence); Identity Promotion (adolescence).

References

Arnold, J., & Kuh, G. (1992). *Brotherhood and the bottle: A cultural analysis of the role of alcohol in fraternities.* Bloomington, IN: Center for the Study of College Fraternity.

Bandura, A. (1986). *Social foundations of thought and action: A social cognitive theory.* Englewood Cliffs, NJ: Prentice Hall.

Baumrind, D. (1991). The influence of parenting style on adolescent competence and substance use. *Journal of Early Adolescence, 11*(1), 56–95.

Benedict, R. (1934). *Patterns of culture.* Boston: Houghton Mifflin.

Blumenkrantz, D. (1992). *Fulfilling the promise of children's services: Why primary prevention efforts fail and how they can succeed.* San Fransisco, CA: Jossey-Bass.

Blumenkrantz, D., & Gavazzi, S. (1993). Guiding transitional events for children and adolescents through a modern day rite of passage. *Journal of Primary Prevention, 13,* 199–212.

Campbell, J. (1949). *The hero with a thousand faces.* Princeton, NJ: Princeton University Press.

Catalano, R.F., Berglund, M.L., Ryan, J.A., Lonczak, H.C., & Hawkins, J.D. (1998). *Positive youth development in the United States: Research findings on evaluations of positive youth programs.* Unpublished manuscript, University of Washington, Seattle.

Commission on Substance Abuse at Colleges and Universities. (1994). *Rethinking rites of passage: Substance abuse on America's campuses.* New York: Center on Addiction and Substance Abuse at Columbia University.

Crick, N., & Dodge, K. (1994). A review and reformulation of social-information processing mechanisms in children's social adjustment. *Psychological Bulletin, 115,* 74–101.

Crum, T. (1987). *The magic of conflict.* New York: Touchstone.

Danish, S., Hale, B., & Petispas, A. (1990). Sport as a context for developing competence. In T. Gullotta & G. Adams (Eds.), *Developing social competency in adolescence. Advances in adolescent development* (Vol. 3, pp. 169–194). Thousand Oaks, CA: Sage.

Dewey, J. (1938). *Experience and education.* New York: Macmillan.

DiClemente, R., Hansen, W., & Ponton, L. (1996). Adolescents at Risk: A generation in jeopardy. In R. DiClemente, W., Hansen, & L. Ponton (Eds.), *Handbook of adolescent health risk behavior* (pp. 1–4). New York: Plenum Press.

Dweck, C. (1986). Motivational processes affecting learning. *American Psychologist, 41*(10), 1040–1048.

Fagan, J., & Wilkinson, D. (1998). Social contexts and functions of adolescent violence. In D. Elliott, B. Hamburg, & K. Williams (Eds.), *Violence in American schools* (pp. 55–93). New York: Cambridge.

Farrell, A.D., Meyer, A.L., & White, K.S. (2001). Evaluation of Responding in Peaceful and Positive Ways (RIPP): Λ school-based prevention program for reducing violence among urban adolescents. *Journal of Clinical Child Psychology, 30*(4), 451–463.

Garbarino, J. (1982). *Children and families in the social environment.* New York: Pergamon.

Gass, M. (1984). Programming the transfer of learning in adventure education. In R. Kraft & M. Sakofs (Eds.), *The theory of experiential education.* Boulder, CO: Association for Experiential Education.

Gray, T., Patterson, J., & Linke, R. (1993). The development of quantitative tools for evaluating the impact of extended stay outdoor education school programs on adolescents—A brief overview. *The Outdoor Educator, March,* 5–10.

Henton, M. (1996). *Adventure in the classroom.* Dubuque, IA: Kendall/Hunt.

Humberstone, B. (1989). Macho or multifarious?: The image and place of outdoor adventure education in the school curriculum. *British Journal of Physical Education, 20*(3), 112–114.

Jones, T. (1998). Research supports effectiveness of peer mediation. *The Fourth R, 48,* 1–27.

Hughes, A. (1993). *Travel guide to The Journey to Adulthood.* Durham, NC: St. Philip's Episcopal Church.

Kolb, D. (1985). *Learning-style inventory.* Boston: McBer.

Leigh, B., & Stacy, A. (1993). Alcohol outcome expectancies: Scale construction and predictive utility in higher order confirmatory models. *Psychological Assessment, 5*(2), 216–229.

Lemerise, E., & Arsenio, W. (2000). An integrated model of emotion processes and cognition in social-information processing. *Child Development, 71,* 107–118.

Levanthal, H., & Keeshan, P. (1993). Promoting healthy alternatives to substance abuse. In S. Millstein, A. Petersen, & E. Nightengale (Eds.), *Promoting the health of adolescents* (pp. 260–284). New York: Simon & Schuster.

Meyer, A.L., Farrell, A.D., Northup, W., Kung, E., & Plybon, L. (2000). *Promoting nonviolence in early adolescence: Responding in Peaceful and Positive Ways.* New York: Kluwer Academic/Plenum.

Meyer, A., & Lausell, L. (1996). The value of including a "Higher Power" in efforts to prevent violence and promote optimal outcomes during adolescence. In B. Hampton, P. Jenkins, & T. Gullotta (Eds.), *Preventing violence in America* (pp. 115–132). Thousand Oaks, CA: Sage.

Mitten, D. (1992). Empowering girls and women in the outdoors. *Journal of Physical Education, Recreation, and Dance, February,* 56–60.

Oldfield, D. (1987). The Journey: A creative approach to the necessary crises of adolescence. New York: The Foundation for Contemporary Mental Health.

Priest, S., & Gass, M. (1997). *Effective leadership in adventure programming.* Champaign, IL: Human Kinetics.

Rohnke, K. (1984). *Silver bullets.* Hamilton, MA: Project Adventure.

Shedler, J., & Block, J. (1990). Adolescent drug use and psychological health: A longitudinal inquiry. *American Psychologist, 45*(5), 612–630.

Smith, T. (1996). *Raccoon circles.* Cazenovia, WI: Raccoon Institute.

Taibbi, R. (1991). The uninitiated. *Family Therapy Networker, 14*(4), 30–35.

Tobler, N. (1986). Meta-analysis of 143 adolescent drug prevention programs: Quantitative outcome results of program participants compared to a control or comparison group. *The Journal of Drug Issues, 16*(4), 1–28.

US Department of Education. (2001, April 15). Announcement on the expert panel on safe, disciplined, and drug-free schools. Available: http://www.ed.gov/offices/OESE/SDFS/programs.html

US Department of Health and Human Services. (2000). *Healthy people 2010: National disease prevention goals and objectives.* Washington, DC: Public Health Service, National Institutes of Health.

Retirement Satisfaction, Older Adulthood

Virginia Richardson

INTRODUCTION

Many problems in retirement can be prevented, and many of the benefits of retirement can be attained, if people plan well. This entry reviews retirement satisfaction and the predictors of successful retirement. Definitions are presented first, then relevant theories and research. These are followed by a discussion of important retirement indicators and macro- and micro-interventions that can promote retirement satisfaction.

DEFINITIONS

Most researchers define *retirement* according to whether people have stopped working and receive a pension, public or private (Gendall & Siegel, 1992). These objective definitions often exclude many older women and minority persons who receive no pensions, work without compensation at home, and continue working part-time or intermittently. Broader and more subjective definitions of retirement have emerged in recent years. For example, after Gibson (1987) observed that 40 percent of older Blacks could not afford to retire and that many continued searching for full- or part-time work or declared themselves disabled, she questioned the applicability of traditional definitions of retirement for many African American elderly. She identified the "unretired-retired," who were over the age of 55 and not working but did not consider themselves retired. Zsembik and Singer (1990) reported different perceptions of retirement among Mexican Americans. In a study of Korean Americans, Kim (1992) found three different conceptualizations of retirement—retirement as termination of employment, retirement as leisure, and retirement as grandparenting. Various life circumstances, including a spouse's employment, work history, and self-employment, affect people's definitions of retirement (Szinovacz & DeViney, 1999).

SCOPE

The number of retired men and women has increased substantially over the last 30 years for several reasons. First, more and more people retire early. The percentage of men over the age of 65 who work has declined from 26.8 percent in 1970 to about 17.3 percent in 2000 (Bureau of Labor Statistics, 2000). Similar early retirement trends among men are found in many European countries, especially in France and Germany where early retirement options have become more accessible (O'Rand & Henretta, 1999). In addition, people spend more time in retirement because they are living longer. In 1940, the average man spent 9 years in retirement, about 15 percent of his life span, but by 1990 this increased to at least 14 years of retirement, which is more than 20 percent (US House Select Committee on Aging, 1992). Many retirees will start second careers and meet new friends as their social networks and lifestyles change during this protracted retirement period.

Longer retirements mean that people will experience more varied problems. Most people adjust well to retirement and cope with the many inevitable changes that occur with age, but some—especially those with limited resources—struggle during retirement. The most common retirement problems include poor planning, financial hardship, and involuntary retirement due to family and health problems.

Many retirement problems result from poor planning. Retirees are often surprised and unprepared for the costs involved with long-term care, such as prescription medications, hospitalizations, and nursing homes. Several studies document an association between retirement planning and retirement satisfaction (Monk, 1985). Unfortunately, most people avoid thinking about and planning for retirement. In an analysis of over 3,000 retirees, Richardson (1990) found that only about one third of male retirees compared to about one quarter of female retirees prepared adequately for retirement.

When people retire prematurely they are more susceptible to retirement problems. Peretti and Wilson (1978–1979) found that involuntary retirees had higher suicide rates and expressed greater anomie and alienation than those who retired according to plan. Unemployment, poor health, and family obligations are the most common reasons for involuntary retirement. Several researchers have documented that women consider their family situations more often then men when making decisions about retirement. Hatch and Thompson (1992) looked at the factors that led women to retire and found that having an ill or disabled household member who required assistance was the greatest predictor of their retirements. When retirees stop working because of illness they often become depressed. Approximately 25 percent of cancer patients, 40–65 percent of heart attack survivors, and 10–27 percent of stroke survivors experience some type of depression, and people with diabetes are three times more likely than those without this disease to become depressed (Margolis & Rabins, 1997). Depression is also common among retirees with functional limitations. When illnesses interfere with self-care and activities of daily living, people often become discouraged.

Poverty is, probably, the most serious retirement problem for older women and persons of color. Despite more employed women, older women still have higher poverty rates than older men. Although older women constituted 58 percent of the older population in 1990, they comprised 74 percent of the elderly poor, and with age older women's poverty rates worsen. Fifteen percent of women older than 75 are poor compared to 7.5 percent of men in this age category, and 51 percent of women over 85 live in or near poverty (US Bureau of the Census, 2000a). The situation is especially grave among older women from diverse ethnic backgrounds. Older African American women are twice as likely as older White women to be poor and five times more likely than older White men. White men more often work at jobs that have pensions while the jobs at which many women and minority persons work often lack adequate health and retirement benefits (US Bureau of the Census, 2000b). In 2000, 46 percent of men and only 29 percent of women over the age of 65 received a pension benefit (Purcell, 2000).

Nonmarried women, and especially divorced and separated older women, are particularly vulnerable to economic impoverishment during retirement. Among nonmarried women over the age of 65 in 1998, 27.1 percent were below the poverty line and 39.7 percent were below 125 percent of the poverty line, compared to 19.7 percent and 31.3 percent, respectively, of nonmarried men in this age category (Social Security Administration, 2000). Among nonmarried women over the age of 85, 30.9 percent were below the poverty line and 45.5 percent were below 125 percent of the poverty line. The rates among African American women were even higher. Among unmarried older Black women, 53.8 percent were below the poverty line.

THEORIES AND RESEARCH

Role Theorists, who used mostly cross-sectional research designs, prevailed during the 1970s and early 1980s. These theorists emphasized the centrality of work and marital roles, and viewed role exits, such as widowhood and retirement, as significant sources of distress and unhappiness. *Continuity Theorists*, who typically used longitudinal research methods, conceptualized retirement as an extension of earlier life stages as people tried to maintain previous levels of self-esteem, previous lifestyle patterns, and long-standing values. They found remarkable stability in life satisfaction during retirement, including the initial transition stages (George & Maddox, 1977; Wan & Odell, 1983).

Activity Theorists contended that people adjusted best to retirement when they maintained high levels of activity and continued the same levels of involvement that they experienced in middle age (Havighurst, 1963). Retirees who led active and socially involved lives and who participated in many groups and organizations presumably enjoyed their later years more than those who mostly stayed at home and avoided these activities. Although several studies (e.g., Albrecht, 1951; Havighurst, 1957) have shown strong associations between high levels of activity and well-being, many well-adjusted retirees enjoy their solitude.

Baltes and Smith (1999) and Baltes and Carstensen (1999) proposed a *theory of selective optimization with compensation* as an alternative model for successful aging. They emphasized older persons' resiliencies and compensatory capacities, and believed that as people aged they compensated for age declines and readjusted their priorities, values, and expectations according to more realistic criteria. These theorists maintained that older persons who took advantage of the freedoms and opportunities that retirement offered, reinvested in previously neglected interests, and developed new skills and activities would age successfully.

Critical Gerontologists (e.g., Ovrebo & Minkler, 1993) adopted a broader view of aging that considered the impact of political and socioeconomic influences on aging. They analyzed discriminatory policies and institutional ideologies that accounted for significant retirement gaps between men and women, and between Whites and other minorities in pension coverage, Social Security benefits, and other retirement resources. Their view of retirement is more integrated. They recognize structural *and* individual influences on retirement and the interplay between these.

Feminist Gerontologists (e.g., Hooyman & Gonyea, 1995) have criticized traditional models of retirement for ignoring life-long gender and race inequities. They point to systemic inequities in many women's investments in caregiving. These theorists examine how oppressive institutions,

policies, and ideologies have prevented many older persons from achieving their potential. They are especially interested in the diversity of people's experiences and on how gender, ethnicity, social class, and sexual preference influence people's retirements.

The results from studies on retirement have identified several factors that influence retirement satisfaction. They include socioeconomic status, health, family relations (specifically marriage and caregiving), voluntary retirement, social support, and retirement preparation.

Socioeconomic status, which includes income and occupational status, is the most significant predictor of retirement satisfaction. Richardson and Kilty (1991) found adjustment problems during the six months following retirement among less affluent people who experienced substantial reductions in income and among women of low occupational status. The stresses that these women experience have enormous costs. They result in emotional distress, low self-esteem, and excessive anxiety. People with inadequate incomes during retirement must live more restricted lives, engage in more limited types of leisure, and they worry more about their finances, their health, and access to medical care. More women and minority persons would enjoy their later years if they had adequate funds to invest in the future.

Health is the second most significant predictor of retirement satisfaction (Palmore, Fillenbaum, & George, 1984). Retirees in poor health often have lower morale than those in good health in part because mental and physical well-being are often interrelated. Unhealthy retirees spend more time on health maintenance activities, such as visiting doctors and hospitals, which can interfere with socializing and leisure pursuits. Retirees should continue annual check-ups and routine screenings because many illnesses are preventable.

Marital status is another predictor of retirement satisfaction. Married retirees adjust better and are less susceptible to depression and social isolation than unmarried retirees. Although many couples describe making adjustments immediately following retirement, most revitalize their relationships at this time when work and parental obligations are less demanding. Marital strain, spousal conflict, and lower marital satisfaction are more common when wives continue working after their husbands retire (Szinovacz & Schaffer, 2000). Arber and Ginn (1995) observed that despite trends toward mutual decision-making in marriages, men are more likely than women to pressure their spouses to retire.

Strong social supports also promote retirement satisfaction. Research consistently demonstrates that people with confidantes and close friends adjust better to retirement (Lowenthal & Haven, 1968). Many leisure activities require the company of others. Retirees who maintain friendships outside of work and cultivate broad social ties throughout life usually have various people to socialize with during retirement.

Finally, workers who prepare for retirement adjust better than those who are unprepared; many retirement problems arise from poor planning. Health professionals should encourage people to prepare comprehensively for retirement and consider lifestyle as well as financial issues.

STRATEGIES THAT WORK

Lack of preparation is a major impediment to retirement satisfaction. Preretirement Planning Programs can effectively help potential retirees plan for and adjust better to retirement. Several studies demonstrate an association between those who participate in preretirement planning seminars and satisfaction with retirement (Monk, 1985). Those who prepare have a better idea of their retirement needs, more favorable attitudes toward retirement, higher morale, and fewer longings for the old job than unprepared retirees (Teaff & Johnson, 1983).

Preretirement Planning Programs usually focus on finances, but comprehensive programs cover recreation and hobbies, housing options, advance directives, health care, and successful aging. Trained group leaders usually facilitate discussions, and people with expertise on various topics, such as financial experts, lawyers, health care specialists, housing specialists, accountants, insurance experts, and representatives from the Social Security Administration, Medicare, and state government often speak at these meetings. Many retirees worry about becoming mentally and physically incapacitated and burdening their family members. Retirement planning programs that address long-term care issues can ease these anxieties by encouraging workers to anticipate these problems.

Vocational counseling and on-the-job training can effectively assist older people who must work because of inadequate retirement resources. Many low income older persons will delay retirement, especially if they are healthy enough to remain employed. Work, particularly part-time work, increases retirees' earnings, socializing, and activity levels. Involuntary retirees who become depressed also need help identifying options and employment alternatives. The *Job Training Partnership Act* (JTPA) of 1982 as well as The *Senior Community Service Employment* program were created to help older persons find jobs. These employment programs help elderly persons find jobs at schools, hospitals, parks, and government facilities, although most of these jobs are part-time with low wages (Schulz, 2001). Some private agencies also offer job services for older persons, but few provide training for those who wish to enhance their skills. Contrary to previous assumptions, older workers respond well to training, especially when the training programs are designed specifically for them (Sterns & Doverspike, 1989).

Although most training programs ignore broader influences that affect what jobs people work at, the pay they receive, whether they work continuously or intermittently, and whether they have pensions, older persons who participate in these programs benefit from their involvement and experience high levels of well-being (Kim, 1998).

Retirement policies that expand the options for older persons will help more people retire successfully. Most older persons believe that they must either work full-time at their primary job or retire completely, but when given the option, they often prefer to work fewer hours (Moen, Erickson, Agarwal, Fields, & Todd, 2000). The more options and resources people have when making retirement decisions the more they will feel they retired voluntarily.

The *Phased Retirement Liberation Act*, which was introduced in July 2000, will allow employers greater flexibility in their retirement programs as more and more organizations strive to retain older workers. In a study of several major firms, Graig and Paganelli (2000) found that phased retirement options were already available in a few organizations and that workers *and* employers benefited from gradual retirements, partial retirements, and part-time work. In addition, the elimination of mandatory retirement laws and the end of the earnings test for Social Security eligibility have made it easier for older persons to work in their later years. Nearly three quarters (72 percent) of workers aged 70 and older now work on a part-time basis (National Academy of Aging, 2000). Because retirement is rarely a single event at a single point in time, many people gradually shift from full-time work to part-time or part-year work, sometimes with a different employer or in a different occupation. Prevention approaches that take into account the personal choices people make about their jobs, marriages, and families within the context of systemic influences that affect these decisions, will more successfully emancipate older persons from constraints imposed by involuntary or unplanned retirements.

STRATEGIES THAT MIGHT WORK

Preretirement planning counselors or organizers should also consider the many structural barriers that affect how well people are able to plan for their later years. For example, people need financial resources to prepare for retirement. Workers at low-paying jobs lack adequate funds to invest in retirement, and their employers rarely provide preretirement programs or pension benefits. Preretirement programs can address the needs of low-income retirees by including information on relevant social services and postretirement employment, specifically programs to help older persons find jobs. Companies could create mutual help associations comprised of employees and potential retirees.

Several studies that have evaluated preretirement counseling programs indicate that they effectively facilitate adjustment to retirement. After randomly assigning men to a control group or two experimental preretirement planning groups, Glamser and Dejong (1975) found that those who attended planning programs felt more prepared for retirement and had more plans than members of the control group. Taylor-Carter, Cook, and Weinberg (1997) compared an informal retirement planning group that included planning for leisure time and a more formal planning seminar. They found that those who planned more broadly for retirement had higher levels of self-efficacy than those in the more limited preretirement group. Both groups showed improvements in their expectations about retirement, however.

In an elaborate study comparing four types of preretirement groups, Tiberi, Boyack, and Kerschner (1978) reported that emotionally charged retirement topics elicited more anxiety and negative feelings if participants had no opportunities to process affective material. Shouksmith (1983) also found that some individuals experienced negative feelings after preretirement counseling. Disparate findings about the effectiveness of preretirement planning programs may be attributable in part to differences in designs, samples, and programs; negative outcomes may result if participants are given too little time to process information about retirement. Thus, preretirement planning programs might work best when they include time for participants to share their reactions. Whether an individual or group approach is taken in preretirement counseling, dialogue, expression of affect, any necessary grief counseling, and planning for the future should be emphasized.

People who experience postretirement adjustment problems, such as depression and anxiety, can improve with individual or group counseling. Age-specific interventions, such as cognitive–behavioral therapy and treatments for late life alcoholism, should be accessible to retirees working through mental health issues. Several studies have confirmed the efficacy of cognitive therapy for older persons who are depressed (Thompson, Gallagher, & Breckenridge, 1987). Interpersonal therapy is especially appropriate for older persons who are struggling with loss and grief, interpersonal disputes, role transitions, and interpersonal deficits. Antidepressants also help many depressed older persons, but clinicians must closely monitor the adverse side effects that occur more frequently in this age group. These interventions should be culturally sensitive and include traditional *and* nontraditional outreach strategies to accommodate the growing number of retirees from diverse ethnic backgrounds.

STRATEGIES THAT DO NOT WORK

The dearth of comprehensive preretirement planning programs that offer workers guidance on multiple levels in multiple areas is unfortunate.

Most programs focus solely on financial preparation, which help future retirees anticipate their expenses, such as housing and medical costs. But these programs fail to prepare retirees for transitions they will experience in their families, their social networks and daily routines. Moen, Kim, and Hofmeister (2001) found, for example, that during the initial transition to retirement, marital satisfaction declined and marital conflict increased if one spouse retired and the other remained employed. Planning programs that ignore these broader lifestyle issues will inadequately prepare people for retirement. Generic preretirement planning programs that ignore gender and cultural variations also fail to attract older women and persons of color who generally avoid preretirement seminars (Richardson, 1990). In an analysis of retirement preparation, Szinovacz (1991) found that while financial planning improved retirement satisfaction among men, only planning for activities influenced women's adjustment.

Retirement reforms, such as privatization, will exacerbate current gender and ethnic inequities for several reasons. First, one needs income and resources to invest. Women invest less often because their wages are lower than men's. Second the risks and costs involved in successfully managing private accounts are too high for many older persons, particularly, women and minorities, who more often have discontinuous and unstable work trajectories. Finally, as women spend more and more time at caregiving, which is likely to increase in the next century, they will take more part-time jobs, which rarely provide investment opportunities.

Other proposals to reform retirement include increasing Social Security's survivor benefits, raising benefits for people over the age of 80, and redefining minimum benefits; each has advantages and disadvantages. However retirement policies are changed, experts must consider the effects of proposed changes on older persons over time and within the context of medical and long term care expenditures. Most importantly, they must evaluate the impact any changes might have on divorced or separated and minority persons.

SYNTHESIS

Multilevel interventions that encourage older persons to plan for retirement and concomitantly emphasize reforms in retirement policies will promote retirement satisfaction among a broader constituency of older persons. Such holistic interventions assume that adjustment to retirement is affected by interactions that occur between individuals and their environments, between social and economic factors, and within the private and public spheres. Although many contemporary conceptualizations of retirement are consistent with these ideas, few retirement prevention programs operate on multiple levels or use holistic interventions.

Retirement programs that expand available retirement options, including phased or partial retirement, training for older workers, and caregiving credits, as well as retirement policies that address retirement inequities in wages, pensions, and health care will enhance retirement for many older persons. Unjust gender and ethnic differences in wages, especially during the young adult years, must be eradicated, and women who work in female-dominated professions should receive comparable wages to men who work in similar jobs. Social Security rules that penalize married working women who earn less than their husbands must also be reformed. Special attention must be paid to older women of color who have the least access to pensions despite continuous work histories in full time employment. Systemic inequities that discriminate against women and women's life-long involvement in caregiving must be transformed before retired women can achieve parity with retired men. One strategy that some countries, for example, the United Kingdom, Germany, and Japan, have already instituted is to offer caregiving or homemaker credit to those who stay out of the labor force to raise children or maintain a household (Schulz, 2001).

Most retirement problems are avoidable, but they must be addressed on micro and macro levels. For example, pre-retirement planning, one of the most important predictors of successful retirement, is influenced by one's education, occupational status, income, ethnic background, type of employment, and commitment to work. It is also affected by one's gender, family responsibilities, and work history. The most successful prevention interventions will consider how these multiple influences impact people's planning for retirement. Health professionals must also advocate for large, social structural changes that will take into account the aging population and the increasing number of years that people will spend in retirement.

Baby boomers will reach retirement age in a decade in which experts will thoroughly scrutinize extant policies on work and retirement. Baby boomer retirees, who will be the most healthy, educated, and diverse cohort in history, will demand retirement options that are flexible and gratifying. They will also seek training and educational opportunities that will keep them competitive at work. Social Security reforms will be needed to accommodate the aging population. Additional reforms will also be required because many older women and minorities will remain impoverished despite their advances in the work force. Women will still outlive men and receive fewer and lower retirement benefits in the next century (Anzick & Weaver, 2001).

The historical trends are disheartening. In an analysis of income changes among Social Security beneficiaries in 1982 and 1992, Gregoire, Kilty, & Richardson (in press) found that the most impoverished—Latino, Black and White single females—improved the least while the most affluent—White married men and White married women—gained the most income over a 10-year period.

Experts have proposed various options to correct these inequities. One option involves targeting Social Security benefits to the most vulnerable older women, especially divorced women and women over the age of 80. Another is to universally increase minimum benefits. No reforms will succeed unless they take into account the rising divorce rates, protracted retirements, and long-term care costs (Choudhury, Leonesio, Utendorf, Del Bene, & Gesumaria, 2001; Smeeding, Estes, & Glasse, 2001).

Baby boomers who prepare well for their retirements can avoid many later problems, including ennui, poverty, and expensive long-term care costs. People can boost their retirement satisfaction by planning early and prudently for lifestyle *and* financial changes that inevitably occur in retirement. People can also work to guarantee an adequate income for *all* retirees by advocating for retirement policies that are fair and equitable.

Also see: Age Bias; Caregiver Stress; Chronic Disease, Older Adulthood; Crises of Aging, Depression, Older Adulthood; Health Promotion; Life Challenges; Loneliness/Isolation; Sexuality, Older Adulthood.

References

Albrecht, R. (1951). The social roles of older people. *Journal of Gerontology, 6*, 138–145.

Arber, S., & Ginn, J. (1995). Choice and constraint in the retirement of older married women. In S. Arber & J. Ginn (Eds.), *Connecting gender and ageing* (pp. 69–86). Philadelphia: Open University Press.

Anzick, M., & Weaver, D. (2001). *Reducing poverty among elderly women.* Social Security Administration: Office of Policy and Office of Research, Evaluation, and Statistics Working Paper Series Number 87.

Baltes, P., & Carstensen, L. (1999). Social-psychological theories and their applications to aging: From individual to collective. In V. Bengston & K.W. Shaie (Eds.), *Handbook of theories of aging* (pp. 209–226). New York: Springer.

Baltes, P., & Smith, J. (1999). Multilevel and systemic analyses of old age. In V. Bengston & K.W. Shaie (Eds.), *Handbook of theories of aging* (pp. 153–173). New York: Springer.

Bureau of Labor Statistics. (2000). *Employment & earnings* (Vol. 47[8]). Washington, DC: US Department of Labor.

Choudhury, S., Leonesio, M., Utendorf, K.L., Del Bene, L., & Gesumaria, R. (2001). *Analysis of Social Security Proposals intended to help women: Preliminary results.* Social Security Administration: Office of Research, Evaluation, and Statistics Working Paper Series No. 88.

Gendall, M., & Siegel, J. (1992). Trends in retirement age by sex, 1950–2005. *Monthly Labor Review, July*, 22–29.

George, L., & Maddox, G. (1977). Subjective adaptation of loss of the work role: A longitudinal study. *Journal of Gerontology, 39*, 364–371.

Gibson, R. (1987). Reconceptualizing retirement for black Americans. *Gerontologist, 27*, 691–698.

Glamser, F., & Dejong, G. (1975). The efficacy of preretirement preparation programs for industrial workers. *Journal of Gerontology, 30*, 599–600.

Graig, L., & Paganelli, V. (2000). Phased retirement: Reshaping the end of work. *Compensation and Benefits Management, 16*, 1–10.

Gregoire, T., Kilty, K. & Richardson, V. (in press). Gender and racial inequities in retirement resources. *Journal of Women and Aging.*

Hatch, L.R., & Thompson, A. (1992). Family responsibilities and women's retirement. In M. Szinovacz, D. Ekerdt, & B. Vinick (Eds.), *Families and retirement* (pp. 99–113). Newbury Park: Sage.

Havighurst, R. (1957). The social competence of middle-aged people. *Genetic Psychology Monograph, 56,* 297–375.

Havighurst, R. (1963). Successful aging. In R. William, C. Tibbits, & W. Donahue (Eds.), *Processes of aging* (Vol. 1, pp. 299–320). New York: Atherton Press.

Hooyman, N., & Gonyea, J. (1995). *Feminist perspectives on family care.* Thousand Oaks, CA: Sage.

Kim, J.H. (1998). *The influence of employment on older Korean-American economic self-sufficiency, psychological well-being, status, and social support: Impact evaluation of Senior Community Service Employment Program (SCSEP).* Unpublished doctoral dissertation, University of Southern California.

Kim, M. (1992). *Retirement attitudes, preparations, conceptualizations and behavioral intentions among first-generation Korean Americans in midlife.* Unpublished doctoral dissertation, The Ohio State University, Columbus, Ohio.

Lowenthal, M., & Haven, C. (1968). Interaction and adaptation: Intimacy as a critical variable. *American Sociological Review, 33,* 20–30.

Margolis, S., & Rabins, P. (1997). *The Johns Hopkins White Papers: Depression and Anxiety.* New York: Medletter Associates.

Moen, P., Kim, J., & Hofmeister, H. (2001). Couples' work/retirement transitions, gender, and marital quality. *Social Psychology Quarterly, 64,* 55–71.

Moen, P., Erickson, W., Agarwal, M., Fields, V., & Todd, L. (2000). *The Cornell Retirement and well-being study: Final report.* Syracuse: Syracuse University.

Monk, A. (1985). *Handbook of gerontological services.* New York: Van Nostrand Reinhold.

National Academy on an Aging Society. (2000). *Who are young retirees and older workers.* Washington, DC: Author.

O'Rand, A., & Henretta, J. (1999). *Age and inequality.* Boulder: Westview Press.

Ovrebo, B., & Minkler, M. (1993). The lives of older women: Perspectives from political economy and the humanities. In T. Cole, W. Achenbaum, P. Jakobi, & R. Kastenbaum (Eds.), *Voices and visions of aging: Toward a critical gerontology* (pp. 289–308). New York: Springer.

Palmore, E., Fillenbaum, G., & George, L. (1984). Consequences of retirement. *Journal of Gerontology, 39,* 109–116.

Peretti, P., & Wilson, C. (1978–1979). Contemplated suicide among voluntary and involuntary retirees. *Omega, 9,* 193–201.

Purcell, P. (2000). Older workers: Employment and retirement trends. *Monthly Labor Review, 123,* 19–30.

Richardson, V.E. (1990). Gender differences in retirement planning among educators: Implications for practice with older women. *Journal of Women and Aging, 2,* 27–40.

Richardson, V.E., & Kilty, K.M. (1991). Adjustment to retirement: Continuity vs. discontinuity. *International Journal of Aging and Human Development, 33,* 151–169.

Schulz, J.H. (2001). *The economics of aging* (7th ed.). Westport, CT: Greenwood.

Smeeding, T. Estes, C., & Glasse, L. (1999). *Social Security reform and older women: Improving the system.* Center for Policy Research, Maxwell School of Citizenship and Public Affairs. Syracuse: Syracuse University.

Social Security Adminstration. (2000). *Income of the population 55 or older* (SSA Publication No. 13-11871). Washington, DC: Office of Policy, Office of Research, Evaluation, and Statistics.

Sterns, H., & Doverspike, D. (1989). Aging and the training and learning process. In I.L. Goldstein (Ed.), *Training and development in organizations* (pp. 299–332). San Francisco: Jossey-Bass.

Shouksmith, G. (1983). Change in attitude to retirement following a short preretirement planning seminar. *Journal of Psychology, 114,* 3–7.

Szinovacz, M., & DeViney, S. (1999). The retiree identity: Gender and race differences. *The Journals of Gerontology, 54B,* S207–S218.

Szinovacz, M., & Schaffer, A. (2000). Effects of retirement on marital conflict tactics. *Journal of Family Issues, 21,* 367–389.

Taylor-Carter, M., Cook, K., & Weinberg, P. (1997). Planning and expectations of the retirement experience. *Educational Gerontology, 23,* 273–288.

Teaff, J., & Johnson, D. (1983). Preretirement education: A proposed bill for tution tax credit. *Educational Gerontology, 9,* 31–36.

Thompson, L., Gallagher, D., & Breckenridge, J. (1987). Comparative effectiveness of psychotherapies for depressed elders. *Journal of Consulting and Clinical Psychology, 55,* 385–390.

Tiberi, D., Boyack, V., & Kerschner, P. (1978). A comparative analysis of four preretirement education models. *Educational Gerontology, 3,* 355–374.

US Bureau of the Census. (2000a). *Statistical abstract of the United States: 2000* (120th ed.). Washington, DC: US Government Printing Office.

US Bureau of the Census. (2000b). *The older population in the United States: March 1999.* Available: http://www.census.gov/prod/2000pubs/p20-532.pdf [2001, 1/14/01].

US House Select Committee on Aging. (1992). *Retirement Income for Women.* Washington, DC: Government Printing Office, Hearing before the subcommittee on retirement income and employment of the Select Committee on Aging, House of representatives.

Wan, T., & Odell, B. (1983). Major role losses and social participation of older males. *Research on Aging, 5,* 173–196.

Zsembik, B., & Singer, A. (1990). The problem of defining retirement among minorities: The Mexican-Americans. *The Gerontologist, 30,* 749–757.

S

Schizophrenic Expression, Adolescence

Judy A. McCown

INTRODUCTION AND DEFINITIONS

Schizophrenia is a phenomenon that is infused with confusion, anxiety, and dread. Although the causes of schizophrenia remain unclear, research has made considerable progress, in understanding the symptoms, predicting the progress and identifying effective interventions for this disease. This entry considers possible efforts to prevent the expression of schizophrenia, admittedly an exploration or inference based on what is currently known on this topic.

In 1893, Kraepelin described the symptoms of a baffling syndrome he called "dementia praecox" to denote the early onset and deteriorating course of the disorder (Harms, 1971). The term "schizophrenia" comes from the Greek words meaning "split mind" and many people mistakenly believe that this disorder refers to individuals who have multiple personalities. In fact, the term was intended to refer to the disconnection among thinking, feeling, and behavior (Bleuler, 1950). Schizophrenia is a mental disorder that is manifested by a combination of characteristics that are categorized broadly as positive and negative symptoms. Positive symptoms are more active behaviors and include hallucinations, delusions, disorganized speech and thought, and disorganized or catatonic or bizarre behaviors. Negative symptoms reflect deficits in functioning and include dampening of emotions, decrease in verbal productivity, and inability to initiate or sustain goal-directed activity. Because the manifestation of schizophrenia can be variable from person to person and even within individuals, diagnosis and prognosis of the disorder are challenging.

SCOPE

Schizophrenia is a disease with profound impact on individuals and society. Each year in the United States, 100,000 people are newly diagnosed with schizophrenia (Torrey, 1983). In a 10-country study by the World Health Organization (Jablensky et al., 1992) incidence rates ranged from 0.7 to 1.4 per 10,000 using narrowly defined criteria to 1.6 to 4.2 per 10,000 using more broadly defined diagnostic criteria. Reports of lifetime prevalence rates show variability reflecting the problems of heterogeneity of diagnostic criteria and impact of cultural factors. Using strict criteria, Kendler, Gallagher, Abelson, and Kessler (1996) found a 0.15 percent lifetime prevalence of schizophrenia in the United States. The Irish Roscommon Study (Kendler & Walsh, 1995) found lifetime prevalence rates of 0.54 percent in men and 0.25 percent in women. The Mini Finland Health Survey (Lehtinen et al., 1990) produced a 1.3 percent lifetime prevalence rate. Using contemporary criteria, the results of the Environmental Catchment Area study by the NIMH suggest that the lifetime prevalence rate for the disorder is 1 percent, translating into over 2 million people per year being affected in the United States and Canada (Reiger, Rae, Narrow, Kaelber, & Schatzberg, 1998). When cultural variability is controlled for, this prevalence rate is stable across cultures and ethnic groups, indicating that schizophrenia affects approximately 45 million people worldwide (Jablensky et al., 1992). Men and women are equally affected, although there may be gender differences in the age of onset and in the course of the disease.

Although the lifetime prevalence rate for schizophrenia is lower than other mental disorders, the economic burden incurred as a result of this disease is staggering. In the United States alone, approximately $65 billion per year is spent in direct costs for treatment and in indirect costs evidenced from loss of productivity in those afflicted and their families, social service expenditures, and related criminal justice costs (Noll, 2000). Approximately one fourth of all mental health costs are expended as a consequence of schizophrenia, vastly out of proportion to the percentage of cases in the population.

THEORIES AND RESEARCH

Onset of schizophrenia typically occurs in late adolescence or early adulthood. Males tend to develop symptoms between the ages of 15 and 25 years while females are more likely to become symptomatic between 25 and 35 years of age. The course of this disease is hallmarked by patterns of relapse and remission, with repeated hospitalizations as needed. Longitudinal studies indicate that approximately 50 percent of those afflicted will have poor outcome with lifelong impairment, 20–30 percent will improve with intermittent hospitalizations, and 20–30 percent will experience moderate symptoms which can be managed with medications and out-patient treatment (Breier, Schreiber, Dyer, & Pickar, 1991; Harrow, Sands, Silverstein, & Goldberg, 1997). The course of schizophrenia varies greatly among affected individuals. Development of schizophrenic symptoms may occur acutely or follow a more gradual, insidious progression. Most people will experience more than one episode of pronounced positive symptoms followed by periods of remission in which negative symptoms may continue. Prognosis is variable depending on the age of onset, gender, level of functioning before the first episode, and family history. In general, women tend to have higher premorbid functioning, more affective symptom presentation, and better prognosis than men. Men with schizophrenia are more likely to demonstrate earlier age of onset, more negative symptoms and poorer prognosis (American Psychiatric Association, 2000).

Causes of Schizophrenia

Explanations for the origins of schizophrenia have focused on biological and environmental domains. Some early theories considered degenerative brain abnormalities as a possible explanation for the symptoms of the disease (Bleuler, 1950; Kraepelin, 1911, 1971) while others looked to psychosocial factors such as pathological child rearing and family interaction dysfunction as sources for the development of this disorder (Bateson, Jackson, Haley, & Weakland, 1956; Fromm-Reichmann, 1948; Lidz, Cornelison, & Fleck, 1958). Current research finds no evidence that parenting practices or family problems are causally related to the occurrence of schizophrenia. However, it has been noted that family environment and highly critical and over controlling communication patterns appear to influence the course of the disorder (Leff & Vaughn, 1985).

The consensus of modern research indicates that schizophrenia is a disease of the brain, which is caused by an inherited genetic vulnerability that interacts with certain environmental and psychosocial stressors to produce the symptoms of schizophrenia. The exact mechanism of this process remains unclear but many studies have made significant progress in identifying possible components.

Genetic Factors

Studies of families of individuals afflicted with schizophrenia have demonstrated convincingly that biological relatives of schizophrenics have a greater risk of developing the disease. First-degree relatives of schizophrenics are 10 times more likely to develop schizophrenia than the rate in the general population (Kety, 1987). Furthermore, relatives of afflicted individuals are also at greater risk for other disorders known as the schizophrenic spectrum disorders including schizoaffective disorder, nonaffective psychoses, and schizotypal and paranoid personality disorder (Kendler, McGuire, Gruenberg, Spellman, O'Hare, & Walsh, 1993).

The findings of studies of monozygotic and dizygotic twins who are discordant for schizophrenia allow researchers to explore the roles of genetic and environmental factors in the development of schizophrenia. Monozygotic twins share 100 percent of their genetic material. If genetic factors are solely responsible for the development of schizophrenia, both twins should always develop the disease. However, studies have demonstrated that concordance rates for monozygotic twins vary from 33 to 78 percent. Furthermore, concordance rates for same-sex dizygotic twins range from 8 to 28 percent (Gottesman, 1991). These findings suggest that while vulnerability for schizophrenia is indeed inherited, environmental factors are also important, if not the controlling influence in some cases.

Neurological Factors

Brain-imaging techniques using computed tomography (CT), magnetic resonance imaging (MRI), and positron emission tomography (PET) have suggested several anomalies that appear to be related to schizophrenia. Ventricular enlargement, gross reduction of cerebral gray matter, and reduced metabolism in the frontal lobes are among the findings that have been noted that may be related to positive and negative symptoms in persons with schizophrenia (Andreasen et al., 1992; Bogerts, Lieberman, Ashtari, Bilder, Degreet, & Lerner, 1993; Gur & Pearlson, 1993; Schlaepfer et al., 1994).

Neurodevelopmental theories suggest that schizophrenia may develop as a result of prenatal stressors that occur during the second trimester of pregnancy—a critical time in brain development (Weinberger, 1987). Prevalence studies indicate that a higher proportion of people with schizophrenia are born during winter months. Possible explanations for this seasonal variation point to in-utero exposure to viral infections during the flu-prone months (Pallast, Jongbloet, Straatman, & Zielhuis, 1994). Other possible prenatal risk factors include poor maternal nutrition (Susser & Lin, 1992), poverty (Cohen, 1993), and delivery complications (Dalman, Allebeck, Cullberg, Grunewald, & Koster, 1999), once again connecting environmental events with schizophrenic expression.

Several neurotransmitter systems have been implicated in the development of schizophrenia. The dopamine hypothesis suggests that schizophrenia is the result of overactivity of the dopaminergic neurons (Abi-Dargham, Gil, Kristal, Baldwin, Selby, & Bowers, 1998). However, this explanation is controversial since dopaminergic hyperactivity is noted in other disorders and may, in fact, be related to long-term use of antipsychotic medications (Mackay et al., 1982). Investigations of possible neurotransmitter dysfunction have broadened to examine other neurotransmitters such as the seratonin, noradrenergic, and glutamate systems (Harrison, 1999; Inayama et al., 1996).

Environmental Factors

Besides environmental factors, which may impinge on prenatal neurological development, certain psychosocial variables have been correlated with the development of schizophrenia. Early psychoanalytic theories (Fromm-Reichmann, 1948) suggested that maladaptive mother–child relationships contributed to the escalation of schizophrenic symptoms, but there are no data to support these ideas and this theory is no longer accepted today. However, several studies have noted a strong association between stressful life events and high levels of family conflict and the risk of schizophrenia. The vulnerability model of schizophrenia (Zubin & Spring, 1977) suggests that an inherited predisposition for the disorder is triggered by exposure to significant life stressors. A World Health Organization study (Day et al., 1987) found higher rates of life stress combined with decreased medication compliance in the three weeks preceding the onset of psychotic symptoms.

Although no evidence exists that family environment directly leads to the development of schizophrenia, several studies have noted the correlation between conflicted home environments and relapse. A specific focus of research has been the impact of expressed emotion on schizophrenic functioning. *Expressed emotion* is defined as a familial interaction style characterized by criticism, hostility, emotional over involvement, and controlling behaviors (Leff & Vaughn, 1985). Among adult patients who live with their families or who have frequent contact with their families, expressed emotion is a significant predictor of relapse and re-hospitalization (Kavanaugh, 1992; Kuipers & Bebbington, 1988).

STRATEGIES: OVERVIEW

For decades, schizophrenia was regarded as an unfortunate but inevitable legacy for those predisposed to the disease. However, more recently researchers have been encouraged to explore areas of preventive interventions that may prove fruitful. Prevention strategies are typically categorized with respect to the timing of the intervention and the targeted population. *Primary prevention* interventions are implemented prior to the onset of symptoms. *Secondary prevention* strategies are employed early in the course of an illness and attempt to inhibit the development of chronic disability. *Tertiary prevention* tactics emphasize approaches that enable afflicted individuals to adapt to the limitations of a disorder and to develop strategies to maintain a satisfactory level of functioning. *Population-based interventions* focus on particular groups of people. Universal preventive interventions are intended for the general population and do not require identifying at-risk individuals. *Selective interventions* are aimed at those people who are susceptible to a disorder but who are asymptomatic. *Indicated preventive* interventions are targeted to those who manifest prodromal symptoms or biological markers for a disorder but do not meet the criteria for diagnostic classification (Munoz, Mrazek, & Haggerty, 1996).

Traditionally, prevention strategies in schizophrenia have largely been focused at the secondary and tertiary levels. Early interventions in first episode cases have demonstrated considerable success in truncating the debilitating course of the disease. Well-coordinated treatment programs have evidenced positive outcomes in preserving functioning and preventing relapse in chronic individuals. Several of these approaches will be discussed later in this entry.

In recent years, researchers have begun to seriously explore the efficacy of interventions at the level of primary prevention. Responding to compelling evidence of schizophrenia's devastating severity in personal, societal, and economic domains, concerted efforts are being made to develop models for primary prevention research and to identify prevention strategies to consider.

To productively investigate the efficacy of primary preventive interventions for schizophrenia, accurate identification of the at-risk population is critical. As noted earlier, schizophrenia is a particularly heterogeneous disorder.

Attempts to identify young people who are asymptomatic and who will develop the disease are likely to result in a high rate of false positives. Using an epidemiological approach, Jablensky (2000) proposed a screening model involving two risk criteria—positive family history and deficit performance on neurocognitive measures. However, the reliability of the results from a hypothetical screening program using these criteria was unsatisfactory. Other researchers propose using Meehl's (1962) concept of "schizotaxia" to identify premorbid status. *Schizotaxia* refers to the physiological vulnerability to developing schizophrenia that is demonstrated by mild negative symptoms, reduced brain volume, and abnormal brain activation in first-degree relatives of individuals with schizophrenia. Tsuang, Stone, and Faraone (2000) state that because schizophrenia is a neurodevelopmental disorder, there are a number of features that develop before the first episode of psychosis. They suggest that identification of those features could be used to detect those at risk. Along a similar vein, Olin and Mednick (1996) recommend identifying two types of precursors to psychosis. First, etiologic factors like family history of psychiatric illness, obstetric complications, neurobehavioral deficits, and family dysfunction can be noted. Second, signs of latent mental illness including psychosis-prone personality styles and teacher ratings of social anxiety and withdrawal, inadequate interpersonal/social skills, and behavioral problems can be assessed. They suggest that using a combination of these two risk factors in a screening protocol may be a useful strategy for pinpointing vulnerable individuals.

STRATEGIES THAT WORK

Clear evidence is not yet available.

STRATEGIES THAT MIGHT WORK

Although research into primary prevention for schizophrenia is still in its infancy, a number of possible approaches are being investigated. Some of these strategies are quite controversial and raise serious ethical questions. Other approaches are already being used as secondary and tertiary tactics and may be productive if introduced earlier in the course of the disease and/or as universal or selective methods.

Probably the most debatable strategy involves the prophylactic use of antipsychotic medications. Tsuang et al. (2000) proposed a two-phase research protocol using schizotaxia indicators to evaluate the usefulness of pharmacological interventions. They recommend giving antipsychotic medication to first-degree adult relatives of schizophrenics and assessing the impact on subthreshold symptoms. Preliminary data from a small sample appear promising with

indications of reduced negative symptoms in these subjects. Evidence suggests that intervention during the premorbid phase (i.e., before the onset of psychosis) may allow brain plasticity to be retained (McGlashan & Johannessen, 1996). In a review of the literature and discussion of preliminary data from clinic experience, McGorry (2000) proposed the use of low doses of risperidone and cognitive therapy with an indicated population—high-risk individuals with mild signs of schizophrenia. Early findings suggest that such interventions result in a decrease of psychotic symptoms. However, given the unreliability of screening measures to accurately identify at-risk individuals and a number of other ethical issues, such strategies are extremely controversial.

A less contentious approach to prevention targets psychosocial interventions. Both as primary and secondary interventions, these strategies seem to hold promise. Two areas in particular—problem solving and family relationships—have been investigated at the secondary intervention level and are now being explored as applicable as primary interventions.

Falloon (2000) has proposed a training program for at-risk individuals, schizophrenic patients and their personal resource groups that focuses on combining education about mental illness with the development of effective personal problem-solving skills. With proficient problem-solving skills, more efficient management of life stress is possible. Looking at the development of schizophrenia from a vulnerability/diathesis stress perspective, decreased stress is associated with prevention or delay of symptom onset. Building on a standard model of structured problem solving (D'Zurilla & Goldfried, 1971), Falloon suggests that training in stress management, goal setting, and identification and activation of social support networks can significantly decrease the rate of recurrence of psychotic episodes. In a pilot study of a 6-session intervention program for secondary school-age children, substantial decreases in referrals for psychological and social crises were found and consumer satisfaction with the protocol was high. Although this model has only been tested in one controlled study (Falloon & Pederson, 1985), there are several factors which suggest that it may be applicable as a universal primary prevention strategy which would benefit not only those at risk for schizophrenia but for other mental illness as well. It is a simple program that can be presented within the context of schools or community-based mental health programs. It requires limited resources and has widespread applicability. Several studies are being conducted to explore the efficacy of this prevention model with various selective populations.

A second domain for development of possible primary prevention strategies for selective populations involves family relationships—specifically with respect to expressed emotion (EE). As mentioned previously, family communication patterns characterized by criticism and emotional over-involvement are associated with increased rates of relapse and re-hospitalization of individuals with schizophrenia. Some researchers suggest that high EE may be included as a source of significant stress that may adversely affect vulnerable persons. Patterson, Birchwood, and Cochrane (2000) propose that identifying the early precipitants of EE in families can inform possible interventions. They suggest that family members' feelings of loss, grief, and guilt may be factors in the development of high levels of criticism and emotional over-involvement. They propose that family intervention programs be developed to evaluate the impact of these variables in primary prevention strategies.

Finally, researchers have speculated on the efficacy of universal primary prevention strategies. Because accurate identification of at-risk individuals is fraught with difficulty, tactics, which could be introduced to the general population are being considered. McGrath (2000) suggests that the first step in developing universal interventions should involve identifying "risk-modifying factors" that have causal impact on the etiology of schizophrenia. He proposes that antenatal and perinatal factors such as prenatal infection, birth complications, and prenatal nutrition are the best targets for universal interventions. Suggested population-based options include general improvement of antenatal health care, preconception counseling, smoking cessation programs, mass vaccinations especially for influenza and rubella, and improved maternal nutrition. Such interventions have the added advantage of benefiting a wide range of individuals and being effective in the possible prevention of not only schizophrenia but also other mental and medical illness.

Ethical Considerations in Primary Prevention

Early intervention in the etiologic process of schizophrenia is an important albeit challenging proposition. Although potentially beneficial, primary prevention of schizophrenia carries a number of risks and raises some thorny ethical issues. In a review of contemporary considerations, Rosen (2000) addressed concerns related to research priorities, screening, and assessment.

The reality of the current state of knowledge regarding the etiology and prevention of schizophrenia is that no irrefutable evidence exists that specifies the causes of the disorder or that guarantees that certain interventions will prohibit its development. Given that status, any primary preventive measures must be considered experimental. One of the problems that must be considered is whether or not research is being conducted largely for the sake of scientific inquiry or if there is a priority for clinical application.

As mentioned previously, accurate identification of a selective and indicated population is an ambiguous endeavor. The screening process is imperfect and must be scrutinized for problematic procedures. Because of its deficiencies, screening for schizophrenia may lead to persons being labeled as "at risk" which may lead to stigmatization. Others such as family members, teachers, and physicians who become aware of this status (whether accurate or not) may perceive the individual differently. Furthermore, being labeled as "high-risk" may cause an individual undue anxiety and depression. Screening procedures must be carefully considered to maximize confidentiality. Informed consent in writing should always be obtained.

If screening warrants further assessment, other considerations must be taken into account. Rosen (2000) suggests that ideally the assessment process should be mutually beneficial for both the researcher and the subject. It should preserve participants' sense of privacy, avoid being overly technical and not be too intrusive or too lengthy.

Overall, ethical concerns in primary prevention should focus on respect for the individual. In some cases, individuals may prefer not to know about the potential for developing schizophrenia and this perspective should be honored. Some studies have challenged this expectation (Peterson, 2000; Turner, 2000) demonstrating that many people find assessment feedback helpful and want to be informed as to the disease course, prognosis, and possible treatment. However, given the potentially devastating impact of schizophrenia on an individual's and family's life, every consideration must be made in developing primary preventive interventions. The development of guidelines addressing these and other ethical concerns is an immediate priority even as research proceeds in this area.

Other Prevention Strategies

Although preventing the onset of schizophrenia is the most desirable objective, a number of secondary and tertiary measures have been implemented which demonstrate significant benefits to persons evidencing manifestations of early or first episodes of symptomatology. Schizophrenia is now considered a highly treatable disease. With greater understanding of the etiology of the disorder, early intervention is possible which allows patients, families, and mental health professionals to work collaboratively to effectively manage the course of the symptoms, improve the level of functioning and prevent relapse and extend remission. Treatment of schizophrenia is critical across all phases of the illness—acute episodes, stabilization periods following exacerbations, and maintenance or long-term recovery phases. The efficacy of several treatment interventions has been empirically supported (Drake et al., 2000) and expert recommendations for prevention and treatment have been developed (Lehman & Steinwachs, 1998; Weiden, Scheifler, McEvoy, Frances, & Ross, 1999). The consensus among mental health professionals is that treatment interventions should include a coordinated program of medication, psychotherapy, and social support services.

Medication

The recent report of the Surgeon General of the United States on mental health (US Department of Health and Human Services, 1999) recommends that the first-line of treatment for schizophrenia should be the use of antipsychotic medications. One of the strongest predictors for long-term remission of psychotic symptoms and for prevention of relapse is the consistent use of antipsychotic medication (Lehman & Steinwachs, 1998). Developing an effective medication regimen ideally involves a coordinated effort by the treating physician and the patient. Individual response to medication can vary greatly depending on symptom severity and the phase of the illness. However, stabilization of the troublesome and often distressing symptoms of schizophrenia is important as it allows individuals to participate and respond to other forms of intervention.

Pharmacological treatment of schizophrenia has made significant progress since the introduction of the first antipsychotic medications over 50 years ago. Today, two categories of medication are available—conventional and atypical antipsychotic medications.

Conventional antipsychotic medications such as chlorpromazine and haloperidol have demonstrated effectiveness in reducing positive symptoms by blocking dopamine D2 receptors (Dixon, Lehman, & Levine, 1995). Used for treatment of acute psychotic episodes and for long-term maintenance, these medications unfortunately produce a number of unpleasant side effects such as tremors, muscle rigidity, spasms, and tardive dyskinesia. Approximately 40 percent of patients experience these side effects and compliance with the medication regimen is problematic (US Department of Health and Human Services, 1999). Furthermore, conventional antipsychotics have little effect on the treatment of negative symptoms. For these reasons, these medications are less frequently prescribed. However, for patients who are noncompliant with oral medication recommendations, long-acting injections of conventional antipsychotics are recommended (Lehman & Steinwachs, 1998).

A newer group of medications called atypical antipsychotics have been developed which are reported to be as effective as conventional medications for treatment of positive symptoms with fewer side effects (Kane & Marder, 1993). These medications are called "atypical" because their mechanism is different from earlier medications. It is believed that the atypical antipsychotics work by blocking both the dopamine D2 and serotonin 5-HT2 systems. One of the first of the atypical antipsychotics was clozapine, which has been shown to be particularly effective with treatment-resistant patients. However, clozapine has been associated with the development of agranulocytosis, a decrease in the number of white blood cells needed to fight infection, in approximately 1 percent of patients, so those using this medication must submit to weekly monitoring of blood levels (Meltzer, 1997). Because of this potentially life-threatening complication, clozapine is rarely prescribed until other medications have been found ineffective.

Most recently, risperidone, olanzapine, and quetiapine have been included in the pharmacological armamentarium for treatment of schizophrenia. These atypical antipsychotics are as effective as older medications for the treatment of positive symptoms, do not cause troublesome side effects, and do not require the kind of follow-up associated with clozapine (Lieberman, 1993). Furthermore, these medications seem to be effective in the treatment of negative symptoms, although it has been suggested that this may actually be related to the absence of extrapyramidal symptoms and the decrease in positive symptoms (Marder & Meibach, 1994). The high level of efficacy of these medications combined with lack of unpleasant side effects translates into improved compliance.

If medication conformity is problematic, relapse is much more likely. It is important to determine the reasons for noncompliance and to intervene as soon as possible. If unpleasant side effects are the cause, other medications may be recommended or adjunctive medications may be added to manage the side effects. If the issue is related to the patient's inability or unwillingness to take the medication, a long-acting injectable medication may be offered. In any case, consistent involvement in pharmacological treatment efforts is critical. It is recommended that patients continue on antipsychotic medication for at least one year following stabilization of symptoms before dosage reduction should be considered (Lehman & Steinwachs, 1998). With successful management of symptoms, participation in adjunctive interventions such as psychotherapy and social support services is more likely to be beneficial.

Psychotherapy

Therapeutic intervention can take many forms but consensus among mental health professionals is that treatment should focus on the practical aspects of coping with schizophrenia. Individual and/or group therapy can help patients to learn about the nature of schizophrenia, to develop strategies and skills to monitor and manage medications and to identify the warning signs of relapse. Supportive therapy can provide reassurance to help patients cope with the anxiety and depression that often accompanies living with schizophrenia. Behavioral therapy can be effective in increasing skills necessary for day-to-day functioning in such areas as money management, household chores, and personal hygiene. Cognitive therapy helps patients cope with the stigma of having a chronic mental illness and learn alternative, adaptive ways of responding to everyday demands and situations (Kingdon, Turkington, & John, 1994). Group therapy can be particularly helpful in decreasing social isolation and increasing social support (Scott & Dixon, 1995).

Psychoeducational family interventions can help family members understand what schizophrenia is and how it affects their own family. People with schizophrenia must often rely on family members to assist them in finding appropriate treatment and in accessing support services. Family members often feel overwhelmed and isolated and may need supportive therapy themselves. Family support groups in the community are often very helpful in these circumstances.

Families with high levels of expressed emotion may benefit from cognitive behavioral family therapy that can help them learn to communicate and problem-solve more effectively. In turn, improved communication can help to prevent relapse and lead to improved relationships for all involved (Tarrier, Barrowclough, Porceddu, & Fitzpatrick, 1994). Therapy groups consisting of several families may be helpful in developing a support network for both patients and family members.

Beyond formal therapeutic interventions, some individuals with schizophrenia may benefit from self-help groups. After symptoms have stabilized, participation in a peer support group may provide opportunities for discussion, sharing, and socialization that are especially important in order to maintain adaptive functioning.

Social Support Services

Individuals with schizophrenia may need to seek out various social services to help them manage their illness and maintain a satisfying level of functioning. Available services will vary from community to community but some of the more common systems of care include hospitalization, partial hospitalization, day treatment aftercare, case management, assertive community treatment (ACT), and rehabilitation programs, .

At times of acute exacerbations of psychotic symptoms, persons with schizophrenia may require hospitalization. This becomes particularly important if individuals are experiencing severe hallucinations or delusions and may be suicidal or in danger of harming others. Since approximately 10 percent of people with schizophrenia commit suicide, appropriate response to acute episodes is vital.

Once symptoms are stabilized, follow-up care may include partial hospitalization or day treatment aftercare. Partial hospitalization typically includes intensive treatment several days per week with medication management and individual and group therapy. Day treatment is usually less structured but also serves as a transitional program between acute phase care and maintenance.

Case management and assertive community treatment (ACT) both involve in-home follow up. Individual case managers or multidisciplinary teams work directly with schizophrenic individuals to offer intensive support services. Patients who have had a severe and unstable course of illness often need extensive support to maintain adequate functioning and these types of interventions allow them to avoid hospitalization and have a higher quality of life than would otherwise be possible.

Rehabilitation programs generally focus on helping an individual acquire the skills needed to assume an active role in the community. A review of the literature by Mueser, Drake, and Bond (1997) outlined components of rehabilitation programs that were deemed essential for effective intervention. These included developing specific behavioral goals, focusing on long-term strategies, and providing interventions in naturalistic settings whenever possible. Rehabilitation programs usually provide training in several areas including personal goal setting, development of job, independent living and social skills, assistance with housing arrangements, and development of social support networks (World Health Organization, 1997).

SYNTHESIS

This entry has examined schizophrenia from the perspective of prevention. Although it is a disease, which has a relatively low prevalence rate, its impact is significant in terms of economic burden and decreased quality of life for those afflicted and their families. Research into the etiology of schizophrenia indicates that it is likely caused by the interaction of inherited genetic vulnerability and environmental and psychosocial stressors.

A clearer understanding of causation sets the stage for research into strategies that may help prevent or delay the onset of schizophrenic symptoms, preserve healthy levels of functioning and prevent relapse and re-hospitalization. A significant body of work has been developed regarding secondary and tertiary preventive interventions focusing on a coordinated program of medication, psychotherapy, and social support services. More recently, in response to awareness of the chronic deleterious impact of schizophrenia on individuals and society, researchers have been encouraged to develop models for primary prevention.

Selective and indicated preventive measures require being able to accurately identify at-risk individuals. Because of the heterogeneous nature of schizophrenia, this process is challenging and, at present, very unreliable. Studies are being conducted to develop models for screening and assessment, which will improve reliability. Concurrently, primary intervention models are being investigated which build upon known etiologic theories.

Because the onset of schizophrenia most commonly occurs in late adolescence or early adulthood, primary prevention measures are targeted toward a younger population. One controversial tactic proposes administering antipsychotic medication to at-risk youngsters before the onset of psychotic symptoms. Other research has investigated the use of psychosocial interventions including structured problem-solving training, mental health education, and family communication programs. Universal prevention strategies are also being developed that target prenatal infection, birth complications, and prenatal nutrition as viable avenues for primary preventive interventions.

Although the goal of prevention of schizophrenia is generally accepted as valuable, ethical issues in primary intervention must be considered. Current concerns include the experimental status and unproven efficacy of primary preventive measures, the risk of false positives resulting from inaccurate screening methods, and the repercussions of stigmatization from being labeled "at risk" for schizophrenia.

At the present time, the development of primary prevention models for schizophrenia is in its earliest stages. Serious methodological and ethical consideration is being given to accurate identification of those who are most vulnerable to this devastating disorder. As these efforts bear fruit, early intervention may allow us to circumvent the course of this disease and provide true relief to those afflicted and their families.

Also see: Children, Parents with Mental Illness; Chronic Disease entries; Families with Parental Mental Illness; Family Strengthening entries.

References

Abi-Dargham, A., Gil, R., Kristal, J., Baldwin, R., Selby, J., & Bowers, M. (1998). Increased striatal dopamine transmission in schizophrenia: Conformation in a second cohort. *American Journal of Psychiatry, 155*, 761–767.

American Psychiatric Association. (2000). *Diagnostic and statistical manual of mental disorders* (4th ed., text revision). Washington, DC: Author.

Andreasen, N., Rezai, K., Alliger, R., Swayze, V., Flaum, M., Kirchener, P., Cohen, G., & O'Leary, D. (1992). Hypofrontality in neuroleptic-naive patients and in patients with chronic schizophrenia: Assessment with xenon 133 single-photon emission computed tomography and the Tower of London. *Archives of General Psychiatry, 49*, 943–958.

Bateson, G., Jackson, D., Haley, J., & Weakland, J. (1956). Toward a theory of schizophrenia. *Behavioral Science, 1*, 251–264.

Bleuler, E. (1950). *Dementia praecox or the group of schizophrenias* (J. Zinkin, Trans.). New York: International Universities Press. (Original work published 1911).

Bogerts, B., Lieberman, J., Ashtari, M., Bilder, R., Degreet, G., & Lerner, G. (1993). Hippocampus-amygdala volumes and psychopathology in chronic schizophrenia. *Biological Psychiatry, 33*, 236–246.

Breier, A., Schreiber, J., Dyer, J., & Pickar, D. (1991). National Institute of Mental Health longitudinal study of chronic schizophrenia: prognosis and predictors of outcome. *Archives of General Psychiatry, 48*, 239–246.

Cohen, C. (1993). Poverty and the course of schizophrenia: Implications for research and policy. *Hospital and Community Psychiatry, 44*, 951–958.

Dalman, C., Allebeck, P., Cullberg, J., Grunewald, C., & Koster, M. (1999). Obstetric complications and the risk of schizophrenia. *Archives of General Psychiatry, 56*, 234–240.

Day, R., Neilsen, J., Korten, A., Emberg, G., Dube, K., Gebhart, J., Jablensky, A., Leon, C., Marsella, A., Olatawura, M., Sartorius, N.,

Stromgren., E., Takahashi, R., Wig, N., & Wynne, L. (1987). Stressful life events preceding the acute onset of schizophrenia: A cross-national study from the World Health Organization. *Culture, Medicine and Psychiatry, 11*, 123–206.

Dixon, L., Lehman, A., & Levine, J. (1995). Conventional antipsychotic medications for schizophrenia. *Schizophrenia Bulletin, 21*, 567–577.

Drake, R., Mueser, K., Torrey, W., Miller, A., Lehman, A., Bond, G., Goldman, H., & Leff, H. (2000). Evidence-based treatment of schizophrenia. *Current Psychiatry Reports, 2*(5), 393–397.

D'Zurilla, T., & Goldfried, M. (1971). Problem solving and behavior modification. *Journal of Abnormal Psychology, 78*, 107–126.

Falloon, I. (2000). Problem solving as a core strategy in the prevention of schizophrenia and other mental disorders. *The Australian and New Zealand Journal of Psychiatry, 34*(Suppl.), 185–190.

Falloon, I., & Pederson, J. (1985). Family management in the prevention of morbidity of schizophrenia: The adjustment of the family unit. *British Journal of Psychiatry, 147*, 156–163.

Fromm-Reichmann, F. (1948). Notes on the development of treatment of schizophrenics by psychoanalytic psychotherapy. *Psychiatry, 11*, 263–273.

Gottesman, I. (1991). *Schizophrenia genesis: the origins of madness*. New York: W.H. Freeman.

Gur, R., & Pearlson, G. (1993). Neuroimaging in schizophrenia research. *Schizophrenia Bulletin, 19*, 337–353.

Harms, E. (1971). Emil Kraepelin's dementia praecox concept: An introduction. In: Kraepelin, E. *Dementia praecox and paraphrenia* (R. Barclay, Trans.). Huntington, New York: Krieger (Original work published 1911).

Harrison, P. (1999). The neuropathology of schizophrenia: A critical review of the data and their interpretation. *Brain, 122*, 593–624.

Harrow, M., Sands, J., Silverstein, M., & Goldberg, J. (1997). Course and outcome for schizophrenia versus other psychotic patients: A longitudinal study. *Schizophrenia Bulletin, 23*, 287–303.

Inayama, Y., Yoneda, H., Sakai, T., Ishida, T., Nonomura, Y., Kono, Y., Takahata, R., Koh, J., Sakai, J., Takai, A., Inada, Y., & Asaba, H. (1996). Positive association between a DNA sequence variant in the serotonin 2A receptor gene and schizophrenia. *American Journal of Medical Genetics, 67*, 103–105.

Jablensky, A. (2000). Prevalence and incidence of schizophrenia spectrum disorders: implications for prevention. *The Australian and New Zealand Journal of Psychiatry, 34*(Suppl.), S26–S38.

Jablensky, A., Sartorius, N., Ernberg, G., Anker, M., Korten, A., Cooper, J., Day, R., & Bertelsen, A. (1992). Schizophrenia: Manifestations, incidence and course in different cultures. A World Health Organization ten-country study. *Psychological Medicine, 20*(Suppl.), 1–97.

Kane, J., & Marder, S. (1993). Psychopharmacologic treatment of schizophrenia. *Lancet, 346*, 820–825.

Kavanaugh, D. (1992). Recent developments in expressed emotion and schizophrenia. *British Journal of Psychiatry, 160*, 601–620.

Kendler, K., Gallagher, T., Abelson, J., & Kessler, R. (1996). Lifetime prevalence, demographic risk factors, and diagnostic validity of non-affective psychosis as assessed in a US community sample. *Archives of General Psychiatry, 53*, 184–192.

Kendler, K., McGuire, M., Gruenberg, A., Spellman, M., O'Hare, A., & Walsh, D. (1993). The Roscommon family study: II. The risk of non-schizophrenic nonaffective psychoses in relatives. *Archives of General Psychiatry, 50*, 645–652.

Kendler, K., & Walsh, D. (1995). Gender and schizophrenia: Results of an epidemiologically-based family study. *British Journal of Psychiatry, 167*, 1022–1031.

Kety, S. (1987). The significance of genetic factors in the etiology of schizophrenia: Results from the national study of adoptees in Denmark. *Journal of Psychiatric Research, 21*, 423–429.

Kingdon, D., Turkington, D., & John, C. (1994). Cognitive behaviour therapy of schizophrenia. *British Journal of Psychiatry, 164,* 581–587.

Kraepelin, E. (1971). *Dementia praecox and paraphrenia* (R. Barclay, Trans.). Huntington, New York: Krieger (Original work published 1911).

Kuipers, L., & Bebbington, P. (1988). Expressed emotion research in schizophrenia: Theoretical and clinical applications. *Psychological Medicine, 18,* 893–909.

Leff, J., & Vaughn, C. (1985). *Expressed emotion in families.* New York: Guilford Press.

Lehman, A., & Steinwachs, D. (1998). Translating research into practice: The Schizophrenia Patient Outcomes Research Team (PORT) treatment recommendations. *Schizophrenia Bulletin, 24,* 1–10.

Lehtinen, V., Joukamaa, M., Lahtela, K., Raitasalo, R., Jyrkinen., E., Maatela, J., & Aromaa, A. (1990). A prevalence of mental disorders among adults in Finland: Basic results from the Mini Finland Health Survey. *Acta Psychiatrica Scandinavica, 81,* 418–425.

Lidz, T., Cornelison, A., & Fleck, S. (1958). The transmission of irrationality. *Archives of Neurology and Psychiatry, 79,* 305–316.

Lieberman, J. (1993). Understanding the mechanism of action of atypical antipsychotic drugs. A review of compounds in use and development. *British Journal of Psychiatry, 22*(Suppl.), 7–18.

Mackay, A., Iversen, L., Rossor, M., Spokes, E., Bird, E., Arregui, A., Creese, I., & Snyder, S. (1982). Increased dopamine and dopamine receptors in schizophrenia. *Archives of General Psychiatry, 39,* 991–997.

Marder, S., & Meibach, R. (1994). Risperidone in the treatment of schizophrenia. *American Journal of Psychiatry, 151,* 825–835.

McGlashan, T., & Johannessen, J. (1996). Early detection and intervention with schizophrenia: Rationale. *Schizophrenia Bulletin, 22*(2), 201–222.

McGorry, P. (2000). The nature of schizophrenia: Signposts to prevention. *The Australian and New Zealand Journal of Psychiatry, 34*(Suppl.), S14–S21.

McGrath, J. (2000). Universal interventions for the primary prevention of schizophrenia. *The Australian and New Zealand Journal of Psychiatry, 34*(Suppl.), S58–S64.

Meehl, P. (1962). Schizotaxia, schizotypy, schizophrenia. *American Psychologist, 17,* 827–838.

Meltzer, H. (1997). Treatment-resistant schizophrenia—The role of clozapine. *Current Medical Research Opinion, 14,* 1–20.

Mueser, K., Drake, R., & Bond, G. (1997). Recent advances in psychiatric rehabilitation for patients with severe mental illness. *Harvard Review of Psychiatry, 5,* 123–137.

Munoz, R., Mrazek, P., & Haggerty, R. (1996). Institute of Medicine report on prevention of mental disorders. Summary and commentary. *American Psychologist, 51*(11), 1116–1122.

Noll, R. (2000). *The encyclopedia of schizophrenia and other psychotic disorders* (2nd ed.). New York: Facts on File.

Olin, S., & Mednick, S. (1996). Risk factors of psychosis: Identifying vulnerable populations premorbidly. *Schizophrenia Bulletin, 22*(2), 223–240.

Pallast, E., Jongbloet, P., Straatman, H., & Zielhuis, G. (1994). Excess seasonality of births among patients with schizophrenia and seasonal ovopathy. *Schizophrenia Bulletin, 20,* 269–276.

Patterson, P., Birchwood, M., & Cochrane, R. (2000). Preventing the entrenchment of high expressed emotion in first episode psychosis: Early developmental attachment pathways. *The Australian and New Zealand Journal of Psychiatry, 34*(Suppl.), 191–197.

Peterson, D. (2000). The ethics of research into schizophrenia prevention: A carer's perspective. *The Australian and New Zealand Journal of Psychiatry, 34*(Suppl.), 201–203.

Reiger, D., Rae, D., Narrow, W., Kaelber, C., & Schatzberg, A. (1998). Prevalence of anxiety disorders and their comorbidity with mood and addictive disorders. *British Journal of Psychiatry, 34*(Suppl.), 24–28.

Rosen, A. (2000). Ethics of early prevention in schizophrenia. *The Australian and New Zealand Journal of Psychiatry, 34*(Suppl.), 208–212.

Schlaepfer, T., Harris, G., Tien, A., Peng, L., Lee, S., Federman, E., Chase, G., Barta, B., & Pearlson, G. (1994). Decreased regional cortical gray matter volume in schizophrenia. *American Journal of Psychiatry, 151,* 842–848.

Scott, J., & Dixon, L. (1995). Psychological interventions for schizophrenia. *Schizophrenia Bulletin, 21,* 621–630.

Susser, E., & Lin, S. (1992). Schizophrenia after prenatal exposure to the Dutch Hunger Winter of 1944–1945. *Archives of General Psychiatry, 49,* 983–988.

Tarrier N., Barrowclough, C., Porceddu, K., & Fitzpatrick, E. (1994). The Salford Family Intervention Project: Relapse rates of schizophrenia at five and eight years. *British Journal of Psychiatry, 165,* 829–832.

Torrey, E. (1983). *Schizophrenia: A family manual.* New York: Harper and Row.

Tsuang, M., Stone, W., & Faraone, S. (2000). Towards the prevention of schizophrenia. *Biological Psychiatry, 48*(5), 349–356.

Turner, G. (2000). Presymptomatic screening for schizophrenia: A geneticist's perspective. *The Australian and New Zealand Journal of Psychiatry, 34*(Suppl.), 204–207.

US Department of Health and Human Services. (1999). *Mental health: A report of the surgeon general.* Rockville, MD: Author.

Weiden, P., Scheifler, P., McEvoy, J., Frances, A., & Ross, R. (1999). Expert consensus treatment guidelines for schizophrenia: A guide for patients and families. *Journal of Clinical Psychiatry, 60*(Suppl. 11), 3–80.

Weinberger, D. (1987). Implications of normal brain development for the pathogenesis of schizophrenia. *Archives of General Psychiatry, 44,* 660–669.

World Health Organization. (1997). Psychosocial rehabilitation: A consensus statement. *International Journal of Mental Health, 26,* 77–85.

Zubin, J., & Spring, B. (1977). Vulnerability—A new view of schizophrenia. *Journal of Abnormal Psychology, 8,* 103–126.

School Absenteeism, Childhood

Fabricio E. Balcazar and
Christopher B. Keys

INTRODUCTION

The problem of school absenteeism in childhood has been identified in the literature as a potential precursor of serious academic problems and eventual dropout during adolescence. This is why it is important to intervene early. This entry reviews the issues associated with the definition of school absenteeism, as well as various intervention models that have been developed to address the problem. Most effective intervention models include a combination of school-based and community-based approaches. It should be recognized that these models do require systemic changes at the family, school, and community levels.

The studies suggest that the complex contexts of the children, their families, their schools, and their communities are not only part of the problem but also part of the solution.

DEFINITIONS

Most children may miss a few days of school each year due to common illnesses and other excusable circumstances. These events usually do not have serious consequences to the child, and teachers provide the supports to avoid academic problems. On the other hand, the problem of *school absenteeism* occurs when some children fail to attend school regularly and their absences affect their academic performance. *School absenteeism* has typically being associated with students' refusal to attend school or with truancy (Cooper, 1986). The difference between these two terms is subtle and perhaps best characterized in terms of the reasons for not attending school. Issues associated with *school refusal* include children with serious social and emotional problems, fears and/or stress (Robinson & Rotter, 1991). Increasingly, and particularly in large urban school districts, children are refusing to attend school because of fears of violence (Massey, 1998). In some cases, school absenteeism is also related to teasing (Freedman, 1999), or the onset of serious medical problems or disability (US Department of Education, 1994).

Truancy is another form of school absenteeism associated with a series of educational and/or emotional difficulties that result in a pattern of school non-attendance that eventually leads the student to be forced to repeat grades or drop out. Irving and Parker-Jenkins (1995) also suggest that, in some cases, truancy is a manifestation of school-generated problems, such as boredom and underachievement. One important difference in the classification of students with school refusal problems versus truants is the response from schools and parents. In general, students who experience refusal to attend school receive treatment and accommodations, while truants are typically punished, often with unsuccessful results.

SCOPE

School absenteeism can lead to children falling behind their peers in their academic work, which can lower their self-esteem and, in some cases, result in having to repeat a grade. This forced retention can have additional negative social consequences for the child, in some cases exacerbating the problem and leading to continued poor academic performance and dropout. Absenteeism is detrimental to students' achievement, promotion, self-esteem, and employment potential (DeKalb, 1999). Robins and Ratcliff (1978, cited by DeKalb, 1999) conducted a longitudinal study of African American male

students and found that 75 percent of those who were often truant in elementary school and truant in high school failed to graduate. Truancy is indeed a predictor of early school desertion, which in turn has been associated with reduced earning potential in adulthood and other poor outcomes such as early pregnancy and juvenile delinquency. In fact, Garry (1996) reported that the Los Angeles County Office of Education identifies truancy as the most important predictor of juvenile delinquency. She added that police departments across the United States report that many students not in school during regular hours are committing crimes, including vandalism and shoplifting. Truancy seems to increase the risk of incarceration or dropping out from school.

Incidence and Prevalence Cases Per Year. School absenteeism is typically determined in terms of daily records of school attendance. The problem has been extensively studied in several countries (for instance, see Hyman, 1990 and Reid, 1984, for a sample of analyses of the problem in the United Kingdom; Desnoyers & Pauker, 1988, in Canada; Gill, 1997, in Ireland; and Fergusson, Horwood, & Shannon, 1986, in New Zealand). In the United States, there are some problems with the national database because states utilize different criteria in their reports. For example, until the 1990–1991 school year, California included excused absences in their report, while other states did not (National Center for Education Statistics, 1999). During the 1996–1997 school year, there were a total of 46,127,194 children enrolled in public elementary and secondary schools in the United States. The average daily attendance for that year was 42,261,976 (not including excused absences); thus, an average of 8.38 percent of the enrolled students or 3,865,218 were missing from school in any given day (National Center for Education Statistics, 1999).

Very large school districts in the United States have average daily attendance records that are lower than the national average. For example, in 1996, the New York City Public School System reported an average of 15 percent absentees (almost 150,000 unexcused children) per day; the Los Angeles Public School District reported a 10 percent absenteeism rate (62,000 unexcused children); and the Chicago Public Schools reported an average of 9.4 percent absentees (40,000 unexcused children) per day (Garry, 1996). The trend in Chicago, however, seems to be gradually improving since the 1993–1994 school year, when the daily attendance average was 88.2 percent to an average of 90.2 percent during the 1998–1999 school year. Unfortunately, the national reports do not separate elementary and secondary students. In the Chicago Public School System, where these data were available, the average daily attendance rate for elementary students was 92.1 percent (which was below the state average of 93.6 percent), with high school students having a lower attendance rate of 83 percent in the

1998–1999 school year. If representative, these data suggest that absenteeism problems increase for adolescents.

Potential Costs to Society. Experts agree (e.g., DeKalb, 1999; Garry, 1996) that school absenteeism can be the beginning of a series of events that may lead to early school leaving and in many cases criminal activity, with the accompanying consequences of minimum wage jobs and limited career opportunities. Truant students are at higher risk of being drawn into behavior involving drug and alcohol use, or violence. Wish, Gray, and Levine (1996), reported that 51 percent of female juvenile detainees not in school at the time of their arrest tested positive for drugs. There are additional costs to students and their families when youth get pregnant or become involved in the juvenile justice system. Garry (1996) argued that truancy generates multiple costs to society at various levels: School districts lose hundreds of millions of dollars each year in Federal and State funds that are reimbursements based on daily attendance records. Businesses also lose money because they pay more to train uneducated workers. Finally, taxpayers pay higher taxes to cover increased welfare, law enforcement, and prison costs, and to offset the lower revenue resulting from dropouts who are underemployed.

THEORIES

The problem of school absenteeism—whether it be related to school refusal or truancy—can be conceptualized from an ecological perspective, which considers that the behaviors of the children cannot be understood without consideration of the ecological context in which such behavior takes place (Kelly, 1979). School refusal problems associated with fears and school-related anxiety have been effectively analyzed and treated with systematic desensitization and cognitive-behavioral interventions (Robinson, Rotter, Fey, & Robinson, 1991). In the case of truancy, multiple factors and experiences appear to contribute to the problem. For instance, Traux (1985) used a literature review to develop a general profile of the habitually absent student or truant, and identified key factors that influence such absenteeism. He found that older and less popular students were most likely to be absent. Peer pressure not to attend school, disorganized classroom and school environments, lack of parental involvement, and lower socio-economic status of the community seemed to be the strongest predictors of school absenteeism. He also found some evidence that habitually absent students were characterized by lower academic achievement rates, lower IQ scores, and lower grades.

Several researchers (e.g., Barnes, 1998; Fine, 1986) have found that a central factor influencing school absenteeism and dropout is the lack of engagement or bonding between students and their schools. Based on that premise, Hawkins (1997) has connected his social development model of healthy and health-risk behaviors to academic success. He argues that increasing student commitment and attachment to school is critical for promoting academic achievement and preventing absenteeism and dropout. He argues that the children's ability to bond to school is the result of three principles: First, it is important that the school environment provides the child multiple opportunities for active involvement in his/her own educational process (active learning). Second, it is important that the child experience multiple opportunities to use and develop appropriate social, emotional, and cognitive skills in the school. Third, it is important that the students be consistently reinforced for appropriately using their social, emotional, and cognitive skills. These principles suggest important elements of prevention interventions by increasing the connections and engagements between the students and their school environments. These principles are common to most successful intervention programs in this area.

RESEARCH

Cooper (1986) noted that most absenteeism research has either concentrated on school refusal or truancy. School refusal has been explained frequently in terms of problems with emotional and social development. Truancy, on the other hand has been described in terms of dissatisfied youth, and much attention has been given to the home background. Cooper argued that school refusers often feel lonely in spite of belonging to protective and often indulging families. He also found that these same feelings were not strongly expressed by adolescent truants, with the evidence pointing to a more neglectful, non-caring family environment.

Some researchers have examined multiple personal and contextual factors that appear to influence chronic absenteeism among students. For example, Reid (1984) conducted an investigation of the social, psychological, and educational factors involved in persistent school absenteeism involving 384 third, fourth, and fifth grade students from Wales, UK. The participants were divided into three equal groups (*n* = 128 each), representing an experimental group of school absentees and two control groups matched for sex and age. The participants were evaluated in a number of factors, and the findings showed that persistent absentees came from socially disadvantaged backgrounds and enjoyed less permanent economic security at home than controls. Forty-six percent of absentees reported having committed undetected offenses (e.g., vandalism). Self-concept was lower among persistent absentees than among controls, and absentees displayed greater alienation from school than did controls. In addition, absentees tended to report more negative perceptions about school, had fewer career aspirations, and disliked subjects that are more difficult like math and English. They had a more pessimistic view about the possibility of improving their school performance and tended to disagree with the controls about the appropriateness of the punishment imposed for absenteeism in the school. In a previous study, Reid (1981) found that students with high absenteeism rates reported not having anybody to turn to in the school to discuss their personal problems, which accentuated their feelings of alienation. In addition, a great proportion of school absentees were inclined to blame their institutions, rather than personal or psychological factors, for their behavior (Reid, 1983).

Hansen, Sanders, Massaro, and Last (1998) examined possible relations among socio-demographic, clinical, and familial variables and level of school absenteeism in children with anxiety-based school refusal. Participants were 76 children referred to treatment for anxiety-based school refusal who exhibited a great deal of variability in the severity of the symptoms, from occasional absences to pervasive school absenteeism. Regression analyses revealed that older age, lower levels of fear, and families with little involvement in school activities were primary predictors of greater levels of school absenteeism.

Lee (1999) conducted an ethnographic study of students with low achievement and absentee records at risk of dropping out from an inner city high school and found several additional contextual factors at play. The students complained that their teachers' lectures were boring and inhibited interactions between teachers and students. Students felt that teachers did not express themselves well, which negatively influenced their desire to participate in class. The students felt unchallenged and disengaged in the school. It is precisely this lack of engagement that has been cited in several studies of dropout students as a central factor influencing students' decision to drop (e.g., Barnes, 1998; Jordan, Lara, & McPartland, 1996). At the same time, many minority youth attending low-income inner city schools are confronted with teachers who have very low expectations of their students' success, and therefore are unsupportive or unchallenging (Fine, 1986). In fact, some minority students feel discriminated against based on teachers' negative stereotypes or perceptions and said that teachers did not seem to care for them (Lee, 1999).

In sum, the problem of school absenteeism is closely related to personal and contextual factors that seem to contribute to its origins and maintenance over time. Children who refuse to attend school due to fears or anxiety often find a more supportive response from school personnel and their families, and therapy or counseling become the avenue to address the problem. Children who miss school for no "apparent reason" are often called truants. However, their persistent absenteeism has many reasons. We concur with researchers who argue that truancy is a manifestation of school-generated problems that interact with negative contextual factors in the lives of many children. This conceptualization requires interventions to re-structure the school environment and re-define the role of the parents and other community members in the education of the children.

STRATEGIES THAT WORK

As the previous section suggests, effective intervention strategies to reduce and/or prevent school absenteeism must include multiple components in order to address the personal and contextual factors of the problem. Several models of educational reform have been developed to address common school performance issues and be a part of an overall school-improvement plan. The following are brief descriptions of four models that illustrate how the principles discussed by Hawkins (1997) can be incorporated into classroom, school, and family activities to prevent later academic and absenteeism problems.

Success for All

This model is designed to raise the achievement of the students in low-performing schools (Madden, Slavin, Karweit, Dolan, & Wasik, 1991). It is predicated on the premise of early academic success, which increases self-esteem and bonding with the school environment (reducing the risk of truancy). It uses everything known from research on effective instruction, to prevent and intervene in the development of learning problems in the early years (pre-k to sixth grade). The model promotes the development of pro-social skills by encouraging cooperation and mutual support. Specific elements of the program include: (1) cooperative learning (this is the central tenet of this model; students work together in teams—helping one another—with an emphasis on accountability, common goals, and recognition of team success); (2) tutors (who give one-on-one assistance to students who are failing, particularly during the first grade); (3) facilitators (who work with teachers and families to make sure every child is making adequate progress); (4) assessments every 8 weeks (to determine students' progress and re-assign student reading levels, tutoring, and supports as necessary); and (5) family support teams (a team of school administrators works with families to promote parent involvement, develop plans to address issues of tardiness and absenteeism, and make referrals to needed community services). This program has been experimentally evaluated and implemented in many schools across the United States. Compared to control group members, Success for All participants score about 3 months higher in first grade and

1.1 years higher in fifth grade on standard reading measures. Grade retention and placements in special education have also declined significantly. Discipline and attendance problems in schools that start implementing this model have also decreased compared with records prior to the program implementation (Madden, Slavin, Karweit, Dolan, & Wasik, 1993).

Adaptive Learning Environments Model (ALEM)

This model was developed by the Laboratory for Student Success at Temple University and has been evaluated and replicated over the last 20 years (Wang, 1992). The model emphasizes individual differences among students, recognizing that students learn in different ways, at different rates, and with differing amounts of instructional support. The implementation of the model includes the following components: (1) individualized progress plans (which include highly structured prescriptive components for basic skills mastery, and exploratory components to allow the students to try self-direction and problem solving while fostering personal and social development). (2) A diagnostic-prescriptive monitoring system (which assesses students' mastery of the subject matter). (3) A classroom instruction-management system (which provides classroom supports to students and team teaching; the program also includes peer-teaching and cooperative learning). (4) A databased professional development program (which provides ongoing training and technical assistance to meet the implementation needs of individual teachers). (5) A school-based restructuring process (which provides school and classroom organizational support and re-deployment of school resources to achieve and sustain the program implementation goals). (6) An active program of family involvement (which is targeted to meet the individual needs and issues of each child). The teacher circulates among the students, instructing and providing corrective feedback. Learning tasks are broken down into incremental steps, frequently providing opportunities for evaluation. Multiple replications of the model indicate positive changes that lead to intended academic, attitudinal, and social competence outcomes. Students tend to be highly task-oriented, and teachers spend more time in instruction-related activities. Students also demonstrate high levels of self-responsibility in managing their behaviors and the classroom learning environment, decreasing both discipline and absenteeism problems (Sobehart, 1991; Wang & Zollers, 1990).

Consistency Management and Cooperative Discipline Model

This model is based on the assumption that the responsibility for learning and classroom organization should be shared by students and teachers (Freiberg, 1998).

The program provides consistent messages to students about what it means to be self-disciplined and evaluates school climate and discipline referrals throughout the school year. The teacher creates a consistent but flexible learning environment and joins with students to establish a cooperative plan for classroom rules, use of time, and academic learning, that governs the classroom in a democratic framework. Students are partners and stakeholders in the classroom, from creating a classroom constitution to establishing new student job responsibilities for some 50 tasks that teachers usually take upon themselves. The model was first implemented in the Houston School District at the elementary school level. Evaluations of the model have shown sustained academic gains over 3 years of follow up; significant reductions in student discipline referrals to the office, including unexcused absences (48–80 percent fewer referrals than in previous years); and more direct instruction time (an average of 36 more minutes a day due to fewer discipline problems and greater student cooperation). Replications of the model have shown that when students and teachers see each other as partners, the instructional climate improves for both teachers and students (Freiberg, Stein, & Huang, 1995).

The School Transitional Environmental Project (STEP)

This program is a preventive intervention for students experiencing problems in their transition into middle school and high school (Felner et al., 1993). The program employs a school restructuring and transformation approach to prevent problems associated with school transition, and create a school environment that enhances development. Key elements of the model include: (1) reorganizing the school social system. The school environment is re-arranged so program participants' classrooms are located in close physical proximity, and all program participants share the same core classes as a team. This reorganizing is done to minimize the flux and complexity that the students typically confront in a large school. This change provides a stable and consistent set of classmates and peers at school. (2) Restructuring the homeroom teacher's role and increasing teacher support. The homeroom teacher helps students choose classes and serves as an advisor; provides counseling for academic and personal problems; follows up on student absences and tardiness; and meets with parents. Long-term follow-up results of an experimental evaluation of the program indicated a 50 percent reduction in dropout rates among participating students and an average of 9 percent fewer absences in the STEP school compared with the control school in grades 9 through 11 (16 percent average absences in the STEP school, 25 percent in the control school).

STRATEGIES THAT MIGHT WORK

There are a growing number of secondary prevention programs (i.e., children are referred after violating their State's mandatory school attendance policies) that first recognize that parents must be involved and held responsible for their children's school attendance; and second, provide intensive monitoring, counseling, and family-support services to help the truants and their families (Garry, 1996). These programs are designed to help the youth graduate from school and are often implemented as diversion from juvenile court petitions. The following is a brief description of a representative sample of such programs.

Truancy Prevention and Diversion Program

Sheldon (1987) reported the findings from an experimental evaluation of a voluntary truancy prevention and diversion program implemented by the Douglas County Juvenile Court in Kansas since 1977. This program utilizes undergraduate college students to mentor students who have violated the compulsory school attendance law of the state. Volunteer mentors are required to complete several university courses designed to teach them the skills they will need to work with youth and their families, including a course in juvenile law. The mentors receive college credit for their work. Mentors meet with students regularly for a period of 45 school days, offering counseling and skills training (e.g., conflict resolution, problem solving) as needed. At the end of the period, the participant youth, the family, the mentor, and a representative from the district attorney's office meet. The mentor is asked to make a recommendation about further action. Alternatives include graduation from the program, placement in an additional diversion program, or filing of a petition alleging that the student is in need of care. The representative from the district attorney then makes a determination. An evaluation of the program compared a sample of 58 participants (ages 8–15) with a random sample of 13 truant students who received traditional school procedures. The results indicated that the program significantly reduced unexcused absences, and participants increased their grade point averages. Only 3 of the 58 participating students were returned to the truancy program after completion.

Truancy Diversion Program

Stewart and Ray (1984) evaluated a truancy diversionary program in which parents were given the option of enrolling the child in an informal program of intervention or attending a formal court hearing for truancy. The principal of the local school referred children for truancy violations. There were 335 individuals, ages 13–25, who participated in the program, and their results were compared with a comparable sample of 159 individuals who were referred to the court before the initiation of the program. The results showed no decrease in subsequent return to court for criminal offences for the individuals in the diversion group. However, they were significantly less likely to return to court for truancy than the comparison group.

The Adolescent Diversion Program

Davidson and Redner (1988) reported an experimental evaluation of the adolescent diversion program, which was started in 1973 in Champaign-Urbana, Illinois. This program, like the truancy prevention and diversion program of Sheldon (1987), utilized college students as change agents during an 18-week period in which the college students interacted 6–8 hr per week with the youth in the experimental group. Youths were referred to the program prior to their formal involvement with the juvenile justice system (diversion). There were a total of 73 youth assigned randomly to either the experimental ($n = 49$) or control ($n = 24$) condition. The intervention consisted of developing a good relationship with the youth, behavioral contracting, and child advocacy. The contract included modifying relationships with parents or teachers. The advocacy component included specifying areas of personal need, locating individual or organizational resources to meet those needs, and transferring the advocacy skills to the youth. The results of a 2-year follow-up indicated significantly lower recidivism rates among participants in the program (45 percent of the youth in the experimental group, and 96 percent of the youth in the control group had one or more petitions). Additional evaluations of the program have shown consistent results (Eby, Mekan, Scofield, Legler, & Davidson, 1995).

Project Helping Hand

Started in 1989 in Atlantic City, New Jersey, this program encourages parents to work with the schools to keep their children in class (US Department of Education, 1996). The program provides counseling to parents and elementary students at risk for developing chronic truancy problems. Students with 5–15 days of unexcused absences are required to participate. After an assessment of the situation of the youth and the family, a counselor meets with the family and school personnel to develop a plan to improve the child's attendance and address family needs. Participants can receive weekly counseling for up to 8 weeks. Counselors use multiple resources, including group-study teams, tutoring, parent–teacher conferences, and cooperative agreements among parents, youth, and schools. Counselors can refer families to programs including housing, food stamps, day care, medical, substance abuse, psychiatric, parent support, and single parent assistance. They also strive to use extended family members as a support system and involve the family in the school as often as possible. Counselors do home visits when family members fail to keep appointments to encourage cooperation. If the family continues to resist participation, the case may be referred to family court. The counselor continues to make phone or in-person contact with the family on a monthly basis after school attendance improves and the case is closed. The program reports an average recidivism of 17 percent among the 300 or so participating students per year.

Save the Kids Partnership

This is a broad-based coalition of citizens and businesses in Arizona, started in 1994, involving 10 cities and 15 school districts serving more than 63,000 students in the Phoenix area (US Department of Education, 1996). The program targets 6–16 year olds who have 3 days of unexcused absences. Parents discuss with school officials the situation and outline measures to ensure the student's attendance. If the child continues to be truant (5 days of unexcused absences), the case is forwarded to the city prosecutor to request that criminal charges be filed against the parents. In lieu of criminal proceedings, the prosecutor can offer families a deferred prosecution diversion program designed to strengthen family relationships and encourage youth to go to school. The program includes an evaluation of the children and the family, and requires parents to attend a parenting skills support group, while the youth receive counseling and are required to attend school. If parents and/or students fail to comply with the program, the case may be referred to court. If they complete the program, the case is closed. Evaluation of the program in 12 elementary and 2 high schools indicated a 72 percent attendance increase after initial notification to parents, and only 28 percent of the cases were referred for prosecution. Of those students in the diversion program, 92 percent completed the program and did not repeat the truancy offense.

STRATEGIES THAT DO NOT WORK

Many harsh disciplinary practices and school policies implemented to punish school absenteeism seem to have the opposite effect, particularly when these policies are applied in the absence of any other comprehensive program and support for students and families. Many students with serious attendance records end up as "push outs" or dropouts (Bowditch, 1993; Fine, 1986). Adolescents do not respond well to threats or punishment. For example, Duckworth and

DeJung (1989) collected questionnaire data regarding class cutting practices from 5,799 students enrolled in six urban high schools in Great Britain and found that the general climate of student opinion regarding cutting is uninhibited and opposed to penalties to the point where negative academic and disciplinary consequences do not enter into students' decisions about class attendance. The authors suggest that a change in the climate of opinion may be necessary to reduce the impact of class cutting. Hyman (1990) also found that schools tend to be ineffective in dealing with the problem of class cutting and absenteeism because too often disciplinarians act out a limited series of punishments without having a theoretical base for understanding why a particular approach does not work. They tend to ignore the system or culture in which misbehavior occurs.

Some efforts to increase enforcement of truancy laws have shown mixed results. Ekblom (1979) reported an evaluation of an experimental truancy patrol program implemented in Bristol, England for a week. The police officers stopped any youth they saw in the streets during school hours. Results showed a lower rate of daytime offenses by truants, but the study did not show any improvements in school attendance of the youth detained or whether the patrols caused any other children to return to school or stay at home. The author concluded that police patrols require many more resources than most police forces are willing or able to commit.

Finally, Reyes and Jason (1991) evaluated an intervention with 77 primarily low-income Latino students who were at risk of dropping out due to absenteeism and academic achievement records in an inner city high school. An additional sample of 77 students served as comparison group. The program used an ecological approach to modify relevant aspects of the school environment to improve students' attendance and achievement. First, the program worked with school administrators and teachers to re-define the role of the homeroom teacher so that students could have better communication and guidance from a teacher who would get to know them personally over the academic year. Second, the system of class rotation was rearranged so that the same group of students could take the same core classes together (e.g., math, English, social studies), again increasing familiarity and the possibility that the students would build personal relationships, develop a peer support network, and enhance their sense of belonging. Finally, they organized a regular feedback system to communicate with parents about their children school performance. Unfortunately, the program students did not demonstrate significant differences in GPA, absenteeism, test scores, or rate of course failure when compared with the students in the control group. The authors considered various explanations for their failure. First, the complexities of the large school environment may make it impossible for a small demonstration project to affect the culture and the climate of the school. Second, many students need early intervention, and efforts at the high school level may be too little too late to be of real help.

SYNTHESIS

Table 1 summarizes the elements that characterize successful school interventions to prevent school absenteeism based on this literature review. These elements combined, represent the state-of-the-art technologies needed to address the problem. As we mentioned, the problem of school absenteeism has serious consequences for the students, families, schools, and society at large. It is often the beginning of a downward spiral of failure and alienation from society that traps the youth in a labyrinth of hopelessness. It has been recognized that appropriate social and emotional development paired with an engaging, nurturing, and supportive school environment can prevent the problem. Systemic school reform efforts play an important role in transforming schools into places where children would want

Table 1. Interventions to Prevent School Absenteeism

School-based models	Community-based models
Elementary School	
Cooperative learning	Behavioral contracts with students
Tutors/mentors	and family members
Appropriate diagnostic and	Intensive supervision by case worker
frequent monitoring of	Development of a plan (goal setting)
academic progress	to improve school attendance with
Individualized learning plans	active parent and student involvement
Team teaching	Group or individual therapy and
Peer teaching	counseling as needed
Ongoing training and	Social skills development
technical assistance to teachers	Parenting skills development training
Re-allocation of school	Referral to appropriate social services
resources to meet the	including housing, food stamps,
demands of the new program	health care, mental health services,
Active student involvement	day care, substance abuse treatment,
in school activities (academic	family support, and other support
and non-academic)	groups as needed
Active student involvement	Home visits by case workers
in classroom management	Anti-truancy legislation
and discipline	Deferred prosecution diversion
Family support	program
Family involvement in	Truant processing center
school activities	Filling misdemeanor charges
High School	against the parents
Reorganization of the social and	
physical environment to	
increase familiarity	
Restructuring of the homeroom	
teacher's role to increase student	
support	
Tutors/mentors	

to be—where they would be allowed to explore, learn, and develop. Early intervention and the creation of appropriate school ties with the child and the family are central to the development of positive academic performance. The models described here demonstrate exemplary practices to prevent academic failure and promote positive school attachment.

Families also play a central role in efforts to prevent school absenteeism. Parents have to take responsibility for getting their children to school. Schools need to recognize, however, that they are often unwelcoming places. It is unfortunate that many educational models are not consistently applied in school systems and that many students are not exposed to educational practices and models that have been experimentally evaluated and validated. Unfortunately, schools of education do not necessarily do a good job of preparing teachers with innovative visions about the possibilities of changing education, classroom relations, teachers' roles, the roles of the students and their families, or even the physical environment of the school and classroom. Antiquated instructional methods are stubbornly preserved by teachers who do not seem to care about their students and by students who do not know any better.

We argue that students, their families, and even teachers should demand better education, resources, and opportunities to learn and develop appropriately. The right for an education should not be simply the access to a desk and a locker in the school. It is the right to be educated, to learn and develop as a knowledgeable and responsible citizen that counts. We are all responsible for the mediocrity of our schools. It is up to parents and their supporters to demand reform and demand that more empirically validated educational models become accessible to every school and every child.

ACKNOWLEDGMENTS

Special thanks to Tina Ritzler and Cleo Jacobs for their assistance in collecting relevant information to prepare this document.

Also see: School entries, Intellectual Growth; Academic Success; Bullying; Literacy.

References

Barnes, H. (1998). *Early school leaving in Latino youth with disabilities: The impact of personal and contextual factors.* Unpublished Masters Thesis, University of Illinois at Chicago, Chicago, IL.

Bowditch, C. (1993). Getting rid of troublemakers: High school disciplinary procedures and the production of dropouts. *Social Problems, 40,* 493–509.

Cooper, M. (1986). A model of persistent school absenteeism. *Educational Research, 28,* 14–20.

Davidson, W.S., & Redner, R. (1988). The prevention of juvenile delinquency: Diversion from the juvenile justice system. In R. Price,

E. Cowen, R. Lorion, & J. Ramos-McKay (Eds.), *Fourteen ounces of prevention: A casebook for practitioners* (pp. 123–137). Washington, DC: American Psychological Association.

DeKalb, J. (1999). *Student truancy* (ERIC Digest No 125). Eugene, OR: ERIC Clearinghouse on Educational Management (ERIC Document Reproduction Service No. ED 429 334).

Desnoyers, J., & Pauker, J.D. (1988). *School attendance and non-attendance in Canada and the United States: Survey of methods and programs to increase school attendance, decrease absenteeism and deal with dropout.* Toronto, Ontario, Canada: Ontario Department of Education, MGS Publication Services.

Duckworth, K., & DeJung, J. (1989). Inhibiting class cutting among high school students. *High School Journal, 73*, 188–195.

Eby, K., Mekan, J., Scofield, M., Legler, R., & Davidson, W.S., (1995). The adolescent diversion Program. In R.R. Ross (Ed.), *Going straight: Effective delinquency prevention and offender rehabilitation* (pp. 120–132). Ottawa, Canada: Air Training.

Ekblom, P. (1979). Police truancy patrols. In J. Burrows, P. Ekblom, & K. Heal (Eds.), *Crime prevention and police in England* (pp. 80–88). Mystic, CT: Pendragon House.

Felner, R.D., Brand, S., Adam, A.M., Mulhall, P.F., Flowers, N., Sartain, B., & DuBois, D.L. (1993). Restructuring the ecology of the school as an approach to prevention during school transitions: Longitudinal follow-ups and extensions of the school transitional environment project (STEP). *Prevention in Human Services, 10*, 103–136.

Fergusson, D.M., Horwood, L.J., & Shannon, F.T. (1986). Absenteeism amongst primary schools children. *New Zealand Journal of educational studies, 21*, 3–12.

Fine, M. (1986). Why urban adolescents drop into and out of public high school. *Teachers College Record, 87*, 393–409.

Freedman, J.S. (1999). *Easing the teasing: How parents can help their children.* Champaign, IL: ERIC Clearinghouse on Elementary and Childhood Education (ERIC Document Reproduction Service No. ED 431 555).

Freiberg, H.J. (1998). Consistency management & cooperative discipline: From tourist to citizens in the classrooms. In H.J. Freiberg (Ed.), *Beyond behaviorism: Changing the classroom management* (pp. 75–97). Boston, MA: Allyn & Bacon.

Freiberg, H.J., Stein, T., & Huang, S. (1995). The effects of classroom management intervention on students achievement in inner-city elementary schools. *Educational Research and Evaluation, 1*, 33–66.

Garry, E.M. (1996, October). Truancy: First step to a lifetime of problems. *Juvenile Justice Bulletin.* Washington, DC: Office of Juvenile Justice and Delinquency Prevention, US Department of Justice.

Gill, P.E. (1997). Interaction effects and absence from school. *Scandinavian Journal of Educational Research, 21*(3), 147–156.

Hansen, C., Sanders, S.L., Massaro, S., & Last, C.G. (1998). Predictors of severity of absenteeism in children with anxiety-based school refusal. *Journal of Clinical Child Psychology, 27*, 246–254.

Hawkins, J.D. (1997). Academic performance and school success: Sources and consequences. In R.P. Weissberg, T.P. Gullotta, R.L. Hampton, B.A. Ryan, & G.R. Adams (Eds.), *Healthy children 2010: Enhancing children wellness* (pp. 278–305). Thousand Oaks, CA: Sage.

Hyman, I. (1990). Class-cutting: An ecological approach. In R.M. Gupta, P. Coxhead et al. (Eds.), *Intervention with children* (pp. 107–129). London: Routledge.

Irving, B.A., & Parker-Jenkins, M. (1995). Tracking truancy: An examination of persistent non-attendance amongst disaffected school pupils and positive support strategies. *Cambridge Journal of Education, 25*, 225–235.

Jordan, W.J., Lara, J., & McPartland, J.M. (1996). Exploring causes of early dropout among race-ethnic and gender groups. *Youth & Society, 28*, 62–94.

Kelly, J.G. (1979). *Adolescent boys in high school: A psychological study of coping and adaptation.* Hillsdale, NJ: Erlbaum.

Lee, P.W. (1999). In their own voices: An ethnographic study of low-achieving students within the context of school reform. *Urban Education, 24*, 214–244.

Madden, N.A., Slavin, R.E., Karweit, N.L., Dolan, L.J., & Wasik, B.A. (1991). Success for all. *Phi Delta Kappan, 72*, 593–599.

Madden, N.A., Slavin, R.E., Karweit, N.L., Dolan, L.J., & Wasik, B.A. (1993). Success for all: Longitudinal effects of a restructuring program for inner-city elementary schools. *American Educational research Journal, 30*, 123–148.

Massey, M.S. (1998). *Early childhood violence prevention.* Champaign, IL: ERIC Clearinghouse on Elementary and Childhood Education (ERIC Document Reproduction Service No. ED 424 032).

National Center for Education Statistics. (1999). *Digest of education statistics: Elementary and secondary education (Chapter 2).* Washington, DC: US Department of Education.

Reid, K.C. (1981). Alienation and persistent school absenteeism. *Research in Education, 26*, 31–40.

Reid, K.C. (1983). Retrospection and persistent school absenteeism. *Educational Research, 25*, 110–115.

Reid, K.C. (1984). Some social, psychological and educational aspects related to persistent school absenteeism. *Research in Education, 31*, 63–82.

Reyes, O., & Jason, L. (1991). An evaluation of a high school dropout prevention program. *Journal of Community Psychology, 19*, 221–230.

Robinson, E.H., & Rotter, J.C. (1991). *Coping with fears and stress.* Ann Arbor, MI: ERIC Clearinghouse on Counseling and Personnel Services (ERIC Document Reproduction Service No. ED 341 888).

Robinson, E.H., Rotter, J.C., Fey, M., & Robinson, S.L. (1991). Children fears: Toward a preventive model. *The School Counselor, 38*, 187–202.

Sheldon, J.B. (1987). Legal and ethical issues on the behavioral treatment of juvenile and adult offenders. In E.K. Morris & C.J. Braukmann (Eds.), *Behavioral approaches to crime and delinquency: A handbook of application, research and concepts* (pp. 543–575). New York: Plenum Press.

Sobehart, H.C. (1991). Implementing ALEM: An encouraging first year. In J.C. Lindle (Ed.), *Pennsylvania educational leadership yearbook 1990–1991* (pp. 12–19). Lancaster: Pennsylvania Association for Supervision and Curriculum Development.

Stewart, M.J., & Ray, R.E. (1984). Truants and the court: A diversionary program. *Social Work in Education, 6*, 170–192.

Traux, C.T. (1985). *Student absenteeism: Explanations, problems, and possible solutions.* Arlington, VA: National Criminal Justice Reference Service (NCJRS No 149 503).

US Department of Education (1996). *Manual to combat truancy* [on-line]. Washington, DC: Safe and Drug free Schools Office. Available: www.ed.gov/pubs/truancy/

US Department of Education. (1994). *National agenda for achieving better results for children and youth with serious emotional disturbance.* Washington, DC: US Department of Education, Office of Special Education Programs (ERIC Document reproduction Service No. ED 376 690).

Wang, M.C. (1992). *Adaptive education strategies: Building on diversity.* Baltimore, MD: Paul H. Brookes.

Wang, M.C., & Zollers, N.J. (1990). Adaptive instruction: An alternative service delivery approach. *Remedial and Special Education, 11*, 7–21.

Wish, E.D., Gray, T.A., & Levine, E.B. (1996). *Recent drug use in female juvenile detainees: Estimates from interviews, urinalysis, and hair analysis* [on-line]. College Park, MD: Center for Substance Abuse Research, University of Maryland. Available: www.cesar.umd.edu/

School Drop-Outs, Adolescence

Peter W. Dowrick

INTRODUCTION

Dropping out of school is an important concern for most young people, leading to under-employment and a lower quality of life. While methods of preventing dropout are widely reported, few have been evaluated.

DEFINITIONS

The term *drop out* is widely used in education-related circles in reference to youth who do not finish high school, or it can be used to refer to the phenomenon itself (usually one word, *dropout*). This raises the question of what does it mean to finish? In the United States, students are expected to complete 12 grades from the age of 6 years. Depending on their marks, the students' high school can award a certificate of completion or a "graduation diploma," usually about the age of 17 or 18. This system differs in other parts of the world. For example, in western European countries and other developed countries, the last 3 years of high school are widely considered optional. There are external (national) examinations, at different levels, in these years. So a student may earn a *school certificate*, or *university entrance*, or *O level* and *A level* credentials, leaving school with a employable qualification, usually aged 15–18 years. Thus "dropping out" is used more generally used to refer to leaving school before attaining any recognized credentials, or before reaching the desired level to fulfill appropriate, potential employment opportunities.

SCOPE

The US Department of Education reports 5 percent (National Center for Educational Statistics [NCES], 1999) as the annual "event" dropout rate, referring to the percentage of students in 10th–12th grade who left school without a certificate. However, a better measure is "status" dropout (12 percent) which represents the percent of 16–24-year-olds who left school incomplete, regardless of when they left. Rates are significantly lower now than in the 1970s, but have changed little in the last decade.

Rates vary considerably across schools and social conditions. In small high schools in stable communities, over 90 percent of students finish; in large high schools in less stable, low-income communities, fewer than 50 percent complete school. Half of students identified with learning disabilities or conduct disorders drop out of school. Dropout rates vary across the major ethnic/linguistic groups (in ascending order): Asian American: Euro-American; African American; Latino; and Native American, with Native Americans four times as likely to drop out as Asian Americans. The rates for youth in low-income families are three times that of other youth. Girls are more likely to graduate than boys, and this difference increases among settings/groups most at risk.

Internationally, success in school is highly dependent on what the country can afford and on government priorities. Many European countries, plus Canada, New Zealand, Australia, Japan, South Korea, Israel and others have rates comparable to the United States—often better, because of the potential to gain a good exit-outcome at an earlier age. But there are other differences in incidence. For example, many countries do not have free and accessible high schools. In these places, high school attendance may be as low as 5 percent of any age group, favoring the rich and males.

There are costs to individuals in the loss of quality of life, and to society in national productivity. Those who finish high school are more likely to get jobs, to gain higher education of their choice, and to participate in the democratic process. Youth who drop out have lower incomes and are at greater risk of criminal activity. It has been estimated in the United States that the financial costs to society per dropout, range from $200,000 to $2,000,000 (Cohen, 1998).

THEORIES

Youth leave school because of poor grades; failure; repeating a grade; poor attendance; low self-determination; and dislike of school (Vallerand, Fortier, & Guay, 1997). Other reasons include misconduct, family, and community factors (Rosenthal, 1998). Although intelligence is an indicator for dropping out, low IQ and learning disabilities are not as predictive as other factors listed earlier. At-risk groups include students from low-income neighborhoods, with parents who dropped out, and where teachers have low expectations. In short, students drop out when: (1) they do not like school, (2) the incentives to stay are weak, and (3) sometimes there are strong short-term incentives to leave. Theories for dropping out of school tend to relate to the risk and protective factors associated with these three issues or circumstances.

First, it is useful to consider why children dislike school. Important reasons include not succeeding and experiencing negative social outcomes. Both reasons often associated with learning disabilities and behavioral disorders. While in other nations "learning disabilities" refers to overall cognitive deficits, in the United States, the term refers to an uneven development where core academics, especially literacy, are adversely affected, but other learning may show promise. This type of learning disorder may contribute to frustration and a dislike of school (Tobler, 2000). Emotional and behavioral disorders, especially conduct disorders, have been identified as primary risk factors for leaving school (Rylance, 1997). The associated theoretical basis involves the creation of a vicious cycle in which the institutional response to an aberrant behavior feeds back into the emotional condition making it worse. Another risk factor is speaking non-standard English (or whatever is the language of instruction). This makes learning more difficult and may create an impression of less intelligence, or dispose teachers and others to interact less favorably (Worrell, 1997).

Next, dropping out is likely when the incentives to stay are weak. One associated risk/protective factor is the value placed on education by the student's family. Youth are at risk if family members have little education and do not take positive steps to offset that circumstance. Incentives to stay in school are few if individuals see no future or only bleak futures ahead. Clearly, failing and expecting failure are interrelated. Indeed, the importance of self-belief has a strong theoretical basis (Bandura, 1993). Schools have a responsibility for encouraging self-efficacy that encompasses teacher expectations, beliefs about whether failing students are worth the effort, and the quality of the home-school relationship. It is not just a case of seeing low probability of academic success but of seeing inevitability of a bleak future no matter what is achieved at school, or of simply not seeing a future, good or bad (Dowrick, 1999).

Lastly, there may be immediate needs or short-term opportunities out of school, which students will weigh against the choice of staying in school (Jordan, Lara, & McPartland, 1996). These opportunities can range from earning almost a living wage in a fast food franchise, to selling illicit drugs. Girls may leave because of pregnancy. Youth in poor families may feel a responsibility to secure a paid job.

These theories have evolved in developed nations with resources and a perceived value of education. In countries whose economies cannot support 10–15 years of public education for all children, "theories of dropout" are simply that education is not available, not considered widely appropriate, or not valued by the society.

RESEARCH

Research on Disliking School

Most students who drop out do not like school. Their reason for not liking school is not succeeding in school

(Battistich & Hom, 1997). To illustrate, Finn and Rock (1997) studied 1,800 ethnically diverse low-income high school students from 1,000 schools. They measured "school engagement" for students identified as succeeding in school (vs. dropping out), while eliminating other personal and family differences. School engagement roughly equates to liking school. They found significant differences in the levels of engagement, with evidence for disliking school being a strong predictor of dropping out.

Other research with high school dropouts from US middle-income families demonstrates how multiple factors have a part to play. For example, a study of "middle class dropouts" found high rates of mental health disorders, substance abuse, dysfunctional families, learning disorders, and difficulties with school authority or other relationships at school (Franklin & Streeter, 1995).

Learning disabilities represent one of the most cited risk factors for dropping out, with as many as 50 percent of youth with a learning disability leaving school without a credential (Rylance, 1997). Nevertheless, the profiles of learning disabled students who drop out are very similar to those of students who complete high school but do not go on to postsecondary education. Indeed, there is little evidence that learning disability, by itself, is a pathway to dropout. Rather, it is when learning disabilities are combined with other factors like poor support from family, school, or community that negative outcomes result. In the Finn and Rock (1997) study, school engagement was found to be a protective factor that offset learning and behavior disorders.

Many studies have examined the overrepresentation of youth with emotional and behavioral disorders (EBD) in dropout statistics. Youth with EBD have lower grades, fail more courses, and drop out of school more often than students in any other category (Wood & Cronin, 1999; Rylance, 1997). These youth also experience the worst post-school outcomes, such as unemployment and incarceration.

In many countries, immigrants who speak another language are more likely to drop out of school. Studies in Canada report dropout rates up to 75 percent for second language learners. These rates correlate inversely with proficiency in the language of instruction. In a study of students in the eastern US, Worrell (1997) reports ethnicity, poverty, and limited English proficiency as risk factors for dropping out.

Research on Incentives to Stay in School

There is evidence from low-income communities that family importance placed on education is a protective factor. Studies have indicated a positive influence of parental involvement on youth staying in school, even with low student academic achievement (Jimerson, Egeland, Sroufe, & Carlson, 2000).

There is also research related to the importance of self-efficacy. Having a specific positive image of the future can be crucial to remaining engaged in an unpleasant situation (Dowrick, 1999). Collective school efficacy (administrators and teachers' beliefs that they can get good academic outcomes) is just as important as the self-beliefs of students. To illustrate, a comparison across 79 elementary schools showed that students from "disadvantaged" backgrounds, based on family income, education, and ethnicity, performed significantly better in schools exhibiting high levels of belief that they could produce high standards of academic achievement in these students (Bandura, 1993).

Research on Incentives to Leave

While overall dropout rates have remained stable in the last decade, rates have increased for children in families receiving public assistance. This suggests a possible modeling effect or a response to the need to earn more money by leaving school to take a job. A study by McCaul, Donaldson, Coladarci, and Davis (1992) cited rural students' main reasons for leaving school to get a job or to get married; urban students most frequently reported leaving school to support families or because friends were dropping out.

Evidence from drug abuse research suggests the potential influence of peer and financial incentives. Approximately 17 percent of teenagers in US urban centers were involved in drug dealing in the 1990s (Centers & Weist, 1998). While reliable evidence for youth income from these activities is meager, drug related earnings might be four times those of other income earning opportunities in these neighborhoods.

STRATEGIES THAT WORK

The best dropout prevention strategies are comprehensive in two senses of the phrase. First, they include school, family, community, and individual elements. Second, they identify and address specific risk and protective factors relevant to the individuals and the setting. Effective programs fall into three overlapping categories. They are programs designed to:

1. *Improve school climate* by affecting teacher–student relationships; or school–family relationships; or (smaller) school size. That is, the feeling of size or attractiveness of curriculum.
2. *Improve school outcomes* by school-wide academic overhaul; or school-wide improvement of social behavior; or after school and recreational programs.
3. *Address risk and protective factors*, focusing on at-risk communities; or at-risk students, with

additional support for academic success; or risky behaviors (drug use, aggression, etc.).

Although hundreds of such programs have been tried, few have been documented as "proven" by the criterion of this encyclopedia. That is, has the program worked successfully three times or meets some other recognized criteria. Two examples of documented effective strategies are described below.

One program to *improve school climate* by affecting adult–student relationships is *Check and Connect* (Sinclair, Christenson, Evelo, & Hurley, 1998). It features mentoring, monitoring, and building effective transitions from middle to high school. Its evaluation demonstrates that it has lowered dropout rates. It also addresses risk factors for students with learning disabilities and emotional disorders.

This program has five features of note. First, an adult with good cooperative skills is assigned to a group of 25 students as a mentor/monitor. Next, the mentors check on factors like attendance, conduct, and academics known to affect engagement with school. Third, the mentors provide regular support and encouragement for all students. Mentors also provide structured student training in problem solving for risky situations (e.g., tardiness). Fourth, where monitoring suggests elevated risk, students are provided with additional guidance that includes involving parents. On the basis of this guidance, students can access academic support, recreational or community opportunities. Finally, the system is started in seventh grade, continued in the eighth grade and into high school (ninth grade).

Results indicate positive outcomes for attendance and assignment completion, with modest effects on grades, conduct, and self-reported attitude toward school (Sinclair et al., 1998).

One program developed to improve school outcomes and address some specific risk factors, is the *Seattle Social Development Project*. It is a multi-year effort directed at teachers, parents, and children. Compared with controls, children in a 6-year evaluation showed greater school commitment and class participation; girls experimented less with drugs; boys improved their school work and social skills (O'Donnell, Hawkins, Catalano, Abbott, & Day, 1995).

The program is designed to decrease *risk factors* like academic failure, low commitment to school, early conduct disorders, family management problems, and involvement with antisocial peers. It is also designed to improve *protective factors* such as positive social bonds to school and family and belief in family and school values.

The program begins in first grade and continues through sixth grade. Teachers are trained in proactive classroom management, interactive teaching, cooperative learning, and problem solving. This approach improves predictability, the amount of praise, modeling, and appropriate student involvement. Children are provided with individual social skills interventions, but not with extra tutoring, after school opportunities, or with in-school support by community members. Parents are offered training in behavior management, monitoring of risk for drug involvement, and homework support—although it has been difficult to attract high levels of parent participation. Recently, the program has been extended to middle school and early high school.

Study results have been good but modest. Teachers learned new practices. Apparently some of the children at risk benefited academically, and some avoided or reduced their predicted involvement with substance abuse.

Some programs have been developed to address conduct issues that have shown positive effects on completing high school qualifications. For example, *First Step to Success* (Walker, Stiller, Severson, Feil, & Golly, 1998) is intended to address childhood aggression in schools, thus improving the school climate and academic success of all students. Another documented program with similar goals is the *Effective Behavior Supports* model (Lewis, Sugai, & Colvin, 1998).

STRATEGIES THAT MIGHT WORK

Recent efforts in dropout prevention programs are based on indirect data (e.g., smaller high schools correlate with better outcomes) or address the reduction of risk factors (e.g., gang membership) without reporting dropout outcomes. The best of these promising efforts combine at least two of the following eight elements.

1. *Smaller Learning Communities in Schools.* High school size of around 600 pupils correlates with the lowest rates of dropout. Given that many high schools now have enrollments of 1,500 to 5,000, the US Department of Education has called for initiatives to restructure these large schools with "freshman academies," career tracks, or block scheduling to reduce the negative effects of size.

2. *Intervening Early is Advocated.* For example, teaching literacy should be implemented before a child starts to fail at other subjects (Dowrick, Power, Manz, Ginsburg-Block, Leff, & Kim-Rupnow, 2001). For teenagers at risk, most of whom read below fifth grade level, it is never too early and never too late to help. The preferred timing of

interventions has been moving to earlier ages (Dryfoos, 1998).

3. *Focus on School Activities in School Locations.* Classrooms and after school programs are essential to succeeding well enough academically to improve adult prospects and to feel good about going to school.

4. *Extra-Curricular Activities and Involvement of Outside Organizations (On-Campus).* This is needed to provide recreational and prevention programs. School staff can collaborate or contract with local agencies, private foundations, and postsecondary institutions to provide expertise and person power beyond school resources (Mahoney & Cairns, 1997).

5. *Community and Vocational Programs (Off-Campus).* As well as internships to give meaning to schoolwork, some health and mental health services, if not available on site, may have a potential contribution. Job placements, community service, cross-age tutoring (with employment-style responsibilities and rewards) can make participation in school more meaningful.

6. *Parent Involvement.* This is effective when there are specific roles such as paid classroom and playground aides, voting membership of committees, and advising based on individual expertise. These responsibilities require support and training to be effective (Martin, 1994).

7. *Peer Involvement.* This can also be achieved in ways comparable to those described for parents. Youth can develop educational roles that eventually serve themselves and others. For example, students who lack reading skills can develop those skills at the same time serving as peer coaches for other students (Topping & Ehly, 1998).

8. *Mentorship with (Intensive) Individualization.* Promising programs use community members, senior citizens, and others to provide students with mentors. Mentoring appears helpful, but individualized assistance of greater intensity may be necessary to make a difference in educational outcomes for youth most at risk (VanDenBerg & Grealish, 1996).

Promising strategies are similar internationally, except where the issues are strikingly different. For example, in one part of Namibia the goal is ensure that children stay in school at least 3 years and learn basic reading skills. Here they use a community responsive approach to reduce discrimination by teachers and to accommodate the local language and culture (Pfaffe, 1995).

STRATEGIES THAT DO NOT WORK

There is little evidence that small-scale or unitary approaches have much promise for preventing students from leaving school. For example, providing only additional academic support for failing students has little effect on dropout rates. This situation is illustrated in a report by Hamovitch (1999) who discusses the failure of an after-school compensatory program for low-income African American students. He attributes the program's failure to an emphasis on tutorials after school (more of the school day), without incorporating either local culture or needs.

SYNTHESIS

Strategies to prevent dropping out must: (1) improve pupils' appreciation of school, (2) increase incentives to stay, and (3) decrease incentives to leave. This can be achieved using a hierarchical approach that makes schools an inviting place for students (and community members), improves the outcomes of school-related activities, and addresses a locally prioritized list of risk and protective factors. It makes sense to put local effort and federal funds into the following:

1. Assess schools in terms of items (1)–(3) above and where deficient take action. If school climate is good, but the outcomes (e.g., grades; lost games) are poor, then that suggests a focus on supporting agreed-upon objectives of attainment. If the school is enjoyable and successful, then it may be valuable to focus on specific problems with individuals.
2. There a number of programs that are widely implemented but lack data. There has been little research that addresses the causal relationships between school improvement efforts and any outcomes that are measured.
3. Recognize that different programs for at-risk children and youth have considerable overlap. We would benefit from a synthesis of programs designed to address drug abuse, delinquency, violence, truancy, teen pregnancy.
4. Over the past 15 years in the United States, an effort has gone into addressing dropout and related issues for students with disabilities. The synthesis of findings has remarkably little overlap with the recommendations for general education. Clearly, schools and students could benefit from efforts that take into account all areas of program evaluation.
5. Recognize that creating a good school is basic: a healthy environment and effective teaching. There have been strides in creating effective curriculums (design and expectations), how it is taught, and school-wide reform that could be more consistently and conscientiously applied.

There are also improvements that could be made with the stroke of a legislator's pen or by school board action. These include:

1. Reducing the size of high schools. Is it really much more expensive to build three campuses of 900 students than to maintain one campus for 2,700?
2. In the United States, changing the hours of the school day to begin earlier and end later.

Internationally, there are considerable differences in how dropping out is perceived. Broadly speaking, in the Americas effort has gone into academics, vocational preparation, and encouraging cooperative behavior among students. In Europe, emphasis has been placed on improving attitudes and developing friendships. In Asia and Africa, the effort has been focused on increasing opportunities to attend school.

ACKNOWLEDGMENT

Preparation of this article was partially supported by US Department of Education (Office of Elementary and Secondary Education), although no endorsement is implied of the views expressed herein. I thank Julie Holmes for her support in documenting relevant literature.

Also see: School entries; Identity Promotion; Academic Success; Literacy; Violence Prevention, Childhood; Bullying.

References

Bandura, A. (1993). Perceived self-efficacy in cognitive development and functioning. *Educational Psychology, 28*, 117–148.

Battistich, V., & Hom, A. (1997). The relationship between students' sense of their school as a community and their involvement in problem behaviors. *American Journal of Public Health, 87*, 1997–2001.

Centers, N.L., & Weist, M.D. (1998). Inner city youth and drug dealing: A review of the problem. *Journal of Youth & Adolescence, 27*(3), 395–411.

Cohen, M.A. (1998). The monetary value of saving high-risk youth. *Journal of Quantitative Criminology, 14*, 5–33.

Dowrick, P.W. (1999). A review of self modeling and related applications. *Applied and Preventive Psychology, 8*, 23–29.

Dowrick, P.W., Power, T.J., Manz, P.H., Ginsburg-Block, M., Leff, S.S., & Kim-Rupnow, S. (2001). Community responsiveness: Examples from under-resourced urban schools. *Journal of Prevention and Intervention in the Community, 21*(2), 71–90.

Dryfoos, J.G. (1998). *Safe passage: Making it through adolescence in a risky society.* New York: Oxford University Press.

Finn, J., & Rock, D. (1997). Academic success among students at risk for school failure. *Journal of Applied Psychology, 82*, 221–234.

Franklin, C., & Streeter, C.L. (1995). Assessment of middle class youth at-risk to dropout: School, psychological and family correlates. *Children & Youth Services Review, 17*(3), 433–448.

Hamovitch, B. (1999). More failure for the disadvantaged: Contradictory African-American student reactions to compensatory education and urban schooling. *Urban Review, 31*(1), 55–77.

Jimerson, S.R., Egeland, B., Sroufe, L.A., & Carlson, B. (2000). A prospective longitudinal study of high school dropouts: Examining multiple predictors across development. *Journal of School Psychology, 38,* 525–549.

Jordan, W.J., Lara, J., & McPartland, J.M. (1996). Exploring the causes of early dropout among race-ethnic and gender groups. *Youth & Society, 28*(1), 62–94.

Lewis, T.J., Sugai, G., & Colvin, G. (1998). Reducing problem behavior through a school-wide system of effective behavioral support: Investigation of a school-wide social skills training program and contextual interventions. *School Psychology Review, 27,* 446–459.

Mahoney, J.L., & Cairns, R.B. (1997). Do extracurricular activities protect against early school dropout? *Developmental Psychology, 33,* 241–253.

Martin, C.J. (1994). *Schooling in Mexico: Staying in or dropping out.* Brookfield, VT: Ashgate.

McCaul, E.J., Donaldson, G.A., Coladarci, T., & Davis, W.E. (1992). Consequences of dropping out of school: Findings from high school and beyond. *Journal of Educational Research, 85,* 198–207.

National Center for Educational Statistics (NCES). (1999). *Dropout rates in the United States: 1998.* Washington, DC: US Department of Education.

O'Donnell, J., Hawkins, J.D., Catalano, R.F., Abbott, R.D., & Day, L.E. (1995). Preventing school failure, drug use, and delinquency among low-income children: Long-term intervention in elementary schools. *American Journal of Orthopsychiatry, 65,* 87–100.

Pfaffe, J.F. (1995). The Village Schools Project: Ju/'hoan Literacy Programme and community-based education in Nyae Nyae, Namibia. *School Psychology International, 16,* 43–58.

Rosenthal, B.S. (1998). Non-school correlates of dropout: An integrative review of the literature. *Children & Youth Services Review, 20,* 413–433.

Rylance, B.J. (1997). Predictors of high school graduation or dropping out for youths with severe emotional disturbances. *Behavioral Disorders, 23*(1), 5–17.

Sinclair, M.F., Christenson, S.L., Evelo, D.L., & Hurley, C.M. (1998). Dropout prevention for youth with disabilities: Efficacy of a sustained school engagement procedure. *Exceptional Children, 65,* 7–21.

Tobler, N.S. (2000). Lessons learned. *Journal of Primary Prevention, 20,* 261–273.

Topping, K., & Ehly, S. (1998). *Peer-assisted learning.* Mahwah, NJ: Lawrence Erlbaum.

Vallerand, R.J., Fortier, M.S., & Guay, F. (1997). Self-determination and persistence in a real-life setting: Toward a motivational model of high school dropout. *Journal of Personality & Social Psychology, 72,* 1161–1176.

VanDenBerg, J.E., & Grealish, E.M. (1996). Individualized services and supports through the wraparound process: Philosophy and procedures. *Journal of Child & Family Studies, 5*(1), 7–21.

Walker, H., Stiller, B., Severson, H., Feil, E., & Golly, A. (1998). First Step to Success: Intervening at the point of school entry to prevent antisocial behavior patterns. *Psychology in the Schools, 35,* 259–269.

Wood, S.J., & Cronin, M.E. (1999). Students with emotional/behavioral disorders and transition planning: What the follow-up studies tell us. *Psychology in the Schools, 36,* 327–345.

Worrell, F.C. (1997). Predicting successful or non-successful at-risk status using demographic risk factors. *High School Journal, 81*(1), 46–53.

School Violence, Adolescence

Michael J. Furlong, Jill D. Sharkey, and Tisa C. Jimenez

INTRODUCTION

The Prevention of School Violence. Throughout much of the 1970s and 1980s educators in the United States marginally addressed the issue of school violence. By the mid-1990s, however, a cluster of school shootings occurring in suburban and rural schools caught the American public's attention and raised school violence to the top concern about public education (Furlong & Morrison, 2000). By way of contrast, in Norway (Olweus, 2001), England (Smith, Shu, & Madsen, 2001), Australia (Owens, Slee, & Shute, 2001), and other countries the term school violence has typically not been used because these countries have focused on the prevention of bullying and harassment behaviors on school campuses. More recently in the United States, the recognition that a number of the school shooters had a previous school history of bully victimization, has begun to merge school safety interests across national boundaries (Juvonen & Graham, 2001; Olweus, Limber, & Mihalic, 1999; Nansel, Overpeck, Pill, Ruan, Simons-Morton, & Scheidt, 2001).

Because the issue of school safety is a community concern, in the United States much of the early responses to violent acts came from public health and juvenile justice agencies (Furlong & Morrison, 2000). Although the perspectives of these disciplines are important, in this entry we focus on school violence prevention from the educator's perspective. As Morrison, Furlong, and Morrison (1994) have argued, schools must come to own the problem of school violence. The following sections present an overview taking an educational focus to the problem of school violence by: (a) discussing what is known about the occurrence of violence on school campuses, (b) reviewing exemplary and promising prevention programs that have a clear school-based process, (c) discussing unsupported school violence prevention strategies, and (d) commenting on the elements of the best practices in school violence prevention.

DEFINITIONS AND SCOPE

It is widely recognized (Larson, Smith, & Furlong, 2002) that the most useful information about the incidence of school violence is derived from the periodic compilation of school safety related data taken from each school district, and preferably each school site. All safe school planning models (Dwyer & Osher, 2000; Stephens, 1998) emphasize the importance of gathering data that informs each school of its specific safety needs and assets. These sources of information typically include school crime incident reports, school disciplinary reports, and student surveys. Kingery and Coggeshall (2001) compared the three most prominent student surveys conducted in the United States (the Center for Disease Control and Prevention's Youth Risk Behavior Surveillance Survey [YRBS]; the US Department of Justice National Crime Victimization Survey, School Supplement [NCVS]; and the University of Michigan's Monitoring the Future Survey [MTF]). They concluded that the incidence of school violence derived from these surveys was affected by the degree of anonymity they afforded. In addition, the items used in these surveys to assess school violence were developed in a hodge-podge fashion during the 1990s and have not been well linked to an objective definition of school violence (Small & Tetrick, 2001). With this caution in mind, the following brief summary of school violence trends is presented taken from the YRBS administrations in 1993, 1995, 1997, and 1999 (see Furlong, Morrison, Austin, Huh-Kim, & Skager, 2001, for a review of the YRBS):

1. Since 1993, there has been a 21.3 percent reduction in the incidence of reporting physical fights on school campuses among boys. In 1999, 18.5 percent of high school males indicted they had a physical fight in the past 12 months. In contrast, only 9.8 percent of females indicated that they had been in a physical fight; however, this was a 14.0 percent increase.

2. Among high school males (9.2–9.5 percent) and females (5.4–5.8 percent) there were slight increases in the percentages of students reporting that they had been threatened or injured by someone with a weapon at school.

3. A most promising trend indicated that students reported carrying weapons to school far less often in 1999 than in 1993. For males, weapon possession decreased by 34.5 percent (17.9–11.0 percent). Similarly, female weapon possession decreased by 45.1 percent (5.1–2.8 percent).

Related to these broad school violence indicators, information about school associated deaths has been compiled by the National School Safety Center (see www.nssc1.org). This database reveals that school associated deaths peaked in 1992–1993 and have decreased by 63 percent through the 2000–2001 school year. Nonetheless, the occurrence of tragic school shootings involving multiple victims motivates schools to continue to search for effective methods to reduce school violence. One development that has emerged from the

United States's experience of school shootings has been an increased appreciation for the effects of chronic bullying on school campuses, an issue that has long been acknowledged outside of the United States (Olweus, 2001). Although bullying incidence varies by school, community, and nation, it is now generally acknowledged that it is a common and widespread phenomenon that has deleterious effects on both the victims' and perpetrators' academic and social-emotional development (Hawker & Boulton, 2001; Smith et al., 2001). One recent study in the United States that used the World Health Organization's Health Behavior in School-Aged Children Survey found that nearly 30 percent of students in grades 6–10 reported being a bully or victim, or both.

THEORY

Building an Educational Foundation for Violence Prevention

Extreme forms of physical violence on school campuses are less frequent than in other social settings (Small & Tetrick, 2001); however, given the common occurrence of low-level violence on school campuses (e.g., fighting, verbal abuse, and social isolation) action is needed. There are several preliminary steps educators can take to promote healthy development for all children before implementing more detailed programs to meet specified school violence reduction objectives. Grant and Van Acker (2000) describe four developmental needs of students that are needed for them to feel safe and secure in the school setting. First, safety is necessary. Not only does safety encompass physical security, but more importantly, the psychological health of students. In addition to being victimized by peer name-calling and fighting, other sources of harm may be present on a school campus. In some unfortunate circumstances, students may even be subjected to harmful experiences by teachers, such as discussing student behavior in public and exclusionary disciplinary policies. Second, positive regard and belonging are necessary, and must be actively fostered in those who initially feel isolated or rejected from individuals at school. Exclusionary disciplinary practices in school may also send a message to students that they are not welcomed. When prosocial avenues to support are tenuous, students may find that friendships with other antisocial youth are more rewarding, and consequently grow increasingly distant from their teachers and prosocial peers. Third, students must feel competent to meet the demands required of them. Lacking feelings of competence, some students may turn to disruptive behaviors in order to avoid challenging tasks. Finally, students have the basic need for power, control, and efficacy; that is, to feel in charge of their lives. When feelings of powerlessness arise in school, a student may react aggressively in order to gain power through dominance. Efforts to prevent school violence would be well served to consider these four development needs prior to implementing specific programs and plans.

Although schools should focus on the well being of all students, youths differ in the amount of intervention necessary to maximize their healthy development. Recognizing the importance of interpersonal bonding to positive outcomes, a five-level system may be useful in conceptualizing school violence prevention efforts (Furlong, Pavelski, & Saxton, 2002). Universal prevention programs are appropriate for the majority of students in order to *Reaffirm* relationships. For students who are not responsive to such programs, but are still somewhat involved in school, there is a need to *Reconnect* relationships. A third level involves the need to *Reconstruct* relationships with those students who have disengaged from school, and may already have histories of antisocial behaviors. Another marginalized group of students in need of intensive intervention are those who have been victimized at school and for whom there is a need to *Repair* school relationships. Finally, schools need to *Protect* their students from acts of school violence committed by individuals outside the school campus.

School Safety Plan: The Foundation of Violence Prevention

In order to combat and prevent the threat of school violence, effective programs begin with a comprehensive effort to create safe schools. A safe school is a place where students can go to learn and where teachers can teach, both without the experience of fear or intimidation, physical or psychological. The safe school has a peaceful environment that fosters growth, collaboration, and mutual respect among and between students and teachers. The blueprints for this design will vary between schools based upon the particular needs, priorities, and interests of the students, their families, the teaching staff, as well as the available resources within the school and the surrounding community. As such, a well considered safe school plan must involve long-term planning and commitment, comprise both school site and district wide planning components, and foster a diverse collaborative team approach (Stephens, 1998). The individuals on this planning team should incorporate key members of the community including law enforcement officials, teachers, administrators, counselors, school staff, security and custodial personnel, as well as parents and students. The team should also reflect the cultural diversity of the school and community in order to assure that decisions being made are sensitive to the needs of the school and community it represents. The safe school plan should be continuously monitored, reevaluated, and modified when necessary by the members of the team (Stephens, 1998). The plan should focus on interagency and local business support to enhance not only efforts in violence prevention and student safety but also to increase educational opportunities and standards for all students. Stephens

suggests that the ingredients for creating a safe school plan should include the following: (a) placing school safety on the educational agenda, (b) developing a safe school planning team, (c) conducting a site assessment, (d) developing a plan of where a school wants to be (e.g., setting goals), (e) involving students and parents, (f) reviewing the law, (g) formulating a crisis response plan, (h) continuing development, and (i) conducting a continuing evaluation.

In addition to an efficient and structured safety planning process, school violence prevention needs to address core-motivating principles. These principles assist safety-planning teams to articulate which prevention programs have the potential to address site-specific needs. Schools that choose to actively develop a comprehensive plan must also attend to many difficult and serious questions (Furlong et al., 2002). Which problems are most likely to affect the school? How has violence affected the school climate and culture? Are possible prevention efforts "research based" programs that have proven effectiveness? Given the assumption that the educators at a specific school site have engaged in a thoughtful safe school planning process, the remaining sections of this entry focus on: (a) exemplary and promising practices that reduce school violence and (b) practices that fail to prevent the occurrence of school violence.

STRATEGIES: OVERVIEW

Only recently have empirical studies focused on the effectiveness of programs to reduce violence specifically on school campuses, as opposed to youth violence in general, juvenile delinquency, or other forms of antisocial behavior. Although it has been assumed that positive effects of youth violence prevention programs would generalize to school settings, this has waited for empirical verification. Selecting specific programs appropriate for the prevention of school violence continues to remain a challenging task (Bates, Furlong, Saxton, & Pavelski, 2001) because of the small number of studies completed to date. Derzon and Wilson (1999), in fact, in a meta-analysis of school violence prevention studies notes that there have been more conceptual articles written about how to prevent school violence than actual empirical studies of program effectiveness. As such, it remains difficult to determine with absolute certainty which prevention programs are most appropriate or effective and for which type of students, schools, or communities (Bates et al., 2001). In an effort to move schools toward an outcome-based school violence prevention model, The US Departments of Education and Justice have recommended a comprehensive three-level approach (Dwyer & Osher, 2000; see Figure 1). The foundation and first level of this approach involves school-wide prevention in order to build positive discipline and academic success for all students.

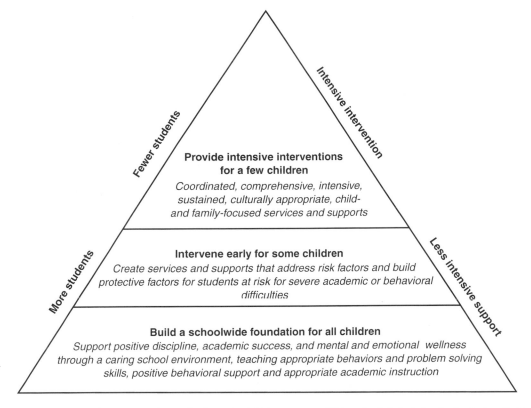

Figure 1. Safe school prevention hierarchy from the US Department of Education's Safe Schools: An Action Guide.

The second level entails efforts in early intervention appropriate for all students, while the third level includes intensive and coordinated services for students who are most at-risk of participating in or being a victim of school violence (Dwyer & Osher, 2000). Exemplary school violence prevention programs typically target one of these three levels of prevention.

STRATEGIES THAT WORK

The USDE expert panel required that exemplary programs have at least one evaluation with demonstrated effects on violent behavior, substance abuse, or conduct problems for a minimum of one year. Programs in this category had to receive a rating of 3 (on a 0–3 scale) on criterion one, a 2 (or higher) on criterion two through seven, and receive a 3 on at least three of the criteria one through seven (US Department of Education, 2001).

The panel's choice of exemplary programs emphasized primarily drug and alcohol prevention. Programs specifically designed for the sole purpose of violence prevention appear to have taken more time to evolve in comparison to more widely implemented substance prevention programs. However, each of the exemplary programs does address aspects of the recommended levels of violence prevention discussed previously (Dwyer & Osher, 2000). Four out of

the nine programs selected as exemplary by the expert panel included: Second Step, the Life Skills Training program, the Bullying Prevention Program, the Strengthening Families Program, and Striving Together to Achieve Rewarding Tomorrows (CASASTART). These exemplary programs are a combination of substance abuse prevention programs and violence prevention programs implemented in schools settings.

Second Step

This program is a school based, social skills curriculum for students from preschool through junior high school (Frey, Hirschstein, & Guzzo, 2000). The program aims at teaching students effective social skills in order to reduce impulsive and aggressive behaviors while increasing students' social competence. Some 20 lessons are provided per grade level ranging from 20 to 50 min in length (depending upon the grade level). Second Step emphasizes three key goals in each lesson: empathy, impulse control, and anger management. Teachers are provided with photo lesson cards, lesson outlines, reproducible homework sheets, overhead transparencies, and a video. In a recent evaluation conducted by the Harborview Injury Prevention and Research Center at the University of Washington, the Second Step curriculum was found to decrease students' aggressive behavior while increasing more prosocial behaviors within the school setting (Grossman et al., 1997).

Life Skills Training (LST)

The LST program (Botvin, Mihalic, & Grotpeter, 1998) is an effective substance abuse and violence prevention program. The program is geared toward middle or junior high school students and consists of 15 units, which focus on five sequential components. Students are taught ways to: (a) increase their self-esteem and self-confidence, (b) developing more effective ways of dealing with social anxieties, and (c) increase their knowledge regarding the consequences of substance abuse. LST aims at teaching the necessary skills to combat peer pressure involving smoking, drinking, and using drugs. The literature has shown there to be a strong link between school violence and substance use (Grunbaum, Basen-Engquist, & Pandey, 1998). This explains how programs designed to reduce substance use in turn reduce the incidence of school violence. Research on this effectiveness of the program has found a decrease in risk-taking behaviors, with increases in knowledge related to drugs and alcohol. The program has also been shown to cut tobacco, alcohol, and illicit drug use by 87 percent with effects lasting at least up to 6 years (Botvin et al., 1998).

Bullying Prevention Program

The program focuses on school-wide prevention of bullying (Olweus et al., 1999). *Bullying* is defined as aggressive behavior, repeated over time, occurring within an interpersonal relationship, and where there exists an imbalance of power (Olweus et al., 1999). The program can be implemented within an elementary, middle school, or high school campus and involves specific school-wide, classroom based, and individualized student components. At the school-wide level, the prevalence of bullying is assessed and a school conference day is designated to discuss the occurrence of bullying on the school campus. Within the classroom, rules specifically addressing bullying behavior are discussed and established with students' involvement. Individual students who are thought to be at high-risk of participating in or becoming a victim of bullying at school are involved in additional interventions with their parents and various school personnel (e.g., teachers, counselor, and mental health professionals). Results have shown a reduction in student reports of bullying, antisocial behavior (e.g., vandalism, fighting, theft, and truancy), and improvements in discipline, positive social relationships, and positive attitudes toward school (Olweus et al., 1999).

Strengthening Families Program

This program is a violence prevention developed for Project Family at the Institute for Social and Behavioral Research at Iowa State University (Kumpfer, Molgaard, & Spoth, 1996). Primarily implemented by outside agencies, the curriculum has also been used within school districts and designed to support parents, youth and whole families through a skills building curriculum. The curriculum includes the following components: strengthening parenting skills, building families' strengths, and preventing teen substance abuse. The program consists of seven sessions with four additional booster sessions of two hours each. Initially, parents and youth are met with separately and later participate in the learning process as a whole family. Ethnically diverse families and youth from both rural and urban settings have successfully participated in this program. In a study following 446 families from 6th through the 10th grades, youth attending the program demonstrated significantly lower rates of marijuana, alcohol, and tobacco use in addition to fewer conduct problems in school when compared to youth not involved in the study. In addition, parents involved in the study showed an increase in positive feelings toward their child, and demonstrated gains in child management skills (e.g., effective monitoring, rule setting and consistent discipline).

Striving Together to Achieve Rewarding Tomorrows (CASASTART)

This approach is a substance abuse and delinquency prevention program. CASASTART provides intensive services for at-risk youth involved in serious drug use and violence at school and in the community (see: http://www.casacolumbia.org). Developed by the National Center on Addiction and Substance Abuse at Columbia University, CASASTART is a neighborhood-based school-centered program. The program depends upon a collaborative effort between law enforcement, schools, and social service agencies in order to provide participating students with services in the following areas: tutoring, mentoring, family services, after-school activities, counseling, community policing, juvenile justice intervention, and other incentives. Case managers are assigned to work one-on-one with 15 families in order to coordinate services, make referrals, and develop case plans. In a program evaluation, CASASTART participants associated themselves less with delinquent peers, reported significantly lower levels of violent offenses, demonstrated higher levels of positive peer influences and were less likely to use drugs. The program is currently being implemented in 19 sites in the United States.

STRATEGIES THAT MIGHT WORK

The programs selected by the expert panel and designated as promising programs were required to have at least one evaluation showing an effect on violent behavior, substance use, conduct problems or one or more risk and protective factors associated with these behaviors (US Department of Education, 2001). In all, the expert panel selected 33 promising programs. Only six of the 33 programs are described below and are categorized according to elementary, middle school and secondary programs.

Elementary School Programs: Providing Alternative Thinking Strategies (PATHS)

This a curriculum developed by Greenberg, Kusché, and Mihalic (1998). The curriculum is used by teachers and counselors and is intended to improve students' skills in '...emotional literacy, positive peer relations, and problem-solving' (Greenberg et al., 1998, p. 7). PATHS focuses on improving students' abilities to: (a) increase self control, (b) recognize and interpret similarities and differences in others' points of view, (c) become aware of how feelings can affect one's behaviors and the behaviors of others, and (d) understand and implement problem solving skills in order to prevent and resolve conflicts. The curriculum is composed of three major units including self-control, feelings and relationships, and interpersonal cognitive problem-solving. Controlled studies with children in both general and special education programs have shown significant increases in students' abilities to understand social problems, decrease the percentage of aggressive and violent solutions, as well as develop alternative solutions to problems and conflicts. Teachers have reported a decrease in students' internalizing symptoms (e.g., sadness and anxiety), as well as externalizing symptoms (e.g., aggressive and disruptive behavior).

Open Circle

This curriculum was developed by The Reach Out to Schools: Social Competency Program (see: http://www.wellesley.edu/opencircle). It addresses such topics as: listening to others, voicing one's ideas and feelings, coping with teasing, recognizing discrimination, learning how to appropriately express one's anger, learning how to calm down, reaching consensus with others, as well as learning effective problem solving strategies. The individual lessons are conducted twice per week for 15–30 min per day. During lessons, the students and teacher form a circle facing one another, leaving an additional chair available for anyone else who decides to join the group. Open Circle has included more than 200,000 children in over 221 schools. This curriculum provides teachers with lessons, supplementary resources, parent letters, suggestions for homework, and additional reading. Program evaluations have shown significant gains in students' specific interpersonal and problem solving skill development, in addition to gains in individual responsibility. An evaluation conducted in 1996 found that according to teacher reports, students in the program experienced fewer problem behaviors and had a greater number of social skills in comparison to students whom had not participated in the program.

Middle School Programs: I Can Problem Solve (ICPS)

This prevention program, one of the oldest, addresses interpersonal, cognitive, problem-solving skills and was developed by Spivack and Shure (Shure, 1992). This self-contained program contains 77 lessons including games, stories, and role-plays. The lessons provide teachers with specific scripts, reproducible illustrations, and a list of additional materials supporting the program's goals and objectives. ICPS has been shown to effectively help children acquire interpersonal problem solving skills. Fifth grade students who had been trained in the ICPS program when compared to students trained in an alternative program, showed improvement in alternative solution thinking, consequential thinking and means–ends thinking in addition to notable progress in positive, and prosocial behaviors. Research and program evaluations on ICPS have been conducted with children from diverse ethnic and economic backgrounds in addition to students with special needs. This program has been extended to include components appropriate for students in the preschool, kindergarten, and primary grades.

Lions-Quest Skills for Adolescence

Quest International developed this specialized life skills and drug prevention program for students in sixth through eighth grades (Sprunger & Pellaux, 1989). The program works on character development, communication and decision-making skills, as well as community service learning. This program seeks to: (a) help youth develop more positive and responsible behaviors; (b) involve members of the community, family and school in program implementation; and (c) build students' citizenship skills, while providing youth with ongoing support, resources and guidance. Evaluations of the Lions-Quest program have shown effective change in students' knowledge, attitudes, and beliefs surrounding violent behavior and substance abuse. Participating students reported significantly lower rates of beer, liquor, and chewing tobacco use when compared to nonparticipating students. Additional Lions-Quest curricular programs available for the elementary (Skills for Growing) and secondary (Skills for Action) grades have been also shown to be effective.

Secondary School Programs: Community of Caring

This project addresses destructive attitudes in teens through a total community approach (see: http://www.communityofcaring.org). The program emphasizes the values of caring, responsibility, respect, trust, and family while showing how these values can be acknowledged and included in everyday life. Students who participate in the program are able to increase their self-confidence, responsibility, and decision-making skills. Students' families involve themselves in the program by planning, implementing, and setting goals along with school personnel and students. Community service is an additional component of the program. Through community service, students apply what they have learned in the classroom, benefiting both the community as well as the participating students. Evaluations of Community of Caring have noted increases in academic performance, reduced numbers of pregnancies, and fewer unexcused absences.

Teenage Health Teaching Modules (THTM)

The philosophy of this program views health as a particular condition allowing individuals to live to their full potential and involving areas of physical, mental, emotional, spiritual, and social skills (see: http://www.edc.org/thtm). Students work on building such skills as decision-making, goal setting, health advocacy, and self-management. An evaluation of THTM found positive effects on students' attitudes, health knowledge and self-reported behaviors. In a large-scale study involving approximately 5,000 students, and 150 teachers, THTM showed positive effects on students' attitudes and health-related knowledge. High school students who had participated in the THTM program reported reductions in tobacco, alcohol and drug use. THTM has also been successfully implemented in the intermediate grades (sixth through ninth).

STRATEGIES THAT DO NOT WORK

It is extremely important to review strategies that do not work in preventing school violence, as these strategies are often a natural reaction to the threat of physical danger. As discussed previously, fostering a safe school environment is essential to the successful integration of all students into the school environment. However, strategies such as building perimeter fences, hiring security guards, constructing metal detectors, profiling, and implementing zero tolerance policies are all reactions to the fear of violence that oftentimes alienate students rather than act as effective means of preventing school violence. Rather than view schools as a place to control and reform wayward youth, schools should take responsibility for their role in shaping the lives of the students they serve in a more thoughtful and protective manner.

Brotherton (1996) investigated the effect of inner-city schools' practice of social control in order to prevent acts of violence on their campuses. These inner-city schools all struggled with gang violence on their school campuses. The first strategy implemented by the schools was to bring in police surveillance in order to collect data about gang relationships. This knowledge was useful to school personnel, but when used to guide prevention efforts it focused attention on suppression techniques and did not necessarily address a specific school's most pressing school safety needs. In addition, the schools brought guards onto campus, built fences around the perimeter of the school, and formed an alliance between police, teachers, and administrators. This approach served to alienate some students from their teachers, contributed racial and ethnic stereotypes of gang members, and restricted educational access to those students who did commit delinquent acts (Brotherton, 1996). Students in this study stated that these interventions made school another unsafe place where they felt scrutinized and punished by authorities. Post intervention evidence suggested that gang graffiti and intergang fights were just as prevalent as before the interventions. Brotherton (1996) states that such police presence in the schools may foster a 'battle for respect' between marginalized students and the police. In their attempt to control these youth, the police presence on school campus may actually promote feelings of alienation and distrust in the students they are trying to serve and protect. These are possible unintended outcomes that should be considered on a school-by-school basis.

With the recent incidents of shootings on school campuses, federal and state legislators have created policies that requires specific consequences for serious offenses, such as mandatory expulsion for causing physical injury to another, weapon possession, drug possession, or robbery (Morrison, Anthony, Storino, Cheng, Furlong, & Morrison, 2001). It has been argued that such a policy actually has the opposite effect intended, exacerbating antisocial behavior on campus (Hyman & Perone, 1998). Through a review of expulsion practices, the ultimate consequence of zero tolerance policy, Morrison and colleagues (2001) discuss the outcome of such a discipline policy. They found that very few students who were expelled presented a danger to other students or staff and that there is an overrepresentation of minority students and students with special needs among those so punished. These authors note that such strict discipline policies may serve to further alienate students who have already been struggling in school, and may contribute to antisocial behavior for these youth. Zero tolerance is not an educational intervention, and has no empirical support (Skiba & Petersen, 1999). Rather than use reactive strategies to student misbehavior, schools should consider using approaches specific to the needs of each student (Morrison et al., 2001).

Another recently promoted strategy to prevent school shootings has been to profile potential school shooters by reviewing the characteristics of those youths that have committed such acts. The goal of profiling is to be able to predict which youths are likely to commit a school shooting, and single out likely candidates. However, the odds that a child will die in school (by homicide or suicide) are no more than one in a million (Hyman & Perone, 1998). This makes singling out a student as a potential school shooter a psychometric impossibility, and thus, potentially harmful to the large number of misidentified students. Profiling has typically been used in order to determine the perpetrator of a crime after it has occurred. Setting criteria in order to profile an outcome is an inherently biased social decision, and not something that can be accurately determined. The March 2001 issue of *Psychology in the Schools* provides a thorough review of the limitations and possibilities of violence assessment (Furlong, Kingery, & Bates, 2001). In brief, measures of violence potential should only be used to provide intervention services to all youths in need. School violence prevention should not be limited to a small percentage of aggressive youth, but reflect a system wide focus (Furlong et al., 2001).

SYNTHESIS

Helping students to develop effective strategies to cope with teasing, taunting, and other forms of harassment provides a critical component of school violence prevention. The reasoning is that schools can and should make every effort to create a positive, supportive learning climate at school, but despite even the best efforts, it may be inevitable that some students in some unsupervised contexts will be victimized by bullies or other acts of violence. Students need to be prepared to have the internal resources with which to make the most effective response. The most effective response may vary by the chronological age and developmental maturity of the student. Among early elementary-age students getting support from a friend and telling a teacher have been associated with the long-term reduction of victimization (Kochenderfer Ladd & Ladd, 1997, 2001). In contrast, middle-school students may be better served by taking a "whatever-no-big-deal" response (Salmivali, Karhunen, & Lagerspertz, 1996). At all ages, however, helpless/passive or aggressive responses are associated with continued victimization (Smith et al., 2001).

What has been lacking in school violence prevention has been overarching conceptual rationales to drive these efforts. Early on, Morrison et al. (1994) argued that school violence prevention efforts might be enhanced if the definition of school violence is expanded to include the notion of the prevention of harm in the school setting. If this conceptual reframing is made, then school violence prevention efforts then become: (a) more integrated within the broader school mission of educating students and (b) allows school safety promotion efforts to move beyond addressing risk of extreme physical harm to other sources of harm in the school setting: non-malicious physical dangers, bullying, harassment, and ineffective education practices. This linking of violence prevention efforts to threats of harm in the school setting increases the chances that schools will embrace violence prevention as an educational, not just a security, priority (Morrison, Furlong, Morrison, & D'Incau, in press).

Additionally, the amount of conceptual thinking about violence prevention has focused more on the development of programs to change the dysfunctional and potential dangerous behaviors of specific students and less so on the context in which these behaviors occur (Astor, Meyer, & Behre, 1999). One common theme that has emerged in the school violence prevention literature that merits consideration is the integration of concepts and research from the risk and resiliency literature (see Morrison et al., 1994) to drive the development, implementation, and refinement of violence prevention programs. This is based on the recognition that while an important goal of violence prevention programs is to reduce the incidence of violence (indeed if any program cannot show this outcome, then it should not be used), ultimately violence reduction alone is not a sufficient objective. The penultimate goal is to enhance the social–emotional competence of students so that they will be safer at school AND so that they can live more purposeful, effective lives everywhere. As such, the recent past and future of school violence prevention will increasingly involve programs that provide a solid basis in strategies that enhance students' internal resources and external assets (Morrison et al., in press; Smith et al., 2001).

Also see: School entries; Violence Prevention; Childhood; Bullying.

References

Astor, R.A., Meyer, H.A., & Behre, W.J. (1999). Unknown places and times: Maps and interviews about violence in high schools. *American Educational Research Journal (AERJ), 36*, 3–42.

Bates, M.P., Furlong, M.J., Saxton, J.D., & Pavelski, R. (2001). Research needs for school crisis prevention programs. In S. Brock, P. Lazarus, & S. Jimerson (Eds.), *Best practices in school crisis response*. Bethesda, MD: National Association of School Psychologists.

Botvin, G.J., Mihalic, S.F., & Grotpeter, J.K. (1998). *Blueprints for violence prevention, book five: Life skills training*. Boulder, CO: Center for the Study and Prevention of Violence.

Brotherton, D.C. (1996). The contradictions of suppression: Notes from a study of approaches to gangs in three public high schools. *The Urban Review, 28*, 95–117.

Derzon, J.H., & Wilson, S.J. (1999). *An empirical review of school-based programs to reduce violence* [on-line]. Washington, DC: Hamilton Fish Institute. Available: http://hamfish.org/pub/schoolint.pdf

Dwyer, K., & Osher, D. (2000). *Safeguarding our children: An action guide*. Washington, DC: US Departments of Education and Justice, American Institutes for Research.

Frey, K.S., Hirschstein, M.K., & Guzzo, B.A. (2000). Second Step: Preventing aggression by promoting social competence. *Journal of Emotional & Behavioral Disorders, 8*, 102–112.

Furlong, M.J., Kingery, P.E., & Bates, M.P. (2001). Introduction to special issue on the appraisal and prediction of school violence, *Psychology in the Schools, 38*, 89–92.

Furlong, M.J., & Morrison, G.M. (2000). The SCHOOL in school violence: Definitions and facts. *Journal of Emotional and Behavioral Disorders, 8*, 71–82.

Furlong, M.J., Morrison, G.M., Austin, G., Huh-Kim, J., & Skager, R. (2001). Using student risk factors in school violence surveillance reports: Illustrative examples for enhanced policy formation, implementation, and evaluation. *of Law and Policy, 23,* 271–295.

Furlong, M.J., Pavelski, R.E., & Saxton, J.D. (2002). The prevention of school violence. In S. Brock, P. Lazarus, & S. Jimerson (Eds.), *Best practices in school crisis response.* (131–149). Bethesda, MD: National Association of School Psychologists.

Grant, S.H., & Van Acker, R. (2000). Do schools teach aggression? Recognizing and retooling the interactions that lead students to aggression. *Reaching Today's Youth, 5,* 27–32.

Greenberg, M.T., Kusché, C., & Mihalic, S.F. (1998). *Blueprints for violence prevention, book ten: Promoting Alternative Thinking Strategies (PATHS).* Boulder, CO: Center for the Study and Prevention of Violence.

Grossman, D.C., Neckerman, H.J., Koepsell, T.D., Liu, P.Y., Asher, K.N., Beland, K., Frey, K., & Rivera, F.P. (1997). Effectiveness of a violence prevention curriculum among children in elementary school: A randomized controlled trial. *Journal of the American Medial Association, 277,* 1605–1611.

Grunbaum, J., Basen-Engquist, K., & Pandey, D. (1998). Association between violent behaviors and substance use among Mexican-American and non-Hispanic White high school students. *Journal of Adolescent Health, 23,* 153–159.

Hawker, D.S., & Boulton, M.J. (2001). Subtypes of peer harassment and their correlates. In J. Juvonen & S. Graham (Eds.), *Peer harassment in school: The plight of the vulnerable and victimized* (pp. 378–419). New York: Guilford Press.

Hyman, I.A., & Perone, D.C. (1998). The other side of school violence: Educator policies and practices that may contribute to student misbehavior. *Journal of School Psychology, 36,* 7–27.

Juvonen, J., & Graham, S. (Eds.). (2001). *Peer harassment in school: The plight of the vulnerable and victimized.* New York: Guilford Press.

Kingery, P.M., & Coggeshall, M.B. (2001). Surveillance of school violence, injury, and disciplinary actions. *Psychology in the Schools, 38,* 117–112.

Kochenderfer Ladd, B., & Ladd, G.W. (1997). Victimized children's responses to peers' aggression: Behaviors associated with reduced and continued victimization. *Development and Psychopathology, 9,* 59–73.

Kochenderfer Ladd, B., & Ladd, G.W. (2001). Variations in peer victimization: Relations to children's maladjustment. In J. Juvonen & S. Graham (Eds.), *Peer harassment in school: The plight of the vulnerable and victimized* (pp. 25–48). New York: Guilford Press.

Kumpfer, K.L., Molgaard, V., & Spoth, R. (1996). The Strengthening Families Program for the prevention of delinquency and drug use. In R.D. Peters & R.J. McMahon (Eds.), *Preventing childhood disorders, substance abuse, and delinquency* (pp. 241–267). Thousand Oaks, CA: Sage.

Larson, J., Smith, D., & Furlong, M (2001). School violence. In A Thomas & J. Grimes (Eds.), *Best Practices in School Psychology-IV* (pp. 1081–1097). Bethesda, MD: National Association of School Psychologists.

Morrison, G.M., Anthony, S., Storino, M., Cheng, J., Furlong, M.J., & Morrison, R.L. (2001). School expulsion as a process and as event: Before and after effects on children at-risk for school discipline. In R.J. Skiba & G.G. Noam (Eds.) *New Directions in Mental Health/New Directions in Youth Development (special issue on zero-tolerance).*

Morrison, G.M., Furlong, M.J., & Morrison, R.L. (1994). School violence to school safety: Reframing the issue for school psychologists. *School Psychology Review, 23,* 236–256.

Morrison, G.M., Furlong, M.J., Morrison, R.L., & D'Incau, B. (2000). The safe school: Moving beyond crime prevention to school empowerment. In J. Conoley & A. Goldstein (Eds.), *School violence prevention: A practical handbook* (2nd ed.). New York: Guilford Press.

Nansel, T.R., Overpeck, M., Pill, R.S., Ruan, J., Simons-Morton, B., & Scheidt, P. (2001). Bullying behaviors among US youth: Prevalence and association with psychosocial adjustment. *Journal of the American Medical Association, 285,* 2094–2100.

Olweus, D. (2001). Peer harassment: A critical analysis and some important issues. In J. Juvonen & S. Graham (Eds.), *Peer harassment in school: The plight of the vulnerable and victimized* (pp. 3–20). New York: Guilford Press.

Olweus, D., Limber, S., & Mihalic, S.F. (1999). *Blueprints for violence prevention, book nine: Bullying prevention program.* Boulder, CO: Center for the Study and Prevention of Violence.

Owens, L., Slee, P., & Shute, R. (2001). Victimization among teenage girls: What can be done about indirect harassment. In J. Juvonen & S. Graham (Eds.), *Peer harassment in school: The plight of the vulnerable and victimized* (pp. 215–241). New York: Guilford Press.

Salmivali, C., Karhunen, J., & Lagerspertz, K.M.J. (1996). How do victims respond to bullying? *Aggressive Behavior, 22,* 99–109.

Shure, M.B. (1992). *I Can Problem Solve: An interpersonal cognitive problem-solving program: Intermediate elementary grades.* Champaign, IL: Research Press.

Skiba, R., & Petersen, R. (1999). Zero-tolerance: Can punishment lead to safe schools? *Phi Delta Kappan, 80,* 372–376, 381–382.

Small, M., & Tetrick, K.D. (2001). School violence: An overview. *Juvenile Justice, School Violence an Overview, 8,* 3–12.

Smith, P.K., Shu, S., & Madsen, K. (2001). Characteristics of victims of school bullying: Developmental changes in coping strategies. In J. Juvonen & S. Graham (Eds.), *Peer harassment in school: The plight of the vulnerable and victimized* (pp. 332–351). New York: Guilford Press.

Sprunger, B., & Pellaux, D. (1989). Skills for adolescence: Experience with the international Lions-Quest program. *Crisis Hogrefe & Huber Publishers, 10,* 88–104.

Stephens, R.D. (1998). Safe school planning. In D.S. Elliott, B.A. Hamburg, & K.R. Williams (Eds.), *Violence in American schools* (pp. 253–289). United Kingdom: Cambridge University Press.

US Department of Education. (2001). *1999 Guidelines for submitting safe, discipline, and drug-free schools programs for designation as promising or exemplary* [On-line]. Available: http://www.ed.gov/offices/OERI/ORAD/KAD/expert_panel/drug-free.html

Self-Esteem, Early Childhood

David L. DuBois

INTRODUCTION

Self-esteem has been defined as "the evaluation which an individual makes and customarily maintains with regard to himself [or herself]; it expresses an attitude of approval or disapproval" (Rosenberg, 1965, p. 5). At what age, however, do young children first begin to express coherent evaluations of their own worth and abilities consistent with this definition? Related to this concern, what factors constitute important influences on the development of self-esteem during early childhood (i.e., approximately ages 3–7)? Do young children who exhibit high levels of self-esteem, in turn, demonstrate healthier overall adjustment and less susceptibility to disorder? Informed by an understanding of answers to these questions, what results can be anticipated for interventions that seek to promote self-esteem during early childhood? Furthermore, what types of programs appear to be most effective and how might these be modified and strengthened in the future?

SCOPE

Measuring the self-esteem of young children presents special challenges because of developmental limitations that may exist in their abilities to both form and communicate an internal sense of self (Cassidy, 1990; Harter, 1999). Findings from several recent studies demonstrate, however, that children as young as $3\frac{1}{2}$ years of age possess psychologically meaningful conceptions of themselves (Eder, 1990; Measelle, Ablow, Cowan, & Cowan, 1998; Verschueren, Marcoen, & Schoefs, 1996). These conceptions, moreover, are multidimensional. Thus, in addition to a sense of being generally (un)worthy and (un)lovable, children as early as age 5 begin to harbor more differentiated views of their competence or adequacy related to academic, social, and physical domains (Marsh, Craven, & Debus, 1991). Young children also manifest varying degrees of feelings of self-worth through their behavior, with those high in "behaviorally presented self-esteem" tending to exude confidence, curiosity, initiative, and independence (Harter, 1999). These considerations indicate that it is not sufficient to simply know the overall feelings that a young child expresses about himself or herself as a person (often referred to as "global self-esteem"). Equally important may be whether the child possesses a positive sense of self related to specific areas such as school, peer relations, and physical abilities, and whether he or she conveys a high level of self-esteem to others through his or her behavior.

It is not unusual for young children to report unrealistically positive or even "perfect" views of themselves (Cassidy, 1990). This tendency can be attributed to developmental limitations such as the predominance of "all-or-none" thinking among young children and their failure to make use of comparisons to others (Harter, 1999). Highly negative self-perceptions are nevertheless reported by a small subset of young children, many of whose socialization histories involve abuse, maltreatment, or neglect (Harter, 1999). In studies conducted in both the United States and other Western countries, it has been found that more than one third of young children include at least some negative statements about themselves when given the opportunity to do so across a range of differing areas (Cassidy, 1990; Verschueren et al., 1996; Verschueren, Buyck, & Marcoen, 2001). This result is consistent with the multidimensionality of young children's self-esteem. It also suggests that unfavorable evaluations of the self in one or more localized areas are fairly common at this stage of development (Harter, 1999). Furthermore, even among young children whose self-descriptions are suggestive of uniformly high self-esteem, significantly less positive feelings of worth may be

evident in observations of their behavior by others such as parents or teachers (Cassidy, 1990).

Because self-esteem is important for healthy development (Harter, 1999), there may be significant costs when young children do not develop a strong sense of self-worth. These include greater risk for mental health problems, which can necessitate utilization of expensive services such as psychological testing, therapy and counseling, and residential treatment. Further costs may be associated with negative outcomes linked to poor self-esteem during childhood and adolescence, such as academic underachievement, juvenile crime, substance use, and health concerns (e.g., eating disorders). A lack of positive self-esteem developed early in childhood thus may contribute to increased levels of demand on a wide range of educational, social, and health care services and ultimately detract from the ability of youth to develop into productive members of society. From a more positive perspective, cultivating a strong sense of self-esteem in young children may facilitate healthy development and significantly reduce reliance on outside sources of support. To the extent that a collective esteem is fostered among all developing youth, a further benefit may be an enhanced overall quality of life within the surrounding community (Beane, 1994).

Several considerations point to early childhood as a time when efforts to enhance self-esteem may be especially beneficial. Many of the developmental tasks of young children such as starting formal schooling and establishing friendships with peers necessitate increased independence from primary caregivers. Children who have a positive conception of themselves and their abilities may be better prepared to cope effectively with these new types of situations and demands (Harter, 1999). Self-representations established in early childhood also represent an important foundation for views and feelings about the self throughout later stages of development (Cassidy, 1990). Efforts to promote a strong, healthy sense of self at this age therefore have the potential to yield dividends that accrue across the entire life span. Relatedly, the ages of onset for most negative outcomes that have been linked to low levels of self-esteem (e.g., substance use) are concentrated during subsequent stages of development. In this respect, esteem-enhancement programs for young children thus fit the definition of primary prevention. For this reason, they may offer greater potential for reducing incidence rates of future disorder than those focused on later points in development.

THEORIES

In normal development, self-esteem is derived from both a sense of personal competence or efficacy and a perception of being accepted and valued by others (Harter, 1999). These underpinnings of self-esteem have their earliest foundation in representations of the self that grow out of attachment relationships with primary caregivers (Cassidy, 1990). The extent to which young children experience parents or other important caregivers as concerned for their well-being may promote generalized feelings of being lovable and valued by others. Similarly, the opportunities that parent figures provide young children to explore the world around them, and their favorable responses to these efforts, provide the earliest basis for a sense of competence and mastery (Harter, 1999). Young children's feelings of self-worth also may be influenced to a significant degree, however, by the quality of their relationships with other adults (e.g., teachers) and peers and by their success in meeting adaptive demands in settings outside the home (e.g., preschool). To the extent that young children's needs for feelings of self-worth are met through their behavior and experiences in these areas, they may be motivated to engage in similar positive interactions with others and strivings for learning and mastery in the future as a way of maintaining a high level of self-esteem. Processes of self-esteem and healthy development that become closely intertwined in this way at an early age may help to set in motion long-term trajectories of overall positive adjustment throughout childhood and adolescence (DuBois & Tevendale, 1999).

There also, however, is a wide array of self-protective or self-enhancing strategies that young children may engage in to aid their efforts to maintain a sense of self-esteem. As described by Kaplan (1986),

> Self-protective/self-enhancing responses ... are oriented toward the goal of (1) forestalling the experience of self-devaluing judgments and consequent distressful self-feelings (self-protective patterns) and (2) increasing the occasions for positive self-evaluations and self-accepting feelings (self-enhancing patterns). (p. 174)

Kaplan (1986) distinguished three general forms of self-protective/self-enhancing responses relating to self-referent cognition, personal need-value systems, and behavior. With relevance to each of these categories, young children may attempt to protect or enhance their self-esteem by seemingly "filtering out" or ignoring less flattering information about themselves in their thinking, discounting the value or importance of activities in which they are less successful, and seeking out greater contact with persons who respond to them more positively (Harter, 1999). In many respects, these tendencies are not surprising. It is the rare child, after all, who can be expected to unfailingly accept in stride criticism or "corrective feedback", experience success in all endeavors, and universally be liked and well-regarded. Some degree of reliance on self-protective/self-enhancing strategies thus seems an inevitable and functional necessity for maintaining a robust sense of self-worth beginning at the earliest stages of development (Harter, 1999).

Self-protective/self-enhancing strategies provide insight into how differing levels of self-esteem may be linked to problems in adjustment (Kaplan, 1986). This is, in part, because strategies that children with low self-esteem use to protect or restore feelings of self-worth can be both counterproductive and maladaptive. Some young children lacking in self-esteem, for example, may display problem behavior at home or school in an effort to increase the attention they receive from others in these settings. Such children may further attempt to act out or aggress against others (e.g., peers) whom they experience as contributing to their lowered sense of worth (Kaplan, 1986). Other young children may exhibit generalized patterns of avoidance or withdrawal in response to feelings of inadequacy in one or more areas of their lives (Cassidy, 1990). Although interpretable as efforts to protect against exposure to future threats to self-esteem, this type of response may nevertheless increase their susceptibility to development of emotional disorders such as depression and anxiety. An extreme desire to "escape" from painful negative feelings of self-regard may contribute to suicidal thoughts and behaviors being displayed by some preschool-age children despite their very young age (Harter, 1999).

It is important to note, that even self-protective/self-enhancing strategies used by young children that are successful in maintaining or raising their self-esteem may create significant problems for other areas of their adjustment. Within the educational realm, for example, children who experience learning difficulties may be able to protect their overall feelings of self-worth by disavowing the value or importance of success in school (Harter, 1999). Doing so, however, is likely to substantially restrict the opportunities of such children for future academic achievement. Other young children may engage in denial or related forms of maladaptive coping to the point of cultivating excessively unrealistic or inflated self-concepts. For these children, high self-esteem may come with the price of limitations in self-awareness and difficulties getting along with others that detract significantly from their overall adjustment (Harter, 1999). In the long-run, the negative consequences associated with problematic self-protective/self-enhancing strategies may well even come full circle to undercut whatever gains in self-esteem were possible initially with the strategies involved at earlier points in development (DuBois & Tevendale, 1999).

RESEARCH

Research findings support the view that parent–child relationships are an important factor influencing the development of self-esteem among young children. The highest levels of self-esteem are found for those children who exhibit secure attachments to both parents (Verschueren & Marcoen,

1999). Accordingly, mothers and fathers each should be regarded as having a significant contribution to make in promoting their young children's feelings of self-worth. Conditions conducive to learning and safe exploration in the home environment also are associated with more positive self-concepts for preschool-age children. The likely multiply-determined nature of feelings of self-worth in early childhood, furthermore, is suggested by a wide range of other factors having been linked to variations in self-esteem during this stage of development. These include quality of relationships with teachers and peers, physical skills and abilities, and indicators of cognitive competence (Verschueren et al., 1996).

A positive sense of self at an early age has been found to promote the favorable adjustment of young children as they progress further in their development and schooling (Verschueren et al., 2001). Consistent with the multidimensionality of young children's self-esteem noted previously, there is evidence that strengths and weaknesses in distinct areas of self-evaluation can have significant implications for their adjustment. These types of views seem especially likely to influence aspects of functioning that are conceptually related to the area of self-esteem involved. In one recent study of young children, for example, a favorable academic self-concept was associated with better school performance, whereas self-perceptions of social competence and peer acceptance were linked to lower levels of aggression-hostility (Measelle et al., 1998). Negative views of the self in each domain, however, were associated with greater reported levels of depression-anxiety. It thus appears that, as is the case at other points in development, a pervasive tendency toward unfavorable self-evaluation across multiple areas in early childhood may heighten vulnerability to significant emotional disturbance (DuBois & Tevendale, 1999; Harter, 1999).

There also is evidence that processes providing the underlying bases for self-esteem among young children are an important consideration. Kindergarteners providing positive ratings of their self-concepts, but nominated as low in social or academic competence by teachers, were found to exhibit significant levels of negative classroom behavior and perform relatively poorly on tests of academic achievement (Strain et al., 1983). A recent study of second and third graders similarly found that inflated (i.e., unrealistically high) self-concepts were characteristic of students demonstrating the highest levels of aggression (Hughes, Cavell, & Grossman, 1997, cited in DuBois & Tevendale, 1999). These results are consistent with research conducted with older age groups in their suggestion that high levels of self-esteem lacking a realistic or adaptive basis are most likely to *detract* from, rather than facilitate, the overall adjustment of young children (DuBois & Tevendale, 1999; Harter, 1999).

To summarize, research indicates that healthy self-esteem during early childhood is promoted by a combination of both social acceptance and competence or mastery experiences within home, school, and peer settings. Young children who possess a high overall level of self-esteem, in turn, exhibit more positive functioning in a variety of other areas. Positive self-evaluations in specific domains also appear to contribute to favorable adaptation in early childhood. The extent to which young children rely on various self-protective/self-enhancing strategies to sustain or increase their self-esteem, however, is an important consideration. In the extreme, such tendencies can result in inflated or maladaptive bases for feelings of self-worth, undermining the potential benefits associated with a high level of self-esteem in early childhood.

STRATEGIES: OVERVIEW

Several literature reviews have considered the effectiveness of esteem-enhancement programs for children. Two are particularly noteworthy because of their use of meta-analytic procedures (Haney & Durlak, 1998; Hattie, 1992). Meta-analysis provides an objective method of quantitatively assessing the overall magnitude of effect produced by a given type of intervention on one or more outcome measures (e.g., self-esteem). Meta-analytic procedures also can be used to investigate differences in effect size along any dimension of interest that varies across studies (e.g., participant characteristics, program features, type of evaluation methodology).

In the meta-analyses of esteem-enhancement programs, Hattie (1992) reported an average effect size of 0.31 for programs targeting children (positive effect sizes indicate that programs were successful in raising participants' levels of self-concept or self-esteem). Haney and Durlak (1998) similarly found an average effect size of 0.27 across 120 evaluations of esteem-enhancement programs for children and adolescents. Overall, results indicate that children participating in programs typically have experienced small to moderate gains in self-esteem.

An association between the magnitude of positive program effects and age of participants was not found by Haney and Durlak (1998). Only a small number of programs ($n = 5$) targeted young children (ages 3–5 years), however, thus limiting the ability to evaluate program effectiveness for this particular age group. The other meta-analysis (Hattie, 1992) did not report comparative effect sizes for programs targeting children of varying ages. Accordingly, although both reviews report important findings, the extent to which results are applicable to promotion of self-esteem in early childhood specifically is a significant issue requiring clarification in future research. Several more recent interventions targeting young children (discussed below), however, have been found to be effective in enhancing self-esteem at this stage of development. These results provide a basis for optimism with regard to generalization of findings from programs conducted with older youth.

Haney and Durlak (1998) also examined whether children and adolescents participating in esteem-enhancement programs exhibit positive change in other areas of their adjustment. The areas considered were behavior (usually as determined by direct observation or teacher rating scales), personality/emotional functioning (typically reports by youth of their levels of anxiety or depression), and academic performance (grades and performance on standardized tests). Positive outcomes were evident in each of these domains. Programs producing the largest favorable effects on other areas of adjustment, furthermore, tend to be those in which participants experience the greatest increases in self-concept or self-esteem (Haney & Durlak, 1998). This result is important because it establishes a direct association between effective esteem-enhancement activities and overall improvements in child adjustment.

The extent to which interventions produce lasting increases in self-esteem (i.e., those that remain evident following completion of participation) is a further significant concern. It is possible, for example, that some positive effects observed are attributable to "euphoria" or good feelings at the end of programs and that these dissipate relatively quickly thereafter (Harter, 1999). Each meta-analysis reported some evidence of sustained effects of esteem-enhancement programs at follow-up (Haney & Durlak, 1998; Hattie, 1992). Only a few evaluations, however, addressed this concern. The authors thus cautioned that available findings did not provide a basis for drawing conclusions about the durability of program outcomes. A further limitation is that most follow-up intervals were relatively brief, rarely extending more than a few months past the end of programs. In an exception to this trend, assessments of self-esteem or self-concept have been included in a few long-term follow-up studies of early intervention programs such as Head Start. Overall, results have provided only limited evidence of effects of program participation on self-esteem at later points in development. It should be noted, however, that most of the interventions involved were not designed with the specific goal of enhancing self-esteem.

A final general concern is whether programs are effective in strengthening the self-esteem of all participating youth. The most substantial positive effects of interventions have been found for youth who enter programs already exhibiting low self-esteem or other types of pre-existing problems (Haney & Durlak, 1998; Hattie, 1992). In accordance with this trend, a majority of the programs found to enhance self-esteem in early childhood have targeted children believed to be "at-risk" for low self-esteem on the basis of either individual characteristics (e.g., developmental delay) or environmental considerations (e.g., poverty). By contrast, existing enhancement strategies have yielded only modest improvements in the self-esteem or self-concept of children for whom indicators of pre-existing vulnerability are lacking (Haney & Durlak, 1998; Hattie, 1992). Factors contributing to this pattern may include greater malleability of low or negative self-views as well as ceiling effects on measures of self-esteem for those exhibiting normal functioning. The content and design of programs, however, also is a significant consideration. Interventions to date have been geared almost exclusively toward raising children's overall feelings of self-worth. As a result, other potentially important concerns have received little attention. These include efforts to strengthen self-evaluations in specific areas as well as attempts to ensure that young children rely on healthy strategies to sustain their sense of self-worth (DuBois & Tevendale, 1999). If such factors were addressed more consistently, it might prove feasible to extend program benefits to a broader spectrum of children.

STRATEGIES THAT WORK

Both meta-analyses investigated trends in effectiveness across differing types of esteem-enhancement programs. Hattie (1992) found programs to be similar in their effectiveness regardless of whether they sought to increase self-esteem directly (e.g., curriculum) or by indirect methods (e.g., enhancing academic achievement). Haney and Durlak (1998) made a distinction between interventions that had a primary goal of changing self-esteem or self-concept (referred to as "SE/SC interventions") and those that did not have this specific aim but nonetheless did assess change in self-esteem or self-concept as a program outcome (i.e., "non-SE/SC interventions"). Less than half of the studies included in their review were evaluations of SE/SC interventions. The average effect size for these programs (0.57) was substantially higher than that of non-SE/SC interventions (0.10). Programs in which enhancement of self-esteem or self-concept was a primary goal (i.e., SE/SC interventions) also were associated with better overall adjustment outcomes for participants than those without this emphasis (Haney & Durlak, 1998).

Haney and Durlak (1998) found, furthermore, that programs with a well-defined basis in theory or prior research were substantially more effective than those without this type of foundation. Remarkably, this factor alone predicted nearly one third of the overall variation in program outcomes. Developmental theory, it will be recalled, emphasizes both: (a) experiences of competence or mastery and (b) a sense of being valued and accepted by significant others as key normative sources of self-esteem during early childhood. It is noteworthy, therefore, that some of the most promising results have been reported for esteem-enhancement efforts designed to provide young children with such experiences.

Several of these have been incorporated into existing early intervention programs with the aim of increasing their capacity to influence self-esteem and related outcomes. The *Values-for-Life* curriculum (Taylor, Turner, Underwood, Franklin, Jackson, & Stagg, 1994), a program designed to help teachers implement instructional routines to promote the socioemotional development of young children, is illustrative in this regard. Instructional activities designed specifically to enhance self-esteem focus on providing learning opportunities, stimulating inquisitiveness and language use, and giving reinforcement. In evaluation research, this program was found to produce significant gains in young children's self-esteem when implemented both in differing Head Start programs and various other types of child care centers (Taylor et al., 1994). Results also indicated co-occurring positive effects on children's objectively assessed skills in cognitive, social, and physical areas of development. Furthermore, Head Start children selected randomly to receive the curriculum in one evaluation study were rated as superior in their self-esteem to those who received only "regular" Head Start classes. This suggests that programs with a specific focus on esteem-enhancement can add significantly to the benefits associated with typical early intervention services.

Several programs oriented toward physical skill development also have been found to have favorable effects on the self-esteem of young children. In one such program (Alpert, Field, Goldstein, & Perry, 1990), preschoolers participated in 30 min of aerobic exercises on a daily basis for 8 weeks. Compared to children in a randomly assigned control group, those in the program exhibited significant increases in both self-esteem and cardiovascular fitness and agility (Alpert et al., 1990). Similar results have been reported for programs providing young children with training in perceptual-motor skills and those encouraging use of physical activity as a means of self-expression (e.g., pre-ballet). The effectiveness of such programs parallels the demonstrated capacity of physically oriented interventions to also produce substantial gains in self-esteem when implemented at later points in development (Hattie, 1992).

STRATEGIES THAT MIGHT WORK

There is a beginning of empirical evidence of other effective strategies for enhancing the self-esteem of young children. This includes promising indications of success for early intervention programs that seek to actively involve and support families. The strategies used in these programs are consistent with research highlighting the significance of positive parent–child relationships and a stimulating home environment for development of healthy self-esteem in early childhood. Some programs, for example, have had success utilizing home-based methods of teaching and instruction with young children. Others reporting favorable results have increased access of families to community-based resources as a means of supplementing more traditional, curricular-based esteem-enhancement activities. Several further programs have focused on parent training and education. These interventions show encouraging signs of being able to enhance the self-esteem of parents as caregivers, thus affording a potentially powerful route to promoting a positive sense of self in their young children.

There also is evidence that it may be useful to tailor the design of programs to meet the specific needs of children with differing characteristics and backgrounds. Young children provided with instruction in the language of their cultural or ethnic group (i.e., heritage language instruction), for example, were found to exhibit improvements in both personal and collective self-esteem compared to those receiving instruction only in a second language (Wright & Taylor, 1995). Similar positive results have been reported when adapting the curricula of early intervention programs (e.g., Head Start) to incorporate content and activities consistent with the cultural backgrounds of children and their families. Esteem-enhancement strategies geared toward the needs of young children exhibiting differing types of individual and environmental risk factors also demonstrate promise. Examples include school-based tutoring and mentoring services for those with learning disabilities and provision of after school programming for those in "latchkey" home situations.

Most programs to date reflect a focus on enhancing overall feelings of self-worth. Despite this trend, some interventions have strengthened young children's more circumscribed evaluations of themselves in particular areas or domains. The specific dimensions of self-concept or self-esteem affected typically have had direct relevance to aims of the program. These include gains in academic self-esteem within educationally oriented interventions, increased perceptions of physical competence in motor skills training programs, and growth in the social self-concepts of young children whose parents have received instruction in effective childrearing practices. Other interventions, such as the Values-for-Life program described earlier, also have been found to enhance presented or behavioral manifestations of self-esteem in young children. Cumulatively, results indicate that greater attention to strengthening distinct facets of self-esteem would be useful in both the design and evaluation of esteem-enhancement interventions for young children.

STRATEGIES THAT DO NOT WORK

Certain types of interventions, furthermore, do not seem likely to be effective for enhancing the self-esteem of young children. Based on literature reviewed in preceding sections, programs that lack a theory- or research-driven approach to promoting self-esteem during early childhood would fall into this category. There is little evidence, for example, to expect early intervention programs such as Head Start to produce substantial gains in the self-esteem of young children when implemented in their usual form without incorporation of activities that specifically address the goal of esteem-enhancement. There also are several reasons to question the value of programs directed solely to the goal of enhancing overall feelings of self-worth. These include the demonstrated capacity of interventions to be successful in promoting other distinct facets of self-esteem in early childhood. Developmental tendencies of young children (e.g., all or none thinking) also may in some instances interact with program activities focused narrowly on the goal of enhancing overall self-esteem so as to produce unrealistically positive self-perceptions that have limited adaptive value (Harter, 1999). Of related note are the modest and not necessarily long-lived effects of interventions to date on the self-esteem of young children. This suggests that even the most promising approaches to esteem-enhancement for this age group may not have strong or sustained positive effects if they continue to be implemented in relative isolation from one another.

SYNTHESIS

A synthesis of available findings points instead to the need for an integrated, multi-faceted approach to promoting self-esteem in early childhood. Programs developed within this type of framework can be expected to be most effective when enhancement of self-esteem is an explicit goal and relevant theory and research informs intervention activities. In other words, achieving gains in self-esteem should be a clearly defined aim of the program, and there should be a well-reasoned set of strategies in place for achieving this objective. It will be recalled, however, that indirect approaches to esteem-enhancement have been found to work at least as well as those that are more direct in their orientation (e.g., self-esteem curricula; Hattie, 1992). Rather, what appears most important is: (a) that interventions be designed in ways that clearly take advantage of existing, literature-based knowledge of self-esteem and its role in early childhood development and (b) that a clear set of expected linkages be established between whatever program activities are implemented and positive changes in feelings of self-worth.

Within these general parameters, it may be desirable for programs to include several types of interrelated components. First, opportunities should be made available for young children to derive self-esteem from developmentally normative sources. Core program elements in this area could encompass a wide range of strategies focused on skill-building and strengthening of significant relationships. These include, for example, components designed to promote secure attachments to parental figures and the presence of other esteem-enhancing conditions in the home environment. Similar efforts within school settings could focus on use of age-appropriate instructional strategies to increase opportunities for positive learning experiences. Based on available research, activities designed to promote physical fitness and motor skills development during early childhood also merit consideration.

Second, to complement these types of components, interventions should include efforts to address adaptive use of self-protective/self-enhancing strategies by young children. Core intervention elements in this area might involve use of psychoeducational activities to increase awareness of both young children's universal need for self-esteem and potential types of problematic self-protective/self-enhancing tendencies for this age group (e.g., denying personal shortcomings, disengaging from important areas such as school, exhibiting negative behavior to gain the attention of others). This type of component could be directed toward parents and other significant adults in the lives of young children (e.g., teachers). It does not seem unreasonable, however, to expect that children themselves could absorb at least a general understanding of the messages involved with the use of a developmentally sensitive approach.

Third, consistent with available research (Haney & Durlak, 1998), interventions should include components designed to directly address the developing self-esteem of young children. Numerous esteem-enhancement curricula have been designed for this purpose. In some instances, there are promising signs of effectiveness for these types of curricula when incorporated into established early intervention programs such as Head Start. Based on available theory and research, however, it would be useful to expand their focus to more strongly reflect the multidimensionality of young children's self-esteem (DuBois & Tevendale, 1999). Thus, in addition to the current emphasis on enhancing overall feelings of self-worth, curricula could be broadened to include materials and activities oriented toward enhancing their self-evaluations for particular areas or domains (e.g., school). Of further value might be elements designed to increase the capacity of young children to demonstrate signs of high self-esteem in their outward behavior (i.e., presented self-worth).

Fourth, several considerations argue for including additional program components geared directly toward strengthening relevant areas of young children's adjustment (as opposed to relying solely on achieving such gains via enhancements in self-esteem). A close relation exists between gains in self-esteem in programs and growth occurring in emotional, behavioral, academic, and physical domains of children's functioning (Haney & Durlak, 1998). Increases in self-esteem are likely to contribute to positive changes in these other areas and vice-versa. Consequently, when both types of goals are a part of interventions, desired outcomes may be more readily attained (DuBois & Tevendale, 1999). Strategies to increase adjustment in differing areas might be usefully adapted from early childhood prevention and health promotion programs that already exist in the literature.

Fifth, attention should be given to adapting program elements in each of the preceding areas to address the needs of young children with differing characteristics and backgrounds. To date, efforts of this nature have focused on increasing program sensitivity to the cultural and ethnic backgrounds of participating children and their families. Other approaches, however, also merit consideration. These include the use of strategies tailored to the needs of individual children within differing areas of programs. In promoting normative developmental sources of self-esteem, individualized components might include family support services for children living in troubled home environments or specialized skills training for those exhibiting signs of developmental delay. An individualized orientation also might be useful in activities focusing directly on enhancement of self-esteem. Strategies in this area might be adapted to take into account differences among children in their pre-existing levels of self-esteem, patterns of strength and weakness across multiple areas of self-evaluation, and varying degrees of behaviorally presented feelings of self-worth.

Sixth, programs should be designed to maximize the likelihood of lasting benefits for participating children. Efforts need to be directed toward ensuring that interventions are of sufficient duration and intensity to produce sustained gains in self-esteem and, further, that these will be substantial enough to have practical value for health promotion and prevention of disorder. Currently, most programs seeking to strengthen the self-esteem of young children rely on time-limited and relatively isolated modes of intervention (e.g., exposure to a single curriculum). More promising would seem to be a multimodal approach. By addressing multiple facets of the emerging skills and day-to-day experiences of young children, and doing so over extended periods of time, interventions may be better able to create long-term positive effects on self-esteem and other areas of adjustment. A comprehensive psychosocial approach in which there is attention to both "inner" and "outer" forces affecting development of self-esteem in early childhood is likely to necessary for interventions to meet this need (Hamachek, 1994).

In summary, programs to promote self-esteem in early childhood represent a promising strategy for health promotion and prevention. Esteem-enhancement interventions show encouraging indications of being able to produce positive changes in young children's self-esteem as well as accompanying improvements in other important areas of their functioning. Emerging "best practice" guidelines, furthermore, offer a useful starting point to build on these results. Future advances are most likely to occur through a mutually informing process of basic research, innovations in program design, and strategic implementation and dissemination efforts.

Also see: Self-Esteem entries.

References

Alpert, B., Field, T., Goldstein, S., & Perry, S. (1990). Aerobics enhances cardiovascular fitness and agility in preschoolers. *Health Psychology, 9*, 48–56.

Beane, J.A. (1994). Cluttered terrain: The schools' interest in the self. In T.M. Brinthaupt & R.P. Lipka (Eds.), *Changing the self: Philosophies, techniques, and experiences* (pp. 69–87). Albany: State University of New York Press.

Cassidy, J. (1990). Theoretical and methodological considerations in the study of attachment and the self in young children. In M.T. Greenberg, D. Cicchetti, & E.M. Cummings (Eds.), *Attachment in the preschool years: Theory, research, and intervention* (pp. 87–119). Chicago: University of Chicago Press.

DuBois, D.L., & Tevendale, H.D. (1999). Self-esteem in childhood and adolescence: Vaccine or epiphenomenon? *Applied and Preventive Psychology, 8*, 103–117.

Eder, R.A. (1990). Uncovering young children's psychological selves: Individual and developmental differences. *Child Development, 61*, 849–863.

Hamachek, D. (1994). Changes in the self from a developmental/psychosocial perspective. In T.M. Brinthaupt & R.P. Lipka (Eds.), *Changing the self: Philosophies, techniques, and experiences* (pp. 21–68). Albany: State University of New York Press.

Haney, P., & Durlak, J.A. (1998). Changing self-esteem in children and adolescents: A meta-analytic review. *Journal of Clinical Child Psychology, 27*, 423–433.

Harter, S. (1999). *The construction of the self: A developmental perspective.* New York: Guilford.

Hattie, J. (1992). *Self-concept.* Hillsdale, NJ: Lawrence Erlbaum.

Kaplan, H.B. (1986). *Social psychology of self-referent behavior.* New York: Plenum.

Marsh, H.W., Craven, R.G., & Debus, R. (1991). Self-concept of young children 5 to 8 years of age: Measurement and multidimensional structure. *Journal of Educational Psychology, 83*, 377–392.

Measelle, J.R., Ablow, J.C., Cowan, P.A., & Cowan, C.P. (1998). Assessing young children's views of their academic, social, and emotional lives: An evaluation of the Self-Perception Scales of the Berkeley Puppet Interview. *Child Development, 69*, 1556–1576.

Rosenberg, M. (1965). *Society and the adolescent self-image.* Princeton, NJ: Princeton University Press.

Strain, P.S., Kerr, M.M., Stagg, V., Lenkner, D.A., Lambert, D.L., Mendelsohn, S.R., & Franca, V.M. (1983). Relationships between self-concept and directly observed behaviors in kindergarten children. *Psychology in the Schools, 20*, 498–505.

Taylor, J., Turner, S., Underwood, C., Franklin, A., Jackson, E., & Stagg, V. (1994). Values for Life: Preliminary evaluation of the educational component. *Journal of Black Psychology, 20*, 210–233.

Verschueren, K., Buyck, P., & Marcoen, A. (2001). Self-representations and socioemotional competence in young children: A 3-year longitudinal study. *Developmental Psychology, 37*, 126–134.

Verschueren, K., Marcoen, A., & Schoefs, V. (1996). The internal working model of the self, attachment, and competence in five-year-olds. *Child Development, 67,* 2493–2511.

Verschueren, K., & Marcoen, A. (1999). Representation of self and socio-emotional competence in kindergartners: Differential and combined effects of attachment to mother and father. *Child Development, 70,* 183–201.

Wright, S.C., & Taylor, D.M. (1995). Identity and the language of the classroom: Investigating the impact of heritage versus second language instruction on personal and collective self-esteem. *Journal of Educational Psychology, 87,* 241–252.

Self-Esteem, Childhood

David L. DuBois

INTRODUCTION

Self-esteem is one of the most widely discussed markers of positive mental health for developing children. In recent years, researchers have made significant progress addressing questions about the basic nature of self-esteem, the factors that most influence its development during childhood, and the conditions under which high levels of self-esteem promote healthy overall adjustment and reduce susceptibility to disorder. Informed by an understanding of answers to such questions, what results can be anticipated for interventions that seek to promote self-esteem during childhood? Furthermore, what types of programs appear to be most effective and how might these be modified and strengthened in the future?

DEFINITION

Self-esteem has been defined as "the evaluation which an individual makes and customarily maintains with regard to himself [or herself]; it expresses an attitude of approval or disapproval" (Rosenberg, 1965, p. 5). Recent work has demonstrated that self-esteem is best viewed as multidimensional and thus complex and multi-faceted in its underlying structure (Harter, 1999). During childhood (approximately ages 7–12), youth reliably distinguish between different areas in the views and feelings that they have about themselves. These include their experiences in major settings of child development (i.e., school, family life, and peer group) as well as other salient areas of concern such as physical appearance, athletic ability, and behavioral conduct (Harter,

1999). Further distinct facets of self-esteem for children may include: (a) separate positive and negative dimensions of self-evaluation (i.e., feelings of self-pride and self-derogation, respectively); (b) stability of feelings about the self across time and situations; and (c) presented feelings of self-worth evident in observable behavior (as opposed to those experienced and reported by children themselves). To adequately describe the self-esteem of the typical school-age child, it thus may not be sufficient to simply know the overall feelings that he or she expresses about himself or herself as a person (usually referred to as "global self-esteem" or "feelings of self-worth"). Equally important may be whether the child feels satisfied with himself or herself in specific areas such as school, peer relations, and physical appearance, harbors feelings of self-pride (as opposed to merely an absence of feelings of self-dislike), is able to sustain feelings of worth on a consistent, day-to-day basis, and conveys a high level of self-esteem to others through his or her behavior.

SCOPE

Studies in the United States, Canada, and other Western countries indicate that approximately 10 percent of school-age children report a level of self-esteem that is low in the sense of reflecting unfavorable views or feelings about the self. As children grow older and approach adolescence, they appear to be at greater risk for experiencing low self-esteem. Longitudinal studies have found as many as one in five youth to experience marked declines in self-esteem upon entering adolescence, despite having reported positive feelings of self-worth in childhood (DuBois & Tevendale, 1999). Even among children who do report overall feelings of self-worth, a significant number (perhaps even a majority) are apt to have liabilities in one or more specific facets of their self-esteem (Harter, 1999). Profiles of domain-specific self-esteem reported by school-age children, for example, often include negative self-views or feelings relating to one or more areas (e.g., school). Studies similarly suggest a substantial amount of day-to-day instability or "ups and downs" in many children's self-esteem. Reports of high self-esteem by any given child, furthermore, are no guarantee that others who know the child well such as parents, teachers, or peers will not have a much different and less positive impression of the youth's feelings of self-worth (DuBois & Tevendale, 1999).

Because self-esteem is presumed to be important for healthy development, there may be significant costs when children do not possess a strong sense of self-worth (DuBois, Burk-Braxton, & Tevendale, 2002). These include risk for mental health problems, which can necessitate utilization of expensive services such as psychological testing, therapy or counseling, and residential treatment. Further costs may be associated with negative outcomes linked to poor self-esteem such as academic underachievement, juvenile crime, substance use, and health concerns (e.g., obesity). These may require use of costly educational, social, and medical services and ultimately are likely to detract from the ability of youth to develop into productive members of society. From a more positive perspective, cultivating a strong sense of self-esteem in children may do a great deal to facilitate their healthy development and reduce the need for outside supportive services. To the extent that a collective esteem is fostered among all developing youth, a further benefit may be an enhanced overall quality of life within the surrounding community (Beane, 1994).

Several considerations point to childhood specifically as a time when efforts to enhance self-esteem may be beneficial. First, a strong sense of self-worth may function as a valuable resource that enables children to cope more effectively with stressful situations and other adversities they encounter in differing areas of their lives (Sandler, 2001). Second, the formative years of childhood may be important in establishing patterns in self-esteem that are then continued at later stages of development. Children who have low self-esteem, in particular, often continue to exhibit negative self-regard during adolescence and even adulthood (DuBois & Tevendale, 1999). Third, as already pointed out, there is a well-documented risk for declines in self-esteem in early adolescence, the period of transition between childhood and adolescence. Strengthening feelings of self-worth prior to this point in development thus may have significant value in terms of preventing later drops in self-esteem and associated onset of adjustment problems during the teenage years.

THEORIES

According to the *Additive Model of Self-Worth* proposed by Harter (1999), self-esteem during normal development is derived from both (a) a sense of personal competence or efficacy in multiple areas of importance and (b) a perception of being accepted and valued by significant others. This model represents a synthesis of the views of previous theorists who emphasized perceptions of competence as a major determinant of feelings of self-worth during development, and those who advocated instead a more socially based perspective which focused on how a child saw himself or herself viewed and regarded by significant others (often referred to as the "looking-glass-self" model). These theoretical views highlight the manner in which children's feelings of self-worth often may be fueled by experiences of accomplishment or success that they have in school and other age-appropriate pursuits (e.g., a favorite sport or hobby). They call equal attention to the esteem-enhancing

potential of patterns of conduct by children that are likely to generate positive feedback from important persons in their lives such as parents, teachers, and peers. The *Self-Esteem Motive*, proposed by numerous theorists (see Harter, 1999), further assumes that developing children will tend to seek out experiences that help them to maintain positive feelings of worth. Children who are able to derive self-esteem in the ways just described thus may be encouraged to seek out additional competence-building experiences and to continue their positive relationships with others. In this manner, opportunities to obtain feelings of self-worth through normative and age-appropriate forms of activity may help to set in motion self-reinforcing trajectories of both high self-esteem and positive adjustment during childhood (DuBois & Tevendale, 1999).

However, there are also a wide array of self-protective or self-enhancing strategies that children can engage in to aid their efforts to maintain a sense of self-esteem (Sandler, 2001). As described by Kaplan (1986, p. 174),

> Self-protective/self-enhancing responses ... are oriented toward the goal of (1) forestalling the experience of self-devaluing judgments and consequent distressful self-feelings (self-protective patterns) and (2) increasing the occasions for positive self-evaluations and self-accepting feelings (self-enhancing patterns).

Kaplan (1986) distinguished three general forms of self-protective/self-enhancing responses relating to self-referent cognition, personal need-value systems, and behavior. The use of self-protective/self-enhancing strategies in each of these areas is quite commonplace at all points in development, including childhood (Harter, 1999; Kaplan, 1986). Individual children may, for example, attempt to protect their self-esteem by seemingly "filtering out" negative or less flattering information from their self-concepts, by "discounting" the value or importance of pursuits in which they are less successful, and by selectively seeking out greater association with peers or adults who hold more positive views of them. In many respects, these tendencies are not surprising. It is the rare child, after all, who can be expected to unfailingly accept in stride criticism or "corrective feedback", achieve success in all endeavors, and universally be liked and well-regarded. Some degree of reliance on self-protective/self-enhancing strategies thus seems an inevitable and functional necessity for maintaining a robust sense of self-worth during childhood (Harter, 1999).

Self-protective/self-enhancing strategies also, however, provide insight into how differing levels of self-esteem may be linked to problems in adjustment (Kaplan, 1986). This is, in part, because strategies used by children with low self-esteem to attempt to protect or restore feelings of self-worth can be both counterproductive and maladaptive (Sandler, 2001). According to Kaplan's (1986) *General Theory of*

Deviant Behavior, children whose self-esteem has been affected adversely by experiences at school or in their families or peer group may then begin to display problem behavior in a misguided effort to earn greater acceptance or admiration from others. Such children also may receive personal satisfaction from acting out or aggressing against those perceived to be responsible for their lowered sense of worth (Kaplan, 1986). Other children may respond to feelings of low self-regard with generalized patterns of avoidance or withdrawal in an effort to minimize exposure to future threats to self-esteem. This, however, makes them more susceptible to developing serious emotional disorders such as depression and anxiety. A desire to "escape" painfully negative feelings of self-regard also may lead some children to experiment with drug use and, in extreme instances, to show suicidal tendencies (Harter, 1999).

It is important to note, furthermore, that even self-protective/self-enhancing strategies used by children that are successful in maintaining or raising their self-esteem still may create significant problems for other areas of their adjustment. Within the educational realm, for example, children who experience learning difficulties may protect their overall feelings of self-worth by attaching limited or even no value to how well they do in school. Doing so, however, may substantially restrict their opportunities for future academic achievement. Children who enhance their perceptions of themselves to the point of having excessively unrealistic or inflated self-concepts provide a further illustration. When this occurs, high self-esteem is likely to come with the price of limitations in self-understanding and difficulties getting along with others that detract significantly from adjustment (Harter, 1999). In the long-run, unfavorable consequences may well even come full circle to undercut whatever gains in self-esteem were possible initially with the self-protective/self-enhancing strategies involved.

RESEARCH

Research supports the view that experiences of both mastery or success and social acceptance are important normative sources of self-esteem in childhood (Harter, 1999). Consistent with the multidimensional view of self-esteem described earlier, perceptions of personal competence and approval from others in multiple differing domains have been demonstrated to make distinct contributions to children's feelings of self-worth. These include views that they have about themselves relating to school work, involvement in athletics and other types of extracurricular activities (e.g., music or art), their physical appearance, and their relationships with parents, peers, teachers, and other significant adults (Harter, 1999).

Research findings also indicate, as expected, that children with low self-esteem are at greater risk for negative adjustment (DuBois & Tevendale, 1999). Children lacking in feelings of self-worth are more prone to exhibiting symptoms of depression and anxiety, interpersonal difficulties such as loneliness and rejection by peers, involvement in delinquent behavior, and a variety of other types of concerns such as eating disorder symptomatology, experimentation with substance use, obesity, and suicidal tendencies. Conversely, high levels of self-esteem for children are linked to a wide range of favorable outcomes. These include positive mood and happiness, adaptive classroom behavior and academic achievement, physical fitness and desirable health practices, and greater overall life satisfaction. It also has been demonstrated in longitudinal studies that levels of self-esteem reported by children can predict future trends in their adjustment status, including those evident during later stages of development (DuBois & Tevendale, 1999). In a few of these investigations, childhood self-esteem has been tied to levels of functioning well into adulthood. In one such study, higher levels of self-criticism reported at age 12 predicted poorer adult adjustment at age 31, including less positive personal/social adjustment, fewer years of education completed, and, for males, lower occupational status (Zuroff, Koestner, & Powers, 1994). These associations remained significant when controlling for childhood measures of both IQ and family socioeconomic status.

It should be noted that evidence of health-enhancing benefits for high levels of self-esteem during childhood has not been obtained in all studies. The associations found, even when "statistically significant," also have not necessarily always been large or strong enough to be of practical importance (DuBois & Tevendale, 1999). Such findings could be seen as detracting from the rationale for investing time and resources in esteem-enhancement programs for children.

To date, however, most research has limited itself to a view of self-esteem as unidimensional and undifferentiated. This approach is at odds with a more refined, multidimensional understanding of children's self-esteem. The relatively few studies that have addressed this concern indicate that strengths and weaknesses in multiple, distinct facets of self-esteem have implications for children's adjustment that are at least as important as those associated with the extent to which they experience overall feelings of self-worth (DuBois & Tevendale, 1999; Harter, 1999). These findings highlight the significance of how children evaluate themselves in specific areas or domains. Such views seem especially likely to influence aspects of functioning that are conceptually related to the area of self-esteem involved. A favorable academic self-concept during elementary school has been found to facilitate better school performance, for example, whereas pre-adolescent girls who report a negative body-image are at greater risk for developing symptoms of eating disorders. Overall profiles of children's self-esteem across such areas also may be important. A pervasive pattern of negative self-evaluation across all domains, for example, has been linked to risk to clinically significant depressive symptomatology and suicidal ideation.

Additional findings point to the importance of whether peer-salient and adult-salient sources of self-esteem are each well-represented in profiles (Harter, 1999). Even though affording high overall feelings of self-worth, profiles favoring peer-salient sources of self-esteem to the relative exclusion of adult-salient sources have been found to be associated with increased risk for both behavioral problems (e.g., delinquency) and poor school performance (DuBois & Tevendale, 1999). Those reflecting the opposing pattern of relative strength for adult-salient as compared to peer-salient sources seem to increase susceptibility to emotional difficulties such as depression and anxiety. In further preliminary research, liabilities in other specific facets of self-esteem have been similarly linked to adjustment problems for children (DuBois & Tevendale, 1999). These include short-term patterns of volatility in feelings of self-worth as well as indications of low self-esteem that are evident to observers, but not reported by the child.

There is also evidence that processes providing the underlying bases for acquiring and maintaining self-esteem are an important consideration. Several studies have identified groups of children with notably inflated (i.e., positively biased) views of themselves, presumably resulting from their excessive reliance on various types of self-protective/self-enhancing strategies. When compared to peers whose self-perceptions have a greater basis in reality, these children consistently have been revealed to be more poorly adjusted (DuBois & Tevendale, 1999; Harter, 1999). Furthermore, as the transition to adolescence approaches, it has been found that some children do indeed seek out affiliation with deviant or antisocial peer groups as a means of attempting to enhance their feelings of self-worth. Doing so, as expected, increases risk for these children exhibiting problem behavior themselves (Kaplan, 1986).

To summarize, available research indicates that children's self-esteem is promoted by both competence or mastery experiences and rewarding social ties within multiple areas of their development. There is evidence that a high overall level of self-esteem, in turn, can have an important role in promoting positive mental health and in preventing the emergence of adjustment problems during childhood (and potentially at later stages of development as well). The nature and patterning of multiple, distinct facets of children's self-esteem, however, appears to be a further key factor influencing numerous aspects of their well-being and functioning. So too does the extent to which they rely on various types of potentially problematic self-protective/self-enhancing strategies to enhance and maintain a favorable sense of self-regard.

STRATEGIES: OVERVIEW

Several literature reviews have considered the effectiveness of esteem-enhancement programs for children. Two are particularly noteworthy because of their use of meta-analytic procedures (Haney & Durlak, 1998; Hattie, 1992). Meta-analysis provides an objective method of quantitatively assessing the overall magnitude of effect produced by a given type of intervention on one or more outcome measures (e.g., self-esteem). Meta-analytic procedures also can be used to investigate differences in effect size along any dimension of interest that varies across studies (participant characteristics, program features, type of evaluation methodology, etc.).

In the meta-analyses of esteem-enhancement programs, Hattie (1992) reported average effect sizes of 0.31 for programs targeting children and 0.20 for those geared toward pre-adolescents (positive effect sizes indicate that programs were successful in raising participants' levels of self-concept or self-esteem). Haney and Durlak (1998) similarly found an average effect size of 0.27 across 120 evaluations of esteem-enhancement programs for children and adolescents. An association between the magnitude of positive program effects and age of participants was not found. It was noted, however, that this possibility could not be assessed adequately based on available data. Overall, the size of the positive effects reported in esteem-enhancement programs to date are in the small to medium range when compared to other types of psychological, educational, and behavioral interventions (Haney & Durlak, 1998). They are indicative of gains in self-esteem that are moderate rather than large in magnitude.

Haney and Durlak (1998) also examined whether changes in self-concept/self-esteem experienced by youth in programs were associated with positive changes in other areas of their adjustment. These included behavior (usually as determined by direct observation or teacher rating scales), personality/emotional functioning (typically reports by youth of their levels of anxiety or depression), and academic performance (grades and performance on standardized tests). Positive outcomes were evident in each area. Desirable adjustment outcomes, furthermore, are most apparent for programs that produce the largest increases in participants' levels of self-concept or self-esteem (Haney & Durlak, 1998). This result is important because it establishes a direct association between effective esteem-enhancement activities and overall improvements in children's adjustment.

The extent to which interventions produce lasting increases in self-esteem that remain evident after participation has ended also is a significant concern. It is possible, for example, that some of the positive effects observed are attributable to "euphoria" or good feelings at the end of programs and that these dissipate relatively quickly thereafter (DuBois et al., 2002). Each meta-analysis reported limited evidence of sustained effects at follow-up (Haney & Durlak, 1998; Hattie, 1992). Because so few evaluations addressed this concern, the authors cautioned that available findings did not provide a basis for drawing conclusions about the durability of program outcomes. An additional limitation is that, in most instances, follow-up intervals have been relatively brief, rarely extending more than a few months past the end of program participation. There are, however, a few exceptions in which the durability of effects for interventions enhancing self-concept or self-esteem in childhood has been assessed over longer periods of time with encouraging results (see "Strategies that work" below).

A final general concern is whether programs are effective in strengthening the self-esteem of all participating youth. The most substantial positive effects of interventions have been found for youth who enter programs already exhibiting low self-esteem or other types of pre-existing problems (Haney & Durlak, 1998; Hattie, 1992). By contrast, only limited improvements have been apparent for youth lacking in such indications of vulnerability. Factors contributing to this trend may include greater malleability of low or negative self-views as well as ceiling effects on measures of self-esteem for those exhibiting normal functioning. The content and design of programs, however, also is a significant consideration. Interventions to date have been geared predominantly toward raising overall levels of self-esteem. As a result, other potentially important concerns have received little attention. These include efforts to strengthen self-evaluations in specific areas as well as attempts to ensure that children rely on healthy strategies to sustain a sense of self-worth (DuBois & Tevendale, 1999). If such factors were addressed more consistently, it might prove feasible to extend program benefits to a broader spectrum of children.

STRATEGIES THAT WORK

Both meta-analyses investigated trends in effectiveness across differing types of esteem-enhancement programs. Hattie (1992) found the effectiveness of programs to be similar regardless of whether they sought to increase self-esteem directly (e.g., curriculum) or by indirect methods (e.g., enhancing academic achievement). Haney and Durlak (1998) made a distinction between interventions that had

a primary goal of changing self-concept or self-esteem (i.e., referred to as "SE/SC interventions") and those that did not have this specific aim but nonetheless did assess change in self-concept or self-esteem as a program outcome (i.e., "non-SE/SC interventions"). Less than half of the studies included in their review were evaluations of SE/SC interventions. The average effect size for these programs (0.57) was substantially higher than that of non-SE/SC interventions (0.10). Programs in which enhancement of self-esteem or self-concept was a primary goal (i.e., SE/SC interventions) also were associated with better overall adjustment outcomes for participants than those without this emphasis (Haney & Durlak, 1998).

Haney and Durlak (1998) found, furthermore, that programs with a well-defined basis in theory or prior research were substantially more effective than those without this type of foundation. Remarkably, this factor alone predicted nearly one third of the overall variation in program outcomes. Developmental theory (i.e., Harter's *Additive Model of Self-Worth*), it will be recalled, emphasizes both (a) a sense of competence or mastery and (b) a perception of being accepted and valued by significant others as key normative sources of self-esteem during childhood. It is noteworthy, therefore, that interventions oriented toward enhancing these sources of self-esteem in different "real world" settings of children's lives have reported some of the most encouraging results. This is particularly true with regard to evidence of producing effects on children's self-esteem that are lasting and that radiate to other areas of their adjustment.

Mentoring programs (e.g., Big Brothers/Big Sisters) are one such type of intervention. The typical mentoring program seeks to establish a supportive one-to-one relationship between each participating youth and a caring adult volunteer. Mentor and youth see each other on a regular basis (e.g., weekly) and may engage in a variety of different activities ranging from informal social outings to helping the youth with school work. Programs, furthermore, usually are designed with the expectation that mentors will maintain their relationships with youth for some minimal period of time (e.g., one year). Positive effects of mentoring programs on the self-esteem of children have been reported in several studies.

Beneficial effects of adult mentoring on children's self-esteem also are suggested by positive outcomes that have been found to be associated with participation in various types of community-based youth development organizations (Roth, Brooks-Gunn, Murray, & Foster, 1998). In these programs (e.g., Boys & Girls Clubs), adult mentoring or guidance typically occurs on a small group basis in combination with a variety of other activities oriented toward skill-building, recreation, and cultural enrichment. Interestingly, there is evidence that mentoring and other types of "experiential" components in such programs can enhance the effectiveness of more traditional, curriculum-based approaches to promoting children's self-esteem. In a recent evaluation of *Across Ages* (Aseltine, Dupre, & Lamlein, 2000), a substance abuse prevention program for middle school-age youth, those who received the mentoring and community service components of the intervention in combination with its positive youth development curriculum (which includes lessons focused on building self-esteem) were found to demonstrate the most positive changes in self-confidence. There is similar evidence of increased effectiveness when esteem-enhancement programs incorporate additional components designed specifically to improve children's relationships with significant others such as parents, teachers, and peers (Gurney, 1987). The preceding types of interventions also have been found to have co-occurring favorable effects on other important areas of children's adjustment such as school performance and problem behavior involvement.

Outcomes relating to prevention and health promotion for mentoring and other community-based interventions may be attributable (at least in part) to their role in strengthening developmentally normative bases for self-esteem in childhood. The utility of such programs as tools for esteem-enhancement is by no means guaranteed, however, but rather can be expected to depend on a variety of factors. These range from use of "best practices" in their design to the quality and intensity of each individual child's experience (Roth et al., 1998). Findings from a national study of youth receiving mentoring through *Big Brothers/Big Sisters* programs are illustrative (Grossman & Rhodes, 2002). In this research, positive changes in overall feelings of self-worth, social and scholastic areas of self-concept, and several other indicators of functioning were found only for youth whose mentoring relationships lasted at least one full year. By contrast, at the other end of the continuum, when mentoring relationships ended after less than 3 months, youth showed significant *declines* in self-esteem and other indicators of functioning relative to those in a control group.

Promising exemplars of effective esteem-enhancement programs for children also exist within the realm of education. One of these is the *School Development* program (Haynes & Comer, 1996). This program focuses on systemic reform of elementary and middle school environments through the institution of a school planning and management team, student and staff support team, and an intensive parent outreach and involvement program. Notably, there is evidence that this program has not only immediate positive effects on children's self-esteem, but also produces gains in feelings of self-worth that are sustained after children leave the environments of the host schools (Cauce, Comer, & Schwartz, 1987). The School Development Program (and other similar school reform efforts), furthermore, have been found to be effective vehicles for promoting co-occurring gains in other areas of children's adjustment, including academic achievement and psychosocial functioning (DuBois et al., 2002).

Similar benefits have been reported for interventions geared toward physical activity (Hattie, 1992; Hattie, Marsh, Neill, & Richards, 1997). Outcomes reported again have included lasting increases in self-esteem as well as gains in other important areas of functioning (e.g., physical fitness levels). Noteworthy examples include exercise programs as well as outdoor activity programs such as *Outward Bound*. In the latter, small groups of participants engage in challenging outside activities as a means of building self-confidence and interpersonal skills (e.g., cooperation, leadership). These types of programs typically have been geared toward older youth (e.g., adolescents). Positive results for interventions emphasizing physical activity and skill development, however, have been reported in controlled evaluations for children as young as preschoolers (Alpert, Field, Goldstein, & Perry, 1990).

STRATEGIES THAT MIGHT WORK

There is beginning empirical evidence of several other effective strategies for enhancing children's self-esteem. Most programs to date have focused on enhancing overall feelings of self-worth. Relatively little information is thus available concerning the potential to promote more specific facets or dimensions of children's self-esteem. Preliminary efforts to address this issue, however, have yielded encouraging results. These interventions have reported gains in several differing areas of children's self-perceptions, including those relating to academic, family, and physical domains (Hattie, 1992). The specific dimensions of self-evaluation targeted typically have had direct relevance to aims of the program, such as academics in educational interventions and physical abilities or appearance in programs emphasizing exercise and fitness activities. Gains in domain-specific areas of self-evaluation have been found, in turn, to be linked to significant growth in related areas of children's functioning such as physical fitness and academic performance. Other distinct facets of children's self-esteem (e.g., presented feelings of self-worth) may have been strengthened as well, but have been largely ignored in programs.

Some interventions, however, do show promise of having a desirable influence on the motivations and behaviors that guide children's efforts to maintain a sense of self-worth (i.e., self-protective/self-enhancing strategies; DuBois et al., 2002). *Multisystemic Therapy* (so called because changes are sought in multiple developmental contexts such as peers, school, and family), for example, has proven successful in limiting the associations of older children and adolescents with delinquent peers, thus addressing one possible maladaptive route for attempts to bolster feelings of self-worth (recall, in this regard, Kaplan's *General Theory of Deviant Behavior* described previously). Youth development programs and educational interventions similarly have been found to increase children's involvement and motivation in school, thus enhancing the extent to which they are oriented toward deriving self-esteem within this important context (Roth et al., 1998).

Programs tailored specifically toward the needs of children with differing characteristics and backgrounds represent a further promising trend (DuBois & Tevendale, 1999). Positive results have been reported, for example, when using Afrocentric methods to enhance the identity and self-esteem of African American youth. An empowerment perspective similarly has been indicated to be useful for guiding efforts to promote a stronger sense of agency and self-worth among girls. An *individualized* approach to esteem-enhancement also has been discussed as a useful strategy for addressing the differing intervention needs of particular children within programs (Harter, 1999). The possible advantages of such an approach, however, have not yet received systemic evaluation.

STRATEGIES THAT DO NOT WORK

Certain types of interventions, furthermore, seem unlikely to be effective for enhancing children's self-esteem. Based on findings reviewed in preceding sections, programs that lack a clear theory- or research-driven approach would fall into this category. There also is reason to seriously question the effectiveness of programs in which the predominant or exclusive emphasis is on use of curricular based strategies to enhance overall feelings of self-worth. Such an approach is characteristic of the majority of programs attempted to date (Haney & Durlak, 1998). These types of interventions by themselves, however, seem likely to produce only relatively modest and short-lived gains in the self-esteem or self-concepts of participants. As noted, an important factor limiting the effectiveness of purely curricular programs may be the absence of more experientially based components, especially those that are oriented toward providing a sustained, normative basis for children's self-esteem within real world settings.

Programs also may be relatively ineffective when there is a narrow focus on enhancing children's overall feelings of self-worth. Such an approach may fail, for example, to strengthen important underlying dimensions of children's self-esteem. It also does not address the appropriateness of children's uses of various types of self-protective/self-enhancing strategies. In addition to limiting potential for

positive outcomes, these omissions create the risk of high levels of self-esteem being established that have such a weak or unrealistic foundation that they *detract* from rather than facilitate the adjustment of some children participating in programs (DuBois & Tevendale, 1999).

SYNTHESIS

A synthesis of available findings indicates that an integrated, multifaceted approach offers the most promising strategy for enhancing self-esteem in childhood. As noted, programs are more effective when the intention of changing self-esteem is an explicit goal and relevant theory and research informs their content. In other words, it should not be assumed that gains in self-esteem (and any related areas of adjustment) will occur unless this is a clearly defined aim of the program and there is a well-reasoned set of strategies in place for achieving such an objective. It is important to recall in this regard, however, that indirect approaches to esteem-enhancement (e.g., environmentally oriented programs) have been found to work at least as well as those that are more direct in their orientation (Hattie, 1992). Rather, whatever the program's orientation, what is needed is a general approach of actively taking advantage of existing, literature-based knowledge of self-esteem and its role in child development. A key aim in doing so should be to establish a clear set of expected linkages between program activities and positive changes in children's feelings of self-worth (Bartholomew, Parcel, & Kok, 1998).

Within these general parameters, it would seem desirable for programs to include several types of interrelated components. First, opportunities should be made available for children to derive self-esteem from developmentally normative sources. Core program elements in this area could include any of a wide range of strategies focused on skill-building and positive relationship development. Examples include promotion of positive learning experiences in the school setting, facilitation of involvement in age-appropriate extracurricular activities, and work with parents to ensure esteem-enhancing experiences in the home environment.

Second, to complement these types of components, interventions should incorporate efforts to encourage children's responsible use of self-protective/self-enhancing strategies. Core intervention elements in this area might emphasize a psychoeducational approach in which children are made aware of the universal human need for self-esteem (i.e., Self-esteem motive) and how it can influence their thoughts, attitudes, and behaviors. Special consideration could be given to risks associated with specific types of self-protective/self-enhancing strategies that may be relied on by children. These include tendencies to deny personal weaknesses, form negative opinions about important areas of their development (e.g., school), and associate with problem peer groups.

Third, consistent with available research (Haney & Durlak, 1998), interventions should include components designed to directly address the self-esteem of children. It seems that a wide variety of affective and cognitive–behavioral techniques can be of benefit for promoting overall feelings of self-worth during childhood (Hattie, 1992). As noted, however, to yield optimal results it also may be important to include components that target specific facets of dimensions of children's self-esteem. One useful approach could be simply to increase children's awareness and appreciation of significant aspects of their self-esteem other than overall feelings of self-worth. Such efforts could occur in conjunction with strategies geared toward actively strengthening multiple, distinct facets of self-esteem (Harter, 1999). Efforts to promote self-evaluations relating to specific areas or domains of children's lives are particularly promising. In doing so, attention should be given to helping participants to establish well-balanced profiles of domain-specific self-esteem across all major areas of child development. Programs that address this concern may lessen the potential for deficits in one or more localized areas of children's self-esteem (e.g., body-image) to contribute to negative adjustment outcomes. Other dimensions of self-esteem found to be related to children's adjustment also should receive consideration in future programs (DuBois & Tevendale, 1999). Training in coping skills, for example, might be used to reduce children's susceptibility to potentially damaging short-term fluctuations and instability in their feelings of self-worth. Components to help ensure that children manifest high levels of self-esteem in their outward behavior (i.e., presented self-worth) represent another promising avenue.

Fourth, several considerations point to the value of program components that are geared directly toward promoting targeted areas of child adjustment (as opposed to relying solely on achieving such goals via enhancements in self-esteem). A close relation exists between gains in self-esteem in programs and improvements occurring in emotional, behavioral, academic, and physical domains of children's functioning (Haney & Durlak, 1998). Increases in self-esteem are likely to contribute to positive changes in these other areas and vice versa. Consequently, when components to achieve both types of goals are included in programs, desired outcomes may be more readily attained (DuBois & Tevendale, 1999). Strategies to strengthen adjustment in differing areas might be adapted from programs already in existence to prevent specific forms of disorder and promote general health and well-being during childhood.

Fifth, attention should be given to modifying core program elements in each of the preceding areas to address the needs of children with differing characteristics and backgrounds. Currently, the rationale for use of specialized approaches to esteem-enhancement is most well-established with respect to participant differences along group dimensions such as gender and ethnicity. Individualized strategies geared to the needs of particular children, however, also merit investigation (Harter, 1999). These could prove useful in several areas of programs. In promoting normative developmental sources of self-esteem, for example, individualized components might include family support services for children living in troubled home environments or specialized skills training for those exhibiting marked deficits in key areas of personal competence. The multidimensionality of school-age children's self-esteem indicates that an individualized orientation also might be useful in activities focused directly on enhancement of self-esteem. Strategies in this area might be tailored to differences among children in their pre-existing levels of self-esteem, patterns of strength and weakness across specific areas of self-evaluation, and varying degrees of behaviorally presented feelings of self-worth.

Sixth, programs should be designed to maximize the likelihood of lasting benefits for participants. Efforts should be made to ensure that interventions are of sufficient duration and intensity to produce sustained gains in self-esteem and, furthermore, that these will be substantial enough to have practical value for purposes of health promotion and prevention of disorder. A theme among interventions with the most promising signs of effectiveness is an emphasis on using environmental and experientially based methods to increase the ongoing opportunities of children to demonstrate competence and form rewarding relationships with others in areas important to their overall development. Accordingly, whenever possible, the predominant use of time-limited, structured curricula for promoting children's self-esteem should be broadened to incorporate more sustained, environmentally oriented modes of intervention (e.g., mentoring). In other words, a comprehensive psychosocial approach is needed in which there is attention to both "inner" and "outer" forces affecting children's self-esteem (Hamachek, 1994). Sustainability also may be increased by implementing programs in ways that are integrated with the practices of existing organizations and institutions that serve the needs of children (Schorr, 1988). This may allow esteem-enhancement interventions to be maintained on a long-term basis without the involvement of original program developers, thereby making it possible for large numbers of youth to benefit over extended periods of time.

In summary, interventions to enhance self-esteem during childhood represent a promising strategy for health promotion and prevention. Existing programs have been demonstrated to produce positive changes in school-age children's self-esteem as well as accompanying improvements in other areas of their functioning. An emerging set of "best practice" guidelines for programs, furthermore, offers a useful starting point to build on these results. Future advances are most likely to occur through a mutually-informing process of basic research, innovations in program design, and strategic implementation and dissemination efforts.

Also see: Self-Esteem Entries.

References

Alpert, B., Field, T., Goldstein, S., & Perry, S. (1990). Aerobics enhances cardiovascular fitness and agility in preschoolers. *Health Psychology, 9*, 48–56.

Aseltine, R.H., Dupre, M., & Lamlein, P. (2000). Mentoring as a drug prevention strategy: An evaluation of Across Ages. *Adolescent and Family Health, 1*, 11–20.

Bartholomew, L.K., Parcel, G.S., & Kok, G. (1998). Intervention mapping: A process for developing theory- and evidence-based health education programs. *Health Education Behavior, 25*, 545–563.

Beane, J.A. (1994). Cluttered terrain: The schools' interest in the self. In T.M. Brinthaupt & R.P. Lipka (Eds.), *Changing the self: Philosophies, techniques, and experiences* (pp. 69–87). Albany: State University of New York Press.

Cauce, A.M., Comer, J.P., & Schwartz, D. (1987). Long-term effects of a systems-oriented school prevention program. *American Journal of Orthopsychiatry, 57*, 127–131.

DuBois, D.L., Burk-Braxton, C., & Tevendale, H.D. (2002). Esteem-enhancement interventions during early adolescence. In T.M. Brinthaupt & R.P. Lipka (Eds.), *Understanding early adolescent. self and Identity, Applications and interventions* (pp. 321–371). Albany: State University of New York Press.

DuBois, D.L., & Tevendale, H.D. (1999). Self-esteem in childhood and adolescence: Vaccine or epiphenomenon? *Applied and Preventive Psychology, 8*, 103–117.

Grossman, J.B., & Rhodes, J.E. (2002). The test of time: Predictors and effects of duration in youth mentoring programs. *American Journal of Community Psychology, 30*, 321–371.

Gurney, P.W. (1987). Self-esteem in the classroom II: Experiments in enhancement. *School Psychology International, 8*, 21–29.

Hamachek, D. (1994). Changes in the self from a developmental/ psychosocial perspective. In T.M. Brinthaupt & R.P. Lipka (Eds.), *Changing the self: Philosophies, techniques, and experiences* (pp. 21–68). Albany: State University of New York Press.

Haney, P., & Durlak, J.A. (1998). Changing self-esteem in children and adolescents: A meta-analytic review. *Journal of Clinical Child Psychology, 27*, 423–433.

Harter, S. (1999). *The construction of the self: A developmental perspective.* New York: Guilford.

Hattie, J. (1992). *Self-concept.* Hillsdale, NJ: Lawrence Erlbaum.

Hattie, J., Marsh, H.W., Neill, J.T., & Richards, G.E. (1997). Adventure education and outward bound: Out-of-class experiences that make a lasting difference. *Review of Educational Research, 67*, 43–87.

Haynes, N., & Comer, J.P. (1996). Integrating schools, families, and communities through successful school reform: The School Development Program. *School Psychology Review, 25*, 501–506.

Kaplan, H.B. (1986). *Social psychology of self-referent behavior.* New York: Plenum.

Rosenberg, M. (1965). *Society and the adolescent self-image.* Princeton, NJ: Princeton University Press.

Roth, J., Brooks-Gunn, J., Murray, L., & Foster, W. (1998). Promoting healthy adolescents: Synthesis of youth development program evaluations. *Journal of Research on Adolescence, 8*, 423–459.

Sandler, I. (2001). Quality and ecology of adversity as common mechanisms of risk and resilience. *American Journal of Community Psychology, 29*, 19–61.

Schorr, L.B. (1988). *Within our reach: Breaking the cycle of disadvantage.* New York: Anchor.

Zuroff, D.C., Koestner, R., & Powers, T.A. (1994). Self-criticism at age 12: A longitudinal study of adjustment. *Cognitive Therapy and Research, 18*, 367–385.

Self-Esteem, Adolescence

David L. DuBois

INTRODUCTION AND DEFINITIONS

Self-esteem has been defined as "the evaluation which an individual makes and customarily maintains with regard to himself [or herself]; it expresses an attitude of approval or disapproval" (Rosenberg, 1965, p. 5). Self-esteem in adolescence is multidimensional and thus both complex and multifaceted in its underlying structure (Harter, 1999). Specific dimensions of adolescent self-esteem are quite varied and may include: (a) levels and patterns of self-evaluations across multiple areas or domains; (b) positive and negative tendencies corresponding to feelings of self-pride and self-derogation, respectively; (c) both "trait" and "state" aspects, the latter including short-term stability across time and situations; (d) presented feelings of self-worth evident in observable behavior (rather than only those reported directly by adolescents themselves); (e) "true" self-esteem (derived from actions consistent with one's genuine personal identity) versus "contingent" self-esteem (based on efforts to conform to the views and expectations of others); and (f) explicit and implicit self-esteem (aspects of self-evaluation that are or are not part of conscious awareness, respectively).

To adequately describe the self-esteem of the typical adolescent, it thus is not sufficient to simply know how the youth says that he or she feels about himself or herself overall as a person (usually referred to as "global self-esteem" or "feelings of self-worth"). Equally important may be whether the youth feels satisfied with himself or herself in specific areas such as school, peer relations, or physical appearance, harbors feelings of self-pride (as opposed to merely an absence of feelings of self-dislike), is able to remain in a more or less consistent "state" of high self-esteem, conveys feelings of self-worth outwardly in his or her behavior, is guided primarily by "true" self desires rather than the opinions of others, and is free of feelings of inferiority or self-doubt possibly existing outside personal awareness.

SCOPE

Studies of adolescents in the United States, Canada, and other Western countries indicate that between 10 and 15 percent of youth in this age range report a level of self-esteem that is low in the sense of reflecting unfavorable views or feelings about the self. Notably, as many as one in five youth experience marked declines in self-esteem upon entering adolescence, despite having reported positive feelings of self-worth in late childhood (DuBois & Tevendale, 1999). A similar trend exists for older children already exhibiting low self-esteem to continue to report unfavorable self-regard as they progress into adolescence. Furthermore, even among the remainder of adolescents who do report overall feelings of self-worth, a significant number (perhaps even a majority) can be expected to manifest liabilities in one or more distinct facets of their self-esteem (DuBois, Burk-Braxton, & Tevendale, 2002). Adolescents' profiles of self-evaluation across multiple areas of their lives, for example, frequently include negative views in one or more domains (Harter, 1999). As many as one third of adolescents also report substantial short-term instability in "state" aspects of their self-esteem. Reports of high self-esteem by any given adolescent, moreover, are no guarantee that others who know the youth well such as parents, teachers, or peers will not have a much different and less positive impression of his or her feelings of self-worth.

Because self-esteem is presumed to be important for healthy development, there may be significant costs when adolescents do not possess a strong sense of self-worth. These include greater risk for mental health problems, which can necessitate utilization of expensive services such as psychological testing, therapy or counseling, and residential treatment. Further costs may be associated with negative outcomes linked to poor self-esteem in adolescence such as school dropout, juvenile crime, substance use, and sexually-transmitted diseases. A lack of positive self-esteem at this stage of development thus has the potential to result in costly involvement in educational, social, and health care services and ultimately detract from the ability of youth to become productive members of society. From a more favorable perspective, a strong sense of self-esteem may promote healthy adjustment in adolescence and thus significantly reduce reliance on outside supportive services. To the extent that a collective esteem is fostered among all adolescents, a further benefit may be an enhanced overall quality of life in the surrounding community (Beane, 1994).

Several considerations also point to adolescence as a time when efforts to enhance self-esteem may be particularly

beneficial. Because of the rapid change and multifaceted demands that are characteristic of adolescence, high levels of stress often are experienced. A strong sense of self-worth may function as a valuable resource that facilitates effective coping with these challenges. Of further note is the increased level of complexity and abstraction in thinking that is a hallmark of adolescence. Thought processes, in particular, tend to become focused more inwardly on issues of relating to the self during this stage of development (e.g., identity formation). With these cognitive shifts, the ability to engage in positive forms of self-reflection may take on special significance. Adolescence, moreover, is a time of growing independence and autonomy from parents and other authority figures. It thus may be important to have secure and positive feelings about oneself at this age as a foundation for making healthy decisions and engaging in appropriate behavior without the benefit of adult guidance.

THEORIES

In normal development, self-esteem is derived from both a sense of personal competence or efficacy and a perception that one is accepted and valued by others (Harter, 1999). For many adolescents, feelings of self-worth thus may stem from experiences of mastery or success they have in school and various extracurricular activities as well as from age-appropriate patterns of conduct that generate positive validation from parents, peers, and other important persons in their lives (e.g., teachers). To the extent that experiences in these areas become established as viable routes to self-esteem, adolescents may actively seek to continue them through further efforts to demonstrate competence and maintain positive relationships with others. Processes of self-esteem and healthy development may become closely intertwined in this way and help to sustain long-term trajectories of positive adjustment (DuBois & Tevendale, 1999).

Adolescents also have at their disposal, however, a wide array of self-protective or self-enhancing strategies that may be used to help acquire and maintain a sense of self-worth. As described by Kaplan (1986),

> Self-protective/self-enhancing responses are oriented toward the goal of (1) forestalling the experience of self-devaluing judgments and consequent distressful self-feelings (self-protective patterns) and (2) increasing the occasions for positive self-evaluations and self-accepting feelings (self-enhancing patterns). (p. 174)

Kaplan (1986) distinguished three general forms of self-protective/self-enhancing responses relating to self-referent cognition, personal need-value systems, and behavior. Each may be evident in adolescents' attempts to protect or enhance their self-esteem. Possibilities include seemingly "filtering out" less flattering feedback or information about themselves in their thinking, discounting the value or importance of pursuits in which they are less successful, and seeking to affiliate with those who express the most positive views of them (Harter, 1999; Kaplan, 1986). In many respects, these tendencies are not surprising. It is the rare youth, after all, who can be expected to unfailingly accept in stride critical or "corrective" feedback from others, achieve success in all endeavors, and universally be liked and well-regarded. Some degree of reliance on self-protective/ self-enhancing strategies thus seems an inevitable and functional necessity for maintaining a robust sense of self-worth during adolescence (Harter, 1999).

Self-protective/self-enhancing strategies nevertheless also provide insight into processes through which liabilities in self-esteem may be linked to adjustment problems during adolescence (Kaplan, 1986). This is in part because certain strategies adolescents rely on to maintain a high level of self-esteem may be both counterproductive and maladaptive. When faced with esteem-threatening experiences at school or home, for example, some adolescents may attempt to bolster their sense of worth by becoming involved with more accepting, but delinquent peer groups (Kaplan, 1986). Such youth also may be at risk for engaging in anti-social behavior because of a desire to act out against the persons or institutions (e.g., school) perceived to be responsible for their lowered self-esteem (Kaplan, 1986). Other adolescents may respond to feelings of low self-regard with generalized patterns of avoidance or withdrawal in an effort to minimize exposure to future threats to self-esteem. This, however, may heighten their susceptibility to developing serious emotional disorders such as depression and anxiety. A desire to "escape" from painfully negative feelings of self-regard also may encourage some adolescents to become involved in drug use and, in relatively extreme instances, to exhibit suicidal thoughts and behaviors.

It is important to note, furthermore, that even when self-protective/self-enhancing strategies used by adolescents are successful in raising their self-esteem, these still may create significant problems for their adjustment. Within the educational realm, for example, adolescents experiencing academic difficulties may be able to protect their self-esteem by devaluing the importance of school. Doing so, however, is likely to restrict their opportunities for achievement in school even further. In other instances, adolescents may enhance their perceptions of themselves to the point of having excessively unrealistic or inflated self-concepts. Under these circumstances, high self-esteem may come with the price of limitations in self-awareness and increased difficulty getting along with others that detract significantly from overall adjustment (Harter, 1999). In the long run,

unfavorable consequences may well even come full circle to undercut whatever gains in self-esteem were possible initially with the self-protective/self-enhancing strategies involved (DuBois & Tevendale, 1999).

RESEARCH

Research supports the view that both (a) experiences of mastery or success and (b) social acceptance are important normative sources of self-esteem during adolescence (Harter, 1999). In one study (Luster & McAdoo, 1995), over 80 percent of adolescents reported high self-esteem when at least four of five positive indicators in these areas were evident— examples of the favorable indicators were success in school and a strong sense of being supported and approved of by parents. Whether or not adolescents enjoy supportive ties with peers and a sense of physical competence (including a positive body-image) also have been identified in research as salient influences on their levels of self-esteem (Harter, 1999).

High levels of self-esteem during adolescence are linked, in turn, to a variety of indicators of favorable adjustment, including positive mood and happiness, life satisfaction, physical fitness, and academic achievement (DuBois & Tevendale, 1999). Conversely, adolescents lacking in feelings of self-worth have been found to be more prone to depression and anxiety, interpersonal difficulties (e.g., loneliness, rejection by peers), and involvement in delinquent behavior in numerous studies. Other adolescent concerns linked to low self-esteem include substance abuse, gang membership, high-risk sexual activity, signs of possible eating disorders, and suicidal tendencies.

It is important to note, however, that all studies have found evidence of health-enhancing benefits for high levels of self-esteem in adolescence. The associations found, even when "statistically significant," also have not necessarily always been large or strong enough to be of practical importance (DuBois & Tevendale, 1999). These trends could be seen as detracting from the rationale for investing time and resources in efforts to promote self-esteem in adolescence.

To date, however, most research has limited itself to a view of the self-esteem of adolescents as unidimensional and undifferentiated. This approach is at odds with the more refined, multidimensional understanding of adolescents' self-esteem described earlier. The relatively small number of studies that have addressed this concern indicate that strengths and weaknesses in multiple, distinct facets of self-esteem have implications for the adjustment of adolescents that are at least as important as those associated with the extent to which they report overall feelings of self-worth (DuBois & Tevendale, 1999; Harter, 1999). Findings from several of these investigations highlight the significance of how adolescents evaluate themselves in specific areas or domains. Such views seem especially likely to influence aspects of functioning that are conceptually related to the area of self-esteem involved. Examples include a favorable academic self-concept facilitating better school performance and a negative body-image increasing risk for the development of an eating disorder (DuBois & Tevendale, 1999). Profiles of individual adolescents' self-esteem across differing areas also are a significant consideration (Harter, 1999). One pattern indicated to seriously compromise adolescent adjustment, not surprisingly, is a pervasive pattern of negative self-evaluation across all domains. It also appears to be detrimental when profiles do not include feelings of pride in reference to areas that are both "peer-salient" (e.g., peer friendships) and "parent-salient" (e.g., school performance; Harter, 1999). Liabilities in other specific dimensions or facets of self-esteem also have been linked to adjustment difficulties in adolescence (DuBois & Tevendale, 1999). These include: (a) short-term fluctuations or volatility in feelings of self-worth (i.e., "state" self-esteem); (b) manifestations of low self-esteem perceived by observers, but not necessarily adolescents themselves (i.e., presented self-worth); (c) separate tendencies toward lack of favorable self-regard (i.e., positive self-esteem) and presence of self-derogation (i.e., negative self-esteem); and (d) "false self" behavior reflecting an excessive desire to conform to external pressures or demands.

There is also evidence that processes providing the underlying bases for acquiring and maintaining self-esteem in adolescence are an important consideration (DuBois & Tevendale, 1999). When developmentally normative sources of feelings of self-worth are predominant (i.e., age-appropriate competencies and positive relationships with others), it appears that this can be instrumental in promoting positive adjustment and protecting against the emergence of disorder. Conversely, certain patterns in the use of self-protective/self-enhancing strategies have been linked to increased risk for adjustment problems during adolescence. Several studies, for example, have identified adolescents with notably inflated (i.e., positively biased) views of themselves, presumably resulting from their excessive reliance on various types of self-protective/self-enhancing strategies. When compared with peers whose self-perceptions have a greater basis in reality, such youth consistently have been revealed to be more poorly adjusted (DuBois & Tevendale, 1999; Harter, 1999). In other relevant research, it has been established that some adolescents do indeed seek out affiliation with deviant peer groups as a means of attempting to enhance feelings of self-worth. Doing so, as predicted, increases their risk for becoming involved themselves in delinquent behavior (Kaplan, 1986).

To summarize, competence/mastery experiences and social acceptance constitute important normative sources of self-esteem during adolescence. A high overall level of self-esteem, in turn, may promote positive mental health and help to prevent the emergence of adjustment problems often experienced by this age group. Equally compelling, however, is evidence that the nature and patterning of multiple, distinct facets of self-esteem is a key factor influencing adjustment outcomes in adolescence. Also noteworthy are self-protective/self-enhancing strategies that adolescents may rely on to sustain or increase their self-esteem. Such tendencies may result in inflated or maladaptive bases for feelings of self-worth and thus undermine the benefits associated with high levels of self-esteem during this stage of development.

STRATEGIES: OVERVIEW

Several literature reviews have considered the effectiveness of esteem-enhancement programs for adolescents. Two of these are particularly noteworthy because of their use of meta-analytic procedures (Haney & Durlak, 1998; Hattie, 1992). Meta-analysis provides an objective method of quantitatively assessing the overall magnitude of effect produced by a given type of intervention on one or more outcome measures (e.g., self-esteem). Meta-analytic procedures also can be used to investigate differences in effect size along any dimension of interest that varies across studies (participant characteristics, program features, type of evaluation methodology, etc.).

In the meta-analyses of esteem-enhancement programs, Hattie (1992) reported an average effect size of 0.23 for programs in which adolescents were the participants (positive effect sizes indicate that programs were successful in raising participants' levels of self-concept or self-esteem). Haney and Durlak (1998) similarly found an average effect size of 0.27 across 120 evaluations of esteem-enhancement programs for children and adolescents. An association between the magnitude of program effects and age of participants was not found. Overall, results indicate that adolescents participating in programs typically have experienced small to moderate gains in self-esteem.

In their meta-analysis, Haney and Durlak (1998) also examined whether youth participating in esteem-enhancement programs have exhibited positive change in other areas of their adjustment. The areas considered were behavior (usually as determined by direct observation or teacher rating scales), personality/emotional functioning (typically reports by youth of their levels of anxiety or depression), and academic performance (grades and performance on standardized tests). Positive outcomes were evident in each of these domains. Programs producing the largest favorable effects on other areas of adjustment, furthermore, tend to be those in which participants experience the greatest increases in self-concept or self-esteem (Haney & Durlak, 1998).

This result is important because it establishes a direct association between effective esteem-enhancement activities and overall improvements in adolescent adjustment.

The extent to which interventions produce lasting increases in self-esteem (i.e., those that remain evident following completion of participation) is a further significant concern. It is possible, for example, that some of the positive effects observed are attributable to "euphoria" or good feelings at the end of programs and that these dissipate relatively quickly thereafter (DuBois *et al.*, 2002). Each meta-analysis reported some evidence of sustained effects of esteem-enhancement programs at follow-up (Haney & Durlak, 1998; Hattie, 1992). Because so few evaluations addressed this concern, however, the authors cautioned that available findings did not provide a basis for drawing conclusions about the durability of program outcomes. An additional limitation is that, in most instances, follow-up intervals have been relatively brief, rarely extending more than a few months past the end of program participation. There are, however, a few exceptions in which the durability of effects for interventions enhancing self-concept or self-esteem in adolescence has been assessed over longer periods of time with encouraging results (see "Strategies that work" and "Strategies that might work" below).

A final general concern is whether programs are effective in strengthening the self-esteem of all participating youth. The most substantial positive effects of interventions have been found for youth who enter programs already exhibiting low self-esteem or other types of pre-existing problems (Haney & Durlak, 1998; Hattie, 1992). By contrast, only limited improvements have been evident for youth lacking in such indications of vulnerability. Factors contributing to this pattern may include greater malleability of low or negative self-views as well as ceiling effects on measures of self-esteem for those exhibiting normal functioning. The content and design of programs, however, also is a significant consideration. Interventions for adolescents to date have been geared predominantly toward raising their overall levels of self-esteem. As a result, other potentially important concerns have received little attention. These include efforts to strengthen different dimensions of adolescents' self-esteem as well as attempts to ensure that they rely on healthy strategies to acquire and sustain feelings of self-worth (DuBois & Tevendale, 1999). If such factors were targeted to a greater extent, it might prove feasible to extend program benefits to a broader spectrum of youth.

STRATEGIES THAT WORK

Both meta-analyses investigated trends in effectiveness across differing types of esteem-enhancement programs.

Hattie (1992) found the effectiveness of programs to be similar regardless of whether they sought to increase self-esteem directly (e.g., curriculum) or by indirect methods (e.g., enhancing academic achievement). Haney and Durlak (1998) made a distinction between interventions that had a primary goal of changing self-esteem or self-concept (referred to as "SE/SC interventions") and those that did not have this specific aim but nonetheless did assess change in self-esteem or self-concept as a program outcome (i.e., "non-SE/SC interventions"). Less than half of the studies included in their review were evaluations of SE/SC interventions. The average effect size for these programs (0.57) was substantially higher than that of non-SE/SC interventions (0.10). Programs in which enhancement of self-esteem or self-concept was a primary goal (i.e., SE/SC interventions) also were associated with better overall adjustment outcomes for participants than those without this emphasis (Haney & Durlak, 1998).

Haney and Durlak (1998) found, furthermore, that programs with a well-defined basis in theory or prior research were substantially more effective than those without this type of foundation. Remarkably, this factor alone predicted nearly one third of the overall variation in program outcomes. Developmental theory, it will be recalled, emphasizes both (a) experiences of competence or mastery and (b) a sense of being valued and accepted by significant others as key normative sources of self-esteem during adolescence. It is noteworthy, therefore, that interventions oriented toward enhancing these sources of self-esteem in different "real world" settings of adolescents' lives have reported some of the most encouraging results. This is particularly true with regard to evidence of producing effects on adolescents' self-esteem that are lasting and that radiate to other areas of their adjustment.

Mentoring programs (e.g., Big Brothers/Big Sisters) are one such intervention. The typical mentoring program seeks to establish a supportive one-to-one relationship between each participating youth and a caring adult volunteer. Mentor and youth see each other on a regular basis (e.g., weekly) and may engage in a variety of different activities ranging from informal social outings to helping the youth with school work. Programs, furthermore, usually are designed with the expectation that mentors will maintain their relationships with youth for some minimal period of time (e.g., one year). Positive effects of mentoring on the self-esteem of adolescents have been reported in several studies.

Beneficial effects of adult mentoring on adolescents' self-esteem also are suggested by positive outcomes found to be associated with participation in various types of community-based youth development organizations (Roth, Brooks-Gunn, Murray, & Foster, 1998). In these programs (e.g., Boys & Girls Clubs), adult mentoring or guidance typically occurs on a small group basis in combination with a variety of other activities oriented toward skill-building, recreation, and cultural enrichment. Interestingly, there is evidence that mentoring and other types of "experiential" components in such programs can enhance the effectiveness of more traditional, curriculum-based approaches to promoting adolescents' self-esteem. In a recent evaluation of *Across Ages* (Aseltine, Dupre, & Lamlein, 2000), a substance abuse prevention program for young adolescents, those who received both the mentoring and community service components of the intervention in combination with its positive youth development curriculum (which includes lessons focused on building self-esteem) demonstrated most positive changes in self-confidence. There is similar evidence of increased effectiveness when esteem-enhancement programs incorporate components designed specifically to improve children's relationships with significant others such as parents, teachers, and peers (Gurney, 1987). The preceding types of interventions also have been found to have co-occurring favorable effects on other important areas of adolescents' adjustment, such as school performance and levels of problem behavior involvement.

Outcomes relating to prevention and health promotion for mentoring and other community-based interventions may be attributable (at least in part) to their role in strengthening developmentally normative bases for self-esteem in adolescence. The utility of such programs as tools for esteem-enhancement is by no means guaranteed, however, but rather can be expected to depend on a variety of factors. These range from use of "best practices" in their design to the quality and intensity of each individual child's experience (Roth et al., 1998). Findings of a recent study of young adolescents receiving mentoring through *Big Brothers/Big Sisters* programs illustrate this concern (Grossman & Rhodes, 2002). In this research, positive changes in overall feelings of self-worth, social and scholastic areas of self-concept, and several other indicators of functioning were found only for youth whose mentoring relationships lasted at least one full year. By contrast, at the other end of the continuum, when mentoring relationships ended after less than 3 months, youth showed significant *declines* in self-esteem and other indicators of functioning relative to those in a control group (Grossman & Rhodes, in press).

School restructuring and reform initiatives have proven to be another effective mechanism for increasing self-esteem in adolescence. These include the *School Transitional Environment Program* (STEP), an intervention designed to facilitate entrance into new school environments (Felner, 1999). This program seeks to: (a) reduce adaptational demands of coping with flux and complexity in new school settings; (b) increase support and guidance from school staff and other students; and (c) increase students' sense of

connectedness and belonging within the new school. To help accomplish these goals, students participating in the program are kept together in "teams" for homeroom and core classes within the same part of the school building; additionally, the role of program teachers is restructured such that they meet regularly in an active advisory role with students and establish contact with their parents. An initial study of STEP's effectiveness, conducted in a large urban high school, found that it produced significant gains in multiple areas of students' self-concepts during the first year of their transition from junior high school relative to a matched control sample (Felner, 1999). Subsequently, a 5-year longitudinal follow-up study documented sustained positive effects of the program, including a reduction of nearly 50 percent in the school dropout rate. Subsequent research has replicated favorable results for STEP with other populations, including students making the transition into middle and junior high schools. The latter groups of students were found to demonstrate higher levels of both overall feelings of self-worth and school and family dimensions of self-esteem specifically relative to non-STEP students (Felner, 1999).

Programs with a physical activity emphasis also have well-documented effectiveness for enhancing the self-esteem of adolescents. Illustrative in this regard are adventure education programs such as *Outward Bound*. In these programs, participants are assigned a variety of mentally and/or physically challenging tasks that are personally demanding and that require effective group problem-solving under the guidance of a trained leader. In a recent meta-analysis of evaluations of *Outward Bound* and other adventure education programs (Hattie, Marsh, Neill, & Richards, 1997), it was found that participants experienced immediate gains in both general and domain-specific aspects of self-concept (e.g., physical ability) as well as co-occurring improvements in other areas of functioning such as physical fitness, leadership skills, and academic achievement. Notably, program effects on self-esteem and self-concept also were found to *increase* substantially in size over periods of follow-up assessment that averaged nearly 6 months (Hattie et al., 1997). These types of programs thus appear to have the capacity to set in motion processes for enhancing self-esteem that continue to be influential even after formal program involvement has ended. Again suggesting the importance of intervention duration or intensity, the size of follow-up effects was found to become larger as the length of programs increased (Hattie et al., 1997).

STRATEGIES THAT MIGHT WORK

There is also beginning empirical evidence of other effective strategies for enhancing the self-esteem of adolescents.

Programs tailored specifically toward the needs of adolescents with differing characteristics and backgrounds are one promising trend (DuBois & Tevendale, 1999). Some programs, for example, have obtained positive results when using culturally specific intervention strategies, such as Afrocentric methods of enhance the identity and self-esteem of African American adolescents. In a similar manner, an empowerment perspective has been indicated to be useful for guiding efforts to promote a stronger sense of agency and self-worth among adolescent girls.

Most programs to date have focused on enhancing overall feelings of self-worth. Despite this trend, there are promising indications that interventions also can strengthen domain-specific facets or dimensions of adolescents' self-esteem (Hattie, 1992). This potential is illustrated by findings reported for interventions described previously. The specific dimensions of self-esteem or self-concept affected often have had direct relevance to aims of the program. These include improvements in academic self-esteem within educational interventions (e.g., STEP) and in perceptions of physical competence for programs involving exercise and fitness activities (e.g., Outward Bound). Gains in such areas of self-concept or self-esteem for youth in programs have been found, moreover, to be associated with co-occurring positive changes in related aspects of their functioning such as academic performance and physical fitness.

There is also some evidence that interventions can have a desirable influence on the underlying processes that provide the basis for adolescents' self-esteem (DuBois et al., 2002). *Multisystemic Therapy* for juvenile offenders (so called because changes are sought in multiple developmental contexts such as peers, school, and family) has proven successful in limiting the associations of these youth with delinquent peers, thus addressing one possible maladaptive route for attempts to bolster feelings of self-worth. Programs seeking to modify educational environments similarly have shown effectiveness for increasing adolescents' levels of motivation to succeed in school. Under these circumstances, youth may be significantly less likely to devalue the importance of school as a maladaptive approach to attempting to protect their self-esteem.

STRATEGIES THAT DO NOT WORK

Certain types of interventions, furthermore, do not seem likely to be effective for enhancing the self-esteem of adolescents. Based on findings already described, programs that lack a well-articulated, theory- or research-based approach to promoting self-esteem during adolescence clearly would fall into this category. There is also reason to seriously question the effectiveness of programs in which there is a predominant or exclusive emphasis on using curricular-based strategies to enhance feelings of self-worth within this stage of development. Despite constituting the overwhelming majority of programs that have been attempted (Haney & Durlak, 1998), these types of interventions by themselves seem likely to produce only modest or relatively short-lived gains in the self-esteem of participants. An important factor limiting the effectiveness of purely curricular programs may be the absence of more experientially based components, especially those that are oriented toward providing a sustained, normative basis for adolescents' self-esteem within real world settings. Curricular programs also may be relatively ineffective when there is a narrow focus on enhancing only adolescents' overall feelings of self-worth. Such an approach may fail, for example, to strengthen important underlying dimensions of the self-esteem of adolescents. It also does not address the appropriateness of adolescents' uses of various types of self-protective/self-enhancing strategies. In addition to limiting potential for positive outcomes, the preceding types of omissions create the risk of high levels of self-esteem being established that have such a weak or unrealistic foundation that they *detract* from rather than facilitate the adjustment of some adolescents participating in programs (DuBois & Tevendale, 1999).

SYNTHESIS

A synthesis of available findings indicates that an integrated, multifaceted approach offers the most promising strategy for promoting self-esteem in adolescence. Within this type of framework, programs can be expected to be effective only when the intention of enhancing self-esteem is an explicit goal and the content of intervention activities is informed by relevant theory and research. In other words, strengthening of self-esteem should be a clearly defined aim of the program and there should be a well-reasoned set of strategies in place for achieving this objective. It should be kept in mind, however, that indirect approaches to esteem-enhancement (e.g., mentoring) have been found to work at least as well as those that are more direct in their orientation (e.g., self-esteem curricula; Hattie, 1992). Rather, whatever the program's orientation, what is needed is an approach of actively taking advantage of existing, literature-based knowledge of self-esteem and its role in development. A key aim in doing so should be to establish a clear set of expected linkages between program activities and positive changes in adolescents' feelings of self-worth (Bartholomew, Parcel, & Kok, 1998).

Within these general parameters, it may be desirable for interventions to include several types of interrelated components. First, opportunities should be made available to derive self-esteem from developmentally normative sources during adolescence. Core program elements in this area could encompass any of a wide range of strategies focused on skill-building and positive relationship development. Examples include elements designed to strengthen parent–adolescent relationships, facilitate adjustment to school transitions, and increase involvement in age-appropriate extracurricular activities. Because they are particularly salient sources of self-esteem in adolescence, program activities in this area should incorporate opportunities for participants to establish supportive ties with peers as well as a sense of physical competence (including a positive body-image).

Second, to complement these types of efforts, interventions should incorporate components that encourage adolescents' responsible use of self-protective/self-enhancing strategies. Core intervention elements in this area might emphasize a psychoeducational approach in which youth are made aware of the universal human need for self-esteem and how this need can influence their thoughts, attitudes, and behaviors. Special consideration could be given to risks associated with specific types of self-protective/self-enhancing strategies that may be relied on by adolescents. These might include tendencies to deny personal weaknesses, form negative opinions about important areas of development (e.g., school), and associate with problem peer groups.

Third, consistent with available research (Haney & Durlak, 1998), interventions should include components designed to directly address the self-esteem of adolescents. It seems that a wide variety of affective and cognitive–behavioral techniques can be useful in raising overall feelings of self-worth during this period of development (Hattie, 1992). As noted, however, to yield optimal results it may be important also to include components that address more specific facets or dimensions of adolescents' self-esteem. One useful approach in this regard could be to simply increase the awareness and understanding that adolescents have of the significance of aspects of their self-esteem other than overall feelings of self-worth. Such efforts could occur in conjunction with strategies geared toward strengthening multiple, distinct facets of their self-esteem. Efforts to promote self-evaluations relating to specific areas or domains of adolescents' lives are particularly promising. In doing so, attention should be given to helping participants to establish well-balanced profiles of domain-specific self-esteem across all major areas of adolescent development (DuBois & Tevendale, 1999). Programs that address this concern may lessen the potential for deficits in more localized aspects of adolescents' self-esteem (e.g., body-image) to contribute to negative adjustment outcomes. Other dimensions of self-esteem found to be related to adolescent adjustment also should receive consideration in future programs (DuBois & Tevendale, 1999). Training in coping skills, for example, might be used to reduce adolescents' susceptibility to

potentially damaging short-term fluctuations and instability in their feelings of self-worth. Other components could be geared toward helping ensure that adolescents manifest a high level of self-esteem in their outward behavior (i.e., presented self-worth) and that their feelings of worth are based on a well-developed personal identity, relatively free from pressures for conformity (i.e., "true" self-esteem).

Fourth, several considerations argue for programs incorporating components geared directly toward promoting targeted areas of adolescent adjustment (as opposed to relying solely on achieving such goals via enhancements in self-esteem). A close relation exists between promotion of self-esteem in programs and improvements occurring across emotional, behavioral, academic, and physical domains of functioning (Haney & Durlak, 1998). Increases in self-esteem are likely to contribute to positive changes in these other areas and vice versa. Consequently, when strategies to achieve both types of goals are a part of interventions, desirable outcomes may be more readily attained (DuBois & Tevendale, 1999). Strategies to strengthen adjustment in differing areas might be adapted from programs already in existence to prevent specific forms of disorder and promote general health and well-being during adolescence (as detailed elsewhere in this volume).

Fifth, attention should be given to the benefits of modifying program elements in each of the preceding areas to address the needs of adolescents with differing characteristics and backgrounds. Currently, the rationale for use of specialized approaches to esteem-enhancement is most well-established with respect to participants varying along group dimensions such as gender and ethnicity. Other approaches, however, also merit consideration. Among these is the use of strategies tailored to the needs of individual adolescents within differing areas of programs (DuBois et al., 2002). In promoting normative developmental sources of self-esteem, for example, individualized components might include mentoring relationships for adolescents in need of positive adult role models or specialized training in exercise and nutrition for those with poor fitness. The complex, multidimensional processes underlying feelings of self-worth in adolescence suggest that an individualized orientation also might be useful in activities focused directly on enhancement of self-esteem. Strategies in this area might be tailored to differences in pre-existing levels of self-esteem of participants as well as varying patterns of strength and weakness that are evident across multiple, distinct facets of their self-esteem.

Sixth, programs should be designed to maximize the likelihood of lasting benefits for participants. Efforts should be made to ensure that interventions are of sufficient duration and intensity to produce sustained gains in self-esteem and, furthermore, that these will be substantial enough to have practical value for purposes of health promotion and prevention of disorder. Currently, most programs seeking to strengthen the self-esteem of adolescents rely either on only one primary strategy or a limited number of relatively isolated modes of intervention. As suggested previously, an integrated, multimodal approach seems more promising. A theme among interventions with the most promising signs of effectiveness is an emphasis on using environmental and experientially based methods to increase the ongoing opportunities of adolescents to demonstrate competence and form rewarding relationships with others in areas important to their overall development. Accordingly, whenever possible, the predominant use of time-limited, structured curricula for promoting adolescents' self-esteem should be broadened to incorporate more sustained, environmentally oriented modes of intervention (e.g., mentoring). In other words, a comprehensive psychosocial approach is needed in which there is attention to both "inner" and "outer" forces affecting self-esteem in adolescence (Hamachek, 1994).

In summary, interventions to promote self-esteem in adolescence represent a promising strategy for health promotion and prevention. Existing programs have been demonstrated to produce positive changes in adolescents' self-esteem as well as accompanying improvements in other important areas of their functioning. An emerging set of "best practice" guidelines for programs, furthermore, offers a useful starting point to build on these results. Future advances are most likely to occur through a mutually informing process of basic research, innovations in program design, and strategic implementation and dissemination efforts.

Also see: Self-Esteem entries.

References

Aseltine, R.H., Dupre, M., & Lamlein, P. (2000). Mentoring as a drug prevention strategy: An evaluation of Across Ages. *Adolescent and Family Health, 1*, 11–20.

Bartholomew, L.K., Parcel, G.S., & Kok, G. (1998). Intervention mapping: A process for developing theory- and evidence-based health education programs. *Health Education Behavior, 25*, 545–563.

Beane, J.A. (1994). Cluttered terrain: The schools' interest in the self. In T.M. Brinthaupt & R.P. Lipka (Eds.), *Changing the self: Philosophies, techniques, and experiences* (pp. 69–87). Albany: State University of New York Press.

DuBois, D.L., Burk-Braxton, C., & Tevendale, H.D. (2002). Esteem-enhancement interventions during early adolescence. In T.M. Brinthaupt & R.P. Lipka (Eds.), *Understanding early adolescent. self and identity: Applications and interventions* (pp. 321–371). Albany: State University of New York Press.

DuBois, D.L., & Tevendale, H.D. (1999). Self-esteem in childhood and adolescence: Vaccine or epiphenomenon? *Applied and Preventive Psychology, 8*, 103–117.

Felner, R.D. (1999). An ecological perspective on pathways of risk, vulnerability, and adaptation: Implications for preventive interventions. In S.W. Russ & T.H. Ollendick (Eds.), *Handbook of psychotherapies*
with children and adolescents: Issues in clinical child psychology (pp. 483–503). New York: Kluwer Academic/Plenum.

Grossman, J.B., & Rhodes, J.E. (2002). The test of time: Predictors and effects of duration in youth mentoring relationships. *American Journal of Community Psychology, 30*, 199–206.

Gurney, P.W. (1987). Self-esteem in the classroom II: Experiments in enhancement. *School Psychology International, 8*, 21–29.

Hamachek, D. (1994). Changes in the self from a developmental/psychosocial perspective. In T.M. Brinthaupt & R.P. Lipka (Eds.), *Changing the self: Philosophies, techniques, and experiences* (pp. 21–68). Albany: State University of New York Press.

Haney, P., & Durlak, J.A. (1998). Changing self-esteem in children and adolescents: A meta-analytic review. *Journal of Clinical Child Psychology, 27*, 423–433.

Harter, S. (1999). *The construction of the self: A developmental perspective*. New York: Guilford.

Hattie, J. (1992). *Self-concept*. Hillsdale, NJ: Lawrence Erlbaum.

Hattie, J., Marsh, H.W., Neill, J.T., & Richards, G.E. (1997). Adventure education and outward bound: Out-of-class experiences that make a lasting difference. *Review of Educational Research, 67*, 43–87.

Kaplan, H.B. (1986). *Social psychology of self-referent behavior*. New York: Plenum.

Luster, T., & McAdoo, H.P. (1995). Factors related to self-esteem among African-American youths: A secondary analysis of the High/Scope Perry Preschool data. *Journal of Research on Adolescence, 5*, 451–467.

Rosenberg, M. (1965). *Society and the adolescent self-image*. Princeton, NJ: Princeton University Press.

Roth, J., Brooks-Gunn, J., Murray, L., & Foster, W. (1998). Promoting healthy adolescents: Synthesis of youth development program evaluations. *Journal of Research on Adolescence, 8*, 423–459.

Sexual Assault, Adolescence

Paul A. Schewe

INTRODUCTION AND DEFINITIONS

Adolescence is the developmental period marked by the onset of puberty and the beginning of romantic (dating) attachments. Unfortunately for some adolescents, their earliest sexual experiences are marked by humiliation, coercion, aggression, or violence. Sexual aggression among adolescents takes on many forms ranging from *sexual harassment* (unwanted sexual advances, joking ...) to *rape* (oral, anal, or vaginal penetration with a non-consenting partner). Until recently, most rape prevention efforts were directed at college populations, and the majority of these programs targeted women, primarily teaching avoidance and self-defense skills (Parrot, 1990). Very little was known about adolescent dating, and less still about sexual violence in adolescence. As our knowledge of adolescent sexual assault has advanced, and our primary prevention efforts have expanded, more and more programs have begun to target younger audiences. This entry covers the research on sexual assault in adolescence and reviews existing outcome evaluations in an effort to define the state-of-the-art in rape prevention efforts for adolescents and young adults.

SCOPE

Middle School

Data from middle school students indicate that between 28 and 45 percent of students have experienced some form of sexual harassment by a peer or group of peers (Cascardi, Avery-Leaf, & O'Brien, 1998; Connolly, McMaster, Craig, & Pepler, 1997). Represented by these data are students from a Canadian urban community of primarily European descent and a US urban community of predominantly African American students. Only one published study reports rates of sexual aggression among middle school students with 1–5 percent of students reporting perpetration of sexual aggression and 7–15 percent reporting sexual victimization (Foshee, Linder, Bauman, & Langwick, 1996).

High School

Data from high school students indicate that the rate of sexual violence in a multiethnic, economically diverse sample was 15.7 percent (Bergman, 1992). Females consistently report higher rates of sexual victimization than do males; one study found that 17.8 percent of high school females reported experiencing forced sexual activity, compared to 0.3 percent of males (Molidor & Tolman, 1998). Similarly, Bennett and Fineran (1998) found that 16 percent of high school girls reported being the victim of sexual violence, while only 1 percent said that they had perpetrated sexual violence. For boys, the rates were 6 and 4 percent, respectively, for victimization and perpetration of sexual violence.

College

The rate of sexual violence among young adults has been well-documented. Survey research among American college women indicates that as many as half report being victims of some form of sexual abuse and 27 percent report being victims of rape (15 percent) or attempted rape (12 percent; Koss, 1988). Gavey (1991) found a very similar rate (25.3 percent) using Koss' survey in New Zealand. Moreover, 25 percent of the men in Koss' (1988) survey indicated that they had behaved sexually with a woman against her will. Finally, Denmare, Briere, and Lips (1988) found that 22 percent of undergraduate males reported at least some future likelihood of raping.

The Costs of Sexual Aggression

The National Center for Injury Prevention & Control's Rape Fact Sheet (www.cdc.gov/ncipc/factsheets/rape.htm) indicates that victims of rape often manifest long-term symptoms of chronic headaches, fatigue, sleep disturbance, recurrent nausea, decreased appetite, eating disorders, menstrual pain, sexual dysfunction, and suicide attempts (Resnick, Acierno, & Kilpatrick, 1997). Victims of date rape are 11 times more likely to be clinically depressed, and 6 times more likely to experience social phobia than are non-victims. Psychological problems are still evident in cases as long as 15 years after the assault (Kilpatrick, Best, Saunders, & Veronen, 1988). In a longitudinal study, sexual assault was found to increase the odds of substance abuse by a factor of 2.5 (Kilpatrick, Acierno, Resnick, Saunders, & Best, 1997). The adult pregnancy rate associated with rape is estimated to be 5 percent and estimates of the occurrence of sexually transmitted diseases resulting from rape range from 3.6 to 30 percent (Resnick et al., 1997). A study examining the use of health services over a 5-year period by female members of a health maintenance program found that the number of visits to physicians by rape victims increased 56 percent in the year following the crime, compared to a 2 percent utilization increase by non-victims (Koss, Koss, & Woodruff, 1991). The National Public Services Research Institute estimated the lifetime cost for each rape with physical injuries that occurred in 1987 to be $60,000 (Miller, Cohen, & Rossman, 1993).

THEORIES AND RESEARCH

Feminist Theory

Feminist scholars (Dobash & Dobash, 1994; Yllo, 1993) highlight the importance of patriarchal social structure in the etiology of male violence toward female partners. This sociological perspective emphasizes the relationship between gender-based power inequities in the culture at large and male abuses of power and control within intimate relationships. While it is clear that changing these inequities in the culture at large with a short-term school-based curriculum may not be possible, a feminist approach targets attitudes and beliefs as the key to preventing intimate partner violence. Specifically, individuals' attitudes toward interpersonal violence, adherence to traditional gender roles, and the behavioral expression of power and control in one's relationships are targeted for individual change.

A Socio-Biological Approach

Finkelhor, Araji, Baron, Browne, Peters, and Wyatt (1986) has proposed a model to account for child sexual abuse that could be adapted to account for adolescent sexual assault. He proposes that four components must be present before sexual offenses can occur. The first component can be termed "motivation to sexually offend" which includes deviant arousal (sexual arousal to aggression or sexual violence) or blockage from more appropriate sources of sexual satisfaction. The second component entails overcoming internal inhibitions. A variety of personal and social factors, such as feelings of guilt or fear of criminal sanctions, ordinarily work together to inhibit sexual offending. Perceptions of social tolerance for the behavior, distorted ideas or myths about rape, drug or alcohol abuse, and perceptions of the low probability of negative sanctions all work against the normal mechanisms that inhibit sexual offending. The third factor involves overcoming external inhibitions. Bystanders and witnesses will generally not tolerate sexually offensive behavior. Offenders overcome external inhibitions by isolating their victims either by design or accident (Finkelhor et al., 1986). Lastly, the offender must overcome the target's resistance. An offender may overcome the victim's resistance through persuasion or coercion, by taking advantage of the victim's relative powerlessness, or by using threats of violence or other sanctions (Finkelhor et al., 1986; Walker, Bonner, & Kaufman, 1988).

Cognitive–Behavioral Theory

A cognitive–behavioral explanation of sexual assault is evident in most explicit and implicit theories of rape. Cognitive distortions justifying rape (aka "rape myths") are targeted more often than any other construct in pro-grams designed to prevent rape (Schewe, 2002). Supporting the use of rape myth interventions are data indicating that cognitive distortions justifying rape are the most common immediate precursor to rape (Scully & Marolla, 1985). On the behavioral side, repeated pairings of sex and violence might account for the development of deviant arousal to violence, while a lack of skills (communication skills, anger management skills, ability to cope with rejection, etc.) might prevent adolescents from developing healthy sexual relationships. With regard to classical conditioning, consider the age that boys are often exposed to their first horror movie; often right around puberty. In these movies, there is the almost obligatory nude/shower/slasher scene; for pubescent adolescent boys, a perfect pairing of sexual arousal and violence. If Pavlov were interested in creating a sex offender, he would not have to go any further than his local video store.

STRATEGIES THAT WORK

Rape Myths

A review of recent literature reveals that rape myth acceptance is the most common construct addressed in rape prevention programming. A variety of irrational beliefs are associated with rape and sexual offending (Burt, 1980; Hildebran & Pithers, 1989; Muehlenhard & Linton, 1987), making rape myths an ideal target for prevention programming. For example, Pithers, Kashima, Cumming, Beal, and Buell (1988) analyzed the case records of 64 incarcerated rapists and found that cognitive distortions justifying rape (i.e., *rape myths*) were the second most frequent immediate precursor to rape (anger was the first). In published evaluations of rape prevention programs over the last 15 years, rape myths were frequently targeted in successful intervention programs and were rarely targeted in unsuccessful programs (Schewe, 2002).

Recommendations for Interventions

Effective interventions targeting rape myths have been as minimal as the presentation of brief written material (Malamuth & Check, 1984) to as thorough as a 2-hr workshop targeting only empathy and rape myths (Lee, 1987). One warning is that a rape myths intervention (a presentation of false beliefs about rape along with corrective information) should not be confused with the presentation of factual information alone. Factual information such as legal definitions of rape, descriptions of victims and offenders, and descriptions of rape trauma syndrome have been found to have no effect on students' attitudes about rape nor their empathy for victims of rape (Borden, Karr, & Caldwell-Colbert, 1988; Lenihan, Rawlins, Eberly, Buckley, & Masters, 1992; Schewe & O'Donohue, 1993b).

Victim Empathy

Victim empathy is a cognitive–emotional recognition of a rape victim's trauma (Hildebran & Pithers, 1989). Programs that target victim empathy attempt to help students develop an understanding of the experiences of a rape victim and typically involve both an understanding of the victim's experience of the actual rape as well as the aftermath of rape (shame, guilt, depression, pregnancy, and social sanctions—what has been called by some as the "second assault," Williams & Holmes, 1981). The idea behind these interventions is that students who understand the horrible experience of rape would never inflict that type of pain on anyone, and would be more likely to help/believe a person who reports that they have been raped.

Examination of the evaluation literature reveals strong support for including victim empathy in rape prevention programs. Of the 10 programs that targeted victim empathy, 8 programs reported clear positive effects (Schewe, 2002). Notably, the only program to report clear long-term positive effects of an intervention included victim empathy as a key component of the program (Foubert, 2000). The two exceptions provide useful information for developers of prevention curricula. In Berg's study of 54 college males, she found that men who were asked to empathize with a female rape victim reported a greater likelihood of sexual aggression than men who were asked to empathize with an adolescent male who was victimized by another adolescent male (Berg, Lonsway, & Fitzgerald, 1999). In a similar study, Ellis, O'Sullivan, and Sowards (1992) found that when mixed-gender groups of undergraduates were asked to consider a situation where a close friend told them that she was raped, women became more rejecting of rape myths, but men became *less* rejecting of them. Review of the other empathy programs reveals that having males empathize with other male victims of rape was a key part of many of the more successful programs (Schewe, 2002).

Recommendations for Interventions

Typical victim empathy interventions involve having participants listen to survivors' stories of rape, engage in written exercises describing a victim's experiences, or imagine themselves as a victim of rape. Whenever males are in the audience, empathy-inducing exercises should absolutely include at least one scenario where the victim is a male. In order to reflect the reality of male rape, the perpetrator should also be male.

Self-Defense Strategies

Teaching women self-defense strategies appears to be an effective tool in helping students avoid rape. An evaluation of a model mugging course found that 46 of 48 women assaulted after taking the course fought back sufficiently to avoid harm (Peri, 1991). Other studies cite beneficial psychological consequences for women taking self-defense classes as compared to a no-treatment control group (Cohen, Kidder, & Harvey, 1978). Furthermore, there is fairly strong evidence concerning the types of strategies that are effective in deterring an attacker. Ullman and Knight (1993) examined police reports and court testimonies of 274 women who were either raped or avoided rape by subsequently incarcerated violent stranger rapists. They found that women who fought back forcefully were more likely to avoid rape; that women who screamed or fled when confronted with weapons experienced less severe sexual abuse; and that increased physical injury was associated with pleading, crying, reasoning, and

the women's use of drugs or alcohol. In two prevention programs that included a discussion of self-defense strategies (Hanson & Gidycz, 1993; Women against Rape, 1980), both programs were effective in either decreasing the incidence of victimization or increasing confidence in the use of self-defense strategies and willingness to confront a perpetrator.

Recommendations for Interventions

When discussing effective rape avoidance strategies, it is important to discuss some of the social barriers that may prevent women from using effective defense strategies. For example, students might be too embarrassed to yell or scream, or may be afraid of losing a friend if they fight back, or may be so shocked that someone they trust is attacking them that they are unable to react.

STRATEGIES THAT MIGHT WORK

Avoidance of High-Risk Situations

Early research identifying "high-risk" situations for sexual assault (use of alcohol, hitchhiking, attending parties, dating in isolated locations, being involved with older teenage men) (Muehlenhard & Linton, 1987; Ullman, 1997) suggests that educating women to avoid these high-risk situations could be an important part of efforts to reduce the incidence of rape among program participants. One program addressing this construct found that they were able to successfully increase women's perceptions of their vulnerability to rape and increase their intentions to avoid "risk-taking" behaviors (Gray, Lesser, Quinn, & Bounds, 1990). Hanson and Gidycz's (1993) risk reduction program was successful in decreasing women's involvement in situational factors associated with rape, and was successful in decreasing victimization among women who did not have a history of sexual victimization.

Recommendations for Interventions

There are two major cautions for educators attempting to incorporate information regarding high-risk situations into their curricula. One caution is that these programs should not be used for male or mixed-gender audiences. In the course of a program that highlights women's awareness of high-risk situations and perceptions of vulnerability, women in the audience may learn that date rape occurs very frequently, that most rapes go unreported to police, and that they should avoid alcohol and isolated dating locations. Men in the same audience may learn that rape is a common experience, that if they do commit rape the chances of being caught are very slim, and that if they get a woman intoxicated and take her to an isolated location, their chances of being caught are even more slim. Given the differences in the information that men and women need concerning rape, it is important that more programs are developed exclusively for each gender, and programs that attempt to target both sexes should be very careful when selecting information to present. A second caution is that information regarding high-risk situations might unintentionally increase victim blaming. Educators implementing such programs have the difficult job of teaching women about situations where sexual assault is more likely to occur, while at the same time instilling the belief that rape is never the survivors' fault, regardless of her prior behavior.

Negative Consequences for Perpetrators

Perceived rewards, costs, and low probability of punishment can be viewed as contributory factors of rape (Bandura, 1973; Scully & Marolla, 1985). Decision-making theory asserts that people weigh the costs and benefits of their actions, along with the probabilities of potential outcomes, when deciding which course of action to take. Breslin, Riggs, O'Leary, and Arias (1988) found that male undergraduates who committed acts of dating violence anticipated fewer negative consequences than nonaggressive students. Scully and Marolla (1985) used information from interviews with 114 incarcerated rapists to suggest that most rapists viewed rape as a rewarding, low risk act.

Decision theories suggest that information that changes men's perceptions of rape such that they begin to view it as: (1) less rewarding than consensual sex, both short term and long term, (2) more costly than consensual sex (i.e., imprisonment, guilt, loss of job, etc.), and (3) more likely to lead to negative consequences (i.e., high probability of getting caught or feeling guilt) might be beneficial in preventing attempted rapes. However, out of the rape prevention programs evaluated in the literature, only three addressed the negative consequences of raping for men (Intons-Peterson, Roskos-Ewoldsen, Thomas, Shirley, & Blut, 1989; Schewe & O'Donohue, 1996; Schewe & Shizas, 2000). Of these three, two evidenced positive outcomes, while in a third, a combination of outcome expectancies and victim empathy was less effective than a program targeting rape myths.

Communication Training/Assertiveness/ Limit Setting

Miscommunication has been implicated as a cause of date rape for many years. Results of one study involving prison inmates suggest that rapists are particularly poor at interpreting negative cues from women in first date situations when compared incarcerated non-rapists (Lipton, McDonel, & McFall, 1987). Muehlenhard postulates that men interpret women's behavior more sexually than do women, and that this misunderstanding can lead to sexual offending (Muehlenhard & Linton, 1987). Muehlenhard and Andrews (1985) studied men's reactions to a woman's stating directly that she did not want to do anything more than kiss. The researchers found that this direct form of limit setting decreased men's ratings of how much the woman wanted to have sex; it decreased men's ratings of how likely they would be to try sexual behaviors beyond kissing; it decreased men's ratings of how much she led the man on; and it decreased men's ratings of how justified the man was to engage in petting after the woman said "no" (Muehlenhard & Andrews, 1985). The construct of "communication skills" has been included along with other interventions in at least three different rape prevention programs that have been evaluated and published. Each of these programs have indicated some level of success in changing knowledge and attitudes, although communication skills were not evaluated specifically as an outcome measure (Foubert & McEwen, 1998; Gilbert, Heesacker, & Gannon, 1991; Proto-Campise, Belknap, & Woolredge, 1998).

STRATEGIES THAT DO NOT WORK

Knowledge/Rape Awareness Programs

The type of information covered in this class of interventions include the definitions of rape, legal terms, statistics regarding the prevalence of rape, ways that society condones/perpetuates rape, descriptions of typical perpetrators or victims, descriptions of the rape trauma syndrome, gender roles, gender differences, and information on local resources for victims of rape. These programs appear to operate on the premise that the more students understand and know about rape, the less likely it is that they will become victims or perpetrators. However, perhaps the clearest message that comes from the evaluation literature is that these programs rarely work. When these programs do report success, often the success is based on increases in knowledge or changes in attitudes among females, with little or no change among male participants, the population for whom change is most essential.

SYNTHESIS

Using Multiple, Interactive Presentation Methods

In order to maximize learning among students, use several presentation methods. Students' memory for information will be enhanced when they hear it, see it, write it, read it, speak it, and do it. In Mary Heppner, Humphrey, Hillenbrand-Gunn, and DeBord's (1995b) study that compared a standard video and lecture presentation to an interactive drama, she found that students in the interactive drama condition were more motivated to hear the message, were more able to recognize consent and coercion, and were more likely to demonstrate behavioral changes. Generalizing from this study and from the literature on persuasion and attitude change, interactive presentations should be more effective than lecture only. Try engaging students in discussions that draw upon their own experiences. Have students engage in role-plays to practice skills that they have learned or to help them understand the perspective of another person. Written exercises also help to cement memories and reinforce what was learned. Homework assignments that involve parents can give parents the opportunity to reinforce at home what their child has learned at school. Also, try using videotaped presentations that capture students' attention. In several interventions, videos alone were as effective as alternate treatments or video plus discussion, and were more effective than discussion alone (Anderson, Stoelb, Duggan, Heiger, Kling, & Payne, 1998; Harrison, Downes, & Williams, 1991; Mann, Hecht, & Valentine, 1988).

More Sessions

Practical limitations often only allow a single session, and almost all of the programs reviewed for this entry were single session interventions. However, as a general rule, more sessions will be better than fewer sessions. In Mary Heppner, Neville, Smith, Kivlighan, and Bershuny's (1999) evaluation of a 3-session rape prevention program, the strongest predictor of whether male participants would change and stay changed over a 5-month period was how many of the sessions they attended. Some curricula developers have overcome some of the practical barriers to multiple sessions by designing their curricula to meet state guidelines for Health Education. In this way, the *Safe-T for Teens* program has replaced the existing health education classes in several middle schools with their own 30-hr curricula that emphasizes healthy relationship skills and sexual abuse prevention.

Single-Gender Audience

As noted above, some of the information included in rape prevention programs is more appropriate for one gender or the other. Many authors have cited strong arguments for addressing single-gender audiences in rape prevention programs (Berkowitz, 1992; Lonsway, 1996; Schewe & O'Donohue, 1993a), and a few have specifically addressed a program's impact on single gender versus co-ed classrooms. Kline (1993) found greater positive changes for males in a single-gender group as compared to males in a co-ed group.

Furthermore, both males and females in the single-gender groups reported a more positive group experience than those in the mixed-gender groups. When possible, single-gender curricula should be developed. However, because of practical constraints (schools often are not willing or able to split up classrooms), mixed-gender curricula should be developed that avoid blaming men, blaming victims, or unintentionally teach males how to rape and get away with it.

Developmentally Appropriate Interventions

Regarding age, it is important to know where your audience is developmentally with regard to dating and sexuality. With younger students, frank discussions about sex, rape, and dating may not be appropriate, and parents and school administrators may frown on such presentations. With younger students, a focus on increasing healthy relationships skills (communication skills, anger management skills, etc.) may be better than a more direct presentation targeting rape-related beliefs and attitudes. Another developmentally appropriate way to address younger audiences is to focus on sexual harassment (teasing, name calling, gender discrimination) rather than sexual assault. Many of the interventions used in rape prevention programs can be easily modified to address sexual harassment, and sexual harassment is an easier topic to address in mixed-gender audiences, because males and females are more equally likely to be victims and/or perpetrators, especially at younger ages.

Specifically Targeting the Race/Ethnicity of the Audience

Mary Heppner and colleagues' (1999) study is the only one to date that has tested the effects of including culturally relevant material in a prevention program. This study compared the effects of a "color-blind" intervention to one that subtly but purposefully integrated African American content and process into the intervention. The results indicate that "Black students in the culturally relevant treatment condition were more cognitively engaged in the intervention than their peers in the traditional treatment condition" (Heppner et al., 1999, p. 16). "Cultural relevance" included having a Black group facilitator, including incidence and prevalence figures for both Black and White populations, specifically targeting race-related rape myths and facts, and including culture-specific information concerning the recovery process of Black and White women.

Exploiting Cognitive Dissonance

The cognitive dissonance literature informs us that *changing behavior* can be an effective way of changing attitudes. Rape prevention programming can take advantage of this knowledge by having students engage in activities that are the opposite of supporting rape. Such activities might include participating in anti-rape discussions, making anti-rape posters or artwork, performing in a dramatic presentation, or convincing a hypothetical person not to use force in sexual relations. The cognitive dissonance literature suggests that students who engage in anti-rape activities should show a positive shift in their attitudes concerning rape.

Male–Female Co-presenters

Both educators and researchers appear to hold a variety of beliefs about the gender of the presenter as it relates to the audience. Some believe that male presenters will have the greatest impact on male audiences, while females will have the greatest impact on female audiences. Others believe the exact opposite. Still others believe that a male/female team of presenters works best for all audiences because of the team's ability to model healthy male–female relationships. Unfortunately, only one published study has specifically addressed the gender of the presenters in their experimental design. Jones and Muehlenhard (1990) found that the gender of presenters (male, female, or male/female team) had no impact on the outcome of a prevention program to a mixed-gender audience.

EFFORTS THAT SHOULD NOT BE UNDERTAKEN

Confrontation

The one study that specifically examined a "confrontational" format in a rape prevention program found that confrontation resulted in a greater tolerance for rape among men (Fischer, 1986). In Mary Heppner and colleagues' (1995a) study, they found that one-third of the men reacted to the program in a bored or negative manner. In her next two studies, she and her colleagues worked to reduce male defensiveness by letting men know that they are leaders in their schools and that they can be part of the solution, and by reinforcing men for getting training. Other rape educators, in an attempt to be as non-confrontational as possible, have adopted a "bystander approach" of teaching students how to help survivors of sexual assault. The true goal of these rape prevention programs, changing participants' attitudes and beliefs about rape, is left unstated. The only rape prevention program to document positive changes that were largely maintained at a 7-month follow-up used this approach to attitude change (Foubert, 2000).

Limitations of this Literature Review

One limitation of this review is that it was based only on reports of rape prevention evaluations that have been published in scientific journals. One bias in these journals is that studies with negative outcomes are less likely to be published. For researchers and rape advocates developing curricula, the lessons that can be learned from unsuccessful programs are at least as important, and may be more important, than the lessons learned from programs documenting success.

An important qualifier of this review is that the programs evaluated focused on the *primary prevention* of rape (preventing new instances of rape), and not *secondary prevention* (preventing re-victimization or targeting at-risk populations). Because of this focus on primary prevention, several important constructs such as "what a person should do if s/he has been raped" and "important community resources" were not addressed. However, because some individuals in any audience will have already experienced sexual assault, these constructs should certainly be integrated into any primary prevention program.

While our knowledge of how to prevent rape is still in its infancy, the number of people dedicated to eradicating rape and improving the quality of rape prevention programs continues to expand. This entry has presented a list of lessons that have been learned from the hard work of educators and researchers. The most effective sexual assault prevention programs will consider the needs of each gender specifically, will avoid confrontation, will provide multiple sessions in an engaging, interactive format, will strive to change behavior, will be tailored to the ethnicity and developmental stage of the audience, will teach female participants self-defense skills and how to avoid high-risk situations, will primarily target rape myths and victim empathy, and may also teach communication skills and highlight the negative consequences that raping holds for perpetrators.

At this time, there are many agencies providing school-based prevention services with little solid evidence of effectiveness. In order to progress as a field, more research regarding effective interventions is necessary.

Also see: Violence Prevention, Childhood.

References

Anderson, L.A., Stoelb, M.P., Duggan, P., Heiger, B., Kling, K.H., & Payne, J.P. (1998). The effectiveness of two types of rape prevention programs in changing the rape-supportive attitudes of college students. *Journal of College Student Development, 39*, 131–142.

Bandura, A. (1973). *Aggression: A social learning analysis.* Englewood Cliffs, NJ: Prentice Hall.

Bennett, L., & Fineran, S. (1998). Sexual and severe physical violence among high school students: Power beliefs, gender, and relationship. *American Journal of Orthopsychiatry, 68*(4), 645–652.

Berg, D.R., Lonsway, K.A., & Fitzgerald, L.F. (1999). Rape prevention education for men: The effectiveness of empathy-induction techniques. *Journal of College Student Development, 40*(3), 219–234.

Bergman, L. (1992). Dating violence among high school students. *Social Work, 37*, 21–27.

Berkowitz, A. (1992). College men as perpetrators of acquaintance rape and sexual assault: A review of recent research. *Journal of American College Health, 40*, 175–181.

Borden, L.A., Karr, S.K., & Caldwell-Colbert, A. (1988). Effects of a university rape prevention program on attitudes and empathy toward rape. *Journal of College Student Development, 29*(2), 132–136.

Breslin, F.C., Riggs, D.S., O'Leary, K.D., & Arias, I. (1988). *The impact of interpersonal violence on dating violence: A social learning analysis.* Unpublished.

Burt, M. (1980). Cultural myths and supports for rape. *Journal of Personality and Social Psychology, 38*(2), 217–230.

Cascardi, M., Avery-Leaf, S., & O'Brien, M.K. (1998). *Dating violence among middle school students in a low income urban community.* Paper Presented at 727 Grantee Meeting, Centers for Disease Control and Prevention, Atlanta, GA.

Cohen, E.S., Kidder, L., & Harvey, J. (1978). Crime prevention versus victimization: The psychology of two different reactions. *Victimology, 3*, 285–296.

Connolly, J.A., McMaster, L., Craig, W., & Pepler, D. (1997). *Dating, puberty, and sexualized aggression in early adolescence.* Paper presented at the Annual Meeting of the Association for the Advancement of Behavior Therapy, Miami, FL.

Denmare, D., Briere, J., & Lips, H.M. (1988). Violent pornography and self-reported likelihood of sexual aggression. *Journal of Research in Personality, 22*, 140–153.

Dobash, R.E., & Dobash, R.P. (1994). *Violence against wives: A case against patriarchy.* NY: Free Press.

Ellis, A.L., O'Sullivan, C.S., & Sowards, B. (1992). The impact of contemplated exposure to a survivor of rape on attitudes toward rape. *Journal of Applied Social Psychology, 22*, 889–895.

Finkelhor D., Araji, S., Baron, L., Browne, A., Peters, S., & Wyatt, G. (Eds.). (1986). *A sourcebook on child sexual abuse.* Beverly Hills, CA: Sage.

Fischer, G.J. (1986). College student attitudes toward forcible date rape: Changes after taking a human sexuality course. *Journal of Sex Education and Therapy, 12*, 42–46.

Foshee, V.A., Linder, G.F., Bauman, K.E., & Langwick, S.A. (1996). The Safe Dates project: Theoretical basis, evaluation design, and selected baseline findings. *American Journal of Preventive Medicine, 12*, 39–46.

Foubert, J.D., & McEwen, M.K. (1998). An all-male rape prevention peer education program: Decreasing fraternity men's behavioral intent to rape. *Journal of College Student Development, 39*(6), 548–555.

Foubert, J.D. (2000). The longitudinal effects of a rape-prevention program on fraternity men's attitudes, behavioral intent, and behavior. *Journal of American College Health, 48*(4), 158–163.

Gavey, N.J. (1991). Sexual victimization among Auckland University students: How much and who does it? *New Zealand Journal of Psychology, 20*(2), 63–70.

Gilbert, B., Heesacker, M., & Gannon, L. (1991). Changing the sexual aggression-supportive attitudes of men: A psychoeducational intervention. *Journal of Counseling Psychology, 38*(2), 197–203.

Gray, M., Lesser, D., Quinn, E., & Bounds, C. (1990). Effects of rape education on perception of vulnerability and on reducing risk-taking behavior. *Journal of College Student Development, 31*(2), 217–223.

Hanson, K.A., & Gidycz, C.A. (1993). Evaluation of a sexual assault prevention program. *Journal of Consulting and Clinical Psychology, 61*, 1046–1052.

Harrison, P.J., Downes, J., & Williams, M.D. (1991). Date and acquaintance rape: Perceptions and attitude change strategies. *Journal of College Student Development, 32*(2), 131–139.

Heppner, M.J., Good, G.E., Hillenbrand-Gunn, T.L., Hawkins, A.K., Hacquard, L.L., Nichols, R.K., DeBord, K.A., & Brock, K.J. (1995a). Examining sex differences in altering attitudes about rape: A test of the elaboration likelihood model. *Journal of Counseling and Development, 73*, 640–647.

Heppner, M.J., Humphrey, C.F., Hillenbrand-Gunn, T.L., & DeBord, K.A. (1995b). The differential effects of rape prevention programming on attitudes, behavior, and knowledge. *Journal of Counseling Psychology, 42*, 508–518.

Heppner, M.J., Neville, H.A., Smith, K., Kivlighan, D.M., & Bershuny, B.S. (1999). Examining immediate and long-term efficacy of rape prevention programming with racially diverse college men. *Journal of Counseling Psychology, 46*(1), 16–26.

Hildebran, D., & Pithers, W. (1989). Enhancing offender empathy for sexual-abuse victims. In D. Laws (Ed.), *Relapse prevention with sex offenders* (pp. 236–243). New York: Guilford Press.

Intons-Peterson, M.J., Roskos-Ewoldsen, B., Thomas, L., Shirley, M., & Blut, K. (1989). Will educational materials reduce negative effects of exposure to sexual violence? *Journal of Social and Clinical Psychology, 8*, 256–275.

Jones, J., & Muehlenhard, C. (1990, November). *Using education to prevent rape on college campuses.* Presented at the Annual Meeting of the Society for the Scientific Study of Sex, Minneapolis, MN.

Kline, R.J. (1993). The effects of a structured-group rape-prevention program on selected male personality correlates of abuse toward women. *Dissertation Abstracts Online.*

Kilpatrick, D.G., Acierno, R., Resnick, H.S., Saunders, B.E., & Best, C.L. (1997). A 2-year longitudinal analysis of the relationships between violent assault and substance use in women. *Journal of Consulting and Clinical Psychology, 65*(5), 834–847.

Kilpatrick, D.G., Best, C.L., Saunders, B.E., & Veronen, L.J. (1988). Rape in marriage and in dating relationships: How bad is it for mental health? *Annals of New York Academy of Sciences, 528*, 335–344.

Koss, M.P., Koss, P.G., & Woodruff, W.J. (1991). Deleterious effects of criminal victimization on women's health and medical utilization. *Archives of Internal Medicine, 151*, 342–347.

Koss, M. (1988). Hidden rape: Sexual aggression and victimization in a national sample of students in higher education. In A. Burgess (Ed.), *Rape and sexual assault II* (pp. 3–25). New York: Garland.

Lenihan, G., Rawlins, M., Eberly, C.G., Buckley, B., & Masters, B. (1992). Gender differences in rape supportive attitudes before and after a date rape education intervention. *Journal of College Student Development, 33*, 331–338.

Lonsway, K.A. (1996). Preventing acquaintance rape through education: What do we know? *Psychology of Women Quarterly, 20*, 229–265.

Lee, L. (1987). Rape prevention: Experimental training for men. *Journal of Counseling and Development, 66*, 100–101.

Lipton, D.N., McDonel, E.C., & McFall, R.M. (1987). Heterosocial perception in rapists. *Journal of Consulting and Clinical Psychology, 55*, 17–21.

Malamuth, N.M., & Check, J.V.P. (1984). Debriefing effectiveness following exposure to pornographic rape depictions. *The Journal of Sex Research, 20*, 1–13.

Mann, C.A., Hecht, M.L., & Valentine, K.B. (1988). Performance in a social context: Date rape versus date right. *Central States Speech Journal, 3/4*, 269–280.

Miller, T.R., Cohen, M.A., & Rossman, S.B. (1993). Victim costs of violent crime and resulting injuries. *Health Affairs, 12*(4), 186–197.

Molidor, C., & Tolman, R.M. (1998). Gender and contextual factors in adolescent dating violence. *Violence Against Women, 4*(2), 180–194.

Muehlenhard, C.L., & Andrews, S.L. (1985, November). *Sexual aggression in dating situations: Do factors that cause men to regard it as more justifiable also make it more probable?* Presented at the Annual Meeting of the Association for the Advancement of Behavior Therapy, Washington, DC.

Muehlenhard, C.L., & Linton, M.A. (1987). Date rape and sexual aggression in dating situations: Incidence and risk factors. *Journal of Counseling Psychology, 34,* 186–196.

Parrot, A. (1990). Do rape education programs influence rape patterns among New York State college students? *Presented at the 1990 Annual Meeting of the Society for the Scientific Study of Sex*, Minneapolis, Minnesota.

Peri, C. (1991, March). Below the belt: Women in the martial arts. *Newsletter of the National Women's Martial Arts Federations*, 6–14.

Pithers, W.D., Kashima, K., Cumming, G.F., Beal, L.S., & Buell, M. (1988). Relapse prevention of sexual aggression. In R. Prentky & V. Quinsey (Eds.), *Human sexual aggression: Current perspectives* (pp. 244–260). New York: New York Academy of Sciences.

Proto-Campise, L., Belknap, J., & Wooldredge, J. (1998). High school students' adherence to rape myths and the effectiveness of high school rape-awareness programs. *Violence Against Women, 4,* 308–328.

Resnick, H.S., Acierno, R., & Kilpatrick, D.G. (1997). Health impact of interpersonal violence 2: Medical and mental health outcomes. *Behavioral Medicine, 23,* 65–78.

Schewe, P.A. (2002). Guidelines for developing rape prevention and risk reduction interventions. In P. Schewe (Ed.), *Preventing violence in relationships: Interventions across the life span.* Washington, DC: American Psychological Association.

Schewe, P.A., & O'Donohue, W.T. (1993a). Rape prevention: Methodological problems and new directions. *Clinical Psychology Review, 13,* 667–682.

Schewe, P.A., & O'Donohue, W.T. (1993b). Sexual abuse prevention with high risk males: The roles of victim empathy and rape myths. *Violence and Victims, 8*(4), 339–351.

Schewe, P.A., & O'Donohue, W.T. (1996). Rape prevention with high risk males: Short-term outcome of two interventions. *Archives of Sexual Behavior, 25*(5), 455–471.

Schewe, P.A., & Shizas, N. (2000, May). *Rape prevention with college age males: Short-term outcomes of a video-taped intervention vs. a peer-mediated group discussion.* Presented at the National Sexual Violence Prevention Conference, Dallas, TX.

Scully, D., & Marolla, J. (1985). "Riding the bull at Gilley's": Convicted rapists describe the rewards of rape. *Social Problems, 32*(3), 251–263.

Ullman, S.E. (1997). Review and critique of empirical studies of rape avoidance. *Criminal Justice and Behavior, 24*(2), 177–204.

Ullman, S.E., & Knight, R.A. (1993). The efficacy of women's resistance strategies in rape situations. *Psychology of Women Quarterly, 17,* 23–38.

Walker, C.E., Bonner, B.L., & Kaufman, K.L. (1988). *The physically and sexually abused child: Evaluation and treatment.* New York, NY: Pergamon Press.

Williams, J.E., & Holmes, K.A. (1981). *The second assault: Rape and public attitudes.* Westport, CT: Greenwood Press.

Women Against Rape. (1980). A rape prevention program in an urban area: Community action strategies to stop rape. *Signs, 5,* 238–241.

Yllo, K. (1993). Through a feminist lens. In R.J. Gelles, & D.R. Loseke (Eds.), *Current controversies in family violence.* Newbury Park, CA: Sage.

Sexual Harassment, Adulthood

Meg A. Bond

INTRODUCTION

Sexual harassment is a serious barrier to the personal, social, and financial well-being of women, yet it is so pervasive as to be considered normative and so widely accepted as to be rendered almost invisible. Women have been sexually harassed since they first started working outside the home (Fitzgerald, 1993). Yet, the unwanted sexualization of work, academic, or otherwise non-sexual relationships was not actively labeled as a problem until the late 1970s when Catherine MacKinnon declared that "... lacking a term to express it, sexual harassment [has been] literally unspeakable, which [has] made a generalized, shared and social definition of it inaccessible. The unnamed [however] should not be mistaken for the nonexistent" (1979, p. 27). MacKinnon's analysis was ground breaking, and over the last two decades, the phenomenon has indeed been labeled, acknowledged in several countries with a legal definition, and received significant attention from media, researchers, and activists. This entry summarizes some of the recent literature by first addressing issues of definition and scope of the problem, and then turning to ways that sexual harassment is explained by various theoretical approaches. The second half of the entry describes intervention strategies, both those that appear to be promising and those that have shown only minimal effectiveness.

DEFINITIONS

The formal definition of *sexual harassment* adopted by the US Equal Employment Opportunity Commission (EEOC) is "unwelcome sexual advances, requests for sexual favors, and other verbal or physical conduct of a sexual nature" (1) when such behavior becomes a condition of employment, (2) when it affects employment decisions, and/or (3) when "such conduct has the purpose of effect of unreasonably interfering with an individual's work performance or creating an intimidating, hostile or offensive work environment" (EEOC, 1980). In 1981, the US Education Department's Office of Civil Rights adopted a similar definition for the academic community that added learning environments to the third condition.[1] Other countries have also taken proactive steps to define and prohibit sexual harassment (e.g., policies adopted by the Canadian Human Rights Commission in 1983, included under England's 1975 Sex Discrimination Act in 1986, and addressed by the Rubinstein report conducted by the European Parliament in 1987).

Definitions adopted by researchers have generally been compatible with these legal definitions in terms of the emphasis on unwanted verbal and physical behavior of a sexual nature that interferes with the victim's work and/or well-being. Legal and research-based definitions both stress the subjective experience of the victim as a defining feature of sexual harassment. There remains, however, a lack of broad consensus among researchers (and even less among the general public) about whether the definition should factor in a power differential between the harasser and the target, the context (or location) of the behavior, or specific job-related consequences.

Legal definitions distinguish between two types of sexual harassment: (1) *quid pro quo harassment* and (2) hostile work environment (also referred to as *gender harassment*). *Quid pro quo harassment* (which literally means "this for that") involves subtle and overt bribery or coercion for sexual attentions and includes inappropriate sexual advances that can range from unwanted flirtation or repeated requests for dates to more direct pressure, threats, or actual physical assault. *Gender harassment* refers to generalized sexist remarks and behavior which are not necessarily designed to elicit sexual cooperation yet contribute to an environment in which women feel intimidated, unsafe, devalued, or otherwise isolated. While the general public is often reluctant to see gender harassment as problematic, the US Supreme Court has affirmed that both types of sexual harassment violate Title VII and thus are illegal. Researchers have also attempted to develop typologies, with the most empirically validated approach being to delineate three types: *gender harassment, unwanted sexual attention*, and *sexual coercion* (Gelfand, Fitzgerald, & Drasgow, 1995). This three-part distinction is useful in further clarifying aspects of quid pro quo harassment (unwanted attention and coercion). While related, each of the three types of harassment involves somewhat different dynamics and thus different implications for prevention.

SCOPE

Extent of the Problem

The exact number of women being harassed at any point in time is difficult to measure for several reasons

including reluctance to report, lack of public consensus regarding what constitutes harassment, and fear of retaliation. Experts estimate that fewer than 5 percent of victims ever file a formal complaint or report their experiences to someone in authority (Fitzgerald et al., 1988). There are also few large-scale formal studies. However, based on what investigations are available, researchers in the United States, Canada, and Europe estimate that about half of all women will experience some form of sexual harassment at work and/or school at some point during their lifetimes (see Gruber, Smith, & Kauppinen-Toropainen, 1996, for cross-national comparisons). When definitions include sexist comments and jokes, some studies show incidence rates that exceed 70 percent. If we then also include secondary victims (i.e., people who are aware of and concerned about the harassment of friends and coworkers), the percentage of people personally affected by sexual harassment rises even further. Research has consistently shown that gender harassment is the most common form of sexual harassment, followed by unwanted sexual attention, and then by sexual coercion.

Sexual harassment is a much more pervasive and debilitating problem for women than for men. Men are sometimes harassed, and these incidents should not be overlooked. However, the vast majority of harassment incidents involve male harassers and female targets. In studies where men do report sexual harassment, their harassers are also typically men. Not only do incidence rates differ dramatically by gender, but women and men also tend to have quite different definitions and perceptions of sexual harassment. Women tend to consider harassment a more serious problem; they recognize a wider variety of behaviors as sexual harassment; and they experience unwanted sexual attention and gender harassment as more threatening, inappropriate, and uncomfortable than do men. Major studies indicate that almost all of the people who describe serious job-related consequences of sexual harassment are women. Given the significant gender differences and their implications for prevention, this entry focuses primarily on the harassment of women.

Costs

There are serious emotional, physical, occupational, and economic costs associated with sexual harassment. The documented effects of sexual harassment on women workers include depression, anxiety, lowered self-confidence, and debilitating stress-related physical symptoms (e.g., headaches, tiredness, sleep disturbances, loss of appetite, weight loss). Sexual harassment can affect work performance, morale, motivation, and absenteeism. Sexual harassment can also result in the deterioration of interpersonal relationships with coworkers and supervisors, lowered job

---

[1] In 1993, the EEOC clarified that gender harassment is "verbal or physical contact that denigrates or shows hostility or aversion" (p. 51269).

satisfaction, fewer opportunities for advancement, and reduced commitment to the organization. Many women who are harassed at work either choose to or are forced to change jobs as a result. Women students who have been sexually harassed in academic settings often experience similar physical and emotional reactions. In addition, many change their courses, majors, and even career directions to avoid further harassment. Some drop out of school altogether. The effects of sexual harassment on individual women can be significant and enduring.

The costs for the organizations, schools, or other settings that women frequent are also significant. Not only do organizations risk potentially costly lawsuits, but they can also lose millions of dollars due to absenteeism, turnover, lost productivity, and health care costs associated with sexual harassment. Additional indirect costs include harm to teamwork, loss of trust among coworkers, loss of faith in leaders, and loss of commitment to the organization. (See Koss, Goodman, Brown, Fitzgerald, Keita, & Russo, 1994, for a summary of research on the consequences of sexual harassment.)

THEORIES AND RESEARCH

Various models have been proposed to explain why sexual harassment occurs. Some basic models include: (1) *biological models* which suggest that most of what gets labeled sexual harassment is a natural expression of heterosexual attraction and that cases of extreme sexual harassment are the result of a few very misguided or "sick" individuals, (2) *organizational models* that emphasize the role of setting factors such as climate, structures, authority relations, and policies, and (3) *sociocultural models* that hold that sexual harassment is a reflection of our patriarchal system and societal beliefs that devalue women and support male expressions of dominance. (For reviews of these three types of models, see Tangri, Burt, & Johnson, 1982, and O'Donohue, Downs, & Yeater, 1998.)

The *biological model* has been widely dismissed given evidence that most sexual harassment does *not* occur between men and women who might be considered "eligible" or likely for a relationship together (i.e., both unattached or similar in age, attitudes, and status). Few targets of the sexual attention express mutual interest, and most suffer negative emotional and/or job consequences as a result. Nor do harassers typically direct their unwanted advances toward only one person. The notion that more serious sexual harassment is the result of a few perverse men is contradicted by the high base rate of the problem.

There is, however, evidence for some individual differences among those who tend to be involved in harassment situations. Harassers tend to be married men who hold traditional beliefs about gender roles and hold higher status positions than their targets. It also appears that some women are at higher risk for harassment than others are. Several studies find that young, unmarried women who live in urban settings and hold lower status work positions are the most frequent targets. These findings are open to multiple interpretations and some sampling and measurement problems. In fact, several other studies find that women of relatively high professional status are also frequent targets—even by men with less organizationally defined status (e.g., students, patients, and customers). Peer harassment is also quite common. There is mixed evidence regarding whether experiences of sexual harassment vary based on the race or ethnicity of the recipient. Some studies find no differences in incidence across racial groups, while other studies do find such differences. Whether numerical rates vary or not, the sexual harassment of women of color is so inextricably linked with racial stereotyping and racism that their experiences of harassment are often qualitatively different than the experiences of White women (Mecca & Rubin, 1999). Unfortunately, we know relatively little about the intersection of sexual and racial harassment since many studies of sexual harassment (particularly early ones) do not even inquire about race. There is evidence that lesbians, in particularly those who are open about their sexual orientation, face considerably more sexual harassment than other women do (Schneider, 1991).

There is general support for the assumptions underlying both *organizational* and *sociocultural models*. For example, many studies indicate that local norms and organizational values can set the stage for sexual harassment. Sexual harassment is more likely to occur in settings where there is perceived tolerance for sexist behavior, general norms that condone sexual relationships among workers, and no standards or policies that explicitly prohibit sexual harassment. It is more common when there is general disrespect for employees and coworkers, there is a lack of support for women's professional development, and management is seen as less responsive. (For an overview of climate studies, see Fitzgerald, Drasgow, Hulin, Gelfand, & Magley, 1997.)

There is also considerable evidence that sexual harassment is likely to occur in settings dominated by men (*power stratification*) and occupations traditionally associated with men (*numerical dominance* and *occupational culture*). Such findings support the notions behind the sociocultural model that sexual harassment is both an expression of women's inequality and a method for enforcing it. In terms of findings related to male dominance as expressed through *power stratification*, women in female-dominated roles (e.g., clerical) are at risk for sexual harassment due to their lack of power relative to their typically male supervisors and/or to the sexualization of their work activities through a dynamic termed "*sex role spill over*" (Gutek, 1985). Additional support for this model is provided by findings that there is less sexual harassment in organizations with higher percentages of women in management positions.

In terms of dynamics related to *numerical dominance*, we know that women in traditionally male occupations (e.g., military, trades, police, and security positions) report more sexual harassment than do women in female-dominated settings. In such occupations, women's minority status makes them more visible, and the association of maleness with the job and work environment contributes to an unwelcoming culture. Sexual harassment with its emphasis on gender and sexuality are effective reminders to women that they are outsiders who do not belong. There is also evidence that women who simply have more routine contact with men—regardless of actual type of job—will be subjected to more inappropriate sexualized attention which underlines the importance of immediate work group dynamics as critical mediators of occupational norms (see Gruber, 1998).

Fitzgerald et al. (1997) have proposed a model that looks at both organizational and societally related factors, which is supported by one of the very few existing longitudinal studies of the antecedents and consequences of sexual harassment (Glomb, Munson, Hulin, Bergman, & Drasgow, 1999). Their research suggests that sexual harassment is a function of *organizational climate* (operationalized as perceptions of organizational tolerance for sexual harassment) and the *job gender context* (i.e., gender traditional vs. nontraditional as well as gender ratio of work group). The longitudinal study found that perceptions of organizational tolerance for sexual harassment that coincided with experiences of sexual harassment at one point in time were predictive of rates of sexual harassment 2 years later. This work not only begins to develop a multilevel model, but it also documents the enduring and reciprocal relationship between organizational climate, gendered work roles, and rates of harassment.

The various findings that delineate individual, organizational, as well as societal contributors support the need for models that incorporate interactions among all levels of analysis. Models that consider the characteristics of individuals involved, relationship dynamics and power differentials, as well as organizational and societal factors that set the stage for harassment are critical for guiding prevention efforts. Some work has been done to develop more comprehensive systemic or ecological models, but most work to date has not fully elucidated how organizational factors and job characteristics interact with individual differences *and* are embedded in the broader context of gendered relations, stratification, and societal beliefs about gender roles (see Bond, 1995, for a discussion of an ecological model

and Pryor, LaVite, & Stoller, 1993, for a description of a person–environment interactional model).

STRATEGIES THAT WORK

There is no clear evidence of a single approach to the prevention of sexual harassment that is effective across a variety of settings.

STRATEGIES THAT MIGHT WORK

The majority of interventions aimed at the prevention of sexual harassment involve the development of organizational policies, grievance procedures, and awareness training. According to a Bureau of National Affairs study, 97 percent of companies have sexual harassment policies (National Council for Research on Women, 1995). The importance of these interventions is supported by survey research that indicates correlations between policy conditions and rates of sexual harassment. For example, women who are more aware of workplace grievance procedures are less likely to have experienced sexual harassment. Organizations in which leaders are perceived as proactive in addressing sexual harassment have fewer problems with harassment than organizations where leaders are seen as indifferent, passive, or even encouraging of sexist behaviors (Pryor et al., 1993). There appears to be less harassment in settings where women believe harassers will face negative consequences for their behavior (Fitzgerald, 1993). There is little empirical guidance for delineating specific elements of effective sexual harassment policies. However, there is general agreement based on survey research, practical experience, and legal precedents that policies should include: a clear and understandable definition of sexual harassment, descriptions of disciplinary actions for individuals who do harass, accessible reporting and complaint procedures for both formal and informal resolution, and protection from retaliation.

Broad surveys repeated before and after policy changes support the claim that the implementation of "zero tolerance" policies and proactive educational initiatives have reduced incidents of sexual harassment in such settings as the US Department of Defense and the LA Police Department (Gruber, 1998). However, the few attempts made to systematically evaluate the effectiveness of such approaches have yielded mixed results. One of the earliest published evaluations indicated that the primary measurable change following a sexual harassment awareness training

---

[2] The majority of which were established after 1980 when the EEOC published guidelines.

program at the University of Michigan was in participants' ability to recognize appropriate reactions to harassing behavior (i.e., how to help victims but not in how to prevent problematic behavior; Beauvais, 1986). A comprehensive sexual harassment program at the University of Hawaii at Manoa (UHM) that included educational components, advocacy, and supportive counseling (Hippensteele & Pearson, 1999) showed some preventive potential in raising faculty recognition of sexual harassment as a campus-wide problem (immediately post-seminar). While increasing recognition of more subtle forms of behavior like jokes or comments as potentially harassing is a positive change, the impact on actual rates of harassment and/or the overall treatment of women is unknown. In fact, there is generally discouraging evidence about the long term, sustainable impact of educational approaches. One carefully conducted study of two approaches to sexual harassment prevention training at University of Missouri-Columbia found that neither type of workshop effected *any* significant change among participants' attitudes, feelings, or behaviors at 10-weeks follow-up (Cohen, 1995).

Thus, among those evaluation reports that do exist, there is no strong evidence pointing to the effectiveness of a particular single approach to the prevention of sexual harassment. An optimistic note is provided by the results of one large scale survey of almost 2,000 Canadian women that indicated that there is less harassment when organizations sponsor prevention programs with multiple components (e.g., policies, plus training, plus complaint procedures) than when programs involve only passive education (e.g., simply providing employees with information about sexual harassment) (Gruber, 1998). Similarly, Koss et al. (1994) argue that for prevention training programs to be effective, they must include strong management or institutional support and should focus on attitude and behavior change in addition to education about sexual harassment definitions and policies.

STRATEGIES THAT DO NOT WORK

Under ideal conditions, strong policies supported by proactive educational efforts can serve as deterrents to future incidents of sexual harassment. If conveyed with conviction and the support of organizational leaders, they can help create an overall climate intolerant of sexual harassment. However, most sexual harassment policies focus primarily on definition and punitive action steps. The adversarial relations between women and men that can result from these approaches do not forward the general cause of sexual harassment prevention. Backlash and retaliation too frequently accompany increased attention to regulations regarding sexual harassment.

Similarly, educational and awareness campaigns that accompany policies—including training for employees and managers on how to define or identify problems as well as training for victims on how to report or avoid harassment—often focus more on reducing legal liability than on fostering conditions that actually protect women and prevent harassment. Important limitations of many training programs are that they receive minimal support from organizational leaders and are not integrated into institution-wide initiatives. Too often "prevention" in policy and training initiatives refers to the avoidance of costly charges of sex discrimination as opposed to focusing on more qualitative and substantive changes in organizational behavior or the development of alternatives to sexual harassment. Such approaches to policy and training rarely promote respectful interactions among coworkers and do not necessarily foster equality, reduce sexism, or prevent misogynist actions.

The reliance on policies alone for prevention can bring with it other dilemmas. More specifically, it is not clear that formal complaint mechanisms can deter any but the most blatant quid pro quo variety of sexual harassment. In other words, somewhat ironically, it is the least frequent form of sexual harassment that is the form most likely to be addressed through current organizational policy approaches. Many of the most pervasive and thus insidious forms of harassment are less likely to be addressed by standard policies. Gender harassment can be quite devastating and isolating even when it may not reach the critical or egregious levels that would be required for institutional or legal punitive action. Additionally, the existence of sexual harassment policies can create the illusion that the problem has been addressed. This illusion, when combined with the lack of public consensus regarding what constitutes harassment, can contribute to the accusation that people who raise continued concerns about sexist behavior and/or gender harassment are over-reacting. In sum, policy and education may play a useful role in raising awareness and establishing some guidelines for interpersonal behavior. However, they are clearly not sufficient to prevent sexual harassment since they typically do little to challenge broader gender inequalities in work and academic settings.

SYNTHESIS

Primary prevention requires us to identify and address risk factors while also creating environmental and structural changes to promote women's active and equal participation in all aspects of organizational life. For many organizations and institutions, this goal requires some fundamental shifts in how they operate. To effectively prevent sexual harassment, we need a wide range of strategies to ensure gender equality including: (1) improvements in organizational culture, (2) broader gender representation throughout organizations, and (3) changes in societal beliefs about gender and gender roles.

Organizational Culture

Given the evidence that local norms are so closely associated with incidence of sexual harassment, it stands to reason that efforts to prevent sexual harassment should include the development of new, shared organizational values (organizational culture) that visibly support equity and the nonsexist, nonsexualized treatment of all people. As discussed above, some of the research on organizational contributors to sexual harassment has focused on values specific to harassment and degree of tolerance for such behavior; thus interventions that promote strong clear messages from leaders about unacceptable behaviors would seem useful. Other findings encourage us to go further and emphasize the more global treatment of workers and/or students. For example, rates of harassment have been linked to supports for women's professional development and to the overall "professional" atmosphere of the work place.

In the spirit of such findings, I would argue that prevention of sexual harassment can be supported by promoting generally respectful work and academic environments in which: (1) interdependencies between people are recognized and participants are required to be accountable for their impact on others, (2) diversity is supported such that organizational procedures and standards incorporate a value for varied backgrounds, styles, and approaches to work (whether based on gender, race, ethnicity, sexual orientation, disability or other typically dis-equalizing bases), (3) the salience of gender is reduced such that gendered expectations and stereotypes do not intrude into job design, evaluations, and support from peers, and (4) there is collective awareness that contextual influences and qualities of the environment shape organizational behavior (including recognition of how privilege and power differences influence behavior) (Bond, 1995). These qualities of an organizational culture would support the empowerment of women to be fully equal participants with their male cohorts.

Some of the challenge here is to infuse these perspectives throughout the fabric of the organization or institution. Some approaches might include: (1) engaging key leaders as partners in organizational culture change, (2) communicating the expectation that supervisors will model professional, respectful, egalitarian behavior, (3) socializing new members by emphasizing values and standards for behavior in all orientation processes, (4) regularly addressing issues of respectful treatment in settings where groups of people come together, and (5) including respectful, nonsexist treatment and support for diversity as performance criteria in teaching and job evaluations.

Gender Representation in Organizations

Attempts to foster empowering organizational cultures would be empty without the parallel effort to actually elevate women's status in the workplace by increasing the representation of women in all ranks. Throughout the US workforce, most women work in sex-segregated jobs, which are typically of lower status than their male counterparts. Even when women do occupy management positions, they tend to be in lower and mid-level positions that have little authority over others (Blau, Ferber, & Winkler, 2001). And yet, it is work sites with more equal numbers of women and men at all levels that tend to have fewer problems with sexual harassment than male-dominate settings. Thus, aggressive recruitment, more equitable hiring practices, and increased mentoring and support for women's development are critical to the prevention of sexual harassment. Helping women move into jobs traditionally held by men, moving women into management positions, and adopting policies that reduce barriers to women's professional involvement (e.g., supports for balancing family and work roles) can be helpful. Work toward equity for women in all aspects of organizational or academic life is a critical element in the prevention of sexual harassment.

Beliefs about Gender and Gender Roles

Prevention of sexual harassment can also be enhanced by addressing social stereotypes and myths about masculinity, femininity, gender roles, and appropriate ways of relating across gender lines. Deeply held beliefs about proper roles for women and men as well as hostility toward equality for women are associated with incidence of sexual harassment. Some have described sexual harassment as a problem of role definition where gender role expectations spill over into work role expectations. In addition, there are findings that both men and women with more traditional gender role beliefs are more likely to blame women for their own harassment. Research indicates that girls become targets of sexual harassment in the forms of gender harassment and unwanted sexual advances at such a young age that it leads many to see this treatment as acceptable. In essence, as a result of this socialization, the sexualization of male–female interactions and bold expressions of male sexual attention become "normative" and thus something men perpetuate and women endure without question.

Prevention efforts that challenge traditional gender role specifications are critical. Such efforts would seem most useful if implemented at young ages such that rigid values about gender roles never set in for girls and boys. They would be most constructive if they involved work with families, schools, churches, and other institutions of socialization. They would ideally work to expand acceptance of a wide range of behaviors, values, aspirations, and roles in relationships for both genders—including acceptance of gay and lesbian orientations. It would be important to address intersections of race and gender in challenging stereotyped expectations and tracking. Consciousness raising training can also be useful later in the life cycle when sponsored by organizations and academic institutions and focused directly on interpersonal relations within work and learning environments. Some such training can focus on stereotyping and gendered notions of acceptable behavior. It can also focus on bridging differences by increasing empathy and the ability of participants to understand how others might experience and perceive common work interactions quite differently.

In sum, sexual harassment, in its multiple forms, is a common experience for women. It can have devastating effects on women's health and well-being, as well as serious negative outcomes for organizations and institutions where women work and attend school. The most common approaches to prevention have been the development of sexual harassment policies and the delivery of training programs to increase awareness of the problem. While such approaches form an important foundation for any prevention effort, they have limitations and are simply not enough. Further efforts that focus on changing organizational cultures to be more inclusive and supportive of women, altering hiring and promotion strategies such that women are represented at all ranks within organizations, and even starting earlier to challenge rigid gender role specifications are all suggested as more primary interventions important to the prevention of sexual harassment.

Also see: Aggressive Behavior, Adolescence.

References

Beauvais, K. (1986). Workshops to combat sexual harassment: A case study of changing attitudes. *Signs: Journal of Women in Culture and Society, 12,* 130–145.

Blau, F.D., Ferber, M.A., & Winkler, A.E. (2001). *The economics of women, men, and work* (4th ed.), Upper Saddle River, NJ: Prentice-Hall.

Bond, M.A. (1995). Prevention and the ecology of sexual harassment: Creating empowering climates. *Prevention in Human Services, 12*(2), 147–173.

National Council for Research on Women (1995). *Sexual Harassment: research and resources* (3rd ed.). New York: Author.

Canadian Human Rights Commission (CHRC). (1983). *Unwanted sexual attention and sexual harassment.* Montreal: Minister of Supply and Services of Canada.

Cohen, B. (1995). *Evaluation of workshops to counter sexual harassment.* Dissertation, University of Missouri-Columbia.

Equal Employment Opportunity Commission (EEOC). (1980). Guidelines on discrimination because of sex. *Federal Register, 45,* 74676–74677.

Fitzgerald, L.F. (1993). Sexual harassment: Violence against women in the workplace. *American Psychologist, 48*(10), 1070–1076.

Fitzgerald, L.F., Drasgow, F., Hulin, C.L., Gelfand, M.J., & Magley, V.J. (1997). Antecedents and consequences of sexual harassment in organizations: A test of an integrated model. *Journal of Applied Psychology, 82*(4), 578–589.

Fitzgerald, L.F., Shullman, S.L., Bailey, N., Richards, M., Swecker, J., Gold, Y., Ormerod, M., & Weitzman, L. (1988). The incidence of sexual harassment in academia and the workplace. *Journal of Vocational Behavior, 32,* 152–175.

Gelfand, M., Fitzgerald, L., & Drasgow, F. (1995). The structure of sexual harassment: A confirmatory analysis across cultures and settings. *Journal of Vocational Behavior, 47,* 164–177.

Glomb, T.M., Munson, L.J., Hulin, C.L., Bergman, M.E., & Drasgow, F. (1999). Structural equation models of sexual harassment: Longitudinal explorations and cross sectional generalizations. *Journal of Applied Psychology, 84,* 14–28.

Gruber, J.E., Smith, M., & Kauppinen-Toropainen, K. (1996). Sexual harassment types and severity: Linking research and policy. In M. Stockdale (Ed.), *Sexual harassment in the workplace: Perspectives, frontiers, and response strategies* (pp. 151–173). Thousand Oaks, CA: Sage.

Gruber, J. (1998). The impact of male work environments and organizational policies on women's experiences of sexual harassment. *Gender and Society, 12*(3), 301–320.

Gutek, B.A. (1985). *Sex and the workplace: Impact of sexual behavior and harassment on women, men, and organizations.* San Francisco: Jossey-Bass.

Hippensteele, S., & Pearson, T.C. (1999). Responding effectively to sexual harassment. *Change, 31*(1), 48–54.

Koss, M.P., Goodman, L.A., Brown, A., Fitzgerald, L.F., Keita, G.P., & Russo, N.F. (1994). *No safe haven: Male violence against women at home, at work, and in the community.* Washington, DC: American Psychological Association.

MacKinnon, C. (1979). *The sexual harassment of working women.* New Haven, CT: Yale University.

Mecca, S.J., & Rubin, L.J. (1999). Definitional research on African American students and sexual harassment. *Psychology of Women Quarterly, 23,* 813–817.

O'Donohue, W., Downs, K., & Yeater, E.A. (1998). Sexual harassment: A review of literature. *Aggression and Violent Behavior, 3*(2), 111–128.

Pryor, J.B., LaVite, C., & Stoller, L.M. (1993). A social psychological analysis of sexual harassment: The person/situation interaction. *Journal of Vocational Behavior, 42,* 68–83.

Schneider, B.E. (1991). Put up and shut up: Workplace sexual assaults. *Gender and Society, 5,* 533–548.

Tangri, S., Burt, M., & Johnson, L. (1982). Sexual harassment at work: Three explanatory models. *Journal of Social Issues, 38,* 33–54.

Sexuality, Childhood

D. Kim Openshaw

INTRODUCTION

No other term conjures up such delight and apprehension as does the word, "sex." Over the past three decades, information regarding sexuality has been proliferated, primarily through various media. While this may be seen as positive progress in dispelling myths surrounding sexuality, it has not provided the information or the skills necessary to promote healthy sexuality in children, which is the concern of this entry.

DEFINITIONS AND SCOPE

Sexuality "consists of all the sensations, emotions and cognitions that an individual associates with physical sexual arousal and that usually give rise to sexual desire and/or behavior" (McAnulty & Burnette, 2001). Sexuality is developmental in nature, beginning prior to birth and continuing across the life cycle. At the time of puberty, these feelings, thoughts, and behaviors take on a more adult nature and lead to the possibility of reproduction. Healthy sexual development takes place without harm to the individual(s), whereas destructive sexuality produces harmful outcomes (such as in cases of rape or incest). By definition, sexuality suggests that any kind of bodily touch may be pleasurable (erogenous), just as may be the beliefs about touch, or the feelings about the people involved in that touching.

Sexuality is a self-reinforcing experience. No one has to tell a child to be sexual. As he or she experiences sensations, thoughts, and behaviors which bring about pleasure, some of these will eventually take on an adult sexual nature. What is important to understand, however, is that cultures differ widely in what is accepted as normative sexual experiences. This entry focuses on western societies, and those experiences that lead, over time, to the development of healthy sexuality.

THEORIES

Numerous theories have attempted to explain human sexuality. Evolutionary theories have examined sexuality in terms of proximate versus ultimate causes of behavior (Symons, 1979), gender differences in sexuality (Oliver & Hyde, 1993), parental investment (Trivers, 1972), and courtship strategies. Psychoanalytic approaches have examined the source of sexual energy or drive and stages of psychosexual development, most relevant here being the latency stage. More recently object-relations theory has addressed attachment and its relationship to intimacy across the life cycle (Simpson & Rholes, 1998). Learning approaches examine how children recognize, select, imitate, and incorporate information into intra- and interpersonal behaviors (Brody, 1997). Finally, sociologists believe that human sexual behavior is best understood through an examination of the socialization processes within the context of cultural beliefs and norms (Reiss, 1986).

RESEARCH

A review of the literature suggests that there is *no* specific theory, or group of theories, which directly address the promotion of healthy sexuality in children and youth. A first step toward such a theory would be to understand the normative development of sexuality in children. Such an understanding helps in the development of models for promoting healthy sexuality in childhood and later.

Normative Development in Human Sexuality

For the purposes of this entry, Erikson's (1963) life stage model, in which earlier achievements become the basis for later ones, is used. Unfortunately there is minimal information regarding what is considered "normal" and "healthy" sexual development. Red-tape (i.e., Federal guidelines making it very difficult to conduct such research in the United States) and concern that asking about sexuality might be interpreted as exploiting children or introducing them to sexual ideas has interfered with our understanding of healthy sexuality in early childhood and youth. One landmark study, however, provides data for children aged 2–5 (see Table 1), 6–9 (see Table 2), and 10–12 (see Table 3) years (Friedrich, Fisher, Broughton, Houston, & Shafran, 1998).

Sexual Development in Infancy

During *infancy* sexual knowledge is grounded in sensorimotor intelligence and primitive cognition. Studies suggest that young infants respond to a variety of physical sensations, manifesting signs of sexual arousal including erections in infant males, and vaginal lubrication and clitoral erections in infant females. Although there is no socio-sexual erotic meaning associated with these sensations, these positive, sensual behaviors are self-reinforcing and promote interest in sexuality.

Initially, pleasurable sensations are experienced in the context of the caregiver. It is suggested that this aspect of development facilitates bonding and attachment, two emotionally based phenomena which serve the infant throughout life in the area of intimacy. On the other hand, if the caregiver deprives the infant of a warm, comforting and safe-environment, long-term negative consequences may be observed in the context of relationships.

Making meaning out of the reflexive sexual behavior most often occurs in the context of caregiver reaction. Caregivers who respond in a comforting and explanatory style encourage a positive and healthy attitude toward sexuality. Conversely, caregivers who act in disdain and horror, project a message of disappointment and shame, which may become internalized and associated with, not only the infants' sexual sensations, but their sexual anatomy as well.

Reactive responses encourage the child to conceal, suppress, or substitute the behavior and its attendant emotions.

Sexual Development in Early Childhood

This stage of life begins at about the age of 2 and ends near age 5. By age 2 children are walking, talking, and exploring. Their exploration is not limited to the environment within which they live, but applies to themselves and others as well. Caregivers observing children are well aware of the interest that these young children have in their anatomy. Genital stimulation is perceived as a source of pleasure, and is not associated with erotic or adult sexual meaning *unless* propelled precociously into the realm of adult sexuality through exposure to some aberrant sexual behavior such as sexual abuse or pornography. If this occurs, confusion surrounds sexual sensations and anatomy, often breeding guilt and shame as the child grows in knowledge and understanding of sexuality. Coping with these emotional consequences relies heavily on the resiliency of the child, along with the perceived support from their environment (Openshaw, 1999).

At first, genital exploration and stimulation is solitary. As time progresses and the child becomes increasingly social, the behavior may move into sexual games such as, "You show me yours and I will show you mine." As the child matures physically, intellectually, emotionally and socially, these games increase in sophistication from exposure (e.g., playing doctor) to imitation of behaviors depicting sexual roles (e.g., playing house) and behavior (e.g., simulated intercourse). Table 1 outlines some of the more common sexual behaviors noted in children aged 2–5.

During early childhood, attitudes regarding sexuality continue to be significantly affected by the caregiver's response to sexual behavior. Three styles of caregiving

Table 1. Common Sexual Behaviors of Children 2–5 as Reported by Mothers by Gender

	% Males		% Females
Touches genitals at home	60.2	Touches genitals at home	43.8
Touches breasts	42.4	Touches breasts	43.7
Touches genitals in public	26.5	Masturbates with hand	15.8
Masturbates with hand	16.7	Touches genitals in public	15.1
Shows sex parts to adults	15.4	Shows sex parts to adults	13.8
Shows sex parts to children	9.3	Touches other child's sex parts	8.8
Touches adult's sex parts	7.8	Shows sex parts to children	6.4
Puts mouth on breasts	5.7	Masturbates with toy/object	6.0
Knows more about sex	5.3	Knows more about sex	5.3
Touches other child's sex parts	4.6	Puts mouth on breasts	4.3

Source: Friedrich et al., 1998

response are noted: authoritative, conservative, and rigid. Authoritative caregivers clarify the anatomy and physiology of the body at a developmental level appropriate to the child, while educating the child in terms of the social and moral aspects of sexuality. Authoritative caregivers foster three significant outcomes:

1. Age-appropriate and accurate information about the anatomical structures of the body and how they work (physiology). Communication utilized by these caregivers includes empathy and unconditional love, which fosters a safe environment for future discussion, while promoting a sense of mutuality.
2. A principle-based foundation that supports the values of the family and society and provides the child with a decision-making methodology.
3. Clarification of expectations about the appropriateness of sexual behaviors in various contexts.

At the opposite extreme is the rigid caregiver. Such individuals tend to respond emotionally, often publicly chastising the child for his/her behavior. Reactive behavior fosters secretiveness, guilt, and shame, while enhancing curiosity. Alternative avenues for discovering and exploring sexuality may be sought out by these children including paraphilic behaviors such as voyeurism (i.e., secretly attempting to view others), exhibitionism (i.e., exposing themselves), and frottage (i.e., rubbing up against another person or object for sexual pleasure).

A midline, conservative, approach is held in the belief that children should be taught about sexuality, but an uncertainty about when, where, and by whom such information should be revealed. These caregivers encourage knowledge about anatomy and physiology, but limit such information to body parts which do not include genitalia, believing that such information can only "spur on" curiosity and eventually spiral out of control into immoral sexual behavior, unwanted pregnancy, and/or contraction of STIs. Conservative caregivers, while well meaning, are often uncomfortable with their own sexuality.

Sexual Development in School-Aged Children

It is important for caregivers and other significant adults to differentiate between that which is truly sexual *exploration*, and that which is *perpetration* (i.e., gaining sexual satisfaction from a victim or displaying dominance over another) at this age (6–9). Making this differentiation necessitates that the adult examine the behavior with the following factors being taken into consideration:

1. *Age Difference.* The greater the difference in age, the more likely the behavior will not be regarded as exploratory.

2. *Aggressive Components Included in Sexual Behavior.* When the sexual behavior moves out of the realm of "showing," and begins to include aggression (e.g., insertion of objects into the vagina or rectum) or coercion—regardless of whether it is overt [i.e., "If you don't, I will let my dog bite you."] or covert [i.e., stops playing with the person until they ask why, then again requests sexual behavior as a condition of play]—the behavior can no longer be regarded as exploratory.
3. *Exploitive and Manipulative Behavior.* When one person exploits or manipulates (e.g., "I will give you a prize …") another to gain compliance to a sexual outcome, the behavior is regarded as perpetration (Table 2).

The sexual behaviors demonstrated by a child as he or she matures are noted in Table 3. From these data, we infer that

1. Sexuality will take place regardless of whether the child has been provided sexual information.
2. Sexuality can be either exploratory, serving the purpose of satisfying curiosity, or for perpetration.
3. Parents or other caregivers may either choose to be the individual who provides their children with sexual information, or others will—maybe even those who are less informed.
4. Healthy sexuality is promoted in a context of principle-based knowledge appropriate to the age of the child.

This leads to a general hypothesis that children who have been provided age-appropriate and accurate sexual information are less likely to act out sexually than those who have received no sexual information, street knowledge of sexuality, or media-based sexual information.

Sexual Development in Middle School-Aged Children

Table 3 highlights key developmental issues pertinent for caregivers of pre-teens to know and understand if they are to develop with healthy sexual ideas, and attitudes, feelings, and behaviors. Middle school age children, while undergoing the visible anatomical and physiological changes brought on by puberty are concomitantly experiencing cognitive changes which affect their sense of morality. Moving away from rule-bound thinking into the ability to hypothesize, assume, generate logic, and engage in social cognition

Table 2. Sexual Behavior of School-Age Children

Age	Sexual behavior	Purpose	Physical or psycho-emotional impact
6–7-year-olds	Basic understanding of anatomic differences between the sexes Strong sense of modesty about body exposure Natural curiosity resulting in playing sexually based games such as "doctor" and "house" that permit sexual exploration Games may include touching, kissing, rubbing, or inserting objects into the rectum or vagina Sexual experimentation may include the same or opposite sex	*Seeking* knowledge about how similar or different one is from the same and opposite sex *Expanding* one's limits and testing to see just how far one is able to extend beyond the "forbidden." This allows the child to gain an understanding about, for example: What they can and cannot do. Who will find out. How they will react. Their own response to the behavior.	*Childhood* sex play has not been found to be harmful when abuse, manipulation, and aggression are absent *Childhood* sex play has been viewed as a valuable psychosocial experience in developmental terms, fostering self and other awareness. *Psychological* harm can come from harsh parental reaction *Remember*, from the child's point of view, play is play
8–9-year-olds	Masturbation in private (less random) Masturbation in heterosexual or homosexual pairs or groups Sexual play with animals Oral or anal sex Sexual contact between siblings The infamous question, "Where did I come from?" is noted in this age group Repeating of sexual jokes is a common behavior as they revel in testing the limits	*Sexual behavior* can no longer be perceived as merely "play" *Erotic arousal* may be accompanied by sexual fantasies *Erotic meaning* is being attached to sexual behavior and material *In public* these youth may state they are "grossed" out by displays of sexual behavior; yet in private they have their own fascination with it	*Sexual experiences* may be infrequent and less important than other events but may include the entire range of possible acts *These youth* have an awareness of the erotic element of sexual activities *Feelings* of "sacred privacy" emerge *Empathy*, though more based in concrete "right" and "wrong" is noted

Source: Friedrich et al., 1998; Masters, Johnson, & Kolodny, 1986

Table 3. Sexual Behavior of Middle School-Age Pre-Teens

Age	Sexual behavior	Purpose	Physical or psycho-emotional impact
10–12-year-olds	Increased association with peers Puberty begins to manifest, usually first in girls (10.5) and then in boys (11.5) Girls will begin menstruation Boys will experience ejaculation either through masturbation or nocturnal emission Forms of sexual harassment may be noted, though not necessarily attended to	They may begin to experiment with sexual behavior to "discover" their own sexuality Puberty sets in motion the anatomical and physiological changes necessary for adult sexual functioning Sexuality can take on a variety of dimensions ranging from erotic pleasure, to increased self-awareness, to perpetration	These youth have alternating periods of disinhibition and inhibition Learning self-mastery is an important personal focus within the context of social cognition, which allows them to respect others and integrate empathy skills The meaning of sexuality moves from merely erogenous and intrapersonal, to erotic and interpersonal

Source: Friedrich et al., 1998; Masters et al., 1986

enables the pre-teen to empathize and make informed decisions regarding their behavior.

This sketch of sexual development provides the basis for developmentally appropriate instruction and training to facilitate healthy sexuality in childhood and beyond.

STRATEGIES THAT WORK

There are no rigorous research data that describe an effective program for promoting healthy sexuality in children.

STRATEGIES THAT MIGHT WORK

Caregivers may wonder, even if they know the basics of human development and sexuality, how to proceed in teaching their children effectively. The National Guidelines Task Force (1996) of the Sexuality Education and Information Council of the United States (SEICUS) has produced a 50-page document entitled, *Guidelines for Comprehensive Sexuality Education*, 2nd ed. This document provides sexuality information around six key concepts, namely, human development, relationships, personal skills, sexual behavior, sexual health, and society and culture. These guidelines are organized developmentally, with Level I focusing on ages 5–8, and Level II addressing ages 9–12. This information can be accessed on the Internet at http://www.seicus.org/pubs/guidelines/guidelines.pdf.

STRATEGIES THAT DO NOT WORK

Strategies that are not developmentally appropriate will be ineffective. Further, any strategy which is not culturally sensitive, regardless of how well it is formulated, will not only be ineffective but possibly harmful (Carkhuff & Anthony, 1993).

SYNTHESIS

In my opinion, the best available material on promoting healthy sexuality in children is contained in *Guidelines for Comprehensive Sexuality Education*. These guidelines focus on four primary goals (p. 6), namely:

1. Providing accurate human sexuality *information* (e.g., growth and development, human reproduction, anatomy, physiology, etc.).
2. Providing ways for children, youth, and adolescents to *question, explore*, and *assess* their sexual attitudes, values, and insights.
3. Helping children, youth, and adolescents effectively use critical *interpersonal skills* (e.g., communication, assertiveness, resisting peer pressure, etc.).
4. Helping children, youth, and adolescents exercise sexual *responsibility*.

The above information is organized around six key concepts and associated topics, subconcepts, and developmental messages which are organized according to age levels (e.g., Level I is 5–8 year olds, Level II is for 9–12, Level III 12–15, and Level IV 15–18). The six sexuality concept (p. 8) areas include:

1. *Human development* (e.g., appreciation of one's own body, interacting with both genders in respectful and appropriate ways);
2. *Relationships* (e.g., viewing the family as a valuable source of support, avoiding exploitative or manipulative relationships);
3. *Personal skills* (e.g., identifying and living ones values, practicing effective decision making);
4. *Sexual behavior* (e.g., expressing one's sexuality in ways congruent with one's values, discriminating between life-enhancing sexual behaviors and those that are harmful to self and/or others);

5. *Sexual health* (e.g., effective use of contraceptive methods, preventing sexual abuse);
6. *Society and culture* (e.g, demonstrating respect for people with different sexual values).

These general guidelines provide parents with information from which they can then seek out specific knowledge, developmentally appropriate to their child/youth, and become sufficiently informed so as to present a healthy sexual education to their children.

Also see: Abuse and Neglect entries; Family Strengthening, Childhood; Peer Relationships, Childhood.

References

Brody, S. (1997). *Sex at risk*. New Brunswick, NJ: Transaction.

Carkhuff, R.R., & Anthony, W.A. (1993). *The skills of helping*. Amherst, MA: Human Resource Developmental Press.

Erikson, E.H. (1963). *Childhood and society* (2nd ed.). New York: Norton.

Friedrich, W.N., Fisher, J., Broughton, D., Houston, M., & Shafran, C.R. (1998). Normative sexual behavior in children: A contemporary sample. *Pediatrics, 101*, 1–13.

Masters, W.H., Johnson, V.E., & Kolodny, R.C. (1986). *Masters and Johnson on human sex and loving*. Boston, MA: Little, Brown & Company.

McAnulty, R.D., & Burnette, M.M. (2001) *Exploring human sexuality: Making healthy decisions*. Needham Heights, MA: Allyn & Bacon.

National Guidelines Task Force. (1996). *Guidelines for comprehensive sexuality education* (2nd ed.). Washington, DC: Sexuality Information and Education Council of the United States.

Oliver, M.B., & Hyde, J.S. (1993). Gender differences in sexuality: A meta-analysis. *Psychological Bulletin, 114*, 29–51.

Openshaw, D.K. (1999). "Resiliency in children." In C. Smith (Ed.), *The encyclopedia of parenting theory and research* (pp. 357–359). Westport, CT: Greenwood Press.

Reiss, I.L. (1986). *Journey into sexuality: An exploratory voyage*. Englewood Cliffs, HJ: Prentice-Hall.

Simpson, J.A., & Rholes, W.S. (1998). *Attachment theory and close relationships*. New York: Guilford Press.

Symons, D. (1979). *The evolution of human sexuality*. New York: Oxford University Press.

Trivers, R.E. (1972). Parental investment and sexual selection. In B. Campbell (Ed.), *Sexual selection and the descent of man* (pp. 136–179). Chicago: Aldine.

Sexuality, Adolescence

Willa M. Doswell

INTRODUCTION AND DEFINITIONS

Adolescence often begins with the onset of puberty. It is a critical developmental period during which children achieve reproductive capability. For more than 1 billion adolescents worldwide, these years set the template for adult sexuality. During this time, adolescents need to learn those behaviors, which are healthy and those which are not. The World Health Organization defines *sexual health* as "the integration of the physical, emotional, intellectual, and social aspects of sexual being in ways that are positively enriching, and that enhance personality, communication and love" (http://www.siecus.org/pubs/cnct/cnct0001.html). In early adolescence the following decisions about sexual behavior are made: (1) When to become sexually active; (2) How to express one's sexuality; (3) Whether and how one should control one's reproductive abilities; (4) Who are the people with whom one expresses one's sexuality; and (5) How one uses sex in relationships (Wyatt, 1997).

There exists a need to identify more effective reproductive health and promote healthy sexual behavior in the adolescent population worldwide. Primary prevention programs can assist adolescents in successfully negotiating this lifestage.

SCOPE

Today's adolescents confront a society where childhood years and activities are diminished by adult-like activities. The urban hip-hop youth culture of music, dress, and attitudes is a dominant influence on American and other first world adolescent societies. In North America, African American youth, particularly girls, ages 9–12, are an important target of that culture, and are especially vulnerable to these trends due to their earlier pubertal development (Herman-Gidden et al., 1997; Stanton, Li, Cottrell, & Kaljee, 2001). Early pubertal development, and boy–girl or same sex interest are increasing across the American preadolescent population, and may be occurring worldwide.

While the US teen pregnancy rate declined 17 percent between 1990 and 1999, 78 percent of the pregnancies that did occur were unplanned. Additionally every year approximately 3 million US teens, (about 1 in 4) are infected with an STD. In a single act of unprotected sex with an infected partner, an adolescent female has a 1 percent risk of acquiring HIV, a 50 percent risk of genital herpes and a 50 percent chance of acquiring gonorrhea (Allen Guttmacher Institute, 1999). According to a 1999 surveillance report from the Center for Disease Control, adolescents between the ages of 10–19 years are at greatest risk of contracting sexually transmitted diseases (STDs) for 4 reasons: (1) they are more likely to have multiple sex partners; (2) they engage in unprotected sexual intercourse; (3) they may select partners who are at higher risk of being infected; and (4) adolescent females have a higher physiologic susceptibility to selected STDs (center for Disease Control, 1999) (http://www.cdc.gov/nchstp/dstd/stats-trends/1999survrpt.htm).

Efforts to help minimize the adoption of risky sexual behavior, and to promote effective prevention behaviors must employ theoretically based health promoting interventions. Many successful programs are based on theories that have been well tested in intervention research over the past 10–25 years.

THEORIES

Theory of Reasoned Action

The Theory of Reasoned Action (TRA) (Fishbein & Ajzen, 1975) posits that attitude toward a specific behavior and subjective norms concerning the behavior co-predict the intent to perform behavior X and its subsequent performance. *Attitude* refers to a favorable or unfavorable disposition toward behavior X. *Subjective norms* refers to perceived social pressure from significant others to carry out behavior X. *Intention* refers to willful intent to perform behavior X, and *behavior* refers to the actual performance of a specific behavior; in this case, accelerated sexual behavior. These theoretical linkages are supported by independent studies (Basen-Engquist & Parcel, 1992; Burak, 1994).

Theory of Planned Behavior (TPB)

The theory of planned behavior is Ajzen's extension of the theory of reasoned action (Ajzen, 2000) According to the TPB, human behavior is guided by three considerations: beliefs about the likely outcomes of the behavior, and the evaluations of these outcomes (*behavioral beliefs*), belief about the normative expectations of others, motivation to comply with these expectations (*normative beliefs*), beliefs about the presence of factors that may facilitate or impede performance of the behavior, and the perceived power of these factors, (*control beliefs*). In combination, attitude toward the behavior, subjective norm, and perception of behavioral control lead to the formation of a behavioral intention. Finally, given a sufficient degree of actual control over the behavior, people are expected to carry out their intentions when the opportunity arises. This theory has been used successfully in adolescent sexual behavior research (Jemmott, Jemmott, & Fong, 1998, 1999; Rannie & Craig, 1997).

Health Belief Model

The Health Belief Model (HBM) hypothesizes that an individual is more likely to engage in a recommended health behavior if the individual feels: (1) susceptible to a health problem (*perceived susceptibility*); (2) perceives its complications to be serious (*perceived severity*); (3) considers the recommended behavior(s) to be beneficial in maintaining health or preventing complications (*perceived benefits*); and (4) that the benefits of following the recommended health behaviors outweigh the consequences of not following the recommended behavior or the possible barriers to adopting those behaviors (*perceived barriers*) (Becker & Maiman, 1980; Becker, Rankin, & Rickel, 1998). Specific studies have examined adolescent sexual behavior using the HBM (Charon-Prochownik, 2001; Guthrie et al., 1996; Laraque, McClean, Brown-Peterside, Ashton, & Diamond, 1997; Lollis, Johnson, & Antoni, 1997).

Problem Behavior Theory

Problem behavior theory (Donovan, Jessor, & Costa, 1991; Jessor & Jessor, 1977) is a social-psychological framework developed to explain adolescent involvement in multiple problem behaviors as well as conventional behaviors. The theory rests upon the relationships among three major systems: the personality system, the perceived environment system, and the behavior system. The personality system is conceptualized as having three component structures: (1) *motivational instigation* viewed as values placed on goals and expectation of attaining the goals; (2) *personal beliefs* referred to as restraints on engaging in nonconformity or constraints against engaging in problem behaviors; and (3) *personal control* referred to as control against nonnormative behavior (Jessor & Jessor, 1977). Problem-behavior theory accounts for between a third and a half of the variance in different problem behaviors (including risky sexual behavior), and conventional behaviors in national samples of adolescents (Albrecht, Payne, Stone, & Reynolds, 1998; Costa, Jessor, Fortenberry, & Donovan, 1995; Stanton et al., 2001).

Trans-Theoretical Model of Change

The trans-theoretical model of change by Prochaska, DiClemente, and Norcross (1992) has four major constructs: stages of change, processes of change, self-efficacy, and decisional balance. *Stages of change* refer to a five-stage model of human behavior change, specifically intentional behavior. *Pre-contemplation*, the first stage, is defined as a stage in which individuals engage in little change behavior. *Contemplation*, stage 2, refers to a stage in which individuals are thinking about changing behavior without making a commitment to actions necessary for actual change to occur. Individuals in contemplation must decide to take action and initiate preliminary actions to move forward to the next stage. *Preparation* is defined as stage 3 in which individuals make definite plans to change a behavior in the near future. *Action*, the next stage, refers to the stage in which individuals make a commitment to change the problem behavior and take actions consistent with the commitment. The final stage, *maintenance*, is the stage in which individuals have successfully incorporated the behavior change into their lives for at least 6 months. There is not yet widespread use of this theory in adolescent sexual behavior research.

Social Cognitive Theory (SCT)

This theory hypothesizes that *self-efficacy*, the conviction that one can successfully execute the specific behavior required to produce the specific outcome, determines the amount of effort a person will expend on a task, and the length of time a person will persist (Bandura, 1997). The use of this theory is promising in studies examining sexual behavior interventions in adolescents (Jemmott et al., 1998; Schaalma, Kok, Bosker, & Parcel, 1996).

RESEARCH

Some of the most significant descriptive research has come from the Guttmacher Institute Reports, the Sexuality and Education Council of the United States, (SIECUS, 1994), the Add Health Study, and the Youth Risk Behavior Surveillance System (YRBSS). These studies have identified the at-risk youth, sexuality knowledge gaps, socio-environmental and contextual variables that influence adolescent sexual behavior, and the prevalence of sexual behavior in adolescent populations. The Add health study (Bearman, Jones, & Udry, 1997) is the largest and one of the most nationally representative studies to examine social contextual influences on sexual and other risk behaviors in a national racially and socio-economically diverse sample of adolescents, ages 12–18 years. Data was gathered from 20,000 adolescents, their parents, siblings, friends, romantic partners, fellow students, and school administrators. The YRBSS (Kann et al., 2000), a study that monitored health risk behaviors in a national sample representing 33 states and 16 local agencies, found that substantial morbidity and social problems among adolescence were due to the practice of risky sexual behaviors. These findings have guided policies and programs in achieving national health objectives for 2010.

Experimental research has focused on preventive interventions. Interventions to delay the onset of early sexual behavior must include components and processes that make them efficacious, a criteria recently endorsed by the US Surgeon General's report on sexual health (2001) (http://www.surgeongeneral.gov/library/sexualhealth/glancetable.htm).

Research on adolescent sexual behavior in Canada and Europe has been modest in amount and mainly descriptive. England has the highest teenage pregnancy rate among 15–19 year olds in Western Europe (Adler, 1997). Oakley et al. (1995) conducted a methodological review of sexual health education intervention studies in England, and out of 270 studies, 73 of which were interventions, only 12 met the criteria for being methodologically sound. Researchers in the Netherlands have evaluated the effects of an AIDS/STD curriculum administered to 9th and 10th graders and reported that a theory-based curriculum had a positive impact on changing attitudes about consistent condom use in sexual intercourse (Schaalma et al., 1996). Although the adolescent population is smaller in countries such as France than in the United States, they have similar problems with teenage pregnancy and STDs (Tursz, 1997).

Dine and Wolf (1995) identify three areas of concern in research on adolescent sexual behavior. They are the inconsistency of study variable definitions as to what constitutes sexual behavior and risky sexual behavior, the inadequacy of self-report instruments, and the use of retrospective research designs. These factors do not allow control of extraneous and mediating variables within the adolescent's contextual environment. Additionally, research on the promotion of healthy sexual development is too focused on prevention of negative outcomes, without a corresponding teaching of what is healthy sexual development, what types of heterosexual relationships adolescents should have, and what types of sexual expression are appropriate from early through middle to late adolescence.

Many intervention programs do not have effectively designed evaluations, and many only measure short-term outcomes of 12 months or less. Additionally, many have not used comparable operational definitions or measures of sexual behavior and other program outcomes. The pedagogy used in these programs is often not well-defined, grounded in theory, and does not include relevant input from the cultural context of adolescent participants.

STRATEGIES THAT WORK

Five successful well-tested sexual behavior intervention programs endorsed by the Center for Disease Control (CDC), presented in Table 1, are representative of important efforts in this field.

The first program targets high school youth in rural, urban, and suburban schools (Mains, Iverson, Bernspach, Collins, McGlain, & Rugg, 1994). The 14-week intervention has demonstrated that youth are able to assess their own vulnerability for HIV infection, describe the characteristics and risks for other sexually transmitted diseases, identify reasons for delaying sex and principles of safe sex, and demonstrate effective refusal skills to use in risky situations. In the second effort, Jemmott et al. (1998) developed a

Table 1. CDC Supported Sexual Behavior Intervention Programs

Program name	Target subjects	Type of program	Program length
Get Real About AIDS (Mains et al., 1994)	Ages 14–18	Delay Sex/ AIDS education	14 sessions
Be Proud! Be Responsible! (Jemmott et al., 1998)	Ages 13–18/ males only	Teach condom use/Abstinence	15-h session
Reducing the Risk (Kirby et al., 1991)	Ages 14–15	Abstinence education	17 sessions
Becoming a Responsible Teen (St. Lawrence et al., 1995)	Ages 14–18	Sex Education/ HIV/AIDS Education in condom use	8 sessions
Focus on Kids (Stanton et al., 1996)	Ages 13–15	Education in condom use	8 sessions

culturally sensitive condom use intervention, and an alternative abstinence intervention, for early adolescent African American males. They found that safe sex was a more effective intervention with sexually active youth, although both interventions were effective for up to 6 months. Next, Kirby, Barth, Leland, and Fetro (1991) program, *Reducing the Risk*, provided an intervention integrated into the schools' health promotion curriculum in comparison to a standard health education curriculum alone. Program findings were a greater increase in parent–child communication about abstinence and contraception, an increase in knowledge about contraception, and a more realistic perception of the sexual activity of their peers.

The *Becoming a Responsible Teen* program taught assertiveness/refusal skills, condom use and general sexuality knowledge. Program participants were less likely to engage in early sexual intercourse when compared with control group participants, and twice as likely to remain abstinent one year later (St. Lawrence, Brasfield, Jefferson, Alleyne, O'Bannon, & Shirley, 1995). The *Focus on Kids* program is an HIV and AIDS prevention 8-session intervention that taught a curriculum focusing on condom-use and abstinence and some prevention of substance abuse content (Stanton, Li, Ricardo, Galbraith, Feigelman, & Kaljee, 1996). Using an interactive computer for testing at baseline and 6 months after the intervention, the researchers found that adolescents participating in the intervention were more likely than the control group in their intention to use a condom at the next sexual intercourse, perceived greater peer-use of condoms, and recognized increased personal vulnerability to HIV. These five programs are theory-based

and include boys and girls, frequently across racial/ethnic groups (White, African American, and Latino). What is a noticeable shortcoming about the programs is that few of them begin during the preadolescent years.

STRATEGIES THAT MIGHT WORK

Promising Theoretical Models

The Information-Motivation-Behavior skills (IMB) model states that for people to change their behavior they must have three things: *information* about the problem behavior, *motivation* to change the problem behavior, and a *behavioral repertoire* to accomplish the change (Fisher & Fisher, 1992). This theory might be useful for sexual behavior research in adolescent populations, but clear evidence of effectiveness has not yet been established. The *Developmental Assets* framework (Leffert, Benson, & Roehkepartian, 1997), drawn from research on resilience categorizes 40 assets as either *external*, those necessary to provide safety and support, or *internal*, those provided by communities' nurturance of children in order to promote healthy behaviors. The fact that this conceptual model does not have well developed theoretical propositions at this time limits its applicability as a research model.

In this time of greater examination of health disparities, the following two new theories may contribute to the research on adolescent sexual behavior among ethnically and racially diverse groups. *The Theory of Mediated Action* (TMA) proposes a new way of examining cultural and contextual influences on the their sexual behavior. To the fundamental components of the theory of reasoned action's constructs of attitude, subjective norms, and behavioral intention, the TMA adds the role of information processing to predict behavior. This theory has potential usefulness in examining the influence of the media on sexual behavior and health. A second theory proposed by Taylor, the *theory of cultural alienation* (Doswell, 2000; Taylor, Obechina, & Harrison, 1998) posits that African Americans (and presumably members of other diverse groups) living in a societal context of racial discrimination and prejudice, may begin to internalize the negative stereotypes of their particular racial or ethnic group resulting in specific adverse health, social, and educational outcomes. These negative outcomes may result in risky sexual behavior, teen pregnancy, and other dysfunctional behaviors. The concept of cultural alienation has been operationalized into a measure of internalized racism (Taylor & Grundy, 1996), and has been tested with some adult and adolescent populations. Taylor proposes an intervention strategy, *Values for Life*, as a potential remedy to the problem of cultural alienation, by positing seven values and five target areas of health promotion behavior to decrease cultural alienation (Taylor, Turner, & Lewis, 1999).

The effectiveness of abstinence-based programs is in question. A review by Thomas (2000) identified nine abstinence-based programs conducted in the United States. These programs were divided into abstinence-only and abstinence plus interventions with the latter including safe sex practice knowledge in the curriculum. Only a small percentage of these programs had attempted any type of rigorous formal evaluation of their efficacy and those findings were, at best, inconclusive. *Postponing Sexual Involvement* (PSI), a peer-led middle school abstinence program showed that abstinent preadolescents were more likely to continue an abstinent commitment following the completion of the program. Early evaluation of PSI found that participants who were virgins, were significantly more likely to continue to postpone sexual activity through the end of the ninth grade than were control students (Howard & McCabe, 1990). Although this program has been replicated elsewhere, there is not a substantive empirical literature that documents replication of these initial findings. While *Best Friends* (1996), an abstinence-based program for youth in grades 6 through 12, has reported lower sexual involvement rates for program participants, a more thorough empirical evaluation of the impact, knowledge and behavior and behavior change remains to be undertaken.

STRATEGIES THAT DO NOT WORK

As discussed elsewhere in this volume, it is known that knowledge only programs do not change behavior.

SYNTHESIS

Descriptive research in the United States has focused on describing adolescent sexual behavior, primarily among Caucasian and African American adolescents, while the intervention research has focused on providing knowledge about sexuality and sexual behavior, interventions to reduce intention, or provide safe sex information for those determined to be sexually active, and the adoption of negotiating and social skills to avoid peer pressure to engage in early or inappropriate sexual behavior. There have been several interventions developed over the past 5 years, and the target of this research has been high school age adolescents; programs are beginning to include middle school, and a few upper elementary school.

Research suggests that primary prevention programs can be successful. Yet, even the most successful have either not tested outcomes beyond the first year or have noted a decline in positive outcomes at that time point. Abstinence programs have been found to be either ineffective or inconclusive (due to a lack of rigorous evaluation) especially among sexually active females.

Miller, Benson, and Galbraith's (2001) review of research examining parental influences on adolescent sexual behavior indicates that there is remarkable consensus on the positive influence of parental support, supervision and parent/teen communication on adolescent sexual behavior (across racial groups). In coming years, this important parental role needs to be better incorporated into program efforts.

In the year 2000 there were 70.4 million adolescents in the United States, making up 26 percent of the population, and 31 percent of the American child/preadolescent and adolescent population were members of diverse groups. The fastest growing segments of the adolescent population are Latino youth, representing 16 percent of US adolescents, with African Americans representing 14 percent, and Caucasians representing 64 percent of the US adolescent population at this time.

Though the number of pregnancy prevention intervention programs have increased over the past 7 years, many of these programs do not address the cultural/contextual factors that influence sexual behavior and sexual health. Research examining adolescent sexual behavior needs to consider the societal contexts for special groups who experience racial and social discrimination, and how internalized racism may influence their sexual health and behavior.

Research in the United States is beginning to focus on adolescents across cultural and racial groups. This focus needs to continue, with consideration to theories that explain and account for racial and cultural attitudes and practices about adolescent sexual behavior that differ from Western European attitudes, culture, and practices. The empirical literature is sparse on ethnic/racial differences in decision-making, sexual values, attitudes and beliefs, and family and cultural values about sexual behavior.

Cohen (1996) indicates that research must focus on the cultural and social contextual settings in which adolescents live, including the study of homeless adolescents, and those who have a lesbian or gay sexual orientation. There is also a need for researchers of specific cultural groups and sexual orientations to examine and conduct sexuality research because of their familiarity with these contexts. Although sexual behavior has been examined in diverse populations in the United States, it has not been examined in middle and upper income diverse populations extensively. This is a promising area for research, to see if problems are similar, but take a different trajectory.

The literature indicates that interventions with the greatest success need to be theoretically based, culturally relevant, developmentally appropriate, target high-risk groups, and contain effective intervention components that are implemented before dysfunctional behavior appears.

A priority research area for the 21st century is for the development of age-appropriate, and culturally relevant interventions to reduce risky and early sexual behavior among children in middle childhood, particularly in racially and ethnically diverse groups.

Marks, Murray, Evans, and Willig (2000) suggest that future research include how the results of sexuality research are disseminated and utilized by the target populations. They suggest further expansion in theory production around the concepts of sexual desire, fantasy, sexual pleasure and attraction, how the sexual experience is subjectively experienced, and what constitutes sexual pleasure.

There is a need to conduct more bio-behavioral research, which examines the relevance of biologic markers of puberty and sexual behavior in relation to the adoption of either healthy or early and risky sexual behavior. Giedd, Blumenthal, Jeffries, Castellanos, Liu, & Zijdenbos, (1999) report that the prefrontal cortex of adolescent brains is not mature, yet is the center for self-control judgment, emotional regulation, organization, and planning. Research needs to be conducted on what effective sexual health interventions can be developed that take prefrontal lobe immaturity into account. Additionally, adolescent sexual behavior research needs to be conducted using new theoretical paradigms that incorporate physiological explanations and mechanisms such as the self-regulation paradigm.

Although empirical and theoretical research affirm that knowledge of sexuality is not enough to promote healthy sexual behavior, more research is needed on how gaps in that knowledge contribute to risky sexual behavior, and the interplay of knowledge, attitudes, norms and intention lead to a path of healthy or risky sexual behavior. The promotion of healthy sexual development is too focused on prevention of negative outcomes, without a corresponding teaching of what is healthy sexual development, what types of heterosexual relationships adolescents should have, and what types of sexual expression are appropriate from early through middle to late adolescence.

Because sexual behavior research in the international community is not as extensive as in the United States, there is a need for more research in countries that have a higher incidence of early and risky sexual behavior. Specifically the cultural contexts of these countries in relation to sexual development and behavior, how the acculturation and adoption of American customs, music, mores contribute to risky sexual behavior in established and developing countries need more examination. Theories based on the cultural contexts and historical background of international communities needs to be developed.

Psychometrically sound instruments to describe and measure healthy and risky sexual behavior, developed in America, need to be translated into the languages of international communities and examined for relevance in those countries. There is a need to examine how parents from different cultural contexts and socioeconomic backgrounds are best taught how to help their adolescents have a healthy sexual behavior trajectory. Theories examining adolescent sexual behavior need to account for the media's influence on adolescent sexual behavior by including a component examining the adolescent's processing and interpretation of the sexual information and how that may influence his or her intentional or actual sexual behavior.

The area of adherence to behavioral interventions needs greater study. Adherence research literature has been based on a handful of well-respected and well-tested measures from pharmacological clinical trials of chronic illnesses, but not in relation to at-risk adolescent sexual behavior (Dunbar-Jacob & Schlenk, 2000). Finally, sexual health education and intervention research to prevent the occurrence of sexual activity, early teen pregnancy, and sexually transmitted diseases may need to begin with children as early as 8 or 9 years of age, because poor decision making, early pubertal development, modeling of peer and sibling early sexual behavior and sexual risk-taking compromises sexual health, especially in early adolescence (Doswell & Vandiestienne, 1996).

ACKNOWLEDGMENT

The author wishes to acknowledge the work of Kathy Kane, doctoral student, University of Pittsburgh School of Nursing in the retrieval of the literature upon which this publication is based.

Also see: Self-Esteem, Adolescence; Abuse and Neglect, Adolescence; Life Skills; Peer Relationships, Adolescence; Pregnancy, Adolescence; Risk-Taking; Social Inoculation

References

Albrecht, S., Payne, L., Stone, C., & Reynolds, C. (1998). A preliminary study of the use of peer support in smoking cessation interventions for pregnant adolescents. *Journal of the American Academy of Nurse Practitioners, 10*(3), 119–125.

Adler, M. (1997). Sexual health—a health of the nation failure. *British Medical Journal, 31*(4), 1743–1747.

Ajzen, I. (2000). *Theory of Planned Behavior (TpB)*. Available: http://www.unix.oit.umass.edu/aizen/tpb.html

Allen Guttmacher Institute. (1999). *Teenage pregnancy: Overall trends and state-by-state information*. New York: Author.

Bandura, A. (1997). Toward a unifying theory of behavior change. *Psychological Review, 84*, 191–215.

Basen-Engquist, K., & Parcel, G.S. (1992). Attitudes, norms, and self-efficacy: A model of adolescents' HIV-related sexual risk behavior. *Health Education Quarterly, 19*(2), 263–277.

Bearman, P., Jones, J., & Udry, R. (1997). *The national longitudinal study of adolescent health: Research design* [wwwdocument]. Available: http://www.cpc.unc.edu/addhealth

Becker, M.H., & Maiman, L.A. (1980). Strategies for enhancing patient compliance. *Journal of Community Health, 6*, 113–135.

Becker, E., Rankin, E., & Rickel, A. (1998). *High-risk sexual behavior.* New York: Plenum Press.

Best Friends Foundation. (1996). *Best friends.* [Brochure]. Washington, DC: Author.

Burak, L.J. (1994). Examination and prediction of elementary school teachers' intentions to teach HIV/AIDS education. *AIDS Education & Prevention, 6*(4), 310–321.

Center for Disease Control. (1999). Available: http://www.cdc.gov/nchstp/dstd/stats-trends/1999survrpt.htm

Cohen, M. (1996). Great transitions, preparing adolescents for a new century. *Journal of Adolescent Health, 19*, 2–5.

Costa, F., Jessor, R., Donovan, J., & Fortenberry, J. (1995). Early initiation of sexual intercourse: The influence of psychosocial unconventionality. *Journal of Research on Adolescents, 5*(1), 93–121.

Charon-Prochownik, D. (2001). Reproductive health beliefs and behaviors in teens with diabetes: application of the expanded health belief model. *Pediatric Diabetes, 2*, 30–39.

Dine, C., & Wolf, E. (1995). School sexuality education and adolescent risk-taking behavior. *Journal of School Health, 65*(3), 91–95.

Donovan, J.E., Jessor, R., & Costa, F.M. (1991). Adolescent health behavior and conventionality-unconventionality: An extension of problem-behavior theory. *Health Psychology, 10*(1), 52–61.

Doswell, W. (2000). Promotion of sexual health in the American cultural context: Implications for health promotion in school age African-American girls. *Journal of the National Black Nurses Association, 11*(1), 51–57.

Doswell, W., & Vandestienne, G. (1996). The use of focus groups to examine pubertal concerns in preteen girls: Initial findings and implications for practice and research. *Issues in Comprehensive Pediatric Nursing, 19*, 103–120.

Dunbar-Jacob, J., & Schlenk, E. (2000). Patient adherence to treatment. In A. Baum, T. Revenson, & J. Singer (Eds.), *Handbook of health psychology* (pp. 571–580). Hillsdale, NJ: Lawrence Erlbaum Associates.

Duffy, K.G. & Wong, F.Y. (2002). *Community Psychology.* Boston: Allyn & Bacon.

Fishbein, M., & Ajzen, I. (1975). *Belief, attention, intention and behavior: An introduction to theory and research.* Reading, MA: Addison-Wesley.

Fisher, J.D., & Fisher, W.A. (1992). Changing AIDS-risk behavior. *Psychological Bulletin, 111*(3), 455–474.

Giedd, J.N., Blumenthal, J., Jeffries, N.O., Castellanos, F.X., Liu, H., & Zijdenbos, A. (1999). Brain development during childhood and adolescence: A longitudinal MRI study. *Nature Neuroscience, 2*, 861–863.

Guthrie, B., Wallace, J., Doerr, K., & Janz, N. et al. (1996). Girl talk: Development of an intervention for prevention of HIV/AIDS and other sexually transmitted diseases in adolescent females. *Public Health Nursing, 13*(5), 318–330.

Herman-Gidden, M., Slora, E., Wasserman, R., Bourdony, C., Bhapkan, M., Koch, G., & Hasemeier, C. (1997). Secondary sexual characteristics and menses in young girls seen in office practice: A study from the pediatric research in office settings network. *Pediatrics, 89*(4), 505–510.

Howard, M., & McCabe, J.B. (1990). Helping teenagers postpone sexual involvement. *Family Planning Perspectives, 22*(1), 21–26.

Jemmott, J.B., III, Jemmott, L.S., & Fong, G.T. (1998). Abstinence and safer sex HIV risk-reduction interventions for African American adolescents: A randomized controlled trial. *Journal of the American Medical Association, 279*(19), 1529–1536.

Jemmott, J.B., III, Jemmott, L.S., & Fong, G.T. (1999). Abstinence and safer sex HIV risk-reduction interventions for African American adolescents: A randomized controlled trial. *Journal of the American Medical Association, 279*(19), 1529–1536.

Jessor, R., & Jessor, S. (1977). *Problem behavior and psychosocial development: A longitudinal study of youth.* New York: Academic Press.

Kann, L., Kinchen, S., Williams, B., Ross, J., Lowry, R., Grunbaum, J., & Koble, L. (2000). Youth risk behavior surveillance—United States, 1999. *Morbidity & Mortality Weekly Report, 49*(SS-5), 1–94.

Kirby, D., Barth, R.P., Leland, N. & Fetro, J.V. (1991). Reducing the risk: Impact of a new curriculum on sexual risk-taking. *Family Planning Perspectives, 23*(6), 253–263.

Laraque, D., McClean, D., Brown-Peterside, P., Ashton, D., & Diamond, B. (1997). Predictors of reported condom use in central Harlem youth as conceptualized by the health belief model. *Journal of Adolescent Health, 21*, 318–327.

Leffert, N., Benson, P.L., & Roehkepartian, J.L. (1997). Starting out right: Developmental assets for children. Minneapolis, MN: Search Institute.

Lollis, C., Johnson, E., & Antoni, M. (1997). The efficacy of the health belief model for predicting condom usage and risky sexual practices in university students. *AIDS Education & Prevention, 9*(6), 551–563.

Mains, D.S., Iverson, D.C., Bernspach, S.W., Collins, D., McGlain, J., & Rugg, D. (1994). Preventing HIV infection among adolescents: Evaluating a school-based program. *Preventive Medicine, 23*, 409–417.

Marks, D., Murray, M., Evans, B., & Willig, C. (2000). *Healthy Psychology.* Thousand Oak, CA: Sage.

Miller, B., Benson, B., & Galbraith, K. (2001). Family relationships and adolescent pregnancy risk: A research synthesis. *Developmental Review, 21*, 1–38.

Oakley, A., Fullerton, D., Holland, J., Arnold, S., France-Dawson, M., Kelley, P., & McGrellis, S. (1995). Sexual health education interventions for young people: A methodological review. *British Medical Journal, 310*, 158–203.

Prochaska, J., DiClemente, C., & Norcross, J. (1992). In search of how people change: Applications to addictive behaviors. *American Psychologist, 47*(9), 1102–1114.

Rannie, K., & Craig, D.M. (1997). Adolescent females' attitudes, subjective norms, perceived behavioral control, and intentions to use latex condoms. *Public Health Nursing, 14*(1), 51–57.

St. Lawrence, J.S., Brasfield, T.L., Jefferson, K.W., Alleyne, E., O'Bannon, R.E., & Shirley, A. (1995). Cognitive-behavioral intervention to reduce African-American adolescents' risk for HIV infection. *Journal of Consulting and Clinical Psychology, 63*(2), 221–237.

Schaalma, H., Kok, G., Bosker, R., & Parcel, G. (1996). Planned development and evaluation of AIDS/STD education for secondary school students in the Netherlands: Short-term effects. *Health Education Quarterly, 23*(4), 469–487.

Sexuality in Educational Communities in the United States (SIECUS). (1994). *Annotated bibliographies of sexuality education curricula: A SIECUS annotated bibliography* [on-line]. New York: SIECUS. Available: http://www.siecus.org/pubs/cnct0001.html

Stanton, B.F., Li, X., Ricardo, I., Galbraith, J., Feigelman, S., & Kaljee, L. (1996). A randomized, controlled effectiveness trial of an AIDS prevention program for low-income African-American youths. *Archives of Pediatrics and Adolescent Medicine, 150*, 363–372.

Stanton, B., Li, X., Cottrell, L., & Kaljee, L. (2001). Early initiation of sex, drug-related risk behaviors, and sensation-seeking among urban, low-income African-American adolescents. *Journal of the National Medical Association, 93*(4), 129–138.

Taylor, J., & Grundy, C. (1996). Measuring black internalization of white stereotypes about blacks: The Nadanolization Scale. In R.L. Jones (Ed.), *Handbook of tests and measurements for black populations.* Berkeley, CA: Cobb & Henry.

Taylor, J., Obiechina, C., & Harrison, S. (1998). Toward a psychology of liberation and restoration: Answering the challenge of cultural alienation. In R.L. Jones (Ed.), *African American Mental health.* Hampton, VA: Cobby & Henry.

Taylor, J., Turner, S., & Lewis, M. (1999). Valucation: definition, theory and methods. In R.L. Jones (Ed.), *Advances in African American Psychology.* Hampton, VA: Cobb & Henry.

Thomas, M. (2000). Abstinence-based programs for prevention of adolescent pregnancies. *Journal of Adolescent Health, 26,* 5–17.

Tursz, A. (1997). Problems in conceptualizing adolescent risk behaviors: International comparisons. *Journal of Adolescent Health, 21,* 116–127.

US Surgeon General's report on sexual health. (2001). Available: http://www.surgeongeneral.gov/library/sexualhealth/glancetable.htm

Wyatt, G. (1997). *Stolen women: Reclaiming our sexuality, taking back our lives.* New York: John Wiley and Sons.

Sexuality, Older Adulthood

Mark A. Yarhouse

INTRODUCTION

A persistent stereotype of older adults is that they have little sexual desire and are involved in little or no sexual behavior. Research suggests that while there is a decline in sexual activity as people age (Laumann, Gagnon, Michael, & Michaels, 1994), older adults are more sexually active than the stereotype suggests. Unfortunately, it is this kind of stereotyping behavior that may keep health professionals from promoting healthy sexuality in older adults and may keep older adults from enjoying sexual expression as they age (Yarhouse, 2000).

DEFINITIONS

Health professionals can consider how to promote healthy sexuality in older adults. *Sexuality,* broadly defined, refers to a person's gender identity as either male or female, his or her desire or attraction to others, and associated behaviors that express that desire, including hugging, kissing, sexual intercourse, masturbation or mutual masturbation, and petting or the manual or oral stimulation of external sex organs (such as the clitoris, vagina, breasts, and penis). *Sexual intercourse,* a more common expression of sexual desire, refers most often to penile–vaginal intercourse that typically culminates in ejaculation in the male and orgasm, which is an emotional and physical "release" of energy experienced by both males and females. Also, menopause is considered by some experts to be the "most salient marker of aging in women" (Leiblum & Segraves, 2000, p. 423), and can lead to *vaginal atrophy* or diminished vaginal lubrication and changes to the vaginal wall. However, there is no necessary change in sexual interest or behavior because of these age-related developments.

In terms of sexual dysfunction in females, other important terms include *anorgasmia,* which refers to the inability to achieve orgasm (*primary* anorgasmia refers to lifelong/global anorgasmia, while *secondary* anorgasmia refers to situational/acquired difficulties); *dyspareunia* or painful intercourse; and *vaginismus,* which refers to involuntary muscle contractions that preclude vaginal penetration by the penis or fingers. Terms associated with sexual dysfunction in males include *premature ejaculation,* which refers to a lack of control over ejaculation during intercourse; *retarded ejaculation,* which has been recently conceptualized as male anorgasmia or an inability to achieve orgasm; and *erectile dysfunction* or impotence, which refers to the inability to achieve or maintain an erection.

Healthy sexuality and sexual expression is presumed to be between consenting adults, free from disease, discomfort, and dysfunction, satisfying by subjective self-report, and consistent with the cultural, religious and personal values of the particular older adult.

SCOPE

Research on sexuality and sexual behavior among older adults supports the view that older adults continue to experience sexual desire. In a study of 100 older adults, Bretshneider and McCoy (1988) reported that that both men (88 percent) and women (71 percent) fantasized about being intimate with the opposite sex, and that 63 percent of men reported engaging in sexual intercourse; 72 percent reported masturbating; and 82 percent reported caressing/touching without intercourse. Among women, 30 percent reported engaging in sexual intercourse; 40 percent reported masturbating; and 64 percent reported caressing/touching without intercourse.

In a study of 335 older adults in Italy (age range of 65–106 years), 39 percent were interested in sex and 31 percent were still sexually active (Buono et al., 1998). In a national study of married persons age 60 and over, about half of the sample and nearly one fourth of those over age 76, reported having had at least one sexual relation in the month prior to the study (Marsiglio & Donnelly, 1991). Additional studies support the view that many older adults are generally knowledgeable about sexuality and are interested in sexual behavior (e.g., Starr & Weiner, 1981; Steinke, 1994).

Health professionals may be interested to identify what keeps older adults from enjoying a healthy sex life. In the national study mentioned above, frequency of sexual behavior was not influenced by gender or race, nor by their spouse's health status (Marsiglio & Donnelly, 1991). Buono et al. (1998) reported that marital status predicted sexual activity and interest and appears to be especially salient for women. This has been reported in several studies (e.g., Malatesta, Chambless, Pollack, & Cantor, 1988) and may have to do with the tendency among women to have fewer lifetime sexual partners than men or a cohort difference related to this particular age group of women.

Malatesta et al. (1988) reported on 100 elderly widows and found that younger widows identified three major "sexual barriers": (1) body image changes, (2) lack of available men, and (3) limited monetary resources to facilitate social outings. Interestingly, Malatesta et al. found that nonsexual activities, such as "conversations with a man" and "going places with a man" were an important part of happiness and quality of life (p. 59). Also, a variety of activities met the "affectional and sexual needs" of elderly widows, including "activities [with] children and grandchildren," "wearing attractive clothing," and "expressing … spirituality" (p. 59).

Yet there are important age-related changes that both elderly males and females experience, and some of these changes can affect sexual behavior. Among women, normal, age-related changes influence their reproductive system, including menopause at about age 50–55 and the accompanying diminution of estrogen and progesterone production (Whitbourne, 1996). Normal age-related changes also include the sagging of breasts and some changes to the genitalia, such as pubic hair becoming coarser and the labia majora and minor becoming thinner (Whitbourne, 1996; cf., Leiblum & Segraves, 2000). One of the more common complaints among older women who are sexually active is pain during intercourse due to the thinning and drying of the vaginal wall.

Likewise, although males are still capable of reproducing into old age, they do experience a decrease in the number of viable sperm produced. Normal, age-related changes also include fewer and softer penile erections (Schiavi, Schreiner-Engel, Mandeli, Schanzer, & Cohen, 1990), a slowing of the sexual response cycle (from *desire* to *excitement* to *orgasm* to *resolution*), and a longer refractory period, which is the time needed to achieve another erection and orgasm (Whitbourne, 1996). Concerning erectile dysfunction, incidence rates increase with age: in one study of 1,709 randomly sampled men was 12.4 cases per 1,000 man-years (ages 40–49), 29.8 cases per 1,000 (ages 50–59), and 46.4 cases per 1,000 (ages 60–69) (Johannes, Araujo, Feldman, Derby, Kleinman, & McKinlay, 2000). In addition to age, increased risk of erectile dysfunction was related to lower education and health factors, such as diabetes and heart disease.

Older adults may also be at risk of sexually transmitted diseases (STDs). Murphree and DeHaven (1995) reported on 995 women and, although nonrepresentative of the general population (63 percent were black, about 40 percent were single, and 65 percent had an income below $15,000 per year), there was some evidence to rebut the assumption that "every older adult is in a monogamous, long-term relationship" (p. 237). However, it is generally recognized that nonmonogamy places older women and men at risk for STDs, and that older adults in particular have limited knowledge of or experience with condoms that might provide for safer sex practices than non-condom use. In a recent study of 32 HIV infected older adults, Gordon and Thompson (1995) reported that most older adults with HIV became infected through sexual intercourse (38 percent) or injection drug use (16 percent), and a disproportionate percentage of infected persons self-identified as homosexual or bisexual ($n = 10$ or 31 percent). The authors recommended sexual education for those with a history of STDs or who practice behaviors that put them at risk for infection.

THEORIES

The major theory of sexual functioning and intervention is cognitive-behavioral, which will be discussed in greater detail. However, other approaches, such as psychodynamic and systems models, have also been developed. In a *dynamic approach*, various defense mechanisms, such as denial, minimization, or repression, are identified. That which operates at the unconscious level is brought to consciousness by working through the conflicts underlying symptom expression. In contrast, *systems approaches* tend to focus on the sexual dyad, so that problems in expressions of healthy sexuality reflect more fundamental symptoms of dysfunction in the couple's relationship.

Cognitive-behavioral approaches are founded on learning theory where problems in sexual expression are conditioned fear reactions or reinforced behaviors where anxiety often precludes a person's or couples' ability to enjoy healthy sexuality and sexual behavior. Cognitive-behavioral interventions, such as sensate focus (non-demand caressing), are tailored to the needs of a couple and often emphasize relaxation, which is incompatible with anxiety. Additional interventions include providing education about sexual anatomy and physiology, assigning bibliotherapy resources, challenging and replacing irrational thoughts with rational thoughts about sexuality and sexual expression, promoting changes in attitudes, and encouraging positive exchanges with one's partner that enhance sexual functioning.

Cognitive-behavioral theorists have produced the most research to support their theory of sexual functioning. This has been true for individual and couple interventions (Cranston-Cuebas & Barlow, 1990), as well as group interventions that focus on psychoeducation, self-esteem building, assertiveness training, or self-exploration and directed masturbation (Mills & Kilmann, 1982; Robinson, Faris, & Scott, 1999). These findings will be applied in the following section of strategies.

STRATEGIES THAT WORK

Despite widespread acknowledgement of the increased numbers of older adults in the United States and throughout the world, there is remarkably little published with the specific intention of promoting healthy sexuality in older adults. Selected studies are organized by the following categories: psychoeducational programs, pharmacology and over-the-counter aids, sexual counseling and adult sex education, and alternative interventions.

Psychoeducational Programs

In one of the few studies specifically focused on promoting healthy sexuality in older adults, Goldman and Carroll (1990) reported on a psychoeducational curriculum as an adjunct to interventions to treat erectile dysfunction. According to the researchers, those who participated in the workshop reported increased knowledge of sexual issues and sexual satisfaction at post-test as compared to controls.

Robinson et al. (1999) reported on the use of a psychoeducational group that reduced fears related to sexual behavior following cancer treatment. Again, the curriculum was offered in a medical setting as an adjunct to treatment. Older women who participated in the psychoeducational program also reported an increase in sexual knowledge.

White and Catania (1982) provided a psychoeducational intervention to older adults, family members of the elderly, and nursing home staff who work with older adults. The curriculum included educational material on sexuality and normal aging. The results of this sexual health promotion curriculum were that knowledge of sexuality and aging and attitudes about sexuality and aging changed from knowledge and attitudes held prior to the training and as compared to the control group. Participants reported increased knowledge of sexuality and aging and a more open or permissive attitude with respect to sexuality and sexual behavior.

Interestingly, White and Catania (1982) believed that staff and family should be involved in psychoeducational program to promote healthy sexuality in older adults because staff and family often play key roles in facilitating or limiting access to or privacy with respect to sexual behavior among older adults. Obtaining physical privacy and private time are complicated in institutional settings, and their absence reflects the asexual stereotype that even professionals hold about older persons. The authors conclude that the change in knowledge and attitudes may be helpful to older adults seeking sexual activities, and their findings seem to support this conclusion, as there was a reported 400 percent increase in both sexual intercourse and masturbation among older adults who participated in the program.

In an older study, Rowland and Haynes (1978) reported on a sexual enhancement psychoeducational curriculum specifically designed for elderly couples. Ten married couples (age range 51–71) participated in one of three psychoeducational groups. Participants were provided educational materials on sexual functioning among older adults, followed by skill-based modules on communication training and sexual techniques to increase sexual enjoyment. Results at posttest and 1-month follow-up indicated increases in sexual satisfaction, frequency of specific sex practices, and marital and life satisfaction.

Pharmacology and Over-the-Counter Aids

As a compliment to psychoeducational programs, medical advances, such as the introduction of sildenafil (Viagra), have had an impact on promoting sexual functioning, particularly for males. Sildenafil, however, is contraindicated for men with some forms of heart disease. Although there is no parallel oral pharmacological agent for females, some anecdotal reports of the benefits of sildenafil to women are being researched and can be considered strategies that might work.

Age-related changes, such as declining levels of estrogen in women and testosterone in women and men, can be compensated for with estrogen and testosterone replacement therapies. Also, because some medications (e.g., hypotensive agents, Beta-blockers) taken by older adults can lead to diminished sexual desire or ejaculatory problems, these may be discontinued or replaced with alternative pharmacological agents (Leiblum & Rosen, 2000).

There are many over-the-counter aids to sexual expression for older persons and others. Lubricants can lessen vaginal dryness, and body lotions and oils can enhance sexual performance. Vibrators can provide stimulation where physical facility may be lacking. There are also adult sex education videos that can inform and encourage new ways of sexual expression.

Health professionals should note that these medical advances can be introduced in a multidisciplinary approach to addressing healthy sexuality in older persons and are typically offered in conjunction with sex education and therapy.

Sex Counseling and Adult Sex Education

Sex education with older adults, according to Leiblum and Segraves (2000), often involves recognizing important cohort differences in attitudes toward sexuality and sexual expression. For example, they discuss how older adult males often think sexual behavior has to include penile vaginal intercourse, whereas younger males may more readily recognize or have assumed a broader sexual repertoire.

Sexual counseling and education to older persons without manifest sexual problems is similar in many ways to sex therapy with younger adults. There is a gray area between offering primary preventive services and early intervention (treatment) services, and one may flow into the other. Following a sex history, education can be provided about normal aging and health professionals can be aware to rule out possible chronic diseases and effects on sexual functioning of medications to treat chronic diseases (which assumes a collaborative relationship with the older adult's physician). Counseling often includes standard exercises such as sensate focus, directed masturbation, and specific homework assignments tailored to the needs of an individual or couple.

For some of the more common presenting concerns, Heiman and Meston (1997) summarize the research on sex therapy outcomes (not necessarily of older adults) and note the following: directed masturbation is preferred in the treatment of primary anorgasmia, with sensate focus enhancing the effects; use of vaginal dilators and relaxation for vaginismus; systematic desensitization and sensate focus for erectile dysfunction; and the "squeeze" technique (applying firm pressure just below the glans of the penis during sexual arousal but before ejaculation) for premature ejaculation. According to Heiman and Meston, there does not appear to be enough research available to specify efficacious treatments for desire disorders, dyspareunia, and retarded ejaculation.

STRATEGIES THAT MIGHT WORK

Alternative Interventions

Complimentary and alternative medicine are also beginning to be studied as to their sexual health-promoting qualities. However, caution is advised in using these alternatives until satisfactory research is available. According to Bartlik and Goldberg (2000), complimentary and alternative medicines considered to date have included caffeine (which enhances dopaminergic stimulation), L-Arginine (stimulates penile erections), and Yohimbine (increases blood flow to penis) for males and dehydroepiandrosterone (DHEA) (often used with menopausal women) for females. Promising for both genders are Damiana (increases genital engorgement), Dong Quai, Ginkgo biloba (increases genital blood flow but increases the risk of blood thinning), Ginseng, Ma huang (may stimulate nerve endings), Muira Puama, Royal jelly, and Sarsaparilla root.

In light of an increased awareness of cultural and religious diversity in the United States, multidisciplinary educational strategies may be enhanced by tailoring them to the specific cultural contexts that provide the valuative framework out of which older adults make decisions concerning their sexual behavior. For example, religiously affiliated older adults (and the current cohort of older adults is more religious than younger adults) may benefit from curricula that is consistent with their religious beliefs and values about the purpose and design of human sexuality and sexual behavior. One's culture or religion may prescribe specific behaviors, such as sexual intercourse in marriage or various nonsexual activities (Christenson & Gagnon, 1965), such as close companionship and fellowship with family members, and these have been found to be sexually satisfying to older adults (Malatesta et al., 1988). It should be noted that this may be a cohort difference and not an age difference.

STRATEGIES THAT DO NOT WORK

There has been insufficient research on promoting healthy sexuality in older adults to identify strategies that do not work. As more research is conducted in this important area—simply in response to the sheer number of persons who will be age 65 and over in the coming years—there will undoubtedly be greater clarity as to which strategies are especially helpful and which strategies do not work.

SYNTHESIS

Taken as a whole, it appears as though the best efforts to promote healthy sexuality in older adults will take two parallel approaches: first, to the general audience of older people (and society in general) that sexuality may be a renewable resource of personal or interpersonal pleasure throughout the older years that contributes to ongoing quality of life. Second, that sexuality in older adults needs to be tailored to the unique needs and interests of the individual within his or her cultural context. What the research supports to date would be centered on education regarding normal aging and the effects of aging on sexual interest and functioning as an important component in a psychoeducational curriculum.

A synthesis, then, would include education about: (a) normal changes associated with aging including information on the four stages of the sexual response cycle; (b) the impact of injuries on sexual functioning (e.g., pelvic fracture); (c) the potential impact on sexual functioning of disease and chronic illness, such as arteriosclerosis and diabetes mellitus; (d) the effects on sexual functioning of medications such as diuretics and antihypertensives used to treat conditions more common among older adults. As appropriate, adult sex education and counseling emphasizing standard interventions, such as sensate focus, bibliotherapy, directed masturbation, and other intervention strategies, would compliment this education curriculum and would be prepared to refer for medications that may improve sexual functioning (e.g., sildenafil). A synthesized approach would also include family members and staff of residential facilities to facilitate healthy sexuality among those living in institutionalized settings, with suitable times and places set aside for these and other personal uses.

Older adults may also benefit from intervention modules that address high-risk behaviors, including behaviors that put them at risk of STDs, such as AIDS. These behaviors include nonmonogamous sexual intercourse, homosexual behavior (including same-sex behavior among women, who, when they do engage in sex with men, are more likely to be sexually active with bisexual males), and intravenous drug use. Framed positively, safer sex practices include sex in a monogamous relationship with a partner who is not infected with an STD, sexual caressing/touching, and mutual masturbation.

Finally, efforts to promote healthy sexuality in older adults can recognize the effects on older adults of living in a youth-driven culture. Health professionals can promote positive messages that encourage older adults to see themselves as having sexual desires that can find expression through behaviors that are consistent with their personal, cultural, and religious beliefs and values.

Also see: Marital Satisfaction; Marital Enhancement, Health Promotion.

References

Bartlik, B., & Goldberg, J. (2000). Female sexual arousal disorder. In S.R. Leiblum & R.C. Rosen (Eds.), *Principles and practice of sex therapy* (3rd ed., pp. 85–117). New York: Guilford.

Bretschneider, J.G., & McCoy, N.L. (1988). Sexual interest and behavior in healthy 80- to 102-year olds. *Archives of Sexual Behavior, 17*(2), 109–129.

Buono, M.D., Zaghi, P.C., Padoani, W., Scocco, P., Urciuoli, O, Pauro, P., & de Leo, D. (1998). Sexual feelings and sexual life in an Italian sample of 335 elderly 65 to 106-year-olds. *Archives of Gerontology and Geriatrics, 6,* 155–162.

Christenson, C.V., & Gagnon, J.H. (1965). Sexual behavior in a group of older women. *Journal of Gerontology, 20,* 351–356.

Cranston-Cuebas, M.A., & Barlow, D.H. (1990). Cognitive and affective contributions to sexual functioning. *Annual Review of Sex Research, 1,* 119–161.

Goldman, A., & Carroll, J.L. (1990). Educational intervention as adjunct to treatment of erectile dysfunction in older couples. *Journal of Sex & Marital Therapy, 16*(3), 127–141.

Gordon, S.M., & Thompson, S. (1995). The changing epidemiology of human immunodeficiency virus infection in older persons. *Journal of the American Geriatric Society, 43,* 7–9.

Heiman, J.R., & Meston, C.M. (1997). Empirically validated treatment for sexual dysfunction. *Annual Review of Sex Research, 8,* 148–194.

Johannes, C.B., Araujo, A.B., Feldman, H.A., Derby, C.A., Kleinman, K.P., & McKinlay, J.B. (2000). Incidence of erectile dysfunction in men 40 to 69 years old: Longitudinal results from the Massachusetts male aging study. *Journal of Urology, 163*(2), 460–467.

Laumann, E.O., Gagnon, J.H., Michael, R.T., & Michaels, S. (1994). *The social organization of sexuality.* Chicago: University of Chicago Press.

Leiblum, S.R., & Rosen, R.C. (Eds.). (2000). Principles and practice of sex therapy (3rd ed.). New York: Guilford.

Leiblum, S.R., & Segraves, R.T. (2000). Sex therapy with aging adults. In S.R. Leiblum & R.C. Rosen (Eds.), *Principles and practice of sex therapy* (3rd ed., pp. 423–448). New York: Guilford.

Malatesta, V.J., Chambless, D.L., Pollack, M., & Cantor, A. (1988). Widowhood, sexuality and aging: A life span analysis. *Journal of Sex & Marital Therapy, 14*(1), 49–62.

Marsiglio, W., & Donnelly, D. (1991). Sexual relations in later life: A national study of married persons. *Journal of Gerontology, 46*(6), 338–344.

Mills, K.H., & Kilmann, P.R. (1982). Group treatment of sexual dysfunctions: A methodological review of the outcome literature. *Journal of Sex and Marital Therapy, 8,* 259–296.

Murphree, D.D., & DeHaven, M.J. (1995). Does grandma need condoms? Condom use among women in a family practice setting. *Archives of Family Medicine, 4,* 233–238.

Robinson, J.W., Faris, P.D., & Scott, C.B. (1999). Psychoeducational group increases vaginal dilation for younger women and reduces sexual fears for women of all ages with gynecological carcinoma treated with radiotherapy. *International Journal of Oncology, Biology, Physiology, 44*(3), 497–506.

Rowland, K.F., & Haynes, S.N. (1978). A sexual enhancement program for elderly couples. *Journal of Sex & Marital Therapy, 4*(2), 91–113.

Schiavi, R.C., Schreiner-Engel, P., Mandeli, J., Schanzer, H., & Cohen, E. (1990). Healthy aging and male sexual function. *American Journal of Psychiatry, 147*(6), 766–771.

Starr, B., & Weiner, M. (1981). *The Starr-Weiner report on sex and sexuality in the mature years.* New York: McGraw-Hill.

Steinke, E.E. (1994). Knowledge and attitudes of older adults about sexuality and ageing: A comparison of two studies. *Journal of Advanced Nursing, 19,* 477–485.

Whitbourne, S.K. (1996). Psychological perspectives on the normal aging process. In L.L. Carstensen, B.A. Edelstein, & L. Dornbrand (Eds.), *The practical handbook of clinical gerontology* (pp. 3–35). Thousand Oaks, CA: Sage.

White, C.B., & Catania, J.A. (1982). Psychoeducational intervention for sexuality with the aged, family members of the aged, and people who work with the aged. *International Journal of Aging and Human Development, 15*(2), 121–138.

Yarhouse, M.A. (2000). Review of social cognition research on stereotyping: Application to psychologists working with older adults. *Journal of Clinical Geropsychology, 6*(2), 121–131.

Sexually Transmitted Diseases, Adolescence

Alison Moriarty Daley

INTRODUCTION AND DEFINITIONS

Sexually transmitted diseases (STDs) are a group of infections passed from partner to partner during unprotected sexual activity. Several of these infections present significant threats to the health of teens and young adults worldwide and may cause lifelong sequelae for infected individuals. The adolescent population has the highest incidence of many STDs (Centers for Disease Control and Prevention [CDC], 1998), while the prevalence of trichomoniasis, human papillomavirus, and herpes simplex virus type 2 in the adolescent population is uncertain because these infections are not reportable. The actual incidence of STDs in teens may be even higher because the rates are based on the total population of 15- to 19-year-olds, not just those who are sexually active (Berman & Hein, 1999; Panchaud, Singh, Feivelson, & Darroch, 2000).

DEFINITIONS

Gonorrhea (Neisseria gonorrhoeae) is a bacterial infection with a prevalence of 3–18 percent in adolescent females and 3–9 percent in adolescent males in the United States (Stewart & Hofmann, 1997). The incidence of gonorrhea among teens increased by 13 percent from 1997 to 1999 (CDC, 2000). Gonorrhea initially causes an endocervical infection in women of whom as many as 80 percent remain asymptomatic. Symptoms typically develop 2–5 days following exposure, infected females experience purulent, thick vaginal discharge, swollen lymph nodes, dyspareunia (pain during sexual intercourse), lower abdominal pain, fever, urinary frequency, and dysuria (burning with urination). Male adolescents with gonorrhea typically experience dysuria, copious purulent penile discharge, and swollen inguinal lymph nodes. Asymptomatic infections are less common in males, however this occurs in 10–40 percent of those affected (Stewart & Hoffman, 1997).

Chlamydia (Chlamydia trachomatis), causes reproductive tract infections and has an overall prevalence of 5–10 percent in teens (CDC, 2000). About 40 percent of all reported cases of chlamydia occur in individuals 15- to 19-years-old (CDC, 2000); the majority of teens are asymptomatic (75 percent of women, 50 percent of males). The number of chlamydial infections has decreased in response to several screening programs across the country, however high rates of infection are still present in areas where enhanced screening programs are not available (CDC, 2000). Women infected with chlamydia most commonly experience a watery endocervical discharge and cervical bleeding. Males experience a discharge from the urethra and dysuria.

If endocervical gonorrhea or chlamydia is not treated, either infection can ascend into the upper reproductive tract and cause pelvic inflammatory disease (PID), an infection of the uterus, fallopian tubes, ovaries, and peritoneum. Two thirds of all cases of PID occur in women less than 24 years old and account for 60 out of every 10,000 hospital admissions (Stewart & Hofmann, 1997). Teens are at greater risk for developing PID than women of any other age group because they are more likely to delay seeking treatment. The teen usually experiences symptoms in the first half of the menstrual cycle, which include: cramps, lower abdominal pain, abnormal vaginal bleeding, discharge, fever, nausea/vomiting, dysuria, malaise, weakness and fainting (Stewart & Hofmann, 1997). Potential consequences of PID include infertility, ovarian abscess, chronic pelvic pain, and an increased incidence of ectopic pregnancy (Youngkin, 1995). Untreated gonorrhea or chlamydial infection in males can cause epididymitis, an infection of the epididymis caused by the retrograde spread of bacteria from the urethra via the vas deferens. The teen experiences dull achy scrotal pain and urethral discharge. Male and female adolescents can also develop either infection in the rectum or throat if exposed through anal or oral sex.

Human papillomavirus (HPV) is thought to be the most common STD among adolescents. More than one million individuals are infected annually, 46 percent of women under the age of 25 have HPV (CDC, 2000). Actual infection rates among males are not available but rates are thought to resemble closely those of women (CDC, 2000). There are approximately 30 different types of HPV that effect the genital tract (CDC, 2000). HPV infection may be asymptomatic or present with visible genital warts and has been implicated as a precursor of cervical, penile, and rectal cancer. Visible warts are usually multiple, pink to brown, skin tag-like lesions of varying size. The risk of contracting HPV is associated with unprotected sex, younger age at sexual debut (because of the increased potential number of lifetime sexual partners and cervical ectopy), tobacco use, pregnancy, and an altered immune system (Carson, 1997).

Herpes simplex virus type 2 (HSV-2) is an incurable viral infection characterized by painful clusters of ulcers of the genitals, perianal area, mouth, lips and throat. This infection appears to be more common in women (1 in 4) than men (1 in 5) and effects approximately one million people annually (CDC, 2000). The most dramatic increase in infection rates occurred in teens and young adults between 1970 and 1990 (CDC, 2000). The CDC (2000) reports that 15–20 percent of teens are infected with HSV-2 prior to becoming adults. Fleming et al. (1997) found that less than 10 percent of those infected with HSV-2 and who tested positive for the virus via blood antibody tests knew they had the virus. Once infected with the virus, an individual experiences an initial outbreak 2–20 days following exposure that may include: painful ulcers, swollen tender inguinal lymph nodes, dysuria, painful defecation, fever, malaise, headache, myalgia, urinary retention, constipation, aseptic meningitis, and sacral anesthesia (Emans, Laufer, & Goldstein, 1998). Symptoms may last up to 3 weeks before resolving.

Subsequent episodes of HSV-2 can be triggered by physical or emotional stress, exposure to sunlight, or other infections and the symptoms are often less intense and shorter in duration. HSV-2 can be passed even in the absence of the ulcers, which makes condom use with every sexual encounter essential in preventing the spread of the virus.

Trichomoniasis (Trichomonas vaginalis) is an infection of the vagina or urethra caused by a motile protozoan. The incidence and prevalence of this infection are unknown. It is estimated that 50 percent of all those infected are asymptomatic (Stewart & Hoffman, 1997). Symptoms appear about 7 days (4–20 days) following exposure and typically include a frothy, greenish-yellow, malodorous discharge accompanied by intense vaginal itching, urinary frequency, burning with urination, post-coital bleeding, or dyspareunia. Recent research has reported an increase risk of acquiring HIV for those infected with Trichomonas vaginalis (Sorvillo & Kerndt, 1998).

Syphilis (Treponema pallidum) is an infection caused by a spirochete. The overall incidence of syphilis is low in the United States, however, 10 percent of all infections occur in the adolescent population (Panchaud et al., 2000). Infection with syphilis progresses, in stages, if it is not diagnosed and treated. The initial stage occurs about three weeks following exposure and is characterized by a painless, raised, sharply demarcated genital ulcer called a chancre and is accompanied by painless inguinal lymph nodes. If not treated the chancre with resolve in 2–6 weeks. The second stage begins 2 weeks to 6 months following resolution of the chancre and lasts 10–14 days. Typical symptoms include: fever, malaise, headache, sore throat, arthralgias, prominent lymph nodes, enlarged liver or spleen, hair loss, and a polymorphic rash anywhere on the body including palms, soles, or oral mucosa. An untreated individual with syphilis usually experiences a latency period that may last 15 years and then one third of patients will develop destructive lesions of the heart, bone, skin, or brain.

SCOPE

A recent study looked at the incidence of syphilis, gonorrhea, and chlamydia among adolescents in developed countries (Panchaud et al., 2000). Overall, the incidence of these infections has decreased in the general population and among adolescents worldwide since 1990. However, in the Russian Federation the incidence of syphilitic infections has risen dramatically to 211 cases per 100,000 15- to 19-year-olds compared to 0.6/100,000 in Canada and 6.4/100,000 in the United States (Panchaud et al., 2000). Gonnococcal infections disproportionally affect adolescents more than any other age group and range from lower rates in Belgium (0.6/100,000), Sweden (1.8/100,000), and 59.4/100,000 in Canada to an incidence of 571.8/100,000 in the United States

and 596.5/100,000 in the Russian Federation (Panchaud et al., 2000). Chlamydial infections are also common in the adolescent population with rates of 12.2/100,000 in Belgium, 563.3/100,000 in Canada and the highest rate of 1,131.6/100,000 in the United States (Panchaud et al., 2000).

THEORIES AND RESEARCH

Developmental, physiological, and behavioral factors have been found to place adolescents at risk for acquiring a sexually transmitted disease.

Developmental Factors

Adolescents present a challenge to health care providers as they move from concrete thinking to formal operational thought. Formal operational thought is the ability to think abstractly and allows the teen for the first time to think about the possible outcomes of a behavior, envision the future, and transfer information learned in one situation to another, different situation (Inhelder & Piaget, 1958). Early in adolescence most teens are not capable of appreciating the consequences of behavior because they have not yet developed this ability. The inability to envision the future makes it difficult for a teen to anticipate when he or she may engage in sexual activity, obtain condoms, carry them, and finally remember to use the condom at the time of sexual activity.

Another thought process called the "personal fable," the belief that one's experience is special and unique, leads the adolescent to believe that he or she is invulnerable to harm (Elkind, 1984). For example, a teen may understand that people are infected with a STD while engaging in unprotected sex, however many may not believe that they could become infected from the same activity. By late adolescence, most teens have developed the capacity for abstract thought and are able to fully contemplate the possible consequences of behavior and understand how current behaviors may affect future outcomes. It should be emphasized that teens progress through these cognitive stages at various rates and some individuals never truly achieve the capacity for abstract thought (Ingersoll, 1992).

Physiologic Factors

Immaturity of an adolescent's cervix may place her at an increased risk for acquiring a STD. The cervix consists of two different types of epithelial cells: squamous and columnar. The junction between the two types of cells is called the squamocolumnar junction. During adolescence the columnar cells regress into the endocervix. The squamous cells, which are more resistant to infection, remain prominent on the ectocervix and may provide some protection against STDs. Younger teens, who have not completed the physiologic transformation of the endocervix to squamous epithelium, are potentially more vulnerable to acquiring a STD during unprotected sex (Beach, 1992).

Behavioral Factors

National trends indicate that the age of initiation of sexual activity is decreasing and the percent of teenagers who are sexually active at specific ages has increased over the last several decades. The most recent Youth Behavior Risk Survey indicates that 38.6 percent of 9th graders and 64.9 percent of 12th graders are sexually active. Approximately, 8 percent of teens reported initiating sexual activity before the age of 13 and 16.2 percent of high school students reported four or more sexual partners during their lifetime (Kann et al., 2000). However, only 58 percent of teens (50.7 percent females, 65.5 percent males) reported using a condom during the last act of sexual intercourse.

STRATEGIES THAT WORK

Condom Availability Programs

School-based condom availability programs appeared in the United States in the early 1990s in an effort to reduce the number of unintended teen pregnancies and STDs. The American Academy of Pediatrics, American College of Obstetricians and Gynecologists, American School Health Association, and the National Medical Association have recommended that condoms be available to teens through comprehensive school health programs (American Academy of Pediatrics, 2001; Epner, 1996). The availability of condoms in schools has met with mixed reaction. Proponents of school-based condom availability programs maintain that unrestricted access to free condoms will reduce unprotected sexual acts and encourage discussion between partners about condom use. Opponents argue that such programs condone and encourage sexual behavior (Schuster, Bell, Berry, & Kanouse, 1998).

Kirby and Brown (1996) conducted telephone interviews to determine the number of school-based condom availability programs in US public schools, the characteristics of these schools, and their condom programs. The results of this study indicated that as of January 1995, at least 431 (2.2 percent) public schools in 50 school districts, made condoms available in school, 92 percent were in high schools, 72 percent were located in regular academic schools, and 28 percent in alternative schools. Condoms were made available to students, usually by more than one source: nurses (54 percent), teachers (52 percent), counselors (47 percent), principals (27 percent), bowls or baskets (5 percent), vending machines (3 percent), and other students (2 percent). Most programs required

parental consent and counseling prior to distributing condoms. A majority of the schools imposed limits on the number of condoms a student could receive at one time. Schools that had a greater number of staff distributing condoms, that did not restrict the number of condoms a student could receive at one time, made condoms available in baskets or bowls, or had a comprehensive K-12 sex education program provided more condoms per student per year (Kirby & Brown, 1996).

Subsequent studies have sought to determine the impact condom availability programs have had on teens' self-reported sexual behavior and condom use patterns. Guttmacher, Lieberman, Ward, Fruedenberg, Radosh, and Jarlais (1997) studied the relationship between condom use and sexual behavior in New York City (NYC) public high schools following the implementation of a condom availability program as compared to a similar population of Chicago students without a program. The NYC Board of Education implemented a system-wide condom availability program in 1991. As part of this initiative, public high schools were required to assemble an HIV/AIDS team; teach at least six HIV/AIDS educational classes in each grade per year; identify a resource room for HIV/AIDS information and condom distribution which would be open a minimum of 10 class periods a week; name and inform students of at least one male and female volunteer who would staff the resource room; and provide an information session for parents addressing HIV/AIDS (Guttmacher et al., 1997).

Results demonstrated that the proportion of new (in school for < 1 year) and continuing (in school ≥1 year) students who reported any sexual activity in New York and Chicago were the same (new students 47 percent, continuing students 60 percent) and that these groups had a comparable increase in sexual activity as they got older. Therefore, condom availability did not increase sexual activity. This study also found that continuing NYC students were more likely than Chicago students (61 vs. 56 percent; $p < 0.01$) to report the use of a condom at last sexual intercourse. The results were even more pronounced among a sub-group of higher-risk continuing students, those that reported three or more partners in the previous six months, than the entire sample of continuing students (higher risk group OR = 1.85, $p < 0.01$; entire sample OR = 1.36, $p < 0.01$).

Schuster et al., (1998) also studied the effects of a condom availability program on teens from a Los Angeles County high school. Analysis of the results revealed that no significant difference in the percentage of male or female students who reported engaging in vaginal intercourse, had vaginal sex in the previous year or had a history of vaginal sex with three or more partners. However, results indicated the condom availability program had a significant impact on two groups: (1) those students who had not yet engaged in vaginal intercourse at the onset of the program and (2) male students. The percentage of male students who reported engaging in vaginal intercourse in the previous year and reported using condoms "every time" increased significantly from 37 to 50 percent ($p = 0.005$). The percentage of males who reported condom use at first vaginal intercourse also rose significantly from 46 to 56 percent ($p = 0.02$). The number of sexually inexperienced students, who anticipated that they would use a condom if they were to become sexually active, increased from 62 to 90 percent among males and 73 to 94 percent among females ($p > 0.001$ for males and females) at the 1-year follow-up. Female students had no significant change in reported condom use.

The impact of school condom availability was also examined by Furstenburg, Geitz, Teitler, and Weiss (1997) in nine high school drop-in centers in Philadelphia following the implementation of a policy aimed at reducing teen pregnancies, STDs, and HIV. Health Resource Centers (HRCs) were established in the schools to provide health referrals, reproductive health information, and condoms to students.

Results from two samplings demonstrated a decrease in the percent of teens reporting they had ever had sex, from 64 to 58 percent in schools that had HRCs in comparison to those schools that did not have the program (56–59 percent). Students reporting sex in the previous 4 weeks also declined among students in schools with HRCs (32–29 percent) versus non-HRC schools (24–26 percent). Unprotected sex decreased in the HRC schools from 8 to 6 percent, while the comparison schools had no change (5 percent) (Furstenburg et al., 1997).

These researchers then examined the sexual behaviors of students in schools with the highest rate of HRC use. In these schools, 53–57 percent of students reported using HRC services. The percent of students that reported ever engaging in sexual intercourse decreased from 75 to 66 percent from 1991–1993. By comparison, non-program schools had an increase in those reporting sexual activity (56–59 percent). Finally, reported condom use increased most dramatically in high use HRC schools from 37 to 50 percent, than in lower use schools (57–61 percent) or schools without this program (62–65 percent).

Educational Programs

Sex and HIV education programs have been shown to successfully delay the onset of sexual activity and increase the use of condoms/contraceptives in sexually active teens (Kirby, 2001). A recent report, Emerging Answers (Kirby, 2001), has identified 10 common characteristics of effective sex and HIV education programs. The curricula of these programs share the following characteristics:

1. Focus on reducing one or more sexual behaviors that lead to unintended pregnancy or HIV/STD infection.
2. Are based on theoretical approaches that have been demonstrated to influence other health-related behavior of specific important sexual antecedents to be targeted.
3. Deliver and consistently reinforce a clear message about abstaining from sexual activity and/or using condoms or other forms of contraception.
4. Provide basic, accurate information about risks of teen sexual activity and ways to avoid intercourse or use methods of protection against pregnancy and STDs.
5. Include activities that address social pressures that influence sexual behavior.
6. Provide examples of and practice with communication, negotiation, and refusal skills.
7. Employ teaching methods designed to involve participants and have them personalize the information.
8. Incorporate behavioral goals, teaching methods, and materials that are appropriate to the age, sexual experience, and culture of the students.
9. Last a sufficient amount of time (i.e., more than a few hours).
10. Select teachers or peer leaders who believe in the program and then provide them with adequate training.

The programs discussed in this section have been identified as possessing the characteristics identified by Kirby (2001).

Jemmott, Jemmott, and Fong (1998) evaluated the effects of abstinence and safer-sex HIV reduction strategies on a group ($n = 659$) of sixth and seventh grade teens (mean age 11.8 years; 53 percent male) in Philadelphia. The teens were randomized into one of three groups: (1) abstinence HIV intervention; (2) safer-sex HIV intervention; or (3) health promotion control group. The intervention consisted of eight one-hour modules presented on two consecutive Saturdays and incorporated themes from the *Be Proud! Be Responsible!* curriculum. Confidential questionnaires were administered before the intervention and then at 3, 6, and 12 months following the program. The goal was to determine the self-reported sexual behaviors of these teens and their beliefs about condoms, abstinence, and HIV-risk reduction.

Jemmott et al. (1998) found that teens in the safer-sex HIV intervention had the most favorable outcomes—a reduction in reported unprotected sexual activity and an increase in condom use. Specifically, teens in this group were more likely to report consistent condom use (defined as the use of a condom with every act of sexual intercourse) at the 3-month follow-up than the teens in the control or abstinence groups. The teens that were sexually experienced at baseline and were in the safer-sex HIV group reported less unprotected sexual intercourse than the other groups. These teens also had a significantly higher frequency of condom use and reported fewer days on which they were sexually active than the teens in the control group (Jemmott et al., 1998). At the 3-month follow-up, the safer-sex group had a significantly higher knowledge of condom use, believed more strongly that condoms are effective in preventing pregnancy, STDs, and HIV, reported a higher amount of confidence that they could have condoms available as needed, and believed more strongly that condoms would not interfere with sexual pleasure than the other groups (Jemmott et al., 1998). Teens in the abstinence intervention were less likely to report sexual activity only at the 3-month follow-up than the safer-sex or control groups.

Kirby, Barth, Leland, and Fetro (1991) studied the effect of the *Reducing the Risk* curriculum on students in 13 California high schools. The goal of the curriculum was to reduce unprotected sex in this population by encouraging teens not to have sex or by increasing contraceptive use. The curriculum, which is based on the social learning, social inoculation, and cognitive behavioral theories, was incorporated into an existing health education course and consisted of 15 classes. Students were surveyed prior to and immediately after the program and at 6- and 18-month follow-ups.

Kirby and colleagues (1991) found that 37 percent of the total sample had initiated sexual intercourse prior to the implementation of the "Reducing the Risk" curriculum. However, by the 18-month follow-up, there were significant differences between the treatment and control groups. About 29 percent of the treatment group and 38 percent ($p < 0.05$) of the control group, who were sexually inexperienced at the pretest, had initiated sexual activity in 18 months following the program. This represents a reduction in the initiation of sexual intercourse by 24 percent in the treatment group. The groups also differed significantly when asked if they had engaged in unprotected sex. Same 11 percent of both groups reported they had engaged in unprotected sex at the pretest. By 18 months, 13 percent of the treatment group and 23 percent ($p < 0.05$) of the control group reported engaging in unprotected sex. Of those who were sexually inexperienced at pretest, 9 percent of the treatment group and 16 percent ($p < 0.05$) of the comparison group reported a history of unprotected sex by 18 months, and 13 percent of the control group (vs. 7 percent treatment) reported engaging in unprotected sex most or all of the time.

Hubbard, Giese, and Rainey (1998) replicated Kirby et al.'s (1991) study. This time the "Reducing the Risk" curriculum was implemented in five rural and urban Arkansas school districts during the required one-semester health education classes.

An analysis was completed to determine the impact the "Reducing the Risk" curriculum had on the sexually inexperienced students at the 18-month follow-up. There was an increase of those students reporting sexual activity in both groups. However, fewer students in the intervention group (28 vs. 43 percent) became sexually active. Of those students who became sexually active during the study, 89 percent of the intervention group and 46 percent ($p > 0.05$) of the comparison group reported that they used strategies to prevent STD/HIV and pregnancy.

STRATEGIES THAT MIGHT WORK

STD Urine Screening Programs

Most adolescents do not receive routine screening for STDs and may have undetected infections, which can be passed unknowingly to others. In particular, Chlamydia trachomatis infections have been reported to be asymptomatic in up to 80 percent of those infected. Several studies have examined screening as a strategy to prevent the transmission of asymptomatic STDs.

Rietmeijer et al. (1997) examined the feasibility of screening for Chlamydia trachomatis infection among high-risk male youth. Research assistants collected urine specimens from male subjects less than 26 years old in nontraditional settings like high schools, recreation centers, and a STD/HIV prevention outreach facility. Of 486 urine samples collected during the project, 32 (6.6 percent) were positive for Chlamydia trachomatis. These infected males were significantly more likely to report having engaged in vaginal sex with a partner in the last 30 days.

Gaydos et al. (1998) collected specimens from 13,204 female Army recruits between 17 and 39 years old to determine the prevalence of Chlamydia trachomatis infection. The results of this study showed that the highest rate of chlamydial infection occurred in the 17-year olds and declined sharply as age increased. Recruits less than 25 years old had a prevalence of 10 percent in comparison to the 26- to 39-year-olds who had a prevalence of 3.6 percent. Other factors that were associated with increased prevalence of chlamydia were vaginal sex, having had more than one sex partner in the previous 90 days, sex with a new partner in the previous 90 days, inconsistent use of condoms, and a past history of an STD.

Other studies by Burstein, Gaydos, Diener-West, Howell, Zenilman, and Quinn (1998) and Cohen, Nsuami, Martin, and Farley (1999) had similar success in identifying asymtomatic youth with STDs. Urine screening for STDs has promise for the detection of asymptomatic infections in teens. Issues of cost and outreach to high-risk populations remain to be addressed.

STRATEGIES THAT DO NOT WORK

Abstinence only programs have not demonstrated a positive impact on sexual behavior among teens (Kirby, 2001). Few programs have been evaluated and their findings presented in the literature (Kirby, Korpi, Barth, & Cagampang,

1997; St. Pierre, Mark, Kaltreider, & Aikin, 1995; Weed, Olsen, DeGatson, & Prigmore, 1992). However, an intensive review of federally funded abstinence-only programs is currently underway and results may indicate more favorable results of this type of program.

The largest of the published abstinence-only studies evaluated the impact of the *Postponing Sexual Involvement* (PSI) curriculum (Kirby et al., 1997) on a cohort of ethnically diverse, California junior high school teens (12–13 years old, mean age 12.8 years). The curriculum was presented in five one-hour classroom sessions presented by either peer-leaders or adults. The program curriculum focused on postponing sexual intercourse via the social influence theory. It taught students to recognize peer/social pressure and skills to resist sexual pressure. Data were collected prior to the curriculum and at two follow-ups (3- and 17-months).

Self-reported sexual activity rates ranged from 9.7 to 11 percent across groups at baseline. Kirby and colleagues (1997) found no significant impact on delaying sexual activity, frequency of engaging in sexual intercourse, or the number of sexual partners students reported at either the 3- or 17-month follow-up. There was also no significant difference between the intervention and control group's reported use of condoms.

SYNTHESIS

Sexually transmitted infections present a significant threat to the health of teens worldwide. Efforts to prevent infections in teens have taken a variety of forms and produced promising results. Specifically, school-based condom availability programs have demonstrated success in increasing the use of condoms (Furstenberg et al., 1997; Guttmacher et al., 1997), delaying the onset of sexual activity (Furstenberg et al., 1997), and increasing the use of condoms at sexual debut (Schuster et al., 1998). In addition, condom availability programs have not increased the sexual activity among teens as feared by opponents of these programs (Furstenberg et al., 1997; Guttmacher et al., 1997). Educational programs have demonstrated success in delaying the onset of sexual activity among sexually inexperienced students and increasing the reported use of condoms and contraceptives among sexually active teens (Hubbard et al., 1998; Jemmott et al., 1998; Kirby et al., 1991). Research has also shown that students that have participated in these education programs have a greater knowledge of condom use and STDs, are more likely to report confidence in their ability to refuse sex, and use strategies learned to prevent STDs, HIV and pregnancy (Hubbard et al., 1998; Jemmott et al., 1998). Urine screening for gonorrhea and chlamydia has potential for preventing the transmission of STDs and the sequelae of untreated infections (Burstein et al., 1998;

Cohen et al., 1999; Gaydos et al., 1998; Rietmeijer et al., 1997). This is especially important because the vast majority of teens who were diagnosed with gonorrhea and chlamydial infection were asymptomatic (Burstein et al., 1998; Cohen et al., 1999).

Unfortunately, despite the successes that have been demonstrated with various populations of teens, no single approach seems to work with the majority of adolescents. Particular attention needs to be focused on girls who appear to be the most difficult reach. In addition, research has shown, that once a teen is sexually active it is difficult to change current risky behaviors to safer-sex practices. Primary prevention efforts need to begin earlier, many programs are for teens in junior high school, however, many teens have already initiated sexual activity prior to exposure to prevention efforts.

Health care providers, educators, and parents need to educate young people about the benefits of delaying sexual activity, maintaining safer-sex practices, recognizing symptoms of infection, and effectively accessing appropriate health care services. In addition, serious efforts are needed to treat infected sexual partners and limit the spread of these infections.

Also see: Marital Satisfaction; Marital Enhancement; Health Promotion.

References

American Academy of Pediatric Committee on Adolescence. (2001). Condom use by adolescents. *Pediatrics, 107,* 1463–1468.

Beach, R. (1992). Female genitalia: Examination and findings. In S. Friedman, M. Fisher, S.K. Schonberg: *Comprehensive adolescent health care* (pp.956–989). St Louis, MI: Quality Medical.

Berman, S., & Hein, K. (1999). Adolescents and STDs. In: K. Holmes et al. (Eds.), *Sexually Transmitted Diseases* (3rd ed.). New York: McGraw Hill.

Burstein, G., Gaydos, C., Diener-West, M., Howell, M., Zenilman, J., & Quinn, T. (1998). Incident Chlamydia trachomatis infections among inner-city adolescent females. *Journal of the American Medical Association, 280,* 521–526.

Carson, S. (1997). Human papillomatous virus infection update: Impact on women's health. *The Nurse Practitioner, 22,* 24–37.

Centers for Disease Control and Prevention (CDC). (1998). 1998 guidelines for the treatment of sexually transmitted diseases. *Morbidity and Mortality Weekly Report, 47,* 1–116.

Centers for Disease Control and Prevention (CDC). (2000). *Tracking the hidden epidemics: Trends in STDs in the United States 2000.* Centers for Disease Control and Prevention, 1–31. Available: CDC website.

Cohen, D., Nsuami, M., Martin, D., & Farley, T. (1999). Repeated school-based screening for sexually transmitted diseases: A feasible strategy for reaching adolescents. *Pediatrics, 104,* 1281–1285.

Elkind, D. (1984). *All grown up and no place to go.* Reading, MA: Addison-Wesley.

Emans, S.J., Laufer, M., & Goldstein, D. (1998). *Pediatric and adolescent gynecology* (4th ed.). New York: Williams & Wilkins.

Epner, J. (1996). *Policy compendium on reproductive health issues facing adolescents.* Chicago: American Medical Association.

Fleming, D., McQuillan, G., Johnson, R., Nahmias, A., Aral, S., Lee, F., & St. Louis, M. (1997). Herpes simplex virus type 2 in the United States, 1976 to 1994. *New England Journal of Medicine, 337,* 1105–1111.

Furstenberg, F., Geitz, L.M., Teitler, J., & Weiss, C. (1997). Does condom availability make a difference? An evaluation of Philadelphia's health resource centers. *Family Planning Perspectives, 29,* 123–127.

Gaydos, C.A., Howell, M.R., Pare, B., Clark, K., Ellis, D., Hendrix, R.M., Gaydos, J.C., McKee, K.T., & Quinn, T. (1998). Chlamydia trachomatis infections in female military recruits. *The New England Journal of Medicine, 339,* 739–744.

Guttmacher, S., Lieberman, L., Ward, D., Freudenberg, N., Radosh, A., & Jarlais, D. (1997). Condom availability in New York City public schools: Relationships to condom use and sexual behavior. *American Journal of Public Health, 87,* 1427–1433.

Hubbard, B., Giese, M., & Rainey, J. (1998). A replication study of Reducing the Risk, a theory-based sexuality curriculum for adolescents. *Journal of School Health, 68,* 243–247.

Ingersoll. G. (1992). Psychological and social development. In E. McAnarney, R. Kreipe, D. Orr, & G. Comerci (Eds.), *Textbook of adolescent medicine.* Philadelphia: W. B. Saunders Company.

Inhelder, B., & Piaget, J. (1958). *The growth of logical thinking from childhood to adolescence.* New York: Basic Books.

Jemmott, J.B., Jemmott, L.S., & Fong, G.T. (1998). Abstinence and safer sex HIV risk-reduction interventions for African American adolescents: A randomized controlled trial. *Journal of the American Medical Association, 279,* 1529–1536.

Kann, L., Kinchen, S., Williams, B., Ross, J., Lowry, R., Grunbaum, J., Kolbe, L., & State and Local YRBSS Coordinators. (2000). Youth risk behavior surveillance—United States, 1999. *Morbidity and Mortality Weekly Report, 49* (No. SS-5).

Kirby, D. (2001). *Emerging answers: Research findings on programs to reduce teen pregnancy.* Washington, DC: National Campaign to Prevent Teen Pregnancy.

Kirby, D., Barth, R., Leland, N., & Fetro, J. (1991). Reducing the Risk: Impact of a new curriculum on sexual risk-taking. *Family Planning Perspectives, 23,* 253–263.

Kirby, D., & Brown, N. (1996). Condom availability programs in US schools. *Family Planning Perspectives, 28,* 196–202.

Kirby, D., Korpi, M., Barth, R., & Cagampang, H. (1997). The impact of the Postponing Sexual Involvement curriculum among youths in California. *Family Planning Perspectives, 29,* 100–108.

Panchaud, C., Singh, S., Feivelson, D., & Darroch, J. (2000). Sexually transmitted diseases among adolescents in developed countries. *Family Planning Perspectives, 32,* 24–32.

Rietmeijer, C., Yamaguchi, B., Ortiz, C., Montstream, B., LeRoux, T., Ehert, J., Judson, F., & Douglas, J. (1997). Feasibility and yield of screening urine for Chlamydia trachomatis by polymerase chain reaction among high-risk male youth in field-based and other non-clinic settings: A new strategy for sexually transmitted disease control. *Sexually Transmitted Diseases, 24,* 429–435.

Schuster, M., Bell, R., Berry, S., & Kanouse, D. (1998). Impact of a high school condom availability program on sexual attitudes and behaviors. *Family Planning Perspectives, 30,* 67–72, 88.

Sorvillo, F., & Kerndt, P. (1998). Trichomonas vaginalis and amplification of HIV-1 transmission. *Lancet, 315,* 213–214.

Stewart, D., & Hofmann, A. (1997). Infections of the male and female reproductive tracts. In A. Hoffman & D. Greydanus (Eds.), *Adolescent medicine* (3rd ed., pp. 493–519). Stamford, CT: Appleton & Lange.

St. Pierre, T., Mark, M., Kaltreider, D., & Aikin, K. (1995). A 27-month evaluation of sexual activity prevention program in Boys and Girls Clubs across the nation. *Family Relations, 44,* 69–77.

Weed, S., Olsen, J., DeGatson, J., & Prigmore, J. (1992). *Predicting and changing teen sexuality rates: A comparison of three Title XX programs.* Washington, DC: Office of Adolescent Pregnancy Programs.

Youngkin, E.Q. (1995). Sexually transmitted diseases: Current and emerging concerns. *Journal of Obstetric, Gynecologic, and Neonatal Nursing, 24,* 743–758.

Single-Parent Families, Childhood

Elizabeth A. Sharp and Mark A. Fine

INTRODUCTION

In recent decades, family formation patterns in the United States have changed considerably. One dramatic change has been the rise in the number of single-parent families. Approximately half of all children in the United States will live in a single-parent family for some portion of their childhood. Given this high prevalence, it is important to examine issues related to the adjustment of children living in single-parent families.

DEFINITIONS

Several terms are frequently used in discussions of single-parent families. One such term is *family structure*, which is typically conceptualized in terms of parents' marital status and the number of parents present in the household. There are several classifications of family structure, such as: *intact* or *nuclear families* (two first-married parents married to each other with their child living in the same household); *stepfamilies* (a biological parent, stepparent, and a (step)child living in the same household); and *single-parent families* (an unmarried parent with at least one child living in the same household). Important distinctions also have been made between *single-parent families* and *single-parent households*. A *single-parent family* includes a single parent and his/her child living in the same household with no other parent actively involved in the child's life due to death, divorce, sperm donation, or other circumstances. In contrast, a *single-parent household* is defined as a single parent and his/her child living in the same household, but another parent may remain involved (at some level) in the child's life. This distinction is important because the presence and involvement of another parent often leads to both positive (e.g., more financial and social support) and negative consequences (e.g., increased levels of parental conflict). Because the majority of studies tend to group these together, however, it is impossible to distinguish between single-parent households and single-parent families for the purpose of the present entry. Thus, we will use the term *single-parent families* in the more general sense to refer to both single-parent households and single-parent families. Another important term is *family processes*, which refers to interactions between and among family members, including but not limited to the quality of parent–child relationships, parental conflict, affection, support, and parental monitoring.

In addition to the aforementioned terms, there are a few concepts that are particularly important to understanding the development of children living in single-parent families. Of these, *fluidity* and the *formation* of single-parent families are especially salient. *Fluidity* refers to the movement of children in and out of single-parent families. In the United States, 50–60 percent of American children will spend at least part of their childhood in a single-parent family and many of these children will live in a variety of single-parent and two-parent households during their childhood and teenage years (Hetherington, Bridges, & Insabella, 1998). For example, one study examined trajectories of children born to unmarried mothers and found that only one in five lived their entire childhood in a single-parent family (Aquilino, 1996). Thus, it is misleading to think that children in single-parent families have spent their entire lives in this type of family; most have transitioned into and out of a number of different family arrangements.

Another important consideration is the manner in which single-parent families are formed. There are several pathways that can lead to the formation of single-parent families including divorce, widowhood, and non-marital births. In general, most single-parent families are formed through divorce (57 percent), followed by non-marital childbirths (33 percent), and parental death (6 percent) (Rawlings & Saluter, 1995). These various pathways often influence child adjustment. For example, children raised in widowed single-mother families have higher levels of education, occupational status, and happiness in adulthood than do children reared in single-mother families formed following divorce. These outcomes are thought to be related to differing circumstances of these groups of women; divorced single mothers are more financially stressed and employed in lower occupational positions than are widowed single mothers (Biblarz & Gottainer, 2000).

SCOPE

In the past several decades, there has been a substantial increase in the number of children living in single-parent families throughout the world (Burns & Scott, 1994). In the United States, for example, single-parent families are the fastest growing family type, with an increase from 13 percent of children living in single-parent families in 1970 to 22 percent in 1995 (US Bureau of the Census, 1996) to over 25 percent in 1999 (Kleist, 1999). Similarly, in Canada and Sweden, 12.3 and 20 percent, respectively, of all households were single-parent families during the mid-to-late 1990s (Statistics Canada, 1996; Statistics Sweden, 2000).

Unique Challenges for Single-Parent Families

There are several unique challenges for the majority of single-parent families. One major challenge faced by many single parents, particularly women, is a lack of financial resources. Single parents are disproportionately poor, with single mothers and their children comprising a considerably large segment of the poor. Single mothers also tend to have lower incomes and educational levels than single fathers (Hetherington et al., 1998). Within single-parent families, children residing in cohabiting households with one parent and one other adult are less likely to live in poverty than children living only with a single parent, but they are not as economically well off as children who live in married couple families (Manning & Lichter, 1996).

As a consequence of low socioeconomic status, single-parent families are often vulnerable to stressful life conditions (e.g., daily hassles, lack of adequate child care) due to the limited availability of social, emotional, and financial resources that can potentially buffer these types of stressors. As a result, single mothers have reported that the most stressful aspect of single parenting is the continuous pressure of adult responsibilities without relief (Hetherington et al., 1998).

THEORIES

Several theories have been used to understand single-parent families. Of these, structural functionalism, Bronfrenbrenner's ecological model, family systems theory, and social exchange theory will be discussed. *Structural functionalism* is a macro-level theory that examines the relationship between families and society. Specifically, this theory looks at how families fulfill necessary tasks for their survival, emphasizing the importance of family structure. This theory suggests that families need to have two parents in order to function properly, with the father fulfilling the instrumental role (i.e., breadwinner) and the mother assuming the expressive role (i.e., homemaker; Parsons & Bales, 1955). These highly segregated roles are thought to help families provide physical and emotional support for their members. Without such roles being performed in the pre-scripted manner, families are viewed as dysfunctional. If structural functionalism theory were applied to single-parent families, this type of family would be viewed as inherently dysfunctional. However, it is important to note that this theory has been heavily criticized and has received minimal, if any, empirical support in its ability to help us understand nonnuclear families.

The *ecological model* emphasizes the context in which individual development occurs (Bronfenbrenner, 1979). Specifically, four levels of environmental context have been identified as influential in the development of individuals and families: microsystems are direct and immediate influences on daily life (e.g., families and schools); mesosystems involve the relations between microsystems (e.g., the inter-actions between family and school experiences); exosystems include indirect influences on individuals through social set-tings in which the individual does not have an active role (e.g., the employment setting of a parent may impact how the parent interacts with his/her child); and the macrosystem involves the culture and its norms (e.g., federal policies). The major assumption of this theory is that all levels mutually and interactively influence and are influenced by the individual. Identifying contextual influences has been very helpful in furthering our understanding of child outcomes related to liv-ing in a single-parent family. For example, researchers have examined a child's environment from all levels, such as the macro-level (e.g., welfare reform), the employment setting of the mother (exosystem), the relationship between the mother and child care provider (mesosystem), and the relationship between the mother and child (micro-level).

Family systems theory suggests that families are sys-tems with members functioning together to make decisions, achieve goals, and solve problems. Reciprocal relations characterize family systems; thus, each member influences and is influenced by other family members as well as by the external environment. Boundaries both within and outside families are important indicators of family functioning. In general, this theory assumes that appropriate boundaries between parent and children are necessary for healthy func-tioning. In the case of single-parent families, there is an increased likelihood that the boundaries between parent and child can be blurred, with the child serving as the parent's confidant in the absence of another adult.

Another theory that has been used to understand single-parent families is *social exchange theory*. This theory suggests that individuals make decisions based on a cost–benefit analysis. That is, people seek to maximize their rewards and minimize costs. In terms of single-parent fami-lies, this theory suggests that, in certain circumstances, sin-gle parents may reach the conclusion that the cost/benefit ratio favors staying in a single-parent family as opposed to

some other family arrangement. Thus, this theory alerts us to the possibility that single parents remain in their present family circumstance by choice and may actually prefer to function without the aid of a marital partner.

RESEARCH

One of the greatest concerns for researchers, practi-tioners, and those living in single-parent families is child adjustment. Understanding the effects of single-parent status on child outcomes is a complex issue because of the fluidity of children's living situations, the multiple pathways for the formation of single-parent families, and the unique challenges faced by single parents. The following section provides a brief overview of the findings related to child out-comes in single-parent families.

Some research suggests that children who live in single-parent families fare worse, in general, than children who grow up in first-married households (Hetherington et al., 1998). For example, children in intact families fare better, on average, on socioemotional adjustment, academic per-formance, and global well-being (Acock & Demo, 1994). Consistent with findings in the United States, there has been evidence that small, but reliable, differences in adjustment between children living in two-parent families and children living in single-parent families exist cross-culturally. An extensive review of research related to children and families in the United Kingdom, Australia, and New Zealand found that family structure itself is not a strong predictor of child adjustment (see Demo & Cox, 2000).

One reason living in a single-parent family may not be a strong indicator of adjustment is related to the influences of family demographic and process variables on child out-comes. It is important to emphasize that many of the studies that have found negative outcomes for children living in single-parent families have not taken into account a variety of factors that may partially explain these negative outcomes, such as the relative impact of poverty (Edin & Lein, 1997), living in an abusive household (Furstenberg & Cherlin, 1991), and unhealthy family processes (Kurdek, Fine, & Sinclair, 1995). In other words, scholars have found that these other factors may be stronger predictors of child out-comes than single-parenthood per se. Therefore, while family structure appears to have some unique effects on child outcomes even when controlling for these other factors, the other variables explain larger proportions of variability in children's well-being than does the type of family the child lives in (Fine, 2000). However, at the same time, other researchers caution not to completely dismiss these small differences, as some of these are meaningful (Simons & Associates, 1996).

Frequency and timing of changes in family households for a child also have important implications for child adjustment. Recent research suggests that multiple parenting transitions (three or more parental divorces and/or remarriages), especially during later childhood, are associated with particularly negative outcomes for children (Demo & Cox, 2000).

To add to the complexity of this issue, there is even some indication that living in a single-parent family may have beneficial effects for some adolescents. For example, one study found that, although White and Latino adolescents from two-parent families were less likely to use drugs than were those from single-parent families, African American youth living in two-parent families were more likely to use drugs than were their counterparts living in single-parent mother-headed families (Amey & Albrecht, 1998).

Another study of African American adolescents found that family structure was not related to youth outcomes. Instead, the quality of family relationships predicted adolescent development. In particular, a supportive, positive, and controlled family environment, and having an involved, non-residential father were associated with fewer behavioral and psychological problems of youth (see Fine, 2000). These findings are consistent with other research suggesting that African American children may not be as negatively influenced by living in a single-parent family as are White children (Fine, 2000).

Given that there is considerable variation in child outcomes in single-parent families, factors other than family structure per se are thought to influence child adjustment. Because such factors are related to conditions in single-parent families (e.g., decreased financial resources, increased stress), it might be most useful to conceptualize living in single-parent families as a risk factor for poor adjustment outcomes and to focus on protective factors that may serve to minimize stress for members of single-parent families. For example, a child's high self-esteem, a positive parent–child relationship, and social support are related to positive outcomes for children living in single-parent families (Garmezy, 1985).

STRATEGIES THAT WORK

Overall, there has been limited evaluation research of intervention programs aimed at single-parent families. Part of this is because of the dearth of programs developed for single-parent families as a collective group and a lack of evaluative research on the programs that do exist. In general, the majority of programs are specifically aimed at single-parent families formed as a result of divorce. Although the evaluations of these programs have often yielded mixed results, there are some promising findings.

Parent education programs are typically based on the model of authoritative parenting. These programs educate parents on child development issues, effective communication, and the importance of responsivity and discipline. Two such programs are *Parent Effectiveness Training* (PET) *and Systematic Training for Effective Parenting* (STEP; Brock, Oertwein, & Coufal, 1993). The PET program emphasizes flexibility and conflict resolution and has been found to help parents become more accepting of their children's behaviors and to endorse more egalitarian attitudes (Hamner & Turner, 1990). The STEP program underscores the functions of children's misbehavior, emphasizes providing logical consequences for children's misbehavior, and recommends consistent family meetings. Some positive outcomes related to the STEP program include improved parent–child interaction, parental attitudes, and parental perceptions of child behavior (American Guidance Service, 1991).

STRATEGIES THAT MIGHT WORK

Divorce-related interventions tend to be time-limited, educational programs for either parents, children, or both parents and children. Although programs vary, many emphasize understanding the developmental needs of children, improving communication, conflict resolution, and enhancing the parent–child relationship, as well as expanding support networks. Interventions developed for parents are thought to help children in indirect ways, as parents' adjustment to divorce is a strong predictor of child outcomes. Research reveals that such interventions can lead to improved mother–child relationships, but child-related program effects have been inconsistent, with some positive outcomes (e.g., less aggression for children in intervention groups than children not receiving the intervention), but no differences on other dimensions (e.g., depression, anxiety; see Grych & Fincham, 1997).

There are also some promising and mixed results for child-focused interventions. These interventions typically emphasize children's perceptions of divorce (e.g., that they are not responsible for causing the divorce), coping strategies, and increasing the size and quality of children's support networks. Findings indicate that children participating in these programs exhibit better overall adjustment. However, other research suggests that these programs may have limited impact on children. For example, one study found that, although children receiving treatment were rated by parents as having better overall adjustment compared to their counterparts not in treatment, teacher ratings did not indicate any treatment effects (Alpert-Gillis, Pedro-Carroll, & Cowen, 1989).

Interventions including parents and children tend to focus on typical responses for parents and children experiencing divorce, the parent–child relationship, responsive and consistent parenting, and effective communication techniques for both parents and children to reduce and manage conflict. Evaluations of this type of intervention have not shown that the parent–child focus is more effective than either parent-focused or child-focused interventions alone (see Grych & Fincham, 1997).

In addition to the divorce-related interventions, in recent years there have been some programs aimed at never-married single-parents. One type of program that has gained increased attention in recent years is based on home-visiting models. Home-visiting models emphasize the importance of home visitors frequently meeting with parents in the parent's residence, while sharing parenting information, making referrals, and providing resources. Evaluation studies of six programs using the home-visiting model indicated that benefits for parents and children were only found for a subset of families and these benefits were often only modest in magnitude (Culross & Behrman, 1999).

Home-visiting programs that use an ecological framework, aimed at helping single-parent families on multiple levels, tend to be the most effective. The newly developed *Early Head Start* program for children under the age of 3 years is an example of such an intervention. Based on Bronfenbrenner's ecological model, the Early Head Start program attempts to provide the child with developmentally stimulating experiences and a supportive environment through encouraging positive parenting, connecting parents with social networks, and encouraging parents to finish and/or enroll in education or job training programs. Preliminary results from an experimental evaluation design suggested that children enrolled in Early Head Start have shown more favorable outcomes at 24 months of age than their nonenrolled counterparts. For example, Early Head Start children scored higher on cognitive development, language, and literacy than did children not enrolled in Early Head Start (US Department of Health and Human Services, 2001).

STRATEGIES THAT DO NOT WORK

On a broad level, existing federal policies aimed at single-parent families are inadequate. In particular, policies related to the allocation of financial resources to single-parent families need improvement. As previously mentioned, socioeconomic status is one of the strongest predictors of child outcomes, accounting, for example, for about half of the variability in children's achievement (Simons & Associates, 1996). As noted earlier, single-parent families are disproportionately poor, particularly single mothers.

One reason single mothers remain poor is because only a quarter of single mothers actually receive the full amount of child support awards (Lin, 2000). As evidence of the importance of child support, several studies suggest that child support payments from non-residential fathers positively influence children's outcomes (see Lin, 2000). Unfortunately, efforts to increase child support payments have been met with only limited success. On the positive side, one study found that child support compliance was increased by withholding father's wages and when fathers felt that their child support obligations were fair.

Other financial constraints of single-parent families are related to federal policies such as welfare reform. The Personal Responsibility Act, with its purpose of ending dependence on welfare, was implemented in 1997. Although this goal has been partially achieved with a reduced number of single-parent families that are dependent on welfare, the quality of lives for many of these families has not improved. Three major welfare-reform-related challenges face the majority of single parents living in poverty; these include finding an adequate job, receiving appropriate job training (DeBord, Canu, & Kerpelman, 2000), and having access to quality and affordable child care (Hagen, 1999). In terms of job availability and training, research suggests that a lack of skills restricts wages for those obtaining jobs through welfare programs, and that most single mothers in this situation will remain in poverty even though they are working (Burtless, 1997). Furthermore, approximately one third of unemployed poor mothers are not working because of child-care-related problems.

SYNTHESIS

Because approximately half of the children in the United States will live in a single-parent family for at least some portion of their childhood, understanding and supporting single-parent families is crucial. Toward this end, we believe that addressing the unique challenges faced by single-parent families through a systemic and comprehensive approach is the most promising way to support these families. The most effective interventions meet children's and parent's needs on multiple levels, including adequate federal policies, supportive community networks, and the parent–child relationship. In addition, recognizing the considerable variation among single-parent families, it is important to develop several intervention strategies that specifically target the unique needs of particular types of single-parent families.

Two major challenges many single-parent families face include financial constraints and stressful life conditions related to limited time and support. In response to these challenges, federal policies need considerable modification. In particular, two important recommendations would be the development of uniform standards for child support to fully enforce routine child support withholdings and the creation of "safety nets" for families.

We suggest that US policy enact uniform standards for child support (rather than allowing for extensive state-to-state variation) and fully implement routine child support withholdings. Doing so would enhance the normative nature of child support obligations similar to the federal income tax or social security system. Consequently, fathers may be more likely to see their child support obligations as fair when they realize that most other fathers are also fulfilling their child support obligations (see Lin, 2000). Nevertheless, we acknowledge that there are very serious challenges that have made it difficult to increase compliance with child support awards. Further, increasing child support award compliance can only benefit those children and families for whom paternity has been established and/or that have fathers with the financial means to pay child support.

In terms of the welfare reform issues, work supports for single-parent families, including affordable, available, and quality child care as well as education, job training, and transportation are clearly needed. In the relatively recent post-welfare reform era, these work supports would address some of the major issues these families face while providing important "safety nets."

In addition to addressing policy-level issues, intervention strategies also need to focus on community-level supports. A variety of supportive programs should be available for single-parent families, including parent education programs. The vast majority of parent education interventions have been developed for children living in single-parent families formed following parental divorce. As a result, intervention programs have focused on single-parent families that may have more financial resources and, in some ways, have less need for systematic interventions. Therefore, it may be helpful to provide more educational programs and other types of support for single-parent families formed for reasons other than divorce. Such programs might address, for example, the unique needs of never-married single-parents, such as how to raise a child without a co-parent.

Furthermore, it may be important to develop multiple prevention programs designed to meet a variety of single-parent families' needs. For example, there should be programs targeted to high-risk single-parent families, as well as interventions designed for single-parent families already experiencing problems (e.g., those with children who have developmental delays and/or behavioral problems). At risk single-parent families may need intervention strategies such as information about parenting, child care after work, financial management assistance, or available resources in the community. In contrast, families already experiencing problems may need counseling and/or intensive home visits from service providers.

Also see: Parenting, Single Parent.

References

Acock, A., & Demo, D. (1994). *Family diversity and children's well-being.* Thousand Oaks, CA: Sage.

Alpert-Gillis, L.J., Pedro-Carroll, J.L., & Cowen, E.L. (1989). The children of divorce intervention program: Development, implementation, and evaluation of a program for young urban children. *Journal of Consulting and Clinical Psychology, 57*, 583–689.

American Guidance Service. (1991). *STEP research studies.* Circle Pines, MN: Author.

Amey, C.H., & Albrecht, S.L. (1998). Race and ethnic differences in adolescent drug use: The impact of family structure and the quantity and quality of parental interaction. *Journal of Drug Issues, 28*, 283–298.

Aquilino, W.S. (1996). The life course of children born to unmarried mothers: Childhood living arrangements and young adult outcomes. *Journal of Marriage and the Family, 58*, 293–310.

Biblarz, T.J., & Gottainer, G. (2000). Family structure and children's success: A comparison of widowed and divorced single-mother families. *Journal of Marriage and the Family, 62*, 533–548.

Brock, G.W., Oertwein, M., & Coufal, J.D. (1993). Parent education theory, research, and practice. In M.E. Arcus, J.D. Schvaneveldt, & J.J. Moss (Eds.), *Handbook of family life education* (Vol. 2, pp. 87–110). Newbury Park, CA: Sage.

Bronfenbrenner, U. (1979). Contexts of child rearing: Problems and prospects. *American Psychologist, 34*, 844–850.

Burns, A., & Scott, C. (1994). *Mother-headed families and why they have increased.* Hillsdale, NJ: Erlbaum.

Burtless, G.T. (1997). Welfare recipients' job skills and employment prospects. *The Future of Children, 7*(1), 39–51.

Culross, P.L., & Behrman, R.E. (1999). Home visiting: Recent program evaluations—Analysis and recommendations. *The Future of Children, 9*, 23–26.

DeBord, K., Canu, R.F., & Kerpelman, J. (2000). Understanding a work-family fit for single-parents moving from welfare to work. *Social Work, 45*, 313–324.

Demo, D.H., & Cox, M.J. (2000). Families with young children: A review of research in the 1990s. The changing demography of America's families. *Journal of Marriage and the Family, 62*, 876–895.

Edin, K., & Lein, L. (1997). *Making ends meet: How single mothers survive welfare and low-wage work.* New York: Russell Sage Foundation.

Fine, M. (2000). Divorce and single-parenting. In C. Hendrick & S.S. Hendrick (Eds.), *Close relationships: A sourcebook* (pp. 139–152). Thousand Oaks, CA: Sage.

Furstenberg, F.F., & Cherlin, A.J. (1991). *Divided families: What happens to children when parents part.* Cambridge, MA: Harvard University Press.

Garmezy, N. (1985). Stress-resistant children: The search for protective factors. In J.E. Stevenson (Ed.), *Recent research in developmental psychopathology* (pp. 213–233). Oxford: Pergamon Press.

Grych, J.H., & Fincham, F.D. (1997). Children's adaptation to divorce: From description to explanation. In S.A. Wolchik & I.N. Sandler (Eds.), *Handbook of children's coping: Linking theory and intervention* (pp. 159–193). New York: Plenum Press.

Hagen, J.L. (1999). Time limits under temporary assistance to needy families: A look at the welfare cliff. *Affilia, 14*, 294–314.

Hamner, T.J., & Turner, P.H. (1990). *Parenting in contemporary society (2nd ed.).* Englewood Cliffs, NJ: Prentice Hall.

Hetherington, E.M., Bridges, M., & Insabella, G.M. (1998). What matters? What does not? Five perspectives on the association between marital transitions and children's adjustment. *American Psychologist, 53*, 167–184.

Kleist, D.M. (1999). Single-parent families: A difference that makes a difference? *The Family Journal: Counseling and Therapy for Couples and Families, 7*, 373–378.

Kurdek, L.A., Fine, M.A., & Sinclair, R.J. (1995). School adjustment in sixth graders: Parenting transitions, family climate, and peer norms effects. *Child Development, 66*, 430–445.

Lin, I. (2000). Perceived fairness and compliance with child support obligations. *Journal of Marriage and the Family, 62*, 388–398.

Manning, W.D., & Lichter, D.T. (1996). Parental cohabitation and children's economic well-being. *Journal of Marriage and the Family, 58*, 998–1010.

Parsons, T., & Bales, R.F. (1955). *Family, socialization and interaction process*. Glencoe, IL: Free Press.

Rawlings, S.W., & Saluter, A. (1995). *Household and family characteristics: March 1994* (US Bureau of the Census. Current Population Reports, P-20, No. 483). Washington, DC: US Government Printing Office.

Simons, R.L., & Associates. (1996). *Understanding differences between divorced and intact families: Stress, interaction, and child outcome*. Thousand Oaks, CA: Sage.

Statistics Canada. (1996). *Microdata file of economic families, 1973 and 1996*.

Statistics Sweden. (2000). *Children and their families: Demographic reports*.

US Bureau of the Census. (1996). *Statistical abstract of the United States*. Washington, DC: US Government Printing Office.

US Department of Health and Human Services. (2001). *Building their futures: How early head start programs are enhancing the lives of infants and toddlers in low-income families*. Washington, DC: Author.

Social Competency, Adolescence

Janet F. Gillespie

INTRODUCTION

Adolescence is a time of growth, challenge, and change. Parents, educators, and adolescents have long tried to do what they can, not only to survive, but to make the most of that major life transition that occurs from age 10–18 (Arnett, 2000). The adolescent years are transforming at all levels: physical, emotional, social, cognitive, and behavioral. Helping professionals have searched for ways for adolescents to acquire the skills necessary to face these many changes. What *is* the best way to promote a high quality of life for adolescents? Can the skills that protect adolescents be taught? The possibilities for both the method and the teacher are many. Positive outcomes may be facilitated by a teen's academic counselor, coach, or parent, among others, or by a girl/boyfriend. Healthy adjustment, however, is the quintessential two-way street. Social competency can only be obtained using resources both from "without" (the environment and all persons in it) and "within" (the adolescent's existing skills, capabilities, and capacity for change).

DEFINITIONS

To promote healthy functioning in adolescents is to facilitate *social competence*—the ability to adapt to change, regulate one's emotions as changes occur, and successfully solve interpersonal problems and challenges (Anderson & Messick, 1974; Goleman, 1995). Alternatively, social competence can be more simply thought of as the ability to show capable behavior whenever one is interacting with other people (McFall, 1982). Cowen (1980) sees use of strategies to promote competency, and prevent emotional disturbance as *primary prevention*. More recently, the term *health promotion* has been used to emphasize strengths and positive aspects of health and development (Durlak & Wells, 1997). Accordingly, health promotion efforts are aimed at creating programs that foster well-being through a variety of techniques, such as teaching cognitive skills that aid effective coping and help ensure mastery of essential life tasks that go with a given age period. The goal is to help adolescents build strengths (resiliencies) that protect them from unhealthy choices and enable them to make life-affirming ones.

SCOPE

The scope of the challenge that adolescents face is vast. Adolescents have always had to cope with the bodily changes of puberty, and the reality of "growing up"; but the risks they face in doing so changed significantly in the 20th century, and remain changed today. Dryfoos (1994) has termed these risks the "new morbidities" for American youth, in contrast to the "old morbidities" of previous generations: chronic and contagious illnesses, and nutritional deficiencies. Although those older "morbidities" have not been completely eradicated, the new, more pervasive threats for American and European youth today are drugs, violence, early sexual activity, and depression. These factors now constitute the biggest risks to adolescents' healthy functioning as they deal with issues of independence, identity formation, and physical, cognitive, and emotional development. Linked to the presence of such threats is the reality that adolescents must often confront strong peer pressure in the context of these risks—pressure to smoke, try alcohol and other drugs, or become sexually active. Many are not able to refuse.

Studies of *epidemiology*, or distribution and prevalence of the "new morbidities," show that approximately 25 percent of US students have smoked a cigarette before age 13 (Duffy & Wong, 2000). Nearly 15 percent of 13–14-year-olds, and 25 percent of 15–16-year-olds surveyed have reported binge drinking (consuming five or more alcoholic drinks at one "sitting") (Bachman, Johnston, O'Malley, & Schulenberg, 1996). The use of drugs other than alcohol has increased as well; the 1997 Youth Risk Behavior Surveillance System found 47 percent of students had tried marijuana, nearly 10 percent before age 13 (Center for Disease Control and Prevention [CDC], 1998). These trends are not limited to the United States. The Canadian Ontario Student Drug Use Survey's (OSDUS) 1997 results showed that 75 percent of high school students had used alcohol, with 60 percent drinking within the past year (Adlaf, Ivis, & Smart, 1997). OSDUS findings also showed 30 percent of high school students trying marijuana at some point, and 25 percent reporting its use within the past year.

Sexually transmitted diseases (STDs), including HIV (nonexistent as a health threat in previous generations), are also a serious health risk to older adolescents, with the US having the highest overall infection rates for its citizens in the industrialized world. Additionally, levels of emotional distress (both depression and mood disorders, as well as anxiety), are also thought to affect more adolescents than ever before (Dryfoos, 1994). It is estimated that between 7 and 8 percent of high school students have attempted suicide, with approximately half of these attempts requiring medical attention (CDC, 1998). Ohberg, Lonnqvist, Sarna, and Vuori (1996) report that in Finland, the European country with the highest rates of suicide and attempted suicide, the rates of suicide (particularly for male adolescents) doubled from 1947 to 1991. Finally, school adjustment and achievement remain a huge concern in education; US dropout rates average 20 percent (Baker & Sansone, 1990).

THEORIES

Decades of scientific study of human development yield valuable theoretical contributions that relate to the promotion of social competency in adolescence. The discipline of *developmental psychology*, for example, contributes several important principles. Developmental psychology's tenets include the *organizational principle*, which holds that development is a series of re-organizations, or re-ordering, of one's behavior in relationship to the demands of the essential tasks in a given developmental period (Carlson & Sroufe, 1995). An example of the organizational principle could be an adolescent's slowly reviewing and revising his or her views about school and having to attend school. As a child, the adolescent might have viewed school and homework assignments very negatively—as nothing more than time away from play. Changing that perspective to view academic excellence, social opportunities, and extracurricular activities as worthwhile allow the adolescent to begin to change his or her behavior as well and move toward greater involvement in school activities, greater investment in receiving good grades, and initiation of dating and romantic relationships. The organizational perspective

also suggests that the rewards of such successful negotiation of "life tasks" is progress toward a healthy, happy adulthood, as success in one stage increases the likelihood of smooth progress toward the next stage and a positive resolution of the next set of milestones. Alternatively, difficulty in coping with adolescent life tasks can result in emotional distress that persists during adolescent and adult years, as incompetence at one stage can predispose one to continued delays in development and/or competence.

Developmental psychologists also view development as a series of *transactions* between the adolescent and those in his or her environment. Each (adolescent and environment) can affect the other in positive and negative ways. The teenager is not a passive recipient of the real-world impact of different choices. He or she can influence or be influenced by other adolescents, teachers, parents, or people in the larger community. This concept is similar to Bronfenbrenner's (1977) *ecological* view of development, which describes multiple spheres of influence representing an adolescent's immediate family, peer group, and wider community. Community and environmental psychologists have also utilized the ecological concept to define goodness of fit, or *person–environment fit*, which refers to the appropriateness of the fit between individuals and the setting in which they find themselves. Thus, a so-called "problem" adolescent might be showing behaviors that are adaptive in one setting, but very unhelpful in another.

Another useful theoretical lens through which to view efforts to improve adolescents' social competency is known as *transition theory*. Felner and Adan (1988) wrote that life transitions can be the springboard for the development of problems that would not have occurred had the proper supports been in place to ease the transition. With guidance, transitions also can be fertile ground for positive change rather than negative change. Finally, *cognitive theories of stress, adjustment, and cognitive skills* relate to adolescents' social competency. Researchers in child adjustment have long surmised that social competence can be "operationalized" or specifically defined as a set of core cognitive skills that are distinct from intelligence as measured by IQ. Indeed, social problem-solving theory holds that those who are better at thinking of ways to solve social problems are at less risk for psychological problems because they possess greater social competence. Finally, cognitive theorists believe that behavior is determined in large part by what a person thinks about the *causes* of events in one's life; behavioral adjustment can be changed for the better by helping people think differently about themselves and the world. The research of Seligman (1991) has proven that those with an optimistic outlook on life get better grades, experience better peer relationships, suffer fewer health problems, and may even improve their life expectancy.

RESEARCH

Exemplary research done in the area of adolescent social competence promotion has taken three major forms. The first is scholarship of a conceptual nature that presents a helpful "lens" through which to view notions of adolescent social competence. The second type of research is *applied* clinical and community research; conducting preventive interventions with real activities and participants, measuring their effects upon the students who were enrolled, and drawing conclusions regarding the program's success. The third type of research is evaluative reviews of others' programmatic efforts; that is, using statistical methods to evaluate the outcomes of programs to determine what works best. An example of the first type of research, conceptual foundations is Gullotta, Adams, and Montemayor's (1990) collection of articles that discuss concepts pertaining to social competence promotion. For example, Bloom (1990) clarified target areas for preventive efforts by classifying the components of social competence in adolescence into categories of *personal* factors (physical and sexual maturation and accompanying thoughts, feelings, and behaviors), *interpersonal* factors (such as the increased importance of peers, and an adolescent's changing views of his or her parents), *social* factors (such as changes in relationships with school personnel and authority figures), and *intercultural* changes (mass media developments such as the Internet, wireless communication, and movies/TV targeted specifically to teens would all figure significantly in this area). Together with these components go personal, interpersonal and social, and environmental factors that may influence resolution of the tasks of adolescence and the success of potential interventions.

Price, Cowen, Lorion, and Ramos-McKay (1988) described 14 evidence-based prevention programs, including several programs for adolescents. These include detailed information on the activities presented; a sound method for indicating the program's success; and measurable, significant changes in behavior that remained with the participants after the program ended.

The third type of research relevant to adolescents' social competency has focused upon using statistics to identify which approaches are most successful. *Meta-analysis* is a statistical method used to calculate effect sizes, numerical values using standard scores that indicate how much participants changed for the better at the end of a program. It is used to compare large groups of prevention program examples that may have differed in number of students enrolled and types of measures used to evaluate program effectiveness. Durlak and Wells (1997), and Tobler, Roona, Ochshorn, Marshall, Streke, and Stackpole (2000), presented meta-analytic reviews which examined success rates for primary prevention programs for behavior problems and substance abuse prevention. A third review, edited by Mrazek and Haggerty (1994), did not use meta-analysis, but rather reviewed the levels of behavioral change shown by pupils enrolled. Taken together, these studies give proof for the value of efforts at social competence promotion with adolescents, as all concluded that certain primary prevention programs are effective, and that it helps adolescents as much, if not more, than more traditional means of intervention (i.e., waiting until problems appear). Moreover, primary prevention is cost-effective and more economical than delivering services to adolescents already showing symptoms. Finally, the personal costs saved (in preventing depression, loneliness, school alienation, and physical illness) are of vital importance. In sum, research in adolescent social competence promotion has helped us see which kinds of programs should be developed, offered on a large scale, and continued based upon their rates of success.

STRATEGIES THAT WORK

The high quality reports described earlier examined hundreds of programs developed to promote social competency in children and adolescents. Several of the most successful will be described here. All are *evidence-based*, or proven to have an impact by using more than one "real-world" index of change (such as school records of grades, absences, visits to school counselors). Also, these programs measured program success with actual self-report, such as questionnaires administered to both enrolled students and teachers. This type of assessment allowed the participants to give information on how well they retained, and benefited from, the material that the programs presented.

The first program is the *Social-Competence Promotion Program for Young Adolescents* (SCPP-YA) (Weissberg & Greenberg, 1998). This middle-school program is conducted in classrooms where a specially trained teacher leads discussions on issues of relevance to teens such as resisting peer pressure, making decisions about sexual behavior, and coping with stress at school. Forty-five sessions are held, emphasizing social problem-solving skills and strategies for decision-making and stress management. In the discussion groups, students learn the steps of social problem-solving, which are to stop and think, to identify what the problem is, to generate possible solutions, and to evaluate their alternatives before trying one out. A "stop light" analogy is used to begin the 5-step social problem-solving process, which is then practiced by the students in role plays. The SCPP-YA has been successful. Students learned better problem-solving strategies that involved less confrontation and conflict, and they were observed putting these new ways into use at their schools. Also, their teachers reported that the students felt better about themselves, were more aware of the need to avoid drugs and sexual acting-out, and dealt with their day-to-day school problems more effectively.

The *Life Skills Training (LST)* program of Botvin and Tortu (1988) sought to prevent drug use in seventh graders, and students were followed up through eighth and ninth grades. The program is based on the idea that substance abuse is the result of many different personal and social factors. LST relies on five modules, or clusters of group meetings, that include the presentation of information on drugs, decision-making skills, self-image improvement, techniques to manage anxiety, and social skills training (including "refusal skills") to help overcome shyness and peer pressure to try cigarettes, drugs, or alcohol. Botvin and Tortu's findings, after implementing the program with seventh graders, showed up to 75 percent fewer students smoking cigarettes (compared to students who were not enrolled), and significantly fewer trying alcohol or marijuana.

The *School Transition Environmental Project* (STEP) by Felner and Adan (1988) was conducted in schools in New Haven, Connecticut. It was designed to prevent students from encountering problems that often occur in middle school or high school such as lowered grades and greater rates of absences. The long-term goal was to decrease rates of dropping out of school at age 16. STEP was based on the premise that a major reason that students do drop out is their negative experience of school at the time of the transition from elementary school to junior high and later high school. As guided by this theory, the major program elements of STEP are to make the school environment less complex and anxiety-provoking, and more welcoming to entering students. For example, one element of the program is changing of the role and availability of home room teachers and guidance counselors so that students receive more individual attention. This was accomplished in part by allowing enrolled STEP students to take all of their classes only with other STEP participants and locating classrooms near each other in the same wing of the building. Home room teachers were also put "in charge" as the main contact for problems encountered by the student and communications with parents. Furthermore, home room teachers incorporated counseling sessions into home room periods. The first evaluation of STEP was done in a large, urban high school with ninth grade students. The results showed that STEP students showed fewer absences from school, smaller decreases in academic performance, and improved self-concepts in comparison to students who had not received the program.

A different approach to competency-building during school transitions is the *School Transition Project* (STP) of Jason and colleagues in Chicago, Illinois (Jason et al., 1992). The STP was designed for sixth graders and emphasized home and school tutoring components, a series of informational sessions for teachers to give them information on the pressures on youth that accompany school transition, and a sixth grade "peer leader" who led welcoming orientation sessions for students at the new school. After the program was over, STP students showed higher academic achievement, felt better about themselves, and more readily participated in school activities. Furthermore, these behavioral gains were maintained at a 1-year follow-up assessment of their behavior.

STRATEGIES THAT MIGHT WORK

All of the social competency programs reviewed thus far have been school based. This reflects the nature of program efforts over the last 20 years. Schools are considered prime settings for intervention, as in that setting one is reaching the largest numbers of adolescents at one time and in one place. Other settings and other approaches, however, most notably those that include parents, hold promise as well. One program that involved early adolescents is *Project CARE* (Hostetler & Fisher, 1997), which encouraged family involvement and had as one of the program goals the improvement of family communication between enrolled fourth graders and their parents. Other goals were to decrease absences and suspensions from school and improve grades, decrease drug use or experimentation, and boost involvement in positive school activities. Although the program did not achieve significant changes in all of these areas, students who participated did derive benefits. They showed higher rates of participation in extracurricular activities and community service than did a comparison group that received no program.

Dusenbury (2000) provided recommendations for drug prevention programs with older children and adolescents that seek to involve the children's parents as a major component. These programs, she noted, need group leaders who share cultural and ethnic similarities to the parents, should always afford parents as much respect as that given the program leaders, must make the program as accessible to parents as possible, and should encourage parents' attendance by providing incentives and reminders of group meetings.

Other strategies that show promise for competency training draw upon existing community-based youth support structures in addition to schools. These settings could include 4-H, Boys & Girls Clubs, and adolescents' workplaces for part-time jobs. Finally, there is growing evidence to support widening all adolescents' participation in existing social structures such as churches, youth sports teams, afterschool programs, and schools offering a unique curriculum (i.e., those high schools that offer a specific job training track—e.g., medical technician apprenticeships; or schools for the arts).

STRATEGIES THAT DO NOT WORK

Gillespie and Ikhlas (1998) reviewed community-based groups for children and adolescents and concluded that some of the most frequently-tried methods in the 1980s appeared to be least effective. Usually, these methods consist of information presentation only, with no active participation on the part of the adolescents assigned to the program. One such method, *Drug Abuse Resistance Education* (DARE), consisted of visits to schools by law enforcement officers who lectured on the dangers of drug and alcohol abuse. Unfortunately, outcome studies (Ennett, Tobler, Ringwalt, & Flewelling, 1994) of DARE's effectiveness were disappointing. Similar outcomes were obtained with the "Just Say No" public service announcement campaigns begun in the 1980s. It would appear that to tell adolescents—i.e., to present didactic, information-giving approaches only—will not sell (convince) them of the value in resisting the temptation to try drugs or alcohol. DARE programs were not without their unique benefits, however. Although it was not a primary goal of the programs, anecdotal evidence shows that DARE improves students' views of law enforcement officers and increases their trust in the police. Data have also shown that single, "one shot" presentations to large groups of students rarely have a lasting impact. Programs that are successful incorporate continuing contact with the adolescents, in many cases including follow-up components through later grades.

SYNTHESIS

This entry has examined strategies for promoting social competency in adolescents. Taken together, these contributions suggest a need for flexibility and innovation in developing interventions, a sensitive ear and eye for noting relevance of interventions to diverse cultural and ethnic groups, and a realization that strategies that work well for children will inevitably need to be tailored to the unique needs of older children and adolescents. The most successful programs of those presented engage adolescents in enthusiastically interactive discussions, allow them to select examples that hold the most meaning and relevance for their lives, provide lots of feedback on their practicing of new skills learned, and remain sensitive to the adolescents' contributions and ideas in defining topics to be included. Durlak and Wells (1997) summarized the characteristics of programs that are most successful as including a focus upon positive and protective factors, encouraging adolescents' participation by providing social support, using peers as role models for positive behaviors, and, perhaps most importantly, paying keen attention to how well the goals of the program were carried out (assessment of *program implementation*).

Tobler (2000) gave recommendations for smoking and drug prevention programs. She emphasized that programs should include information on short-term negative consequences as well as long-term ones; should teach more than one type of refusal-related interpersonal skill, and should avoid lecturing or teacher-centered class discussions. Indeed, it seems clear that *social and emotional learning* (Elias et al., 1997) should become a part of school curricula early in students' school careers and be continued throughout adolescence. Finally, more effort should be paid to other areas of adolescent adjustment. Rare, so far, are the programs that focus upon adolescent dating violence, or lack of contact with extended family. This "dichotomy of target behaviors" (i.e., focusing upon what *not* to do as opposed to pursuing optimal goals) needs much more attention. Practitioners and researchers alike need to explore ways to maximize adolescents' meaningful integration into the adult world. While it is true that one of the prime tasks of adolescence is separation from parents, separation must not equal alienation. The positive benefits of adult–teen teamwork and combined efforts in areas such as community service (e.g., "Make a Difference Day") are ripe for future study and are just beginning to be explored. Taken together, all of these efforts may someday allow attainment of the highest goal of promotion of social competency: parent–child and individual–societal cooperation as co-equals when the adolescent is an adult.

Also see: Social and Emotional Learning entries; Sport; Social Inoculation.

References

Adlaf, E.M., Ivis, F.J., & Smart, R.G. (1997). *Ontario student drug use survey: 1977–1997* (Addiction Research Foundation Research Document No. 136). Toronto: Addiction Research Foundation.

Anderson, S., & Messick, S. (1974). Social competency in young children. *Developmental Psychology, 10*, 282–293.

Arnett, J.J. (2000). Emerging adulthood: A theory of development from the late teens through the twenties. *American Psychologist, 55*, 469–480.

Baker, J., & Sansone, J. (1990). Interventions with students at risk for dropping out of school: A high school responds. *Journal of Educational Research, 83*, 181–186.

Bloom, M. (1990). The psychosocial constructs of social competency. In T.P. Gullotta, G.R. Adams, & R. Montemayor (Eds.), *Developing social competency in adolescence* (pp. 11–27). Newbury Park, CA: Sage.

Botvin, G.J., & Tortu, S. (1988). Preventing adolescent substance abuse through life skills training. In R.H. Price, E.L. Cowen, R.P. Lorion, & J.R. McKay (Eds.), *Fourteen ounces of prevention: A casebook for practitioners* (pp. 98–110). Washington, DC: American Psychological Association.

Bronfenbrenner, U. (1977). Toward an experimental ecology of human development. *American Psychologist, 52*, 513–531.

Carlson, E.A., & Sroufe, L.A. (1995). Contribution of attachment theory to developmental psychopathology. In D. Cicchetti & D.J. Cohen (Eds.), *Developmental psychopathology: Vol. 1. Theory and methods* (pp. 581–617). NY: Wiley.

Centers for Disease Control and Prevention. (1998, August 14). Youth risk behavior surveillance—United States, 1997. *Morbidity and Mortality Weekly Report, 47*(SS-3), 1–89.

Cowen, E.L. (1980). The wooing of primary prevention. *American Journal of Community Psychology, 8,* 258–284.

Dryfoos, J.G. (1994). *Full-service schools: A revolution in mental health and social services for children, youth and families.* San Francisco: Jossey-Bass.

Durlak, J.A., & Wells, A.M. (1997). Primary prevention mental health programs for children and adolescents: A meta-analytic review. *American Journal of Community Psychology, 25,* 115–152.

Dusenbury, L. (2000). Family-based drug abuse prevention programs: A review. *Journal of Primary Prevention, 20,* 337–352.

Elias, M.J., Zins, J.E., Weissberg, R.P., Frey, K.S., Greenberg, M.T., Haynes, N.M., Kessler, R., & Shriver, T.P. (1997). *Promoting social and emotional learning: Guidelines for educators.* Alexandria, VA: Association for Supervision and Curriculum Development.

Ennett, S.T., Tobler, N.S., Ringwalt, C.L., & Flewelling, R.L. (1994). How effective is drug abuse resistance education? A meta-analysis of Project DARE outcome evaluations. *American Journal of Public Health, 84,* 1394–1400.

Felner, R.D., & Adan, A.M. (1988). The school transitional environment project: An ecological intervention and evaluation. In R.H. Price, E.L. Cowen, R.P. Lorion, & J. Ramos-McKay (Eds.), *Fourteen ounces of prevention: A casebook for practitioners* (pp. 111–122). Washington, DC: American Psychological Association.

Gillespie, J.F., & Ikhlas, M. (1998). Groups in the community context. In K.C. Stoiber & T.R. Kratochwill (Eds.), *Handbook of group intervention for children and families* (pp. 29–46). Needham Heights, MA: Allyn & Bacon.

Goleman, D. (1995). *Emotional intelligence.* NY: Bantam.

Gullotta, T.P., Adams, G.R., & Montemayor, R. (1990). Developing social competency in adolescence. In T.P. Gullotta, G.R. Adams, & R. Montemayor (Series Eds.), *Advances in adolescent development* (vol. 3). Newbury Park, CA: Sage.

Hostetler, M., & Fisher, K. (1997). Project C.A.R.E.: A substance abuse prevention program for high-risk youth: A longitudinal evaluation of program effectiveness. *Journal of Community Psychology, 25,* 397–419.

Mrazek, P.J. & Haggerty, R.J. (1994). *Reducing risks for mental disorder: Summary.* Washington, DC: National Academy Press.

Jason, L.A., Weine, A.M., Johnson, J.H., Warren-Sohlberg, L., Filippelli, L.A., Turner, E., & Lardon, C. (1992). *Helping transfer students: Strategies for educational and social readjustment.* San Francisco: Jossey-Bass.

McFall, R.M. (1982). A review and reformulation of the concept of social skills. *Behavioral Assessment, 4,* 1–33.

Ohberg, A., Lonnqvist, J., Sarna, S., & Vuori, E. (1996). Violent methods associated with high suicide mortality among the young. *Journal of the American Academy of Child and Adolescent Psychiatry, 35,* 144–153.

Price, R.H., Cowen, E.L., Lorion, R.P., & Ramos-McKay, J. (1988). *Fourteen ounces of prevention: A casebook for practitioners.* Washington, DC: American Psychological Association.

Seligman, M.E.P. (1991). *Learned optimism.* NY: Alfred A. Knopf.

Tobler, N.S., Roona, M.R., Ochshorn, P., Marshall, D.G., Streke, A.V., & Stackpole, K.M. (2000). School-based adolescent drug prevention programs: 1998 meta-analysis. *Journal of Primary Prevention, 20,* 275–336.

Tobler, N.S. (2000). Lessons learned. *Journal of Primary Prevention, 20,* 261–274.

Weissberg, R.P., & Greenberg, M. (1998). School and community competence enhancement and prevention programs. In W. Damon (Series Ed.), I.E. Siegel & K.A. Renninger (Vol. Eds.), *Handbook of child psychology: Child psychology in practice* (5th ed., vol. 4, pp. 877–954). NY: Wiley.

Social and Emotional Learning, Early Childhood

Susanne A. Denham

INTRODUCTION

Emotional literacy is as vital as any other type of learning and is central to children's ability to interact and form relationships with others—their social competence. Broadly stated, aspects of emotional competence developing through the lifespan include emotional expression and experience, understanding emotions of self and others, and the regulation of emotion. Children become increasingly emotionally competent over time. Growing evidence suggests that such emotional competence contributes not only to children's social competence and well-being during the early childhood years, but also to later outcomes, such as school adjustment and mental health (Denham, 1998; Saarni, 1999). In this entry, the importance of both emotional and social competence (subsumed as social emotional learning, or SEL), along with related risk and resilience factors and programming to promote SEL during early childhood, are outlined.

DEFINITIONS

Emotional competence has recently been acknowledged for its central role in the development of pathways to social competence, to school success, and to mental health and risk, from foundations laid during preschool and early primary grades (Peth-Pierce, 2000). Emotional competence includes expressing emotions that are, or are not, experienced, regulating emotions in ways that are age and socially appropriate, and decoding these processes in others (Halberstadt, Denham, & Dunsmore, 2001). More specifically, emotionally competent children purposefully express a broad variety of emotions without incapacitating intensity or duration. They understand the emotions of themselves and others, and they regulate their emotion when it is "too much" or "too little."

Social competence can be defined as effectiveness in interaction, the result of organized behaviors that meet short- and long-term developmental needs (Rose-Krasnor, 1997). Social competence in the early years has been recognized as key to school success. In the case of preschoolers, socially competent behaviors are organized around the developmental tasks of positive engagement and self-regulation during peer interaction. Following these guiding principles in evaluating social competence, investigators seek information about very specific abilities, behaviors, and motivations, such as initiation of peer interaction, response to provocation, cooperativeness, empathy, inhibition of aggression, and positive demeanor.

SEL refers to the constituents of both emotional and social competence, as promoted by parents, early childhood educators, and preventionists. Thus, the specific abilities we want to promote include all the elements of emotional and social competence listed earlier. The skills of emotional competence are essential for social competence. More attention is given to emotional competence in the following.

SCOPE

The presence of emotional or social competence in preschool and early gradeschool years is related to contemporaneous and later success in school—both with peers and academically (Denham, 1998). Such social success, indexed by peer status (i.e., overall popularity, rejection, or isolation), friendship, and school success, is in turn related to later well-being and successful negotiation of the developmental tasks of adulthood.

Children lacking emotional and social competence enter school at risk for both concurrent and continuing difficulties, such as low peer status, aggression, and early onset conduct disorder (CD) and internalizing disorder. Externalizing and internalizing behavior disorders cause untold difficulty for parents, teachers, the children themselves, and the society as a whole (Campbell & Ewing, 1990). In particular, in promoting SEL, we are concerned with children who exhibit early externalizing behavior problems. First, although many children are oppositional and defiant during the preschool years, when such behaviors are frequent, intense, or persistent (beyond the normal developmental course), they are symptomatic. The prevalence of oppositional defiant disorder (ODD) is from 2 to 16 percent of young children. Manifestations of this pattern of noncompliance are usually evident before age 8.

Aggression plays a pivotal role in continuity from ODD to CD (Loeber, Lahey, & Thomas, 1991). In contrast to ODD, CD includes persistent, more serious forms of behavior difficulties, in which the basic rights of others or age-appropriate societal norms or rules are violated. Thus, although society tolerates sporadic oppositional behavior at young ages, it rarely accepts these more serious symptoms of CD. In general, onset of ODD wanes with age, whereas onset of CD increases, and its diagnosis supersedes that of oppositional disorder where both patterns are present. Children with CD may display aggression to people and animals and/or destroy property. Their aggression is often of a more serious nature than that of ODD children. They often are deceitful and may steal or exhibit other serious rule violations, such truancy, runaway, or curfew violation. The prevalence of CD overall is 6–16 percent cross-nationally. Males and children living in urban settings are over-represented.

CD is related to costly and damaging social problems (e.g., delinquency, substance use, adult mental disorder). Early onset CD, the form which most concerns us here, is exhibited prior to 10 years of age, as early as 5 or 6 years. Although most incidents of CD remit, early onset, as opposed to later onset, is more likely to be persistent and more likely predicts antisocial personality disorder in adulthood.

We are also concerned with internalizing behavior problems. In contrast with ODD and CD, diagnosable dysthymia, depression, and anxiety disorders affect fewer children, as little as 1–3 percent for dysthymia and depression and 5 percent for anxiety disorders (with some nations, such as Finland, reporting somewhat higher prevalence). Even when episodes remit, however, they often recur and interfere with children's competent functioning. In comparison to externalizing problems, fewer prevention programs exist for internalizing problems.

Are young children with diagnosable externalizing and internalizing problems lacking in emotional and social competence? The literature on these problems repeatedly mentions emotional factors. Moreover, such emotion-related descriptors often predict continuity of such behavior problems, although the connection is studied regrettably implicitly (but see Jenkins & Oatley, 2000; Lemerise & Dodge, 2000). Expressing under-regulated anger, misperceiving others (including their emotional expressive and situational cues), and lacking sympathy for others' feelings are hallmarks of emotional competence deficits and, at extreme levels, are markers of externalizing difficulties. Expressing under-regulated anxiety and sadness are hallmarks of emotional competence deficits and, at extreme levels, are markers of internalizing difficulties. When emotional competence is hampered in these ways, it is difficult for children to demonstrate social competence. It is easy to see why the child lacking emotional competence cannot meet, for example, the twin challenges of smoothly joining peers at play while simultaneously responding benignly to provocation.

THEORIES AND RESEARCH

What Specific Risk Factors Compromise SEL in Early Childhood?

Many factors can thwart preschoolers' development of social and emotional competence (Davis, 1999; Peth-Pierce,

2000). These include both intrapersonal and interpersonal/contextual risk factors. Intrapersonal risk factors include gender-related vulnerabilities. Starting from 4 years of age, boys are more likely than girls to engage in physical aggression and antisocial behavior. In contrast, girls show more continuity of internalizing symptoms even during early childhood. Another intrapersonal risk, related to emotional expressiveness, involves temperament. Early temperaments characterized by high levels of negativity when aroused, or by behavioral inhibition and shyness, place young children at risk for externalizing and internalizing difficulties, respectively. Temperamentally difficult 3-year-olds grow up to be impulsive, unreliable, and antisocial, with more conflicts in their social networks and at work. Temperamentally inhibited 3-year-olds were more likely to be unassertive and depressed, with fewer sources of social support. Lack of temperamental attentional control (i.e., attention focusing and shifting), especially in interaction with temperamental negativity, is associated with long-term social dysfunction. Cognitive deficits also play a role, both those that are more general, such as low IQ and delayed language development, and those that are more specific, such as deficiencies in planning and interpersonal problem-solving abilities (potentially related to emotion understanding). Davis (1999) specifically cites deficits in emotional competence, including emotion regulation and delay of gratification, as intrapersonal risk factors. Similarly, lack of relational competence—the abilities to recruit support when needed, to be well thought of in the peer group, and to make and sustain friendships—renders the important tasks of grade school more difficult to attain. Children already rejected in kindergarten are the least adjusted to school by sixth grade. Peer rejection is one of the strongest predictors of eventual school dropout.

Interpersonal/contextual risk factors also are many and varied. They include the following:

1. *Low socioeconomic status* is a marker for multiple risk factors, including lower maternal education; homelessness; unexplained separations from parents; hunger; lack of daily routines; and exposure to violent and otherwise unsafe, chaotic neighborhoods, maltreatment, or neglect.
2. *Absence of a secure attachment relationship* with a caregiver or multiple caregivers leaves a young child at a distinct disadvantage. Such a child has no one person on whom he or she can count in times of distress as a fundamental support for learning and growing and to aid in forming a positive view of their own worth.
3. *Parents' own punitive or inconsistent parenting practices*, and/or their own psychopathology, are related to emotional and social competence problems in their children.
4. Other *family stressors*, such as marital conflict, lack of social support, and parents' experience of daily hassles, also add to the probability of such problems as early as $3^1/_2$ years, particularly when these stressors are cumulative.
5. There is some evidence that *intrapersonal and interpersonal risks, in combination*, are also important. For example, the interaction of negative emotionality and parental conflict may be a particularly potent predictor of internalizing disorders at the end of the preschool period. Analogously, the interaction of early externalizing and parental punitiveness predict later externalizing disorder.

Protective factors exist which can moderate the deleterious effects of existent risk factors. These include intrapersonal and interpersonal/contextual factors and parallel the enumerated risk factors. Intrapersonally, the confident child with an "easy" temperament, who exhibits relatively high cognitive functioning, is relationally competent enough to have friends (or be able to make them when exposed to peers), and has an early history of functioning well with respect to developmental milestones, has a better chance of also marshaling the component skills of emotional and social competence by kindergarten entry. Regarding interpersonal/contextual protective factors, parental investment and involvement in the child's development is a key advantage. Concomitant with this positive involvement is the presence of the child's caring relationship with at least one adult. As Peth-Pierce (2000) has noted, children's early relationships are the foundation for their emotional and social competence during the preschool and early primary years. Social support for the child and parents also can be crucial and adds to the benefits of positive parenting practices.

Durlak and Wells (1997), in their meta-analysis of mental health prevention programs, assert that clear goals (e.g., maximizing emotional and social competence) and targeted risk and protective factors, many of which offer the opportunity for change, are necessary for the success of prevention programs.

Halberstadt, Denham, and Dunsmore (2001) propose a theoretical model of *affective social competence*, which includes skills of sending, receiving, and experiencing emotions. Feelings are experienced, inferred, and talked about within social interactions and relationships and elaborated into expectancies that guide future interactions. Although sending (expressing), receiving (understanding), experiencing (closely related to regulating) are considered to be distinct component skills, all are interrelated within the ongoing flow of social interaction and relationships (i.e., they are not called for at different times, but simultaneously). All are situated within particular contexts (e.g., the particular sets of skills needed in interacting with a father who has had a bad day are different from those necessary when approaching a friend with a new scooter). In addition, self-factors such as temperament, demeanor, and self-esteem moderate the component skills. Finally, cultural issues are important to consider, because differing groups value differing dimensions of emotional life.

In this theory, we refer to *experience of emotions* as not only the awareness and recognition of one's own emotions but also as the effective regulation of one's emotional expression in the context of an ongoing social interaction. What happens when children (or anyone, for that matter) experience emotion? First, there is arousal. Sometimes this arousal is limited to lower, more primitive brain systems. When a boy falls, emotion and its attendant behavior ensue automatically. As higher brain functioning becomes increasingly involved in emotional experience, children create an increasingly complicated network of desires and outcomes they want to attain. Arousal gives the child key information about these ongoing goals and coping potential, but the information needs to be understood, not just reacted to. How does a shy boy's "stomach butterflies" affect his goal of joining play, if at all? What does this arousal mean? Before he feels any emotion, or others notice any, the boy must attend to the event, comprehend, and interpret it. Such goal-related interpretations lead not only to felt emotions but also to actions associated with each specific emotion and new changes in arousal. Does the boy try to "deal with" his jitters? Do his regulation attempts work, so he really is calmer, with better chances for social success?

We postulate important abilities within this element of emotional competence. The first ability is the simple recognition that one is experiencing an emotion. The valence of the emotion possibly is registered at this level of skill. This low-level awareness enables higher level abilities of understanding: "What emotional signal am I sending to these other persons?" "How do my emotional signals affect them?" Next, one must comprehend one's emotional experience within the constraints of the emotion-scripts that are active and the ongoing social context. Knowledge of feeling rules may guide children in selecting aspects of their emotional experiences upon which to focus.

Understanding one's own emotions within the social context also includes realizing that inner and outer emotional states may differ (i.e., sending more, fewer, or different affective messages than those which are felt, based on others' expectations: "I know I feel really scared, but I need to be calm."). Such attunement to one's own emotions may yield interpersonal benefits as well. Children's similarities of emotional experience allow them to predict and read others' emotions.

With respect to regulation or management of emotional experience, we consider those emotions that are aversive or distressing, those that are positive but possibly overwhelming, and those that need to be amplified for either intra- or interpersonally strategic reasons. To succeed at such emotion regulation, several abilities are key. One must experience clear rather than diffuse feelings to know what to regulate. Managing "false" signals is also crucial, as in the case of the boy who had a sudden "tummy rumble" as he neared the others but ignored it as not pertinent. One also can use false self-signals to facilitate communication and achieve a goal. Consider the falling boy who feels mad at himself as well as hurt. Maybe he can "use" his anger to motivate a quick, albeit hobbling, recovery. Children learn to retain or enhance those emotions that are relevant and helpful, to attenuate those that are relevant but not helpful, and to dampen those that are irrelevant. Moderating emotional intensity when it threatens to overwhelm, enhancing it when necessary to meet a goal, and shifting between emotion states via coping help children to maintain genuine and satisfying relationships with others.

Another key element of emotional competence is *emotional expressiveness*, the sending of affective messages. These emotions must be expressed in keeping with the child's goals but also in accordance with the social context. For the emotionally competent child, the goals of self and of others must be taken into account and coordinated. Thus, emotional competence includes expressing emotions in a way that is advantageous to moment-to-moment interaction and relationships over time. First, emotionally competent individuals are aware, at least at some level, that an affective message needs to be sent in a given context. But what affective message should be sent for interaction to proceed smoothly? Children slowly learn which expressions of emotion facilitate specific goals. Second, children must also come to determine the appropriate affective message for the given social context. What is appropriate in one setting or with one person may not be appropriate elsewhere. Third, children must also learn how to send the situationally appropriate, intended message convincingly. Method, intensity, and timing of sending an affective message are crucial to its meaning and its eventual success or failure. Showing slight annoyance for a short while over a best friend's winning a game is different from remaining very angry for days. As well, one must keep in mind the constraints of display rules. Finally, and most difficult, one must consider characteristics of interaction partners and their interpersonal interchange.

At times it is necessary to manage "false" affective signals sent to others. There are times when real affective messages are not appropriate. Some are relevant to the situation but not the context, and some irrelevant ones need to be masked. For example, disappointment and even rage at being reprimanded by a parent may be relevant but imprudent to express. Anxiety when playing a new game is probably irrelevant to the goal of having fun and needs to be suppressed.

Understanding emotion lies at the heart of emotional competence, with both experiencing and expressing emotions contributing to understanding, and understanding contributing to both other aspects. There are four components of this element of emotional competence. An initial appraisal that another person is sending affective information is necessary. Missing such information definitely puts one at a disadvantage. For example, if a girl misses the muted expressions of annoyance on her friend's face, she may gloat about her new toy. Once perceived, the other individual's affective message, and its intensity, must be interpreted. Ability to use emotion language is also crucial.

Realizing that inner and outer emotional states may differ, and that different individuals have differing emotional "styles," is also important. One must be able to ignore false affective messages or accept them as real, whichever is more advantageous. Conversely, managing others' true signals can be tricky, too. A child must: (1) pick up real, relevant, helpful messages; (2) ignore real but irrelevant messages; and (3) somehow deal with real and relevant but not helpful messages. In terms of real but not helpful messages, children have to decide whether to censor certain expressions that are momentary "blips."

One more theoretical perspective is informative here. *Social information processing theory*—encoding information from the social surround, interpreting it, forming goals, selecting and enacting what the child considers the most favorable response—now includes emotional information and content at every step (Lemerise & Arsenio, 2000). Children are constantly attempting to understand their own and others' behavior, and emotions play a role in this understanding. In the *encoding and interpreting* steps, the child takes in the important information from others' behavior, emotions, intentions, and the likely effect of the others' behavior, as well as his/her own arousal level, the intensity of the emotions felt, and his/her relationship with others. In the next step, *clarification of goals*, the child formulates goals which are themselves focused arousal states that function to motivate him or her to produce outcomes. When a child cannot regulate her emotion, she may focus on external goals, such as revenge, or may retreat into passivity, neither of which promotes social competence. A child who more successfully regulates emotions is more able to focus on competence-related, perhaps even relationship-enhancing, goals. The child's perception of the other's emotions may also affect the goals chosen. In the last step, *response generation, evaluation, decision*, access to and choice of responses differ depending on the child's goals. If the child is mired in under-regulated anger and hurt, then pre-emptive cognitive processing may take place rather than the effortful processing needed to choose a socially competent behavioral response.

Rose-Krasnor's (1997) recent theorizing is useful in this regard. She puts forward a *prism model* in which the topmost level (Theoretical) defines the construct of social competence as effectiveness in interaction, the result of organized behaviors that meet short- and long-term developmental needs. In the case of preschoolers, socially competent behaviors would be organized around the developmental tasks of positive engagement and self-regulation during peer interaction. Within this theoretical view of social competence, it is also necessary to decide whether to focus on the self-domain or the other domain. Are we interested in accessing the child's success in meeting personal goals or in interpersonal connectedness? To this end, the middle level of the prism (Index) reflects success in both intra- and interpersonal goals, for example, qualities of relationships, group status, and social self-efficacy. The bottom level of Rose-Krasnor's model (Skills) includes very specific social, emotional, cognitive abilities, behaviors, and motivations that are primarily individual.

Organizational views of competence are also important. *Organizational* theorists emphasize the dynamic involvement of biological factors, affect, cognition, and behavior, along with the multiply important contexts in which the child is involved, to describe and explain competent behavior— "developmental tasks"—at differing age levels. At the preschool/primary grade level, the developmental tasks include managing emotional communication and maintaining positive engagement with peers (Parker & Gottman, 1989). The prevention of dysfunction and the promotion of SEL require attention to these multiple contributors to the child's growth.

STRATEGIES: OVERVIEW

It makes intuitive sense, following the theoretical perspectives already detailed, that facets of emotional competence should contribute to success in interacting with one's peers (i.e., social competence) and serve as a platform for later well-being, success in school, and ultimately vocation and adult relationships. Accumulating evidence suggests that this is true. Emotions are central in the task of maintaining positive engagement—dealing with negative conflict, remaining emotionally regulated in the face of arousal, taking pleasure in interaction, and understanding one's partner's cues (see Denham, 1998).

Emotional expressiveness

At its simplest level, this aspect of emotional competence refers to the individual child's profile of frequency, intensity, and/or duration of basic and complex emotions—happiness, sadness, anger, fear, guilt, and empathy, for example. Preschoolers' expression of specific emotions, especially their enduring patterns of expressiveness, relates to their peer status and to their teachers' evaluation of their friendliness and aggression. *Positive* affect is important in the initiation and regulation of social exchanges and for communication during socially directed acts. Sharing positive affect may facilitate the formation and persistence of friendships. Peers like happier children, and their teachers see them as friendly and cooperative. Conversely, *negative* affect can be quite problematic during social interaction. Preschoolers, who show larger proportions of negative affect, particularly anger, are often seen by both teachers and peers as troublesome and difficult. Specifically, angrier preschoolers are rated as disliked by their peers and as aggressive, independent, unfriendly, and uncooperative by their teachers. Young children who respond to the emotional needs of others, sharing positive affect and reacting prosocially rather than antisocially to others' distress, are more likely to succeed in the peer arena. Teachers and peers alike view preschoolers who react both empathically and prosocially to peers' emotions as more socially competent.

Emotion Knowledge

As noted earlier, emotion knowledge yields information about emotional expressions and experience in the self and others which is used to understand and interpret events in the environment. Such information refers not only to one's own and others' expressions and experience of emotions but also to situations that elicit emotion; the duration and intensity of emotions; display rules; simultaneous emotions; person-specific aspects of emotions (e.g., one playmate likes preschool; another feels sad when he arrives); and effective strategies of emotion regulation.

Children's understanding of emotion in themselves and in others develops in important ways during the 2nd and 3rd years. From 2 years of age on, young children are interested in emotions. In spontaneous conversations, they talk about and reflect upon their own and others' feelings and discuss causes and consequences of their own and others' emotional experiences and expressiveness (Dunn, 1994). Throughout the rest of the preschool period, children come to understand many aspects of the expression and situational elicitation of basic emotions (with negative emotions slowly emerging as separate). Toward the end of the period, they begin to comprehend complex dimensions of emotional experiences, such as the possibility of simultaneous emotions, but often show this understanding best when child-friendly methods are used. Through the early years of elementary school, much understanding is consolidated regarding simultaneity of emotions, display rules, personalized emotional experiences, and varied emotion regulatory strategies (Denham, 1998).

Although there are developmental progressions in the various aspects of emotion knowledge, with knowledge of expressions and situations preceding other sorts of understanding, there also are marked individual differences in these developments. These relatively stable individual differences are correlated with differences in children's experiences of family discourse concerning feelings, causes, and consequences, and with differences in family relations (Dunn, 1994). Such emotion knowledge often is associated with aspects of social competence. For example, children who understand emotions more proficiently respond more appropriately to others (including more prosocial reactions to others' emotions, as when one playmate is angry about another's purported "cheating"), better regulate their own emotions, and are more liked by peers. Disruptive, hard-to-manage preschoolers often show deficits in this aspect of emotional competence.

Emotion Experience and Regulation

Emotion regulation is the ability to modify the intensity, duration, or even valence of emotional expression and/or experience by emotion-related, cognitive, or behavioral means. Children who regulate emotions capably are more well-liked and seen as functioning well socially by teachers across a range of ages from preschool to the end of gradeschool.

Socialization of Emotional Competence

If emotional competence is intimately related to social competence and mental health, then the question of its cultivation must be answered by creating effective prevention programs. Three mechanisms describe such socialization: modeling emotional expressiveness, teaching about emotion, and reactions to children's emotions (Denham, 1998). Each of these mechanisms can influence children's emotional expression, understanding, and regulation, as well as social functioning. Of course, parents are not the only socializers of emotional competence. Others are important from preschool on. Specifically, with regard to modeling, exposure to parents' and others' broad but not overly negative emotions helps children learn about emotions and come to express similar profiles. In particular, whether in families or classrooms, adult negative emotion is deleterious to young children's emotion knowledge and profile of expressiveness. Parents' and others' reactions to children's emotions are also related to understanding, expression, and regulation of emotions. As well, parents and others' *teaching* about emotions promote emotional competence. For example, in one study of children in child care transitions

(Dunn, 1994), preschoolers remembered both sadness and fear during these times, as well as the support given them by teachers and friends, to help them feel better. In terms of promoting SEL, teacher/caregiver training should include a focus on ways of sustaining adult–child interchanges about emotions. More broadly, secure, warm relationships with parents and/or teacher are vital to young children's emotional and social competence (Mardell, 1992).

STRATEGIES THAT WORK

Because of the crucial nature of early childhood SEL, and the considerable risk associated with their lack, there has been a call for primary prevention programs targeted at preschoolers' emotional and social competence needs. For those at special risk, and for children in general, the learning of emotional and social competence should not be left to chance. In fact, theoretical and empirical evidence of risk and potential reviewed so far suggest the utility of universal prevention to assist in lowering the incidence and prevalence of related problems (e.g., aggression, depression, anxiety, impulsiveness, antisocial behavior) and increasing the probability of successful management of social–emotional developmental tasks. Nonetheless, there have been few large-scale efforts to provide programs focusing on these goals for preschool children. Unfortunately, early childhood educators' concern with social–emotional development often remains implicit rather than being made explicit through specific interventions. Many preventionists, despite acknowledging the utility of early programming, institute programs only when children reach school age (Weissberg & Greenberg, 1998).

What overarching principles can inform prevention programs to promote SEL and deter early behavior problems and their sequelae? Durlak and Wells' recent meta-analysis (1997) asserts that a prevention approach works for a wide range of ages, from toddlers to adolescents, with the following provisos. Programs must work from a theoretical perspective and implement specific strategies to alter developmental trajectories. Specific risk and protective factors already enumerated should be targeted as far as is possible. Multiple components and intervening in multiple contexts are necessary to facilitate both person-centered and environmental change by involving peers, parents, teachers, and school climate. To be effective, programs should span multiple years. Realistically, it takes time to assist development and change existing behavior patterns. To be able to evaluate the effectiveness of programs, experimental or quasi-experimental designs should be utilized, and the fidelity and dosage of implementation must be specified. Finally, "the earlier the better" are the watchwords for primary prevention of deficits in SEL.

There are few programs that fully and directly address SEL during early childhood. Four exist that meet many of the Durlak and Wells' requisites and have met with some success. Two of these include specific parent-training components, addressing compliance and oppositionality problems common in families with preschool children, and focusing mainly on social skills training when working directly with children. First, a bimodal prevention program for disruptive kindergarten boys included social problem solving and cognitive–behavioral training for the children, along with parent training in child development and parenting practices for mothers (Tremblay, Pagani-Kurtz, Masse, Vitaro, & Pihl, 1995). Mothers were trained to monitor their children's behavior and to give children positive reinforcement for prosocial behavior. Another set of program components emphasized training parents to discipline effectively without using abusive punishment, teaching them family crisis management techniques, and encouraging transfer from lessons to home. The child component of the program focused on altering participants' social acceptance as well as their peers' behavior so that participants would be less inclined to turn to antisocial activities. To this end, boys were exposed to prosocial skills and self-control training as well as problem-solving lessons, and they spent time during lunch periods with prosocial peers and professionals in small groups. This program has shown beneficial effects into adolescence.

Webster-Stratton's (1998) combination of training mothers about positive discipline and effective parenting skills, and training their Head Start 4-year-olds in social skills is also effective. For example, mothers who have experienced Webster-Stratton's program, in comparison with those who have not, make fewer critical remarks and commands, use less harsh discipline and more positive parenting, and are more involved in their children's education. Their children, exposed to a program to strengthen their prosocial and social skills, exhibit fewer conduct problems, less noncompliance, less negative affect, and more positive affect. In this program, home–school consistency and parent involvement are also promoted. Training includes a 4-day workshop for parents, with ongoing weekly supervision, vignettes on video, role-plays, activities and stories, and homework. Implementation of the training program is tracked via weekly checklists of group process, parent interest, and participation. These improvements were largely maintained after one year.

Two other programs center more specifically on aspects of emotional competence addressed here. The *Second Step* program (Frey, Hirschstein, & Guzzo, 2000) is a self-named "violence prevention" program spanning preschool through Grade 9. Grounded in social learning theory, it includes key units on the promotion of empathy, social problem solving (also including ignoring distractions, interrupting politely, dealing with wanting something that's not yours), impulse control, and anger management (including triggers for anger, calming down, self-talk, reflection, keeping out of a fight, and dealing with teasing). The empathy unit especially stresses many aspects of emotion knowledge (identifying feelings, looking for similarities and differences or changes in feelings, predicting feelings, and communicating feelings). Both general competencies and domain-specific skills (e.g., resisting peer pressure to victimize unpopular peers) are addressed. Practice in these skills is achieved through modeling followed by role-plays and discussion. The program is supported by the organization and management of the classroom.

Finally, Denham and Burton's (1996; Burton & Denham, 1999) program includes core teacher/center training in ways to foster the elements of social and emotional competence we have enumerated here. All children participating in this program showed gains on both teacher-report and observed indices of social competence although those at most risk (i.e., with the greatest evidence of disruptive and/or anxious behavior) benefited most.

First, creating attachment relationships is vital (Burton & Denham, 1999; Mardell, 1992). Secure attachment with a primary caregiver can buffer preschoolers from emotional competence deficits, altering vulnerability and enhancing resilience. The securely-attached child feels confident to explore the social world and to seek emotional closeness with others during stress or arousal. A consistently-responsive adult also provides the child with a model for competent social interaction upon which to build other relationships. Children may even seek psychological proximity to teachers when their prior attachment history is insecure. Such relationships are promoted in this prevention program through use of "floor time," a means of building a warmth and intimacy between caregiver and child.

Second, for teachers and caregivers of young children who are already demonstrating signs of emotional and social competence deficits, positive behavior management must be an integral part of SEL programs. Fortunately, positive discipline can also further the goals of SEL. Bergin and Bergin (1999) advocate the use of persistent persuasion until the child complies, without increasing the level of power assertion or using coercive threats. The overuse of power assertion can damage adult–child relationships and fails to promote the child's internal motivation. In fact, power assertive behavior management can actually entrain the child in aggression and raise the expectancy level for coercion.

In the use of persistent persuasion, coercive elements are veiled, if not nonexistent. Such ambiguity increases the child's tendency to attribute their compliance to self-motivation. Affective aspects of this discipline are also

important. Explaining to the child why one is pleased or displeased with his or her behavior, with feeling, is associated with emotional competence (Berkowitz & Grych, 2000). Thus, some felt anxiety, in the context of the warm relationship, motivates the child to comply.

Thinking about the effect of one's actions on others also requires understanding one's own feelings. Emotion understanding is, then, the third component of this program. With such knowledge, children can learn to regulate emotions by attaching a label to feelings inside and bringing them to consciousness. Recognizing her own feelings, she can also begin to empathize with others' feelings. The intervention emphasized didactic activities in understanding and labeling emotions, in order to provide the child with the use of these feeling words with which to label affect in self and others, and in recognizing that actions can cause emotions.

Once feelings are recognized and labeled, the child must learn to regulate the expression of those feelings into socially acceptable channels. In this program, then, children are taught a validated method of controlling negative feelings, the Turtle Technique. They learn to imagine that they are turtles retreating into their shells when they feel scared or hurt or angry, pulling their arms close to their bodies, putting their heads down, and closing their eyes. They then relax their muscles to cope with tension. This gives them time to regulate feelings, reflect on them, and decide how to react to their causes.

Experience in talking through affect-laden social problems and concerns also enhances the child's ability to solve problems that occur with peers. Thus, the fourth component of the program was instruction in interpersonal cognitive problem solving (ICPS). This approach improves an individual's ability to think through interpersonal conflicts through the habit of generating multiple options, evaluating these options, and using step-by-step means to reach their goal. Denham and Almeida's (1987) meta-analysis of then-extant evaluation research on ICPS programs revealed that these programs do result in successful ICPS skills acquisition in preschool-aged children. Also, on average, children's behavior does change in a prosocial direction. In this program, ICPS techniques were expanded to include emphasis on prosocial alternative solutions with aggressive children.

Finally, the complex interplay of factors that influence development is unique to each child. Accordingly, it is important for optimum transfer, as well as for efficient use of time and resources, that work with each child be individualized in a way that utilizes all program components but tailors information from each to meet the child's particular needs during emotional and social events. Teachers are taught to investigate the history of the child and use that information to facilitate effective interventions. In particular, dialoguing involves identifying the problem "in vivo" and talking about the feelings of all parties related to the problem. Burton and Denham (1999; see also Denham & Almeida, 1987) found that including discussion of feelings in the dialoguing process, both one's own and those of the other parties involved, was a critical aspect of their program.

STRATEGIES THAT MIGHT WORK

Several large-scale early childhood education programs include some, but not all, aspects that are deemed crucial for SEL prevention programs. First, Head Start Mental Health Curriculum components include some of the above but are not organized similarly and do not appear as extensive (US DHHS, 1996, 1997). Although its major components address other issues, some aspects of the HighScope preschool curriculum may augment the SEL components above (e.g., the self-confidence enhancement involved in choosing a "center" at which to play, the empowerment and practice in relating experience symbolically involved in reporting on one's experiences). Some of these elements could be incorporated profitably into comprehensive SEL prevention programs.

Parent involvement works in other prevention programs (see Tremblay et al., 1995; Webster-Stratton, 1998; also Strayhorn & Weidman, 1991; Weissberg & Greenberg, 1998) and needs even more systematic evaluation and inclusion in SEL programs. The active engagement of parents can provide opportunities to facilitate SEL within the home, a domain that is particularly relevant for preschool children whose social world is only beginning to expand. It is also important that parenting programs have been effective specifically in strengthening parents with multiple risk factors.

Further, classroom climate, school ecology and neighborhood issues are very important. We believe that early childhood classrooms can be "caring communities," in which affective bonds develop between the child and the community, promoting acceptance and internalization of community mores. To this end, SEL concepts should be generalized across children's daily activities and integrated with other important themes of learning (Elias et al., 1997). Further, not only teachers, but all key adults in the school environment (e.g., center directors, bus drivers, teachers' aides), should be trained in SEL strategies.

Recent empirical evidence suggests promise for comprehensive SEL strategies that include classroom climate as well parent training and teacher training. Hawkins, Catalano, Morrison, O'Donnell, Abbott, and Day's (1992) work upheld hypothesizes that (1) training teachers to teach and manage classrooms in ways that promote greater opportunities for active student and involvement and recognition for positive participation in the classroom, (2) training parents to manage families in ways that increase opportunities and recognition for positive involvement in the family and school, and (3) providing children with skills for social interaction, would strengthen children's bonds of commitment to education and attachment to family and school. In turn, stronger bonding to school and family was associated with children's improved academic achievement and the decreased likelihood that they would engage in disapproved of behaviors. Thus, we need to reach beyond the classroom to influence the lives of all of the adults with whom children have contact. This concept has particular relevance for early childhood education.

STRATEGIES THAT DO NOT WORK

Short-term programs do not work. Most programs begun now, as opposed to those of the 1970s and 1980s, try to heed this caveat. Isolated behavior modification programs are unlikely to succeed in promoting long-lasting SEL. Behavioral interventions are often methodologically rigorous, showing high effectiveness, but there are definite concerns about ecological validity, particularly in reference to generalization of the behavior change as well as its simplistic nature (cf. Bergin & Bergin, 1999). Similarly, social skills training alone (i.e., teaching children to increase their competence in specific skills but not from a emotional competence/resilience perspective) may work, but only in the short term.

SYNTHESIS

Many kernels of effective SEL programming in early childhood have been introduced. Making these possibilities explicit within early childhood education, rather than implicit, is a priority that we can no longer postpone. Although there is much evidence-based research to support the importance of early social and emotional competence, as well as growing support for specific SEL practices during early childhood, more focused attention on effective SEL programming and successful implementation is needed. Our children deserve this care.

Also see: Social and Emotional Learning entries.

References

Bergin, C., & Bergin, D.A. (1999). Classroom discipline that promotes self-control. *Journal of Applied Developmental Psychology, 20,* 189–206.

Berkowitz, M.W., & Grych, J.H. (2000). Early character development and education. *Early Education and Development, 11,* 56–72.

Burton, R., & Denham, S.A. (1999). "Are you my friend?": A qualitative analysis of a social–emotional intervention for at-risk four-year-olds. *Journal of Research in Childhood Education, 12,* 210–224.

Campbell, S., & Ewing, L.J. (1990). Follow-up of hard-to-manage preschoolers: Adjustment at age 9 and predictors of continuing symptoms. *Journal of Child Psychology and Psychiatry, 31,* 871–889.

Davis, N.J. (1999). *Resilience: Status of the research and research-based programs*. Working draft. Rockville, MD: Center for Mental Health Services. http://www.mentalhealth.org/consumersurvivor/5-28resilience.htm, 7/24/01.

Denham, S.A. (1998). *Emotional development in young children*. New York: Guilford Press.

Denham, S.A., & Almeida, M.C. (1987). Children's social problem-solving skills, behavioral adjustment, and interventions: A meta-analysis evaluating theory and practice. *Journal of Applied Developmental Psychology, 8*, 391–409.

Denham, S.A., & Burton, R.A. (1996). A social-emotional intervention for at-risk 4-year-olds. *Journal of School Psychology, 34*, 225–245.

Dunn, J. (1994). Understanding others and the social world: Current issues in developmental research and their relation to preschool experiences and practice. *Journal of Applied Developmental Psychology, 15*, 571–583.

Durlak, J.A., & Wells, A.M. (1997). Primary prevention mental health programs for children and adolescents: A meta-analytic review. *American Journal of Community Psychology, 26*, 115–152.

Elias, M.J., Zins, J.E., Weissberg, R.P., Frey, K.S., Greenberg, M.T., Haynes, N.M., Kessler, R., Schwab-Stone, M.E., & Shriver, T.P. (1997). *Promoting social and emotional learning: Guidelines for educators*. Alexandria, VA: ASCD.

Frey, K.S., Hirschstein, M.K., & Guzzo, B.A. (2000). Second step: Preventing aggression by promoting social competence. *Journal of Emotional and Behavioral Disorder, 8*, 102–110.

Halberstadt, A., Denham, S.A., & Dunsmore, J. (2001). Affective social competence. *Social Development, 10*, 79–119.

Hawkins, J.D., Catalano, R.F., Morrison, D.M., O'Donnell, J., Abbott, R.D., & Day, L.E. (1992). The Seattle Social Development Project: Effects of the first four years on protective factors and problem behaviors. In J.McCord & R.E. Tremblay (Eds.), *Preventing antisocial behavior: Interventions from birth through adolescence* (pp. 139–161). New York: Guilford.

Jenkins, J.M., & Oatley, K. (2000). Psychopathology and short-term emotion: The balance of affects. *Journal of Child Psychology and Psychiatry, 41*, 463–472.

Lemerise, E., & Arsenio, W.F. (2000). An integrated model of emotion processes and cognition in social information processing. *Child Development, 71*, 107–118.

Lemerise, E.A., & Dodge, K.A. (2000). The development of anger and hostile interactions. In M. Lewis & J.M. Haviland-Jones (Eds.), *Handbook of emotions* (pp. 594–606). New York: Guilford.

Loeber, R., Lahey, B.B., & Thomas, C. (1991). Diagnostic conundrum of oppositional defiant disorder and conduct disorder. *Journal of Abnormal Psychology, 100*, 379–390.

Mardell, B. (1992). A practitioner's perspective on the implications of attachment theory for daycare professionals. *Child Study Journal, 22*, 201–232.

Parker, J.G., & Gottman, J.M. (1989). Social and emotional development in a relational context: Friendship interaction from early childhood to adolescence. In T.J. Berndt & G.W. Ladd (Eds.), *Peer relationships in child development*. New York: Wiley.

Peth-Pierce, R. (2000). *A good beginning: Sending America's children to school with the social and emotional competence they need to succeed*. Chapel Hill, NC: The Child Mental Health Foundations and Agencies Network. http://www.nimh.nih.gov/childhp/fdnconsb.htm, 7/24/01.

Rose-Krasnor, L. (1997). The nature of social competence: A theoretical review. *Social Development, 6*, 111–135.

Saarni, C. (1999). *Emotional competence*. New York: Guilford Press.

Strayhorn, J.M., & Weidman, C.S. (1991). Follow-up of one year after parent–child interaction training: Effects on behavior of preschool children. *Journal of the American Academy of Child and Adolescent Psychiatry, 30*, 138–143.

Tremblay, R.E., Pagani-Kurtz, L., Masse, L.C., Vitaro, F., & Pihl, R.O. (1995). A bimodal preventive intervention for disruptive kindergarten boys: Its impact through mid-adolescence. *Journal of Consulting and Clinical Psychology, 63*, 560–568.

US DHHS, ACYF, ACF, Head Start Bureau (1996). *Promoting mental health*. Washington, DC: US Government Printing Office.

US DHHS, ACYF, ACF, Head Start Bureau (1997). *Supporting children with challenging behaviors: Relationships are key*. Washington, DC: US Government Printing Office.

Webster-Stratton, C. (1998). Preventing conduct problems in Head Start children: Strengthening parenting competencies. *Journal of Consulting and Clinical Psychology, 66*, 715–730.

Weissberg, R.P., & Greenberg, M.T. (1998). School and community competence-enhancement and prevention programs. In I.E. Sigel & A. Renninger (Eds.), *Handbook of child psychology: Child psychology in practice* (5th ed., Vol. 4, pp. 955–998). New York: John Wiley.

Social and Emotional Learning, Childhood

Joseph E. Zins, Maurice J. Elias, and Keith J. Topping

INTRODUCTION

Children and youth throughout the world face significant social and emotional demands in their lives every day. For most that includes functioning in school, dealing with peer and media pressure, working cooperatively and productively with others, making responsible value judgments and decisions regarding their health and behavior, and contributing as members of their family and community. Many must deal with the uncertainty that accompanies the threat or actuality of violence, terrorism, or war. To be successful in these endeavors they must acquire the necessary and appropriate knowledge, critical understanding, skills, attitudes, beliefs, and values. There is increasing evidence that systematically teaching children social and emotional skills helps provide the foundation for their cognitive and behavioral development. A balanced education emphasizing the integration of academic, social, and emotional learning can enhance school performance and more generally promote the positive development of youth. Becoming competent in these areas enhances the likelihood that children and adolescents will be on a positive trajectory to become knowledgeable, responsible, caring, productive, nonviolent, and ethical citizens (Elias et al., 1997).

DEFINITIONS

Many terms have been used to refer to aspects of *social and emotional learning* (SEL), including character education, positive youth development, and social competence promotion. Although there are more similarities than differences in the terms, SEL has achieved widespread recognition and acceptance as a broad, scientifically based, umbrella concept. It provides a common framework that can be applied to programs with many diverse outcomes.

SEL is defined as the integration and coordination of affect, cognition, and behavior concerning functioning in the social world. Skills and knowledge in four major domains are developed: (a) life skills and social competencies; (b) health-promotion and problem prevention skills; (c) coping skills and social support for use with transitions and crises; and (d) positive, contributory service (Elias et al., 1997).

SEL is embodied in a wide variety of efforts, ranging from informal activities in an individual classroom to coordinated, school-district wide programs. Examples include classroom management strategies emphasizing positive behavior supports; social skills education such as social problem solving and assertiveness training; alcohol, tobacco, and other drug prevention and resistance programs; conflict resolution and violence prevention; health education and promotion; and character or citizenship education. Usually steps are taken to create a supportive organizational climate to bolster to these efforts.

SCOPE

A growing number of young people in the United States, Canada, the United Kingdom, and other western counties either are experiencing or are at risk for developing significant social, behavioral, and health problems. Many of these students are facing a similar situation with respect to succeeding in school. These difficulties must be framed against the backdrop of disruptions in the socialization process in a rapidly changing world.

Mental health needs have long surpassed the capacity to provide them (Albee, 1959). It is estimated that about 25 percent of those between 10 and 17 years of age are vulnerable to the negative consequences of engaging in multiple high-risk behaviors. Examples of the outcomes of these behaviors include suicide, school failure, STDs, substance abuse, physical injury, unwanted teen pregnancy, and delinquency, which result in tremendous costs for these individuals and society (Dryfoos, 1990). Yet, less than a quarter of the children and youth who have mental health problems severe enough to warrant treatment receive appropriate services (Tuma, 1989). Further, efforts must also be directed toward those who may be at lower levels of risk so that they do not begin to engage in negative behaviors.

Results of the annual Youth Risk Behavior Surveillance System (YRBSS; CDC, 1999) provide further evidence of the extent of the problem. For example, between 1991 and 1999 there were increases in frequent cigarette use, episodic heavy drinking, and lifetime marijuana use, and fewer young people used birth control during their most recent sexual intercourse. Numbers of children, who felt unsafe going to school, attempted suicide, currently used alcohol, and currently were sexually active continued to be unacceptably high. Improvements had been made in the percentages who used seat belts and bicycle safety helmets, carried a weapon to school, seriously considered suicide, and ever had sexual intercourse, but these behaviors continue to be a concern.

These points make it clear that our traditional, individual treatment-oriented approaches are not adequate to meet the growing needs of today's children and adolescents. More emphasis needs to be shifted toward systemic prevention and promotion activities.

THEORIES AND RESEARCH

A number of studies have identified similar individual, family, school, and community factors that are associated with attainment of positive outcomes (e.g., success in school) and avoidance of negative outcomes (e.g., interpersonal violence) for children and youth. These factors include acquisition of social-emotional skills, developing strong bonds with healthy adults, and maintaining involvement in positive activities. Positive developmental pathways can be constructed and problems prevented as a result (Hawkins, Catalano, & Miller, 1992). Accordingly, SEL efforts are directed toward reducing risk and/or toward enhancing protective mechanisms and increasing resilience. *Modifiable risk factors* are continuing life or contextual circumstances that are likely to lead to maladaptive behaviors. Examples of those that can be reduced include keeping weapons and drugs out of schools and minimizing opportunities for students to be exposed to violence through the media. *Protective mechanisms* may mitigate the effects of being exposed to risk (Rutter & Smith, 1995). For instance, orientation programs for students entering high school may help them meet other students, learn what to expect in this new environment, and teach them relevant study skills. Consequently, they are more likely to experience success within this more personal, supportive, and nurturing environment.

Zins, Elias, Greenberg, and Weissberg (2000, p. 76) note that, "Being socially and emotionally competent involves the ability to adapt and integrate behaviors (actions), cognition (thinking), and emotions (feeling) to achieve specific goals. It also includes understanding, managing, and expressing the social and emotional aspects of daily living to attain success in the academic, interpersonal, and health areas."

Examples of skills associated with social-emotional competence that can be addressed include (Payton, Wardlaw, Graczyk, Bloodworth, Tompsett, & Weissberg, 2000):

- being aware of and regulating feelings;
- perceiving the perspectives of others accurately;
- analyzing social norms;
- possessing a high sense of self-efficacy;
- engaging in safe, healthy, and ethical behaviors;
- being fair, just, charitable, and compassionate;
- respecting others and appreciating differences;
- identifying problems correctly;
- setting positive and realistic goals;
- developing positive and informed problem solutions;
- listening and attending to others;
- communicating clearly, both verbally and non-verbally;
- cooperating with children and adults;
- resolving conflicts peacefully;
- asserting oneself;
- resisting negative pressure; and
- identifying the need for assistance and knowing how to access it.

More recently, the attention of SEL researchers has been expanded to include examination of factors related to school success. There is substantive recognition that social and emotional learning and academic performance are causally related. Increasingly, researchers are finding evidence suggesting that the promotion of social and emotional competence has a positive effect on children's school success, and that succeeding in school during childhood can be a key aspect of social and emotional well being (Zins, Weissberg, Wang, & Walberg, in press).

STRATEGIES THAT WORK

A number of analyses of school-based prevention programs have been conducted in recent years focusing on areas such as preventing and reducing substance abuse, conduct problems, delinquent behavior, and other forms of problem behaviors. General agreement has emerged that some of these programs are effective in reducing these maladaptive behaviors (Dryfoos, 1990), and that progress is being made in delineating characteristics associated with strategies that work. Meta-analytic studies have been informative in identifying effective programs and key elements for success.

Wilson, Gottfredson, and Najaka (2001) conducted a meta-analysis of 165 studies of school-based preventive interventions, ranging from individual counseling and behavior modification to school-wide changes in management practices. They found that self-control or social competency promotion instruction using cognitive-behavioral and behavioral instructional methods and noninstructional programs consistently were effective in reducing alcohol and drug use, dropout and nonattendance, and other conduct problems. The cognitive-behavioral and behavioral training involved repeated exposure to new behaviors through modeling, coupled with practice and performance feedback, along with extended use of cues to elicit behavior over long periods or across settings. In addition to these techniques, environmentally focused interventions (e.g., classroom management, reorganization of classes, and school management interventions) were especially effective in decreasing delinquency and drug use. Finally, they found instructional prevention programs based on sound learning principles to be more effective.

Tobler and Stratton's (1997) meta-analysis of 120 school-based drug prevention programs led them to conclude that the method of program delivery was an important factor related to effectiveness for adolescents. They ranked programs on a continuum from those involving no or little interaction (e.g., didactic presentations) to those that involved substantial interaction among group members, and concluded that interactive programs consistently were more effective than non-interactive ones. There have been several major reviews of prevention and competence enhancement programs conducted in recent years. Illustrative of the reviews are one from the Centers for Disease Control ("Programs that Work" project, available at www.cdc.nccdph/dash), and another from the Collaborative for Academic, Social, and Emotional Learning (CASEL), available at www.casel.org. The CDC report identified programs meeting specific criteria for effectiveness derived from the scientific literature and thus were considered "Programs That Work," while CASEL provides an ongoing and updated listing of programs reviewed and rated primarily around features related to guidelines established by CASEL (Elias et al., 1997) for effective implementation and, where available, information about their outcomes.

A large number of programs were included in the CDC and CASEL reviews. Two examples of programs identified as ones that work by CDC and also included in the CASEL review are *Life Skills Training* (available from Princeton Health Press, 115 Wall Street, Princeton, NJ 08540; 800/636-3415; E-mail: Sales@phplifeskills.com) and *Get Real About AIDS* (available from AGC/United Media, 560 Sherman Avenue, Suite 100, Evanston, Illinois 60201; 800/323-9084; E-mail: agc@mcs.net).

Life Skills Training, which also was selected for prevention excellence by the US Department of Education, Drug Strategies, Inc., and the Center for Substance Abuse Prevention, is a substance abuse prevention/competency enhancement program that addresses the major psychological and social factors related to substance use. The program is designed to help students develop the skills to deal with social (peer) pressure for substance abuse; improve their self-esteem, self-mastery, and self-confidence; cope with social anxiety; and understand the consequences of substance use. Among the contents are lessons on decision making, dealing with media influences, skills building activities (resolving conflict, assertiveness, social skills, communication skills, coping with anxiety and anger), and information about smoking, alcohol, and marijuana. It consists of 15 lessons that are implemented in the first year of middle or junior high school, along with booster sessions in the two subsequent grades. A new version of the program includes similar content for 24 classes spread over third through fifth or fourth through sixth grades.

The *Get Real about AIDS (2nd ed.)* gives students accurate content information (i.e., HIV/AIDS and STDs) and social skills such as assertiveness and self-control related to sexual behaviors. In addition, it promotes safety, fun, and healthy behaviors as alternatives to risky ones. The program presents a strong anti-drug message and emphasizes the benefits of abstinence from sex at all grade levels, but also addresses the concerns of students who already are sexual active. Cooperative learning is used as an instructional technique, and notably there also are activities that extend the program to the family and the community. An important component of the program is teacher training, which provides teachers with the latest content information and the opportunity to explore their own attitudes and beliefs related to teaching the material. Although the CDC review covered only the high school version, the curriculum also includes materials for upper elementary and middle-level age groups.

STRATEGIES THAT MIGHT WORK

There are many promising programs available that have a solid conceptual foundation, provide sequential, multi-year instruction, and have an extensive array of lessons, but lack an evidence base. An example is the Responsive Classroom (www.responsiveclassroom.org), which is an approach to teaching and learning for grades kindergarten through grade eight developed by the Northeast Foundation for Children. It encourages safe, challenging, and joyful schools and classrooms to help children develop academically, socially, and emotionally. Among its seven guiding principles are that the social curriculum is as important as the academic curriculum, and that how children learn is as important as what they learn. Further, it is based on the belief that the greatest cognitive growth occurs through social interaction, and accordingly it teaches cooperation, assertion, responsibility, empathy, and self-control skills. In addition, it has a strong school–family component. Finally, it utilizes the following specific teaching strategies and elements: Morning Meeting; Rules and Logical Consequences; Guided Discovery; Academic Choice; Classroom Organization; and Family Communication Strategies (see their website for explanations of these components). Although there are many anecdotal and other suggestions of the effectiveness of the Responsive Classroom, there have not been peer-reviewed studies published to date.

STRATEGIES THAT DO NOT WORK

The research literature and our experiences indicates that many schools use the SEL instruction over a short period of time, in only a single grade, and separate from related school and community endeavors; or these schools do not use evidence-based programs. The research is clear: such programs have a limited impact on children's social and emotional development, and the benefits do not generalize to multiple prevention domains. Moreover, it is unlikely that they will protect children against the many negative influences and pressures they will experience throughout their school careers and in their lives outside of school.

Similar limited results have been associated with programs that primarily involve didactic instruction or focus on giving information without the active involvement of students (Tobler & Stratton, 1997). The meta-analysis by Wilson et al. (2001) found consistently negative effects with non-cognitive behavioral counseling, social work, and other therapeutic interventions. And, finally, programs that are directed solely at children independent of their school's culture, their families, and the broader community, also are less effective (Greenberg, Weissberg, Elias, & Zins, in press).

A well-known example of the above points is the *Drug Abuse Resistance Education* (DARE) program. Thousands of schools throughout the United States have implemented the program in response to the need to prevent drug abuse and violence, yet many are probably unaware of the research on its effectiveness. The preponderance of the empirical studies have found that DARE has no long-term effects on drug use (Dukes, Stein, & Ullman, 1997). Moreover, in a ten-year follow-up investigation researchers found no more successful outcomes in those exposed to DARE compared to those who received a standard drug-education curriculum (Lynam et al., 1999). Similar negative outcomes have been found with other prevention programs that rely on a school-based social influence approach (Peterson, Kealey, Mann, Marek, & Sarason, 2000). Efforts are currently underway to revise the DARE program.

Also see: Social and Emotional entries.

SYNTHESIS

Social and emotional education is directed toward enhancing student's prosocial development, and it can take a variety of forms and be directed toward various goals. Although different approaches have been found to have positive outcomes, there are several elements that are essential to effective practice. First, these activities must be delivered in a planned, systematic manner. Second, they should be coordinated throughout the school and related settings on an integrated, programmatic basis. Thus, efforts in individual classrooms must be supported by school-wide, community-based and family elements to be most effective. Additionally, there may be cultural variations in the definition of social and emotional competence, and it is important that the program goals are salient and appropriate for the participants, not merely reflecting the values of the program directors or funders.

Next, program implementation and outcomes need to be monitored to insure a high level of integrity. Effectiveness cannot be assumed. Topping, Holmes, and Bremner (2000) reviewed the effectiveness of school-based programs for the promotion of social competence in the United Kingdom and concluded that the evidence suggested that behaviorally-based and cognitive-behavioral/self-management programs tended to be effective more consistently, social skills training and peer-mediated programs less consistently, and counseling and therapeutic programs least consistently. A number of programs that were in widespread use did not have a significant evaluation literature, and others were well evaluated but not particularly well known or widely used.

Finally, as part of a school's overall service delivery system, SEL programs need to be directed toward students who are at low or moderate risk, as well as those who are experiencing significant problems, because SEL instruction is necessary for *all* children regardless of risk status. Converging evidence across many fields suggests that socialization for SEL in home and school contexts must take its place as a standard promotion and prevention strategy to help children and adolescents meet the challenges of living healthy, socially conscious, engaged, and enriched moral and ethical lives in the 21st century.

References

Albee, G.W. (1959). *Mental health manpower trends.* New York: Basic Books.

Centers for Disease Control and Prevention (CDC). (1999). *Youth risk behavior trends: From CDC's 1991, 1993, 1995, 1997, and 1999 Youth Risk Behavior Surveys.* Silver Spring, MD: Author. National Center for Chronic Disease Prevention and Health Promotion Division of Adolescent and School Health's Information Service.

Dryfoos, J. (1990). *Adolescents at risk: Prevalence and prevention.* New York: Oxford University Press.

Dukes, R.L., Stein, J.A., & Ullman, J.B. (1997). Long-term impact of Drug Abuse Resistance Education (DARE). *Evaluation Review, 21,* 483–500.

Elias, M.J., Zins, J.E., Weissberg, R.P., Frey, K.S., Greenberg, M.T., Haynes, N.M., Kessler, R., Schwab-Stone, M.E., & Shriver, T.P. (1997). *Promoting social and emotional learning: Guidelines for educators.* Alexandria, VA: Association for Supervision and Curriculum Development.

Greenberg, M.T., Weissberg, R.P., Elias, M.J., & Zins, J.E. (in press). Promoting positive youth development through school-based social and emotional learning. *American Psychologist.*

Hawkins, J.D., Catalano, R.F., & Miller, J.Y. (1992). Risk and protective factors for alcohol and other drug problems in adolescence and early adulthood: Implications for substance abuse prevention. *Psychological Bulletin, 112,* 64–105.

Lynam, D.R., Milich, R., Zimmerman, R., Novak, S.P., Logan, T.K., Martin, C., Leukefeld, C., & Clayton, R. (1999). Project DARE: No effects at 10-year follow-up. *Journal of Consulting and Clinical Psychology, 67*(4), 590–593.

Payton, J.W., Wardlaw, D.M., Graczyk, P.A., Bloodworth, M.A., Tompsett, C.J., & Weissberg, R.P. (2000). Social and emotional learning: A framework for promoting mental health and reducing risk behaviors in children and youth. *Journal of School Health, 70,* 179–185.

Peterson, A.V., Jr., Kealey, K.A., Mann, S.L., Marek, P.M., & Sarason, I.G. (2000). Hutchinson Smoking Prevention Project: Long term randomized trial in school-based tobacco use prevention—Results on smoking. *Journal of the National Cancer Institute, 92,* 1979–1991.

Rutter, M., & Smith, D.J. (1995). *Psychosocial disorders in young people: Time trends and their causes.* London: Wiley.

Tobler, N.S., & Stratton, H.H. (1997). Effectiveness of school-based drug prevention programs: A meta-analysis of the research. *The Journal of Primary Prevention, 18,* 71–128.

Topping, K.J., Holmes, E.A., & Bremner, W.G. (2000). The effectiveness of school-based programs for the promotion of social competence. In R. Bar-On & J.D.A. Parker (Eds.), *The handbook of emotional intelligence* (pp. 411–432). San Francisco: Jossey-Bass.

Tuma, J. (1989). Mental health services for children: The state of the art. *American Psychologist, 44,* 188–199.

Wilson, D.B., Gottfredson, D.C., & Najaka, S.S. (2001). School-based prevention of problem behaviors: A meta-analysis. *Journal of Quantitative Criminology, 17,* 247–272.

Zins, J.E., Elias, M.J., Greenberg, M.T., & Weissberg, R.P. (2000). Promoting social and emotional competence in children. In K.M. Minke & G.C. Bear (Eds.), *Preventing school problems— promoting school success: Strategies and programs that work* (pp. 71–100). Bethesda, MD: National Association of School Psychologists.

Zins, J.E., Weissberg, R.P., Wang, M.L., & Walberg, H.J. (Eds.). (in press). *Building school success through social and emotional learning.* New York: Teachers College Press.

Social and Emotional Learning, Adolescence

Maurice J. Elias, Jeffrey S. Kress, and Deborah Neft

INTRODUCTION

A complete understanding of adolescent health and well-being must include systematic attention to their social and emotional competence. This entry summarizes current knowledge in this area, the relationship of social and emotional competencies to indicators of problem behavior, and principles to guide best practices for promoting social and emotional learning in schools, homes, and other contexts in which adolescents are socialized.

DEFINITIONS

Attempts to define social competence have a rich and controversial history. The William T. Grant Consortium on the School-Based Promotion of Social Competence (1994) believes that *social competence* involves the capacity to integrate cognition, affect, and behaviors to achieve specified social tasks and positive developmental outcomes. It is comprised by a set of core skills, attitudes, abilities, and feelings given functional meaning by the contexts of culture, neighborhood, and situation. Thus, *social competence* can be viewed in terms of "life skills for adaptation to diverse ecologies and settings." This perspective incorporates the possibility that in certain cultures, neighborhoods, and situations, so-called "undesirable" behaviors (e.g., aggressive, selfish, or passive behavior) may be required if one is to be perceived as "well adjusted" or to avoid being subject to harm. Also, it implies that behaviors that may appear to reflect a lack of competence may instead be adaptations to idiosyncratic or harmful ecological circumstances.

If one accepts this distinction, it follows that an understanding of how the skills of social and emotional competence link to judgments of adjustment requires a detailed knowledge of: (a) the social contexts surrounding individuals and (b) the meanings they attach to their life, roles, relationships, and future. Expressions of competence may take unpopular forms, an issue that must continue to draw the attention of researchers who focus on peer relationships and social competence. For example, a child with competencies

in studying and academic work will, in some environments, be perceived as less well adjusted by peers than someone with skills in interpersonal aggression.

Ultimately, a perspective on social competence must reflect the ever-increasing complexity of our society. The application of skills occurs across a variety of life tasks, social contexts, and what we have come to view as sociocultural/linguistic contexts. This implies, for example, that one should be prepared to examine differences within national subgroups as one would consider differences between nations; from this perspective, we are less likely to overestimate the parameters of generalization of knowledge, attitudes, and skills to these subgroups than is currently the case. Illustratively, for a high school teacher in Texas, it would be unwise to assume that there is a strong "American" consensus between a Mexican American child in Texas and a Puerto Rican American child in his or her class; rather, this is a non-trivial empirical question.

Nevertheless, there appears to be an array of skills that comprise social and emotional competencies for everyday living: knowledge of feelings in self and others; self-regulation of behavior, cognition, and affect; the encoding of relevant social cues and to the norms of a social context; perspective-taking, reading intentions, and empathy; short and long-term goal setting and planning; the generation of effective solutions to interpersonal problems; the realistic anticipation of consequences of, and potential obstacles to, one's actions and delay of immediate gratification; the translation of social decisions into effective verbal and nonverbal interpersonal and group behavior and relationship-maintenance skills, including teamwork and leadership skills; and the expression of a positive sense of self-efficacy and optimism about outcomes.

The social-emotional competence construct has additional heuristic value in its relationship to the concept of risk and protective factors. Rutter (1987) identified specific "mechanisms" which serve a protective function to individuals even when they are in circumstances that most would find to be harmful. These mechanisms are based in certain key skills, such as planning, anticipating consequences, reacting to obstacles, and the ability to form and maintain caring relationships (Salovey & Sluyter, 1997).

SCOPE

There is abundant evidence that despite increases in material possessions and improvements on many indicators of health and safety, the mental health and well-being of adolescents is not showing corresponding improvement.

Cigarette Smoking

In 1996, it was estimated that unless current trends changed, some 30–40 percent of the 2.3 billion children and teenagers in the world would become smokers in early adult life (Peto, Lopez, Boreham, Thun, Heath, & Doll, 1996). The Centers for Disease Control survey in 1999 showed that 64 percent of American high school students smoked at least once; 28.5 percent were current smokers and 29.1 percent smoked six cigarettes on the days that they smoked (Centers for Disease Control and Prevention [CDC], 2000). The same survey was given to students aged 15–18 in Budapest; 46 percent of the Hungarian students reported current smoking, and 23.5 percent of them smoked 11 cigarettes on the days that they smoked (Kiss, Ferenczi, Végh, & Lun, 2000). According to the Centre for Addiction and Mental Health's 1999 Ontario Student Drug Use Survey, 29 percent of Canadian students have smoked more than one cigarette during the past year and 23 percent smoked daily. Studies on 15–19-year-old South Americans in the 1990s revealed that 57 percent of boys and 40 percent of girls smoked cigarettes in Peru and 41 percent of boys and 28 percent of girls did in Cuba (Burt, 1996).

Alcohol

In the United States, the majority of high school students have tried alcohol, 81 percent having had at least one drink in their lifetime. Even more alarming, 13 percent drove a vehicle one or more times after drinking alcohol, and 32 percent reported episodic heavy drinking during the past month (Kahn et al, 2000). The 1999 Ontario Student Drug Use Survey showed that 73 percent of Canadian adolescents have drank alcohol during their lifetime. Some 20 percent of the drinkers drank weekly, 42 percent of the students consumed five or more drinks on a single occasion, and 16 percent of licensed drivers reported driving within an hour of consuming two or more drinks. In England, a survey of students aged 11–15 showed that 23 percent of boys and 18 percent of girls drank alcohol in the last week (Goddard & Higgins, 1999).

Drugs

Among US adolescents, 27 percent used marijuana during the past month and 10 percent had ever used cocaine (Kahn et al., 2000). The Ontario study showed that among Canadian teens, 9 percent of users (3 percent of all students) used cannabis daily during the past year and 17 percent used four or more drugs. In the United Kingdom, a survey of illicit drug use among cohort of 15- and 16-year-old students showed that a third of girls and 40 percent of boys had used illicit drugs. A total of 37 percent used cannabis, 19 percent used glues and solvents, 9 percent used amphetamines, and 5 percent used Ecstasy (Plant, 2000).

Juvenile Crime

In 1997, approximately one in five arrest in the United States made by law enforcement agencies involved persons under the age of eighteen. Juveniles accounted for: 37 percent of burglary arrests, 30 percent of robbery arrests, 24 percent of weapon arrests, 14 percent of drug arrests, and 5 percent of violent crimes (Snyder & Sickmund, 1999). In Canada, the juvenile crime rate has been falling since 1991; however, the youth violent crime rate in 1998 was still 77 percent higher than a decade ago (Statistics Canada, 1999). In 1998, juvenile crime accounted for 25 percent of all criminal cases, including 12 percent of all murders, 17 percent of serious assault, 36 percent of robbery and violent theft, 40 percent of cases of breaking and entering, and 13 percent of all drug offences (INTERPOL, International Crime Statistics, 1998).

THEORIES

Understanding these adolescent difficulties from the perspective of social and emotional competence results from a convergence of a number of theoretical approaches. Foremost, it is grounded in *social learning theory* (Rotter, 1954), which states that behavior is a function of generalized and specific expectancies, reinforcement history, and expectancies about outcomes, locus of control, and the trustworthiness of the environment. This theory clearly anticipates the current movement toward positive psychology, although without the explicit biological basis. Two other influential perspectives are *developmental theory* and, within that, *identity theory*. From these points of view, we focus on the competencies of the growing organism and therefore see the optimal development of those competencies at any age as a developmental right. During adolescence, competencies, deficiencies, preferences, tendencies, attitudes, and values all become organized and mobilized by the development of a sense of identity. Cognitively, children are able to focus on the future and ask the question, Who am I and what can I become? with a sense of reality and potential commitment. It is clear that cultural and socioeconomic factors place constraints on the possible answers that children can envision. Yet, it is also noteworthy that the rise of global mass media serves to create identity images linked to wealth, status, and consumption, many of which are incompatible with local culture or realistic opportunity. Some believe that one result of this, which is still being played out, is the continued decline of youth on indicators of well-being despite their increasing material advantages.

Emotional intelligence and social-emotional learning (EQ/SEL) theory seeks to integrate the previous with advancing knowledge about the development of the brain and the importance of emotion in all aspects of social functioning, including academic and vocational (Goleman, 1995; Salovey & Sluyter, 1997). Research suggests three fundamental tenets of the theory:

1. Positive, caring relationships form the foundation of all learning.

2. Our emotions affect how and what we learn.
3. Goal setting and problem solving provide direction and energy for learning.

Corollaries to this are that promoting social and emotional competence in adolescence requires attention in five areas (Elias, Tobias, & Friedlander, 2000):

1. *Appreciation.* Adolescents need to know that they are appreciated by those around them, that they are loved and valued and that they matter.
2. *Belonging.* They want to belong to schools and families that stand for something, that have meaning, and can be a source of pride and nourishment. In the absence of positive opportunities, teenagers will join gangs and antisocial peer groups to engender the sense of belonging.
3. *Competencies and Confidence.* To enact key roles, children need competencies, the specific skills of emotional intelligence noted earlier, and they also need the confidence to use those skills constructively.
4. *Contributions.* Teenagers also derive great satisfaction from being able to be useful, to make contributions to others, to mentor, to teach, to coach, to have parts in meaningful activities, to engage in service learning, and civic and faith-based social participation. They need to enact what Brendtro, Brokenleg, and Van Bockern (1990) call the "Spirit of Generosity," that part of us that gets satisfaction by giving and comes to value this feeling, and the appreciation that comes with it, as a rival to substance use.
5. *Chance.* Finally, teenagers need opportunity structures, context in which to enact their skills and to get their developmental needs met and their sense of identity confirmed and expanded.

STRATEGIES: OVERVIEW

Given the scale of problems related to adolescent development, it is no surprise that a myriad of programs are put forth as "solutions" to the issues of substance use, delinquency, incarceration, and dropout. However, many of the programs and curricula are market-driven, rather than based on a firm theoretical and empirical research. Further, programs may focus on a specific problem area rather than addressing broader EQ/SEL issues in the school. For example, behavior modification and social skills training have both been shown to increase social competence in targeted interventions (Topping et al., 2000). However, given the complex nature of EQ/SEL and the promotion of these competencies, it is important to view EQ/SEL interventions as a systemic change, rather than as a specific program to be run.

Successful EQ/SEL interventions, while often packaged as unitary "programs," can easily be seen as an integrated and cohesive amalgam of interventions aimed at various ecological levels (e.g., individual students, the climate of the school as a whole) and varying degrees of problem behavior, across grade levels and throughout the school day. In fact, a set of guidelines for EQ/SEL programming developed by the Collaborative for Academic, Social, and Emotional Learning (CASEL, an organization founded in 1994 with the mission to establish research-based social and emotional learning as an essential part of education from preschool through high school, in order to educate children to be knowledgeable, responsible, nonviolent, healthy, and caring) and the Association for Supervision and Curriculum Development explicitly recommend a comprehensive approach to programming (Elias et al., 1997). Programs based on the core components of EQ/SEL have been developed and implemented in different districts nationwide over the last two decades. The specific focus of these interventions may differ (i.e., violence, health, drug use) but all aim at promoting prosocial skills in students. Recently, efforts have been made to empirically test some of the programs, and the results look promising.

STRATEGIES THAT WORK

The *Resolving Conflicts Creatively Program* (RCCP) began in the late 1980s as a joint venture of Educators for Social Responsibility and the New York Public School system, and is a research-validated, comprehensive EQ/SEL program. In the middle and high school, every student receives direct instruction in skills such as caring communication, expression of feelings, and peaceful conflict resolution and negotiation. This forms the groundwork for ways to incorporate RCCP skills and ideas into improving the climate within a school. Student-led peer mediation allows for students with difficulties to address these in a prosocial arena. Evaluation has shown that educators in RCCP schools report a variety of positive outcomes in their students, including increased use of conflict resolution skills, and increased self-esteem and awareness of feelings. Further, reductions were found for physical violence, in- and out-of school suspension and dropout rate.

In urban schools, Aber, Jones, Brown, Chaudry, and Samples (1998) found that receiving a high number of RCCP lessons significantly slowed the increase of aggressive thoughts and behaviors over time. Students who received an average of 25 lessons over the school year had significantly slower growth in self-reported hostile attributions, aggressive fantasies, and aggressive problem-solving strategies, as well as in teacher-reported aggressive behavior, compared to children receiving a low number of lessons or no lessons at all. Additionally, students receiving approximately 25 lessons received significantly increased ratings on prosocial skills and emotional control by their teacher and showed greater improvement on standardized academic achievement tests compared to the other two groups. This evaluation and similar efforts to build social competence in a largely African American middle school population (Weissberg & Elias, 1993) highlight several important themes in understanding research on SEL programming: (a) successful programs may not eliminate, or even decrease, aggressive behavior, but may serve to slow the rise; (b) when not used as intended and carried out with fidelity, programs are unlikely to achieve their expected results; and (c) even successful programs will not work equally well for all children.

The *Teenage Health Teaching Modules* (THTM) also have been evaluated and shown to be successful. THTM is a comprehensive health curriculum for students in grades 6–12 that focuses on teaching adolescents the skills to act in ways to improve their immediate and long-term health. THTM consists of a series of modules that concentrate on essential health skills: risk assessment, self-assessment, communication, decision-making, goal setting, health advocacy, and healthy self-management. Also reinforced in the modules are the issues of protection, responsibility, interdependence, and respect. A large-scale controlled study conducted with 5,000 middle and high school students in schools in seven states showed that THTM had a positive effect on the health-related attitudes and knowledge of the students; high school students reported positive changes in many health behaviors, including substance use (Errecart, Walberg, Ross, Gold, Fiedler, & Kolbe, 1991).

The *Reconnecting Youth* program targets students at-risk for dropping out of high school. Once identified, these adolescents participate in a five-month intervention consisting of daily hour-long lessons. Reconnecting Youth has three main objectives: (a) to increase school performance, (b) to decrease drug involvement, (c) to decrease suicide risk by decreasing specific risk factors (i.e., depression) and increasing specific protective factors (i.e., self-esteem). A research study investigating the effects of Reconnecting Youth on 600 high school students in Seattle, Washington found a 60 percent decrease in hard drug use, a 20 percent increase in their Grade Point Averages, increased personal control (including anger management), and more positive relationships with teachers, friends, and family members (Eggert, Nicholas, & Owen, 1995).

Perhaps the approach that has a presence in the largest number of countries worldwide is the collaboration between Quest International and Lions Clubs International. *Skills for Adolescence* and *Skills for Action* (Quest International, 2000) both have been subject to several quasi-experimental

evaluations. The former program has shown benefits in reduction of substance use and improvements in anger management and attitudes toward resisting problem behaviors. Skills for Action, across 27 high schools in seven states in the United States, was effective in preventing expected developmental increases in a range of negative lifestyle behaviors, including school dropout, as well as improving academic skills, social competencies, and alliance with positive community values.

STRATEGIES THAT MIGHT WORK

An emerging area of EQ/SEL that holds great promise involves the overlap of EQ/SEL and issues of spiritual development. The *Passages* program, developed by Kessler (2000) and her colleagues, builds on the adolescent search for meaning and connectedness. In approaching spirituality from an intra- and inter-personal perspective, rather than from the point of view of a particular religious doctrine, a variety of classroom-based experiences address themes of connection to self and others, emotional expression, and self-reflection. Activities often revolve around a rite of passage to mark and strengthen the emerging adolescent identity and to serve as an initiation into adulthood.

Facing History and Ourselves (FHAO) provides an intriguing example of how a time-limited, content area-based program can contribute to EQ/SEL promotion. Taught as part of a social studies and civics programs in secondary schools, FHAO studies the rise of Nazism in Germany and the Holocaust and other examples of human genocide in order to prompt students to "reflect critically on their beliefs, behaviors, and responsibilities toward one another" (Fine, 1991, p. 48). Reports from teachers who have implemented the program point toward changes in teens' attitudes regarding stereotypes, and improved interpersonal and moral reasoning. Further, teachers report that they themselves became better listeners and more adept at dealing with complex social issues in the classroom (Brabeck, Kenny, Stryker, Tollefson, & Sternstrom, 1994). It is clear that such a program can be integrated into a school-wide SEL effort.

Berman (1997) and Pasi (2001) have pioneered whole school approaches that have integrated Service Learning and Citizenship Education with an infusion of EQ/SEL activities throughout their schools, including and especially in high schools. While their approaches have not received experimental evaluation (which would be highly challenging to design), their work is fully consistent with guidelines for effective EQ/SEL efforts put forward by CASEL and they have accumulated numerous indicators of improvement, including students' commitment to school, morale, positive climate, and reduced problem behaviors. Additional descriptions of promising approaches for use with adolescents, including the Responsive Classroom and Social Decision Making and Social Problem Solving, can be found in Cohen (1999).

STRATEGIES THAT DO NOT WORK

Several studies illustrate what strategies do not work to promote social and emotional competence in adolescence. As a strategy, interventions need to be comprehensive, multicomponent, and longitudinal. A literature review and series of site visits to empirically supported programs found that enduring success and likelihood of generalization were related to programs being multicomponent, multimodal, multiyear, and comprehensive (Elias et al., 1997). Promoting social and emotional competence requires attention to both "person" and "environmental" variables and the interrelationship of the two. Further, there must be a coherent theoretical structure that organizes and integrates the various components (Dalton, Elias, & Wandersman, 2001).

Weissberg and Greenberg's (1997) thorough review of programs directed at children and adolescents suggests the importance of a skill focus, which involves presenting a skill, defining a rationale, practicing component parts and skill integration, and preparing for generalization and transfer of learning in addition to ensuring that displays of the skill will be reinforced in the adolescent's environment (Elias & Tobias, 1996).

Finally, Gager and Elias (1997) examined the implementation of exemplary school-based social and emotional competence programs in a variety of settings. They found that model programs were as likely to succeed as they were to fail, and that fidelity of implementation was the critical factor. That is, if programs are not implemented with care, given a chance to grow, linked with the mandates and culture of their settings, focused on student strengths, and supported by implementers, administrators, and parents, they are less likely to succeed. There is no strategy that is "implementation proof," though there are approaches that are unlikely to be successful regardless of implementation fidelity.

SYNTHESIS

In practice, the promotion of social and emotional competence in adolescence occurs in contexts that are more complex and with fewer resources than is often true for the experimental studies used to validate specific approaches. Hence, CASEL has worked to develop guidelines for those wishing to promote social-emotional competence in youth, especially in school settings. These guidelines are designed for use when experimental testing is not feasible and yet, action is needed. CASEL is continually updating its information at the web site, www.CASEL.org, through its process of Program Review.

We envision increased attention and interest in adolescents across countries and cultures, as they share the importance of seeing youth as resources, both in the present and as preparation for continuing social institutions. Promoting their social and emotional competence can be viewed as a significant "missing piece" that is a necessary complement to efforts to improve adolescent health and academic abilities and an essential adjunct to selected and indicated interventions once problems have emerged. Over the next decades, secondary level education must become accountable for preparing adolescents with the social and emotional skills needed to enact adult roles in the family, workplace, and civic life. Educators will need to be systematically prepared to help build adolescents' EQ/SEL skills and systematic evaluation of adolescents' health and social-emotional and life skills, as well as problem behaviors, should become an ongoing focus of school and/or community concern. Without feedback, we are likely to make assumptions that could put the well-being of our youth at risk.

Also see: Social and Emotional entries.

References

Aber, J.L., Jones, S.M., Brown, J.L., Chaudry, N., & Samples, F. (1998). Resolving conflict creatively: Evaluating the developmental effects of a school-based violence prevention program in neighborhood and classroom context. *Development & Psychopathology, 10*(2), 187–213.

Berman, S. (1997). *Children's social consciousness and the development of social Responsibility*. Suny Series: Democracy and Education.

Brabeck, M., Kenny, M., Stryker, S., Tollefson, T., & Sternstrom, M. (1994). Human rights education through the "Facing History and Ourselves" program. *Journal of Moral Education, 23*, 333–347.

Brendtro, L., Brokenleg, M., & Van Bockern, S. (1990). *Reclaiming youth at risk: Our hope for the future*. Bloomington, IN: National Educational Service.

Burt, M.R. (1996). *Why should we invest in adolescents?* Presentation at the Conference on Comprehensive Health of Adolescents and Youth in Latin America and the Caribbean, July 9–12, 1996. Pan American Health Organization, Washington, DC.

Centers for Disease Control and Prevention (CDC). (2000). CDC surveillance summaries, October 13, 2000. *Morbidity and Mortality Weekly Report, 49* (SS-10).

Cohen, J. (Ed.). (1999). *Educating hearts and minds: Social emotional learning and the passage into adolescence*. New York: Teachers College Press.

Consortium on the School-Based Promotion of Social Competence. (1994). The school-based promotion of social competence: Theory, research, practice, and policy. In R.J. Haggerty, L.R. Sherrod, N. Garmezy, & M. Rutter (Eds.), *Stress, risk, and resilience in children and adolescents: Processes, mechanisms, and interventions* (pp. 268–316). New York: Cambridge University Press.

Dalton, J., Elias, M.J., & Wandersman, A. (2001). *Community psychology: Linking individuals and communities*. Belmont, CA: Wadsworth.

Eggert, L.L., Nicholas, L.J., & Owen, L.M. (1995). *Reconnecting youth: A peer group approach to building life skills*. Bloomington, IN: National Educational Service.

Elias, M.J., & Tobias, S. (1996). *Social problem solving interventions in the schools*. New York: Guilford.

Elias, M.J., Tobias, S.E., & Friedlander, B.S. (2000). *Raising emotionally intelligent teenagers: Parenting with love, laughter, and limits*. NY: Harmony/Random House.

Elias, M.J., Zins, J.E., Weissberg, K.S., Greenberg, M.T., Haynes, N.M., Kessler, R., Schwab-Stone, M.E., & Shriver, T.P. (1997). *Promoting social and emotional learning: Guidelines for Educators*. Alexandria, VA: Association for Supervision and Curriculum Development.

Errecart, M.T., Walberg, H.J., Ross, J.G., Gold, R.S., Fiedler, J.L., & Kolbe, L.J. (1991). Effectiveness of Teenage Health Teaching Modules. *The Journal of School Health, 61*(1), 26.

Fine, M. (1991). Facing history and ourselves: Portrait of a classroom. *Educational Leadership, 49*(4), 44–49.

Gager, P.J., & Elias, M.J. (1997). Implementing prevention programs in high-risk environments: Application of the resiliency paradigm. *American Journal of Orthopsychiatry, 67*(3), 363–373.

Goddard, E., & Higgins, V. (1999). *Smoking, drinking and drug use among young teenagers in 1998. Volume 1: England*. London: SO.

Goleman, D. (1995). *Emotional intelligence*. New York: Bantam.

INTERPOL, International Crime Statistics. (1998). Available: http://www.interpol.int/Public/Publications/sci/contents1998.asp

Kahn, L., Kinchen, S.A., Williams, B.I., Ross, J.G., Lowry, R., Grunbaum, J., & Kolbe, L.J. (2000). Youth Risk Behavior Surveillance—United States 1999. *Morbidity and Mortality Weekly Report, 49*(SS5).

Kessler, R. (2000). *The soul of education: Helping students find connection, compassion, and character at school*. Alexandria, VA: Association for Supervision and Curriculum Development.

Kiss, É., Ferenczi, F., Végh, E., & Lun, K. (2000). Prevalence of cigarette smoking among secondary school students—Budapest, Hungary, 1995 and 1999. *Morbidity and Mortality Weekly Report, 49*(20), 438–441.

Pasi, R. (2001). *Challenging and caring schools: Social and emotional learning in education*. Alexandria, VA: Association for Supervision and Curriculum Development.

Peto, R., Lopez, A.D., Boreham, J., Thun, M., Heath, C., & Doll, R. (1996). Mortality from smoking worldwide. *British Medical Bulletin, 52*, 12–21.

Plant, M. (2000). Drug use has declined among teenagers in United Kingdom. *British Medical Journal, 320*(7248), 1536–1544.

Quest International. (2000), *Report for the US Department of Education Expert Panel on safe, disciplined, and drug-free schools: Skills for adolescence and skills for action*. Newark, Ohio: Quest International.

Rotter, J.B. (1954). *Social learning and clinical psychology*. Englewood Cliffs, N.J.: Prentice-Hall.

Rutter, M. (1987). Psychosocial resilience and protective mechanisms. *American Journal of Orthopsychiatry, 57*, 316–331.

Salovey, P., & Sluyter, D. (Eds.). (1997). *Emotional development and emotional intelligence: Educational implications*. New York: Basic Books.

Snyder, H.N., and Sickmund, M. (1999). *Juvenile offenders and victims: 1999 National Report*. Washington, DC: Office of Juvenile Justice and Delinquency Prevention.

Statistics Canada. (1999). Available: http://www.statcan.ca/Daily/English/991221/d991221c.htm

Topping, K., Holmes, E.A., & Bremner, W. (2000). The effectiveness of school-based programs for the promotion of social competence. In R. Bar-On & J.D.A. Parker (Eds.), *The handbook of emotional intelligence* (pp. 411–432). San Francisco: Jossey-Bass.

Weissberg, R.P., & Elias, M.J. (1993). Enhancing young people's social competence and health behavior: An important challenge for educators, scientists, policy makers, and funders. *Applied & Preventive Psychology, 3*, 179–190.

Weissberg, R., & Greenberg, M.T. (1997). Community and school prevention. In I. Sigel and A. Renninger (Eds.), *Handbook of child psychology Vol. 4: Child psychology in practice* (5th ed., pp. 877–954). New York: John Wiley.

Social Inoculation

Richard I. Evans and J. Greg Getz

This entry describes the development of the social inoculation model of health-risk behavior prevention (Evans, 1998, 2001). It connects this approach to its major derivative elaborations and extensions. Lastly, it articulates a set of generic strategies for the creation of primary prevention programs that may have utility at various stages of the life course.

DEVELOPMENT OF THE SOCIAL INOCULATION MODEL

American culture might be described as creatively pragmatic in developing solutions to social problems. In no arena is this more evident than in the application of scientific knowledge to health issues. Beginning in the 1970s, an explosion of interest in physical and mental health issues emerged in the social sciences. Some social scientists were on the cutting edge of theoretical and empirical efforts to understand the relationships between various health-risk and health-protective factors at the biological, psychological, social, and cultural levels of analysis. Sensitivity to the importance of considering multiple levels of analysis resulted in the ubiquitous, interdisciplinary advocacy of conceptualizing health outcomes in terms of biopsychosocial models. This creative ferment in the expanding field of health psychology/behavioral medicine was context for the development of the social inoculation model for the prevention of health risking behavior among adolescents.

Empirical Refutation of Conventional Wisdom: Fear Arousal or Risk Information Alone Do Not Promote Health Behavior

Two assumptions embodied by early efforts at health-risk behavior prevention and intervention programs were that high fear arousal alone and/or the provision of accurate information alone regarding the negative health consequences of a particular behavior would induce sufficient motivation for behavioral change. Empirical research challenged both of these presumptions.

Early findings of the Social Psychology/Behavioral Medicine Research Group at the University of Houston (Evans, Rozelle, Lasater, Demobroski, & Allen, 1968; Evans, Rozelle, Noblitt, & Williams, 1975) were consistent with those of Janis's and Feshbach's (1953) seminal study of tooth brushing among young adolescents that demonstrated high fear arousal alone to be ineffective in motivating long-term, health-enhancing behavioral change. Leventhal, Singer, and Jones (1965) came to a similar conclusion in a study addressing subjects' responses to persuasive strategies to obtain tetanus inoculations. Our findings suggested that exposing young adolescents to explicit instructions and the modeling of oral hygiene behavior without fear induction resulted in significantly more long-term effective oral hygiene behavior.

Also demonstrated as ineffective in altering health behavior was the assumption embodied in "information only" prevention efforts that merely providing adolescents with correct information about a health-risking behavior such as cigarette smoking or alcohol and other drug use would effectively prevent those behaviors (Edmundson, McAlister, Murray, Perry, & Lichtenstein, 1991). Regardless of delivery mode (didactic lecture, videotapes, posters, pamphlets, guest-expert speaker, etc.), research has shown this approach to effect little or no behavioral change relative to control group behavior (Goodstadt, 1978; Thompson, 1978).

The Social Inoculation Model as an Approach to Prevention of Adolescent Cigarette Smoking

Sensitive to empirical findings challenging conventional wisdom regarding effective prevention/intervention efforts and to the dangers of under-theorizing complex behavioral issues, we embarked upon a research agenda in the early 1970s exploring adolescent cigarette smoking. Prevalence rates of smoking showed that school-based prevention efforts were relatively ineffective. Such programs rarely, if ever, were rigorously grounded in behavioral or social science. They seemed predicated on assumptions already refuted in the literature. Namely, it had been demonstrated that high fear arousal or correct information alone would seldom motivate long-term health-enhancing behavior. Development of the social inoculation approach began with an effort to understand adolescent smoking behavior from the subject's point of view. Focused interviews were conducted with a large population of seventh-grade students to determine the range of beliefs, attitudes, and perceptions of social influences that might motivate initiation of tobacco smoking and subsequent acceleration to regular use (Evans,

Table 1. Possible Coping Responses to Increasing Levels of Peer Pressure to Smoke

Perceived peer pressure level	Coping response	Behavioral example
Low	Simple refusal	Just say no!
Moderate	Persistent refusal	Keep saying no!
	delay decision	Not now … maybe later.
	make excuses	Coach would kill me!
High	Avoidance	Walk away … get out!
	counter-pressure	I thought you were my friend … why do you want to give me cancer?

Raines, & Hanselka, 1984). As a result of these interviews, we began to develop a set of heuristic assumptions regarding the causes of adolescent tobacco use. We identified: (1) sources of social influence (e.g., parents, siblings, friends, peers, celebrities or other public figures, general social norms); (2) mechanisms of social influence (e.g., direct peer pressure, indirect effects of role modeling); and (3) states or traits enhancing or mitigating susceptibility to social influences to smoke tobacco (e.g., predisposition toward risk-taking, anti-smoking attitudes, resistance self-efficacy). The pilot social inoculation program that emerged from these considerations (Evans, Rozelle, Mittelmark, Hansen, Bane, & Havis, 1978) involved an effort to communicate correct information about the consequences of tobacco smoking *combined* with two crucial programmatic innovations. The first innovation was instruction in how to recognize various modalities of social influence to smoke, and the second was instruction, and rehearsal of specific social influence resistance techniques. The latter has come to be known generically as *resistance skills training*. It was recognized that different intensities of social pressure might require qualitatively different resistance strategies. Table 1 exemplifies this point for three intensities of one modality of social influence, that is, direct peer pressure.

The resistant response, "just say no", was suggested initially by middle school students during focused interview sessions. This phrase was intended as one possible response to low level peer pressure only (Evans, 2002). Its politicization and employment as a media catch phrase exemplifies how focusing, out of context, on one small component of a multi-faceted prevention program can encourage a simplistically formulaic approach to the prevention of substance abuse.

Prevention/Intervention and the Ubiquity of Dual Theories: Problematic Behavior and Program Implementation

Another lesson learned during the development of the social inoculation approach to adolescent tobacco smoking was that any prevention or intervention program should explicitly involve two theories. Too often at least one of these theories has been implicit and, hence, not rigorously articulated by the researchers involved. These are a theory of the *problematic behavior* and a theory of *effective program implementation*. Regarding the former, the social inoculation approach drew primarily upon social learning theory (Bandura, 1977, 1982; Evans, 1989) in suggesting that children might acquire smoking-related attitudes and behaviors not only as a direct result of reinforcement but also via the process of vicarious learning. Less likely to be explicitly theory-based than the problem behavior in question is the process of implementing the prevention program.

McGuire's Information-Processing Communication Model

Sensitized to the notion that an academic understanding of health and health-risk behaviors was an issue orthogonal to successfully inducing health behavior or refraining from health-risk behavior among subjects in a target population. We drew on McGuire's (1961, 1968) stage-process, information processing communication model (Table 2) in addressing program design.

Attending to a message and, if comprehended, accepting it partly depends upon the subjects' attitudes toward the source of information (Laswell & Casey, 1946). Instead of adult authority figures who could be perceived as representing arbitrary constraint for subjects, our messages were delivered by adolescent (i.e., same age) narrators selected on the basis of their perceived acceptability or attractiveness by the subjects. The narrators acted as peer brokers of scientific information rather than as authority figures whose message might have been discounted by adolescents. It was found that peers were more persuasive than adults were. Their credibility was enhanced by prefacing comments with such phrases as "the researchers have found..." or, "the researchers have asked me to tell you...."

Regarding comprehension, messages were developed employing standard educational methodology for reading level assessment. They were pretested with students at the resource schools. Subject feedback assured that language used was clearly understood by the target audience. We enlisted students from the study population to assist in writing scripts and to act out role-played situations that were videotaped for presentation to student audiences. In this way, the materials presented to students were personalized

Table 2. McGuire's Information Processing Communication Model

Attention > Comprehension > Acceptance > Retention > Action

(Evans, Raines, & Owen, 1990). Formative process evaluation indicated that peer audiences found such scenes to be realistic.

THEORETICAL MODELS RELATING TO PREVENTION INTERVENTIONS

As might be inferred from the discussion thus far, the social inoculation approach to prevention was developed with simultaneous, explicit attention to empirical characteristics of the study population at hand and to the theoretical propositions of Bandura's Social Learning Theory (1977) and McGuire's Information Processing Communication Model (1968). The rapid development of health psychology and behavioral medicine in the 1970s resulted in considerable cross-fertilization as prevention researchers made efforts to apply general, empirically grounded theory from the behavioral and social sciences in their program designs. While space here precludes a detailed discussion of all relevant paradigms, some prominent ones whose assumptions are implicit in the social inoculation approach will be noted.

Five distinct yet overlapping theoretical paradigms have been central regarding efforts to understand health and illness-related behavior (Fishbein, Triandis, Kanfer, Becker, Middlestadt, & Eichler, 2001). They are Bandura's extended *Social Cognitive Theory*, Becker's *Health Belief Model*, Fishbein's *Theory of Reasoned Action*, Kanfer's *Self-Regulation/Self-Control Theory*, and Triandis' *Subjective Culture and Interpersonal Relations* approach. These theoretical perspectives converge on a set of eight conditions necessary for the performance of any volitional behavior. The first three conditions are essential for an action to be performed. They are: (1) a strong intention or commitment to engage (or not to engage) in a particular action; (2) absence of environmental barriers that would make the action impossible; and (3) possession of the skills necessary to engage in the action. The next five conditions can be regarded as either influencing directly the strength of intention or the strength of the action. Another possibility is that these conditions moderate the relation between intention and action. These conditions are: (4) the person has a positive attitude toward the action (its benefits are perceived to outweigh its costs); (5) the person perceives the action to be consistent with social norms; (6) the person perceives the action to be consistent with his or her self-image; (7) the person's emotional reaction to performing the action is positive; and (8) the person realistically perceives that he or she has the capability to perform the action, that is, self-efficacy.

Collectively these conditions embody a model of semi-volitional behavior in general and health behavior in particular. From a prevention standpoint, the social inoculation approach can be understood as an effort to manipulate each of the variables in this model to facilitate health behavior and inhibit health-risking behavior. For example, consider the active avoidance of cigarette smoking as an example of a school-based prevention program goal (Evans et al., 1978). Communication of accurate information via peer leaders about the health consequences of smoking is an effort to influence attitudes toward smoking (costs outweigh the benefits) and intentions not to smoke. Communicating accurate information about the proportion of students' peers who smoke and engage in deviant or antisocial behaviors is an effort to sensitize students to social norms that militate against smoking and thus to strengthen the intention not to smoke. Resistance skills training and rehearsal aims to first, give students the social skills to successfully resist social influences to smoke, and second, to build their smoking resistance self-efficacy, that is, their perception that they can successfully translate intentions not to smoke into action assertive enough to counter any intensity of social influence to smoke. The intention here is not to imply that the social inoculation model was developed exclusively as a deductive exercise in applied social psychology—quite the contrary. We are merely suggesting that this approach has been adopted and extended by other researchers, such as Botvin (1995) in the context of life skills training, because it resonated constructively with advances in social psychological theory occurring at the same historical moment.

STRATEGIES FOR CONSTRUCTION OF POST-ADOLESCENT PREVENTION INTERVENTIONS THROUGHOUT THE LIFE COURSE

In ignoring the necessity of developing an empirical basis for a social inoculation preventive program (Evans, 1976), many studies produced too general, "cookie cutter" applications. This has unfortunately characterized prevention efforts such as *Drug Abuse Resistance Education* (DARE) that fail to be situationally effective for all or any sub-populations targeted by the program (Ennett, Tobler, Ringwalt, & Flewelling, 1994). Simply applying the conceptual base and content of the social inoculation model will prove to be of questionable value unless a field-generated knowledge base can be introduced into a process of formative evaluation. To review this procedure as outlined above, step one requires access to a representative sample of the projected target population for the prevention program. For example if the program is directed at individuals who are past mid-life, a series of focused interviews should be conducted even as was done during the development of the social inoculation model with children and adolescents.

Failure to comply with prescribed drug regimens is a significant example of a health-risk behavior pertinent throughout the life span. We shall utilize this issue of compliance to exemplify extension of the social inoculation model to health issues other than cigarette smoking and beyond adolescence.

Respondents should be queried regarding their knowledge of the prescribed drug effects and related treatment format. Next respondents should be queried regarding problems or pressures they experience in attempting to comply with regimens. The following are examples of possible problems: side effects of the drug; compliance while traveling in different time zones; memory lapses that may at times preclude adherence to recommended ingestion frequency; multiple chronic health problems; assigned multiple drug regimens; fears associated with potential negative drug interaction effects; media reports or scientifically unsupported on-line of studies that question the efficacy of drugs that have been prescribed by a physician; and so on.

Once establishing perceived barriers to compliance with a physician-prescribed drug regimen through such focused interviews, some content of prevention strategy may emerge. Another important focus of such interviews would be the elicitation of effective coping strategies actually employed by the respondents. So in keeping with the social inoculation approach, in the prevention program these subjects would be first informed about these pressures and provided with strategies to cope.

In the application of the social inoculation model to the prevention of substance abuse in children and adolescents, peer pressure or models of health-risking behavior were often appropriate. For older persons, data from focused interviews might reveal different, strong correlates or predictors of health risking behavior. Illustrating this is the prior example of non-compliance with a drug use regimen. Such non-compliance might result from misinformation through the media, memory deficits, or a variety of other situational influences. Each target population for a preventive intervention should be assessed in this way by the program developer consistent with the emphasis placed on formative evaluation in the social inoculation approach. This procedure has been employed in developing many current interventions applied across ethnic groups, gender, and other demographic categories (Botvin, 1995). As indicated earlier, "cookie cutter" strategies for prevention fail to address critical group differences that can obviate the effectiveness of the program. In fact, the criticism based on conventional wisdom made by many politicians or lay spokespersons that prevention is less fruitful than punitive strategies, does not take into consideration that prevention programs often lack the dosage intensity and target specificity necessary to be effective in the long term.

Another essential element is the engendering of perceived behavior control (Ajzen et al., 1985), that is, self-efficacy (Bandura, 1977, 1992). Engendering resistance skills within adolescent subjects implies a shift toward greater self-efficacy in *not* engaging in health-risking behaviors. With regard to compliance with drug regimens, an example might involve communicating to elderly, memory-impaired patients techniques for accomplishing certain behaviors. For example, tactics aimed at accomplishing the systematic ingestion of prescribed drugs might entail setting an alarm for the same time every day, keeping medications in a large container in plain view rather than in a drawer or cabinet. Learning and rehearsing such actions can simultaneously habituate the behavior and build self-efficacy regarding its accomplishment.

Many other examples of prevention content could be explored in other behavioral arenas such as exercise, diet, use of alcohol or other drugs, coping with depression, and life stress events such as loss of spouse or other significant others critical for social support.

Lastly, it should be noted that hopeful and optimistic attitudinal dispositions regarding health behavior, enhanced health self-efficacy, and commitment to persist in health constructive behavior are merely health-specific elements of the multifaceted construct of resiliency. Although some factors within the domain of resiliency may be hard-wired and not amenable to change, other factors are more modifiable in the context of preventive intervention efforts. Thus the social inoculation approach can be regarded as an early, health-specific effort at resiliency enhancement.

PREVENTIVE INTERVENTION ACROSS THE LIFE COURSE AS AN APPLICATION OF SCIENTIFIC EPISTEMOLOGY

From an historical perspective Thomas Kuhn's analysis (1962) of the process of science including paradigmatic change noted that paradigm shifts begin almost imperceptibly with empirical anomalies that multiply until conventional theories are perceived to longer account for them satisfactorily. Although we would hardly claim to be the precursors of a paradigm shift in primary prevention research, attending to empirical anomalies (i.e., the limited long-term impact of fear arousal and "information only" messages) motivated the development of the social inoculation approach. Subsequent elaboration of this particular approach to preventive interventions was merely an application of the scientific method insofar as we oscillated back and forth between the induction of theoretical constructs and propositions, and the deductive testing of those propositions.

Short of an actual paradigm shift, progress within any particular science (Kuhn's "normal science") depends upon the development of data-grounded theory combined with sensitivity to empirical anomalies that might signal the need for revision of one's working theoretical model. The science

of health risk behavior prevention is no exception to this rule. The suggestions made above for extending the social inoculation approach to other health risk behaviors across the life course (e.g., medical non-compliance) and across diverse study populations (e.g., the elderly) are essentially recommendations for this refinement of the internal and external validity of prevention-oriented theoretical models.

Moving into the commercial and political world of persuasive communication the increasing use of focus groups, even if less than objectively or competently conducted, are often a key element in major decision-making. As pressures are mounting for the behavioral and social sciences to become more applied in nature there is a danger that the legitimate demand for accountability may result in the too casual attention to theoretical grounding of prevention strategies. Assessing the determinants of long-term failure or success of a prevention program is difficult to accomplish and does not easily provide an answer to "where do we go from here?"

Also see: Social Competence; Family Strengthening entries.

References

Ajzen, I. (1985). From intentions to actions: A theory of planned behavior. In J. Kuhl and J. Beckmann (Eds.), *Action control: from cognition to behavior* (pp. 11–39). New York: Springer-Verlag.

Bandura, A. (1977). *Social learning theory*. Englewood Cliffs, NJ: Prentice-Hall.

Bandura, A. (1992). Exercise of personal agency through the self-efficacy mechanism. In R. Schwarzer (Ed.), *Self-efficacy: Thought control of action* (pp. 3–38). Washington, DC: Hemisphere.

Botvin, G.J. (1995). Drug abuse prevention in school settings. In G.J. Botvin, S. Schinke, & M.A. Orlandi (Eds.), *Drug abuse prevention with multiethnic youth* (pp. 169–192). Thousand Oaks: Sage.

Edmundson, E., McAlister, A., Murray, D., Perry, C., & Lichtenstein, E. (1991). Approaches directed to the individual. In *Strategies to control tobacco use in the United States: A blueprint for public health in the 1990s.* (Publication No. 92-3316, pp. 147–199.) Washington, DC: National Institutes of Health.

Ennett, S.T., Tobler, N.S., Ringwalt, C.L., & Flewelling, R. (1994). How effective is drug abuse resistance education? A meta-analysis of Project DARE outcome evaluations. *American Journal of Public Health, 84*, 1394.

Evans, R.I. (1976). Smoking in children: Developing a social psychological strategy of deterrence. *Preventive Medicine, 5*, 122–127.

Evans, R.I. (1989). The evolution of challenges to researchers in health psychology. *Health Psychology, 8*, 631–639.

Evans, R.I. (1998). An historical perspective on effective prevention. In W.J. Bukoski & R.I. Evans (Eds.), *Cost-benefit/cost-effectiveness research on drug abuse prevention: Implications for programming and policy* (National Institute on Drug Abuse Research Monograph Series No. 176). NIH Institutes of Health, Superintendent of Documents, US Government Printing Office.

Evans, R.I. (2001). Social influences in etiology and prevention of smoking and other health threatening behaviors in children and adolescents. In A. Baum, T.A. Revenson, & J.E. Singer (Eds.), *Handbook of health psychology* (pp. 459–468). Mahwah, NJ: Lawrence Erlbaum.

Evans, R.I. (2002). Just say no. In L. Breslow (Ed.), *Encyclopedia of public health* (p. 1354). New York: Macmillan.

Evans, R.I., Raines, B.E., & Hanselka, L.L. (1984). Developing data-based communications in social psychological research: Adolescent smoking prevention. *Journal of Applied Social Psychology, 14*, 289–295.

Evans, R.I., Raines, B.E., & Owen, A.E. (1990). *Adolescent health promotion: The Galveston Project.* Final report to the Bureau of Health Care Delivery and Assistance, Division of Maternal and Child Health.

Evans, R.I., Rozelle, R.M., Lasater, T.M., Dembroski, T.M., & Allen, B.P. (1968). New measure of effects of persuasive communications: A chemical indicator of toothbrushing behavior. *Psychological Report, 23*, 731–736.

Evans, R.I., Rozelle, R.M., Mittelmark, M.B., Hansen, W.B., Bane A.L., & Havis, J. (1978). Deterring the onset of smoking in children: Knowledge of immediate physiological effects and coping with peer pressure, media pressure and parent modeling. *Journal of Applied Social Psychology, 8*, 126–135.

Evans, R.I., Rozelle, R.M., Noblitt, R., & Williams, D.L. (1975). Explicit and implicit persuasive communication over time to initiate and maintain behavior change: A new perspective utilizing a real-life dental hygiene program. *Journal of Applied Social Psychology, 5*, 150–156.

Fishbein, M., Triandis, H.C., Kanfer, F.H., Becker, M., Middlestadt, S., & Eichler, A. (2001). Factors influencing behavior and behavior change. In A. Baum, T.A. Revenson, & J.E. Singer (Eds.), *Handbook of health psychology* (pp. 3–17). Mahwah, NJ: Lawrence Erlbaum.

Goodstadt, M.S. (1978). Alcohol and drug education: Model and outcomes. *Health Education Monograph, 6*, 263–279. Washington, DC: National Institutes of Health.

Janis, I.L., & Feshbach, S. (1953). Effects of fear-arousing communications. *Journal of Abnormal & Social Psychology, 48*, 78–92.

Kuhn, T. (1962). *The structure of scientific revolutions.* Chicago: University of Chicago Press.

Laswell, H.D., & Casey, R.D. (1946). *Propaganda, communmication, and public opinion.* Princeton, NJ: Princeton University Press.

Leventhal, H., Singer, R.P., & Jones, S. (1965). Effects of fear and specificity of recommendations upon attitudes and behavior. *Journal of Personality & Social Psychology, 2*, 20–29.

McGuire, W.J. (1961). The effectiveness of supportive refutational defenses in immunizing and restoring beliefs against persuasion. *Sociometry, 24*, 184–197.

McGuire, W.J. (1968). The nature of attitudes and attitude change. In G. Lindzey & E. Aronson (Eds.), *Handbook of social psychology* (pp. 136–314). Reading, MA: Addison-Wesley.

Thompson, E.L. (1978). Smoking education programs, 1960–1976. *American Journal of Public Health, 68*, 250–257.

Sport, Childhood

Steven Danish, Ken Hodge,
Ihirangi Heke, and Tanya Taylor

INTRODUCTION

Considerable evidence exists to support the positive physical and mental health benefits that accrue from participation in sport and physical activity (ISSP, 1992; US Surgeon General Report, 1996). There are many reasons young athletes give for participating in sport: having fun, seeking affiliation, demonstrating power, improving skills, pursuing excellence, exhibiting aggression, having something to do, experiencing thrills or excitement, being independent, receiving rewards, fulfilling parental expectations, and winning. However, while there are multiple motives, the most common are to improve skills (i.e., develop physical competency through a task orientation), to have fun, and to be with friends or make new friends (i.e., develop social competency through peer relations) (Athletic Footwear Association, 1990; Weiss & Petlichkoff, 1989). Thus, if sport is to be an attractive activity for youth, it must provide opportunities for competency building and enjoyment.

DEFINITIONS

What exactly is sport and is it the same as physical activity? *Sport* is defined as an "institutionalized competitive activity that involves vigorous physical exertion or use of relatively complex physical skills" (Coakley, 1994, p. 21). *Physical activity* is defined as "any bodily movement produced by skeletal muscles that results in energy expenditure" (Willis & Campbell, 1992, p. 10). The element of "competition" is a key aspect that differentiates sport from other physical activities. *Competition* is a "situation in which a comparison of an individual's performance is made with some standard of excellence, in the presence of others who are aware of the criteria (standard), ... and can evaluate the comparison process" (Martens, 1975, p. 74). It is important to note that in the definition of competition, comparisons need not be made with others' performance. The standard on which competition can be based is one's actual or expected performance. However, it is the experience of competition that provides many potential opportunities for psychological development through participation in sport.

SCOPE

There are several reasons to focus on physical activity and sport as vehicles for promoting healthy lifestyles. First, the impact of sport on our society is pervasive (Coakley, 1994). It is a major source of entertainment for both the young and the old. Only family, television, and school involve children's time more than sport (Institute for Social Research, 1985). Ewing, Seefeldt, and Brown (1996) estimated that there are 48,374,000 children in the 5–17 age range participating in sport in the United States. Twenty-two million or 45 percent of the children and youth are involved in community-based sport organizations such as Little

League Baseball and Pop Warner Football. Almost 2.5 million or 5 percent are paying to participate in sport activities such as ice skating and swimming; 14.5 million or 30 percent participate in recreational sports programs; 451,000 participate in intramural sports in middle, junior, and senior high school; and 12 percent of all children play interscholastic sports. By far the largest number of youth participate in non-school-based sports programs. Therefore, if we expect to reach children with healthy lifestyle messages, we should consider trying to reach them where they are and want to be—involved in physical activity and sport (Danish, 2000; Hodge & Danish, 1999). Unfortunately, as the number of youth participating in sport increases in the United States, there has been a concomitant decrease in school-based intramural sports and physical education. In fact, physical education is no longer a mandated activity in any of the 50 states.

Second, sport is a significant factor in the development of physical well-being as well as in one's self-esteem, identity, and feelings of competence (Bloom, 2000; Fejgin, 1994). Bloom (2000) identifies a number of components of psychosocial competence. These components are to be able to play well, think well, work well, love well, and serve well. The concept "be well" should also be added to Bloom's list. Sport *can* be an ideal vehicle for learning many of these competencies.

Third, sport skills and healthy lifestyle skills are learned in the same way—through demonstration, modeling, and practice (Orlick & McCaffrey, 1991).

Despite the increase in the number of youth active in sports and its potential benefits, there are also downsides to sport participation. First, too much involvement in sport can lead to overtraining problems such as being prone to injury. Because youth are beginning participation earlier and earlier, burnout is possible as well, especially when parents and coaches require more and more practice. Second, too great an investment in sports may lead youth, especially boys, to avoid learning other skills or participating in other activities, and as a result, seek security instead of fully searching for their identity (Petitpas & Champagne, 1988). Third, because of its inherently competitive nature, sport tends to reinforce an orientation toward ego goals rather than task goals. Researchers have concluded that the later is most adaptive for psychosocial development (Roberts, 1993). If sport is to be a positive force for development, it must facilitate the attainment of both task and ego goals. This balance is often difficult to achieve because the focus in sport is predominantly on winning and social comparison criteria. This is especially true for boys in sport. Indeed, it has been suggested that sport is *the* social context in which young boys use social comparison processes to determine their status with their peers and to determine their self-esteem (Veroff, 1969).

THEORIES AND RESEARCH

If sport is to be viewed as contributing to the healthy development of youth, the skills learned in sport must be seen as not only enhancing sport performance but as promoting life development. The *sport skills* become *life skills* because they can be transferred from one life domain (e.g., sport) to another (e.g., school or career) (Danish, Petitpas, & Hale, 1993; Hodge, Cresswell, Sherburn, & Dugdale, 1999). For example, many of the skills learned in sport (e.g., motivation, commitment, coping with pressure, concentration, teamwork) are transferable to other life domains such as education, relationships, and jobs.

These life skills are cognitive (e.g., concentration), affective (e.g., self-esteem), and behavioral (e.g., goal setting). To be successful in sport and life it is not enough to know what to avoid (i.e., not losing), one must know how to succeed (i.e., to reach goals) (Danish, 1997; Hodge & Danish, 1999). Life skills involve learning ways to say *yes* to health-enhancing behaviors (e.g., managing emotions, developing a support team, overcoming roadblocks), as opposed to learning to *just say no* to health-compromising behaviors (e.g., alcohol, drugs, gangs, truancy). The focus enables youth to acquire a sense of personal control over themselves and be equipped to make better "life" decisions and thus enhance their physical and mental health.

Sport is an ideal environment for this learning to take place. Kleiber and his colleagues (Kleiber & Kirshnit, 1991; Kleiber & Roberts, 1981) have observed that sport is a forum, a structured test, for learning character values such as responsibility, conformity, persistence, risk taking, courage, and self-control. Moreover, because sport is so important to youth, it is an environment where they spend time willingly. This is not always true for time spent at school and it is well known that we learn best when we are in environments where we want to be.

For the positive health benefits to accrue, physical activity and sport have to be organized appropriately so that each participant is able to reach her or his personal goals and derive satisfaction from doing so (Danish et al., 1993). Successful and satisfying goal accomplishment is regarded as a powerful mediator of psychosocial development. One of the advantages of using sport examples to signify goal accomplishment is that the goals in sport are typically tangible, short term, and easily measured. This gives a youngster a better opportunity to see the value in goal setting and to experience success in setting and achieving goals. Lifestyle goals such as developing good nutritional habits, avoiding tobacco and alcohol, or attaining academic and job skills are often less tangible and clear-cut. Additionally, because these lifestyle goals typically require a longer time period to achieve, youth tend to lose sight of their goal and fail to fully appreciate the worth of goal setting and the life skill benefits of successful goal accomplishment.

The American College of Sport Medicine (ACSM, 1988) issued an opinion statement that regular participation in physical activity provides physical and mental health benefits for people of all ages. Existing research identifies the health benefits of regular physical activity for the general population (US Surgeon General Report, 1996). The US Surgeon General Report (1996) and the ACSM (1988) recommend that children accumulate 30 min or more of moderate intensity physical activity over a course of most days of the week. Significant health benefits can be obtained with only a moderate amount of physical activity, but greater benefits can occur through longer duration and more intense physical activity.

Physical activity is important for the health of muscles, bones, and joints. In addition to reducing the risk of developing chronic illnesses, the US Surgeon General Report (1996) notes that regular participation in physical activity appears to reduce symptoms of depression, anxiety, improve mood, and enhance the ability to perform daily tasks throughout life (see also ISSP, 1992).

Although the body of research on the health benefits of physical activity for children is somewhat limited, there is some compelling evidence of its worth (Rowland, 1996). For example, there is mounting evidence that vigorous and frequent physical activity plays an important role in the process of growth and development for children (Cooper, 1996). Additionally, physical activity serves as a buffer against the increasing incidence of obesity and Type 2 diabetes among children. The observation that exercise is one of the major physiological stimuli of growth hormone indicates the physiological importance of physical activity in the daily life of the developing child. In addition, there is considerable evidence that regular physical activity is important for the development of motor skill acquisition (Fagard, 1996) and bone mass (Bailey, 1996) in the developing child. Finally, there is some evidence that patterns of physical activity during childhood may affect the incidence and morbidity of disease (e.g., coronary artery disease) later in life (Cooper, 1996).

If physical activity for children is to affect health beneficially, the most likely means is by initiating exercise habits that will be maintained throughout life (ACSM, 1988; Blair, Clark, Cureton, & Powell, 1989). The development of these habits usually begins with activities that the participating child finds enjoyable. These activities often involve participating in sport.

In summary, physical activity and sport have considerable potential as both a vehicle for, and a means of, promoting physical and mental health for children. In addition, many youth are already engaged in sport and participate in recreational activities that have the potential for positive consequences regarding physical and mental health.

STRATEGIES: OVERVIEW

As prevention specialists and youth workers have begun to understand the value of sport and physical activity as a means of enhancing development, there have been a number of programs that have purported to teach life skills, character education, and other positive attributes. Most of these programs describe what is being done, not how they are being done. Few programs have been effectively evaluated. Even fewer programs purporting to be effective have been replicated. Without information about how the program was implemented or whether the program was effective, it is difficult to describe strategies that work.

A critical issue in designing effective programs is to make certain that they serve the children, not only for the present, but for the future. The effect that a particular experience has on future learning is called transfer of learning or transfer of training. There are a number of strategies that can enhance the transfer. They include: designing conditions to enhance transfer at the beginning of the activity; creating similarities between the environment of the activity and the environment where the transfer is to occur; providing opportunities to practice transfer during the activity; providing opportunities to reflect on the experiences; involving peers who have successfully completed the activity; involving significant others in the learning process; and providing follow-up experiences to reinforce learning (Gass, 1985).

STRATEGIES THAT WORK

For a program to be considered in this category, it would need to be implemented more than once with a variety of children of different genders and ethnic groups. Additionally, a program would have to be implemented and evaluated by someone other than the program developer. Given these basic criteria, no program has sufficient evidence to be placed in this category. As noted above, one of the most significant problems in determining the effectiveness of different programs is that there is minimal documentation on what the implementation process is. Frequently, meta-analyses are conducted on an intervention strategy such as adventure programming (Hattie, Marsh, Neill, & Richards, 1997). Unfortunately, these kind of analyses tend to lump programs together with the same name (e.g., adventure programs) that may differ dramatically in such factors as the length and structure of the program, the leadership style, the skill level of the leader, and various participant characteristics among others. For these reasons, we are not comfortable identifying any program that meets the criterion of an evidence-based program that works well.

STRATEGIES THAT MIGHT WORK

During the last 10 years, programs have been developed that involve sports. Initially, the programs used sport as a metaphor for learning life skills. However, there are now programs that integrate sport activities and skills to learn life's lessons, sometimes somewhat seamlessly, so that the transfer of the skills is easily done.

The *Going for the Goal* (GOAL) program (Danish, 1997) conducted both in the United States and New Zealand is an example of a "sport as a metaphor for life skills program." GOAL is a 10-session, 10-hr program. The life skills taught in GOAL are how to: (1) identify short-term (about two-month) goals that are positively stated, specific, important to the goal setter, and under the goal setter's control; (2) focus on the process (not the outcome) of attaining these goals; (3) use a general problem-solving model; (4) identify health-compromising behaviors that can impede goal attainment; (5) identify health-promoting behaviors that can facilitate goal attainment; (6) seek and create social support; and (7) transfer the skills learned from one domain to another.

GOAL is taught by well-trained high school student-leaders chosen by their schools for their academic performance, leadership qualities, and extracurricular involvement. Following the training, the student-leaders teach the skills to middle/junior high school students during school. The ratio is approximately 2–3 high school student-leaders to 15 middle/junior high school students.

In the United States, GOAL (Danish et al., 1998) has been taught in 28 sites to over 20,000 students. Across two studies of ethnically diverse US middle school students, participants learned the information the Program teaches and had better school attendance (as compared to a control group). Additionally, they reported being able to achieve the goals they set, had less of an increase in getting drunk, smoking cigarettes, drinking beer and liquor than the control group (for boys only); and decreased their involvement in violent and other problem behavior as compared to a control group (for boys only) (Danish, 1997).

The GOAL Program was adapted and modified for the New Zealand context and an evaluation study was completed to examine the effectiveness of GOAL with New Zealand children. The most important modification was to make the sport metaphor more prominent by using examples and quotes from famous New Zealand athletes. Hodge et al. (1999) evaluated the effectiveness of the GOAL Program in changing intrinsic motivation for schoolwork and self-esteem for a group of New Zealand adolescents. The results revealed that the GOAL Program was successful in developing self-esteem and intrinsic motivation for schoolwork among a group of at-risk 12-year-old children. There was a significant increase in both global and academic self-esteem

for the GOAL group, but no change for the contrast group over the 10-week intervention period and 2-month follow-up. With respect to intrinsic motivation (IM) for schoolwork, there was a significant increase in both IM-enjoyment and IM-effort for the GOAL group, but no change for the contrast group over the 10-week intervention period and 2-month follow-up. Interviews conducted also revealed positive changes as the following quote from one of the New Zealand GOAL leaders indicated:

> It was actually [great to] ... see some of the kids change a bit, because some of them were like real trouble kids when they came to us, but now they're actually settling down and they're doing the work. ... The Principal ... said quite a few of them have changed and they're actually doing their work in class, they're not being trouble kids [and] they're loving it. ... It sort of makes you feel good, because you sort of think "oh yeah I had a part in changing that kid's life", and so it's good. (16-year-old GOAL Leader)

Sports United to Promote Education and Recreation (SUPER) (Danish, Fazio, Nellen, & Owens, 2001), *Teaching Responsibility through Physical Activity* (Hellison, 1995), *Rugby Advantage Program* (RAP) (Hodge, Heke, & McCarroll, 2000), and the *First Tee Life Skills* program (Danish, 2001) are examples of integrated sport and life skills programs.

SUPER is a series of sports-based life skills. Sessions are taught like sports clinics with participants involved in three sets of activities: learning the physical skills related to a specific sport; learning life skills related to sports in general and how these skills are applicable outside of sport; and playing the sport. Skill modules are adapted to fit the specific sport and time. Each of the three activities lasts between 20 and 45 min to teach.

SUPER has been taught by college men's and women's basketball teams, trained to teach the program, to middle school students. The program takes place once per week for 12 weeks after school. The middle school students are placed in teams of approximately 10 with 2 college student-athletes serving as their coaches. During the 90-min sessions, there are three stations; basketball fundamentals, basketball games, and life skill teaching. Some of the same skills as in GOAL are taught but the examples are related to basketball. Others focus on managing emotions and learning positive self-talk.

Student-athlete coaches are taught how to use Sport Observation System (SOS). The SOS involves focusing on *how* youth participate and not just on *how well* they perform. Understanding "how" provides information on the mental skills participants have in dealing with coaching/teaching and may be indicative of how they will respond to other forms of instruction such as school and job training. The SOS is presented in Table 1.

Table 1. The Sport Observation System

- How attentive are participants when given instructions or observing demonstration?
- What happens when they cannot perform an activity to their expectations?
- Do they initiate questions when they do not understand something, or do they wait for someone else to talk first?
- Do they initiate conversation with others, or do they wait for someone else to talk first?
- How do they respond when they have a good or a bad performance?
- How do they respond when others have a good or a bad performance?
- How do they respond when someone gives them praise or criticism?
- Do they give up when they don't do well, or do they persist?
- Do they compete or cooperate with teammates?

SUPER student-athlete leaders are asked to speak to the members of their team about what they observe. A "life skills card" is given to each middle school participant at the end of the program. The report card provides feedback to the participants on the "how" *and* "how well" they have done. In an initial evaluation of the program, etc. participants knew more about how to set goals (Brodeur, Fazio & Danish, in preparation).

Hellison (1995) has developed a program for teachers and coaches to teach responsibility through physical activity. Teaching Responsibility through Physical Activity was developed in Chicago but has been implemented elsewhere (Hellison, Cutforth, Kallusky, Martinek, Parker, & Stiehl, 2000). The model consists of five levels of what it means for students to be responsible and what they need to be responsible for: (a) respect the rights and feelings of others; (b) understand the role of effort in improving oneself in physical activity and life; (c) be self-directed and responsible for one's own well-being; (d) be sensitive and responsible for the well-being of others; and (e) apply what you have learned in different non-physical activity/sport settings. Cummings (1997) examined the impact of the program on school attendance, grades, and dropout rates. She found that the control group had a 34 percent school dropout rate as opposed to no one dropping out of the program group. No differences were found between the groups with respect to school attendance or grades.

RAP (Hodge et al., 2000) is a sport-specific program that utilizes unique aspects of this sport to teach life skills to young rugby players. RAP consists of 15 workshops that teach general life skills. The name of the program, the "Rugby Advantage Program", comes from a rugby rule called the "advantage rule." In this rule, the referee has the discretion *not* to call a penalty if a mistake/rule infraction by one team provides an opportunity for the other team to gain an advantage. In other words, the referee can allow play to continue if the non-offending team gains an "advantage" of possession or field position. The rule has some excellent life skills metaphors: the need to "play on" after a mistake; to re-group

and make the best of a difficult situation; and, most importantly, to accept that mistakes and errors are part of a positive life skill mindset. Working hard to improve one's level of play inevitably results in some short-term mistakes and failures but these "failures/mistakes" are part of the learning process for long-term success. No data are yet available on this program.

The First Tee is a national initiative launched in November 1997 to create affordable and accessible golf facilities for youth from 8 to 18. By the end of 2001, 100 sites will be operational. A national teaching and certification program has been developed that includes learning golf skills, golf rules and etiquette, and life skills. The goal of the First Tee Life Skills Program (Danish, 2001) is to "grow the child as we grow the game of golf" by building an effective golf and life skills instructional program—one that will propel participating young people on a successful life trajectory. As with other life skills programs, the goal is to teach life skills that can be applied to golf and other life domains in a structured format that provides opportunities for practice both on- and off- the golf course.

Twelve life skill modules have been developed that are integrated with the teaching of the other First Tee programming—golf instruction, golf rules instruction, and golf etiquette instruction. Life skills content is divided into three areas: interpersonal skills, self-understanding, and goal setting.

An initial evaluation was held at The First Tee National Youth Golf and Leadership Academy. A total of 119 youth, ages 14–17, from 22 states attended. During this week-long experience, the developers of the Academy hoped to affect the personal values (e.g., concern with the welfare of others), emotional intelligence (e.g., empathy, effective interpersonal skills), and leadership ability (e.g., helping others set goals and develop plans to reach these goals) of participants. Each participant completed a pre- and post-survey to measure the amount of change that occurred on a number of instruments (Danish, Brunelle, Fazio, & Hogan, 2000).

The Academy seemed to have a positive effect on the participants. Many of the changes were associated with the specific leadership and life skills that the participants formally learned and practiced during the week. They felt more competent to lead others and to set and achieve their goals. Additionally, there were changes in some of the values and attitudes measured; this was surprising because attitudes and values are more resistant to change and more likely to evolve over time and through experience. For example, participants felt more concern for others, felt that they understood better the importance of effective communications and felt more able to act responsibly (Danish et al., 2000). Although these results were very preliminary, it does appear that teaching life skills through golf may be an effective primer for continued growth, both in skills and values.

Although the life skill programs described above have been taught to individuals who live in their country's dominant culture, a life skill program loosely based on the GOAL and SUPER programs is being developed by and for an indigenous population in New Zealand. The *Hokowhitu* program (Heke, 2001) is a sport-based drug and alcohol intervention program designed by New Zealand Maori for New Zealand Maori. The Hokowhitu Program will train young Maori students to use skills learned in sport as a model for learning life skills related to deciding whether to engage in drug and alcohol use. As with GOAL and SUPER, older peers will be the teachers.

What is especially unique about this program is its cultural context. Maori are enlisted as active partners in producing a program that is relevant and valid within their community. Research has determined that most intervention programs are inappropriate and ineffective because many of the fundamental aspects of non-indigenous programs are based on non-indigenous cultural paradigms, often ill-suited to indigenous people (Blair, Heke, & Siata'ga, 1996). Until recently, Maori have been strongly encouraged to adopt non-indigenous intervention programs. However, now they want to use Maori perspective. The indigenous/cultural basis of the Hokowhitu Program is termed Kaupapa Maori. As an indigenous approach to education and intervention, Kaupapa Maori signifies the need for any intervention with Maori to be initiated, determined, and validated in terms of the worldview of Maori (Bishop, 1996; Smith, 1992).

One aspect this program shares with other programs is its use of sport. For many Maori, sporting achievement is a source of widely accepted mana (pride) and social prestige (Best, 1976). To take an area of natural strength and abundant resource, as in sporting ability, and build upon these attributes as a means of positive change will be important.

Thus, the aim of the Hokowhitu Program is to integrate both the life skills and Kaupapa Maori ideologies so that a sport-based, life skills intervention can be developed that will prove effective with adolescent Maori. Just as important, however, will be sense of self-determination that will exist—Maori determining what is best for Maori and teaching a program that will work alongside Maori culture.

These programs have the potential to be both valuable and effective for children. What is needed is more carefully documented evaluation efforts.

STRATEGIES THAT DO NOT WORK

Some intervention specialists believe that participating in sport itself is sufficient to promote healthy development. Others feel that if sport participation is combined with lectures, about the dangers of alcohol and drugs, managing anger, and staying in school by well-known athletes, the result will be positive healthy development. We believe both approaches are inadequate and without empirical evidence.

Teaching sport skills without teaching the skills for enhancing healthy development sends the wrong message. There is nothing about a ball or a sport venue that teaches how to be physically and mentally healthy. Lectures are not effective either. Children are active individuals. Their life experiences suggest they learn best by doing rather than by talking. It is said that individuals remember only 10 percent of what they are told. Being told what not to do is common fodder for them and, although the messenger may be important to them, the message often has a limited impact.

In other words, although physical activity and sport provide many opportunities for positive physical and psychological health benefits, the potential benefits of participation in physical activity and sport are not transmitted through mere participation in games (Danish et al., 2001). Indeed, if these benefits available though sport are to be realized, they must be purposely planned, structured, and taught (Weiss, 1995).

SYNTHESIS

Plato (1920) said, "The moral value of exercises and sports far outweigh the physical value (p. 46)." It is one thing to believe that sport can achieve these values, it is still another thing to make sure such an outcome is achieved. Some of the research presented indicates that there are programs that have the potential, yet totally unrealized, to enhance children's commitment to education, health, and personal well-being while helping them to be better athletes. These programs also are enjoyable.

For such benefits to be realized, there must be a recognition among educators, coaches, sport administrators, parents, and prevention specialists that such outcomes can be attained through sport and physical activity. This recognition does not presently exist. No state mandates physical education for elementary or secondary students. Related school-based extracurricular activities such as intramural sports are becoming increasingly rare. Many after-school organizations are placing more and more of their energies in the more skilled athletes (Edmundson, 2000).

Even when organizations, usually those that are community-based, develop sport programs designed to promote positive youth development, they often fail. For programs to be effective, they need clearly defined outcomes and a specific set of activities designed to achieve these outcomes. Learning the skills necessary to enhance development must be taught, not caught. The programs must be designed so that they can be implemented in a variety of sport and activity settings. Moreover, the programs should be able to be adapted for use with different cultures. If needed, the individuals implementing the program should be trained. In other words, personal growth outcomes from participating in programs will not happen accidentally; they must be planned.

Programs must not only be better thought through and implemented; they must be better evaluated. We must develop evaluation plans based on program objectives. Therefore, we must include evaluation planning at the outset. It will be important to identify the "active ingredients" or components of successful programs. We must assess the effectiveness of the program on different populations and in different settings. We must examine both the proximal and distal outcomes of the intervention.

However, the development of evidenced-based programs will not be sufficient. We must reach organizations that conduct sport and physical activity programs for children, both school-based and after-school-based, to adopt these programs. Sport is a well-established institution worldwide with well-developed mores and traditions. Many individuals and organizations believe that sport teaches life skills and there may be resistance. Collaborating with national organizations, including professional sports organizations to disseminate effective programs may be necessary.

Sport can be an essential element in personal growth when programs are designed to enhance life's lessons. This is especially true when youth are taught to compete against themselves; more specifically, when competition is focused on maximizing one's own potential and achieving one's own goals. In other words, participation in sport is best when the focus is on knowing oneself as opposed to proving oneself.

Also see: Social Competency; Self-Esteem entries; Academic Success; Nutrition and Physical Activity; Adolescence; Physical Fitness, Adulthood.

References

ACSM. (1988). American College of Sports Medicine opinion statement on physical fitness in children and youth. *Medicine and Science in Sport and Exercise, 20,* 422–423.

Athletic Footwear Association. (1990). *American youth and sports participation.* North Palm Beach, Florida.

Bailey, D. (1996). The role of physical activity in the regulation of bone mass during growth. In O. Bar-Or (Ed.), *The child and adolescent athlete: Volume VI of the encyclopaedia of sports medicine* (pp. 138–152). Oxford: Blackwell Science.

Best, E. (1976). *Games and pastimes of the Māori.* Wellington: A.H. Shearer, Government Printer.

Bishop, R. (1996). *Whakawhānaungatanga: Collaborative research stories.* Palmerston North: Dunmore Press.

Blair, S., Clark, D., Cureton, K., & Powell, K. (1989). Exercise and fitness in childhood: Implications for a lifetime of health. In C. Gisolfi & D. Lamb (Eds.), *Perspectives in exercise science and sports medicine: Youth, exercise, and sport* (pp. 401–430). Indianapolis: Benchmark.

Blair, S., Heke, I., & Siata'ga, P. (1996). *Evaluation of adventure based counselling.* Education Department: University of Otago.

Bloom, M. (2000). The uses of theory in primary prevention practice: Evolving thoughts on school and after-school activities as influences of social competence. In S.J. Danish & T. Gullotta (Eds.), *Developing competent youth and strong communities through after-school programming.* Washington, DC: CWLA Press.

Brodeur, S., Fazio, R., & Danish, S. *The SUPER program: A pilot evaluation.* In preparation.

Coakley, J. (1994). *Sport in society: Issues and controversies* (5th ed.). St Louis: Times Mirror/Mosby.

Cooper, D. (1996). Cardiorespiratory and metabolic responses to exercise: Maturation and growth. In O. Bar-Or (Ed.), *The child and adolescent athlete: Volume VI of the encyclopaedia of sports medicine* (pp. 54–73). Oxford: Blackwell Science.

Cummings, T. (1997) *Testing the effectiveness of Hellison's personal and social responsibility model.* Unpublished Master's thesis; California State University, Chico.

Danish, S. (1997). Going for the goal: A life skills program for adolescents. In T. Gullotta & G. Albee (Eds.), *Primary prevention works* (pp. 291–312). Newbury Park: Sage.

Danish, S.J. (2000). Youth and community development: How after-school programming can make a difference. In S.J. Danish & T. Gullotta (Eds.), *Developing competent youth and strong communities through after-school programming* (pp. 275–301). Washington, DC: CWLA Press.

Danish, S.J. (2001). The first tee: Teaching youth to succeed in golf and life. In P.R. Thomas (Ed.), *Optimising performance in golf* (pp. 67–75). Brisbane, Australia: Australian Academic Press.

Danish, S., Brunelle, J., Fazio, R., & Hogan, C. (2000). *The First Tee National Youth Golf and Leadership Academy: First Evaluation Report.* Richmond; VA: Life Skills Center. Unpublished report.

Danish, S., Fazio, R., Nellen, V., & Owens, S. (2001). Teaching life skills through sport: Community-based programs to enhance adolescent development. In J. Van Raalte & B. Brewer (Eds.), *Exploring sport and exercise psychology* (2nd ed., pp. 205–225). Washington, DC: American Psychological Association.

Danish, S., Meyer, A., Mash, J., Howard, C., Curl, S., Brunelle, J., & Owens, S. (1998). *Going for the goal: Leader manual and student activity book* (2nd ed.). Department of Psychology, Virginia Commonwealth University.

Danish, S., Petitpas, A., & Hale, B. (1993). Life development intervention for athletes: Life skills through sports. *The Counseling Psychologist, 21,* 352–385.

Edmundson, K. (2000). Issues in after-school youth development programming. In S.J. Danish & T. Gullotta (Eds.), *Developing competent youth and strong communities through after-school programming.* Washington, DC: CWLA Press.

Ewing, M., Seefeldt, V., & Brown, T. (1996). *The role of organized sport in the education and health of American children and youth.* Unpublished paper commissioned by the Carnegie Corporation, New York.

Fagard, J. (1996). Skill acquisition in children: A historical perspective. In O. Bar-Or (Ed.), *The child and adolescent athlete: Volume VI of the encyclopaedia of sports medicine* (pp. 74–91). Oxford: Blackwell Science.

Fejgin, N. (1994). Participation in high school sports: A subversion of school mission or contribution to academic goals? *Sociology of Sport Journal, 11,* 211–230.

Gass, M. (1985). Programming the transfer of learning in adventure education. *Journal of Experimental Education, 8*(3), 18–24.

Hattie, J., Marsh, H., Neill, J., & Richards, G. (1997). Adventure education and outward bound: Out-of-class experiences that make a lasting difference. *Review of Educational Research, 67*(1), 43–87.

Heke, I. (2001). *The Hokowhitu Program: Designing a sporting intervention to address alcohol and substance abuse in adolescent Maori.*

Unpublished manuscript, University of Otago, Dunedin, New Zealand.

Hellison, D. (1995). *Teaching responsibility through physical activity*. Champaign, IL: Human Kinetics.

Hellison, D., Cutforth, N., Kallusky, J., Martinek, T., Parker, M., & Stiehl, J. (2000). *Youth development and physical activity*. Champaign, IL: Human Kinetics.

Hodge, K., & Danish, S. (1999). Promoting life skills for adolescent males through sport. In A. Horne & M. Kiselica (Eds.), *Handbook of counselling boys and adolescent males* (pp. 55–71). Thousand Oaks, CA: Sage.

Hodge, K., Heke, J.I., & McCarroll, N. (2000). *The Rugby Advantage Program (RAP)*. Unpublished manuscript, University of Otago, Dunedin, New Zealand.

Hodge, K., Cresswell, S., Sherburn, D., & Dugdale, J. (1999). Physical activity-based lifeSkills programmes: Part II—Example programmes. *Physical Education NZ Journal, 32*, 12–15.

Institute for Social Research. (1985). *Time, goods & well-being*. Ann Arbor, Michigan: University of Michigan Press.

ISSP. (1992). Physical activity and psychological benefits: A position statement from the International Society of Sport Psychology. *Journal of Applied Sport Psychology, 4*, 94–98.

Kleiber, D.A., & Kirshnit, C.E. (1991). Sport involvement and identity formation. In L. Diamant (Ed.), *Mind-body maturity: Psychological approaches to sports, exercise, and fitness* (pp. 193–211). New York: Hemisphere.

Kleiber, D.A., & Roberts, G.C. (1981). The effects of sport experience in the development of social character: An exploratory investigation. *Journal of Sport Psychology, 3*, 114–122.

Martens, R. (1975). *Social psychology and physical activity*. New York: Harper & Row.

Orlick, T., & McCaffrey, N. (1991). Mental training with children for sport and life. *The Sport Psychologist, 5*, 322–334.

Petitpas, A.L., & Champagne, D.E. (1988). Developmental programming for intercollegiate athletes. *Journal of College Student Development, 29*(5), 454–460.

Plato. (1920). Protagoras. In A. Cubberly (Ed.), *Readings in the history of education* (p. 46). New York: Houghton-Mifflin.

Roberts, G. (1993). Motivation in sport: Understanding and enhancing the motivation and achievement of children. In R. Singer, M. Murphey, L.K. Tennant (Eds.), *Handbook of research on sport psychology* (pp. 405–420). New York: Macmillan.

Rowland, T. (1996). Athleticism, physical activity and health in the early years: A question of persistence. In O. Bar-Or (Ed.), *The child and adolescent athlete: Volume VI of the encyclopaedia of sports medicine* (pp. 153–160). Oxford: Blackwell Science.

Smith, G.H. (1992). Tane -Nui-a Rangi's Legacy. ... Propping up the sky ... (Kaupapa Māori as Resistance and Intervention). Paper Presented at NZARE/AARE Joint Conference. Deakin University, Australia.

US Surgeon General Report. (1996). *Physical activity and health: A report of the Surgeon General*. Atlanta, GA: US Department of Health and Human Services, Centers for Disease Control and Prevention, National Center for Chronic Disease Prevention and Health Promotion.

Veroff, J. (1969). Social comparison and the development of achievement motivation. In C.P. Smith (Ed.), *Achievement-related motives in children* (pp. 46–101). New York: Russell Sage.

Weiss, M. (1995). Children in sport: An educational model. In S. Murphy (Ed.), *Sport psychology interventions* (pp. 39–69). Champaign, IL: Human Kinetics.

Weiss, M., & Petlichkoff, L. (1989). Children's motivation for participation in and withdrawal from sport: Identifying the missing links. *Pediatric Exercise Science, 1*, 195–211.

Willis, J., & Campbell, L. (1992). *Exercise psychology*. Champaign, IL: Human Kinetics.

Stepfamilies, Childhood

Blair J. Carter

INTRODUCTION

Remarriages and stepfamilies have become an increasingly popular area of study for scholars in child and human development, psychology, sociology, family studies, and other disciplines (Coleman, Ganong, & Fine, 2000). However, the study of family structures and processes has not generally been a central focus for epidemiologists, health educators, and other public health scientists and practitioners. This entry examines how public health scientists and practitioners may design programs that promote the development of children and adolescents who are living or who have lived in stepfamilies.

DEFINITIONS

Remarriages and *stepfamilies* are related, but not identical, terms. For example, not all remarriages result in the formation of a stepfamily. Many remarriages are childfree at the time of the remarriage. Some of these remarriages result in the birth of children into the remarried family while others remain childfree. In either case, these resulting remarried families are technically not stepfamilies. Stepfamilies may, therefore, be properly conceptualized as a subset of remarried families in which at least one of the adults comes in to the remarriage with a child (or children) from a previous committed relationship (usually marriage). Although some scholars (e.g., Ganong & Coleman, 1994) use the terms interchangeably, I will use the terms to describe distinctly different concepts and realities.

SCOPE

Incidence and Prevalence

Demographers have rarely studied remarriages and stepfamilies. Therefore, our knowledge of the demography of such families is limited. As the public health consequences of family structures and processes are established and disseminated, this limitation may be overcome; then, more varied demographic analyses may begin to play a larger role in the study and design of interventions for remarriages, stepfamilies, and other kinds of family units.

One exception to this lack of demographic research is a frequently cited paper by Glick (1989). Although dated, his analysis serves as an estimate of the incidence and prevalence of remarriages and stepfamilies in the United States. Glick (1989) used US Census Data for his 1980 estimates and Current Population Survey for his 1987 estimates of the point prevalence (i.e., the total number at a particular time) of remarriage and stepfamilies living in the United States. Estimates of incidence (i.e., new cases) are even more difficult to obtain but new population surveys may reduce this problem in the future. In 1987 there were approximately 64.49 million families of which about half (31.9 million) had children under the age of 18 living at home. Just fewer than 80 percent (24.65 million) of these families with children under 18 were married couple families. A little over 20 percent (5.24 million) of the married couple families with children under 18 were remarried families. Of the 5.24 million remarried families with children under age 18, 4.3 million were stepfamilies and 940,000 were not stepfamilies. These 940,000 families consisted of remarried couples that had children in their remarriage but had no children from their previous relationships. This group of almost one million families has not been the subject of previous investigations and will be excluded from following. Thus, we might estimate that about one third of the 4.3 million stepfamilies with children under 18 years, or somewhat less than 1.5 million families, have children aged 6–12 years, and another third have adolescents (12–18 years). (This is an upper limit because we do not know the degree to which stepfamilies with children may be double counted. That is, how many of these stepfamilies would have more than one stepchild living in the household. The more frequent this situation occurs, the larger the overestimation of stepfamilies with children would be.)

Another way of looking at prevalence is to look at the number of children aged 6–12 living in stepfamilies. Glick (1989) found that about 9.75 million, or nearly 15.6 percent of the total of 62.51 million children living in the United States in 1987, were members of remarried families. Of these, about 8.78 million (or 90 percent) were living in stepfamilies. About two thirds (5.85 million) of these children living in stepfamilies were stepchildren and the other third (2.93 million) were half-siblings born subsequent to the remarriage. If we assume that one third of the 8.78 million children in stepfamilies are children aged 6–12, we come up with an estimate of close to 1 million children living in stepfamilies. (This estimate, which uses the individual child as the unit of analysis, is not subject to the same problem of overestimation as the preceding estimate using stepfamilies as the unit of analysis. That is, double counting is not a problem when the child, rather than the stepfamily, is the unit of analysis.) Likewise, our estimates would be another third

adolescents, or about three million young persons between the ages of 12 and 18.

Estimates for Canada, and other western countries, suggest that the incidence and prevalence rates are somewhat, but not substantially, lower than in the United States (Levin & Sussman, 1997). Many Catholic countries and many non-western and less-developed countries have significantly lower rates of divorce and remarriage.

Individual, Family, and Societal Costs

There are few cost–benefit or cost-effective analyses on this topic reported in the scientific literature. However, in very general terms, there is both clinical (Visher & Visher, 1996) and empirical (Amato, 1994) support for suggesting that individual members of stepfamilies, and stepfamily systems as a whole, may bear costs that devolve from the structure and processes of the families in which they live.

In a meta-analysis of 21 studies reporting on children living in stepfamilies, Amato (1994) found that children in stepfamilies performed more poorly than children in "intact two-parent" families on five outcome domains. The total mean effect size for all outcomes (stepfamily vs. intact nuclear family) was -0.17 ($p < 0.001$). This effect size, Amato suggests, though statistically significant, may not be meaningful for individual- or family-level decision-making. However, from a community or population-based perspective, a mean effect size of -0.17 implies that the average child living in a stepfamily scores about as well as the 43rd percentile of children from intact nuclear families. Using this same logic, from a public health perspective, the studies reporting conduct/behavior problems had a mean effect size of -0.32 ($p < 0.001$), and the studies examining psychological adjustment had a mean effect size of -0.37 ($p < 0.001$). This implies that the average child living in a stepfamily performed at the 37th percentile on conduct/behavior problems and at the 36th percentile on psychological adjustment when compared with children from intact nuclear families. Therefore, the average child living in a stepfamily did as poorly on conduct/behavior and psychological adjustment outcomes as almost the lowest one third of the children living in intact nuclear families.

The other three areas, academic achievement, self-esteem, and social relations, had mean effect sizes ranging from -0.007 to -0.16 and were also statistically significant. However, it is in the findings regarding conduct/behavior problems and social adjustment that we find effect sizes that demand the attention of primary prevention professionals. In short, there appears to be a consensus that children and adolescents living in stepfamilies experience more behavior and adjustment problems than young people living in intact nuclear families (Coleman et al., 2000; Zill, Morrison, & Coiro, 1993).

Visher and Visher (1996) and other clinicians who have worked with stepfamilies (Pasley, Dollahite, & Ihinger-Tallman, 1993; Walsh, 1992) have reported additional problems. Ganong and Coleman (1986, 1987, 1994) reported that family dynamics, transitional adjustment, incomplete institutionalization of the stepfamily (Cherlin, 1978), emotional responses, and stepfamily expectations are common concerns of clinicians working with stepfamilies.

THEORIES AND RESEARCH

Much of the work on stepfamilies remains atheoretical. However, in a comprehensive review of clinical and empirical literatures on stepfamilies, Ganong and Coleman (1986, 1987) found that clinicians, more than researchers, used a *family systems framework*. Coleman et al. (2000) suggested that progress had been made in the development of theoretical explanations for stepfamily effects on stepchildren. These authors provide references for those interested in how *systems theory, role theory, gender theory, exchange theory, social ecological theory*, and a *life course perspective* have influenced the study of stepfamilies and their members. However, they suggest that "… most explanations for stepparent effects on stepchildren could be categorized as variants of stress models, (step)parent involvement rationales, (step)parent role models, and selection" (p. 1293). *Stress models* identify the particular responses available to stepfamilies experiencing the specific stresses and strains inherent in such families. The diverse kinds of rationales and involvements associated with stepparent roles (Cherlin, 1978) are central to models of stepparent involvement and roles. The differential selection of families for studies of stepfamilies is also important to understand. Stepfamilies participating in studies may have characteristics that are not representative of stepfamilies in general.

Kuller (1999) proposed the concept of "circular epidemiology." This concept speaks to the concern that certain areas of epidemiological study are basically providing more and more information about increasingly unimportant areas of investigation. The use of limited resources to investigate questions in areas where answers are abundant is a poor use of resources. Much of the research on stepfamilies is of this kind. For example, once we "know" that certain outcomes are more likely to occur in a particular type of family structure (e.g., stepfamily) than in another type of family structure (e.g., intact nuclear family), we in the primary prevention community need to apply that knowledge to improve the health of families and their members. Additional knowledge may be obtained from family and public health investigators while current knowledge is being applied. This process, sometimes termed "action research,"

helps to overcome the limitations of circular investigations—whether undertaken by epidemiologists, health educators, family scholars, or others interested in improving the health of stepfamilies and their individual members.

STRATEGIES: OVERVIEW

The possibilities for intervening to promote the health of stepfamilies and their members are almost endless. However, in practice, the paucity of interventions is noteworthy and the dearth of evaluations of those few interventions is even more problematic. In short, very little has been tried and, when tried, even less has been satisfactorily evaluated.

Most of the research on stepfamilies has been noninterventional. The idea of intervening in a systematic manner to promote the health of stepfamilies in general, and the children or adolescents living in them in particular, has not taken hold in the scholarship of students of such families. Therefore, this entry will make some inferences from the literature on the promotion of healthy development in general, with appropriate caveats.

STRATEGIES THAT WORK

There is no information available regarding any rigorous research on programs that work to promote the healthy development of children and adolescents who are living in stepfamilies.

STRATEGIES THAT MIGHT WORK

The following material is based on inferences from the few existing studies involving various systems that make up stepfamily life—the larger social systems in which stepfamilies exist, the family systems themselves, and then several subsystems such as the marital dyad or stepparent/stepchild units.

Larger social systems can be more sensitive to the needs of stepfamilies. For example, Ganong (1993) describes some ways in which the leadership, staff, and membership of state 4-H organization perceived and interacted with stepfamilies relative to nuclear intact families and single parent families. Some suggestions for interventions are provided including several ways in which 4-H staff may be sensitized to the needs of stepfamilies and their members, such as the inclusion of step- and biological parents and siblings in events when appropriate, and the incorporation of phrases related to diverse family structures (including stepfamilies) in printed materials. These types of programs and materials may be useful with stepfamilies in other contexts, such as health service organizations, and other youth-oriented groups (like the YMCA, YWCA, Big Brothers/Big Sisters) and religious organizations.

Likewise, Crosbie-Burnett and Skyles (1989) have provided recommendations for educational policy changes in schools and universities (see also, Fine, 1997). These policies might enhance the relationships between the schools and the stepfamilies they serve. For example, interventions may include policies adopted for use by state departments of education, district school superintendents, local school boards, and for teachers, counselors, social workers, nurses, and others directly involved with the education of stepchildren. Educational workshops, reviews of existing curricula and policies, analysis of student outcomes by family structure type, and obtaining input from parents in stepfamilies are all possible ways of intervening on behalf of stepfamilies with children in schools. Assuming that these policy changes received positive empirical support, they could offer another method to promote the health of stepchildren.

Legal systems may be involved with stepfamilies (Mahoney, 1997). Currently, the legal system in the United States and many other countries provides little protection for the rights of stepfamily members. Examples of areas where changes in the legal system might be beneficial include child support, estate planning, and stepparent visitation and custody following divorce. Examples of how other countries, for example, Great Britain (Fine, 1997), have modified their laws provide possible models for state and federal legislators in the United States. These kinds of macro interventions should be carefully evaluated because of their possibilities for extensive affects on society.

There are no research reports of successful primary prevention programs targeting stepfamilies as a system. Hughes and Schroeder (1997) reviewed four family life education programs targeted at entire stepfamilies, but none of these programs were evaluated. Two of the programs addressed family dynamics (although they contained little content covering non-residential parents). Other content covered in one or more of the four programs were stepfamily transition issues, stepfamily strengths, and expectations of stepfamily members. Family life education programs in general might be promising for stepfamilies as they are with any kind of family, talking about predictable issues of discipline, how to enhance academics, how to deal with concerns around budding sexuality. What would be especially helpful is research on whether stepfamilies need to make any special efforts as they face these ordinary challenges of growing children.

Interventions with stepfamily sub-systems (e.g., marital dyads, (step)parent–child dyads) have not been the target of specific health promotion or primary prevention efforts. Hughes and Schroeder (1997) reviewed programs that inter-

vened directly with children, but none were evaluated. However, several features of classroom programs suggest for further investigation. First, all students in a classroom were involved; stepchildren were not singled out. Second, these programs taught children about stepfamilies, clarifying stereotypes and presenting positive views of this kind of family. These programs were "well received" by the over 2,000 student participants, but being well received is not the same as being effective. These features represent a beginning point for developing processes and content for further development.

STRATEGIES THAT DO NOT WORK

Hughes and Schroeder (1997) reviewed family life programs directed toward adults. Most of these programs were not evaluated and had serious design problems (such as no control groups). Of those that were partially evaluated, none showed much promise. Information concerning non-residential parents, legal, and financial issues impacting stepfamilies was generally absent or given little attention. Most of these programs dealt with parenting issues as opposed to general stepfamily dynamics. Such approaches may not be fruitful paths for future prevention programming unless the content is increased to include additional information of use in understanding the entire family system.

SYNTHESIS

It is difficult to present a multidimensional program based on the best available information, when there essentially is little information available. Therefore, I offer several ideas to begin to build a basis for promoting the healthy development of children and adolescents living in stepfamilies.

First, young people have certain basic needs that must be met in order to develop and thrive, regardless of the family structure in which they live. These basic needs are discussed in detail in other entries in this encyclopedia, but (at a minimum) they include loving, supportive, involved, committed, and authoritative (not authoritarian) parents.

The next question is what is distinctive about stepfamilies that require special attention to the needs for health promotion and primary prevention for the young people who live in them? For example, family life education programs for stepfamilies need to address issues related to the separation of one parent from the primary family (at least part of the time) and the presence of another adult/authority figure in the stepfamily, for example, the "wicked stepmother" myth (Skeen, Robinson, & Covi, 1985). Also, in complex stepfamilies, there are also special issues related to "instant" siblings and new relatives, and the various challenges arising from the complex relationships among them, as well as relatives and friends from the former family.

What follows are some beginning points on promoting the healthy development of children living in stepfamilies. They are based on current theoretical perspectives (e.g., stress theory) and on the few hints we have from the empirical literature (Skeen et al., 1985).

1. Stepparents should develop age-appropriate relationships with stepchildren that are warm and understanding without expecting that the stepchildren will immediately return that warmth or understanding. Patience is an important virtue for stepfamily members in general, and for stepparents in particular. Adolescence, it is worth remembering, is a time of growing independence and deepened connection with peers, whether in a biological or a stepfamily context.

2. Biological parents and stepparents should set reasonable boundaries and rules. They should also be supportive of one another in enforcing these decisions consistently. The use of family meetings (when the children are old enough to understand and participate) should be held to discuss the rules and the reasons for them. These rules should benefit all stepfamily members and not merely be for the benefit of the biological and stepparents. For example, there should be rules respecting the children's privacy.

3. The fact that the biological parents are divorced does not imply that the children are divorced from the non-resident parent. Stepparents need to understand and respect the strength of these attachments. Stepparents also need to understand the ambivalence that children will likely experience in their old and new relationships and develop the patience to allow the children time and space to maintain these relationships. The relationships with non-resident parents are particularly important to understand and support.

4. The new marriage partners need to work to keep that relationship strong and vibrant and should not neglect their relationship because of temporary problems and issues related to the children in the stepfamily. The new marital relationship is the basis for the healthy development of the children in the stepfamily.

These suggestions reflect our current knowledge of healthy stepfamilies. However, further research and theory development should help us develop additional specific knowledge that will help us promote the healthy development of children living in stepfamilies. Matthews and Hudson (2001) have provided guidelines of the evaluation of parent training programs. These guidelines use a "CIPP protocol" that suggests that a total evaluation consists of Context, Input, Process, and Product (or outcomes) evaluations. This may be a useful set of guidelines for those responsible for evaluating interventions with (step)parents in particular and, with

slight modifications, stepfamily supra-systems and stepfamilies in general.

Also see: Family Strengthening entries; Marital Satisfaction.

References

Amato, P.R. (1994). The implications of research findings on children in stepfamilies. In A. Booth & J. Dunn (Eds.), *Stepfamilies: Who benefits? Who does not?* (pp. 81–87). Hillsdale, NJ: Erlbaum.

Cherlin, A. (1978). Remarriage as an incomplete institution, *American Journal of Sociology, 84*, 634–650.

Coleman, M., Ganong, L., & Fine, M. (2000). Reinvestigating remarriage: Another decade of progress. *Journal of Marriage and the Family, 62*, 1288–1307.

Crosbie-Burnett, M., & Skyles, A. (1989). Stepchildren in schools and colleges: Recommendations for educational policy changes. *Family Relations, 38*(1), 69–94.

Fine, M. (1997). Stepfamilies from a policy perspective: Guidance from the empirical literature. In I. Levin & M.B. Sussman (Eds.), *Stepfamilies: History, research, and policy* (pp. 249–264). New York: Haworth.

Ganong, L.H. (1993). Family diversity in a youth organization: Involvement of single-parent families and stepfamilies in 4-H. *Family Relations, 42*, 286–292.

Ganong, L.H., & Coleman, M. (1986). A comparison of clinical and empirical literature on children in stepfamilies. *Journal of Marriage and the Family, 48*, 309–318.

Ganong, L.H., & Coleman, M. (1987). Effects of parental remarriage on children: An update and comparison of theories, methods, and findings from clinical and empirical research. In K. Pasley & M. Ihinger-Tallman (Eds.), *Remarriage and stepparenting today: Current research and theory* (pp. 94–140). New York: Guilford.

Ganong, L.H., & Coleman, M. (1994). *Remarried family relationships*. Thousand Oaks, CA: Sage.

Glick, P.C. (1989). Remarried families, stepfamilies, and stepchildren: A brief demographic profile. *Family Relations, 38*, 24–27.

Hughes, R., & Schroeder, J.D. (1997). Family life education programs for stepfamilies. In I. Levin & M.B. Sussman (Eds.), *Stepfamilies: History, research, and policy* (pp. 281–300). New York: Haworth.

Kuller, L. (1999). Invited commentary: Circular epidemiology. *American Journal of Epidemiology, 150*, 897–903.

Levin, I., & Sussman, M.B. (Eds.). (1997). *Stepfamilies: History, research, and policy*. New York: Haworth.

Mahoney, M. (1997). Stepfamilies from a legal perspective. In I. Levin & M.B. Sussman (Eds.), *Stepfamilies: History, research, and policy* (pp. 231–247). New York: Haworth.

Matthews, J.M., & Hudson, A.M. (2001). Guidelines for evaluating parent training programs. *Family Relations, 50*, 77–86.

Pasley, K., Dollahite, D.C., & Ihinger-Tallman, M. (1993). Bridging the gap: Clinical applications of research findings on the spouse and stepparent roles in remarriage. *Family Relations, 42*, 315–322.

Skeen, N.P., Robinson, B.E., & Covi, R.B. (1985). Stepfamilies: A review of the literature with suggestions for practitioners. *Journal of Counseling and Development, 64*(2), 121–125.

Visher, E.B., & Visher, J.S. (1996). *Therapy with stepfamilies*. New York: Bruner/Mazel.

Walsh, W.M. (1992). Twenty major issues in remarriage families. *Journal of Counseling and Development, 70*, 709–715.

Zill, N., Morrison, R., & Coiro, M.J. (1993). Long-term effects of parental divorce on parent–child relationships, adjustment, and achievement in young adulthood. *Journal of Family Psychology, 7*, 91–103.

Substances (Children of Substance Abusers), Childhood

James G. Emshoff, Jeannette Johnson, and Laura Jacobus

INTRODUCTION

Children of alcoholics (COAs) and other substance-abusing parents are considered to be at high risk because there is a greater likelihood that they will develop alcoholism or substance abuse, as well as a range of other psychosocial problems. Children of substance-abusing parents (COSAPs) are especially vulnerable to the risk for maladaptive behavior because they have combinations of many risk factors present in their lives. The single most potent risk factor is their parent's substance-abusing behavior. This single risk factor can place children of substance abusers (COSAs) at biological, psychological, and environmental risk. Research reports that COAs and other substance abusers are at risk for cognitive, psychological, biological, or neuropsychological deficits. Not surprisingly, the findings of these diverse studies are inconsistent; thus, a unified concept of risk for alcoholism or substance abuse has not yet emerged. This entry reviews primary prevention efforts to promote healthy development in COSAPS.

DEFINITIONS

The term "children of alcoholics" was established earlier in the literature and is perhaps better recognized by researchers and practitioners. However, despite variations of impact upon children as a function of the substance abused by parents, there are more similar dynamics than differences. Thus, we will refer to the more generic term of COSAPs.

SCOPE

Eigen and Rowden (2000) provide a refined estimate of the prevalence of COAs. They distinguish between children of current alcoholics (of which there are 11 million, representing 17 percent of our youth under 18), children whose parents have been alcoholics at sometime during the child's life (of which there are 14 million, or 22 percent of our youth

population) and children whose parents were alcoholics at some point in their lives (17.5 million, or 27 percent of the population under 18). No precise estimates of the number of COSAPS could be located. However, the number of individuals addicted to illicit substances is approximately 42 percent of the number addicted to alcohol (NIDA, 1999). Thus, if none of these additional addicts was also an alcoholic, we could extrapolate the above prevalence estimates by 42 percent. However, this extrapolation would need to be attenuated by the proportion of illicit drug addicts who are also alcoholics.

Substance abuse is a major public health problem that affects millions of people and places enormous financial and social burdens on society. It destroys families, damages the economy, victimizes communities, and places extraordinary demands on the education, criminal justice, and social service systems. A study by the Office of Management and Budget estimated the substance abuse costs to the United States at $300 billion a year, including government antidrug programs and the costs of crime, health care, accidents, and lost productivity (Falco, 1993).

The scientific and practitioner literature regarding COSAPs has been developed primarily in the United States. However, it is obvious that these issues and dynamics are as international in scope as substance abuse itself. In understanding the global issues of COSAPS, it is important to have both an understanding of the epidemiology of the use of various substances in different countries, as well as an understanding of how culture affects family dynamics, and how these dynamics interact with the presence of parental addiction.

THEORIES AND RESEARCH

Risk Theory

Risk and protective theory states that a person's probability of engaging in substance abuse is predictable from the combination of risk and protective factors s/he is exposed to. These factors exist at the individual, family, community, and macro levels. Data clearly support a familial disposition toward alcoholism. A relationship between parental substance abuse and subsequent alcohol problems among their children has been extensively documented. The literature on COAs far outweighs the literature on children of other drug abusers. Relatively little is known about children of heroin addicts, cocaine abusers, or poly-drug abusers (Johnson, Boney, & Brown, 1990–1991). Children of addicted parents are at greater risk for later dysfunctional behaviors and they, too, deserve significant attention to prevent intergenerational transmission of drug abuses later in life.

Children of substance-abusing parents are at great risk for behavioral problems and physiological damage when exposed in-utero to their mother's drug addiction. Some of these problems may last well through maturation. We currently lack the necessary longitudinal data allowing any firm conclusions about the long-term effects of parental substance abuse. Even if children are not exposed to chemicals in-utero, they are at greater risk for childhood behavioral problems if their parents are involved in the drug culture.

Anthony (1974) suggested the possibility that all COSAs could not be grouped into a single, unitary entity. Similar experiences affect children differently due to individual differences in, for example, temperament, intelligence, and environmental resources, with the result that there is no single profile of COSAs.

Resilience Theory

Among these subgroups of COSAPs are those who, despite all odds, enjoy good health from birth, experience a positive environment at home, and develop normally into socialized, competent, and self-confident individuals. Certain individuals, often referred to as "resilient," may be more competent than others in adapting to stressful living environments. Such a child is able to compensate and cope with the various negative biological or environmental influences in his/her life. Certain individuals may be able to manipulate their environment by choosing roles and goals in life that stabilize their developmental process and bring them the positive reinforcement they need to develop a positive self-image, and eventually a relatively healthy life. Other individuals may be able to master and conceptualize the environment in such a way as to choose positive behaviors in life that compensate for whatever problems are present.

Genetic Research

Reviews of the literature of COSAPs (Johnson & Leff, 1999) have typically categorized the research into four basic groups of studies. The first group includes those that emphasize the heritability of alcoholism. Many studies of related individuals (e.g., families, twins, or adopted out siblings) support a genetic theory of alcoholism transmission. In particular, the greater influence of the biologic versus the adoptive family in the development of alcoholism has fostered the idea of genetic transmission. In one representative study, male adoptees with alcoholic biologic fathers were four times as likely to become alcoholic than those without, although relationships with alcohol misuse in the adoptive parents were not observed (Cadoret, Cain, & Grove, 1980). Goodwin (1985) reported that the prevalence of alcoholism among both male (25 percent) and female (5–10 percent)

relatives of alcoholics exceeded the estimated population prevalence for alcoholics that are 3–5 percent for men and 0.1–1 percent for women. The pathway by which the genetic diathesis is expressed is currently a subject of great interest.

Teratogenic Effects

The second group of studies consists of those investigating the teratogenic effects of maternal alcohol and other drug (AOD) use. These studies report strong relationships between in-utero AOD use on the one hand and later childhood problems such as minor physical anomalies, hyperactivity, mental retardation, and EEG anomalies (Jones & Smith, 1973). Jones and Smith (1973) first described *Fetal Alcohol Syndrome* as a cluster of four characteristics occurring in the offspring of mothers who drank excessively during pregnancy: central nervous system dysfunction, abnormal facial features, behavioral deficits, and growth deficiency.

Family Systems Theory and Research

A third group of studies highlight different aspects of the addicted family environment and family interaction. Family studies view children from a family illness perspective with regard to the dynamics of the illness and its effects on family functioning. Family studies involve two separate areas of research: the impact of addiction upon family functions and the impact of addiction on the adult COSAPs specifically. These studies typically conclude that the transmission of alcoholism is complex and involves multiple genetic, psychological, sociological, and cultural interactions (Adger, 2000).

Developmental Theory and Research

A fourth group of studies center on various biological and psychosocial characteristics of children of differing maturational stages who grow up in addicted families. These studies attempt to isolate biological and psychological variables that differentiate children at risk for alcoholism. Isolating biological mechanisms that may distinguish populations at high or low risk for alcoholism has involved a variety of techniques. COAs are differentiated from children of nonalcoholics, for example, on the basis of EEG, event-related potentials, enhanced antagonistic placebo response, and endocrine deviations (Children of Alcoholics, 1997). Despite many promising leads, this line of research has not yet successfully identified a premorbid biological marker that will accurately predict those who become alcoholic from those who do not.

Although there are a number of general strategies that have proven successful with COSAP populations, and there is a substantial literature documenting the success of certain substance abuse prevention programs for the general youth population, there is limited information based on well-designed evaluations regarding prevention programs designed specifically for COSAPs. Kumpfer (1999) notes that many programs utilize self-developed measurement tools whose psychometric properties are unknown. The vast majority of these instruments are used only once, prohibiting the comparability of results across studies (Johnson, Rolf, Tiegel, & McDuff, 1996). Replication of findings is rarely attempted, let alone achieved.

Kumpfer also notes that many evaluations fail to be sensitive to the fact that prevention programs may be differentially successful with different types of children. Thus, in order to demonstrate the true effectiveness of an intervention, evaluations should examine not only the overall effectiveness of programs, but also the ways in which different subpopulations of participants responded to the intervention. Additionally, because many prevention programs are designed to address a number of risk factors, the results of prevention programs may not be immediately apparent and may not be manifest until several years after the intervention has completed. In order to effectively measure these outcomes, researchers must investigate and utilize more effective ways to collect longitudinal information with this population.

STRATEGIES THAT WORK

It seems premature to endorse any strategy as conclusively effective based on solid evidence. Nevertheless, it is likely that the firmer literature on substance abuse prevention is likely to be relevant here. As such, it seems reasonable to emphasize programs that are interactive and skill-based, as described below.

STRATEGIES THAT MIGHT WORK

Despite these numerous design and measurement issues, several prevention programs have documented considerable success with COSAP populations. Listed below is a brief overview of several of these programs.

Focus on Families Program

The Focus on Families Program (Catalano, Haggerty, Fleming, Brewer, & Gainey, 2000) is a family-based program that targets chemically dependant parents and their children. By providing families with parent-management skills and at-home case-management services, the Focus on Families Program attempts to reduce the risk of relapse by parents and prevent substance abuse among their children.

Evaluations have indicated that parents participating in the program demonstrate increased general problem-solving skills and drug-refusal skills at a 24-month follow-up assessment than did parents in a control group. Parents also reported using significantly less heroin at the completion of the program and at the 12-month follow-up, as well as less cocaine at the 12-month follow-up. The evaluation also revealed a trend level reduction in both drug use and delinquent behaviors among the children at the 24-month follow-up. Although this program did not demonstrate statistically strong changes in child behaviors, the evaluators suggested that the sample of children used in the evaluation might have been too young for the program to demonstrate efficacy in reducing problem behaviors (Catalano, Gainey, Fleming, Haggerty, & Johnson, 1999).

Children Are People Too (CAP)

The CAP Program is an 8–10 week curriculum that was designed to address psychosocial difficulties among COSAP populations. Although the content of the program usually relies on the child having continued access to a drug-free adult, the program was recently revised for use with children who did not have access to such an adult (Dore, Nelson-Zlupko, & Kaufman, 1999). The revised program also included an increased emphasis on children's feelings, perceptions of their parents' behavior, and an emphasis on the connections between drug use and violence.

This revised curriculum led to increased (but statistically insignificant) levels of social acceptance, self-worth, and internal locus of control among children participating in the program (Dore et al., 1999). Teacher observations also suggested that children improved on several dimensions of classroom behavior. Despite these generally positive trends, the only change that was statistically significant was a decreased likelihood of children participating in a physical attack. Although the revised curriculum may indeed have merit for use with COSAP populations, the researchers suggested that the duration of the intervention itself was simply too short to have any real, lasting effect on children's behavior.

Creating Lasting Connections (CLC)

The CLC Program (Johnson et al., 1996) is designed to address a number of risk and resiliency factors that are associated with AOD use among high-risk youth. Although this program is not specifically targeted at COSAPs, an unspecified number of participants identified themselves as COSAPs and the program addresses many of the family dynamics and behaviors relevant to COSAPs.

The CLC Program attempts to increase family resilience to AOD by: increasing parents knowledge of AOD issues, improving family management skills, communication skills, providing positive role-modeling of alcohol use, increasing community involvement with their children, and utilizing community services if the need arises. In addition, the CLC Program attempts to increase youth resilience by improving communication and refusal skills, family bonding, community involvement, and use of community services when situation warranted. Families participating in the program also receive follow-up care for one year.

Evaluations of the CLC Program (Johnson et al., 1996) have utilized an experimental design. Evaluations have indicated that parents participating in the program demonstrate increased knowledge about AOD information, and family use of community services. In addition, the program demonstrated some success in increasing youth resiliency by increasing the utilization of community services when need arose, increasing bonding with family members, improving communication skills, and increasing community involvement under some conditions. As a result of these successful prevention efforts, The Center for Substance Abuse Prevention, and the National Prevention Network has selected the CLC Program as 1 of 16 exemplary prevention programs.

Stress Management and Alcohol Awareness Program (SMAAP)

The SMAAP is an 8-week, 1-hr per week, school-based prevention program that targets COSAPs. The program, which is administered in a small-group format, utilizes a variety of strategies including discussion, modeling, and role-play exercises to address issues that are relevant to COSAP populations. The program specifically addresses issues such as self-esteem, alcohol-related education, and emotion and problem-focused coping strategies (Roosa, Gensheimer, Ayers, & Shell, 1989). A revision of SMAAP (Short et al., 1995) included a component that specifically addressed misconceptions COSAPs have about alcohol consumption.

Evaluations of SMAAP program have indicated that program participants are more likely than non-participants to demonstrate increased knowledge, social support, as well as emotion-focused coping behaviors. The evaluation also highlighted a possible unintended negative side effect of the program. Participation in the program led to significant increase in the expected tension release resulting from alcohol use. Past research has demonstrated that positive alcohol expectancies may be related to increased alcohol consumption among adolescents (Simons-Morton, Haynie, Crump, Saylor, Eitel, & Yu, 1999). This may suggest particularly troubling unintended effects for adolescent COSAP populations, who have been shown to have elevated alcohol expectancies to begin with (Colder, Chassin, Stice, & Curran, 1997; Wiers, Gunning, & Sergeant, 1998).

Students Together and Resourceful (STAR)

STAR is an intervention that is based on a community psychology orientation. One goal was to provide students with accurate information concerning alcohol, alcoholism, and family reactions to alcoholism in order to understand the etiology of alcoholism and to reduce self-blame. A secondary goal was to increase social competence and both the quantity and quality of peer relations. Group exercises were designed to facilitate the identification, acceptance, and expression of feelings. A related goal was that of improving the social network of participants. Specific skills such as problem-solving, decision-making, stress management, and refusal skills were emphasized. In short, the intervention was designed to do what parents normally do: help children learn to live with themselves in their environments, to establish good relationships, and to make constructive decisions and follow them through.

One strength of this program was its use of a wait list control group who received the intervention at a later time. The analyses consisted of comparisons between the control and treatment groups over time, strengthening the argument that outcomes were a result of the intervention. Participants were successful in establishing stronger social relations, a sense of control, and improved self-concept. Participants reported increases in the number of friends, peer involvement, and perceived social support. Participants also reported decreased loneliness and depression (Emshoff, 1990).

Children of Drug Abusers and Alcoholics (CODA)

CODA is an early intervention program for high-risk children aged 4–10 who live with at least one parent (or guardian) addicted to alcohol and/or other drugs. The program consisted of two 12-week components, one for children and one for families. Children were involved in small group activities involving art and play therapy activities. One evening each week children participated with their parent or guardian in a family interaction group in which the families engaged in unstructured art and play therapy activities. Results demonstrated improved competence and behavior as measured by the Child Behavior Checklist (CBCL). However, the evaluation results should be interpreted with caution due to the lack of a control group (Springer, Phillips, Phillips, Cannady, & Kerst-Harris, 1992).

Strengthening Families Program

The Strengthening Families Program (SFP) is a family intervention that has been shown to reduce risk factors, increase resilience, and decrease alcohol, tobacco, and drug use among elementary-aged COSAs (Kumpfer, DeMarsh, & Child, 1989). The basic intervention consists of a parent-training program and social-skills training for the children as well as a family relationship enhancement program. Typically the program is conducted in churches or community centers in brief sessions of two or three hours.

Kumpfer, Molgaard, and Spoth (1996) offer several suggestions for successful implementation of family-focused interventions. It is crucial that focus groups include members who are representative of the target population. Innovative recruitment strategies should include outreach to community agencies, schools, churches, housing authorities, and youth service agencies, among others, in an attempt to involve hard-to-reach families.

The SFP has been modified for a variety of cultural groups including rural and urban African American COSAs, Hawaiian COSAs, Latino COSAs, and rural preteens. Evaluation studies showed that the basic program with minor cultural revisions was more effective than a substantially revised program (Kumpfer et al., 1996). The authors concluded that the core content of the program should not be deleted when making cultural revisions. As a result of positive outcomes of SFP replications, NIDA has chosen SFP as one of three model substance abuse prevention programs for dissemination.

Alateen

Alateen is a program for COAs based on the Alcoholics Anonymous 12-Step Program of Recovery. Very little evaluation data on the effectiveness of Alateen is available. Hughes (1977) found that Alateen participants had more positive scores on a mood state and self-esteem scale than COAs who did not participate in Alateen. Peitler (1980) compared Alateen to group counseling and no treatment in sons of alcoholics aged 4–16. Group counseling had more positive effects than Alateen in improving self-worth and reducing withdrawal and anti-social tendencies.

CASPAR

The Cambridge and Somerville Program for Alcoholism Rehabilitation (CASPAR) is a pioneer in the COA prevention field offering a range of prevention and intervention services. Classroom teachers and CASPAR staff conduct classes on AODs for primary through twelfth grade students. The goal of this approach is to prevent the development of substance abuse and related problems in a general population of children. CASPAR also has programs for high risk groups of youth at all grade levels. Groups are conducted by adult staff in school and community settings (e.g., housing developments and recreation centers), and by trained peer leaders in after-school groups in junior high schools (Davis et al., 1994). Students can then either self-refer or be referred by parents, teachers, community agencies, other students, or CASPAR personnel.

Evaluation data have provided interesting findings. Students participated in either COA-specific groups or a basic education group. COAs in the basic alcohol education groups consistently reported that they learned useful information and indicated they would drink differently, and were drinking less as a result of participation than non-COAs or children in the COA group. However, children in the alcoholic families group reported more positive learning experiences. Although COAs seemed to gain more from groups dealing directly with parental alcoholism, more children were willing to attend the basic education group where they could avoid self-identification as a COA, and were still able to learn useful information (DiCicco, Davis, Hogan, MacLean, & Orenstein, 1984).

Although prevention programs that are targeted to COSAPs use a variety of strategies, there are some elements that are relatively common across programs. These common components include information about AODs, problem-focused and emotion-focused coping behaviors, and social and emotional support. Not only are these strategies common among program that may work, they are theoretically linked to the needs of COSAPs, which adds plausibility to their effectiveness. In addition, these same strategies have been used in prevention programs for other, more general audiences that have produced more definitive positive outcomes.

Information about Alcohol and Other Drugs

Prevention programs for COSAPs often include a component that helps children learn about substance-related issues in a developmentally appropriate manner. Although many children may benefit from this information, this type of education may be especially important for COSAPs, as they are more likely than other children to have misconceptions concerning the positive effects of drinking on cognitive and social performance (Brown, Creamer, & Stetson, 1987; Colder et al., 1997). Although the amount and type of information that a child is able to handle will vary depending on the child's developmental level and maturity, programs can help to clear up some of the misconceptions that COSAPs often hold about addiction.

Another common component of prevention programs is to help COSAPs understand their risk status in a developmentally appropriate manner. Prevention programs can help COSAPs to understand that although they may be at increased risk for a variety of psychosocial problems including alcoholism, having an addicted parent does not ensure that they will become addicted themselves. However, it is important to convey the information that these children are at higher risk for alcoholism and substance abuse and that the risk of transition from casual use to addiction is higher for them. Children who are aware of their risk status drink significantly less (in both quantity and frequency) than do COSAPs who are unaware of this information (Kumpfer, 1989).

Skill Building

The majority of prevention programs targeted at COSAPs include a component that involves teaching emotion-focused and problem-focused coping skills (Nastasi & DeZolt, 1994). Emotion-focused coping skills may be especially important for COSAPs to acquire because they often do not have control over their parent's drinking habits. By addressing these issues indirectly, COSAPs may be able to regain some sense of control over their lives. Additionally, COSAPs often benefit from problem-focused coping skills training in which the children learn strategies for living with an addicted parent, such as avoiding driving with an intoxicated parent and explaining parental behaviors to their friends. Other skills often addressed in COSAP prevention programs include communication, stress management, decision-making, and peer resistance (Price & Emshoff, 2000).

Social Support

Social support may be especially important for COSAPs, who often face substantial stresses with relatively little support. By offering COSAPs additional sources of support, programs may assist these children in dealing with the difficult issues that they face on a daily basis. Furthermore, there is evidence that children may benefit not only from receiving support, but also from offering support. Some research with other populations demonstrates that programs that allow participants to both provide and receive support have the most positive outcomes (Maton, 1987).

Incorporating Prevention into Existing Practice Settings

Another promising primary prevention strategy is to incorporate screening and referral for familial substance abuse into the normal procedures used by those that see children on a regular basis. Toward that end, the National Association of Children of Alcoholics, assisted by the Office of National Drug Policy, the Center for Substance Abuse Prevention, as well as other leading health organizations have developed a set of core competencies for use within primary-care health settings (Adger, McDonald, & Wenger, 1999). Pediatricians are in an opportune position to conduct a brief screening to assist in the early identification of COSAPs and

to provide information and referrals that may help to prevent future difficulties (Werner, Joffe, & Graham, 1999). Although many health care providers still believe that substance-abuse problems are the domain of mental health professionals, a growing number of health-care providers are becoming involved in the identification and referral of COSAPs to appropriate services. One product of this collaboration has been the development of a set of core competencies for pediatricians dealing with children in substance-abusing families

STRATEGIES THAT DO NOT WORK

The literature does not directly speak of what strategies do not work with COSAPs. However, we can interpolate from meta-analyses which have identified ineffective strategies for prevention of substance abuse in children, in general (Tobler, 2000). These strategies include non-interactive programs, passive delivery, and programs that do not include a focus on interpersonal skills. Given the specific needs of COSAPS (e.g., interpersonal skill development, becoming proactive rather than reactive), it is likely that these general findings are applicable to COSAPs, despite the lack of specific empirical validation of these findings for this population.

SYNTHESIS

To date, there is no single program that has been tested with sufficient rigor, using psychometrically sound instruments, with multiple replications, over extended periods of time, and diverse samples of COSAPs to warrant its identification as THE model preventive program. However, a number of programs and practitioners have provided convergent evidence regarding some principles of intervention that seem worthy of consideration.

Successful prevention programs that are targeted to COSAP populations share many of the same characteristics of successful prevention programs designed for other populations. Prevention programs that are of a longer duration, offer participants an opportunity to participate in some form of follow-up care or "booster" sessions, and have characteristics that allow intervention results to be generalized to everyday settings are more likely to demonstrate success than interventions that do not share these characteristics (Botvin, Baker, Filazzola, & Botvin, 1990; Lochman, 1992). In addition, the programs that have promising findings for COSAPs all seem to have some balance among *information, skill-building, and support*.

Programs targeted at this population must remain cognizant of the fact that COSAPs represent a remarkably heterogeneous group. Thus, prevention programs targeted to COSAP populations should avoid utilizing a narrow focus.

A broad range of strategies that address a number of different risk and protective factors and the diverse needs and characteristics of COSAPs is recommended.

One dimension of diversity is the range of outcomes experienced by COSAPs. While COSAP status implies risk, it does not imply a pre-determined, inescapable outcome. The resilience and normality of many COSAPs must be recognized. Prevention programs targeted at COSAP populations must be developed with sensitivity to the negative impact of assuming pathology and the consequent effects of labeling on COSAP populations. One way to diminish these negative effects is to design programs to be delivered to all children, not only COSAPs. This approach has the added benefit of allowing programs to reach COSAPs who would not ordinarily be identified as such. By allowing larger number of individuals access to these programs, researchers can ensure that their prevention services are received by all affected children, while also reducing the stigma attached to their delivery. The use of non-stigmatizing settings (e.g., schools, community centers, and churches) may also reduce the stigma attached to receiving COSAP services.

Because peers exert such a powerful influence on substance-use decisions (Hawkins, Catalano, & Miller, 1992), interventions that are broadly targeted to include both COSAPs and their peers may prove to be more effective prevention strategies than those that utilize more narrowly targeted groups. Interventions that are designed to target COSAP populations may also prove more successful and more easily generalized when peers are included as facilitators. Past research has demonstrated that substance abuse prevention programs in which peers instruct and practice program components with participants are better generalized than are programs that do not incorporate the use of peers (Botvin et al., 1990).

Continued and expanded research is imperative. We need to know more about the differences between COSAPs and children from other dysfunctional families and stressful environments. The epidemiology and etiology of diverse subpopulations of COSAPs need to be explored. The development and evaluation of prevention programs could benefit by attention to many of the issues described in this entry. Despite these limitations, there is no doubt that the effort and concern focused on this population has improved the lives of many children.

Also see: Substances Entries.

References

Adger, H. (2000). Children in alcoholic families: Family dynamics and treatment issues. In S. Abbott (Ed.), *Children of alcoholics: Selected readings* (Vol. II). Rockville, MD: National Association of Children of Alcoholics Press.

Adger, H., McDonald, D.I., & Wenger, S. (1999). Core competencies for involvement of health care providers in the care of children and adolescents affected by substance abuse. *Pediatrics, 103*(5), 1083–1084.

Children of Alcoholics [Special issues]. (1997). *Alcohol and Health Research world, 21*(3), 241–247.

Anthony, E. (1974). *The child in his family. Children at psychiatric risk* (Vol. 3). New York, NY: Wiley & Sons.

Botvin, G.J., Baker, E., Filazzola, A.D., & Botvin, E.M (1990). A cognitive-behavioral approach to substance abuse prevention: One-year follow-up. *Addictive Behaviors, 15*(1), 47–63.

Brown, S.A., Creamer, V.A., Stetson, B.A. (1987). Adolescent alcohol expectancies in relation to personal and parental drinking patterns. *Journal of Abnormal Psychology, 96*, 117–121.

Cadoret, R.J., Cain, C.A., & Grove, W.M. (1980). Development of alcoholism in adoptees raised apart from alcoholic biologic relatives. *Archives of General Psychiatry, 37*, 561–563.

Catalano, R.F., Gainey, R.R., Fleming, C.B., Haggerty, K.P., & Johnson, N.O. (1999). An experimental intervention with families of substance abusers: One-year follow-up of the focus on families project. *Addiction, 94*(2), 241–254.

Catalano, R.F., Haggerty, K.P., Fleming, C.B., Brewer, D.B., & Gainey, R.R. (2000). *Children of substance abusing parents: Current findings from the focus on families project.* Unpublished draft.

Colder, C.R., Chassin, L, Stice, E.M., & Curran, P.J. (1997). Alcohol expectancies as potential mediators of parent alcoholism effects on the development of adolescent heavy drinking. *Journal of Research on Adolescence, 7*(4), 349–374.

Davis, R.B., Wolfe, H., Orenstein, A., Bergamo, P., Buetens, K., Fraster, B., Hogan, J., MacLean, A., & Ryan, M. (1994). Intervening with high risk youth: A program model. *Adolescence, 29*(116), 763–774.

DiCicco, L., Davis, R.B., Hogan, J., MacLean, A., & Orenstein, A. (1984). Group experiences for children of alcoholics. *Alcohol Health and Research World, 8*, 20–24.

Dore, M.M., Nelson-Zlupko, L., & Kaufman, E. (1999). "Friends in need": Designing and implementing a psychoeducational group for school children in need from drug-involved families. *Social Work, 44*(2), 179–190.

Eigen, L.D., & Rowden, D.W. (2000). A methodology and current estimate of the number of children of alcoholics in the United States. In S. Abbott (Ed.), *Children of alcoholics: Selected readings* (Vol. II). Rockville, MD: National Association of Children of Alcoholics Press.

Emshoff, J.G. (1990). A preventive intervention with children of alcoholics. *Prevention in Human Services, 7*(1), 225–253

Falco, M. (1993). *Demand reduction. Proceedings of the inaugural symposium on crime and punishment in the United States* (pp. 243–249). Washington, DC: United States Sentencing Commission.

Goodwin, D.W. (1985). Alcoholism and genetics: The sins of the fathers. *Archives of General Psychiatry, 42*, 171–174.

Hawkins, J.D., Catalano, R.F., & Miller, J.Y. (1992). Risk and protective factors for alcohol and other drug problems in adolescence and early adulthood: Implications for substance abuse prevention. *Psychological Bulletin, 112*(1), 64–105.

Hughes, J.M. (1977). Adolescent children of alcoholic parents and the relationship of Alateen to these children. *Journal of Consulting and Clinical Psychology, 45*, 946–947.

Johnson, J.L., Boney, T.Y., & Brown, B.S. (1990–1991). Evidence of depressive symptoms in children of substance abusers. *International Journal of Addictions, 25*(4-A), 465–479

Johnson, J.L., & Leff, M. (1999). Children of substance abusers: Overview of research findings. *American Academy of Pediatrics, 103*(5), Part 2 of 2, 1085–1099.

Johnson, J.L., Rolf, J.E., Tiegel, S., & McDuff, D. (1996). Developmental assessment of children of alcoholics. In S. Abbott (Ed.), *Children of alcoholics: Selected readings*. Rockville, MD: National Association of Children of Alcoholics Press.

Johnson, K., Strader, T., Berbaum, M., Bryant, D., Bucholtz, G., Collins, D., & Noe, T., (1996). Reducing alcohol and other drug use by strengthening community, family and youth resiliency: An evaluation of the Creating Lasting Connections Program. *Journal of Adolescent Research*, 11, 36–67.

Jones, K.L., & Smith, D.W. (1973). Recognition of the fetal alcohol syndrome in early infancy. *Lancet, 2*, 999–1001.

Kumpfer, K.L. (1989). Promising prevention strategies for high-risk children of substance abusers. *OSAP High Risk Youth Update*, 2, 1–3.

Kumpfer, K.L. (1999). Outcome measures of interventions in the study of children of substance-abusing parents. *Pediatrics, 5*(2), 1128–1144.

Kumpfer, K.L., DeMarsh, J.P., & Child, W. (1989). *Strengthening families program: Children's skills training curriculum manual, parent training manual, children's skill training manual, and family skills training manual (Prevention services to children of substance-abusing parents)*. Social Research Institute, Graduate School of Social Work, University of Utah.

Kumpfer, K.L., Molgaard, V., & Spoth, R. (1996). The strengthening families program for the prevention of delinquency and drug use. In R.D. Peters & R.J. McCahon (Eds.), *Preventing childhood disorders: Substance abuse and delinquency* (pp. 241–267). Newburg, CA: Sage.

Lochman, J.E. (1992). Cognitive-behavioral intervention with aggressive boys: Three year-follow-up and preventive effects. *Journal of Consulting and Clinical Psychology, 60*(3), 426–432.

Maton, K.I. (1987). Patterns and psychological correlates of material support within a religious setting: The bi-directional hypothesis. *American Journal of Community Psychology, 15*, 185–207.

Nastasi, B.K., & DeZolt, D.M. (1994). *School interventions for children of alcoholics*. New York: The Guilford Press

NIDA. (1999). *National Household Survey on Drug Abuse (NHSDA)*. Substance Abuse and Mental Health Services Administration (SAMHSA), Department of Health and Human Services, Washington, DC.

Peitler, E.J. (1980). A comparison of the effectiveness of group counseling and Alateen on the psychological adjustment of two groups of adolescent sons of alcoholic fathers. *Dissertation Abstracts International, 41*, 1520-B.

Price, A., & Emshoff, J.G. (2000). Breaking the cycle of addiction: Prevention and treatment with children of alcoholics. In S. Abbott (Ed.), *Children of alcoholics: Selected readings* (Vol. II). Rockville, MD: National Association of Children of Alcoholics Press.

Roosa, M.W., Gensheimer, L.K., Ayers, L.K., & Shell, R. (1989). A preventive intervention for children in alcoholic families: Results of a pilot study. *Family Relations, 38*, 295–300.

Short, J.L., Roosa, M.W., Sandler, I.N., Ayers, T., Gensheimer, L., Baver, B., & Yu, L. (1995). Evaluation of a preventive intervention for a self-selected sub-population of children. *American Journal of Community Psychology, 23*, 223–247.

Simons-Morton, B., Haynie, D.L., Crump, A.D., Saylor, K.E., Eitel, P., & Yu, K. (1999). Expectancies and other psychosocial factors associated with alcohol use among early adolescent boys and girls. *Addictive Behaviors, 24*(2), 229–238

Springer, J.F., Phillips, J.L., Phillips, L., Cannady, L.P., & Kerst-Harris, E. (1992, June). CODA: A creative therapy program for children in families affected by abuse of alcohol or other drugs [OSAP Special issue]. *Journal of Community Psychology*, 55–74.

Tobler, N.S. (2000). Lessons learned. *The Journal of Primary Prevention, 20*(4), 261–274.

Werner, M.J., Joffe, A., & Graham, A.V. (1999). Screening, early identification, and office-based intervention with children and youth living in substance-abusing families. *Pediatrics, 5*(2), 1099–1112.

Wiers, R.W., Gunning, W.B., & Sergeant, J.A. (1998). Do young children of alcoholics hold more positive or negative alcohol-related expectancies than controls? *Alcoholism Clinical and Experimental Research, 22*(8), 1855–1863.

Substances, Childhood

Ty Partridge and Brian Flay

INTRODUCTION

Childhood substance use is a significant public health concern. The majority of research and prevention efforts are targeted at middle-school and high-school students, because this is where substance use is most manifest. The roots of the problem likely lay much earlier in the developmental process, yet the prevention issues of adolescence do not translate directly to the needs of childhood substance use prevention. In the ensuing entry, we articulate several theoretical constructs that are useful for constructing and evaluating the prevention of childhood substance use. Additionally, we provide a targeted review of the literature highlighting both empirical successes and significant research needs.

DEFINITIONS

Biosocial Heterochrony refers to differences in the rate of timing of both biological and social events in the course of development.

Precocious Puberty is the onset of puberty that is significantly earlier than the population average. For girls this tends to be around 9–10 years of age and for boys 11–12 years of age.

SCOPE

US Population. Relative to adolescent research, there is a relative dearth of epidemiological data regarding childhood substance use in the United States. However, we do have some estimates regarding the extent of childhood substance use. By and large, childhood substance use is restricted to alcohol, tobacco, marijuana, and the use of inhalants. Alcohol and tobacco are the most widely used substances in this age group. Monitoring the Future (Johnston, O'Malley, & Bachman, 1999) reported retrospective data for their eighth grade sample that asked about substance use as far back as the fourth grade. Alcohol use prevalence rates were reported to be approximately 10 percent in the fourth grade. There was a steady increase in prevalence each year until students reached the seventh grade. Estimated prevalence rates were 20, 27, and 47 percent for the fifth, sixth, and seventh grades, respectively. The eighth grade prevalence, approximately 50 percent, indicated a flattening trend. A similar pattern was found for tobacco use. Prevalence rates were 10, 17, 28, and 43 percent for the fourth, fifth, sixth, and seventh grades, respectively. Again, the eighth grade rate of 48 percent indicated a leveling off. By the eighth grade use of inhalants and marijuana were at approximately equal levels with prevalence rates of about 20 percent for each substance. However, inhalant use was higher in younger children and leveled off more quickly than marijuana use. Inhalant prevalence rates were 5, 10, 12, and 17 percent for the fourth, fifth, sixth, and seventh grades. Marijuana rates, on the other hand, were around 1 percent for the fourth and fifth grades, but jumped to 5 percent by sixth grade and then increased to 15 percent by the seventh grade.

While the Monitoring the Future data have indicated an overall reduction in the lifetime prevalence of early adolescent substance use, there have been indications that the age of first use for alcohol, tobacco, and marijuana have been decreasing over the last decade (Lloyd, 1996). This is of substantial importance because earlier age of first use considerably increases the risks of long-term use, as well as other negative outcomes (Fergusson, Lynskey, & Howard, 1994).

Australian Population.   Similar to the United States, alcohol, tobacco, and marijuana are the most common substances used by youth in Australia. According to a 1990 survey, by age 12 approximately 8 percent of females and 13 percent of males had reported drinking alcohol in the past week (world health organization [WHO], 1999). A recent study of 12 and 13 year old youth found that approximately 6 percent were regular smokers (Tang et al., 1998). Further, marijuana is the most common illicit substance used by Australian youth. Indeed, approximately 10 percent of youth between the ages of 13 and 14 report using marijuana at some point in their lifetime (WHO, 1998). Thus, the overall pattern of substance use among Australian youth is similar to that of the US population. Also similar to the United States, however, is a relative lack of research on substance use in populations younger than age 12.

THEORIES

Traditionally, substance use prevention programs have drawn either from *social learning theory* or health beliefs models (Orlandi, 1996). The former recognizes the influence of salient role models such as parents, peers, siblings, and other individuals with whom a given child identifies (e.g., teachers, athletes, celebrities, etc.). A *health beliefs model* suggests that adolescent substance use is influenced by perceived normative attitudes toward, and expectancies about the consequences of substance use. These two theoretical perspectives are not mutually exclusive, however, and are likely complementary. As such, more recent prevention-oriented theoretical frameworks have synthesized these two approaches. Indeed, the growing trend in prevention theory is a move toward *integration of micro-theories* (Orlandi, 1996). While social learning theory and health beliefs models form the core of these integrated theoretical perspectives, the most promising theories are also incorporating theoretical notions related to biological and personality factors, affective and cognitive factors, interpersonal and social skills, and ecological contextual factors such as family structure, school-environments, and community organization.

The *theory of triadic influence* (TTI) is one model based on these integrative theoretical frameworks (Flay & Petraitis, 1994). TTI is comprised of two primary dimensions. One dimension refers to three general sources of influence: biological/personality influences, social context influences, and culture/ecological influences. The second dimension refers to the causal proximity to substance use behavior of different events in a given domain of influence. TTI suggests seven distinct levels of causal proximity. The developmental dynamics of TTI are captured in the heuristic language of streams referring to the three sources of influence and tiers referring to the levels of causal proximity. Causal influence from each stream can be thought of as flowing down the levels of causal proximity, each funneling toward behavior. Further, the interdependencies between the three streams of influence are captured in cross-stream influences. For example, the biological stream influences the social stream and the social stream influences the biological stream. Finally, TTI allows for iterative influences such that engaging in trial behaviors such as initial experimentation with tobacco, alcohol, or other substances provides feedback upstream changing the state of more distal variables in each of the three streams of influence.

TTI is a more general theoretical statement that addresses not only substance use, but also health risk behavior in general, and further, applies to a broad age range including younger children as well as adolescents. Therefore, in addressing substance use in a pre-adolescent population some special considerations need to be made explicit.

First, individual differences in rates of biological and social development (biosocial heterochrony) play an important role in childhood substance use. The predominant instance of heterochrony in substance use is precocious puberty (Brooks-Gunn & Graber, 1994). There are two traditional hypotheses regarding the role of precocious puberty (Tschann, Adler, Irwin, Millstein, Turner, & Kegeles, 1994). The early-maturation hypothesis suggests that precocious puberty increases risk for engaging in substance use behavior through increased social pressure and exposure to substance use without the requisite social skills to successfully address these pressures. The maturation-deviance hypothesis suggests that off-time development increases social and emotional stress, thereby increasing the likelihood of substance use as a coping mechanism. The effects of precocious puberty on substance use can also be interpreted from a developmental contextual framework (Stattin & Magnusson, 1990).

Second, special consideration needs to be given to the distinction between prevention efforts targeting children who are beginning to experiment with and use substances prior to adolescence and prevention efforts geared toward experimental and regular substance use in adolescence. Substance use, particularly alcohol and tobacco, are somewhat normative during adolescence; however, during childhood such behavior is more indicative of pathology. Thus, whereas peer influences seem to be the predominant consideration in adolescence they are of less importance during childhood (Bush, Weinfurt, & Iannotti, 1994).

The majority of successful adolescent prevention programs incorporate social skills training, particularly emphasizing refusal skills. In younger children, especially those in primary grades, such social skill training needs to take into account the less mature nature of these children's social cognitive skills. Social skills of younger children tend to be more rote, less flexible, and social rules tend to be much more parochial.

Developmental timing issues are of substantial theoretical import in conceptualizing childhood substance use programs (Cicchetti & Cohen, 1995). Multiple sources of influence and temporal dependencies in developmental processes predict that earlier trial use and/or regular use orients the child's developmental context toward a state that supports an escalation toward long-term regular substance use, and in some cases illicit poly-drug use as well as a host of other negative developmental outcomes. Conversely, the later the onset of trial substance use, the more likely the larger developmental context will be oriented such that trial behavior will be experimental and of short duration, substantially reducing the risk of chronic use.

RESEARCH

The current trend in substance use prevention theory toward multi-domain interactional frameworks is drawn from earlier work in developmental systems theory (Damon & Lerner, 1998; Ford & Lerner, 1992). Empirical evidence supporting this trend is voluminous and the cited sources provide a more appropriate venue for review. One noteworthy point needs to be emphasized here, however, regarding the implications for developmental systems approaches to childhood and adolescent substance use etiology. Because of the multiple domains of influence and the contextual nature of the meaning of any given risk or protective factor, there are multiple etiological pathways (Cicchetti & Cohen, 1995). This suggests that empirical findings can be inconsistent across studies and at times contradictory, but nevertheless useful in different contexts. While many of these issues are beyond the scope of the current entry, we will address those issues that are of special consideration for childhood substance use.

First, the issue of precocious puberty is often underaddressed in prevention curricula. However, there is ample evidence that it plays an important role. Stattin and Magnusson (1990) report extensive findings indicating that precocious pubescent girls are much more likely than their normative pubescent peers to engage in a wide range of risk behaviors, prominent among them substance use. Further, there is evidence to suggest that the effects of precocious puberty on substance use are not purely biological in nature, but rather represent the convergence of multiple sources of influence in a single biopsychosocial event (Brooks-Gunn & Graber, 1994). For example, precocious pubescent girls may get caught in a vicious cycle of mutually reinforcing influences that stabilizes early smoking behavior. The confluence of distorted body image, early weight gain associated with early pubescence, and the perceived weight reduction properties of cigarettes have been shown to lead to early initiation of smoking in pre-adolescent girls (Crisp, Sedgwick, Halek, Joughin, & Humphrey, 1999). There is somewhat mixed evidence for the influence of precocious puberty on males (Tschann et al., 1994), but this is a much more difficult population to study.

The second area of special consideration for the prevention of childhood substance use is the role of the family versus peers as the predominant influence on substance use behavior. For example, perceived family use has been shown to be a stronger influence relative to perceived peer use on substance use behaviors among fourth and fifth grade students. However, this relationship was reversed by the seventh grade (Bush et al., 1994). Furthermore, a deviant peer group is a major predictor of adolescent substance use, but parent–child conflict, the quality of mother–child interactions, and several other parental factors have been shown to predict belonging to a deviant peer group (Fergusson & Horwood, 1999).

In addition to the identification of multiple etiologies derived from the adoption of developmental systems theoretical perspectives, the timing of onset becomes much more critical (Cicchetti & Cohen, 1995). As noted by Fergusson et al. (1994) in a sample of Australian children, exposure to alcohol between the ages of 6 and 11 increased the likelihood of becoming a regular alcohol user during adolescence by 3.5 to 7 times.

STRATEGIES THAT WORK

Much as in the case of childhood substance use epidemiology, there is a substantial lack of research on effective prevention programs aimed at elementary school aged children. The 1999 school drug prevention resource guide, *Making the grade: A guide to school drug prevention programs* (Drug Strategies, 1999) identified nine elementary school-oriented drug prevention programs, none of which has been systematically evaluated. Further, many of the prevention programs being implemented at these younger ages are revisions of programs originally designed for middle-school and high-school students. However, it seems likely that there are some universal program elements that should be common to both pre-adolescent and adolescent designs.

First and foremost, these programs need to address multiple domains of influence—ranging from the biological to the immediate psychosocial context to the larger family, school, neighborhood, and community contexts. Second, similar to adolescent prevention programs, curricula that utilize an interactive teaching format also to be of more benefit. Third, school-based programs must take into account teacher acceptance of the program and provide teacher training on implementation. Prevention materials should minimize interference with regular classroom activities (Tobler & Stratton, 1997).

As noted above, there are some special considerations regarding the elements of an elementary school-aged prevention program. First, there needs to be a shift in focus, emphasizing more family relations and support and less emphasis on peer factors. However, this should gradually shift during the transition from primary grades to fourth and fifth grades. Second, more emphasis should be given to general substance use education regarding effects and consequences than to social refusal skills. Social refusal skills tend to be less effective in younger children as a result of the time lag between learning the skill and the situations in which those skills are used (Herrmann & McWhirter, 1997; Shope, Copeland, Kamp, & Lang, 1998; Wynn, Schulenberg, Maggs, & Zucker, 2000). Again, this relative shift in focus should gradually transition during the fourth and fifth grade years. Finally, more

emphasis should be given to aiding children who have started to either experiment and/or regularly use substances in finding effective treatment resources. Given that early and middle childhood substance use is often indicative of one or more comorbid conditions, special efforts need to be made to address the needs of these children.

It should be noted that the aforementioned considerations do not represent a fundamental deviation from the standard prevention technology paradigm. We find this noteworthy because it highlights the lack of alternative approaches to prevention programs for substance use. While there have been some best practices guidelines generated from existing adolescent research (Drug Strategies, 1999), these guidelines have not been tested against a substantially distinct alternative. For example, many of the core theoretical principles derived from general developmental systems theory have not been translated into a change technology for substance use.

Growing Healthy is a comprehensive health education curriculum developed by the National Center for Health Education (Connell, Turner, & Mason, 1985). The program curriculum is designed for children in kindergarten through sixth grade. The basic design of the program involves anywhere from 43 to 51 sessions per year, with each year's lessons focusing on a single health topic. Substance use education and social/refusal skills are incorporated into the overall curriculum design. Further, there is a special curriculum unit directly addressing tobacco use. In addition to the comprehensiveness of this program, two features make it especially attractive. First, the training materials are highly detailed and quite extensive; thus, program fidelity is likely to be relatively high. Second, there is a strong family involvement component utilizing multiple methods of incorporating parents. These include curriculum activities requiring parental assistance (i.e., homework, workshops, and presentations), targeted family training, and utilization of family members as program volunteers.

There has been one independent evaluation involving a sample of 30,000 students in grades 4 through 7 (Connell et al., 1985). This evaluation found that the experimental group had lower rates of smoking in ninth grade than controls. Further, experimental subjects had higher scores on important mediator variables including general health information and attitudes regarding health risk behavior.

The *Know Your Body* program sponsored by the American Health Foundation is another empirically tested program designed for students in grades ranging from kindergarten through 12th grade (Resnicow, Cross, & Wynder, 1993). This program is also a more general health oriented program, but emphasizes substance use knowledge and mediating variables such as self-esteem, social skills, coping skills, and explicit refusal skills. The program is packaged in a 10 module curriculum requiring between 40 and 50 total sessions. This program may be difficult to implement due to the substantial time and training requirements, but there are specific measures included to assess program fidelity. Parental involvement activities are similar to those of the Growing Healthy program. There have been recent revisions of the elementary school components, which have yet to be empirically validated. The curriculum does distinguish between the primary grades (k–3) and intermediate grades (4–6), which is an attractive feature.

Although, the new revisions have not been empirically validated at this point, the program designers have conducted several evaluations of the original program curriculum. The most substantial of these evaluations involved a sample of 1,100 children starting in the fourth grade. Similar to the Growing Healthy program, the experimental group had significantly lower rates of smoking at a ninth grade follow-up. Further, there were significant program effects for substance use knowledge and information, as well as attitudes toward health risk behaviors (Resnicow et al., 1993).

STRATEGIES THAT MIGHT WORK

Despite the limited number of empirically validated prevention programs for childhood substance use, there are some promising programs that may have a substantial impact. Many of these programs do not focus on substance use per se, but rather emphasize changes in variables thought to mediate late-childhood and adolescent substance use. This may lend these programs a greater potential for the prevention of childhood substance use given the low-rates of actual childhood substance use and the lack of immediate salience of direct substance abuse prevention messages. Further, a subset of these programs utilizes a substantially different change technology than the standard designs. Thus, they represent a testable alternative to the best practice guidelines derived from prevention programs designed for adolescents. These programs can loosely be organized into three general groups: school-based programs, family systems-oriented programs, and integrated school-family oriented programs.

School-Based Programs

The *Good Behavior Game* is a classroom behavior management program. The aim of this program is to reduce aggressive/disruptive behavior in the classroom. However, aggressive and disruptive behaviors figure prominently in the etiology of early substance use, especially cigarette smoking. As such, it has been hypothesized that use of the Good Behavior Game can reduce early substance use by targeting this important mediator. In a test of this hypothesis,

Kellam and Anthony (1998) reported on an epidemiological randomized field trial involving 2,311 first-graders attending Baltimore area elementary schools. This study showed a significantly reduced risk of smoking by age 14 for children who participated in the Good Behavior Game versus controls. This effect was significantly stronger for boys than for girls, but this finding is consistent with gender differences in the etiological role of aggression in smoking.

The *Be A Star* program is a substance use program aimed at high-risk children. The focus of this program is to build on factors thought to be associated with resilience to community and family risk factors associated with substance use. The program consists of weekly group meetings structured as an after-school program. In one study, it was found that students ranging in age from 5 to 12 years participating in the Be A Star program increased their scores in 16 of 18 resilience domains (Pierce & Shields, 1998). Further these increases were significantly greater than those achieved by control students participating in traditional after-school programs.

Family Systems-Based Programs

Given the empirical evidence that parents are a primary influence on childhood substance use behaviors, programs that focus on improving child–parent relationships may be of considerable value (Briggs, Miller, Sayles, Tovar, & Davenport, 1997). One such program is the *Preparing for the Drug Free Years (PDFY)* program. PDFY is a parenting education curriculum targeting parent–child communication and improved parent–child interactions. This program has been shown to be effective at improving parent–child relations in families of children ranging in age from 8 to 14 years (Kosterman et al., 1997).

Early childhood home visitation programs may also decrease childhood and adolescent substance use by improving general family functioning. The most thoroughly investigated home visitation program utilizes nurses as home visitors. The program is designed to provide parent education and support as well as increase positive parent–child interactions. Analyses of a 15-year follow-up to a randomized control trial of this program suggest significant improvement in family functioning and a reduction in both substance use by adolescence and a range of mediating variables (Olds et al., 1998).

Integrative Programs

The *Fast Track (Families And Schools Together)* program is one of the few relatively well-researched approaches that attempts to draw on the strengths of traditional school-based prevention approaches and family oriented approaches. The core program involves a school-based intervention along with a parenting skills group, parent–child interaction training, and a home visitation program. The Fast Track program is targeted primarily to children who display conduct problems in kindergarten; however, by improving family functioning and reducing general delinquent behavior, the program may well reduce substance use both during childhood and early adolescence (McMahon & Slough, 1996).

Another integrative approach is the *Positive Action* program (Flay, Allred, & Ordway, in press). The core principles of Positive Action suggest that through an improvement in self-concept a host of negative behaviors can be prevented. Improved self-concept is achieved, however, via interventions targeted at psychosocial education, school climate, family functioning, and community factors. Similar to the results of the Good Behavior Game, evaluative data on the Positive Action program suggest that it is effective in improving important substance use mediator variables such as school achievement and conduct problems (Flay et al., 2001). Additionally, there is some preliminary evidence to suggest that the Positive Action program in elementary school reduces substance use in middle school (Positive Action, Inc., 2000).

STRATEGIES THAT DO NOT WORK

Here again we must preface our comments with a disclaimer regarding a lack of necessary research. As noted above, very few elementary-school targeted prevention programs have been evaluated, and among those that have been, no substantial long-term effects have been documented. While a few elementary school programs are efficacious in the short-term, by twelfth grade these effects have eroded unless there have been follow-up programs (Peterson, Kealey, Mann, Marek, & Sarason, 2000). As such, it seems clear that isolated "single-shot" interventions are ineffective. Elementary school prevention programs must be incorporated into a systematic prevention regime that extends from middle school through high school. This is especially relevant given the limited long-term effects of early prevention programs targeting substance use behaviors (Peterson et al., 2000; Resnicow & Botvin, 1993).

We would be remising not to mention programs such as *Drug and Alcohol Resistance Education* (DARE). DARE is a school-based resistance skill program and is one of the more widespread substance use prevention programs currently being implemented. However, DARE has been shown on multiple occasions to be ineffective at even short-term reduction of substance use (e.g., Ennett, Tobler, Ringwalt, & Flewelling, 1994).

SYNTHESIS

Substance use issues in childhood are generally understudied. Because early adolescence is where the majority of substance use occurs, that developmental period

has traditionally been the focus of both research and intervention. There is a growing recognition that substance use prevention should occur as early as grades k–3, however. This shifting trend is derived from both growing evidence that onset of substance use behaviors is occurring at younger ages and theoretical understanding of the importance of putting children on a path early in their development that discourages long-term use of particular substances.

The foremost theoretical underpinnings of current prevention thinking are derived from work in developmental systems theory. The two key concepts that have been incorporated into prevention theory are that: (a) childhood substance use is multifaceted in nature resulting in multiple etiological pathways; and (b) preventive intervention is highly sensitive to developmental timing. As such, both intra-individual factors such as neurochemistry, affective/cognitive traits, and personality/temperament profiles; as well as contextual factors including, caregivers, siblings, peers, community institutions, media, and national funding and policy mandates all play a vital role in the development of youth substance use. Further, the relative importance of any of these individual factors is dependent upon both the current states of all of the other salient factors listed above and the sequence of events across all etiological factors for a given developmental history.

The significant advance in developmental and prevention theory in recent years has not yet resulted in widespread behavior change technology, however. The most preventive interventions are still targeted at early adolescent recipients and are largely school-based health education models. There are a few programs directly targeting substance use that have recognized the multidimensional influences involved in substance use etiology. These programs have begun to involve parents, schools, and communities in a much more explicit way and are showing promising early evaluations. Many of these programs were originally designed for middle-school children. There are, however, a number of programs that have been designed specifically for younger children and are targeted directly at variables that mediate later substance use behaviors. What is most intriguing about these programs is that many of them utilize a different change technology than the more traditional substance use prevention programs. Of particular note are programs that focus on family-systems, as well as programs that utilize a home visitation designs.

Given current empirical findings, theoretical constructs, and available prevention technology, we believe that a viable childhood substance use program must be, at a minimum, comprised of the following components. It must recognize local contextual influences such as peer and family influences. It also must address school, community infrastructure and policies, and media influences. Thus, prevention technology needs to extend beyond the classroom walls into the family and community functions that support youth substance use. Childhood prevention programs initially should emphasize substance use knowledge and health risk beliefs and transition to refusal skills and alternative behavior approaches as the children get older.

Tacit in the above recommendation is the need for programs to develop with and follow youth from childhood through adolescence. Single exposure programs are clearly insufficient. Finally, prevention programs should be sensitive to the fact that youth substance use arises out of a complex set of interactions across multiple variables that are sensitive to developmental history. As such, programs need to be flexible in addressing the many different pathways through which children come to use substances. However, we must emphasize the caveat that there is still a great need for both basic research and prevention/intervention trials with early childhood cohorts.

Also see: Substances entries.

References

Briggs, H.E., Miller, D.B., Sayles, R., Tovar, D.D., & Davenport D.C. (1997). Correlates of substance abuse among youth: A note for professionals, service providers and families. *Community Alternatives: International Journal of Family Care, 9*, 109–142.

Brooks-Gunn, J., & Graber, J.A. (1994). Puberty as a biological and social event: Implications for research on pharmacology. *Journal of Adolescent Health, 15*, 663–671.

Bush, P.J., Weinfurt, K.P., & Iannotti, R.J. (1994). Families versus peers: Developmental influences on drug use from grade 4–5 to grade 7–8. *Journal of Applied Developmental Psychology, 15*, 437–456.

Cicchetti, D., & Cohen, D.J. (1995). Perspectives on developmental psychopathology. In D. Cicchetti & D.J. Cohen (Eds.), *Developmental psychopathology Vol. 1: Theory and methods* (pp. 3–20). New York: John Wiley & Sons.

Connell, D.B., Turner, R.R., & Mason, E.F. (1985). Summary of findings of the School Health Education Evaluation: Health promotion effectiveness, implementation, and costs. *Journal of School Health, 55*, 316–321.

Crisp, A., Sedgwick, P., Halek, C., Joughin, N., & Humphrey, H. (1999). Why may teenage girls persist in smoking? *Journal of Adolescence, 22*, 657–672.

Damon, W., & Lerner, R. (1998). *Handbook of child psychology (Vol. 1).* New York: John Wiley & Sons.

Drug Strategies. (1999). *Making the grade: A guide to school drug prevention programs.* Washington, D.C.

Ennett, S.T., Tobler, N.S., Ringwalt, C.L., & Flewelling, R.L. (1994). How effective is drug abuse resistance education? A meta-analysis of Project DARE outcome evaluations. *American Journal of Public Health, 84*, 1394–1401.

Fergusson, D.M., & Horwood, L.J. (1999). Prospective childhood predictors of deviant peer affiliations in adolescence. *Journal of Child Psychology & Psychiatry & Allied Disciplines, 40*, 581–592.

Fergusson, D.M., Lynskey, M.T., & Horwood, L.J., (1994). Childhood exposure to alcohol and adolescent drinking patterns. *Addiction, 89*, 1007–1016.

Flay, B.R., Allred, C.G., & Ordway, N. (in press). Effects of the Positive Action program on achievement and discipline: Two matched-control comparisons. *Prevention Science, 2*, 71–89.

Flay, B.R., & Petraitis, J. (1994). The theory of triadic influence: A new theory of health behavior with implications for preventive interventions. In G. S. Albrecht (Ed.), *Advances in medical sociology Vol. IV: A reconsideration of models of health behavior change* (pp. 19–44). Greenwich, CN: JAI Press.

Ford, D.H., & Lerner, R.M. (1992). *Developmental systems theory: An integrative approach.* Newbury Park, CA: Sage.

Herrmann, D.S., & McWhirter, J.J. (1997). Refusal and resistance skills for children and adolescents: A selected review. *Journal of Counseling and Development, 75*, 177–187.

Johnston, L.D., O'Malley, P.M., & Bachman, J.G. (1999). *Monitoring the future: National survey results on drug use, 1975–1999.* US Department of Health and Human Services.

Kellam, S.G., & Anthony, J.C. (1998). Targeting early antecedents to prevent tobacco smoking: Findings from an epidemiologically based randomized field trial. *American Journal of Public Health, 88*, 1490–1495.

Kosterman, R., Hawkins, J.D., Spoth, R., Haggerty, K.P. et al. (1997). Effects of a preventive parent-training intervention on observed family interactions: Proximal outcomes from preparing for the drug free years. *Journal of Community Psychology, 25*, 337–352.

Lloyd, J. (1996). Alcohol and young people: A case for supporting education about alcohol in primary and secondary schools. *Educational Review, 48*, 153–161.

McMahon, R.J., & Slough, N.M. (1996). Family-based intervention in the Fast Track program. In R.D Peters, R.J. McMahon et al. (Eds.), *Preventing childhood disorders, substance use, and delinquency* (pp. 90–110). Thousand Oaks, CA: Sage.

Olds, D., Henderson, C.R., Cole, R. Eckenrode, J., Kitzman, H. Luckey, D., Pettitt, L., Sidora, K. et al. (1998). Long-term effects of nurse home visitation on children's criminal and antisocial behavior: 15-year follow-up of a randomized control trial. *Journal of the American Medical Association, 280*, 1238–1244.

Orlandi, M.A. (1996). Prevention Technologies for Drug involved youth. In C.B. McCoy, L.R. Metsch et al. (Eds.), *Intervening with drug-involved youth* (pp. 81–100). Thousand Oaks, CA: Sage.

Positive Action, Inc. (2000). *Evaluations of the Positive Action program: Summary of findings 1978–2000.* Twin Falls, ID: Author.

Peterson, A.V., Kealey, K.A., Mann, S.L., Marek, P.M., & Sarason, I.G. (2000). Hutchinson Smoking Prevention Project: Long-term randomized trial in school-based tobacco use prevention—Results on smoking. *Journal of the National Cancer Institute, 92*, 1979–1991.

Pierce, L.H., & Shields, N. (1998). The Be a Star community-based after-school program: Developing resiliency factors in high-risk preadolescent youth. *Journal of Community Psychology, 26*, 175–183.

Resnicow, K., & Botvin, G. (1993). School-based substance use prevention programs: Why do effects decay? *Preventive Medicine, 22*, 484–490.

Resnicow, K., Cross, D., & Wynder, E. (1993). The Know Your Body program: A review of studies. *Bulletin of the New York Academy of Medicine, 70*, 188–207.

Shope, J.T., Copeland, L.A., Kamp, M.E., & Lang, S.W. (1998). Twelfth grade follow-up of the effectiveness of a middle school-based substance abuse prevention program. *Journal of Drug Education, 28*, 185–197.

Stattin, H., & Magnusson, D. (1990). *Pubertal maturation in female development: Paths through life Vol. 2.* Hillsdale, NJ: Lawrence Erlbaum Associates.

Tang, C.K., Rissel, C., Bauman, A., Fay, J., Porter, S., Dawes, A., & Steven, B. (1998). A longitudinal study of smoking in year 7 and 8 students speaking English or a language other than English at home in Sydney. *Tobacco Control, 7*, 35–40.

Tobler, N.S., & Stratton, H.H. (1997). Effectiveness of school-based drug prevention programs: A meta-analysis of the research. *Journal of Primary Prevention, 18*, 71–128.

Tschann, J.M., Adler, N.E., Irwin, C.E., Millstein, S.G., Turner, R.A., & Kegeles, S.M. (1994). Initiation of substance use in early adolescence: The role of pubertal timing and emotional distress. *Health Psychology, 13*, 326–333.

World Health Organization (WHO). (1998). *Cannabis: A health perspective and research agenda.*

World Health Organization (WHO). (1999). *Global status report on alcohol.*

Wynn, S.R., Schulenberg, J., Maggs, J.L., & Zucker, R.A. (2000). Preventing alcohol misuse: The impact of refusal skills and norms. *Psychology of Addictive Behaviors, 14*, 36–47.

Substances, Childhood (Meta-Analysis)

Andrei Streke, Michael Roona, and Diana Marshall

INTRODUCTION

This entry examines what research can tell us about school-based and family-based programs for children 5–12 years old related to the use of alcohol, tobacco, and other drugs (ATOD). Our purpose is not to provide an exhaustive review but to evaluate effectiveness of these two different types of programs to prevent the use of ATOD in childhood.

DEFINITIONS

We synthesize the research about school-based and family-based ATOD programs by computing effects sizes for each measured substance use outcome associated with each prevention program and averaging these effect sizes across similar measures and types of programs. We define *effect size* as a standardized measure of difference between intervention and comparison groups. *ATOD* is an acronym for prevention programs targeting alcohol, tobacco, or other drugs. The specific technique we use to systematically assess program effects in the ensemble of available studies is called *meta-analysis*, which involves controlling for differences in sample sizes and other factors that influence statistical findings when averages are computed.

SCOPE

The economic cost of substance use in the United States and Canada is substantial. Health care expenditures due to tobacco use in the United States have been estimated to range from $50 to $73 billion annually (Centers for Disease Control and Prevention, 2000). Medical care, lost productivity, and other consequences of alcohol and illicit drug use in the United States have been estimated to cost over $275 billion. Approximately 70 percent of these costs are due to lost productivity caused by incarceration, illness, or premature death. Less than 15 percent are associated with prevention and treatment (US Department of Health and Human Services [USDHHS], 1998).

Canadian reports indicate the cost of substance abuse was more than $18.45 billion in 1992: $11.7 billion for indirect costs, such as productivity losses; $4.06 billion for direct health care costs; $1.75 billion for direct law enforcement costs; $545 million in other direct costs; $231 million for prevention and research; $53.8 million for administrative costs for transfer payments; and $20.1 million for losses in the workplace (Canadian Centre on Substance Abuse,1996a).

Two major US surveys target the 12 years and older population. Monitoring the Future (US Department of Health and Human Services [USDHHS], 2000) surveys youth in the eighth grade (13–14 year olds) and higher grades. The National Household Survey on Drug Abuse (US Substance Abuse and Mental Health Services Administration [SAMHSA], 1999) targets 12 year olds and older. Thus, determining the incidence and prevalence of drug use by children under 12 years is difficult. Monitoring the Future, however, asks eighth graders to retrospectively recall their early experiences with ATOD use. These retrospective reports indicate that by the end of sixth grade (ages 11–12) one quarter had smoked a cigarette and one quarter had imbibed alcohol. In addition, one in twelve had smoked marijuana by the end of sixth grade. Smokeless tobacco use and inhalant use also begin early (grade 6 and grade 5, respectively) (USDHHS, 2000, p. 213).

Like US surveys, major Canadian surveys target 12 year olds and older (Canadian Centre on Substance Abuse, 1995). The large Atlantic Canada initiative samples 7th, 9th, 10th and 12th graders (Canadian Centre on Substance Abuse, 1996b). Another large Canadian study, done in 1993 and 1995 and again in 1997, targeted students in grades 9 through 12. The results of this survey showed first drinking at age 13; first drug use at 14, with marijuana being the most used; and cigarettes first used at 13 years (Canadian Centre on Substance Abuse, 1997, pp. 2–4).

THEORIES

ATOD prevention programs for children are based to varying degrees on social learning theory, social control theory, and human ecology theory.

Social learning theory focuses on the importance of role models in shaping behavior. It posits that children learn from significant others in two ways: direct modeling of the behavior of peers or adults, and reinforcement of beliefs, attitudes, and behavior through social approval or disapproval (Bandura, 1977). Peers and others who do not use drugs and who disapprove of doing so can positively influence the lives of vulnerable children.

Social control theory posits that bonding or attachment to positive social groups or institutions, such as family and school, protects young people against substance abuse and delinquency (Hirschi, 1969). Poor bonding results from harsh discipline and lack of supervision that contributes to a failure to identify with parental and societal values regarding substance use.

Human ecology theory (Bronfenbrenner, 1979) emphasizes the role of social contexts in determining behavior. It suggests that an adolescent's interactions with social, school, and family environments ultimately influence substance abuse and other antisocial behaviors. Compared to social control theory, which emphasizes interactions between agents, human ecology theory puts more emphasis on interactions between structural forces, such as the domains of family, school, community, and the larger societal or global environments.

Evaluations of ATOD prevention programs for 5–12 year olds, like national surveys targeting this age group, rarely measure substance use. Rather, these employ risk and protective factors to measure program success. Researchers believe that it is necessary both to reduce risks and to enhance protective factors to maximize the prevention of adolescent substance abuse.

Risk factors encompass individual realms (like biology, behavior, and personality), family risk mechanisms, and environmental and contextual risk factors. Among the plethora of risk factors that have been associated with future substance use, aggression and its correlates (e.g., attention deficit hyperactivity disorder (ADHD), conduct disorder, oppositional defiant disorder) have been researched extensively. The diagnostic criteria for these "disruptive behavior disorders" include signs and symptoms of aggressive behavior, and commonly an aggressive child or adolescent is diagnosed as having either one or more of these disorders. The presence of these specific psychiatric disorders among children and adolescents is believed to be associated with a heightened risk for subsequent alcohol and drug abuse and adult antisocial personality.

RESEARCH

The causal relationship between the hypothesized risk factors and adolescent substance use or abuse has not been established. However, evidence that such a causal relationship exists has been inferred based on longitudinal observations of children possessing risk factors who later go on to use or abuse substances as adolescents.

The findings of the Woodlawn study (Kellam, Brown, Rubin, & Ensminger, 1983) indicate that aggressiveness during first grade (when children are 6–7 years old), especially when coupled with shyness, increases the likelihood of males' use of beer, hard liquor, marijuana, and cigarettes. Gittelman, Mannuzza, Shenker, and Bonagura (1985) found a correlation between hyperactivity and substance use. They tested adolescents who, at the time of referral to the study, were 9 years old and tested relatively high for hyperactivity. Their results indicate that a major risk factor for the development of antisocial behavior and drug use is the occurrence of ADHD symptoms. Substance use disorders followed the onset of conduct disorder in the overwhelming majority of cases.

Lerner and Vicary (1984) found that subjects who had "difficult" temperaments at 5 years of age also tend to be more severe users of tobacco, alcohol, and marijuana in adulthood. The authors posit, therefore, that temperament characteristics play a role in the development of later substance abuse. Shedler and Block (1990) assessed 101 children on a wide range of psychological measures when they were 3, 4, 5, 7, 11, 14, and 18 years old. They found that for most youth, substance use is not problematic, but that the frequent drug user is a troubled adolescent who is "interpersonally alienated, emotionally withdrawn, and manifestly unhappy and who expresses his or her maladjustment through undercontrolled, overtly antisocial behavior" (p. 617).

Shedler and Block (1990) also found that frequent substance use in adolescence is related to the quality of mother/child interaction in early childhood. The quality of parenting provided to children at age 5 discriminated between frequent and experimental users of marijuana by age 18. Mothers of frequent users were relatively cold and underprotective, pushing their children to perform without offering them adequate support. Parental disciplinary techniques, such as a lack of inconsistent discipline or excessively harsh punishment, have also been linked to the risk for substance abuse (Kandel & Andrews, 1987). Other risk factors include low parental educational aspirations for children, and unclear or unrealistic parental expectations for children's behavior (Hawkins, Catalano, & Miller, 1992).

In addition, parental and sibling behaviors and attitudes have been linked to children's drug use. Children from a family with a history of alcoholism run a higher risk of having substance abuse problems (Hawkins et al., 1992). Children are more likely to become substance abusers in adolescence when parents use illegal drugs, are heavy users of alcohol, or are tolerant of their children's use of drugs (Cotton, 1979;

Goodwin, 1985). Brook, Whiteman, Gordon, and Brook (1988) found that siblings are also role models for younger children. In fact, they found the drug behavior and attitudes of older brothers are more strongly related to a younger brother's use than is parental modeling of substance abuse.

Many studies have shown that conflict among family members is a potent predictor of delinquency and antisocial behavior, including substance abuse (McCord, 1979; Porter & O'Leary, 1980; Simcha-Fagan, Gerstein, & Langner, 1986). Physical abuse also has been identified as a risk factor for adolescent substance abuse as well as for other antisocial behaviors. The earlier the age when physical abuse is experienced, the greater the potential for negative effects (Hawkins et al., 1992).

STRATEGIES

Effectiveness of Family-Based ATOD Prevention Programs: A Meta-Analytic Overview

Family life provides the context within which young children cultivate behaviors that lay the foundation for adolescent development. The aim of family-based ATOD prevention programs is to positively affect a child's ability to resist drug use behaviors by strengthening family bonds and/or improving family skills. A meta-analysis of family-based ATOD intervention evaluations conducted in 1999 provides some evidence regarding the effectiveness of family-based prevention programs (Tobler Research Associates, 1999).

Tobler and her colleagues assessed substance use prevention programs meta-analytically by computing effect sizes for ATOD use when possible. Effect sizes for aggression and conduct disorder also were computed for family-based programs.

To interpret effect sizes, values of −0.1, 0.0, 0.1, and 0.2 are used as reference points. An effect size of 0.1 is the smallest clinically meaningful indicator that a program is effective and an effect size of 0.2 designates moderate effectiveness. An effect size around 0 points to program ineffectiveness and an effect size of −0.1 indicates that the program is counterproductive. When effect sizes based on all measured outcomes (including conduct disorder, aggression, and substance use) are averaged, the overall effect of the 44 family-based programs is found to be 0.25. The program effect on conduct disorder for the 28 evaluations that measured it is 0.29 and the program effect on aggression for the 35 evaluations that measured it also is 0.29. These are moderate effect sizes. The relationship between these beneficial program effects and ATOD use is questionable, however; the program effect on substance use for the 12 family-based evaluations that measured it is a mere 0.05.

Tobler and her colleagues (1999) classified non-court mandated family-based programs into the following categories: Group Skills, Group Therapy, Intensive Individual Counseling, and Low Intensity Individual Counseling. Group Skills programs include modeling and use of role-plays, general behavior management skills, behavior modification, feedback and reinforcement of new skills, token economy, or use of appropriate punishment. In Group Therapy programs, the clinician focuses on family communication patterns and helps families shift the perception of the problem from blaming to caring. These programs are administered in different sessions.

In Intensive Individual Counseling, the family unit is seen separately, most often in the home. The clinician focuses on issues specific to the family; counseling is supportive and the clinician helps the family obtain concrete services, such as housing, health care, other counseling, and government assistance. The clinician may visit on a weekly basis for as long as 6 months, and is on call for daily emergencies. Home-based counseling includes parent skills training, parent therapy, and case management, often provided by visiting nurses.

Low Intensity Individual Counseling programs are more time-limited. They usually are no more than 3 months, and the clinician may use a form of structural, strategic, or functional family therapy.

This classification scheme of program types employed by Tobler and her colleagues is quite compatible with the Prevention Enhancement Protocols System (PEPS) approach developed by a panel of experts for the Center for Substance Abuse Prevention (1998). PEPS approach 1 (Parent and Family Skills Training) includes individual families and groups of families out-of-home (in clinic or classroom) and is well matched to Tobler's Group Skills category. Similarly, the Intensive Individual Counseling category compares to PEPS approach 2 (Family In-Home Support). PEPS approach 3 (Family Therapy) includes only individual counseling, but combines home-based services with out-of-home services and compares to Tobler's Low Intensity Individual group (Tobler Research Associates, 1999).

Comparison of program types does not yield much differentiation when effect sizes based on all measured outcomes are averaged. The Group Therapy programs are not significantly different from the Group Skills programs. Nor are the Intensive Individual programs more effective than the Low Intensity Individual programs when effect sizes based on all outcome measures are averaged. Combining Group Skills and Group Therapy programs into a "Group" category, and the Intensive Individual Counseling and Low Intensity Individual programs into an "Individual" category allows these broad formats to be compared. The mean difference between Individual and Group programs is not statistically significant. Thus, dividing family-based programs into these categories yields no further information due to the paucity of evaluated programs and their small size.

Effectiveness of School-Based ATOD Prevention Programs: A Meta-Analytic Overview

In contrast to family-based programs, dividing universal school-based ATOD prevention programs into categories based on their content and process is quite informative. Interactive programs, in which students actively participate in the learning process, are more effective prevention programs than non-interactive programs that use a didactic approach to teaching. The effect size for overall drug use for the 47 elementary school-based programs is 0.07; but the 26 interactive programs are significantly more effective than the 21 non-interactive programs (0.13 vs. 0.02). The contrast between the 14 interactive and the 7 non-interactive programs evaluated using higher quality research designs is ever more striking: 0.20 vs. 0.03.

The group of more effective interactive interventions consists of three distinct types of programs: Social Influences (SI), Comprehensive Life Skills (CLS), and System-Wide Change (SWC).

Social Influences programs focus primarily on interpersonal skills development. They include a knowledge component, emphasize refusal skills training, and may include a limited affective component. Students learn about media influences on an individual's choice to use or not use drugs, as well as normative expectations. Emphasis is placed on resisting pro-drug social influences. One well-known program, *Project SMART* (Self-Management and Resistance Training), targets all three gateway drugs for sixth and seventh graders. Project SMART has shown small favorable effects on tobacco use, moderate favorable effects on alcohol use, but no effect on marijuana use (Johnson, Graham, Hansen, Flay, McGuigan, & Gee, 1987). It has been argued that Social Influences programs do not appear to be entirely appropriate for younger children, since children in elementary school lack the cognitive experiences for understanding what social influence means, particularly the subtle ways in which people can be pressured into trying drugs (Ellickson, 1995). The rational cognition approach to decision making, upon which Social Influences programs are based, largely ignores the influence of affect on substance use among youth.

Comprehensive Life Skills programs have content similar to that of the Social Influences programs, but add life skills training that includes the development of communication, assertiveness, coping, problem-solving and goal-setting skills, as well as, a more broad affective component. These incorporate strategies for improving general personal competence as well as the capacity to identify and resist social pressures. Schinke and Gilchrist (1983) have tested this approach with fifth and sixth graders and demonstrated modest favorable effects on tobacco use.

System-Wide Change programs are interactive comprehensive approaches that are supported by family and/or community, or aim to alter the "business as usual" school environment and/or engage students in the learning process. The *Child Development Project* (Battistich, Schaps, Watson, & Solomon, 1996) is a good example of this type of program. It has demonstrated small beneficial effects on alcohol and tobacco use, but no effect on marijuana use.

The 16 elementary school Social Influences programs meta-analyzed by the authors for this article yield an average ATOD effect size of 0.11. The eight Comprehensive Life Skills programs yield an average ATOD effect size of 0.25. The two System-Wide Change programs yield an average ATOD effect size of 0.13. These average ATOD effect sizes may be misleading, however, because few interventions measure the use of substances other than tobacco at the elementary school level. For cigarettes, the mean difference between Comprehensive Life Skills and Social Influences programs is 0.26. Because our earlier work shows interactive program effectiveness decreases as the number of program youth increases (Tobler, Roona, Ochshorn, Marshall, Streke, & Stackpole, 2000), adjustments should be made to account for program size differences. Controlling for program size differences between Social Influences and Comprehensive Life Skills interventions reduces the mean difference in program effectiveness to 0.21, but has no effect on the statistical significance of the superiority of CLS programs at the elementary school level.

The finding that students in the Comprehensive Life Skills group showed significantly less increase in tobacco use relative to comparison students than students in the Social Influences group is consistent with the findings of Tobler et al. (2000).

Effectiveness of Family-Based Programs Relative to School-Based Universal Programs

At first glance, family-based programs appear to be nearly four times more effective (0.25) than school-based programs (0.07). However, some caution should be exercised before drawing that conclusion. First, compared to family-based programs, many universal school-based drug prevention programs have been implemented on a very large scale. Because our earlier work shows interactive program effectiveness decreases as the number of program youth increases (Tobler et al., 2000), some adjustment has to be made before comparison. To enable some reasonable point of reference, we computed the effectiveness of the

86 smallest school-based programs. The average effect size for this group (0.18 for drug use only) is higher than the average effect size for all school-based programs and is much closer to the average effect size for the group of 44 family-based programs (0.25).

Second, universal school-based interventions generally target more heterogeneous populations than family-based programs. For the subset of 30 interactive school-based interventions targeting more homogeneous special populations, the average effect size is 0.21. Thus, adjusted for program size and heterogeneity of the population, effect sizes for school-based and family-based programs appear to be of the same order and signify moderate effectiveness.

Finally, the overall effect size of 0.25 for family-based programs is based on all measured outcomes including conduct disorder, aggression, and substance use. The program effect on substance use only is a mere 0.05, which is compatible to the 0.07 for school-based elementary school interventions. This finding, combined with the failure of one type of family-based program to demonstrate its superiority leads us to conclude that family-based programs are less effective than school-based Comprehensive Life Skills programs.

Unfortunately, we have been unable to determine what type of family-based program is most effective at preventing ATOD use, but for school-based universal programs, interactive programs are more effective than non-interactive ones, and Comprehensive Life Skills programs outperform Social Influences programs for all substances combined and for cigarette outcomes. This relative ineffectiveness of Social Influences programs at preventing cigarette use in the short term appears to persist in the long term. The longitudinal Hutchinson Smoking Prevention Project (Peterson, Kealey, Mann, Marek, & Sarason, 2000) found no effect on smoking prevalence at grade 12 for students who began an 8-year comprehensive Social Influences program in third grade. Peterson et al. (2000) questioned "the social-influences approach as presently conceived and applied to smoking prevention in the school/classroom setting, including those school-based interventions that comply with CDC's 'best practices' guidelines for comprehensive tobacco control programs" (p. 1988).

Other longitudinal studies have demonstrated favorable long-term effects, however. The Perry Pre-School evaluators measured outcomes when the 3–4 year old preschool students reached ages 14, 19 and 27 years old. Among 27 year olds, intervention effects were found to be moderately favorable for smoking and alcohol use. In addition, the program group averaged a significantly lower number of lifetime criminal arrests (2.3 vs. 4.6 arrests) and adult criminal arrests (1.8 vs. 4.0). There also were fewer frequent

offenders (7 vs. 35 percent) in the program group and fewer arrests for adult felonies, significantly fewer arrests for adult misdemeanors, and noticeably fewer juvenile arrests. There were fewer arrests for drug-making or drug-dealing crimes. Shorter probation or parole sentences also were found in the program group (Schweinhart, Barnes, & Weikart, 1993, p. 83).

The Montreal Longitudinal Study of Disruptive Boys followed kindergarten boys through adolescence. The study linked preschool aggressive behavior to later deviant behavior, including substance use. Two modes of intervention, parent training and child training, were directed at variables that had been postulated to be causes of delinquency (i.e., poor parenting and aggressive behavior). At the 8-year follow-up, when the subjects were 14 years old, alcohol use and illicit drug use were markedly lower in the intervention group than in the comparison group. In addition, treated boys were less involved in deviant gangs and significantly less involved in delinquency (stealing, vandalism, and substance use) than untreated boys (Tremblay, Masse, Pagani, & Vitaro, 1996).

SYNTHESIS

School-based programs have constituted the bulk of ATOD prevention efforts in the past and are likely to do so in the future. For universal school-based programs, interactive programs are more effective than non-interactive ones. School-based prevention programs that use non-interactive lecture formats hardly work. Interactive school-based programs seem to work quite well for some substances at some grade levels but work less well or not at all for other substances or grade levels. For example, the Comprehensive Life Skills model holds the most promise as a substance abuse prevention strategy at the elementary school level. It outperforms Social Influences programs for all substances combined and for cigarette outcomes. However, as with most substance abuse prevention programs, the model has been tailored to junior high school (sixth graders and above). There is little evidence in our meta-analyses of what might constitute effective prevention programs for younger children.

We have been unable to determine what type of family-based program is most effective at preventing ATOD use. We do know, however, that family-based ATOD program effects are comparable with those for elementary school-based interventions. Although the exact combination of school-based and family-based components is not apparent, we advocate supplementing universal school programs with family-focused interventions, especially for selective and indicated populations. Ultimately, as the System-Wide Change approach suggests, the key part of the prevention effort may be at the community level, where social norms and environmental determinants of individual behavior can be affected. For this SWC approach to work, all segments of the community must become involved: parents, schools, community groups, health professionals, the faith community, businesses, and government officials. However, there has been little evaluation of the ways in which community strategies can be joined with school-based and family-based efforts and the ways in which the effectiveness of prevention can be enhanced through such multicomponent activities, thus more research is needed.

Also see: Substances Entries.

References

Bandura, A. (1977). *Social learning theory*. Englewood Cliffs, NJ: Prentice-Hall.

Battistich, V., Schaps, E., Watson, M., & Solomon, D. (1996). Prevention effects of the Child Development Project: Early findings from an ongoing multisite demonstration trial. *Journal of Adolescent Research, 11*(1), 12–35.

Bronfenbrenner, U. (1979). *The ecology of human development: Experiments by nature and design*. Cambridge, MA: Harvard University Press.

Brook, J.S., Whiteman, M., Gordon, A.S., & Brook, D.W. (1988). The role of older brothers in younger brothers' drug use viewed in the context of parent and peer influences. *Journal of Genetic Psychology, 151*, 59–75.

Canadian Centre on Substance Abuse. (1995). *Horizons Three: Young Canadians' alcohol and other drug use: Increasing our understanding* [on-line]. Available: http://www.ccsa.ca

Canadian Centre on Substance Abuse. (1996a). *The costs of substance abuse in Canada* [on-line]. Available: http://www.ccsa.ca

Canadian Centre on Substance Abuse. (1996b). *Atlantic Student Drug Use Surveys executive summaries from the reports* [on-line]. Available: http://www.ccsa.ca

Canadian Centre on Substance Abuse. (1997). *Highlights report: 1997 AFM student survey on alcohol and other drugs* [on-line]. Available: http://www.ccsa.ca

Center for Substance Abuse Prevention. (1998). *Preventing substance abuse among children and adolescents: Family-centered approaches. Reference guide* (DHHS Publication No. SMA 3223-FY98). Washington DC: US Government Printing Office.

Centers for Disease Control and Prevention. (2000). Youth tobacco surveillance—United States, 1998–1999. *CDC Morbidity and Mortality Weekly Report, 10/13/00*(SS10), 1–93.

Cotton, N.S. (1979). The familial incidence of alcoholism: A review. *Journal of Studies on Alcohol, 40*, 89–116.

Ellickson, P. (1995). Schools. In R.H. Coombs & D.A. Ziedonis (Eds.), *Handbook on drug abuse prevention* (pp. 93–120). Boston: Allyn and Bacon.

Gittelman, R., Mannuzza, S., Shenker, R., & Bonagura, N. (1985). Hyperactive boys almost grown up. Vol. I. Psychiatric status. *Archives of General Psychiatry, 42*(10), 937–947.

Goodwin, D.W. (1985). Alcoholism and genetics: The sins of the fathers. *Archives of General Psychiatry, 42*, 171–174.

Hawkins, J.D., Catalano, R.F., & Miller, J.Y. (1992). Risk and protective factors for alcohol and other drug problems in adolescence and early adulthood: Implications for substance abuse prevention. *Psychological Bulletin, 112*, 64–105.

Hirschi, T. (1969). *Causes of delinquency*. Berkeley, CA: University of California Press.

Johnson, C.A., Graham, J., Hansen, W., Flay, B., McGuigan, K., & Gee, M. (1987). *Project SMART after three years: An assessment of sixth-grade and multiple-grade implementations*. Unpublished manuscript, USC-IPR, Pasadena, CA. (Available from: C. Anderson Johnson, Ph.D., USC-IPR, 35 North Lake Avenue, Suite 200, Pasadena, CA 91101.)

Kandel, D.B., & Andrews, K. (1987). Processes of adolescent socialization by parents and peers. *International Journal of the Addictions, 22*, 319–342.

Kellam, S., Brown, C.H., Rubin, B.R., & Ensminger, M.E. (1983). Paths leading to teenage psychiatric symptoms and substance use: Developmental epidemiological studies in Woodlawn. In S.B. Guze, F.J. Earls, & J.E. Barrett (Eds.), *Childhood psychopathology and development* (pp. 17–47). New York: Raven.

Lerner, J., & Vicary, J. (1984). Difficult temperament and drug use: Analyses from the New York Longitudinal Study. *Journal of Drug Education, 14*(1), 1–8.

McCord, J. (1979). Some child-rearing antecedents of criminal behavior in adult men. *Journal of Personality and Social Psychology, 37*, 1477–1486.

Peterson, A.V., Kealey, K.A., Mann, S.L., Marek, P.M., & Sarason, I.G. (2000). Hutchinson Smoking Prevention Project: Long-term randomized trial in school-based tobacco use prevention—results on smoking. *Journal of the National Cancer Institute, 92*(24), 1979–1991.

Porter, B., & O'Leary, K.D. (1980). Marital discord and childhood problems. *Journal of Abnormal Child Psychology, 8*, 287–295.

Schinke, S., & Gilchrist, L. (1983). Primary prevention of tobacco smoking. *Journal of School Health, 53*(7), 416–419.

Schweinhart, L., Barnes, H., & Weikart, D. (1993). *Significant benefits: The high/scope perry preschool study through age 27*. Ypsilanti, MI: High/Scope Educational Research Foundation.

Shedler, J., & Block, J. (1990). Adolescent drug use and psychological health: A longitudinal inquiry. *American Psychologist, 45*(5), 612–630.

Simcha-Fagan, O., Gerstein, J.C., & Langner, T. (1986). Early presursors and concurrent correlates of illicit drug use in adolescents. *Journal of Drug Issues, 16*, 7–28.

Tobler Research Associates. (1999). *Meta-analysis of family-based drug prevention programs: Technical report*. Bethesda, MD: Center for Substance Abuse Prevention.

Tobler, N., Roona, M., Ochshorn, P., Marshall, D., Streke, A., & Stackpole, K. (2000). School-based adolescent drug prevention programs: 1998 meta-analysis. *The Journal of Primary Prevention, 20*(4), 275–336.

Tremblay, R., Masse, L., Pagani, L., & Vitaro, F. (1996). From childhood physical aggression to adolescent maladjustment: The Montreal Prevention Experiment. In R.D. Peters & R.J. McMahon (Eds.), *Preventing childhood disorders, substance abuse, and delinquency* (pp. 268–298). Thousand Oaks, CA: Sage.

US Department of Health and Human Services (USDHHS). (1998). *The Economic Costs of Alcohol and Drug Abuse in the United States 1992*. (NIH Publication No. 98-4327). Washington DC: National Institute on Drug Abuse.

US Department of Health and Human Services (USDHHS). (2000). *Monitoring the future national survey results on drug use, 1975–1999. Vol. I: Secondary school students*. (NIH Publication No. 00-4802). Washington DC: National Institute on Drug Abuse.

US Substance Abuse and Mental Health Services Administration (SAMHSA), Office of Applied Studies. (1999). *National household survey on drug abuse: Population estimates 1998* (DHHS Publication No. SMA 99-3327). Rockville, MD: Author.

Substances, Adolescence

Christopher L. Ringwalt and
Mallie J. Paschall

INTRODUCTION

Substance abuse is an international problem of epidemic proportions that has particularly devastating effects on youth because the early initiation of alcohol, tobacco, or other drug use within this population has been repeatedly linked to abuse and related problem behaviors among adults. However, there is a steadily growing body of research evidence that adolescent substance use is preventable, through a mix of strategies that seek to decrease both their interest in consuming substances and the availability of substances in their social and physical environments. In this entry we begin by defining "substance use" and other key terms, continue by describing what is known of the epidemiology of substance use in adolescent populations, and conclude with discussions of theory- and evidence-based strategies designed to prevent substance use, as well as promising but as of yet unproven approaches.

DEFINITIONS

In this entry, *substances* will refer to alcohol and tobacco as well as other drugs; collectively these are known by the acronym ATODs. Because the use of *any* substance by children or adolescents is illegal and considered harmful, most prevention specialists focus their attention on either the prevention of first use or, to a lesser extent, substance use cessation. However, some prevention specialists who serve older adolescents believe that the prevention of occasional or experimental use may be futile, and instead address their strategies to the reduction of harm associated with use.

Risk factors are attitudes, behaviors, or social or physical characteristics and conditions that increase or mediate the likelihood that individuals will use drugs. Risk factors are typically sorted into a variety of biochemical and psychosocial domains, as are *protective factors*, which moderate or block the effects of risk factors (Hawkins, Catalano, & Miller, 1992) and collectively build resilience. *Resilience* may be defined as a generalized resistance to engaging in a range of risk behaviors, and includes the capacity to recover expeditiously from adverse life events and the ability to function effectively even in the presence of stressful conditions (Center for Substance Abuse Prevention [CSAP], 2000).

SCOPE

The Monitoring the Future Study, the United State's preeminent annual survey of ATOD use by 12th graders, has been conducted by the University of Michigan since 1975, and provides an excellent opportunity to observe patterns of use over time. Key trends in use by 12th graders are displayed in Table 1. Annual surveys of 8th and 10th graders were added in 1991.

After manifesting a nearly 50 percent increase in the smoking rates by 8th, 10th, and 12th graders between 1991 and 1996, rates of smoking gradually declined. Alcohol use by adolescents has also declined over the past decade. During the 90s, the use of marijuana and other drugs peaked in 1996 and has remained fairly stable among high school seniors, while it has decreased among 8th graders.

Estimates of the cost of ATOD use to the Unites States vary widely, and are generally based on lost productivity and the direct and indirect costs of mortality and morbidity. According to the National Institutes of Health, alcohol abuse and alcoholism cost $148 billion in 1992, and drug abuse and dependence cost $98 billion (Samber, 1998). In contrast, in 1993 the total cost of ATOD use to society was $400 billion (Center for Addiction and Substance Abuse [CASA], 1993). A more recent estimate of the cost of alcohol abuse to society is $250 billion in health care, public safety, and social welfare expenditures (Join Together Online, 1999).

In Canada, the Ontario Student Drug Use Survey (Center for Addiction and Mental Health [CAMH], 2000) of youth in odd-numbered grades 7–13 constitutes the longest ongoing study of ATOD use, and has been administered biennially since 1979. The annual rate of 12-month alcohol use decreased from 76.3 percent in 1977 to 59.6 percent in 1997. Cigarette use declined from 30.4 to 27.6 percent, and

Table 1. Trends in ATOD use by 12th graders from 1975 to 2000

	1975	1980	1985	1990	1995	2000
Tobacco						
Lifetime	73.6	71.0	68.8	64.4	64.2	62.5
30-day	36.7	30.5	30.1	29.4	33.5	31.4
Alcohol						
Lifetime	90.4	93.2	92.2	89.5	80.7	80.3
30-day	68.2	72.0	65.9	57.1	51.3	50.0
Other drugs						
Lifetime	55.2	65.4	60.6	47.9	48.4	54.0
30-day	30.7	37.2	29.7	17.2	23.8	24.9

Source: Tables 4 and 6. The University of Michigan, News and Information Services. News Release, Thursday, December 14, 2000.

marijuana use from 25.8 to 24.9 percent. These comparisons mask a downward trend in use of all substances until 1991, followed by a gradual rise since that time. Costs of substance abuse to Canadian society in 1995 have been expressed in terms of percent of total mortality, and admissions to hospitals, for any cause: alcohol (3.1, 2.7 percent); tobacco (16.5, 6.5 percent); and illicit drugs (0.4, 0.2 percent) (Single, Rehm, Robson, & Van Truong, 2000).

Trends of adolescent substance use in other countries are more difficult to determine, because youth surveys have been conducted only sporadically. Lifetime prevalence of marijuana use among 15 and 16 year olds in France increased from 11.9 to 23.0 percent from 1993 to 1997 and increased over a similar period in the mid-90s in Greece (3.0–10.2 percent) and Denmark (18.0–24.4 percent) (European Monitoring Centre for Drugs and Drug Addiction [EMCDDA], 2000).

THEORIES

A number of models and theories currently address the etiology of adolescent ATOD use, of which the most salient is the *Risk and Protective Factor framework*, the key terms of which are defined above. There is now a substantial body of evidence linking risk factors to adolescent substance use and related problems (Bry & Krinsley, 1990; Newcomb & Felix-Ortiz, 1992). Most of the research in this area, which has now been repeatedly summarized (CSAP, 1998, 2000; Hawkins et al., 1992), has identified and assessed the strength of psychosocial factors in the following domains: the individual, family, school, peer, community, and larger environment. In the individual domain, substance use has been linked to values, beliefs about, and attitudes towards substances; genetic susceptibility; early ATOD use; sensation seeking or preferences for novel or unusual situations; and various psychological disorders including antisocial, aggressive and other problem behavior. In the family domain ATOD use has been associated with familial substance use, poor parenting practices including harsh or inconsistent discipline, poor intra-familial communication, and inadequate supervision and monitoring of children's behaviors and peer associations. In the peer domain substance use has been linked to social isolation and association with ATOD-using peer networks. In the school domain ATOD use has been linked to poor academic performance and truancy, as well as a disorderly and unsafe school climate, and lax school policies concerning substance use. ATOD use has been linked to association with ATOD-using and otherwise deviant peers, as well as low acceptance by peers (i.e., social isolation). In the community and environmental domains, ready access to ATODs has been associated with use, as has lack of recreational resources (especially during the after school hours).

Protective factors have also been identified in these various domains. Among those most frequently cited in the individual domain are religiosity or spirituality, commitment to academic achievement, and strong life skills, social competencies, and belief in self-efficacy. Protective factors in the family and school domains include strong intra-familial bonds and positive family dynamics, and positive attachment to school. Association with peers in structured activities has also been identified as a buffering factor. In the community and environmental domains, strongly held adult values antithetical to substance use constitute protective factors, as do clearly communicated and consistently enforced regulations concerning use.

Other theories have also been tapped to explain the etiology of adolescent substance use (for a review, see Petraitis, Flay, & Miller, 1995). Motives for using ATODs may include rebelliousness, pleasure- or sensation-seeking, autonomy, modeling of adult behavior, stress relief, or social bonding with peers (Paglia & Room, 1999). *Social Control Theory* (Elliott, Huizinga, & Menard, 1989; Hirschi, 1969) lays out the processes by which adolescents come to associate with substance using peers as a result of neighborhood disorganization, low attachment to families, and deviant social values. The *Social Development Model* (Hawkins & Weis, 1985) suggests that weak conventional bonds to society, as well as to conventional, pro-social role models (especially parents), promote substance use. The value-expectancy *Theory of Reasoned Action* (Fishbein & Ajzen, 1975) has been used to explain substance use as a function of adolescents' attitudes towards substances and their understanding of the social norms concerning use. *Problem Behavior Theory* (Jessor, Donovan, & Costa, 1991) suggests that substance use may be one of a variety of problem behaviors that mark the progression of adolescents from childhood to adulthood, and thus constitute a rite of passage. Substance use is considered particularly likely among adolescents with weak attachments to parents who disapprove of such use, and correspondingly strong attachments to deviant peers. We note that most of the social science theories that have been postulated to explain the etiology of substance use concern its initiation, and do not address the vexing issue of why some young adults discontinue use while others progress from occasional or recreational use to problem use. To address these issues some researchers (Fishbein, 2000a) are beginning to investigate the biological determinants of differential addiction.

RESEARCH

At present the United States accounts for the great majority of research into the prevention of substance use, most of which has been conducted within the past three decades and has been sponsored by the National Institutes of Health (Paglia & Room, 1999). Much of this research has been conducted under carefully controlled, experimental conditions. The examples summarized below have been selected to represent some of the domains investigated, and not because they constitute the "best" studies in those domains.

The Efficacy of School-Based Substance Use Prevention Programs. In 1986, Tobler published the first of a series of meta-analyses of the results of short-term evaluations of 143 universal school-based drug prevention strategies, which was most recently updated in 1998 to include a total of 207 programs. Meta-analysis is a statistical technique designed to synthesize results of comparable studies in a systematic manner, through quantifying program effects in a standard metric. The relative outcomes of treatment versus control (or comparison) groups for these evaluations, which were conducted over the course of two decades, were typically framed in terms of self-reported past month ATOD use. Tobler, Roona, Ochshorn, Marshall, Streke, and Stackpole (2000) systematically coded information pertinent to outcome measures, intervention components, participant and program characteristics, implementation factors, and evaluation methodology and instrumentation. They utilized a classification system based on a combination of 34 major program content areas organized into seven major domains: knowledge, affective, drug refusal skills, generic skills, safety skills, extracurricular activities, and others. Programs were also classified on a four-point continuum from didactic to interactive. Weighted categorical and regression analyses were used to determine program attributes most closely and consistently associated with program success. Didactic, lecture-oriented programs designed to increase knowledge and enhance self-esteem showed small effects, while interactive programs targeting the development of interpersonal skills demonstrated greatest effects, although these effects attenuated when the programs were implemented under large scale, real world conditions.

The Efficacy of a School-Based Tobacco Prevention Program. Peterson, Kealey, Mann, Marek, and Sarason (2000) published the results of a longitudinal evaluation of a smoking prevention project in Washington State, which was based on a social influences approach to tobacco use prevention. The program was implemented when children were in the third grade and continued at regular intervals over the next 10 years until they completed or left high school. The intervention comprised the following key components: skills for identifying and resisting inducements to smoke, information correcting erroneous beliefs about the extent of youth smoking, enhancing motivations to be smoke-free, promoting self-efficacy to resist smoking, and involving the family in smoking prevention. Between 5 and 10 lessons were taught each year from the 3rd through the 10th grades,

inclusive. High school students who smoked were also given tobacco cessation materials. Altogether, approximately 8,400 youth were enrolled in 40 school districts in Washington State that were randomly assigned to a treatment or control group. Evaluators re-interviewed 94 percent of the original sample upon completion of school and again 2 years later. No differences were found between youth in the experimental or control school districts for daily smoking, amount of current smoking, or cumulative smoking. As the authors point out, the failure of this multi-year intervention that complied with generally held "best practices" casts a shadow over the social influences approach, and suggests the need to rethink the theoretical justification for such approaches (Clayton, Scutchfield, & Wyatt, 2000) and the relative advantages of involving families and communities in prevention efforts.

Reducing Alcohol Use by Minors through Environmental Strategies. Wagenaar et al. (1998) have sought to reduce underage drinking by changing and/or enforcing local alcohol policies. In a 3-year community-based study in Minnesota they sought to: change community norms that promote underage drinking, reduce the number of alcohol outlets selling to minors, and reduce the amount of alcohol given or resold to minors from family or acquaintances. Study results showed an increase in the proportion of alcohol outlets that checked buyers' identification. There was a commensurate increase in merchants' beliefs that they might be penalized for selling to minors. Study results also revealed that minors were less likely to attempt to purchase alcohol and to report difficulties in securing alcohol, as well as a reduction among young adults in drinking in bars and taverns. In another study, O'Malley and Wagenaar (1991) compared adolescent alcohol use and collisions attributed to alcohol in states with high and low legal drinking ages, and examined changes in these outcomes among states that raised their legal drinking age to 21. They found that in states with lower drinking ages adolescents consumed more alcohol, and continued to consume more as they entered adulthood. Raising the drinking age had the effect of reducing adolescents' alcohol consumption and time spent in bars; the proportion of car crashes attributed to alcohol were similarly reduced. A more recent study by Wagenaar, O'Malley, and LaFond (2001) also found that reducing the legal blood alcohol limit lowered rates of drinking and driving among individuals under the age of 21.

STRATEGIES THAT WORK

As suggested earlier, universal school-based ATOD prevention strategies have amassed the greatest amount of evaluative evidence based on scientifically controlled studies.

Of these, the *Life Skills Training* program (Botvin, Baker, Dusenburg, Botvin, & Diaz, 1995) has received the most attention. This universal classroom curriculum addresses a wide range of risk and protective factors through teaching personal and social skills in conjunction with normative education and drug resistance skills. The program involves a 3-year prevention curriculum targeting middle-school students; 15 lessons are delivered in the first year and 10 and five booster sessions in the second and third years, respectively. The curriculum has been extensively evaluated over the course of the last 20 years. Evaluative results indicate that this curriculum can reduce substance use by at least 50 percent (relative to adolescents in control groups). With the aid of the booster sessions, significant effects persisted up to six years following initial baseline assessment. There are preliminary indications that this curriculum is also effective with minority youth (Botvin, Griffin, Diaz, & Ifill-Williams, 2001).

Also of note is *Project Alert* (Ellickson, Bell, & McGuigan, 1993). Project Alert is designed to help adolescents develop non-drug norms and reasons not to use, as well as to resist pro-drug pressures, to understand the consequences of using drugs, to establish school-wide norms antithetical to drug use, to counter advertising inducing substance use, and to support others' decisions not to use. The curriculum also addresses the prevention of inhalant use and smoking cessation. Teaching strategies include guided classroom discussions and small group activities to generate peer interaction and modeling through presentations from teachers and older peers (through videotapes), and utilizes role-playing to give students the opportunity to practice resistance skills. Parents are also encouraged to become involved in the initiative through homework assignments. The project has been tested and validated in a number of ethnic populations of adolescents, and has demonstrated effectiveness in reducing marijuana and tobacco (but not alcohol) use.

Biglan, Ary, Smolkowski, Duncan, and Black (2000) recently published the results of an experimental evaluation of a comprehensive community-wide initiative to prevent adolescent tobacco use. Sixteen communities were randomly assigned to one of two conditions: a school-based prevention curriculum alone or the curriculum in combination with a community-based program. The curriculum, titled *Program to Advance Teen Health* (PATH), comprised five sessions over a one week period, and include the health-related effects of smoking, refusal skills designed to counter inducements to use tobacco or illegal drugs, video presentations modeling these skills, public pledges concerning tobacco use, and peer-led discussions and skill rehearsal activities. The community-based program comprised media advocacy, youth anti-tobacco activities, communications to adolescents' families about tobacco use, and strategies designed to reduce adolescents' access to alcohol. These latter strategies

included developing community support, educating employees of establishments selling alcohol, rewarding and publicizing employees who declined sales to minors, providing reminders to employees who did sell to minors, and providing information to store owners concerning their sales to minors. The researchers found that relative to the school-only condition, the combined school and community condition significantly affected seventh and ninth grade adolescents' weekly cigarette use after 5 years.

The *Iowa Strengthening Families* program (Spoth, Redmond, & Lepper, 1999) involves 21 2-hr competency-training sessions, seven each of which are delivered to adolescents, their parents, and both together. Parent sessions include viewing and discussing videotapes that portray negative and positive interactions with youth, skill-building activities, clarifying expectations of normal adolescent development and behavior, effective behavior management, responding appropriately to strong emotions, and effective communication techniques. Youth sessions include content similar to that delivered to their parents, but also involves opportunities to learn peer refusal skills as well as stress management and other social skills. Family sessions include a mix of the above strategies, and focus on the development and consistent implementation of rules, encouraging communication and good behavior, appreciating parents, building family communication, and conflict resolution. Together, families also engage in a variety of activities designed to build their cohesiveness and to involve their adolescents constructively in family affairs. In a study of 446 families of sixth graders randomly assigned to a treatment or control group, the investigators found that youth and their families attending the program had significantly lower rates of substance use and school-related conduct problems. Parents showed gains in parenting skills and child-management skills. Further, differences between program and control youth actually became more pronounced over time, a most unusual finding in a field that typically manifests rapidly attenuating effects.

The *Reconnecting Youth* program (Eggert, Thompson, Herting, Nicholas, & Dicker, 1994) is an indicated strategy that targets high school students who manifest poor academic achievement or who are at high risk for dropping out and other problem behaviors, including substance abuse and suicide ideation. The purpose of the program is to help students build resiliency, manage their anger more effectively, build self-esteem, enhance personal control of their lives, and develop interpersonal communication skills. The program builds on a foundation of social support and life skills training to which is added social activities in small groups and opportunities to bond to the school, as well as monitoring for potentially suicidal behaviors. Research results indicate improvements in affected students' school performance and reductions in substance use and involvement with deviant peers.

Inferences. In school settings, educational interventions targeting *individual* behavior that combine strategies that teach educational and personal skills are considered the most effective school-based approach to date. This approach, which typically includes practicing strategies designed to resist peer inducements to use substances, is often combined with exercises that include values clarification and that disabuse adolescents of exaggerated beliefs about the extent to which their peers are using drugs. Decision-making, problem-solving, and goal setting may also be taught. "Media literacy" lessons, designed to inoculate youth against the effects of advertising by the alcohol and tobacco industries, have increased adolescents' sophistication concerning the industries' efforts to manipulate consumers. These content areas are particularly effective if taught utilizing interactive techniques, and include cooperative learning, discussions, group exercises, peer leadership, and role playing (CSAP, 1998; Drug Strategies, 1999). For indicated populations of high-risk youth, extensive involvement in structured activities, led by charismatic and caring adults, show some signs of positive effects. Such strategies should be sensitive to the multidimensional nature of youth problems and include tailored interventions that affect these domains simultaneously.

In the *family* domain, educational approaches that target the entire family or that involve parents and adolescents in complementary prevention curricula have yielded positive results, especially if they are adapted to the family's particular cultural characteristics and target the families of high-risk youth. Effective programs have targeted parenting skills, parental monitoring and supervision, intra-familial communication patterns and the establishment of consistently applied disciplinary techniques and practices. Indicated interventions often require a substantial investment in family therapy or counseling, coupled with case management. As with school-based curricula, effective parenting is best taught through a combination of coaching, modeling, and role-playing.

In the *peer* domain, structured group activities, including recreation and competitive athletics, artistic expression, and supervised alternative events, offer an opportunity for socialization in settings that not only are ATOD-free but also require sobriety for successful performance. Such activities also assist youth in developing social bonds with peers who do not use substances and to promoting group norms antithetical to ATOD use. The more effective of these programs require an extended and intensive commitment.

In the *school* domain, effective interventions may focus both on increasing the academic competencies of the adolescent through tutoring and mentoring, and changing the structure and climate of the school to enhance youths' satisfaction with their academic experience. Considerable attention is now being paid to improving classroom teaching and behavioral management techniques, reducing teacher–student ratios, involving parents more closely in their children's education, and addressing the attitudes of teachers and administrators towards youth. The development of effectively and consistently administered school policies addressing ATOD use by both students and school personnel is also considered important. Finally, prevention specialists are encouraging schools to integrate anti-substance use messages into their curricula in all school grades, and to ensure that their prevention curricula are comprehensive and developmentally appropriate.

In the *community* and *environmental* domains, attention is increasingly being paid to the development and enforcement of public policies and ordinances that inhibit adolescent substance use (CSAP, 1998; Pacific Institute for Research and Evaluation, 1999). These include efforts targeting tobacco and alcohol outlets, including restrictions on their location and density and restricting alcohol and tobacco advertising. Schools are also establishing drug-free zones that establish substantial penalties for the sales or use of substances. Restrictions on tobacco use in enclosed environments have been very effective in reducing tobacco use and exposure to second-hand smoke, and in changing norms concerning the acceptability of tobacco use. Also effective are strategies promoting responsible behavior by alcohol servers and clerks in alcohol and tobacco outlets, which include instruction on pertinent laws and penalties for infractions (including liability for adolescents' subsequent behavior), as well as recognizing underage consumers and recognizing false identification. Such strategies are most effective when combined with the vigorous enforcement of laws governing sales to minors, including using underage youth to buy alcohol and tobacco products in "sting" operations. Increasing excise taxes on alcohol and tobacco products has also been associated with reductions in use, as has linking apprehension for infractions of laws related to purchasing and consuming ATODs to suspension or revocation of drivers licenses. Other preventive measures that target youth drivers include "zero tolerance" laws linking evidence of breath alcohol to driving privileges. Some communities have successfully mounted special law enforcement campaigns that target contexts where alcohol may be served to adolescents (e.g., fraternity parties).

STRATEGIES THAT MIGHT WORK

A number of other preventive interventions that show considerable promise are as of yet unproven in terms of their potential to prevent ATOD use in adolescence. Some are developing from our rapidly growing understanding of neurocognition and physiological processes that are closely related to addiction (Fishbein, 2000b; Giancola, 2000). These underlying factors may explain why some youth have relatively poor decision-making abilities, are prone to risk taking, and tend to act impulsively when confronted with opportunities to use substances. Youth with such deficits may not benefit from the universal prevention strategies described above, and may need more targeted interventions.

Preventive interventions such as FAST Track, Positive Alternative Thinking Strategies (PATHS), and the Good Behavior Game target young children who exhibit poor social skills and abnormal externalizing behavior, and/or who live in high-risk environments (Greenberg, Domitrovich, & Bumbarger, 1999). The *FAST Track* program integrates universal and targeted models of prevention, and is intended to provide a comprehensive longitudinal model for the prevention of conduct disorders in childhood and problem behaviors in adolescence (Conduct Problems Prevention Research Group, 1992). The universal intervention includes teacher consultation in the use of a series of grade-level versions of the PATHS curriculum throughout the elementary years. The targeted intervention package includes a series of interventions that involve the family (home visiting, parenting skills, case management), the child (academic tutoring, social skills training), the school, peer group, and community. Targeted children and families are identified by a multi-stage screening for externalizing behavior problems during kindergarten in schools in neighborhoods with high crime and poverty rates. The first three years of FAST Track evaluation have indicated significant reductions in special education referrals and aggression both at home and at school for targeted children (Greenberg et al., 1999).

The *PATHS* curriculum was developed to promote social/emotional competence among high-risk elementary school students through cognitive skill building, with an emphasis on teaching students to identify, understand, and self-regulate their emotions. Several randomized trials have shown the PATHS curriculum to be effective in improving children's problem-solving skills, emotional understanding, conduct problems, adaptive behavior, and cognitive abilities related to social planning and impulsivity (Greenberg et al., 1999).

The *Good Behavior Game* is a team-based classroom program designed to improve children's social adaptation to the classroom related to rules and authority. The classroom is divided into three heterogeneous teams that compete for rewards based on not violating established classroom standards for behavior. The Good Behavior Game has been shown to reduce teacher and peer ratings of aggressive behavior, as well as teacher ratings of shy behavior, in

first grade students, and has also been shown to reduce aggression and tobacco use in middle-school students (Kellam & Anthony, 1998; Kellam, Ling, Merisca, Brown, & Ialongo, 1998).

Targeted school-based interventions, such as *Positive Adolescent Choices Training* (PACT) (Yung & Hammond, 1998), also have been developed for adolescents in high-risk environments. PACT was developed for African American middle-school students in low-income urban communities who have engaged in violent behavior in school. PACT includes approximately 38 50-min sessions that focus on nonviolent conflict-resolution skills. Skills are taught with a videotaped program, "Dealing with Anger: A Social Skills Training Program for African American Youth." Youth who participated in the PACT program demonstrated improvements in all social-cognitive target areas, and were less likely to be suspended from school than youth in a comparison group. However, no studies have yet been conducted to assess the effects of PACT on adolescent ATOD use.

Other community-based approaches also show promise. Adolescent involvement with religious and youth-oriented institutions offer youth opportunities to become engaged in prosocial activities with non-drug using peers in contexts in which norms antithetical to ATOD use can be communicated. It is generally recognized that to be effective such involvement should be relatively long-term, but even single events can publicize the community's commitment to prevention (CSAP, 1998). The development of active coalitions of public and voluntarily agencies dedicated to ATOD prevention can mobilize, coordinate, and focus prevention efforts, as well as avoid duplication and fragmentation of services. Strong grassroots anti-drug efforts can also be very effective in dislocating drug dealers and taking direct action against alcohol and tobacco outlets that constitute public nuisances.

A number of promising preventive interventions have been developed for elementary and middle school youth who live in high-risk environments and have exhibited externalizing problem behaviors (e.g., aggression) that are known to be associated with underlying neurocognitive and physiological abnormalities (Fishbein, 2000b; Giancola, 2000). Such abnormalities may predispose youth to ATOD use and addiction, but may be modified by targeted social-cognitive skill-building interventions in childhood or adolescence. Additional research is needed, however, to assess the effects of these targeted interventions on adolescent ATOD use.

STRATEGIES THAT DO NOT WORK

The results of two decades of evaluative research have yielded considerable information suggesting the lack of effectiveness of a number of approaches to adolescent ATOD use prevention (CSAP, 1998). Scare tactics, designed to frighten adolescents into avoiding drugs, are often recognized as such by their target audiences and can even be counter-productive. Efforts to raise self-esteem as a drug prevention strategy have long been discredited given the lack of association between self-esteem and ATOD use. Strategies designed to increase knowledge and convey information about the risks and dangers of drug use, including media campaigns, are generally recognized to be failures, in part because of the lack of association between knowledge and use. Indeed, all largely didactic approaches to prevention education, such as *Project Drug Abuse Resistance Education* (DARE), are now widely understood to be ineffective (Ennett, Tobler, Ringwalt, & Flewelling, 1994; Tobler, 1986), especially if they concentrate on long-term risks. Mass media campaigns are of dubious value, especially if they are brief, aired in contexts that are unlikely to reach their target audience, and uncoordinated with a comprehensive, community-wide strategy. Also ineffective are media campaigns that demonstrate substance use and use scare tactics to discourage use. While such campaigns may affect knowledge and awareness, they have had little impact on attitudes and behaviors.

SYNTHESIS

The field of ATOD prevention has made substantial progress over the course of the last two decades. Because of the very high investment in both prevention practice and research targeting adolescents in middle school settings, we now know about as much as we are likely to know about effective programming in this environment, although we have much to learn about how prevention should be delivered to high school students.

Unfortunately, even the most effective and comprehensive school-based strategies, and even those that reinforce their messages across grade levels, are only slightly more effective than school-based programs that are now generally discredited. There is now a consensus among both practitioners and researchers that school-based programs, by themselves, are insufficient, and should be part of a broad array of prevention approaches (Dusenbury, 2000). However, little is known about how best to mount an integrated set of strategies addressing both supply and demand reduction in the family and community, as well as the individual, domains.

It is also likely that elaborate, multi-lesson curricula like *Life Skills Training and Project* ALERT will not survive in school environments that are subjected to increasing pressures to teach primarily to standardized tests of educational achievement. In response, researchers are turning their attention to determining the irreducible components of effective prevention strategies, and which combinations of these components are critical for what types of evaluations. In addition, researchers are beginning to track exactly how teachers adapt curricula for their own use, and why, recognizing that such adaptations are not only inevitable but may in some situations be desirable.

The prevention field has hardly begun to address some very big and important questions. As of this writing, the notion that current laws in the United States pertaining to marijuana and other drugs that are illegal for adults may be not only ill-advised but destructive has yet to be empirically investigated. Case studies of the experience of nations that have decriminalized non-addictive drugs are clearly needed, to determine their effects on both adult and youth use. By the same token, we need further research concerning the long-term effects of measures that various countries have taken to reduce the accessibility and increase the costs of both alcohol and tobacco products.

We also know relatively little about prevention in two key settings, namely college campuses and worksites. College-aged youth—that is, young adults—are at the greatest risk of any time in their lives for heavy or binge drinking. Many college campuses have cultures that are at least covertly supportive of alcohol consumption, and administrators who treat the issue with benign neglect. While we believe that most drinking on college campuses occurs in neighborhood bars and residential contexts such as fraternities, relatively little has been done to develop and implement demonstration programs that increase enforcement of, and penalties for, selling or otherwise supplying liquor to underage students.

The workplace also presents a promising venue for ATOD prevention, especially in those industries that hire young adults or in which the sobriety of employees is essential for their own and the public's safety. A number of innovative strategies are now being implemented and assessed, among them the use of trained and supervised peer helpers to whom troubled employers can turn for confidential advice. In a related approach that also capitalizes on peer interventions, workers in a high-risk transportation industry have been encouraged to confront co-workers who may be impaired in a manner that both reduces the threat of an accident and protects the co-worker from a punitive managerial response. Some industries are also training supervisors and managers to be alert to the early signs of substance abuse and to make effective use of company Employee Assistance Programs (EAPs).

The Internet represents a largely untapped frontier for prevention, and offers several indisputable advantages. First, it is easily accessible to a substantial and growing proportion of adolescents, at least in developed nations. Second, it is interactive, and thus inherently engaging, in nature. Third, prevention websites can offer immediate, tailored, and completely confidential feedback in response to completed health risk appraisals. Fourth, such websites can provide contact information for appropriate local resources for those in need of assistance. Interactive websites are now being developed to disseminate prevention messages to school- and college-aged populations, but the effects of this mode of communication will not be known for some time.

Also see: Substances entries.

References

Biglan, A., Ary, D.V., Smolkowski, K., Duncan, T., & Black, C. (2000). A randomized controlled trial of a community intervention to prevent adolescent tobacco use. *Tobacco Control, 9*, 24–32.

Botvin, G.J., Baker, E., Dusenburg, L., Botvin, E.M., & Diaz, T. (1995). Long-term followup results of a randomized drug abuse prevention trial in a white middle-class population. *Journal of the American Medical Association, 273*(14), 1106–1112.

Botvin, G.J., Griffin, K.W., Diaz, T., & Ifill-Williams, M. (2001). Drug abuse prevention among minority adolescents: Posttest and one-year follow-up of a school-based preventive intervention. *Prevention Science, 2*(1), 1–13.

Bry, B., & Krinsley, K. (1990). Adolescent substance abuse. In E. Feindler & G. Kalfus (Eds.), *Adolescent behavior therapy handbook* (pp. 219–232). New York: Springer & Krinsley.

Center for Addiction and Mental Health (CAMH). (2000). *Ontario student drug use survey. Executive summary [on-line]*. Available: www.camh. net/understanding/ont_study_drug_use.html. Accessed on January 2, 2001.

Center for Addiction and Substance Abuse (CASA), Columbia University. (1993). *The cost of substance abuse to America's Health Care System, Report 1: Medicaid hospital costs*. New York: Columbia University.

Center for Substance Abuse Prevention (CSAP), Division of Knowledge Development and Evaluation. (1998). *Science-based practices in substance abuse prevention: A guide*. Washington, DC: Substance Abuse and Mental Health Services Administration, Center for Substance Abuse Prevention, Division of Knowledge Development and Evaluation. Working Draft.

Center for Substance Abuse Prevention (CSAP), National Center for the Advancement of Prevention, (2000). *2000 Annual summary: Effective prevention principles and programs*. Rockville, MD: Author.

Clayton, R.R., Scutchfield, F.D., & Wyatt, S.W. (2000). Editorial: Hutchinson Smoking Prevention Project: A new gold standard in prevention science requires new transdisciplinary thinking. *Journal of the National Cancer Institute, 92*(24), 1964–1965.

Conduct Problems Prevention Research Group. (1992). A developmental and clinical model for the prevention of conduct disorders: The FAST track program. *Development and Psychopathology, 4*, 509–527.

Drug Strategies. (1999). *Making the grade: A guide to school drug prevention programs*. Washington, DC: Author.

Dusenbury, L. (2000). Implementing a comprehensive drug abuse prevention strategy. In W.B. Hansen, S.M. Giles, & M. Fearnow-Kenney (Eds.), *Increasing prevention effectiveness* (chap. 13, pp. 269–280). Greensboro, NC: Tanglewood Research.

Eggert, L.L., Thompson, E.A., Herting, J.R., Nicholas, L.J., & Dicker, G.C. (1994). Preventing adolescent drug abuse and high school dropout through an intensive school-based social network development program. *American Journal of Health Promotion, 8*(3), 202–215.

Ellickson, P.L., Bell, R.M., & McGuigan, K. (1993). Preventing adolescent drug use: Long-term results of a junior high program. *American Journal of Public Health, 83*, 856–861.

Elliott, D.S., Huizinga, D., & Menard, S. (1989). *Multiple problem youth: Delinquency, substance use, and mental health problems*. New York: Springer-Verlag.

Ennett, S., Tobler, N.S., Ringwalt, C.L., & Flewelling, R.L. (1994). How effective is Drug Abuse Resistance Education? A meta-analysis of Project DARE outcome evaluations. *American Journal of Public Health, 84*, 1394–1401.

European Monitoring Centre for Drugs and Drug Addiction (EMCDDA). (2000). Table: Lifetime prevalence of use of different illegal drugs among 15- to 16-year old students in recent nation-wide school surveys in some EU countries. In: *Evaluating the treatment of drug abuse in the European Union [on-line]*. Available: www.emcdda.org/publications/ publications_monographs.shtml. Accessed on January 3, 2001.

Fishbein, D.H. (Ed.). (2000a). *The science, treatment, and prevention of antisocial behaviors: Application to the criminal justice system*. Kingston, NJ: Civic Research Institute.

Fishbein, D.H. (2000b). The importance of neurobiological research in the prevention of psychopathology. *Prevention Science, 1*, 89–106.

Fishbein, M., & Ajzen, I. (1975). *Belief, attitude, intention and behavior: An introduction to theory and research*. Reading, MA: Addison-Wesley.

Giancola, P.R. (2000). Neuropsychological functioning and antisocial behavior: Implications for etiology and prevention. In D. Fishbein (Ed.), *The science, treatment and prevention of antisocial behavior* (pp. 11-1–11-16). New Jersey: Civic Research Institute.

Greenberg, M.T., Domitrovich, C., & Bumbarger, B. (1999). *Preventing mental disorders in school-age children: A review of the effectiveness of prevention programs*. Report prepared for the Center for Mental Health Services, Substance Abuse and Mental Health Services Administration, US Department of Health and Human Services.

Hawkins, J.D., Catalano, R.F., & Miller, J.Y. (1992). Risk and protective factors for alcohol and other drug problems in adolescence and early adulthood: Implications for substance abuse prevention. *Psychological Bulletin, 112*(1), 64–105.

Hawkins, J.D., & Weis, J.G. (1985). The social development model: An integrated approach to delinquency prevention. *Journal of Primary Prevention, 6*, 73–97.

Hirschi, T. (1969). *Causes of delinquency*. Berkeley: University of California Press.

Jessor, R., Donovan, J.E., & Costa, F.M. (1991). *Beyond adolescence: Problem behavior and young adult development*. Cambridge, England: Cambridge Unviersity Press.

Join Together OnLine. (1999). *Alcohol abuse costs society $250 billion per year [on-line]*. Available: www.jointogether.org/sa/wire/features/ reader.jml. Accessed January 2, 2001.

Kellam, S.G., & Anthony, J.C. (1998). Targeting early antecedents to prevent tobacco smoking: Findings from an epidemiologically-based randomized field trial. *American Journal of Public Health, 88*, 1490–1495.

Kellam, S.G., Ling, X., Merisca, R., Brown, C.H., & Ialongo, N. (1998). The effect of the level of aggression in the first grade classroom on the course and malleability of aggressive behavior into middle school. *Development and Psychopathology, 10*, 165–185.

Newcomb, M.D., & Felix-Ortiz, M. (1992). Multiple protective and risk factors for drug use and abuse: Cross-sectional and prospective findings. *Journal of Personality and Social Psychology, 63*(2), 280–296.

O'Malley, P.M., & Waganeer, A.C. (1991). Effects of minimum drinking age laws on alcohol use, related behaviors and traffic crash involvement among American youth: 1976–1987. *Journal of Studies on Alcohol, 52*, 478–491.

Pacific Institute for Research and Evaluation (PIRE). (1999). *Strategies to reduce underage alcohol use: Typology and brief overview*. Washington, DC: US Department of Justice, Office of Justice Programs, Office of Juvenile Justice and Delinquency Prevention (Award No. 98-AH-F8-0114).

Paglia, A., & Room, R. (1999). Preventing substance use problems among youth: A literature review and recommendations. *Journal of Primary Prevention, 20*(1), 3–50.

Peterson, A.V., Kealey, K.A., Mann, S.L., Marek, P.M., & Sarason, I.G. (2000). Hutchinson Smoking Prevention Project: Long-term randomized trial in school-based tobacco use prevention—results on smoking. *Journal of the National Cancer Institute, 92*(24), 1979–1991.

Petraitis, J., Flay, B.R., & Miller, T.Q. (1995). Reviewing theories of adolescent substance use: Organizing pieces in the puzzle. *Psychological Bulletin, 117*(1), 67–86.

Samber, S. (1998). The economic costs to society of alcohol and drug abuse. *The NCADI reporter [on-line]*. May 14, 1998. Available: www.health. org:80/newsroom/rep/79.htm. Accessed January 2, 2001.

Single, E., Rehm, J., Robson, L., & Van Truong, M. (2000). The relative risks and etiologic fractions of different causes of death and disease attributable to alcohol, tobacco and illicit drug use in Canada. *Canadian Medical Association Journal, 162*, 1669–1675.

Spoth, R., Redmond, C., & Lepper, H. (1999). Alcohol initiation outcomes of universal family-focused preventive interventions: One- and two-year follow-ups of a controlled study. *Journal of Studies on Alcohol, 13*, 103–111.

Tobler, N.S. (1986). Meta-analysis of 143 adolescent drug prevention programs: Quantitative outcome results of program participants compared to a control or comparison group. *Journal of Drug Issues, 16*(4), 537–567.

Tobler, N.S., Roona, M.R., Ochshorn, P., Marshall, D.G., Streke, A.V., & Stackpole, K.M. (2000). School-based adolescent drug prevention programs: 1998 meta-analysis. *The Journal of Primary Prevention, 20*(4), 275–336.

University of Michigan, News and Information Services. (2000). *"Ecstasy" use rises sharply among teens in 2000; use of many other drugs stays steady, but significant declines are reported for some.* For release at 10 A.M. EST, Thursday, December 14, 2000, Ann Arbor, MI.

Wagenaar, A.C., Gehan, J.P., Jones-Webb, R., Wolfson, M., Toomey, T.L., Forster, J.L., & Murray, D.M. (1998). *Communities mobilizing for change on alcohol: Experiences and outcomes from a randomized community trial.* Paper presented at the Fourth Symposium on CommunityAction Research and the Prevention of Alcohol and Other Drug Programs: A Kettil Bruun Society Thematic Meeting, Russell, New Zealand.

Wagenaar, A.C., O'Malley, P.M., & LaFond, C. (2001). Lowered legal blood alcohol limits for young drivers: Effects on drinking, driving, and driving-after-drinking behaviors in 30 states. *American Journal of Public Health, 91*(5), 801–804.

Yung, B., & Hammond, R. (1998). Breaking the cycle: A culturally sensitive prevention program for African American children and adolescents. In J. Lutzker (Ed.), *Handbook of child abuse research and treatment* (pp. 319–340). New York, NY: Plenum.

Substances, Adolescence (Meta-Analysis)

Michael Roona, Andrei Streke, and Diana Marshall

INTRODUCTION AND DEFINITIONS

Prevention programs targeting alcohol, tobacco, or other drugs are often referred to as *ATOD programs*. Most formal, structured ATOD programs for adolescents are implemented in schools and most school-based programs target the entire population of students in a specific grade without singling out subpopulations based on risk factors. If relatively few students in the school are known to be "at-risk" of using or abusing substances, these interventions targeting the entire population are known as universal interventions. If most of the students in the schools are "at-risk" or if the programs target subpopulations within the schools possessing risk factors predictive of substance use or abuse (e.g., children of substance abusing parents), then the interventions are known as selective interventions. Programs like student assistance programs that often target drug involved but asymptomatic subpopulations are known as indicated interventions.

In this entry, we synthesize the research about school-based ATOD programs by computing *effect sizes*, which are standardized measures of differences between intervention and comparison groups, for each measured substance use outcome associated with each prevention program and averaging these effect sizes across similar measures and types of programs. The specific technique we use to systematically assess program effects in the ensemble of available studies is called *meta-analysis*, which involves controlling for differences in sample sizes and other factors that influence statistical findings when averages are computed.

SCOPE

Alcohol is used by 100 million Americans, tobacco is used by 60 million Americans, marijuana is used by 10 million Americans, cocaine is used by 5 million Americans, and heroin is used by one half million Americans. Annually, 650 tobacco users, 150 alcohol users, 80 heroin users, 4 cocaine users, and 0 marijuana users die per 100,000 Americans who use each substance (Ostrowski, cited in Meier, 1994). (Cocaine use has decreased to 1.5 million since Ostrowski published these figures in 1989, but relative mortality rates remain stable.)

Among eighth graders in the United States surveyed over the past decade for the Monitoring the Future study (2000), half reported having used alcohol at some point in their lives, and one quarter reported having gotten drunk. Forty percent reported having smoked a cigarette, 20 percent reported having smoked marijuana, and 15–20 percent reported having used an illicit drug other than marijuana. Among twelfth graders, 80 percent reported having imbibed alcohol and 60 percent reported having gotten drunk. Sixty percent also reported having smoked a cigarette, and over half reported having used an illicit drug. Across grade levels, approximately three quarters of those who reported having engaged in these behaviors during their lifetimes reported having done so in the past year, and 60 percent of those reported having done so within the past 30 days.

THEORIES

The two theories that have had the most significant impact on the development and implementation of science-based adolescent ATOD interventions over the past quarter century are social learning theory (Bandura, 1977) and problem behavior theory (Jessor & Jessor, 1977). *Social learning theory* posits that adolescents learn from others in two important ways: (1) direct modeling of the behavior of peers or adults and (2) reinforcement of beliefs, attitudes, and behavior. Lessons designed to undermine adolescents' misguided beliefs regarding the frequency and/or quantity of substance use by their peers, which are common to most science-based drug education programs, constitute curriculum components motivated by social learning theory.

Problem behavior theory posits that adolescents use substances for functional purposes (i.e., substance use fulfills a need for the adolescent). From this perspective, substance use is seen as a way of coping with (real or anticipated) failure, boredom, social anxiety, unhappiness, rejection, social isolation, low self-esteem, or lack of self-efficacy. Many lessons designed to teach social or life skills and some lessons designed to foster prosocial development or promote social competency constitute curriculum components motivated largely (though not exclusively) by problem behavior theory.

Problem behavior theory focuses on deficits or shortcomings of adolescents. Social learning theory, at least when applied to correct normative perceptions regarding peer drug use, also largely focuses on deficits of adolescents. Because these two theories frame substance use as a manifestation of individual deficits, they are compatible with an ideological position held by many funders of drug education programs (who significantly guide our understanding for action), namely, that drug education programs should promote abstinence (or at the very least not tolerate use). According to this view, abstinence is a moral imperative and the normative perceptions that drug education programs seek to correct are both descriptive and prescriptive.

Because all substance use is wrong and a consequence of individual deficits, the distinction between use and abuse is blurred by these theoretical and ideological lenses. Preventing ATOD *use* is seen as the best way to prevent harm to individuals and reduce the cost to society associated with ATOD *abuse*. In addition, when ATOD prevention programs express concern about the use of substances other than tobacco or alcohol, they generally treat preventing the use of these "gateway" substances as the key to preventing the abuse of other drugs. Stages in the development of adolescent substance use and the critical turning points associated with transitions from non-use to first use of a substance, from onset of use to occasional experimentation with the same or other substances, from occasional experimentation to regular use of one or more substances, and from regular use to abuse, are ignored. Hence, multiple opportunities to prevent adolescents from advancing to the substance abuse stage are missed.

An alternative perspective frames experimentation with substance use as *normative behavior* for adolescents who are developmentally prone to experiment with many lifestyles and their attendant behaviors. Most of these experimental users will never become abusers. Those who do will become abusers because they lack sufficient developmental assets to ensure resilience in the face of risk or adversity. Fostering resilience is seen as a way to reduce substance abuse (Brown, D'Emidio-Caston, & Benard, 2000). Taking this perspective further, harm reductionists argue that substance use per se is not problematic. What is problematic is the harm that might befall an adolescent under the influence and the prospect that experimental use will evolve into abuse for a small percentage of adolescents. Hence, rather than try to prevent the onset of use or adolescent experimentation, harm reduction oriented drug education programs focus on preventing harm and the transition to substance abuse (Rosenbaum, 1999).

RESEARCH

The experimental use of licit and illicit substances by adolescents in America is the norm. As the prevalence data from the Monitoring the Future study presented above indicate, by the time they reach twelfth grade, most adolescents not only will have consumed alcohol, but they will have gotten drunk. Most also will have smoked a cigarette and used an illicit drug. Most of the adolescents who engaged in these behaviors at least once during their lifetimes also will have done so in the past year, and most of those who engaged in these behaviors during the past year will have done so within the past 30 days.

The good news is that most of these adolescent substance users do not grow up to be substance abusers. Furthermore, they may mature into better adjusted adults than adolescents who abstain. In one of the few prospective longitudinal studies of the psychological antecedents of adolescent drug use that involved study subjects who were recruited as nursery school students, Shedler and Block (1990) concluded that "it is difficult to escape the inference that [drug] experimenters are the psychologically healthiest subjects, healthier than either abstainers or frequent users" (p. 625). Because this study was a prospective study involving such young subjects, Shedler and Block were able to relate psychological differences among abstainers, experimental users, and frequent drug users to the quality of parenting provided, thereby providing encouragement to researchers and practitioners implementing family-focused ATOD prevention programs.

The finding that most adolescent substance use does not evolve into persistent use appears to be corroborated by other longitudinal studies of adolescents. The Program of Research on the Causes and Correlates of Delinquency involving study sites in Rochester, NY, Denver, CO, and Pittsburgh, PA found that "most problem behaviors (including drug use) are intermittent or transitory" (Huizing, Loeber, Thornberry, & Cothern, 2000, p. 2). Unfortunately for universal ATOD prevention programs grounded in Jessor's problem behavior theory or designed to address the childhood psychological health antecedents of adolescent substance abuse found by Shedler and Block, preliminary findings presented by Huizing et al. (2000) indicate that "a large proportion of persistent serious delinquents are not involved in persistent drug use, nor do they have persistent school or mental health problems" (p. 5). Jessor's theory implies that similar factors foster a wide range of adolescent problem behaviors (e.g., delinquency, early sexual experience, and drug use). It is a general theory that allows for the classification of adolescents along a dimension of deviance susceptibility that will predict their use of drugs. If Jessor's theory and the antecedents found by Shedler and Block are shown by Huizing et al. (2000) to lack predictive validity, then the theoretical foundations of ATOD prevention programming may need to be rebuilt.

The claim that the theoretical foundations of ATOD prevention programming need to be rebuilt has been advanced by researchers who published a study that "is destined to become the gold standard in [ATOD] prevention science" (Clayton, Scutchfield, & Wyatt, 2000, p. 1964). Peterson, Kealey, Mann, Marek, and Sarason (2000) argue as a result of long-term evidence from their rigorously designed large-scale evaluation of an ATOD intervention "that, given this major failure of the social influences approach despite the extensive nature of the intervention, the remedy should not be more of the same (e.g., starting earlier, lasting longer, or combining unproven components with other approaches). It may be time for an altogether new approach that incorporates different theories, different intervention strategies, different venues, and/or different providers ... that can effectively gain the attention and trust of youth, especially those at high risk ... [because] current school program 'best practices' are not strong enough" (p. 1988).

STRATEGIES: OVERVIEW

The finding of Peterson et al. (2000) demonstrating that "there is no evidence of an intervention impact on the prevalence of daily smoking [or other smoking outcome measures] at grade 12, either for girls or boys" (p. 1984) reinforces concerns about the long-term effects of school-based ATOD interventions for children and adolescents. Given a limited body of longitudinal research and the fact that the few longitudinal studies generally have not demonstrated effectiveness at preventing ATOD use, the following discussion focuses exclusively on first year program effects, that is, effects on study subjects within the first year. Favorable effects within the first year should be construed as evidence that prevention programs have delayed the onset of use or suspended use behaviors for some youths, not prevented use.

The ability of prevention programs to delay the onset of substance use was assessed meta-analytically by computing effect sizes for each substance use outcome measured by a program evaluator, averaging these effect sizes to derive an overall measure of program effectiveness regarding ATOD use for each program, and then averaging the average effect sizes across groups of programs clustered according to program type, which is defined both in terms of program content and process. In addition, for types of programs that demonstrated effectiveness delaying the onset of substance use when program effects on all measured substance use outcomes were averaged, the average effects of the programs on specific substance use outcomes were contrasted. The 207 evaluated programs yielded 2,035 drug use effect sizes associated with 689 measured drug use outcomes for five types of Non-Interactive programs and three types of Interactive programs.

Non-interactive programs use didactic teaching methods that emphasize conveying information to students. *Interactive programs* provide adolescents with the opportunity to exchange ideas with their teacher and their classmates and to try out new roles or explore alternative ways to address potential future drug-related predicaments. The interactive programs include those that focus on Social Influences (SI), those that teach Comprehensive Life Skills (CLS), and those that promote System-Wide Change (SWC). SI programs focus primarily on interpersonal skills development. They may include a limited affective component, but they tend to emphasize a rational cognition approach to decision-making and largely ignore the influence of affect on substance use decision-making by youth. They emphasize resisting pro-drug social influences, including the subtle indirect pressures to use drugs. Students are shown that they tend to overestimate the frequency and/or quantity of substance use by their peers in order to reduce the pressure students feel to conform their behavior with mistaken perceptions of high levels of use. Students also may learn how media influences shape an individual's drug use decisions. CLS programs have content similar to that of the SI programs but add life skills training that includes the development of communication, assertiveness, coping, and goal-setting skills, as well as a broader affective component. SWC programs try to transform the school atmosphere, engage students more fully, and/or involve the students' families and/or community.

STRATEGIES THAT WORK

For all drugs combined, the effects of the interactive school-based programs measured within the first year are small but clinically and statistically significant. The interactive programs produced an average effect size of 0.15 (Tobler, Roona, Ochshorn, Marshall, Streke, & Stackpole, 2000). Furthermore, when this overall impact is disaggregated, the effect size associated with the interactive programs is 50 percent greater for at-risk than for universal populations (0.21 vs. 0.14), indicating that the significant but modest overall average effect size for these programs may fail to capture their true value, because the programs appear to have a more pronounced impact on at-risk youth.

Interactive programs, however, require an approach to teaching that is not the norm in American classrooms. In fact, we found mental health clinicians to be significantly more effective than teachers as prevention program implementers. We presumed clinicians are more effective because they are professionally trained to conduct interactive groups effectively, but in a study of instructor characteristics associated with the integrity of role plays, Sobol, Rohrbach, Dent, Gleason, Brannon, Johnson, and Flay (1989) found no statistically significant relationship between role play integrity and "professional background, preparedness for program delivery, beliefs regarding the effectiveness of the program, [or] knowledge of key program concepts" (p. 64). However, they did find "high performers were more animated, articulate, organized, enthusiastic, and confident ... [and] felt more effective in the use of the Socratic method, and reported a less authoritarian teaching style than low performers" (p. 64). Presumably, anyone with these characteristics who is willing to focus on the perceptions and experiences of adolescents in a non-judgmental way can lead effective interactive groups. In fact, it may be that interaction with caring adults is more important than the content of the interaction. In a study that evaluated mentoring as a drug prevention strategy, Aseltine, Dupre, and Lamein (2000) found that mentoring in conjunction with a standard school-based life skills curriculum to be more effective than the curriculum by itself or no intervention at all.

STRATEGIES THAT MIGHT WORK

Of the three types of interactive programs, the SWC programs have the highest first year effect size for all drugs combined (0.27), followed by the CLS (0.17), and SI (0.12) programs. When those interventions that were evaluated using lower quality research designs are excluded, the pattern remains the same but the effect sizes become 0.22, 0.17, and 0.14, respectively. However, relatively few SWC interventions have been evaluated, and none of those evaluation designs involved randomized assignment or a sufficient number of schools, so the most we can say given the limited available evidence is that these are promising interventions that might effectively delay, prevent, or reduce the use or abuse of some substances.

A substantially greater body of evidence about CLS and SI programs has been amassed, however, allowing for a refined quantitative analysis of the literature about the 113 CLS and SI interventions that measured their impact on substance use behaviors during the first year. While CLS programs appear to be more effective than SI programs when all substances and all grade levels are combined, differential effects for different substance use outcomes exist at the elementary, junior high,[1] and high school levels. For all drugs combined, CLS programs appear to be more effective than SI programs at the elementary and senior high school levels, but not at the junior high school level. This is largely because the effects of SI programs are neither statistically nor clinically significant at the elementary and senior high levels (but the CLS effects are), whereas at the junior high level, the SI and CLS programs have effect sizes that are quite close (0.103 and 0.129, respectively).

When the effects of the SI and CLS programs on cigarette use are examined, a similar pattern is found. CLS programs are found to be more effective than SI programs at the elementary and senior high school levels (where the SI programs are ineffective). At the junior high school level, a statistically significant difference is found favoring the CLS programs, but when the difference is adjusted to take into account the smaller size of the CLS programs, the difference disappears. Given evidence that program effectiveness decreases as program size increases (Tobler et al., 2000), this adjustment for sample size results in a more accurate estimate of the difference in program effect.

---

[1] Interventions delivered exclusively to sixth graders, even if those sixth graders were in a middle school, are coded as elementary school programs. Interventions delivered to sixth graders and at least one higher grade in a middle school are coded as junior high school programs. Thus, in some cases, evaluation data provided by sixth graders contributes to the elementary school average effect size and in others to the junior high school average effect size.

No CLS program evaluations measured marijuana use at the elementary school level within the first year. The relationship between the effectiveness of SI and CLS programs on marijuana use at the junior high and senior high levels, however, parallels the relationship found for all drugs combined and for cigarettes. At the high school level, the two SI program evaluations that measured marijuana use demonstrated no effect whereas the two CLS program evaluations that measured marijuana use demonstrated an effect that was statistically and clinically significant. At the junior high school level, however, the 12 SI program evaluations and the 8 CLS program evaluations that assessed intervention effects on marijuana use demonstrated statistically and clinically beneficial effects that were not statistically different.

The effects of SI and CLS programs on alcohol use are quite different. At the high school level, the SI programs are still ineffective and the CLS programs show promise, but at the junior high school level, the CLS programs range from ineffective to counter productive, depending on the alcohol use measure. No elementary CLS evaluations measure alcohol use.

Concerns about binge drinking and other forms of alcohol abuse motivate some program evaluators to measure alcohol use in multiple ways. We reviewed evaluations of 21 SI and 11 CLS programs at the junior high school level as well as 8 SI and 4 CLS programs at the senior high school level that assessed program effects on alcohol use. Of these, 17 SI and 8 CLS programs at the junior high level as well as 4 SI and 2 CLS programs at the senior high level were evaluated using measures that determined whether any alcohol was consumed recently. Of these, evaluations of five SI and seven CLS programs at the junior high level and one SI and one CLS program at the high school level also included measures of heavy alcohol use. For a small number of programs, therefore, effects on both use and abuse can be contrasted.

For all alcohol use measures combined, effects of the SI programs at the junior high school level were statistically greater than zero and they approached a clinically significant effect size of 0.1. The CLS programs, however, had no effect at the junior high school level. At the high school level, the reverse was true. The SI programs demonstrated no effect but the CLS programs demonstrated clinically and statistically significant benefits. When heavy alcohol use measures are excluded, the pattern demonstrating the superiority of SI programs at the junior high school level and the superiority of CLS programs at the high school level remains, but the effectiveness of the interventions drops considerably. The junior high SI programs are found to be statistically greater than zero but not large enough to be clinically meaningful (0.06) and the CLS programs are found to be clinically and statistically counterproductive (−0.10). At the high school level, the magnitude of the difference in effect sizes between the SI and CLS programs remains large

(0.23), but the loss of power due to the small sample size in the two remaining CLS interventions precludes the possibility of that difference being statistically significant.

While the CLS programs appear to be promising alcohol use prevention programs at the high school level, neither the SI nor the CLS programs appear to prevent alcohol use at the junior high school level. Furthermore, at the junior high school level, the CLS programs appear to be counterproductive when the outcome measured is any alcohol use. When heavy alcohol use is measured, the CLS programs yield positive effects that would be clinically significant if they were statistically significant and the SI programs demonstrate statistically and clinically significant effects that are quite large. Evaluations of the five SI interventions that measured both any alcohol use and heavy alcohol use dramatically demonstrate the importance of knowing what you want to prevent and how to measure it. These SI interventions had an effect size of 0.05 (which is neither statistically nor clinically significantly greater than zero) and would be considered ineffective if their goal was to prevent alcohol use. If, however, the goal of these SI interventions was to prevent alcohol abuse, then these programs would be considered quite effective, given a statistically significant effect size of 0.25. This group of similar interventions that measured both use and abuse is five times more effective at preventing abuse than at preventing use. Furthermore, the magnitude of the effect on abuse is one of the largest seen for a drug use outcome measure in a meta-analysis of universal ATOD program evaluations.

STRATEGIES THAT DO NOT WORK

The non-interactive school-based programs produced an average effect size of 0.05, which is neither clinically nor statistically different from zero. Furthermore, when this overall impact is disaggregated and effects on at-risk and universal populations are contrasted, the effect sizes indicate that the non-interactive programs are potentially counterproductive with at-risk populations (−0.05), despite their potential to be minimally effective when implemented universally (0.07). While the difference between the effects of non-interactive programs on at-risk and universal populations is both clinically and statistically significant, the effect sizes themselves are neither clinically nor statistically different from zero. What is noteworthy is that the more effective interactive programs (0.15 overall) had a more pronounced effect on at-risk populations (0.21), whereas the non-interactive programs are clearly not effective with at-risk populations. The best known and most widely evaluated of these non-interactive programs is DARE, which overwhelmingly has been shown to be ineffective. However, as of this writing DARE is in rehab and the phoenix that arises from the ashes may be effective.

SYNTHESIS

School-based prevention programs that use scare tactics or non-interactive lecture formats do not work. Other school-based programs seem to work quite well for some substances at some grade levels but work less well or not at all for other substances or grade levels. Unfortunately, in this era of high stakes educational testing, schools are not likely to implement separate programs for tobacco, alcohol, and other drugs in addition to programs trying to prevent violence, pregnancy, academic failure, or other social problems, because such programs require too much class time. SWC programs seem to offer the greatest promise, but many are not only labor-intensive but costly, so they are unlikely to be widely implemented. The most promising school-based approaches in this era of high stakes educational testing are likely to be those that reinforce the academic mission of public schools by focusing on student success as a prevention tool. Universal approaches include prosocial schooling, resilience education, and the development of protective schools.[2] Promising adjunct school-based programs for selective and indicated (i.e., "at-risk") youth include student assistance programs that provide necessary counseling services and harm reduction programs that provide adolescents with the skills required to avoid dangerous behaviors like drinking and driving. In addition, mentoring and other after-school programs that provide youth with the opportunity to interact with caring adults may prevent substance use or reduce abuse.

In their review of the literature over a decade ago, Newcomb and Bentler (1989) pointed out that "the distinction between use and abuse of drugs … is critical … for considering psychological intervention" (p. 242). Evidence presented herein indicates that the distinction between use and abuse also is critical for defining program effectiveness. Recommending one set of prevention strategies over another, therefore, entails specifying prevention program goals and objectives clearly and recognizing when pursuing one set of goals might hinder achievement of other more worthwhile goals.

To identify ATOD prevention program goals and objectives, we should begin with an assessment of needs. Evidence from the Monitoring the Future study indicates that most adolescents experiment with both licit and illicit substances, and one might argue this constitutes evidence that ATOD prevention programs should strive to prevent substance use. However, as Newcomb and Bentler (1989) noted: "Adolescence is a period of experimentation, exploration, and curiosity. In this society, drug use has become one aspect of this natural process to the extent that

a teenager is deviant (from a normative perspective) if he or she has not tried alcohol, cigarettes, or marijuana by the completion of high school" (p. 246). Furthermore, in most cases this adolescent experimentation does not result in significant adverse health consequences.

Setting aside for the moment the ideological motivations for prevention programs and the fact that it is illegal for adolescents to use tobacco, alcohol, or illicit substances and focusing strictly on public health concerns, we are inclined to see the prevention of tobacco use as a top priority because tobacco is more addictive than alcohol and far more addictive than marijuana and because mortality and morbidity are much higher for tobacco than for any other substance (with the possible exception of inhalants, about which reliable data are scarce).

On the other hand, alcohol and marijuana play such prominent roles in American culture generally and American youth culture specifically that creating school-based programs to prevent their use seems misguided. Furthermore, attempts to prevent use can have disastrous unintended consequences. Raising the drinking age, for example, has reduced the prevalence of alcohol use among underage college students but increased the prevalence of binge drinking among underage students who now drink to get drunk when they have an opportunity to imbibe alcohol (Wechsler, Kuo, Lee, & Dowdall, 2000). Preventing adolescents from frequently binge drinking, playing drinking games, and most importantly, driving while drunk, seem like more important public health objectives than preventing use of alcohol, especially given evidence culled from the 1997 National Household Survey on Drug Abuse indicating that less than 3 percent of 12–14 year olds and a mere 12 percent of 15–17-year-olds consume over 80 percent of the alcohol imbibed by youths in their age groups (Pacific Institute for Research and Evaluation, 2000). Given evidence that prevention programs can reduce the prevalence of drunken driving (Tobler & Stratton, 1997) and alcohol abuse, but generally are not effective at reducing alcohol use, harm reduction oriented prevention programs seem to be in order for alcohol.

Harm reduction oriented prevention programs also may be in order for tobacco. While our meta-analytic findings indicate that interactive prevention programs reduce tobacco use in the short term and Botvin, Baker, Dusenbury, Botvin, and Diaz (1995) demonstrated favorable longer term tobacco use prevention effects, the best long-term evidence indicates no beneficial prevention effects. Hence, the claim by Peterson et al. (2000) that "current school program 'best practices' are not strong enough to deter adolescent tobacco use … [so] a new round of theory development and empirical basic research appears essential" (p. 1988) seems worth heeding. One new approach built on a public health framework that may provide a mechanism for focusing on the

---

[2] Program developers include the Developmental Studies Center in Oakland, CA; the Center for Educational Research and Development in Berkeley, CA; and the University of Arizona's College of Education, respectively.

critical transition from infrequent use to regular use is harm reduction. This approach should be rigorously evaluated using appropriate measures that capture information about critical transitions between stages of use.

Replication studies involving the *Life Skills Training* program developed by Botvin and his colleagues and other interventions that go beyond the "best practices" referred to by Peterson et al. (2000) are underway and may corroborate earlier findings of long-term effectiveness. Until they do, prosocial schooling and other approaches that create protective schools and provide adolescents with sufficient developmental assets to ensure resilience should be considered, as should student assistance programs that provide necessary counseling services and harm reduction programs that provide adolescents with the skills required to avoid dangerous behaviors like drinking and driving.

Also see: Substances Entries.

References

Aseltine, R.H., Dupre, M., & Lamlein, P. (2000). Mentoring as a drug prevention strategy: An evaluation of *Across Ages. Adolescent and Family Health, 1*(1), 11–20.

Bandura, A. (1977). *Social learning theory.* Englewood Cliffs, NJ: Prentice-Hall.

Botvin, G.J., Baker, E., Dusenbury, L., Botvin, E.M., & Diaz, T. (1995). Long-term follow-up results of a randomized drug abuse prevention trial in a white middle-class population. *Journal of the American Medical Association, 273*(14), 1106–1112.

Brown, J.H., D'Emidio-Caston, M., & Benard, B. (2000). *Resilience education.* Thousand Oaks, CA: Corwin/Sage.

Clayton, R.R., Scutchfield, F.D., & Wyatt, S.W. (2000). Hutchinson Smoking Prevention Project: A new gold standard in prevention science requires new transdisciplinary thinking. *Journal of the National Cancer Institute, 92*(24), 1964–1965.

Huizing, D., Loeber, R., Thornberry, T.P., & Cothern, L. (2000). *Co-occurrence of delinquency and other problem behaviors.* Washington, DC: US Department of Justice.

Jessor, R., & Jessor, S.L. (1977). *Problem behavior and psycho-social development: A longitudinal study of youth.* New York: Academic.

Meier, K.J. (1994). *The politics of sin: Drugs, alcohol, and public policy.* Armonk, NY: M.E. Sharpe.

Monitoring the Future. (2000). *Data Tables.* [WWW document]. http://www.monitoringthefuture.org/data/00data.html#2000data-drugs

Newcomb, M.D., & Bentler, P.M. (1989). Substance use and abuse among children and teenagers. *American Psychologist, 44*(2), 242–248.

Pacific Institute for Research and Evaluation. (2000). *Insights from the 1997 national household survey on drug abuse: Underage drinking patterns and consequences.* Rockville, MD: Author.

Peterson, A.V., Kealy, K.A., Mann, S.L., Marek, P.M., & Sarason, I.G. (2000). Hutchinson Smoking Prevention Project: Long-term randomized trial in school-based tobacco use prevention—Results on smoking. *Journal of the National Cancer Institute, 92*(24), 1979–1991.

Rosenbaum, M. (1999). *Safety first: A reality-based approach to teens, drugs, and drug education.* San Francisco: The Lindesmith Center.

Shedler, J. & Block, J. (1990). Adolescent drug use and psychological health: A longitudinal inquiry. *American Psychologist, 45*(5), 612–630.

Sobol, D.F., Rohrbach, L.A., Dent, C.W., Gleason, L., Brannon, B.R., Johnson, C.A., & Flay, B.R. (1989). The integrity of smoking prevention curriculum delivery. *Health Education Research, 4*(1), 59–67.

Tobler, N.S., Roona, M.R., Ochshorn, P., Marshall, D.G., Streke, A.V., & Stackpole, K. (2000). School-based adolescent drug prevention programs: 1998 meta-analysis. *The Journal of Primary Prevention, 20*(4), 275–336.

Tobler, N., & Stratton, H. (1997). Effectiveness of school-based drug prevention programs: A meta-analysis of the research. *The Journal of Primary Prevention, 18*(1), 71–128.

Wechsler, H., Kuo, M., Lee, H., & Dowdall, G.W. (2000). Environmental correlates of underage alcohol use and related problems of college students. *American Journal of Preventive Medicine, 19*(1), 24–29.

Substances, Adult

Ray Daugherty and Carl Leukefeld

INTRODUCTION

This entry presents approaches for preventing alcohol and drug problems among adults. After relevant terms are defined and selected theories reviewed, evidence-based research is reported to synthesize approaches for adult prevention. Finally, five conditions are presented to personalize adult prevention within a Lifestyle Risk Reduction approach.

DEFINITIONS

Risk Factors are biological, psychological, or social factors that *increase* the risk for development of problems if present, and *decrease* the risk if removed or neutralized. A risk factor contributes to causation and, in prevention, is directly targeted to reduce risk. However, absence of risk factors does not imply zero risk.

Risk Indicator are factors that may be associated with increased risk, but actually results from a third risk factor(s) that influences the development of both the problem and the risk indicator. Changing the risk indicator will not reduce risk. In prevention, a risk indicator is used to identify people who need more intensive, or targeted, prevention.

A *Standard Drink* is a measure for one alcoholic beverage based only on alcohol content. In the United States and Sweden this amount is $1/2$ oz (1.5 cl) of pure alcohol. In Canada and the United Kingdom it is 1 cl ($2/3$ oz) and is referred to as a "standard unit."

Low-Risk Choices are the number of standard drinks for which there is little/no evidence of increased risk. In Canada this amount is defined as 3–4 units a day for men, 2–3 for women. The United States Department of Agriculture defines it as no more than one standard drink per day for women or no more than two for men. Prevention Research Institute defines low-risk as 0–2 standard drinks if drinking daily, and 0–3 if drinking less than daily for those who have no biological risk factors; 0–2 standard drinks and not daily for those with one biological risk factor; and zero for those with two or more biological risk factors.

High-Risk Choices refers to the number of standard drinks that increases risk for alcohol-related problems. This would be any amount above the low-risk amount.

Heavy Episodic Drinking is called "binge drinking" in the prevention literature and is generally defined as five standard drinks in a row. Sometimes it is defined as four drinks in a row for women.

Peak Drinking refers to the largest number of standard drinks consumed in any one day within a specified period of time.

SCOPE

Sales data indicate that per capita consumption of alcohol is 6.8 L in the United States, 6.5 in Canada, and 5.3 in Sweden, with "off the books" consumption in Sweden adding another 2 L. Evidence from the United States suggests that 24 percent of males and 15 percent of females qualify for a *DSM IV* dependence diagnosis at some point in life, with 6.3 percent and 4.4 percent qualifying within the past 12 months. Evidence from Sweden suggests a lifetime alcohol dependence rate of 19 percent for Swedish males and 3 percent for females.

Data on drinking among young adults in college illustrates a danger of assuming that prevention approaches developed for children will carry forward into adulthood. For example, between 1989 and 1993 in the United States, alcohol use among high school seniors dropped by 20 percent and the percent engaging in heavy episodic drinking fell from 41 to 28 percent (Johnston, O'Malley, & Bachman, 1996). Advocates of zero tolerance prevention believed that a reduction in drinking by teens would translate into reduced drinking and problems as those teens moved into adulthood. Data on abstaining supports this prediction, but data on heavy use does not. Abstaining among young adult college males increased from 3 percent in 1977 to 9 percent in 1989 and 21 percent in 1999. Among females abstaining increased from 4 to 15 to 19 percent in the same time period. However, heavy drinking increased simultaneously. Drinking for the purpose of getting drunk among males increased from 20 percent in 1977 to about 43 percent in 1999. Among females the increase was from 10 to 43 percent. College males who reported getting drunk 1–3 times in a month increased from 25 percent in 1977 to 41 percent in 1989. By 1999, 54 percent reported getting drunk *more* than 3 times per month, up from 45 percent in 1993. (Survey questions changed between 1989 and 1993.) For females the increase was from 14 to 37 percent for 1–3 times per month between 1977 and 1989. Between 1993 and 1999, the percent of women getting drunk more than three times per month increased from 19 to 25 percent. By 1999, heavy episodic drinking in males was at 50 percent and for women, 40 percent (Wechsler & Isaac, 1992, Wechsler, Lee, Kuo, & Lee, 2000).

THEORIES

Reducing alcohol and drug problems among adults requires more than simply applying strategies and theories to adults that were developed for prevention with youth. Life span-focused prevention faces the reality that in most cultures, alcohol use is legal for adults. Thus, recognition of personal choice plays a more central role in effective prevention. Lifetime prevention goals not only include increasing the prevalence of abstinence, but also reducing high-risk consumption. Thus, the zero-tolerance philosophies that have characterized youth prevention in the 1980s and 1990s are not relevant to most adults and young adults. Several theories are, or could be, used to guide our understanding of how to prevent alcohol and drug problems with adults.

Environmental Theories: Two Environmental Theories Are Currently Finding Relevance to Adult Prevention

The *Distribution of Consumption Theory* (Moore & Gerstein, 1981), initially proposed by Ledermann (1956), stimulated interest in the use of policy measures to reduce per capita consumption of alcohol. The theory posits that alcohol consumption is proportionally distributed across a population in a way that stays in relative balance. Thus, when per capita consumption increases or decreases, it changes proportionately the same in light, moderate, and heavy consumers. The logical extension of this theory is that policy measures (such as taxation, limiting outlets, limiting sales hours) that are capable of reducing per capita consumption will lower consumption among those drinking high-risk quantities as well as low-risk quantities, thus reducing problems.

Another environment theory, *Social Norms Approach or "Social Marketing Strategies"* (Haines & Spear, 1996;

Perkins & Berkowitz, 1986), suggests that most people perceive that others hold higher risk attitudes and behaviors regarding alcohol and drugs than are actually true. This misperception creates an erroneous climate that encourages and supports high-risk drinking and drug use beyond the level that is supported by the actual norms. Consequently, moving the perception of the norm closer to the actual norm facilitates reduced consumption.

Biological Theories. Emerging biological theories attempt to explain the well-documented role that heredity plays in the etiology of alcohol and drug problems. Each has the potential to be useful for guiding prevention strategies. To date the theories include Cloninger's (1987) *Neurogenetic Adaptive Mechanisms Theory*, Schuckit's (1994) *Low Sensitivity Theory*, and Begleiter and Porjesz's (1999) *Neurological Disinhibition Theory*. Thus far, only Schuckit's theory has been applied to prevention with adults.

Schuckit suggests that alcohol abuse and dependence are related to inherited low sensitivity to the effects of alcohol. Low sensitivity means that a person demonstrates a less intense response to alcohol when compared to most people. People with low sensitivity have less internal feedback that they are drinking a high-risk amount in that they become less intoxicated. They also tend to have a positive biological reaction to alcohol (drinking feels good!) and to interpret their low sensitivity positively (I can really handle it!). Rather than seeing their low sensitivity as a risk, they are likely to see it as a protection (because I can handle alcohol well, I am not likely to experience problems with alcohol). Thus, they tend to consume more and become vulnerable to the effects of that heavy consumption. The theory suggests that prevention efforts could succeed by helping people who have low-sensitivity reframe their biological reaction as an indicator of risk rather than an indication that they are protected by their ability to "handle" alcohol. To facilitate that, Schuckit developed a paper and pencil test, the SRE (Self-Rating of Effects of Alcohol), to help adults identify whether they have low sensitivity (Schuckit, Smith, Tipp, Wiesbeck, & Kalmijn, 1997).

Psychosocial Theories. The predominate theories guiding youth-focused prevention are psychosocial theories (Petraitis & Flay, 1995) and practitioners often apply them to adults. The predominant theories are the *Social Development Model* (best known as Risk and Resiliency), the *Social Influences Model*, and the *Personal and Social Skills Model*.

The *Social Development Model,* articulated primarily by Hawkins and Catalano (1992), identifies both individual and environmental risk and protective factors that increase or decrease the risk for drug use and problems developing. Those with the fewest risk factors and most protective factors are least likely to use drugs. The model emphasizes the role of bonding to family, school, and community. According to the model, bonding occurs when there is an opportunity to be an active contributor to a group, when a person has the skills needed to successfully contribute, and when the group has a system of consistent recognition. If a person bonds to groups that promote traditional values such as nonuse of drugs, then the elements are likely to be present that will discourage use.

The *Social Influences Model* (Hansen, Johnson, Flay, Graham, & Sobel, 1988) suggests that drug use occurs primarily in response to social influences, that can be countered through activities such as: peer resistance training, correction of normative expectations, inoculation against mass media messages, information about parental and other adult influences, and peer leadership.

Botvin (1990) brought together some of the most salient elements of other models to create the *Personal and Social Skills Model*. This model takes each of the elements of the Social Influences Model and adds skill development in areas such as problem solving and decision-making.

Theories that Overlap with Treatment. Two approaches are applied both to treatment populations and prevention audiences.

Miller and Rollnick (1991) developed principles for *Motivational Interviewing* primarily for treatment populations. Therapists use motivational interviewing principles to discover and build on client desire for and commitment to change. This approach also includes some activities that are similar to social norms approaches and have been used in prevention settings in the United States, Canada, Sweden, and other countries.

Marlatt (1998) and others have proposed *Harm Reduction* strategies both for treatment and prevention. These strategies are based on the assumption that many people will not discontinue use of alcohol and drugs, but that other behaviors can be modified to reduce associated problems. Designated driver and needle exchange programs are harm reduction strategies that have received a great deal of discussion. Harm reduction strategies are becoming increasingly used in parts of the European Union and, more recently, in the United States.

Integrative Theories. Two models combine biological, psychological, and social factors into integrated theories of prevention.

In the *Public Health Model*, problems occur in an interaction among the agent (alcohol or drugs), the host (the individual), and the environment (the setting that brings the two together). An effective intervention aimed at any one of these three elements can prevent the problem. The Public Health Model is generic to all health problems and provides a general framework for preventive action on any specific problem. To develop specific strategies for any problem it is necessary to combine the Public Health Model with another problem specific model. For example, the Public Health Model is frequently combined with the Distribution of Consumption Model to guide policy efforts to prevent alcohol problems.

While the Public Health Model is purposefully nonspecific and applies across health problems, the *Lifestyle Risk Reduction Model* (Daugherty & Leukefeld 1998; Daugherty & O'Bryan 1986, 1996) is specific to problems with a lifestyle component and suggests that it is important to delineate the role played by each factor in order to understand how to more effectively intervene. In this model, the core interaction determining most alcohol and drug problems is the interaction between the individual's biology and the quantity and frequency of the alcohol or drug use. Biology establishes a threshold at which a biological outcome will occur such as intoxication, addiction, or liver damage, and the quantity/frequency choices regarding alcohol or drug use determine whether that threshold will be reached. This interaction of biology and choice determines the degree of intoxication, and thus risk for impairment problems, as well as the degree of physiological damage or risk for health problems. Psychosocial factors primarily play the role of influencing whether the person will use alcohol or drugs, and, if so, how much and how often. According to this model, prevention strategies will be most effective if they first establish a sense of personal vulnerability, establishing the belief that high-risk choices are likely to cause either alcohol/drug-related health or impairment problems for the individual. Proponents of the model suggest that an understanding of biological risk is useful in establishing a sense of personal vulnerability. People then must have clear guidance on how to estimate personal risk and identify choices that are low-risk and receive psychosocial support for making low-risk choices. This model can be used to explain all types of alcohol and drug problems except for those legal or social problems that are completely independent of quantity of use. For example, mere possession of alcohol by a minor, or an illegal substance at any age can result in legal or social problems.

RESEARCH

A review of alcohol and drug research points out the nature versus nurture question and the interaction of various factors. What influences are genetic, what are more environmental or psychological in origin; and how might they interact? Research is beginning to yield answers.

A substantial body of research has established that heredity plays an important role in both alcohol and drug dependence (Hesselbrock, 1995). For example, it has been estimated that about 60 percent of the risk for alcoholism is genetic, with similar figures for tobacco and illegal drugs.

Family incidence studies first established that those who develop alcoholism have a disproportionately high percentage of relatives with alcoholism. Family studies only establish that alcoholism tends to be familial without any indication of the relative role played by heredity or environment. Adoption studies better distinguish between the two since adoption separates the parents who contribute genes from those who contribute to the family environment. Adoption studies in three countries show that the biological children of alcoholics experience about a four times greater incidence of alcoholism as adults even when raised with nonalcoholic adoptive parents. Conversely, children raised with alcoholic adoptive parents do not experience any increased incidence of alcoholism as adults. International twin research (not separated twins) confirms that heredity plays a significant role not only in alcohol dependence but also with marijuana, cocaine, nicotine, and most other drugs of abuse (Kendler, Karkowski, Neale, & Prescott, 2000; Kendler & Prescott, 1998). Twin research adds an additional clarification in demonstrating that heredity alone does not explain the risk for alcohol or drug dependence.

Several psychological traits are more common among people who develop alcoholism, however the development, and thus the influence, of psychological traits overlap with both heredity and the environment. Research with separated twins indicates that as much as 50–60 percent of personality may be genetically determined with the remainder coming from environmental interactions. Cloninger (1987) offers evidence that three personality dimensions/traits play a role in risk for alcoholism: novelty seeking, harm avoidance, and reward dependence. While a high percentage of people who have alcoholism have these traits, a low percentage of people who have the traits develop alcoholism. Since the traits are not useful predictors of who will develop alcoholism, Cloninger's theory has limited usefulness for prevention. Research using the MAC scale of the MMPI (Levenson, Aldwin, Butcher, DeLabry, Workman-Daniels, & Bosse, 1990) identified such traits as sociability, rebelliousness, and reward seeking as being especially important in influencing heavy alcohol consumption. The researchers noted that these traits also form a description of a person who might be inclined to become an entrepreneur or engage in other exciting or exceptional behaviors. Similarly, research strongly supports that the degree of sensation seeking is an important influence on drinking and drug taking behavior.

A high percentage of people with alcoholism also qualify for another psychiatric diagnosis. However, research raises questions as to which of these diagnosis might precede alcoholism and contribute to its development versus which result from the alcoholism. For example, Vaillant's (1995) 50-year natural history study indicated that in most cases, people who developed alcoholism were not psychiatrically different than the rest of the population prior to onset. One clear exception to this is antisocial personality disorder, which precedes and co-exists with alcoholism in about one fifth of people with alcoholism, and may play a larger role in drug dependence (Hesselbrock et al., 1984). Those who score higher on scales measuring rebellion are also more likely to use more alcohol or drugs (Kandel, 1982). The conduct disorder/antisocial personality subpopulation seems to be responsible for a disproportionate share of the social problems experienced by alcohol and drug dependent persons, particularly in the criminal justice system.

While comprising only a small portion of cases of alcoholism, the genetic factors in the antisocial subpopulation may be strong enough to confuse other findings if not controlled. For example, Cloninger identified a subtype of alcoholism ("Type 2") as having a very high genetic component (nine times increased risk in adoption research) and being characterized by early onset and high levels of legal problems. Later studies indicate that this subtype is an overlap of alcoholism and antisocial personality disorder (Penick, Powell, Nickel, Read, Gabrielli, & Liskow, 1990). Begleiter and Porjesz (1999) demonstrated that children of alcoholics are more likely to have a low P300 evoked brain potential. This EEG response is central to their theory on brain disinhibition and alcohol. However, Hesselbrock has found that the low P300 is specific to those with both a family history of alcoholism and antisocial personality disorder. Perhaps both Cloninger's theory and Begleiter and Porjesz's theory may be most applicable to the antisocial subpopulation.

The research supporting Schuckit's (1994) theory on low sensitivity to alcohol excluded those with a family history of antisocial personality disorder and thus may be more relevant to preventing the approximately 80 percent of cases of alcoholism that are not linked to that disorder. Schuckit (1999) found that about 60 percent of those who had low response to alcohol as a young adult and had a family history of alcoholism, qualified for a diagnosis of alcohol abuse or dependence by about age 30.

Genetic risk for alcohol and drug problems seems to be shared across biological and psychological risk factors. While at this point in time genetic risk cannot be directly modifiable for prevention purposes, it may be possible to use genetic information to modify psychological risk. For example, both Schuckit's theory on low response and the Lifestyle Risk Reduction Model suggest that one goal of prevention should be to *alter perception of risk*, especially for those who exhibit biological risk factors.

A growing body of research demonstrates the importance of perception of risk in altering alcohol and drug behavior. For example, Bachman, Johnston, and O'Malley (1998) found that perception of risk provides a better explanation of the temporal changes in marijuana use when compared to the generic psychosocial risk factors that are more commonly the focus of alcohol and drug prevention

programs using the Social Development Model. Their study indicated that when perception of risk increased, drug use decreased even among students who had the strongest psychosocial risk indicators. Similarly, Bailey, Flewelling, and Rachal (1992) reported that general psychosocial risk indicators were good predictors of who would initiate marijuana use, but perception of risk and biological response were better predictors of who would continue or discontinue use. More recently, Feldman, Harvey, Holowaty, and Shortt (1999) found that concern about the impact on health (one measure of perception of risk) is a leading reason that young adults offer for not using alcohol. Swedish research (Sjöberg, 1998) indicates that people respond differently to measures of personal risk and general risk, and that personal perception of risk is a more powerful predictor of behavior.

A question for prevention, then, would be, "How can prevention programs be used to alter perception of risk?" Lifestyle risk reduction advocates suggest that sharing information on biological risk is one way to establish perception of risk. People may believe that they can maintain personal control over psychological or social risks, but are unlikely to have the same belief about biology. It seems possible that a different kind of perception of risk may be at work in the success of social marketing strategies. When people over-estimate use in their environment, it may provide a sense of "safety in numbers." When social marketing methods change perception of the norm, they may also shatter this sense of security.

Research indicates that alcohol use is very unevenly distributed in the population. In the United States, the heaviest drinking 30 percent of the population drinks 90 percent of all of the alcohol (Greenfield & Rogers, 1999). In Sweden, the heaviest drinking 30 percent drinks 70 percent of the alcohol (H. Leifman [personal communication to Ray Daugherty, 2001, Addiction Research Centre, University of Stockholm]). Daugherty and O'Bryan (1996) suggested that heavy drinkers are unaware that their drinking is so far outside of the norm because they tend to drink with those who drink similarly to them, creating the illusion that their drinking is normal. Miller and Rollnick (1991) suggest that *motivational interviewing techniques* can be used to allow heavy drinkers to discover how different their drinking is from the norm. In Canada, Sweden, and the United States, Motivational Interviewing has been used successfully for indicated prevention with heavy drinking adults in a variety of health care and other settings.

The environment may also be modified to reduce the risk for alcohol and drug problems. For example, Lederman and others provide substantial data supporting his theory that alcohol consumption remains in a rather constant pattern of distribution throughout a society and that policy control measures that change per capita consumption will reduce alcohol consumption in all groups (Moore & Gerstein, 1981). For example, per capita consumption seems especially sensitive to changes in price, and sales polices that alter availability such as number of outlets and hours of sale.

Findings have accumulated about risk factors using the Social Development Model and the Social Skills Model. While these research-based models are often discussed as though they apply to all people and all ages, this research focused on early alcohol and drug users and may not apply to others; consequently it is important to distinguish between risk factors and risk indicators. For example, early age of use has been identified as a risk factor in the Social Development Model and this finding has influenced the direction of many prevention programs. However, considerable evidence suggests that early onset of use is most accurately viewed as a risk indicator rather than a risk factor (Daugherty & Leukefeld, 1998; Prescott & Kendler, 1999). This important distinction implies that, contrary to popular theories, delaying onset of use during adolescence may not reduce alcohol and drug problems during adulthood. Instead, current data indicate that early users are at increased risk for later problems due to inherited proneness to disinhibited behavior that increases risk both for early use and later problems (McGue, Iacono, Legrand, Malone, & Elkins, 2001a,b). By identifying early users for intensive, indicated prevention we may well succeed in decreasing the risk for problems in adulthood. That is yet to be demonstrated.

STRATEGIES THAT WORK

Compared to the number of prevention studies with youth, there are relatively few with adults. Of the prevention strategies that have been tested with adults, *policy measures* have the longest history of effectiveness in influencing adult drinking. Sweden, Canada, and the United States have all used a public health approach with Sweden having the longest history and greatest success. For example, per capita consumption in Sweden dropped by 17 percent from 1976 to 1982 following implementation of policy measures designed to reduce consumption. From 1979 to 1982, deaths from cirrhosis declined by 28 percent in men and 29 percent in women and pancreatitis mortality by 30 percent in men and 36 percent in women (Romelsjo & Agren, 1985). Ironically, membership in the European Union will require Sweden to lower its taxes on alcohol and liberalize sales policies by 2004. It has been estimated that these changes will lead to significant increases in consumption.

In the United States most policy actions are left to individual states or local municipalities. There is evidence that one national effort, a 21 purchase age, led to decreased consumption and driving fatalities among high school students, but may have been associated with increased consumption among young adults of college age (Allen, Sprenkel, & Vitale, 1994).

STRATEGIES THAT MIGHT WORK

Young adults in college have been the targets of numerous prevention efforts. Haines and Spear (1996) and Perkins and Berkowitz (1986) both offered data that supports Social Marketing Theory. Their findings indicate that most people believe that levels of drinking and drug use, and attitudes about use, are more high risk than is actually the case and that this distortion seems to influence higher levels of consumption. Haines and Spear (1996) reported a drop from 43 to 34 percent in heavy episodic drinking following a 5-year *social marketing* campaign. However, Carter and Kahnweiler (2000) found that this approach did not work with fraternity members.

Agostinelli, Brown, and Miller (1995) applied *motivational interviewing* techniques with heavy drinking college students in a brief intervention and found statistically significant decreases after 6 weeks. Marlatt, Baer, and Larimer (1995) combined motivational interviewing techniques and harm reduction philosophies in a semester-long program that reduced drinking with college students.

Thompson applied a *Lifestyle Risk Reduction* curriculum to half of the first year students at one university, using the other half as a control group. She found reductions in high-risk drinking accompanied by simultaneous changes in attitudes. A lifestyle risk reduction education approach has been used for indicated prevention with adult DUI offenders. For example, a study by the Iowa Alcohol and Drug Research Consortium found that posttest attitudes on perception of risk were predictive of lower recidivism rates three years later. A study conducted by a team from Emory University found that changes in perception of risk were maintained virtually unchanged over a 3-year follow-up period. The recidivism rate was about 50 percent lower in the offenders who received the curriculum, in spite of that group having a higher percentage with previous arrests; a strong predictor of recidivism (Thompson, 1996).

STRATEGIES THAT DO NOT WORK

Strategies that have been effective with youth may not be effective with adults. For example, Brochu and Souliere (1988) tested *Botvin's Lifeskills* curriculum with adults and found no impact on behavior, although the same curriculum had positive findings with middle school students.

SYNTHESIS

Given the small number of strategies that have been applied to adult prevention, the success (at least with alcohol) could be considered remarkable. Policy measures, social marketing, motivational interviewing, and lifestyle risk reduction education have all shown promise for altering alcohol behaviors with adults. Wider use of integrative theory to pull together the best of each approach may further enhance effectiveness.

The Public Health Model provides a beginning framework with a vocabulary and structure that is widely recognized. However, as noted earlier, the Public Health Model is generic and must be combined with a problem-specific model to identify specific prevention strategies. Any of the theories described earlier could be used for that purpose, specifically the Distribution of Consumption Model or The Lifestyle Risk Reduction Model.

In using the *Lifestyle Risk Reduction Model*, it is important to distinguish between the approach and the programs that are based on the approach (such as the PRIME for Life program [1996], or the Talking About Alcohol and Drugs Series [1986]). As noted above, the approach suggests that the central interaction that leads to alcohol and drug problems is the level of biological risk interacting with the quantity and frequency of alcohol or drug consumption. Social and psychological factors primarily establish risk by influencing whether, how much, and how often the person uses alcohol or drugs. The approach suggests that five conditions are necessary for effective prevention.

Condition One—It Could Happen to Me; My Choices Matter

People increase personal perception of risk by coming to believe that alcohol and drug problems could happen to them and that quantity and frequency of alcohol and drug intake are the only controllable factors standing between them and a problem.

A prevention strategy that establishes the first condition will help people understand that their risk for alcohol and drug problems is real and personal. Commonly held beliefs suggest that alcohol and drug problems occur because of the type of person one is, rather than the type of choices a person makes. The common image of a person with alcohol or drug problems is a person who is a "weak-willed, immoral, loser with low self-esteem." If I hold these beliefs I am likely to think that my drinking or drug use is of little consequence as long as I am not "that kind of person." In addition, people with low sensitivity to alcohol believe they are protected by their ability to drink a lot without experiencing problems, rather than seeing their low sensitivity as a sign of risk. In addressing these misperceptions, it is useful to help people think in terms of total risk as a combination of personal biological risk plus the risk inherent in personal choices. Because I cannot change my biological risk, I must change my personal choices if I want to avoid problems. Condition

One focuses on attitudes and beliefs regarding perception of risk. It addresses the risk factor of "attitudes supportive of use" and incorporates Schuckit's theory on low sensitivity.

Condition Two—I Know What to Do to Reduce Risk

People learn how to estimate their level of biological risk and learn what specific quantity and frequency behaviors are high risk and low risk.

A strategy that establishes Condition Two teaches people how to identify signs of increased biological risk and give specific guidance on low-risk choices. For alcohol, it becomes important to define a standard drink and give specific low-risk guidelines on how many drinks constitute a low-risk versus a high-risk choice. These guidelines should be research-based and should include abstinence as well as other quantities and frequencies of drinking that are not associated with increased risk for problems.

A lifestyle risk reduction approach suggests that it is important to establish Condition One before addressing Condition Two. Until people believe that their risk is real, personal, and directly related to their choices, they are not likely to take low-risk guidelines seriously. For some health problems such as heart disease, Condition One is quite well established, at least in the United States. Thus, widespread publication of heart disease low-risk guidelines can be useful. It may not be useful for a problem for which people widely believe that they do not have personal risk or that the problem happens because of emotional or character problems rather than lifestyle choices. A lifestyle risk reduction approach also suggests that while it is possible to change behavior implementing only Conditions One and Two, the most effective prevention incorporates Conditions Three, Four, and Five. Condition Two can integrate tools such as Schuckit's Self-Rating of Effects questionnaire to help measure biological risk. Those using this model will want to identify ways of assisting people in assessing the biological risk that may be indicated in their family history.

Condition Three—People Around Me Support Low-Risk Choices

People experience environmental support for low-risk choices from norms, expectations, laws, policies, and messages from informal and formal groups such as family, friends, media, workplace, religious groups, school, community, and government.

Strategies that implement Condition Three either alter the environment, or the individual's perception of the environment, in a way that supports low-risk choices. Lifestyle risk reduction theory suggests that activities addressing Condition Three can be effective all by themselves, but will be most effective if Conditions One and Two are established first or concurrently. A variety of existing strategies help establish Condition Three. Policy measures designed to change per capita consumption help create a legal/policy environment that supports low-risk choices by keeping prices high and reducing availability. Social Marketing approaches do not change the environment but make people more aware of the degree of support that exists in the environment. Motivational Interviewing strategies can help heavy drinkers understand the degree to which their drinking exceeds community or national norms.

Condition Four—I Want to Make Low-Risk Choices

People develop personal commitment to making low-risk choices and hold attitudes, values, and self-concepts that support low-risk choices.

Strategies that establish Condition Four will be more personal in nature. Am I the kind of person who would make low-risk choices? What do I value more, fun with high-risk choices, or things such as health, family, or security that may be endangered by my high-risk choices? Some of the techniques in Motivational Interviewing can be used to build personal support for low-risk choices. While bonding is often emphasized in youth-focused prevention, in adult-focused prevention, it may be more important to develop understanding of how high-risk choices jeopardize relationships and bonds that already exist.

Condition Five—I Have the Skills I Need

People develop skills that will allow them to implement low-risk choices in their daily lives.

Strategies that accomplish Condition Five are likely to be relatively time intensive. Attention needs to be paid to the skills that will be useful for nondependent adults to make and maintain low-risk choices. Both lifestyle risk reduction programs and motivational interviewing approaches have targeted skills involved with making and implementing a plan to change behavior. Lifestyle risk reduction approaches have also included an analysis of skills that may have been affected by state dependent learning when making high-risk choices, and development of a plan for overcoming them.

A lifestyle risk reduction approach not only articulates the Public Health Model, but also integrates a number of theories and models. However, all five conditions should be addressed. A prevention effort that addresses only policy measures would be acting consistently with Condition Three but that would not be considered a lifestyle risk reduction activity by itself. However, policy measures that are part of a comprehensive prevention strategy that addresses all five conditions would be part of a lifestyle risk reduction approach. We can accomplish more effective prevention of alcohol and drug problems with adults by using multiple strategies and targeting all five conditions.

Also see: Substances entries.

References

Agostinelli, G., Brown, J.M., & Miller, W.R. (1995). Effects of normative feedback on consumption among heavy drinking college students. *Journal of Drug Education, 25*(1), 31–40.

Allen, D.N., Sprenkel, K.G., & Vitale, P.A. (1994). Reactance theory and alcohol consumption laws; Further confirmation among collegiate alcohol consumers. *Journal of Studies on Alcohol, 55*, 34–40.

Bachman, J.G., Johnston, L.D., & O'Malley, P.M., (1998). Explaining recent increases in students' marijuana use: Impacts of perceived risk and disapproval, 1976 through 1996. *American Journal of Public Health, 88*(6), 887–892.

Bailey, S.L., Flewelling, R.L., & Rachal, J.V. (1992). Predicting continued use of marijuana among adolescents: The relative influence of drug-specific and social context factors. *Journal of Health and Social Behavior, 33*, 51–66.

Begleiter, H., & Porjesz, B. (1999). What is inherited in the predisposition toward alcoholism? A proposed model. *Alcoholism: Clinical and Experimental Research, 23*, 1125–1135.

Botvin, G.J. (1990). Substance abuse prevention: Theory, practice, and effectiveness. In M. Tonry & J.Q. Wilson (Eds.), *Drugs and crime*. Chicago: The University of Chicago Press.

Brochu, S., & Souliere, M. (1988). Long-term evaluation of a life skills approach for alcohol and drug abuse prevention. *Journal of Drug Education, 18*, 311–331.

Carter, C.A., & Kahnweiler, W.M. (2000) The efficacy of social norms approach to substance abuse prevention applied to fraternity men. *Journal of American College Health, 49*, 66–71.

Cloninger, C.R. (1987) Neurogenetic adaptive mechanisms in alcoholism. *Science, 236*, 410–416.

Daugherty, R., & Leukefeld, C. (1998.) *Reducing the risks for substance abuse: A life span approach*. New York and London: Plenum Press.

Daugherty, R., & O'Bryan, T. (1986). *Talking about alcohol and drugs series*. Lexington, Kentucky: Prevention Research Institute.

Daugherty, R., & O'Bryan, T. (1996). *PRIME for life series*. Lexington, Kentucky: Prevention Research Institute.

Feldman, L., Harvey, B., Holowaty, P., & Shortt, L. (1999). Alcohol use beliefs and behaviors among high school students. *Adolescent Health, 24*, 48–58.

Greenfield, T.K., & Rogers, J.D. (1999). Who drinks most of the alcohol in the US? The policy implications. *Journal of Studies on Alcohol, 60*, 78–89.

Haines, M., & Spear, S.F. (1996). Changing the perception of the norm: A strategy to decrease binge drinking among college students. *Journal of American College Health, 45*, 134–140.

Hansen, W., Johnson, C.A., Flay, B., Graham, J., & Sobel, J. (1988). Affective and social influences approaches to the prevention of multiple substance abuse among seventh grade students. *Preventive Medicine, 17*, 135–154.

Hawkins, J.D., & Catalano, R.F. (1992). *Communities that care: Action for drug abuse prevention*. San Francisco: Jossey-Bass.

Hesselbrock, B.M. (1995). The genetic epidemiology of alcoholism. In H. Begleiter & B. Kissin (Eds.), *Alcohol and alcoholism: Vol. 1. The genetics of alcoholism* (pp. 17–39). New York: Oxford University Press.

Hesselbrock, M., Hesselbrock, V., Babor, T., Stabenau, J., Meyer, R., & Weidenman, M. (1984). Antisocial behavior, psychopathology and problem drinking in the natural history of alcoholism. In D. Goodwin, K. VanDusen, & S. Mednick (Eds.), *Longitudinal research in alcoholism* (pp. 197–214). Boston: Kluwer Nihoff.

Johnston, L.D., O'Malley, P.M., & Bachman, J.G. (1996). *National survey results on drug use from the monitoring the future study, 1975–1995.* Washington, DC: National Institute on Drug Abuse, US Department of Health and Human Services.

Kandel, D. (1982). Epidemiological and Psychosocial Perspectives on Adolescent Drug Use. *Journal of the American Academy of Child Psychiatry, 21,* 328–347.

Kendler, K.S., Karkowski, L.M., Neale, M.C., & Prescott, C.A. (2000). Illicit psychoactive substance use, heavy use, abuse, and dependence in US population-based sample of male twins. *Archives of General Psychiatry, 57,* 261–269.

Kendler, K.S., & Prescott, C.A. (1998). Cannabis use, abuse, and dependence in a population-based sample of female twins. *American Journal of Psychiatry, 155,* 1016–1022.

Ledermann, S. (1956). Cited in *Alcohol and public policy: Beyond the shadow of prohibition.* Report of the Panel on Alternative Policies affecting the Prevention of Alcohol Abuse and Alcoholism. (1981). M.H. Moore & D.R. Gerstein (Eds). Washington, DC: National Academy Press.

Levenson, M.R., Aldwin, C.M., Butcher, J.N., DeLabry, L., Workman-Daniels, K., & Bosse, R. (1990). The MAC scale in a normal population: The meaning of "false positives." *Journal of Studies on Alcohol, 51,* 457–462.

Marlatt, G.A. (1998). *Harm reduction.* New York: The Guilford Press.

Marlatt, G.A., Baer, J.S., & Larimer M. (1995) Preventing alcohol abuse in college students: A harm-reduction approach. In G.M. Boyd, J. Howard, & R.A. Zucker (Eds.), *Alcohol problems among adolescents.* New Jersey: Lawrence Erlbaum.

McGue, M., Iacono, W.G., Legrand, L.N., & Elkins, I. (2001a). Origins and consequences of age at first drink. II. Familial risk and heritability. *Alcoholism: Clinical and Experimental Research, 25,* 1166–1173.

McGue, M., Iacono, W.G., Legrand, L.N., Malone, S., & Elkins, I. (2001b). Origins and Consequences of age at first drink. I. Associations with substance-use disorders, disinhibitory behavior and psychopathology and P3 amplitude. Familial risk and heritability. *Alcoholism: Clinical and Experimental Research, 25,* 1156–1165.

Miller, W.R., & Rollnick, S. (1991) *Motivational interviewing: Preparing people to change addictive behavior.* New York and London: Guilford Press.

Moore, M.H., & Gerstein, D.R. (1981). *Alcohol and public policy: Beyond the shadow of prohibition.* Washington, DC: Committee on Substance Abuse and Habitual Behavior, National Academy Press.

Penick, E.C., Powell, B.J., Nickel, E.J., Read, M.R., Gabrielli, W.F., & Liskow B.I. (1990). Examination of cloninger's type I and type II alcoholism with a sample of men alcoholics in treatment. *Alcoholism: Clinical and Experimental Research, 14,* 623–629.

Perkins, H.W., & Berkowitz, A.D. (1986). Perceiving the community norms of alcohol use among students: Some research implications for campus alcohol education programming. *The International Journal of the Addictions, 21*(9 & 10), 961–976.

Petraitis, J., & Flay, B. (1995). Reviewing theories of adolescent substance use: Organizing pieces in the puzzle. *Psychological Bulletin, 117*(1), 67–86.

Prescott, C.A., & Kendler, K.S. (1999). Age at first drink and risk for alcoholism: A noncausal association. *Alcoholism: Clinical and Experimental Research, 23*(1), 101–107.

Romelsjo, A., & Agren, G. (1985) Has mortality related to alcohol decreased in Sweden? *Bristish Medical Journal, 291*(6489), 167–170.

Schuckit, M.A. (1994). A clinical model of genetic influences in alcohol dependence. *Journal of Studies on Alcohol, 55,* 5–17.

Schuckit, M.A. (1999). Biological, psychological, and environmental predictors of the alcoholism risk: A longitudinal study. *Journal of Studies on Alcohol, 59,* 485–494.

Schuckit, M.A., Smith, T.L., Tipp, J.E., Wiesbeck, G.A., & Kalmijn, J. (1997). The relationship between self-rating of the effects of alcohol and alcohol challenge results in ninety-eight young men. *Journal of Studies on Alcohol, 58,* 397–404.

Sjöberg, L. (1998). Risk perception of alcohol consumption. *Alcoholism: Clinical and Experimental Research, 22*(7), 277S–284S.

Thompson, M.L. (1996) A review of prevention research institute programs. *A report to the division of substance abuse.* Kentucky Cabinet for Human Resources, Frankfort, Kentucky.

Vaillant, G. (1995). *The natural history of alcoholism revisited.* Cambridge, MA: Harvard University Press.

Wechsler, H., & Isaac, N. (1992). "Binge" drinkers at Massachusetts colleges. *Journal of the American Medical Association, 267,* 2929–2931.

Wechsler, H., Lee, J.E., Kuo, M., & Lee, H. (2000) College binge drinking in the 1990s: A continuing problem. *Journal of American College Health, 48,* 199–210.

Substances, Older Adulthood

Waldo C. Klein

INTRODUCTION

The use of alcohol is a normal part of contemporary adult life in the United States and elsewhere around the world. In addition, older people consume a disproportionate share of pharmaceutical medications—both prescribed and over the counter (OTC). For older people, striking the balance among these substances to produce maximally positive outcomes can be complex. Developmental changes alter physiological functions in ways that can render lifelong behavior patterns inappropriate or dysfunctional. Interactions among alcohol, medications, social behaviors, or other circumstances that may include the seemingly benign, even unnoticeable, may lead to dramatic and even life threatening outcomes.

Managing these realities is not so simple as managing the substances themselves, for indeed, even as the problems exist, so too exist the obvious positive benefits associated with the substances. As will be discussed, alcohol has been shown to have beneficial effects for some people when consumed in moderate levels. This entry highlights the appropriate use and misuse of alcohol with an eye to preventing predictable problems related to alcohol use, protecting existing responsible lifestyle patterns and promoting future healthful choices.

DEFINITIONS

Alcohol includes any form of processed alcohol that is intended as a social beverage—beer, wine, or distilled spirits. It is important when talking with seniors to be explicit in including all forms of alcohol. For various social and cohort reasons, wine and beer are sometimes not included affirmatively by seniors when responding to the question, "Do you drink?" Also, it is important to understand the equivalency in alcohol content among the forms a standard *"drink"* may take—a 12-ounce beer, a 5-ounce glass of wine, and a "shot," "mixed drink," "high ball," or "cocktail" made with 1.5 ounces of a distilled spirit. Each contains approximately 12–14 grams of alcohol.

Alcoholism is a widely used term that is variously defined but that generally refers to a physiological or psychological dependence on alcohol. Because of the varying definitions in use, it is advised that the assessment criteria by which the diagnosis of *alcoholism* is made always be explicit.

Alcohol dependence refers to a physiological addiction to the drug alcohol. Detoxification and medically managed withdrawal from alcohol is required as a part of the treatment for alcohol dependence.

In the context of this entry, *problem drinking* refers to any drinking behavior that results in behaviors that are deemed problematic to the drinker or to others within the drinker's social environment. The resultant problems may be of a social, psychological, or physical nature. As such, the drinking behavior may be one of several interactive factors that contribute equally to a problematic situation.

Low risk drinking refers to any alcohol consumption pattern that does not lead to problems or does not exceed recommended guidelines for older adults. For people of age 65 and older, the Consensus Panel for Substance Abuse Among Older Adults of the Center for Substance Abuse Treatment has recommended no more than one drink per day, with a maximum of two drinks on any drinking occasion (New Year's Eve, weddings), with somewhat lower limits for women (Blow, 1998).

At risk drinking refers to any drinking behavior that heightens an individual's statistical likelihood of experiencing negative consequences as a result of alcohol consumption whether or not those consequences are experienced. This includes alcohol consumption patterns that exceed the recommended levels but may also reflect special circumstances in one's social environment or the heightened possibility of interaction effects.

Interaction effects refer to any effects that result from the combined use of alcohol and other drugs—prescribed, OTC or illicit. The effects may exacerbate or mitigate the intended effect of one or another of the consumed substances.

Problems with alcohol include the full range of problems that can result from the consumption of alcohol in combination with other substances including medications or in social circumstances that might cause problematic circumstances to arise. These problems may be no more attributable to the consumption of alcohol per se than they are to the social circumstance or the use of the other substance. Rather, the problem arises out of the *specific combination* of socio-environmental dynamics in play and should be recognized and addressed as such. For example, "drinking and driving" at any age is a problematic combination. The problem, however, is neither drinking nor driving alone. So it is with other situations involving seniors. Unfortunately, not all "situations" are as discretionary as driving, nor managed as easily as having a "designated driver" or calling a cab.

SCOPE

It is difficult to describe the prevalence of the potential problem with alcohol use among older people since data are not systematically maintained. In a way parallel to saying that anyone who enjoys the benefits of driving an automobile may also experience the negative consequences of a traffic accident, older adults who consume alcohol experience some potential risk of its negative consequences even as they enjoy its potential benefits. Risks associated with alcohol use among older people include increased heart problems, strokes from bleeding, falls and fractures, adverse reactions with other medications, impaired driving, memory problems, sleep problems, stomach problems, and liver problems (Barry, Oslin, & Blow, 2001). The risk of these untoward outcomes is increased for older adults by virtue of basic changes in the aging body and the way that alcohol is processed and may potentially interact with other drugs that older people commonly take. As we age, several physiological changes take place in our bodies. These are important changes for older adults to understand, because they help to explain the differences in the way that alcohol will be experienced.

There is a general shift in the lean body mass to fat ratio reducing the fluid volume that is available for the distribution of water-soluble drugs including alcohol—a smaller quantity of alcohol produces a higher proportional content than previously would have been the case (Vogel-Sprott & Barrett, 1984). The blood–brain barrier appears to become increasingly permeable with aging producing an increased sensitivity to the central nervous system effects of alcohol (Lamy, 1988). Older adults are the largest consumers of prescription and OTC drugs in the country and at least 100 prescription drugs that are commonly taken by seniors can interact with alcohol (Walker, 1996). Hence, the likelihood of one experiencing an alcohol–drug interaction increases among older adults. For all of these reasons, if one is to prevent problems with alcohol use among older adults, the preventive action must be focused on drinking patterns that fall well outside of the behaviors that have been traditionally labeled "problem drinking," "alcohol abuse," or "alcoholism." The convergence of preventive activity should be on empowering older adults to recognize the complex role of alcohol in their contemporary lifestyle and to make appropriate healthful decisions.

As indicated, alcohol consumption carries with it potential benefits as well. These include decreased risk of heart disease, decreased risk of stroke by blockage, and increased sociability (Barry et al., 2001). Two points should be clarified with respect to these benefits. First, based on a review of the findings of 25 studies, the protective benefits of alcohol consumption appear to derive equally to all forms of beverage alcohol (Rimm, Klatsky, Grobbee, & Stampfer, 1996). Some earlier studies had identified the "French paradox"—low levels of cardiovascular disease in spite of high levels of smoking and high dietary fat intake—and suggested the moderate intake of red wine with meals as a protective factor. While the ethanol content of the wine may indeed be a protective factor, the impact of the flavonioids (unique to the red wine) are probably quite small (LoBuono, 2000). Second, the benefits of drinking are not so substantive or universal that older adults who do not drink or who drink infrequently should be encouraged to begin or increase their drinking. People may choose not to drink for many reasons—financial, personal taste, family history of drinking problems—and these personal choices should be respected. The evidence in support of the benefits of drinking alcohol is not so strong as to overturn the personal choices not to drink.

In addition to these potential risks and benefits associated with drinking alcohol, it is important to understand the degree to which the behavior is commonplace among older adults. A recent study of community residing older adults found that 62 percent reported drinking (Mirand & Welte, 1996). Estimates for the prevalence of "problem drinking" are much lower but help to confirm that the use of alcohol among older adults is indeed common. Based on an extensive review of community surveys, hospital surveys, and nursing home surveys published between 1995 and 1998, Johnson (2000) found prevalence rates for "problem drinking" among older adults ranging from 2 to 53 percent. At least some of the variance in these estimates is due to the variation is the specific population studied, definitional problems (see *alcoholism* above), or other methodological differences. Common estimates of "alcohol dependence" and "heavy drinking" (often defined as more than two drinks per day) are in the range of 10 percent of older persons.

However, estimates of "problem drinking" substantially underestimate the proportion of older people who are at risk of problems related to the *use of alcohol* for at least two reasons. First, as suggested above, problems with the use of alcohol are more commonly interactive and stem from circumstances reaching far beyond the consumption of alcohol itself. Because research tends to look at more narrow problem definitions specified in terms of frequency or quantity of alcohol consumption, interaction problems or difficulties such as falls or secondary health effects that might arise related to alcohol consumption are seldom recorded. When they are, these secondary effects of alcohol consumption are found to be high indeed (Adams, Yuan, Barboriak, & Rimm, 1993). These effects may involve pharmaceutical interactions or complications with other familiar physical challenges common among older adults such as hypertension, diabetes, or depression. Second, the hugely growing number of seniors in the United States and virtually all other post-industrialized countries of the world represent a new cohort of seniors for whom patterns of alcohol and (potentially) other drug use may be quite different than the current population of seniors on whom the present set of utilization and prediction models has been developed (Patterson & Jeste, 1999).

In summary, while the concern of the interactive effects of alcohol is not completely unique for older persons, it does emerge as a much greater concern because of the changed way that alcohol is processed in the aging body, the increase number of pharmaceuticals taken by older adults, and because of the increased number of comorbidities (hypertension, depression, decreased bone density, increased risk of stroke, etc.) that an aging person is likely to experience. Drinking patterns that may never have been problematic may become problematic as one ages. The slight sway brought on by a glass of sherry in the evening can couple with a modest gait problem to produce a disastrous hip fracture. Without knowledge or intent, interactions with alcohol occur that may render other medications useless, or excessively potent. In short, the use and misuse of alcohol and other drugs among older people creates a very substantial problem that is largely unrecognized by older people themselves or by the professionals who serve them. The costs of this problem are uncalculated but can be seen in the real dollar costs of lost productivity among younger seniors, increased acute health care costs among all seniors, and increased long-term care needs among older seniors. Beyond these costs lie the even more difficult to quantify value of informal supports provided by family as they care for the direct and indirect consequences of alcohol and its interactive effects.

THEORIES

There are no theories on promoting appropriate alcohol use in the elderly per se. However, the principle preventive recommendations made in this entry are for the use of a strategy increasingly known in the alcohol literature as brief intervention, which was developed from the concepts of motivational psychology and the cognitive behavioral self-control literature (Miller & Rollnick, 1991; Miller & Taylor, 1980). As discussed below, the use of the brief intervention with alcohol has been evaluated systematically over the past 20 years. Most importantly for those interested in primary prevention and older adults, in the last few years research on the use of the brief alcohol intervention has been extended to its use with nonproblematic older adult drinkers.

RESEARCH

Major streams of research concerning alcohol and older adults have focused on the physiological effects of alcohol in the aging body (see Lamy, 1988), the consequences of heavy drinking by elderly persons (e.g., Finlayson & Hurt, 1998), and treatment of older alcoholics (e.g., Dupree & Schonfeld, 1998). Unfortunately, prevention research is scarce. Understanding the interplay of alcohol with physiological changes that naturally occur with aging is, however, important to developing primary prevention strategies for older adults.

From a preventive perspective, the goal of any alcohol screen should be to assist in identifying drinking behaviors that have the potential of putting an individual at risk of negative consequences. In that light, the drinking quantity, frequency, as well as the context and other substances being consumed should be considered. The National Institute on Alcohol Abuse and Alcoholism (NIAAA) Physicians' Guide To Helping Patients with Alcohol Problems (NIAAA, 1995) provides an excellent set of non-threatening questions to ascertain basic information about alcohol consumption. Contrary to the popular notion, all people who drink do not have a tendency to underreport their drinking if asked in a nonjudgmental manner (Barry et al., 2001). Thus, screening for basic levels of alcohol consumption, especially for the purposes of promoting primary prevention behaviors by the older adult, does not neces-sarily involve elaborate or time consuming assessment instrumentation.

However, if a screening tool is needed to establish the presence of a clinically significant problem with alcohol (i.e., alcohol dependence), the practitioner should be certain to use an instrument that has been validated for use for older adults. The Michigan Alcohol Screening Test—Geriatric Version (Blow, Brower, Schulenberg, Demo-Dananberg, Young, & Beresford, 1992) is recommended.

Brief Intervention

When alcohol screening reveals clinically significant drinking problems, appropriate *treatment* referrals should be made. However, when nonproblematic drinking patterns are identified that may place an individual at risk of future negative consequences due to any of the unique circumstances that can arise for older adults, preventive intervention should be undertaken. For nonproblematic older drinkers, the brief intervention introduced above has the strongest base of empirical support for use as a primary prevention tool. Fleming and Manwell (1999) have provided an excellent review of the over 20 empirical studies that have investigated the use of brief interventions to reduce alcohol consumption. Brief interventions involve a focused approach—typically only one or two face-to-face interactions—by a health care professional during a regular office visit to bring attention to the level of alcohol consumption by a client with the intention of reducing the client's drinking quantity or frequency. Although the majority of these studies have been based in clinical settings, some have been performed exclusively in community-based settings. The studies have been conducted across a range of diverse populations, ages, and have included both genders.

The brief intervention treatment has generally involved five essential steps: (1) assessment and direct feedback; (2) negotiation and goal setting; (3) behavioral modification techniques; (4) self-help information materials on alcohol use, its associated problems, and behavior modification exercises; and (5) follow-up and reinforcement (Fleming & Manwell, 1999). Generally the primary intervention visit is conducted in the context of a routine office visit with follow-up involving an additional visit or even a phone call. Drinking diaries or additional follow-up calls can be used to further reinforce positive behaviors. Results have been positive—10–30 percent of non-dependent problem drinkers reduced their drinking to moderate levels after a brief intervention (Fleming, Barry, Manwell, Johnson, & London, 1997).

Brief interventions of this nature represent a particularly valuable tool in prevention because they are not the kind of intervention that must wait until a problem is fully apparent to be utilized—they are legitimately prevention. Unlike traditional approaches to alcohol *treatment*, brief intervention can be used with an older person whose alcohol consumption has not been a problem but who may now face the possibility of a problem with, for example, an interaction with new medications and alcohol. A health professional is working *with* a client to anticipate predictable problems and put behaviors into place that will prevent foreseeable problems.

STRATEGIES: OVERVIEW

As we consider the best available solutions for the prevention of problems with alcohol for older adults, we are well-served to remind ourselves of what our goal *is not*. It is not about the best treatment approaches for people who have identified problems with alcohol (i.e., dependence or addiction). This is not to say that people who experience dependence or addiction cannot benefit from further preventive effort—they can. Prevention and harm reduction are for everyone. Rather, the treatment approach that is appropriate when addiction/ dependence is involved seeks to prevent additional harm from the existing problem state and goes beyond the intent of this entry. The goal here is to identify the strategy that can reduce the potential for harm to the substantial majority of older adults who currently consume alcohol at nonproblematic levels. To that end, we turn our attention to the empirical evidence in support of strategies that work, that might work, and for which there is no evidence of effectiveness.

STRATEGIES THAT WORK

As suggested earlier, there is empirical support for the efficacy of brief interventions by physicians in primary practice to motivate individuals to reduce the quantity and frequency of their drinking. A study of particular interest to readers of this entry randomized 158 older adults (65+) into intervention and control groups (Fleming, Manwell, Barry, Adams, & Stauffacher, 1999). The intervention involved two 10–15-min counseling sessions with a primary care physician that included advice, education, and client contracting. At each of the follow-up assessments, clients who received the intervention showed significant reductions in alcohol use, binge drinking, and the number of individuals drinking more than 21 drinks per week. These positive results were even larger than had been found with non-elderly groups in brief intervention trials.

It is important to note that the use of such brief interventions does not require that an individual be "diagnosed" as a "problem drinker" or meet any external criteria for a drinking behavior. Quite to the contrary. *Any drinking behavior* that might place an individual at risk of harm—including low risk behaviors—can be the focus of a brief intervention, not because the drinking is a problem in and of itself, but because it contributes to the potential of a problem occurring. Thus, the use of the brief intervention approach avoids the moralizing ("Drinking is wrong… You are bad…") that often accompanies alcohol treatment. Instead, it relies on a cognitive approach to harm reduction and is supported by an impressive accumulation of empirical evidence.

Guidelines and training materials for talking with clients and screening for alcohol problems have been prepared by the NIAAA (1995) and are available on the web at www.niaaa.nih.gov/publications/physicn.htm. This document provides clear steps for initiating discussions about alcohol and drinking with clients. Indicators and basic assessment procedures for drinking are outlined. In spite of the reference to "alcohol problems" in the publication title, the guidelines are equally appropriate for initiating sensitive discussion with nonproblematic drinkers as well.

Following guidelines of this type, the brief intervention approach could be incorporated into the standard routine for an annual physical. Given the emerging recognition of the way that alcohol is implicated in acute care hospitalizations (Adams et al., 1993) and the costs involved, it seems reasonable that Medicare would seize this opportunity for prevention as well as fiscal saving by reimbursing the cost of this well-validated intervention for reducing alcohol consumption.

STRATEGIES THAT MIGHT WORK

One strategy involves an increase in routine alcohol screening for older adults. These screenings could take two forms. The first could parallel the use of brief interventions through the use of primary health care providers. One of the priorities of the Healthy People 2000 guidelines is to increase the proportion of primary care providers who offer alcohol screening and counseling to 75 percent (Barry et al., 2001).

A second approach to increasing alcohol screening could involve the sort of voluntary mass screenings that one currently sees in senior centers, drug stores, and other public places for cholesterol screenings. In these alcohol screenings, however, seniors could take a simple self-assessment. As with any self-assessment, accurate results would depend on the willingness of the individual to be forthright with information; however, that is also true when individuals are working directly with helping professionals. In large-scale public screenings, it would be desirable to have professional staff or trained volunteers available to consult with individuals or to arrange for follow-up appointments as indicated by senior interest. Screenings done in either of these settings could be viewed as a part of a general "system check up" in the same sense that many people currently screen their weight, blood pressure, and cholesterol. Clearly, a major goal of such screenings would be self-education and awareness.

A final strategy involves the use of general public information and education about responsible senior drinking. The availability of senior-specific alcohol information is relatively new and not widespread. Like the "safer sex" message for HIV infection and other sexually transmitted diseases, the public health message for responsible drinking among seniors has not yet been widely communicated. Frankly, as we have a new population of seniors, we have a new population of senior professionals and we are all learning together. Most senior programmers know that "bingo is on the way out." Perhaps the time has come to assess the impact of "responsible drinking" programming and education.

STRATEGIES THAT DO NOT WORK

Prevention strategies that do not work, can be grouped into three categories: moralizing temperance strategies, strategies that fail to consider the unique aspects of aging, and strategies that target traditional "at risk" individuals. Support for these comments is not found in empirical research but rather drawn piecemeal from experience, the anecdotes of colleagues, and the practice literature. Each will be considered. First, moralizing and temperance. People have had a long history with intoxicating beverage—a very long history. While there have been ebbs and flows in our patterns of consumption, abstinence has rarely played well or for long. Moderation may be good moral policy but there appears little in our collective human history that suggests that we can deliver the desired individual behaviors based on the moral argument alone.

The second group of prevention strategies that is likely to fail are those that do not take into account the many unique aspects of aging in contemporary society. To be an older person is to be—whether one likes it or not, admits it or not—different than a younger person. Bodies change; experiences change; many other things change. That said, aging is a developmental stage of tremendous diversity—"old people" are arguable less alike than "non-old" people. No prevention strategy that depends on a workplace setting, or a senior center, or any other monolithic approach can succeed uniformly. The age span covered by people considered in this entry is 30 or more years! Given what we have come to know about changes in aging physiology, the propensity for interaction between alcohol and many common medications taken by older adults, and the comorbidities of alcohol and chronic ailments familiar to aging, our goal should be to screen every unique older adult, for example, as a part of regular physical exams.

The final group of prevention strategies likely to fail are those that target older individuals who are identified as "at risk" for alcohol problems. Available research generally identifies these individuals as consuming two or more drinks a day (already exceeding the NIAAA guidelines for older adults). I want to quickly qualify my inclusion of these prevention efforts as "failures," for I do so only in the sense that we have already failed by missing the opportunity to intervene at an earlier point and thus preventing the heightened potentiality for damage that has already occurred. If our goal is prevention of the problems that result from the complex interplay of alcohol with changing physiology, complex health care including multiple medications, managing chronic conditions and living full social lives, waiting until one thinks he or she might be drinking "too much" is waiting too long. Successful prevention of problems with alcohol among older persons must involve regular screening for all seniors before they are identified as being "at risk."

SYNTHESIS

A number of points require emphasis in preventing problems with alcohol misuse among older persons. First, beverage alcohol consumption is a normal part of an adult lifestyle in American society. Second, beverage alcohol consumption carries with it both positive and negative attributes. Third, the negative attributes of beverage alcohol consumption are for many seniors largely interactive with other circumstances including physiological and social. Fourth, a substantial portion—perhaps a substantial majority—of all drug and alcohol misuse among seniors is unintentional and unrecognized by professionals, by informals, and by seniors themselves.

The good news is that each of these points can be addressed in the context of a brief intervention conducted by a physician, during a regularly scheduled appointment for any number of other unrelated purposes. Alcohol screening is effective and takes little time. For the purposes of primary prevention, the purpose is not to assess drinking frequency/quantity against some standard, but rather to assess the ways in which alcohol might be interacting with other dimensions in the individual's life to create the potential for problems. Client contracts, reinforcing "homework" and follow-up calls have been shown to be remarkably effective in reducing both the frequency of drinking and the amount of alcohol consumed.

Perhaps the ultimate prevention technique is to "just say no" and avoid the use of alcohol or other drugs altogether. Of course, that approach appears not to have produced uniformly effective results with adolescents relating to drugs or sexual concerns and it is not likely to work well with seniors either. When one considers the additional complexities that the goal of the prevention message in this case is not abstinence but rather the *problems* associated with the use of alcohol, the "just say no" message is clearly inappropriate. Instead, the best science leads us to the conclusion that the most appropriate approach to preventing predictable problems with alcohol and other drug use among older adults involves a combination of screening every person and the provision of appropriate education for successful aging (Klein & Bloom, 1997).

Also see: Substances entries.

References

Adams, W., Yuan, Z., Barboriak, J., & Rimm, A. (1993). Alcohol-related hospitalizations of elderly people. *Journal of the American Medical Association, 270,* 1222–1225.

Barry, K., Oslin, D., & Blow, F. (2001). *Alcohol problems in older adults.* New York: Springer.

Blow, F. (1998). *Substance abuse among older adults* (Treatment Improvement Protocol (TIP) Series 26. DHHS Publication No. 98-3179). Substance Abuse and Mental Health Services Administration. CSAT: Rockville, MD.

Blow, F., Brower, K., Schulenberg, J., Demo-Dananberg, L., Young, J., & Beresford, T. (1992). The Michigan alcoholism screening test—Geriatric version (MAST-G): A new elderly-specific screening instrument. *Alcoholism: Clinical and Experimental Research, 16*, 372.

Dupree, L., & Schonfeld, L. (1998). Older alcohol abusers: Recurring treatment issues. In E. Gomberg, A. Hegedus, & R. Zucker (Eds.), *Alcohol problems and aging* (pp. 339–358) (NIH Publication No. 98-4163). Bethesda, MD: National Institutes of Health.

Finlayson, R., & Hurt, R. (1998). Medical consequences of heavy drinking by the elderly. In E. Gomberg, A. Hegedus, & R. Zucker (Eds.), *Alcohol problems and aging* (pp. 193–212) (NIH Publication No. 98-4163). Bethesda, MD: National Institutes of Health.

Fleming, M., Barry, K., Manwell, L., Johnson, K., & London, R. (1997). Brief physician advice for problem alcohol drinkers: A randomized controlled trial in community-based primary care practices. *Journal of the American Medical Association, 277*, 1039–1045.

Fleming, M., & Manwell, L. (1999). Brief intervention in primary care settings: A primary treatment method for at-risk, problem, and dependent drinkers. *Alcohol Research and Health, 23*(2), 128.

Fleming, M., Manwell, L., Barry, K., Adams, W., & Stauffacher, E. (1999). Brief physician advice for alcohol problems in older adults: A randomized community-based trial. *Journal of Family Practice, 48*, 378.

Johnson, I. (2000). Alcohol problems in old age: A review of recent epidemiological research. *International Journal of Geriatric Psychiatry, 15*, 575–581.

Klein, W., & Bloom, M. (1997). *Successful aging: Strategies for healthy living.* New York: Plenum Press.

Lamy, P. (1988). Actions of alcohol and drugs. *Generations, 12*(4), 9–13.

LoBuono, C. (2000, March 15). Dealing with the alcohol controversy. *Patient Care*, 211–225.

Miller, W., & Rollnick, S. (1991). *Motivational interviewing.* New York: Guilford Press.

Miller, W., & Taylor, C. (1980). Relative effectiveness of bibliotherapy, individual and group self-control training in the treatment of problem drinkers. *Addictive Behaviors, 5*, 13–24.

Mirand, A., & Welte, J. (1996). Alcohol consumption among the elderly in a general population, Erie County, New York. *American Journal of Public Health, 86*, 978–984.

National Institute on Alcohol Abuse and Alcoholism. (1995). *The physicians' guide to helping patients with alcohol problems* (NIH Publication No. 95-3769). Bethesda, MD: NIH.

Patterson, T., & Jeste, D. (1999). The potential impact of the baby-boom generation on substance abuse among elderly persons. *Psychiatric Services, 50*, 1184–1188.

Rimm, E., Klatsky, A., Grobbee, D., & Stampfer, M. (1996). Review of moderate alcohol consumption and reduced risk of coronary heart disease: Is the effect due to beer, wine, or spirits? *British Medical Journal, 312*, 731–736.0

Vogel-Sprott, M., & Barrett, P. (1984). Age, drinking habits and the effects of alcohol. *Journal of Studies on Alcohol, 45*, 517–521.

Walker, B. (1996). *Injury prevention in the elderly: Preventing falls.* Gaithersburg, MD: Aspen.

Suicide, Childhood

Morton M. Silverman

INTRODUCTION

Suicide is a self-inflicted injury with the intent to die. For many, it is hard to believe that children have a well-formed concept of death and, furthermore, a true intention to die. It is also difficult to imagine that children have the wherewithal to plan for their own deaths by intentionally engaging in self-destructive behaviors. Nevertheless, children aged 5–12 years do die by suicide, necessitating a real need to develop preventive interventions targeted to this age group.

Suicidal behaviors are complex behavioral expressions emanating from multiple etiologies (psychological, biological, genetic, sociological, economic, etc.) (Silverman & Felner, 1995). Commonly agreed upon definitions for this range of suicidal behaviors still elude us (O'Carroll, Berman, Maris, Moscicki, Tanney, & Silverman, 1996). This is particularly true when trying to understand the suicidal behaviors when they occur in children. Because suicide is a relatively low base rate disorder, and because it rarely occurs in children below the age of 11, it has been very difficult to enumerate the common risk factors most often associated with suicidal behavior in this age group (US Public Health Service, 1999). Developing effective preventive interventions to combat this lethal behavior has been a challenge.

DEFINITIONS

Defining *suicide* is a complex endeavor. Pfeffer (1986) has suggested that the definition of suicide needs to be clarified somewhat for youth. She has provided the following perspective: "It is not necessary for a child to have an understanding of the finality of death but it is necessary to have a concept of death, regardless of how idiosyncratic it may be. Therefore, suicidal behavior in children can be defined as self-destructive behavior that has the intent to seriously damage oneself or cause death" (p. 14).

SCOPE

In the United States, the suicide rate and suicide attempt rate is higher among young boys than among young girls (Peters, Kochanek, & Murphy, 1998). This may be due to the males' propensity to resort to impulsive, violent, irreversible methods of suicide, whereas female suicide attempters often use less lethal methods (Brent & Kolko, 1990). Native American males have the highest child suicide rates in the United States, followed by White males and then Black males (Wallace, Calhoun, Powell, O'Neil, & James, 1996).

Although suicide may be rare among children, suicidal behavior is not. Studies have shown high rates of nonfatal suicidal behaviors and ideation among children, especially those who are psychiatric patients (Pfeffer, Klerman, Hurt, Kakuma, Peskin, & Siefker, 1993). Researchers suggest that both rates of suicidal behavior and suicide are underreported in all age groups, but particularly in children (O'Carroll, 1989). In 1997, it was estimated that nearly 1 percent of school-aged children attempted to harm themselves and even more contemplated self-harm (Goldman & Beardslee, 1999). In addition, an undetermined number of traumatic injuries and "accidental" self-poisonings are believed to be suicidal in their intent. Many families conceal evidence of their children's suicidal behavior because of the associated social stigma (Greene, 1994).

The percentage of international suicides for the 5–14 year old age group is: males 0.7 percent, females 0.9 percent, and total 0.8 percent. For the United States, in 1996, the percentage of suicide for the 5–14 year old age group was: males 0.01 percent (225), females 0.01 percent (77), total 0.01 percent (302), or less than 1 per 100,000 (CDC, 1997). Because suicides are so rare under the age of 10 in the United States, the commonly reported age range for childhood fatalities due to suicide is 10–14 years. In 1998, there were 317 suicides in the 10–14 year old age group, making it the third leading cause of death for this age group. Unintentional injuries (1710) were first and malignant neoplasms was second (526). Homicide was fourth (290) (National Center for Health Statistics [NCHS], 2000).

In the United States, the rate for suicide among white males and other males (non-Caucasian, non-African American) age 10–14 years is much higher than for African American males, and all female racial groups. The overall male suicide rate, aged 10–14 years, is about 3 times higher than the comparable female suicide rate (Peters et al., 1998). Use of guns and firearms is the leading cause of suicidal death in the United States for all age groups (Peters et al., 1998). Specifically, the suicide rate for injury by firearms for the 5–14 year old group is 0.4 per 100,000 compared to 7.5 per 100,000 for 15–24 year olds. Males aged 5–14 years have a firearm suicide rate of 0.7 per 100,000, compared to 0.2 per 100,000 for similar-aged females. In the last decade, the rate of suicide among 5–14 year olds has increased and reflects a trend of escalating suicide rates among youth. In 1998, the rate of suicide for 5–14 year olds continued to increase, in contrast to a reduced suicide rate for 15–24 year olds from 1995 to 1998.

The costs of completed and medically treated youth suicide acts (ages 0–20 years) in the United States were calculated by state in 1996 and reported in 1998 dollars (Cox & Miller, 1999). Injury costs primarily fell into three categories: medical costs, future earnings, and quality of life. The total medical costs (emergency services as well as funeral costs) amounted to $945 million. The total future earnings figure (victim's lost wages, family members missed work) amounted to $2.85 billion. The quality of life estimate (pain, suffering) came to $11.84 billion. The total was $15.64 billion.

What is much more difficult to calculate is the emotional and psychological cost to parents, siblings, relatives, friends, and schoolmates, when a child dies by suicide. Studies have suggested that the bereavement process is especially intense, painful, and prolonged when a child dies by suicide (Callahan, 2000).

THEORIES

There are many theories that attempt to explain why individuals die by suicide, but few are applicable to the very young. Several studies indicate that although prepubertal children frequently experience serious suicidal thoughts and impulses, this age group may be protected against suicide by their cognitive immaturity. Consequently, young children may be unable to plan or execute a fatal suicide act (Brent & Kolko, 1990).

From a cognitive developmental perspective, researchers generally agree that a child's understanding of death develops gradually and changes over time (Mishara, 1999). The more experiences children had related to death (e.g., death of an animal or pet, or death education at school), the more mature their concept of death in general (Normand & Mishara, 1992). A recent study by Mishara (1999) obtained detailed information about what children 6–12 years old know and think about suicide. Most children (by age 8–9) understand the concept of "killing oneself." They are all able to name at least one means of committing suicide and generally cite methods frequently used in completed suicides.

Many children in Grades 1 and 2 and almost all children in the higher grades recognize that death is permanent and final. Children develop their knowledge about suicide based upon discussions with other children, television depictions of suicide as a heroic act, and direct experience with the suicidal death of a family member or friend. What children learn about suicide at a young age may stay with them as they develop into teenagers and adults. Mishara concluded that these results also suggest that it may not be appropriate to ignore self-injurious behavior in children and suicide threats because of the belief that children do not understand enough about death or suicide to engage in "true" suicidal behavior. This study indicates that children generally know enough to knowledgeably commit suicide with a realization that this will result in permanent death. Even so, children often do not have a realistic view of life and death issues, and their concepts of the future and of time may be quite confused.

One theory suggests that the suicidal act is the result of impulses and aggressive drives that are out-of-the-control of the individual and may often occur without warning. This theory is based on a *stress-diathesis model*, suggesting that a neurobiological imbalance of neurotransmitters in the central nervous system may account for the impulsive act (Mann & Stoff, 1997). At the other end of the theoretical spectrum is the conceptualization of suicide as a behavior in *response to frustrated psychological needs* that produces intolerable psychological pain (Shneidman, 1996). Suicide becomes a solution to ending the intolerable psychological pain caused by unmet or frustrated needs, such as love, respect, attention, caring, sense of identity, sense of community, hope, etc.

Orbach, Mikulincer, Blumenson, Mester, and Stein (1999) posit that the subjective experience of problem irresolvability in children and adolescents leads to suicidal behavior. This experience can be defined as one's sense of lack of control over life, resulting from the belief that other powerful people, usually parents, present them with unrealistic problems within the family domain and exert pressure on the youngsters to solve them. The *problem irresolvability model* posits that family dynamics of suicidal youngsters include excessive demands, achievement pressures, and family conflicts. However, this model suggests an additional paradoxical aspect of the irresolvable problem. Not only is the youngster pressured to resolve difficult problems, but at the same time he or she is actively prevented from solving them, even when the youngster tries to do so. This paradoxical behavior is rooted in the family's need to scapegoat a family member in order to keep it from total deterioration or as a means to cover up other serious familial problems (Orbach, 1988).

The emotional atmosphere created in such families is one of oppression and rejection, hurting the youngster's sense of competence and self-esteem (Orbach, Lotem-Peleg, & Kedem, 1995). The model suggests that the subjective experience of problem irresolvability is strongly associated with hopelessness, depression, anxiety, and other negative affect.

RESEARCH

Children with certain psychiatric disorders (e.g., depression, conduct disorder, specific developmental disorders, and adjustment disorder) are more vulnerable to suicidal behavior. Depression is a major symptom present in suicidal children. The severity of depression in children has been found to be positively associated with the severity of suicidal tendencies (Brent & Kolko, 1990). Evidence shows that a high proportion of child psychiatric patients present serious suicidal ideation or behavior (Pfeffer, 2000). The extent of preoccupation with death, recent aggression, and previously stressful experiences (e.g., loss) has also been found to be significantly related to suicide behavior in children. Suicidal children often report feeling sad, hopeless, and worthless (Pfeffer, 1986).

A variety of early negative life events have been related to the etiology of subsequent suicidal behavior, including: (1) child maltreatment, (2) family instability, and (3) poor general family environment (Yang & Clum, 1996). Childhood maltreatment, including physical abuse, sexual abuse, and neglect has been related to suicidal behavior. Family instability, defined as parental separation, divorce, absence, and death, has also been related to an individual's suicidal behavior. Finally, poor general family environment, defined as deficient parenting skills, negative parent–child relationships, and parental discord and violence, has been related to suicidal behavior (Yang & Clum, 2000).

Research exists linking early negative life events to impaired cognitive functioning, as reflected by such constructs as: (1) self-esteem, (2) locus of control, (3) hopelessness, and (4) problem-solving deficits. Cognitive deficits have been found to predict a variety of suicidal behavior, including ideation, attempts, and suicide status. Furthermore, these relationships have been found obtained over both the short-term and long-term (Yang & Clum, 2000). Suicidal children have been found to demonstrate a limited ability to find solutions to interpersonal problems. They are less able to consider alternatives and come up with new ideas or solutions to problems. Suicidal, compared to nonsuicidal, children appear less able to generate active cognitive coping strategies (e.g., self-comforting statements and instrumental problem solving) in the face of stressful life events (Weishaar & Beck, 1990).

Suicidal children have poor reality testing, are impulsive, feel hopeless, and have problems in emotional and social problem solving (Pfeffer, 2000). The combined deficits in cognitive abilities, adaptive functioning, and present life event stresses increase vulnerability to suicidal behavior among children. Social adjustment, measured as children's competence in carrying out appropriate social role behavior, has been shown to be aberrant in these children (Pfeffer et al., 1993). In fact, this is a hallmark of risk for childhood suicidal behavior and often an important precipitant of suicide attempts in children. For example, loss of a friendship due to arguments, or failure in academic achievement and fear of retribution from parents, are common ingredients for an acute suicidal episode (Pfeffer, 2000).

Shneidman (1996) has noted that the common consistency in suicide is not the precipitating event but life-long coping patterns. Children who kill themselves experience a steady toll of threat, stress, failure, challenge, and loss that gradually undermines their adjustment process (Leenaars & Wenckstern, 1991). One event, however, that has frequently been identified as a possible precipitating event is the death of a parent (Pfeffer, 1986). Indeed, when the death occurs by suicide, everyone in the family is at risk. However, availability of a lethal agent to carry out suicidal intent appeared to be the most important factor for impulsive suicide attempters (Brent & Kolko, 1990).

The families of suicidal children often show a high incidence among first-degree relatives of suicidal behavior, substance abuse, depression, and violence (Brent et al., 1994). Affective illness in families extracts a considerable toll from all members, including children. Early and chronic life event stresses are associated with prepubertal suicidal behavior (Pfeffer et al., 1993). Events that lead to family instability, such as moves, death, loss of relatives, and illness of significant caretakers, may increase the likelihood for suicidal behavior among prepubertal children.

In summarizing the research literature, Goldman and Beardslee (1999) suggest that some reasons that children engage in suicidal behaviors are: (1) an attempt to regain control in their lives; (2) retaliation or revenge against real or perceived wrongs; (3) reunion fantasies; (4) relief or escape from unbearable pain; (5) they see themselves as the family scapegoat; (6) to distract the family from other issues (e.g., divorce); and (7) acting out a covert or overt desire of the parent to be rid of the child.

In the United States, one in ten children and adolescents suffer from mental illness severe enough to cause some level of impairment (Burns et al., 1995). Yet, in any given year, it is estimated that about one in five of such children receive specialty mental health services. In March 2000, the White House held a follow-up meeting to its historic "White House Conference on Mental Health," held in June, 1999 (US DHHS, 1999). This follow-up meeting specifically addressed the need to improve the diagnoses and treatment of children with emotional and behavioral conditions (US Public Health Service, 2000).

In September 2000, US Surgeon General Satcher convened a conference on "Children's Mental Health: Developing a National Action Agenda." Satcher noted that children and families are suffering because of missed opportunities for prevention and early intervention, fragmented services, and low priorities for resources. Overriding these problems is the issue of stigma that continues to surround mental illness (and suicide) (US Public Health Service, 2000). He emphasized the need to improve early recognition and appropriate identification of mental disorders in children within all systems serving children, and improve access to services by removing barriers faced by families with mental health needs, with a specific aim to reduce disparities in access to care.

STRATEGIES: OVERVIEW

There is a tendency in our society to deny suicide and especially the possibility of child suicide. In order to prevent child suicide, we must first acknowledge that children do have suicidal thoughts and they might act upon these thoughts.

Gould and Kramer (2001) argue that suicide prevention strategies should be evidence-based and have two general goals: case finding with accompanying referral and treatment, and risk factor reduction. They list the following case-finding strategies: school-based suicide awareness curricula, screening, gatekeeper training, and crisis centers and hotlines. Under risk factor reduction strategies they list: restrictions of lethal means, media education, postvention/crisis interventions, and skills training (e.g., symptom management and competency enhancement for youth).

Another approach is to focus solely on protective factors, inasmuch as it is often very difficult to significantly change risk factors. Protective factors can include an individual's genetic or neurobiological makeup, attitudinal and behavioral characteristics, and environmental attributes. Protective factors include effective and appropriate clinical care for mental, physical and substance abuse disorders; easy access to a variety of clinical interventions and support for help seeking; restricted access to highly lethal methods of suicide; family and community support; support from ongoing medical and mental health care relationships; learned skills in problem solving, conflict resolution, and nonviolent handling of disputes; cultural and religious beliefs that discourage suicide and support self-preservation instincts (US Public Health Service, 1999).

STRATEGIES THAT WORK

At the present time, there are no rigorous evaluation studies that provide information on strategies that work to prevent suicide in school-aged children. There are many programs that hold promise for the future; I will explore some of these below.

STRATEGIES THAT MIGHT WORK

Evidence is mounting that a focus on family systems and community support building might prove to be effective preventive interventions. Approaches include parent education training, healthy family functioning, conflict resolution training, communication skills building, improving access to health care, and access to crisis hotlines (Workman & Prior, 1997).

The Australian Institute of Family Studies conducted an evaluation of their National Youth Suicide Prevention Strategy in 2000 (Mitchell, 2000). They evaluated the strategy according to "six maps of program logic": (1) primary prevention and cultural change; (2) early intervention; (3) crisis intervention and primary care; (4) treatment, support and postvention; (5) access to means/injury prevention; and (6) system level activities. They identified "four maps of achievements": (1) primary prevention and cultural change; (2) early intervention; (3) crisis intervention and primary care; and (4) treatment, support and postvention. For these four "maps," they evaluated the public health elements of each effort and concluded that they have the highest promise of success.

Many of the suicide preventive interventions directed at the adolescent and young adult groups might be applicable and, where suitably modified, appropriate for children and preadolescents. These include: (1) means restriction strategies (limited access to lethal means; firearm disposal or containment; restricted access to alcohol or other drugs); (2) gatekeeper training (health and mental health professionals); (3) health communication campaigns (increase risk assessment techniques for health professionals; community health awareness campaigns); (4) school gatekeeper training (school nurses, counselors, teachers, coaches); (5) postvention response (interventions directed at survivors of loved ones who die by suicide); and (6) psychotherapeutic interventions (family, psychopharmacology, psychoeducation, group therapy) (Grossman & Kruesi, 2000).

The State of Oregon developed a *Youth Suicide Prevention* program beginning in 1997 (Bloodworth, 2000). They will soon report on their evaluation of the program. The 15 strategies, which represent an overview of possible interventions, are to:

1. Develop and implement public education campaigns to increase knowledge about symptoms of depression and suicide, response skills, and resources; increase help-seeking behavior; and decrease stigma associated with treatment for behavioral health problems.
2. Promote efforts to reduce access to lethal means of self-harm.
3. Educate youth and young adults about suicide prevention.
4. Reduce harassment in schools and communities.
5. Provide media education to reduce suicide contagion.
6. Provide education for professionals in health care, education, and human services.

7. Provide gatekeeper training to create a network of people trained to recognize and respond to youth in crisis.
8. Implement screening and referral services.
9. Increase effectiveness of crisis hot lines.
10. Enhance crisis services.
11. Establish and maintain crisis response teams.
12. Improve access to affordable behavioral health care.
13. Provide skill-building support groups to increase protective factors and involve families.
14. Support suicide survivors by fostering the development of bereavement support groups.
15. Improve follow-up services for suicide attempters.

The plan emphasizes three key prevention approaches: (1) community education, (2) integration of systems serving high risk youth, and (3) access to a full range of health care that includes mental health and alcohol and drug treatment services.

STRATEGIES THAT DO NOT WORK

There is little evidence for what strategies do not work with children. However, there is evidence from adolescent suicide prevention studies that certain strategies are not effective. They include: (1) scare tactic approaches; (2) and health awareness programs that focus solely on suicide prevention (Shaffer, Garland, Vieland, Underwood, & Busner, 1991).

SYNTHESIS

Addressing the problem of childhood suicide requires recognition of the variable signs and symptoms of depression in children and understanding the demographic, familial, biological, and psychological risk factors for suicide. Depression is a treatable mental disorder. The task of preventing depression and suicide in children remains to be achieved.

The most important need for the prevention of suicide in children seems to be a greater awareness, recognition, and response to children in need and in times of crisis. This increased sensitivity to the potential for childhood self-injurious behaviors ultimately rests with parents, educators, school personnel, health care professionals, mental health professionals, clergy, first responders (firefighters, police, emergency technicians), and even children themselves. Suicide is preventable. Resources for providing effective interventions must be available that are affordable, accessible, and age-appropriate. The locus of intervention for children must be targeted first to the family, community (religious organizations and school), and pediatrician's office.

Inasmuch as childhood suicide is a multidimensional disorder with a multicausal and multifactorial etiology, the prevention of suicide in children must encompass a comprehensive, coordinated, and collaborative approach. A biopsychosocial framework seems appropriate to such a challenging enterprise. What with childhood suicide rates being low (albeit underreported), prevention efforts must be sustained and maintained over long periods of time before a reduction in the rate can be measured and attributed to ongoing preventive initiatives. A comprehensive strategy may well encompass two approaches: direct prevention approaches and system level approaches. Direct prevention approaches include: the provision of information and training to parents, teachers, and other people having direct contact with children; restricting access to the means of committing suicide; crisis intervention and primary care (because the time frame for action is so brief in immature children); and sensitivity to cultural issues related to suicide or depression.

System level approaches include: policy and planning activities; ongoing research and evaluation; improved and expanded communications and media training; education and training of community gatekeepers and health care professionals; networking and collaboration between and among community organizations and institutions; and community development.

However, it is fairly certain that we will not see a substantial change in the suicide rate if we do not address the common risk factors that have been shown to contribute to a multitude of childhood disorders and dysfunctions. Such well-known and common risk factors for childhood disorders include:

- substance misuse and abuse
- precocious sexual activity
- exposure to violence and crime
- involvement in the juvenile justice system
- being in foster care
- dysfunctional family functioning
- emotional, sexual and/or physical abuse
- marital discord and divorce
- undiagnosed and/or untreated psychiatric disorders
- homelessness
- chronic physical illness
- poor or no access to health care
- underachievement in school
- poor social adjustment
- poor coping strategies
- lack of mentorship
- lack of religious or community affiliation
- an absence of hope
- a sense of a future

(Dryfoos, 1990; US DHHS, 2001). To this list, I would add access to lethal means of self-injury as a risk factor being specific for childhood suicide.

As a society, we may well not be able to eliminate all the risk factors that increase the potential for suicidal behavior. However, we surely can agree that the enhancement of resilience or protective factors are at least as essential as risk reduction in preventing suicide. Such a dual-pronged strategy, sustained over time, will most likely achieve the outcome we seek.

Also see: Suicide entries.

References

Bloodworth, R. (2000). *The Oregon plan for youth suicide prevention: A call to action.* Oregon Department of Human Services: Injury Prevention and Epidemiology Program.

Brent, D.A., & Kolko, D.J. (1990). The assessment and treatment of children and adolescents at risk for suicide. In S.J. Blumenthal & D.J. Kupfer (Eds.), *Suicide over the life cycle.* Washington, DC: American Psychiatric Press.

Brent, D.A., Perper, J.A., Moritz, G., Liotus, L., Schweers, J., Balach, L., & Roth, C. (1994). Familial risk factors for adolescent suicide: A case-control study. *Acta Psychiatrica Scandinavica, 89,* 52–58.

Burns, B.H., Costello, E.J., Angold, A., Tweed, D., Stangl, D., Farmer, E.M.Z., & Erkanli, A. (1995). Children's mental health service use across service sectors. *Health Affairs, 14*(3), 147–159.

Callahan, J. (2000). Predictors and correlates of bereavement in suicide support group participants. *Suicide and Life-Threatening Behavior, 30*(2), 104–124.

CDC. (1997). Rates of homicide, suicide, and firearm related death among children—26 industrialized countries. *Morbidity and Mortality Weekly Report, 46*(5), 101–105.

Cox, K., & Miller, T (1999). *Costs of completed and medically treated youth suicide acts by state, 1996.* Report of the Children's Safety Network Economics and Insurance Resource Center, The Pacific Institute for Research and Evaluation.

Dryfoos, J. (1990). *Adolescents at risk: Prevalence and prevention.* NY: Oxford University Press.

Goldman, S., & Beardslee, W.R. (1999): Suicide in children and adolescents. In D. G. Jacobs (Ed.), *The Harvard medical school guide to suicide assessment and intervention* (pp. 417–442). San Francisco, CA: Jossey-Bass.

Gould, M.S., & Kramer, R.A. (2001). Youth suicide prevention. *Suicide and Life-Threatening Behavior, 31*(Suppl.), 6–31.

Greene, D.B. (1994). Childhood suicide and myths surrounding it. *Social Work, 39*(2), 230–232.

Grossman, J.A., & Kruesi, M.J.P. (2000). Innovative approaches to youth suicide prevention: An update of issues and research findings. In R.W. Maris, S.S. Canetto, J.L. McIntosh, & M.M. Silverman (Eds.), *Review of suicidology, 2000* (pp. 170–201). NY: The Guilford Press.

Leenaars, A.A., & Wenckstern, S. (1991). Suicide in the school-age child and adolescent. In A.A. Leenaars (Ed.), *Life span perspectives of suicide: Time-lines in the suicide process* (pp. 95–107). NY: Plenum Press.

Mann, J.J., & Stoff, D.M. (1997). A synthesis of current findings regarding neurobiological correlates and treatment of suicidal behaviors. *Annals of the New York Academy of Sciences, 836,* 352–363.

Mishara, B.L. (1999). Conceptions of death and suicide in children ages 6–12 and their implications for suicide prevention. *Suicide and Life-Threatening Behavior, 29*(2), 105–118.

Mitchell, P. (2000). *Valuing young lives: evaluation of the National Youth Suicide Prevention Strategy.* Commonwealth of Australia: Australian Institute of Family Studies (Melbourne, Australia).

National Center for Health Statistics (NCHS). (2000). *Mortality data tapes*. Hyattsville, MD: DHHS: Centers for Disease Control, NCHS.

Normand, C., & Mishara, B.L. (1992). The development of the concept of suicide in children. *Omega Journal of Death and Dying, 25*(3), 183–203.

O'Carroll, P.W. (1989). A consideration of the validity and reliability of suicide mortality data. *Suicide and Life-Threatening Behavior, 19*(1), 1–16.

O'Carroll, P.W., Berman, A.L., Maris, R.W., Moscicki, E.K., Tanney, B.L., & Silverman, M.M. (1996). Beyond the tower of babel: A nomenclature for suicidology. *Suicide and Life-Threatening Behavior, 26*(3), 237–252.

Orbach, I. (1988). Children who don't want to live. San Francisco: Jossey-Bass.

Orbach, I., Lotem-Peleg, M., & Kedem, P. (1995). Attitudes toward the body in suicidal, depressed, and normal adolescents. *Suicide and Life-Threatening Behavior, 25*, 211–221.

Orbach, I., Mikulincer M., Blumenson, R., Mester, R., & Stein, D. (1999). The subjective experience of problem irresolvability and suicidal behavior: dynamics and measurement. *Suicide and Life-Threatening Behavior, 29*(2), 150–164.

Peters, K.D., Kochanek, K.D., & Murphy, S.L. (1998). *Deaths: Final data for 1996*. National Vital Statistics Reports, Vol. 47, No. 9. Hyattsville, MD: National Center for Health Statistics.

Pfeffer, C.R. (1986). *The suicidal child*. New York: Guilford.

Pfeffer, C.R. (2000). Suicidal behaviour in children: An emphasis on developmental influences. In K. Hawton & K. van Heeringen (Eds.), *The international handbook of suicide and attempted suicide* (pp. 237–248). London: John Wiley and Sons.

Pfeffer, C.R., Klerman, G.L., Hurt, S.W., Kakuma, T., Peskin, J.R., & Siefker, C.A. (1993). Suicidal children grow up: Rates and psychosocial risk factors for suicide attempts during follow-up. *Journal of the American Academy of Child and Adolescent Psychiatry, 32*, 106–113.

Shaffer, D., Garland, A., Vieland, V., Underwood, M.M., & Busner, C. (1991). The impact of a curriculum-based suicide prevention program for teenagers. *Journal of the American Academy of Child and Adolescent Psychiatry 27*, 675–687.

Shneidman, E.S. (1996). *The suicidal mind*. NY: Oxford University Press.

Silverman, M.M., & Felner, R.D. (1995). Suicide prevention programs: issues of design, implementation, feasibility, and developmental appropriations. *Suicide and Life-Threatening Behavior, 25*(1), 92–103.

US DHHS. (1999). *Mental health: A report of the surgeon general*. Rockville, MD: US DHHS, SAMHSA, CMHS, NIH, NIMH.

US DHHS. (2001). *National strategy for suicide prevention: Goals and objectives for action*. Rockville, MD: Public Health Service.

US Public Health Service. (1999). *The Surgeon General's call to action to prevent suicide*. Washington, DC: USPHS/DHHS.

US Public Health Service. (2000). *Report of the Surgeon General's Conference on children's mental health: A national action agenda*. Washington, DC: DHHS/USPHS/NIH Publication No.: NIH 00-4919.

Wallace, L.D.J., Calhoun, A.D., Powell, K.E., O'Neil, J., & James, S.P. (1996). *Homicide and suicide among Native Americans, 1979–1992*. (Violence Surveillance Summary Series, No. 2) Atlanta, GA: CDC.

Weishaar, M.E., & Beck, A.T. (1990). Cognitive approaches to understanding and treating suicidal behavior. In S.J. Blumenthal & D.J. Kupfer (Eds.), *Suicide over the life cycle*. Washington, DC: American Psychiatric Press.

Workman, C.G., & Prior, M. (1997). Depression and suicide in young children. *Issues in Comprehensive Pediatric Nursing, 20*, 125–132.

Yang, B., & Clum, G.A. (1996). Effects of early negative life experiences on cognitive functioning and risk for suicide: A review. *Clinical Psychology Review, 16*, 177–195.

Yang, B., & Clum, G.A. (2000): Childhood stress leads to later suicidality via its effect on cognitive functioning. *Suicide and Life-Threatening Behavior, 30*(3), 183–198.

Suicide, Adolescence

John Kalafat

INTRODUCTION AND SCOPE

In the United States, for people 15–24 years old, suicide is the third leading cause of death, behind unintentional injury and homicide. In 1996, the rate among children aged 10–14 was 1.6/100,000, the rate for youth aged 15–19 was 9.7 per 100,000, and the rate for youth aged 20–24 was 14.5/100,000. From 1980 to 1996, the rate of suicide among persons aged 15–19 years increased by 14 percent and among persons aged 10–14 years by 100 percent. The risk for suicide among young people is greatest among young White males; however, from 1980 to 1996, suicide rates increased most rapidly among young Black males (105 percent). Males under the age of 25 are much more likely to commit suicide than their female counterparts. The 1996-gender ratio for people aged 15–19 was 5:1 (males: females), while among those aged 20–24 it was 7:1. Among persons aged 15–19 years, firearm-related suicides accounted for 63 percent of the increase in the overall rate of suicide from 1980 to 1996. Various surveys consistently indicate that about ten percent of youths have made suicide attempts, and the attempt to completion ratio for youths has been estimated at between 20:1 and 50:1.

Although there is international variation in suicide mortality, the global picture for the last few decades has mirrored the increasing trends in the United States. For example, rates for 15–24 year old males and females, respectively, in 1990 were: Canada (24.6, 5.0), Australia (26.6, 4.7); other countries ranged from lower rates such as Greece (5.2, 1.1) and Armenia (3.7, 1.2) to higher rates such as Finland (50.9, 11.0) and New Zealand (38.0, 6.7).

Apart from the costs involved in providing a range of services to those who exhibit suicidal behavior and those around them, another measure of cost is the years of productive life lost. In 1998, it was estimated that across all ages at a global level economic losses from suicidal behavior amount to about 1.8 percent of the total economic burden due to disease. This was equal to the burden of wars and homicide (World Health Organization, 2000).

DEFINITIONS

The first definition issue is to agree that what are we trying to prevent is suicide attempts and completions.

A *suicide completion* is defined as death from injury where there is explicit or implicit evidence that the injury was self-inflicted and that the decedent intended to kill him/herself. A *suicide attempt* is defined as an action resulting in nonfatal injury, or potentially self-injurious behavior with a nonfatal outcome, where there is explicit or implicit evidence that the injury was self-inflicted and that the survivor intended at some (nonzero) level to kill him/herself (O'Carroll, Berman, Maris, Moscicki, Tanney, & Silverman, 1996).

Suicide is best conceptualized along a trajectory that starts with conditions consisting of a combination of substantial risk and limited protective factors; and, leads to thoughts, plans, attempts, and completion. By definition, prevention occurs before the fact, so intervention can occur at any point along this trajectory, beginning with broad-based programs that address risk and protective factors generic to a number of destructive behaviors, and moving to programs that target conditions that are progressively more specific, first to the individual, and then to the disorder, moving closer to full manifestation of suicidal behavior. Within this framework, the last stage that at least technically qualifies as prevention is in providing effective treatment for suicide attempters.

Risk and protective factors are characteristics of individuals and/or their environments that increase or decrease, respectively, the probability of suicidal behavior. Risk factors associated with youth suicide include:

- Previous attempt(s)
- Current, ideation, intent, and plan (resolve)
- Exposure to suicide
- Affective disorder
- Hopelessness
- Substance abuse
- Personality disorders (conduct, borderline)
- Family functioning and history (high conflict, low support, abuse, mental illness, suicide)
- Social relationships (isolation, withdrawal, low support)
- Ineffective coping mechanisms, rigid cognitive and problem solving style
- Reluctance to seek help
- Services that are psychologically, culturally, and temporally inaccessible.

It must be noted that these are not sensitive predictors in that the best will yield over 80 percent false positive rates. Also, aside from the first three, these risk factors are not specific to suicide, in that they are associated with a broad array of other disorders, which are themselves often employed as predictors of youth suicide. Again, suicide is not a disease caused by specific agents, but is multiply determined and is comorbid with other disorders and destructive behaviors.

Protective factors that have been associated with a variety of destructive behaviors are:

- Personal characteristics such as positive disposition and problem solving ability
- Contact with a caring adult
- A sense of connection with school or community based on opportunities to participate and make contributions.

These characteristics can attenuate the likelihood of destructive behavior, even by those who experience one or more risk factors. Some prospective studies have found them to be more powerful predictors of outcomes than risk factors (Jessor, Van Den Bos, Vanderryn, Costa, & Turbin, 1995).

Suicide is often preceded by *precipitants*. These are stressful events that do not cause suicide, but may prompt it in vulnerable individuals. Studies have found that these events often precede completed suicide. These events may not seem great in themselves. They simply have particular meaning to a youth who is already at risk for suicide. These stressors include:

- Getting into trouble with authorities (e.g., school, police); not knowing and afraid of the consequences.
- Disappointment and rejection such as dispute with boy/girlfriend, failing in school, failure to get a job, or rejection from college.
- Anxiety over impending change.
- Shortly before or after anniversary of death of friend or relative.
- Knowing someone who committed or attempted suicide.
- Conflict with family.

THEORIES

Various approaches to suicide prevention stem from different theoretical frameworks such as medical or disease, public health, operational, crisis, community, and ecological models. Suicide is neither a disease nor the manifestation of a specific disease. Rather, suicidal behaviors arise from complex interplays of developmental, individual, environmental, and, at times, biological circumstances. Therefore, an eclectic approach that combines elements from different models to address as many of these circumstances as is feasible seems best suited to address suicide.

Thus, the NIMH (1995) concluded that there is no justification for the dispute among those who advocate preventive interventions aimed at reduction of the incidence of specific risk factors such as mental disorders, those aimed at more general risk factors, and those aimed at promoting health or protective factors. This applies to advocates for universal, selective, and indicated approaches to be described below. In fact, NIMH pointed out connections among these approaches such as the possibility that failure to respond to a universal intervention might itself be an important indication for including individuals in more intense, targeted interventions.

Also, a position paper for the Third National Injury Control Conference (Department of Health and Human Services [DHHS], 1992) stated:

> Having recognized that no single type of intervention is likely to be universally effective, we can turn our attention to a much more appropriate question: Which combination of the many potential interventions is likely to be most effective (as well as feasible) in preventing violent injuries? ... Which are likely to be effective across different types of violent injuries? Which of the potential interventions are feasible and most likely to be adopted? (p. 169)

Therefore, different theoretical frameworks can inform a variety of prevention approaches. The *public health model* acknowledges the importance of both a high-risk approach which seeks to identify and protect susceptible individuals, and a *population approach* which addresses the broader social and environmental factors that influence suicidal behavior. This model combines four interactive components: surveillance, epidemiological research, design and evaluation of interventions, and implementation of programs (Potter, Powell, & Kachur, 1995). The *operational model* defines a set of interventions based on their targets (Institute of Medicine [IOM], 1994). The terms for these interventions are *universal*, which are targeted at an entire population that has not been selected on the basis of manifestation of suicidal behavior; *selective*, which are targeted at populations known or thought to be at elevated risk for suicidal behavior (also described as characterized by shared exposure to some epidemiologically determined risk factor); and, *indicated*, which are targeted at specific individuals who are known to be at high risk for suicidal behavior (or have made suicide attempts). The *community model* reminds us to attend to the contexts of our interventions and to develop feasible programs that are likely to be adopted and retained because they fit with the culture and resources of institutions such as schools. The *ecological approach* combines many features of other models and calls for interventions that address both individual and systemic or environmental levels and the interaction between them (Felner & Felner, 1989). Thus, in

a recent United Nations report (Department for Policy Coordination and Sustainable Development, 1996) on the prevention of suicide:

> The representative, commenting on the keynote address [delivered by M. Silverman] expressed support for the emphasis upon community-based and population-focused prevention models. There was an increasing convergence toward a belief that individuals must be helped not only by specialists but primarily in the supportive context of their social surroundings. (1996, p. 4)

RESEARCH

A summary of the empirical research in the area of youth suicide must conclude that the causes for this problem are not yet known, there is a dearth of empirical suicide prevention trials, and there is a dearth of empirical suicide prevention trials (Clark & Gould, 1998; NIMH, 1995). At the same time, evidence is accumulating about precipitants for youth suicide; several risk factors that distinguish suicidal youth from other young people; and, protective factors that have been demonstrated to attenuate other destructive behaviors such as poor school performance and dropout, substance abuse, and delinquency. Recent research evidence suggests an accumulative risk model of suicidal behavior in which the individual's risk of suicidal behavior rises markedly with the number of risk factors to which s(he) has been exposed. This suggests that suicidal behavior is not simply a consequence of current mental disorder, nor current life stressors, but, rather represents the culmination of adverse life course sequences in which risk factors have accumulated from a variety of domains. The overlap of suicide risk and protective factors with those of other youth psychosocial and mental health problems suggests not only that they may share overlapping pathways and processes but also that they may be addressed by common interventions. There is also empirical work that suggests an array of specific interventions that will be reviewed next.

STRATEGIES THAT WORK

Clear evidence of effectiveness is not yet available.

STRATEGIES THAT MIGHT WORK

Several reports, many developed for national and state plans (Beautrais, 1998; Clark & Gould, 1998; Eggert, Thompson, Randell, & McCauley, 1995; Kalafat, 1997;

Youth Suicide Prevention, 1998) review the conceptual and empirical bases for a set of prevention approaches that span both the range from early interventions addressing broad risk and protective factors to interventions addressing suicidal behaviors per se, and the range from universal to indicated interventions. None currently meet the criterion of clearly empirically validated approaches, but many can be described as promising in that they are theoretically well supported, but not yet proven; draw upon empirical support for prevention of related problems; or, in a few cases, are in the early stages of building empirical bases.

Strategies can be grouped into three complementary, interrelated categories as depicted in Table 1. The reports cited previously contain primary citations regarding the empirical bases for these interventions, and, given space limits, only a brief statement of the conceptual and/or empirical bases for the strategies is provided here. Of course, research on risk and protective factors, and

prevention and treatment approaches remains a critical strategy in this area.

1. Suicidal individuals are characterized by problem solving deficits, and youth who participated in social problem solving curricula responded more effectively to stressors, and were less likely to engage in vandalism, aggression, and alcohol use, as compared to controls (Kalafat, 1997).
2. Youth sense of bonding and connection with schools and communities and caring adults has been found to be associated with less problem behaviors such as alcohol and drug use, delinquency, sexual activity, and suicide risk (Kalafat, 1997).
3. Adolescents' prosocial competencies and provision of help have been found to be inversely related to several problem behaviors. Some adolescents, particularly males do not respond in helpful way to troubled peers (Kalafat, 1997).
4. Adolescents, particularly males, are notoriously reluctant to seek help and to comply with treatment (Clark & Gould, 1998; Kalafat, 1997).
5. Public awareness campaigns have been included in several state and national plans, but empirical evidence of their efficacy is currently lacking.
6. There is growing literature on the need for, strategies for developing, and impacts of coordinated service systems for children and youth (Illback, Cobb, & Joseph, 1997).
7. There is evidence that sensationalized reporting of suicides and media depicting suicidal behavior can lead to suicidal acts on the part of vulnerable youth. The Centers for Disease Control has developed guidelines for media reporting in this area (Centers for Disease Control, 1994).
8. There is evidence that access to firearms and other lethal means is associated with increased risk for suicide and that stricter handgun control laws may reduce suicide rates (Clark & Gould, 1998).
9. There is some evidence that physical barriers and call boxes located on bridges where there have been suicides by jumping have reduced the incidence of suicide at those sites (Clark & Gould, 1998).
10. Research indicates that youth are more likely to use hotlines than other services, although the majority of callers are females. Improved accessibility and staff training is recommended for this strategy. School-based crisis teams provide the necessary rapid, coordinated response to troubled youth (Eggert et al., 1995).

Table 1. Suicide Prevention Strategies

Enhance Individual and Environmental Protective Factors
1. Enhance individual interpersonal, problem solving, decision-making skills.
2. Enhance individual sense of connection to schools and communities through provision of opportunities and reinforcement for participation and contribution.
3. Promote social norms of caring and mutual support.
4. Promote acceptability of seeking help for oneself or others (also called reduce stigma of help seeking and mental illness).
5. Promote public awareness of suicide and resources for responding to it.
6. Promote coordination and collaboration among service agencies.
7. Increase physical, temporal, cultural, psychological, and financial accessibility to mental health services.

Identify and Address Risk Factors
8. Promote appropriate media reporting of suicide.
9. Reduce access to lethal means.
10. Erect physical barriers to common suicide sites.
11. Improve availability of and access to crisis services in communities and schools.
12. Improve professional training in treatment of mental disorders such as depression, anxiety, and substance abuse.

Identify and Treat Suicidal Individuals
13. Train adults and peers for first response to at risk youth.
14. Train community and school gatekeepers to identify, respond to, and refer at risk youth.
15. Improve professional training in risk assessment, treatment, and management of suicidal individuals.
16. Improve surveillance (including follow up research) for attempts and completions.
17. Where appropriate and feasible conduct screening for major risk factors and suicidality.
18. Provide support and follow up after suicide (postvention).
19. Provide skill building, support, and connection for suicidal youth.

11. Research indicates that many youth in need fail to access mental health services. There is a growing national movement of school-based mental health services aimed at meeting this need and evidence that these programs can attenuate problem behaviors (Illback et al., 1997).

12. Research indicates that peers are usually the first to know of an at-risk youth, but the majority of them are reluctant to tell an adult, particularly school-based adults, about their troubled peers. Recent controlled studies provide evidence that school curricula that focus on awareness of and obtaining adult help for troubled peers may increase the likelihood of this appropriate response (Kalafat, 1997).

13. Gatekeeper training has been included in a variety of state and national plans and controlled studies have shown increased knowledge and skill levels of participants (Eggert et al., 1995).

14. Professionals lack training in this area, and empirical evidence for the impact of treatment on suicidal behavior is needed (Clark & Gould, 1998).

15. Surveillance is the first step in the public health model for addressing disorders. Surveillance with regard to suicide completions has improved, but meaningful attempt data are lacking. Recent initiatives have included improved E (external cause) coding for hospital information that promises to improve attempt data.

16. Suicidal youth will self identify in screening programs, but these programs require expert interviewers as current instruments lack predictive validity (Goldston, 2000). Youths will also identify as suicidal at one time and not at a close follow-up time and vice versa, so single screenings are not sufficient. Thus, screening becomes expensive for such settings as schools. In addition, active parental consent adds to the cost of this strategy, and the medical model upon which screening is based is at odds with current school cultures.

17. Postvention programs seek to provide support for surviving family and community members and identify vulnerable youths who may be at risk for "copycat" suicide. Considerable consensus exists for postvention procedures, but empirical studies as to the impact of this strategy are lacking (Gould & Kramer, 2001).

18. Controlled evaluations of school-based indicated programs for identified at-risk youth that emphasize skill building, group support, and connection with school have provided evidence for enhanced self-efficacy and reduced suicidal risk (Kalafat, 1997).

These strategies have been listed separately, but, again, it may be most effective to combine sets of them into multifaceted, ecological programs that can be feasibly implemented by schools and communities. Ultimately, durable environmental influences may supercede the effects of interventions directed toward more proximal individual-based factors, but we are not at that point now.

Schools are seen as the nexus for most of these comprehensive strategies because most youths are found in schools, schools have a mandate to educate and protect youth, and school environments have a profound effect on youths' functioning and development. Also, there is an increasing number of school-based or school-linked integrated health, mental health, and social service systems that provide a context for multifaceted prevention approaches (Dryfoos, 1994).

As has been noted, none of these strategies can be considered empirically validated. Efforts to evaluate the proximal impacts of each of them, and the distal impacts of integrated sets of them must proceed. In the meantime, promising conceptually grounded approaches such as gatekeeper training and public awareness should continue.

Multifaceted, long-term strategies do not lend themselves to traditional experimental research designs, and present significant challenges to evaluators seeking to identify the active ingredients of prevention programs. Moreover, in order to detect the impact of programs on suicide rates, they must be disseminated with fidelity in a number of sites over a sufficient period of time.

To date, reports containing descriptions and outcome data for three comprehensive suicide prevention programs that can be described as community/ecological programs are available.

Two are school-based programs and one is a United States Air Force (USAF) program that was modeled after school-based programs. The school programs were developed and implemented by a county (New Jersey) community mental health center (Kalafat & Ryerson, 1999) and a county (Florida) public school Department of Crisis Management (Zenere & Lazarus, 1997). Each program was systematically disseminated and sustained over a period of 15 years covered by the reports in all secondary schools in urban/suburban counties that had an average of approximately 130,000 school-age youth. Each aimed to prepare schools and communities to identify, respond to, and obtain help for at-risk youth, as well as other health topics such as substance abuse, coping, and self-efficacy. The Florida program included additional health promotion programming for elementary schools. Each was comprehensive in that they promoted linkages among school and community services, and included school-based crisis teams, community crisis response capability, administrative polices and procedures, training for school personnel, parents, students, and, to a lesser extent, community gatekeepers. Follow-up studies showed a reduction in county youth suicide rates associated with the dissemination of the programs that was not replicated for the states or nationally for the same time periods (Kalafat, 2000).

The USAF explicitly conceptualized suicide as a community, rather than medical, problem and organized the program around the concept of the Competent Community (Litts, 2000). Two characteristics of competent communities are:

1. Leaders who are committed and engaged.
   - Community leaders and school officials must clearly and consistently convey the vision that in this community/school, we care deeply about the safety and positive development of all of our members.
2. Members who:
   - Share responsibility for the general welfare of the community and its members: In this community/school, we take care of each other.
   - Have collective competence in responding to suicide as a threat to the integrity of the community and the safety of its members: In this community/school, we know how to come to the assistance of those in need.

The USAF chain of command was mobilized to actively promote the concepts of mutual support, acceptance of responsibility for one's subordinates and peers, and destigmatizing help seeking through a series of policies and messages. In addition, the initiative included a surveillance database, re-engineering of human services to emphasize prevention and integrated services, annual screening and unit behavioral health surveys, gatekeeper training, and training of mental health and health professionals. In the time period after program implementation, suicide rates for USAF members decreased significantly from 16.4 to 9.4. This decline was not matched in the other service branches (MMWR, 1999).

The decline in suicide rates associated with these school and military programs cannot be directly attributed to the programs. Taken together, they meet some of the epidemiological criteria for supporting the possibility of causal relationships, including consistency of findings across studies, temporal sequence of exposure and outcome, and logical plausibility of the relationship (Potter et al., 1995); and, they provide encouraging initial support for comprehensive, community-oriented prevention approaches.

WHAT DOES NOT WORK

Experience over the past 20 years in prevention in general and youth suicide in particular has also identified what does not work, including:

- Low dosage or one-time interventions, particularly those involving large assembly presentations.
- Promoting myths about suicide or school-based programs such as talking about it with youths will stimulate suicidal behavior. There is no evidence to support this myth.
- Poorly implemented programs. Even well-designed programs will fail when they are not implemented with fidelity or by inexperienced personnel. Research has shown relationships between program implementation and outcomes (Kalafat, 2000).
- Programs that cannot or will not be implemented in given settings due to cost or conflicts with community values.
- Media that depicts suicidal behavior or feature previous attempters.
- Programs that promote one particular strategy rather than a combination of complementary strategies.

SYNTHESIS

The elements of an integrated, multidimensional youth suicide prevention strategy summarized in Table 1 cannot be implemented in communities all at once, and consideration must be given to appropriate sequencing or prioritizing. Some strategies logically precede others. For example, ensuring that mental health professionals and service systems are prepared to respond effectively to at-risk or suicidal individuals must occur before efforts to improve identification and referral and reduce the stigma of mental illness and help seeking are initiated. Surveillance methods must be in place in order to assess the impact of programs on suicidal behavior.

An example from the school-based suicide prevention initiatives can illustrate this. Comprehensive school programs start with *administrative consults* to ensure linkages with community services and the presence of policies and procedures for responding to suicidal phenomena. This is followed by *general training* for all adults in the school for responding to troubled and at-risk students. Next, *parents* receive similar training and are apprised of the school program. When these have been accomplished, classes folded into the health curricula to train *students* to respond to and obtain adult help for troubled peers. When such programs were implemented, it was often discovered that community service providers were not well trained to respond to referrals of high-risk students, or crisis services response systems were inadequate. Moreover, school-based adults were temporally and or/ culturally and psychologically inaccessible to students. Thus, changes in the organization of schools (such as reducing disciplinary roles of school counselors) and additional faculty/staff training was required; and, additional training for and integration of community services was required.

In sum, an ecological approach that takes into account the interrelationships among strategies and between persons and environments is called for. This is a daunting task that requires collaboration among community service systems, families, and schools. Models for such collaboration exist in the growing movement to address family, individual, and community risk and protective factors that affect youths' ability to succeed in school (Dryfoos, 1994; Illback et al., 1997), and such collaborations are now required components in some federal requests for prevention program proposals. The fact that suicide shares risk and protective factors with other youth psychosocial problems makes it likely that such efforts will have an impact on a variety of problem areas, and thus may increase their cost effectiveness as well as the likelihood that schools and communities will sustain them.

The competent community may serve as an effective organizing framework for integrating the strategies that have been identified for addressing youth suicide.

References

Beautrais, A. (1998). *A review of evidence: In our hands-the New Zealand youth suicide prevention strategy.* Wellington, New Zealand: Ministry of Health.

Clark, D.C., & Gould, M. (1998). *Youth suicide prevention: A national strategy.* Paper prepared for Advancing the National Strategy for Suicide Prevention: Linking Research and Practice Conference. Reno, Nevada.

Centers for Disease Control and Prevention. (1994). Suicide contagion and the reporting of suicide: Recommendations from a national workshop. *Morbidity and Mortality Weekly Report, 43,* (No. RR-6), 13–18.

Department for Policy Coordination and Sustainable Development. (1996). *Prevention of suicide: Guidelines for the formulation and implementation of national strategies.* NY: United Nations: Author.

Department of Health and Human Services (DHHS). (1992). *The third national injury control conference* (DHHS Publication No. 1992-634-666). Washington, DC: US Government Printing Office.

Dryfoos, J. (1994). *Full service schools.* San Francisco: Jossey-Bass.

Eggert, L.L., Thompson, E.A., Randell, B.P., & McCauley, E. (1995). *Youth suicide prevention plan for Washington State.* Olympia, WA: Washington State Dept. of Health.

Felner, R.D., & Felner, T.W. (1989). Primary prevention programs in the educational context: A transactional-ecological framework and analysis. In L.A. Bond & B.E. Compas (Eds.), *Primary prevention and promotion in the schools* (pp. 13–49). Newbury Park, CA: Sage.

Goldston, D. (2000). *Assessment of suicidal behaviors and risk among children and adolescents.* Technical report submitted to NIMH under Contract No. 263-MD-909995.

Gould, M.S., & Kramer, R.A. (2001). Youth suicide prevention. *Suicide and Life-Threatening Behavior, 31*(Suppl.), 6–31.

Illback, R.J., Cobb, C.T., & Joseph, H.M. (1997). *Integrated services for children and families.* Washington, DC: American Psychological Association.

Institute of Medicine (IOM). (1994). *Reducing risk for mental disorder: Frontiers for preventive intervention research.* Washington, DC: National Academy Press.

Jessor, R., Van Den Bos, J., Vanderryn, J., Costa, F.M., & Turbin, M.S. (1995). Protective factors in adolescent problem behavior: Moderator effects and developmental change. *Developmental Psychology, 31,* 923–933.

Kalafat, J. (1997). The prevention of youth suicide. In R.P. Weissberg, T.P. Gullotta, B.A. Ryan, & G.R. Adams (Eds.), *Healthy children 2010: Enhancing children's wellness* (pp. 175–213). Thousand Oaks, CA: Sage.

Kalafat, J. (2000). Issues in the evaluation of youth suicide prevention initiatives. In T. Joiner & D. Rudd (Eds.), *Suicide science: Expanding boundaries.* Boston: Kluwer Academic.

Kalafat, J., & Ryerson, D.M. (1999). The implementation and institutionalization of a school-based youth suicide prevention program. *Journal of Primary Prevention, 19,* 157–175.

Litts, D. (2000). *U. S. Air Force suicide prevention: A community based public health approach.* Presentation at public hearing on the National Suicide Prevention Plan. Boston, MA.

MMWR. (1999). *Suicide prevention among active duty Air Force personnel-United States, 1990–1999. 48*(46), 1053–1057. Atlanta, GA: Author.

NIMH Committee on Prevention Research. (1995). *A plan for prevention research for the National Institute of Mental Health* (A report to the National Advisory Mental Health Council). Washington, DC: Author.

O'Carroll, P.W., Berman, A.L., Maris, R.W., Moscicki, E., Tanney, B.L., & Silverman, M. (1996). Beyond the tower of Babel: A nomenclature for suicidology. *Suicide and Life-Threatening Behavior, 26,* 237–252.

Potter, L., Powell, K.E., & Kachur, P.S. (1995). Suicide prevention from a public health perspective. *Suicide and Life-Threatening Behavior, 25,* 82–91.

World Health Organization. (2000). *Preventing suicide: A resource guide for general physicians.* Geneva: Department of Mental Health: Author.

Youth suicide prevention: A framework for British Columbia. (1998). University British Columbia: Author.

Zenere, F.J., III, & Lazarus, P.J. (1997). The decline of youth suicidal behavior in an urban, multicultural public school system following the introduction of a suicide prevention and intervention program. *Suicide and Life-Threatening Behavior, 4,* 387–403.

Suicide, Adulthood

Brian L. Mishara

INTRODUCTION

Each year, more people die by suicide worldwide than in the combined effect of all wars, armed conflicts and terrorist attacks; and suicide rates are increasing annually (World Health Organization, 2000). Suicide is the eighth leading cause of death in the United States (Murphy, 2000) and contrary to popular belief, death by suicide is not primarily a phenomenon associated with youth. Overall in the world, as in the United States, the highest suicide rates are in the adult population and the elderly; in Canada, the highest suicide rates are in those aged 20–64.

DEFINITIONS AND SCOPE

Although it seems evident that suicide should be defined as when a persons kills himself or herself, the application of such a simple definition is often problematic. Data on deaths by suicide, called *completed suicides* (the term *"successful* suicides" is now considered politically incorrect), come from official statistics as reported by the coroner or medical examiners office in each state or province. There are significant variations in the reliability of these reports, with a general consensus that official statistics underestimate true suicide rates. In the United States in 1998, there were 11.3 completed suicides per 100,000 population per annum and in 1997, 12.3 in Canada. As is the case in most of the world, more men than women die by suicide: there are about four male completed suicides for each female in North America.

Although deaths by suicide are rare, nonlethal suicide attempts are much more common. There are at least one hundred attempts for each completed suicide. Women attempt suicide much more often then men. This sex difference has been explained by various hypotheses, including male preferences for more lethal methods, men having more severe mental health problems, and the greater reluctance by men to seek help and use social support.

If one limits the study of attempted suicide to those that involve a hospitalization, we find that there are approximately five persons hospitalized for a suicide attempt for each completed suicide (National Center for Health Statistics, 1998). However, if we rely upon self-reports of whether or not a person made a serious suicide attempt, survey data indicate that about 0.7 percent of the US population reports having attempted suicide (Crosby, Cheltenham, & Sacks, 1999). Since having attempted previously is an important risk factor in predicting completed suicides, in North America, suicide is often conceptualized along a continuum from "mild ideation" to serious intentions, attempts, and completed suicide. However, in Europe, the term "parasuicide" is used to describe suicide attempts and it is often assumed that those who attempt suicide constitute an etiologically different group with less psychopathology than suicide completers.

THEORY AND RESEARCH

Suicide has been explained by sociologists, psychologists, geneticists, biologists, anthropologists, psychiatrists, and even political analysts and economists. The classic book by Durkheim (1897) often inspires sociologists who explain variations in population suicide rates based upon a number of sociocultural factors. Psychological approaches by Freud as well as many contemporary theorists (Shneidman, 1993) explain the dynamics of suicidal tendencies based upon cognitions or intrapsychic conflicts. Some theories of suicide are "justified" by empirical data and the research literature abounds with studies of suicide rate differences based on race, economics, family situation, and literally hundreds of other variables. Despite these findings, the reality of the situation is that no subgroup of the population is spared from suicide. Despite all these correlational studies, none of the biological, socioeconomic, psychiatric, or psychological factors explain a sufficient proportion of the variance to accurately predict the future suicidal risk of individuals (Clark, 1990). For this reason there is a general consensus among those who plan prevention programs that suicide is multi-determined.

If one compares all the risk factors, the most important is being a male, and this factor is followed by having a psychiatric disorder. Although the methodologies are controversial, the vast majority (over 80 percent, if drug and alcohol abuse are included as a "psychiatric disorder") of persons who die by suicide have either been diagnosed as having a psychiatric disorder or can be classified as having had a psychiatric disorder on the basis of retrospective psychological autopsy studies (Lesage, 1994). In interpreting this finding, one must keep in mind that suicide completers still constitute a very small proportion of all persons with psychiatric disorders. Thus, this factor alone has little predictive power. Furthermore, it would be erroneous to conclude on the basis of this correlation that a psychiatric disorder "causes" suicide, just as it would be erroneous to conclude that being a male causes suicide.

What Is Being Prevented

At first blush, it would appear that primary prevention of suicide would involve actions which result in a decrease in suicide mortality. However, because of the infrequency of suicide completions, many approaches aim for a reduction in suicide attempts or reduction in ideation, assuming that reducing these will result in a decrease in suicide mortality. This assumption is based upon the untested implicit assumptions that suicidal behavior may be classified on a continuum from ideations to attempts and completed suicides.

Ethical Issues

Some contend that one should not engage in suicide prevention because individuals have a right to determine the nature and timing of their own death. This argument is in opposition to beliefs, policies, and laws in some locations that oblige citizens to prevent the death of any person in danger. Those who support the "right to suicide" usually base their belief on the view that the "choice" of suicide is the result of a rational decision-making process. However, rational decision-making is rarely observed as part of the process leading to a suicide. Most suicides involve a desperate attempt to stop what is seen as an interminable and unbearably painful life situation. The severity of the pain (called "psychache" by Shneidman, 1993) precludes logical decision-making. Reasoning is often illogical. The suicide victim's preoccupation with suicide as the solution appears at times to be the result of constricted cognitive abilities rather than a rational process.

Methodological Challenges

By definition primary prevention programs should involve actions that result in decreased rates of suicide at some future time. However, it is extremely difficult to link any future changes in suicide rates to earlier actions because of the innumerable concurrent socioenvironmental changes. Furthermore, research methods that involved experimental and control groups are impractical or unethical: it is rarely possible to intervene with one group without having others become aware of the intervention. Even more important, it is considered unethical to help some persons who are at risk of ending their own life and ignore others whose lives are also in danger. Because of these problems, controlled studies are almost non-existent.

STRATEGIES THAT WORK

Limiting Access to Means

Most people who commit suicide use one of several common methods. These include: firearms, hanging, ingesting medications or poisons, and to a lesser extent jumping from high places, asphyxiation from carbon monoxide as well as some locally available methods such as being hit by a train or a subway car. Research on firearms control provides the most conclusive proof that control of access to means may prevent deaths by suicide. Studies in the United States indicate that households with a firearm have over 6 times the risk of a completed suicide than households without a firearm. Changes in legislation controlling access to firearms appear to be related to parallel changes in suicide rates. The effectiveness of controlling access to means may be justified by the fact that this can decrease impulsive suicidal behavior. In a crisis situation, if a means of killing oneself is immediately and readily available, there is a greater risk that a person will impulsively commit suicide. However, if one must take hours, days, or weeks to procure the chosen means, there is a high probability that the extent of the crisis will be diminished by that time.

Subway systems, such as in Singapore and in Lyon, in which access to the tracks is barred by an automatic door system do not have suicides. In England, creating so-called "suicide pits" between the rails in stations which allow persons to fall underneath the train appear to significantly decrease deaths by suicide. A number of other methods of reducing subway suicides are being tested, including that in Japan of putting mirrors opposite the platform so potential jumpers can see themselves, reducing the speed of the entrance of trains in the stations, computerized analyses of television monitors which provide automatic signals of suspicious activities to train drivers coming into a station (in Montreal), as well as providing telephone help lines and suicide prevention posters in stations.

Similarly, one may prevent access to certain high-risk areas, including some bridges. Studies by Seiden (1978) of suicides at the Golden Gate Bridge in San Francisco indicate that people who are intercepted before they jump generally do not kill themselves afterwards by another means.

There is currently an international movement to install carbon monoxide detectors which stop the motor in all new vehicles. It is also being recommended that automobile exhaust pipes be shaped in a manner which would make it difficult to attach the type of standard hoses which are often used in suicides. The cost of these vehicular modifications would be minimum, but action on the part of government regulating agencies appears to be slow moving.

Influencing Media Reporting on Suicide

Many years of research focus upon the complex issue of media reports increasing the risk of death by suicide. Recent reviews show that media reports often increase the risk of suicide among persons whose characteristics are similar to those of the victim, or when the report is about an admired celebrity (Stack, 2000). Depictions of suicidal deaths are related to increased suicide rates, regardless of what is said or done after the death is depicted. One of the most impressive instances of an intervention limiting media reports was in the Vienna subway where for several years suicidal deaths in the media received much public attention and subway suicides became increasingly frequent. Once the Austrian suicide prevention association convinced reporters to stop reporting on subway suicides, subway suicide rates diminished greatly and there was no concurrent increase in suicides by other methods.

Recently, there has been an emphasis upon the way suicides are reported rather than the fact of reporting or not. Studies indicate clearly that the extent to which suicides are given attention or "glamorized" influences the extent of its impact.

Physician Training

Studies show that at least one out of five persons consult a physician in the month before they kill themselves. There is much speculation about the reasons for this consultation. Some skeptics feel that this is simply an attempt to obtain lethal medications. However, these consultations are generally viewed as an attempt to seek help. Training programs for general practitioners may be justified by the effects of the educational program given by the Swedish Committee for the Prevention and Treatment of Depression to all the general practitioners of the Island of Gotland. This was evaluated based upon baseline data before the program as compared to data obtained after the training. Besides finding a 30 percent decrease in the frequency of sick leave for depressive disorders and an increase in the prescription of antidepressants (paralleled by a decrease in the prescription of major tranquillizers, sedatives, and hypnotics), they found a significant decrease in the frequency of suicide on the island (Rutz, von Knorring, & Walinder, 1989). However, 3 years after the project ended, inpatient care for depressive disorders increased, the suicide rate returned almost to the baseline values while levels of prescription of antidepressants did not change (Rutz et al., 1992). It was concluded that educational programs can have significant effects on suicide, but they need to be repeated if long-term effects are to be expected. This research is frequently cited as "proof" that greater prescription of antidepressants and increased identification and medical treatment of depressive disorders may prevent suicides. However, since suicide rates increased 3 years after the training, but prescriptions of antidepressants did not decrease, the author of this entry wonders if the positive effects of the educational program may be also due to increased communication with physicians when they were made more aware of the specific needs of suicidal and depressed clients.

STRATEGIES THAT MIGHT WORK

Broad-Based Mental Health Promotion Approaches

Suicide is related to a variety of socio-environmental and economic factors which also increase the risk of other problems. For example, it appears that people with drug-abuse problems and victims of abuse are at greater risk of suicide. Preventing drug-related problems and diminishing abuse has wide ranging benefits, with suicide prevention being just one of many. Many programs which improve people's health and well-being have positive effects in preventing suicide.

Educational Approaches

Persons who are suicidal rarely keep their thoughts and feelings to themselves. They usually give indications of their suicidal intentions to others. These indications are usually in the form of verbalizations, sometimes explicit and sometimes less direct (e.g., "I don't think I can go on living like this"). Thus, several health promotion strategies focus upon educating individuals and groups about suicide. The implicit hypothesis underlying these activities is that if individuals learn more about suicide, particularly how to identify when someone is suicidal, to respond appropriately and to know how and where to refer to help, this will prevent suicide.

In some instances, these strategies focus upon the general population, for example, in a broad public campaign such as a *Suicide Prevention Week*. For example, the Quebec Suicide Prevention Week has been happening for 11 years. Each year, during the week, there are regular television and radio announcements with a well-known spokesperson as well as numerous regional activities. The effects of the Quebec Suicide Prevention Week campaign over 3 years were evaluated, using a social marketing model (Daigle, Brisoux, Beausoleil, Raymond, & Charbonneau, 2001). The researchers identified the messages that the campaign for the week attempted to convey and assessed the effectiveness of this activity in conveying those messages. In a survey of the target population of adult men before and after this activity, they found that 43 percent of men recalled being exposed to the campaign and 24 percent were able to recall specific target messages. Whether or not remembering the messages is actually related to behavioral changes and suicide prevention remains to be seen.

Among those who call to suicide prevention centers, as many as 10–15 percent of callers are friends and family members of persons who are suicidal who request help or information about what they should do for their suicidal friend or relative. These so-called "third party" callers are often supported on the phone and given instructions about identifying suicide risk and how to talk about the problem and refer a suicidal person for help. Five different pilot programs which involve offering more intensive help and training to third party callers are currently being evaluated by the author of this entry at Suicide-Action Montreal including family therapy with the suicidal person, face-to-face meetings and education sessions, continued telephone support, and group information sessions.

National Suicide Prevention Programs

Given the multi-determined nature of suicide, when countries try to reduce suicide rates, they generally take an approach that involves a wide variety of concurrent actions. The first countries in Europe to produce national suicide prevention strategies were Finland in 1957, Norway in 1993, and Sweden in 1995. These programs focused on mobilizing professionals in various areas throughout the country to develop suicide prevention activities locally.

The Finnish national program *Suicide Can Be Prevented* first focused on having professionals from all sectors involved by joining the suicide prevention network (Hakanen & Upanne, 1996). When a survey questionnaire was sent to 6,000 professionals, 1,800 replied and 1,200 said that they had some kind of activity or interest in the program and 1,100 said they had joined the contact network as a representative of their unit. Most persons who joined (40–60 percent) were professionals in the health sector and other sectors involved included schools, church, police, and rescue services. There were 200 local suicide prevention projects developed as part of this program, of which 42 percent were specifically concerned with preventing suicides. About 25 percent concerned handling and treatment of crisis situations, including support for the relatives of suicide victims. There were also some general health promotion programs, for example, 7 percent involved supporting people's coping skills.

There are no outcome data from the Finnish national program, and even if there were, these data would be difficult to interpret. However those who participated in the program felt that their actions can prevent suicides and there appears to be great enthusiasm for participation in the programs. Respondents reported improvement in understanding suicidal risk factors, enhanced multi-sector and multi-professional involvement in suicide prevention, improved recognition of needs and greater respect for suicide prevention activities. There was more discussion of suicide matters with clients and among colleagues and increases in the development of prevention methods.

The *Quebec Provincial Suicide Prevention Strategy* (Government of Québec, 1998) began in 1998. The first goal of the Quebec strategy is to provide and consolidate essential services and end the isolation of caregivers throughout the province who are confronted with suicidal individuals or involved in suicide prevention activities. Each region is mandated to identify a person or organization responsible for local leadership and to involve all regional agencies and individuals interested and involved in suicide prevention in developing a regional action plan. The strategy leaves it to each region to determine who is going to be involved in which essential activities. The regional goals include the improvement of professional skills by training all practitioners in the diagnosis of depression, in adjustment problems and in treatment strategies, and specific training in working with suicidal persons and people who are bereaved by suicide. Furthermore, each region should provide for a series of services for persons who are suicidal ranging from telephone help for those who want to discuss their problems to specific intervention strategies with individuals in crisis or who are hospitalized after an attempt. In addition, each region should develop specific prevention strategies for groups at greater risk of suicide. General priorities for these strategies for high-risk groups include: men at risk of suicide, particularly men with problems of substance abuse or dependency (drugs, alcohol, other), men and young people with mental disorders, men in prison, and men presenting a number of risk factors. Another high-risk group for attempts is young women between the ages of 14 and 19 with multiple risk factors as well as men and women who have made previous suicide attempts.

The Quebec program encourages voluntary and non-professional organizations to be intimately involved in the planning and implementation of the Provincial Suicide Prevention Strategy at the regional level. In addition, this strategy calls for mental health promotion strategies and prevention programs among young people. These include school programs to reinforce personal and social skills and to promote a favorable environment for the adoption of healthy lifestyles, and the development of suicide prevention programs in schools. The strategy also calls for the development of regional response teams to work with schools in cases of suicide and attempted suicide. In addition to these regional activities, the strategy involves a number of actions to reduce access and to minimize risks associated with the means of suicide. This includes greater control of firearms in the home of persons at risk of suicide, protecting bridges and other dangerous sites, restricting access to stocks of medications frequently associated with suicide attempts, and attempts to change the regulations concerning motor vehicle manufacturing to equip cars with devices that would switch off the motor when there is a dangerous level of carbon monoxide in the vehicle.

In addition to the specific regional actions, there is a provincial action to attempt to counteract the trivialization and the sensationalization of suicide by developing a sense of community and media responsibility. These actions include support of a Quebec National Suicide Prevention Week which has been run for several years by the Quebec Association of Suicidology. Furthermore, the Quebec Government funded a number of pilot projects in order to evaluate and develop different specific methods of suicide prevention throughout the province. Unfortunately, evaluation data on the Quebec program are not yet available.

Telephone Help Lines

Despite the proliferation of crisis intervention services throughout the world, there is little concrete data indicating that these services are generally helpful or are effective in preventing suicide. Mishara and Daigle (2000) conclude that there is some evidence from different sources that the presence of a suicide prevention or crisis telephone help line may reduce suicide rates in the population which is characteristic of callers, but more research is needed. Their own studies found short-term positive effects on callers which were related to certain intervention styles (Mishara & Daigle, 1997). Since telephone help lines have a rapidly increasing clientele (and they have branched out into Internet services), it is crucial to identify their effects and more specifically which intervention methods or approaches may be proven useful in preventing suicide.

STRATEGIES THAT DO NOT WORK

As with all evaluative research, programs which are failures are rarely diffused and evaluative research showing no results are rarely published in journals on suicidology. Clinical experience as well as naturalistic observations of suicide prevention programs around the world indicate that there are no simple short-term prevention strategies which appear to have a significant or long lasting effect on population suicide rates. Therefore, a combination of strategies has been adopted in all national suicide prevention programs.

Legislature to make suicide illegal and punishing attempters is not related to decreased suicide rates. Furthermore, rates do not increase when suicide is decriminalized, although more accurate reporting on suicides may be encouraged. Furthermore, legislation in the Netherlands allowing for the practices of euthanasia and assisted suicide with terminally ill persons has not resulted in either an increase or a decrease in suicide rates in that country.

It is clear from research on media influences that publicizing suicides, even when the publicity purports to be dissuasive by decrying a horrible or wasteful death, often has the inverse effect of increasing the probability of imitation behavior. Furthermore, advances in psychiatry, and particularly the use of psychotropic medications to treat mental disorders, while they certainly may save some lives, have not resulted in significant declines in suicide rates in the late 20th century. Therefore, a strictly medical approach to the problem does not appear to be warranted.

SYNTHESIS

Given the methodological and ethical difficulties, we have very little evidence that any primary prevention programs have had a significant effect upon population suicide rates. Also, since suicide is a relatively infrequent phenomenon and is multi-determined, simple causal models are impossible. Despite these problems, many actions appear to be effective in decreasing suicide. For example, the training of physicians in Gotland appears to have had a short-term effect in reducing suicide. But, there is always the risk that this was a Hawthorne effect. That is, it is possible that doing anything to focus attention on depression or suicide will be effective in preventing suicide. We simply do not have the data to reach definitive conclusions at this time and it looks like the necessary research data to even approximate conclusions is not going to appear in the near future.

The lack of conclusive research has not stopped people from engaging in a wide variety of suicide prevention activities. This may be explained by the fact that, although there is no conclusive research evidence that suicide prevention activities decrease populations suicide rates, there are thousands of volunteers and professionals around the world who have had the personal subjective experience of having saved someone's life. Second, there is a pervasive general impression that one cannot wait until conclusive research evidence is available to engage in the primary prevention of suicide. Deaths by suicide are simply far too devastating a phenomenon worldwide for individuals, agencies, and governments to simply sit back and do nothing. For this reason, planners and strategists scrutinize the available meager evidence of effectiveness and continue to try different programs. In many cases these programs have at least a firm theoretical basis. However, far more often they are developed on the basis of personal experiences and clinical impressions. Also, since suicide prevention programs generally do some good for people, they can be encouraged whether or not they actually prevent suicides.

There have been no miraculous breakthroughs in suicide prevention in the known history of the human race. It appears that certain primary prevention strategies may prevent some suicides in some populations or at least may prevent increases in suicide as risk factors exert their effects. The late 20th century development of new medications to treat depression and other mental disorders has certainly helped some individuals and prevented some suicides. However there is no clear evidence that the use of these medications has significantly decreased suicide rates. However, the risk of suicide appears to decrease when access to means is limited. Nevertheless, it is impossible to control access to all suicide methods. There is research evidence that psychotherapy by a skilled therapist will decrease the risk of a suicide in high-risk clients based on case-controlled studies. Nevertheless, the increased availability of psychotherapy in the past decades has not stemmed increases in suicide rates for adults.

An important debate in suicidology is whether or not there is a need for specific suicide prevention programs or that the primary prevention of suicide can be accomplished by more general health promotion programs. Many of the wide-ranging health promotion strategies which are the topic areas of the other entries in this book may help prevent suicide. We probably need both general health promotion activities to prevent distress and programs with a specific suicide content. Furthermore, in certain high-risk groups, we may be able to develop very specific programs. Although these high-risk groups, such as Native populations and men in prisons, are extremely challenging, it may be that because of the possibility of access to the entire high-risk population, programs for these target groups may offer the potential to be more successful.

Perhaps the positive effects of prevention programs are masked by an increase in socio-environmental and cultural risk factor for suicide. The implications of this optimistic view of the effects of prevention activities (and pessimistic view of overall progress in society) suggest that we need to continue all of the various programs now available and increase research efforts to evaluate their effectiveness. A more pessimistic view would suggest that we have yet to develop sufficiently effective primary prevention strategies for suicide and that more creative approaches need to be taken.

Perhaps it is a question of dosage: most programs are limited to a few hours of training or brief exposure to educational messages. Effective primary prevention program may need to involve very intensive long lasting activities which are provided to a large proportion of a population and which may take many years to evaluate.

Also see: Suicide entries.

References

Clark, D. (1990). Suicide risk assessment and prediction in the 1990s. *Crisis, 11*(2), 104–112.

Crosby, A.E., Cheltenham, M.P., & Sacks, J.J. (1999). Incidence of suicidal ideation and behavior in the United States, 1994. *Suicide and Life-Threatening Behavior, 29*(2), 131–140.

Daigle, M., Brisoux, J., Beausoleil, L., Raymond, S., & Charbonneau, L. (2001). *Progrès vers une semaine de prévention du suicide plus utile.* 62ᵉ congrès de la Société Canadienne de psychologie, Université Laval, Québec.

Durkheim, E. (1897). *Le suicide: Étude de sociologie.* Paris: Alcan.

Government of Québec. (1998). Help for life: Quebec's strategy for preventing suicide. Quebec: Ministère de la Santé et des Services sociaux.

Hakanen, J., & Upanne, M. (1996). Evaluation strategy for Finland's suicide prevention project. *Crisis, 17*(4), 167–174.

Lesage, A. (1994). Suicide and mental disorders: A case-control study of young men. *American Journal of Psychiatry, 151*(7), 1063–1068

Mishara, B.L., & Daigle, M. (1997). Effects of different telephone intervention styles with suicidal callers at two suicide prevention centers: An empirical investigation. *American Journal of Community Psychology, 25*(6), 861–895.

Mishara, B.L., & Daigle, M. (2000). Helplines and crisis intervention services: Challenges for the future. In D. Lester (Ed.), *Suicide prevention: Resources for the millennium* (pp. 153–171). Philadelphia: Brunner/Mazel.

Murphy, S.L. (2000). Deaths: Final data for 1998, *National Vital Statistics Reports, 48*(11). Hyatts.

National Center for Health Statistics. (1998). *National hospital discharge survey 1996–1998. Public Use data file and documentation.* ftp://ftp.cdc.gov/pub/Health_Statistics/NCHS/Datasets/NHDS

Rutz, W., von Knorring, L., & Walinder, J. (1989). Frequency of suicide on Gotland after systematic postgraduate education of general practitioners. *Acta Psychiatrica Scandinavica, 80,* 151–154.

Rutz, W., von Knorring, L., & Walinder, J. (1992). Long-term effects of an educational program for general practitioners given by the Swedish Committee for the Prevention and Treatment of Depression. *Acta Psychiatrica Scandinavica, 85,* 83–88.

Seiden, R.H. (1978) Where are they now? A follow-up study of suicide attempters from the Golden Gate Bridge. *Suicide and Life-Threatening Behavior, 8*(4), 203–216.

Shneidman, E. (1993). *Suicide as psychache. A clinical approach to self-destructive behavior.* Jason-Aronson.

Stack, S. (2000). Media impacts on suicide: A quantitative review of 293 findings. *Social Sciences Quarterly, 81*(4), 975–988.

World Health Organization. (2000). Statistics on suicide worldwide. Publicuse datasets. Geneva: Author.

Suicide, Older Adulthood

Brian L. Mishara

INTRODUCTION

This entry considers suicide and its prevention in persons over 65. Contrary to popular beliefs that suicide is a phenomenon of youth, in developed countries persons over age 65 usually have the highest suicide rates, and worldwide suicide statistics indicate a dramatic increase in suicide rates with advanced age (World Health Organization [WHO], 2000). This association between suicide and old age is evident in the United States where the highest suicide rate for all age-gender-race groups is in White men over age 85 (Murphy, 2000). White men over 85 had in 1996 a suicide rate of 65.4 per 100,000 population, which is almost six times the rate for all other age groups. Despite the association between increased suicide risk and advanced age, few primary prevention programs focus upon older persons.

DEFINITIONS

The definitions of *completed suicide, attempted suicide,* and *suicidal ideation* in the chapter on Suicide in Adulthood are the same as used with the elderly. However, in this chapter it would be useful to add definitions of *assisted suicide* and *euthanasia*. *Euthanasia* involves actions that cause a premature death, which are initiated by another person, with or without the victim's consent. Withdrawing and withholding life-sustaining treatment can fall into this category, as well as direct actions, which result in death. Furthermore, the motivations for euthanasia and the nature of prevention activities in terminally ill persons appear to be different from the dynamics of suicide (Mishara, 1999). However, *assisted suicide* warrants some attention in this entry.

In Europe, *assisted suicide* is generally understood to be when another person (usually a physician) provides the means of killing oneself (e.g., by providing lethal medication). *Assisted suicide* is also used to describe the situation when another person provides information as to how to end one's life. Individuals then use those means to end their lives by themselves. If one accepts this definition, then *assisted suicide* constitutes a specific instance of suicidal behavior which should be covered in this chapter. However, in North America many people are confused by the term *assisted suicide*. This confusion stems from the fact that some, for example Dr. Jack Kevorkian, claimed that their direct action to end another person's life was not murder or the specific form of "humane" killing called "*euthanasia*," but rather was a case of "*assisted suicide*" because the other person requested that the person end their life. As argued elsewhere (Mishara, 1998), whenever another person initiates the actions that result in death, this cannot be considered killing oneself or a form of suicide. This must be identified in one of the categories of actions by another which result in death, that is, murder, mercy killing, or the specific form of killing for humane reasons which is called *euthanasia*.

SCOPE

Suicide Statistics. In the United States suicide rates increase with age with the highest rates being for persons over age 85 (Murphy, 2000). However in Canada, the peak rates are from age 20 to 64 (but remain high for men over age 65). The elderly made up 12.7 percent of the 1998 population in the United States but commit 19 percent of the suicides. There are more elderly women than men in developed countries, since the life expectancy of women is longer than the life expectancy of men. Nevertheless, in the United States 84 percent of elderly suicides are by men and elderly men's rates are seven times those of elderly women. In the general population, when we consider all age groups combined, there are at least 100 attempts for each completed suicide. However, over age 65 there are only four attempts for each completed suicide. Thus, although older adults attempt suicide less often than in other age groups, they have a much greater likelihood of dying from an attempt.

In the United States the elderly most frequently use firearms with 78 percent of men and 36 percent of women using this method. Despite common beliefs that the elderly who commit suicide are often terminally ill, only 2–4 percent of persons over age 65 who die by suicide have been diagnosed with a terminal illness at the time of their death (American Association of Suicidology, 1999) and at least two thirds of older adults in their late sixties, seventies, and eighties were in relatively good health when they died by suicide.

The lower ratio of attempts to completed suicides in the elderly may be interpreted in three different ways: First, because older persons generally have a lower overall physical reserve capacity, attempts which would have non-lethal outcomes in younger and generally healthier individuals may be more likely to result in death. Second, this difference may be explained by the preference among the elderly for more lethal means for suicide, such as firearms. A third interpretation is that older persons are more "certain" of their desire to end their lives and thus are more likely to complete their attempts and are less likely to choose obviously non-lethal methods as a "cry for help." There are data supporting the first two explanations, but the third explanation is controversial and lacks empirical validation.

There is a general consensus that suicide rates for older adults considerably underestimate the extent of suicide in this population and that these underestimates are much more prevalent than for any other age group. In younger age groups, more care is generally taken to correctly classify deaths as due to natural causes, accident, suicide, or homicide. However, there is a tendency to under-investigate possible suicidal deaths in the elderly. This is simply due to the fact that most persons over age 65 have chronic illnesses, which risk foreshortening their lives and elders tend to take several medications on a regular basis. Thus, when an elderly person who suffers from a life threatening illness, such as heart disease is found dead in his bed, it is unlikely that there will be an investigation to determine if the death was due to a medication overdose, or to his not taking necessary medication for the heart disease. When the method of suicide does not involve a violent means, such as hanging or a firearm, there is less likelihood that there will be a detailed investigation unless there are obvious indications that it was a suicide.

Most of the attention in research on suicide in the elderly has focused upon direct actions to end one's life, which can clearly be identified as suicidal. However, there are many indirect or more subtle means of increasing the risk of a premature death which are generally not identified as suicidal behaviors. For example, an older person may not take a medication prescribed for a heart condition despite his knowledge that this will increase the likelihood that he will die. Similarly, an older person may not dress warm enough for cold weather or insist on shoveling snow despite a doctor's warning that strenuous activity is dangerous. One can add to this list many other self-injurious behaviors, such as not sticking to dietary restrictions (e.g., in the case of a diabetic). Some may go so far as to include much more common behaviors which are associated with an eventual risk of premature death, such as smoking cigarettes. Although the suicidology research literature has generally focused upon the more dramatic direct behaviors which immediately result in death, there are indications that a great number of older persons engage in self-injurious behaviors which in the short run do not have lethal outcome, but which greatly increase the probability of dying prematurely nevertheless.

THEORIES

None of the contemporary theories of suicide indicate that suicide in the elderly should be treated as different from other age groups. Suicide is multi-determined and there are no simple explanations that permit the accurate prediction of suicidal behavior in any age group. However, one may examine whether or not various risk factors for suicide may be more or less present in the older population in a specific culture and whether or not prevention strategies need to be specifically adapted to older persons.

One may also ask if the biological, social, psychological, and cultural theories of aging have specific implications for our understanding of suicide in older persons. I summarized those theories in a textbook on aging (Mishara & Riedel, 1994). Although it may be fascinating to interpret suicidal behavior on the basis of these theories, there is simply no empirical proof that the theories of aging have anything useful to say about suicide. It does not appear that psychological

changes associated with old age are related to suicidal behavior. For example, one could predict that the wisdom from life experiences would protect elders from suicide. However, one can just as easily predict that the realization of decline, personal losses and the approach of death would result in depression and increased risk of suicide. The reality remains that in many countries the suicide rate for older persons is the highest of all age groups but in some other countries it is the lowest. Furthermore, empirical studies of the etiology of suicide in older persons indicate that, although the nature of the losses and stresses may sometimes be age specific (e.g., retirement and entering a nursing home are specific stresses for elders), suicide remains a very rare event and the dynamics of suicide do not appear to be age specific.

Some Characteristics of Suicide in Older Persons. One of the most striking findings concerning elderly suicide is the fact that at least 20 percent of older persons had been seen by a physician within 24 hr of committing suicide, 24 percent had been seen by a physician within a week before their completed suicide, and 75 percent had seen a primary care physician within a month of their suicide (American Association of Suicidology, 1999.) We know very little about the reasons for these consultations, however it is often suggested that these were unsuccessful attempts to seek help. One may conclude that since there were subsequent deaths by suicide, there was inadequate identification of the suicidal risk or depressive symptoms by the physician and that appropriate interventions were not undertaken. According to psychological autopsy studies, between 66 and 90 percent of elderly suicides can be classified as having at least one psychiatric diagnosis, and in about two thirds of cases this diagnosis is of late-onset single episode clini-cal depression (Conwell, 1996). It is estimated that up to 75 percent of depressed older Americans do not receive appropriate treatment for their depression.

In their review of factors related to suicide in seniors, Dyck, Mishara, and White (1998) found that suicide in persons over 65 was related to a number of factors in the social and economic environment, including limited income, retirement, widowhood in men, lack of social support, and media reporting on elderly suicides. Suicide was related to two key factors in the physical environment: placement in a nursing home and the availability of lethal means, particularly a firearm and lethal medications. In the area of personal health practices, alcoholism, and substance abuse are less related to suicide in the elderly than in other age groups. However, misuse and side-effects of prescription and over-the-counter medications are linked to depression and increased suicide risk. Also, help seeking in the current generation of elders is mostly limited to consulting physicians, and the current generation of elders infrequently use mental health services.

As in the case of suicide in adulthood, mental health problems, particularly depression appear to be omnipresent in later life suicides. Therefore, it is important to determine the possible causes of depression in the elderly. It was previously mentioned that older persons generally take several medications. Many of those medications have side effects of depressive reactions, which can increase the risk of suicide (Mishara & Legault, 2000).

Losses are often cited as precipitating of suicide in younger persons as well as the elderly. Losses include death of a spouse, loss of job and the associated loss of role in society, loss of physical abilities, decreased income, and so forth. In all instances, it is important to look at sex differences in reaction to loss. For example, in the United States, widowhood in men dramatically increases the likelihood that a man will die in the year following the death of his spouse. However, women's life expectancies *increase* when their husband dies.

Since losses are omnipresent in old age, one may speculate why more older persons do not end their life by suicide. One explanation is the fact that vulnerability to suicide may be acquired earlier in life and that most persons at risk of ending their lives by suicide would have probably done so long before they reach old age. If one makes it to an advanced age, that may be an indication that the person has the ability to cope with loss and change and the challenges associated with the later part of life.

One cannot discuss suicide in the elderly without bring up the topic of religion. The current generation of elders is more likely to report religious practices and beliefs than younger age groups. Often these beliefs include condemnation of suicide. Sometimes these beliefs are a source of solace when one is faced with a difficult situation which leads one to think about committing suicide. However, in some instances, these religious beliefs may have the paradoxical effect of increasing a person's sense of guilt about his or her suicidal intentions. Rather than preventing the suicide, the sense of guilt for their suicidal thoughts can result in a decrease in their sense of self-worth and thus lead to greater despair and higher suicide risk.

Cohort Differences. Whenever we consider the population of older adults, it is important to note that the current generation of elders is different from past and future generations of older persons. The current generation is different because of their unique life experiences associated with being born and raised at a certain period in the history of the world and in its specific cultural context. These cohort differences, based upon when one is born may result in important changes in the nature of suicide in elders as the next cohort of the baby-boom generation become the older adults in our society. Cohort differences may also have important implications for primary prevention. For example, the current generation of elders rarely calls the suicide prevention help lines. This may be explained by cohort differences: today's elders grew up before telephones were widely available and also were never acculturated to picking up the phone and talking to a stranger to get help. Furthermore, the current generation of elders is more likely to have learned earlier in their lives that seeking help from a psychiatrist or psychologist for "mental" problems is an indication that a person is "crazy" and perhaps could be locked up in a mental institution.

Although older persons rarely use telephone help lines now, this may change in the near future as today's technologically sophisticated adults age. In considering any primary prevention strategies, it is important to keep in mind that the cohort group for which the program is developed may change in future years. As different cohort groups become the older adults in our society our understanding and planning of prevention programs must be adjusted to effectively meet their needs.

Ethical Issues. In the later years, the issue of choosing to die by suicide as an ethical choice becomes a more central issue. Organizations that promote suicide, assisted suicide, and euthanasia in persons who are terminally ill or who suffer from chronic illnesses, such as the Hemlock Society, have hundreds of thousands of members worldwide. These organizations promote the idea that one may rationally choose to end one's life and if one so chooses, he/she should have appropriate means available. Survey studies consistently show that the general population considers that the death of an older person who is suffering from a chronic debilitating disease is more acceptable than the death of a healthy or a younger person. In questionnaire studies, people go so far as to characterize many older persons as "better off dead" than to continue living with degenerative disorders. This belief was characterized several years ago by a member of the British Parliament who seriously proposed that all health care services be cut off after age 65.

Regardless of negative attitudes towards aging, the elderly themselves have no general desire to die prematurely. For example, the recent Quebec Health Survey data (Daveluy, Pica, Audet, Courtemanche, & Lapointe, 2000) have shown consistently that the elderly are the happiest of all age groups, are the most pleased of all age groups with their social supports and family relations and that elders experience the least psychological distress of all age groups. Although the elderly generally do not fit the stereotype of being abandoned (there is no evidence that the elderly in America are abandoned by their families or becoming increasingly dependant) nor unhappy, there are obviously some older adults who are sufficiently distressed to end their lives by suicide. However, there is basis for concern that in many instances where the so-called "rational" decisions to kill oneself occur, those decisions are actually highly emotionally charged because of the extent of anguish or depression the person is experiencing. If it is possible by relatively simple interventions to control the pain, prevent the depression, or diminish a person's anxiety by offering comfort from another person, society should provide this care before considering providing means or encouragement for suicide.

Negative Attitudes toward Helping Older Adults. Freud felt that psychotherapy was not indicated for older persons because of the extent of their accumulated subconscious material. Similarly, the beliefs that it is too late to consider primary prevention with older persons are widespread among caregivers and program planners. However, if one examines the outcome studies of psychotherapy, treatment, and prevention projects, regardless of the methods used in the programs, the results indicate clearly that the elderly generally respond as well as and frequently better than younger age groups. Therefore, one of the first challenges in any primary prevention program with older adults is to understand and influence the pervasive attitudes that it is too late to change when one reaches an advanced age and the erroneous beliefs that older persons cannot benefit from prevention programs as well as younger people.

STRATEGIES THAT WORK

Improving Living Conditions and Increasing Health and Welfare Support

Any programs within a society which increase the involvement of older persons in their community, improve their well-being, increase their economic status, and provide better health care are likely to result in decreased suicidal behavior. One of the explanations for the fact that in Quebec, unlike many developed areas of the world, the elderly have a relatively low suicide rate compared to other age groups, is the fact that older people in Quebec benefit from a wide range of social services and health care programs which guarantee a relatively comfortable income, complete health care, including home care services at no cost, and a variety of programs, including outlawing forced retirement based upon age, which may increase participation by elders in their community. However, there is a skeptical interpretation of the relatively low elderly suicide rates in Quebec. The skeptics contend that the current cohort of elders in Quebec had such a difficult time earlier in life that these social, economic, and health programs are more greatly appreciated. However, in the coming years, as the baby-boom generation becomes the older population, their expectations will be much greater and they will continue to have the high suicide rates they experienced in their middle years or they may even become more likely to commit suicide.

When one compares older persons in Quebec with other age groups, it is the elders who have the lowest levels of psychological distress and they are the most content with their relationships with family and social supports, their social life and older persons give more instrumental and emotional support to their children than they receive

(Daveluy et al., 2000). Given the association between suicide in older adults and isolation, low-income, health problems, and depression, it is possible that if the positive services and programs like those provided for the Quebec older population were present in countries with high elder suicide rates, a reduction in those rates may be observed.

STRATEGIES THAT MIGHT WORK

Controlling Access to Means

Because of the large numbers of older persons who use guns as a means of suicide in the United States and elsewhere, gun control is a promising method of suicide prevention. The presence of a firearm in a home increases the likelihood of a death by suicide by 600 percent. If more strict general gun control practices are not possible, another option would be to adopt and publicize laws and procedures which would encourage and allow physicians who are aware that an older person is depressed and at risk of suicide to have all firearms removed from the home. Also, programs that educate family members about the risks of having a firearm available to a depressed or suicidal elder and information about how to have the firearm removed from the home may prevent many suicides.

Elders who use medications to kill themselves often have a large variety of excess medications on hand in their homes. If physicians prescribe and pharmacists dispense medications in smaller quantities and programs are initiated to ensure that unused medications are returned to a pharmacy, many lives may be saved.

Education of Physicians

Since so many older adults who commit suicide consult a physician shortly before their death, it may be useful to train physicians to better recognize depression in older persons and to evaluate suicidal intentions more systematically. The World Health Organization has on its Web site a training document for physicians on identifying suicidal risk and the treatment of suicide and depression. Despite this and other initiatives, there is still a reluctance on the part of many caregivers, including physicians, to do what they are taught in education programs on suicide prevention. They are often reluctant to ask direct questions such as "Have you been thinking of killing yourself?" in order to evaluate if there is significant suicidal risk. It may be that continuing educations programs for physicians and other caregivers will have better results than the distribution of informative booklets. Several ongoing evaluations of physician training programs should provide important additional information on the effectiveness of this approach in preventing suicide in older persons.

Programs for Widowed Men and the Isolated Elderly

The isolated elderly are of particular risk, particularly men who are recently widowed. There are numerous programs to help newly widowed persons adjust to life after losing a spouse. Many of these programs, for example the *Widow-to-Widows* program (Silverman, 1970), which exists in many areas of the United States, involves using widows to help other widows. This successful model might be expanded to serve men. Besides the need for emotional support after the death of a spouse, many widowers need to learn concrete ways of continuing activities in daily life, such as shopping for food, cooking, and doing laundry.

The *Gatekeeper Model* developed in Spokane, Washington (Raschko, 1990) targeted older persons who were living in their own homes, but isolated and lacking social support. Their target population suffered from physical illness, memory impairment, emotional problems, environmental stress, and had difficulties with personal care and daily living. The program involved training workers who come into contact with these high-risk elders to identify problems and ensure that community based services are provided to meet their needs. This program was proactive in that it involved seeking out those elders who have multiple risk factors but whose needs were not being met and linking them with various sources of help. Although there are no outcome evaluation data on suicide risk, this type of program looks promising because it makes use of knowledge of factors related to suicide in older persons.

Telephone Surveillance Programs

De Leo, Carollo, and Dello-Buono (1995) evaluated the effects of a program specifically focused upon suicide prevention in Italy. This program, called *Tele-Help* was provided for 12,136 older persons upon their discharge from hospital. The program included the availability of help for a problem over the phone and each participant was provided with a portable device capable of sending an alarm signal in the event an emergency situation. Having this system in place resulted in a decrease in home visits by general practitioners and a reduced number of hospital admissions. In the 4 years during which the program was in place there was only one suicide, which compares with the expected number of suicides for this population during the same time period of 7.44. It may be that the feeling of security, which this program provided resulted in a decreased level of anxiety and general distress and that this had a preventive effect on suicides.

Prevention with the Terminally Ill and Seriously Chronically Ill

In a monograph summarizing research and evidence on factors effecting the desire of terminally and chronically ill persons to hasten death, Mishara (1999) concluded that although persons who are terminally and chronically ill are at greater risk of suicide, only a small percentage of these persons take their own lives. Research indicates that the etiology of suicide differs greatly with each illness. In the case of cancer, better pain control and palliative care appear to be linked to less suicide risk. However, with most other debilitating diseases, treatment of depression is often cited as the best means of preventing suicides. Although there is no clear evidence that treating depression in persons who are gravely ill actually prevents suicide, there are clinical reports that programs identifying and treating depression have beneficial effects. However, in some instances the source of the depression is a side effect of the medication or physical treatment used to treat the illness or alleviate suffering. In other instance the depression may be a reaction to the social isolation and physical restrictions imposed by the illness. Regardless of its origins, education programs for caregivers and family members which focus upon helping to identify problems and to understand that suicide may be prevented by improving the quality of life of persons who are terminally or seriously chronically ill appear to have positive effects.

STRATEGIES THAT DO NOT WORK

A review of the research and program evaluation literature on the prevention of suicide in older adulthood has not revealed a single report indicating that a program whose goal was the prevention of suicide did not work with older persons. This is in part due to the fact that there are so few primary prevention programs for the elderly, which gather data about suicide as well as the common practice to not publish negative results even if they did exist. We know from research on the prevention of suicide in general that there is no simple prevention strategy which has significant effects on suicide rates; suicide is a multi-determined phenomenon so that any prevention strategy would have to consider multiple risk factors in order to be effective.

Legislation to make suicide illegal and punish attempters does not have a preventive effect. Furthermore, the legal access to euthanasia and assisted suicide in The Netherlands has not resulted in either an increase or a decrease in suicide rates in that country.

It has sometimes been said that having a lethal method for ending one's life available "just in case" a situation becomes unbearable is a means of preventing a premature suicide by people who fear that their lives will become worse in the future.

However, research indicates clearly that having a lethal means for killing oneself readily available significantly increases the likelihood of a death by suicide and has no preventive effect.

SYNTHESIS

We have little empirical data on what works in suicide prevention with older persons. We have a scattering of pilot programs and studies on how to improve the well-being of the elderly which have sometimes been evaluated. However, there is little evidence of their effectiveness in suicide prevention. This is in part due to the fact that suicide is such an infrequent phenomenon that one would have to study programs which effect hundreds of thousands of older persons over a period of several years in order to reach some tentative conclusions. Most pilot programs involve only a few hundred elders. Therefore, their benefits for suicide prevention remain speculative.

Another reason we know so little about the primary prevention of suicide in older adulthood is that most evaluative research in suicide prevention focuses upon young people. There is a pervasive popular belief that suicide is a phenomenon of youth, despite that fact that the data indicate clearly that in most countries, including the United States, the highest risk groups for suicide are the elderly. This lack of interest is compounded by the belief that an older person who commits suicide does so for understandable rational reasons, as opposed to the more frivolous suicides of youth. This belief persists despite research linking suicide in older adulthood to dimensions of the quality of life, which can be easily changed if enough resources are allocated and persistent findings that depressed and seriously ill elders respond as well or better to prevention programs than all younger age groups. Perhaps the first step in developing primary prevention programs for older persons is to realize that people who have managed to survive until old age without taking their own lives have acquired a tremendous amount of life skills on which one can capitalize to develop effective primary prevention programs.

When we consider the current state of knowledge on the prevention of suicide in older adulthood, it is likely that many of the broad-based primary prevention programs described elsewhere in this book which improve the well-being of elders would have a primary prevention effect on suicidal behavior as well. If one were to develop specific primary prevention programs for older persons, the most important high risk group to target is older men and the time when there is the greatest risk is when loss events are experienced, particularly the death of a spouse. Physicians may play a particularly important role in the prevention of suicide since the majority of older persons consult a physician in the month before they commit suicide. Better treatment of depression in the elderly may decrease suicide rates, but older persons frequently experience such important losses that drug treatment of depression alone may not be sufficient.

We live in a society where there is increasing interest and public support for making euthanasia and assisted suicide more readily available, particularly for persons suffering from incurable or debilitating diseases. The vast majority of candidates for euthanasia and assisted suicide are older persons. Even if access to help in ending one's life is not readily available, we may wonder what effects attitudes and beliefs favoring ending life prematurely may have on suicide in older adulthood. We know that media reports that depict suicides often result in increased suicide risks among persons who identify with the victim in the report. One of the least explored areas in the primary prevention of suicide with the elderly is to examine how changes in societal belief systems concerning the encouragement of choosing to die affect suicidal behavior in older persons.

Also see: Suicide Entries Crises of Aging: Health Promotion, Older Adulthood.

References

American Association of Suicidology. (1999). *Elderly suicide fact sheet.* Washington: Author.

Conwell, Y. (1996) Outcomes of depression. *American Journal of Geriatric Psychiatry, 4*(Suppl. 1), S34–S44.

Daveluy, C., Pica, L., Audet, N., Courtemanche, R., & Lapointe, F. (2000). *Enquête sociale et de santé 1998.* Québec: Institut de la Statistique du Québec.

De Leo, D., Carollo, G., & Dello-Buono, M. (1995). Lower suicide rates associated with a Tele-Help/Tele-Check service for the elderly at home. *American Journal of Psychiatry, 152*(4), 632–634.

Dyck, R.J., Mishara, B.L., & White, J. (1998) *Suicide in children, adolescents and seniors: Key findings and policy implications* (vol. 3, pp. 311–373). In National Forum on Health Determinants of Health Settings and Issues.

Mishara, B.L. (1998). The right to die and the right to live: Perspectives on euthanasia and assisted suicide. In A. Leenaars, M. Kral, R. Dyck, & S. Wenckstern (Eds.), *Suicide in Canada* (pp. 441–458). Ottawa: University of Toronto Press.

Mishara, B.L. (1999). Synthesis of research and evidence on factors affecting the desire of terminally ill or seriously chronically ill persons to hasten death. *Omega, International Journal on Death and Dying, 39*(1), 1–70.

Mishara, B.L., & Legault, A. (2000). L'abus de médicaments, d'alcool et de drogues. In P. Landreville, P.Cappeliez, & Jean Vézina (Eds.), *Psychologie clinique de la personne âgée* (pp. 175–196). Ottawa: Presses de l'Université d'Ottawa-Masson.

Mishara, B.L., & Riedel, R. (1994). *Le vieillissement.* Paris: Presses Universitaires de France.

Murphy, S.L. (2000). Deaths: Final data for 1998. *National Vital Statistics Reports, 48*(11), 7–10, 25–50, 65–75.

Raschko, R. (1990). The gatekeeper model for the isolated, at-risk elderly. In N.L. Cohen (Ed.), *Psychiatry takes to the streets* (pp. 195–209). New York: Guilford Press.

Silverman, P.R. (1970). The widow as caregiver. *Mental Hygiene, 54,* 540–547.

World Health Organization (WHO). (2000). *Statistics on suicide worldwide. Public-use datasets.* Geneva: Author.

T

Tobacco, Adolescence

Brian Colwell, Dennis W. Smith, and Steve Sussman

INTRODUCTION

American society glamorizes negative health behaviors to our youth, like tobacco use. The alluring nature of risky behaviors is often the centerpiece of popular culture, including mass media. These behaviors are often portrayed glamorously through messages in advertisements, reality television, soap operas, and talk shows. These cultural messages appear to be effective, as more than 80 percent of young people in the United States who use tobacco, start before their 18th birthday. Hence, tobacco use prevention is crucial in combating tobacco use. In the absence of effective anti-tobacco interventions, more than 5 million children living today will die prematurely because of their use of tobacco.

DEFINITIONS

Bidis (also known as beedis or beedies) are small brown cigarettes, often flavored, consisting of tobacco hand-rolled in tendu or temburni leaf and secured with a string at one end. They are primarily produced in India and in some Southeast Asian countries, and are imported into the United States (Centers for Disease Control and Prevention [CDC], 2000a).

Kreteks (also known as clove cigarettes) are flavored cigarettes containing tobacco and clove extract (CDC, 2000a).

Spit tobacco refers to chewing tobacco, snuff, or other forms of smokeless tobacco.

SCOPE

In the United States, 3,000 youth begin smoking every day, and the number of teens who have begun smoking daily increased by 73 percent from 1988 to 1996 (CDC, 1999). According to the United States Centers for Disease Control & Prevention (CDC), nearly 90 percent of tobacco users begin using before age 18 (Chassin, Presson, Sherman, & Edwards, 1990). If tobacco use continues unabated, estimates are that 5 million individuals who are currently less than 18 years old will die prematurely due to the effects of tobacco. A small, but significant percentage of youth consumed their first tobacco before age 11. Numbers range from 8.5 percent of high school students that consumed their first cigarette below that age to 3.5 percent who used spit tobacco at that time.

According to the 1999 Youth Tobacco Survey (CDC, 2000a) 29.3 percent of middle school students have ever smoked cigarettes. About 15.4 percent of middle school youth had smoked at least one cigar during their lifetime, and nearly twice as many males (20.1 percent) had used them as females (10.9 percent). Some 7 percent of middle school youth had used spit tobacco, and males (11 percent) were more likely to have used than females (3.3 percent). With regard to the use of bidis, 5.4 percent of the middle school youth had smoked at least one, with males (6.7 percent) more likely to have smoked one than females (4.1 percent). There is a wide disparity in lifetime tobacco use between youth in different states, ranging from a low of 33.4 percent in Nebraska to a high of 60.2 percent in Arkansas.

Among high school youth, 63.5 percent had ever smoked cigarettes, with 41.6 percent replying that they had used cigars in their lifetime. Males (51.1 percent) were much more likely to have ever tried a cigar than females (31.9 percent). Nearly 20 percent of high school students had used some form of spit tobacco, with 28.5 percent of males and 7.6 percent of females having used the product at some time. 14.1 percent of students had used bidis in their lives.

Current Use. In 1999, 27 percent of the males and 23 percent of females over the age of 15 in Canada smoked (Health Canada, 1999). Also 9 percent of male and 11 percent of female youth between the ages of 11 and 15 smoked.

In the United States, the numbers are somewhat higher, although some of the differences may be in definitions. The CDC defines current tobacco use as having used tobacco at least once during the past 30 days and, based on this definition, 12.8 percent of middle school students had used some form of tobacco in the past month. Also 9.2 percent had smoked cigarettes and 6.1 percent had smoked cigars in the past month, while 2.4 percent had used spit tobacco at least once and 1.9 percent had used kreteks. Males were more likely than females to have used all forms of tobacco.

Among high school students, 34.8 percent were current users of any form of tobacco. About 28.5 percent of high school students use cigarettes with 28.7 percent of males and 28.2 percent of females having smoked cigarettes in the past month. Some 15.3 percent of high school students had smoked cigars in the past month, 6.6 percent had used some form of spit tobacco, 5 percent bidis and 5.8 percent kreteks. Interestingly, 2.8 percent had used pipes to smoke tobacco.

Just over 10 percent of middle school students who had ever smoked cigarettes had smoked more than 100 cigarettes, a marker considered by some to be indicative of dependence (Distefan, Gilpin, Choi, & Pierce, 1998). Also 12.3 percent of males and 7.7 percent of females had consumed this many. Just over 30 percent of high school students had smoked this many. About 13.1 percent of high school students had smoked at least one cigarette on 20 or more of the past 30 days. This level is defined by the CDC as "frequent" tobacco use, but is also probably another reliable indicator of daily tobacco use.

While data are sketchy, it is also instructive to look at tobacco use patterns in China, where environmental controls and social prohibition are less powerful in controlling youth access to tobacco, as well as its consumption. In China, 63 percent of males and 3.9 percent of females between the ages of 15 and 69 currently smoke cigarettes. (Yang et al.,

1999). About 23 percent of males and 5 percent of females under the age of 15 currently smoke (Li, Fang, & Stanton, 1999).

Costs to Society. Kaufman and Yach (2000) have noted the tremendous social cost of tobacco worldwide, stating that by the end of the 2020s, tobacco will kill 8.4 million people per year. Economic costs are incalculable.

In the United States, the CDC estimates that tobacco-related health care costs alone in the United States amount to $50 to $73 billion per year (CDC, 1999) while another $50 billion are incurred in indirect costs (CDC, 2000b). Over 430,000 deaths each year in the US (one in every five) are attributable to tobacco use. Despite these figures, the calculation of tobacco-related health care costs among youth is difficult and inexact.

Nevertheless, these are evidence of similar adverse health effects to many youth. These effects include abnormal spriometry and lung function tests and respiratory bronchiolitis. Histologic evidence indicates that, even in young smokers, the small airways are damaged (US Department of Health and Human Services [USDHHS], 1994). Additional evidence indicates an increased risk of atherosclerosis in males aged 15–34 who smoke, reduced levels of physical fitness and diminished exercise performance, and presumed adverse outcomes associated with pregnancy noted in all other age groups.

THEORIES

While there are several correlates for initiating tobacco use in youth. No factors can be identified as causal. Contributing correlates include depression, suicidal ideation, stress at home and school, and a desire to self-medicate. Generally adolescent tobacco users have more positive attitudes toward smoking. Tobacco use tends to cluster with other risky behaviors, including alcohol and marijuana use (Flay, Hu, & Richardson, 1998). Overall, smoking is rarely the sole risky behavior in which a youth participates; it often takes place within the context of other risk-taking behaviors. In the terms of Jessor and Jessor (1977) they are "generally deviance prone."

Interpersonally, youth smoking is correlated with parental tobacco use and acceptance of tobacco use in youth, as well as friend acceptance and use of tobacco products (Flay et al., 1998). Youth who use tobacco, however, discount the idea that this is due to peer pressure (Smith, Colwell, Zhang, Brimer, McMillan, & Stevens, 2001). Nevertheless, there is a strong impact on perceived social norms, as well as immersion in environments in which tobacco use is not only seen as socially acceptable but is modeled as a means of coping with negative affective states.

Flay et al. (1998) also noted that family conflict is predictive of the transition from experimental to regular use among females.

There is a clear pathway through which youth progress in their smoking careers (Leventhal & Cleary, 1980; Sussman, Dent, Burton, Stacy, & Flay, 1995). Flay and his colleagues (1998) have identified four stages through which adolescent smokers progress. In the initial stage, youth form a variety of cognitions, including attitudes, bonding to others and outcome expectancies related to tobacco use. The second stage is one of initial experimentation, leading to a determination of whether the physiological effects are acceptable and social reinforcement from salient others positive. The next stage is one of continued experimentation in settings where the user believes smoking to be socially beneficial. Finally, 2–3 years after first experimentation (Leventhal, Fleming, & Glynn, 1988), the user has adopted a pattern of regular use leading to nicotine dependence and addiction.

Maintaining a smoking habit is dependent on a different set of factors. Evidence indicates that smoking fulfills a variety of needs in smokers' lives (USDHHS, 1988). One primary need is to relieve or avoid physical dysphoria. Similarly, nicotine often serves to enhance psychological coping with uncomfortable emotional states like anger, boredom, and general stress (Smith et al., 2001). Nicotine addiction and associated withdrawal symptoms play a large part in sustaining the behavior with over 80 percent of youth indicating that they needed to continue their tobacco use (Henningfield, Clayton, & Pollin, 1990). Researchers have reported that nicotine is as addictive as cocaine or alcohol (USDHHS, 1994).

Little data exist that describes why youth choose to quit using tobacco. Reasonable assumptions would include health concerns, financial costs, and social sanctions against tobacco users.

RESEARCH

Inoculation theory provides a principle understanding for preventing tobacco use (Evans, 1976; McGuire, 1964). Its application provides youth with a rehearsal to the social pressures for using tobacco use and provides them opportunities to reject those pressures.

More recent interventions have built on the comprehensive *social influences approach* and have added rigor to the trials. These interventions emphasize components, "skills for identifying social influences to smoke, skills for resisting influences to smoke, and information for correcting erroneous normative perceptions regarding smoking (Peterson, Kealey, Mann, Marek, & Sarason, 2000, p. 1980)." Botvin (2000)

reported that such approaches usually produce reductions in tobacco use incidence and prevalence by 30–50 percent.

However, Peterson et al. (2000) noted that the use of a social influences tobacco curriculum in 20 school districts, augmented by increased availability to smoking cessation materials, supplemental curricular materials, and limited school-based (posters & school newspapers) media, was ineffective in reducing tobacco use among youth at grade 12. Responding to this observation, Sussman, Hansen, Flay, and Botvin (2001) disputed this report noting that other researchers have seen positive program effects across a variety of social-influence programs (Tobler, Roona, Ochshorn, Marshall, Streke, & Stackpole, 2000).

Regardless of the effects of an individual curriculum, Clayton, Scutchfield, and Wyatt (2000) have cautioned that a transdisciplinary approach to tobacco control in youth is needed and that consideration of social and cultural factors is critical. These comments echo those of others who maintain not only that individual factors such as knowledge, attitudes, and behavioral intent must be affected by programming, but the social and physical environment must be affected also (McLeroy, Bibeau, Steckler, & Glanz, 1988). This includes modifying proximal social networks, instituting organizational change within relevant community agencies, modifying community efforts at controlling tobacco and reexamining public policy to be supportive of the health behavior of interest.

STRATEGIES: OVERVIEW

According to Novotny, Romano, Davis, and Mills (1992), there are seven essential elements of tobacco use prevention and control strategies. These are surveillance, problem assessment, legislation, health department and community based programs, public information campaigns, technical information collection and dissemination, and coalition building.

This view is echoed in the CDC Best Practices in Comprehensive Tobacco Control Programs—August 1999 (CDC, 1999). In it, the CDC recommends the inclusion of community-based programs to reduce tobacco use, chronic disease programs to reduce the burden of tobacco-related disease, school programs to prevent the onset of smoking in youth, enforcement of existing tobacco statutes (especially minors' access and clean indoor air regulations), aggressive counter-marketing, cessation programs and ongoing surveillance and evaluation of programming.

In *Guidelines for School Health Programs to Prevent Tobacco Use and Addiction* (1994), the CDC identified several principles for school programs to be effective. These include establishing an environment that is supportive of tobacco non-use by prohibiting its use at school facilities and events, encouraging and assisting students and staff to quit using tobacco, and providing appropriate health instruction. The guidelines also recommend providing consistent messages regarding tobacco use from schools, families, and the community and reinforcing community-based efforts to reduce its use. The recommendations include specific school tobacco-related policies such as prohibiting tobacco advertising (including clothing) at school events or in school-related publications and implementing policies that are supportive of tobacco education and cessation.

STRATEGIES THAT WORK

Presently, two school-based curricula meet the standard for inclusion in this section. The first is the program, *Project Toward No Tobacco Use (Project TNT)*. It is a 10-lesson curriculum that is directed at seventh grade students. Previous tests of this curriculum among Whites, Latinos, African Americans and Asian Americans indicated effectiveness in reducing the initiation of cigarette smoking, reducing the frequency of smoking among youth that smoke, and reducing the initiation and frequency of spit tobacco use among youth. The program is 10 lessons in length over a 2- to 4-week period with two booster lessons in the eighth grade.

Project TNT takes a social influences approach to teaching youth about tobacco. While the curriculum focuses on the immediate and long-term effects of tobacco on the health of youth, it is concerned as well with helping youth to understand that the information they hear about tobacco and what they may have been led to believe about smoking may be false (Sussman et al., 1995).

Project TNT was designed as a comprehensive intervention consisting of a physical consequences program, normative social influences program (to counteract pressure to yield to behavioral norms in order to achieve acceptance), and informational social influences program (to counteract overt pressure to share similar attitudes and beliefs of salient peers). The research design utilized a standard care control condition on a group of approximately 7,000 youth from 48 junior high schools. While all single-component programs achieved some effects, and the physical consequences program actually was the strongest of the single component programs, the combined program exerted the strongest effects overall. Followed over 2-years, junior high to high school transition period, with safeguards including use of a Solomon-Four group design, the combined condition, relative to the control, reduced initiation of cigarette and smokeless tobacco use by 26 and 30 percent, respectively, and reduced weekly use of cigarettes and smokeless tobacco by 60 and 100 percent, respectively.

Life Skills Training. Like Project TNT, the Life Skills Training (LST) program is based on a similar approach, although Botvin (2000) now refers to the program as a "competence enhancement" initiative. The program is intended for youth in the sixth and seventh grades, with young people receiving booster sessions in later grades.

Botvin (2000) has reported reductions in tobacco use initiation between 40 and 80 percent with other effects including reduced smoking intentions, increased smoking knowledge, and improved drug refusal skills (Botvin, Batson, Witts-Vitale, Bess, Baker, & Dusenbury, 1989). Botvin, Griffin, Diaz, Miller, and Ifill-Williams (1999) also reports that after 6 years, 44 percent fewer students used tobacco one or more times a month than did control subjects, with the strongest effects among students who were exposed to the most parts of the curriculum.

He states that the approach used by this curriculum is distinctly different from that of other social influences programs because it emphasizes the teaching of generic self-management and social skills rather than substance-specific behavioral skills. The program was designed to counteract social influences to smoke, but includes components intended to build personal capacities like self-esteem, stress management, and assertiveness (Botvin, 2000).

Social skills programs like those just described are not without their critics. Gorman (1998) has argued that the evidence presented in support of the effectiveness of these programs is not compelling. His argument is that investigators selectively focus on significant changes in a small set of salient variables while ignoring other findings that do not demonstrate significant changes in attitudes, knowledge, or behavior. It is wise for those involved in choosing curricula to examine effectiveness data to determine if the curricula may be effective in their community.

STRATEGIES THAT MIGHT WORK

Clayton et al. (2000) noted that the most important questions to ask in regards to prevention programming are what works for a specific population and under what conditions. He extended this line of inquiry by stating that the mechanism of action of the program needed to be clearly examined.

Although social influences approaches to prevention programming have a mixed history of success, they retain conceptual promise. Competence enhancement and comprehensive life skills education approaches have been demonstrated to be more effective than other health education approaches, but the effect sizes remain relatively low and much remains to be learned about what are the best components and how best to deliver them. While some of these programs are promising, questions such as those raised by Gorman (1998) have not been answered fully.

STRATEGIES THAT DO NOT WORK

While what works is still open to some debate among researchers, what does not work in tobacco education is better known. While the use of scare tactics remains popular among adults, there is little evidence to indicate that it has any effectiveness in health education efforts for youth. Kelder, Edmundson, and Lytle (1997) noted that such approaches, "frequently did more to undermine the credibility of adults and authority than to deter drug use" (p. 267). They also note that "affective education" approaches have had little effect on use patterns and may have actually served to increase experimentation.

The method of presentation of a program must be considered as well. As Tobler et al. (2000) reported that program type and size are significant predictors of program effectiveness. Non-interactive, lecture-oriented prevention programs that stress drug knowledge or affective development show small effects. Interactive programs that foster development of interpersonal skills show significantly greater effects that decrease with large-scale implementations. It is an unfortunate, but undeniable, truth that many school-based prevention programs are primarily of the non-interactive, lecture-oriented sort.

SYNTHESIS

The prevention of youth tobacco use requires a variety of coordinated interventions. Using a single intervention will not provide the level of contextual support necessary for youth tobacco use prevention and cessation within a community tobacco control program. School-based interventions like tobacco education (best done within the context of a comprehensive health education curriculum), prohibition of tobacco possession and use on school property or at school functions, and early intervention with youth who use tobacco are important steps. The importance of strong administrative support for school-based tobacco control is vital (Smith, Steckler, McLeroy, & Frye, 1990).

There is an abundance of bad tobacco prevention interventions, including poorly and atheoretically designed curricula and fear-based approaches like forcing experimenters to observe autopsy photographs. Occasionally, a well-designed, tested, and proven curriculum may be disseminated, but teachers are often ill-prepared to implement it. In other instances, teachers may alter the curriculum with inappropriate materials and methods, reducing its effectiveness.

There are cases of effective curricula, with good training components, not being maintained. As staff turnover occurs and the "institutional memory" of an appropriate training is lost, teachers may not know how to best use the curriculum. Another common threat to effective tobacco instruction is "pro-innovation bias". That is, newer is better—unfortunately, this is not always true.

Finally, influencing behavior can be achieved by limiting tobacco access through retail sales controls and taxes. Policies that remove tobacco vending machines from places to which youth have access, placing all tobacco products behind counters or in locked cabinets in stores, and vigorous enforcement of retail sales bans on providing tobacco to youth all constitute environmental support for maintenance of a tobacco-free lifestyle among youth. High sales taxes have also been demonstrated to have a significant impact on youth consumption.

The goal of youth tobacco prevention must include delaying the onset of first experimentation with tobacco, delay in onset of regular smoking, and development and implementation of effective cessation interventions before dependence develops.

Also see: Substances entries.

References

Botvin, G.J. (2000). Preventing drug abuse in schools: Social and competence enhancement approaches targeting individual-level etiologic factors. *Addictive Behaviors, 25*(6), 887–897.

Botvin, G.J., Batson, H., Witts-Vitale, S., Bess, V., Baker, E., & Dusenbury, L. (1989). A psychosocial approach to smoking prevention for urban black youth. *Public Health Reports, 104*, 573–582.

Botvin, G.J., Griffin, K.W., Diaz, T., Miller, N., & Ifill-Williams, M. (1999). Smoking initiation and escalation in early adolescent girls: One-year follow-up of a school-based prevention intervention for minority youth. *Journal of the American Medical Women's Association, 54*, 139–143.

Centers for Disease Control and Prevention (CDC). (1999). *Best practices for comprehensive tobacco control programs—August 1999.* Atlanta: US Department of Health and Human Services, Centers for Disease Control and Prevention, National Center for Chronic Disease Prevention and Health Promotion, Office on Smoking and Health.

Centers for Disease Control and Prevention (CDC). (2000a, October 13). CDC surveillance summaries. *MMWR, 49* (No. SS-10).

Centers for Disease Control and Prevention (CDC). (2000b). *Targeting Tobacco Use: The Nation's Leading Cause of Death At-a-glance, 2000.* Atlanta: US Department of Health and Human Services, Centers for Disease Control and Prevention, National Center for Chronic Disease Prevention and Health Promotion, Office on Smoking and Health.

Chassin, L., Presson, C.C., Sherman, S.J., & Edwards, D.A. (1990). The natural history of cigarette smoking: Predicting young adult smoking outcomes from adolescent smoking patterns. *Health Psychology, 9*(6), 701–716.

Clayton, R.R., Scutchfield, F.D., & Wyatt, S.W. (2000). Hutchinson Smoking Prevention Project: A new gold standard in prevention science requires new transdisciplinary thinking. *Journal of the National Cancer Institute, 92*(24), 1964–1965.

Distefan, J.M., Gilpin, E.A., Choi, W.S., & Pierce, J.P. (1998). Parental influences predict adolescent smoking in the United States, 1989–1993. *Journal of Adolescent Health, 22*(6), 466–474.

Evans, R.I. (1976). Smoking in children: Developing a social psychological strategy of deterrence. *Preventive Medicine, 5*, 122–127.

Flay, B.R., Hu, F.B., & Richardson, J. (1998). Psychosocial predictors of different stages of cigarette smoking among high school students. *Preventive Medicine, 27*(5), A9–A18.

Gorman, D.M. (1998). The irrelevance of evidence in the development of school-based drug prevention policy, 1986–1996. *Evaluation Review, 22*(1), 118–146.

Guidelines for school health programs to prevent tobacco use and addiction. (1994). *MMWR, 43*(RR-2), 1–18, 02/25/1994.

Health Canada. (1999). 10. Other Tobacco Products. CTUMS (Canadian Tobacco Use Monitoring Survey), Wave 1, February–June 1999.

Henningfield, J.E., Clayton, R., & Pollin, W. (1990). Involvement of tobacco in alcoholism and illicit drug use. *British Journal of Addiction, 85*(2), 279–292.

Jessor, R., & Jessor, S.L. (1977). *Problem behavior and psychosocial development: A longitudinal study of youth.* New York: Academic Press.

Kaufman, N., & Yach, D. (2000). Tobacco control—challenges and prospects. *Bulletin of the World Health Organization, 78*(7), 867.

Kelder, S.H., Edmundson, E.W., & Lytle, L.A. (1997). Health behavior research and school and youth health promotion. In D.S. Gochman (Ed.), *Handbook of health behavior research IV: Relevance for professionals and issues for the future.* New York: Plenum Press.

Leventhal, H., & Cleary, P.D. (1980). The smoking problem: A review of the research and theory in behavioral risk modification. *Psychological Bulletin, 88*(2), 370–405.

Leventhal, H., Fleming, R., & Glynn, K. (1988). A cognitive-developmental approach to smoking intervention. In S. Maes, C.D. Spielberger, P.B. Defares, & I.G. Sarason (Eds.), *Topics in health psychology: Proceedings of the first annual conference on health psychology.* New York: John Wiley and Sons.

Li, X., Fang, X., & Stanton, B. (1999). Ever cigarette smoking in Beijing among middle school students: Cigarette smoking among schoolboys in Beijing, China. *Journal of Adolescence, 22*(5), 621–625.

McGuire, W.J. (1964). Inducing resistance to persuasion. In L. Berkowitz (Ed.), *Advances in experimental social psychology,* New York: Academic Press.

McLeroy, K.R., Bibeau, D., Steckler, A., & Glanz, K. (1988). An ecological perspective on health promotion programs. *Health Education Quarterly, 15*(4), 351–376.

Novotny, T.E., Romano, R.A., Davis, R.M., & Mills, S.L. (1992). The public health practice of tobacco control: Lessons learned and directions for the states in the 1990s. *Annual Review of Public Health, 13*, 287–318.

Peterson, A.V., Kealey, K.A., Mann, S.L., Marek, P.M., & Sarason, I.G. (2000). Hutchinson Smoking Prevention Project: Long-term randomized trial in school-based tobacco use prevention—results on smoking. *Journal of the National Cancer Institute, 92*(24), 1979–1991.

Smith, D.W., Colwell, B., Zhang, J.J., Brimer, J., McMillan, C., & Stevens, S. Theory-based development & testing of an adolescent tobacco-use awareness program. *American Journal of Health Behavior, 28*(2), 137–144.

Smith, D.W., Steckler, A.B., McLeroy, K.R., & Frye, R. (1990). Tobacco prevention in North Carolina public schools. *Journal of Drug Education, 20*(3), 257–268.

Sussman, S., Dent, C.W., Burton, D., Stacy, A.W. & Flay, B.R. (1995). *Developing school-based tobacco use prevention and cessation programs.* Thousand Oaks, CA: Sage.

Sussman, S. Hansen, W.B., Flay, B.R., & Botvin, G.J. (2001). Hutchinson Smoking Prevention Project: Long-term randomized trail in school-based tobacco use prevention—results on smoking. *Journal of the National Cancer Institute, 93*(16), 1267.

Tobler, N.S., Roona, M.R., Ochshorn, P., Marshall, D.G., Streke, A.V., & Stackpole, K.M. (2000). School-based adolescent drug prevention programs: 1998 meta analysis. *Journal of Primary Prevention, 20*, 275–336.

US Department of Health and Human Services (USDHHS). (1988). *The health consequences of smoking. Nicotine addiction: A report of the Surgeon General.* Atlanta: Author, Centers for Disease Control and Prevention, National Center for Chronic Disease Prevention and Health Promotion, Office on Smoking and Health.

US Department of Health and Human Services (USDHHS). (1994). *Preventing tobacco use among young people: A report of the Surgeon General.* Atlanta: Author Centers for Disease Control and Prevention, National Center for Chronic Disease Prevention and Health Promotion, Office on Smoking and Health.

Yang, G., Fan, L., Tan, J., Qi, G., Zhang, Y., Samet, J.M., Taylor, C.E., Becker, K., & Xu, J. (1999). Smoking in China: Findings of the 1996 National Prevalence Survey. *Journal of the American Medical Association, 282*(13), 1247–1253.

V

Violence Prevention, Early Childhood

Jannette Rey and Garret D. Evans

INTRODUCTION

Despite a consistent, downward trend in juvenile violent crime in the late 1990s, violence continues to be a primary public health problem for our nation's youth, with estimates of a 22 percent increase in violence arrests for youth ages 10–17 by the year 2010 (Snyder, Sickmund, & Bilchik, 1999). While these trends are generally evident across the nation, children living in impoverished communities continue to be at greatest risk. These factors coupled with the effects of violence on society in general point to a need for effective, early preventive interventions.

DEFINITIONS

Violence has been described in various ways depending on discipline, setting, and developmental stage. A severe conduct problem, *violence* is sometimes included under the heading of delinquency in criminology circles, *antisocial behavior* in developmental and social psychology, and as *conduct disorder* in clinical psychology and psychiatry.

Study in the area of violence prevention has been guided by recommendations for more extensive research regarding the influences, trajectories, and frameworks for understanding antisocial behavior. In this entry, we discuss the nature of violence prevention in early childhood including the pathways that lead to poor outcomes and the risk and protective factors that influence these trajectories. Next, we provide an overview of effective violence preventive interventions for this population. The terms violence and antisocial behavior will be used in a broad manner so as to incorporate the developmental and severity variations inherent in current explanatory and intervention models.

SCOPE

Features of antisocial behavior continue to be the most commonly referred presenting problems. Results of three longitudinal projects (i.e., Denver Youth Survey, Pittsburgh Youth Study, and Rochester Youth Development Study) highlight trends of serious violent behavior patterns in children as young as 10 years. The costs of antisocial and aggressive behavior to society encompasses aspects such as the costs of treating delinquent youth, costs as a result of later adult criminality in terms of damage to goods and property, and finally the costs of incarceration. While there are few if any sex differences across most types of conduct problems for infants and toddlers (Keenan & Shaw, 1997), the development of antisocial behavior in boys has been found to follow two distinct trajectories—onset in childhood or onset in adolescence. This pattern has not been clearly demonstrated for girls and, instead, research has found that severe antisocial behavior in females is most commonly tracked to adolescent-onset (Silverthorn & Frick, 1999).

THEORIES AND RESEARCH

Risk Factors and Correlates of Youth Violence

A number of robust and reliable correlates of juvenile violent behavior and overall delinquency have been identified in the empirical literature (Dahlberg, 1998; Hawkins, Herrenkohl, Farrington, Brewer, Catalano, & Harachi, 1998). These key factors include individual variables, family variables, peer/school variables, and community/environmental variables. Current research suggests that risk factors exist across multiple domains, a combination of risks is multiplicative in terms of its impact, common risk factors precede diverse behavioral outcomes, risks differentially impact development at different stages, and risk factors are consistent across racial, cultural, and socioeconomic groups. Protective factors, however, can help prevent maladaptive development or can also reduce the impact of biological or environmental risks. A risk-focused approach to violence prevention, then, seeks to reduce identified risk factors and enhance protective factors across all domains.

Child Variables

Certain individual factors are risk factors for violence. Prenatal factors, such as fetal exposure to alcohol and other drugs, may affect the development of conduct problems and heredity factors may account for some ODD and CD in children (Mason & Frick, 1994). Infant temperament, particularly difficult or oppositional temperament, has been found to have a direct relationship to later antisocial and coercive behavior whereby difficult infant temperament transforms to oppositional behaviors during early childhood (e.g., argumentativeness). Studies examining the interaction of temperament and parenting, however, suggest that the relationship may not be as direct as previously conceptualized, particularly for low-risk samples. Instead, multiple dimensions of temperament may combine to yield a child's vulnerability to risk for later aggression and violence.

The age of onset of conduct problems is a key factor in the stability of aggression and conduct problems. Research in the area of antisocial behavior suggests that childhood aggressive behavioral patterns are well-formed by age 8 and become less responsive to treatment and more characteristic of a chronic disorder (Kazdin, 1995). Specifically, childhood-onset patterns of conduct problems appear to begin with severe oppositional and argumentative behavior, then progressing to more severe antisocial behavior patterns. This pattern of emergence of early problematic behavior, *life-course persistent*, is associated with poorer outcomes and more serious violent and antisocial behaviors (Moffitt & Caspi, 2001).

Cognitively-based risk factors for violence include a child's belief that aggression is an acceptable and effective strategy for conflict resolution and a biased social information processing style whereby actions of others are inaccurately interpreted as hostile (Crick & Dodge, 1994). Deficits in the young child's ability to regulate behavior and/or emotional responding can also increase the risk of poor psychosocial adaptation and the development of aggressive behavior (Eisenberg, 2000). Higher intelligence in young children, however, may serve as a protective factor in that higher verbal ability in young childhood, associated with higher intelligence levels, promotes better socialization by parents and the child's own ability to interact with the environment to attain goals (Keenan & Shaw, 1997).

Family Variables

Parenting practices and family management have been identified as the primary determinant of child antisocial behavior, particularly for families in which there is an identified history of parental mental illness, high risk of harsh discipline practices, or domestic violence (Widom, 1997). Parents who lack emotion regulation skills also influence healthy child socioemotional development, particularly during the critical period of early childhood, increasing the risk of poor behavioral control and later development of conduct problems (Hay, Zahn-Waxler, Cummings, & Iannotti, 1992).

Families with domestic violence (witnessing or victimization) are characterized by high levels of discord, alcohol and other drug use, social isolation, psychological distress, and higher probability of child abuse (Fantuzzo, Depaola, Lambert, & Martino, 1991). Parents with the highest levels of stress are at the highest risk of abusing their children. Abused children have been found to initiate fewer positive peer interactions and, instead, display higher rates of aggressive, antisocial behavior with peers. Children as young as 5 years who witness family violence have been found to endorse more beliefs about violence as an appropriate means of conflict resolution than nonwitnessing children and social cognitive processing styles that increase the likelihood of antisocial behaviors (e.g., hostile attributional styles, external locus of control, poor understanding of social cues) (Dadds & Powell, 1991). Where family stress is high, parental support and cognitive stimulation of the child is also compromised. Parent- and child-related protective factors include healthy parental attachment, high parental supervision, and high caregiver attention. In addition, family harmony, father involvement, and school bondedness have been found to be key protective factors.

Peer/School Variables

In the "peer influence model," children with deviant friends are at an increased risk for the development of delinquent behavior than those with nondeviant friends (Farrington et al., 1990). However, while the presence or absence of deviant friends for very young children has not been demonstrated as predictive of later conduct problems, it may be that this association serves as a moderating role and increases risk as time goes on for those children already at-risk for the development of severe behavioral problems. Research has also identified a strong association between rejection status during early childhood (i.e., kindergarten) and significant rates of externalizing behaviors during early childhood and beyond (Kraatz-Keiley, Bates, Dodge, & Pettit, 2000). Childhood victims of aggression are more likely to experience repeated victimization and its negative effects on emotional development when effective alternative skills are not adopted.

Community Variables

Many children and youth are exposed to violence on a daily basis either through witnessing violence first hand in their communities and/or through media exposure to violence. For urban children, studies have shown that over 80 percent of children in these environments are witnesses to chronic violence. While the family environment has been shown to moderate some effects of witnessed violence on children's antisocial behavior, the degree of community violence witnessed remains a strong indicator for the development of aggressive behavior. Poor neighborhoods are often characterized by high crime, poor parental monitoring of their children, and fewer resources in general (McLoyd, 1998). Research examining community characteristics and childhood conduct problems suggests that differences in conduct problems between children living in disadvantaged neighborhoods and those who do not are evident as early as age 5 (Brooks-Gunn, Duncan, Klebanov, & Sealand, 1993). Further, families living in disadvantaged neighborhoods also increase the risk of exposure to delinquent peers in their child's school. The relationship between exposure to violence through the media and subsequent aggression and violence is less clear. In a meta-analysis, Friedlander (1993) asserts that direct models of interpersonal violence are likely to influence violent behavior over that of indirect, media models. Environmental protective factors include prosocial peer groups and supportive communities with low incidence of violence.

Violence and its Development

The relationship between violence and aggression has been investigated over several decades. Aggression has been identified in children as young as 1 year of age, with instrumental aggression peaking in toddlerhood and hostile aggression becoming more prevalent in preschool-aged children. There are distinct deficit patterns in cognitive processing related to each type of aggression. The development of negative biases, for example, may underlie the hostile attributions identified in children with behavior problems (Dodge, 1991). Children with difficulties in encoding social cues are more likely to exhibit reactive aggression, while children with limited response skills are more likely to exhibit proactive aggression. For children with poor abilities in behavioral responding, accidental aggression is more commonly observed.

Childhood psychopathology has been described as stemming from specific interactions between the child and environment whereby the child's age, type and number of risk factors, and context within which development occurs can influence the expression of pathology. Social interactional models of antisocial behavior development suggest that repeated exposure to violence increases the likelihood that children will view violent behavior as effective and normative. The *social development model* is a related explanatory model for the initiation and persistence of antisocial behavior in youth (Catalano & Hawkins, 1996). Specifically, the degree to which a youth experiences bonding (i.e., attachment to others, moral commitment) and is exposed to an environment that does not support antisocial behavior is linked to reduced likelihood of adolescent delinquent behavior and drug use. Further, the process by which youth are able to bond is influenced by social competence, opportunity, and recognition for prosocial behavior.

Attachment theory describes how positive parent–infant attachment may promote a motivational set for social interaction and readiness to comply with caregivers' requests. Where early interactions are marked by maternal unresponsiveness or inaccessibility and the reciprocal nature of the parent–child interaction is hindered, the child is less responsive or motivated to respond to the mother's requests. Conversely, the child may utilize aggressive behavior to regulate parental proximity for unresponsive caregivers or establish predictability in responsiveness on the part of the caregiver. Patterson's *coercion model* is widely known and incorporates principles from social learning theory to explain how family interactional patterns can produce conduct problems in children (Dishion, Patterson, & Kavanagh, 1992). In this model, a coercive cycle develops as the parent and child attempt to gain control of the interaction utilizing aversive behaviors (e.g., child's whining). The repetition of this cycle often results in increasingly problematic child conduct problems and the parenting characterized by permissive, inconsistent, or overly harsh discipline. Relatedly, the transactional model and social–ecological theory describe the reciprocal impact that parents and children have that can influence later behavior (Bronfenbrenner, 1979).

STRATEGIES OVERVIEW

In recent years, there has been an increasing emphasis on reducing juvenile violence by intervening in the early childhood years with comprehensive prevention programs that focus on improving parenting practices and enhancing parent–child bonds, teaching caregivers and children effective ways to resolve conflicts in a non-aggressive manner, and improving home–school linkages. However, the literature regarding the effectiveness of violence prevention programs with young children is in an early stage of development with limited longitudinal examinations.

STRATEGIES THAT WORK

Given that many of the key risk factors for violence are family-related, improving family functioning is especially important for young children whose primary contacts are with their caregivers in the home. Parent management/parenting education programs during the infancy period include home visitation services and selected family therapies that are designed to teach parents effective family management skills, to adopt realistic developmental expectations for their children, and to improve family communication, problem solving and child nurturing skills. The *Prenatal/Early Infancy Project* (Olds et al., 1998) is an effective preventive intervention designed to teach or enhance mothers' healthy beliefs and expectations about maternal/infant health care, enhance parent–infant bonding, and build mother's skills in maintaining a healthy pregnancy and their infant's health. Program components include home visitation by a nurse, health education, job and educational counseling, parent training, and linkages to social service agencies. Outcome data indicate significant reductions in child behavior problems and for several risk factors including parental neglect, academic failure, and child health problems (Olds et al., 1998). Similarly, the *Carolina Abecedarian Project* (Ramey & Campbell, 1994) and the *Infant Health and Development Program* (McCarton, Brooks-Gunn, Wallace, & Bauer, 1997) are educational intervention for mothers and their high-risk infants. Again, interventions consist of an infant development curriculum, parent training activities throughout preschool age, home visits by the classroom teacher, and follow-up home visits. Outcome data indicate that these programs were effective in significantly reducing behavior problems for participating children and that these impacts were persistent in follow-up examinations.

Unique opportunities for socialization with peers and promotion of prosocial behaviors via quality child care can help prevent the development of violence. Classroom-based programs have yielded significant results for the reduction of conduct problems and later delinquency when combined with family-focused interventions. The *High/Scope Perry Preschool Program* is one such intervention that was designed for preschool-aged children (ages 3 and 4 years) at-risk for school failure (Schweinhart, Barnes, & Weikart, 1993). The intervention includes a 2-year school-based curriculum to promote school commitment and academic interest and weekly home visits by the child's classroom teacher to enhance home–school linkages and bonding. Longitudinal follow-up data indicate that children who participated in the program were less likely to be adjudicated, demonstrated greater literacy and school attendance, and achieved higher employment levels than controls. *First Step to Success* (Walker, Kavanagh, Stiller, Golly, Severson, & Feil, 1998) is a preventive intervention for preschool-aged and kindergarten children with early signs of antisocial behavior patterns. The program is comprised of a 6-week home component and a school component consisting of 30 program days that target promotion of those competencies that increase social and behavioral adjustment. The school-based intervention is an adapted version of the *CLASS program for Acting-out Children* and is guided by behavioral principles for the promotion of adaptive academic and social behaviors. Similarly, HomeBase, the home-based intervention, involves consultation to parents in behavioral practices to promote social competence in the home setting. Outcome data indicate that participating children demonstrate fewer aggressive behaviors and better social competence at post-treatment as reported by teachers and these effects were maintained at 1- and 2-year follow-up (Golly, Stiller, & Walker, 1998). In *The Incredible Years Parents and Teachers Series* (Webster-Stratton, 1992), caregivers receive training in the use of effective behavior management practices, strategies to enhance positive child–caregiver interactions and prosocial competence. Through the use of videotape vignettes, caregivers participate in guided discussions regarding the strategies they viewed and discuss or practice alternatives. The parent component consists of approximately 24-hr course over 12–14 weeks while the teacher component is comprised of a 6-day workshop series. The efficacy and effectiveness of the Parent series for the treatment of childhood conduct problems has been demonstrated in a number of empirical investigations (Scott, Doolan, Aspland, Spender, & Jacobs, 2001). Further, behavior gains have been found at both post-treatment and 1-year follow-up. The Teacher Series also yielded significant reductions in child conduct problems, improved academic and social performance, and improved teacher discipline strategies as compared to controls. In fact, behaviors in children whose teachers and parents had participated in the program demonstrated the greatest improvements.

STRATEGIES THAT MIGHT WORK

The following programs have demonstrated some evidence of effectiveness. Current parent training programs are largely based on the work of Patterson, Reid, Jones, and Conger (1975) as well as Hanf and these *behavioral parent training programs* are designed to address family risk factors related to the development of antisocial behavior. Program goals commonly involve teaching parents ways to improve their parenting and interactions with their children, promote prosocial behaviors, support academic success and commitment, and improve parent–school linkages. Other parent training programs have utilized a group-based model, where parents utilize videotapes of parent–child interactions toward the development of their skills and, more recently, self-administered parent training models accompanied by consultation (Webster-Stratton, 1992). Selected empirically supported parenting programs include *Living with Children* (Patterson et al., 1975), *Parent–Child Interaction Therapy* (Eyberg, Boggs, & Algina, 1995), *Helping the Noncompliant Child* (Forehand & McMahon, 1981), *Synthesis Training* (Wahler, Cartor, Fleischman, & Lambert, 1993), and *Dare to Be You* (Miller-Heyl, MacPhee, & Fritz, 1998). While the empirical evidence is mixed regarding the generalization of treatment effects from the home to the school setting, those programs that address parental stressors have demonstrated additional gains in overall family functioning.

Promising school-based preventive interventions that target cognitive or academic development and performance have increased in recent decades. *Interpersonal Cognitive Problem Solving* (ICPS) programs (Shure, 1997) is a preventive intervention designed for children of various ages and targeting early aggression and antisocial behavior through the building of cognitive problem solving ability to improve social adjustment and interpersonal competence. ICPS is a 12-week school-based curriculum that involves daily lesson with didactic and group interaction discussions. Outcome data indicate that participating children demonstrated significant improvement in their interpersonal cognitive problem-solving skills as measured by formal assessment and improved behavioral control as reported by their teachers. Follow-up evaluations have found treatment maintenance one and two years post-treatment (Shure, 1997). *Positive Schools* (Luiselli, Putnam, & Handler, 2001) is an application of a behavioral systems perspective model of prevention designed to prevent violence, improve student social outcomes, and improve student achievement. Program components include staff training and mentoring in the development of school-wide, classroom-wide, and individual behavior support plans. Preliminary outcome data have suggested significant reductions in school-wide disciplinary problems, increased student academic engagement and performance, improved school and classroom environments, and improved staff, parent, and student satisfaction.

Child-care sites are often the settings in which children are first identified as displaying early and persistent antisocial behavior. *Project Head Start* is an example of a longstanding early prevention intervention program to increase exposure to a cognitively stimulating learning environment for economically disadvantaged children (Zigler & Styfco, 2001). Although lacking in randomized controlled experimental trials, several studies have found lower rates of enrollment in special education services for Head Start preschoolers as compared to non-Head Start peers. Another approach needing further study is The *Primary Mental Health Project* (PMHP) (Cowen, Hightower, Pedro-Carroll, Work, Wyman, & Haffey, 1996). The PMHP is a preventive intervention for at-risk young children where paraprofessional staff are coordinated by a school-based mental health professional to provide both structured therapeutic play and within classroom environments. Although the program has been extensively studied, well-designed randomized control trials have yet to be conducted, thus limiting its empirical support.

Finally, because many disruptive children are deficient in social skills and problem solving ability, child-focused efforts to reduce disruptive behaviors are largely comprised of interventions to improve child social cognitive skills (Reid, 1993). While association with prosocial peers can enhance a child's development of social problem solving skills, child-focused prevention strategies have been found to be more effective when combined with parenting education practices.

STRATEGIES THAT DO NOT WORK

In general, programs that have failed to demonstrate effectiveness in preventing violence focused exclusively on the child in terms of skill building with little attention given to altering the child rearing environment.

SYNTHESIS

Effective programs in violence prevention are characterized by their use of developmentally and theory-based interventions that target skill enhancement in light of violence-related risk factors. Further, the effectiveness of programming is enhanced when the intervention is comprised of multimodal components that promote collaboration and support between home and school settings. Notably, the most effective delinquency prevention programs were targeted at early childhood populations, family-oriented, and resource-strengthening (Yoshikawa, 1995).

Given that childhood is a period in which aggressive and antisocial behaviors can develop and become stabilized, interventions applied during the early childhood can help to mitigate the impact of chronic exposure to violence and adversity. The re-conceptualization of many "social problems" as health risk behaviors (e.g., violence and substance abuse) has added to an increased emphasis on the provision of school-based violence prevention efforts. The information presented suggests that, when school preventive interventions are delivered in combination with parent-focused programs, the impact on child conduct problems is enhanced. Continued efforts toward longitudinal assessment of violence preventive interventions are warranted. In this way, both the science and practice of violence prevention can be expanded in useful and relevant directions.

Also see: Violence Prevention entries; Family Strengthening entries; Media Habits; Self-Esteem, Early Childhood.

References

Bronfenbrenner, U. (1979). Contexts of child rearing: Problems and prospects. *American Psychologist, 34,* 844–850.

Brooks-Gunn, J., Duncan, G.J., Klebanov, P.K., & Sealand, N. (1993). Do neighborhoods influence child and adolescent development? *American Journal of Sociology, 99,* 353–395.

Catalano, R.F., & Hawkins, J.D. (1996). The social development model: A theory of antisocial behavior. In J.D. Hawkins (Ed.), Delinquency and crime: Current theories. *Cambridge criminology series* (pp. 149–197). New York: Cambridge University Press.

Cowen, E., Hightower, A.D., Pedro-Carroll, J.L., Work, W.C., Wyman, P., & Haffey, W.G. (1996). *School-based prevention for children at risk: The Primary Mental Health Project.* Washington, DC: American Psychological Association.

Crick, N.R., & Dodge, K.A. (1994). A review and reformulation of social information-processing mechanisms in children's social adjustment. *Psychological Bulletin, 115,* 74–101.

Dadds, M.R., & Powell, M.B. (1991). The relationship of interparental conflict and global marital adjustment to aggression, anxiety, and immaturity in aggressive and nonclinic children. *Journal of Abnormal Child Psychology, 19,* 553–567.

Dahlberg, L.L. (1998). Youth violence in the United States: Major trends, risk factors, and prevention approaches. *American Journal of Preventive Medicine, 14,* 259–272.

Dishion, T.J., Patterson, G.R., & Kavanagh, K.A. (1992). An experimental test of the coercion model: Linking theory, measurement, and intervention. In J. McCord & R.E. Tremblay (Eds.), *Preventing antisocial behavior: Interventions from birth through adolescence* (pp. 253–282). New York: The Guilford Press.

Dodge, K.A. (1991). Emotion and social information processing. In J. Garber & K.A. Dodge (Eds.), The development of emotion regulation and dysregulation. *Cambridge studies in social and emotional development* (pp. 159–181). New York: Cambridge University Press.

Eisenberg, N. (2000). Emotion, regulation, and moral development. *Annual Review of Psychology, 51,* 665–697.

Eyberg, S.M., Boggs, S.R., & Algina, J. (1995). Parent–child interaction therapy: A psychosocial model for the treatment of young children with conduct problem behavior and their families. *Psychopharmacology Bulletin, 31,* 83–91.

Fantuzzo, J., DePaola, L.M., Lambert, L., & Martino, T. (1991). Effects of interparental violence on the psychological adjustment and competencies of young children. *Journal of Consulting and Clinical Psychology, 59,* 258–265.

Farrington, D.P., Loeber, R., Elliott, D.S., Hawkins, J.D., Kandel, D.B., Klein, M.W., McCord, J., Rowe, D.C., & Tremblay, R.E. (1990). Advancing knowledge about the onset of delinquency and crime. In B.B. Lahey & A.E. Kazdin (Eds.), *Advances in clinical child psychology* (Vol. 13, pp. 283–342). New York: Plenum Press.

Forehand, R.L., & McMahon, R.J. (1981). *Helping the noncompliant child: A clinician's guide to parent training.* New York: Guilford Press.

Friedlander, B.Z. (1993). Community violence, children's development, and mass media: In pursuit of new insights, new goals, and new strategies. *Psychiatry: Interpersonal and Biological Processes, 56,* 66–81.

Golly, A.M., Stiller, B., & Walker, H.M. (1998). First Step to Success: Replication and social validation of an early intervention program. *Journal of Emotional and Behavioral Disorders, 6,* 243–250.

Hawkins, J.D., Herrenkohl, T., Farrington, D.P., Brewer, D., Catalano, R.F., & Harachi, T.W. (1998). A review of predictors of youth violence. In R. Loeber & D.P. Farrington (Eds.), *Serious & violent juvenile offenders: Risk factors and successful interventions* (pp. 106–146). Thousand Oaks, CA: Sage.

Hay, D.F., Zahn-Waxler, C., Cummings, E.M., & Iannotti, R.J. (1992). Young children's views about conflict with peers: A comparison of the daughters and sons of depressed and well women. *Journal of Child Psychology and Psychiatry and Allied Disciplines, 33,* 669–683.

Kazdin, A.E. (1995). Conduct disorder. In F.C. Verhulst & H.M. Koot (Eds.), *The epidemiology of child and adolescent psychopathology* (pp. 258–290). New York: Oxford University Press.

Keenan, K., & Shaw, D. (1997). Developmental and social influences on young girls' early problem behavior. *Psychological Bulletin, 121,* 95–113.

Kraatz-Keiley, M., Bates, J.E., Dodge, K.A., & Pettit, G.S. (2000). A cross-domain growth analysis: Externalizing and internalizing behaviors during 8 years of childhood. *Journal of Abnormal Child Psychology, 28,* 161–179.

Luiselli, J.K., Putnam, R.F., & Handler, M.W. (2001). Improving discipline practices in public schools: Description of a whole-school and district-wide model of behavior analysis consultation. *The Behavior Analyst Today, 2,* 18–27.

Mason, D.A., & Frick, P.J. (1994). The heritability of antisocial behavior: A meta-analysis of twin and adoption studies. *Journal of Psychopathology and Behavioral Assessment, 16,* 301–323.

McCarton, C.M., Brooks-Gunn, J., Wallace, I.F., & Bauer, C.R. (1997). Results at age 8 years of early intervention for low-birth-weight premature infants: The infant health and development program. *Journal of the American Medical Association, 277,* 126–132.

McLoyd, V.C. (1998). Socioeconomic disadvantage and child development. *American Psychologist, 53,* 185–204.

Miller-Heyl, J., MacPhee, D., & Fritz, J.J. (1998). DARE to be you: A family-support, early prevention program. *Journal of Primary Prevention, 18,* 257–285.

Moffitt, T., & Caspi, A. (2001). Childhood predictors differentiate life-course persistent and adolescence-limited antisocial pathways among males and females. *Development and Psychopathology, 13,* 355–375.

Olds, D., Pettitt, L.M., Robinson, J., Henderson, C., Eckenrode, J., Kitzman, H., Cole, B., & Powers, J. (1998). Reducing risks for antisocial behavior with a program of prenatal and early childhood home visitation. *Journal of Community Psychology, 26,* 65–83.

Patterson, G.R., Reid, J.B., Jones, R.R., & Conger, R.W. (1975). *A social learning approach to family intervention* (Vol. 1). Eugene, OR: Castalia.

Ramey, C.T., & Campbell, F.A. (1994). Poverty, early childhood education, and academic competence: The Abecedarian experiment In

A.C. Huston (Ed.), *Children in poverty: Child development and public policy* (pp. 190–221). New York: Cambridge University Press.

Reid, J.B. (1993). Prevention of conduct disorder before and after school entry: Relating interventions to developmental findings. *Development and Psychopathology, 5*, 243–262.

Schweinhart, L.J., Barnes, H.V., & Weikart, D.P. (1993). *Significant benefits: The High/Scope Perry preschool study through age 23* (Vol. 12). Ypsilanti, MI: High/Scope.

Scott, S., Doolan, M., Aspland, H., Spender, Q., & Jacobs, B. (2001). Multicentre controlled trial of parenting groups for child antisocial behaviour in clinical practice. *British Medical Journal.*

Shure, M.B. (1997). Interpersonal cognitive problem solving: Primary prevention of early high-risk behaviors in the preschool and primary years. In G.W. Albee & T.P. Gullotta (Eds.), *Primary prevention works. Issues in children's and families' lives* (Vol. 6, pp. 167–188). Thousand Oaks, CA: Sage.

Silverthorn, P., & Frick, P.J. (1999). Developmental pathways to antisocial behavior: The delayed-onset pathway in girls. *Development and Psychopathology, 11*, 101–126.

Snyder, H., Sickmund, M., & Bilchik, S. (1999). *Juvenile offenders and victims: 1999 National Report* (p. 63). Washington, DC: Office of Juvenile Justice and Delinquency Prevention.

Wahler, R.G., Cartor, P.G., Fleischman, J., & Lambert, W. (1993). The impact of synthesis teaching and parent training with mothers of conduct-disordered children. *Journal of Abnormal Child Psychology, 21*, 425–440.

Walker, H.M., Kavanagh, K., Stiller, B., Golly, A., Severson, H.H., & Feil, E.G. (1998). First step to success: An early intervention approach for preventing school antisocial behavior. *Journal of Emotional and Behavioral Disorders, 6*, 66–80.

Webster-Stratton, C. (1992). Individually administered videotape parent training: "Who benefits?" *Cognitive Therapy and Research, 16*, 31–52.

Widom, C. (1997). Child abuse, neglect, and witnessing violence. In D.M. Stoff & J. Breiling (Eds.), *Handbook of antisocial behavior* (pp. 159–170). New York: John Wiley & Sons.

Yoshikawa, H. (1995). Long-term effects of early childhood programs on social outcomes and delinquency. *Future of Children, 5*, 51–75.

Zigler, E., & Styfco, S.J. (2001). Can early childhood intervention prevent delinquency? A real possibility. In A.C. Bohart & D.J. Stipek (Eds.), *Constructive & destructive behavior: Implications for family, school, & society* (pp. 231–248). Washington, DC: American Psychological Association.

Violence Prevention, Childhood

Sharon G. Portwood and Robert G. Waris

INTRODUCTION

An apparent onslaught of widely publicized incidents of youth violence, including homicides committed by very young children, has contributed to a recognition of youth violence as a serious public health problem. While much attention has focused on violence in adolescence, prevention efforts are increasingly targeting the childhood roots of violent behavior.

DEFINITIONS

Violence has been defined as "an act carried out with the intention of, or an act perceived as having the intention of, physically hurting another person" (Steinmetz, 1987, p. 729). Thus, violence is distinguished from accidental injury or mere threats. *Serious violence* typically encompasses criminal offenses, including homicide, *aggravated assault* (i.e., an unlawful attack in which the offender uses or threatens to use a weapon or the victim sustains severe bodily injury), robbery, and rape, as well as gang fights. Criminal acts perpetrated by an individual under age 18 may also be characterized as *juvenile delinquency*, a topic examined separately elsewhere in this volume.

SCOPE

Two general strategies have been employed in measuring violence among children and youth: (1) official crime statistics compiled by law enforcement agencies (e.g., number of arrests), and (2) self-report data (e.g., survey responses). The available law enforcement statistics on violence among young people tend to center on adolescents; however, some figures nonetheless encompass violent acts committed by younger children. For example, for 1998, the United States Federal Bureau of Investigation (1999) reported arrests of children under age 15 in connection with 139 murders/non-negligent homicides; 1,384 forcible rapes; 5,848 robberies; 17,192 aggravated assaults; and 4,199 arsons. Nonetheless, given persuasive evidence that the majority of crimes committed by young people do not come to the attention of law enforcement, there is widespread consensus that self-report data, while subject to both intentional and unintentional inaccuracies in reporting, offer the best measure of violent behavior (US Department of Health and Human Services [DHHS], 2001). These data indicate that contrary to the perceptions of many, following a dramatic increase (i.e., approximately 50 percent) in the rate of self-reported serious assaults between 1983 and 1993, incident rates have remained essentially level through 1998.

Data obtained from youth in England/Wales, the Netherlands, Spain, and Italy through the International Self-Report Delinquency Study (Junger-Tas, Terlouw, & Klein, 1994) evidence prevalence rates for violent behavior ranging from 16 to 26 percent. In comparison, the Monitoring the Future Survey, administered to high school seniors annually since 1975, indicates an approximately 30 percent prevalence rate among American youth (DHHS, 2001). One obvious difference between the United States and these other countries that may account for this discrepancy is the accessibility of firearms. Not only did the United States have the highest rate of gun-related youth deaths from 1990 to 1995 among the 26 industrialized countries examined, but the rate for children younger than age 15 was five times higher than that of the other countries combined (Centers for Disease Control and Prevention, 1997).

Not surprisingly, a substantial proportion of violence among children and youth occurs in the school setting. Although data from the Centers for Disease Control and Prevention in partnership with the US Departments of Education and Justice evidence that the number of school homicides declined throughout the 1990s, the number of multiple homicides has increased. Contrary to public perception, the rate of nonfatal injuries at school has remained relatively stable, hovering at about 8 to 13 per 1,000 students (DHHS, 2001). However, risk of victimization appears to be distributed unequally, with higher rates of victimization among males and African American students. In contrast with overall school violence rates, rates of drug use and physical fighting have remained high. Although there has been a recent decline in gangs, gang members appear to commit the majority of serious youth violence; violence rates are higher in schools with gangs (DHHS, 2001). The high cost of this violence is manifest in the emotional, physical, and economic consequences to victims, perpetrators, families, schools, and the larger community.

THEORIES

Attempts to identify the "cause" of violent behavior in children have prompted debate regarding the relative influence of individual, family, and environmental factors. While some studies (e.g., Duyme, 1989) point to genetic and perinatal factors, others (e.g., Loeber & Stouthamer-Loeber, 1986) focus on ineffective parenting as the source of violence in children. Either of these factors may precipitate aggressiveness and/or a lack of social skills in children that contributes to violent behavior. Regardless of whether the individual is predisposed to aggressive responses biologically and/or learns them through life experience, violent behavior may be exacerbated or inhibited through societal responses.

According to basic principles of *operant learning*, the primary mechanism for learning violent behavior is a long-term shaping of a person's aggressive behavior by environmental reinforcement and punishment of early versions or indicators of later violent behavior. For example, being instructed by parents to "stick up for yourself" may lead to the reinforcement of fighting behaviors, as would being punished for not fighting for one's rights. Beating one's opponent may also provide reinforcement for future fighting to obtain whatever it is one wants, from the psychological feeling of personal triumph to the social admiration and reputation one gets from being successfully violent.

However, reinforcement may be complex. Bandura's (1989) social *cognitive learning theory* suggests that it is nether the individual nor his or her environment alone that is responsible for aggressive behavior; rather, aggression can only be explained by a complex set of reciprocal, interactive relationships among the individual (e.g., developmental factors, cognition, personality), the behavior, and the environment. In contrast with operant learning, Bandura's model of reciprocal triadic determinism views the individual as interacting with both the stimulus (i.e., the external and social environment) and the response (i.e., the behavior). From this theory, it follows that in order to prevent aggressive behavior, all three determinants must be addressed.

While all theories of aggression do not focus on those pathways that are promoted by socializing agents in the environment (e.g., the cognitive-neoassocianistic and cognitive-excitation approaches), there is a general consensus that environmental factors are a key component in those developmental trajectories from aggression to violence. The environment provides a number of situational factors that may facilitate violent behavior, including media representations of violence, the availability of weapons, easy access to drugs and alcohol (which serve as disinhibitors), and discrimination and stereotyping based on race, ethnicity, and gender. When children are exposed to violence, they are exposed to a set of norms that justify violence. Interventions that fail to address these social factors can obtain only limited success.

The *public health approach* currently being applied to the prevention of violence encompasses not only the reduction of those factors that place children at *risk* of violent behavior, but also the enhancement of *protective* factors that can serve to mediate the impact of risks to which children are exposed. While not causes, per se, risk factors are useful in predicting the onset, continuity, or escalation of violence. The process of determining effective prevention is complex given that factors that constitute risks at one developmental stage may not persist into later stages. Thus, many propose that the key to effective prevention is not only to identify risk and protective factors, but also to determine when they emerge over the course of development.

RESEARCH

There is intensifying concern that the precursors to the violence that is documented in the adolescent years actually begin much earlier, during elementary school. Based on longitudinal research, in addition to a late-onset trajectory, in which youth do not become violent until adolescence, there is an early-onset trajectory in which children commit their first serious violent act prior to the onset of puberty. In contrast with children in the late-onset group, those in the early-onset group are characterized by higher offense rates and more serious offenses in adolescence; similarly, they evidence a higher level of continuing violence into adulthood (DHHS, 2001). In fact, antisocial behavior patterns and high levels of aggression early in a child's life are among the best predictors of later violent and delinquent behavior (Hawkins & Catalano, 1992). Such behavior patterns appear to become refined and more harmful over time. Little serious violence has been observed in children younger than age 10 (only 0.2 percent of 1997 arrests for serious violent crime involved a child in this age group); rather, the onset of serious violence most often occurs between the ages of 12 and 20 (DHHS, 2001). Nonetheless, others (e.g., Eron, 1990) have suggested that aggressive behavior crystallizes by age 8, indicating the importance of primary prevention efforts that target young children.

Research indicates that violence is influenced by numerous risk and protective factors at the individual, family, school, and community levels. At the individual level, aggression and being male are perhaps the primary risk factors for violent behavior. Other temperamental traits such as high activity level, insensitivity to the feelings of others, high susceptibility to boredom, lack of physical fear, a tendency to seek excitement, and below average intelligence, have been identified as factors that place a child at risk for aggression (Garbarino, 1999). Research has further indicated that for those children who exhibit conduct disorder, the risk of serious violence is greater than for those individuals whose chronic bad behavior does not emerge until adolescence (Garbarino, 1999). The reason that childhood-onset of conduct disorder is more severe than late-onset is unclear.

Research has also produced a solid body of evidence that factors beyond the individual child can serve to prompt or exacerbate aggressive behavior. In his well-known "Bobo doll" study, Bandura (1971) demonstrated that when exposed to adults who displayed aggressive behavior with the doll, children closely imitated these models and treated the doll in a similarly aggressive manner. In contrast, children who did not view the adult behaving aggressively rarely perpetrated any aggressive actions against the doll. Given these findings, it is perhaps not surprising that researchers have found that the use of harsh, inconsistent discipline by parents is most likely to lead to aggressive patterns of behavior in children (Garbarino, 1999). Likewise, a lack of parental responsiveness and/or abusive behavior can lay the foundation for aggressive behavior in children. For example, Garbarino (1999) proposes a developmental trajectory in which abused

children: (1) become hypersensitive to negative social cues, (2) become oblivious to positive social cures, (3) develop a repertoire of aggressive behaviors that are easily accessed and invoked, and (4) conclude that aggression is a successful way of getting what they want. Similarly, Karr-Morse and Wiley (1999) presented a persuasive review of research indicating that violent behavior is linked to abuse and neglect in the first two years of life, when the foundations for trust, empathy, conscience, and lifelong learning are established. Poor parent–child relationships and, in particular, harsh, lax, or inconsistent discipline have been shown to be somewhat predictive of later violence (DHHS, 2001).

Research has shown significant correlations between children's viewing television violence and aggressive behavior; the more a child witnesses violence on television, the more aggressive that child becomes. Longitudinal research has demonstrated that the effects of continued exposure to televised violence are even greater over extended periods of time (Eron, Huesmann, Lefkowitz, & Walder, 1996). While theoretically more dangerous given their interactive nature, video games have yet to be researched fully (DHHS, 2001).

Research in the field of developmental psychopathology demonstrating that some children exposed to multiple risk factors may escape their impact has also led to an interest in researching protective factors. However, as noted in the report of the US Surgeon General (DHHS, 2001), "[t]o date, the evidence regarding protective factors against violence has not met the standards established for risk factors" (chap. 4, section 5, p. 1). Nonetheless, early data indicate that: (1) the formation of secure relationships with parents or other adults and (2) commitment to school may serve an important protective function (DHHS, 2001).

STRATEGIES: OVERVIEW

Violence prevention strategies have generally sought to address individual risk factors associated with violence (e.g., aggressive behavior, conduct problems), environmental risk factors, or both through skill- and competency-building, parent training, behavior management, teaching strategies, and/or both school- and community-based programs. In recent years, there have been several initiatives, most notably those sponsored by the Office of the US Surgeon General and the Center for Substance Abuse Prevention (CSAP) of the Substance Abuse and Mental Health Services Administration (SAMHSA) that have highlighted not only specific programs that work (model programs) or might work (promising programs), but also the particular components of these programs that appear to contribute to their success.

STRATEGIES THAT WORK

Many prevention programs aimed at violence in childhood are delivered in the school setting. Foremost among those school-based strategies that evidence a positive, consistent effect on reducing violence, delinquency, and related risk factors are behavior management programs. Those behavioral approaches that appear to be most effective in preventing youth violence on a universal level encompass behavior monitoring; reinforced school attendance, academic performance, and school behavior; and behavioral techniques for classroom management (DHHS, 2001). Among the best strategies for enhancing classroom behavior are the establishment of clear rules and directions, use of praise and approval, modeling of positive behavior, shaping, token reinforcement, self-specification of contingencies, and self reinforcement (O'Leary & O'Leary, 1977). Negative reinforcement strategies, specifically, ignoring misbehavior and using disciplinary techniques such as timeouts and fines (in token economies), have also been shown to be effective.

Illustrative of the successful implementation of behavioral classroom management techniques is the *Good Behavior Game*. A 2-year randomized trial with 1,000 urban first graders demonstrated that after 1 year of participation, students were viewed as significantly less aggressive by teachers and peers. Improvement, as demonstrated by a reduction in teacher ratings of aggressive behavior, was also observable during key transitions (i.e., in first grade and middle school) (Kellam, Rebok, Ialongo, & Mayer, 1994). Program effects were most profound among those males who had exhibited higher levels of aggression in first grade.

Classroom behavior management techniques are also an essential component of the *Bullying Prevention Program* designated as a model program by CSAP (2001). (Note that the topic of bullying prevention is treated in more detail elsewhere in this volume.) Developed by Dan Olweus, the program is designed to restructure the social environment by involving teachers, parents, and students themselves in setting firm limits to unacceptable behaviors. Limits are balanced with the consistent use of non-hostile, non-corporal restrictions on rule violations. In evaluating 42 elementary and junior high schools in Norway over a 2-year period, Olweus (1997) found a 50–70 percent decrease in the frequency of bully/victim problems 2 years post-intervention. Although somewhat weaker, positive effects have also been obtained in the United States, the United Kingdom, and Germany (CSAP, 2001).

Taking an environmental approach, many commentators have suggested that violence committed by children is a consequence of the violence they themselves experience in the form of child maltreatment. Thus, it has been proposed that one effective method of decreasing violence is to reduce the incidence of child abuse and neglect. (See "Prevention of physical and sexual abuse and neglect in childhood" in this volume.) Parent training using *Multi-systematic Therapy* (MST) has been effectively applied to abusive and neglectful parents of elementary school-aged children. Brunk, Henggler, and Whelan (1987) randomly assigned abusive and neglectful families to either MST or traditional behavioral parent training. At posttest, parents who received either treatment demonstrated a decline in emotional disturbance, overall stress, and severity of identified problems. However, MST was more successful in reforming parent–child behavior patterns that differentiate maltreating parents from non-abusive parents. In the post-program period, MST parents restricted their child's behavior more successfully, maltreated children showed less passive non-compliance, and neglecting parents became more receptive to their child's behavior.

Other studies indicate that risks for violence can be reduced during the elementary grades by combined interventions with parents, teachers, and children themselves. Successful interventions have focused on promoting academic success, cognitive-emotional development, and behavioral self-regulation. The *Seattle Social Development Project* (SSDP) (later named the Skills, Opportunities, and Recognition [SOAR] Program) is a multi-component intervention designed to prevent delinquency and other problem behaviors through enhancing elementary school students' connectedness to school and family and reducing early risk factors for violence (e.g., academic failure, alcohol and drug use). SSDP provides parent-training, a social competence component for students, and a package of classroom behavior management and instruction methods. Evaluations of SSDP show a reduction in aggression, antisocial and externalizing behaviors, and self-destructive behaviors at the end of second grade among children who have participated in the program during first and second grade (Hawkins, Catalano, Morrison, O'Donnell, Abbott, & Day, 1992). In follow-ups at age 18, participants demonstrated significant improvement in attachment and commitment to school and school achievement, as well as a reduction in self-reported violent acts (DHHS, 2001). Program benefits for both general and high-risk populations have been confirmed through replication studies (DHHS, 2001). SSDP/SOAR has been recognized as a model program by both the CSAP (2001) and the US Surgeon General (DHHS, 2001).

Other programs have sought to affect children's behavior both at home and at school by integrating individual, school, parent, family, and community components into a comprehensive prevention strategy. The *Positive Action Program*, designated as a model program by CSAP, is one such comprehensive program, which incorporates a variety of strategies, including positive classroom management; active learning; a detailed curriculum with daily lessons that teach specific positive actions in the physical, intellectual, and social/emotional areas; a school climate program; parent support and involvement; and community involvement in schools. Data from more that 100 diverse elementary schools have shown consistent positive effects on student behavior (e.g., discipline suspensions, crime, and violence), performance (i.e., attendance and achievement), and self-concept (CSAP, 2001).

Across the Ages is a program that combines community service, problem-solving, resistance skills training, and parental involvement with elders mentoring youth. Evaluation data indicating improvements in school attendance and bonding to school, adults, and community, particularly among those students with a highly involved mentor, have prompted CSAP to designate Across Ages as a model program (CSAP, 2001).

STRATEGIES THAT MIGHT WORK

Additional school-based programs that focus on reducing risk by promoting social skills to students might prove effective in preventing violence. One such program is *I Can Problem Solve*, which has been used effectively with students in preschool, kindergarten, fifth grade, and sixth grade. The program provides training in problem-solving skills (i.e., strategies for resolving interpersonal problems) to students in small group sessions over a 3-month period. Evaluation data indicate improvements in classroom behavior and problem-solving skills for up to 4 years postintervention, particularly with students living in poor, urban areas (DHHS, 2001). A similar program, the *Promoting Alternative Thinking Strategies* (PATHS) curriculum, has been presented to students, including special education students, from their entry into elementary school through grade 5. Three times a week, students participate in 20- to 30-min lessons that focus on emotional competence (e.g., expression, understanding, and regulation), self-control, social competence, positive peer relations, and interpersonal problem-solving skills. Evaluation data indicate that PATHS reduces aggressive behavior, anxiety and depression, conduct problems, and lack of self-control (DHHS, 2001).

Two family-based, rather than school-based programs that combine student skill-training with parent training have also been designated as promising programs by the Office of the Surgeon General. The first of these is the *Iowa Strengthening Families* program, which includes seven weekly sessions of parent and child training aimed at improving parenting skills and family communication among sixth-graders and their families. Similarly, *Preparing for the Drug-Free Years* seeks to promote health and protective parent–child interactions through family competency

and youth skills training. The program consists of five sessions, four of which include only parents. Both programs have been implemented in rural, midwestern communities and have evidenced positive effects on child–family relationships, as well as alcohol, tobacco, and drug use, for up to 4 years. A third promising program, *Linking the Interests of Families and Teachers* (LIFT), combines parent training with school-based skills training for students in first and fifth grade. The classroom component consists of 20 1-hr sessions over 10 weeks. Also included is a peer component designed to encourage positive social behavior during playground activities. The parent-training component consists of weekly parent group meetings over 6 weeks. All components focus on reducing children's antisocial behaviors, involvement with delinquent peers, and drug and alcohol use. Evaluation data indicate that student participants exhibit positive effects in all of these areas, including less physical aggression on the playground and enhanced social skills, as well as a reduction in other risk factors for violence (e.g., association with delinquent peers, alcohol use) (DHHS, 2001).

There is also a great deal of optimism around community-based strategies that seek to prevent youth violence at the universal level and, more specifically, positive youth development programs. Mentoring programs, in particular, enjoy widespread support. While a lack of conclusive evaluation data precludes the designation of well-known programs such as Boys and Girls Clubs and Big Brothers/Big Sisters of America as model programs, they may be effective in reducing youth violence and violence-related outcomes (DHHS, 2001).

STRATEGIES THAT DO NOT WORK

Peer counseling, peer mediation, and peer leaders are among the school-based primary prevention programs that have consistently failed to demonstrate their effectiveness in scientific studies (DHHS, 2001). Nonpromotion to succeeding grades (i.e., "holding students back") has also been shown to be ineffective, with some studies actually indicating that nonpromotion has a negative effect on students' achievement, attendance, behavior, and attitudes toward school, factors that could serve a protective function in regard to violence (DHHS, 2001).

Likewise, strategies that aim to prevent violence through "shock" dispositional programs, such as *Scared Straight*, have not proven effective. Aimed primarily at juveniles who commit low-level delinquent acts, Scared Straight and other jail visitation programs are based on the premise that viewing jail conditions first-hand and having inmates relate their personal experiences with prison life will shock young people into rehabilitation before they become involved in more serious crimes. Despite its media popularity, which began with the 1978 television debut of a documentary of the same name, Scared Straight has produced no scientific evidence of its effectiveness. Although producers of the original documentary claimed that of the 8,000 youth who had participated in the program, 80 percent had been "scared straight," researchers later discovered that the majority of these participants had visited the prison as part of a field trip and had never committed a crime. When only those participants who had been referred by the justice system were contrasted with a comparison group, those who visited the prison were actually *more* likely to reoffend (Petrosino, Turpin-Petrosino, & Fincknauer, 2000).

SYNTHESIS

As noted by the Office of the Surgeon General in its recent report on youth violence (DHHS, 2001), "researchers know much more today than they did two decades ago, when some declared that 'nothing works' to prevent violence" (chap. 5, p. 1). A major theoretical advance in designing effective primary prevention programs has been the application of a developmental framework to the prediction and prevention of antisocial behaviors, such as early childhood violence. While additional research is needed to clarify the interaction of a variety of causal factors that differ by age and different risk patterns, there are strong indicators of several effective primary prevention strategies.

Employing meta-analysis and reviews of the evaluation research, the US Surgeon General sought to identify best practices for preventing youth violence; however, it was noted that one critical limitation of these results was a potential failure to identify whether programs were effective for some populations, but not others (e.g., females but not males). Applying scientific standards (i.e., sound experimental design, evidence of significant deterrent effects, and replication of effects at multiple sites or in clinical trials), the Surgeon General concluded that few programs could be designated as highly effective or "model" programs. A substantially larger number met minimal effectiveness standards, qualifying them as "promising programs". Moreover, many of these programs might qualify as model programs, but they currently lack rigorous evaluation data. As noted by Tolan and Guerra (1994), evaluation efforts are needed not, only to identify effective strategies, but also to determine those strategies that may actually increase or exacerbate violent behavior.

Based on current research, the most effective primary prevention strategies include skills training, behavior monitoring and reinforcement, behavioral techniques for classroom management, building school capacity, continuous progress programs, cooperative learning, and positive youth development programs. Overall, successful strategies may target individual risk factors, environmental risk factors, or both. Such successful anti-violence programs involve families, communities and schools; are instituted across grade levels; contain a strong staff development component; and are tailored to the participants of the program. It is also recommended that, in order to be successful, programs should involve interactive teaching techniques (Murray, 1998).

While a great deal of information is available from which effective prevention strategies can be identified, scarce resources continue to be allocated to ineffective programs. Ineffective universal prevention strategies include peer counseling, peer mediation, peer leaders, and nonpromotion to succeeding grades (DHHS, 2001). Likewise, approaches that employ "scare tactics," focus on overburdened teachers, and only impart information (without the follow-through necessary to effect behavior change) do not work. It is not enough to institute a "one-shot" intervention; rather, in order to prevent violence, interventions need to be comprehensive.

Also see: Violence Prevention entries; Aggressive Behavior, Childhood; Anger Regulation entries; Bullying, Media Habits; Self-Esteem, Childhood.

References

Bandura, A. (1971). *Social learning theory*. Morristown, NJ: General Learning.

Bandura, A. (1989). Social cognitive theory. In R. Vasta (Ed.), Six theories of child development. *Annals of Child Development* (Vol. 6, pp. 1–60). Greenwich, CT: JAI Press.

Brunk, M., Heggeler, S.W., & Whelan, J.P. (1987). A comparison of multi-systematic therapy and parent training in the brief treatment of child abuse and neglect. *Journal of Consulting and Clinical Psychology, 63*, 569–578.

Centers for Disease Control and Prevention. (1997). Rates of homicide, suicide, and firearm-related death amoung children: 26 industrialized countries. *Morbidity and Mortality Weekly Report, 46*, 101–105.

Center for Substance Abuse Prevention (CSAP). (2001). *2001 Annual report of science-based prevention programs*. Washington, DC: US Department of Health and Human Services.

Duyme, M. (1989). Antisocial behaviors and postnatal environment: A French adoption study. *Journal of Child Psychology and Psychiatry, 7*, 285–291.

Eron, L.D. (1990). Understanding aggression. *Bulletin of the International Society for Research on Aggression, 12*, 5–9.

Eron, L., Huesmann, L.R., Lefkowitz, M.M., & Walder, L.O. (1996). Does television violence cause aggression? In Greenberg, D.F. (Ed.), *Criminal careers, Vol. 2. The international library of criminology, criminal justice, and penology* (pp. 311–321). Brookfield, VT: Dartmouth.

Federal Bureau of Investigations. (1999). *Crime in the United States*. Washington DC: US Department of Justice.

Garbarino, J. (1999). *Lost boys: Why our sons turn violent and how we can save them*. New York: The Free Press.

Hawkins, J.D., & Catalano, R.F. (1992). *Communities that care*. San Francisco: Jossey-Bass.

Hawkins, J.D., Catalano, R.F., Morrison, D., O'Donnell, J., Abott, R., & Day, L.E. (1992). The Seattle Social Development Project: Effects of the first four years on protective factors and problem behaviors. In J. McCord & R.E. Tremblay (Eds.), *Preventing antisocial behavior: Interventions from birth through adolescence*. New York: The Guilford Press.

Junger-Tas, J., Terlouw, G.J., & Klein, M.W. (1994). *Delinquent behavior among young people in the western world: First results of the international self-report delinquency study*. Amsterdam: Kugler.

Karr-Morse, R., & Wiley, M.S. (1999). *Ghosts from the nursery: Tracing the roots of violence*. New York: Grove/Atlantic.

Kellam, S.G., Rebok, G.W., Ialongo, N., & Mayer, S.L. (1994). The course and malleability of aggressive behavior from early first grade into middle school: Results of a developmental epidemiological-based prevention trial. *Journal of Child Psychology and Psychiatry, 35*, 259–281.

Loeber, R., & Stouthamer-Loeber, M. (1986). Family factors as correlates and predictors of juvenile conduct problems and delinquency. In M. Tonry & N. Morris (Eds.), *Crime and justice: An annual review of research* (pp. 29–149). Chicago, IL: University of Chicago Press.

Murray, B. (1998, July). What works in violence prevention. *APA Monitor, 29*, 17.

O'Leary, K.D., & O'Leary, S.G. (1977). *Classroom management: The successful use of behavior modification* (2nd ed.). New York: Pergamon Press.

Olweus, D. (1997). Bullying/victim problems in school: Facts and intervention. *European Journal of Psychology of Education, 12*, 495–510.

Petrosino, A., Turpin-Petrosino, C., & Finckenauer, J.O. (2000). Well meaning programs can have harmful effects! Lessons from experiments of programs such as Scared Straight. *Crime and Delinquency, 46*, 354–379.

Steinmetz, S.K. (1987). Family violence: Past, present, and future. In M.B. Sussman & S.K. Steinmetz (Eds.), *Handbook of marriage and the family* (pp. 725–765). New York: Plenum.

Tolan, P., & Guerra, N. (1994). *What works in reducing adolecent violence: An empirical review of the field*. Boulder, CO: The Center for the Study and Prevention of Violence.

US Department of Health and Human Services (USDHHS). (2001). *Youth violence: A report of the Surgeon General [on-line]*. Available: http://www.surgeongeneral.gov/library/youthviolence/report/html

Contributors

Inquiries for further information should be directed to the editors, Thomas R. Gullota <tpg@cfapress.org> and Martin Bloom <bloom@uconn.edu>

Adams, Gerald, R. PhD, is Distinguished Professor of Teaching in the Department of Family Relations and Applied Nutrition, University of Guelph, Ontario, Canada, and Editor of the *Journal of Adolescent Research.* His research program intertwines adolescent development, personal and social identity formation, and social and applied primary prevention. He is also Co-Section Editor for Adolescence in this *Encyclopedia of Primary Prevention and Health Promotion.*

Albee, George W., PhD, is Professor Emeritus of Psychology, University of Vermont, and Courtesy Professor, Florida Mental Health Institute. The Editors of this *Encyclopedia* note that his many contributions to primary prevention have spanned over a half century, not the least of which is the development of the Vermont Conference on Primary Prevention of Psychopathology, and the many volumes emerging from those conferences.

Alexander, Kristi, PhD, is Associate Professor at the Department of Psychology and Family Studies at US International University, San Diego, California.

Amico, K. Rivet., PhD, is Assistant Research Professor, at the Center for HIV Intervention and Prevention, in the University of Connecticut's Department of Psychology.

Archibald, Andrea B., PhD, is a Research Scientist at the Center of Children and Families, Teachers College, Columbia University. Her work focuses on the health and development of adolescent girls.

Arcus, Doreen, PhD, is Assistant Professor, Department of Psychology, University of Massachusetts at Lowell, with research interests in child development.

Ayers, Tim S., PhD, is Assistant Director of the Program for Prevention Research at Arizona State University, where he has been involved with the development and evaluation of preventive interventions for children.

Balcazar, Fabricio E., PhD, is Associate Professor, Department of Disability and Human Development, Department of Psychology, University of Illinois at Chicago. His research focuses on developing and evaluating strategies that low-income minority individuals with disabilities, and their families, can use to improve their quality of life.

Barber, Bonnie L., PhD, is Associate Professor of Family Studies and Human Development, at the University of Arizona in Tucson. Her interests are in developmental psychology.

Begun, Audrey, PhD, has conducted research in adolescent substance abuse prevention and the evaluation of intimate partner violence prevention, at the University of Wisconsin at Milwaukee, School of Social Work, where she is a Professor.

Belyea, Monica J., MPH, RD, is Extension Instructor in Residence, Senior Nutrition Awareness Project, University of Connecticut/ University of Rhode Island Family Nutrition.

Bernstein, Avis, PhD, is Assistant Professor at the University of Miami School of Medicine. As a clinical psychologist, she has facilitated support groups for caregivers , and services on the executive committee for the Miami Area Geriatric Education Center.

Bertera, Elizabeth M., PhD, LCSW, BCD, is Assistant Professor at the School of Social Service, Catholic

University of America in Washington, DC, with research and practice interests in gerontology, minority health, and social support. She is on the Editorial Board of the *Journal of Gerontological Social Work*.

Bingenheimer, Jeffrey B. is a doctoral student at the University of Michigan School of Public Health.

Bishop, Brian, PhD, is a community psychologist, School of Psychology, Curtin University, Perth, Australia, where he teaches community and cross-cultural psychology and conducts research on community-based interventions and community health.

Blakely, Craig, PhD, MPH, is Professor and Head, Department of Health Policy and Management, School of Rural Public Health, at Texas A & M Health Science Center. He is also Co-Editor on the Infancy and Young Children section of the *Encyclopedia of Primary Prevention and Health Promotion*.

Blank, Michael, B., PhD, is with the Center for Mental Health Policy and Services Research, and is Assistant Professor of Psychology in Psychiatry at the University of Pennsylvania, School of Medicine. He also has an appointment at the Penn School of Nursing, and is a Senior Fellow at the Leonard Davis Institute of Health Economics.

Bloom, Martin, PhD, is Editor of the *Journal of Primary Prevention*, Co-Editor of this *Encyclopedia of Primary Prevention and Health Promotion*, and Professor at the University of Connecticut. He is interested in theory, research, and practice in primary prevention.

Bond, Lynne, PhD, is Professor of Psychology at the University of Vermont, and is the recent winner of the Albee Award for Distinguished Contributions to Primary Prevention. She is also Section Editor on Children for the *Encyclopedia of Primary Prevention and Health Promotion*.

Bond, Meg A., PhD, is Professor of Psychology, at the University of Massachusetts, Lowell. She is Co-Director of the Center for Women and Work, and her current research involves an analysis of organizational approaches to diverse employees and the dynamics around gender and race.

Borg, Jr., Mark B., PhD, is Executive Director, Interpersonal Empowerment Institute; Associate Director of Psychology, Fifth Avenue Center for Counseling and Psychotherapy, New York City.

Bothell, Joan is editor and writer at the Environmental Research Institute, University of Connecticut.

Botvin, Gilbert J., PhD, is Professor of Public Health, Director of Cornell's Institute for Prevention Research, and Professor of Psychiatry at Weill Medical College of Cornell University. He is also Editor of *Prevention Science*.

Bowen, Gary L., PhD, is the Kenan Distinguished Professor of Social Work, the University of North Carolina, at Chapel Hill.

Boyce, Thomas E., PhD, is Assistant Professor of Psychology and Director, Center for Behavioral Safety Research at University of Nevada, Reno.

Braun, Kathryn L., Dr. PH, is Professor of Public Health, and Director, Center on Aging, John A. Burns School of Medicine, University of Hawaii. Her interests include cultural issues in end-of-life decision-making.

Bray, Melissa A., PhD, is Assistant Professor of School Psychology at the University of Connecticut. Her research interests include interventions for communication, behavior, and health-related disorders.

Britto, Pia Rebello PhD, is Research Scientist at the Center for Children and Families: Advancing Policy, Education, and Development, at Teachers College, Columbia University.

Brookins, Craig C., PhD, is Associate Professor of Psychology, and Director, Africana Studies, Multidisciplinary Studies, North Carolina State University, Raleigh. His research focus is on the African Diaspora.

Brooks-Gunn, Jeanne, PhD, is Virginia and Leonard Marx Professor and Co-Director of the Center for Children and Families, at Teachers College, Columbia University. She is also Co-Director of the Columbia University Institute for Child and Family Policy.

Brown, Jeffrey, MD, MPH. is the General Pediatrics Division Director at Denver Health and is an Associate Professor in the Section of Academic Pediatrics in the Department of Pediatrics at the University of Colorado School of Medicine in Denver.

Brown, Margaret, PhD, coordinates a children, youth, and family at-risk initiative with the Cooperative Extension, and provides consultation on home visitor training and parent education and support programs, at the University of Delaware.

Browne, Colette V., Dr. PH, MSW, MEd, is Associate Professor of Social Work at the. University of Hawaii, and is faculty affiliate with the University of Hawaii Center on Aging. Her areas of scholarship include feminist gerontology, ethnogerontology, and gerontology curricula development.

She is also Co-Section Editor on Older Persons for the *Encyclopedia of Primary Prevention*.

Bryan, Angela, PhD, is Assistant Professor, Department of Psychology, Institute of Behavioral Science, University of Colorado. She has received funding by NIAAA to study the relationship between alcohol use and HIV risk among adolescents on probation. abryan@psych.colorado.edu C-9.

Buchanan, Jeffrey is a clinical psychology graduate student at the University of Nevada, Reno. His interests include investigating psychological treatments for caregivers of elderly individuals.

Bush, Kevin R., PhD, is Assistant Professor in Child and Family Development at the University of Georgia. His research interests include parent–adolescent relationships within and across cultures.

Caldwell, Kathryn, PhD, is a training consultant on a project that teaches child care providers about the social–emotional needs of young children. She is affiliated with the University of Washington, Department of Family and Child Nursing.

Cantwell, Anne-Marie is a doctoral candidate in the Department of Family Relations and Human Development, College of Social and Applied Human Sciences, University of Guelph, Ontario, Canada.

Carey, Michael P., PhD, is Professor of Psychology and Director of the Center for Health and Behavior at Syracuse University, where he investigates sexual health, including HIV prevention.

Carter, Blair, MBA, MPH, PhD, is Research Program Analyst, Adolescent Health Risk Study, Medical Quality Assurance, Texas Department of Human Services, State Headquarters. He founded the Center for the Advancement of Family Epidemiology and Services and has worked in academic and applied public health settings in Texas, California, and Mexico.

Chafouleas, Sandra M., PhD, is Assistant Professor, Department of Educational Psychology, University of Connecticut.

Chalmers, David, PhD, is Associate Professor and Deputy Director, Injury Prevention Research Unit, University of Otago Medical School, Department of Preventive and Social Medicine, Dunedin, New Zealand. His research has focused on childhood injury prevention, with emphasis on playground injury.

Colwell, Brian, PhD, CHES, is Associate Professor, Department of Social and Behavioral Health, Texas A&M.

Connell, Christian M., PhD, is Associate Research Scientist in the Division of Prevention of Community Research at the Yale University School of Medicine. His research focuses on the promotion of social, behavioral, and academic competence in low-income and at-risk populations.

Cornman, Deborah, H., PhD, a clinical psychologist and behavioral scientist, is Associate Director for the Center for HIV Intervention and Prevention (CHIP) at the University of Connecticut.

Couch, Sarah C., PhD, RD, Assistant Professor of Nutrition, Department of Health Sciences, University of Cincinnati.

Crowley, Angela A., PhD, APRN, CS, PNP, is Associate Professor at Yale University School of Nursing. Her research interests focus on the health and development of children and families in primary care and early care settings.

Daley, Alison Moriarty, MSN, RN, CS, PNP, is Assistant Professor, Yale University School of Nursing, and PNP at the Yale-New Haven Hospital Adolescent Clinic.

Danish, Steven J., PhD, Director, Life Skills Center, and Professor of Psychology, Preventive Medicine and Community Health at Virginia Commonwealth University.

Daugherty, Ray, PhD, founded the Prevention Research Institute, a nonprofit organization. Over one million people in the United States and Scandinavia have received one of the eight curricula he co-authored, based on the Lifestyle Risk Reduction Model.

Dawson, Kimberley A., PhD, is Associate Professor, Department of Kinesiology and Physical Education, at Wilfrid-Laurier University, Waterloo, Ontario, Canada. Her research focuses on the influence of perceived control on health behavior, including exercise.

Dawson-McClure, Spring R. is a doctoral student in psychology, at Arizona State University, with research interests in understanding ways that parents facilitate children's adaptation to stressors, including parental divorce.

Deckelbaum, Richard J., MD, CM, FRCP(C) is Robert R. Williams Professor of Nutrition, and Director of the Institute of Human Nutrition, Columbia University. He also serves as a Professor of Pediatrics and Director in the Division of Gastroenterology and Nutrition, Department of Pediatrics, Columbia University.

Dela cruz, Georgia G., DMD, MPH, is a Dental Officer in the US Army, stationed at the Center for Health Promotion and Preventive Medicine, Aberdeen Proving Grounds, MD.

Denham, Susanne A., PhD, is Professor at George Mason University, Fairfax, Virginia. Her work centers on social–emotional development. She is also Co-Editor of the journal, *Social Development*.

Doswell, Willa M., RN, PhD, FAAN, is Assistant Professor, University of Pittsburgh School of Nursing, where she serves as Adolescent Scholarship Group Coordinator, Associate Director for Dissemination at an NINR-funded Center for Research in Chronic Disorders.

Downs, Chris, PhD, Director of Developmental Research , Casey Family Programs, Seattle Washington, where he is involved in many research projects related to youth development, self-sufficiency, and well-being. He is also interested in social competence, adolescent sexuality, and interpersonal stereotyping.

Dowrick, Peter W., PhD, is Professor of Disability Studies and Graduate Studies in Psychology, University of Hawaii at Manoa. He has 25 years experience in US, European, and Pacific countries in psychology and other disciplines, with special interests in video self-modeling.

Doyle, Charlotte, PhD, is Professor of Psychology, at Sarah Lawrence College, Bronxville, New York. Her research area is on the creative process in children and adults, and along with her other professional publications are five picture books for children.

Dubois, David L., PhD, is Associate Professor of Psychology (Clinical-Community Psychology) at University of Illinois at Chicago.

Duffy, Michael, PhD, ABPP, is Professor of Counseling Psychology at Texas A&M University also specializing in clinical geropsychology.

Dumka, Larry E., PhD, is Associate Professor of Marriage and Family Therapy in the Department of Family Resources and Human Development, Arizona State University. His research focuses on developing and testing family strengthening interventions for ethnically diverse low-income families.

Durlak, Joseph A., PhD, is Professor of Psychology, Loyola University in Chicago. He has written two books on prevention, and co-edited a third.

Elias, Maurice J., PhD, Department of Psychology, Rutgers University, and Leadership Team Vice Chair for the Collaborative for Academic, Social, and Emotional Learning.

Emshoff, James G., PhD, is the Director of the Community Psychology Program at Georgia State University, Atlanta. Most of his work has focused on the evaluation of preventive interventions, including those focused on children of alcoholics.

Erchul, William P., PhD, is Professor of Psychology, and Director of the School Psychology Program at North Carolina State University. He studies interpersonal processes and outcomes within school-based consultation.

Evans, Garret D., PsyD, is Associate Professor of Clinical Psychology and Director of the National Rural Behavioral Health Center at the University of Florida.

Evans, Richard I., PhD, is Distinguished University Professor and Director, Social Psychology Program and Social Psychology/Behavioral Medicine Research Group at the University of Houston. The editors of this *Encyclopedia* note that he has conducted pioneering prevention research related to social influence and resistance.

Falciglia, Grace A., EdD, MPH, RD, is Professor of Nutrition, and Chairperson of the Department of Health Sciences, Program in Dietetics and Nutrition Science at the University of Cincinnati.

Farrington, David P., PhD, is Professor of Psychological Criminology in the Institute of Criminology at the University of Cambridge, England.

Feinberg, Mark E., PhD, is Research Associate in the Prevention Research Center, College of Health and Human Development, Pennsylvania State University.

Feldman, David B. is a graduate student in Clinical Psychology at the University of Kansas. His interests involve positive psychology.

Ferland, Francine, PhD, (Laval University). She has conducted considerable research on preventing problem gambling, and has produced two videos on this topic.

Fernandez, Ephrem, PhD, is Associate Professor, Psychology Department, Southern Methodist University, and special faculty at the University of Texas Southwestern Medical Center.

Ferrer-Wreder, Laura, PhD, is Assistant Professor of Psychology at Penn State Capital College, with research interests in creating preventive/promotive interventions for youth.

Fine, Mark A., PhD, is Professor and Chair, Department of Human Development and Family Studies, University of Missouri at Columbia. He is Editor of the *Journal of Social and Personal Relationships*. His research interests are in family transitions, early intervention program evaluation, social cognition, and relationship stability.

Finkel, Julia J. is a doctoral student in Community Psychology at the University of Missouri at Kansas City. Her interests are in prevention-oriented policy and programming for children, youth, and families.

Fintor, Louis, PhD, is at McGill University, Montreal, Quebec, Canada. He has worked in the cancer prevention area for more than a decade, and has held cancer research positions at the US National Cancer Institute and the US Centers for Disease Control.

Fisher, Jane E., PhD, is Professor of Psychology at the University of Nevada. Her interests include bereavement, prevention of elder abuse, and interventions for caregivers.

Flay, Brian, D Phil, is Distinguished Professor of Public Health, School of Public Health, University of Illinois at Chicago. His research involves why youth engage in health-compromising behaviors, and on school/community interventions to prevent substance use, violence, unsafe sex, and low academic achievement.

Fogel, Joshua, PhD, is a psychologist with clinical interests in health psychology, including primary prevention of cardiovascular disease, cancer, and Internet communication use. He is at Johns Hopkins University, Bloomberg School of public Health, Baltimore, M.D.

Forbes-Jones, Emma L., MA, is a doctoral student in Clinical Psychology at the University of Rochester, with research interests in risk and protective factors in the development of aggression, and in preventive programs with at-risk children and adolescents.

Ford, Briggett C., PhD, MPH, is a post-doctoral research fellow in the School of Social Work at the University of Michigan, Ann Arbor. Dr. Ford's research examines the epidemiology of mental disorder and the mental health consequences of exposure to violence for African American women.

Freres, Derek R., BA, is Project Coordinator for the Penn Resiliency Project at the University of Pennsylvania. This is a school-based program on the prevention of depression for adolescents.

Fried, Carrie S., MA, is a graduate student in Psychology at the University of Virginia. Her research focuses on the development of empathy and the prevention of youth violence.

Fuligni, Allison Sidle, PhD, is Research Scientist at the Center for Children and Families: Advancing Policy, Education, and Development, at Teachers College, Columbia University.

Furlong, Michael J., PhD, is Professor and Program Leader in the Department of Clinical, Counseling, and School Psychology, at the University of California at Santa Barbara. He has conducted research in the areas of school safety and violence prevention.

Garcia, Victor F., MD, is Director of the Trauma Service at Cincinnati Children's Hospital Medical Center, and also principal investigator on several pediatric injury-related studies.

Garrod, Emily, PhD, Clinical Director, Interpersonal Empowerment Institute; Adjunct Assistant Professor, John Jay College of Criminal Justice; Clinical Supervisor, Saint Vincent's Hospital, Department of Psychiatry, New York City.

Gavazzi, Stephen M., PhD, is Associate Professor, Department of Human Development and Family Science, Ohio State University. He is also Research Coordinator for the John Glenn Institute's Center for Learning Excellence. His research involves family-based programming efforts.

Geller, E. Scott, PhD, is Professor of Psychology and Director of the Center for Applied Behavior Systems at Virginia Polytechnic Institute. He is associate editor of *Environment and Behavior*, and past editor of the *Journal of Applied Behavior Analysis*, and fellow of the American Psychological Association.

Getz, J. Gregory, PhD, is Associate Professor of Sociology and Assistant Chair in the Department of Social Sciences, at the University of Houston, Downtown. His research areas include the sociology and social psychology of health and illness, with a focus on adolescent substance use.

Gillespie, Janet F., PhD, is Associate Professor of Psychology, Coordinator of Graduate Studies in Psychology, SUNY Brockport.

Gillham, Jane E., PhD, is Co-Director of the Penn Resiliency Project at the University of Pennsylvania, and Visiting Assistant Professor of Psychology at Swarthmore College.

Gironda, Melanie, PhD, is Lecturer in the Department of Social Welfare, University of California at Los Angeles. Her research involves social aspects of older persons without children, and loneliness among aging populations.

Godenzi, Alberto, PhD, is Dean and Professor of the Graduate School of Social Work at Boston College. He was Chair of the Department of Social Work and Social Policy at the University of Fribourg, Switzerland. His research interests include violence against women.

Graber, Julia A., PhD, is Associate Professor in the Department of Psychology, University of Florida at Gainsville. She studies biopsycho-social changes during the transition to adolescence.

Griffin, Kenneth W., PhD, MPH, is Assistant Professor of Public Health at Cornell University Medical College.

Gullotta, Thomas P., MA, MSW, is the CEO of Child and Family Agency of Southeastern Connecticut and has written extensively on families and adolescents. He is Editor Emeritus of the *Journal of Primary Prevention*. He has also been the Book Series Editor for *Advances in Adolescent Development and Prevention in Practice*. Presently, he edits *Issues in Chidren's and Families' Lives* and is the Co-Editor of this encyclopedia.

Gupta, Giri Raj, PhD, is Professor of Sociology at Western Illinois University, Macomb, Illinois. His areas of interest are marriage and the family, sociological theory, and mental health. He edited a six-volume series on Indian Sociology.

Gustafson, Elaine, MSN, RN, CS. PNP, is Assistant Professor at the Yale University School of Nursing, and at Fair Haven Community Health Center where she practices as a pediatric nurse practitioner.

Hampton, Robert, PhD, is Associate Provost for Academic Affairs, and Dean for Undergraduate Studies, the University of Maryland at College Park. His research interests include partner violence, family abuse, community violence, stress and social support, and social change. He is one of the founders of the National Institute on Violence in the African American Community.

Hansson, Robert O., PhD, is Professor of Psychology, University of Tulsa. His research interests include bereavement, loss, and coping in aging families.

Harper, Gary W., PhD, MPH, is Associate Professor, Department of Psychology, DePaul University, Chicago. He is also the Director of the Community-Clinical Doctoral Training Program at DePaul.

Hearne, Shelley, PhD, is Director, Trust for America's Health, Baltimore, Maryland. She is also Johns Hopkins Visiting Scholar, member of the EPA's Children's Health Advisory Committee, and former director, Pew Environmental Health Commission.

Heiby, Elaine M., PhD, Professor and Director, Clinical Studies, Department of Psychology, University of Hawaii.

Heke, Ihirangi, MEd and PhD, finalist, is a practicing sport psychologist, player, and coach in several sports, and specializes in Maori driven health and social initiatives in New Zealand.

Henderson, Deborah is a graduate student in clinical psychology at the University of Nevada, Reno. Her research interests concern the treatment and prevention of elder abuse.

Hodge, Ken, PhD, is Senior Lecturer in sport psychology at the School of Physical Education, University of Otago, New Zealand. His research focuses on the psychosocial effects of participation in sports.

Hooyman, Nancy R., PhD, is Professor and Dean Emeritus at the University of Washington School of Social Work. She is the author of a number of books in gerontology, family caregiving, and feminist perspective on gender and justice.

Horne, Arthur M., PhD, is Department Head and Director of Training, in the Department of Counseling and Human Development Services, at the University of Georgia. He has been active in other areas as well, including marriage and family therapy, group work, and violence reduction in schools.

Hosek, Sybil G., PhD, is doing post-doctoral work in the Department of Adolescent Psychiatry at Cook County Hospital in Chicago, where she will continue her research and clinical work with HIV-infected youth.

Hughes, Tegwyn L., D.D.S., is a pediatric dentist who is completing a PhD, in epidemiology at the University of North Carolina, with a specialty in dental public health.

Irving, Lori M. (deceased), PhD, was Associate Professor of Psychology, Washington State University at Vancouver, and Coordinator, Columbia River Eating Disorder Network.

Iscoe, Ira., PhD, is the Ashbel Smith Professor of Psychology Emeritus, at the University of Texas at Austin. He directed various prevention programs including community psychology training and the Institute for Human Development.

Jacobus, Laura L., MA, is a graduate student in the community psychology program at Georgia State University in Atlanta, Georgia.

Jimenez, Tisa C. is a doctoral student in Special Education, Disability and Risk Studies/School Psychology Credential Program at the University of California, Santa Barbara, California.

Johnson, Blair, T. PhD, is Director for the Center for HIV Intervention and Prevention at the Department of Psychology, University of Connecticut. His areas of interest include the prevention of HIV transmission, social influence, and research methods.

Johnson, Jeannette, PhD, is the Director of the Center for Child and Adolescent Research at the State University of New York at Buffalo.

Judd, Brian M. is Research Assistant at Casey Family Programs, Seattle, Washington. His research interests include the development of LGBT youth, how entertainment media affect the perception of reality, and what we can learn about children from their stories and drawings. He will be entering the doctoral program in Psychology at Washington State.

Kalafat, John, PhD, is Associate Professor, Graduate School of Applied and Professional Psychology, Rutgers University. He will become President of the American Association of Suicidology in April, 2002.

Kameoka, Velma A., PhD, is Professor of Psychology at the University of Hawaii.

Katz, David L., MD, MPH, is Associate Clinical Professor of Public Health and Medicine at Yale University School of Medicine, and Director of the Yale Prevention Research Center.

Kaufman, Joy S., PhD, is Assistant Professor of Psychology in Psychiatry in the Division of Prevention and Community Research at the Yale University School of Medicine. She is also Director of Program and Service System Evaluation at the Consultation Center.

Kehle, Thomas J., PhD, is Professor and Director of the School Psychology Program, University of Connecticut.

Kelly, James G., PhD, is Emeritus Professor, University of Illinois at Chicago, and now Lecturer, University of California, Davis. The editors of this *Encyclopedia* note that he is one of the founders of the field of community psychology, and has made many contributions to this area, as well as in primary prevention.

Kennedy, Cara L. is a clinical psychology graduate student at Arizona State University, where she is interested in prevention and intervention efforts for community-level change.

Kennedy, Nancy, Dr PH, with almost 30 years of experience in mental health and substance abuse, works currently with the federal Center for Substance Abuse Prevention.

Keys, Christopher B., PhD, is Professor and Chair of the Psychology Department, and Professor of Disability and Human Development, University of Illinois at Chicago. His research interests focus on the empowerment of people of color with disabilities and their families in low-income communities.

Kirby, Douglas, PhD, is Senior Research Scientist at ETR Associates, in Scotts Valley, California. He has conducted and reviewed many studies of programs to reduce adolescent sexual risk-taking behavior.

Kiyak, H. Asuman, PhD, is Director of the Institute on Aging, Professor of Oral and Maxillofacial Surgery, Adjunct Professor of Psychology at the University of Washington. Her research focuses on methods to improve oral health knowledge and practices among older adults.

Klein, Waldo, PhD, MSW, is Associate Professor at the University of Connecticut, School of Social Work. His research interests include work on substance use and abuse with older adults, as well as long-term care policy. Dr. Klein is also Co-Section Editor for Older Adults for the *Encyclopedia of Primary Prevention and Health Promotion*.

Kliewer, Wendy, PhD, is Associate Professor of Psychology at Virginia Commonwealth University. Her research focuses on parental contributions to children's coping and adjustment to stressful events.

Kotch, Jonathan, MD, MPH, is Professor and Associate Chair for Graduate Studies in the Department of Maternal and Child Health, School of Public Health, University of North Carolina. He is a board certified specialist in both pediatrics and preventive medicine. Dr. Kotch is also Co-Section Editor for Infants and Young Children for the *Encyclopedia of Primary Prevention and Health Promotion*.

Kress, Jeffrey S., PhD, is Senior Research Associate at the William Davidson Graduate School of Jewish Education, the Jewish Theological Seminary in New York. His interests include religious and spiritual identity, social–emotional learning, and program development.

Ladouceur, Robert, PhD, is Professor of Psychology, and Director to the Center for the Prevention and Treatment of Gambling, at Ecole de Psychologie, Universite Laval, Ste-Foy, Quebec, Canada. His research interests focus on gambling.

Lammi-Keefe, Carol J., PhD, RD, Professor and Department Head, Department of Nutritional Sciences, University of Connecticut. Her research interests focus on nutrition for both the elderly and for the pregnant woman and the neonate.

Ledford, Cynthia H., MD, is Assistant Professor of Clinical Medicine at Ohio State University College of Medicine and Public Health. She practices primary care, internal medicine, and pediatrics in the fifth fattest city in the United States.

Lee, Jeong Rim is a doctoral student in Human Development and Family Studies at Texas Tech University.

Lee, Judy H. is a graduate student in the Clinical Studies Program at the University of Hawaii conducting research on the assessment of depression and secondary depression. Her interests include multicultural issues in psychopathology and prevention protocols for depression.

Leukefeld, Carl, PhD, is Professor of Psychiatry and Behavioral Science as well as Director of the Center of Drug and Alcohol Research at the University of Kentucky.

Levine, Michael P., PhD, is Professor of Psychology, Department of Psychology, Kenyon College, and former board member of Eating Disorders Awareness and Prevention, Inc.

Liu, Chien, PhD, is Associate Professor of Sociology at Wagner College, Staten Island, NY. His research focuses on marriage and family, social institutions, and social/economic development in China.

Lombardo, Sylvie A. is a doctoral student in clinical-community psychology at Wayne State University. Her research interests include at-risk youth, cross-cultural issues, and homeless and other marginal groups.

Lorente, Carolyn Cass, PhD, is an instructor at George Washington University. Her research interests are in identity development and youth prevention programming.

Lorion, Raymond P., PhD, is Professor and Chair, Psychology in Education Division in the Graduate School of Education, University of Pennsylvania. His extensive work includes conceptualization, design, implementation, and evaluation of the prevention of emotional and behavioral disorders in youth and in the development of programs to promote wellness and optimal development.

Lubben, James, DSW, MPH, is Professor of Social Welfare and Urban Planning, University of California at Los Angeles, School of Public Policy and Social Research. His research examines social support networks among aging populations.

MacEntee, Michael I., PhD, LDS(I), FRCD(C), is Professor and Chair of the Division of Prosthondontics in the Faculty of Dentistry, University of British Columbia, Vancouver, Canada. His research addresses the measurement, distribution, impact, and management of oral disorders in elderly populations.

Macik, Felicia K., DO, is Assistant Professor of Family and Community Medicine at the Texas A&M College of Medicine/Brazos Family Medicine Residency.

Maddux, James E., PhD, is Professor in the Department of Psychology, and Associate Chair for Graduate Studies, George Mason University, Fairfax, VA. His research focuses on the role of goals and self-efficacy beliefs in motivation, emotion, and psychological well-being.

Magarian, Lucia holds a Master of Science in Family Studies and a Master of Fine Arts in Creative Writing. She is a licensed clinical marriage and family therapist as well as a playwright and poet.

Mancini, Jay A., PhD, is Professor of Human Development at Virginia Polytechnic Institute and State University, in Blacksburg, Virginia.

Marsh, Kerry L., PhD, is Associate Research Professor, Department of Psychology, University of Connecticut. Her research interests focus on studies of persuasion, motivational influences on social cognition, and HIV prevention.

Marshall, Diana, PhD, is Research Assistant at the Tobler Research Center, Social Capital Development Corporation, Albany, New York, which specializes in substance abuse prevention and youth development.

Martin, James A., PhD, is Associate Professor of Social Work at Bryn Mawr College.

Matthieu, Monica is a doctoral student at Columbia University School of Social Work. Her research interests are in the areas of mental health, prevention, and trauma.

McConatha, Jasmin Tahmaseb, PhD, is Professor of Psychology, West Chester University in Pennsylvania. Her work has focused on factors affecting well-being in later adulthood.

McCown, Judy A., PhD, is Associate Professor of Psychology, at the University of Detroit Mercy, where she has studied information processing in schizophrenia.

Meyer, Aleta L., PhD, Assistant Professor of Psychology, Virginia Commonwealth University. She uses her human development and family studies background in research on positive peer development.

Milewski, Theresa Myung Hee, MA, is a community psychologist with longstanding interests in adoption, foster care, and child welfare.

Miller, Brent C., PhD, is currently Vice President for Research at Utah State University, at Logan, where he was formerly Head of the Department of Family and Human Development.

Mishara, Brian L., PhD, is Professor of Psychology and Director of the Centre for Research and Intervention on Suicide and Euthanasia, University of Quebec, Montreal.

Montgomery, Marilyn J., PhD, is Assistant Professor of Psychology at Florida International University. Her research interests include identity development, adolescent relationship beliefs, and psychosocial intervention.

Mowbray, Carol T., PhD, is Professor and Associate Dean for Research at the School of Social Work, University of Michigan. Her research focuses on mental health services.

Mulroy, Maureen T., PhD, is Associate Professor in the School of Family Studies and serves as the human development specialist for the Cooperative Extension System at the University of Connecticut.

Mulsow, Miriam, PhD, is Assistant Professor, and Graduate Program Director, Human Development and Family Studies, Texas Tech University at Lubbock, Texas.

Neft, Deborah is a doctoral student in Clinical Psychology at Rutgers University. She has experience in youth camping, peer education, sexual assault prevention, and school consultation and program development.

Neighbors, Harold W., PhD, is Associate Professor at the Department of Health Behavior and Health Education, School of Public Health, University of Michigan. His research focuses on racial/ethnic differences in the distribution, diagnosis, and treatment of mental disorder.

Newcomb, Patricia M., PhD, is full time faculty at Rochester General Hospital's OB/GYN Residency Program, coordinates didactics, and directs the residency's clinic site. Research interests are leiomyomas and risks to pregnancy.

Nguyen, Viet, MD, is a pediatrician specializing in pediatric rehabilitation. Currently, he is a master's student in Public Health at the University of North Carolina.

O'Connor, Erin, MA, is a doctoral student in Human Development at the Harvard School of Education.

O'Neal, Keri K. is a doctoral candidate in Human Development and Family Studies at Texas Tech University.

Openshaw, D. Kim, PhD, LCSW, is Associate Professor, Family and Human Development, Utah State University at Logan, where he teaches human sexuality.

Orpinas, Pamela, PhD, MPH, is Associate Professor, Department of Health Promotion and Behavior, University of Georgia. Her research interests focus on the prevention of school violence.

Oyserman, Daphna, PhD, is Associate Professor and Associate Research Scientist, Research Center for Group Dynamics, Institute for Social Research, University of Michigan. Her research interests relate to how race/ethnicity, culture, and social context frame self-concept and understanding, and how these influence mental health.

Park, Elizabeth, PhD, practices family therapy and conducts participatory program evaluations and staff training with child and family human service agencies.

Parker, Robyn, PhD, is Senior Research Officer, Australian Institute of Family Studies, Melbourne. She conducts the Institute's Positive Family Relationships program, focusing on couple relationships, and is currently undertaking (with Michele Simons) a national study of relationship education service activities.

Parks, Carlton, W. PhD, is Professor and Coordinator, Multicultural Community-Clinical Psychology, at the California School of Professional Psychology, Alliant International University, Los Angeles.

Partridge, Ty, PhD, is Assistant Professor of Psychology at Wayne State University. His research interests include the integration of biology, behavior, and ecology in development, with special emphasis on temperament; and a study of analytic methods related to developmental systems theory.

Paschall, Mallie J., PhD, is Research Scientist with the Pacific Institute for Research and Evaluation, with interests in the etiology and prevention of substance abuse among adolescents and young adults.

Pedro-Carroll, JoAnne, PhD, is Director of Program Development at the Children's Institute, and Associate Professor of Psychology and Psychiatry at the University of Rochester. She is the founder and Director of the Children of Divorce Intervention Program.

Peterson, Gary W., PhD, is Professor and Department Head of Child and Family Studies, the University of Tennessee at Knoxville. His research examines parent–adolescent relationships and the development of youthful social competence within and across cultures.

Pettit, Gregory S., PhD, is Alumni Professor in the Department of Human Development and Family Studies, Auburn University. He is Associate Editor of *Developmental Psychology*.

Pierce, Michelle B. is at the University of Connecticut, Family Nutrition Program, Storrs Agricultural Experimental Station.

Piran, Niva, PhD, is Professor in the Department of Education, University of Toronto, and Eating Disorders Consultant to the Canadian National Ballet School.

Portwood, Sharon G., JD, PhD, is Assistant Professor of Psychology and Women's and Gender Studies, at the University of Missouri, Kansas City. Her research interests reflect her training and practice in law, community psychology, and developmental psychology. These interests focus on violence prevention, especially with children, youth, and women.

Ramos, Jessica M., BA, is staff member for the *Encyclopedia of Primary Prevention and Health Promotion*, without whose meticulous efforts this project would not have gone as smoothly as it has.

Reis, Sally M., PhD, is Department Head and Professor of Educational Psychology at the University of Connecticut. She also serves as a Principal Investigator at the National Resource Center on the Gifted and Talented. She was a teacher for 15 years, mostly working with gifted and talented students. She is past-president of the National Association for Gifted Children.

Renzulli, Joseph S., PhD, is Board of Trustee Distinguished Professor at the Neag Center for Gifted Education and Talent Development, School of Education, University of Connecticut.

Repetto, Paula B. is a doctoral candidate in the Department of Health Behavior and Health Education at the University of Michigan where she is working on health promotion among children and adolescents.

Reppucci, N. Dickon, PhD, is Professor of Psychology, and Director of Community Psychology at the University of Virginia. His research interests include community psychology, preventive interventions, and children and the law.

Rey, Jannette, PhD, is a Senior Educational Consultant in the Centers for Applied Research and Professional Development at The May Institute, Inc., in Norwood, Massachusetts.

Richardson, Virginia, PhD, is Professor at the College of Social Work, and Director of Aging Research at Ohio State University.

Riley, Lori has a BA and MS from West Chester University. She has worked extensively in the area of aging and is currently the activities director at the West Chester Senior Center.

Ringwalt, Christopher L., Dr PH, is Center Director, Pacific Institute for Research and Evaluation, Chapel Hill, North Carolina. His research interests include the epidemiology and etiology of adolescent risk behavior, and the evaluation of risk behavior prevention programs.

Roberts, Clare, PhD, is a clinical psychologist who teaches graduate level child clinical psychology and conducts research on the prevention of mental health problems in children. She is with the School of Psychology, Curtin University, Perth, Australia.

Roberts, Michael C., PhD, ABPP, is Professor and Director of the Clinical Child Psychology Program at the University of Kansas. His interests include children's services and prevention.

Rohrbeck, Cynthia A., PhD, is on the faculty of Psychology at George Washington University.

Roona, Michael, PhD, is Executive Director, Tobler Research Center, Social Capital Development Corporation, Albany, New York.

Rose, Hilary A., PhD, is Assistant Professor, Department of Human Development, Washington State University, Pullman, Washington. Her research interests include bullying, risk/resiliency, and gender.

Roth, Jodie L., PhD, is Research Scientist with the Center for Children and Families, Teachers College, Columbia University.

Rozier, R. Gary, DDS, MPH, is Professor of Health Policy and Administration, University of North Carolina.

Sackey, Brigid, PhD, is Cultural Anthropologist and Head of the African Religions and Philosophy section, the Institute of African Studies, University of Ghana-Legon.

Sandler, Irwin N., PhD, is Professor and Director of the Program for Prevention Research, Department of Psychology, Arizona State University, where he is involved in research on resilience, bereaved children, and children of divorce.

Schinke, Steven P., PhD, is Professor of Social Work, Columbia University School of Social Work, where he develops and tests preventive interventions for at-risk children and adolescents. He is also with the National Center for the Advancement of Prevention in New York City.

Schmidt, Melinda G., MA, is a doctoral candidate in Community Psychology at the University of Virginia. She is studying issues related to decision-making in adolescence, risk, and protective factors for delinquency, aggression, and violence, and juvenile justice.

Schumm, Walter R., PhD, CFLE, is Professor, School of Family Studies and Human Services, Kansas State University, where he teaches and writes in the area of family studies.

Schewe, Paul A., PhD, is a clinical/community psychologist at the University of Illinois at Chicago, whose work focuses on sexual assault and teen dating violence prevention efforts, as well as other interventions to promote positive individual and community development. He is a home-schooling father of three.

Sharkey, Jill D. is a doctoral candidate in the Special Education, Disability and Risk Studies/ School Psychology Credential Program, at the University of California, Santa Barbara, California.

Sharp, Elizabeth A. is a doctoral student in the Department of Human Development and Family Studies, at the University of Missouri at Columbia. Her research interests include early childhood intervention, divorce education, marital expectations, and relationship obligations.

Shatté, Andrew J., PhD, is Vice President of Research and Development with Adaptive Learning Systems and is on the research and teaching faculty at the University of Pennsylvania.

Sheehan, Nancy W., PhD, is Director of the Center on Aging and Human Development, and Associate Dean in the School of Family Studies at the University of Connecticut. Her interests include the impact of planned residential environments on elders' well-being.

Sherif, Bahira, PhD, is Assistant Professor, Department of Individual and Family Studies, University of Delaware. She is interested in issues of intergenerational relationships, and diversity and gender issues in families.

Shore, Milton F., PhD, ABPP, is a clinical child psychologist. He is a recipient of the Distinguished Professional Contribution to Public Service Award of the American Psychological Association for his many contributions while in the federal government.

Silliman, Benjamin, PhD, CFLE, Associate Professor, 4-H Youth Development, North Carolina State University, Raleigh. His area of interest includes research and educational works on marriage education, including many posted at www.marriagealive.com.

Silverman, Morton M., MD, is Associate Professor of Psychiatry and Director of the Student Counseling and Resource Service, and Associate Dean of Students at the University of Chicago.

Simons, Michele, PhD, is Lecturer at the University of South Australia. Her interests are related to the field of relationship education and pre-marriage education.

Smith, Dennis W., PhD, FASHA, is Associate Professor and Chair, Department of Health and Human Performance, University of Houston.

Smith, Douglas C., PhD, is Associate Professor and Acting Chair of the Department of Counselor Education, University of Hawaii. His research and teaching deal with children's social and emotional development.

Snyder, C. Rick, PhD, is Professor of Psychology at the University of Kansas. His interests are in positive psychology in general, and hope in particular.

Stokes, Julie, PhD, is a Consultant Clinical Psychologist, and founder of Winston's Wish, a community-based, national service for bereaved children and young people in the United Kingdom.

Streke, Andrei, PhD, is a doctoral candidate, and also a Research Associate at the Social Capital Development Corporation, Albany, New York.

Stroebe, Margaret S., PhD, is Associate Professor of Psychology at Utrecht University, The Netherlands. She recently co-edited (with Robert Hansson, Wolfgang Stroebe, & Henk Schut) the *Handbook of Bereavement Research*.

Sussman, Steve, PhD, is Professor of Preventive Medicine and Psychology at the University of Southern California. Dr. Sussman conducts research in the prediction, prevention, and cessation of tobacco and other drug abuse and empirical program development.

Tadmor, Ciporah S., PhD, is Medical Psychologist, at the Rambam Medical Center, Haifa, Israel, where she had developed and implemented research on primary prevention programs for populations at risk in the general hospital setting. She also serves as adjunct lecturer at the Faculty of Medicine, Technion, Israel Institute of Technology.

Taylor, Tanya, MSc, is a doctoral student in the Counseling Psychology Program at Virginia Commonwealth University, with research interests in life skill development in adolescence.

Tebes, Jacob Kraemer, PhD, is Associate Professor of Psychology in Psychiatry, and Child Study at the Yale University School of Medicine. He is also Co-Director of the Yale Division of Prevention and Community Research and Deputy Director of the Consultation Center, with interests in prevention research methodology, program and services evaluation, resilience, and the prevention of adolescent substance abuse.

Topping, Keith, J., PhD, directs postgraduate educational psychology and is Director of the Centre for Paired Learning at the University of Dundee, Scotland. He specializes, and writes extensively, in peer assisted learning, parents as educators, computer-assisted learning, and social, emotional, and behavioral learning.

Toro, Paul A., PhD, Associate Professor, Research Group on Homelessness and Poverty, Department of Psychology, Wayne State University. His extensive research interests and publications include the evaluation of longitudinal interventions on samples of homeless people.

Tuchfarber, Barbara, RN, MS, is a pediatric injury epidemiologist with Cincinnati Children's Hospital Medical Center. Her research focus is evaluation of pediatric injury prevention programs.

Unger, Donald G., PhD, is Associate Professor in the Department of Individual and Family Studies at the University of Delaware. His research focuses on family support, families with young children with disabilities, and the development and evaluation of community-based preventive interventions with families.

Vallbona, Carlos, MD, FACPM, is Distinguished Service Professor of Family and Community Medicine and Physical Medicine and Rehabilitation at Baylor College of Medicine in Houston, Texas.

Wade, Nathaniel G. is a doctoral candidate in counseling psychology at Virginia Commonwealth University. His research interests include the psychology of forgiveness, religion, and spirituality.

Walls, Angus WG, PhD, BDS, FDSRCS, is Professor, Restorative Dentistry at the University of Newcastle upon Tyne, United Kingdom. He conducts research on oral health and well-being in older adults.

Waris, Robert G. MA, is a doctoral student in Community Psychology at the University of Missouri at Kansas City. His research interests include program evaluation, youth mentoring, and youth antisocial behaviors such as violence, bullying, and substance use.

Webb, Kinari is a medical student at Yale University, School of Medicine. She is interested in international health and has studied the relationship between malnutrition and cognitive development.

Welsh, Brandon C., PhD, is Assistant Professor, Department of Criminal Justice, University of Massachusetts at Lowell.

Whitney, Grace-Ann C., PhD, is Developmental Psychologist and the Director of Connecticut's Head Start State Collaboration Office where she works to integrate Head Start with various state initiatives, such as health care for low-income families.

Whitten, Kathleen is a doctoral candidate in developmental psychology specializing in adoption at the University of Virginia. She has published extensively on health and family relationships.

Williams, Jason, MS, is a Research Specialist, Casey Family Programs, Seattle, Washington. His research and professional interests include abuse and neglect, eating disorders, coping skills and resiliency, psychometrics, and self-harm.

Wolchik, Sharlene, A., PhD, is Professor of Psychology at Arizona State University. Her research focuses on designing and evaluating preventive interventions for children of divorce and bereaved children.

Wolpe, Paul Root, PhD, is a Fellow at the Center of Bioethics at the University of Pennsylvania where he holds appointments in the Departments of Psychiatry and Sociology. He is Director of the Program in Psychiatry and Ethics at Penn and also Chief of Bioethics for the National Aeronautics and Space Administration (NASA).

Wood, David Lee, MD, MPH, is Clinical Associate Professor, University of South Florida and Medical Director, Medicaid Program, Delmarva Foundation for Medical Care. He is also Board Certified in both Pediatrics and Preventive Medicine. He is a health services researcher and quality improvement expert currently working with a Peer Review Organization to improve health services to poor children and families.

Worthington, Jr., Everett, PhD, is Professor and Chair of Psychology at Virginia Commonwealth University. He is a licensed Clinical Psychologist in Virginia, and does research on forgiveness, marriage, and religion.

Wyman, Peter, A., PhD, is Director of the Rochester Child Resilience Project, which has investigated competence and adaptation among at-risk children and families since 1987. He is also Associate Professor, Department of Psychiatry and of Clinical and Social Sciences in Psychology at the University of Rochester.

Yapchai, Courtney J. is a doctoral student in child-clinical psychology at Wayne State University, with research interests in preventive and therapeutic services for the homeless and other at-risk children and families.

Yarhouse, Mark A., PsyD, School of Psychology and Counseling, Regent University, Virginia Beach, Virginia. He teaches human sexuality and community psychology.

Yeh, Ming-Chin, PhD, is Research Associate, Yale University Prevention Research Center, with expertise in nutritional epidemiology and community nutrition interventions.

Yodanis, Carrie, PhD, is a head researcher at the University of Fribourg, Switzerland. A sociologist, she studies women, inequality, violence, and work in families.

Zimmerman, Marc A., PhD, is Professor in the Department of Health Behavior and Health Education at the University of Michigan School of Public Health. His research includes work in empowerment and adolescent health.

Zins, Joseph E., PhD, is Professor at the University of Cincinnati, Teachers College, and Editor of the *Journal of Educational and Psychological Consultation*. He is on the Leadership Team of the Collaborative for Academic, Social, and Emotional Learning.

Index

This index contains the names of authors of entries only. Titles of all entries are given in boldface, as are the standard categories used across entri₍ (definitions, research, scope, strategies that work, strategies that might work, strategies that do not work, synthesis, and theories), in order that readers ca. quickly identify major indexing terms.

00006

ISBN 0-306-47296-1